Thyroid Cancer

Leonard Wartofsky • Douglas Van Nostrand
Editors

Thyroid Cancer

A Comprehensive Guide to Clinical Management

Third Edition

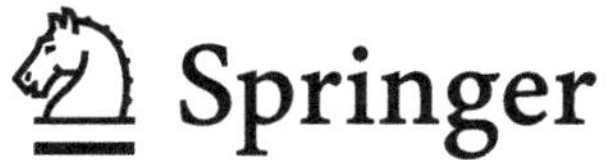

Editors
Leonard Wartofsky, MD, MACP
Department of Medicine
MedStar Washington Hospital Center
Georgetown University School of Medicine
Washington, DC, USA

Douglas Van Nostrand, MD, FACP, FACNM
Director
Nuclear Medicine Research
MedStar Research Institute
and Washington Hospital Center
Georgetown University School of Medicine
Washington Hospital Center
Washington, DC, USA

ISBN 978-1-4939-3312-9 ISBN 978-1-4939-3314-3 (eBook)
DOI 10.1007/978-1-4939-3314-3

Library of Congress Control Number: 2016935400

Printed on acid-free paper

This Springer imprint is published by Springer Nature
The registered company is Springer Science+Business Media LLC New York

To my past and present students, residents, technologists, staff, colleagues, and patients, who give me purpose.

Douglas Van Nostrand, MD

Dedicated to the memory of my mentor and colleague, Dr. Sidney H. Ingbar, and to memory of the authors of the Forewords to the first two editions of this book, Ernest L. Mazzaferri and E. Chester Ridgway, good friends and colleagues and highly skilled clinicians in the management of thyroid cancer. And to all of our patients who struggle under the cloud of an uncertain future with their malignancies.

Leonard Wartofsky, MD

Foreword to Second Edition

Cancer remains a major health problem for our society as we enter the new millennium. In 2002 there were approximately 550,000 deaths in the United States from cancer, which remains the second leading cause of mortality in our society behind heart disease. Each one accounts for approximately 25 % of the deaths in the United States on an annual basis. The most common cancers to appear in 2005 remain prostate, breast, lung and colon which will generate between 150,000 and 250,000 new cases this year. Likewise, the most common causes of death from cancer during this same period will be lung, colon, breast and prostate which will cause approximately 160,000, 50,000, 40,000, and 30,000 deaths, respectively.

In comparison, thyroid cancer is a relatively uncommon cancer. In 2005 we expect approximately 26,000 new cases and approximately 1500 thyroid cancer deaths will occur in the same period. Interestingly, thyroid cancer is the eighth most common cancer in women, similar in prevalence to ovarian cancer and melanoma. Moreover, American Cancer Society statistics indicate that thyroid cancer is currently the cancer in women with the greatest rate of increased incidence. Fortunately, for most thyroid cancers the five year survival rate has always been outstanding and is continuing to slowly improve. In the 1970s, the five year survival rate for differentiated thyroid cancer was approximately 92 % and in 2005 it is expected to be 97 %. This is to be compared with 99 %, 88 %, 63 %, and 15 % for the five year survival rates of prostate, breast, colon, and lung, respectively. Thus, thyroid cancer is important, not only because it is one of the top 10 cancers in women, but because it is amenable to early diagnosis, accurate and specific therapies, and excellent survival rates. Despite these salutary characteristics of thyroid cancer, it is problematic to both patients and their physicians because of its high, but nonfatal, recurrence rates that approximate 30 % for differentiated thyroid cancer over a 40 year followup period. Although not resulting in death, these recurrences result in additional interventions for the patient and the necessity for long-term followup.

In the second edition of Thyroid Cancer, Drs. Leonard Wartofsky, Douglas Van Nostrand, and their skilled and expert group of contributing authors have presented a wealth of new information on the problem of thyroid cancer. One would hope that all new editions to existing textbooks would bring as much new information to the subject as Dr. Wartofsky has provided in his new edition. The number of chapters has increased from 52 to 91. The text is again organized according to thyroid cancer type: papillary carcinoma followed by follicular carcinoma, medullary thyroid carcinoma, thyroid lymphomas, and anaplastic cancers. However, new General Considerations sections on Thyroid Cancer and, in particular, on Nuclear Medicine aspects of thyroid cancer, now introduce the entire text with improved organization and wonderfully expanded new information on the molecular pathogenesis, oncogenic determinants and staging of thyroid cancer. This new edition could serve as a textbook for nuclear medicine physicians, with the importance of nuclear medicine in thyroid cancer emphasized and expanded with clearly articulated chapters on radiation exposure, whole-body imaging with iodine isotopes, and on the emergence of important new isotopic imaging techniques such as PET scanning of thyroid malignancies. More and more we are recognizing that one basic standard dose for radioiodine therapy may not be appropriate for all patients, and hence the chapters on "dosimetry" during either thyroxine withdrawal or after recombinant human TSH provide convincing rationale and arguments for this valuable method for determining maximal safe radioactive iodine dosing.

The Thyroid Nodule section has been expanded to emphasize the importance of thyroid ultrasound as a diagnostically critical element for not only the performance of fine needle aspiration biopsy, but also for the diagnosis of thyroid nodules and followup surveillance of thyroid cancer patients for recurrence in cervical lymph nodes. Clearly, the newer ultrasonographic modalities and their use by endocrinologists have been one of the reasons why more thyroid nodules are being detected, which in turn, results in the higher number of thyroid cancer cases seen today than five and ten years ago. Doubtless, the above-mentioned observed improvements in remission and cure rates must relate to this earlier diagnosis.

Recombinant human thyrotropin or Thyrogen®, had just been approved for the diagnostic followup of differentiated thyroid cancer in 1999 at the time of the first edition of this book. In the intervening five years recombinant thyrotropin has emerged as one of the most important discoveries leading to improved diagnosis and followup of thyroid cancer. The new text details and expands our collective experiences in the use of recombinant thyrotropin as well as illuminates the promise for this reagent in remnant ablation treatment of thyroid cancer, and its dramatic potential for augmenting thyroglobulin testing and even its incremental value when utilized prior to PET scanning. Ongoing prospectively designed studies in the United States and Europe are providing intriguing results for these indications that will likely alter our management algorithms for diagnosing and treating thyroid cancer in the future.

Finally, the new edition ends with some very insightful predictions about the future for nuclear medicine as well as genetic and chemotherapeutic approaches to thyroid cancer. I particularly liked the very informative last new section on resources for patients including low iodine diets, and the listings of books, multiple Internet web sites, and recommendations for patients who have recently been treated with radioactive iodine. Drs. Wartofsky, Van Nostrand, and their colleagues should be very proud of this new edition and its formidable amount of new information. The physicians treating thyroid cancer will find this text comprehensive and accurate. The field of thyroid cancer will be enriched and our patients will be the beneficiaries of this new second edition of Thyroid Cancer.

E. Chester Ridgway, MD, MACP

Foreword to First Edition

As the 20th century draws to a close, it seems like a propitious time to look back upon the advances we have made in understanding thyroid carcinoma, since our knowledge today will certainly serve to light the path of discovery in the next century. Gazing at the world through a small looking glass focused on thyroid carcinoma seems an appropriate way to begin thinking about the clinical management of this group of diseases. What are the important things that we have learned in recent years that form the basis of our current clinical knowledge? How can we best use that information in the care of our patients? Dr. Leonard Wartofsky's new and sharply focused text, Thyroid Cancer, promises to answer this hypothetical set of questions in a succinct and clinically relevant way.

It sometimes seems that thyroid carcinoma is a neglected orphan among human cancers, which is at the root of some important issues. Thyroid carcinomas comprise a diverse group of malignancies ranging from indolent microscopic papillary carcinomas that pose no threat to survival to anaplastic carcinomas that are the most vicious carcinomas afflicting humans. Yet, because of its low incidence, there have been no prospective randomized clinical trials of the treatment of thyroid carcinoma. Furthermore, none are likely to be done, given the prolonged survival and relatively low mortality rates associated with the majority of these cancers. Nonetheless, patients often suffer greatly from this disease: many have serious recurrences and some die from relentlessly progressive and untreatable cancer. This is a disease that knows no boundaries, striking young and old alike. Unfortunately, management paradigms derive from retrospective studies, and few new drugs have been added to our therapeutic armamentarium. One would thus anticipate a deep void in our understanding of these tumors. Despite these shortcomings, the 20th century has seen major advances in our understanding of their etiology, pathophysiology, and management. The good news is that the advances have been rapidly translated into improved outcomes for many patients with thyroid carcinoma. For example, data from the National Cancer Institute shows that, although the incidence of thyroid carcinoma has increased significantly—almost 28 %—since the early 1970s in the United States, cancer-specific mortality rates during this same period have dropped significantly—by almost 21 %. In my view this results from the earlier diagnosis of the cancer, which allows the full impact of effective therapy, and which I believe has dramatically altered the clinical course of these tumors.

One of the dazzling success stories in medicine in the last half of this century is that with medullary thyroid carcinoma, a truly orphan tumor afflicting relatively few people. First identified in 1959 as a discrete entity, this tumor was identified before calcitonin was known to exist and before the mystery of the multiple endocrine neoplasia syndromes had been completely unraveled. The pieces of the puzzle fell together at lightning speed over a few decades. The Ret protooncogene mutations recently identified in this tumor will serve as the portal to our eventual complete understanding of its biology and are already the keystone to its diagnosis in members of afflicted kindreds. Now children with this genetic defect can be identified with molecular testing well before medullary thyroid carcinoma becomes clinically manifest or is identifiable by any other test, resulting in thyroidectomy that cures the disease. What a wondrous group of developments to pass on to the patients and physicians of the next century! This work serves as a model for the scientific investigation of malignant tumors.

We are also acquiring a clearer view of the molecular biology of well-differentiated—papillary and follicular—thyroid carcinomas. Ret rearrangements found in papillary carcinomas of humans have been shown to produce the tumor in transgenic mice, underscoring the central role of Ret in the pathogenesis of papillary carcinoma. Study of familial papillary thyroid carcinoma—now recognized to occur in a small but important subset of patients in whom it may be transmitted as an autosomal dominant trait—undoubtedly will provide important new information. These and other exciting discoveries, such as the identification of the sodium-iodide symporter in laboratory animals and humans, portend more basic discoveries that will generate currently unimaginable diagnostic and therapeutic tools. The latest example of this success in the laboratory is recombinant human TSH, which was recently introduced into clinical practice and already is dramatically improving and simplifying the care of patients with differentiated thyroid carcinoma.

During the past 50 years we have learned much about the important etiologic role of ionizing radiation in thyroid carcinoma. Introduced at the turn of the 20th century by Roentgen, external radiation soon became routine practice in the United States for many benign clinical conditions ranging from "statushymicolymphaticus" to acne. It took over 50 years, however, to understand that the thyroid gland of children is extremely sensitive to the carcinogenic effects of ionizing radiation and that this therapy itself caused papillary thyroid carcinoma, often decades after the exposure. Studies of the Japanese survivors of the atomic bombings of Nagasaki and Hiroshima first documented thyroid carcinoma as a consequence of radioactive fallout. Nonetheless, the notion was long held that internal radiation of the thyroid from ingested radioactive iodine was not a thyroid carcinogen. The outbreak of papillary thyroid carcinoma among children exposed to radioactive iodine fallout from the nuclear reactor accident in Chernobyl, however, abruptly closed the door on this notion. This accident placed a deadly exclamation mark after the statement that small doses of radioiodine indeed are carcinogenic to the thyroid glands of infants and children, and sparked renewed concerns about the above-ground nuclear weapons testing program in Nevada between 1950 and 1960, during which radioactive iodine fallout rained down on nearly the entire continental United States. The National Cancer Institute estimates that a substantial excess of thyroid carcinomas has probably occurred and perhaps will continue to occur as a result of this exposure. How clinicians will deal with this information, including what tests should be done, is under discussion, but national screening studies are not likely to be done.

We also have learned much about the pathology of thyroid carcinoma during the 20th century. The early observations about the prognostic implications of tumor size and invasion through the thyroid capsule are now well accepted. In addition, pathologists now recognize a number of histologic variants of papillary and follicular carcinoma that have important implications that must be carefully factored into the assessment of a tumor's prognosis. Other important advances in our understanding of thyroid pathology have occurred in this decade. What was once considered small-cell anaplastic thyroid carcinoma is now recognized as thyroid lymphoma—known to be a rare complication of Hashimoto's disease—which nevertheless seems to be occurring with increasing frequency. While we were busy discovering thyroid lymphoma, the incidence of anaplastic thyroid carcinoma has been quietly declining, probably as a result of early diagnosis and treatment of well-differentiated tumors that often serve as its forerunner. All of us breathe a quiet sigh of relief at this improvement. Now it is well appreciated that a tumor's prognosis cannot be fully assessed until its final histology has been carefully studied, sometimes both histologically and immunochemically, to uncover the dark secrets of its origin. This has therapeutic implications.

I think much of our success in reducing mortality from thyroid carcinoma stems from early diagnosis. Thirty years ago the main diagnostic tests to identify a malignant nodule were thyroid hormone suppression and radionuclide imaging. Now the standard of care in a clinically euthyroid patient is to perform a fine-needle aspiration biopsy of the nodule before any other tests are done. Though it remains a less than perfect test, the study of fine-needle cytology has prevented unnecessary surgery in many patients while increasing the yield of carcinoma among those undergoing thyroidectomy. I think fine-needle aspiration of nodules has saved more lives than is generally acknowledged—by preventing long periods of thyroid hormone suppression—while malignant nodules sometimes became wildly metastatic. There is evidence that long delays in therapy significantly increase cancer-specific mortality rates of papillary and follicular thyroid carcinoma. The key to fine-needle aspiration diagnosis is to understand the diagnostic details of the cytology report and to act accordingly.

Much of the current debate on thyroid carcinoma has revolved around the extent of initial therapy, both surgical and medical, that is necessary for patients with differentiated thyroid carcinoma. Almost everyone believes that some differentiated thyroid carcinomas require minimal therapy, whereas others require more aggressive management. The problem lies in defining aggressive tumors. Several staging systems and prognostic scoring systems have been devised to discriminate between low-risk patients who are anticipated to have a good outcome with minimal therapy and higher risk patients who require aggressive therapy to avoid morbidity or mortality from thyroid carcinoma. However, most of the prognostic systems do not identify the variants of papillary and follicular carcinoma that have remarkably different behaviors. Most prognostic scoring systems have been created with multiple regression analysis to find predictive combinations of factors, but almost none include therapy in the analysis. Moreover, almost all of them have considered cancer mortality as the endpoint of therapy, ignoring tumor recurrence or disease-free survival. This becomes problematic in defining risk because patients under age 40 typically have low cancer mortality rates, but experience high rates of tumor recurrence. Because most recurrences are in the neck and are easily treated, some clinicians regard them as trivial problems—but my patients find this notion incomprehensible. Most patients are devastated by a recurrence of tumor, regardless of its site. The greatest utility of prognostic scoring systems lies in epidemiological studies and as tools to stratify patients for prospective therapy trials, but they are least useful in determining treatment for individual patients.

In the past few decades most have come to believe that near-total or total thyroidectomy is the optimal treatment for thyroid carcinomas, even for patients at relatively low risk of mortality from their carcinomas. The main reason not to do total thyroidectomy is that it is associated with higher complication rates than those of lobectomy. However, there is now evidence documenting what most of us have known for a long time: surgeons with the most experience have the lowest complication rates, regardless of the extent of the thyroidectomy. Given the low frequency of this disease, a compelling argument can be made to refer patients to centers with highly experienced surgeons for their initial management.

Follow up of differentiated thyroid carcinomas and medullary thyroid carcinoma is greatly facilitated by sensitive serum tests—thyroglobulin and calcitonin—and the use of a variety of scanning techniques. I believe that what we term recurrence of tumor is actually persistent disease that previously fell below the radar of our older, less-sensitive detection tools. With newer sensitive tests including, for example, thyroglobulin measured by messenger RNA, we now have the opportunity to identify and treat thyroid cancers at an earlier and more responsive stage. Perhaps the most vivid example of this is the identification of diffuse pulmonary metastases among patients with high serum thyroglobulin levels and negative diagnostic imaging studies, which are only seen on posttherapeutic whole-body scans done after large therapeutic doses of 131I. Whether this enhances survival continues to be debated, but I think there are compelling reasons to suggest that it does improve outcome.

Thus many relatively new observations and management tools that have largely been developed in the last half of this century are being brought to the bedside to substantially enhance our ability to improve the outcome of most patients with thyroid carcinoma. Many challenges remain, however. More effective therapy is urgently needed for patients with widely metastatic disease that is unresponsive to current therapies. We need to understand more about the molecular predictors of recurrence and death from thyroid cancer. Nonetheless, our present state of knowledge provides clinicians a wide variety of diagnostic and therapeutic modalities to effectively manage this group of cancers. I believe the knowledge contained in Thyroid Cancer will give the practicing clinician the necessary information to provide patients with the latest and best diagnostic and therapeutic techniques.

Ernest L. Mazzaferri, MD, MACP

Foreword

Over the last decade, the epidemiology, clinical presentation, strategies for diagnosis, approaches to treatment, and natural history of differentiated thyroid cancer (DTC) have undergone an astonishing transformation. Indeed, it is difficult to think of another malignancy, or even another disease entity, that has undergone such a sea change than DTC. The incidence of DTC is rising faster than any malignancy; when the last edition of this text was published in 2006, DTC wasn't even among the top ten cancers in the US population. Now, according to recent American Cancer Society statistics, it is the fifth most common cancer diagnosis in women. While a number of reasons have been proposed to explain this remarkable acceleration in incidence, most experts believe that the majority of the increase is not due to known causal factors, such as radiation and other environmental exposures, but instead to the proliferation of imaging (e.g., neck sonography, CT scans, and MRI) and, perhaps, an increase in "screening" by primary care physicians doing increased numbers of thyroid physical examinations. Thus, although a true rise in disease incidence cannot be ruled out, increased diagnostic scrutiny has likely led to the detection of a hidden reservoir of smaller thyroid nodules, some of which are cancerous. In turn this has led to a surge in the number of fine needle aspiration biopsies being performed, the development of a new cytologic scheme for categorizing thyroid nodules, the rise of molecular diagnostic testing, and a record number of thyroidectomies being performed annually. This "epidemic" has also led to more postoperative radioiodine administrations, more laboratory testing, and the need for overextended clinicians to monitor thousands more thyroid cancer patients, typically for decades, if not for life.

It is also important to remember that while the vast majority of the increase in thyroid cancer incidence is among patients with lower stages of disease, the death rate from thyroid cancer has also increased, albeit much less dramatically, over the last decade. Somewhat ironically perhaps, while the scope of thyroid cancer care in the twenty-first century has shifted to diagnosing and treating increasingly lower risk disease, major advances in basic cancer genetics and in targeted chemotherapy have enhanced the prospects of the minority of patients at the other end of the clinical spectrum, who are afflicted with advanced or life-threatening thyroid malignancy.

The thyroid cancer epidemic has also led to an expansion of basic and clinical research directed at improving the care of patients with thyroid nodules and thyroid cancer, much of which has been published since the appearance of the previous edition of this text: a quick literature search revealed that about 15,000 papers related to "thyroid cancer" or "thyroid neoplasia" have been published since 2006. Based on this new knowledge, a paradigm shift has occurred in traditional thyroid cancer management from "total thyroidectomy and radioiodine therapy for all," to a more nuanced, evidence-based, individualized approach to care. Sadly, randomized clinical trials (RCTs), the pinnacles in the hierarchy of evidence-based medicine, are still few and far between in this field, although several recent widely publicized RCTs may be a signal that things are changing for the better. At the same time that our scientific knowledge is advancing, clinical epidemiologic studies have also described inexplicable and troubling differences in thyroid cancer management across geography, age, sex, race, physician specialty, and patient socioeconomic status. This variation in care has led some professional groups such as the American Thyroid Association, the National Comprehensive Cancer Network, and the European Thyroid Association to publish clinical practice guidelines, as one of their main objectives, to improve outcomes for thyroid cancer patients by minimizing the well-documented and seemly irrational variability in thyroid cancer treatment.

The new edition of this important text could not come at a more auspicious time. The rapid expansion of knowledge about the molecular underpinnings of thyroid cancer that has occurred over the last few years has led to new diagnostic tests, novel approaches to imaging, important clinical studies that have questioned standardized therapeutic dogma, and therapeutic advances that have led to the promise of control of heretofore untreatable advanced disease. This volume covers these topics and much more, with chapters written by the field's most authoritative experts. Of course, there is still a vast amount that we do not know about thyroid cancer, from basic tumor biology to the most appropriate diagnostic tools and initial therapies, to the most cost-effective follow-up strategies. Nevertheless, the third edition of *Thyroid Cancer* covers the current state of the art with encyclopedic breadth and depth. It will be an invaluable asset to any clinician involved in the care of patients with thyroid neoplasia, and the final section in the text will be a useful resource for patients with thyroid cancer and their families.

The Johns Hopkins University School of Medicine
Baltimore, MD, USA

David S. Cooper

Preface

This third edition of *Thyroid Cancer: A Comprehensive Guide to Clinical Management* yet again marks the publication of markedly updated and expanded volume that covers all aspects of the etiology, pathogenesis, diagnosis, initial treatment, and long-term management of all varieties of thyroid cancer. Like the earlier editions, it will serve as a valuable reference source for pathologists, endocrine surgeons, endocrinologists, nuclear medicine physicians, and oncologists. This edition again presents updated and extensive topics related to nuclear medicine, the inclusion of which recognizes the key role played by nuclear medicine physicians in the management of thyroid cancer patients. With Dr. Douglas Van Nostrand as coeditor of this volume, there are chapters dedicated to expert and extensive discussion of isotopes, isotope uptake, and scanning procedures including SPECT/CT, radioiodine ablation (with or without recombinant human TSH), stunning, dosimetry (with or without recombinant human TSH), Octreotide and FDG-PET scanning, and other alternative imaging modalities. There is a valuable reference atlas of scan images and illustrations and a scholarly summary of the side effects of radioiodine and how to avoid or minimize adverse effects of treatment. In addition to an updated section on ultrasonography of the thyroid gland, new sections on ultrasonography of cervical lymph nodes and imaging for thyroid cancer employing computerized tomography (CT), positron emission tomography (PET), and magnetic resonance imaging (MRI) have been added.

When the first edition was published in 2000, it was intended to meet the needs of practicing physicians for up-to-date clinically relevant information concerning the diagnosis and management of patients with thyroid cancer. The book received considerable acclaim and filled a void in the endocrine literature as a guide and reference source on the topics covered. Much has occurred in the field in the past 8 years since the second edition of 2006 that justifies the publication of this, an updated and extensively expanded, third edition. The topics of all of the new chapters are too lengthy to list here, and the reader is referred to the *Table of Contents*. We are especially pleased to now have new chapters on the role of genetics in the development of familial non-medullary thyroid cancer, as well as a section on alternative approaches to management of thyroid cancer. Again, the various chapters are written by highly knowledgeable experts, including many who are new to this edition. The authors provide not only the most current review of their respective areas, but also their own recommendations and approach. In this regard, the reader is forewarned that in many cases these approaches, albeit rooted in available data, may be empiric rather than based upon clear-cut results of well-controlled clinical trials. Nevertheless, controversial issues are examined and evidence-based recommendations are presented when available. As we were going to press, so were the newly revised guidelines for the management of thyroid cancer of the American Thyroid Association, and reference to these new guidelines has been included where feasible.

In addition, there are updated chapters on our current state of knowledge of the molecular changes in thyroid cancer, molecular markers, and aspects of how targeted therapies are being developed. New therapeutic trials of redifferentiation agents to restore the sodium iodide symporter when lacking and more traditional chemotherapies are discussed, with referral sources listed for entry of patients into Phase 1–3 clinical trials. Happily, most patients with well-differentiated thyroid cancer have an excellent prognosis when managed early and appropriately. But contributing authors also present their approaches to the management of more difficult cases, those with extensive bone metastases, those with negative isotope scans but high serum thyroglobulin, and those patients with positive antithyroglobulin antibodies that interfere with measurement of serum thyroglobulin.

Thyroid cancer is fortunately rare in children, but special problems apply to the pediatric population when it does occur in children. The sections on both differentiated thyroid cancer and medullary thyroid cancer in children have been updated with particular attention to the need for cautious approaches to radioiodine scanning and treatment to minimize radiation exposure when radioiodine is indicated. Thyroid cancer occurring under special or unique circumstances is well covered, such as during pregnancy, in thyroglossal duct cysts and struma ovarii, as well as the special problem related to radioiodine therapy for the end-stage renal patient with thyroid cancer. The rationale and methods for the use of low iodine diets are presented with practical guidelines for the patient, as are radiation safety guidelines (for both physicians and patients) for radioiodine therapy with sample formats and worksheet documents and a list of resources for more information for patients. And finally, newer locally ablative techniques to destroy metastatic foci are discussed such as ethanol instillation and laser and radiofrequency ablation.

In general, the same format as used in the earlier two editions is again employed, that of separating each type of thyroid cancer and having authors separately address clinical presentation, diagnosis, surgery, pathology, follow-up, treatment, and prognosis for each tumor. This arrangement allows the reader to quickly refer to the specific cancer in his or her patient, with everything and anything that they need to know in one place in a concise, readable format. This format works well in most but not all cases, with some obvious overlap in the management of the two well-differentiated cancers, papillary and follicular, and so some discussions of these two tumors is combined when appropriate. Separate sections deal with Hürthle cell cancer, thyroid lymphoma, and more rare and unusual tumors of the thyroid. Given the publication deadlines for manuscript submission, the most current reference citations possible are provided in the bibliography of each chapter.

I am indebted to the skilled and professional support staff of Springer, especially Jessica Gonzalez and Kevin Wright. I thank our outstanding group of authors for their expert and well-written contributions and my coeditor, Douglas Van Nostrand, for his invaluable expertise and assistance with this project. We hope that the result will provide useful information to physicians managing patients with thyroid cancer for years to come.

Washington, DC, USA Leonard Wartofsky, MD, MACP

Contents

Editors

Douglas Van Nostrand, MD, FACP, FACNM. Dr. Van Nostrand is the Director of Nuclear Medicine Research, MedStar Research Institute, and MedStar Washington Hospital Center. He received his BS from Duke University (1969) and his MD from Emory University (1973). He completed his residency in Internal Medicine at Wilford Hall Medical Center (1976) and his fellowship in Nuclear Medicine at the National Naval Medical Center (1978). He is board certified in both Internal Medicine and Nuclear Medicine. He was previously the Director of Nuclear Medicine at Malcolm Grow Medical Center (1979–1980), Walter Reed Army Medical Center (1980–1987), Good Samaritan Hospital (1987–1999), and MedStar Washington Hospital Center (1999–2015). He became Director of Nuclear Medicine Research Institute in January 2016 and is Professor of Medicine at Georgetown University School of Medicine. He is Past President of the Mid-Eastern Chapter of the Society of Nuclear Medicine, Past Vice President and Past President–Elect of the Medical Staff of the MedStar Good Samaritan Hospital, Past Chair of the Department of Continuing Medical Education at MedStar Good Samaritan Hospital and MedStar Washington Hospital Center. He has won numerous awards, including United States Air Force Commendations Medal; Fellow American College of Physicians; "A" Professional Designator Award, USA; United States Army Meritorious Service Medal; Fellow American College of Nuclear Physicians; Mentor of the Year Award by the America College of Nuclear Medicine, and the MedStar Washington Hospital Center Department of Medicine, Barbara; and Wm. James Howard Award for Outstanding Academic Achievement. He has been actively involved in thyroid cancer diagnosis and treatment for over 35 years. He has published more than 200 articles and 9 books including this medical textbook, and *Thyroid Cancer: A Guide for Patients* edited by D Van Nostrand, L Wartofsky, G Bloom, and K Kulkarni, which has been translated into Spanish and Chinese. His major area of research is thyroid cancer and nuclear medicine. He lectures and presents on radioiodine imaging and therapy of differentiated thyroid cancer through the year at many facilities, locally, regionally, nationally, and internationally.

Leonard Wartofsky, MD, MACP. Dr. Wartofsky is Emeritus Chairman of the Department of Medicine at MedStar Washington Hospital Center and a Professor of Medicine at Georgetown University School of Medicine as well as at the Uniformed Services University of the Health Sciences, and Schools of Medicine of George Washington University, Howard University, and University of Maryland. He holds MS, MD, and MPH degrees from GWU and trained in internal medicine at Barnes Hospital, Washington University, St. Louis, and in Endocrinology at the Thorndike Memorial Laboratory on the Harvard University Service, Boston City Hospital under Dr. Sidney H. Ingbar. While serving at Walter Reed Army Medical Center, he was Director of the Endocrinology Division and then Chair, Department of Medicine, and Consultant in Medicine to the Surgeon General. He has been elected to several highly honorific medical societies, including the American Society for Clinical Investigation, Association of American Physicians, Association of Professors of Medicine, and as Governor of the American College of Physicians (ACP). He is a past President of both the American Thyroid Association (ATA) and the Endocrine Society. Among his numerous other military and civilian awards are the Distinguished Educator Award of the Endocrine Society, Distinguished Laureate of the ACP, Distinguished Alumnus Achievement Award of GWU School of Medicine, the Robert H. Williams Leadership Award of The Endocrine Society, the Delbert A. Fisher Research Scholar Award of The Endocrine Society, the Gold-Headed Cane Award of MedStar Washington Hospital Center, the Washington University/Barnes Hospital House Staff Outstanding Achievement Award, and the Lewis E. Braverman Distinguished Lectureship Award of the ATA for 2014. Dr. Wartofsky's major clinical and research interest is in the management of patients with thyroid cancer, and he is the Author or Coauthor of over 400 articles or book chapters in the medical literature. He has served as editor of several endocrine volumes, including coediting this book with Dr. Van Nostrand and another on thyroid cancer for patients. He was the Editor-in-Chief of *The Journal of Clinical Endocrinology and Metabolism* from 2010 to 2014 and is now Editor-in-Chief of *Endocrine Reviews*.

Contributors

Ejigayehu G. Abate, MD Division of Endocrinology & Metabolism, Mayo Clinic, Jacksonville, FL, USA

Department of Medicine, Mayo Clinic, Jacksonville, FL, USA

Elmo R. Acio, MD Division of Nuclear Medicine, Department of Medicine, MedStar Washington Hospital Center, Washington, DC, USA

Sheba Asghar, MD Division of Endocrinology, Metabolism and Lipids, Emory University School of Medicine, Atlanta, GA, USA

Frank B. Atkins, PhD Division of Nuclear Medicine, MedStar Washington Hospital Center, Georgetown University School of Medicine, Washington, DC, USA

Anca M. Avram, MD Division of Nuclear Medicine, Department of Radiology, University of Michigan, Ann Arbor, MI, USA

BIG505G University Hospital, Ann Arbor, MI, USA

James R. Baker Jr., MD Michigan Nanotechnology Institute for Medicine and Biological Science, University of Michigan, Ann Arbor, MI, USA

Douglas W. Ball, MD Departments of Medicine, Oncology, and Radiology, Johns Hopkins University School of Medicine, Baltimore, MD, USA

Zubair W. Baloch, MD, PhD Department of Pathology and Laboratory Medicine, University of Pennsylvania Medical Center, Perelman School of Medicine, Philadelphia, PA, USA

Andrew J. Bauer, MD Division of Endocrinology and Diabetes, Department of Pediatrics, The Children's Hospital of Philadelphia, The Perelman School of Medicine, The University of Pennsylvania, Philadelphia, PA, USA

Victor J. Bernet, MD Division of Endocrinology, Mayo Clinic, Jacksonville, FL, USA

Gary Bloom ThyCa: Thyroid Cancer Survivors' Association, Inc., Olney, MD, USA

James D. Brierley, MBBS, FRCP, FRCR, FRCPC Department of Radiation Oncology, Princess Margaret Hospital, University of Toronto, Toronto, ON, Canada

Henry B. Burch, MD, FACE Endocrinology Division, Uniformed Services University of the Health Sciences, Walter Reed National Military Medical Center, Bethesda, MD, USA

Stephen J. Burgun, MD Department of Medicine, University Hospitals, Case Western Reserve University, Chardon, OH, USA

Kenneth D. Burman, MD Divisions of Endocrinology, Washington Hospital Center and Georgetown University Hospital, Washington, DC, USA

Nancy Marie Carroll, MD Department of Surgery, MedStar Washington Hospital Center, Washington, DC, USA

Stewart C. Davidson, MBBS Northeast Nuclear Medicine, Mooloolaba, QLD, Australia

Gerard M. Doherty, MD, FACS Department of Surgery, Boston Medical Center, Boston University, Boston, MA, USA

D. Robert Dufour, MD Clinical Pathology, Veterans Affairs Medical Center, Washington, DC, USA

Rossella Elisei, MD Endocrine Unit, Department of Clinical and Experimental Medicine, University Hospital of Pisa, Pisa, Italy

Gennady Ermak, PhD Division of Molecular and Computational Biology, Ethel Percy Andrus Gerontology Center, Los Angeles, CA, USA

Giuseppe Esposito, MD Division of Nuclear Medicine, MedStar Georgetown University Hospital, Washington, DC, USA

James A. Fagin, MD Department of Medicine, Memorial Sloan-Kettering Cancer Center, New York, NY, USA

Lorraine M. Fig, MBChB, MPH Department of Nuclear Medicine, University of Michigan, Ann Arbor, MI, USA

James J. Figge, MD, MBA, FACP Department of Biomedical Sciences, School of Public Health, State University of New York, Albany, NY, USA

Department of Medicine, St. Peter's Health Partners, Albany, NY, USA

Gen*NY*Sis Center for Excellence in Cancer Genomics, State University of New York, Rensselaer, NY, USA

Stephanie A. Fish, MD Department of Medicine, Memorial Sloan-Kettering Cancer Center and Weill Cornell Medical College, New York, NY, USA

Leah Folb, MD Endocrinology, Medical Clinic of Houston, L.L.P., Houston, TX, USA

Gary L. Francis, MD, PhD Division of Pediatric Endocrinology, Department of Pediatrics, Children's Hospital of Richmond Virginia Commonwealth University, Richmond, VA, USA

Andrea Frasoldati, MD, PhD Endocrinology Unit, Arcispedale S. Maria Nuova - IRCCS, Reggio Emilia, Italy

John E. Freitas, MD Department of Radiology, St. Joseph Mercy Health System, Ypsilanti, MI, USA

Carlos Alberto Garcia, MD Division of Nuclear Medicine, Department of Medicine, MedStar Washington Hospital Center/Georgetown University, Washington, DC, USA

Onelio Geatti, MD Servizio di Medicina Nucleare, Ospedale Maggiore, Trieste, Italy

Stephen K. Gerard, MD, PhD Department of Nuclear Medicine, Department of Pathology, Seton Medical Center, Daly City, CA, USA

Gregory Gerasimov, MD, PhD Thyroid Division, Endocrinology Research Center, Moscow, Russian Federation

John Glenn, PhD Radiation Safety, Georgetown University Hospital, Washington, DC, USA

Ravinder K. Grewal, MD Nuclear Medicine Service, Department of Radiology, Memorial Sloan Kettering Cancer Center, New York, NY, USA

Milton D. Gross, MD Division of Nuclear Medicine, Department of Radiology, University of Michigan Medical School, Ann Arbor, MI, USA

Nuclear Medicine and Radiation Safety Service, Department of Veterans Affairs Health Systems, Washington, DC (field based) and Ann Arbor, MI, USA

Sigurdis Haraldsdottir, MD Division of Medical Oncology, Department of Internal Medicine, The Ohio State University Comprehensive Cancer Center, Columbus, OH, USA

Laszlo Hegedüs, MD, DMSc Department of Endocrinology and Metabolism, Odense University Hospital and University of Southern Denmark, Odense, Funen, Denmark

Robert Hobbs, PhD Department of Radiation Oncology, Johns Hopkins University School of Medicine, Baltimore, MD, USA

Andrei Iagaru, MD Department of Radiology, Nuclear Medicine, Stanford University Medical Center, Stanford School of Medicine, Stanford, CA, USA

Ayman Jarwan, MD Department of Nuclear Engineering and Radiological Sciences, University of Michigan, Ann Arbor, MI, USA

James Jelinek, MD, FACR Department of Radiology, MedStar Washington Hospital Center, Washington, DC, USA

Timothy A. Jennings, MD Department of Pathology and Laboratory Medicine, Albany Medical Center, Albany, NY, USA

Nikolai A. Kartel, PhD Molecular Genetics Laboratory, The Institute of Genetics and Cytology of the National Academy of Sciences of Belarus, Minsk, Republic of Belarus

Kimberlee J. Kearfott, ScD Department of Nuclear Engineering and Radiological Sciences, University of Michigan, Ann Arbor, MI, USA

Gauri R. Khorjekar, MD Division of Nuclear Medicine, Department of Medicine, MedStar Washington Hospital Center, Washington, DC, USA

Ian David Kirkwood, MBBS Department of Nuclear Medicine, Royal Adelaide Hospital, Adelaide, SA, Australia

Joanna Klubo-Gwiezdzinska, MD, PhD Combined Divisions of Endocrinology, National Institutes of Health, Bethesda, MD, USA

Kanchan Kulkarni, MD Division of Nuclear Medicine, MedStar Washington Hospital Center, Washington, DC, USA

David A. Liebner, MD Division of Medical Oncology, Department of Internal Medicine, The Ohio State University, Columbus, OH, USA

Department of Biomedical Informatics, The Ohio State University, Columbus, OH, USA

Virginia A. LiVolsi, MD Department of Pathology and Laboratory Medicine, University of Pennsylvania Medical Center, Perelman School of Medicine, Philadelphia, PA, USA

Gregory Lund, MD Denver Endocrinology Diabetes & Thyroid Center, Swedish Medical Center, Englewood, CO, USA

Michael T. McDermott, MD Division of Endocrinology, Metabolism and Diabetes, Department of Medicine, University of Colorado, Aurora, CO, USA

Iain Ross McDougall, MD, PhD, FRCP Department of Radiology, Nuclear Medicine, Stanford University Hospital and Clinics, Stanford, CA, USA

Andreas Moraitis, MD Section on Endocrinology and Genetics, Program in Developmental Endocrinology and Genetics, *Eunice Kennedy Shriver* National Institute of Child Health and Human Development, National Institutes of Health, Bethesda, MD, USA

Sogol Mostoufi-Moab, MD, MSCE Divisions of Oncology and Endocrinology, Department of Pediatrics, The Children's Hospital of Philadelphia, Philadelphia, PA, USA

Barbara Mensah Onumah, MD Medicine – Section of Endocrinology, MedStar Washington Hospital Center, Washington, DC, USA

Claudio Maurizio Pacella, MD Department of Diagnostic Imaging and Interventional Radiology, Regina Apostolorum Hospital, Rome, Albano Laziale, Italy

Enrico Papini, MD, FACE Endocrinology Unit, Regina Apostolorum Hospital, Rome, Albano Laziale, Italy

Hee-Myung Park, MD Department of Radiology, Indiana University Hospital, Indianapolis, IN, USA

Nikita Pozdeyev, MD, PhD Division of Endocrinology, Metabolism and Diabetes, Department of Medicine, University of Colorado, Aurora, CO, USA

Matthew D. Ringel, MD Division of Endocrinology, Diabetes and Metabolism, Department of Internal Medicine, Wexner Medical Center, The Ohio State University, Columbus, OH, USA

Richard J. Robbins, MD Department of Medicine, The Methodist Hospital, Houston, TX, USA

Karen C. Rosenspire, MD, PhD Department of Radiology, Wayne State University, Detroit, MI, USA

Vittoria Rufini, MD Institute of Nuclear Medicine, Agostino Gemelli University Polyclinic, Rome, Italy

Anna M. Sawka, MD, PhD Division of Endocrinology and Metabolism, Department of Medicine, University Health Network – University of Toronto/Toronto General Hospital, Toronto, ON, Canada

Arthur B. Schneider, MD, PhD Section of Endocrinology, Diabetes and Metabolism, University of Illinois at Chicago, Chicago, IL, USA

Mark Schneider, MD Cardiovascular/Metabolic, Boehringer Ingelheim, Chicago, IL, USA

Kristoffer Seelbach, MD Endocrinology Division, Department of Medicine, The Methodist Hospital and Institute for Academic Medicine, Houston, TX, USA

George Sgouros, PhD Department of Radiology and Radiological Science, School of Medicine, Johns Hopkins University, Baltimore, MD, USA

Manisha H. Shah, MD Division of Medical Oncology, Department of Internal Medicine, The James Cancer Hospital and Solove Research Institute, Columbus, OH, USA

Brahm Shapiro, MBChB, PhD Radiology (Nuclear Medicine), Formerly, University of Michigan Health System, Ann Arbor, MI, USA

Division of Nuclear Medicine, Department of Radiology, University of Michigan Medical School, Ann Arbor, MI, USA

Nuclear Medicine and Radiation Safety Service, Department of Veterans Affairs Health Systems, Washington, DC (field based) and Ann Arbor, MI, USA

Barry M. Shmookler, MD Department of Pathology, Washington Hospital Center and Medlantic Research Institute, Washington, DC, USA

Merica Shrestha, MD Endocrinology Service, Dwight David Eisenhower Army Medical Center, Ft. Gordon, GA, USA

Jennifer A. Sipos Department of Endocrinology, The Ohio State University, Columbus, OH, USA

Monica C. Skarulis, MD National Institute of Diabetes, Digestive and Kidney Diseases, NIH Clinical Center, Bethesda, MD, USA

Robert C. Smallridge, MD Division of Endocrinology & Metabolism, Mayo Clinic, Jacksonville, FL, USA

Department of Medicine, Mayo Clinic, Jacksonville, FL, USA

Department of Cancer Biology, Mayo Clinic, Jacksonville, FL, USA

Louis O. Smith III , MD Department of Radiology, Washington Hospital Center, Washington, DC, USA

James M. Smith, PhD Division of Environmental Health, Emory University, Rollins School of Public Health, Atlanta, GA, USA

Nikolaos Stathatos, MD Department of Medicine, Massachusetts General Hospital, Thyroid Associates, Boston, MA, USA

Constantine A. Stratakis, MD, D(med)Sci Section on Endocrinology and Genetics, Program in Developmental Endocrinology and Genetics, *Eunice Kennedy Shriver* National Institute of Child Health and Human Development, National Institutes of Health, Bethesda, MD, USA

Shannon D. Sullivan, MD, PhD Department of Endocrinology & Metabolism, MedStar Washington Hospital Center, Washington, DC, USA

Richard W. Tsang, MD, FRCP(C) Department of Radiation Oncology, Princess Margaret Hospital, University of Toronto, Toronto, ON, Canada

Robert Michael Tuttle, MD Department of Medicine, Memorial Sloan Kettering Cancer Center, New York, NY, USA

Douglas Van Nostrand, MD, FACP, FACNM Nuclear Medicine Research, MedStar Research Institute and Washington Hospital Center, Georgetown University School of Medicine, Washington Hospital Center, Washington, DC, USA

Richard J. Vetter, PhD, CHP Biophysics, Mayo Clinic and Medical School, Rochester, MN, USA

Steven G. Waguespack, MD Endocrine Neoplasia and Hormonal Disorders, The University of Texas MD Anderson Cancer Center, Houston, TX, USA

Su He Wang, MD, PhD Department of Internal Medicine, University of Michigan, Ann Arbor, MI, USA

Leonard Wartofsky, MD, MACP Department of Medicine, MedStar Washington Hospital Center, Georgetown University School of Medicine, Washington, DC, USA

Jason A. Wexler, MD Department of Internal Medicine/Section of Endocrinology, MedStar Washington Hospital Center, Georgetown University Medical Center, Washington, DC, USA

Ka Kit Wong, MBBS, FRACP Division of Nuclear Medicine, Department of Radiology, University of Michigan Health System, Ann Arbor, MI, USA

Mingzhao Xing, MD, PhD Department of Medicine/Endocrinology and Metabolism, Johns Hopkins Hospital, Baltimore, MD, USA

Richard Young, MD Department of Radiology, Washington Hospital Center, Washington, DC, USA

Marina S. Zemskova, MD Diabetes, Obesity and Endocrinology Branch, National Institutes of Health, National Institute of Diabetes, Digestive and Kidney Diseases, Bethesda, MD, USA

Part I

General Considerations I: Thyroid Cancer

Anatomy and Physiology of the Thyroid Gland: Clinical Correlates to Thyroid Cancer

1

Nikolaos Stathatos

Detailed knowledge of thyroid gland anatomy and physiology is extremely important for any physician that manages thyroid disorders, including thyroid malignancies. The thyroid gland is a relatively small butterfly-shaped organ located in the lower neck, anteriorly to the trachea. A large number of ectopic sites of thyroid tissue have been described, including thyroglossal duct cysts, lingual thyroid, or struma ovarii. The thyroid gland is in close proximity to several important structures, such as the recurrent laryngeal nerves, the parathyroid glands, as well as the large cervical blood vessels like the carotid artery and the jugular vein.

The function of the thyroid gland is to provide adequate amounts of thyroid hormone, a hormone with clinically important actions practically in every system in the human body. Its main functional unit is the thyroid follicle, a single cell-layered cystic unit that contains colloid. Thyroglobulin is the main component of colloid and it represents the large-molecular-weight protein in which the thyroid hormones, thyroxine (T4) and triiodothyronine, (T3) are stored.

The molecular biology of thyroid function has been studied extensively with identification of important cellular elements such as the thyroid-stimulating hormone receptor and the sodium–iodide symporter. These advances have significantly improved our understanding of thyroid physiology and have allowed us to identify potential therapeutic targets for diseases such as thyroid cancer.

To better understand the biology of thyroid malignancies, it is extremely important to have a thorough understanding of the thyroid's relationship to its surrounding structures, both anatomically and functionally. This would allow a clinician to understand the behavior of thyroid cancers in regard to issues of local invasion, regional spread to cervical lymph nodes, and distant metastasis. This short review focuses on some aspects of thyroid anatomy and physiology that are clinically relevant to the diagnosis and management of thyroid cancer.

Thyroid Anatomy, Histology, and Embryology

The thyroid gland is a butterfly-shaped organ located anteriorly to the trachea at the level of the second and third tracheal rings. Its name originates from the Greek term "thyreos," which means shield (named after the laryngeal thyroid cartilage). It consists of two lobes connected by the isthmus in the midline. Its bilaterality is important because the presence of malignant cells on one or both sides can significantly alter the management of the patient, e.g., requiring more extensive surgery, such as bilateral neck dissections if there is local extension of the tumor. Each lobe is about 3–4 cm long, about 2 cm wide, and only a few millimeters thick. Because of its very close anatomic relationship to the rounded trachea, nodules arising from the posterior aspect of the gland are usually inaccessible to the examining fingers and therefore often missed on a routine clinical examination. The isthmus is 12–15 mm high and connects the two lobes. Occasionally, a pyramidal lobe is located in the midline, superior to the isthmus (Fig. 1.1). It represents a remnant of the thyroglossal duct, as the primitive thyroid gland descends from the base of the tongue to its final location in the neck during embryonic development. Anatomic variations of the thyroid gland occur and are encountered in clinical practice; one of the more common is thyroid hemiagenesis [1], with only one lobe and an isthmus of the gland. Hemiagenetic thyroid lobes are susceptible to the same abnormalities as are normal thyroid glands, including nodules and thyroid cancer.

N. Stathatos, MD (✉)
Department of Medicine, Massachusetts General Hospital, Thyroid Associates, 15 Parkman Street, Boston, MA 02114, USA
e-mail: nstathatos@partners.org

L. Wartofsky, D. Van Nostrand (eds.), *Thyroid Cancer*, DOI 10.1007/978-1-4939-3314-3_1

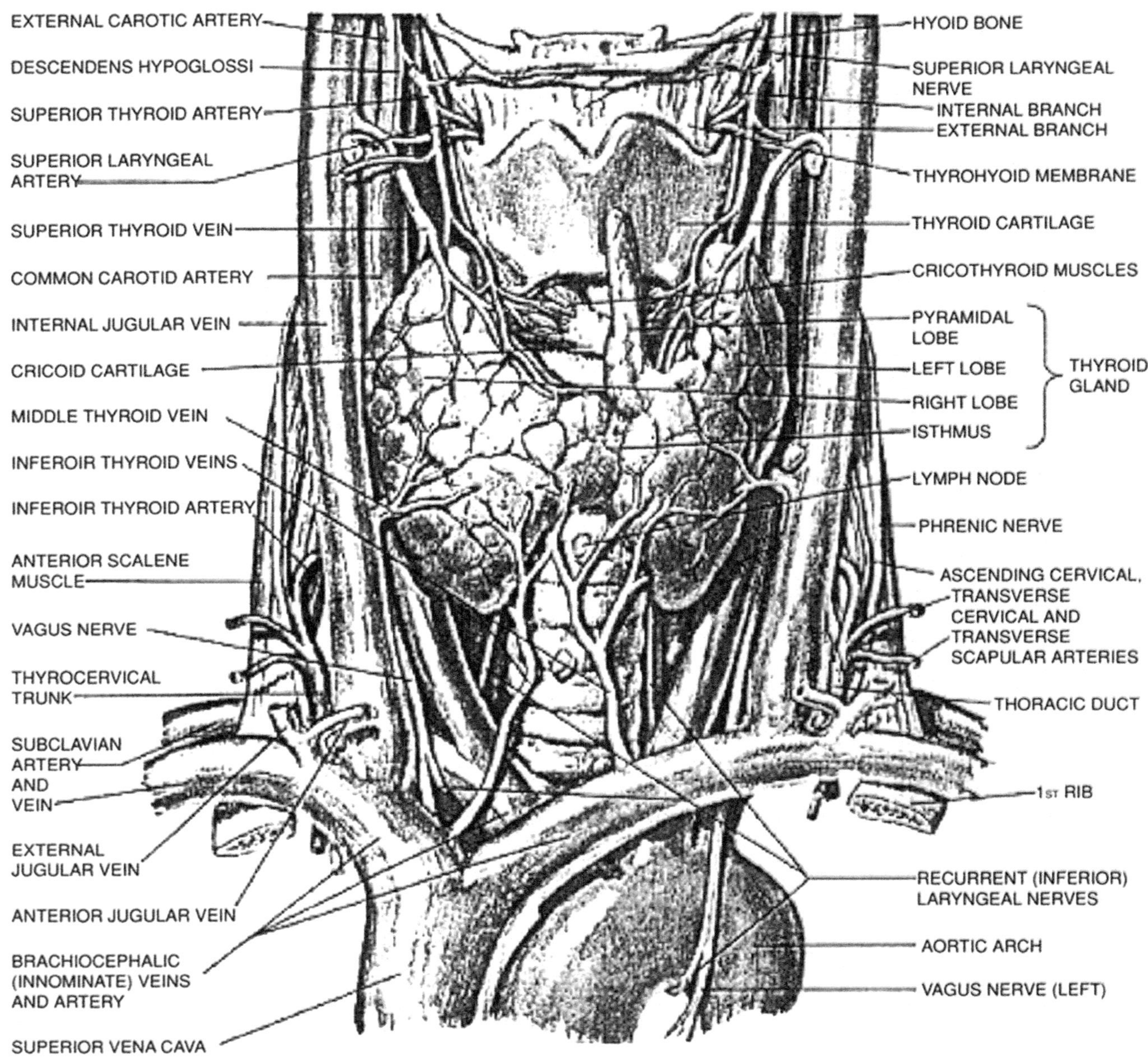

Fig. 1.1 Thyroid anatomy. Thyroid relations with surrounding cervical structures

A fibrous capsule covers the thyroid gland. Nodules within the parenchyma of the gland may also have a capsule or pseudocapsule. Surgical pathology reports may refer to tumor invasion "through the capsule," and for staging purposes, prognosis, and management, it is important to know if this represents extension through the capsule of the gland into the surrounding perithyroidal tissues. Several key structures are located in relation to the capsule and should be considered in the context of surgery on the thyroid gland, such as the parathyroid glands and the recurrent laryngeal nerve. This is particularly significant with total thyroidectomy in patients with thyroid cancer. The small parathyroid glands are located in the posterior aspect of this capsule. Their identification and preservation is critical during surgery and can be particularly difficult with invasive cancers that require extensive surgery for complete resection, including modified lymph node dissections. Also, close monitoring of their function by measurements of serum total and ionized calcium in the early postoperative period is important to avoid or adequately treat surgical hypoparathyroidism in a timely manner.

The recurrent laryngeal nerves provide an essential part of the innervation of the larynx, and any injury can result in symptoms that range from a hoarse voice to stridor and the need for a tracheostomy. They originate from the vagus nerve at the level of the aortic arch and turn superiorly toward the tracheoesophageal groove. Several anatomic variations have been described; on the right side the recurrent laryngeal nerve runs laterally to the tracheoesophageal groove [2, 3]. It runs close to the inferior thyroid artery and can be found anteriorly, posteriorly, or in between the branches of the blood vessel. Several surgical approaches have been proposed to try to identify and preserve this nerve during surgery of the thyroid gland. Most investigators recommend identifying the nerve before ligating the artery to prevent inadvertent injury to the nerve, but there are variations in proposed methods to achieve this. As the nerve travels superiorly in or laterally to the tracheoesophageal groove, it is located directly posterior to the thyroid gland itself and can be adherent to it. This requires special attention by the thyroid surgeon to prevent damage to the nerve as the thyroid lobe is removed. Another variation is a division of the recurrent laryngeal nerve before entering the larynx [2, 3]. In less than 1 % of cases, an anomalous nonrecurrent nerve has been reported, originating from the cervical potion of the vagus nerve (also called the "inferior laryngeal nerve"), instead of the recurrent laryngeal nerve. This nerve is usually seen on the right side of the neck [4].

The gland's blood supply comes from two sets of arteries on each side. The superior thyroid arteries originate from the external carotid arteries. They descend to the superior poles of the thyroid gland and are accompanied by the superior laryngeal nerve. This nerve originates from the inferior vagus ganglion. As it approaches the larynx, it divides into the external and internal branches. The internal branch supplies sensory innervation to the supraglottic larynx, and the external branch innervates the cricothyroid muscle [5]. The surgeon should ligate the superior thyroid artery as close to the thyroid gland as possible to try to avoid damaging any branches of the superior laryngeal nerve. Clearly, the type of symptoms a patient will develop postoperatively is highly dependent on the experience and skill of the surgeon and the type of nerve injury. Unfortunately, it is not rare that the surgeon may have to sacrifice one of the recurrent laryngeal nerves in an en bloc resection because cancer has directly invaded the nerve.

Anatomy and Physiology

The inferior thyroid artery is a branch of the thyrocervical trunk, and as noted, this artery is in close proximity with the recurrent laryngeal nerve. Occasionally, the thyroidea ima artery also provides blood supply to the thyroid gland and may originate from either the thyrocervical trunk or the arch of the aorta. The venous drainage of the thyroid gland consists of three sets of veins: the superior, middle, and inferior. The superior and middle thyroid veins drain into the internal jugular veins, and the inferior veins anastomose with each other anteriorly to the trachea and drain into the brachiocephalic vein. The lymphatic drainage of the thyroid gland mainly involves the deep cervical lymph nodes in the central compartment. This area is usually dissected by the surgeons performing thyroidectomies for malignant disease to minimize the chance of residual malignancy in the neck. A few lymphatic vessels also drain to the paratracheal lymph nodes.

Another important aspect of thyroid anatomy is the potential presence of thyroid tissue at locations that are considered "ectopic." To better understand this, a short description of the embryonic development of the thyroid gland is necessary. The primitive thyroid gland develops in the first month of gestation in the pharyngeal floor and elongates caudally, forming the thyroglossal duct. As the duct descends to its final location in the neck, it comes in contact with the ultimobranchial pouch of the fourth pharyngeal pouch—the origin of the C cells that produce calcitonin. Their final resting place is at the lower part of the upper one third of the adult thyroid gland. Once the thyroid gland reaches its destination at the base of the neck, the thyroglossal duct regresses and usually disappears, leaving a remnant of only the foramen cecum at the base of the tongue. Sometimes, its distal part near the thyroid gland persists and forms the pyramidal lobe of the thyroid gland. Occasionally, the thyroglossal duct remains and presents (most often during childhood) as a neck mass. This mass usually represents a benign thyroglossal duct cyst, but cases of primary thyroid malignancy have been described at any place along the track of the duct's migration [6]. In addition to these ectopic sites for thyroid tissue and thyroid malignancy, benign ectopic thyroid tissue has been described in many different parts of the human body. These include the base of the tongue [7–10], intralaryngeal [11], intratracheal [12], submandibular [13], carotid bifurcation [14], intracardiac [15, 16], ascending aorta [17], gallbladder [18], porta hepatis [19], intramesenteric [20], and ovarian [21]. Thyroid cancer has been described in many of these sites as well, e.g., at the base of the tongue or in the ovary (struma ovarii) [16, 22–25], but whether some of these tumors are primary or secondary is a matter of debate.

Another aspect of ectopic thyroid tissue relates to the presence of thyroid follicular elements in cervical lymph nodes. Significant controversy exists in the literature about whether the thyroid tissue deposits are indeed benign or representative of metastatic disease [26]. Nevertheless, the presence of ectopic thyroid tissue—benign or malignant—can confuse the clinical perspective and may require a different therapeutic approach to adequately treat thyroid cancer and to follow the patient optimally.

The thyroid gland has a characteristic histology and distinctions between benign and malignant thyroid tissue are important to appreciate. The main histological structure is the thyroid follicle (Fig. 1.2), which consists of a single layer of epithelial cells—the thyroid follicular cells—surrounded by

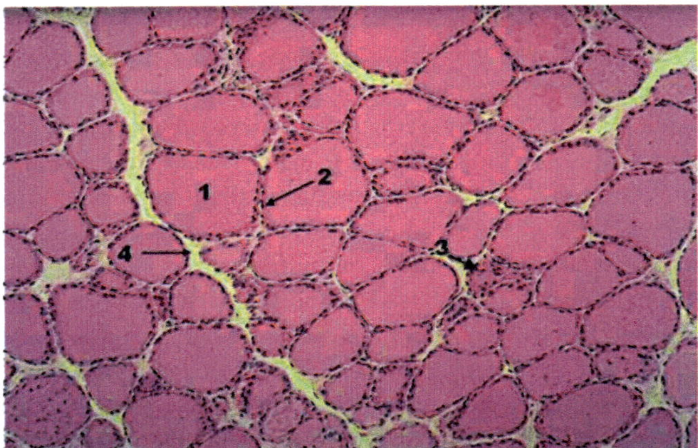

Fig. 1.2 Histology of normal adult thyroid gland: (*1*) colloid of a thyroid follicle; (*2*) follicular cells. Single-layer cells forming a follicle; (*3*) parafollicular cells (C cells); (*4*) connective tissue septum

a basement membrane. The follicle is filled with a colloid material that contains thyroglobulin, the precursor macromolecule and storage protein for the thyroid hormones: thyroxine (T4) and triiodothyronine (T3). The size of these follicles varies significantly—even within a single thyroid gland—but is usually about 200 μm. Every 20–40 follicles are separated from the rest by connective tissue septa. Although most authorities believe that the thyroid cells are monoclonal in origin, emerging evidence [27] suggests that different parts of the thyroid originate from different precursors, most interestingly with different malignant potentials. The differences could be reflected by those groups of thyroid follicles separated by the connective tissue septa. Blood vessels and supporting connecting tissue are seen in between the follicles, as well as groups of C cells (also called "parafollicular cells") that produce calcitonin. As mentioned above, these cells are concentrated in the lower part of the upper third of the thyroid gland and nodules in that part of the thyroid gland may be more suspicious for medullary thyroid cancer.

Thyroid Physiology

The main function of the thyroid gland is to provide adequate amounts of thyroid hormone for the proper regulation of a large number of bodily functions, e.g., energy expenditure and metabolic rate. Thyroid hormone is an iodinated hormone and thus requires the ability of the thyroid gland to concentrate iodine from the circulation and organify it for incorporation into the thyroid hormone molecules. The amount of thyroid hormone produced by the thyroid gland is tightly regulated in the human body under normal conditions. This process is very complex and requires several steps, both within and outside of the thyroid gland. Each step may have clinical relevance to thyroid cancer.

First, as thyroid cancer cells are derived from normal noncancerous thyroid cells, they use the same cellular mechanisms to function, depending on their level of differentiation. As a result, some of the physiologic functions of normal thyroid cells are used to identify, characterize, or ultimately treat thyroid cancer. For example, one of the most critical properties of a thyroid cell is its ability to trap iodine from the circulation, most often against a concentration gradient. Thus, radioactive iodine can be employed to destroy thyroid cancer cells. The uptake of iodine is accomplished by the sodium–iodide symporter (NIS), located at the basal membrane of the thyrocyte (Fig. 1.3). This active, energy-requiring process can concentrate iodide in the thyrocyte some 20–40-fold above its level in the circulation and is accomplished by the transport of sodium into the cell. Notably, similar iodide transport mechanisms are also present in other tissues, such as the salivary gland. Thus, because salivary tissue will actively transport radioactive iodine when administered, patients may suffer from radiation-induced sialadenitis or xerostomia when treated with radioactive iodine for thyroid cancer.

For organification of the iodide, the enzyme thyroid peroxidase (TPO), together with hydrogen peroxide, is required to organify the inorganic iodide and incorporate it into a tyrosine residue within thyroglobulin. This occurs in the apical membrane of the thyroid cell, facing the colloid (Fig. 1.3). Each tyrosine molecule can take up as many as four iodide atoms, forming the different types of thyroid hormone. Another important transporter in this system called pendrin has also been identified [28]. It is located at the apical membrane of thyrocytes (Fig. 1.3). It is an important regulator of inorganic iodide efflux into the lumen of the thyroid follicle where organification takes place as described above. Mutations of this gene have been described in the Pendred syndrome. A partial defect of iodide organification leads to the development of goiters in some of these patients [29].

Once the thyroid hormone has been synthesized, it is stored in linkage within the thyroglobulin molecule in the colloid of thyroid follicles. Under stimulation by thyrotropin (TSH), the gland receives the signal that thyroid hormone release is needed, and fragments of thyroglobulin enter the thyrocyte (pinocytosis) and are cleaved by endopeptidases in the endosomes and lysosomes. Thyroxine and triiodothyronine are produced and released into the circulation. Under normal conditions, the thyroid gland output consists of mainly thyroxine (~90 % or ~75–100 μg/day) and a small amount of triiodothyronine (~10 % or 6 μg/day).

Thus, the processes of iodide uptake and thyroid hormone synthesis are largely regulated by TSH, a pituitary hormone that stimulates both of these thyroid functions. As described in detail elsewhere in this volume, either endogenous TSH stimulation prompted by thyroid hormone withdrawal or exogenous recombinant human TSH is critical in the

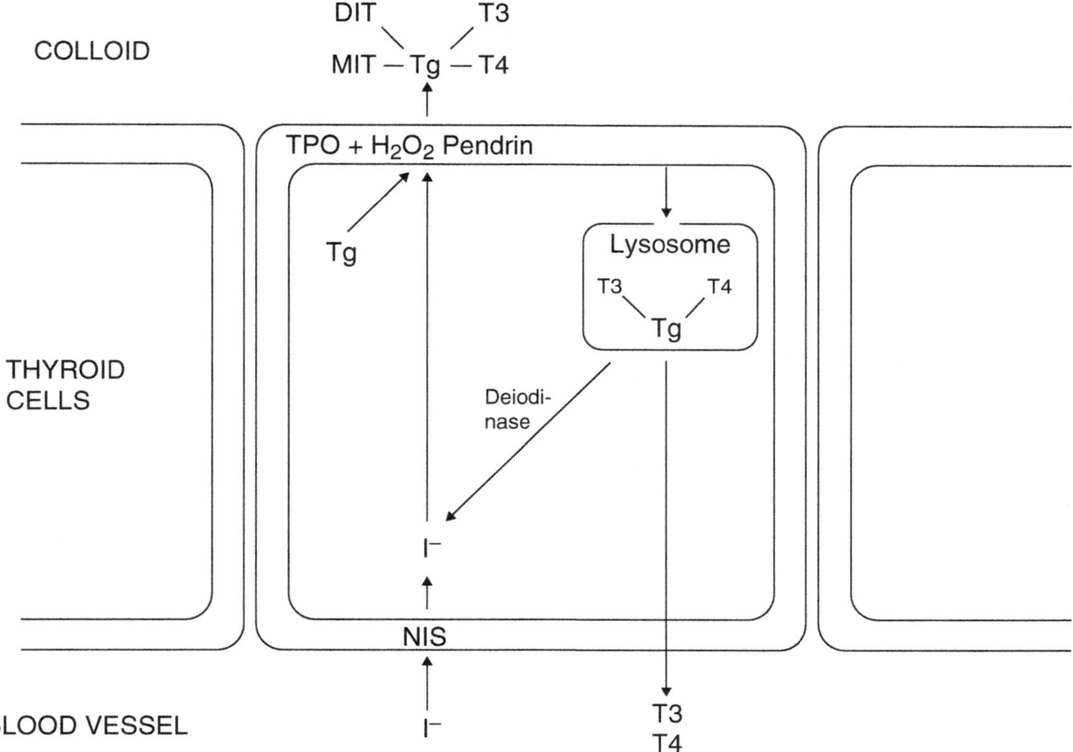

Fig. 1.3 Organification of iodide and synthesis and release of thyroid hormone. *NIS* sodium–iodide symporter, *Tg* thyroglobulin, *TPO* thyroid peroxidase, *MID* monoiodotyrosine, *DIT* diiodotyrosine, *H2O2* hydrogen peroxide, *T3* triiodothyronine, *T4* thyroxine, *I* iodide

diagnosis and treatment of thyroid cancer. On the contrary, as TSH has mitogenic activity, its chronic suppression by thyroxine therapy is critical to the prevention of thyroid cancer growth. Recent evidence suggests a potential role of TSH stimulation in thyroid oncogenesis. Higher TSH values, even within the normal range, are an independent predictor of malignancy for thyroid nodules [30, 31].

Another important aspect of molecular thyroid physiology is the effect that iodine has on thyroid function. As discussed previously, the thyroid gland actively concentrates iodine from the circulation which is used to synthesize thyroid hormone. It is a well-known that iodine deficiency causes goiters, and often when iodine-deficient patients are given iodine, production of excessive amounts of thyroid hormone, hyperthyroidism, is possible, at least transiently. This response is called the "Jod-Basedow phenomenon" [32]. The mechanism for this phenomenon is unclear, but it is thought that it is either because of rapid iodination of poorly iodinated thyroglobulin or the "fueling" of a subclinical autonomous functioning thyroid tissue, as in a "hot" nodule or in Graves' disease [33]. Alternatively, if there is an excess of iodine present in thyrocytes, the sodium–iodide symporter and TPO are inhibited to prevent excessive amounts of thyroid hormone from being synthesized. This inhibition is referred to as "the Wolff–Chaikoff phenomenon" [34]. A high concentration of inorganic iodide is needed for this effect. This inhibition of iodide organification is temporary because the inhibition of iodide transport by the NIS depletes intracellular iodine, allowing the system to reset with new iodide organification—this is called the "escape from the Wolff–Chaikoff effect."

Several molecules discussed have significant clinical utility in the daily management of thyroid cancer. Measurement of the TSH receptor, thyroglobulin, antithyroglobulin antibodies, and thyroperoxidase (TPO) can be used to determine if a neoplasm is of thyroid origin. Multiple other relevant molecules have been described, such as thyroid transcription factors (TTF) 1 and 2, galectin 3, and oncofetal fibronectin. Assessment of the presence of such proteins may be particularly important in the evaluation of material obtained by fine-needle aspiration of suspected metastatic lesions. See Chap. 3 for a more detailed description of molecular thyroid markers.

Finally, there are several elements of thyroid molecular physiology that are poorly understood but may play a significant role in thyroid cell function as well as in thyroid oncogenesis. One such element is the retinoid receptor system. Retinoids are vitamin A derivatives that regulate growth and differentiation of many cell types by binding to specific nuclear receptors. In thyroid cells, these molecules are involved in the regulation of important regulatory factors, such as thyroglobulin and the NIS [35]. There is evidence to suggest that activation of these nuclear receptors may induce some degree of redifferentiation of thyroid cancer cells and make them more susceptible to conventional thyroid cancer treatments such as radioactive iodine [36].

References

1. Burman KD, Adler RA, Wartofsky L. Hemiagenesis of the thyroid gland. Am J Med. 1975;58(1):143–6.
2. Monfared A, Saenz Y, Terris DJ. Endoscopic resection of the submandibular gland in a porcine model. Laryngoscope. 2002;112(6):1089–93.
3. Moreau S, de Goullet Rugy M, Babin E, Salame E, Delmas P, Valdazo A. The recurrent laryngeal nerve: related vascular anatomy. Laryngoscope. 1998;108(9):1351–3.
4. Abboud B, Aouad R. Non-recurrent inferior laryngeal nerve in thyroid surgery: report of three cases and review of the literature. J Laryngol Otol. 2004;118(2):139–42.
5. Miller FR, Netterville JL. Surgical management of thyroid and parathyroid disorders. Med Clin N Am. 1999;83(1):247–59, xi.
6. Naghavi SE, Jalali MM. Papillary carcinoma of thyroglossal duct cyst. Med Sci Monit: Int Med J Exp Clin Res. 2003;9(7):CS67–70.
7. Tang ZH, Li WY. Diagnosis of ectopic thyroid in the tongue root by 99mTcO4(-) and 131I radionuclide thyroid imaging: report of one case. Di 1 jun yi da xue xue bao = Acad J First Med Coll PLA. 2003;23(10):1041–2.
8. Thomas G, Hoilat R, Daniels JS, Kalagie W. Ectopic lingual thyroid: a case report. Int J Oral Maxillofac Surg. 2003;32(2):219–21.
9. Boer A, Polus K. Lingual thyroid: a rare disease resembling base of tongue neoplasm. Magy Onkol. 2002;46(4):347–9.
10. Chiu TT, Su CY, Hwang CF, Chien CY, Eng HL. Massive bleeding from an ectopic lingual thyroid follicular adenoma during pregnancy. Am J Otolaryngol. 2002;23(3):185–8.
11. Jimenez Oliver V, Ruiz Rico R, Davila Morillo A, Fernandez Ruiz E, del Ruiz Portal JM, Perez Arcos JA, Rodriguez Baro G. Intralaryngeal ectopic thyroid tissue. Report of one case and review of the literature. Acta Otorrinolaringol Esp. 2002;53(1):54–9.
12. Byrd MC, Thompson LD, Wieneke JA. Intratracheal ectopic thyroid tissue: a case report and literature review. Ear Nose Throat J. 2003;82(7):514–8.
13. Ulug T, Ulubil SA, Alagol F. Dual ectopic thyroid: report of a case. The J Laryngol Otol. 2003;117(7):574–6.
14. Hollander EJ, Visser MJ, van Baalen JM. Accessory thyroid gland at carotid bifurcation presenting as a carotid body tumor: case report and review of the literature. J Vasc Surg. 2004;39(1):260–2.
15. Larysz B, Jedrzychowska-Baraniak J, Nikodemska I, Sell M. Ectopic thyroid tissue in the heart – a case report. Kardiol Pol. 2003;59(8):149–51.
16. Chosia M, Waligorski S, Listewnik MH, Wiechowski S. Ectopic thyroid tissue as a tumour of the heart – case report and review of the literature. Pol J Pathol. 2002;53(3):173–5.
17. Williams RJ, Lindop G, Butler J. Ectopic thyroid tissue on the ascending aorta: an operative finding. Ann Thorac Surg. 2002;73(5):1642–3.
18. Ihtiyar E, Isiksoy S, Algin C, Sahin A, Erkasap S, Yasar B. Ectopic thyroid in the gallbladder: report of a case. Surg Today. 2003;33(10):777–80.
19. Ghanem N, Bley T, Altehoefer C, Hogerle S, Langer M. Ectopic thyroid gland in the porta hepatis and lingua. Thyroid. 2003;13(5):503–7.
20. Gungor B, Kebat T, Ozaslan C, Akilli S. Intra-abdominal ectopic thyroid presenting with hyperthyroidism: report of a case. Surg Today. 2002;32(2):148–50.
21. Ribeiro-Silva A, Bezerra AM, Serafini LN. Malignant struma ovarii: an autopsy report of a clinically unsuspected tumor. Gynecol Oncol. 2002;87(2):213–5.
22. Perez JS, Munoz M, Naval L, Blasco A, Diaz FJ. Papillary carcinoma arising in lingual thyroid. J Craniomaxillofac Surg. 2003;31(3):179–82.
23. Massine RE, Durning SJ, Koroscil TM. Lingual thyroid carcinoma: a case report and review of the literature. Thyroid. 2001;11(12):1191–6.
24. Kao SY, Tu H, Chang RC, Yang AH, Chang KW, Lee CH. Primary ectopic thyroid papillary carcinoma in the floor of the mouth and tongue: a case report. Br J Oral Maxillofac Surg. 2002;40(3):213–5.
25. Klubo-Gwiezdzinska J, Manes RP, Chia SH, Burman KD, Stathatos NA, Deeb ZE, Wartofsky L. Clinical review: ectopic cervical thyroid carcinoma – review of the literature with illustrative case series. J Clin Endocrinol Metab. 2011;96(9):2684–91.
26. Meyer JS, Steinberg LS. Microscopically benign thyroid follicles in cervical lymph nodes. Serial section study of lymph node inclusions and entire thyroid gland in 5 cases. Cancer. 1969;24(2):302–11.
27. Jovanovic L, Delahunt B, McIver B, Eberhardt NL, Grebe SK. Thyroid gland clonality revisited: the embryonal patch size of the normal human thyroid gland is very large, suggesting X-chromosome inactivation tumor clonality studies of thyroid tumors have to be interpreted with caution. J Clin Endocrinol Metab. 2003;88(7):3284–91.
28. Scott DA, Wang R, Kreman TM, Sheffield VC, Karniski LP. The Pendred syndrome gene encodes a chloride-iodide transport protein. Nat Genet. 1999;21(4):440–3.
29. Bizhanova A, Kopp P. Genetics and phenomics of Pendred syndrome. Mol Cell Endocrinol. 2010;322(1–2):83–90.
30. Boelaert K, Horacek J, Holder RL, Watkinson JC, Sheppard MC, Franklyn JA. Serum thyrotropin concentration as a novel predictor of malignancy in thyroid nodules investigated by fine-needle aspiration. J Clin Endocrinol Metab. 2006;91(11):4295–301.
31. Zafon C, Obiols G, Baena JA, Castellvi J, Dalama B, Mesa J. Preoperative thyrotropin serum concentrations gradually increase from benign thyroid nodules to papillary thyroid microcarcinomas then to papillary thyroid cancers of larger size. J Thyroid Res. 2012;2012:530721.
32. Stanbury JB, Ermans AE, Bourdoux P, Todd C, Oken E, Tonglet R, Vidor G, Braverman LE, Medeiros-Neto G. Iodine-induced hyperthyroidism: occurrence and epidemiology. Thyroid. 1998;8(1):83–100.
33. Ermans AM, Camus M. Modifications of thyroid function induced by chronic administration of iodide in the presence of "autonomous" thyroid tissue. Acta Endocrinol. 1972;70(3):463–75.
34. Wolff J, Chaikoff IL. Plasma inorganic iodide as a homeostatic regulator of thyroid function. J Biol Chem. 1948;174(2):555–64.
35. Kurebayashi J, Tanaka K, Otsuki T, Moriya T, Kunisue H, Uno M, Sonoo H. All-trans-retinoic acid modulates expression levels of thyroglobulin and cytokines in a new human poorly differentiated papillary thyroid carcinoma cell line, KTC-1. J Clin Endocrinol Metab. 2000;85(8):2889–96.
36. Van Herle AJ, Agatep ML, Padua 3rd DN, Totanes TL, Canlapan DV, Van Herle HM, Juillard GJ. Effects of 13 cis-retinoic acid on growth and differentiation of human follicular carcinoma cells (UCLA R0 82 W-1) in vitro. J Clin Endocrinol Metab. 1990;71(3):755–63.

Epidemiology of Thyroid Cancer

2

James J. Figge

Incidence

Thyroid cancer is the most common endocrine malignancy, accounting for 3.6 % of all new malignant tumors (excluding basal and squamous cell skin cancers and in situ carcinomas except urinary bladder) diagnosed annually in the United States (1.7 % of cancers in men; 5.6 % in women; [1]. Annual incidence rates vary by geographic area, age, and sex [2–8]. The age-adjusted annual incidence (from 2006 to 2010) in the United States is 122 new cases per million [2], with a higher incidence in women (182/million) than men (61/million) [2]. Approximately 60,220 new cases of thyroid cancer are now diagnosed annually in the United States with a female to male ratio close to 3:1 [1]. Worldwide, incidence rates are highest in certain geographic areas, such as Sao Paulo, Brazil (149/million women and 39/million men) [5], Hawaii (223/million women and 63/million men) [2, 6], New Jersey (246/million women and 82/million men) [2, 7], Utah (247/million women and 75/million men) [2], and Connecticut (257/million women and 85/million men) [2, 4], probably as a result of local environmental influences. Rates in Poland are among the lowest recorded: 14 per million women and 4 per million men [8]. Thyroid cancer is very rare in children under age 15 [9]. The annual US incidence in children ages 10–14 is ten per million girls and three per million boys [2]. The annual incidence of thyroid cancer increases with age, peaking between 199 and 243 per million by the fifth through eighth decades [2].

J.J. Figge, MD, MBA, FACP (✉)
Department of Biomedical Sciences, School of Public Health, State University of New York, Albany, NY, USA

Department of Medicine, St. Peter's Health Partners, Albany, NY, USA

Gen*NY*Sis Center for Excellence in Cancer Genomics, State University of New York, One Discovery Drive, Rensselaer, NY, USA
e-mail: jfigge@albany.edu

The incidence of thyroid cancer has increased over a period of several decades in the United States, as well as many other countries worldwide, particularly among women [2–4, 10–32]. For example, in Connecticut, the annual age-standardized incidence in women has progressively increased from 13 per million in 1935–1939, to 36 per million in 1965–1969, to 45 per million in 1985–1989, reaching 58 per million in 1990–1991, and 257 per million in 2006–2010 [2, 4]. The corresponding figures for men are 2 per million, 18 per million, 21 per million, 26 per million, and 85 per million, respectively [2, 4]. Davies and Welch [26] analyzed the National Cancer Institute's Surveillance, Epidemiology, and End Results (SEER) database and showed that the increasing incidence of thyroid cancer in the United States between 1973 and 2002 was almost exclusively attributable to an increase in the incidence of papillary thyroid cancer. According to their analysis, 49 % of the increase was restricted to cancers measuring 1 cm or smaller, and 87 % of the increase consisted of cancers measuring 2 cm or smaller [26]. The precise reasons for the increase are not clearly understood but might be related, at least in part, to the introduction of improved diagnostic methodology (e.g., ultrasound, thyroid scans, and fine-needle aspiration biopsy) and improvements in cancer registration [4, 25, 26]. Hence, Davies and Welch concluded that "increased diagnostic scrutiny," reflecting an increased detection of subclinical disease, is the most likely reason for the apparent increase in thyroid cancer incidence. This is consistent with the epidemiologic concept of "overdiagnosis," which postulates that an increasing number of diagnoses reflect more effective detection of a subclinical reservoir of cancers, which, if left undetected, would not have caused symptoms or death [27]. Moris et al. [27] have provided further evidence from the SEER database demonstrating that markers for higher levels of health care access are associated with higher papillary thyroid cancer incidence rates, thus supporting the hypothesis that overdiagnosis explains much of the increase in thyroid cancer incidence. Some of these papillary carcinomas

L. Wartofsky, D. Van Nostrand (eds.), *Thyroid Cancer*, DOI 10.1007/978-1-4939-3314-3_2

represent "incidentalomas," in the sense that they were detected as incidental findings during the course of an evaluation for an unrelated issue, such as a carotid ultrasound or a chest CT scan.

However, other detailed analyses of the SEER database have partially refuted the overdiagnosis hypothesis [28–33]. Devesa's group [28] compared thyroid cancer types by race/ethnicity, gender, and age and concluded that a detection effect cannot completely explain the observed increases in thyroid cancer incidence [28]. Age-specific incidence curves by gender for papillary carcinoma are notably similar across all SEER racial/ethnic groups despite known disparities among the groups in access to healthcare technologies such as ultrasound [28]. For papillary carcinoma, the age-specific rates for whites, Asians, and Hispanics are nearly identical, but the rates for black women and men are slightly lower across all age groups [28]. Additionally, ethnic variations in thyroid cancer incidence are minimal in cases of nonpapillary histology, arguing against differences in diagnostic scrutiny [28]. Li et al. [29] considered socioeconomic status (SES) as a surrogate for access to technology. In analyzing the SEER registry, Li et al. [29] confirmed higher thyroid cancer incidence rates in high- vs. low-SES counties, but only for tumors up to 4.0 cm. For larger tumors (>4.0 cm), the thyroid cancer incidence increased similarly for both high- and low-SES counties. Furthermore, Li et al. [29], Yu et al. [30], Chen et al. [31], Enewold et al. [32], and Morris and Myssiorek [33] have documented an increasing incidence of large (e.g., >4.0 cm) as well as small papillary thyroid carcinomas in the SEER database. Between 1992 and 2005, 50 % of the overall increase in papillary carcinoma incidence rates in SEER was due to papillary microcarcinomas (1.0 cm or less), 30 % to cancers 1.1–2 cm, and 20 % to cancers greater than 2 cm [32]. Among white females, the rate of increase for papillary cancers greater than 5 cm in diameter almost equals that for the smallest papillary cancers [32]. If the early detection hypothesis were entirely correct, then one would expect to see a decreasing, and not increasing, incidence of larger papillary cancers [30]. Thus, the "increased diagnostic scrutiny" hypothesis regarding clinical application of more sensitive diagnostic procedures cannot completely explain the observed increases in papillary thyroid cancer incidence. It is most likely that overdiagnosis contributes significantly to the observed increase in thyroid cancer incidence, but there is a true increase as well. Hence, other relevant factors must exist.

Radiation has been proposed as major factor to explain the increasing incidence of thyroid cancer. In the United States, the increased incidence between 1935 and 1975 may be a consequence of therapeutic radiation treatments administered to the head and neck region of children [11, 34]. However, elevations in thyroid cancer incidence were documented in other countries where childhood radiation treatments were never commonly employed [15, 17, 21]; therefore, other factors must also be involved. Exposure to fallout from nuclear weapon testing has been suggested as an influence in Europe, but epidemiological data indicate that there are still more important factors [16]. In the United States, a committee of the US National Academy of Sciences Institute of Medicine and National Research Council [35] estimated that an excess of 11,300 thyroid cancer cases could be attributed to exposure to fallout from the Nevada atomic bomb testing of the 1950s. Fallout from the Chernobyl accident in Connecticut, Utah, Iowa, and in parts of Europe has been suggested as another factor [24, 36]. Increasing population exposure to medical and dental diagnostic X-rays, particularly CT scans, has been postulated to be a factor [7, 29, 37, 38]. Finally, exposure to environmental pollutants has been proposed as a contributing factor [38]. The incidence of thyroid cancer is no longer rising in certain countries, such as Norway and Iceland [17–19], but it continues to rise in the United States [2].

Prevalence

Thyroid cancer prevalence rates vary widely by geographic area, patient population, and method of survey. Autopsy rates ranging from 0.03 % to over 2 % have been reported [39–46]. Mortensen and colleagues [39] reported on 1,000 consecutive routine autopsies and found a 2.8 % prevalence rate of thyroid carcinoma. The high cancer prevalence can be attributed to the meticulous histological evaluation protocol [39]. On routine clinical assessment, 61 % (17/28) of the cancers originated from thyroid glands that were apparently normal [40]. Similar prevalence rates (2.3–2.7 %) were reported by Bisi and colleagues [41] and Silverberg and Vidone [42]. The high prevalence rates reported in the latter two studies may have also been influenced by the highly selected inpatient populations studied and may not reflect the prevalence in the general population.

Small foci of papillary thyroid carcinoma, measuring 1 cm or less in diameter, can be classified as "papillary microcarcinomas" [47] and occur frequently in autopsy material (reviewed in ref. 48). Most papillary microcarcinomas measure between 4 and 7 mm [49]. These can be subdivided into "tiny" (5–10-mm diameter) and "minute" carcinomas (<5-mm diameter; [47, 50–53]). The term "occult" carcinoma has no pathological meaning and should be abandoned in favor of these more precisely defined terms, as advocated by LiVolsi [47]. Papillary microcarcinomas are usually detected by meticulous sectioning of the thyroid at 2–3-mm intervals, with detailed microscopic examination of each section. The highest prevalence rate of papillary thyroid microcarcinoma (≤1-cm diameter) was reported from Finland [54], with 33.7 % of 101 cases harboring this finding.

Rates over 20 % have been reported from Japan [55, 56], whereas the rate of papillary microcarcinoma is much lower in Sweden (6.4 %; [44]) and in Olmsted County, Minnesota (5.1 %; [57]). Minute papillary carcinomas (<5 mm) are rarely detected on physical exam and are believed to exhibit a relatively benign clinical course. However, there are occasional reports of distant metastases (e.g., pulmonary metastases) that arise from minute papillary carcinomas [58]. Mazzaferri has published an excellent review of the natural history of papillary microcarcinomas [59].

Thyroid cancer prevalence rates are significantly greater than incidence figures, reflecting that substantial numbers of patients survive several decades or longer. Data in the Connecticut registry show a prevalence rate of 677 cases per million in women and 237 cases per million in men [60]. These data refer only to clinically apparent disease and are therefore lower than the rates in many autopsy series [39–46].

Mortality

The annual mortality from thyroid cancer is low—five deaths per million individuals per year [2], presumably reflecting the good prognosis for most thyroid cancers. Mortality rates are lowest in individuals under age 50 and increase sharply thereafter [2]. There are about 1,850 deaths from thyroid cancer annually in the United States [1], accounting for 0.32 % of all cancer deaths (0.26 % of cancer deaths in men; 0.38 % in women).

Although the incidence of thyroid cancer has been increasing over time in both men and women, mortality has decreased over the past 50 years [2]. The reduced mortality is due to earlier diagnosis, improved treatment, and decreased incidence of anaplastic carcinoma. For example, 5-year relative survival rates for thyroid cancer have increased from 80 % in 1950–1954 to 98 % in 2003–2009 [2].

Distribution by Histological Type

The relative proportion of differentiated (follicular and papillary) thyroid cancers in a given geographic area depends on the dietary iodine intake [61]. Papillary cancers predominate in iodine-sufficient areas. For example, in Iceland, which has ample iodine intake, the proportions were 85 % with papillary and 15 % with follicular cancer from 1955 to 1984 [19]; in Bavaria, Germany, an iodine-deficient area, the proportions were 35 % papillary and 65 % follicular during 1960–1975 [61]. The introduction of iodine supplementation in an endemic goiter region results in an increased proportion of papillary cancers [62], coupled with an improved outcome relating to life expectancy [63].

In the United States, approximately 87 % of invasive thyroid cancers are papillary carcinomas [2, 64]. Papillary cancer has a peak incidence in the fourth through eighth decades of life and affects women three times more frequently than men [28]. Follicular carcinoma accounts for about 6 % of US cases [2, 64] and has a peak incidence in the seventh and eighth decades [28]. The tumor is two to three times more common in women than men. Medullary carcinomas comprise nearly 2 % of thyroid carcinomas [2]. Of these, 80 % are sporadic and 20 % are familial. The hereditary familial forms are classified under the multiple endocrine neoplasia type IIA (MEN IIA) syndrome, or the MEN IIB syndrome [65]. The sporadic form presents mostly in the fifth and sixth decades of life and affects females 1.5 times more than males [66]. Classical MEN IIA-related medullary carcinomas present in the first and second decades, and MEN IIB-associated medullary cancers present during the first decade of life [65]. Familial medullary thyroid carcinomas arising in families without pheochromocytomas or primary hyperparathyroidism (FMTC, now recognized to be a variant of MEN IIA) present in the sixth decade and beyond [65]. Familial forms of medullary carcinoma occur with equal frequency in females and males. Anaplastic cancers account for just under 1 % of cases [2]. The incidence of anaplastic cancer has recently declined—a factor that has contributed to the reduction in overall thyroid cancer mortality. The peak incidence of anaplastic cancer is in the seventh decade and beyond; the female to male ratio is approximately 1.5:1 [28]. Lymphomas represent about 5 % of thyroid malignancies, with a mean age of 60–65 at the time of presentation [67, 68]. Females predominate at all ages: in patients under age 60, the ratio is 1.5:1; in patients over age 60, the ratio ranges from 3 to 8:1 [67, 68].

Factors Associated with Thyroid Cancer Risk

There are several strong associations between thyroid cancer incidence and certain risk factors.

1. Thyroid cancer incidence increases with age.
2. Thyroid cancer is more common in females than males. The female predominance suggests that hormonal factors may be involved. Some studies suggest that biological changes that occur during pregnancy may increase the risk of thyroid carcinoma [69–71].
3. Several genetic syndromes are associated with follicular cell-derived thyroid carcinomas: familial adenomatous polyposis (including Gardner syndrome), phosphatase, and tensin homolog deleted on chromosome ten (*PTEN*)-hamartoma tumor syndrome (including Cowden syndrome and Bannayan-Riley-Ruvalcaba syndrome), Carney complex type I, Pendred syndrome, Werner syn-

drome, and several familial papillary thyroid carcinoma (fPTC) syndromes (pure fPTC, with or without oxyphilia, fPTC with papillary renal cell carcinoma, and fPTC with multinodular goiter) [72–74]. Familial cancer syndromes that include medullary thyroid carcinoma (MTC) are multiple endocrine neoplasia IIA (MEN IIA) and MEN IIB. Pure familial MTC syndrome (FMTC) is now recognized to be a variant of MEN IIA.

4. Radiation exposure in childhood is the only factor that has been shown unequivocally to cause thyroid cancer.
5. A history of goiter and a history of benign nodules/adenomas are the strongest risk factors for thyroid cancer, apart from radiation in childhood (see discussion below).
6. Strong evidence indicates that individuals with Hashimoto's thyroiditis have an increased chance to develop thyroid lymphoma [75].

Epidemiology

In addition to these well-established associations, there are postulated risk factors for thyroid carcinoma that remain unproven. These include iodine deficiency and endemic goiter [76], which may result in prolonged stimulation of thyroid tissue by elevated thyroid-stimulating hormone (TSH) levels. Data on this postulated relationship are inconsistent [71, 76–86]. A major study comparing goiter prevalence and the effect of iodine supplementation with thyroid cancer rates in the United States failed to support a link between endemic goiter and thyroid cancer [86]. Graves' disease has also been postulated to be associated with an increased incidence of thyroid cancer. This hypothesis is of interest because of the TSH-like activity of thyroid-stimulating immunoglobulins. However, the data remain inconclusive [87–101], with reported cancer rates ranging from 0.06 % [90] to as high as 8.7 % [92] in glands affected by Graves' disease. Lower rates were reported in older studies [87–90], and several more recent studies [94–96] show rates in the range of 5.1–7.0 %. The possibility that other benign diseases of the thyroid could increase the risk of cancer has also been considered [71, 75, 77, 81, 102–106]. Given the strong possibility of ascertainment and recall bias, these data are difficult to interpret. Furthermore, it is well established that pathological examinations of thyroid tissue can reveal a high rate of unsuspected microcarcinomas that may be of little clinical significance. Nevertheless, a recent pooled analysis of 14 case-control studies [107–111] has provided evidence that a large risk of thyroid cancer is associated with a history of goiter (pooled odds ratio [OR] = 5.9 in women; OR = 38.3 in men) or benign nodules/adenomas (OR = 29.9 in women; 18 cases vs 0 controls in men). This evidence was validated by a prospective study from Denmark [112, 113]. Thus, current data suggest that apart from radiation in childhood, goiter and benign nodules/adenomas are the strongest risk factors for thyroid cancer.

References

1. Siegel R, Naishadham D, Jemal A. Cancer statistics. CA Cancer J Clin. 2013;63:11–30.
2. Howlader N, Noone AM, Krapcho M, Garshell J, Neyman N, Altekruse SF, Kosary CL, Yu M, Ruhl J, Tatalovich Z, Cho H, Mariotto A, Lewis DR, Chen HS, Feuer EJ, Cronin KA ,editors. SEER Cancer Statistics Review, 1975–2010, National Cancer Institute. Bethesda. http://seer.cancer.gov/csr/1975_2010/, based on Nov 2012 SEER data submission, posted to the SEER web site, Apr 2013.
3. Verby JE, Woolner LB, Nobrega FT, Kurland LT, McConahey WM. Thyroid cancer in Olmsted County. J Natl Cancer Inst. 1969;43:813–20. 1935–1965.
4. Polednak AP. Trends in cancer incidence in Connecticut, 1935–1991. Cancer. 1994;74:2863–72.
5. Veiga LH, Neta G, Aschebrook-Kilfoy B, Ron E, Devesa SS. Thyroid cancer incidence patterns in Sao Paulo, Brazil, and the U.S. SEER program, 1997–2008. Thyroid. 2013;23(6):748–57.
6. Goodman MT, Yoshizawa CN, Kolonel LN. Descriptive epidemiology of thyroid cancer in Hawaii. Cancer. 1988;61:1272–81.
7. Roche LM, Niu X, Pawlish KS, Henry KA. Thyroid cancer incidence in New Jersey: time trend, birth cohort and socioeconomic status analysis (1979–2006). J Environ Public Health. 2011;2011(2011):850105.
8. Whelan SL, Parkin DM, Masuyer E. Patterns of cancer in five continents. IARC Sci Publ. 1990;102:1–159.
9. Parkin DM, Stiller CA, Draper GJ, Bieber CA. International incidence of childhood cancer. IARC Sci Publ. 1988;87:1–401.
10. Weiss W. Changing incidence of thyroid cancer. J Natl Cancer Inst. 1979;62:1137–42.
11. Pottern LM, Stone BJ, Day NE, Pickle LW, Fraumeni Jr JF. Thyroid cancer in Connecticut, 1935–1975: an analysis by cell type. Am J Epidemiol. 1980;112:764–74.
12. Carroll RE, Haddon Jr W, Handy VH, Wieben EE. Thyroid cancer: cohort analysis of increasing incidence in New York State, 1941–1962. J Natl Cancer Inst. 1964;33:277–83.
13. Waterhouse J, Muir C, Correa P, Powell J. Cancer incidence in five continents, vol. 3. Lyon: International Agency for Research on Cancer; 1976.
14. Waterhouse J, Muir C, Shanugaratnam K. Cancer incidence in five continents, vol. 4. Lyon: International Agency for Research on Cancer; 1982.
15. Pettersson B, Adami H-O, Wilander E, Coleman MP. Trends in thyroid cancer incidence in Sweden, 1958–1981, by histopathologic type. Int J Cancer. 1991;48:28–33.
16. dos Santos SI, Swerdlow AJ. Thyroid cancer epidemiology in England and Wales: time trends and geographical distribution. Br J Cancer. 1993;67:330–40.
17. Akslen LA, Haldorsen T, Thoresen SO, Glattre E. Incidence pattern of thyroid cancer in Norway: influence of birth cohort and time period. Int J Cancer. 1993;53:183–7.
18. Glattre E, Akslen LA, Thoresen S, Haldoren T. Geographic patterns and trends in the incidence of thyroid cancer in Norway 1970–1986. Cancer Detect Prev. 1990;14:625–31.
19. Hrafnkelsson J, Jonasson JG, Sigurdsson G, Sigvaldason H, Tulinius H. Thyroid cancer in Iceland 1955–1984. Acta Endocrinol. 1988;118:566–72.

20. Staunton MD, Bourne H. Thyroid cancer in the 1980's: a decade of change. Ann Acad Med Singapore. 1993;22:613–6.
21. Levi F, Franceschi S, Te VC, Negri E, La Vecchia C. Descriptive epidemiology of thyroid cancer in the Swiss canton of Vaud. J Cancer Res Clin Oncol. 1990;116:639–47.
22. Leenhardt L, Grosclaude P, Chérié-Challine L. Increased incidence of thyroid carcinoma in France: a true epidemic or thyroid nodule management effects? Report from the French Thyroid Cancer Committee. Thyroid. 2004;14:1056–60.
23. Burke JP, Hay ID, Dignan F, Goellner JR, Achenbach SJ, Oberg AL, Melton III LJ. Long-term trends in thyroid carcinoma: a population-based study in Olmsted County, Minnesota, 1935–1999. Mayo Clin Proc. 2005;80:753–8.
24. Mangano JJ. A post-chernobyl rise in thyroid cancer in Connecticut, USA. Eur J Cancer Prev. 1996;5:75–81.
25. Roush GC, Holford TR, Schymura MJ, White C. Cancer risk and incidence trends: the Connecticut perspective. New York: Hemisphere Publishing; 1987.
26. Davies L, Welch HG. Increasing incidence of thyroid cancer in the United States, 1973–2002. JAMA. 2006;295(18):2164–7.
27. Morris LG, Sikora AG, Tosteson TD, Davies L. The increasing incidence of thyroid cancer: the influence of access to care. Thyroid. 2013;23(7):885–91.
28. Aschebrook-Kilfoy B, Ward MH, Sabra MM, Devesa SS. Thyroid cancer incidence patterns in the United States by histologic type, 1992–2006. Thyroid. 2011;21(2):125–34.
29. Li N, Du XL, Reitzel LR, Xu L, Sturgis EM. Impact of enhanced detection on the increase in thyroid cancer incidence in the United States: review of incidence trends by socioeconomic status within the surveillance, epidemiology and end results registry, 1980–2008. Thyroid. 2013;23(1):103–10.
30. Yu GP, Li JC, Branovan D, McCormick S, Schantz SP. Thyroid cancer incidence and survival in the national cancer institute surveillance, epidemiology, and end results race/ethnicity groups. Thyroid. 2010;20:465–73.
31. Chen AY, Jemal A, Ward EM. Increasing incidence of differentiated thyroid cancer in the United States, 1988–2005. Cancer. 2009;115:3801–7.
32. Enewold L, Zhu K, Ron E, Marrogi AJ, Stojadinovic A, Peoples GE, Devesa SS. Rising thyroid cancer incidence in the United States by demographic and tumor characteristics, 1980–2005. Cancer Epidemiol Biomarkers Prev. 2009;18(3):784–91.
33. Morris LG, Myssiorek D. Improved detection does not fully explain the rising incidence of well-differentiated thyroid cancer: a population-based analysis. Am J Surg. 2010;200:454–61.
34. Sarne D, Schneider AB. External radiation and thyroid neoplasia. Endocrinol Metab Clin North Am. 1996;25:181–95.
35. Committee on Thyroid Screening Related to I-131 Exposure, Institute of Medicine, Committee on Exposure of the American People to I-131 from the Nevada Atomic Bomb Tests, National Research Council. Exposure of the American people to iodine-131 from Nevada nuclear-bomb tests: review of the National Cancer Institute Report and Public Health Implications. Washington, DC: National Academies Press; 1999.
36. Cardis E, Krewski D, Boniol M, Drozdovitch V, Darby SC, Gilbert ES, Akiba S, Benichou J, Ferlay J, Gandini S, Hill C, Howe G, Kesminiene A, Moser M, Sanchez M, Storm H, Voisin L, Boyle P. Estimates of the cancer burden in Europe from radioactive fallout from the Chernobyl accident. Int J Cancer. 2006;119(6):1224–35.
37. Brenner D, Elliston C, Hall E, Berdon W. Estimated risks of radiation-induced fatal cancer from pediatric CT. AJR. 2001;176:289–96.
38. Pellegriti G, Frasca F, Regalbuto C, Squatrito S, and Vigneri R. Worldwide increasing incidence of thyroid cancer: update on epidemiology and risk factors. J Cancer Epidemiol. 2013; 2013(2013): Article ID 965212.
39. Mortensen JD, Bennett WA, Woolner LB. Incidence of carcinoma in thyroid glands removed at 1000 consecutive routine necropsies. Surg Forum. 1954;5:659–63.
40. Mortensen JD, Woolner LB, Bennett WA. Gross and microscopic findings in clinically normal thyroid glands. J Clin Endocrinol Metab. 1955;15:1270–80.
41. Bisi H, Fernandes VS, de Camargo RY, Koch L, Abdo AH, de Brito T. The prevalence of unsuspected thyroid pathology in 300 sequential autopsies, with special reference to the incidental carcinoma. Cancer. 1989;64:1888–93.
42. Silverberg SG, Vidone RA. Carcinoma of the thyroid in surgical and postmortem material: analysis of 300 cases at autopsy and literature review. Ann Surg. 1966;164:291–9.
43. VanderLaan WP. The occurrence of carcinoma of the thyroid gland in autopsy material. N Engl J Med. 1947;237:221–2.
44. Lennart Bondeson L, Otto Ljungberg O. Occult thyroid carcinoma at autopsy in Malmö, Sweden. Cancer. 1981;47:319–23.
45. Sobrinho-Simões MA, Sambade MC, Vicente Gonçalves V. Latent thyroid carcinoma at autopsy: a study from Oporto, Portugal. Cancer. 1979;43(5):1702–6.
46. Solares CA, Penalonzo MA, Xu M, Orellana E. Occult papillary thyroid carcinoma in postmortem species: prevalence at autopsy. Am J Otolaryngol. 2005;26(2):87–90.
47. LiVolsi VA. Papillary neoplasms of the thyroid. Am J Clin Pathol. 1992;97:426–34.
48. Ain KB. Papillary thyroid carcinoma. Endocrinol Metab Clin North Am. 1995;24:711–60.
49. Vickery Jr AL, Carcangiu ML, Johannessen JV, Sobrinho-Simoes M. Papillary carcinoma. Semin Diagn Pathol. 1985;2:90–100.
50. Kasai N, Sakamoto A. New subgrouping of small thyroid carcinomas. Cancer. 1987;60:1767–70.
51. Naruse T, Koike A, Kanemitsu T, Kato K. Minimal thyroid carcinoma: a report of nine cases discovered by cervical lymph node metastases. Jpn J Surg. 1984;14:118–21.
52. Noguchi M, Tanaka S, Akiyama T, Miyazaki I, Michigishi T, Tonami N, et al. Clinicopathological studies of minimal thyroid and ordinary thyroid cancers. Jpn J Surg. 1984;14:110–7.
53. Yamashita H, Nakayama I, Noguchi S, Murakami N, Moriuchi A, Yokoyama S, et al. Thyroid carcinoma in benign thyroid diseases: an analysis from minute carcinoma. Acta Pathol Jpn. 1985;35:781–8.
54. Harach HR, Franssila KO, Wasenius V-M. Occult papillary carcinoma of the thyroid—a "normal" finding in Finland: a systematic autopsy study. Cancer. 1985;56:531–8.
55. Fukunaga FH, Yatani R. Geographic pathology of occult thyroid carcinomas. Cancer. 1975;36:1095–9.
56. Sampson RJ. Prevalence and significance of occult thyroid cancer. In: DeGroot LJ, editor. Radiation-associated thyroid carcinoma. New York: Grune & Stratton; 1997. p. 137–53.
57. Sampson RJ, Woolner LB, Bahn RC, Kurland LT. Occult thyroid carcinoma in Olmsted country, Minnesota: prevalence at autopsy compared with that in Hiroshima and Nagasaki, Japan. Cancer. 1974;34:2072–6.
58. Strate SM, Lee EL, Childers JH. Occult papillary carcinoma of the thyroid with distant metastases. Cancer. 1984;54:1093–100.
59. Mazzaferri EL. Managing small thyroid cancers. JAMA. 2006;295:2179–82.
60. Feldman AR, Kessler L, Myers MH, Naughton MD. The prevalence of cancer: estimates based on the Connecticut tumor registry. N Engl J Med. 1986;315:1394–7.
61. Lohrs U, Permanetter W, Spelsberg F, Beitinger M. Investigation of frequency and spreading of the different histological types of thyroid cancer in an endemic goiter region. VerhDtsch Ges Pathol. 1977;61:268–74.
62. Harach HR, Escalante DA, Onativa A, Lederer Outes J, Saravia Day E, Williams ED. Thyroid carcinoma and thyroiditis in an

endemic goiter region before and after iodine prophylaxis. Acta Endocrinol. 1985;108:55–60.

63. Farahati J, Geling M, Mader U, Mortl M, Luster M, Muller JG, et al. Changing trends of incidence and prognosis of thyroid carcinoma in lower Franconia, Germany, from 1981–1995. Thyroid. 2004;14:141–7.
64. Mazzaferri EL. Thyroid cancer. In: Becker KL, editor. Principles and practice of endocrinology and metabolism. 3rd ed. Philadelphia: Lippincott, Wiiliams & Wilkins; 2001. p. 382–402.
65. Ledger GA, Khosla S, Lindor NM, Thibodeau SN, Gharib H. Genetic testing in the diagnosis and management of multiple endocrine neoplasia type II. Ann Intern Med. 1995;122:118–24.
66. Emmertsen K. Medullary thyroid carcinoma and calcitonin. Dan Med Bull. 1985;32:1–28.
67. Mazzaferri EL, Oertel YC. Primary malignant lymphoma and related lymphoproliferative disorders. In: Mazzaferri EL, Samaan NA, editors. Endocrine tumors. Cambridge, MA: Blackwell Scientific; 1993. p. 348.
68. Anscombe AM, Wright DH. Primary malignant lymphoma of the thyroid-a tumor of mucosa-associated lymphoid tissue: review of seventy six cases. Histopathology. 1985;9:81–97.
69. Kravdal O, Glattre E, Haldorsen T. Positive correlation between parity and incidence of thyroid cancer: new evidence based on complete Norwegian birth cohorts. Int J Cancer. 1991;49:831–6.
70. Glattre E, Kravdal O. Male and female parity and risk of thyroid cancer. Int J Cancer. 1994;58:616–7.
71. Ron E, Kleinerman RA, Boice Jr JD, LiVolsi VA, Flannery JT, Fraumeni Jr JF. A population-based case-control study of thyroid cancer. J Natl Cancer Inst. 1987;79:1–12.
72. Richards ML. Familial syndromes associated with thyroid cancer in the era of personalized medicine. Thyroid. 2010;20(7):707–13.
73. Laury AR, Bongiovanni M, Tille JC, Kozakewich H, Nosé V. Thyroid pathology in *PTEN*-hamartoma tumor syndrome: characteristic findings of a distinct entity. Thyroid. 2011;21(2): 135–44.
74. Nosé V. Thyroid cancer of follicular cell origin in inherited tumor syndromes. Adv Anat Pathol. 2010;17(6):428–36.
75. Holm LE, Blomgren H, Lowhagen T. Cancer risks in patients with chronic lymphocytic thyroiditis. N Engl J Med. 1985;312:601–4.
76. Wegelin C. Malignant disease of the thyroid gland and its relation to goiter in men and animals. Cancer Rev. 1928;3:297.
77. Franceschi S, Fassina A, Talamini R, Mazzolini A, Vianello S, Bidoli E, et al. Risk factors for thyroid cancer in northern Italy. Int J Epidemiol. 1989;18:578–84.
78. Franceschi S, Talamini R, Fassina A, Bidoli E. Diet and epithelial cancer of the thyroid gland. Tumori. 1990;76:331–8.
79. Kolonel LN, Hankin JH, Wilkens LR, Fukunaga FH, Hinds MW. An epidemiologic study of thyroid cancer in Hawaii. Cancer Causes Control. 1990;1:223–34.
80. Glattre E, Haldorsen T, Berg JP, Stensvold I, Solvoll K. Norwegian case-control study testing the hypothesis that seafood increases the risk of thyroid cancer. Cancer Causes Control. 1993;4:11–6.
81. Preston-Martin S, Jin F, Duda MJ, Mack WJ. A case-control study of thyroid cancer in women under age 55 in Shanghai (People's Republic of China). Cancer Causes Control. 1993;4:431–40.
82. Hallquist A, Hardell L, Degerman A, Boquist L. Thyroid cancer: reproductive factors, previous diseases, drug intake, family history and diet: a case-control study. Eur J Cancer Prev. 1994;3:481–8.
83. Franceschi S, Levi F, Negri E, Fassina A, LaVecchia C. Diet and thyroid cancer: a pooled analysis of four European case-control studies. Int J Cancer. 1991;48:395–8.
84. Correa P, Llanos G. Morbidity and mortality from cancer in Cali, Columbia. J Natl Cancer Inst. 1966;36:717–45.
85. Franssila K, Saxen E, Teppo L, Bjarnason O, Tulinius H, Norman T, Ringertz N. Incidence of different morphological types of thyroid cancer in the Nordic countries. Acta Pathol Microbiol Scand A. 1981;89:49–55.
86. Pendergrast WJ, Milmore BK, Marcus SC. Thyroid cancer and thyrotoxicosis in the United States: their relation to endemic goiter. J Chronic Dis. 1961;13:22–38.
87. Beahrs OH, Pemberton JJ, Black BM. Nodular goiter and malignant lesions of the thyroid gland. J Clin Endocrinol. 1951;11:1157–65.
88. Pemberton J, Black BM. The association of carcinoma of the thyroid gland and exophthalmic goiter. Surg Clin North Am. 1948;28:935–52.
89. Olen E, Klinck GH. Hyperthyroidism and thyroid cancer. Arch Pathol. 1966;81:531–5.
90. Sokal JE. Incidence of malignancy in toxic and non-toxic nodular goiter. JAMA. 1954;154:1321–5.
91. Carnell NE, Valente WA. Thyroid nodules in Graves' disease: classification, characterization, and response to treatment. Thyroid. 1998;8:647–52.
92. Shapiro SJ, Friedman NB, Perzik SI, Catz B. Incidence of thyroid carcinoma in Graves' disease. Cancer. 1970;26:1261–70.
93. Wahl RA, Goretzki P, Meybier H, Nitschke J, Linder M, Roher HD. Coexistence of hyperthyroidism and thyroid cancer. World J Surg. 1982;6:385–90.
94. Farbota LM, Calandra DB, Lawrence AM, Paloyan E. Thyroid carcinoma in Graves' disease. Surgery. 1985;98:1148–53.
95. Behar R, Arganini M, Wu TC, McCormick M, Straus FH, DeGroot LJ, Kaplan EL. Graves' disease and thyroid cancer. Surgery. 1986;100:1121–7.
96. Pacini F, Elisei R, Di Coscio GC, Anelli S, Macchia E, Concetti R, et al. Thyroid carcinoma in thyrotoxic patients treated by surgery. J Endocrinol Invest. 1988;11:107–12.
97. Ozaki O, Ito K, Kobayashi K, Toshima K, Iwasaki H, Yashiro T. Thyroid carcinoma in Graves' disease. World J Surg. 1990;14:437–40.
98. Belfiore A, Garofalo MR, Giuffrida D, Runello F, Filetti S, Fiumara A, et al. Increased aggressiveness of thyroid cancer in patients with Graves' disease. J Clin Endocrinol Metab. 1990;70:830–5.
99. Hales IB, McElduff A, Crummer P, Clifton-Bligh P, Delbridge L, Hoschl R, et al. Does Graves' disease or thyrotoxicosis affect the prognosis of thyroid cancer. J Clin Endocrinol Metab. 1992;75:886–9.
100. Cady B. Papillary carcinoma of the thyroid. Semin Surg Oncol. 1991;7:81–6.
101. Shu X, Ji J, Li X, Sundquist J, Sundquist K, Hemminki K. Cancer risk in patients hospitalized for Graves' disease: a population-based cohort study in Sweden. Br J Cancer. 2010;102:1397–9.
102. Goldman MB, Monson RR, Maloof F. Cancer mortality in women with thyroid disease. Cancer Res. 1990;50:2283–9.
103. Levi F, Franceschi S, La Vecchia C, Negri E, Gulie C, Duruz G, Scazziga B. Previous thyroid disease and risk of thyroid cancer in Switzerland. Eur J Cancer. 1991;27:85–8.
104. Preston-Martin S, Bernstein L, Pike MC, Maldonado AA, Henderson BE. Thyroid cancer among young women related to prior thyroid disease and pregnancy history. Br J Cancer. 1987; 55:191–5.
105. Wingren G, Hatschek T, Axelson O. Determinants of papillary cancer of the thyroid. Am J Epidemiol. 1993;138:482–91.
106. McTiernan AM, Weiss NS, Daling JR. Incidence of thyroid cancer in women in relation to previous exposure to radiation therapy and history of thyroid disease. J Natl Cancer Inst. 1984;73:575–81.
107. Negri E, Ron E, Franceschi S, Dal Maso L, Mark SD, Preston-Martin S, et al. A pooled analysis of case-control studies of thyroid cancer. I. Methods. Cancer Causes Control. 1999;10:131–42.
108. Negri E, Dal Maso L, Ron E, La Vecchia C, Mark SD, Preston-Martin S, et al. A pooled analysis of case-control studies of thyroid cancer. II. Menstrual and reproductive factors. Cancer Causes Control. 1999;10:143–55.

109. La Vecchia C, Ron E, Franceschi S, Dal Maso L, Mark SD, Chatenoud L, et al. A pooled analysis of case-control studies of thyroid cancer. III. Oral contraceptives, menopausal replacement therapy and other female hormones. Cancer Causes Control. 1999;10:157–66.
110. Franceschi S, Preston-Martin S, Dal Maso L, Negri E, La Vecchia C, Mack WJ, et al. A pooled analysis of case-control studies of thyroid cancer. IV. Benign thyroid diseases. Cancer Causes Control. 1999;10:583–95.
111. Preston-Martin S, Franceschi S, Ron E, Negri E. Thyroid cancer pooled analysis from 14 case-control studies: what have we learned? Cancer Causes Control. 2003;14:787–9.
112. Mellemgaard A, From G, Jorgensen T, Johansen C, Olsen JH, Perrild H. Cancer risk in individuals with benign thyroid disorders. Thyroid. 1998;8:751–4.
113. From G, Mellemgaard A, Knudsen N, Jorgensen T, Perrild H. Review of thyroid cancer cases among patients with previous benign thyroid disorders. Thyroid. 2000;10:697–700.

Molecular Pathogenesis of Thyroid Cancer and Oncogenes in Thyroid Cancer

3

Nikita Pozdeyev, Gregory Lund, and Michael T. McDermott

Oncogenes and Tumor Suppressor Genes

Throughout their lifespan, somatic cells can be thought of as progressing through three overlapping transitional stages. Stem cells initially proliferate by undergoing repetitive cell division, causing a rapid expansion of immature tissue mass. Subsequently, these cells differentiate into mature cells that deliver the functions characteristic of their particular phenotype. Later, they grow senescent and undergo programmed cell death or apoptosis. Tumor development (or neoplasia) results from stimuli that augment cellular proliferation or impair cell differentiation and/or apoptosis. A diverse set of signaling and effector proteins is involved in the precise regulation of this complex series of events. Mutations in the genes encoding these proteins have been found to underlie the majority of human malignancies [143]. Genes that encode the proteins promoting normal cell proliferation are called proto-oncogenes. Proto-oncogenes develop activating or gain-of-function mutations that result in the production of proteins that are qualitatively overactive or quantitatively excessive and thereby promote over-robust cellular proliferation. These mutated proto-oncogenes are known as oncogenes [25, 36, 50, 61, 91, 93, 143]. Oncogene mutations tend to be dominantly expressed and thus become clinically apparent in the heterozygous state.

N. Pozdeyev, MD, PhD (✉)
Division of Endocrinology, Metabolism and Diabetes, Department of Medicine, University of Colorado, MS 8106, 12801 E. 17th Ave, RC1-South, Room 7103, Aurora, CO 80045, USA
e-mail: nikitapozdeyev@gmail.com

G. Lund, MD
Denver Endocrinology Diabetes & Thyroid Center, Swedish Medical Center, Englewood, CO, USA

M.T. McDermott, MD
Division of Endocrinology, Metabolism and Diabetes, Department of Medicine, University of Colorado, MS 8106, 12801 E. 17th Ave, RC1-South, Room 7103, Aurora 80045, CO, USA

Tumor suppressor genes [50, 70, 89, 102, 142] encode the proteins that serve to restrain excessive cellular proliferation or promote cell differentiation and/or apoptosis. Inactivating or loss-of-function mutations of these tumor suppressor genes can also lead to neoplasia; these tend to be recessive and therefore are clinically consequential only when present in the homozygous or compound heterozygous state.

Cells undergoing unregulated proliferation because of an activated oncogene or inactivated tumor suppressor gene are considered to be transformed. Cancer-causing mutations may be either somatic or germline. Somatic mutations are those that develop in a single cell at any time in life after fertilization. Through survival advantage conferred by the mutation, the transformed cell expands monoclonally into a solitary tumor mass that may eventually invade or metastasize. In contrast, germline mutations originate in a parent and are passed to offspring through a germ cell. Affected offspring have the mutation present diffusely and may thus be susceptible to the development of multiple tumors within a given organ or susceptible to tumors in multiple organs throughout the body. Most known inherited cancer syndromes result from germline mutations in tumor suppressor genes. Accordingly, individuals are born heterozygous at a critical locus but are initially unaffected because of the normal gene at the homologous locus. However, if a somatic mutation later in life inactivates the normal homologous locus, the individual is rendered unable to make any normal suppressor protein and begins to develop cancer.

The complex system that regulates cellular proliferation, differentiation, and apoptosis has many checks and balances. Although a single genetic mutation may initially transform a cell permitting the monoclonal expansion of its progeny, it is unlikely that a single mutation alone could result in the development of highly malignant tumor behavior. Yet, it appears that the unregulated proliferation of a transformed cell predisposes it to develop additional mutations. These, in turn, provide further selective survival advantages by promoting

L. Wartofsky, D. Van Nostrand (eds.), *Thyroid Cancer*, DOI 10.1007/978-1-4939-3314-3_3

ever-accelerating cell proliferation, tissue invasion, and distant metastases. Indeed, experimental evidence indicates that multiple activated oncogenes and inactivated tumor suppressor genes are often found in highly malignant and metastatic tumors [8, 141].

Similar to other cancer types, thyroid cancer initiation and progression occurs through accumulation of genetic and epigenetic alterations, including activating and inactivating somatic and germline mutations in proto-oncogenes and tumor suppressor genes. Somatic mutations in follicular cells occur early in carcinogenesis and trigger malignant transformation.

Pathways Affected in Thyroid Neoplasia

Molecular defects resulting in oncogenic transformation frequently occur in pathways controlling cell proliferation and survival. Thyroid cancer mutations develop most often in genes encoding components of the MAPK/ERK and PI3K/AKT pathways (Fig. 3.1). The MAPK/ERK pathway is activated in response to a diverse array of stimuli, such as mitogens, growth factors, and pro-inflammatory cytokines, and it regulates cell proliferation, differentiation, apoptosis, and survival. Genetic alterations in the MAPK/ERK pathway result in constitutive activation of signaling and can therefore be pro-tumorigenic.

The PI3K/AKT pathway promotes cell cycle progression (reviewed in [118]) and is a key regulator of survival during cellular stress. Activation of growth factor receptor protein tyrosine kinases results in autophosphorylation of tyrosine residues, PI3K recruitment to the cell membrane, and allosteric activation of the catalytic subunit encoded by a gene *PIK3CA*. This leads to production of the second messenger phosphatidylinositol-3,4,5-triphosphate (PIP_3) which then recruits a subset of signaling proteins, including protein kinase AKT, to the membrane. AKT inactivates pro-apoptotic factors such as BAD and procaspase-9. AKT positively regulates G1/S cell cycle progression acting through mTOR and increased cyclin D1 activity. AKT also controls the IκB kinase complex of the pro-survival NFκB pathway. Both MAPK/ERK and PI3K/AKT pathways converge at the level of RAS.

Thyroid cancer develops as a result of mutations in growth factor receptor tyrosine kinases signaling through MAPK/ERK and PI3K/AKT. Mutations in RET, TRK, and ALK tyrosine kinases are discussed in detail below. Since these receptors are expressed in normal neuroendocrine parafollicular C-cells, but not in thyroid follicular cells, gene fusions altering their cell-specific expression pattern are necessary to

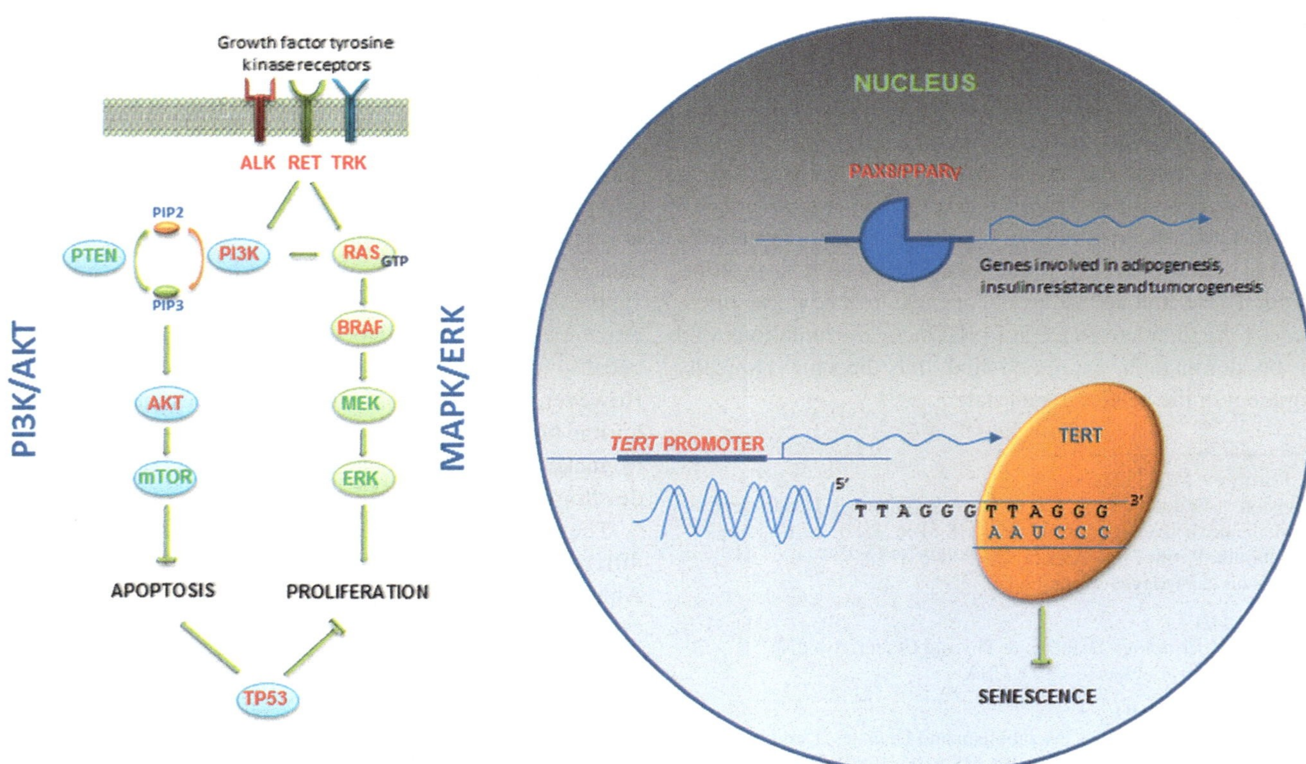

Fig. 3.1 Pathways affected in thyroid cancer. Mutated proteins and genes are highlighted in *red*

cause transformation in thyroid cancer types other than medullary thyroid cancer (MTC).

The *TERT* gene encodes the catalytic subunit of telomerase, the specialized DNA polymerase that lengthens telomeres. Chromosomes are capped by telomeres that replicate incompletely and thus get shorter with each division. Telomere shortening causes replicative senescence, which blocks cell division. Telomerase activity, which prevents telomere shortening and subsequent apoptosis, is absent in non-immortalized cells, including normal follicular cells, but is expressed in the majority of cancers. *TERT* mutations are unique as genetic sequence alterations occur in the promoter region but not in the coding sequence of the gene.

Papillary Thyroid Carcinoma: *BRAF, PIK3CA, RET/PTC, NTRK1*, and *TERT* Mutations

The majority of papillary thyroid carcinomas (PTC) are characterized by mutations in genes for components of the MAPK/ERK pathway: *RET/PTC* and *BRAF*. The *BRAF* gene encodes an intracellular serine-threonine kinase that phosphorylates and activates downstream targets of MAPK/ERK signaling such as MEK. *BRAF* gene mutations are the most prevalent genetic alterations observed in thyroid cancer. A point mutation at nucleotide 1,799 produces a change from a valine to a glutamine at amino acid residue 600 (*BRAF V600E*) of the resulting protein that leads to constitutive BRAF dimerization and chronic activation of the MAPK pathway [27, 83]. Other *BRAF* gene mutations such as *K601E* [138], small in-frame deletions and insertions near codon 600 [20, 21, 74, 137] and even *AKAP9/BRAF* gene fusions [23], have been described, but constitute less than 2 % of all mutations of this gene in a sporadic thyroid cancer. Mutations in *BRAF* have been shown to be unique to PTC and advanced forms of thyroid cancer, poorly differentiated thyroid carcinoma (PDTC), and anaplastic thyroid carcinoma (ATC) that originate from PTC [54, 83, 114]. *BRAF* mutations are found in approximately 45 % of all PTC [5, 27, 54, 83, 114, 116, 135, 150].

Strong evidence indicates that a *BRAF V600E* mutation is associated with a higher risk of recurrence (25–30 % and 10–12 % overall risk for BRAF-mutated and wild-type PTC, respectively). Mutation is linked to higher-risk phenotypes, presence of lymph node metastases, and extrathyroidal extension [5, 97]. However, BRAF mutation is not independently associated with disease mortality and most of the attributable risk is conveyed by histologic analysis. Equally important, BRAF mutation does not affect the prognosis of papillary microcarcinomas, which are associated with 1–2 % risk of recurrence [139, 149]. In addition to promoting tumor cell proliferation/transformation though persistent activation of the MAPK/ERK pathway, a number of mechanisms have been suggested to explain the more aggressive nature of tumors harboring a *BRAF V600E* mutation, such as reduced expression of immune/inflammatory response genes and escape from immune surveillance [134] and silencing of the sodium-iodine symporter gene [154]. Currently, *BRAF* gene testing is not recommended for initial risk stratification in differentiated thyroid cancer, but the field of genetic biomarkers is rapidly evolving.

RET and TRK are receptor tyrosine kinases that signal through MAPK/ERK and PI3K/AKT pathways. Both proteins are present in neuroendocrine C cells but are not expressed in normal thyroid follicular cells. Therefore, activating point mutations in these genes are found in MTC but do not occur in thyroid cancers of follicular cell origin. Instead, chromosomal rearrangements resulting in the formation of chimeric genes consisting of a promoter and a 5′ prime segment of a gene constitutively expressed in follicular cells, and a 3′ segment encoding a kinase domain of RET or TRK occur in follicular cell-derived cancers [66]. Resulting chimeric proteins lead to constitutive stimulation of MAPK/ERK signaling. The most common (>90 %) fusion partners of *RET* are *CCDC6* and *NCOA4* located on the same chromosome 10 producing fusion genes known as *RET/PTC1* and *RET/PTC3* [66, 129] (Table 3.1). The other known *RET* rearrangements (Table 3.1) are interchromosomal. *RET* fusion partner genes encode ubiquitously expressed proteins that contain coiled-coil domains responsible for ligand-independent dimerization of the hybrid protein and constitutive activation of the tyrosine kinase domain of RET. Clonal rearrangements involving the *RET* gene are the second most common genetic alteration seen in PTC, following *BRAF* mutation, and are seen in 10–20 % of patients [83, 128].

TRK oncogenes arise from chromosomal rearrangements involving the *NTRK1* gene. This gene, located on chromosome 1, encodes the high affinity receptor for nerve growth factor that is important for neuronal differentiation and maturation. *TRK* oncogenes contain 5′ sequences from the *TPM3* and *TPR* genes on chromosome 1 and the *TFG* gene on chromosome 3 (Table 3.1). All TRK oncoproteins retain the NTRK1 tyrosine-kinase domain, five tyrosine residues crucial for NTRK1 activity, and are ectopically expressed in thyrocytes. Constitutive dimerization further contributes to upregulated kinase activity [64]. *NTRK1* rearrangements are less frequent in PTC compared to *RET* gene fusions.

Alterations of PI3K signaling in thyroid cancer occur in a number of ways. Mutations affecting genes for the catalytic α-subunit of the kinase PIK3CA [116], AKT (PIP_3 target), and PTEN (PIP_3 phosphatase) are prevalent in undifferentiated forms of thyroid cancer [29, 56, 73, 116, 122, 126]. Genetic alterations of PI3K/AKT pathway are frequently coexisting with mutations in other genes driving malignant transformation, suggesting that these are late events in cancer progression.

Table 3.1 Gene fusions in thyroid cancer.

Rearrangement	Fusion partner	Fusion partner location	Function of the protein encoded by fusion partner gene	Type of thyroid cancer	References
RET/PTC1	*CCDC6*	chr 10	Cellular response to DNA damage	PTC	[66, 117]
RET/PTC2	PRKAR1A	chr 17	Regulatory subunit of type I protein kinase A	PTC	[10]
RET/PTC3	*NCOA4*	chr 10	Ligand-dependent androgen receptor coactivator	PTC, radiation-associated PTC	[105, 129]
RET/PTC4	*NCOA4*	chr 10	Ligand-dependent androgen receptor coactivator	PTC	[52]
RET/PTC5	*GOLGA5*	chr 14	Coiled-coil protein on the Golgi surface	PTC	[85]
RET/PTC6	*TRIM24*	chr 7	Binds chromatin and estrogen receptor to activate estrogen-dependent genes associated with cellular proliferation and tumor development	PTC	[88]
RET/PTC7	*TRIM33*	chr 1	Transcriptional regulator, binding partner of SMAD2 and SMAD3 as a part of canonical TGF-beta pathway	PTC	[88]
RET/PTC8	*KTN1*	chr 14	Anchors elongation factor-1-delta to the endoplasmic reticulum membrane	PTC	[125]
RET/PTC9	*RFG9*	chr 18	Unknown	PTC	[86]
PCM1-RET	*PCM1*	chr 8	Component of centriolar satellites	PTC	[28]
RFP-RET	*TRIM27*	chr 6	Transcription corepressor	PTC	[124]
ELKS-RET	*RAB6IP2*	chr 12	Regulatory subunit of the IKK complex	PTC	[110]
HOOK3-RET	*HOOK3*	chr 8	Microtubule protein	PTC	[22]
TRK	*TPM3*	chr 1	Tropomyosin, a component of the thin filaments of the sarcomere	PTC	[14]
TRK-T1, *TRK-T2*	*TPR*	chr 1	Protein involved in mRNA export	PTC	[63, 65]
TRK-T3	*TFG*	chr 3	Plays role in the function of the endoplasmic reticulum and its associated microtubules	PTC	[62]
PAX8-PPARγ	*PAX8*	chr 2	Thyroid-specific transcription factor essential for thyroid development	FTC, fvPTC	[90]
ETV6-NTRK3	*ETV6*	chr 12	Ets family transcription factor	Radiation-associated PTC	[95]
CREB3L2- PPARγ	*CREB3L2*	chr 7	Member of bZIP family of transcription factors	FTC	[99]
AKAP9-BRAF	*AKAP9*	chr 7	Scaffolding protein for protein kinases and phosphatases	Radiation-associated PTC	[23]
STRN-ALK	*STRN*	chr 2	Ca2+-dependent scaffold protein	ATC, PDTC, PTC	[82]
EML4-ALK	*EML4*	chr 2	Unknown	ATC, PDTC, PTC, radiation-associated PTC	[69, 82]

TERT promoter mutations are relatively infrequent in PTC.

Mutations in *BRAF, RET*, and *RAS* genes(follicular variant of PTC (fvPTC) and follicular thyroid cancer (FTC)) are mutually exclusive, consistent with their roles as driver mutations [83, 135]. In the ThyroSeq cohort, the frequency of the *BRAF V600E* allele was >50 %, supporting its role as a major clonal driver [116]. Alterations of other signaling cascades may rarely coexist with *BRAF* gene mutations. This has been described for *PIK3CA* [73], *TP53* [116], and *TERT* genes [92, 98].

Follicular Variant of Papillary Thyroid Carcinoma: *RAS* Mutations and *PAX8/PPARγ* Rearrangements

The molecular profile of fvPTC is different from classic and tall cell variants, more closely resembling that of the follicular adenoma/carcinoma group of tumors. *RAS* is the most prevalent mutation type in fvPTC [1, 116]. The *PAX8/PPARγ* rearrangement has also been found, though less frequently, in encapsulated fvPTC [123]. *BRAF V600E* mutations are rare in fvPTC [26, 51, 114, 138, 148] although, interestingly, nonclassic mutations in *BRAF* (K601E and small deletion/insertions) are associated with fvPTC [5, 138].

Radiation-Associated Papillary Thyroid Carcinoma: Gene Fusions

Thyroid cancer caused by exposure to ionizing radiation, either therapeutic or as a consequence of nuclear plant accidents, has a distinct genetic background with a greater prevalence of genetic rearrangements. This is plausibly explained by the ability of ionizing radiation to cause double-stranded DNA breaks, facilitating the formation of fusion genes.

Up to 80 % of PTC in patients exposed to ionizing radiation have *RET/PTC* rearrangements (most frequently *RET/PTC3*) [12, 53, 87, 111, 119, 121]. Other fusion genes associated with radiation-induced thyroid cancer are *AKAP9-BRAF* [23], *ETV6-NTRK3* [95], *CREB3L2-PPARG*, and *AGK-BRAF* [121]. *EML4-ALK* gene rearrangements have been found to occur frequently in PTC among atomic bomb survivors [69]; however, this finding was not reproduced in another study [95].

Rearrangement-positive PTCs are associated with greater I131 exposure and possibly iodine deficiency [68, 94, 95]. In contrast, *BRAF* and *RAS* point mutation frequency is negatively correlated with radiation dose [94, 136].

Follicular Adenomas and Follicular Carcinomas: *RAS* and *PAX/PPARγ* Mutations

Three distinct *RAS* genes are known, *HRAS*, *KRAS*, and *NRAS*; these genes encode 21-kDa G-proteins that transmit signals from membrane receptors to the mitogen-activated protein kinase (MAPK) and PI3K/AKT pathways. G-proteins, including RAS, are located at the inner surface of the cell membrane and are bound to GDP in an inactive state. Ligand binding at the corresponding membrane receptor results in activation of RAS through binding to GTP (with the help of guanine nucleotide exchange factor, GEF) and downstream signaling. Intrinsic GTPase activity of RAS is responsible for protein inactivation and signal transduction termination. *RAS* gene point mutations that occur in codons 12, 13, and 61 reduce GTPase activity of the RAS protein, constitutively activating downstream signaling cascades.

RAS mutations have been found in 40–50 % of both follicular adenomas and FTC [44, 96, 115]. Because of their presence in both benign and malignant thyroid lesions, it has been suggested that *RAS* mutations alone may not be sufficient for malignant transformation of thyroid cells but may be an early event in thyroid tumorigenesis predisposing to acquisition of additional genetic or epigenetic alterations that lead to a fully transformed phenotype [115]. This theory is supported by animal studies in transgenic mice with thyroid-specific expression of mutant *KRAS* that develop benign thyroid nodules and follicular adenomas [127].

The *PAX8/PPARγ* fusion protein is created by a t(2; 3)(q13;p25) chromosomal translocation [90, 120]. *PAX8* encodes a transcription factor essential for thyroid development that drives the expression of thyroid-specific genes such as thyroid peroxidase and thyroglobulin. Peroxisome proliferator-activated receptor γ (PPARγ) is a ubiquitously expressed transcription factor that has a role in glucose homeostasis, lipid metabolism, inflammation [3], and tumorigenesis [132].

This *PAX8/PPARγ* rearrangement in thyroid cancer results in an overexpression of a chimeric transcription factor [49]. It was suggested that PAX8/PPARγ functions as a dominant negative suppressor of wild-type PPARγ activities [90], but the exact molecular mechanism of malignant transformation remains to be uncovered. This hypothesis is challenged by a finding that depletion of PPARγ resulted in decreased cell growth of ATC tumors in an animal model [147].

The *PAX8/PPARγ* rearrangement is the second most common genetic alteration in FTC, found in 30–35 % of tumors, and is associated with a more invasive phenotype [37, 49, 101, 113, 115]. An alternative *PPARγ* fusion, *CREB3L2/PPARγ*, has been found in a very small fraction (<3 %) of FTC [99]. With rare exceptions, a *PAX8/PPARγ* mutation is mutually exclusive with a *RAS* mutation.

In mouse model of thyroid cancer caused by the *Pax8/Pparγ* rearrangement, the PPARγ agonist pioglitazone triggers redifferentiation of cancer cells into adipocytes [33]. This finding translated into a clinical trial (NCT01655719) testing the use of pioglitazone for the management of advanced FTC and fvPTC carrying the *PAX8/PPARγ* fusion.

PAX8/PPARγ mutations also occur in benign follicular adenomas [101, 113, 115] but at a lower frequency.

Hurthle cell adenomas and carcinomas have a very low frequency of either *RAS* mutations or *PAX8-PPARγ* rearrangements, suggesting that these tumors are a distinct type of thyroid neoplasm [49, 115].

TERT promoter mutations are more frequent in FTC compared to PTC and occur in 17–36 % of cases [98, 103]. The causative role of *TERT* mutations in development and progression of differentiated thyroid cancer has yet to be proven.

Medullary Thyroid Carcinoma: *RET* Point Mutations

RET is a tyrosine kinase receptor for the glial-derived neurotrophic factor (GDNF) family of ligands: GDNF, neurturin, artemin, and persephin [4, 80]. It is expressed in neuroendocrine calcitonin-producing parafollicular C cells of the thyroid but not in follicular cells. Ligand binding results in dimerization of the RET receptor and autophosphorylation of intracellular tyrosine residues that function as docking sites for adaptor proteins. The RET signaling network is very complex; RAS/ERK, PI3K/AKT, STAT3, c-Src, PLCγ, NFκB, JNK, and other pathways are activated depending on which tyrosine residue is phosphorylated or non-tyrosine-dependent mechanism is activated (reviewed in [30, 76, 145]).

MTC occurs as a component of three distinct dominantly inherited cancer syndromes: multiple endocrine neoplasia type 2A (MEN 2A), associated with pheochromocytoma and primary hyperparathyroidism; multiple endocrine neoplasia type 2B (MEN 2B) that presents with pheochromocytomas, mucosal neuromas, intestinal ganglioneuromas, and functional gastrointestinal disturbances; and familial MTC syndrome (FMTC), in which patients develop MTC only.

In 1993, it was discovered that germline point mutations in the *RET* proto-oncogene cause MEN 2A and MEN 2B as well as FMTC [19, 35, 71, 108].

MEN 2A results from mutations of cysteine codons 609, 611, 618, 620 (exon 10), 630, and 634 (exon 11). Familial MTC is caused by mutations in codons 609, 618, 620 (exon 10), 768, 790, 791 (exon 13), 802, 844 (exon 14), and 891 (exon 15). The genetics of MEN 2B syndrome is less variable with the majority of cases (>95 %) caused by a mutation in codon 918 (exon 16), causing a replacement of methionine with threonine within the catalytic core region of the tyrosine kinase domain [19]. Rarely, MEN 2B is associated with a mutation A883F (exon 15) [59] or double *RET* mutations, such as V804M/Y806C [79] and V804M/S904C [104]. A full list of *RET* mutations and their association with particular syndromes and clinical presentation is available in the 2009 ATA guidelines for the management of MTC [84].

MEN 2A mutations are localized within the cysteine-rich domain of RET and cause ligand-independent dimerization and constitutive kinase activity of the RET protein. MEN 2B mutations that occur within the intracellular tyrosine kinase domain of RET have no effect on receptor dimerization but do cause constitutive activation of intracellular signaling pathways [48]. FMTC mutations affect both cysteine-rich and tyrosine kinase domains.

The existence of clear genotype-phenotype correlations useful for clinical management with respect to screening, surveillance, and prophylaxis has made *RET* genotyping in familial MTC cases a successful application of personalized medicine [41, 84]. For example, patients carrying mutations specific for MEN 2B are considered to have the greatest risk for aggressive MTC; they require prophylactic thyroidectomy as soon as possible within the first year of life and early screening for pheochromocytoma, but not for primary hyperparathyroidism [48, 84]. Early diagnosis followed by an early intervention results in improved outcomes; more than 95 % of patients whose disease was detected at an early stage have remained disease-free [47, 100, 133].

Somatic *RET* mutations are found in approximately 40–78 % of patients with sporadic MTC, occurring sometimes at codons 608, 611, 618, 629, 630, 634, 641, 649, 918, and 922, but most frequently at 918, the codon affected in patients with MEN 2B syndrome [2, 30, 38]. Similar to hereditary MTC syndromes, tumors triggered by somatic codon 918 mutations show more aggressive phenotypes [131, 152, 153]. Somatic *RET* mutations are not consistently distributed within primary tumors and metastases and therefore may occur late in tumor development instead of serving as primary driver events [42, 131].

Mutations in the *RAS* family of small GTPase genes have been identified in sporadic MTC, and *RAS* has been proposed to act as an alternative driver of MTC tumorigenesis [2, 9, 24, 107, 116]. *RET*, *KRAS*, and *HRAS* mutations are mutually exclusive. Exome sequencing has found *RET* or *RAS* mutations in as many as 90 % of sporadic MTC [2].

Poorly Differentiated and Anaplastic Thyroid Carcinoma

The classic model of multistep carcinogenesis suggests that anaplastic carcinomas arise from differentiated carcinomas through accumulated damage to the genome. Most of the mutations described in differentiated cancer (*RET*, *HRAS*, *KRAS*, *NRAS*, *BRAF*, *PIK3CA*, *AKT1*) have also been found in PDTC and ATC, albeit at a varying frequency [116]. PDTC and ATC frequently co-localize with PTC in the same patient, and *BRAF* mutations have been reported in both tumors [7, 114]. This provides molecular evidence supporting the hypothesis that some ATC and PDTC originate from PTC.

While driver mutations in differentiated thyroid cancer are generally mutually exclusive, coexistence of several genetic alterations is common in ATC [116]. For example, *PIK3CA*/*AKT1* mutations found in combination with *BRAF* mutations in dedifferentiated thyroid cancer suggest a synergistic effect of alterations in both pathways for thyroid cancer advancement. *PIK3CA*/*AKT1* mutation status is frequently discordant in lesions originating from primary and advanced metastatic thyroid cancer, suggesting that these mutations occur during tumor progression rather than being primary driver mutations [122].

TERT promoter mutations have been implicated in the progression toward PDTC and ATC. Two mutations, C228T and C250T, have been discovered in the promoter region of the *TERT* gene in thyroid cancer cell lines and tissues. Either of these mutations results in the generation of novel consensus binding sites for ETS transcription factors and causes a several fold increase in *TERT* expression [72, 75]. The frequency of *TERT* promoter mutations is relatively low in differentiated thyroid cancers (9–22 %), but it is much higher in PDTC and ATC (51 %) [92, 103]. *TERT* promoter mutations frequently coexist with mutations in known driver genes, such as *BRAF* and *RAS*, in advanced forms of thyroid cancer. It has been hypothesized that *TERT* promoter mutations occurring in DTC cells harboring driver mutations cause transformation into undifferentiated forms of thyroid cancer. Mechanistically, this makes sense considering that ETS transcription factors are regulated by the MAPK/ERK pathway. This hypothesis remains to be proven experimentally and *TERT* promoter mutations may simply represent a marker of genetic instability, rather than true driver of disease progression.

Mutations in the genes encoding the cell cycle regulator, p53 (*TP53*), and the cell adhesion and Wnt signaling protein, β-catenin (*CTNNB1*), are prevalent in PDTC/ATC but not in differentiated thyroid cancers [32, 34, 46, 55, 57, 78]. *TP53* gene mutations are the most common genetic alterations in ATC [116].

Curiously, *RAS* mutations are prevalent in PDTC but, in contrast to *BRAF* mutations, are associated with the absence of extrathyroidal extension and with longer survival [121].

Anaplastic lymphoma kinase (ALK) is a receptor tyrosine kinase that, like RET and TRK, activates the MAPK/ERK and PI3K/AKT pathways, promoting cell proliferation and survival. *ALK* gene fusions were initially found in anaplastic large-cell non-Hodgkin's lymphomas and are infrequent events in non-small cell lung cancer and inflammatory myofibroblastic tumors. *EML4-ALK* and *STRN-ALK*fusions have been found in thyroid cancer [82]. ALK protein is not expressed in normal thyroid tissue, but the fusion genes are overexpressed in tumors carrying the mutation. *STRN-ALK* fusion results in constitutive autophosphorylation and dimerization of the fusion protein that causes ALK kinase activation and MAPK activation. *STRN-ALK* causes transformation of rat thyroid PCCL3 cells, which causes flank tumors in mice. *ALK* fusions have been found in 1.6 % of PTC, 9 % of PDTC, and 4 % of ATC. The fusion was not found in 36 FTC or in 22 MTC. *ALK* fusions are mutually exclusive with other known thyroid cancer driver mutations.

Point mutations in the tyrosine kinase domain of *ALK* have also been found in ATC [109]. Point mutations resulted in an upregulated kinase activity of ALK, increased phosphorylation of ERK and AKT, and promoted cell transformation. The significance of this finding will depend on whether ALK protein is expressed in ATC.

Clinical Applications

Diagnosis

Cytology examination of fine needle aspiration (FNA) samples classifies 70–75 % of thyroid nodules as benign or malignant with great accuracy. The remaining samples are labeled as indeterminate or inadequate, leading to repeated invasive testing and/or unnecessary diagnostic surgery. Molecular testing was developed as an add-on to FNA when cytology analysis was indeterminate. The best molecular test to exclude malignancy, an ideal "rule-out" test, would have a sensitivity and negative predictive value similar to a benign cytologic diagnosis (94–97 %) [11] and would be most useful for the purpose of avoiding unnecessary surgery for benign thyroid nodules. An ideal "rule-in" test would have a specificity and positive predictive value similar to a malignant cytologic diagnosis (97–99 %).

BRAF V600E mutation positivity has very high specificity (>99 %) and excellent positive predictive value for the diagnosis of thyroid cancer [81]. However, a *BRAF* mutation is only detected in a fraction of malignant lesions, and therefore the sensitivity and negative predictive value of the test is poor. An improved sensitivity was achieved by combining the most frequent driver mutations in a test panel [16, 112]. This panel is now commercially available under the name ThyGenX (Interpace Diagnostics) and includes mutations in the *BRAF*, *HRAS*, *NRAS*, and *KRAS* genes as well as the *RET/PTC1*, *RET/PTC3*, and *PAX8/PPARγ* translocations. A similar test is offered by Quest Diagnostics. While testing for the panel of oncogene driver mutations has improved the presurgical diagnosis of thyroid cancer, its sensitivity (~75 %) is not sufficient to confidently rule out malignancy in thyroid nodules with indeterminate cytology. This is particularly true for Bethesda categories with a low prevalence of malignancy (such as category III, atypia of undetermined significance/follicular lesion of undetermined significance (AUS/FLUS)). However, greater specificity and PPV of oncogene mutation testing together with the prognostic value of certain mutations (aggressive behavior of *BRAF V600E* positive tumors, or tumors with more than one genetic alteration; indolent clinical course of fvPTC due to RAS mutations) may assist in deciding on the extent of the surgery (near total thyroidectomy vs. lobectomy in patients with cytology suspicious for PTC) or decision to do prophylactic central neck dissection.

The development of next-generation sequencing technology has made The Cancer Genome Atlas (TCGA) project feasible and has led to significant advances in the field of thyroid cancer genomics. A number of new likely driver mutations have been discovered, increasing the percentage of tumors with known genetic causes to 93 % (Giordano, personal communication). While probing for more driver mutations will no doubt improve the sensitivity of thyroid cancer molecular testing, it will come at the cost of a greater number of false-positive results since some mutations (such as *RAS* and *PAX8/PPARγ*) are found in benign lesions as well [37, 101, 115].

Another methodological challenge comes from the varying sensitivity of methods used for detection of mutated genes. Ultrasensitive detection methods are capable of identifying mutated alleles present at low frequency (non-clonal alleles). This problem was systematically studied for *RET/PTC* rearrangements, and high-sensitivity RT-PCR was shown to detect non-clonal rearrangements [155]. Highly sensitive methods discovered *RET/PTC* rearrangements in benign thyroid nodules and non-neoplastic thyroid lesions [39, 67, 77, 130, 146]. This problem is acknowledged in 2015 American Thyroid Association Management Guidelines for Adult Patients with Thyroid Nodules and Differentiated Thyroid Cancer (Haugen et al., Thyroid. 2015 Oct 14. [Epub ahead of print]) emphasizing the importance of standardization of molecular testing methodology.

Treatment

Currently, there is no effective therapy for advanced metastatic radioiodine-resistant thyroid cancer. Despite treatment with TSH suppression and local control with surgery and radiation therapy, the disease ultimately progresses causing significant mortality.

Greater understanding of thyroid cancer pathophysiology and the development of new therapies targeting specific molecular defects hold great promise for a pharmacologic cure of advanced thyroid cancer. Pharmacogenomics study how to use genetic and genomic information in clinical practice. This new field of medical science has emerged as a result of advances in molecular characterization of the disease and the development of new so-called targeted drugs aimed at a particular molecular defect. Pharmacogenomics is bringing medicine to a new level when not heterogeneous disease itself, but a molecular defect causing a particular instance of the disease, is targeted by a physician. For example, long-term control of chronic myeloid leukemia is achieved with inhibitors of the chimeric BCR-ABL oncoprotein (imatinib, dasatinib). BRAF inhibitors vemurafenib and dabrafenib produce rapid tumor regression in 80 % of patients with metastatic melanoma caused by *BRAF V600E* mutations. Figure 3.2 illustrates the power of pharmacogenomics. Cell lines from tumors of various origins, including thyroid cancer, were tested for sensitivity to the RAF inhibitor, PLX4720 [58]. Those cell lines that had the *BRAF V600E* mutation, but not the wild type gene, were selectively sensitive to the drug in an *in vitro* proliferation assay.

Unfortunately, the success of targeted therapies in thyroid cancer has been limited so far. In contrast to melanoma, only 25–35 % of patients with radioiodine-resistant metastatic thyroid cancer caused by the *BRAF V600E* mutation respond to BRAF inhibitors [45]. Currently, there are no effective therapies for tumors harboring oncogenic *RAS* mutants. A combination treatment with inhibitors of both the PI3K and MAPK pathway downstream of RAS has shown promise in animal models [6, 43], but this has yet to be tested in human thyroid cancer. The multikinase inhibitor, sorafenib, has been recently approved by the US Food and Drug Administration for the treatment of advanced radioiodine-resistant PTC based on the results of the DECISION trial [13]. Two targeted therapies, vandetanib and cabozantinib, are approved for advanced metastatic MTC. Both drugs are capable of inhibiting mutated RET as well as other targets [18, 151]. Vandetanib and cabozantinib were shown to prolong progression-free survival but not overall survival in phase 3 clinical trials in MTC [40, 144]. It remains controversial whether the presence of a *RET* mutation provided a therapeutic advantage in these trials. In patients who fail treatment with vandetanib or cabozantinib, the National Comprehensive Cancer Network recommends that clinicians consider additional targeted therapies with sorafenib or sunitinib or enrollment in a clinical trial [140]. Of note, sorafenib, sunitinib, and another tyrosine kinase inhibitor, ponatinib,

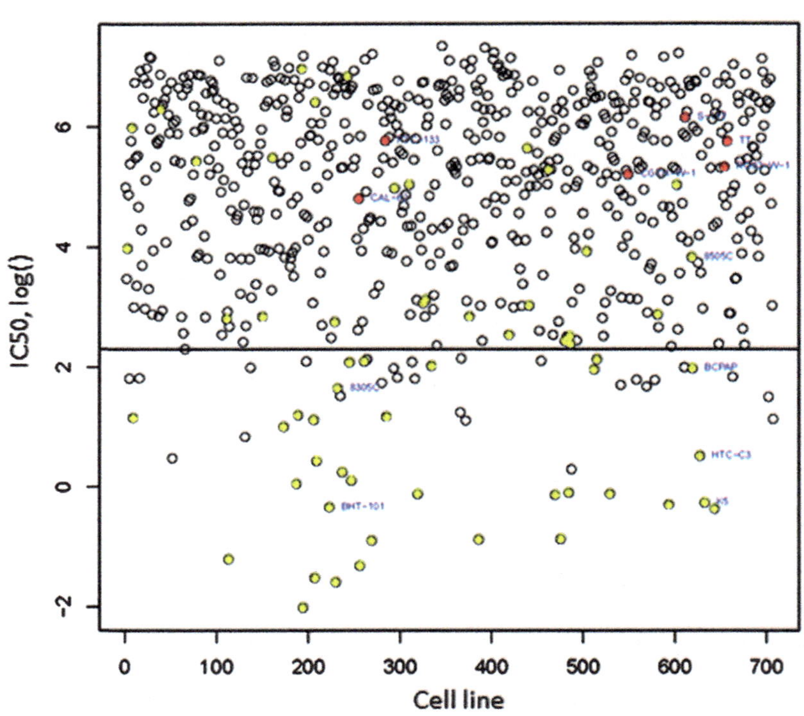

Fig. 3.2 Cell lines carrying the *BRAF V600E* mutation are sensitive to RAF inhibitor PLX4720. IC_{50} is a drug concentration that reduced the cell population by half in an *in vitro* proliferation assay. Thyroid cancer cell lines are named. *Yellow dots* represent cell lines with the *BRAF* mutation. *Red dots* represent thyroid cancer cell lines without the *BRAF V600E* mutation

are capable of blocking phosphorylation of the *RET V804M* mutant, which confers resistance to vandetanib and reduces the effectiveness of cabozantinib [17, 106]. Targeted therapies improve progression-free survival in clinical trials, but ultimately resistance develops and disease progresses in the majority of patients justifying the need for further efforts in developing pathogenesis-based therapies.

While infrequent, activating *ALK* gene mutations may have great therapeutic implications. A dramatic response to an ALK inhibitor, crizotinib, has been reported in a case of ATC with the *ALK* gene rearrangement [60]. Stable disease was achieved with crizotinib treatment in a patient with advanced PTC due to an *EML4-ALK* gene fusion [31]. The efficiency of ALK inhibitors in this subset of thyroid cancer has yet to be tested in a clinical trial.

After this chapter had been submitted for publication, The Cancer Genome Atlas Project dedicated to PTC was completed [15]. Multiplatform analysis of 496 PTC identified putative oncogenic drivers in 98.8 % of cases. New mutations and fusions were found. Higher somatic mutation frequency, the presence of TERT promoter mutations, and BRAF-like molecular signature were associated with advanced age, greater risk of recurrence, and higher MACIS prognostic score. Follicular variant of PTC was found to be distinct on a molecular level, and its reclassification into a follicular thyroid carcinoma group has been suggested.

References

1. Adeniran AJ, Zhu Z, Gandhi M, Steward DL, Fidler JP, Giordano TJ, … Nikiforov YE. Correlation between genetic alterations and microscopic features, clinical manifestations, and prognostic characteristics of thyroid papillary carcinomas. Am J Surg Pathol. 2006;30(2):216–22. Retrieved from http://www.ncbi.nlm.nih.gov/pubmed/16434896.
2. Agrawal N, Jiao Y, Sausen M, Leary R, Bettegowda C, Roberts NJ, … Ball DW. Exomic sequencing of medullary thyroid cancer reveals dominant and mutually exclusive oncogenic mutations in RET and RAS. J Clin Endocrinol Metab. 2013;98(2):E364–9. doi:10.1210/jc.2012-2703.
3. Ahmadian M, Suh JM, Hah N, Liddle C, Atkins AR, Downes M, Evans RM. PPARγ signaling and metabolism: the good, the bad and the future. Nat Med. 2013;19(5):557–66. doi:10.1038/nm.3159.
4. Alberti L, Carniti C, Miranda C, Roccato E, Pierotti MA. RET and NTRK1 proto-oncogenes in human diseases. J Cell Physiol. 2003;195(2):168–86. doi:10.1002/jcp.10252.
5. Basolo F, Torregrossa L, Giannini R, Miccoli M, Lupi C, Sensi E, … Miccoli P. Correlation between the BRAF V600E mutation and tumor invasiveness in papillary thyroid carcinomas smaller than 20 millimeters: analysis of 1060 cases. J Clin Endocrinol Metab. 2010;95(9):4197–205. doi:10.1210/jc.2010-0337.
6. Bedogni B, Welford SM, Kwan AC, Ranger-Moore J, Saboda K, Powell MB. Inhibition of phosphatidylinositol-3-kinase and mitogen-activated protein kinase kinase 1/2 prevents melanoma development and promotes melanoma regression in the transgenic TPRas mouse model. Mol Cancer Ther. 2006;5(12):3071–7. doi:10.1158/1535-7163.MCT-06-0269.
7. Begum S, Rosenbaum E, Henrique R, Cohen Y, Sidransky D, Westra WH. BRAF mutations in anaplastic thyroid carcinoma: implications for tumor origin, diagnosis and treatment. Mod Pathol: Off J U S Can Acad Pathol Inc. 2004;17(11):1359–63. doi:10.1038/modpathol.3800198.
8. Bishop JM. Cancer: the rise of the genetic paradigm. Genes Dev. 1995;9(11):1309–15. Retrieved from http://www.ncbi.nlm.nih.gov/pubmed/7797071.
9. Boichard A, Croux L, Al Ghuzlan A, Broutin S, Dupuy C, Leboulleux S, … Lacroix L. Somatic RAS mutations occur in a large proportion of sporadic RET-negative medullary thyroid carcinomas and extend to a previously unidentified exon. J Clin Endocrinol Metab. 2012;97(10):E2031–5. doi:10.1210/jc.2012-2092.
10. Bongarzone I, Monzini N, Borrello MG, Carcano C, Ferraresi G, Arighi E, … Pierotti MA. Molecular characterization of a thyroid tumor-specific transforming sequence formed by the fusion of ret tyrosine kinase and the regulatory subunit RI alpha of cyclic AMP-dependent protein kinase A. Mol Cell Biol. 1993;13(1):358–66. Retrieved from http://www.pubmedcentral.nih.gov/articlerender.fcgi?artid=358915&tool=pmcentrez&rendertype=abstract.
11. Bongiovanni M, Spitale A, Faquin WC, Mazzucchelli L, Baloch ZW. The Bethesda system for reporting thyroid cytopathology: a meta-analysis. Acta Cytol. 2012;56(4):333–9. doi:10.1159/000339959.
12. Bounacer A, Wicker R, Caillou B, Cailleux AF, Sarasin A, Schlumberger M, Suárez HG. High prevalence of activating ret proto-oncogene rearrangements, in thyroid tumors from patients who had received external radiation. Oncogene. 1997;15(11):1263–73. doi:10.1038/sj.onc.1200206.
13. Brose MS, Nutting CM, Jarzab B, Elisei R, Siena S, Bastholt L, … Schlumberger MJ. Sorafenib in radioactive iodine-refractory, locally advanced or metastatic differentiated thyroid cancer: a randomised, double-blind, phase 3 trial. Lancet. 2014. doi:10.1016/S0140-6736(14)60421-9.
14. Butti MG, Bongarzone I, Ferraresi G, Mondellini P, Borrello MG, Pierotti MA. A sequence analysis of the genomic regions involved in the rearrangements between TPM3 and NTRK1 genes producing TRK oncogenes in papillary thyroid carcinomas. Genomics. 1995;28(1):15–24. doi:10.1006/geno.1995.1100.
15. Cancer Genome Atlas Research Network. Integrated genomic characterization of papillary thyroid carcinoma. Cell. 2014;159(3):676–90.
16. Cantara S, Capezzone M, Marchisotta S, Capuano S, Busonero G, Toti P, … Pacini F. Impact of proto-oncogene mutation detection in cytological specimens from thyroid nodules improves the diagnostic accuracy of cytology. J Clin Endocrinol Metab. 2010;95(3):1365–9. doi:10.1210/jc.2009-2103.
17. Carlomagno F, Guida T, Anaganti S, Vecchio G, Fusco A, Ryan AJ, … Santoro M. Disease associated mutations at valine 804 in the RET receptor tyrosine kinase confer resistance to selective kinase inhibitors. Oncogene. 2004;23(36):6056–63. doi:10.1038/sj.onc.1207810.
18. Carlomagno F, Vitagliano D, Guida T, Ciardiello F, Tortora G, Vecchio G, … Santoro M. ZD6474, an orally available inhibitor of KDR tyrosine kinase activity, efficiently blocks oncogenic RET kinases. Cancer Res. 2002;62(24):7284–90. Retrieved from http://www.ncbi.nlm.nih.gov/pubmed/12499271.
19. Carlson KM, Dou S, Chi D, Scavarda N, Toshima K, Jackson CE, … Donis-Keller H. Single missense mutation in the tyrosine kinase catalytic domain of the RET protooncogene is associated with multiple endocrine neoplasia type 2B. Proc Natl Acad Sci USA. 1994;91(4):1579–83. Retrieved from http://www.pubmedcentral.nih.gov/articlerender.fcgi?artid=43203&tool=pmcentrez&rendertype=abstract.

20. Carta C, Moretti S, Passeri L, Barbi F, Avenia N, Cavaliere A, … Puxeddu E. Genotyping of an Italian papillary thyroid carcinoma cohort revealed high prevalence of BRAF mutations, absence of RAS mutations and allowed the detection of a new mutation of BRAF oncoprotein (BRAF(V599Ins)). Clin Endocrinol. 2006;64(1):105–9. doi:10.1111/j.1365-2265.2005.02401.x.
21. Chiosea S, Nikiforova M, Zuo H, Ogilvie J, Gandhi M, Seethala RR, … Nikiforov Y. A novel complex BRAF mutation detected in a solid variant of papillary thyroid carcinoma. Endocr Pathol. 2009;20(2):122–6. doi:10.1007/s12022-009-9073-3.
22. Ciampi R, Giordano TJ, Wikenheiser-Brokamp K, Koenig RJ, Nikiforov YE. HOOK3-RET: a novel type of RET/PTC rearrangement in papillary thyroid carcinoma. Endocr Relat Cancer. 2007;14(2):445–52. doi:10.1677/ERC-07-0039.
23. Ciampi R, Knauf JA, Kerler R, Gandhi M, Zhu Z, Nikiforova MN, … Nikiforov YE. Oncogenic AKAP9-BRAF fusion is a novel mechanism of MAPK pathway activation in thyroid cancer. J Clin Investig. 2005;115(1):94–101. doi:10.1172/JCI23237.
24. Ciampi R, Mian C, Fugazzola L, Cosci B, Romei C, Barollo S, … Elisei R. Evidence of a low prevalence of RAS mutations in a large medullary thyroid cancer series. Thyroid: Off J Am Thyroid Assoc. 2013;23(1):50–7. doi:10.1089/thy.2012.0207.
25. Cline MJ, Slamon DJ, Lipsick JS. Oncogenes: implications for the diagnosis and treatment of cancer. Ann Intern Med. 1984;101(2):223–33. Retrieved from http://www.ncbi.nlm.nih.gov/pubmed/6331242.
26. Cohen Y, Rosenbaum E, Clark DP, Zeiger MA, Umbricht CB, Tufano RP, … Westra WH. Mutational analysis of BRAF in fine needle aspiration biopsies of the thyroid: a potential application for the preoperative assessment of thyroid nodules. Clin Cancer Res: Off J Am Assoc Cancer Res. 2004;10(8):2761–5. Retrieved from http://www.ncbi.nlm.nih.gov/pubmed/15102681.
27. Cohen Y, Xing M, Mambo E, Guo Z, Wu G, Trink B, … Sidransky D. BRAF mutation in papillary thyroid carcinoma. J Natl Cancer Inst. 2003;95(8):625–7. Retrieved from http://www.ncbi.nlm.nih.gov/pubmed/12697856.
28. Corvi R, Berger N, Balczon R, Romeo G. RET/PCM-1: a novel fusion gene in papillary thyroid carcinoma. Oncogene. 2000;19(37):4236–42. doi:10.1038/sj.onc.1203772.
29. Dahia PL, Marsh DJ, Zheng Z, Zedenius J, Komminoth P, Frisk T, … Eng C. Somatic deletions and mutations in the Cowden disease gene, PTEN, in sporadic thyroid tumors. Cancer Res. 1997;57(21):4710–3. Retrieved from http://www.ncbi.nlm.nih.gov/pubmed/9354427.
30. De Groot JWB, Links TP, Plukker JTM, Lips CJM, Hofstra RMW. RET as a diagnostic and therapeutic target in sporadic and hereditary endocrine tumors. Endocr Rev. 2006;27(5):535–60. doi:10.1210/er.2006-0017.
31. Demeure MJ, Aziz M, Rosenberg R, Gurley SD, Bussey KJ, Carpten JD. Whole-genome sequencing of an aggressive BRAF wild-type papillary thyroid cancer identified EML4-ALK translocation as a therapeutic target. World J Surg. 2014. doi:10.1007/s00268-014-2485-3.
32. Dobashi Y, Sugimura H, Sakamoto A, Mernyei M, Mori M, Oyama T, Machinami R. Stepwise participation of p53 gene mutation during dedifferentiation of human thyroid carcinomas. Diagn Mol Pathol: Am J Surg Pathol Part B. 1994;3(1):9–14. Retrieved from http://www.ncbi.nlm.nih.gov/pubmed/8162258.
33. Dobson ME, Diallo-Krou E, Grachtchouk V, Yu J, Colby LA, Wilkinson JE, … Koenig RJ. Pioglitazone induces a proadipogenic antitumor response in mice with PAX8-PPARgamma fusion protein thyroid carcinoma. Endocrinology. 2011;152(11):4455–65. doi:10.1210/en.2011-1178.
34. Donghi R, Longoni A, Pilotti S, Michieli P, Della Porta G, Pierotti MA. Gene p53 mutations are restricted to poorly differentiated and undifferentiated carcinomas of the thyroid gland. J Clin Invest. 1993;91(4):1753–60. doi:10.1172/JCI116385.
35. Donis-Keller H, Dou S, Chi D, Carlson KM, Toshima K, Lairmore TC, … Wells SA. Mutations in the RET proto-oncogene are associated with MEN 2A and FMTC. Hum Mol Genet. 1993;2(7):851–6. Retrieved from http://www.ncbi.nlm.nih.gov/pubmed/8103403.
36. Druker BJ, Mamon HJ, Roberts TM. Oncogenes, growth factors, and signal transduction. N Engl J Med. 1989;321(20):1383–91. doi:10.1056/NEJM198911163212007.
37. Dwight T, Thoppe SR, Foukakis T, Lui WO, Wallin G, Höög A, … Zedenius J. Involvement of the PAX8/peroxisome proliferator-activated receptor gamma rearrangement in follicular thyroid tumors. J Clin Endocrinol Metab. 2003;88(9):4440–5. doi:10.1210/jc.2002-021690.
38. Elisei R, Cosci B, Romei C, Bottici V, Renzini G, Molinaro E, … Pinchera A. Prognostic significance of somatic RET oncogene mutations in sporadic medullary thyroid cancer: a 10-year follow-up study. J Clin Endocrinol Metab. 2008;93(3):682–7. doi:10.1210/jc.2007-1714.
39. Elisei R, Romei C, Vorontsova T, Cosci B, Veremeychik V, Kuchinskaya E, … Pacini F. RET/PTC rearrangements in thyroid nodules: studies in irradiated and not irradiated, malignant and benign thyroid lesions in children and adults. J Clin Endocrinol Metab. 2001;86(7):3211–6. doi:10.1210/jcem.86.7.7678.
40. Elisei R, Schlumberger MJ, Müller SP, Schöffski P, Brose MS, Shah MH, … Sherman SI. Cabozantinib in progressive medullary thyroid cancer. J Clin Oncol: Off J Am Soc Clin Oncol. 2013;31(29):3639–46. doi:10.1200/JCO.2012.48.4659.
41. Eng C, Clayton D, Schuffenecker I, Lenoir G, Cote G, Gagel RF, … Mulligan LM. The relationship between specific RET proto-oncogene mutations and disease phenotype in multiple endocrine neoplasia type 2. International RET mutation consortium analysis. JAMA: J Am Med Assoc. 1996;276(19):1575–9. Retrieved from http://www.ncbi.nlm.nih.gov/pubmed/8918855.
42. Eng C, Mulligan LM, Healey CS, Houghton C, Frilling A, Raue F, … Ponder BA. Heterogeneous mutation of the RET proto-oncogene in subpopulations of medullary thyroid carcinoma. Cancer Res. 1996;56(9):2167–70. Retrieved from http://www.ncbi.nlm.nih.gov/pubmed/8616867.
43. Engelman JA, Chen L, Tan X, Crosby K, Guimaraes AR, Upadhyay R, … Wong K-K. Effective use of PI3K and MEK inhibitors to treat mutant Kras G12D and PIK3CA H1047R murine lung cancers. Nat Med. 2008;14(12):1351–6. doi:10.1038/nm.1890.
44. Esapa CT, Johnson SJ, Kendall-Taylor P, Lennard TW, Harris PE. Prevalence of Ras mutations in thyroid neoplasia. Clin Endocrinol. 1999;50(4):529–35. Retrieved from http://www.ncbi.nlm.nih.gov/pubmed/10468914.
45. Fagin JA. Clinical Investigator Award Lecture: Thyroid cancer: from genetics to biology to new treatment strategies. ENDO Society Meeting; 2014.
46. Fagin JA, Matsuo K, Karmakar A, Chen DL, Tang SH, Koeffler HP. High prevalence of mutations of the p53 gene in poorly differentiated human thyroid carcinomas. J Clin Invest. 1993;91(1):179–84. doi:10.1172/JCI116168.
47. Frank-Raue K, Buhr H, Dralle H, Klar E, Senninger N, Weber T, … Raue F. Long-term outcome in 46 gene carriers of hereditary medullary thyroid carcinoma after prophylactic thyroidectomy: impact of individual RET genotype. Eur J Endocrinol/Eur Fed Endocr Soc. 2006;155(2):229–36. doi:10.1530/eje.1.02216.
48. Frank-Raue K, Rondot S, Raue F. Molecular genetics and phenomics of RET mutations: impact on prognosis of MTC. Mol Cell Endocrinol. 2010;322(1–2):2–7. doi:10.1016/j.mce.2010.01.012.
49. French CA, Alexander EK, Cibas ES, Nose V, Laguette J, Faquin W, … Kroll TG. Genetic and biological subgroups of low-stage follicular thyroid cancer. Am J Pathol. 2003;162(4):1053–60. doi:10.1016/S0002-9440(10)63902-8.

50. Friend SH, Dryja TP, Weinberg RA. Oncogenes and tumor-suppressing genes. N Engl J Med. 1988;318(10):618–22. doi:10.1056/NEJM198803103181007.
51. Fugazzola L, Mannavola D, Cirello V, Vannucchi G, Muzza M, Vicentini L, Beck-Peccoz P. BRAF mutations in an Italian cohort of thyroid cancers. Clin Endocrinol. 2004;61(2):239–43. doi:10.1111/j.1365-2265.2004.02089.x.
52. Fugazzola L, Pierotti MA, Vigano E, Pacini F, Vorontsova TV, Bongarzone I. Molecular and biochemical analysis of RET/PTC4, a novel oncogenic rearrangement between RET and ELE1 genes, in a post-Chernobyl papillary thyroid cancer. Oncogene. 1996;13(5):1093–7. Retrieved from http://www.ncbi.nlm.nih.gov/pubmed/8806699.
53. Fugazzola L, Pilotti S, Pinchera A, Vorontsova TV, Mondellini P, Bongarzone I, … Demidchik EP. Oncogenic rearrangements of the RET proto-oncogene in papillary thyroid carcinomas from children exposed to the Chernobyl nuclear accident. Cancer Res. 1995;55(23):5617–20. Retrieved from http://www.ncbi.nlm.nih.gov/pubmed/7585643.
54. Fukushima T, Suzuki S, Mashiko M, Ohtake T, Endo Y, Takebayashi Y, … Takenoshita S. BRAF mutations in papillary carcinomas of the thyroid. Oncogene. 2003;22(41):6455–7. doi:10.1038/sj.onc.1206739.
55. Garcia-Rostan G, Camp RL, Herrero A, Carcangiu ML, Rimm DL, Tallini G. Beta-catenin dysregulation in thyroid neoplasms: down-regulation, aberrant nuclear expression, and CTNNB1 exon 3 mutations are markers for aggressive tumor phenotypes and poor prognosis. Am J Pathol. 2001;158(3):987–96. Retrieved from http://www.pubmedcentral.nih.gov/articlerender.fcgi?artid=1850336&tool=pmcentrez&rendertype=abstract.
56. García-Rostán G, Costa AM, Pereira-Castro I, Salvatore G, Hernandez R, Hermsem MJA, … Santoro M. Mutation of the PIK3CA gene in anaplastic thyroid cancer. Cancer Res. 2005;65(22):10199–207. doi:10.1158/0008-5472.CAN-04-4259.
57. Garcia-Rostan G, Tallini G, Herrero A, D'Aquila TG, Carcangiu ML, Rimm DL. Frequent mutation and nuclear localization of beta-catenin in anaplastic thyroid carcinoma. Cancer Res. 1999;59(8):1811–5. Retrieved from http://www.ncbi.nlm.nih.gov/pubmed/10213482.
58. Garnett MJ, Edelman EJ, Heidorn SJ, Greenman CD, Dastur A, Lau KW, … Benes CH. Systematic identification of genomic markers of drug sensitivity in cancer cells. Nature. 2012;483(7391):570–5. doi:10.1038/nature11005.
59. Gimm O, Marsh DJ, Andrew SD, Frilling A, Dahia PL, Mulligan LM, … Eng C. Germline dinucleotide mutation in codon 883 of the RET proto-oncogene in multiple endocrine neoplasia type 2B without codon 918 mutation. J Clin Endocrinol Metab. 1997;82(11):3902–4. doi:10.1210/jcem.82.11.4508.
60. Godbert Y, Henriques de Figueiredo B, Bonichon F, Chibon F, Hostein I, Pérot G, … Soubeyran I. Remarkable response to crizotinib in woman with anaplastic lymphoma kinase-rearranged anaplastic thyroid carcinoma. J Clin Oncol: Off J Am Soc Clin Oncol. 2014. doi:10.1200/JCO.2013.49.6596.
61. Gordon H. Oncogenes. Mayo Clin Proc. 1985;60(10):697–713. Retrieved from http://www.ncbi.nlm.nih.gov/pubmed/2993762.
62. Greco A, Mariani C, Miranda C, Lupas A, Pagliardini S, Pomati M, Pierotti MA. The DNA rearrangement that generates the TRK-T3 oncogene involves a novel gene on chromosome 3 whose product has a potential coiled-coil domain. Mol Cell Biol. 1995;15(11):6118–27. Retrieved from http://www.pubmedcentral.nih.gov/articlerender.fcgi?artid=230863&tool=pmcentrez&rendertype=abstract.
63. Greco A, Miranda C, Pagliardini S, Fusetti L, Bongarzone I, Pierotti MA. Chromosome 1 rearrangements involving the genes TPR and NTRK1 produce structurally different thyroid-specific TRK oncogenes. Gene Chromosome Cancer. 1997;19(2):112–23. Retrieved from http://www.ncbi.nlm.nih.gov/pubmed/9172002.
64. Greco A, Miranda C, Pierotti MA. Rearrangements of NTRK1 gene in papillary thyroid carcinoma. Mol Cell Endocrinol. 2010;321(1):44–9. doi:10.1016/j.mce.2009.10.009.
65. Greco A, Pierotti MA, Bongarzone I, Pagliardini S, Lanzi C, Della Porta G. TRK-T1 is a novel oncogene formed by the fusion of TPR and TRK genes in human papillary thyroid carcinomas. Oncogene. 1992;7(2):237–42. Retrieved from http://www.ncbi.nlm.nih.gov/pubmed/1532241.
66. Grieco M, Santoro M, Berlingieri MT, Melillo RM, Donghi R, Bongarzone I, … Vecchio G. PTC is a novel rearranged form of the ret proto-oncogene and is frequently detected in vivo in human thyroid papillary carcinomas. Cell. 1990;60(4):557–63. Retrieved from http://www.ncbi.nlm.nih.gov/pubmed/2406025.
67. Guerra A, Sapio MR, Marotta V, Campanile E, Moretti MI, Deandrea M, … Vitale M. Prevalence of RET/PTC rearrangement in benign and malignant thyroid nodules and its clinical application. Endocr J. 2011;58(1):31–8. Retrieved from http://www.ncbi.nlm.nih.gov/pubmed/21173509.
68. Hamatani K, Eguchi H, Ito R, Mukai M, Takahashi K, Taga M, … Nakachi K. RET/PTC rearrangements preferentially occurred in papillary thyroid cancer among atomic bomb survivors exposed to high radiation dose. Cancer Res. 2008;68(17):7176–82. doi:10.1158/0008-5472.CAN-08-0293.
69. Hamatani K, Mukai M, Takahashi K, Hayashi Y, Nakachi K, Kusunoki Y. Rearranged anaplastic lymphoma kinase (ALK) gene in adult-onset papillary thyroid cancer amongst atomic bomb survivors. Thyroid: Off J Am Thyroid Assoc. 2012;22(11):1153–9. doi:10.1089/thy.2011.0511.
70. Hartwell LH, Kastan MB. Cell cycle control and cancer. Science (New York, NY). 1994;266(5192):1821–8. Retrieved from http://www.ncbi.nlm.nih.gov/pubmed/7997877.
71. Hofstra RM, Landsvater RM, Ceccherini I, Stulp RP, Stelwagen T, Luo Y, … Romeo G. A mutation in the RET proto-oncogene associated with multiple endocrine neoplasia type 2B and sporadic medullary thyroid carcinoma. Nature. 1994;367(6461):375–6. doi:10.1038/367375a0.
72. Horn S, Figl A, Rachakonda PS, Fischer C, Sucker A, Gast A, … Kumar R. TERT promoter mutations in familial and sporadic melanoma. Science. 2013;339(6122):959–61. doi:10.1126/science.1230062.
73. Hou P, Liu D, Shan Y, Hu S, Studeman K, Condouris S, … Xing M. Genetic alterations and their relationship in the phosphatidylinositol 3-kinase/Akt pathway in thyroid cancer. Clin Cancer Res: Off J Am Assoc Cancer Res. 2007;13(4):1161–70. doi:10.1158/1078-0432.CCR-06-1125.
74. Hou P, Liu D, Xing M. Functional characterization of the T1799-1801del and A1799-1816ins BRAF mutations in papillary thyroid cancer. Cell Cycle (Georgetown, Tex). 2007;6(3):377–9. Retrieved from http://www.ncbi.nlm.nih.gov/pubmed/17297294.
75. Huang FW, Hodis E, Xu MJ, Kryukov GV, Chin L, Garraway LA. Highly recurrent TERT promoter mutations in human melanoma. Science (New York, NY). 2013;339(6122):957–9. doi:10.1126/science.1229259.
76. Ichihara M, Murakumo Y, Takahashi M. RET and neuroendocrine tumors. Cancer Lett. 2004;204(2):197–211. doi:10.1016/S0304-3835(03)00456-7.
77. Ishizaka Y, Kobayashi S, Ushijima T, Hirohashi S, Sugimura T, Nagao M. Detection of retTPC/PTC transcripts in thyroid adenomas and adenomatous goiter by an RT-PCR method. Oncogene. 1991;6(9):1667–72. Retrieved from http://www.ncbi.nlm.nih.gov/pubmed/1717926.
78. Ito T, Seyama T, Mizuno T, Tsuyama N, Hayashi T, Hayashi Y, … Akiyama M. Unique association of p53 mutations with undifferentiated but not with differentiated carcinomas of the thyroid gland. Cancer Res. 1992;52(5):1369–71. Retrieved from http://www.ncbi.nlm.nih.gov/pubmed/1737400.

79. Iwashita T, Murakami H, Kurokawa K, Kawai K, Miyauchi A, Futami H, … Takahashi M. A two-hit model for development of multiple endocrine neoplasia type 2B by RET mutations. Biochem Biophys Res Commun. 2000;268(3):804–8. doi:10.1006/bbrc.2000.2227.
80. Jhiang SM. The RET proto-oncogene in human cancers. Oncogene. 2000;19(49):5590–7. doi:10.1038/sj.onc.1203857.
81. Jia Y, Yu Y, Li X, Wei S, Zheng X, Yang X, … Gao M. Diagnostic value of B-RAF(V600E) in difficult-to-diagnose thyroid nodules using fine-needle aspiration: systematic review and meta-analysis. Diagn Cytopathol. 2014;42(1):94–101. doi:10.1002/dc.23044.
82. Kelly LM, Barila G, Liu P, Evdokimova VN, Trivedi S, Panebianco F, … Nikiforov YE. Identification of the transforming STRN-ALK fusion as a potential therapeutic target in the aggressive forms of thyroid cancer. Proc Natl Acad Sci USA. 2014;111(11):4233–8. doi:10.1073/pnas.1321937111.
83. Kimura ET, Nikiforova MN, Zhu Z, Knauf JA, Nikiforov YE, Fagin JA. High prevalence of BRAF mutations in thyroid cancer: genetic evidence for constitutive activation of the RET/PTC-RAS-BRAF signaling pathway in papillary thyroid carcinoma. Cancer Res. 2003;63(7):1454–7. Retrieved from http://www.ncbi.nlm.nih.gov/pubmed/12670889.
84. Kloos RT, Eng C, Evans DB, Francis GL, Gagel RF, Gharib H, … Wells SA. Medullary thyroid cancer: management guidelines of the American Thyroid Association. Thyroid: Off J Am Thyroid Assoc. 2009;19(6):565–612. doi:10.1089/thy.2008.0403.
85. Klugbauer S, Demidchik EP, Lengfelder E, Rabes HM. Detection of a novel type of RET rearrangement (PTC5) in thyroid carcinomas after Chernobyl and analysis of the involved RET-fused gene RFG5. Cancer Res. 1998;58(2):198–203. Retrieved from http://www.ncbi.nlm.nih.gov/pubmed/9443391.
86. Klugbauer S, Jauch A, Lengfelder E, Demidchik E, Rabes HM. A novel type of RET rearrangement (PTC8) in childhood papillary thyroid carcinomas and characterization of the involved gene (RFG8). Cancer Res. 2000;60(24):7028–32. Retrieved from http://www.ncbi.nlm.nih.gov/pubmed/11156407.
87. Klugbauer S, Lengfelder E, Demidchik EP, Rabes HM. High prevalence of RET rearrangement in thyroid tumors of children from Belarus after the Chernobyl reactor accident. Oncogene. 1995;11(12):2459–67. Retrieved from http://www.ncbi.nlm.nih.gov/pubmed/8545102.
88. Klugbauer S, Rabes HM. The transcription coactivator HTIF1 and a related protein are fused to the RET receptor tyrosine kinase in childhood papillary thyroid carcinomas. Oncogene. 1999;18(30):4388–93. doi:10.1038/sj.onc.1202824.
89. Knudson AG. Antioncogenes and human cancer. Proc Natl Acad Sci U S A. 1993;90(23):10914–21. Retrieved from http://www.pubmedcentral.nih.gov/articlerender.fcgi?artid=47892&tool=pmcentrez&rendertype=abstract.
90. Kroll TG, Sarraf P, Pecciarini L, Chen CJ, Mueller E, Spiegelman BM, Fletcher JA. PAX8-PPARgamma1 fusion oncogene in human thyroid carcinoma [corrected]. Science (New York, NY). 2000;289(5483):1357–60. Retrieved from http://www.ncbi.nlm.nih.gov/pubmed/10958784.
91. Krontiris TG. Oncogenes. N Engl J Med. 1995;333(5):303–6. doi:10.1056/NEJM199508033330508.
92. Landa I, Ganly I, Chan TA, Mitsutake N, Matsuse M, Ibrahimpasic T, … Fagin JA. Frequent somatic TERT promoter mutations in thyroid cancer: higher prevalence in advanced forms of the disease. J Clin Endocrinol Metab. 2013;98(9):E1562–6. doi:10.1210/jc.2013-2383.
93. Latchman DS. Transcription-factor mutations and disease. N Engl J Med. 1996;334(1):28–33. doi:10.1056/NEJM199601043340108.
94. Leeman-Neill RJ, Brenner AV, Little MP, Bogdanova TI, Hatch M, Zurnadzy LY, … Nikiforov YE. RET/PTC and PAX8/PPARγ chromosomal rearrangements in post-Chernobyl thyroid cancer and their association with iodine-131 radiation dose and other characteristics. Cancer. 2013;119(10):1792–9. doi:10.1002/cncr.27893.
95. Leeman-Neill RJ, Kelly LM, Liu P, Brenner AV, Little MP, Bogdanova TI, … Nikiforov YE. ETV6-NTRK3 is a common chromosomal rearrangement in radiation-associated thyroid cancer. Cancer. 2013. doi:10.1002/cncr.28484.
96. Lemoine NR, Mayall ES, Wyllie FS, Williams ED, Goyns M, Stringer B, Wynford-Thomas D. High frequency of ras oncogene activation in all stages of human thyroid tumorigenesis. Oncogene. 1989;4(2):159–64. Retrieved from http://www.ncbi.nlm.nih.gov/pubmed/2648253.
97. Li C, Lee KC, Schneider EB, Zeiger MA. BRAF V600E mutation and its association with clinicopathological features of papillary thyroid cancer: a meta-analysis. J Clin Endocrinol Metab. 2012;97(12):4559–70. doi:10.1210/jc.2012-2104.
98. Leeman-Neill RJ, Kelly LM, Liu P, Brenner AV, Little MP, Bogdanova TI, … Nikiforov YE. ETV6-NTRK3 is a common chromosomal rearrangement in radiation-associated thyroid cancer. Cancer. 2014. doi:10.1002/cncr.28484.
99. Lui W-O, Zeng L, Rehrmann V, Deshpande S, Tretiakova M, Kaplan EL, … Kroll TG. CREB3L2-PPARgamma fusion mutation identifies a thyroid signaling pathway regulated by intramembrane proteolysis. Cancer Res. 2008;68(17):7156–64. doi:10.1158/0008-5472.CAN-08-1085.
100. Machens A, Niccoli-Sire P, Hoegel J, Frank-Raue K, van Vroonhoven TJ, Roeher H-D, … Dralle H. Early malignant progression of hereditary medullary thyroid cancer. N Engl J Med. 2003;349(16):1517–25. doi:10.1056/NEJMoa012915.
101. Marques AR, Espadinha C, Catarino AL, Moniz S, Pereira T, Sobrinho LG, Leite V. Expression of PAX8-PPAR gamma 1 rearrangements in both follicular thyroid carcinomas and adenomas. J Clin Endocrinol Metab. 2002;87(8):3947–52. doi:10.1210/jcem.87.8.8756.
102. Marshall CJ. Tumor suppressor genes. Cell. 1991;64(2):313–26. Retrieved from http://www.ncbi.nlm.nih.gov/pubmed/1988150.
103. Melo M, da Rocha AG, Vinagre J, Batista R, Peixoto J, Tavares C, … Soares P. TERT promoter mutations are a major indicator of poor outcome in differentiated thyroid carcinomas. J Clin Endocrinol Metab. 2014;99(5):E754–65. doi:10.1210/jc.2013-3734.
104. Menko FH, van der Luijt RB, de Valk IAJ, Toorians AWFT, Sepers JM, van Diest PJ, Lips CJM. Atypical MEN type 2B associated with two germline RET mutations on the same allele not involving codon 918. J Clin Endocrinol Metab. 2002;87(1):393–7. doi:10.1210/jcem.87.1.8136.
105. Minoletti F, Butti MG, Coronelli S, Miozzo M, Sozzi G, Pilotti S, … Bongarzone I. The two genes generating RET/PTC3 are localized in chromosomal band 10q11.2. Gene Chromosome Cancer. 1994;11(1):51–7. Retrieved from http://www.ncbi.nlm.nih.gov/pubmed/7529046.
106. Mologni L, Redaelli S, Morandi A, Plaza-Menacho I, Gambacorti-Passerini C. Ponatinib is a potent inhibitor of wild-type and drug-resistant gatekeeper mutant RET kinase. Mol Cell Endocrinol. 2013;377(1–2):1–6. doi:10.1016/j.mce.2013.06.025.
107. Moura MM, Cavaco BM, Pinto AE, Leite V. High prevalence of RAS mutations in RET-negative sporadic medullary thyroid carcinomas. J Clin Endocrinol Metab. 2011;96(5):E863–8. doi:10.1210/jc.2010-1921.
108. Mulligan LM, Kwok JB, Healey CS, Elsdon MJ, Eng C, Gardner E, … Papi L. Germ-line mutations of the RET proto-oncogene in multiple endocrine neoplasia type 2A. Nature. 1993;363(6428):458–60. doi:10.1038/363458a0.
109. Murugan AK, Xing M. Anaplastic thyroid cancers harbor novel oncogenic mutations of the ALK gene. Cancer Res. 2011;71(13):4403–11. doi:10.1158/0008-5472.CAN-10-4041.

110. Nakata T, Kitamura Y, Shimizu K, Tanaka S, Fujimori M, Yokoyama S, … Emi M. Fusion of a novel gene, ELKS, to RET due to translocation t(10;12)(q11;p13) in a papillary thyroid carcinoma. Gene Chromosome Cancer. 1999;25(2):97–103. Retrieved from http://www.ncbi.nlm.nih.gov/pubmed/10337992.
111. Nikiforov YE, Rowland JM, Bove KE, Monforte-Munoz H, Fagin JA. Distinct pattern of ret oncogene rearrangements in morphological variants of radiation-induced and sporadic thyroid papillary carcinomas in children. Cancer Res. 1997;57(9):1690–4. Retrieved from http://www.ncbi.nlm.nih.gov/pubmed/9135009.
112. Nikiforov YE, Steward DL, Robinson-Smith TM, Haugen BR, Klopper JP, Zhu Z, … Nikiforova MN. Molecular testing for mutations in improving the fine-needle aspiration diagnosis of thyroid nodules. J Clin Endocrinol Metab. 2009;94(6):2092–8. doi:10.1210/jc.2009-0247.
113. Nikiforova MN, Biddinger PW, Caudill CM, Kroll TG, Nikiforov YE. PAX8-PPARgamma rearrangement in thyroid tumors: RT-PCR and immunohistochemical analyses. Am J Surg Pathol. 2002;26(8):1016–23. Retrieved from http://www.ncbi.nlm.nih.gov/pubmed/12170088.
114. Nikiforova MN, Kimura ET, Gandhi M, Biddinger PW, Knauf JA, Basolo F, … Nikiforov YE. BRAF mutations in thyroid tumors are restricted to papillary carcinomas and anaplastic or poorly differentiated carcinomas arising from papillary carcinomas. J Clin Endocrinol Metab. 2003;88(11):5399–404. doi:10.1210/jc.2003-030838.
115. Nikiforova MN, Lynch RA, Biddinger PW, Alexander EK, Dorn GW, Tallini G, … Nikiforov YE. RAS point mutations and PAX8-PPAR gamma rearrangement in thyroid tumors: evidence for distinct molecular pathways in thyroid follicular carcinoma. J Clin Endocrinol Metab. 2003;88(5):2318–26. doi:10.1210/jc.2002-021907.
116. Nikiforova MN, Wald AI, Roy S, Durso MB, Nikiforov YE. Targeted next-generation sequencing panel (ThyroSeq) for detection of mutations in thyroid cancer. J Clin Endocrinol Metab. 2013;98(11):E1852–60. doi:10.1210/jc.2013-2292.
117. Pierotti MA, Santoro M, Jenkins RB, Sozzi G, Bongarzone I, Grieco M, … Fusco A. Characterization of an inversion on the long arm of chromosome 10 juxtaposing D10S170 and RET and creating the oncogenic sequence RET/PTC. Proc Natl Acad Sci USA. 1992;89(5):1616–20. Retrieved from http://www.pubmedcentral.nih.gov/articlerender.fcgi?artid=48503&tool=pmcentrez&rendertype=abstract.
118. Porta C, Paglino C, Mosca A. Targeting PI3K/Akt/mTOR signaling in cancer. Front Oncol. 2014;4:64. doi:10.3389/fonc.2014.00064.
119. Rabes HM, Demidchik EP, Sidorow JD, Lengfelder E, Beimfohr C, Hoelzel D, Klugbauer S. Pattern of radiation-induced RET and NTRK1 rearrangements in 191 post-chernobyl papillary thyroid carcinomas: biological, phenotypic, and clinical implications. Clin Cancer Res: Off J Am Assoc Cancer Res. 2000;6(3):1093–103. Retrieved from http://www.ncbi.nlm.nih.gov/pubmed/10741739.
120. Raman P, Koenig RJ. Pax-8-PPAR-γ fusion protein in thyroid carcinoma. Nat Rev Endocrinol. 2014. doi:10.1038/nrendo.2014.115.
121. Ricarte-Filho JC, Li S, Garcia-Rendueles MER, Montero-Conde C, Voza F, Knauf JA, … Fagin JA. Identification of kinase fusion oncogenes in post-Chernobyl radiation-induced thyroid cancers. J Clin Investig. 2013;123(11):4935–44. doi:10.1172/JCI69766.
122. Ricarte-Filho JC, Ryder M, Chitale DA, Rivera M, Heguy A, Ladanyi M, … Fagin JA. Mutational profile of advanced primary and metastatic radioactive iodine-refractory thyroid cancers reveals distinct pathogenetic roles for BRAF, PIK3CA, and AKT1. Cancer Res. 2009;69(11):4885–93. doi:10.1158/0008-5472.CAN-09-0727.
123. Rivera M, Ricarte-Filho J, Knauf J, Shaha A, Tuttle M, Fagin JA, Ghossein RA. Molecular genotyping of papillary thyroid carcinoma follicular variant according to its histological subtypes (encapsulated vs infiltrative) reveals distinct BRAF and RAS mutation patterns. Mod Pathol: Off J U S Can Acad Pathol Inc. 2010;23(9):1191–200. doi:10.1038/modpathol.2010.112.
124. Saenko V, Rogounovitch T, Shimizu-Yoshida Y, Abrosimov A, Lushnikov E, Roumiantsev P, … Yamashita S. Novel tumorigenic rearrangement, delta rfp/ret, in a papillary thyroid carcinoma from externally irradiated patient. Mutat Research. 2003;527(1–2):81–90. Retrieved from http://www.ncbi.nlm.nih.gov/pubmed/12787916.
125. Salassidis K, Bruch J, Zitzelsberger H, Lengfelder E, Kellerer AM, Bauchinger M. Translocation t(10;14)(q11.2:q22.1) fusing the kinetin to the RET gene creates a novel rearranged form (PTC8) of the RET proto-oncogene in radiation-induced childhood papillary thyroid carcinoma. Cancer Res. 2000;60(11):2786–9. Retrieved from http://www.ncbi.nlm.nih.gov/pubmed/10850414.
126. Santarpia L, El-Naggar AK, Cote GJ, Myers JN, Sherman SI. Phosphatidylinositol 3-kinase/akt and ras/raf-mitogen-activated protein kinase pathway mutations in anaplastic thyroid cancer. J Clin Endocrinol Metab. 2008;93(1):278–84. doi:10.1210/jc.2007-1076.
127. Santelli G, de Franciscis V, Portella G, Chiappetta G, D'Alessio A, Califano D, … Manzo G. Production of transgenic mice expressing the Ki-ras oncogene under the control of a thyroglobulin promoter. Cancer Res. 1993;53(22):5523–7. Retrieved from http://www.ncbi.nlm.nih.gov/pubmed/8221693.
128. Santoro M, Carlomagno F, Hay ID, Herrmann MA, Grieco M, Melillo R, … Berger N. Ret oncogene activation in human thyroid neoplasms is restricted to the papillary cancer subtype. J Clin Investig. 1992;89(5):1517–22. doi:10.1172/JCI115743.
129. Santoro M, Dathan NA, Berlingieri MT, Bongarzone I, Paulin C, Grieco M, … Fusco A. Molecular characterization of RET/PTC3; a novel rearranged version of the RETproto-oncogene in a human thyroid papillary carcinoma. Oncogene. 1994;9(2):509–16. Retrieved from http://www.ncbi.nlm.nih.gov/pubmed/8290261.
130. Sapio MR, Guerra A, Marotta V, Campanile E, Formisano R, Deandrea M, … Vitale M. High growth rate of benign thyroid nodules bearing RET/PTC rearrangements. J Clin Endocrinol Metab. 2011;96(6):E916–9. doi:10.1210/jc.2010-1599.
131. Schilling T, Bürck J, Sinn HP, Clemens A, Otto HF, Höppner W, … Raue F. Prognostic value of codon 918 (ATG->ACG) RET proto-oncogene mutations in sporadic medullary thyroid carcinoma. Int J Cancer. J Int Cancer. 2001;95(1):62–6. Retrieved from http://www.ncbi.nlm.nih.gov/pubmed/11241313.
132. Skelhorne-Gross G, Nicol CJB. The key to unlocking the chemotherapeutic potential of PPARγ ligands: having the right combination. PPAR Res. 2012;2012:946943. doi:10.1155/2012/946943.
133. Skinner MA, Moley JA, Dilley WG, Owzar K, Debenedetti MK, Wells SA. Prophylactic thyroidectomy in multiple endocrine neoplasia type 2A. N Engl J Med. 2005;353(11):1105–13. doi:10.1056/NEJMoa043999.
134. Smallridge RC, Chindris A-M, Asmann YW, Casler JD, Serie DJ, Reddi HV, … Aubrey Thompson E. RNA sequencing identifies multiple fusion transcripts, differentially expressed genes, and reduced expression of immune function genes in BRAF (V600E) mutant vs BRAF wild-type papillary thyroid carcinoma. J Clin Endocrinol Metab. 2014;99(2):E338–47. doi:10.1210/jc.2013-2792.
135. Soares P, Trovisco V, Rocha AS, Lima J, Castro P, Preto A, … Sobrinho-Simões M. BRAF mutations and RET/PTC rearrangements are alternative events in the etiopathogenesis of PTC. Oncogene. 2003;22(29):4578–80. doi:10.1038/sj.onc.1206706.
136. Takahashi K, Eguchi H, Arihiro K, Ito R, Koyama K, Soda M, … Hamatani K. The presence of BRAF point mutation in adult papillary thyroid carcinomas from atomic bomb survivors correlates

with radiation dose. Mol Carcinog. 2007;46(3):242–8. doi:10.1002/mc.20277.

137. Trovisco V, Soares P, Soares R, Magalhães J, Sá-Couto P, Sobrinho-Simões M. A new BRAF gene mutation detected in a case of a solid variant of papillary thyroid carcinoma. Hum Pathol. 2005;36(6):694–7. doi:10.1016/j.humpath.2005.04.011.
138. Trovisco V, Vieira de Castro I, Soares P, Máximo V, Silva P, Magalhães J, … Sobrinho-Simões M. BRAF mutations are associated with some histological types of papillary thyroid carcinoma. J Pathol. 2004;202(2):247–51. doi:10.1002/path.1511.
139. Tufano RP, Teixeira GV, Bishop J, Carson KA, Xing M. BRAF mutation in papillary thyroid cancer and its value in tailoring initial treatment: a systematic review and meta-analysis. Medicine. 2012;91(5):274–86. doi:10.1097/MD.0b013e31826a9c71.
140. Tuttle RM, Ball DW, Byrd D, Dickson P, Duh Q-Y, Ehya H, … Hunt JP. NCCN clinical practice guidelines in oncology (NCCN guidelines®) thyroid carcinoma. 2013.
141. Vogelstein B, Kinzler KW. The multistep nature of cancer. Trends Genet: TIG. 1993;9(4):138–41. Retrieved from http://www.ncbi.nlm.nih.gov/pubmed/8516849.
142. Weinberg RA. Tumor suppressor genes. Science (New York, NY). 1991;254(5035):1138–46. Retrieved from http://www.ncbi.nlm.nih.gov/pubmed/1659741.
143. Weinberg RA. How cancer arises. Sci Am. 1996;275(3):62–70. Retrieved from http://www.ncbi.nlm.nih.gov/pubmed/8701295.
144. Wells SA, Robinson BG, Gagel RF, Dralle H, Fagin JA, Santoro M, … Schlumberger MJ. Vandetanib in patients with locally advanced or metastatic medullary thyroid cancer: a randomized, double-blind phase III trial. J Clin Oncol: Off J Am Soc Clin Oncol. 2012;30(2):134–41. doi:10.1200/JCO.2011.35.5040.
145. Wells SA, Santoro M. Targeting the RET pathway in thyroid cancer. Clin Cancer Res: Off J Am Assoc Cancer Res. 2009;15(23):7119–23. doi:10.1158/1078-0432.CCR-08-2742.
146. Wirtschafter A, Schmidt R, Rosen D, Kundu N, Santoro M, Fusco A, … Rothstein JL. Expression of the RET/PTC fusion gene as a marker for papillary carcinoma in Hashimoto's thyroiditis. Laryngoscope. 1997;107(1):95–100. Retrieved from http://www.ncbi.nlm.nih.gov/pubmed/9001272.
147. Wood WM, Sharma V, Bauerle KT, Pike LA, Zhou Q, Fretwell DL, … Haugen BR. PPARγ promotes growth and invasion of thyroid cancer cells. PPAR Res. 2011;2011:171765. doi:10.1155/2011/171765.
148. Xing M. BRAF mutation in thyroid cancer. Endocrine Relat Cancer. 2005;12(2):245–62. doi:10.1677/erc.1.0978.
149. Xing M, Alzahrani AS, Carson KA, Viola D, Elisei R, Bendlova B, … Sykorova V. Association between BRAF V600E mutation and mortality in patients with papillary thyroid cancer. JAMA: J Am Med Assoc. 2013;309(14):1493–501. doi:10.1001/jama.2013.3190.
150. Xu X, Quiros RM, Gattuso P, Ain KB, Prinz RA. High prevalence of BRAF gene mutation in papillary thyroid carcinomas and thyroid tumor cell lines. Cancer Res. 2003;63(15):4561–7. Retrieved from http://www.ncbi.nlm.nih.gov/pubmed/12907632.
151. Yakes FM, Chen J, Tan J, Yamaguchi K, Shi Y, Yu P, … Joly AH. Cabozantinib (XL184), a novel MET and VEGFR2 inhibitor, simultaneously suppresses metastasis, angiogenesis, and tumor growth. Mol Cancer Ther. 2011;10(12):2298–308. doi:10.1158/1535-7163.MCT-11-0264.
152. Zedenius J, Larsson C, Bergholm U, Bovée J, Svensson A, Hallengren B, … Wallin G. Mutations of codon 918 in the RET proto-oncogene correlate to poor prognosis in sporadic medullary thyroid carcinomas. J Clin Endocrinol Metab. 1995;80(10):3088–90. doi:10.1210/jcem.80.10.7559902.
153. Zedenius J, Wallin G, Hamberger B, Nordenskjöld M, Weber G, Larsson C. Somatic and MEN 2A de novo mutations identified in the RET proto-oncogene by screening of sporadic MTC:s. Hum Mol Genet. 1994;3(8):1259–62. Retrieved from http://www.ncbi.nlm.nih.gov/pubmed/7987299.
154. Zhang Z, Liu D, Murugan AK, Liu Z, Xing M. Histone deacetylation of NIS promoter underlies BRAF V600E-promoted NIS silencing in thyroid cancer. Endocrine Relat Cancer. 2014;21(2):161–73. doi:10.1530/ERC-13-0399.
155. Zhu Z, Ciampi R, Nikiforova MN, Gandhi M, Nikiforov YE. Prevalence of RET/PTC rearrangements in thyroid papillary carcinomas: effects of the detection methods and genetic heterogeneity. J Clin Endocrinol Metab. 2006;91(9):3603–10. doi:10.1210/jc.2006-1006.

Molecular Aspects of Thyroid Cancer in Children

4

Andrew J. Bauer and Gary L. Francis

Children with thyroid cancer generally have a more favorable prognosis than adults with similar histology and stage of disease. This chapter reviews data that suggest that the pattern of genetic mutations and/or gene expression in papillary thyroid carcinoma (PTC) in children might differ from those in adults. Additional study is warranted to better define the impact of these factors on the clinical behavior of thyroid cancers in children.

Introduction

PTC and follicular thyroid carcinoma (FTC) share important features in children and adults. The majority of tumors are classic PTC, and about one-third are multifocal in both age groups [1]. Histological variants including tall-cell PTC and poorly differentiated thyroid cancer (PDTC) are found in adults, but their frequency and prognosis are not well described among children [2]. Not as much is known about FTC because it occurs with lesser frequency in both age groups and is very uncommon in children [1]. Despite these similarities, dramatic differences exist in the clinical behavior of thyroid cancers in children and imply that these malignancies might arise through different mechanisms. Most children present with more widespread disease than do adults. At diagnosis, 70 % of childhood PTC has spread beyond the thyroid capsule or into the regional lymph nodes, and 10–28 % already has pulmonary metastases [1–9]. Despite more extensive disease, children are much less likely to die from PTC than are adults [1, 2, 10]. Mortality is generally on the order of 2 % even after 40 or more years [11]. Additionally, following treatment, about half of children with pulmonary metastases develop stable but persistent disease and experience extremely low disease-specific mortality [12, 13]. These are remarkable differences when compared to adults for whom the 10-year mortality approaches 75 % for those with pulmonary metastases [14].

Fewer data exist to compare FTC in children and adults. In one study, disease-free survival for children with PTC and FTC was similar, but the follow-up was short and the number of subjects was small [1]. Finally, poorly differentiated thyroid cancer (PDTC) and anaplastic thyroid cancer (ATC) rarely, if ever, occur in children [2]. This could be a function of time in that most ATCs in adults are thought to arise through dedifferentiation of PTC or FTC over many years [15]. Certainly, the paucity of dedifferentiated thyroid cancers in children improves the overall prognosis, but the prognosis is more favorable for children even when comparing similar histology and extent of disease [1].

Inherited Cancer Syndromes

Approximately 5 % of PTC is inherited with a dominant mode of transmission [16]. Inherited PTC is one feature in a variety of inherited tumor syndromes, including familial adenomatous polyposis, PTEN hamartoma syndrome, DICER1 syndrome, and Carney Complex. Familial Adenomatous Polyposis (FAP) has been linked to germline mutations in the APC gene at chromosome 5q21 [16, 17]. Affected patients develop various intestinal and dermoid tumors, lipomas, and epidermoid cysts that begin as hamartomas around 10–20 years of age and progress to carcinoma [16, 17]. PTC that develops in FAP exhibits a unique (cribriform-morular) histological variant with initiation of tumorigenesis associated with acquisition of a somatic mutation in *APC*, *CTNNB1* (beta-catenin),

A.J. Bauer, MD
Division of Endocrinology and Diabetes, Department of Pediatrics, The Children's Hospital of Philadelphia, The Perelman School of Medicine, The University of Pennsylvania, Philadelphia, PA, USA

G.L. Francis, MD, PhD (✉)
Division of Pediatric Endocrinology, Department of Pediatrics, Children's Hospital of Richmond Virginia Commonwealth University, 1001 E Marshall St, Richmond, VA 23298, USA
e-mail: glfrancis@vcu.edu

L. Wartofsky, D. Van Nostrand (eds.), *Thyroid Cancer*, DOI 10.1007/978-1-4939-3314-3_4

RAS, or a *RET/PTC* rearrangement [18]. PTEN hamartoma tumor syndrome (PHTS) is caused by mutations in the PTEN tumor suppressor gene located on chromosome 10q22-q23 that result in overactivation of protein kinase B (Akt) [19]. Clinical findings include macrocephaly, mucocutaneous lesions, freckling of the glans penis and an increased lifetime risk of thyroid, breast (females), endometrial and renal cancers [20], multiple hamartomas, breast cancer, colon cancer, and nodular goiter. The DICER-1 syndrome is inherited and is associated with missense mutations within the RNase IIIb domain of *DICER 1* (chromosome 14q32.13) with somatic loss of function of the other allele associated with an increased risk for pleuropulmonary blastoma (PPB), Sertoli-Leydig cell tumors, cystic nephroma, multinodular goiter, and differentiated thyroid cancer [21, 22]. Carney complex (spotty skin pigmentation, myxomas, schwannomas, and endocrine overactivity) is caused by a defect in the protein kinase A regulatory subunit type Ia gene located on chromosome 17q22-q24 and can also be associated, albeit rarely (3.8 %), with inherited forms of thyroid cancer [23, 24].

Although these syndromes are uncommon causes of thyroid cancer, they should be considered in any patient with unusual histology or a pedigree that suggests dominant transmission of a multiple tumor syndrome. They also provide evidence for the potential importance of mutations on chromosomes 5 and 10 in thyroid cancers of all ages.

Radiation-Induced Thyroid Cancers

Exposure to ionizing radiation, especially at young age, increases the risk for thyroid neoplasia (benign and malignant) [25]. Radiation-induced thyroid malignancies appear to occur as early as 5 years after exposure and to develop in younger patients when compared to "spontaneous" thyroid cancers for which the peak incidence occurs during adolescence [26, 27]. Generally, radiation-induced thyroid cancers are more likely to be multifocal [28, 29]. They commonly exhibit mutations in the RET proto-oncogene and express higher levels of vascular endothelial growth factor (VEGF) than do other forms of childhood thyroid cancer [30–35]. Radiation-induced PTC in children have been most frequently shown to harbor chromosomal rearrangements between the RET proto-oncogene and regulatory elements of otherwise unrelated genes [35–38]. In radiation-induced PTC of children, this most often generates a specific recombinant gene known as RET/PTC3. Nikiforov et al. found an important spatial geometry that allows ELE1 and RET to recombine following chromosomal breaks that arise from a single radiation track, facilitating the formation of RET/PTC3 [39]. Consequently, the thyroid is particularly vulnerable to radiation-induced cancer, a possibility that is borne out by all studies of children with radiation-induced thyroid cancer [25, 40].

"Spontaneous" Thyroid Cancers

The etiology of "spontaneous" thyroid cancers remains unknown, but emerging evidence supports the hypothesis that thyroid cancers may arise from thyroid stem cells. Pluripotent stem-like cells have been isolated from goitrous thyroid [41–46] and shown to co-express Oct-4, a marker of pluripotent cells, the endodermal markers Gata-4 and HNF4a, and thyroid transcription factor PAX8 [46]. When stimulated with thyrotropin (TSH) these cells differentiate into thyroid cells which express PAX8, thyroglobulin (Tg), sodium-iodide symporter (NIS), thyrotropin receptor (TSHR), and thyroid peroxidase (TPO) and develop self-replication [42]. Compartmentalized p63 staining was shown in a subset of PTC (7/27, 26 %) suggesting that PTC may originate from these stem-like cells [47]. By contrast, FTC may develop from nodules such as follicular adenoma (FA) and nodular goiter (NG). Mutations of the RAS family genes are detected in about 50 % of FTC and are also observed in a small proportion of NG (4 %) and up to 50 % of FA, including those with atypical morphology [48–50]. PAX8/PPARγ rearrangement occurs in 53–63 % of FTC and 8–13 % FA [48, 51].

A variety of genetic alterations have been reported in "spontaneous" thyroid cancers, but RAS, RET/PTC, PAX8/PPARγ, and BRAF represent the four most common genetic alterations in PTC and FTC. All of these mutations lead to either direct (RET/PTC, RAS, BRAF) or indirect (PAX8/PPARγ) constitutive activation of the RET/PTC -> RAS -> RAF -> mitogen extracellular kinase (MEK) -> MAPK/ERK (MAPK) and the phosphatidylinositol 3-kinase (PI3K)/AKT signaling pathways. Activation of this pathway induces cell proliferation, growth, survival, and tumorigenesis [52, 53]. RET/PTC rearrangements [32, 33, 54–60] and BRAF point mutations are common in PTC [58, 61], PAX8/PPARγ is common in FTC [62–64], and N-RAS mutations are found in both FTC and follicular variant PTC (fvPTC) [63, 65–68]. However, RET/PTC [32, 54], RAS [50, 69, 70], and PAX8/PPARγ [71, 72] have also been detected in benign lesions.

BRAF Mutations

BRAF is a serine/threonine kinase that receives a mitogenic signal from RAS and transmits it to the mitogen-activated protein kinase (MAPK) pathway [58, 73, 74]. MAPK activation then leads to more rapid cell division and a distinct survival advantage. Constitutive activation of any effector along the RET/PTC-RAS-BRAF-MAPK pathway is sufficient to increase proliferation and, possibly in concert with other events, induce the malignant phenotype [58, 73, 74].

BRAF mutations are the most common genetic alteration in PTC from adults and are detected in approximately 45 % of PTC (range of 29–87 %) [58, 73, 74]. Although 40 mutations have been identified, 95 % involve nucleotide position

1799 and result in a substitution of valine to glutamate at residue 600 (V600E) [61, 75]. Mutations of BRAF are believed to be both an early event of thyroid tumor induction and an important event in proliferation and progression [58, 65, 73, 74, 76–78].

BRAF mutations appear to be an independent risk factor for PTC progression and recurrence. Xing et al. found significant associations between BRAF mutations and extrathyroidal invasion, lymph node metastasis, and advanced tumor stage [79–82]. In addition, BRAF mutations were more frequently associated with absence of radioactive iodine (RAI) avidity, and perhaps because of the reduced iodine uptake, 25 % of patients with BRAF mutation went on to develop recurrent disease (vs. 9 % without a BRAF mutation) [80, 82, 83]. Kebebew et al. also found a significant association between the BRAF V600E mutation and older age, lymph node metastasis, distant metastasis, higher TNM stage, and recurrent and persistent disease [83]. Elisei et al. showed higher rates of persistent disease and higher mortality rates in the BRAF-positive patients [84]. One potential unifying explanation for the poor prognosis is that constitutive activation of BRAF is associated with repression of NIS and subsequent loss of RAI avidity [85]. Early studies in childhood PTC identified few BRAF mutations [61]. More recent studies, however, report that between 30 and 40 % of pediatric PTC harbor BRAF V600E mutations but, in contrast to adults, the presence of BRAF does not correlate with increased invasive behavior or worse outcome [86–90].

RET/PTC Mutations

About half of all childhood PTCs contain recombination events between the tyrosine kinase domain of the RET proto-oncogene and regulatory elements of other genes [35, 55, 91, 92]. The RET/PTC rearrangements result in over-expression of the RET/PTC chimeric gene and unregulated RET tyrosine kinase activity and are directly transforming in experimental models [93]. The RET/PTC rearrangements occur in children with radiation-induced PTC and spontaneous PTC, but the type of RET/PTC rearrangements may differ [35, 54–56, 60, 94–98].

RET/PTC rearrangements are typically associated with PTCs that have classic papillary morphology and frequent psammoma bodies [99]. They are found in younger and post-radiation exposure patients and are associated with loco-regional lymph node metastasis [100, 101]. RET/PTC is found in approximately 20 % of adult PTC, in 50–80 % of patients with a history of radiation exposure, and in 40–70 % of pediatric patients [55, 102–104]. RET/PTC1 and RET/PTC3 are the most common rearrangements, but detection and/or expression may be heterogeneous within individual tumors [55]. Whereas RET/PTC3 is most common in radiation-induced PTC, RET/PTC1 was detected in 16/34 (47 %) of "spontaneous" PTC [55].

RET expression is associated with nuclear N-RAS and positive ERK staining, supporting a previous in vitro observation that simultaneous activation of several genes may be necessary for tumor formation and progression [69, 105–107]. Transgenic mouse models show the transforming ability of RET/PTC and suggest that RET/PTC may be an early marker of thyroid tumorigenesis [108]. Few studies have correlated the presence or absence of specific RET/PTC mutations with the clinical behavior of PTC in children. A single report failed to find any evidence that RET/PTC mutations are associated with a more or less favorable outcome in children [55]. In contrast, adult PTC harboring an RET/PTC mutation may follow a more aggressive clinical course [100, 102, 104, 109].

RAS

Point mutations in the RAS genes, H-, N-, and K-RAS, occur in a wide continuum of thyroid tumors ranging from FA to FTC (40–53 %), PTC (0–20 %), follicular variant PTC (fvPTC, 17–25 %), and poorly differentiated thyroid cancer (PDTC, 20–60 %) [49, 50, 67, 69, 106, 110]. Vasko et al. found that codon 61 mutation of N-RAS (N2) was more frequently identified in follicular tumors compared to papillary cancers (19 % vs. 5 %, respectively) and that the N2 mutation was more frequently found in malignant compared to benign lesions (25 % vs. 14 %, respectively) [70]. Mutations of the RAS oncogene have been reported with high frequency in adult thyroid cancers but appear to be less frequent in childhood thyroid tumors [55, 111].

PAX8/PPARγ

PAX8/PPARγ rearrangements are found in several different thyroid tumors but are most commonly associated with FTC. In addition, PAX8/PPARγ-positive tumors show more extensive capsular and vascular invasion compared to RAS-positive tumors [112–114]. Freitas et al. found PAX8/PPARγ mutations in 39 % of FTC, 8 % of FA, and 11 % of fvPTC but only rarely in PTC (0.3 %) [115]. Interestingly, RAS mutations and PPARγ rearrangements appear to be mutually exclusive and are uncommon in the same tumor [63]. PAX8/PPARγ is not associated with poorly differentiated foci or PDTC [113].

It is not yet fully understood how PAX8/PPARγ rearrangements participate in thyroid tumorigenesis [116]. In vitro, PAX8/PPARγ appears to act as both a dominant-negative inhibitor of PPARγ and as a partial agonist of PAX8 and PPARγ pathways [64]. On a cellular level, PAX8/PPARγ induces anchorage-independent growth in thyrocytes, decreases apoptosis, and increases proliferation [64, 116–121]. In vivo, there are few data on whether PAX8/PPARγ is able to induce tumorigenesis and/or disease progression. There are discordant reports to suggest that PAX8/PPARγ expression is associated with a less or more aggressive phenotype [117–121]. Recent data have shown an association between PAX8/PPARγ and decreased neovascularization in both a xenograft model and in human FA and FTC [122, 123]. Taken together, PAX8/PPARγ rearrangements appear to be a reliable marker of follicular lesions, more commonly expressed in FTC than FA; however, the mechanism of action and clinical implications have not been fully elucidated.

Other Mutations

Fusion oncogenes involving the neurotrophic tyrosine kinase receptor (NTRK) with nuclear basket protein (TPR) or ets variant 6 (ETV6) were initially reported in pediatric patients exposed to radiation [124]. Recent reports, however, suggest that NTRK fusion oncogenes occur in sporadic DTC. Solid and diffuse follicular variant PTCs are the most common DTC variants with histology showing sclerotic bands, extensive lymphovascular invasion, but with a lack of microcalcifications and lymphocytic infiltration [89, 90]. To date, there are too few reported cases to determine if the presence of NTRK fusion oncogenes is associated with reduced disease-free survival or higher disease-specific mortality.

Poorly differentiated thyroid cancer (PDTC) and ATC occur in adults, but almost never during childhood [2, 125]. Such tumors are often found to have mutations in the p53 tumor suppressor gene [15, 126–128]. Owing to the lack of ATC in children, p53 mutations are expected and confirmed to be rare in childhood thyroid cancers [125, 129–133]. It is highly likely that the reduced incidence of p53 mutations and poorly differentiated thyroid cancers in children contribute to the overall favorable prognosis. However, given their rarity and restriction to poorly differentiated thyroid cancers, p53 mutations are not likely to explain the more positive prognosis in children in comparison to adults with similar histology and extent of disease.

Growth Factors

Although not transforming in and of themselves, several growth factors and cell cycle regulatory proteins have been implicated during the transformation of the normal thyroid into thyroid cancer and have been investigated in children and adults. Generally, expression appears to be a common feature to both age groups, but there are a few important and additional minor quantitative differences.

One major difference involves the expression of insulin-like growth factors (IGFs) and their receptors. IGF-1 has been detected in 90 % of adult PTC and was shown to stimulate the growth of PTC in culture [129–133]. However, there was no relationship between IGF-1 expression and the prognosis for adults [129–133]. The IGF-1 receptor was also expressed by the majority of adult PTC and significantly correlated with tumor size [132, 133]. Vella et al. found that the IGF-1 receptor was expressed only by differentiated thyroid cancers, whereas insulin receptors (IRs) and hybrid receptors (formed between the IGF-1 receptor and IR) were expressed by poorly differentiated thyroid cancers [132, 134]. Ordinarily, these hybrid receptors are only expressed during fetal life and confer the ability to bind IGF-2 [134]. Adult thyroid cancers with increased expression of hybrid IGF-1 receptors/IRs are most often poorly differentiated and have a poor prognosis [132, 134].

Only a few data are available regarding IGF expression in thyroid cancers from children; however, the IGF-1 and IGF-1 receptor were detected in somewhat fewer tumors than in adults (45 % and 43 %, respectively) [135]. Importantly, IGF-1 receptor expression was more intense in invasive, metastatic, recurrent, or persistent tumors. These data support a role for the IGFs, particularly the IGF-1 receptor, in the clinical behavior of thyroid carcinoma.

Another significant protein in thyroid cancer is telomerase. During normal cell division, the terminal ends of the DNA or telomeres are lost, leading to programmed senescence [136–143]. Telomerase is a specific enzyme that replaces telomeric DNA, conferring cellular immortality. In adult thyroid cancers, telomerase activity was increased and associated with a high probability of metastasis [144, 145]. Similar studies also found increased telomerase expression in malignant thyroid tumors in children, suggesting that telomerase expression could allow thyroid cells in either age group to become immortal and accumulate the additional mutations necessary for the full malignant phenotype [141].

The potent angiogenic stimulus, vascular endothelial growth factor (VEGF), and the VEGF receptor (Flt-1) are expressed by childhood thyroid carcinoma, increased in the largest tumors, and most intense in tumors destined to recur [146–148]. In addition, VEGF expression is greater in PTC in children than in adults and even greater in radiation-induced PTC [148, 149]. The importance of VEGF in sustaining thyroid carcinoma has been further demonstrated by abrogating the growth of thyroid cancer xenografts with VEGF monoclonal antibodies [150–152].

Nitric oxide (NO) is another potent stimulus for blood flow and angiogenesis. NO is produced by several isoforms of nitric oxide synthase (NOS) of which endothelial (eNOS) and inducible (iNOS) are potentially important in the thyroid [153–158]. Both iNOS and eNOS have been detected in adult thyroid neoplasms, but there appeared to be no difference between benign and malignant lesions [155, 159]. Other key growth factors are the hepatocyte growth factor/scatter factor (HGF/SF) and HGF/SF receptor (cMET). The overexpression of both components of this autocrine/paracrine loop has been reported in childhood tumors with a higher probability of recurrence [160].

NIS Expression

The level of differentiation of individual tumors has an important role in determining the clinical course. One indicator of differentiated thyroid function is expression of the sodium-iodide symporter (NIS). NIS is also essential for successful therapy with radioactive iodine. The majority of studies have detected NIS expression in adult thyroid cancers [161–164]. A smaller study of childhood PTC documented NIS expression in 35 % of PTC and 44 % of FTC but also found that recurrence developed exclusively from PTC and FTC with undetectable NIS [165]. In addition, the dose of iodine-131 required to achieve remission was greater in patients with PTC that had undetectable NIS. Whether this is a direct reflection of the differentiation level or the ability to concentrate radioactive iodine is not clear from these studies, but the presence of NIS expression may be crucial to promote the favorable long-term survival of children with PTC.

Gene Regulation

Although abundant evidence supports the role for genetic mutations in the induction of thyroid cancers, emerging data also implicate epigenetic regulation of gene expression as important for thyroid malignancies. To our knowledge, however, no studies have yet compared gene regulation in thyroid tumors from adults with those from children leaving unanswered the question as to the potential differences in gene regulation and expression. Nevertheless, important thyroid-specific genes whose expression is altered through methylation include the TSH receptor, thyroglobulin (Tg), and NIS [166, 167]. All of these gene products have important implication in the pathogenesis of advanced tumors, and therapies targeted at re-expression could prove to be clinically beneficial, in particular the ability to improve cell response to radioiodine therapy.

In vitro, demethylating agents have been shown to partially restore the expression of TSHR, and MEK inhibition (U0126 ir siRNA) induces re-expression of NIS in thyroid cells expressing the BRAF V600E mutation [168]. A wide variety of tumor suppressor genes are also hypermethylated in thyroid lesions, both benign and malignant [169–174]. Decreased expression of these genes results in altered growth, angiogenesis, invasion, and metastasis, supporting a role for epigenetic regulation in thyroid cancer progression [175].

MicroRNAs (miRNAs) are small noncoding RNAs that bind cognate messenger RNAs (mRNAs) and function as gene silencers by affecting the stability and degradation of mRNA [176]. Current estimates suggest that approximately one-third of all human gene transcripts contain sites to which miRNA could bind and exert posttranscriptional control. Recent studies have implicated miRNAs in a variety of important human diseases including cancer [177, 178]. Studies in thyroid tumors show that 32 % of all miRNAs are upregulated in thyroid tumors, while 38 % are downregulated by more than a twofold change [179].

From all these studies, miR-221, miR-222, and miR-146 emerge to be implicated in thyroid cancers [180–188]. Changes in expression of miR-146b, miR-221, and miR-222 may be important for PTC induction since their target is the tyrosine kinase KIT [189]. Fewer studies have examined miRNA expression in FTC, but work by Nikiforov et al. found a distinct pattern of miRNA expression in FTC that also included upregulation of miR-221 and miR-222 [190].

Genome-wide microarray data also suggest that a number of genes are potential thyroid cancer markers, to include *MET*, *TFF3*, *SERPINA1*, *TIMP1*, *FN1*, *TPO*, *TGFA*, *QPCT*, *CRABP1*, *FCGBP*, *EPS8*, and *PROS1* [191]. Several reviews of microarray and molecular marker data have been published [115, 192–194]. Microarrays have been used to explore several different questions in thyroid cancer biology, from the molecular signature of specific histological types to distinguishing benign from malignant lesions or prognosis [115, 193–195]. To date, there is no consensus on the number of genes required to accurately determine diagnosis or prognosis, and again, no study has yet compared adult and pediatric cancers with similar histology.

Summary

In conclusion, children with thyroid cancer generally have a more favorable prognosis than adults with similar histology and extent of disease. Although data are limited, there are suggestions that the patterns of mutations in PTC from children differ when compared to those from adults. The Cancer Genome Atlas (TGCA) project defined the genomic landscape of 496 PTCs suggesting that molecular subtypes may afford more accurate prediction of differentiation and clinical behavior [196]. There were no pediatric PTC included in the analysis; however, the increasing use of oncogene profile arrays suggests that within DTC the prevalence of point mutations and gene rearrangements between adult and pediatric patients may be similar. Growth factors and growth factor receptors are expressed by thyroid cancers in both ages but may differ, especially in the expression of the IGFs and IGF receptors. The difference in the growth factors and other unidentified factors within the pediatric age group may explain why pediatric DTC is more likely to maintain differentiation and be associated with lower disease-specific mortality. Recent observations implicating miRNAs in the induction and progression of thyroid cancers have yet to be replicated in children. Further study is warranted to better define the impact of each of these factors on the clinical behavior of thyroid cancers in children. The current data suggest that the difference between benign and malignant thyroid disease is a continuum and that molecular and environmental factors contribute to thyroid mutagenesis.

References

1. Welch Dinauer CA, Tuttle RM, Robie DK, McClellan DR, Svec RL, Adair C, Francis GL. Clinical features associated with metastasis and recurrence of differentiated thyroid cancer in children, adolescents and young adults. Clin Endocrinol (Oxf). 1998;49:619–28.
2. McClellan DR, Francis GL. Thyroid cancer in children, pregnant women, and patients with Graves' disease. Endocrinol Metab Clin N Am. 1996;25:27–48.
3. Fassina AS, Rupolo M, Pelizzo MR, Casara D. Thyroid cancer in children and adolescents. Tumori. 1994;80:257–62.
4. Feinmesser R, Lubin E, Segal K, Noyek A. Carcinoma of the thyroid in children – a review. J Pediatr Endocrinol Metab. 1997;10:561–8.
5. Harness JK, Thompson NW, McLeod MK, Pasieka JL, Fukuuchi A. Differentiated thyroid carcinoma in children and adolescents. World J Surg. 1992;16:547–53; discussion 553–4.
6. Maxon HR. The role of radioiodine in the treatment of childhood thyroid cancer – a dosimetric approach. In: Jacob Robbins M, editor. Treatment of thyroid cancer in childhood. Bethesda: NIDDK, National Institutes of Health; 1992. p. 109–26.
7. Samuel AM, Rajashekharrao B, Shah DH. Pulmonary metastases in children and adolescents with well-differentiated thyroid cancer. J Nucl Med. 1998;39:1531–6.
8. Samuel AM, Sharma SM. Differentiated thyroid carcinomas in children and adolescents. Cancer. 1991;67:2186–90.
9. Yeh SD, La Quaglia MP. 131I therapy for pediatric thyroid cancer. Semin Pediatr Surg. 1997;6:128–33.
10. Gorlin JB, Sallan SE. Thyroid cancer in childhood. Endocrinol Metab Clin N Am. 1990;19:649–62.
11. Hay ID, Gonzalez-Losada T, Reinalda MS, Honetschlager JA, Richards ML, Thompson GB. Long-term outcome in 215 children and adolescents with papillary thyroid cancer treated during 1940 through 2008. World J Surg. 2010;34:1192–202.
12. LaQuaglia M, Black T, Holcomb G, Sklar C, Azizkhan R, Haase G, Newman K. Differentiated thyroid cancer: clinical characteristics, treatment, and outcome in patients under 21 years of age who present with distant metastases. A report from the Surgical Discipline Committee of the Children's Cancer Group. J Pediatr Surg. 2000;35:955–9.
13. Pawelczak M, et al. Outcomes of children and adolescents with well-differentiated thyroid carcinoma and pulmonary metastasis following 131I treatment: a systematic review. Thyroid. 2010;20.
14. Shoup M, Stojadinovic A, Nissan A, Ghossein R, Freedman S, Brennan M, Shah J, Shaha A. Prognostic indicators of outcomes in patients with distant metastases from differentiated thyroid carcinoma. J Am Coll Surg. 2003;197:191–7.
15. Lo CY, Lam KY, Wan KY. Anaplastic carcinoma of the thyroid. Am J Surg. 1999;177:337–9.
16. Ozaki O, Ito K, Kobayashi K, Suzuki A, Manabe Y, Hosoda Y. Familial occurrence of differentiated, nonmedullary thyroid carcinoma. World J Surg. 1988;12:565–71.
17. Camiel MR, Mule JE, Alexander LL, Benninghoff DL. Association of thyroid carcinoma with Gardner's syndrome in siblings. N Engl J Med. 1968;278:1056–8.
18. Giannelli SM, et al. Familial adenomatous polyposis-associated cribriform morular variant of papillary thyroid carcinoma harboring a K-RAS mutation: case presentation and review of molecular mechanisms. Thyroid. 2014;24(7):1184–9.
19. Ringel MD, Hayre N, Saito J, Saunier B, Schuppert F, Burch H, Bernet V, Burman KD, Kohn LD, Saji M. Overexpression and overactivation of Akt in thyroid carcinoma. Cancer Res. 2001;61:6105–11.
20. Ngeow J, Eng C. PTEN hamartoma tumor syndrome: clinical risk assessment and management protocol. Methods. 2015;77–78:11–9.
21. Doros L, Schultz KA, Stewart DR, Bauer AJ, Williams G, Rossi CT, Carr A, Yang J, Dehner LP, Messinger Y, Hill DA. In: Pagon RA, Adam MP, Ardinger HH, Wallace SE, Amemiya A, Bean LJH, Bird TD, Fong CT, Mefford HC, Smith RJH, Stephens K, editors. GeneReviews® [Internet]. Seattle: University of Washington, Seattle; 1993–2016. 24 Apr 2014.
22. Rutter MM, Jha P, Schultz KA, Sheil A, Harris AK, Bauer AJ, Field AL, Geller J, Hill DA. DICER1 mutations and differentiated thyroid carcinoma: evidence of a direct association. J Clin Endocrinol Metab. 2016;101(1):1–5.
23. Bertherat J, Groussin L, Sandrini F, Matyakhina L, Bei T, Stergiopoulos S, Papageorgiou T, Bourdeau I, Kirschner LS, Vincent-Dejean C, et al. Molecular and functional analysis of PRKAR1A and its locus (17q22-24) in sporadic adrenocortical tumors: 17q losses, somatic mutations, and protein kinase A expression and activity. Cancer Res. 2003;63:5308–19.
24. Stratakis CA, Kirschner LS, Carney JA. Clinical and molecular features of the Carney complex: diagnostic criteria and recommendations for patient evaluation. J Clin Endocrinol Metab. 2001;86:4041–6.
25. Veiga LH, Holmberg E, Anderson H, Pottern L, Sadetzki S, Adams MJ, Sakata R, Schneider AB, Inskip P, Bhatti P, Johansson R, Neta G, Shore R, de Vathaire F, Damber L, Kleinerman R, Hawkins MM, Tucker M, Lundell M, Lubin JH. Thyroid cancer after childhood exposure to external radiation: an updated pooled analysis of 12 studies. Radiat Res. 2016;185(5):473–84.
26. Astakhova LN, Anspaugh LR, Beebe GW, Bouville A, Drozdovitch VV, Garber V, Gavrilin YI, Khrouch VT, Kuvshinnikov AV, Kuzmenkov YN, et al. Chernobyl-related thyroid cancer in children of Belarus: a case-control study. Radiat Res. 1998;150:349–56.
27. Pacini F, Vorontsova T, Demidchik EP, Molinaro E, Agate L, Romei C, Shavrova E, Cherstvoy ED, Ivashkevitch Y, Kuchinskaya E, et al. Post-Chernobyl thyroid carcinoma in Belarus children and adolescents: comparison with naturally occurring thyroid carcinoma in Italy and France. J Clin Endocrinol Metab. 1997;82:3563–9.
28. Antonelli A, Miccoli P, Derzhitski VE, Panasiuk G, Solovieva N, Baschieri L. Epidemiologic and clinical evaluation of thyroid cancer in children from the Gomel region (Belarus). World J Surg. 1996;20:867–71.
29. Nikiforov Y, Gnepp DR. Pediatric thyroid cancer after the Chernobyl disaster. Pathomorphologic study of 84 cases (1991–1992) from the Republic of Belarus. Cancer. 1994;74:748–66.
30. Becker DV, Robbins J, Beebe GW, Bouville AC, Wachholz BW. Childhood thyroid cancer following the Chernobyl accident: a status report [published erratum appears in Endocrinol Metab Clin North Am 1996 Jun;25(2):xi]. Endocrinol Metab Clin N Am. 1996;25:197–211.
31. Bongarzone I, Butti MG, Fugazzola L, Pacini F, Pinchera A, Vorontsova TV, Demidchik EP, Pierotti MA. Comparison of the breakpoint regions of ELE1 and RET genes involved in the generation of RET/PTC3 oncogene in sporadic and in radiation-associated papillary thyroid carcinomas. Genomics. 1997;42:252–9.
32. Bounacer A, Wicker R, Caillou B, Cailleux AF, Sarasin A, Schlumberger M, Suarez HG. High prevalence of activating ret

proto-oncogene rearrangements, in thyroid tumors from patients who had received external radiation. Oncogene. 1997;15:1263–73.
33. Bounacer A, Wicker R, Schlumberger M, Sarasin A, Suarez HG. Oncogenic rearrangements of the ret proto-oncogene in thyroid tumors induced after exposure to ionizing radiation. Biochimie. 1997;79:619–23.
34. Dobson C, Gupta S, Patel A, Fenton C, Dinauer C, Tuttle RM, Francis GL. Papillary thyroid carcinoma from Russian children exposed to radiation following the Chernobyl nuclear accident are more likely to contain proliferating non-lymphocytic cells. Lawson Wilkins Pediatric Endocrine Society meeting, Montreal; 2001.
35. Rabes HM, Klugbauer S. Molecular genetics of childhood papillary thyroid carcinomas after irradiation: high prevalence of RET rearrangement. Recent Results Cancer Res. 1998;154:248–64.
36. Beimfohr C, Klugbauer S, Demidchik EP, Lengfelder E, Rabes HM. NTRK1 re-arrangement in papillary thyroid carcinomas of children after the Chernobyl reactor accident. Int J Cancer. 1999;80:842–7.
37. Klugbauer S, Rabes HM. The transcription coactivator HTIF1 and a related protein are fused to the RET receptor tyrosine kinase in childhood papillary thyroid carcinomas. Oncogene. 1999;18:4388–93.
38. Rabes HM, Klugbauer S. Radiation-induced thyroid carcinomas in children: high prevalence of RET rearrangement. Verh Dtsch Ges Pathol. 1997;81:139–44.
39. Nikiforov YE, Koshoffer A, Nikiforova M, Stringer J, Fagin JA. Chromosomal breakpoint positions suggest a direct role for radiation in inducing illegitimate recombination between the ELE1 and RET genes in radiation-induced thyroid carcinomas. Oncogene. 1999;18:6330–4.
40. Nikiforov Y. Spatial positioning of RET and H4 following radiation exposure leads to tumor development. Sci World J. 2001;1:186–7.
41. Cameselle-Teijeiro J, Preto A, Soares P, Sobrinho-Simoes M. A stem cell role for thyroid solid cell nests. Hum Pathol. 2005;36:590–1.
42. Davies TF, Latif R, Minsky NC, Ma R. Clinical review: the emerging cell biology of thyroid stem cells. J Clin Endocrinol Metab. 2011;96:2692–702.
43. Derwahl M. Linking stem cells to thyroid cancer. J Clin Endocrinol Metab. 2011;96:610–3.
44. Klonisch T, Hoang-Vu C, Hombach-Klonisch S. Thyroid stem cells and cancer. Thyroid. 2009;19:1303–15.
45. Lin RY. Thyroid cancer stem cells. Nat Rev Endocrinol. 2011;7:609–16.
46. Thomas T, Nowka K, Lan L, Derwahl M. Expression of endoderm stem cell markers: evidence for the presence of adult stem cells in human thyroid glands. Thyroid. 2006;16:537–44.
47. Reis-Filho JS, Preto A, Soares P, Ricardo S, Cameselle-Teijeiro J, Sobrinho-Simoes M. p63 expression in solid cell nests of the thyroid: further evidence for a stem cell origin. Mod Pathol. 2003;16:43–8.
48. Foukakis T, Au AY, Wallin G, Geli J, Forsberg L, Clifton-Bligh R, Robinson BG, Lui WO, Zedenius J, Larsson C. The Ras effector NORE1A is suppressed in follicular thyroid carcinomas with a PAX8-PPARgamma fusion. J Clin Endocrinol Metab. 2006;91:1143–9.
49. Horie H, Yokogoshi Y, Tsuyuguchi M, Saito S. Point mutations of ras and Gs alpha subunit genes in thyroid tumors. Jpn J Cancer Res. 1995;86:737–42.
50. Nikiforov YE, Nikiforova MN, Gnepp DR, Fagin JA. Prevalence of mutations of ras and p53 in benign and malignant thyroid tumors from children exposed to radiation after the Chernobyl nuclear accident. Oncogene. 1996;13:687–93.
51. Kroll TG, Sarraf P, Pecciarini L, Chen CJ, Mueller E, Spiegelman BM, Fletcher JA. PAX8-PPARgamma1 fusion oncogene in human thyroid carcinoma [corrected] [published erratum appears in Science 2000 Sep 1;289(5484):1474]. Science. 2000;289:1357–60.
52. Saji M, Ringel MD. The PI3K-Akt-mTOR pathway in initiation and progression of thyroid tumors. Mol Cell Endocrinol. 2010;321:20–8.
53. Xing M. Genetic alterations in the phosphatidylinositol-3 kinase/Akt pathway in thyroid cancer. Thyroid. 2010;20:697–706.
54. Elisei R, Romei C, Vorontsova T, Cosci B, Veremeychik V, Kuchinskaya E, Basolo F, Demidchik EP, Miccoli P, Pinchera A, et al. RET/PTC rearrangements in thyroid nodules: studies in irradiated and not irradiated, malignant and benign thyroid lesions in children and adults. J Clin Endocrinol Metab. 2001;86:3211–6.
55. Fenton CL, Lukes Y, Nicholson D, Dinauer CA, Francis GL, Tuttle RM. The ret/PTC mutations are common in sporadic papillary thyroid carcinoma of children and young adults. J Clin Endocrinol Metab. 2000;85:1170–5.
56. Nikiforov YE, Rowland JM, Bove KE, Monforte-Munoz H, Fagin JA. Distinct pattern of ret oncogene rearrangements in morphological variants of radiation-induced and sporadic thyroid papillary carcinomas in children. Cancer Res. 1997;57:1690–4.
57. Pacini F, Elisei R, Romei C, Pinchera A. RET proto-oncogene mutations in thyroid carcinomas: clinical relevance. J Endocrinol Invest. 2000;23:328–38.
58. Soares P, Trovisco V, Rocha AS, Lima J, Castro P, Preto A, Maximo V, Botelho T, Seruca R, Sobrinho-Simões M. BRAF mutations and RET/PTC rearrangements are alternative events in the etiopathogenesis of PTC. Oncogene. 2003;22:4578–80.
59. Sugg SL, Zheng L, Rosen IB, Freeman JL, Ezzat S, Asa SL. ret/PTC-1, -2, and -3 oncogene rearrangements in human thyroid carcinomas: implications for metastatic potential? J Clin Endocrinol Metab. 1996;81:3360–5.
60. Thomas GA, Bunnell H, Cook HA, Williams ED, Nerovnya A, Cherstvoy ED, Tronko ND, Bogdanova TI, Chiappetta G, Viglietto G, et al. High prevalence of RET/PTC rearrangements in Ukrainian and Belarussian post-Chernobyl thyroid papillary carcinomas: a strong correlation between RET/PTC3 and the solid-follicular variant. J Clin Endocrinol Metab. 1999;84:4232–8.
61. Penko K, Livezey J, Fenton C, Patel A, Nicholson D, Flora M, Oakley K, Tuttle RM, Francis G. BRAF mutations are uncommon in papillary thyroid cancer of young patients. Thyroid. 2005;15:320–5.
62. Dwight T, Thoppe SR, Foukakis T, Lui WO, Wallin G, Hoog A, Frisk T, Larsson C, Zedenius J. Involvement of the PAX8/peroxisome proliferator-activated receptor gamma rearrangement in follicular thyroid tumors. J Clin Endocrinol Metab. 2003;88:4440–5.
63. Nikiforova MN, Lynch RA, Biddinger PW, Alexander EK, Dorn 2nd GW, Tallini G, Kroll TG, Nikiforov YE. RAS point mutations and PAX8-PPAR gamma rearrangement in thyroid tumors: evidence for distinct molecular pathways in thyroid follicular carcinoma. J Clin Endocrinol Metab. 2003;88:2318–26.
64. McIver B, Grebe SK, Eberhardt NL. The PAX8/PPAR gamma fusion oncogene as a potential therapeutic target in follicular thyroid carcinoma. Curr Drug Targets Immune Endocrinol Metab Disord. 2004;4:221–34.
65. Brose MS, Volpe P, Feldman M, Kumar M, Rishi I, Gerrero R, Einhorn E, Herlyn M, Minna J, Nicholson A, et al. BRAF and RAS mutations in human lung cancer and melanoma. Cancer Res. 2002;62:6997–7000.
66. Fenton C, Anderson J, Lukes Y, Dinauer CA, Tuttle RM, Francis GL. Ras mutations are uncommon in sporadic thyroid cancer in children and young adults. J Endocrinol Invest. 1999;22:781–9.
67. Hara H, Fulton N, Yashiro T, Ito K, DeGroot LJ, Kaplan EL. N-ras mutation: an independent prognostic factor for aggressiveness of papillary thyroid carcinoma. Surgery. 1994;116:1010–6.
68. Saavedra HI, Knauf JA, Shirokawa JM, Wang J, Ouyang B, Elisei R, Stambrook PJ, Fagin JA. The RAS oncogene induces genomic instability in thyroid PCCL3 cells via the MAPK pathway. Oncogene. 2000;19:3948–54.
69. Kang DY, Kim KH, Kim JM, Kim SH, Kim JY, Baik HW, Kim YS. High prevalence of RET, RAS, and ERK expression in

Hashimoto's thyroiditis and in papillary thyroid carcinoma in the Korean population. Thyroid. 2007;17:1031–8.
70. Vasko V, Ferrand M, Di Cristofaro J, Carayon P, Henry JF, de Micco C. Specific pattern of RAS oncogene mutations in follicular thyroid tumors. J Clin Endocrinol Metab. 2003;88:2745–52.
71. Marques AR, Espadinha C, Catarino AL, Moniz S, Pereira T, Sobrinho LG, Leite V. Expression of PAX8-PPAR gamma 1 rearrangements in both follicular thyroid carcinomas and adenomas. J Clin Endocrinol Metab. 2002;87:3947–52.
72. Puglisi F, Cesselli D, Damante G, Pellizzari L, Beltrami CA, Di Loreto C. Expression of Pax-8, p53 and bcl-2 in human benign and malignant thyroid diseases. Anticancer Res. 2000;20:311–6.
73. Cohen Y, Xing M, Mambo E, Guo Z, Wu G, Trink B, Beller U, Westra WH, Ladenson PW, Sidransky D. BRAF mutation in papillary thyroid carcinoma. J Natl Cancer Inst. 2003;95:625–7.
74. Nikiforova MN, Kimura ET, Gandhi M, Biddinger PW, Knauf JA, Basolo F, Zhu Z, Giannini R, Salvatore G, Fusco A, et al. BRAF mutations in thyroid tumors are restricted to papillary carcinomas and anaplastic or poorly differentiated carcinomas arising from papillary carcinomas. J Clin Endocrinol Metab. 2003;88:5399–404.
75. Xing M, Clark D, Guan H, Ji M, Dackiw A, Carson KA, Kim M, Tufaro A, Ladenson P, Zeiger M, et al. BRAF mutation testing of thyroid fine-needle aspiration biopsy specimens for preoperative risk stratification in papillary thyroid cancer. J Clin Oncol. 2009;27:2977–82.
76. Liu D, Liu Z, Condouris S, Xing M. BRAF V600E maintains proliferation, transformation, and tumorigenicity of BRAF-mutant papillary thyroid cancer cells. J Clin Endocrinol Metab. 2007;92:2264–71.
77. Mitsutake N, Knauf JA, Mitsutake S, Mesa Jr C, Zhang L, Fagin JA. Conditional BRAF V600E expression induces DNA synthesis, apoptosis, dedifferentiation, and chromosomal instability in thyroid PCCL3 cells. Cancer Res. 2005;65:2465–73.
78. Frattini M, Ferrario C, Bressan P, Balestra D, De Cecco L, Mondellini P, Bongarzone I, Collini P, Gariboldi M, Pilotti S, et al. Alternative mutations of BRAF, RET and NTRK1 are associated with similar but distinct gene expression patterns in papillary thyroid cancer. Oncogene. 2004;23:7436–40.
79. Xing M. BRAF mutation in thyroid cancer. Endocrinol Relat Cancer. 2005;12:245–62.
80. Xing M. BRAF mutation in papillary thyroid cancer: pathogenic role, molecular bases, and clinical implications. Endocr Rev. 2007;28:742–62.
81. Xing M. Prognostic utility of BRAF mutation in papillary thyroid cancer. Mol Cell Endocrinol. 2010;321:86–93.
82. Xing M, Westra WH, Tufano RP, Cohen Y, Rosenbaum E, Rhoden KJ, Carson KA, Vasko V, Larin A, Tallini G, et al. BRAF mutation predicts a poorer clinical prognosis for papillary thyroid cancer. J Clin Endocrinol Metab. 2005;90:6373–9.
83. Kebebew E, Weng J, Bauer J, Ranvier G, Clark OH, Duh QY, Shibru D, Bastian B, Griffin A. The prevalence and prognostic value of BRAF mutation in thyroid cancer. Ann Surg. 2007;246:466–70; discussion 470–1.
84. Elisei R, Ugolini C, Viola D, Lupi C, Biagini A, Giannini R, Romei C, Miccoli P, Pinchera A, Basolo F. BRAF (V600E) mutation and outcome of patients with papillary thyroid carcinoma: a 15-year median follow-up study. J Clin Endocrinol Metab. 2008;93:3943–9.
85. Riesco-Eizaguirre G, Rodriguez I, De la Vieja A, Costamagna E, Carrasco N, Nistal M, Santisteban P. The BRAF V600E oncogene induces transforming growth factor beta secretion leading to sodium iodide symporter repression and increased malignancy in thyroid cancer. Cancer Res. 2009;69:8317–25.
86. Henke LE, et al. BRAF V600E mutational status in pediatric thyroid cancer. Pediatr Blood Cancer. 2014;61(7):1168–72.
87. Givens D, et al. BRAF V600E does not predict aggressive features of pediatric papillary thyroid carcinoma. Laryngoscope. 2014;124(9):E389–93.
88. Ballester LY, et al. Integrating molecular testing in the diagnosis and management of children with thyroid lesions. Pediatr Dev Pathol. 2016;19:94–100.
89. Prasad ML, et al. NTRK fusion oncogenes in pediatric papillary thyroid carcinoma in northeast United States. Cancer. 2016;122(7):1097–107.
90. Picarsic JL, et al. Molecular characterization of sporadic pediatric thyroid carcinoma with the DNA/RNA ThyroSeq v2 next-generation sequencing assay. Pediatr Dev Pathol. 2016;19:115–22.
91. Learoyd DL, Messina M, Zedenius J, Guinea AI, Delbridge LW, Robinson BG. RET/PTC and RET tyrosine kinase expression in adult papillary thyroid carcinomas [see comments]. J Clin Endocrinol Metab. 1998;83:3631–5.
92. Martinez Ibanez V, Perez Martinez A, Costa E, Ruiz A, Queizan de la Fuente A, Benlloch C, Marques A. Differentiated thyroid carcinoma in childhood: multicenter review of the club of pediatric oncology. Cir Pediatr. 1993;6:3–6.
93. Buckwalter TL, Venkateswaran A, Lavender M, La Perle KM, Cho JY, Robinson ML, Jhiang SM. The roles of phosphotyrosines-294, -404, and -451 in RET/PTC1-induced thyroid tumor formation. Oncogene. 2002;21:8166–72.
94. Elisei R, Romei C, Soldatenko PP, Cosci B, Vorontsova T, Vivaldi A, Basolo F, Cherstvoy ED, Pinchera A, Pacini F. New breakpoints in both the H4 and RET genes create a variant of PTC-1 in a post-Chernobyl papillary thyroid carcinoma. Clin Endocrinol (Oxf). 2000;53:131–6.
95. Klugbauer S, Lengfelder E, Demidchik EP, Rabes HM. High prevalence of RET rearrangement in thyroid tumors of children from Belarus after the Chernobyl reactor accident. Oncogene. 1995;11:2459–67.
96. Klugbauer S, Lengfelder E, Demidchik EP, Rabes HM. A new form of RET rearrangement in thyroid carcinomas of children after the Chernobyl reactor accident. Oncogene. 1996;13:1099–102.
97. Pisarchik AV, Ermak G, Fomicheva V, Kartel NA, Figge J. The ret/PTC1 rearrangement is a common feature of Chernobyl-associated papillary thyroid carcinomas from Belarus. Thyroid. 1998;8:133–9.
98. Tuttle RM, Becker DV. The Chernobyl accident and its consequences: update at the millennium. Semin Nucl Med. 2000;30:133–40.
99. Basolo F, Giannini R, Monaco C, Melillo RM, Carlomagno F, Pancrazi M, Salvatore G, Chiappetta G, Pacini F, Elisei R, et al. Potent mitogenicity of the RET/PTC3 oncogene correlates with its prevalence in tall-cell variant of papillary thyroid carcinoma. Am J Pathol. 2002;160:247–54.
100. Musholt TJ, Musholt PB, Khaladj N, Schulz D, Scheumann GF, Klempnauer J. Prognostic significance of RET and NTRK1 rearrangements in sporadic papillary thyroid carcinoma. Surgery. 2000;128:984–93.
101. Adeniran AJ, Zhu Z, Gandhi M, Steward DL, Fidler JP, Giordano TJ, Biddinger PW, Nikiforov YE. Correlation between genetic alterations and microscopic features, clinical manifestations, and prognostic characteristics of thyroid papillary carcinomas. Am J Surg Pathol. 2006;30:216–22.
102. Chung KW, Chang MC, Noh DY, Oh SK, Choe KJ, Youn YK. RET oncogene expression of papillary thyroid carcinoma in Korea. Surg Today. 2004;34:485–92.
103. Jarzab B, Handkiewicz-Junak D. Differentiated thyroid cancer in children and adults: same or distinct disease? Hormones (Athens). 2007;6:200–9.
104. Stanojevic B, Dzodic R, Saenko V, Milovanovic Z, Pupic G, Zivkovic O, Markovic I, Djurisic I, Buta M, Dimitrijevic B, et al. Mutational and clinico-pathological analysis of papillary thyroid carcinoma in Serbia. Endocr J. 2011;58:381–93.
105. Liu Z, Hou P, Ji M, Guan H, Studeman K, Jensen K, Vasko V, El-Naggar AK, Xing M. Highly prevalent genetic alterations in receptor tyrosine kinases and phosphatidylinositol 3-kinase/akt and mitogen-activated protein kinase pathways in anaplastic and follicular thyroid cancers. J Clin Endocrinol Metab. 2008;93:3106–16.

106. Melillo RM, Castellone MD, Guarino V, De Falco V, Cirafici AM, Salvatore G, Caiazzo F, Basolo F, Giannini R, Kruhoffer M, et al. The RET/PTC-RAS-BRAF linear signaling cascade mediates the motile and mitogenic phenotype of thyroid cancer cells. J Clin Invest. 2005;115:1068–81.
107. Vasko VV, Saji M. Molecular mechanisms involved in differentiated thyroid cancer invasion and metastasis. Curr Opin Oncol. 2007;19:11–7.
108. Jhiang SM, Cho JY, Furminger TL, Sagartz JE, Tong Q, Capen CC, Mazzaferri EL. Thyroid carcinomas in RET/PTC transgenic mice. Recent Results Cancer Res. 1998;154:265–70.
109. Kjellman P, Learoyd DL, Messina M, Weber G, Hoog A, Wallin G, Larsson C, Robinson BG, Zedenius J. Expression of the RET proto-oncogene in papillary thyroid carcinoma and its correlation with clinical outcome. Br J Surg. 2001;88:557–63.
110. Learoyd DL, Messina M, Zedenius J, Robinson BG. Molecular genetics of thyroid tumors and surgical decision-making. World J Surg. 2000;24:923–33.
111. Suchy B, Waldmann V, Klugbauer S, Rabes HM. Absence of RAS and p53 mutations in thyroid carcinomas of children after Chernobyl in contrast to adult thyroid tumours. Br J Cancer. 1998;77:952–5.
112. Castro P, Rebocho AP, Soares RJ, Magalhaes J, Roque L, Trovisco V, Vieira de Castro I, Cardoso-de-Oliveira M, Fonseca E, Soares P, et al. PAX8-PPARgamma rearrangement is frequently detected in the follicular variant of papillary thyroid carcinoma. J Clin Endocrinol Metab. 2006;91:213–20.
113. Nikiforova MN, Biddinger PW, Caudill CM, Kroll TG, Nikiforov YE. PAX8-PPARgamma rearrangement in thyroid tumors: RT-PCR and immunohistochemical analyses. Am J Surg Pathol. 2002;26:1016–23.
114. Salehian B, Liu Z. Genetic alterations in differentiated thyroid cancers. Endocrinol Metab Immune Disord Drug Targets. 2009;9:257–68.
115. Freitas BC, Cerutti JM. Genetic markers differentiating follicular thyroid carcinoma from benign lesions. Mol Cell Endocrinol. 2010;321:77–85.
116. Eberhardt NL, Grebe SK, McIver B, Reddi HV. The role of the PAX8/PPARgamma fusion oncogene in the pathogenesis of follicular thyroid cancer. Mol Cell Endocrinol. 2010;321:50–6.
117. Aiello A, Pandini G, Frasca F, Conte E, Murabito A, Sacco A, Genua M, Vigneri R, Belfiore A. Peroxisomal proliferator-activated receptor-gamma agonists induce partial reversion of epithelial-mesenchymal transition in anaplastic thyroid cancer cells. Endocrinology. 2006;147:4463–75.
118. Hayashi N, Nakamori S, Hiraoka N, Tsujie M, Xundi X, Takano T, Amino N, Sakon M, Monden M. Antitumor effects of peroxisome proliferator activate receptor gamma ligands on anaplastic thyroid carcinoma. Int J Oncol. 2004;24:89–95.
119. Kroll TG. Molecular events in follicular thyroid tumors. Cancer Treat Res. 2004;122:85–105.
120. Martelli ML, Iuliano R, Le Pera I, Sama I, Monaco C, Cammarota S, Kroll T, Chiariotti L, Santoro M, Fusco A. Inhibitory effects of peroxisome poliferator-activated receptor gamma on thyroid carcinoma cell growth. J Clin Endocrinol Metab. 2002;87:4728–35.
121. Moretti F, Nanni S, Pontecorvi A. Molecular pathogenesis of thyroid nodules and cancer. Baillieres Best Pract Res Clin Endocrinol Metab. 2000;14:517–39.
122. Marlow LA, Reynolds LA, Cleland AS, Cooper SJ, Gumz ML, Kurakata S, Fujiwara K, Zhang Y, Sebo T, Grant C, et al. Reactivation of suppressed RhoB is a critical step for the inhibition of anaplastic thyroid cancer growth. Cancer Res. 2009;69:1536–44.
123. Shimazaki N, Togashi N, Hanai M, Isoyama T, Wada K, Fujita T, Fujiwara K, Kurakata S. Anti-tumour activity of CS-7017, a selective peroxisome proliferator-activated receptor gamma agonist of thiazolidinedione class, in human tumour xenografts and a syngeneic tumour implant model. Eur J Cancer. 2008;44:1734–43.
124. Ricarte-Filho JC, Li S, Garcia-Rendueles ME, et al. Identification of kinase fusion oncogenes in post-Chernobyl radiation-induced thyroid cancers. J Clin Invest. 2013;123:4935–44.
125. Fenton CL, Patel A, Tuttle RM, Francis GL. Autoantibodies to p53 in sera of patients with autoimmune thyroid disease. Ann Clin Lab Sci. 2000;30:179–83.
126. Battista S, Martelli ML, Fedele M, Chiappetta G, Trapasso F, De Vita G, Battaglia C, Santoro M, Viglietto G, Fagin JA, et al. A mutated p53 gene alters thyroid cell differentiation. Oncogene. 1995;11:2029–37.
127. Fagin JA, Matsuo K, Karmakar A, Chen DL, Tang SH, Koeffler HP. High prevalence of mutations of the p53 gene in poorly differentiated human thyroid carcinomas. J Clin Invest. 1993;91:179–84.
128. Moretti F, Nanni S, Farsetti A, Narducci M, Crescenzi M, Giuliacci S, Sacchi A, Pontecorvi A. Effects of exogenous p53 transduction in thyroid tumor cells with different p53 status. J Clin Endocrinol Metab. 2000;85:302–8.
129. Hsiao PJ, Tsai JH. Increased insulin-like growth factor-1 receptors in thyroid tissues of Graves' disease [published erratum appears in J Formos Med Assoc 1995 May;94(5):following 282]. J Formos Med Assoc. 1994;93:925–32.
130. Onoda N, Ohmura E, Tsushima T, Ohba Y, Emoto N, Isozaki O, Sato Y, Shizume K, Demura H. Autocrine role of insulin-like growth factor (IGF)-I in a human thyroid cancer cell line. Eur J Cancer. 1992;11:1904–9.
131. van der Laan BF, Freeman JL, Asa SL. Expression of growth factors and growth factor receptors in normal and tumorous human thyroid tissues. Thyroid. 1995;5:67–73.
132. Vella V, Sciacca L, Pandini G, Mineo R, Squatrito S, Vigneri R, Belfiore A. The IGF system in thyroid cancer: new concepts. Mol Pathol. 2001;54:121–4.
133. Yashiro T, Ohba Y, Murakami H, Obara T, Tsushima T, Fujimoto Y, Shizume K, Ito K. Expression of insulin-like growth factor receptors in primary human thyroid neoplasms. Acta Endocrinol (Copenh). 1989;121:112–20.
134. Vella V, Pandini G, Sciacca L, Mineo R, Vigneri R, Pezzino V, Belfiore A. A novel autocrine loop involving IGF-II and the insulin receptor isoform-A stimulates growth of thyroid cancer. J Clin Endocrinol Metab. 2002;87:245–54.
135. Gydee H, O'Neill JT, Patel A, Bauer AJ, Tuttle RM, Francis G. Differentiated thyroid carcinomas from children and adolescents express Insulin-lIke Growth Factor-1 (IGF-1) and the IGF-1 Receptor (IGF-1-R). Cancers with the most intense IGF-1-R expression may be more aggressive. Pediatr Res. 2004;55:1–7.
136. De Deken X, Vilain C, Van Sande J, Dumont JE, Miot F. Decrease of telomere length in thyroid adenomas without telomerase activity. J Clin Endocrinol Metab. 1998;83:4368–72.
137. Haugen BR, Nawaz S, Markham N, Hashizumi T, Shroyer AL, Werness B, Shroyer KR. Telomerase activity in benign and malignant thyroid tumors. Thyroid. 1997;7:337–42.
138. Kammori M, Takubo K, Nakamura K, Furugouri E, Endo H, Kanauchi H, Mimura Y, Kaminishi M. Telomerase activity and telomere length in benign and malignant human thyroid tissues. Cancer Lett. 2000;159:175–81.
139. Lo CY, Lam KY, Chan KT, Luk JM. Telomerase activity in thyroid malignancy. Thyroid. 1999;9:1215–20.
140. Onoda N, Ishikawa T, Yoshikawa K, Sugano S, Kato Y, Sowa M, Hirakawa-Yong Suk Chung K. Telomerase activity in thyroid tumors. Oncol Rep. 1998;5:1447–50.
141. Straight A, Patel A, Fenton C, Dinauer C, Tuttle RM, Francis G. Thyroid carcinomas that express telomerase follow a more aggressive clinical course for children and adolescents. J Endocrinol Invest. 2002;25:302–8.
142. Umbricht CB, Saji M, Westra WH, Udelsman R, Zeiger MA, Sukumar S. Telomerase activity: a marker to distinguish follicular thyroid adenoma from carcinoma. Cancer Res. 1997;57:2144–7.

143. Yashima K, Vuitch F, Gazdar AF, Fahey 3rd TJ. Telomerase activity in benign and malignant thyroid diseases. Surgery. 1997;122:1141–5; discussion 1145–6.
144. Okayasu I, Osakabe T, Fujiwara M, Fukuda H, Kato M, Oshimura M. Significant correlation of telomerase activity in thyroid papillary carcinomas with cell differentiation, proliferation and extrathyroidal extension. Jpn J Cancer Res. 1997;88:965–70.
145. Saji M, Xydas S, Westra WH, Liang CK, Clark DP, Udelsman R, Umbricht CB, Sukumar S, Zeiger MA. Human telomerase reverse transcriptase (hTERT) gene expression in thyroid neoplasms. Clin Cancer Res. 1999;5:1483–9.
146. Fenton C, Patel A, Dinauer C, Robie DK, Tuttle RM, Francis GL. The expression of vascular endothelial growth factor and the type 1 vascular endothelial growth factor receptor correlate with the size of papillary thyroid carcinoma in children and young adults. Thyroid. 2000;10:349–57.
147. Lennard CM, Patel A, Wilson J, Reinhardt B, Tuman C, Fenton C, Blair E, Francis GL, Tuttle RM. Intensity of vascular endothelial growth factor expression is associated with increased risk of recurrence and decreased disease-free survival in papillary thyroid cancer. Surgery. 2001;129:552–8.
148. Tuttle RM, Fleisher M, Francis GL, Robbins RJ. Serum vascular endothelial growth factor levels are elevated in metastatic differentiated thyroid cancer but not increased by short-term TSH stimulation. J Clin Endocrinol Metab. 2002;87:1737–42.
149. Tuttle RM, Patel A, Francis G, Davis S, Kopecky KJ, Lushnikov E, Abrosimov A, Troshin V, Tsyb A, Fenton, C. Vascular endothelial growth factor (VEGF) and Type 1 VEGF receptor (Flt-1) are highly expressed in Russian papillary thyroid carcinomas. 12th International thyroid congress, Kyoto; 2000.
150. Bauer A, Patel A, Tuttle RM, Ringel M, Francis G. Vascular endothelial growth factor monoclonal antibody inhibits growth of anaplastic thyroid cancer xenografts. Endocrine Society meeting, Denver; 2001.
151. Bauer AJ, Patel A, Terrell R, Doniparthi K, Saji M, Ringel M, Tuttle RM, Francis GL. Vascular endothelial growth factor monoclonal antibody (VEGF-MAb) inhibits growth of papillary thyroid cancer xenografts. Ann Clin Lab Sci. 2003;33:192–9.
152. Bauer AJ, Terrell R, Doniparthi NK, Patel A, Tuttle RM, Saji M, Ringel MD, Francis GL. Vascular endothelial growth factor monoclonal antibody inhibits growth of anaplastic thyroid cancer xenografts in nude mice. Thyroid. 2002;12:953–61.
153. Colin IM, Kopp P, Zbaren J, Haberli A, Grizzle WE, Jameson JL. Expression of nitric oxide synthase III in human thyroid follicular cells: evidence for increased expression in hyperthyroidism. Eur J Endocrinol. 1997;136:649–55.
154. Esteves RZ, van Sande J, Dumont JE. Nitric oxide as a signal in thyroid. Mol Cell Endocrinol. 1992;90:R1–3.
155. Kitano H, Kitanishi T, Nakanishi Y, Suzuki M, Takeuchi E, Yazawa Y, Kitajima K, Kimura H, Tooyama I. Expression of inducible nitric oxide synthase in human thyroid papillary carcinomas. Thyroid. 1999;9:113–7.
156. Millatt LJ, Jackson R, Williams BC, Whitley GS. Nitric oxide stimulates cyclic GMP in human thyrocytes. J Mol Endocrinol. 1993;10:163–9.
157. Millatt LJ, Johnstone AP, Whitley GS. Nitric oxide enhances thyroid peroxidase activity in primary human thyrocytes. Life Sci. 1998;63:L373–80.
158. Motohashi S, Kasai K, Banba N, Hattori Y, Shimoda S. Nitric oxide inhibits cell growth in cultured human thyrocytes. Life Sci. 1996;59:L227–34.
159. Kayser L, Francis D, Broholm H. Immunohistochemical localization of inducible and endothelial constitutive nitric oxide synthase in neoplastic and autoimmune thyroid disorders. APMIS. 2000;108:785–91.
160. Ramirez R, Hsu D, Patel A, Fenton C, Dinauer C, Tuttle RM, Francis GL. Over-expression of hepatocyte growth factor/scatter factor (HGF/SF) and the HGF/SF receptor (cMET) are associated with a high risk of metastasis and recurrence for children and young adults with papillary thyroid carcinoma. Clin Endocrinol (Oxf). 2000;53:635–44.
161. Arturi F, Russo D, Giuffrida D, Schlumberger M. Sodium-iodide symporter (NIS) gene expression in lymph-node metastases of papillary thyroid carcinomas. Eur J Endocrinol. 2000;143:623–7.
162. Arturi F, Russo D, Schlumberger M, du Villard JA, Caillou B, Vigneri P, Wicker R, Chiefari E, Suarez HG, Filetti S. Iodide symporter gene expression in human thyroid tumors. J Clin Endocrinol Metab. 1998;83:2493–6.
163. Caillou B, Troalen F, Baudin E, Talbot M, Filetti S, Schlumberger M, Bidart JM. Na+/I– symporter distribution in human thyroid tissues: an immunohistochemical study. J Clin Endocrinol Metab. 1998;83:4102–6.
164. Lazar V, Bidart JM, Caillou B, Mahe C, Lacroix L, Filetti S, Schlumberger M. Expression of the Na+/I– symporter gene in human thyroid tumors: a comparison study with other thyroid-specific genes. J Clin Endocrinol Metab. 1999;84:3228–34.
165. Patel A, Jhiang S, Dogra S, Terrell R, Powers PA, Fenton C, Dinauer CA, Tuttle RM, Francis GL. Differentiated thyroid carcinoma that express sodium-iodide symporter have a lower risk of recurrence for children and adolescents. Pediatr Res. 2002;52:737–44.
166. Smith JA, Fan CY, Zou C, Bodenner D, Kokoska MS. Methylation status of genes in papillary thyroid carcinoma. Arch Otolaryngol Head Neck Surg. 2007;133:1006–11.
167. Ringel MD, Anderson J, Souza SL, Burch HB, Tambascia M, Shriver CD, Tuttle RM. Expression of the sodium iodide symporter and thyroglobulin genes are reduced in papillary thyroid cancer. Mod Pathol. 2001;14:289–96.
168. Liu D, Hu S, Hou P, Jiang D, Condouris S, Xing M. Suppression of BRAF/MEK/MAP kinase pathway restores expression of iodide-metabolizing genes in thyroid cells expressing the V600E BRAF mutant. Clin Cancer Res. 2007;13:1341–9.
169. Kondo T, Asa SL, Ezzat S. Epigenetic dysregulation in thyroid neoplasia. Endocrinol Metab Clin N Am. 2008;37:389–400, ix.
170. Xing M. Gene methylation in thyroid tumorigenesis. Endocrinology. 2007;148:948–53.
171. Zuo H, Gandhi M, Edreira MM, Hochbaum D, Nimgaonkar VL, Zhang P, Dipaola J, Evdokimova V, Altschuler DL, Nikiforov YE. Downregulation of Rap1GAP through epigenetic silencing and loss of heterozygosity promotes invasion and progression of thyroid tumors. Cancer Res. 2010;70:1389–97.
172. Schagdarsurengin U, Richter AM, Wohler C, Dammann RH. Frequent epigenetic inactivation of RASSF10 in thyroid cancer. Epigenetics. 2009;4:571–6.
173. Guan H, Ji M, Hou P, Liu Z, Wang C, Shan Z, Teng W, Xing M. Hypermethylation of the DNA mismatch repair gene hMLH1 and its association with lymph node metastasis and T1799A BRAF mutation in patients with papillary thyroid cancer. Cancer. 2008;113:247–55.
174. Kondo T, Nakazawa T, Ma D, Niu D, Mochizuki K, Kawasaki T, Nakamura N, Yamane T, Kobayashi M, Katoh R. Epigenetic silencing of TTF-1/NKX2-1 through DNA hypermethylation and histone H3 modulation in thyroid carcinomas. Lab Invest. 2009;89:791–9.
175. Hu S, Liu D, Tufano RP, Carson KA, Rosenbaum E, Cohen Y, Holt EH, Kiseljak-Vassiliades K, Rhoden KJ, Tolaney S, et al. Association of aberrant methylation of tumor suppressor genes with tumor aggressiveness and BRAF mutation in papillary thyroid cancer. Int J Cancer. 2006;119:2322–9.
176. Pillai RS, Bhattacharyya SN, Filipowicz W. Repression of protein synthesis by miRNAs: how many mechanisms? Trends Cell Biol. 2007;17:118–26.

177. Calin GA, Sevignani C, Dumitru CD, Hyslop T, Noch E, Yendamuri S, Shimizu M, Rattan S, Bullrich F, Negrini M, et al. Human microRNA genes are frequently located at fragile sites and genomic regions involved in cancers. Proc Natl Acad Sci U S A. 2004;101:2999–3004.
178. Lu J, Getz G, Miska EA, Alvarez-Saavedra E, Lamb J, Peck D, Sweet-Cordero A, Ebert BL, Mak RH, Ferrando AA, et al. MicroRNA expression profiles classify human cancers. Nature. 2005;435:834–8.
179. Nikiforova MN, Chiosea SI, Nikiforov YE. MicroRNA expression profiles in thyroid tumors. Endocr Pathol. 2009;20:85–91.
180. He H, Jazdzewski K, Li W, Liyanarachchi S, Nagy R, Volinia S, Calin GA, Liu CG, Franssila K, Suster S, et al. The role of microRNA genes in papillary thyroid carcinoma. Proc Natl Acad Sci U S A. 2005;102:19075–80.
181. Pallante P, Visone R, Ferracin M, Ferraro A, Berlingieri MT, Troncone G, Chiappetta G, Liu CG, Santoro M, Negrini M, et al. MicroRNA deregulation in human thyroid papillary carcinomas. Endocrinol Relat Cancer. 2006;13:497–508.
182. Tetzlaff MT, Liu A, Xu X, Master SR, Baldwin DA, Tobias JW, Livolsi VA, Baloch ZW. Differential expression of miRNAs in papillary thyroid carcinoma compared to multinodular goiter using formalin fixed paraffin embedded tissues. Endocr Pathol. 2007;18:163–73.
183. Lassalle S, Hofman V, Ilie M, Bonnetaud C, Puissegur MP, Brest P, Loubatier C, Guevara N, Bordone O, Cardinaud B, et al. Can the microRNA signature distinguish between thyroid tumors of uncertain malignant potential (TT-UMP) and other well-differentiated tumors (WDT) of the thyroid gland? Endocrinol Relat Cancer. 2011;18:579–94.
184. Chen YT, Kitabayashi N, Zhou XK, Fahey 3rd TJ, Scognamiglio T. MicroRNA analysis as a potential diagnostic tool for papillary thyroid carcinoma. Mod Pathol. 2008;21:1139–46.
185. Chou CK, Chen RF, Chou FF, Chang HW, Chen YJ, Lee YF, Yang KD, Cheng JT, Huang CC, Liu RT. miR-146b is highly expressed in adult papillary thyroid carcinomas with high risk features including extrathyroidal invasion and the BRAF (V600E) mutation. Thyroid. 2010;20:489–94.
186. Yip L, Kelly L, Shuai Y, Armstrong MJ, Nikiforov YE, Carty SE, Nikiforova MN. MicroRNA signature distinguishes the degree of aggressiveness of papillary thyroid carcinoma. Ann Surg Oncol. 2011;18:2035–41.
187. Visone R, Pallante P, Vecchione A, Cirombella R, Ferracin M, Ferraro A, Volinia S, Coluzzi S, Leone V, Borbone E, et al. Specific microRNAs are downregulated in human thyroid anaplastic carcinomas. Oncogene. 2007;26:7590–5.
188. Takakura S, Mitsutake N, Nakashima M, Namba H, Saenko VA, Rogounovitch TI, Nakazawa Y, Hayashi T, Ohtsuru A, Yamashita S. Oncogenic role of miR-17-92 cluster in anaplastic thyroid cancer cells. Cancer Sci. 2008;99:1147–54.
189. Marini F, Luzi E, Brandi ML. MicroRNA role in thyroid cancer development. J Thyroid Res. 2011;2011:407123.
190. Nikiforova MN, Tseng GC, Steward D, Diorio D, Nikiforov YE. MicroRNA expression profiling of thyroid tumors: biological significance and diagnostic utility. J Clin Endocrinol Metab. 2008;93:1600–8.
191. Griffith OL, Melck A, Jones SJ, Wiseman SM. Meta-analysis and meta-review of thyroid cancer gene expression profiling studies identifies important diagnostic biomarkers. J Clin Oncol. 2006;24:5043–51.
192. Eszlinger M, Krohn K, Kukulska A, Jarzab B, Paschke R. Perspectives and limitations of microarray-based gene expression profiling of thyroid tumors. Endocr Rev. 2007;28:322–38.
193. Eszlinger M, Paschke R. Molecular fine-needle aspiration biopsy diagnosis of thyroid nodules by tumor specific mutations and gene expression patterns. Mol Cell Endocrinol. 2010;322:29–37.
194. Handkiewicz-Junak D, Czarniecka A, Jarzab B. Molecular prognostic markers in papillary and follicular thyroid cancer: current status and future directions. Mol Cell Endocrinol. 2010;322:8–28.
195. Oler G, Camacho CP, Hojaij FC, Michaluart Jr P, Riggins GJ, Cerutti JM. Gene expression profiling of papillary thyroid carcinoma identifies transcripts correlated with BRAF mutational status and lymph node metastasis. Clin Cancer Res. 2008;14:4735–42.
196. Cancer Genome Atlas Research Network. Integrated genomic characterization of papillary thyroid carcinoma. Cell. 2014;159(3):676–90.

The Role of Genetics in the Development of Familial Nonmedullary Thyroid Cancer

5

Andreas Moraitis and Constantine A. Stratakis

Introduction

In 2010, there were an estimated 44,670 new cases of thyroid cancer and approximately 1,690 deaths related to thyroid cancer [1]. There is no doubt that the incidence of thyroid cancer has been increasing steadily over the past three decades [2]. Increased medical surveillance and more sensitive diagnostic tests are thought to account for some of the increased incidence because most of it has been in subclinical, small (<2 cm), papillary thyroid cancer [2–5]. Most patients have localized or regional disease, which have 5-year survival rates of 100 % and 97 %, respectively. Patients with distant metastases have a 5-year survival rate of only 56 %. The prognosis relates not only to the extent of the disease but also to the type of thyroid cancer. The 10-year survival rates for papillary, follicular, Hurthle cell, medullary, and anaplastic thyroid carcinoma are 93 %, 85 %, 76 %, 75 %, and 14 %, respectively [6]. The survival rates for patients with sporadic medullary thyroid carcinoma (MTC) are lower compared to patients with well-differentiated thyroid cancers (papillary and follicular cancer). Patients with familial medullary thyroid cancer (FMTC) may have higher or lower survival rates than those who have sporadic MTC, depending on the type of familial disease. Finally, patients who have familial nonmedullary thyroid cancer (FNMTC) may have more aggressive tumors with increased rates of extra thyroidal extension, lymph node metastases, and larger tumors in younger patients [7]. The aggressiveness of FNMTC compared with its sporadic counterparts has been reported by a number of studies. In addition, a recent study has found FNMTC to display features of clinical anticipation where individuals in the second generation appear to have more advanced disease at presentation with an earlier age of onset [8]. This variability underscores the importance of diagnosing a familial thyroid cancer accurately. Establishing the diagnosis of a familial thyroid cancer may provide the opportunity for early identification and possible prevention of thyroid cancer in family members. Understanding of the syndromes associated with FNMTC allows the clinician to evaluate and treat the patient for coexisting medical conditions. The relative frequency of different forms of thyroid cancer (sporadic and familial) is shown in Fig. 5.1. Susceptibility genes for FNMTC with as high a frequency as the *RET* gene mutations for hereditary medullary thyroid cancer (MTC) have not yet been identified. Such genes could be of great value to screen at-risk individuals, thereby making early diagnosis and prophylactic thyroidectomy possible as well as selection of appropriate adjuvant therapy that can lead to better outcomes. In familial cases, recommendations vary but include offering total thyroidectomy with prophylactic central node dissection as the first operation, followed by postoperative radioiodine ablation and thyroid hormone suppression regardless of the primary tumor size [8–11]. Prophylactic thyroidectomy in FNMTC remains controversial [11] because there are no reliable molecular screening tools. Identification of molecular markers would permit screening, stratification of management, and potentially treatment of patients at high risk before disease development.

Recognition of FNMTC and Syndromic versus Nonsyndromic FNMTC

Robinson and Orr were the first to present cases of papillary thyroid cancer (PTC) in a pair of monozygotic twins in Kansas [12]. Since then several epidemiological and genetic studies have provided strong evidence for the existence of a genetic component for FNMTC [13–16]. Only 5 % of all

A. Moraitis, MD • C.A. Stratakis, MD, D(med)Sci (✉)
Section on Endocrinology and Genetics, Program in Developmental Endocrinology and Genetics, *Eunice Kennedy Shriver* National Institute of Child Health and Human Development, National Institutes of Health, 10 Center Drive, Building 10-CRC Room 1-3330 MSC 1103, Bethesda, MD 20892, USA
e-mail: stratakc@mail.nih.gov

L. Wartofsky, D. Van Nostrand (eds.), *Thyroid Cancer*, DOI 10.1007/978-1-4939-3314-3_5

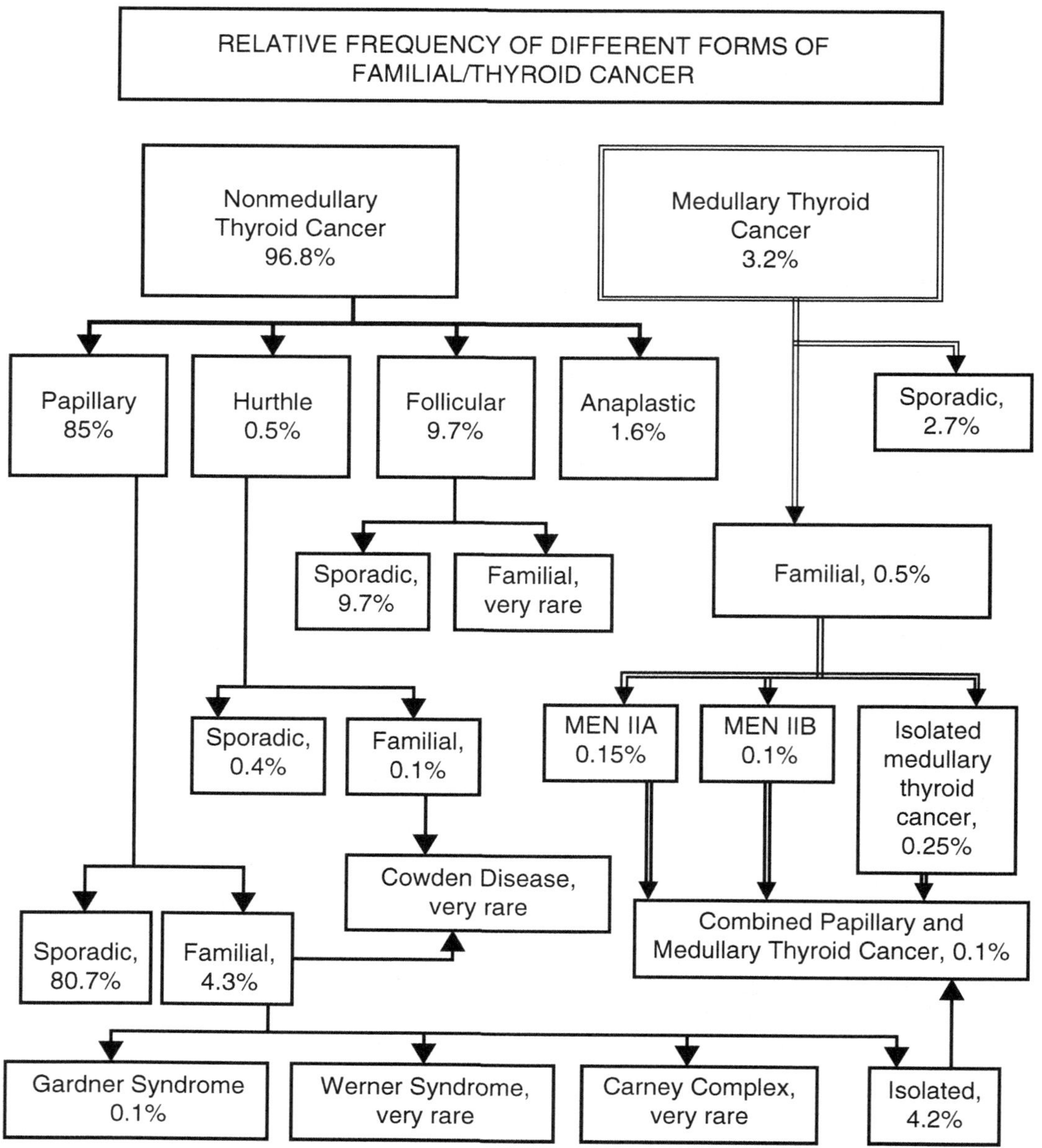

Fig. 5.1 Relative frequency of the different forms of familial/thyroid cancer (Data adapted from the National Cancer Database; Surveillance, Epidemiology, and End Results registry of the National Cancer Institute; and the National Data Bank at the University of California, San Francisco, CA)

nonmedullary thyroid cancers are thought to be of familial origin [9, 15–24]. FNMTC is defined by the presence of well-differentiated thyroid cancer in two or more first-degree relatives. In a retrospective analysis [25] of all the reported cases of differentiated non medullary thyroid cancer in the English literature, Charkes estimates that the disease may be sporadic in 69 % of the families with two affected members, as opposed to 1–4 % in those with three or more affected members. FNMTCs are less aggressive than medullary thyroid cancers (MTCs) but have been reported to be more aggressive than their sporadic counterparts [26]. FNMTC is most often multifocal and has higher rates of recurrence [10]. Those who have more than two direct relatives with FNMTC have been shown to have a decreased survival compared to those who have one or two affected direct relatives [10, 27]. Familial follicular thyroid cancer is categorized into two groups (Table 5.1). The first group accounts for a minority of cases and is called syndromic FNMTC. This group is associated with multiple neoplasia syndromes such as familial adenomatous polyposis and Cowden's syndrome. The second group, nonsyndromic FNMTC, is characterized by familial cases of thyroid cancer without any other neopla-

Table 5.1 Classification of familial follicular cell thyroid cancer (nonmedullary thyroid carcinoma)

Syndromic or familial cancer syndrome with a preponderance of nonthyroidal tumors
1. PTEN hamartoma tumor syndrome (Cowden's syndrome)
2. APC-associated polyposis conditions
3. Carney complex
4. Werner's syndrome
5. Pendred syndrome
6. McCune-Albright syndrome
7. Peutz-Jeghers syndrome
8. Ataxia-telangiectasia syndrome
Nonsyndromic or familial tumor syndrome with a preponderance of follicular cell-derived thyroid tumors
1. Familial papillary thyroid carcinoma
2. Familial multinodular goiter
3. Familial nonmedullary thyroid carcinoma type 1
4. Familial PTC associated with renal papillary neoplasia

sias or in the context of a recognized syndrome. While the genetic loci for syndromic FNMTC have been identified and well documented, the genetics of nonsyndromic FNMTC remain ambiguous.

Syndromic FNMTC

Cowden's Syndrome and the PTEN Hamartoma Tumor Syndromes

The PTEN hamartoma tumor syndromes (PHTS) include disorders of dysfunctional cell growth associated with inherited mutations of the PTEN tumor suppressor gene, found at 10q23.3 [28, 29]. The PHTS syndrome includes Cowden's syndrome (CS), Bannayan-Riley-Ruvalcaba syndrome (BRRS), Proteus syndrome (PS), and Proteus-like syndrome (PLS) [30]. Patients with CS have an increased risk of developing breast, thyroid, and endometrial cancers, benign neoplasias of the same organs, and characteristic mucocutaneous manifestations [31]. BRRS presents with lipomas, macrocephaly, hemangiomas, and pigmented macules of the glans penis [32]. PS and PLS are complex disorders characterized by subcutaneous tumors, hemihypertrophy, and various cutaneous, bone, and vascular anomalies.

PTEN belongs to a subclass of phosphatases called dual-specificity phosphatases that remove phosphate groups from tyrosine as well as serine and threonine. PTEN is a major phosphatase for phosphoinositide-3, 4, 5-triphosphate and thus downregulates the PI3K/Akt pathway. In vitro and human immunohistochemical data suggest that PTEN traffics in and out of the nucleus [33–35]. When PTEN is in the nucleus, it predominantly signals down the protein phosphatase and MAPK pathway to elicit cell cycle arrest [34]. When in the cytoplasm its lipid phosphatase predominantly signals down the AKT pathway to cause apoptosis. A nuclear function of PTEN is to stabilize the genome [36]. Shen et al. [36] found that PTEN is localized in the centromeres and it is physically associated with CENP-C, an integral component of the kinetochore. C-terminal PTEN mutants disrupt the association of PTEN with centromeres and cause centromeric instability. PTEN null cells exhibit spontaneous DNA double-strand breaks.

CS is an autosomal dominant disorder characterized by multiple hamartomas, which can originate from any of the three germ cell layers. CS exhibits variable expressivity, which makes the diagnosis of CS and the accurate measurement of its incidence a challenge. Before the identification of the responsible gene, the incidence of CS was thought to be 1/1,000,000 [28]. However, after the identification of PTEN as the gene for CS, a molecular-based study revealed the incidence to be >1/200,000 [37]. Consensus diagnostic criteria for CS have been developed [38] and are updated each year by the National Comprehensive Cancer Network [39]. Clinical criteria have been divided into three categories: pathognomonic, major, and minor (Table 5.2).

An operational diagnosis of CS is made if an individual meets any of the following criteria:

- Pathognomonic mucocutaneous lesions combined with one of the following:
  1. Six or more facial papules, of which three or more must be trichilemmoma
  2. Cutaneous facial papules and oral mucosal papillomatosis
  3. Oral mucosal papillomatosis and acral keratoses
  4. Six or more palmoplantar keratoses
- Two or more major criteria
- One major and three or more minor criteria
- Four or more minor criteria

In a family in which one individual meets the diagnostic criteria for CS listed above, other relatives are considered to have the diagnosis of CS if they meet any one of the following criteria:

- The pathognomonic criteria
- Any one major criterion with or without minor criteria
- Two minor criteria
- History of Bannayan-Riley-Ruvalcaba syndrome

More than 90 % of individuals affected with CS are believed to manifest a phenotype by the age of 20 years [28, 38]. By the end of the third decade of life, 99 % of affected individuals are believed to have developed at least the mucocutaneous signs of the syndrome, although any of the other clinical features could also be present. The lifetime

Table 5.2 Diagnostic criteria for Cowden's syndrome, NCCN 2010

Pathognomonic criteria
1. Adult Lhermitte-Duclos disease (LDD), defined as the presence of a cerebellar dysplastic gangliocytoma
2. Mucocutaneous lesions
Trichilemmomas (facial)
Acral keratoses
Papillomatous lesions
Mucosal lesions
3. Autism spectrum disorder and macrocephaly
Major criteria
1. Breast cancer
2. Epithelial thyroid cancer (nonmedullary), especially follicular thyroid cancer
3. Macrocephaly (occipital frontal circumference ≥97th percentile
4. Endometrial carcinoma
5. Mucocutaneous lesions
One biopsy-proven trichilemmoma
Multiple palmoplantar keratoses
Multifocal cutaneous facial papules
Macular pigmentation of glans penis
6. Multiple GI hamartomas or ganglioneuromas
Minor criteria
1. Other thyroid lesions (e.g., adenoma, multinodular goiter)
2. Intellectual disability
3. Hamartomatous intestinal polyps
4. Fibrocystic disease of the breast
5. Lipomas
6. Fibromas
7. Genitourinary tumors (especially renal cell carcinoma)
8. Genitourinary malformations
9. Uterine fibroids
10. Autism spectrum disorder

risk [40] of epithelial thyroid cancer can be as high as 10 % in males and females with CS while the general population risk is less than 1 %. Thyroid cancer is the second most common cancer in patients with CS. It is unclear if the age at onset is truly earlier than that of the general population. Histologically, CS-associated thyroid cancer is predominantly follicular carcinoma, although papillary histology has also been rarely reported [40–42]. Medullary thyroid carcinoma is not a true component of CS. However, there has been one case report in the literature of thyroid medullary carcinoma in a teenager with CS [43]. CS has been reported in children as young as 11 years of age [44]. Benign thyroid lesions are the next most common findings in CS, occurring in as many as 75 % of all patients with CS [41, 45]. These lesions include thyroid adenomas, hamartomas, and multinodular goiter. Hashimoto thyroiditis also is seen in CS patients of non-Asian descent. Functional thyroid disorders (i.e., hyper- or hypothyroidism) in the absence of adenomas are not a feature of CS.

PTEN is mutations cause PTEN hamartoma tumor syndrome and definitive diagnosis of CS can be made by identification of *PTEN* mutation. Early studies [46, 47] suggested that up to 85 % of individuals who meet the diagnostic criteria for CS have a detectable *PTEN* mutation. More recently it was found that only 25 % of patients who meet the strict diagnostic criteria for CS have a pathogenic *PTEN* mutation, including large deletions [48]. The discrepancy between the early studies and the more recent study of Tan et al. [48] is likely explained by the early studies analyzing CS that segregated in families and individuals with the most obvious phenotypes. Tan et al. [46] have developed a scoring system for the calculation of point pretest probability of *PTEN* mutation in patients who meet relaxed International Cowden Consortium operational criteria for CS (Table 5.2) (pathognomonic criteria or at least two criteria, either major or minor). At a threshold score of 10 (corresponding to a point pretest probability of approximately 3 %), sensitivity for the diagnosis is 90 %. The authors recommend a threshold Cowden's calculation score of 10 and above for referral to medical genetics for specialist evaluation, this permitting a sensitivity of at least 90 %.

PTEN is a nine-exon tumor suppression molecule that encodes for a 403-amino acid protein. CS was mapped to the 10q22-23 locus in 1996 by Nelen et al. [28] and mutations were first reported in individuals with CS in 1997 by the same group. Germline coding-sequence mutations in *PTEN* are generally reported to be found in 80 % of patients with CS. Approximately two-thirds of these mutations were found in exons 5, 7, and 8 (Table 5.3). Approximately 40 % of all CS germline mutations are located in exon 5, although exon 5 represents only the 20 % of the coding sequence. Genotype-phenotype analysis revealed an association between the presence of germline mutations and malignant breast disease [41].

The genetic testing methods for *PTEN* mutations include sequence analysis, deletion/duplication analysis, and promoter analysis [30]. Missense mutations detected by sequence analysis are found in 25 % of individuals who meet the strict criteria for CS [48]. Examples of mutations detected by sequence analysis may include small intragenic deletions/insertions and missense, nonsense, and splice site mutations. Southern blotting, real-time PCR, MLPA, and other methods of detecting gene copy numbers can each be used to detect large PTEN deletions and rearrangements that are not detectable by PCR-based sequence analysis. Direct sequencing of the promoter region detects mutations that alter the function of the gene in approximately 10 % of those individuals with CS who do not have an identifiable mutation in the *PTEN* coding region [46].

The lack of detectable germline *PTEN* mutations in subsets of patients with CS suggests that additional genetics and epigenetic factors act as phenotypic modifiers in

Table 5.3 Cowden's syndrome management

Women
Education and teaching of breast self-examination (BSE) and regular monthly BSE from age 18 years
Biannual clinical breast examination starting at age 25 years or 5–10 years before the earliest known breast cancer in the family
Annual mammography and breast MRI screening starting at age 30–35 years of 5 years before the earliest known breast cancer in the family (whichever is earlier)
For endometrial cancer screening, participation in a clinical trial is recommended to determine the effectiveness of screening modalities
Risk-reducing mastectomy is an option but it should be discussed on a case by case basis and patients should be counseled regarding degree of protection, extent of cancer risk, and the option of reconstruction
Men and women
Full physical examination with particular attention to the breast and thyroid examination on an annual basis starting at the age of 18 years or 5 years before the youngest age of diagnosis of a component cancer in the family (whoever is earlier)
Thyroid ultrasound scan annually from the age 18 years
Education regarding the signs and symptoms of cancer
Consider annual dermatological examination
Risk to relatives
Advise about possible inherited cancer risk to relatives and recommend referral to geneticist for genetic counseling and consideration of genetic testing for at-risk relatives

Adapted from NCCN guidelines 2010

CS. Pezzolesi et al. [49] have recently suggested that microRNAs, a novel class of negative gene regulators that regulate the expression of several tumor suppressors and oncogenes and contribute to carcinogenesis, may modulate PTEN protein levels. They identified two modifiers miR-19a and miR-21 which are PTEN-targeting miRNAs. The differential expression of these modifiers modulates the PTEN protein levels and the CS phenotypes, irrespective of the patients' mutation status, thus offering an explanation for the lack of correlation of between genotype and phenotype in CS.

Ying et al. [50] showed that a subset of CS who do not have mutations in *PTEN* but have alterations in succinate dehydrogenase complex subunit B (SDHB) or D (SDHD). Mutations in these genes are known to cause familial pheochromocytoma/paragangliomas syndrome. The individuals with *SDHB/SDHD* mutations were shown to have a slightly different cancer profile from the classical CS patients, with an overrepresentation of papillary and papillary renal tumors. The alterations in *SDHB* and *SDHD* described in CS patients, however, have not been formally shown to be causative of familial pheochromocytoma/paraganglioma syndrome.

The management of Cowden's syndrome is summarized in Table 5.3. The key to managing the risks of cancer in CS patients is early identification and diagnoses of CS. Clinicians need to be educated and be vigilant for the signs of CS: obtaining an accurate three-generation family history is important, including both paternal and maternal family histories of cancer. Clinical examination of the thyroid gland, thyroid function tests, as well as thyroid ultrasound scan with fine-needle aspiration or biopsy for suspicious lesions is recommended yearly from age 18 years. The identification of a PTEN mutation is confirmatory for the diagnosis of Cowden's syndrome.

Because CS is underdiagnosed, the actual proportion of simplex cases (defined as individuals with no obvious family history) and familial cases (defined as two or more related affected individuals) cannot be determined. From the literature and the experience of both major CS centers in the USA, the majority of individuals with CS have no obvious family history. As a broad estimate, perhaps 10–50 % of individuals with CS have an affected parent [51]. Although some individuals diagnosed with CS have an affected parent, the family history may appear to be negative because of failure to recognize the disorder in family members, early death of the parent before the onset of symptoms, or late onset of the disease in the affected parent. If a *PTEN* mutation is identified in the proband, the parents should be offered molecular genetic testing to determine if one of them has previously unidentified CS. If no mutation is identified to the proband, both parents should undergo thorough clinical examination to help determine if either parent has signs of CS.

The risk to the siblings of the proband depends on the genetic status of the parents. If the parent of the proband has CS, the risk to siblings is 50 %. If it has been shown that neither parent has the *PTEN* mutation found in the proband, the risk to siblings is negligible, as germline mosaicism has not been reported in CS. If a mutation cannot be identified in the proband, CS can be excluded on the clinical grounds. Normal clinical examination in parents in their 30s done looking specifically for signs of CS would make the risk to the sibs of the proband minimal, since an estimated 99 % of affected individuals have signs by that age.

The risk of the offspring of a proband is 50 % and prenatal diagnosis is possible by DNA extracted from fetal cells obtained by amniocentesis usually performed at approximately 15–18 weeks' gestation or chorionic villus sampling at approximately 10–12 weeks' gestation. The disease-causing allele of an affected family member must be identified before prenatal testing can be performed. Preimplantation genetic diagnosis may be available for families in which the disease-causing mutation has been identified. The risk of other family members of the proband depends on the genetic status of the proband's parents. If a parent is affected, his or her family members are at risk. The proband's relatives who harbor the mutation are in need of ongoing surveillance. Molecular testing is appropriate for at-risk individuals younger than age 18 years, given the possible early disease presentation.

APC-Associated Polyposis Syndromes

The APC-associated polyposis conditions include the overlapping, often indistinguishable phenotypes of familial adenomatous polyposis (FAP), Gardner syndrome, Turcot syndrome, and the attenuated FAP, which has a lower colonic polyp burden and lower cancer risk.

FAP is an autosomal dominant disorder associated with a high risk of multiple intestinal and extra intestinal cancers. FAP is diagnosed clinically in an individual with one of the following:

- One hundred or more colorectal adenomatous polyps (before the age of 40 years)
- Fewer than 100 adenomatous polyps and a relative with FAP

Gardner syndrome is the association of colonic adenomatous polyposis, osteomas, and soft tissue tumors (desmoids tumors, fibromas, epidermoid cysts).

Turcot syndrome is the association of colonic adenomatous polyposis and CNS tumors, usually medulloblastoma.

Attenuated FAP is considered in an individual with one of the following: no family member with more than 100 polyps before the age 30 years and one individual with 10–99 colonic adenomatous polyps diagnosed after the age 30 years and a first-degree relative with colorectal cancer with a few adenomas or at least two individuals with 10–99 adenomas diagnosed after age 30 years.

The main limitation of those criteria is that they do not take into account APC mutation status. A significant proportion of persons with polyposis who do not have an identified APC mutation have biallelic MYH mutations and therefore should be classified as having MYH-associated polyposis (a disorder that is inherited in an autosomal recessive manner). Variable features not included in the diagnostic criteria but potentially helpful in establishing the clinical diagnosis include: gastric polyps, duodenal adenomatous polyps, osteomas, dental abnormalities (especially supernumerary teeth), congenital hypertrophy of the retinal pigment epithelium (CHRPE), soft tissue tumors, desmoid tumors, and associated cancers.

Colorectal adenomatous polyps begin to appear, on average, at age 16 years (range 7–36 years) [52]. By the age 35 years, 95 % of individuals with classic FAP have polyps. Once they appear, the polyps rapidly increase in number, and when colonic expression is fully developed, hundreds to thousands of colonic adenomatous polyps are typically observed. Without complete colectomy, colon cancer is inevitable. The average age of colon cancer diagnosis in untreated patients is 39 years (range 34–43 years) and 7 % of untreated patients with FAP develop colon cancer by age 21 years, 87 % by 45 years, and 95 % by 50 years [53]. Rare cases of asymptomatic individuals in their 50s have been reported [54], with frequently encountered inter- and intrafamilial phenotypic variability [55, 56]. Several extra colonic cancers occur with a higher incidence in individuals with FAP than in the general population [57] (Table 5.4).

Table 5.4 Extra-colonic cancer in patients with FAP

Site	Type of cancer	Lifetime risk of cancer
Small bowel: duodenum or periampulla	Carcinoma	4–12 %
Small bowel: distal to the duodenum	Carcinoma	Rare
Pancreas	Adenocarcinoma	2 %
Thyroid	Papillary thyroid cancer	1–2 %
CNS	Medulloblastoma	<1 %
Liver	Hepatoblastoma	1.6 %
Bile ducts	Adenocarcinoma	Low, but increased

Thyroid cancer in a patient with FAP was first described by Crail in 1964 [58] but the importance of this association was fully appreciated when Camiel et al. [59] reported two sisters with FAP who developed thyroid carcinoma and suggested that thyroid cancer is another manifestation of FAP. In 1987, Plail et al. [60] in a retrospective study including 998 patients with FAP found that thyroid carcinoma occurred at a higher frequency in FAP compared to the general population. Bulow et al. [61] in a large multicenter retrospective study of 3,727 patients from 62 polyposis registers identified 45 patients (1.2 %) with thyroid cancer. FAP-associated thyroid cancer had a striking predominance for females (female-to-male ratio 17/1), 16 patients (36 %) developed thyroid carcinoma at an average of 6 years (range 0–29) before diagnosis of FAP, while 29 developed thyroid carcinoma at diagnosis of FAP or at an average of 6 years (range 0–17) after diagnosis of FAP. Thirty-seven (82 %) had papillary carcinoma and three follicular carcinoma, while the histological type was unknown in five patients. In 29 patients the median size of the tumor was 2.4 cm (range 0.3–6). Carcinoma multicentricity was noted in 20 (44 %) patients, and in three (7 %) patients distant metastases were found. Thyroid cancer was the cause of death for one patient that corresponds to 9 % of all deaths in the series. Iwama et al. [62] in a retrospective study of 1,050 patients with FAP in Japan identified a similar, with Bulow's study, incidence of thyroid carcinoma. The majority of the patients were females and thyroid cancer was diagnosed earlier than intestinal and duodenal tumors. The relative risk for developing thyroid cancer was increased 25 times in females but it was still lower than the FAP European patients (100 times). In 2000, Cetta et al. [63] in a European multicenter study of FAP patients who were diagnosed with thyroid cancer genotype-phenotype correlations were studied. As with prior studies, the incidence of thyroid cancer was 1–2 % in FAP patients. All patients were females and the mean age of diagnosis of thyroid cancer was 24.9 years. All patients had typical papillary carcinoma with at least some areas containing complex and branching papillae, slightly irregular nuclei with a ground glass appearance and frequent grooving. An unusual histological pattern, the so-called cribriform pattern that has been considered typical for FAP-associated tumors, was found in six patients. Three patients had some areas of with the so-called follicular encapsulated variant of the papillary histotype. Three siblings belonging to the same kindred showed three different histological patterns. The specific germline *APC* mutation was detected in 13 of the 15 patients, a cluster of mutations in the 5 portion of exon 5 in FAP-associated thyroid cancer was found, but not a clear-cut genotype-phenotype correlation was detected. In the contrary clear-cut genotype-phenotype correlation has been established for CHRPE, desmoids [55, 64], and number of colon polyps. In the same study a total of 112 patients with FAP-associated thyroid cancer, including data from the literature, were studied. There were 11 men and 101 women. The mean age of diagnosis of thyroid cancer was 24.8 years and 28 years from the world literature and 27.65 years in the entire series of 112 patients. In one third of the cases, thyroid cancer preceded the diagnosis of FAP. Truta et al. [65] recruited 16 unrelated patients with FAP from two registries and investigated the incidence of thyroid cancer. From the two registries, 1.3 % of patients with FAP had thyroid cancer. All patients were females; the mean age of diagnosis of thyroid cancer was 33 years (range 17–55 years) and the mean age of diagnosis of FAP was 29 years. The thyroid tumors were mainly multicentric (69 %) and unilateral (63 %). Papillary thyroid carcinoma was the most common histological type and half of the cases showed the cribriform morular histological subtype. In general, the tumors had nonaggressive histological features, with 10 out of 14 tumors well circumscribed with no invasion of through the capsule. However, four patients had advanced disease, two with positive lymph nodes and two with distant metastases. The patients were followed up for a period of 15 years (range 1–37 years); none of them died of thyroid cancer. In 2007 Herraiz et al. [66] in retrospective analysis of 51 patients with FAP found a higher prevalence of papillary thyroid cancer of 12 %. All patients were females, the mean age of diagnosis of FAP was 28 years, and the mean age of diagnosis of thyroid cancer was 33 years (range 18–51 years). One third of the patients had a diagnosis of thyroid cancer before the diagnosis of FAP, and in one patient the two diagnoses were made simultaneously. Half of them came to attention after they personally noticed an enlarged nodule, while the rest were identified by screening. In all patients with thyroid cancer, a deleterious mutation in the *APC* gene was detected. Papillary thyroid carcinoma was identified in all cases, with five of the six cases being the cribriform morular variant. All of the tumors were multicentric and the thyroid glands contained between two and five tumor foci. The size of the tumors was between 9 and 15 mm and the sonographic characteristics were not highly predictive of malignancy. Also benign-appearing sub-centimeter lesions in some cases found to be malignant in histological examination. It appears that the unusual variant of PTC most often seen in FAP patients is not associated with the typical sonographic features of sporadic PTC. The authors attribute the increased prevalence of thyroid carcinomas in FAP patients in their series to the increased detection of subclinical cases with the use of screening ultrasound and also to the increased rates of thyroid cancer due to environmental factors in the USA. Also a significant risk for thyroid cancer was identified in attenuated FAP kindreds. Follow-up ultrasound examination performed after a mean of 15 months and there were no changes in either the size or the number of the nodules, suggesting that subsequent thyroid ultrasound examinations can be safely performed at intervals greater than 1 year.

A recent prospective study by Jarrar et al. [67] included 192 patients of the Jagelman Registry for hereditary colon cancer. All patients underwent thyroid ultrasound by experienced surgeons and were managed according to the current guidelines for management of thyroid nodules and thyroid cancer. A reference group of individuals with no known history of FAP who underwent the same thyroid workup was analyzed. Within both groups, the majority of patients with an abnormal thyroid ultrasound had a single nodule. As the mean age of patients increased, so did the number of the nodules detected. None of the thyroid nodules detected with thyroid ultrasound screening were palpable and their size was generally small (7±5 mm in FAP patients and 10±8 mm in the reference group). In the FAP group 73 % of the patients had nodules less than 1 cm in size, 4 % of them had FNA, and all of them had benign FNA cytology. The incidence of thyroid cancer in these series was 2.6 %. Among patients with thyroid cancer, 60 % were females; the mean age of patients with thyroid cancer was 44 years (range 35–60 years). None of the patients with thyroid cancer had a prior history of thyroid disease; all of them had extracolonic FAP manifestations at the time of diagnosis with thyroid cancer and none of them belonged to the same family. Eighty percent of the thyroid cancer cases were multifocal and only 20 % showed the typical cribriform morular histological variant. The authors concluded that prior studies likely had underestimated the incidence of thyroid cancer among FAP patients. They showed also that physical examination only, as it had previously suggested, is inadequate to detect thyroid cancer in FAP kindreds and that their findings support the routine use of thyroid ultrasound for thyroid cancer screening in FAP patients. They also found that the risk of thyroid cancer in FAP patients is the same as the risk for duodenal cancer. The younger patient in these series who was found to have a thyroid nodule was 17 years old with the majority of FAP patients diagnosed with thyroid cancer were in their second or early third decades. Finally no statistically significant difference was noted among FAP patients with normal thyroid, benign nodules, and thyroid cancer in terms of the location of the *APC* mutation. It was quite noticeable that only during an initial year of screening, FAP patients with thyroid cancer were identified at a rate that is five times greater than generally reported for a broad population. In the last few decades, the survival of FAP patients has significantly improved by prophylactic GI screening and surgery. FAP patients who are looking forward healthier and longer lives than expected before should receive routine thyroid screening ultrasound that is inexpensive and easy to perform.

The molecular genetic testing for *APC*-associated polyposis conditions can be performed by full gene sequencing, protein truncation testing, duplication/deletion analysis, and linkage analysis. Full gene sequencing of all *APC* exons and intron-exon boundaries appears to be the most accurate clinical test available to detect *APC* mutations. Most of the *APC* mutations are nonsense or frameshift mutations that cause premature truncation of the *APC* protein. The likelihood of detecting an *APC* mutation is highly dependent on the severity of colonic polyposis. Fewer than 30 % of FAP patients with attenuated phenotypes [68] are expected to have an identifiable *APC* mutation. Approximately 20 % of individuals with an apparent de novo APC mutation have somatic mosaicism [69]; thus sequencing of the *APC* gene may fail to detect disease-causing mutations because of weak mutation signals in peripheral blood lymphocytes. Protein truncation testing, which is positive in 80 % of patients with classic FAP, has largely been replaced by more sensitive full gene sequencing techniques. Southern blot analysis, multiplex ligation-dependent probe amplification, and quantitative PCR are used to detect partial and whole-gene deletions or other large rearrangements. Approximately 8–12 % of patients with an APC-associated polyposis condition and 100 or more polyps have a partial or whole *APC* deletion [70–73]. Cytogenetic analysis and/or CGH array is generally pursued only when adenomatous polyposis is accompanied with developmental delays.

Linkage analysis can be considered in families with more than one affected family member belonging to different generations when no disease-causing mutation is identified in an affected individual. The markers used for linkage analysis are highly informative and very tightly linked to the *APC* locus and can be used with greater than 98 % accuracy in more than 95 % of families with an APC-associated polyposis condition [52, 74]. Prenatal diagnosis and preimplantation genetic diagnosis for at-risk pregnancies require prior identification of the disease-causing mutation in the family.

To confirm the diagnosis of FAP in a proband who meets the clinical criteria for FAP, sequence analysis and duplication/deletion analysis of *APC* gene should be performed. If no disease-causing APC mutation is found, molecular genetics for MYH gene should be considered, especially in the FAP attenuated phenotype patients. If no alteration in the *APC* gene is identified in a family with more than one affected relative belonging to different generations, linkage analysis should be considered.

In summary, thyroid cancer in FAP patients is seen more frequently than the general population. Screening with thyroid ultrasound should be offered along with physical examination in all patients above the age 16 years; physical examination alone is not adequate for identification of suspicious lesions. Follow-up thyroid ultrasound in patients with thyroid nodules should be considered at 1-year intervals and FNA should be offered in lesions larger than 9 mm irrespective of the sonographic characteristics of the nodules. If suspicious FNA cytology is identified, total thyroidectomy should be offered due to the multicentricity of the thyroid cancer in FAP patients. Patients with attenuated FAP are at higher risk for thyroid cancer. The cribriform morular histological subtype is usually seen in FAP patients with thyroid cancer, and the identification of this histogical subtype in sporadic cases of thyroid cancer should raise the clinical suspicion of FAP and those cases should be referred for evaluation for colon polyps, though this histological type is not specific to FAP-associated thyroid cancers. Although most of the APC mutations were found in the 5 portion of exon 5 in FAP-associated thyroid cancer, no clear genotype-phenotype correlation can be established between the cribriform histotype and the presence or site of germline APC mutations.

Carney Complex

Carney complex (CNC) is a multiple neoplasia and lentiginosis syndrome inherited in an autosomal dominant manner in approximately half of the reported cases and occurring sporadically in the remaining cases. Dr. J. Aidan Carney first described CNC in 1985, as the combination of myxomas, spotty pigmentation, and endocrine overactivity [75]. CNC is a rare disease. About 500 patients have been registered by the NIH-Mayo Clinic (USA) and the Cochin center (France) [76]. Cumulative reports from these centers, plus information from the Cornell center in New York, indicate that there are about 160 index cases of CNC presently known [77–81]. The manifestations of CNC can be numerous and vary between patients. Even in the same kindred, phenotypic variability can be observed. The most recently reevaluated diagnostic criteria for CNC are listed in Tables 5.5 and 5.6 [82]. A definite diagnosis is given when two or more major manifestations are present.

Table 5.5 Criteria for diagnosis of CNC

Major criteria
1. Spotty skin pigmentation with typical distribution (lips, conjunctiva and inner or outer canthi, vaginal and penile mucosa)
2. Myxoma (cutaneous and mucosal)
3. Cardiac myxoma
4. Breast myxomatosis or fat-suppressed magnetic resonance imaging findings suggestive of this diagnosis
5. Primary pigmented nodular adrenocortical disease (PPNAD) or paradoxical positive response of urinary glucocorticosteroid excretion to dexamethasone administration during Liddle's test
6. Acromegaly as a result of growth hormone (GH)-producing adenoma
7. Large-cell calcifying Sertoli cell tumor (LCCSCT) or characteristic calcification on testicular ultrasound
8. Thyroid carcinoma or multiple, hypoechoic nodules on thyroid ultrasound in a child younger than age 18 years
9. Psammomatous melanotic schwannomas (PMS)
10. Blue nevus, epithelioid blue nevus
11. Breast ductal adenoma
12. Osteochondromyxoma
Supplementary criteria
1. Affected first-degree relative
2. Inactivating mutation of the PRKAR1A gene

Table 5.6 Findings suggestive of or possibly associated with CNC, but not diagnostic for the disease

1. Intense freckling (without darkly pigmented spots or typical distribution)
2. Blue nevus, common type (if multiple)
3. Café-au-lait spots or other "birthmarks"
4. Elevated IGF-I levels, abnormal glucose tolerance test (GTT), or paradoxical GH response to TRH (thyrotropin-releasing hormone) testing in the absence of clinical acromegaly
5. Cardiomyopathy
6. Pilonidal sinus
7. History of Cushing's syndrome, acromegaly, or sudden death in extended family
8. Multiple skin tags or other skin lesions; lipomas
9. Colonic polyps (usually in association with acromegaly)
10. Hyperprolactinemia (usually mild and almost always combined with clinical or subclinical acromegaly)
11. Single, benign thyroid nodule in a child younger than age 18 years; multiple thyroid nodules in an individual older than age 18 years (detected on ultrasound examination)
12. Family history of carcinoma, in particular of the thyroid, colon, pancreas, and ovary; other multiple benign or malignant tumors

The first description of CNC included 40 patients [74]; among them 10 were familial cases, leading to the hypothesis of a genetic origin, at least in a subset of patients. CNC seems to be a genetically heterogeneous disease and linkage analysis has shown that at least two loci are involved: 2p16 and 17q22-24 [83, 84]. The CNC1 gene, located on 17q22-24, has been identified as the regulatory subunit (R1A) of the protein kinase A (PRKAR1A) [85, 86]. PRKAR1A) is a key component of the cAMP signaling pathway that has been implicated in endocrine tumorigenesis. Heterozygous inactivating mutations of *PRKAR1A* have been detected in about 45–65 % of CNC families. In CNC patients with Cushing's syndrome, the frequency of *PRKAR1A* mutations is about 80 %, suggesting that families with PPNAD are more likely to carry a 17q22-24 defect [79]. Interestingly, patients with isolated PPNAD and no familial history of CNC may also carry a germline de novo mutation in PRKAR1A [80]. In the tumors of CNC loss of heterozygosity (LOH) at 17q22-24 may be observed, suggesting that PRKAR1A is a tumor suppressor gene. Somatic mutation of *PRKAR1A* in a patient with PPNAD already carrying a germline mutation may lead to inactivation of the wild-type allele. However, inactivation of the remaining wild-type allele by genetic alteration does not appear to be a constant step in PPNAD and CNC tumor development. In a mouse transgenic model with heterozygous inactivation of PRKAR1A), tumors may develop without allelic loss.

CNC is associated with an increased incidence of thyroid abnormalities. Results of a review of 51 CNC patients [83] showed that 10 % of the patients had thyroid lesions including one carcinoma. Papillary and follicular thyroid carcinomas have also been described with increased frequency in patients with CNC [87–89], leading to the suggestion that thyroid carcinomas in these patients develop in situ from precursor benign lesions in a way similar to the hamartoma/adenoma/carcinoma sequence described elsewhere. Stratakis et al. [83] in a retrospective analysis of 53 CNC patients found increased incidence of thyroid lesions: all 53 patients underwent physical examination and ultrasonography of the thyroid at least annually. If a lesion was present, biannual evaluation was undertaken. Thyroid function tests were determined during each of the follow-up visits over a period of 1.5–2 years. Six patients with thyroid pathology were identified (11.3 %), three of these patients were available for further investigation, and among their relatives six were affected with Carney complex and had thyroid gland investigation. The first patient at the age of 30 years had three hypoechoic thyroid nodules, all measuring less than one centimeter in their biggest diameter; the dominant nodule was biopsied and revealed findings suggestive of follicular variant of PTC. She underwent total thyroidectomy where multiple foci of PTC throughout both lobes were identified, invading the adjacent lymph nodes. This patient received radioiodine treatment and she had been free of disease for 8 years postoperatively. The second patient presented at the age of 28 years with thyroid enlargement; ultrasonography revealed two small hypoechoic lesions one in each lobe. The study was repeated 1 year later and multiple nodules were identified; the dominant nodule (less than 1 cm) was biopsied and the results were suggestive of a follicular adenoma.

Because of continued growth 6 months later, the lesion was re-biopsied and the findings this time were consistent with follicular thyroid carcinoma. The patient underwent total thyroidectomy, which confirmed the diagnosis of FTC with vascular invasion. She received radioiodine treatment and she had remained disease-free for 5 years postoperatively. The third patient at the age of 31 years underwent right hemithyroidectomy for a multinodular enlargement of the thyroid gland that revealed a benign follicular adenoma. At 1-year follow-up, physical examination of the left thyroid lobe was normal but ultrasonography showed two new nodules measuring approximately 5 mm each.

In addition to the three cases mentioned above, 11 more patients were available for prospective evaluation. All patients were clinically and biochemically euthyroid and thyroid autoantibodies were not identified. Among the 11 patients, only 1 (9 %) had a single right-sided thyroid nodule on physical examination. Seven patients were identified with thyroid lesions; overall 21 thyroid lesions identified, the sonographic characteristics of which included well-defined hypoechoic areas measuring from 6.3 to 15 mm with regular borders. Eighty five percent of them had internal echoes suggestive of a solid nodule and the rest appeared cystic. The sonographic characteristics and the thyroid function tests were similar in the familial and the sporadic cases of CNC. Two of the seven patient underwent FNA biopsy (the first patient found to have cytopathology findings consistent with a benign follicular adenoma and the second patient found to have FNA cytopathology findings consistent with Hurthle cell adenoma with atypical follicular cells) underwent hemithyroidectomy that confirmed a benign pathology.

The above study showed that despite clinical and biochemical euthyroidism, ultrasonography revealed thyroid gland lesions in 66 % of the screened relatives affected with the complex and in 60 % of the patients with the sporadic form of the complex who had no previous records of thyroid disease. The prevalence of thyroid nodules was significantly higher compared to the general population especially in pediatric patients. The thyroid pathology was often multifocal and bilateral and was inherited in a manner consistent with autosomal dominant transmission. Among 53 patients with the complex, 2 were identified with thyroid cancer (3.8 %, that is significantly higher compared to the general population); both patients presented at a relatively young age with invasive disease. From previous reports a patient with the complex presented with extensive PTC at the age of 19 years [88] and another underwent thyroidectomy at the age of 13 years for a rapidly growing neoplasm [90]. Finally during a short follow-up period (less than 2 years), new lesions developed in 5 of the 11 patients.

PRKAR1A is the only gene currently known to be associated with CNC [77, 91, 92]. Approximately 20 % of families affected with CNC have been linked to 2p16. It is possible that a third as-yet unidentified locus exists. The genetic testing for CNC includes sequence analysis, deletion/duplication analysis, and linkage analysis for those individuals without an identifiable *PRKAR1A* mutation. In the largest study to date, 114 of 185 (62 %) families studied had an identifiable *PRKAR1A* mutation [92]. The mutation detection frequency increases to 80 % in individuals with CNC presenting with Cushing's syndrome caused by PPNAD [93]. In a study of 36 unrelated individuals with CNC who were negative for *PRKAR1A* point mutations, two large *PRKAR1A* deletions were identified. One patient had thyroid lesions [94].

Predictive testing for young at-risk asymptomatic family members requires prior identification of the disease-causing mutation in the family. Prenatal diagnosis and preimplantation genetic diagnosis (PGD) for at-risk pregnancies require prior identification of the disease-causing mutation in the family. Recommendations for the evaluation of parents of a proband with an apparent de novo mutation include eliciting pertinent family history and physical examination for evidence of cutaneous pigmented spots or lumps or both and for signs of endocrine disease, and imaging and/or biochemical screening. If a mutation in *PRKAR1A* has been identified in the proband, molecular genetic testing of the parents should be considered.

In summary, up to 75 % of individuals with CNC have multiple thyroid nodules, most of which are nonfunctioning thyroid follicular adenomas (there is a single case report of ectopic thymus presenting as a thyroid nodule [95]). Thyroid carcinomas, both papillary and follicular, can occur and occasionally may develop in a person with a long history of multiple thyroid adenomas. Thyroid carcinomas in patients with Carney complex are of particular interest, because this disorder is rarely associated with malignant disorders. The estimated prevalence of thyroid cancer in patients with CNC is approximately 3.8 %; it is usually seen in younger individuals (before the age of 30 years) and it is multifocal with vascular invasion. Screening with thyroid ultrasonography is recommended in all post-pubertal children with established CNC and follow-up as needed based on the initial sonographic findings.

Werner's Syndrome

There are few cases of thyroid cancer in individuals with Werner's syndrome (WS); an autosomal recessive disease characterized by premature segmental aging has a high frequency of association with six rare neoplasms in Japanese patients; only four of these neoplasms also occur excessively in whites. Dr. Werner, as a medical student in the Ophthalmology Clinic at the Royal Christian Albrecht University of Kiel, reported four siblings with scleroderma in association with cataracts as his doctoral dissertation [96]. He described several progeric manifestations observed in the patients in addition to the skin sclerosis and juvenile cataracts. He also assumed a genetic origin of the syndrome without any evidence of their parental consanguinity, as the family had resided in a small Alpine valley and the four siblings showed almost the same clinical signs and symptoms at a similar age. In Japan, Ishida, an ophthalmologist at the University of Kyoto reported the first case of WS in 1917 [97]. He also referred to the progeric phenomenon in the syndrome, though he did not cite Werner's report. In 1934 and 1941, Oppenheimer and Kugel drew attention to the disorder and named it Werner's syndrome [98, 99]. The first mention of cancer in WS, fibro-liposarcoma in this case, was made by Agatston and Gartner in 1939 [100]. In 2000 a total of 1,100 patients with WS had been described all over the world [101]. Japan had the largest number, 810, followed by the USA, 68, and Germany, 51.

Werner's syndrome is caused by the mutations at the *WRN* locus on chromosome 8. The *WRN* gene spans more than 250 kb and consists of 35 exons, 34 of which are coding exons [102] . *WRN* gene encodes one of the RecQ helicase family proteins, WRN, which has ATPase, helicase, exonuclease, and single-stranded DNA annealing activities. *WRN* is ubiquitously expressed in tissues. Helicases separate complementary strands of nucleic acids in a reaction coupled to NTP hydrolysis. RecQ helicases have a common helicase domain with seven conserved motifs, which bind and hydrolyze ATP. WRN helicase activity is structure specific and requires energy from ATP hydrolysis to unwind complementary strands of DNA with a 3_–5_ polarity. Unlike other RecQ helicases, WRN also has intrinsic 3_–5_ exonuclease activity. The preferred DNA substrates of WRN helicase activity, which resemble DNA metabolic intermediates, include forked and Xap structures (intermediates in DNA replication and repair), bubble structures (intermediates in DNA repair and transcription), D-loop and Holliday junction structures (intermediates in DNA recombination), and G-quadruplex DNA and D-loop structures (associated with telomere DNA) [103]. Interestingly, the WRN helicase and exonuclease activities can also work in a coordinated manner on the same substrate. These two catalytic activities of WRN collectively provide access for proteins to the template during replication, recombination, and repair. Consistent with this notion, biochemical and genetic evidence suggest that WRN plays important roles in DNA repair, homologous recombination, replication, and telomere maintenance [104–106].

Ishikawa et al. [107] in a retrospective analysis of 845 Japanese patients with WS, confirmed with molecular analysis, identified 23 cases of thyroid cancer from a series of 150 cancers. Those cancer cases were compared with those of 19,446 tumors in a Japanese national registry of thyroid carcinomas from 1977 to 1991. The average age of patients with thyroid carcinoma was 39 years for those with WS and 49 years for the registry patients. The female-to-male ratio was 2.3:1 and 6.6:1, respectively. The occurrence rates for papillary, follicular, and anaplastic thyroid carcinomas were 35 %, 48 %, and 13 % for Japanese patients with WS and 78 %, 14 %, and 2 % in the general Japanese population. All four cases of follicular carcinoma had germline *WRN* gene mutations in the C-terminal region and the germline mutation for the PTC was in the N-terminal region. These results suggest two possible genotype-phenotype correlation in WS-related thyroid cancer: One concerns thyroid carcinoma histology and the other concerns frequent mutations that occur in the C-terminal region in Japanese patients, but not in white patients with WS. This may account for the higher rates of thyroid carcinoma in Japanese WS patients.

Goto et al. [108] in a retrospective analysis of the National Japanese registry with Werner's syndrome and the reported WS cases around the world till 1995 identified 21 cases of thyroid cancer among Japanese patients with WS and only three patients outside Japan. Fifty percent of the cases included follicular carcinoma, 40 % PTC and 10 % anaplastic. Thirty-three percent of the follicular thyroid cancer cases were associated with multiple primary neoplasia, while papillary thyroid cancer cases were associated with other primary malignancies with a frequency approximating 75 %. Thyroid carcinoma accounted for 14 % of neoplasia in Japanese with WRN as compared with 3 % in non-Japanese.

The diagnosis of WS currently is made with the identification of the cardinal signs along with molecular confirmatory testing. More than 50 different *WRN* disease mutations have been reported thus far [102, 109, 110]. *WRN* gene is the only gene known to be associated with Werner's syndrome. No other loci associated with typical forms of Werner's syndrome have been identified, but it is possible that mutations in genes encoding proteins that interact with WRN may produce a similar phenotype. WS is inherited in an autosomal recessive manner. The parents of a proband are obligate heterozygotes for a disease-causing mutation and, therefore, carry one mutant allele. Although systematic clinical studies have not been reported, heterozygotes do not appear to be at increased risk for any WS-specific symptoms. Carrier testing for WRN mutations using molecular genetic techniques is not offered because it is not clinically available. The optimal time for determination of genetic risk is before pregnancy. No laboratories offering molecular genetic testing for prenatal diagnosis of Werner's syndrome caused by WRN mutations listed in the Gene Tests Laboratory Directory. However, prenatal testing may be available for families in which the disease-causing mutations have been identified in an affected family member.

In summary, WS is associated with an increased incidence of thyroid carcinoma that is usually present in the third to fourth decade of life. Although no prospective studies are currently available, the high prevalence of thyroid carcinoma supports routine thyroid screening in patients with this disorder starting at the beginning of the third decade of life followed by screening thyroid ultrasound as needed.

Pendred Syndrome

Pendred syndrome is an autosomal recessive disorder characterized by sensorineural deafness, euthyroid goiter, temporal bone abnormalities, and a partial defect in iodine organification. It was first described by Vaughan Pendred in 1896 [111]. Pendred syndrome is one of the most common forms of syndromic deafness. The incidence of Pendred syndrome is estimated to be as high as 7.5–10 in 100,000 individuals, thus accounting for up to 10 % of all hereditary hearing loss [112, 113].

Sensorineural deafness is the leading clinical sign of Pendred syndrome [114, 115]. Typically, the hearing loss is profound and prelingual. However, in some individuals, hearing impairment may develop later in childhood and then progress [112, 116]. The hearing loss may fluctuate and it has been shown to progress following even minor head trauma [117, 118]. Deafness is accompanied by malformations of the inner ear, which can be identified by computed tomography or magnetic resonance imaging [119]. These malformations include an enlargement of the endolymphatic system that can be detected as an enlarged vestibular aqueduct (EVA; ≥1.5 mm) on imaging studies. Some patients have a Mondini cochlea, in which the coils of the cochlea are replaced by a single cavity [112, 120]. The Mondini dysplasia is, however, not specific for Pendred syndrome as it can be observed in several other disorders.

The onset and presentation of goiter vary within and between families. It usually develops during childhood and ranges from no enlargement of the thyroid to the development of large goiters [113, 121]. When evaluated with a perchlorate test, all patients with biallelic mutations in the *SLC26A4* gene have a partial iodide organification defect, irrespective of the presence or absence of a goiter [122]. The perchlorate test determines whether iodide is organified normally into thyroglobulin (TG) [123]. Normally, less than 10 % of radioiodide accumulated in thyrocytes are not rapidly organified into thyroglobulin for the purpose of thyroid hormone synthesis (see later). In contrast, patients with Pendred syndrome lose more than 15 %, thus indicating an impaired iodide organification [112, 114]. However, the organification defect is only partial. This differs, for example, from the situation in patients who are homozygous for completely inactivating mutations in thyroid peroxidase that result in a total iodide organification defect [124]. Despite the presence of a partial iodide organification defect, patients with Pendred syndrome only develop hypothyroidism under conditions of a low nutritional iodide intake. Patients from Japan and Korea (countries with a high iodide intake) with documented biallelic mutations in the SLC26A4 gene are always euthyroid [125]. In contrast, patients with Pendred syndrome from iodide-deficient regions may present with congenital hypothyroidism [126]. Many patients have elevated serum levels of thyroglobulin, a finding that correlates with goiter size [127].

Pendrin is a member of the solute carrier family 26A (SLC26A) [128]. With the exception of the motor protein prestin, which is expressed in outer hair cells, all members of this family function as anion exchangers. Pendrin is able to mediate exchange of chloride with bicarbonate, formate, and iodide [129–132]. Pendrin is mostly abundantly expressed in the thyroid, the inner ear, and the kidney [133]. In the thyroid, pendrin is localized at the apical membrane of thyroid follicular cells and appears to be involved in mediating iodide efflux into the follicular lumen [133, 134]. In the inner ear, pendrin is found in the endolymphatic duct and sac, where it acts as a chloride/bicarbonate exchanger. Although the mechanisms regulating iodide uptake at the basolateral membrane of thyroid cells have been extensively explored [135], much less is known about the apical iodide efflux into the follicular lumen. Electrophysiological studies characterizing iodide efflux in inverted plasma membrane vesicles suggested the existence of two apical iodide channels [136]. The expression of pendrin at the apical membrane of thyrocytes and its ability to transport iodide suggest that pendrin may be one of these iodide channels that regulate apical iodide efflux in the thyroid. Moreover, the partial iodide organification defect observed in patients with biallelic *SLC26A4* mutations is consistent with a potential role of pendrin in thyroid hormone biosynthesis. Pendrin was originally proposed to function as a sulfate transporter based on its sequence homology to known sulfate transporters and the presence of a sulfate transporter motif [128]. The physiological role of pendrin in mediating apical iodide transport has, however, been questioned based on the following arguments. Targeted disruption of pendrin in knockout mice does not lead to the development of a goiter or abnormal thyroid hormone levels, at least under conditions of sufficient iodide intake [137]. There are no functional data demonstrating a role of pendrin in iodide transport in vivo. Pendrin has a distinct role as a chloride/bicarbonate exchanger in the kidney [131, 133]. Patients with biallelic mutations in the *SLC26A4* gene have only a mild or no thyroidal phenotype under normal iodide intake conditions [138]; therefore, it is conceivable that other iodide channels and/or transporters are involved in the apical transport of iodide.

Slc26a4 knockout mice have normal thyroid hormone levels but interestingly the follicular pH is reduced suggesting that pendrin is involved in bicarbonate transport at the apical membrane of thyrocytes [139]. The physiological significance of the acidification of the follicular lumen awaits further characterization. The efflux of iodide across the apical membrane of thyrocytes is stimulated by TSH through activation of the cAMP pathway [140–142]. Although TSH regulates apical iodide efflux, it does not stimulate the expression of *SLC26A4* mRNA [135].

The occurrence of malignant thyroid tumors in multinodular goiters is generally considered to be relatively low [143]; it has been estimated to be as high in as 6–8 % in some series [144]. A significantly higher incidence of thyroid cancer of about 17 % (19 cases in 109 reported thyroidectomies) appears to occur in patients with congenital hypothyroidism caused by dyshormonogenesis [145]. Of these 19 patients, six had aggressive metastases to the lung and/or the bone that were resistant to treatment with radioiodine.

Thyroid malignancies have been reported in patients with Pendred syndrome. Thieme [146] reported a 23-year-old deaf man with a large multinodular goiter containing a follicular carcinoma with vascular invasion and tumoral microemboli. Elman [147] described a follicular carcinoma in a 37-year-old deaf woman with multinodular goiter and a positive perchlorate test. Watanabe [148] reported a 42-year-old female patient with a large goiter of approximately 900 g, probable Pendred syndrome, and an undifferentiated thyroid carcinoma that invaded the trachea and the vasculature and that metastasized to the lungs and bones. This patient did not respond to radioiodine therapy and died within 6 months. A rather unusual clinical course was observed by Abs et al. [149] , who followed a 54-year-old patient with Pendred syndrome who had had a subtotal thyroidectomy. The remnant thyroid tissue progressively enlarged, and the patient ultimately showed clinical and biochemical evidence of thyrotoxicosis. A radioiodine scan revealed the presence of a large thyroid gland with extension into the mediastinum and uptake in the ribs, the pelvis, and the femur. Her serum thyroglobulin levels were high. Histopathology of one of her bone metastases revealed a well-differentiated follicular thyroid carcinoma. Camargo et al. [150] reported three cases with Pendred syndrome in a Portuguese family; the index case, who was the offspring of a consanguineous marriage, was found to have an invasive follicular carcinoma with areas of anaplastic transformation. This patient developed a goiter in childhood and she was diagnosed with an invasive follicular carcinoma at the age of 53 years due to a rapid enlargement of the goiter.

All patients with coexisting thyroid carcinomas and Pendred syndrome had no or inadequate treatment with levothyroxine and subsequently developed large goiters, suggesting a possible causal relationship between the long-standing growth stimulation and the development of these malignancies. In some of these patients, the thyroid follicular cancers exhibited aggressive behavior associated with bone and lung metastases. The histological pattern of goitrous tissue from patients with Pendred syndrome typically displays pronounced hyperplasia and multiple nodules, and the pleomorphic histology and the microfollicular pattern may give rise to suspicion of malignancy [151]. However, in contrast to follicular nodules, follicular carcinomas display local and vascular invasion, a criterium that is key in establishing the diagnosis of follicular thyroid cancer [145]. The aggressive behavior of the follicular carcinoma in patients with Pendred syndrome, dyshormonogenesis, or iodine deficiency suggests that the long-standing growth may result in a multistep progression from polyclonal hyperplastic lesion to an increasingly aggressive carcinoma [152]. The observation of anaplastic transformation within the follicular malignancy is in line with this hypothesis, and the clinical course with rapid enlargement of a long-standing goiter and distant metastases to the lung is typical for anaplastic cancer [153].

To date, more than 150 mutations in the *SLC26A4* gene have been reported in patients with Pendred syndrome. The mutations are dispersed throughout the gene. The majority of the *SLC26A4* mutations are missense mutations with a much smaller portion represented by nonsense, splice site, and frameshift mutations [154]. Patients from consanguineous families are homozygous for mutations in the *SLC26A4* gene, whereas compound heterozygous mutations of the gene are found in affected individuals of non-consanguineous families or in sporadic cases. The prevalence of recurring mutations varies among different ethnic groups [155–160]. In a child with severe-to-profound congenital deafness in whom the clinical history and physical examination are consistent with the diagnosis of autosomal recessive nonsyndromic hearing loss, the first test that should be ordered is molecular genetic testing of GJB [161]. If GJB2 molecular genetic testing does not identify two disease-causing mutations, computed tomography (CT) or magnetic resonance imaging (MRI) of the temporal bones should be considered to evaluate for DVA and Mondini dysplasia. The presence of either of these temporal bone anomalies warrants molecular genetic testing of *SLC26A4*. In most children with Pendred syndrome, thyroid enlargement will not be present. Perchlorate testing is not widely available and with molecular genetic testing, not essential to diagnose Pendred syndrome. High-resolution CT or MRI of the temporal bones should be completed in all children with progressive sensorineural hearing loss to evaluate for DVA. If an enlarged vestibular aqueduct is observed, molecular genetic testing of *SLC26A4* is warranted. Carrier testing for at-risk relatives and prenatal and preimplantation genetic diagnosis require prior identification of the disease-causing mutations in the family.

In summary, thyroid disease in Pendred patients may range from minimal enlargement to large multinodular goiter. Most patients remain euthyroid and phenotypic variation is seen between kindreds of the same family. The association of thyroid cancer and Pendred syndrome may be related to untreated congenital hypothyroidism and chronic stimulation by thyroid-stimulating hormone. This process has also been thought to contribute to the progression of follicular thyroid cancer to anaplastic thyroid cancer in Pendred syndrome. The risk of progression from thyroid goiter to cancer is uncommon and likely related to long-standing untreated hypothyroidism. Ultrasound surveillance and routine thyroid examination in a patient who has been found to have hypothyroidism and Pendred syndrome may be helpful for early identification of thyroid cancer. There is no role for routine prophylactic thyroidectomy in patients with Pendred syndrome.

McCune-Albright Syndrome

McCune-Albright syndrome (MAS) is a rare sporadic disease characterized by polyostotic fibrous dysplasia [162], precocious puberty, and café-au-lait pigmentation of the skin. The syndrome may also be associated with autonomous hyperfunction of other endocrine tissues, involvement of non-endocrine tissues [163, 164], and renal phosphate wasting [165].

The underlying molecular mechanism of MAS is an activating mutation in the gene (*GNAS1*) coding for the α-subunit of the stimulatory G protein ($G_S\alpha$) involved in the cAMP cascade. The activating mutation involves substitution at the Arg (201) position (R201), most commonly with cysteine (R201C) or histidine (R201H). This mutation results in inappropriately elevated levels of intracellular cAMP with ensuing endocrine cell hyperfunction and increased cell proliferation [166, 167]. The somatic activating mutation of the GNAS gene which can occur at any stage during postzygotic development leads to a mosaic pattern of distribution among the various organs, as well as within the affected organ, where the mutant allele tends to be more highly represented in areas of increased proliferation [168].

Similar to other endocrine tissues, the thyroid is characterized by the presence of a G-coupled receptor that upon the interaction with its ligand, in this case TSH with the TSH receptor mediates the growth and the endocrine function of the organ. Thus, the sustained increase in intracellular levels of cAMP within the thyroid gland is the result of amplification of the TSH mediated second messenger signaling pathway, causing hypersecretion of thyroid hormones and cell replication. Involvement of the thyroid is highly prevalent in McCune-Albright syndrome, occurring in approximately 30 % of the cases. Case reports represent the vast majority of publications describing thyroid involvement in patients with MAS. Hypothyroidism is a rare occurrence and it is often the result of the treatment of MAS-associated hyperthyroidism or the treatment of pituitary tumors [169]. On the other hand hyperthyroidism is by far the most common thyroid functional abnormality observed in MAS. Classically the onset is within the first decade of life and the course of the disease is indolent [170]. The MAS-associated hyperthyroidism is characterized by the absence of autoimmunity and the presence of exophthalmos should prompt the evaluation of retro-orbital bone disease. There is only one reported case of secondary hyperthyroidism due to a TSH-producing pituitary adenoma in the literature. MAS-associated hyperthyroidism is also characterized by a shifted T3/T4 ratio and relatively often presents as T3 toxicosis with normal or minimally elevated free T4 levels [170, 171].

The diagnostic imaging patterns of MAS-associated thyroid disease have been systemically examined in only a limited number of case series. Clinically euthyroid children with MAS with no clinical evidence (by palpation) of goiter showed ultrasound findings compatible with diffuse cystic multinodular goiter in a review study of 3 MAS cases by Lair-Milan et al. [172]. Ultrasound abnormalities are seen in all patients with biochemical evidence of thyroid dysfunction.

To date, only two cases of thyroid cancer in MAS patients have been described and studied well: the first case, described by Yang et al. [173], was a 41-year-old woman with MAS and a 2 cm thyroid nodule of 10 years duration. She was initially diagnosed with a 1.2 cm firm, round, and mobile thyroid nodule at the age of 30 years. She was treated with levothyroxine for 10 years, the treatment was ineffective, the nodule increased in size, and the FNA was suspicious for PTC. The resected tumor showed 90 % clear cells and 10 % nonclear cells with capsular and vascular invasion. She was initially managed with a hemithyroidectomy followed by a completion thyroidectomy and radioactive iodine treatment. At 4-year follow-up, she was disease-free.

The second case was a 14-year-old Filipino girl who was found to have a 1.5 cm right thyroid nodule with increased vascularity on thyroid ultrasonography and increased uptake on Tc-pertechnetate thyroid scan. She was initially underwent a right hemithyroidectomy that revealed a multifocal PTC. The resected nodule showed a lipid-rich clear cell PTC. A completion thyroidectomy was subsequently performed and no evidence of carcinoma was identified in the surgical specimen from the second surgery. She was received a therapeutic dose of radioactive iodine after the second hemithyroidectomy, and 40 months postoperatively, she was disease-free.

Thyroid tissue from both cases, from areas including the PTC, normal thyroid tissue, and hyperplastic thyroid tissue, were micro-dissected for DNA extraction and PCR amplification. The *GNAS1* mutation was identified in the majority of the malignant cells as well as in the adjacent normal tissue and the hyperplastic tissue. The presence of the mutation in normal thyroid cells indicates that malignancy is likely to have evolved as the result of additional genetic or epigenetic events. Also the histology subtype of the PTC has been described in cases of PTC associated with chronic TSH hyperstimulation as occur in cases of congenital hypothyroidism.

In summary, the appearance of thyroid carcinoma in MAS is an uncommon event. However, there is a need for heightened awareness and observation of the thyroid in MAS patients. This is of particular importance when one considers that both functional and structural thyroid abnormalities are common in MAS. Clinicians can no more assume that all thyroid nodules in MAS are benign and should have a lower threshold to aspirate them to exclude cancer.

Peutz-Jeghers Syndrome

Peutz-Jeghers syndrome (PJS) is a rare, dominantly inherited disease with incomplete penetrance characterized by hamartomatous small bowel polyposis, mucocutaneous hyperpigmentation [174], and increased risk of cancer [175, 176]. PJS belongs to the hamartomatous polyposis syndromes, which are characterized by an overgrowth of cells native to the area in which they normally occur and involve mesenchymal, stromal, and rarely also endodermal and ectodermal components [177].

The incidence of the syndrome ranges from 1 in 8,300 to 1 in 280,000 live births [178, 179]. It is commonly diagnosed in the third decade of life, although one third of the cases are identified in children before the age of 10 years [180] . The first presentation is generally caused by the intestinal complications of the polyps at approximately 10–13 years of age.

The gene responsible for this syndrome is the serine threonine-protein kinase 11/liver kinase B1 (*STK11/LKB1*). *S7K11* is located on chromosome 19p13.3 and encodes for a serine/threonine kinase acting as a tumor suppressor gene. This serine/threonine-protein kinase has a prenylation motif suggesting that it is involved in protein-protein interactions and membrane binding [181]. The predicted protein structure also shows an autophosphorylation domain [182], along with a cyclic AMP-dependent protein kinase phosphorylation site. STK11 expression was shown to cause apoptosis in epithelial cells [183]. The transport of STK11 to the mitochondria appears to be an early step in apoptosis. STK11 colocalizes with p53 during apoptosis and the ability of STK11 to induce apoptosis also depends on p53. These results suggest that signaling through STK11 may be an early event leading to apoptosis through p53 pathways. Tiainen et al. [184] showed that STK11 affects G1 cell cycle arrest and that growth suppression by STK11 is mediated through signaling of cytoplasmic STK11. Inhibition of cellular proliferation by STK11 may occur through induction of WAF1, a cyclin-dependent kinase inhibition [184, 185]. By forming a complex with STRAD and MO25, STK11 was reported to phosphorylate AMPK and several other members of the AMPK-related subfamily of kinases including the microtubule affinity-regulating kinases (MARKs) to regulate cell polarity [186]. Mutations in the C-terminal non-catalytic region decreased mediation of AMP-activated kinase and cell polarity [187–189]. AMPK is an evolutionally conserved Ser/Thr kinase that functions as a key regulator of cellular energy metabolism [190, 191]. Through activation of AMPK by phosphorylation, S7K11 plays a role in energy metabolism [192]. In summary, S7K11 is a multitasking tumor suppressor that has a role in apoptosis, cell cycle arrest, cell proliferation, cell polarity, and energy metabolism.

PJS patients have increased risk for malignancies in the GI tract as well as in several extra intestinal sites including the pancreas, breast, uterus, ovary, and testes [193, 194]. To date only six cases of thyroid cancer in PJS patients have been reported in the literature.

A case of thyroid carcinoma in PJS has been mentioned by Spigelman et al. [195], although they did not describe either the patient's personal history and the histology of the tumor. Reed et al. [196] reported a case of PTC in a 21-year-old woman affected by PJS among a series of patients with thyroid neoplasia and intestinal polyps. Yamamoto et al. [197] described a case of PTC in a 29-year-old Japanese woman with PJS. In this patient, pigmented mucocutaneous lesions were initially reported at 4 years of age, and the diagnosis of PJS was made when the patient was 22 years old, after a small bowel resection performed because of an intussusception caused by hamartomatous polyps. Boardman et al. [198] reported a single thyroid cancer in their series of 26 noncutaneous cancers ascertained among 34 PJS patients. Finally, Zirilli et al. [199] described a 14 mm nodular lesion in the right thyroid lobe of a 25-year-old Caucasian woman affected by PJS. Cytological analysis at FNAB revealed a pattern compatible with PTC, and the histological analysis after total thyroidectomy showed a Hurtle cell variant of PTC, with follicular architecture.

The diagnosis of Peutz-Jeghers syndrome is based on clinical findings. In individuals with a clinical diagnosis of PJS, molecular genetic testing of *STK11 (LKB1)* reveals disease-causing mutations in nearly all individuals who have a positive family history and approximately 90 % of individuals who have no family history of PJS. Such testing is available clinically. In a single individual, a clinical diagnosis of PJS may be made when any *one* of the following is present [200]:

- Two or more histologically confirmed PJ polyps
- Any number of PJ polyps detected in one individual who has a family history of PJS in close relative(s)

- Characteristic mucocutaneous pigmentation in an individual who has a family history of PJS in close relative(s)
- Any number of PJ polyps in an individual who also has characteristic mucocutaneous pigmentation

Currently only mutations in *STK11 (LKB1)* have been identified as a cause for Peutz-Jeghers syndrome (PJS) [201, 202]. The observations of Olschwang et al. [203] suggest that in addition to *STK11*, another genetic locus may predispose to the clinical features of PJS. However, although one child with a PJS hamartoma had a translocation of 19q13.4, no mutations in candidate genes mapping to this breakpoint were identified [204]. In 25 individuals who had PJS but did not have a detectable *STK11* mutation, one had a heterozygous mutation of the DNA repair enzyme MYH that was not observed in 1015 controls [205]. Of note, mutations of MYH ordinarily cause an autosomal recessive form of adenomatous polyposis coli.

Sequence analysis and deletion/duplication studies. In a study of 56 individuals with a clinical diagnosis of PJS in which a combination of sequence analysis to detect point mutations and multiplex ligation-dependent probe amplification (MLPA) to detect large *STK11* deletions was used, *STK11* mutation detection rate was 94 % [206]. A wide variety of mutations have been detected including missense, splicing, and small deletions or insertion deletions. Larger deletions including whole-gene deletion of *STK11* [207] or smaller intragenic deletions [208] can be detected in about 15 % of individuals with PJS. Intragenic homologous recombination has been noted as a mechanism that can lead to deletion of exons 4–7 of *STK11*. One patient with both Peutz-Jeghers syndrome and schizophrenia was found to have a large deletion encompassing exons 2–7 and part of exon 8 [209].

In summary, thyroid cancer is not part of the known spectrum of PJS. In any case, clinicians should be aware that the wide spectrum of cancer diseases possibly occurring in PJS patients could also include differentiated thyroid cancer (DTC), although this is rare. Consequently, US of the thyroid can be recommended to PJS patients even when no clinical sign of thyroid disease is present in the patient's medical history. If thyroid nodules are found at US analysis, their features can help in choosing to perform US-guided FNA biopsy. The management of DTC in a patient with PJS does not differ from the standard guidelines for DTC. Total thyroidectomy as well as radioiodine ablation therapy is recommended, although some concern could be raised about the possible tumorigenic effects of radioiodine therapy in cancer-prone individuals such as patients affected by PJS. Prophylactic thyroidectomy is not indicated in PJS patients, given the relatively low prevalence of PTC, the potential complications of thyroidectomy, and the excellent prognosis for PTC.

Ataxia-Telangiectasia Syndrome

Ataxia-telangiectasia (A-T) is a rare autosomal recessive condition characterized by progressive neuronal degeneration, immunological deficiency, radiosensitivity, and increased risk of cancer. Most cancers in patients with AT are lymphoid type [210, 211]. Serum AFP concentration is elevated above 10 ng/mL in more than 95 % of individuals with A-T. Serum AFP concentration may remain above normal in unaffected children until age 24 months. Intracellular ATM protein is severely depleted in most patients with A-T. To date, this is the most sensitive and specific clinical test for establishing a diagnosis of A-T. Small amounts of ATM protein have been occasionally associated with a milder prognosis, although there are many exceptions to this and the association needs further validation.

The "A-T mutated" (*ATM*) gene was identified in 1995 on chromosome 11q22-23, coding for a protein implicated in genomic homeostasis in case of radio-induced DNA double-strand breaks. The prevalence of A-T in the US is 1:40,000–1:100,000 live births and it is the most common cause of progressive cerebellar ataxia in childhood in most countries. There are two types of A-T, the classic and the nonclassic forms of A-T. The most obvious and troubling characteristic of classic A-T is the progressive cerebellar ataxia. Shortly after learning to walk, children with A-T begin to stagger. The neurologic status of some children appears to improve from age 2 to 4 years; then ataxia begins to progress again; the transient improvement is probably attributable to the rapid learning curve of young children. The ataxia begins as purely truncal but within several years involves peripheral coordination as well. By age 10 years, most children become confined to a wheelchair for the remainder of their lives. Other neurologic manifestations include progressively slurred speech, oculomotor apraxia (inability to follow an object across visual fields), choreoathetosis (writhing movements), and oculocutaneous telangiectasia (usually evident by age 6 years). Immunodeficiencies are present in 60–80 % of individuals with classic A-T; they are variable and do not correlate well with the frequency, severity, or spectrum of infections. The immunodeficiency is not progressive [212–216]. The most consistent immunodeficiency reported in classic A-T is poor antibody response to pneumococcal polysaccharide vaccines [215, 217]. Serum concentration of the immunoglobulins IgA, IgE, and IgG2 may be reduced. Approximately 30 % of individuals with classic A-T who have immunodeficiency have T-cell deficiencies. At autopsy, virtually all individuals have a small embryonic-like thymus.

The risk for malignancy in individuals with classic A-T is 38 %. Leukemia and lymphoma account for about 85 % of malignancies. Younger children tend to have acute lymphocytic leukemia (ALL) of T-cell origin and older children are likely to have an aggressive T-cell leukemia. Lymphomas are usually B-cell types. As individuals with classic A-T are living longer, other cancers and tumors, including ovarian cancer, breast cancer, gastric cancer, melanoma, leiomyomas, and sarcomas, have also been observed.

The nonclassic forms of A-T that are associated with homozygosity or compound heterozygosity for two deleterious ATM mutations include:

- Milder A-T phenotypes including adult-onset A-T [218–223].
- Adult-onset spinal muscular atrophy [224]. This phenotype is also associated with reduced levels of ATM protein.
- A-T$_{Fresno}$, a phenotype that combines features of both Nijmegen breakage syndrome (NBS) and A-T([225, 226].
- Progressive dystonia as the presenting symptom in individuals later diagnosed as having A-T [213, 227, 228]; however, these reports antedated the use of molecular genetic testing to confirm the diagnosis of A-T.
- Early-onset dystonia or hypotonia in some individuals with classic A-T and adult-onset mild ataxia in others associated with homozygosity for the *ATM* mutation, c.6200C>A, seen in the Mennonite population [229].
- A-T variants. Sometimes the A-T-like findings in individuals with diagnostic changes in ATM serine/threonine kinase activity and *ATM* mutations do not meet A-T diagnostic criteria – for example, the combination of progressive ataxia, absence of telangiectasias, normal serum AFP concentration, and normal immune function [230, 231].

The cancer risk of individuals heterozygous for *ATM* disease-causing mutations is approximately four times that of the general population, primarily because of the increased risk for breast cancer [219, 232, 233]. To date only five cases of thyroid cancer in patients with A-T have been reported. Narita et al. [234] reported a case of a 19-year-old female with A-T who developed cerebellar ataxia at the age of 4 years. At the age of 17 years, she was found to have a right-sided ovarian dysgerminoma, operated, received Cobalt-60 radiation, and died of pneumonia 16 weeks after the operation. In autopsy a left thyroid lobe papillary carcinoma, follicular variant, was found. Ohta et al. [235] reported a 18-year-old female with A-T who was found to have differentiated papillary thyroid carcinoma that was successfully treated with surgery. Sandoval et al. [236] reported two cases of thyroid carcinoma: the first case was a 29-year-old woman with A-T who at the age of 21 years had received 4,200 cGy to the left thigh for a pseudolymphoma. At the age of 29 years, she was found to have a papillary transitional cell carcinoma, a large B-cell lymphoma, and a 3 cm follicular thyroid carcinoma with metastasis to the epicardium (autopsy findings). The second case was a 35-year-old male with A-T who was diagnosed with a high-grade lymphoma and died 2 months after he received standard chemotherapy. Autopsy in addition showed a 1.6 cm papillary thyroid carcinoma with metastasis in two cervical lymph nodes. Brasseur et al. [237] described a 9-year-old girl with clinically and genetically confirmed A-T who was diagnosed with a right lobe papillary thyroid carcinoma, follicular variant, with cervical lymph nodes metastasis. She underwent a total thyroidectomy and treatment with radioactive iodine, and 6 months after the diagnosis, she was disease-free.

ATM is the only gene known to be associated with ataxia-telangiectasia. Of the 600 unique mutations reported, approximately 14 large genomic deletions have been described. By convention, these are genomic deletions larger than 500 bp and not those involving single exons only. Only one partial (41-kb) duplication within the *ATM* gene has been described to date [238, 239]. It is unknown how many affected individuals in whom only one *ATM* mutation has been identified by sequence analysis have actually been tested for deletions or duplications by either array CGH or MLPA. Targeted mutation analysis is offered for pathologic alleles common in specific ethnic populations (e.g., c.103C>T). Genetic analysis at 11q23.1 can be used to rapidly identify founder haplotypes that are in linkage disequilibrium with known or unknown pathogenic mutations [240–242].

Ataxia-telangiectasia is inherited in an autosomal recessive manner. The parents are both obligate carriers of an *ATM* gene mutation. Heterozygotes (carriers) appear to be at increased risk for cancer and coronary artery disease [243, 244]. At conception, each sib of an affected individual has a 25 % risk of being affected, a 50 % risk of being an asymptomatic carrier, and a 25 % risk of being unaffected and not a carrier. Once an at-risk sib is known to be unaffected, the risk of his/her being a carrier is two-thirds. Most individuals with A-T do not reproduce due to increased morbidity in young age. Each sib of the proband's parents is at a 50 % risk of being a carrier. Carrier testing is possible if the disease-causing mutations in the family have been identified. This can also be accomplished by linkage analysis (i.e., segregation of affected haplotypes) if an affected family member has also been haplotyped.

In summary, the association between A-T and thyroid cancer has rarely been described, only four adult cases have been reported, and all of them died from a cause not related to thyroid cancer. Although the prevalence is low, screening for thyroid cancer is recommended in all patients with A-T due to the increased overall malignancy risk in these patients. Prophylactic thyroidectomy for A-T patients is not indicated. For heterozygotes though studies have shown an increased risk for breast cancer only, but given the lack of data, clinician should have a low threshold of evaluating with thyroid ultrasound and FNA biopsy thyroid lesions detected in this patient population.

Familial Papillary Thyroid Cancer

An increasing number of case reports, epidemiological analyses, and retrospective clinical studies support the existence of a distinct entity of familial PTC (FPTC) with a strong association with multinodular goiter. Goldgar et al. [245] in a systematic population-based assessment of cancer risk in first-degree relatives of cancer probands from the Utah population database showed an excess of cancers of the same site among relatives, with thyroid and colon cancers and lymphocytic leukemia showing the highest familial risks. These results are supported by a second population-based study carried out in Sweden, suggesting an increased thyroid cancer risk of offspring when one parent has thyroid cancer. This risk is higher when the second parent is affected [246].

Many published pedigrees suggest an autosomal dominant mode of inheritance with reduced penetrance [13, 14, 16, 247, 248], but polygenic inheritance cannot be excluded, which could also explain the rarity of large families with many cases of thyroid cancer. Loh [249] reviewed 15 case reports/series of familial nonmedullary thyroid carcinoma involving kindreds with no obvious associated pathogenetic factors. There were a total of 87 kindreds with 178 affected individuals available for analysis, with a male to female ratio of 1:2.2. The median age group at diagnosis was 30–39 years in both gender groups. Papillary thyroid carcinoma constituted 91 % of the cases, followed by follicular (6 %) and anaplastic (2 %) varieties. There was one case (0.5 %), each of combined papillary and medullary thyroid carcinoma and Hurthle cell carcinoma, respectively. Six of the 15 series observed that patients with familial history generally have more aggressive tumor characteristics compared to the sporadic counterparts. The incidences of multifocality, local invasion, and distant metastases at diagnosis were 49, 32, and 5 %, respectively. The incidences of locoregional recurrence, distant metastases, and deaths were 29, 10, and 5.4 %, respectively, at a mean follow-up period of 11 years.

Couch et al. [250] reported 18 members of an extended pedigree with a form of euthyroid adolescent multinodular goiter. Histological examination showed multiple adenomas with areas of epithelial hyperplasia, hemorrhage, and calcification. In two subjects there were focal areas of epithelial hyperplasia reminiscent of low-grade papillary carcinoma, but capsular and vascular invasion was not found. The pattern of inheritance appeared to be autosomal dominant, with diminished penetrance in males. Austoni [251] described the concordance of papillary thyroid cancer in a pair of monozygotic twins from a mother with a multinodular goiter. Both were diagnosed with T3N0M0 stage PTC in their early 30s. Dzwonkowski et al. [252] reported at the same time two cases of papillary thyroid cancer in HLA identical twins. Both presented at the same age with T4N1MO stage papillary thyroid carcinoma. Samaan [253] reported five cases of PTC, age of diagnosis was 8–39 years, and among those cases two involved a pair of twin sisters. Fischer et al. [254] reported two cases of multifocal T4 papillary thyroid cancer in the same family diagnosed before the age of 25 years.

In 1997, Burgess et al. [16] described 11 cases of PTC in two families associated with multinodular goiter. In the first family, 7 of the 25 members had PTC (6 of these had multinodular goiter) and 11 had multinodular goiter. In the second family, identical male twins and their daughters had PTC. The age of diagnosis was 22–62 years and multifocality was found in 3 out of the 11 cases. Bignell et al. [255] performed a genomic search on a single large Canadian family with 18 cases of nontoxic multinodular goiter in which two individuals also had papillary lesions highly suggestive of papillary carcinoma. A locus on chromosome 14q (MNG1 [multinodular goiter 1]) was identified, with a maximal two-point LOD score of 3.8 at D14S1030 and a multipoint LOD score of 4.88 at the same marker, defined by D14S1062 (upper boundary) and D14S267 (lower boundary). The gene encoding thyroid-stimulating hormone receptor (TSHR), which is located on chromosome 14q, is outside the linked region. However when 37 smaller pedigrees, each containing at least two cases of NMTC was studied to determine the role of this gene in familial nonmedullary thyroid cancer (NMTC); only a very small proportion of familial NMTC was attributable to MNG1.

Canzian et al. [256] identified with linkage analysis the responsible gene, named "TCO" (thyroid tumors with cell oxyphilia), in a French pedigree with multiple cases of multinodular goiter and NMTC. TCO was mapped to chromosome 19p13.2 by linkage analysis with a whole-genome panel of microsatellite markers. Interestingly, both the benign and malignant thyroid tumors in this family exhibit some extent of cell oxyphilia. These findings suggest that the relatives of patients affected with sporadic NMTC with cell oxyphilia should be carefully investigated. Lesueur et al. [257] through an international consortium collected biological samples from NMTC families. Linkage analysis performed on the 56 more informative kindreds collected through the international consortium. Linkage analysis using both parametric and nonparametric methods excluded *MNG1*, *TCO*, and *RET* as major genes of susceptibility to NMTC and demonstrated that this trait is characterized by genetic heterogeneity. McKay et al. [258] performed linkage analysis in 227 patients from families with FNMTC through the international consortium for the genetics of FNMTC. The reconstruction of haplotypes on chromosome 2q21 showed that seven of eight patients with PTC shared a common haplotype extending from D2S436 to D2S1399, with a maximum multipoint LOD score of 1.28 observed for marker D2S1260. Subsequently the relevance of this 2q21 locus to FNMTC was tested using 80 additional informative FNMTC pedigrees, for a total of 191 NMTC patients collected by the international consortium for the genetics of FNMTC. The linkage analysis of the 80 FNMTC pedigrees achieved a maximum multipoint heterogeneity LOD (HLOD) score of 3.07 at marker D2S2271 (a p 0.42; 95 % confidence interval [CI] 0.15–0.70), supporting the notion of an NMTC susceptibility gene on 2q21. This type of FNMTC linked to the chromosomal region 2q21 is called familial nonmedullary thyroid cancer type 1, and it is characterized by PTC without any distinguishing pathologic features and without an obvious increase in frequency on nonthyroidal neoplasms in kindred members. Cavaco et al. [259] performed linkage analysis in 11 members of a Portuguese family affected with benign thyroid lesions and five affected with thyroid carcinomas. Linkage analysis excluded the involvement of the fPTC/PRN, NMTC1, MNG1, and TCO loci. A genome-wide significant evidence of linkage to a single region on chromosome 8p23.1-p22 was obtained, with a maximum parametric haplotype-based LOD score of 4.41 (theta = 0.00). Linkage analysis with microsatellite markers confirmed linkage to 8q23.1-p22, and recombination events delimited the minimal region to a 7.46-Mb span. Seventeen suggestive candidate genes located in the minimal region were excluded as susceptibility genes by mutational analysis. Allelic losses in the 8p23.1-p22 region were absent in seven thyroid tumors from family members, suggesting that the inactivation of a putative tumor suppressor gene may have occurred through other mechanisms.

Musholt et al. [18] after reviewing all series and case reports in the English literature generated predictive criteria that were used for a computer-based chart review of 282 extensively documented PTC cases treated in the Endocrine Surgery Clinic and the Nuclear Medicine Thyroid Clinic at Hannover University Medical School (HUMS). By applying every selection criterion and combinations thereof and evaluating individuals displaying several of these parameters, potential FPTC index patients were selected. Predictive criteria for identification of familial PTC/MNG are summarized in Table 5.7.

The prevalence of FPTC among the Hannover PTC cases evaluated was more than 4 % (11/282). The mean age at diagnosis of malignant thyroid cancer among 11 Hannover FPTC patients was 33 years (median 32 years). Multifocal carcinomas (TXb) were found in four patients, and lymph node metastases were likewise present in four patients at the time of diagnosis. Five tumors showed a partially or predominantly follicular growth pattern. The age of onset or of diagnosis of the thyroid malignancy was relatively constant within families when compared to interfamilial age differences. A father and daughter of one family both suffered

Table 5.7 Predictive criteria for identification of familial PTC/MNG

Exclusion of previous radiation exposure
Exclusion of neoplasia syndromes associated with PTC (e.g., accumulation of colorectal, ovarian, or breast carcinoma in the kindred)
Exclusion of somatic genetic alterations in the tumor DNA (e.g., RET/PTC rearrangements)
Primary criteria
PTC in two or more first-degree blood relatives
Multinodular goiter in at least three first-degree or second-degree relatives of a PTC patient
Secondary criteria
Diagnosis of PTC in patients younger than 33 years
Multifocal or bilateral PTC
Organ-exceeding tumor growth (pT4)
Lymph node metastases (pN1) or distant metastases (M1)
Familial accumulation of adolescent-onset thyroid disease
Hereditary predisposition to PTC is considered if the following is/are present:
Two primary criteria or
One primary criterion plus three secondary criteria

invasive PTC at age 14. In another family, both siblings with invasive, metastasizing PTCs did not exhibit nodular goiters, in contrast to the mother and two sisters harboring MNG. In one family, histological examination of the thyroid glands of all three tumor patients revealed additional encapsulated adenomas, with oncocytic transformation in two cases.

Until more data on the genetic background on FPTC are available leading to early detection of gene carriers in families at risk, identification of index patients relies on clinical data outlined in the predictive criteria mentioned above. Once the hereditary predisposition to PTC is suspected in kindred, thorough clinical examination of all family members with evidence for thyroid pathology seems prudent. Patients with morphologically suspicious lesions demonstrated by sonography or with cold nodules shown by scintigraphy should immediately undergo fine-needle aspiration biopsy; if the cytology is benign, reexamination after 6 months is recommended. Treatment strategies for FPTC patients should consider the genetic background of the disease. Multifocality is an expected feature of the hereditary predisposition to neoplasia. All thyroid follicular cells of FPTC relatives are predisposed to malignant transformation; and consistently, multifocal or bilateral malignant lesions are found in almost half of the affected individuals. In FPTC family members, the thyroid gland should therefore be completely resected if there is a preoperative diagnosis of malignant disease. Because even microcarcinomas associated with FPTC display early lymph node metastasis when compared to sporadic micro-PTCs [260] and because a large number of FPTC patients present with organ-exceeding tumor growth, several authors have recommended aggressive treatment.

This approach would include not only total thyroidectomy but also systematic microdissection of the central lymph node compartment. Postoperative radioiodine ablation reduces the risk of tumor recurrence and facilitates monitoring with thyroglobulin levels.

FPTC family members undergoing surgery for MNG should be treated with at least unilateral lobectomy and ipsilateral central node dissection because the risk of recurrent nerve palsy increases with completion thyroidectomy [261]. In a considerable number of patients belonging to FPTC kindreds, small tumors are identified in nodular goiters only incidentally during histopathologic examination of the surgical specimen. In these cases, completion thyroidectomy and systematic dissection of the central neck compartment should be carried out to prevent residual or recurrent tumor.

Because of the still limited data, however, a more aggressive surgical approach to total thyroidectomy in relatives with benign thyroid disease or to lateral or mediastinal meticulous locoregional lymph node dissection in all FPTC family members with malignant tumors cannot be recommended at this time. Due to the wide-ranging age of onset of the malignant disease, it is reasonable to recommend screening of the family members starting at the second decade of life.

Familial PTC Associated with Renal Papillary Neoplasia

Malchoff et al. [262] investigated the clinical and pathologic characteristics of an unusually large three-generation FNMTC kindred in order to characterize more fully the clinical phenotype. Linkage analysis was performed to determine the chromosomal location of a FNMTC susceptibility gene. Thirty-one members of the multigeneration FNMTC kindred were genotyped using short tandem repeat polymorphisms in close proximity to the chromosomal location of the candidate genes of interest and haplotypes were constructed. Kindred members were reviewed for thyroid neoplasms, premenopausal breast carcinoma, and rare nonthyroidal neoplasms common to more than a single subject. The five subjects with thyroid carcinoma in this family had been identified independently by different primary care physicians without knowledge of the positive family history. PTCs were all greater than 3 cm in diameter at the time of diagnosis. Papillary renal neoplasms (PRN) were present in two of the five affected members with PTC. Mutational analysis by DNA sequencing performed to exclude germline mutations of the MET proto-oncogene, which confer a genetic predisposition to the development of PRC. No mutations were identified in MET exons 12, 13, 16, 17, 18, 19, and 20, which include all known sites of mutations that confer FNMTC susceptibility. Linkage to *RET*, *PTEN*, *TCO*, and *MNG1* genes was excluded. The region of 1q21 was found to be linked to the fPTC/PRN phenotype, when *NTRK1* and *PRCC*, both candidates in this region, were tested for linkage. The genome-wide screen identified this same region as a likely site of linkage. The two highest LOD scores were 2.35 and 1.29 at markers D22S685 and D1S534, respectively. No other LOD scores were greater than 0.9. Haplotype analysis and multipoint analysis using markers surrounding D22S685 suggested that this chromosomal region was unlikely to be linked to the disease phenotype. In contrast, investigation of markers surrounding D1S534 confirmed linkage and defined the limits of the chromosomal region harboring the susceptibility gene.

An association of fPTC with both nodular thyroid disease and PRN was observed in the kindred. There are multiple lines of evidence supporting the likelihood that PRN is part of the FNMTC syndrome in the kindred. The occurrence of PRN in two kindred members strongly suggests a genetic predisposition, since sporadic PRN is extremely rare. An inherited predisposition in this kindred is further supported by the multifocality of papillary renal adenomas. Potential candidate genes located in the chromosomal region of linkage include *N-RAS* and *NTRK1*. Activating RAS mutations have been identified in both benign and malignant thyroid neoplasms. However, they are more common in follicular neoplasms than in papillary neoplasms [263–267]. NTRK1 is rearranged in sporadic PTC, but it is not normally expressed in the thyroid. Therefore, it is unlikely that a germline mutation of NTRK1 would predispose to the development of PTC. A gene that is rearranged in sporadic papillary renal carcinomas, *PRCC*, is in the region of 1q21, although its precise location in this broad region has not yet been determined. This gene is expressed in multiple tissues [268] and is a potential candidate gene for this disorder.

Acknowledgments This work was supported by the *Eunice Kennedy Shriver* National Institute of Child Health and Human Development (NICHD), intramural National Institutes of Health (NIH) project Z01-HD-000642-04 to Dr. C. A. Stratakis.

We thank Dr. Francesco Celi (now at MCV, Richmond,VA) for breast cancer only, but given the reviewing the chapter.

References

1. Jemal A, Siegel R, Xu J, Ward E. Cancer statistics, 2010. CA Cancer J Clin. 2010;60:277–300.
2. US Mortality Files, National Center for Health Statistics, Centers for Disease Control and Prevention; incidence, SEER 9. http://seer.cancer.gov/faststats/selections.php.
3. Leenhardt L, Grosclaude P, Cherie-Challine L. Increased incidence of thyroid carcinoma in France: a true epidemic or thyroid nodule management effects? Report from the French thyroid cancer committee. Thyroid. 2004;14:1056–60.
4. Baloch ZW, LiVolsi VA. Microcarcinoma of the thyroid. Adv Anat Pathol. 2006;13:69–75.
5. Baloch ZW, LiVolsi VA. Pathologic diagnosis of papillary thyroid carcinoma: today and tomorrow. Expert Rev Mol Diagn. 2005;5:573–84.

6. Hundahl SA, Fleming ID, Fremgen AM, et al. National Cancer Data Base report on 53,856 cases of thyroid carcinoma treated in the U.S., 1985–1988. Cancer. 1998;83(12):243–6.
7. Grossman RF, Tu SH, Duh QY, Siperstein AE, Novosolov F, Clark OH. Familial nonmedullary thyroid cancer. An emerging entity that warrants aggressive treatment. Arch Surg. 1995;130(8):892–9.
8. Capezzone M, Marchisotta S, Cantara S, Busonero G, Brilli L, Panayiotou KP, Carli AF, Caruso G, Toti P, Capitani S, Pammolli A, Pacini F. Familial non-medullary thyroid carcinoma displays the features of clinical anticipation suggestive of a distinct biological entity. Endocrinol Relat Cancer. 2008;15:1075–81.
9. Grossman R, Tu S, Duh Q, Siperstein A, Novosolov F, Clark O. Familial nonmedullary thyroid cancer an emerging entity that warrants aggressive treatment. Arch Surg. 1995;130:892–9.
10. Sturgeon C, Clark OH. Familial non medullary thyroid cancer. Thyroid. 2005;15(6):588–93.
11. Sipper RS, Caron NR, Clark OH. An evidence-based approach to familial nonmedullary thyroid cancer: screening, clinical management and follow up. World J Surg. 2007;31:924–33.
12. Robinson D, Orr T. Carcinoma of the thyroid and other diseases of the thyroid in identical twins. Arch Surg. 1955;70:923–8.
13. Lote K, Andersen K, Nordal E, Brennhovd IO. Familial occurrence of papillary thyroid carcinoma. Cancer. 1980;46:1291–7.
14. Ozaki O, Ito K, Kobayashi K, Suzuki A, Manabe Y, Hosoda Y. Familial occurrence of differentiated, nonmedullary thyroid carcinoma. World J Surg. 1988;12:565–71.
15. Houlston RS, Stratton MR. Genetics of non-medullary thyroid cancer. Q J Med. 1995;88:685–93.
16. Burgess JR, Duffield A, Wilkinson SJ, Ware R, Greenawa TM, Percival J, Hoffman L. Two families with an autosomal dominant inheritance pattern for papillary carcinoma of the thyroid. J Clin Endocrinol Metab. 1997;82:345–8.
17. Schlumberger MJ. Papillary and follicular thyroid carcinoma. N Engl J Med. 1998;338:297–306.
18. Musholt TJ, Musholt PB, Petrich T, Oetting G, Knapp WH, Klempnauer J. Familial papillary thyroid carcinoma: genetics criteria for diagnosis, clinical features and surgical treatment. World J Surg. 2000;24:1409–17.
19. Malchoff C, Malchoff D. Familial non-medullary thyroid carcinoma. Semin Surg Oncol. 1999;16:16–8.
20. Pal T, Bogl FD, Chappuis PO, Tsang R, Brierley J, Renard H, Sanders K, Kantemiroff T, Bagha S, Goldgar DE, Narod SA, Goulkes WD. Increased risk for nonmedullary thyroid cancer in the first degree relatives of prevalent cases of nonmedullary thyroid cancer: a hospital-based study. J Clin Endocrinol Metab. 2001;86:5307–12.
21. Orsenigo E, Beretta E, Gini P, Berrecchia F, Invernizzi L, Fiorina P, Carlo VD. A report of six cases of familial papillary thyroid cancer. Eur J Surg Oncol. 2003;29:185–7.
22. Frich L, Glattre E, Akslen LA. Familial occurrence of nonmedullary thyroid cancer: a population based study of 5673 first degree relatives of thyroid cancer patients from Norway. Cancer Epidemiol Biomarkers Prev. 2001;10:113–7.
23. Maxwell EL, Hall FT, Freeman JL. Familial nonmedullary thyroid cancer: a matched-case control study. Laryngoscope. 2004;114: 2182–6.
24. Malchoff C, Malchoff D. Familial non-medullary thyroid carcinoma. Cancer Control. 2006;13:106–10.
25. Charkes ND. On the prevalence of familial non-medullary thyroid cancer in multiply affected kindreds. Thyroid. 2006;16:181–6.
26. Takami H, Ozaki O, Ito K. Familial non medullary thyroid cancer: an emerging entity that warrants aggressive treatment. Arch Surg. 1996;131:676.
27. Triponez F, Wong M, Sturgeon C, et al. Does familial non-medullary thyroid cancer adversely affect survival? World J Surg. 2006;30(5):787–93.
28. Nelen MR, Padberg GW, Peeters EA, Lin AY, van den Helm B, Frants RR, Coulon V, Goldstein AM, van Reen MM, Easton DF, Eeles RA, Hodgsen S, Mulvihill JJ, Murday VA, Tucker MA, Mariman EC, Starink TM, Ponder BA, Ropers HH, Kremer H, Longy M, Eng C. Localization of the gene for Cowden disease to chromosome 10q22-23. Nat Genet. 1996;13(1):114–6.
29. Waite KA, Eng C. Protean PTEN: form and function. Am J Hum Genet. 2002;70(4):829–44. Epub 2002 Mar 1.
30. Eng C. PTEN: one gene, many syndromes. Hum Mutat. 2003; 22(3):183–98.
31. Pilarski R, Eng C. Will the real Cowden syndrome please stand up (again)? Expanding mutational and clinical spectra of the PTEN hamartoma tumor syndrome. J Med Genet. 2004;41(5):32.
32. Gorlin RJ, Cohen Jr MM, Condon LM, Burke BA. Bannayan-Riley-Ruvalcaba syndrome. Am J Med Genet. 1992;44:307–14.
33. Ginn-Peace, Eng C. Increased nuclear phosphatase and tensin homologue deleted on chromosome 10 is associated with G0-G1 in MCF-7 cells. Cancer Res. 2003;63(2):282–6.
34. Chung JH, Ginn-Peace ME, Eng C. Phosphatase and tensin homologue deleted on chromosome 10 (PTEN) has nuclear localization signal-like sequences for nuclear import mediated by major vault protein. Cancer Res. 2005;65(10):4108–16.
35. Minaguchi T, Waite KA, Eng C. Nuclear localization of PTEN is regulated by Ca (2+) through a tyrosil phosphorylation-independent conformational modification in major vault protein. Cancer Res. 2006;66(24):11677–82.
36. Shen, et al. Essential role for nuclear PTEN in maintaining chromosomal integrity. Cell. 2007;128(1):157–70.
37. Nelen MR, van Staveren CG, Peeters EAJ, Ben Hassel M, Gorlin RJ, Hamm H, Lindboe CF, Fryns J-P, Sijmons RH, Woods DG, Mariman ECM, Padberg GW, Kremer H. Germline mutations in the *PTEN/MMAC1* gene in patients with Cowden disease. Hum Mol Genet. 1997;6:1383–7.
38. Eng C. Will the real Cowden syndrome please stand up: revised diagnostic criteria. J Med Genet. 2000;37:828–30.
39. NCCN. Genetic/familial high-risk assessment: breast and ovarian. Clin Pract Guidelines Oncol.
40. Starink TM, van der Veen JP, Arwert F, de Waal LP, de Lange GG, Gille JJ, Eriksson AW. The Cowden syndrome: a clinical and genetic study in 21 patients. Clin Genet. 1986;29(3):222–33.
41. Hanssen AM, Fryns JP. Cowden syndrome. J Med Genet. 1995;32(2):117–9.
42. Longy M, Lacombe D. Cowden disease. Report of a family and review. Ann Genet. 1996;39(1):35–42.
43. Koksal Y, Sahin M, Koksal H, Orhan D, Unal E, Alagoz E. Thyroid medullary carcinoma in a teenager with Cowden syndrome. Laryngoscope. 2007;117(7):1180–2.
44. Tan WH, Baris HN, Burrows PE, Robson CD, Alomari AI, Mulliken JB, Fishman SJ, Irons MB. The spectrum of vascular anomalies in patients with PTEN mutations: implications for diagnosis and management. J Med Genet. 2007;44(9):594–602. Epub 2007 May 25.
45. Harach H, Soubeyran I, Brown A, et al. Thyroid pathologic findings in patients with Cowden disease. Ann Diagn Pathol. 1999;3: 331–40.
46. Marsh DJ, Coulon V, Lunetta KL, Rocca-Serra P, Dahia PL, Zheng Z, Liaw D, Caron S, Duboué B, Lin AY, Richardson AL, Bonnetblanc JM, Bressieux JM, Cabarrot-Moreau A, Chompret A, Demange L, Eeles RA, Yahanda AM, Fearon ER, Fricker JP, Gorlin RJ, Hodgson SV, Huson S, Lacombe D, Eng C, et al. Mutation spectrum and genotype phenotype analyses in Cowden disease and Bannayan-Zonana syndrome, two hamartoma syndromes with germline PTEN mutation. Hum Mol Genet. 1998;7:507–15.
47. Zhou XP, Waite KA, Pilarski R, Hampel H, Fernandez MJ, Bos C, Dasouki M, Feldman GL, Greenberg LA, Ivanovich J, Matloff E,

Patterson A, Pierpont ME, Russo D, Nassif NT, Eng C. Germline PTEN promoter mutations and deletions in Cowden/Bannayan-Riley-Ruvalcaba syndrome result in aberrant PTEN protein and dysregulation of the phosphoinositol-3-kinase/Akt pathway. Am J Hum Genet. 2003;73:404–11.
48. Tan MH, Mester J, Peterson C, Yang Y, Chen JL, Rybicki LA, Milas K, Pederson H, Remzi B, Orloff MS, Eng C. A clinical scoring system for selection of patients for PTEN mutation testing is proposed on the basis of a prospective study of 3042 probands. Am J Hum Genet. 2011;88:42–56.
49. Pezzolesi MG, Platzer P, Waite KA, Eng C. Differential expression of PTEN-targeting microRNAs miR-19a and miR-21 in Cowden syndrome. Am J Hum Genet. 2008;82(5):1141–9.
50. Ni Y, Zbuk KM, Sadler T, Patocs A, Lobo G, Edelman E, Platzer P, Orloff MS, Waite KA, Eng C. Germline mutations and variants in the succinate dehydrogenase genes in Cowden and Cowden-like syndromes. Am J Hum Genet. 2008;83(2):261–8.
51. Marsh DJ, Kum JB, Lunetta KL, Bennett MJ, Gorlin RJ, Ahmed SF, Bodurtha J, Crowe C, Curtis MA, Dasouki M, Dunn T, Feit H, Geraghty MT, Graham JM, Hodgson SV, Hunter A, Korf BR, Manchester D, Miesfeldt S, Murday VA, Nathanson KL, Parisi M, Pober B, Romano C, Eng C, et al. PTEN mutation spectrum and genotype-phenotype correlations in Bannayan- Riley-Ruvalcaba syndrome suggest a single entity with Cowden syndrome. Hum Mol Genet. 1999;8:1461–72.
52. Petersen GM, Slack J, Nakamura Y. Screening guidelines and premorbid diagnosis of familial adenomatous polyposis using linkage. Gastroenterology. 1991;100:1658–64.
53. Heald RJ, Bussey HJ. Clinical experiences at St. Mark's Hospital with multiple synchronous cancers of the colon and rectum. Dis Colon Rectum. 1975;18(1):6–10.
54. Evans DG, Guy SP, Thakker N, Armstrong JG, Dodd C, Davies DR, Babbs C, Clancy T, Warnes T, Sloan P, et al. Non-penetrance and late appearance of polyps in families with familial adenomatous polyposis. Gut. 1993;34:1389–93.
55. Giardiello FM, Krush AJ, Petersen GM, Booker SV, Kerr M, Tong LL, Hamilton SR. Phenotypic variability of familial adenomatous polyposis in 11 unrelated families with identical APC gene mutation. Gastroenterology. 1994;106:1542–7.
56. Rozen P, Samuel Z, Shomrat R, Legum C. Notable intrafamilial phenotypic variability in a kindred with familial adenomatous polyposis and an APC mutation in exon 9. Gut. 1999;45:829–33.
57. Burt RW. Colon cancer screening. Gastroenterology. 2000;119(3): 837–53.
58. Crail HW. Multiple primary malignancies arising in the rectum, brain and thyroid. US Navy Med Bull. 1949;49:123–8.
59. Camiel RM, Mule EJ, Alexander LL, et al. Association of thyroid Carcinoma with Gardner's syndrome in siblings. N Engl J Med. 1968;278(19):1056–8.
60. Plail RO, Bussey HJ, Glazer G, et al. Adenomatous polyposis: an association with carcinoma of the thyroid. Br J Surg. 1987; 74(5):377–80.
61. Bülow C, Bülow S, Leeds Castle Polyposis Group. Is screening for thyroid carcinoma indicated in familial adenomatous polyposis? Int J Color Dis. 1997;12(4):240–2.
62. Iwama T, Mishima Y, Utsunomiya J. The impact of familial adenomatous polyposis on the tumorigenesis and mortality at the several organs. Its rational treatment. Ann Surg. 1993;217(2):101–8.
63. Cetta F, Montalto G, Gori M, et al. Germline mutations of the APC gene in patients with familial adenomatous polyposis-associated thyroid carcinoma: results from a European cooperative study. J Clin Endocrinol Metab. 2000;85(1):286–92.
64. Paul P, Letteboer T, Gelbert L, et al. Identical APC exon 15 mutations result in a variable phenotype in familial adenomatous polyposis. Hum Mol Genet. 1993;2:925–31.
65. Truta B, Allen BA, Conrad PG, et al. Genotype and phenotype of patients with both familial adenomatous polyposis and thyroid carcinoma. Fam Cancer. 2003;2:95–9.
66. Herraiz M, Barbesino G, Faquin W, Chan-Smutko G, Patel D, Shannon KM, Daniels GH, Chung DC. Prevalence of thyroid cancer in familial adenomatous polyposis syndrome and the role of screening ultrasound examinations. Clin Gastroenterol Hepatol. 2007;5(3):367–73. Epub 2007 Jan 26.
67. Jarrar AM, Milas M, Mitchell J, Laguardia L, O'Malley M, Berber E, Siperstein A, Burke C, Church JM. Screening for thyroid cancer in patients with familial adenomatous polyposis. Ann Surg. 2011;253(3):515–21.
68. Lefevre JH, Rodrigue CM, Mourra N, Bennis M, Flejou JF, Parc R, Tiret E, Gespach C, Parc YR. Implication of MYH in colorectal polyposis. Ann Surg. 2006;244:874–9.
69. Hes FJ, Nielsen M, Bik EC, Konvalinka D, Wijnen JT, Bakker E, Vasen HF, Breuning MH, Tops CM. Somatic APC mosaicism: an underestimated cause of polyposis coli. Gut. 2007;57:71–6.
70. Sieber OM, Lamlum H, Crabtree MD, Rowan AJ, Barclay E, Lipton L, Hodgson S, Thomas HJW, Neale K, Phillips RKS, Farrington SM, Dunlop MG, Mueller HJ, Bisgaard ML, Bülow S, Fidalgo P, Albuquerque C, Scarano MI, Bodmer W, Tomlinson IPM, Heinimann K. Whole-gene APC deletions cause classical familial adenomatous polyposis, but not attenuated polyposis or "multiple" colorectal adenomas. Proc Natl Acad Sci U S A. 2002;99:2954–8.
71. Bunyan DJ, Eccles DM, Sillibourne J, Wilkins E, Thomas NS, Shea-Simonds J, Duncan PJ, Curtis CE, Robinson DO, Harvey JF, Cross NC. Dosage analysis of cancer predisposition genes by multiplex ligation-dependent probe amplification. Br J Cancer. 2004;91:1155–9.
72. Aretz S, Stienen D, Uhlhaas S, Pagenstecher C, Mangold E, Caspari R, Propping P, Friedl W. Large submicroscopic genomic APC deletions are a common cause of typical familial adenomatous polyposis. J Med Genet. 2005;42:185–92.
73. Michils G, Tejpar S, Thoelen R, van Cutsem E, Vermeesch JR, Fryns JP, Legius E, Matthijs G. Large deletions of the APC gene in 15% of mutation-negative patients with classical polyposis (FAP): a Belgian study. Hum Mutat. 2005;25:125–34.
74. Burt RW, Ward K, Spirio L, et al. Accurate identification of familial adenomatous polyposis coli using newly developed genetic markers. Gastroenterology. 1992;102:A347.
75. Carney JA, Gordon H, Carpenter PC, Shenoy BV, Go VL. The complex of myxomas, spotty pigmentation, and endocrine overactivity. Medicine (Baltimore). 1985;64:270–83.
76. Stratakis CA, Bertherat J, Carney JA. Mutation of perinatal myosin heavy chain. N Engl J Med. 2004;351:2556–8.
77. Kirschner LS, Sandrini F, Monbo J, Lin JP, Carney JA, Stratakis CA. Genetic heterogeneity and spectrum of mutations of the PRKAR1A gene in patients with the Carney complex. Hum Mol Genet. 2000;9:3037–46.
78. Veugelers M, Wilkes D, Burton K, McDermott DA, Song Y, Goldstein MM, La Perle K, Vaughan CJ, O'Hagan A, Bennett KR, Meyer BJ, Legius E, Karttunen M, Norio R, Kaariainen H, Lavyne M, Neau JP, Richter G, Kirali K, Farnsworth A, Stapleton K, Morelli P, Takanashi Y, Bamforth JS, Eitelberger F, Noszian I, Manfroi W, Powers J, Mochizuki Y, Imai T, Ko GT, Driscoll DA, Goldmuntz E, Edelberg JM, Collins A, Eccles D, Irvine AD, McKnight GS, Basson CT. Comparative PRKAR1A genotype-phenotype analyses in humans with Carney complex and prkar1a haploinsufficient mice. Proc Natl Acad Sci U S A. 2004; 101:14222–7.
79. Groussin L, Kirschner L, Vincent-Dejean C, Perlemoine K, Jullian E, Delemer B, Zacharieva S, Pignatelli D, Carney JA, Luton JP, Bertagna X, Stratakis CA, Bertherat J. Molecular analysis of the

cyclic AMP-dependent protein kinase A (PKA) regulatory subunit 1A (PRKAR1A) gene in patients with Carney complex and Primary Pigmented Nodular Adrenocortical Disease (PPNAD) reveals novel mutations and clues for pathophysiology. Am J Hum Genet. 2002;71:1432–42.
80. Groussin L, Jullian E, Perlemoine K, Leheup B, Luton JP, Bertagna X, Bertherat J. Mutations of the PRKAR1A gene in Cushing's syndrome due to sporadic primary pigmented nodular adrenocortical disease (PPNAD). J Clin Endocrinol Metab. 2002;87:4324–9.
81. Mateus C, Palangié A, Franck N, Groussin L, Bertagna X, Avril MF, Bertherat J, Dupin N. Heterogeneity of skin manifestations in patients with Carney complex. J Am Acad Dermatol. 2008;59: 801–10.
82. Stratakis C, Horvath A. Gene Rev. 2003.
83. Stratakis CA, Carney JA, Lin JP, Papanicolaou DA, Karl M, Kastner DL, Pras E, Chrousos GP. Carney complex, a familial multiple neoplasia and lentiginosis syndrome. Analysis of 11 kindreds and linkage to the short arm of chromosome 2. J Clin Invest. 1996;97:699–705.
84. Casey M, Mah C, Merliss AD, Kirschner LS, Taymans SE, Denio AE, Korf B, Irvine AD, Hughes A, Carney JA, Stratakis CA, Basson CT. Identification of a novel genetic locus for familial cardiac myxomas and Carney complex. Circulation. 1998;98: 2560–6.
85. Kirschner LS, Carney JA, Pack SD, Taymans SE, Giatzakis C, Cho YS, Cho-Chung YS, Stratakis CA. Mutations of the gene encoding the protein kinase A type I-alpha regulatory subunit in patients with the Carney complex. Nat Genet. 2000;26:89–92.
86. Casey M, Vaughan CJ, He J, Hatcher CJ, Winter JM, Weremowicz S, Montgomery K, Kucherlapati R, Morton CC, Basson CT. Mutations in the protein kinase A R1alpha regulatory subunit cause familial cardiac myxomas and Carney complex. J Clin Invest. 2000;106:R31–8.
87. Bier B, Seitz G, Bach R, Volkmer I, Frohlig G. Multiple cutaneous myxomas coinciding with repeated cardiac myxomas. A syndrome. Thorac Cardiovasc Surg. 1989;37:317–9.
88. Ain KB. Papillary thyroid carcinoma. Etiology, assessment, and therapy. Endocrinol Metab Clin N Am. 1995;24:711–60.
89. Radin R, Kempf RA. Carney complex: report of three cases. Radiology. 1995;196:383–6.
90. Schoenberg-Fejzo M. Integrated map of chromosome 17q critical region in multiple sclerosis. Am J Hum Genet. 1999;65:A442.
91. Stratakis CA, Kirschner LS, Taymans SE, Carney JA, Basson CT. Genetic heterogeneity in Carney complex (OMIM 160980): contributions of loci at chromosomes 2 and 17 in its genetics. Am J Hum Genet. 1999;65:A447.
92. Bertherat J, Horvath A, Groussin L, Grabar S, Boikos S, Cazabat L, Libe R, René-Corail F, Stergiopoulos S, Bourdeau I, Bei T, Clauser E, Calender A, Kirschner LS, Bertagna X, Carney JA, Stratakis CA. Mutations in regulatory subunit type 1A of cyclic adenosine 5′-monophosphate-dependent protein kinase (PRKAR1A): phenotype analysis in 353 patients and 80 different genotypes. J Clin Endocrinol Metab. 2009;94:2085–91.
93. Cazabat L, Libè R, Perlemoine K, René-Corail F, Burnichon N, Gimenez-Roqueplo AP, Dupasquier-Fediaevsky L, Bertagna X, Clauser E, Chanson P, Bertherat J, Raffin-Sanson ML. Germline inactivating mutations of the aryl hydrocarbon receptor-interacting protein gene in a large cohort of sporadic acromegaly: mutations are found in a subset of young patients with macroadenomas. Eur J Endocrinol. 2007;157:1–8.
94. Horvath A, Bossis I, Giatzakis C, Levine E, Weinberg F, Meoli E, Robinson-White A, Siegel J, Soni P, Groussin L, Matyakhina L, Verma S, Remmers E, Nesterova M, Carney JA, Bertherat J, Stratakis CA. Large deletions of the PRKAR1A gene in Carney complex. Clin Cancer Res. 2008;14:388–95.
95. Courcoutsakis N, Patronas N, Filie AC, Carney JA, Moraitis A, Stratakis C. Ectopic thymus presenting as a thyroid nodule in a patient with the Carney complex. Thyroid. 2009;19(3):293–6.
96. Werner O. On cataract in conjunction with scleroderma (doctoral dissertation, Kiel University), Kiel: Schmidt and Klaunig; 1904.
97. Ishida R. A case of cataract associated with scleroderma. Nippon Gannka Gakkai Zasshi. 1917;21:1025–32.
98. Oppenheimer BS, Kugel VH. Werner's syndrome – a heredofamilial disorder with scleroderma, bilateral juvenile cataract, precocious graying of hair and endocrine stigmatization. Trans Ass Am Phys. 1934;49:358–70.
99. Oppenheimer BS, Kugel VH. Werner's syndrome, report of the first necropsy and of findings in a new case. Am J Med Sci. 1941;202:629–42.
100. Agatson SA, Gartner S. Precocious cataracts and scleroderma (Rothmund's syndrome; Werner's syndrome). Arch Ophthalmol. 1939;21:492–6.
101. Goto M. Hierarchical deterioration of body systems in Werner's syndrome: implications for normal ageing. Mech Ageing Dev. 1997;98(3):239–54.
102. Yu CE, Oshima J, Wijsman EM, Nakura J, Miki T, Piussan C, Matthews S, Fu YH, Mulligan J, Martin GM, Schellenberg GD. Mutations in the consensus helicase domains of the Werner syndrome gene. Werner's Syndrome Collaborative Group. Am J Hum Genet. 1997;60:330–41.
103. Opresko PL, Cheng WH, von Kobbe C, Harrigan JA, Bohr VA. Werner syndrome and the function of the Werner protein; what they can teach us about the molecular aging process. Carcinogenesis. 2003;24:791–802.
104. Bohr VA. DeWcient DNA repair in the human progeroid disorder, Werner syndrome. Mutat Res. 2005;577:252–9.
105. Nakura J, Wijsman EM, Miki T, Kamino K, Yu CE, Oshima J, Fukuchi K, Weber JL, Piussan C, Melaragno MI. Homozygosity mapping of the Werner syndrome locus (WRN). Genomics. 1994;23:600–8.
106. Huang S, Lee L, Hanson NB, Lenaerts C, Hoehn H, Poot M, Rubin CD, Chen DF, Yang CC, Juch H, Dorn T, Spiegel R, Oral EA, Abid M, Battisti C, Lucci-Cordisco E, Neri G, Steed EH, Kidd A, Isley W, Showalter D, Vittone JL, Konstantinow A, Ring J, Meyer P, Wenger SL, von Herbay A, Wollina U, Schuelke M, Huizenga CR, Leistritz DF, Martin GM, Mian IS, Oshima J. The spectrum of WRN mutations in Werner syndrome patients. Hum Mutat. 2006;27:558–67.
107. Ishikawa Y, Sugano H, Matsumoto T, Furuichi Y, Miller R, Goto M. Unusual features of thyroid carcinomas in Japanese patients with Werner syndrome and possible genotype-phenotype relations to cell type and race. Cancer Sci. 1999;85:1345–52.
108. Goto M, Miller RW, Ishikawa Y, Sugano H. Excess of rare cancers in Werner syndrome (adult progeria). Cancer Epidemiol Biomarkers Prev. 1996;5(4):239–46.
109. Goto M, Imamura O, Kuromitsu J, Matsumoto T, Yamabe Y, Tokutake Y, Suzuki N, Mason B, Drayna D, Sugawara M, Sugimoto M, Furuichi Y. Analysis of helicase gene mutations in Japanese Werner's syndrome patients. Hum Genet. 1997;99: 191–3.
110. Oshima J, Yu CE, Piussan C, Klein G, Jabkowski J, Balci S, Miki T, Nakura J, Ogihara T, Ells J, Smith M, Melaragno MI, Fraccaro M, Scappaticci S, Matthews J, Ouais S, Jarzebowicz A, Schellenberg GD, Martin GM. Homozygous and compound heterozygous mutations at the Werner syndrome locus. Hum Mol Genet. 1996;5:1909–13.
111. Pendred V. Deaf-mutism and goitre. Lancet. 1896;ii:532.
112. Reardon W, Coffey R, Phelps PD, Luxon LM, Stephens D, Kendall-Taylor P, Britton KE, Grossman A, Trembath R. Pendred syndrome – 100 years of under ascertainment? Q J Med. 1997;90: 443–7.

113. Fraser GR. Association of congenital deafness with goitre (Pendred's syndrome) a study of 207 families. Ann Hum Genet. 1965;28:201–49.
114. Morgans ME, Trotter WR. Association of congenital deafness with goiter; the nature of the thyroid defect. Lancet. 1958;1: 607–9.
115. Kopp P, Pesce L, Solis SJ. Pendred syndrome and iodide transport in the thyroid. Trends Endocrinol Metab. 2008;19:260–8.
116. Cremers WR, Bolder C, Admiraal RJ, Everett LA, Joosten FB, van Hauwe P, Green ED, Otten BJ. Progressive sensorineural hearing loss and a widened vestibular aqueduct in Pendred syndrome. Arch Otolaryngol Head Neck Surg. 1998;124:501–5.
117. Colvin IB, Beale T, Harrop-Griffiths K. Long-term follow-up of hearing loss in children and young adults with enlarged vestibular aqueducts: relationship to radiologic findings and Pendred syndrome diagnosis. Laryngoscope. 2006;116:2027–36.
118. Luxon LM, Cohen M, Coffey RA, Phelps PD, Britton KE, Jan H, Trembath RC, Reardon W. Neuro-otological findings in Pendred syndrome. Int J Audiol. 2003;42:82–8.
119. Fugazzola L, Mannavola D, Cerutti N, Maghnie M, Pagella F, Bianchi P, Weber G, Persani L, Beck-Peccoz P. Molecular analysis of the Pendred's syndrome gene and magnetic resonance imaging studies of the inner ear are essential for the diagnosis of true Pendred's syndrome. J Clin Endocrinol Metab. 2000;85: 2469–75.
120. Phelps PD, Coffey RA, Trembath RC, Luxon LM, Grossman AB, Britton KE, Kendall-Taylor P, Graham JM, Cadge BC, Stephens SG, Pembrey ME, Reardon W. Radiological malformations of the ear in Pendred syndrome. Clin Radiol. 1998;53:268–73.
121. Fraser GR, Morgans ME, Trotter WR. The syndrome of sporadic goitre and congenital deafness. Q J Med. 1960;29:279–95.
122. Pryor SP, Madeo AC, Reynolds JC, Sarlis NJ, Arnos KS, Nance WE, Yang Y, Zalewski CK, Brewer CC, Butman JA, Griffith AJ. SLC26A4/PDS genotype-phenotype correlation in hearing loss with enlargement of the vestibular aqueduct (EVA): evidence that Pendred syndrome and non-syndromic EVA are distinct clinical and genetic entities. J Med Genet. 2005;42:159–65.
123. Baschieri L, Benedetti G, Deluca F, Negri M. Evaluation and limitations of the perchlorate test in the study of thyroid function. J Clin Endocrinol Metab. 1963;23:786–91.
124. Kopp P. Thyroid hormone synthesis: thyroid iodine metabolism. In: Braverman L, Utiger R, editors. Wegner and Ingbar's the thyroid: a fundamental and clinical text. Philadelphia: Lippincott Williams & Wilkins; 2005. p. 52–76.
125. Park HJ, Lee SJ, Jin HS, Lee JO, Go SH, Jang HS, Moon SK, Lee SC, Chun YM, Lee HK, Choi JY, Jung SC, Griffith AJ, Koo SK. Genetic basis of hearing loss associated with enlarged vestibular aqueducts in Koreans. Clin Genet. 2005;67:160–5.
126. Gonzalez Trevino O, Karamanoglu Arseven O, Ceballos CJ, Vives VI, Ramirez RC, Gomez VV, Medeiros-Neto G, Kopp P. Clinical and molecular analysis of three Mexican families with Pendred's syndrome. Eur J Endocrinol. 2001;144:585–93.
127. Sheffield VC, Kraiem Z, Beck JC, Nishimura D, Stone EM, Salameh M, Sadeh O, Glaser B. Pendred syndrome maps to chromosome 7q21–34 and is caused by an intrinsic defect in thyroid iodine organification. Nat Genet. 1996;12:424–6.
128. Everett LA, Green ED. A family of mammalian anion transporters and their involvement in human genetic diseases. Hum Mol Genet. 1999;8:1883–91.
129. Scott DA, Karniski LP. Human pendrin expressed in Xenopus laevis oocytes mediates chloride/formate exchange. Am J Physiol Cell Physiol. 2000;278:C207–11.
130. Everett LA. New insights into the role of pendrin (SLC26A4) in inner ear fluid homeostasis. Novartis Found Symp. 2006;273:213–25. discussion 225–230, 261–264.
131. Soleimani M, Greeley T, Petrovic S, Wang Z, Amlal H, Kopp P, Burnham CE. Pendrin: an apical $Cl^-/OH^-/HCO^{3-}$ exchanger in the kidney cortex. Am J Physiol Ren Physiol. 2001;280:F356–64.
132. Scott DA, Wang R, Kreman TM, Sheffield VC, Karniski LP. The Pendred syndrome gene encodes a chloride-iodide transport protein. Nat Genet. 1999;21:440–3.
133. Royaux IE, Suzuki K, Mori A, Katoh R, Everett LA, Kohn LD, Green ED. Pendrin, the protein encoded by the Pendred syndrome gene (PDS), is an apical porter of iodide in the thyroid and is regulated by thyroglobulin in FRTL-5 cells. Endocrinology. 2000;141:839–45.
134. Gillam MP, Sidhaye AR, Lee EJ, Rutishauser J, Stephan CW, Kopp P. Functional characterization of pendrin in a polarized cell system. Evidence for pendrin-mediated apical iodide efflux. J Biol Chem. 2004;279:13004–10.
135. Dohan O, De la Vieja A, Paroder V, Riedel C, Artani M, Reed M, Ginter CS, Carrasco N. The sodium/iodide Symporter (NIS): characterization, regulation, and medical significance. Endocr Rev. 2003;24:48–77.
136. Golstein P, Abramow M, Dumont JE, Beauwens R. The iodide channel of the thyroid: a plasma membrane vesicle study. Am J Physiol. 1992;263:C590–7.
137. Everett LA, Belyantseva IA, Noben-Trauth K, Cantos R, Chen A, Thakkar SI, Hoogstraten-Miller SL, Kachar B, Wu DK, Green ED. Targeted disruption of mouse Pds provides insight about the inner-ear defects encountered in Pendred syndrome. Hum Mol Genet. 2001;10:153–61.
138. Sato E, Nakashima T, Miura Y, Furuhashi A, Nakayama A, Mori N, Murakami H, Naganawa S, Tadokoro M. Phenotypes associated with replacement of his by Arg in the Pendred syndrome gene. Eur J Endocrinol. 2001;145:697–703.
139. Wangemann P, Kim HM, Billings S, Nakaya K, Li X, Singh R, Sharlin DS, Forrest D, Marcus DC, Fong P. Developmental delays consistent with cochlear hypothyroidism contribute to failure to develop hearing in mice lacking Slc26a4/pendrin expression. Am J Physiol Ren Physiol. 2009;297:F1435–47.
140. Nilsson M, Bjorkman U, Ekholm R, Ericson LE. Iodide transport in primary cultured thyroid follicle cells: evidence of a TSH-regulated channel mediating iodide efflux selectively across the apical domain of the plasma membrane. Eur J Cell Biol. 1990;52:270–81.
141. Nilsson M, Bjorkman U, Ekholm R, Ericson LE. Polarized efflux of iodide in porcine thyrocytes occurs via a cAMP-regulated iodide channel in the apical plasma membrane. Acta Endocrinol (Copenh). 1992;126:67–74.
142. Weiss SJ, Philp NJ, Grollman EF. Effect of thyrotropin on iodide efflux in FRTL-5 cells mediated by Ca^{2+}. Endocrinology. 1984;114:1108–13.
143. Bürgi U, Peter HJ, Gerber H. Clinical manifestations and management of nontoxic and diffuse and nodular goiter. In: Braverman LE, Utiger RD, editors. The thyroid. 7th ed. Philadelphia: Lippincott- Raven; 1996. p. 896–900.
144. Pelizzo M, Bernante P, Toniato A, Fassiva A. Frequency of thyroid carcinoma in a recent series of 539 consecutive thyroidectomies for multinodular goiter. Tumori. 1997;83:653–5.
145. Vickery ALJ. The diagnosis of malignancy in dyshormonogenetic goiter. Clin Endocrinol Metab. 1985;10:317–35.
146. Thieme ET. A report of occurrence of deaf-mutism and goiter in four of six siblings of a North American family. Ann Surg. 1957;146:941–8.
147. Elman DS. Familial association of nerve deafness with nodular goiter and thyroid carcinoma. N Engl J Med. 1958;259:219–23.
148. Watanabe I. Dyshormonogenesis. Hokumon to Rinsho (Japanese). 1983;31:627–36.

149. Abs R, Verhelst J, Schoofs E, deSomer E. Hyperfunctioning metastatic follicular thyroid carcinoma in Pendred's syndrome. Cancer. 1991;67:2191–3.
150. Camargo R, Limbert E, Gillam M, Henriques MM, Fernandes C, Catarino AL, Soares J, Alves VAF, Kopp P, Medeiros-Neto G. Aggressive metastatic follicular thyroid carcinoma with anaplastic transformation arising from a long-standing goiter in a patient with Pendred's syndrome. Thyroid. 2001;11(10):981. Mary Ann Liebert, Inc.
151. Mattos P, Bisi H, Medeiros-Neto G. Dyshormonogenetic goiter: a pathological and immunohistochemical study. Endocr Pathol. 1994;5:49–58.
152. Fagin JA. Carcinoma of follicular epithelium. Molecular pathogenesis. In: Braverman LE, Utiger RD, editors. The thyroid. 7th ed. Philadelphia: Lippincott-Raven; 1996. p. 909–16.
153. Ain K. Anaplastic thyroid carcinoma: behavior, biology, and therapeutic approaches. Thyroid. 1998;8:715–26.
154. Kopp P. Pendred syndrome: clinical characteristics and molecular basis. Curr Opin Endocrinol Diabetes. 1999;6:261–9.
155. Park HJ, Shaukat S, Liu XZ, Hahn SH, Naz S, Ghosh M, Kim HN, Moon SK, Abe S, Tukamoto K, Riazuddin S, Kabra M, Erdenetungalag R, Radnaabazar J, Khan S, Pandya A, Usami SI, Nance WE, Wilcox ER, Griffith AJ. Origins and frequencies of SLC26A4 (PDS) mutations in east and south Asians: global implications for the epidemiology of deafness. J Med Genet. 2003; 40:242–8.
156. Coyle B, Reardon W, Herbrick JA, Tsui LC, Gausden E, Lee J, Coffey R, Grueters A, Grossman A, Phelps PD, Luxon L, Kendall-Taylor P, Scherer SW, Trembath RC. Molecular analysis of the PDS gene in Pendred syndrome. Hum Mol Genet. 1998;7: 1105–12.
157. Campbell C, Cucci RA, Prasad S, Green GE, Edeal JB, Galer CE, Karniski LP, Sheffield VC, Smith RJ. Pendred syndrome, DFNB4, and PDS/SLC26A4 identification of eight novel mutations and possible genotype-phenotype correlations. Hum Mutat. 2001; 17:403–11.
158. Tsukamoto K, Suzuki H, Harada D, Namba A, Abe S, Usami S. Distribution and frequencies of PDS (SLC26A4) mutations in Pendred syndrome and nonsyndromic hearing loss associated with enlarged vestibular aqueduct: a unique spectrum of mutations in Japanese. Eur J Hum Genet. 2003;11:916–22.
159. Prasad S, Kölln KA, Cucci RA, Trembath RC, Van Camp G, Smith RJ. Pendred syndrome and DFNB4-mutation screening of SLC26A4 by denaturing high-performance liquid chromatography and the identification of eleven novel mutations. Am J Med Genet A. 2004;124A:1–9.
160. Pera A, Dossena S, Rodighiero S, Gandía M, Bottà G, Meyer G, Moreno F, Nofziger C, Hernández-Chico C, Paulmichl M. Functional assessment of allelic variants in the SLC26A4 gene involved in Pendred syndrome and nonsyndromic EVA. Proc Natl Acad Sci U S A. 2008;105(47):18608–13.
161. Smith RJH, Camp GV. Nonsyndromic hearing loss and deafness, DFNB1 includes: *GJB2*-related DFNB 1 nonsyndromic hearing loss and deafness, GJB6-related DFNB 1 nonsyndromic hearing loss and deafness.
162. Danon M, Crawford JD. The McCune-Albright syndrome. Ergeb Inn Med Kinderheilkd. 1987;55:81–115.
163. Shenker A, Weinstein LS, Moran A, Pescovitz OH, Charest NJ, Boney CM, Van Wyk JJ, Merino MJ, Feuillan PP, Spiegel AM. Severe endocrine and nonendocrine manifestations of the McCune-Albright syndrome associated with activating mutations of stimulatory G protein GS. J Pediatr. 1993;123:509–18. 3.
164. Okamoto S, Hisaoka M, Ushijima M, Nakahara S, Toyoshima S, Hashimoto H. Activating Gs(alpha) mutation in intramuscular myxomas with and without fibrous dysplasia of bone. Virchows Arch. 2000;437:133–7.
165. Collins MT, Chebli C, Jones J, Kushner H, Consugar M, Rinaldo P, Wientroub S, Bianco P, Robey PG. Renal phosphate wasting in fibrous dysplasia of bone is part of a generalized renal tubular dysfunction similar to that seen in tumor- induced osteomalacia. J Bone Miner Res. 2001;16:806–13.
166. Michiels FM, Caillou B, Talbot M, Dessarps-Freichey F, Maunoury MT, Schlumberger M, Mercken L, Monier R, Feunteun J. Oncogenic potential of guanine nucleotide stimulatory factor alpha subunit in thyroid glands of transgenic mice. Proc Natl Acad Sci U S A. 1994;91:10488–92.
167. Collins MT, Shenker A. McCune-Albright syndrome: new insights. Curr Opin Endocrinol Diabetes. 1999;6:119–25.
168. Collins MT, Sarlis NJ, Merino MJ, Monroe J, Crawford SE, Krakoff JA, Guthrie LC, Bonat S, Robey PG, Shenker A. Thyroid carcinoma in the McCune-Albright syndrome: contributory role of activating Gs_ mutations. J Clin Endocrinol Metab. 2003;88(9):4413–7.
169. Bhansali A, Sharma BS, Sreenivasulu P, Singh P, Vashisth RK, Dash RJ. Acromegaly with fibrous dysplasia: McCune-Albright syndrome – clinical studies in 3 cases and brief review of literature. Endocr J. 2003;50(6):793–9.
170. Feuillan PP, Shawker T, Rose SR, Jones J, Jeevanram RK, Nisula BC. Thyroid abnormalities in the McCune-Albright syndrome: ultrasonography and hormonal studies. J Clin Endocrinol Metab. 1990;71(6):1596–601.
171. Brogan P, Khadilkar VV, Stanhope R. Occult T3 toxicosis in McCune-Albright syndrome. Horm Res. 1998;50(2):105–6.
172. Lair-Milan F, Blevec GL, Carel JC, Chaussain JL, Adamsbaum C. Thyroid sonographic abnormalities in McCune-Albright syndrome. Pediatr Radiol. 1996;26(6):424–6.
173. Yang GC, Yao JL, Feiner HD, Roses DF, Kumar A, Mulder JE. Lipid-rich follicular carcinoma of the thyroid in a patient with McCune-Albright syndrome. Mod Pathol. 1999;12:969–73.
174. MacGarrity TJ, Amos C. Peutz-Jeghers syndrome: clinicopathological and molecular alterations. Cell Mol Life Sci. 2006;63:2135–44.
175. Peutz JLA. Very remarkable case of familial polyposis of the membrane of the intestinal tract and nasopharynx accompanied by peculiar pigmentations of the skin and mucous membrane. Ned Maandschr GeneeKd. 1921;10:134–46.
176. Jeghers H, McCusick VA, Katz KH. Generalized intestinal polyposis and melanin spots of the oral mucosa, lips and digits: a syndrome of diagnostic significance. N Engl J Med. 1949;241: 993–1012.
177. Schreibmann IR, Baker M, Amos C, et al. The Hamartomatous polyposis syndromes: a clinical and molecular review. Am J Gastroenterol. 2005;100:476–90.
178. Lindor NM, McMaster ML, Lindor CJ, Greene MH, National Cancer Institute, Division of Cancer Prevention, Community Oncology and Prevention Trials Research Group. Concise handbook of familial cancer susceptibility syndromes – second edition. J Natl Cancer Inst Monogr. 2008;38:1–93.
179. Gammon A, Jasperson K, Kohlmann W, Burt RW. Hamartomatous polyposis syndromes. Best Pract Res Clin Gastroenterol. 2009;23:219–31.
180. Boseto F, Shi E, Mitchell J, Preddy J, Adams S. Gastro duodenal intussusceptions due to Peutz-Jeghers syndrome in infancy. Pediatr Surg Int. 2002;18:178–80.
181. Collins SP, Reoma JL, Gamm DM, Uhler MD. LKB1, a novel serine/threonine protein kinase and potential tumour suppressor, is phosphorylated by cAMP-dependent protein kinase (PKA) and prenylated in vivo. Biochem J. 2000;345(Pt 3):673–80.
182. Mehenni H, Gehrig C, Nezu J, Oku A, Shimane M, Rossier C, Guex N, Blouin JL, Scott HS, Antonarakis SE. Loss of LKB1 kinase activity in Peutz-Jeghers syndrome, and evidence for allelic and locus heterogeneity. Am J Hum Genet. 1998;63:1641–50.

183. Karuman P, Gozani O, Odze RD, Zhou XC, Zhu H, Shaw R, Brien TP, Bozzuto CD, Ooi D, Cantley LC, Yuan J. The Peutz-Jegher gene product LKB1 is a mediator of p53-dependent cell death. Mol Cell. 2001;7:1307–19.
184. Tiainen M, Vaahtomeri K, Ylikorkala A, Makela TP. Growth arrest by the LKB1 tumor suppressor: induction of p21(WAF1/CIP1). Hum Mol Genet. 2002;11:1497–504.
185. Spicer J, Rayter S, Young N, Elliott R, Ashworth A, Smith D. Regulation of the Wnt signaling component PAR1A by the Peutz-Jeghers syndrome kinase LKB1. Oncogene. 2003;22: 4752–6.
186. Lizcano JM, Göransson O, Toth R, Deak M, Morrice NA, Boudeau J, Hawley SA, Udd L, Mäkelä TP, Hardie DG, Alessi DR. LKB1 is a master kinase that activates 13 kinases of the AMPK subfamily, including MARK/PAR-1. EMBO J. 2004;23(4):833–43.
187. Boudeau J, Sapkota G, Alessi DR. LKB1, a protein kinase regulating cell proliferation and polarity. FEBS Lett. 2003;546:159–65.
188. Spicer J, Ashworth A. LKB1 kinase: master and commander of metabolism and polarity. Curr Biol. 2004;14:R383–5.
189. Forcet C, Etienne-Manneville S, Gaude H, Fournier L, Debilly S, Salmi M, Baas A, Olschwang S, Clevers H, Billaud M. Functional analysis of Peutz-Jeghers mutations reveals that the LKB1 C-terminal region exerts a crucial role in regulating both the AMPK pathway and the cell polarity. Hum Mol Genet. 2005;14: 1283–92.
190. Kahn BB, Alquier T, Carling D, Hardie DG. AMP-activated protein kinase: ancient energy gauge provides clues to modern understanding of metabolism. Cell Metab. 2005;1(1):15–25.
191. Sanders MJ, Grondin PO, Hegarty BD, Snowden MA, Carling D. Investigating the mechanism for AMP activation of the AMP-activated protein kinase cascade. Biochem J. 2007;403(1): 139–48.
192. Hawley SA, Boudeau J, Reid JL, Mustard KJ, Udd L, Mäkelä TP, Alessi DR, Hardie DG. Complexes between the LKB1 tumor suppressor, STRAD alpha/beta and MO25 alpha/beta are upstream kinases in the AMP-activated protein kinase cascade. J Biol. 2003;2(4):28.
193. Ayadi-Kaddour A, Bouraoui S, Bellil K, Bellil S, Kchir N, Zitouna MM, Haouet. Colonic adenocarcinoma and bilateral malignant ovarian sex cord tumor with annular tubules in Peutz-Jeghers syndrome. Pathologica. 2004;96:117–20.
194. Brichard B, Chantrain C, Wese F, Gosseye S, Vermylen C. Peutz-Jeghers syndrome and bilateral ovarian tumors in a 14-year-old girl. J Pediatr Hematol Oncol. 2005;27:621–3.
195. Spigelman AD, Murday V, Phillips RKS. Cancer and the Peutz-Jeghers syndrome. Gut. 1989;30:1588–90.
196. Reed MWR, Quayle AR, Harris SC, Talbot CH. The association between thyroid neoplasia and intestinal polyps. Ann R Coll Surg Engl. 1990;72:357–9.
197. Yamamoto M, Hoshino H, Onizuka T, Ichikawa M, Kawakurbo A, Hayakawa S. Thyroid papillary adenocarcinoma in a woman with Peutz-Jeghers syndrome. Int Med. 1992;31:1117–9.
198. Boardman LA, Thibodeau SN, Schaid DJ, Lindor NM, McDonnell SK, Burgart LJ, Ahlquist DA, Podratz KC, Pittelkow M, Hartmann LC. Increased risk for cancer in patients with the Peutz-Jeghers syndrome. Ann Intern Med. 1998;128:896–9.
199. Zirilli L, Benatti P, Romano S, Roncucci L, Rossi G, Diazzi C, Carani C, Ponz De Leon M, Rochira V. Differentiated thyroid carcinoma (DTC) in a young woman with Peutz- Jeghers syndrome: are these two conditions associated? Exp Clin Endocrinol Diabetes. 2009;117:234–9.
200. Beggs AD, Latchford AR, Vasen HF, Moslein G, Alonso A, Aretz S, Bertario L, Blanco I, Bülow S, Burn J, Capella G, Colas C, Friedl W, Møller P, Hes FJ, Järvinen H, Mecklin JP, Nagengast FM, Parc Y, Phillips RK, Hyer W, Ponz de Leon M, Renkonen-Sinisalo L, Sampson JR, Stormorken A, Tejpar S, Thomas HJ, Wijnen JT, Clark SK, Hodgson SV. Peutz-Jeghers syndrome: a systematic review and recommendations for management. Gut. 2010;59:975–86.
201. Hemminki A, Markie D, Tomlinson I, Avizienyte E, Roth S, Loukola A, Bignell G, Warren W, Aminoff M, Hoglund P, Jarvinen H, Kristo P, Pelin K, Ridanpaa M, Salovaara R, Toro T, Bodmer W, Olschwang S, Olsen AS, Stratton MR, de la Chapelle A, Aaltonen LA. A serine/threonine kinase gene defective in Peutz-Jeghers syndrome. Nature. 1998;391:184–7.
202. Jenne DE, Reimann H, Nezu J, Friedel W, Loff S, Jeschke R, Muller O, Back W, Zimmer M. Peutz-Jeghers syndrome is caused by mutations in a novel serine threonine kinase. Nat Genet. 1998;18:38–43.
203. Olschwang S, Boisson C, Thomas G. Peutz-Jeghers families unlinked to STK11/LKB1 gene mutations are highly predisposed to primitive biliary adenocarcinoma. J Med Genet. 2001;38:356–60.
204. Hearle N, Lucassen A, Wang R, Lim W, Ross F, Wheeler R, Moore I, Shipley J, Houlston R. Mapping of a translocation breakpoint in a Peutz-Jeghers hamartoma to the putative PJS locus at 19q13.4 and mutation analysis of candidate genes in polyp and STK11-negative PJS cases. Genes Chromosome Cancer. 2004;41:163–9.
205. Alhopuro P, Phichith D, Tuupanen S, Sammalkorpi H, Nybondas M, Saharinen J, Robinson JP, Yang Z, Chen LQ, Orntoft T, Mecklin JP, Järvinen H, Eng C, Moeslein G, Shibata D, Houlston RS, Lucassen A, Tomlinson IP, Launonen V, Ristimäki A, Arango D, Karhu A, Sweeney HL, Aaltonen LA. Unregulated smooth-muscle myosin in human intestinal neoplasia. Proc Natl Acad Sci U S A. 2008;105(14):5513–8.
206. Aretz S, Stienen D, Uhlhaas S, Loff S, Back W, Pagenstecher C, McLeod DR, Graham GE, Mangold E, Santer R, Propping P, Friedl W. High proportion of large genomic STK11 deletions in Peutz-Jeghers syndrome. Hum Mutat. 2005;26:513–9.
207. Le Meur N, Martin C, Saugier-Veber P, Joly G, Lemoine F, Moirot H, Rossi A, Bachy B, Cabot A, Joly P, Frébourg T. Complete germline deletion of the STK11 gene in a family with Peutz-Jeghers syndrome. Eur J Hum Genet. 2004;12:415–8.
208. De Rosa M, Galatola M, Quaglietta L, Miele E, De Palma G, Rossi GB, Staiano A, Izzo P. Alu-mediated genomic deletion of the serine/threonine protein kinase 11 (STK11) gene in Peutz-Jeghers syndrome. Gastroenterology. 2010;138:2558–60.
209. Kam M, Massare J, Gallinger S, Kinzie J, Weaver D, Dingell JD, Esufali S, Bapat B, Tobi M. Peutz-Jeghers syndrome diagnosed in a schizophrenic patient with a large deletion in the STK11 gene. Dig Dis Sci. 2006;51:1567–70.
210. Taylor A. Ataxia-telangiectasia genes and predisposition to leukemia, lymphoma and breast cancer. Br J Cancer. 1992;66:5–9.
211. Khanna KK. Cancer risk and the ATM gene: a continuing debate. J Natl Cancer Inst. 2000;92:795–802.
212. Boder E. Ataxia-telangiectasia: an overview. In: Gatti RA, Swift M, editors. Ataxia-telangiectasia: genetics, neuropathy, and immunology of a degenerative disease of childhood. New York: Alan R Liss; 1985. p. 1–63.
213. Woods CG, Taylor AM. Ataxia telangiectasia in the British Isles: the clinical and laboratory features of 70 affected individuals. Q J Med. 1992;82:169–79.
214. Gatti RA. Ataxia-telangiectasia. In: Vogelstein B, Kinzler KW, editors. The genetic basis of human cancer. New York: McGraw-Hill; 2002. p. 239–65.
215. Nowak-Wegrzyn A, Crawford TO, Winkelstein JA, Carson KA, Lederman HM. Immunodeficiency and infections in ataxia-telangiectasia. J Pediatr. 2004;144:505–11.
216. Pashankar F, Singhal V, Akabogu I, Gatti RA, Goldman FD. Intact T cell responses in ataxia telangiectasia. Clin Immunol. 2006; 120:156–62.

217. Sanal O, Ersoy F, Yel L, Tezcan I, Metin A, Ozyurek H, Gariboglu S, Fikrig S, Berkel AI, Rijkers GT, Zegers BJ. Impaired IgG antibody production to pneumococcal polysaccharides in patients with ataxia-telangiectasia. J Clin Immunol. 1999;19:326–34.
218. McConville CM, Stankovic T, Byrd PJ, McGuire GM, Yao QY, Lennox GG, Taylor MR. Mutations associated with variant phenotypes in ataxia-telangiectasia. Am J Hum Genet. 1996;59: 320–30.
219. Stankovic T, Kidd AM, Sutcliffe A, McGuire GM, Robinson P, Weber P, Bedenham T, Bradwell AR, Easton DF, Lennox GG, Haites N, Byrd PJ, Taylor AM. ATM mutations and phenotypes in ataxia-telangiectasia families in the British Isles: expression of mutant ATM and the risk of leukemia, lymphoma, and breast cancer. Am J Hum Genet. 1998;62:334–45.
220. Trimis GG, Athanassaki CK, Kanariou MM, Giannoulia-Karantana AA. Unusual absence of neurologic symptoms in a six-year old girl with ataxia-telangiectasia. J Postgrad Med. 2004;50: 270–1.
221. Alterman N, Fattal-Valevski A, Moyal L, Crawford TO, Lederman HM, Ziv Y, Shiloh Y. Ataxia-telangiectasia: mild neurological presentation despite null ATM mutation and severe cellular phenotype. Am J Med Genet A. 2007;143A:1827–34.
222. Saviozzi S, Saluto A, Taylor AM, Last JI, Trebini F, Paradiso MC, Grosso E, Funaro A, Ponzio G, Migone N, Brusco A. A late onset variant of ataxia-telangiectasia with a compound heterozygous genotype, A8030G/7481insA. J Med Genet. 2002;39:57–61.
223. Mitui M, Nahas SA, Du LT, Yang Z, Lai CH, Nakamura K, Arroyo S, Scott S, Purayidom A, Concannon P, Lavin M, Gatti RA. Functional and computational assessment of missense variants in the ATM gene: mutations with increased cancer risk. Hum Mutat. 2009;30:12–21.
224. Hiel JA, van Engelen BG, Weemaes CM, Broeks A, Verrips A, ter Laak H, Vingerhoets HM, van den Heuvel LP, Lammens M, Gabreels FJ, Last JI, Taylor AM. Distal spinal muscular atrophy as a major feature in adult-onset ataxia telangiectasia. Neurology. 2006;67:346–9.
225. Curry CJ, O'Lague P, Tsai J, Hutchison HT, Jaspers NG, Wara D, Gatti RA, Hutchinson HT. ATFresno: a phenotype linking ataxia-telangiectasia with the Nijmegen breakage syndrome. Am J Hum Genet. 1989;45:270–5.
226. Gilad S, Chessa L, Khosravi R, Russell P, Galanty Y, Piane M, Gatti RA, Jorensen TJ, Shiloh Y, Bar-Shira A. Genotype-phenotype relationships in ataxia-telangiectasia (A-T) and A-T variants. Am J Hum Genet. 1998;62:551–61.
227. Bodensteiner JB, Goldlum RM, Goldman AS. Professive dystonia masking ataxia in ataxia-telangiectasia. Arch Neurol. 1980;37: 464–5.
228. Goyal V, Behari M. Dystonia as presenting manifestation of ataxia telangiectasia: a case report. Neurol India. 2002;50:187–9.
229. Yanofsky RA, Seshia SS, Dawson AJ, Stobart K, Greenberg CR, Booth FA, Prasad C, Del Bigio MR, Wrogemann JJ, Fike F, Gatti RA. Ataxia-telangiectasia: atypical presentation and toxicity of cancer treatment. Can J Neurol Sci. 2009;36:462–7.
230. Saunders-Pullman RJ, Gatti R. Ataxia-telangiectasia: without ataxia or telangiectasia? Neurology. 2009;73:414–5.
231. Verhagen MM, Abdo WF, Willemsen MA, Hogervorst FB, Smeets DF, Hiel JA, Brunt ER, van Rijn MA, Majoor Krakauer D, Oldenburg RA, Broeks A, Last JI, van't Veer LJ, Tijssen MA, Dubois AM, Kremer HP, Weemaes CM, Taylor AM, van Deuren M. Clinical spectrum of ataxia-telangiectasia in adulthood. Neurology. 2009;73(6):430–7.
232. Sommer SS, Buzin CH, Jung M, Zheng J, Liu Q, Jeong SJ, Moulds J, Nguyen VQ, Feng J, Bennett WP, Dritschilo A. Elevated frequency of ATM gene missense mutations in breast cancer relative to ethnically matched controls. Cancer Genet Cytogenet. 2002; 134:25–32.
233. Bernstein JL, Teraoka S, Southey MC, Jenkins MA, Andrulis IL, Knight JA, John EM, Lapinski R, Wolitzer AL, Whittemore AS, West D, Seminara D, Olson ER, Spurdle AB, Chenevix-Trench G, Giles GG, Hopper JL, Concannon P. Population-based estimates of breast cancer risks associated with ATM gene variants c.7271T>G and c.1066-6T>G (IVS10-6T>G) from the Breast Cancer Family Registry. Hum Mutat. 2006;27:1122–8.
234. Narita, Tagaki K. Ataxia-telangiectasia with dysgerminoma of right ovary, papillary carcinoma of the thyroid and adenocarcinoma of the pancreas. Cancer. 1984;54:1113–6.
235. Ohta S, Katsura T, Shimada M, et al. Ataxia-telangiectasia with papillary carcinoma of the thyroid. Am J Pediatr Hematol Oncol. 1986;8:255–7.
236. Sandoval C, Schantz S, Posey D, et al. Parotid and thyroid gland cancers in patients with ataxia-telangiectasia. Pediatr Hematol Oncol. 2001;18:485–90.
237. Brasseur B, Beauloye V, Chantrain C, Daumerie C, Vermylen C, Waignein F, Brichard B. Papillary thyroid carcinoma in a 9-year-old girl with ataxia-telangiectasia. Pediatr Blood Cancer. 2008;50(5):1058–60.
238. Cavalieri S, Funaro A, Porcedda P, Turinetto V, Migone N, Gatti RA, Brusco A. ATM mutations in Italian families with ataxia telangiectasia include two distinct large genomic deletions. Hum Mutat. 2006;27:1061.
239. Cavalieri S, Funaro A, Pappi P, Migone N, Gatti RA, Brusco A. Large genomic mutations within the ATM gene detected by MLPA, including a duplication of 41 kb from exon 4 to 20. Ann Hum Genet. 2008;72:10–8.
240. Campbell C, Mitui M, Eng L, Coutinho G, Thorstenson Y, Gatti RA. ATM mutations on distinct SNP and STR haplotypes in ataxia-telangiectasia patients of differing ethnicities reveal ancestral founder effects. Hum Mutat. 2003;21:80–5.
241. Mitui M, Campbell C, Coutinho G, Sun X, Lai CH, Thorstenson Y, Castellvi-Bel S, Fernandez L, Monros E, Carvalho BT, Porras O, Fontan G, Gatti RA. Independent mutational events are rare in the ATM gene: haplotype prescreening enhances mutation detection rate. Hum Mutat. 2003;22:43–50.
242. Coutinho G, Mitui M, Campbell C, Costa Carvalho BT, Nahas S, Sun X, Huo Y, Lai CH, Thorstenson Y, Tanouye R, Raskin S, Kim CA, Llerena J, Gatti RA. Five haplotypes account for fifty-five percent of ATM mutations in Brazilian patients with ataxia telangiectasia: seven new mutations. Am J Med Genet A. 2004;126A: 33–40.
243. Concannon P. ATM heterozygosity and cancer risk. Nat Genet. 2002;32:89–90.
244. Spring K, Ahangari F, Scott SP, Waring P, Purdie DM, Chen PC, Hourigan K, Ramsay J, McKinnon PJ, Swift M, Lavin MF. Mice heterozygous for mutation in Atm, the gene involved in ataxia-telangiectasia, have heightened susceptibility to cancer. Nat Genet. 2002;32:185–90.
245. Goldgar DE, Easton DF, Cannon-Albright LA, Skolnick MH. Systematic population-based assessment of cancer risk in first-degree relatives of cancer probands. J Natl Cancer Inst. 1994;86(21):1600–8.
246. Hemminki K, Vaittinen P. Effect of paternal and maternal cancer on cancer in the offspring: a population-based study. Cancer Epidemiol Biomarkers Prev. 1997;6(12):993–7.
247. Stoffer SS, Van Dyke DL, Bach JV, Szpunar W, Weiss L. Familial papillary carcinoma of the thyroid. Am J Med Genet. 1986;25: 775–82.
248. Kraimps JL, Bouin-Pineau MH, Amati P, Mothes D, Bonneau D, Marechaud R, Barbier J. Familial papillary carcinoma of the thyroid. Surgery. 1997;121:715–8.
249. Loh KC. Familial nonmedullary thyroid carcinoma: a meta-review of case series. Thyroid. 1997;7:107.

250. Couch RM, Hughes IA, DeSa DJ, Schiffrin A, Guyda H, Winter JS. An autosomal dominant form of adolescent multinodular goiter. Am J Hum Genet. 1986;39(6):811–6.
251. Austoni M. Thyroid papillary carcinoma in identical twins [letter]. Lancet. 1988;1:1115.
252. Dzwonkowski P, O'Leary J, Farid NR. Thyroid papillary carcinoma in HLA identical sibs [letter]. Lancet. 1988;2:971.
253. Samaan NA. Papillary carcinoma of the thyroid: hereditary or radiation- induced? [editorial]. Cancer Invest. 1989;7:399.
254. Fischer DK, Groves MD, Thomas Jr SJ, Johnson Jr PC. Papillary carcinoma of the thyroid: additional evidence in support of a familial component. Cancer Invest. 1989;7:323.
255. Bignell GR, Canzian F, Shayeghi M, Stark M, Shugart YY, Biggs P, Mangion J, Hamoudi R, Rosenblatt J, Buu P, Sun S, Stoffer SS, Goldgar DE, Romeo G, Houlston RS, Narod SA, Stratton MR, Foulkes WD. Familial nontoxic multinodular thyroid goiter locus maps to chromosome 14q but does not account for familial nonmedullary thyroid cancer. Am J Hum Genet. 1997;61:1123.
256. Canzian F, Amati P, Harach HR, Kraimps JL, Lesueur F, Barbier J, Levillain P, Romeo G, Bonneau D. A gene predisposing to familial thyroid tumors with cell oxyphilia maps to chromosome 19p13.2. Am J Hum Genet. 1998;63:1743.
257. Lesueur F, Stark M, Tocco T, Ayadi H, Delisle MJ, Goldgar DE, Schlumberger M, Romeo G, Canzian F. Genetic heterogeneity in familial non-medullary thyroid carcinoma: exclusion of linkage to RET, MNG1, and TCO in 56 families: NMTC Consortium. J Clin Endocrinol Metab. 1999;84:2157.
258. McKay JD, Lesueur F, et al. Localization of a susceptibility gene for familial nonmedullary thyroid carcinoma to chromosome 2q21. Am J Hum Genet. 2001;69(2):440–6. Epub 2001 Jul 2.
259. Cavaco BM, Batista PF, Sobrinho LG, Leite V. Mapping a new familial thyroid epithelial neoplasia susceptibility locus to chromosome 8p23.1-p22 by high-density single-nucleotide polymorphism genome-wide linkage analysis. J Clin Endocrinol Metab. 2008;93(11):4426–30. Epub 2008 Sep 2.
260. Lupoli G, Vitale G, Caraglia M, Fittipaldi MR, Abbruzzese A, Tagliaferri P, Bianco AR. Familial papillary thyroid microcarcinoma: a new clinical entity. Lancet. 1999;353:637.
261. Scheumann GF, Seeliger H, Musholt TJ, Gimm O, Wegener G, Dralle H, Hundeshagen H, Pichlmayr R. Completion thyroidectomy in 131 patients with differentiated thyroid carcinoma. Eur J Surg. 1996;162:677.
262. Malchoff CD, Sarfarazi M, Tendler B, Forouhar F, Whalen G, Joshi V, Arnold A, Malchoff DM. Papillary thyroid carcinoma associated with papillary renal neoplasia: genetic linkage analysis of a distinct heritable tumor syndrome. J Clin Endocrinol Metab. 2000;85(5):1758–64.
263. Horie H, Yokogoshi Y, Tsuyuguchi M, Saito S. Point mutations of ras and Gs a subunit genes in thyroid tumors. Jpn J Cancer Res. 1995;86:737–42.
264. Karga H, Lee J-K, Vickery AL, Thor A, Gaz RD, Jameson JL. Ras oncogene mutations in benign and malignant thyroid tumors. J Clin Endocrinol Metab. 1991;73:832–6.
265. Lemoine NR, Mayall ES, Wyllie FS, Williams ED, Goyns M, Stringer B, Wynford-Thomas D. High frequency of ras oncogene activation in all stages of human thyroid tumorigenesis. Oncogene. 1989;4:159–64.
266. Namba H, Rubin SA, Fagin JA. Point mutations of ras oncogenes are an early event in thyroid tumorigenesis. Mol Endocrinol. 1990;4:1474–9.
267. Suarez HG, du Villard JA, Severino M, et al. Presence of mutations in all three ras genes in human thyroid tumors. Oncogene. 1990;5:565–7.
268. Weterman MA, Wilbrink M, Geurts van Kessel A. Fusion of the transcription factor TFE3 gene to a novel gene, PRCC, in t(X;1)(p11;q21)-positive papillary renal cell carcinomas. Proc Natl Acad Sci U S A. 1996;93(15294):15298.

Apoptosis in Thyroid Cancer

6

Su He Wang and James R. Baker Jr.

Introduction

Thyroid cancer can be divided into four types: papillary thyroid carcinoma (PTC) and follicular thyroid carcinoma (FTC), both of which may be classified as differentiated thyroid carcinoma (DTC); anaplastic thyroid carcinoma (ATC), also called undifferentiated thyroid carcinoma (UTC); and medullary thyroid carcinoma (MTC). Estimates will vary, but PTC accounts for about 78 % of thyroid cancer cases, FTC 13 %, MTC 4 %, and ATC 2 % [1]. The etiology of thyroid cancer is not yet fully known. However, it is believed that its development is a multifactor and multistep process. There are several issues that are thought to predispose to thyroid cancer, including radiation, nutrition, sex hormones, environment, and genetics. It appears that all of these factors are related to apoptosis. Radiation is probably one of the most well-studied predisposing factors. The source of radiation is usually traceable, such as from the therapeutic or diagnostic use of radiation and from environmental disasters. The effects are dose dependent and show strong age dependence, with exposure in childhood and adolescence showing almost an order of magnitude higher in the incidence of cancer [2]. Both iodine deficiency and excess iodine can contribute to the development of thyroid cancer [3–5]. Intake of cruciferous vegetables may reduce the risk of thyroid cancer [5]. One of the specific features of thyroid carcinoma is its predilection for women of reproductive age relative to men, suggesting a role of sex hormones in the formation of thyroid cancer. The incidence of thyroid carcinoma is three times more frequent in females than in males [6, 7]. An elevated risk has been documented in women who use estrogens for gynecological reasons, but not in postmenopausal women on low-dose estrogens [8]. Although a responsible gene is not identified for thyroid cancer, its occurrence has been reported in several familial syndromes [9]. Women under 35 years of age with familial adenomatous polyposis, a disease associated with altered apoptosis, have been estimated to have 160-fold higher risk of thyroid cancer than the general population [10].

Apoptosis or programmed cell death is an active process in which a cell dies for the benefit of the whole organism, and this mode of cell death is critical in the development and maintenance of multicellular organisms. Specific morphological features characterize apoptosis. The process starts with chromatin aggregation along the inner walls of the nuclear envelope and is followed by cytoplasmic shrinkage, formation of membrane blebs, extensive DNA degradation, and nuclear pyknosis. Finally, the cell condenses into membrane-bound fragments that are eliminated by surrounding macrophages without an inflammatory reaction. Most of the abovementioned factors are involved in cell proliferation and growth, and they can be directly or indirectly associated with apoptosis.

Although radiation has been reported related to the induction of apoptosis in thyrocytes [11], its carcinogenesis may be more related to its ability to damage DNA and cause mutation in tumor-suppressive genes including p53 [12]. It is reported that high concentrations of iodine increase the rate of Fas-induced apoptosis in thyrocytes, but low concentrations of iodine are able to inhibit apoptosis [13]. Iodine may reduce the sensitivity of papillary thyroid carcinoma cells to apoptotic stimulation via increasing the activity of heme oxygenase (HO) and p21 [14]. A recent study showed that iodine induced the apoptotic pathway in thyroid cancer cells through its involvement in the activation of MAPKs-related p21, Bcl-xL, and mutant p53 regulation [15]. The growth stimulatory effect of estradiol (E2 or 17β-estradiol) has been intensively studied in various estrogen receptor-expressing cells including breast cancer, prostate cancer, and thyroid

S.H. Wang, MD, PhD (✉)
Department of Internal Medicine, University of Michigan,
4037 BSRB 109 Zina Pitcher Place, Ann Arbor, MI 48109, USA
e-mail: shidasui@umich.edu

J.R. Baker Jr., MD
Michigan Nanotechnology Institute for Medicine and Biological Science, University of Michigan, Ann Arbor, MI, USA

L. Wartofsky, D. Van Nostrand (eds.), *Thyroid Cancer*, DOI 10.1007/978-1-4939-3314-3_6

cancer [16–18]. Experimentally, circulating estrogens may activate the estrogen receptor alpha (ERα) on thyroid tissue which increases the incidence of thyroid disease in mice, predisposing them to the development of thyroid cancer, with a higher incidence in female mice [19]. High levels of estrogens may also facilitate the development of thyroid cancers with metastatic phenotypes [20]. Interestingly, the activation of ERα by the ERα agonist PPT promotes, whereas activation of ERβ by the ERβ agonist DPN inhibits, thyroid tumor cell proliferation [21, 22]. The proliferative role of ERα was further supported by a siRNA experiment in which the knockdown of ERα by its siRNA significantly attenuated the PPT-mediated proliferation and growth. The activation of ERα by PPT increased the level of Bcl-2, whereas the activation of ERβ by DPN exerted an opposite effect on its expression in thyroid cancer cells [21], suggesting the involvement of Bcl-2 in ER-mediated regulation of thyrocyte proliferation. These findings appear to support the concepts that the level of ERα is more pronounced in malignant thyroid tissues than in nontumor tissues [23] and that E2/ERα contributes to the increased susceptibility of thyroid tissue to become malignant [19].

Apoptosis and Cancer

The deregulation of apoptosis has been implicated in various clinical disorders, including cancer. Two fundamental lesions are believed to be the underlying pathogenesis of cancer. The first are mutations that give rise to excessive proliferation, and the second is a disruption of apoptotic signaling that allows mutated cells to continue to proliferate and to live beyond their normal lifespan, perpetuating cycles of mutation and oncogenesis. This cycle of mutational activity results in the accumulation of active oncogenes and defective tumor suppressor genes within cells, which makes apoptosis unable to restrict cellular proliferation, and the balance between proliferation and apoptosis is shifted in favor of the former [24].

Apoptosis plays an essential role in the elimination of mutated or transformed cells from the body. During the development of cancer, cancer cells and their precursors must develop highly efficient, and usually multiple, mechanisms to avoid apoptosis. In fact, aborting apoptosis is regarded as one of the hallmarks of cancer cells [25]. A frequent, apparently paradoxical finding in tumors and their precursor lesions is an increased rate of apoptosis, while at the same time, there is an increased resistance to apoptosis as well. The increased apoptosis reflects the enormous pressure on these abnormal cells to undergo programmed cell death, while the increased resistance represents defense mechanisms developed by the mutated cell in an effort to survive. Without the development of apoptotic resistance early during tumorigenesis, the preneoplastic cells would not survive long enough to become invasive cancers. Because apoptosis involves a complex network of interacting checks and balances utilizing several hundreds of genes, cancer cells must develop resistance to apoptosis at multiple levels. To date, two major apoptotic pathways, death receptor-mediated apoptosis and mitochondria-mediated apoptosis, have been described [25, 26] (Fig. 6.1). The death receptor-mediated apoptotic pathway can be achieved by one of several death receptors when bound by the appropriate ligands, including TNF, FasL, and TRAIL. Currently, the most clearly understood aspect of the receptor pathway is the interaction between the Fas receptor and its ligand, FasL, and the activation of the TNF-R1 by TNF. The interaction between the death receptor and its ligand results in receptor aggregation and recruitment of the adaptor molecule Fas-associated death domain (FADD) and caspase-8. Upon recruitment, caspase-8 becomes activated and initiates apoptosis by direct cleavage of downstream effector caspases. UV irradiation, growth factor deprivation, and increased reactive oxygen species cause apoptosis through the mitochondria-mediated apoptotic pathway, which is initiated by the release of apoptogenic factors such as cytochrome c. Cytochrome c forms a multiprotein complex with the adaptor molecule Apaf-1 and procaspase-9. Procaspase-9 is activated upon recruitment to this complex and in turn activates the effector caspases. The receptor and the mitochondria pathways can be interconnected at different levels [27, 28]. Following death receptor stimulation, activation of caspase-8 may result in cleavage of Bid, a BH3 domain-containing protein of the Bcl-2 family, to a truncated form of Bid (tBid). tBid may stimulate cytochrome c release and subsequently initiate a mitochondrial amplification loop.

Apoptosis in Thyroid Carcinogenesis

Solid evidence has indicated that apoptosis plays a significant role in the development of thyroid cancer. An early study on PTC showed that the apoptotic index calculated by the result of TUNEL was directly related to the p53 protein but inversely correlated with the anti-apoptotic molecule, Bcl-2 [29]. It appears that resistance to apoptosis and the ability to proliferate are different among various types of thyroid cancer cells. But they increase with tumor aggressiveness, from PTC to poorly differentiated and undifferentiated thyroid cancers. Among various apoptotic molecules, the Fas/FasL system has been extensively investigated in thyroid cancer. Fas-mediated apoptosis is considered as a key mechanism of T cell-mediated cytotoxicity against neoplastic cells. Thyroid cancer cells express a significant level of Fas, and, upon anti-Fas antibody stimulation in vitro in the presence of interferon gamma and cycloheximide, the cancer cells can undergo apoptosis, suggesting that the Fas on the thyroid cancer cells

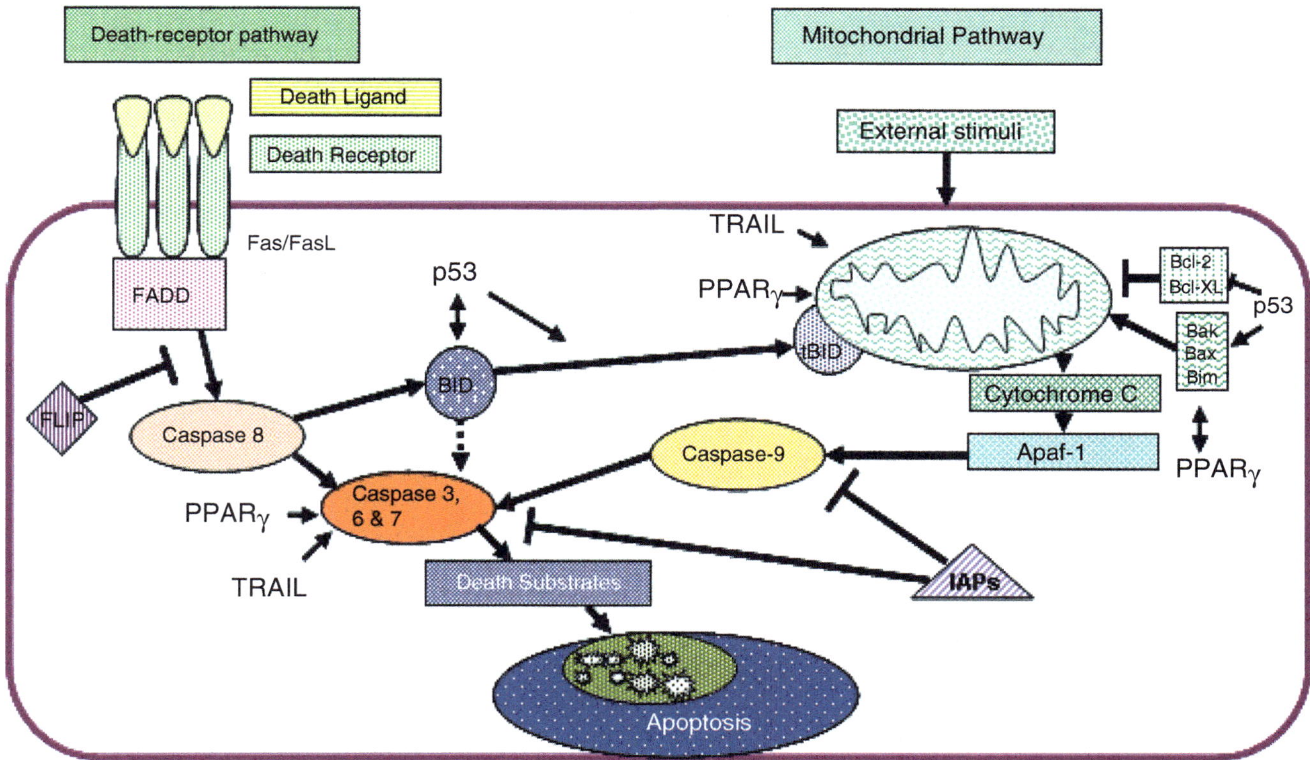

Fig. 6.1 Death receptor-mediated and mitochondria-mediated pathways and the involvement of p53, TRAIL, and PPARγ in the induction of apoptosis in thyroid cancer cells

is functional when there are certain cytokines and protein inhibitors available [30]. Though Fas is functional in thyroid cancer cells, it may not be able to induce apoptosis, and resistance to Fas is found in thyroid cancer cells [31–33]. The mechanism responsible for the resistance is not yet known, but it may be related to decreased numbers of Fas receptors available on the cell surface or to a change in the thyroid cytokine microenvironment. Fas expression has been documented to be lower in thyroid nodules [34]. Studies have indicated the existence of regulators that block apoptosis in thyroid cancer cells, thus pro-inflammatory cytokines may induce apoptosis in noncancer thyroid cells but not in thyroid cancer cells [32, 35]. The levels of Fas and FasL in different thyroid cancer cells may substantially differ, and the expression of Fas has been found to be negatively associated with the advanced stage of thyroid cancer [36]. Furthermore, Fas level is significantly higher in well-differentiated PTC and FTC than in poorly differentiated or undifferentiated PTC and FTC. These observations are consistent with the finding that there is an increasing resistance to apoptosis when thyroid cancer becomes more aggressive [29].

As mentioned before, cancer cells usually develop resistance to apoptosis at multiple levels. One true example is thyroid cancer cells. Thyroid cancer cells cannot only escape apoptosis by either reducing Fas expression on their cell membrane or/and displaying blockers that inhibit the Fas/FasL system [31–33] but can also utilize the Fas/FasL system to downregulate the ability of immune surveillance to kill tumor cells by inducing apoptosis of infiltrating lymphocytes and other immune effector cells [32, 37]. Therefore, FasL expression may correlate with more aggressive types of thyroid cancer [32]. Thyroid cancer cells are not killed by their own FasL because of their inherent resistance to Fas-mediated apoptosis [31–33, 35]. Such FasL-mediated suppression of immune surveillance is called "Fas counterattack" or the "tumor immune privilege" [38, 39].

In addition to the involvement of Fas/FasL death receptor-mediated apoptosis in the development of thyroid cancer, mitochondria-mediated apoptosis, represented by the alternation of Bcl-2 family members, may also play a role in promotion of thyroid cancer cell growth. High levels of Bcl-2 and Bcl-xL, both of which are anti-apoptotic, are found in malignant epithelial cells from PTC, FTC, and ATC [40–42]. Further, the level of pro-apoptotic Bax is reduced in thyroid cancer [42, 43]. The aberrant expression of Bcl-2, Bcl-xL, and Bax is thought to result from a change in the cytokine microenvironment of the thyroid, especially IL-4 and IL-10 [40, 43]. Obviously, the changes in Bcl-2 family members disturb the balance between pro-apoptotic Bax and anti-apoptotic Bcl-2 and Bcl-xL and thus reduce the sensitivity of thyroid cancer cells to apoptotic stimuli. This assumption is in line with the observation that the expression of Bcl-2 is inversely correlated with the apoptotic index in thyroid cancer cells and chemotherapy-induced apoptosis [29, 44].

The function of Bcl-2 and its other family members is closely associated with p53. For example, p53 is able to upregulate pro-apoptotic Bax in a variety of cell types [45, 46]. Unfortunately, evidence directly linking between p53 and Bcl-2 family members in thyroid cancer is lacking. However, apoptosis in poorly differentiated thyroid cancer cells is associated with a high protein level of p53 but a low protein level of Bcl-2 [47]. By overexpression of p53, the proliferation of poorly differentiated thyroid cancer cells is reduced and the cells exhibit malignant behavior [48]. These findings suggest that thyroid cancer cells with a lower level of p53 or lacking p53 are more likely to grow fast and less sensitive to apoptosis. It is believed that mutations of tumor suppressor genes such as p53 are important events in thyroid tumor progression once the early stages of oncogene-driven cell transformation have been established [49]. Some p53 mutants can gain anti-apoptotic functions. For example, mutant p53 (G199V) in anaplastic thyroid cancer cells gains anti-apoptotic function through signal transducer and activator of transcription 3 (STAT3) and thus promotes the growth of tumor cells [50]. Excitingly, the reactivation of p53 mutants can enable thyroid cancer cells to arrest the growth by promoting apoptosis [51]. Peroxisome proliferator-activated receptor gamma (PPARγ) is another important molecule that is involved in apoptosis and tumor development of thyroid cancer. PPARγ is frequently downregulated in thyroid cancer [52, 53]. The mechanism responsible for the PPARγ downregulation is not fully known. However, thyroid hormone receptor beta (TRβ) mutant is able to function as dominant negative inhibitor of PPARγ and thus suppresses the function of PPARγ [53]. In follicular thyroid carcinomas, the downregulation of PPARγ may be caused by a chromosomal translocation that fuses the thyroid-specific transcription factor paired box gene 8 (PAX8) with PPARγ, forming a PAX8-PPARγ fusion protein, PPFP [53–55]. This PPFP can dominantly inhibit expression of the PPARγ-responsive promoter, resulting in enhancement of follicular thyroid cell growth and loss of differentiation that ultimately leads to carcinogenesis [53, 54]. In a transgenic mouse model of thyroidal PPFP expression, it is found that the mice develop thyroid hyperplasia but not carcinoma, suggesting that additional events are required to cause follicular thyroid cancer [55, 56]. Nevertheless, the activation of PPARγ by its ligands has been shown to induce apoptosis, inhibit the growth of thyroid cancer cells, and facilitate the radioiodine treatment of thyroid cancer [57–59]. Therefore, PPARγ activation may counteract the uncontrolled proliferation and thyroid malignant cell growth through induction of apoptosis or promotion of cellular terminal differentiation. It is concluded that the alteration of PPARγ may serve not only as a feature of thyroid cancer development but also as a promising target for cancer therapy.

Though Fas/FasL, Bcl-2 family members, p53, and PPARγ are major players that regulate apoptosis in thyroid cancer cells (Fig. 6.1), a number of new molecules have recently been described to contribute to thyroid cancer development and/or treatment by regulating apoptosis. BAG (Bcl-2-associated athanogene) is found to specifically express in thyroid carcinomas and not in normal thyroid tissue or goiter [60]. The downregulation of BAG3 can significantly sensitize human neoplastic thyroid cells to apoptosis induced by NF-related apoptosis-inducing ligand (TRAIL). TRAIL-induced apoptosis in thyroid cancer cells is also regulated by another novel molecule, DJ-1 [61]. DJ is a cancer-associated protein, which protects cells from multiple toxic stresses. Importantly, DJ-1 is specifically expressed in thyroid carcinomas and not in the normal thyroid tissue. siRNA downregulation of DJ-1 can significantly sensitize thyroid carcinoma cells to TRAIL-induced apoptosis, whereas the forced exogenous expression of DJ-1 significantly suppresses cell death induced by TRAIL [61]. In the study by Siraj et al. [62], TMS1, a tumor suppressor gene that encodes for caspase recruitment domain-containing regulatory protein, is downregulated in a subset of thyroid cancer samples by hypermethylation. Its demethylation can also sensitize thyroid cancer cells to TRAIL-induced apoptosis. A very recent study demonstrates that Ret oncoprotein regulates CD95 (Fas, APO-1)-mediated apoptosis by increasing Fap-1, a potential inhibitor of CD95 (Fas, APO-1) in MTC cells [63]. Therefore, the functional interplay of the Ret mutant with the receptor-mediated apoptosis pathway may provide a mechanism contributing to MTC malignant phenotype and a rational basis for novel therapeutic strategies combining Ret inhibitors and CD95 agonists.

Potential Apoptotic Intervention for Thyroid Cancer

Therapies designed to stimulate apoptosis in target cells play an increasing role in the prevention and treatment of human cancer, including thyroid cancer. For several decades, the classical view of an anticancer drug mechanism has relied on the specific interaction of a drug with its target, and such an interaction can lead to tumor cell death via its direct and injurious effect on the proliferating tumor cells. However, emerging data based on an increasing understanding of the cell cycle control and apoptosis process indicate that, rather than being intrinsically toxic, many anticancer drugs merely stimulate tumor cells to self-destruction via apoptosis. Studies have demonstrated that most, if not all, of currently available anticancer drugs including those that target DNA replication, DNA integrity, mitochondria, and cytokines induce apoptosis in thyroid cancer cells. For example, paclitaxel and manumycin are now known to induce apoptosis in ATC via stimulating p21 expression [64]. UCN-01, a selective protein kinase inhibitor, can significantly induce apoptosis of various types of thyroid cancer cells, probably via inhibiting the expression of Bcl-2, as the overexpression of Bcl-2 can block the UNC-01-activated cell death pathway [65]. Some extracts from traditional Chinese herb medicines have also shown a strong antiproliferative effect via provoking apoptosis in MTC [66].

With the tremendous amount of knowledge gained about apoptosis in thyroid cancer, some promising targets/therapies for certain types of thyroid cancer cells have emerged. Among these targets are aforementioned p53, PPARγ, and TRAIL [51, 57–62]. The major advantage of TRAIL-mediated apoptosis against thyroid cancer is its selective killing of tumor cells without affecting normal thyroid cells [65, 67], thus reducing the possible side effects. Some emerging agents such as histone deacetylase inhibitors [68], Cl-IB-MECA that is adenosine receptor A3 agonist [69], and R-roscovitine that is a novel cyclin-dependent kinase inhibitor [70] have recently shown to either enhance or optimize the TRAIL-induced apoptosis in thyroid cancer cells. In addition to these well-documented targets, the glutathione-dependent redox system may play an important role in the sensitivity to proteasome inhibition-induced apoptosis in thyroid cancer cells [71]. Inhibition of nuclear factor-kappaB is shown to enhance apoptosis of thyroid cancer cells by reducing the levels of MMP-9 and MMP-13 [72]. Resveratrol, a phytoalexin found in grapes and other food products, and rosuvastatin, a statin drug, have been demonstrated to induce apoptosis in thyroid cancer cells by increasing caspase-3 activity [73, 74]. Epigallocatechin-3-gallate (EGCG), a major catechin in green tea, can induce apoptosis of human anaplastic thyroid carcinoma cells through suppression of EGFR/ERK pathway and cyclin B1/CDK1 complex [75].

Conclusion

Apoptosis in thyroid cancer is a multifactor and multistep process, and this process is controlled by a number of different molecules including but not limited to Fas/FasL, Bcl-2 family members, p53, PPARγ, and TRAIL. There is no clear evidence which one is more important than the others in the development of thyroid cancer. It appears that all of them can independently induce or enhance apoptosis in thyroid cancer cells. It is important to understand how they interact with each other since such interactions may greatly optimize the therapeutic targets and enhance apoptosis induced in thyroid cancer cells.

References

1. Hundahl SA, Fleming ID, Fremgen AM, Menck HR. A National Cancer Data Base report on 53,856 cases of thyroid carcinoma treated in the U.S., 1985–1995. Cancer. 1988;83:2638–48.
2. Ron E, Lubin JH, Shore RE, Mabuchi K, Modan B, Pottern LM, Schneider AB, Tucker MA, Boice Jr JD. Thyroid cancer after exposure to external radiation: a pooled analysis of seven studies. Radiat Res. 1995;141:259–77.
3. Laurberg P, Cerqueira C, Ovesen L, Rasmussen LB, Perrild H, Andersen S, Pedersen IB, Carlé A. Iodine intake as a determinant of thyroid disorders in populations. Best Pract Res Clin Endocrinol Metab. 2010;24:13–27.
4. Liu XH, Chen GG, Vlantis AC, van Hasselt CA. Iodine mediated mechanisms and thyroid carcinoma. Crit Rev Clin Lab Sci. 2009;46:302–18.
5. Dal Maso L, Bosetti C, La Vecchia C, Franceschi S. Risk factors for thyroid cancer: an epidemiological review focused on nutritional factors. Cancer Causes Control. 2009;20:75–86.
6. Chen GG, Vlantis AC, Zeng Q, van Hasselt CA. Regulation of cell growth by estrogen signaling and potential targets in thyroid cancer. Curr Cancer Drug Targets. 2008;8:367–77.
7. Rahbari R, Zhang L, Kebebew E. Thyroid cancer gender disparity. Future Oncol. 2010;6:1771–9.
8. Ron E, Kleinerman RA, Boice JD, et al. A population-based case-control study of thyroid cancer. J Natl Cancer Inst. 1987;79:1–12.
9. Nosé V. Familial thyroid cancer: a review. Mod Pathol. 2011;24 Suppl 2:S19–33.
10. Plail RO, Bussey HJ, Glazer G, Thomson JP. Adenomatous polyposis: an association with carcinoma of the thyroid. Br J Surg. 1987;74:377–80.
11. Del Terra E, Francesconi A, Meli A, Ambesi-Impiombato FS. Radiation-dependent apoptosis on cultured thyroid cells. Phys Med. 2001;17 Suppl 1:261–3.
12. Weihrauch M, Bader M, Lehnert G, Wittekind C, Tannapfel A, Wrbitzky R. Carcinogen-specific mutation pattern in the p53 tumour suppressor gene in UV radiation-induced basal cell carcinoma. Int Arch Occup Environ Health. 2002;75:272–6.
13. Feldkamp J, Pascher E, Perniok A, Scherbaum WA. Fas-Mediated apoptosis is inhibited by TSH and iodine in moderate concentrations in primary human thyrocytes in vitro. Hormon Metab Res. 1999;31:355–8.
14. Chen GG, Liu ZM, Vlantis AC, Tse GM, Leung BC, van Hasselt CA. Heme oxygenase-1 protects against apoptosis induced by tumor necrosis factor-alpha and cycloheximide in papillary thyroid carcinoma cells. J Cell Biochem. 2004;92:1246–56.
15. Liu XH, Chen GG, Vlantis AC, Tse GM, van Hasselt CA. Iodine induces apoptosis via regulating MAPKs-related p53, p21, and Bcl-xL in thyroid cancer cells. Mol Cell Endocrinol. 2010;320:128–35.
16. Kim Y, Kim H, Jang SW, Ko J. The role of 14-3-3β in transcriptional activation of estrogen receptor α and its involvement in proliferation of breast cancer cells. Biochem Biophys Res Commun. 2011;414:199–204.
17. Wang X, Clubbs EA, Bomser JA. Genistein modulates prostate epithelial cell proliferation via estrogen- and extracellular signal-regulated kinase-dependent pathways. J Nutr Biochem. 2006;17:204–10.
18. Lee ML, Chen GG, Vlantis AC, Tse GM, Leung BC, van Hasselt CA. Induction of thyroid papillary carcinoma cell proliferation by estrogen is associated with an altered expression of Bcl-xL. Cancer J. 2005;11:113–21.
19. Antico-Arciuch VG, Dima M, Liao XH, Refetoff S, Di Cristofano A. Cross-talk between PI3K and estrogen in the mouse thyroid predisposes to the development of follicular carcinomas with a higher incidence in females. Oncogene. 2010;29:5678–86.

20. Rajoria S, Suriano R, Shanmugam A, Wilson YL, Schantz SP, Geliebter J, Tiwari RK. Metastatic phenotype is regulated by estrogen in thyroid cells. Thyroid. 2010;20:33–41.
21. Zeng Q, Chen GG, van Hasselt CA. Oestrogen mediates the growth of human thyroid carcinoma cells via an oestrogen receptor-ERK pathway. Cell Prolif. 2007;40:921–35.
22. Zeng Q, Chen GG, van Hasselt C. The contributions of oestrogen receptor isoforms to the development of papillary and anaplastic thyroid carcinomas. J Pathol. 2008;214:425–33.
23. Dalla Valle L, Belvedere P, Colombo L. Potential for estrogen synthesis and action in human normal and neoplastic thyroid tissues. J Clin Endocrinol Metab. 1998;83:3702–9.
24. Evan GI, Vousden KH. Proliferation, cell cycle and apoptosis in cancer. Nature. 2001;411:342–8.
25. Gupta S. Molecular signaling in death receptor and mitochondrial pathways of apoptosis. Int J Oncol. 2003;22:15–20.
26. Schultz DR, Harrington Jr WJ. Apoptosis: programmed cell death at a molecular level. Semin Arthritis Rheum. 2003;32:345–69.
27. Sprick MR, Walczak H. The interplay between the Bcl-2 family and death receptor-mediated apoptosis. Biochim Biophys Acta. 2004;1644:125–32.
28. Roy S, Nicholson DW. Cross-talk in cell death signaling. J Exp Med. 2000;192:F21–5.
29. Basolo F, Pollina L, Fontanini G, Fiore L, Pacini F, Baldanzi A. Apoptosis and proliferation in thyroid carcinoma: correlation with bcl-2 and p53 protein expression. Br J Cancer. 1997;75:537–41.
30. Arscott PL, Stokes T, Myc A, Giordano TJ, Thompson NW, Baker Jr JR. Fas (CD95) expression is up-regulated on papillary thyroid carcinoma. J Clin Endocrinol Metab. 1999;84:4246–52.
31. Mitsiades N, Poulaki V, Tseleni-Balafouta S, Koutras DA, Stamenkovic I. Thyroid carcinoma cells are resistant to FAS-mediated apoptosis but sensitive tumor necrosis factor-related apoptosis-inducing ligand. Cancer Res. 2000;60:4122–9.
32. Mitsiades N, Poulaki V, Mastorakos G, Tseleni-Balafouta ST, Kotoula V, Koutras DA, Tsokos M. Fas ligand expression in thyroid carcinomas: a potential mechanism of immune evasion. J Clin Endocrinol Metab. 1999;84:2924–32.
33. Mezosi E, Yamazaki H, Bretz JD, Wang SH, Arscott PL, Utsugi S, Gauger PG, Thompson NW, Baker Jr JR. Aberrant apoptosis in thyroid epithelial cells from goiter nodules. J Clin Endocrinol Metab. 2002;87:4264–72.
34. Andrikoula M, Vartholomatos G, Tsangaris GT, Bafa M, Tzortzatou-Stathopoulou F, Tsatsoulis A. Fas and Bcl-2 protein expression in thyrocytes of patients with nodular goiter. Eur J Endocrinol. 2001;145:403–7.
35. Wang SH, Mezosi E, Wolf JM, Cao Z, Utsugi S, Gauger PG, Doherty GM, Baker Jr JR. IFNgamma sensitization to TRAIL-induced apoptosis in human thyroid carcinoma cells by upregulating Bak expression. Oncogene. 2004;23:928–35.
36. Basolo F, Fiore L, Baldanzi A, Giannini R, Dell'Omodarme M, Fontanini G, Pacini F, Danesi R, Miccoli P, Toniolo A. Suppression of Fas expression and down-regulation of Fas ligand in highly aggressive human thyroid carcinoma. Lab Invest. 2000;80:1413–9.
37. Matiba B, Mariani SM, Krammer PH. The CD95 system and the death of a lymphocyte. Semin Immunol. 1997;9:59–68.
38. Walker PR, Saas P, Dietrich PY. Role of Fas ligand (CD95L) in immune escape: the tumor cell strikes back. J Immunol. 1997;158:4521–4.
39. Hahne M, Rimoldi D, Schroter M, Romero P, Schreier M, French LE, Schneider P, Bornand T, Fontana A, Lienard D, Cerottini J, Tschopp J. Melanoma cell expression of Fas(Apo-1/CD95) ligand: implications for tumor immune escape. Science. 1996;274:1363–6.
40. Stassi G, Todaro M, Zerilli M, Ricci-Vitiani L, Di Liberto D, Patti M, Florena A, Di Gaudio F, Di Gesu G, De Maria R. Thyroid cancer resistance to chemotherapeutic drugs via autocrine production of interleukin-4 and interleukin-10. Cancer Res. 2003;63:6784–90.
41. Xu W, Li X, Chen S, Huang J, Lin S, Lin J, Li Y, Tan X. Expression and distribution of S-100, CD83 and apoptosis-related proteins (Fas, FasL and Bcl-2) in tissues of thyroid carcinoma. Eur J Histochem. 2008;52:153–62.
42. Cvejic D, Selemetjev S, Savin S, Paunovic I, Petrovic I, Tatic S. Apoptosis and proliferation related molecules (Bcl-2, Bax, p53, PCNA) in papillary microcarcinoma versus papillary carcinoma of the thyroid. Pathology. 2008;40:475–80.
43. Vella V, Mineo R, Frasca F, Mazzon E, Pandini G, Vigneri R, Belfiore A. Interleukin-4 stimulates papillary thyroid cancer cell survival: implications in patients with thyroid cancer and concomitant Graves' disease. J Clin Endocrinol Metab. 2004;89:2880–9.
44. Mitsiades CS, Hayden P, Kotoula V, McMillin DW, McMullan C, Negri J, Delmore JE, Poulaki V, Mitsiades N. Bcl-2 overexpression in thyroid carcinoma cells increases sensitivity to Bcl-2 homology 3 domain inhibition. J Clin Endocrinol Metab. 2007;92:4845–52.
45. Häcker S, Karl S, Mader I, Cristofanon S, Schweitzer T, Krauss J, Rutkowski S, Debatin KM, Fulda S. Histone deacetylase inhibitors prime medulloblastoma cells for chemotherapy-induced apoptosis by enhancing p53-dependent Bax activation. Oncogene. 2011;30:2275–81.
46. Lee WT, Chang CW. Bax is upregulated by p53 signal pathway in the SPE B-induced apoptosis. Mol Cell Biochem. 2010;343:271–9.
47. Pohl F, Grosse J, Grimm D, Brockhoff G, Westphal K, Moosbauer J, Koelbl O, Infanger M, Eilles C, Schoenberger J. Changes of apoptosis, p53, and bcl-2 by irradiation in poorly differentiated thyroid carcinoma cell lines: a prognostic marker for the prospect of therapeutic success? Thyroid. 2010;20:159–66.
48. Moretti F, Farsetti A, Soddu S, Misiti S, Crescenzi M, Filetti S, Andreoli M, Sacchi A, Pontecorvi A. p53 re-expression inhibits proliferation and restores differentiation of human thyroid anaplastic carcinoma cells. Oncogene. 1997;14:729–40.
49. Fagin JA. Minireview: branded from the start-distinct oncogenic initiating events may determine tumor fate in the thyroid. Mol Endocrinol. 2002;16:903–11.
50. Kim TH, Lee SY, Rho JH, Jeong NY, Soung YH, Jo WS, Kang DY, Kim SH, Yoo YH. Mutant p53 (G199V) gains antiapoptotic function through signal transducer and activator of transcription 3 in anaplastic thyroid cancer cells. Mol Cancer Res. 2009;7:1645–54.
51. Messina RL, Sanfilippo M, Vella V, Pandini G, Vigneri P, Nicolosi ML, Gianì F, Vigneri R, Frasca F. Reactivation of p53 mutants by p53 reactivation and induction of massive apoptosis in thyroid cancer cells. Int J Cancer. 2012;130:2259–2270.
52. Karger S, Berger K, Eszlinger M, Tannapfel A, Dralle H, Paschke R, Führer D. Evaluation of peroxisome proliferator-activated receptor-gamma expression in benign and malignant thyroid pathologies. Thyroid. 2005;15:997–1003.
53. Aldred MA, Morrison C, Gimm O, Hoang-Vu C, Krause U, Dralle H, Jhiang S, Eng C. Peroxisome proliferator-activated receptor gamma is frequently downregulated in a diversity of sporadic nonmedullary thyroid carcinomas. Oncogene. 2003;22:3412–6.
54. Araki O, Ying H, Furuya F, Zhu X, Cheng SY. Thyroid hormone receptor beta mutants: dominant negative regulators of peroxisome proliferator-activated receptor gamma action. Proc Natl Acad Sci U S A. 2005;102:16251–6.
55. Au AY, McBride C, Wilhelm Jr KG, Koenig RJ, Speller B, Cheung L, Messina M, Wentworth J, Tasevski V, Learoyd D, Robinson BG, Clifton-Bligh RJ. PAX8-peroxisome proliferator-activated receptor gamma (PPARgamma) disrupts normal PAX8 or PPARgamma transcriptional function and stimulates follicular thyroid cell growth. Endocrinology. 2006;147:367–76.
56. Diallo-Krou E, Yu J, Colby LA, Inoki K, Wilkinson JE, Thomas DG, Giordano TJ, Koenig RJ. Paired box gene 8-peroxisome proliferator-activated receptor-gamma fusion protein and loss of phosphatase and tensin homolog synergistically cause thyroid hyperplasia in transgenic mice. Endocrinology. 2009;150:5181–90.

57. Hayashi N, Nakamori S, Hiraoka N, Tsujie M, Xundi X, Takano T, Amino N, Sakon M, Monden M. Antitumor effects of peroxisome proliferator activate receptor gamma ligands on anaplastic thyroid carcinoma. Int J Oncol. 2004;24:89–95.
58. Bonofiglio D, Qi H, Gabriele S, Catalano S, Aquila S, Belmonte M, Andò S. Peroxisome proliferator-activated receptor gamma inhibits follicular and anaplastic thyroid carcinoma cells growth by upregulating p21Cip1/WAF1 gene in a Sp1-dependent manner. Endocr Relat Cancer. 2008;15:545–57.
59. Tepmongkol S, Keelawat S, Honsawek S, Ruangvejvorachai P. Rosiglitazone effect on radioiodine uptake in thyroid carcinoma patients with high thyroglobulin but negative total body scan: a correlation with the expression of peroxisome proliferator-activated receptor-gamma. Thyroid. 2008;18:697–704.
60. Chiappetta G, Ammirante M, Basile A, Rosati A, Festa M, Monaco M, Vuttariello E, Pasquinelli R, Arra C, Zerilli M, Todaro M, Stassi G, Pezzullo L, Gentilella A, Tosco A, Pascale M, Marzullo L, Belisario MA, Turco MC, Leone A. The antiapoptotic protein BAG3 is expressed in thyroid carcinomas and modulates apoptosis mediated by tumor necrosis factor-related apoptosis-inducing ligand. J Clin Endocrinol Metab. 2007;92:1159–63.
61. Zhang HY, Wang HQ, Liu HM, Guan Y, Du ZX. Regulation of tumor necrosis factor-related apoptosis-inducing ligand-induced apoptosis by DJ-1 in thyroid cancer cells. Endocr Relat Cancer. 2008;15:535–44.
62. Siraj AK, Hussain AR, Al-Rasheed M, Ahmed M, Bavi P, Alsobhi SA, Al-Nuaim A, Uddin S, Al-Kuraya K. Demethylation of TMS1 gene sensitizes thyroid cancer cells to TRAIL-induced apoptosis. J Clin Endocrinol Metab. 2011;96:E215–24.
63. Nicolini V, Cassinelli G, Cuccuru G, Bongarzone I, Petrangolini G, Tortoreto M, Mondellini P, Casalini P, Favini E, Zaffaroni N, Zunino F, Lanzi C. Interplay between Ret and Fap-1 regulates CD95-mediated apoptosis in medullary thyroid cancer cells. Biochem Pharmacol. 2011;82:778–88.
64. Yang HL, Pan JX, Sun L, Yeung SC. p21 Waf-1 (Cip-1) enhances apoptosis induced by manumycin and paclitaxel in anaplastic thyroid cancer cells. J Clin Endocrinol Metab. 2003;88:763–72.
65. Wang SH, Phelps E, Utsugi S, Baker Jr JR. Susceptibility of thyroid cancer cells to 7-hydroxystaurosporine-induced apoptosis correlates with Bcl-2 protein level. Thyroid. 2001;11:725–31.
66. Rinner B, Siegl V, Purstner P, Efferth T, Brem B, Greger H, Pfragner R. Activity of novel plant extracts against medullary thyroid carcinoma cells. Anticancer Res. 2004;24:495–500.
67. Ahmad M, Shi Y. TRAIL-induced apoptosis of thyroid cancer cells: potential for therapeutic intervention. Oncogene. 2000;19:3363–71.
68. Borbone E, Berlingieri MT, De Bellis F, Nebbioso A, Chiappetta G, Mai A, Altucci L, Fusco A. Histone deacetylase inhibitors induce thyroid cancer-specific apoptosis through proteasome-dependent inhibition of TRAIL degradation. Oncogene. 2010;29:105–16.
69. Morello S, Sorrentino R, Porta A, Forte G, Popolo A, Petrella A, Pinto A. Cl-IB-MECA enhances TRAIL-induced apoptosis via the modulation of NF-kappaB signalling pathway in thyroid cancer cells. J Cell Physiol. 2009;221:378–86.
70. Festa M, Petrella A, Alfano S, Parente L. R-roscovitine sensitizes anaplastic thyroid carcinoma cells to TRAIL-induced apoptosis via regulation of IKK/NF-kappaB pathway. Int J Cancer. 2009;124:2728–36.
71. Du ZX, Zhang HY, Meng X, Guan Y, Wang HQ. Role of oxidative stress and intracellular glutathione in the sensitivity to apoptosis induced by proteasome inhibitor in thyroid cancer cells. BMC Cancer. 2009;9:56.
72. Bauerle KT, Schweppe RE, Haugen BR. Inhibition of nuclear factor-kappa B differentially affects thyroid cancer cell growth, apoptosis, and invasion. Mol Cancer. 2010;9:117.
73. Truong M, Cook MR, Pinchot SN, Kunnimalaiyaan M, Chen H. Resveratrol induces Notch2-mediated apoptosis and suppression of neuroendocrine markers in medullary thyroid cancer. Ann Surg Oncol. 2011;18:1506–11.
74. Zeybek ND, Gulcelik NE, Kaymaz FF, Sarisozen C, Vural I, Bodur E, Canpinar H, Usman A, Asan E. Rosuvastatin induces apoptosis in cultured human papillary thyroid cancer cells. J Endocrinol. 2011;210:105–15.
75. Lim YC, Cha YY. Epigallocatechin-3-gallate induces growth inhibition and apoptosis of human anaplastic thyroid carcinoma cells through suppression of EGFR/ERK pathway and cyclin B1/CDK1 complex. J Surg Oncol. 2011;107:776–780.

Radiation-Induced Thyroid Cancer

7

James J. Figge, Timothy A. Jennings, Gregory Gerasimov, Nikolai A. Kartel, and Gennady Ermak

Radiation is one of the few accepted risk factors for thyroid cancer. Numerous studies have confirmed that the thyroid gland is one of the most radiation-sensitive human organs and that thyroid cancer is one of the most common radiogenic malignancies. Analysis of these studies is problematic, however, owing to difficulties in dose assessment, long-term follow-up of thousands of exposed subjects, definition and confirmation of pathological diagnoses, and differences in exposure modalities.

The first part of this chapter briefly outlines the nature and methods of the most significant studies to date and analyzes the data available to define the characteristics of the risks of radiation to the thyroid on subsequent development of thyroid cancer. The second part of the chapter presents an update on thyroid cancer in children exposed to fallout from the Chernobyl accident. Terminology used throughout the chapter is defined in Table 7.1.

J.J. Figge, MD, MBA, FACP (✉)
Department of Biomedical Sciences, School of Public Health, State University of New York, Albany, NY, USA

Department of Medicine, St. Peter's Health Partners, Albany, NY, USA

Gen*NY*Sis Center for Excellence in Cancer Genomics, State University of New York, One Discovery Drive, Rensselaer, NY, USA
e-mail: jfigge@albany.edu

T.A. Jennings, MD
Department of Pathology and Laboratory Medicine, Albany Medical Center, Albany, NY, USA
e-mail: jennint@mail.amc.edu

G. Gerasimov, MD, PhD
Thyroid Division, Endocrinology Research Center, Moscow, Russian Federation
e-mail: gerasimov@verizon.net

N.A. Kartel, PhD
Molecular Genetics Laboratory, The Institute of Genetics and Cytology of the National Academy of Sciences of Belarus, Minsk, Republic of Belarus
e-mail: N.Kartel@igc.bas-net.by

G. Ermak, PhD
Division of Molecular and Computational Biology, Ethel Percy Andrus Gerontology Center, Los Angeles, CA, USA
e-mail: ermak@usc.edu

Pathology

Knowledge of the pathology of radiation injury to the thyroid is essential to understanding the data from previous long-term follow-up studies. Thyroid glands exposed to external beam or ^{131}I radiation show a variety of histological abnormalities, most often multinodularity, distorting fibrosis, oncocytic change, and chronic inflammation [1–3]. At higher (>1.5 Gy) doses, hyperplastic nodules may show cytologic atypia, which requires careful scrutiny to distinguish from malignancy [4]. The incidence of benign adenomas in patients who received thyroid irradiation is also greatly increased over nonirradiated individuals, as demonstrated by virtually every study of such populations. Many studies failed to distinguish between benign nodules and carcinoma and are therefore excluded from this discussion.

As early as 1949, Quimby and Werner [5] suggested the possibility of a relationship between radiation and the subsequent development of thyroid carcinoma. Winship and Rosvoll [6] began collecting data on children with thyroid cancer in 1948, and their final report on 878 cases worldwide represents the largest to date. They found a history of radiation in 76 % of 476 children with available records. Most received radiation for enlarged thymus or tonsils and adenoids, with an average thyroid dose of 0.512 Gy and an average interval to diagnosis of 8.5 year; 72 % of the cancers were of papillary type, and 18 % were follicular. Cervical lymph node metastases were present in 74 % of cases, with bilateral neck disease in 32 %. Nearly 20 % had pulmonary involvement, generally at presentation. The authors noted a sharp rise in thyroid cancer incidence in 1945, with the greatest number of cases presenting between 1946 and 1959.

L. Wartofsky, D. Van Nostrand (eds.), *Thyroid Cancer*, DOI 10.1007/978-1-4939-3314-3_7

Table 7.1 Definition of terminology

Term	Definition, conversion factors
Gray (Gy)	Gy is the unit of absorbed dose, the amount of energy imparted by ionizing radiation to a unit mass of tissue; 1 Gy corresponds to 1 J per kg. 1 Gy = 100 rad
Sievert (Sv)	Sievert is the unit of effective dose. When exposure is to mixed radiation (e.g., α and γ), their contribution is weighted to give an equivalent dose. A further weighting is made to account for different susceptibilities of various tissues. 1 Sv = 100 rem
Becquerel (Bq)	Bq is the unit of activity, the number of radioactive transformations taking place per second. 1 curie = 3. 7×10^{10} Bq
Relative risk (RR)	The risk of developing cancer in a radiation-exposed subject compared to the risk in an unexposed individual
Excess relative risk (ERR)	RR = ERR + 1. The ERR is usually specified per Gy. For example, if the ERR is 2.0 per Gy, then the RR would be 3.0 for a 1-Gy exposure, and 5.0 for a 2-Gy exposure
Excess absolute risk (EAR)	Usually expressed per 10,000 person-years per Gy. Defines the increase in the absolute risk of developing cancer as a result of radiation exposure

They attributed the subsequent decline to the curtailment of the practice of head and neck irradiation in children.

A number of additional studies [7, 8] have confirmed that the majority of radiation-induced thyroid carcinomas are well-differentiated papillary adenocarcinomas that more frequently present with extrathyroidal spread and bilateral thyroid lobe involvement but with similar recurrence and mortality rates to tumors in nonirradiated patients. The patients are also younger at diagnosis, usually less than 35 years of age, with an average interval to clinical presentation of 25–30 year. The incidence of radiation-induced thyroid carcinoma appeared to increase from 1940 to at least 1970, but since the discontinuation of widespread use of X-ray therapy in infancy, this trend has decreased [9, 10].

Clinically occult papillary microcarcinomas are generally not included in analysis of these data, but they are often detected by pathologists examining thyroids removed for larger benign nodules. Autopsy studies have demonstrated prevalence rates of papillary microcarcinoma ($\leq$1 cm diameter) of up to 33.7 % in general populations, and ethnic and/or geographic differences exist [11, 12] (see Chap. 2). The prevalence of carcinoma is also dependent on the extent of surgery, the amount of resected thyroid tissue processed for histological assessment, and the absolute number of sections examined by the pathologist [13]. Care is required in evaluating studies with regard to these issues.

Although radiation exposure has a role in the development of clinical papillary carcinoma, the extent of such risk in a given population cannot always be ascertained, as the number of people at risk may be unknown. Currently, it is estimated that 9 % of thyroid cancers may be attributable to radiation [14]. Because radiation-induced thyroid carcinomas rarely include the more aggressive anaplastic and medullary types, its fatality rate is between 3 and 9 % [15].

A small but significant number of patients with anaplastic thyroid carcinoma have had a history of prior exposure to external irradiation or ^{131}I. Such therapy for differentiated thyroid cancer might theoretically induce transformation to an anaplastic carcinoma, but because most cases of anaplastic carcinoma show areas of differentiated tumor, this phenomenon may be an aspect of the natural history of these tumors and may therefore not be a consequence of radiation [16].

Prior Studies

External Radiation

Introduction

From 1920 to 1960, radiation was commonly used to treat a variety of benign conditions, including several head, neck, and upper thoracic sites, which resulted in thyroid gland exposure. In 1950, Duffy and Fitzgerald [17] found that 9 of 28 children with thyroid cancer had received prior irradiation of the thymus as infants. Subsequent reports [18, 19] confirmed the risk of thyroid cancer in children exposed to high-dose radiation and the use of radiation to treat benign disease slowly diminished. Also, the risk of radiation has been analyzed in patients treated for malignant disease, in occupational settings, and in situations of inadvertent exposure.

Atomic Bomb Survivors

A fixed cohort of nearly 80,000 survivors of the atomic bomb exposures in Hiroshima and Nagasaki, Japan, has been followed since 1958 by the Atomic Bomb Casualty Commission and its successor, the Radiation Effects Research Foundation. In a comprehensive report [20] on the incidence and risk estimates for solid tumors diagnosed between 1958 and 1987, the thyroid had one of the highest solid tumor risk estimates in the Life Span Study cohort, with occult tumors excluded. The mean estimated thyroid dose was 0.264 Sv, and a strong linear dose–response was demonstrated. Persons exposed when younger than age 10 year had an excess relative risk (ERR) of 9.46, over three times greater than those in their second decade (see Table 7.2). Although earlier studies [21] suggested otherwise, this report [20] showed that those individuals over the age of 20 year at the time of the blast had no excess of thyroid cancer. Mortality data from the Life Span Study contributed little support for an increased risk of thyroid cancer, because the disease causes so few deaths [22].

Table 7.2 Major cohort studies of external radiation in childhood

Study (Ref.)	No. exposed	Age at exposure	Thyroid dose	Follow-up	ERR/Gy 95 % CI
Atomic bomb [20]	79,972	17.6 years	0.264 Sv	1,950,567 PY	1.15/Sv (0.5–2.1)
Age <10					9.46/Sv (4.1–19)
Hemangioma [25]	14,351	6 months	0.26 Gy	406,355 PY	4.92/Gy
Hemangioma [26]	11,807	5 months	0.12 Gy	370,517 PY	7.5/Gy (0.4–18)
Tonsils and adenoids [27]	4296	4.4 years	0.59 Gy	33 years	3.0/Gy (1–40)
Thymus [33]	2657	5 weeks	1.36 Gy	37.1 year	9.0/Gy (4.2–22)
Tinea [34]	10,834	7.4 years	0.09 Gy	30.2 years	30/Gy

Cervical Tuberculous Adenitis

Tisell and colleagues [23] evaluated 444 patients treated with X-rays for cervical tuberculous lymphadenitis between 1913 and 1951 in Göteborg, Sweden. The mean age at irradiation was 19 years, with almost 50 % of patients between 15 and 24 years of age. The calculated absorbed dose to the thyroid ranged from 0.40 to 50.90 Gy (median: 5.2 Gy; mean: 7.2 Gy); 25 thyroid cancers were found, all but one palpable, with a mean observation time of 43 years. The mean and median latency periods were 40 year to diagnosis. A positive correlation was shown between absorbed dose and the probability of developing carcinoma, even after doses of more than 20 Gy. No significant correlation between age at irradiation and the risk of developing cancer was detected.

Cutaneous Hemangioma

Furst and coworkers [24] conducted follow-up with 18,030 patients with skin hemangioma who were treated with external beam radiation between 1920 and 1959 at the Karolinska Hospital. At the time of therapy, 82 % were less than 1 year of age (median age: 6 months). Treatment methods varied, but the relative risk (RR) of thyroid cancer was only slightly increased (1.18) in the group treated with radium-226 or orthovoltage X-rays. In patients receiving contact X-rays or no radiation, no increased risk was noted. An estimation of absorbed thyroid doses was not made.

A similar analysis [25] of a cohort of 14,351 infants less than 18 months of age (mean: 6 months) irradiated for hemangioma during the period of 1920–1959 in Stockholm covered 406,355 person-years at risk, with a mean follow-up of 39 years. The mean absorbed thyroid dose was 0.26 Gy. The Swedish Cancer Registry documented 17 thyroid cancers. Excess cancers began 19 years after radiation and persisted for at least 40 year following radiation therapy (see Table 7.2).

Another study [26] involved 11,807 infants treated with radium-226 between 1930 and 1965 in Göteborg, Sweden, at a median age of 5 months. The mean absorbed thyroid dose was 0.12 Gy. Follow-up through the Swedish Cancer Registry yielded 15 thyroid cancers (ERR = 7.5/Gy; see Table 7.2).

Tonsils/Adenoids

Extensive data has been reported by Schneider and colleagues [27–30] from long-term follow-up studies of more than 5300 subjects who received external radiation for various benign head and neck abnormalities, principally for enlarged tonsils and adenoids, during 1939–1962. In analyzing 4296 of these individuals with an average age at first exposure of 4.4 years and an average thyroid dose of 0.59 Gy, they found that ERR was 3/Gy for thyroid cancer (see Table 7.2). With a mean follow-up of 33 years, the majority of cases occurred in the interval between 20 and 40 year after radiation therapy, peaking at 25–29 years, with a significant decline in risk with increasing age at exposure [27]. Additional data from this source includes information on the effect of screening, as well as characteristics of the secondary thyroid cancers. The authors documented recurrent malignancy in 13.5 % of the 296 patients with thyroid cancer, nearly all within 10 year after primary tumor resection. Significant risk factors for recurrence were the size of the primary lesion, number of lobes involved, histological type, vessel invasion, and lymph node metastasis [28]. Longer-term follow-up of 118 cases occurring before intensive screening showed recurrences in 23.7 % of this total; 39 % of cancers in children recurred vs 15.6 % in adults. This established an inverse relationship between the frequency of recurrence and the patient's age at surgery (also between the frequency of recurrence and latency period between radiation and surgery). Age at radiation and treatment dose were not related to recurrences [29]. Another aspect explored in this group was the possibility of a radiation sensitivity within the population at risk. Patients with secondary salivary gland and/or neural tumors of the head and neck region had a significantly increased frequency of thyroid cancer compared to patients with neither of these tumors, suggesting that additional factors, such as radiation sensitivity, may account for this increased risk [30].

Acne

Paloyan and Lawrence [31] found that 20 of 224 patients referred for thyroidectomy for solitary nodules had received antecedent radiation for the treatment of acne vulgaris. Of the 20 patients, 12 had thyroid cancer 9–41 years after radiation therapy. Complete records were unavailable, and no statistical analysis was reported.

Thymus

Analysis of radiotherapy's effect for thymic enlargement in infancy on subsequent neoplastic disease was initiated by Hempelmann and colleagues in Rochester, New York, in the 1950s. They established that the risk of cancer was proportional to the thyroid dose and raised concern that persons of Jewish ancestry might be at greater risk [32]. Extended 37-years average follow-up [33] of 2657 of these exposed infants and 4833 of their siblings via mail surveys through 1986 confirmed a linear dose–response relationship, with an ERR of 9/Gy (see Table 7.2). The median age at radiation therapy was 5 weeks, and 95 % were under 34 weeks of age. Estimated thyroid doses ranged from 0.03 to over 10 Gy, with a mean of 1.36 and median of only 0.3 Gy. None of the dose fractionation variables examined (dose per fraction, number of fractions, and interval between fractions) was significant in modifying risk.

Tinea Capitis

A major long-term study [34] of 10,834 subjects who received X-ray therapy for tinea capitis between 1948 and 1960 in Israel was compared with the effects with a similar number of nonirradiated individuals and 5392 nonirradiated siblings. All irradiated subjects were under 16 years old at the time of treatment, with a mean age of 7.4 years. The mean thyroid dose was 0.093 Gy, with the dose highly inversely correlated with age at exposure owing to the proximity of the thyroid to the X-ray fields in smaller children. The Israel Cancer Registry documented 98 thyroid cancers, showing a mean interval of 17.1 years from radiation therapy to diagnosis. A much higher excess risk of thyroid cancer was found than in other studies (Table 7.2), possibly relating to the underestimation of thyroid doses as a result of patient movement. An increased risk in Jewish patients may also have been a factor.

A similar study of 2215 children irradiated for tinea capitis in New York found no thyroid cancers through a mailed questionnaire after an average 20.5-year follow-up [35]. However, there were less than 300 females, and the expected number of thyroid cancers would have been only 2.9 [36]. The mean age at treatment was 7.9 years; the estimated thyroid dose was 0.06 Gy [35].

Previous Malignancy

Tucker and colleagues [37] reported on the experience of the Late Effects Study Group, which followed a roster of 9170 patients surviving any type of malignancy in childhood for over 2 years. The period of risk extended to death, the last follow-up, or the date of developing any form of second malignancy, whether of the thyroid or not. The mean age at initial tumor diagnosis was 7 years, and 45 % of all patients were less than 5 years old. The duration of follow-up beginning 2 years after initial diagnosis was 2–48 years (mean: 5.5 years), with an aggregate follow-up of 50,609 person-years. The radiation dose to the thyroid ranged from 0 to 76 Gy (mean: 12.5; median: 3.6 Gy). The authors documented 23 secondary thyroid cancers through their 13 centers, yielding a 53-fold increased risk over matched controls, and a significantly increased RR was shown among those with early age at initial cancer diagnosis. All the thyroid cancer patients had received at least 1 Gy to the thyroid.

A study of 1787 patients treated for Hodgkin's disease [38] at Stanford University between 1961 and 1989 included 1677 patients who had thyroid radiation, most receiving 44 Gy. The mean age at time of treatment was 28 years (range: 2–82 years). After an average follow-up of 9.9 years, they found six thyroid cancers 9–19 (median: 13) years after therapy began for a RR of 15.6 times expected. The age of these six patients ranged from 5 to 32 years at the time of exposure.

Additional studies [39–43] have assessed the risk of radiation therapy for malignancies on the subsequent occurrence of thyroid and other second cancers. These include investigations of large populations of women treated for uterine cervical cancer and males with testicular malignancy; no increased risk of secondary thyroid cancer has been demonstrated, but one such study in women found a slight insignificant excess (RR =1.1; [39]). In this study, as well as the others, the thyroid gland was outside the field of direct radiation, and the estimated average thyroid dose was 0.15 Gy.

Occupational Exposure

Occupational exposure to low-dose radiation has been analyzed in large studies of workers in the nuclear industry. In a report on mortality among radiation workers in the United Kingdom, thyroid cancer was the only malignancy for which the standardized mortality ratio was raised, but the ERR was low (1.05/Sv; [44]). A similar study of employees of the UK Atomic Energy Authority demonstrated a slight, nonsignificant increase in mortality from thyroid cancer [45]. Additional mortality studies in the United States [46–48] failed to demonstrate excess thyroid cancer deaths among nuclear materials workers.

A study of cancer incidence among medical diagnostic X-ray workers in China [49] found seven thyroid cancers in 27,011 individuals employed between 1950 and 1980, with nearly 700,000 person-years of observation. Thyroid cancers were increased among workers employed for 10 year or more and among those who began such work before 1960. No dosimetry measurements were obtained. A study of more than 143,000 members of the American Registry of Radiologic Technologists [50] from 1926 to 1982, who were evaluated through questionnaires, revealed a total of 220 self-reported thyroid cancers vs an expected number of approx 100 cases. However, these data do not include confirmation of the diagnoses, nor are thyroid dose estimates available.

Mortality analysis by review of death certificates of British radiologists who died between 1897 and 1976 failed to demonstrate an excess of thyroid cancers [51]. Similar mortality data from North American radiologists did not demonstrate any excess deaths from thyroid cancer compared to other specialty physicians during 1920–1969 [52].

Prenatal Exposure

The cancer risk of prenatal irradiation has been analyzed in atomic bomb survivors and from diagnostic imaging. Although some studies have found evidence of an increased incidence of childhood cancer following prenatal abdominal X-ray exposure, thyroid cancer rates have never been shown to increase. Many of these reports have been based on mortality data [53, 54], which would not be expected to show an increase for thyroid cancer, but several have utilized incidence data as well [55–57]. Yet, these studies are confounded by a number of factors, including difficulties in dose estimation and maternal issues that may affect the risk of subsequent malignancy, such as prenatal care, maternal age, sibship position, and prior miscarriage. Follow-up by death records and tumor registries of 1630 of the 2802 individuals surviving in utero exposure from the Japanese atomic bombs disclosed only one thyroid cancer until 1984 [58].

Internal Irradiation

Introduction

Human exposure to ^{131}I has been analyzed in patients treated for hyperthyroidism and at smaller doses (<1 mCi) for diagnostic thyroid scans. Radioactive fallout containing ^{131}I and short-lived radioiodines has also resulted in human thyroid irradiation. Although it is believed that ^{131}I is considerably less effective in producing thyroid abnormalities than X-radiation, one of the best controlled animal studies suggests that the carcinogenic effects are similar [59]. Shorter-lived radioisotopes of iodine are more destructive because of the greater penetration of their beta rays and faster dose rate, but their ability to produce thyroid cancer relative to X-rays is uncertain.

Populations Near Nuclear Facilities

Research from the United States and United Kingdom [60, 61] have investigated the mortality from cancer among people residing near nuclear power plants. Although such analyses are problematic owing to relocation of potentially exposed people, case ascertainment in different areas, information on individual radiation exposures, and various social issues, an increase in thyroid cancer deaths has not yet been reported. The Chernobyl accident is considered separately below.

Hanford Nuclear Site

In 1986, it was revealed that the Hanford Atomic Products Operations in Richland, Washington, had released ^{131}I into the environment over a period of years, the greatest during 1944–1947. The Hanford Thyroid Disease Study [62] reported that the thyroid glands of 3441 people born in the vicinity of the Hanford plant between 1940 and 1946 had been thoroughly examined and thyroid dose reconstruction calculations had been performed. The final Hanford report [62], released in 2002, failed to demonstrate an increased risk of thyroid cancer from exposure to Hanford's ^{131}I atmospheric releases. A review of the study by the National Research Council of the National Academy of Sciences [63] concluded that the imprecision of dose estimates weakened the statistical power of the study. Therefore, although the study did not detect a dose–response relationship, the data are not strong enough to determine whether there is a small incremental risk associated with ^{131}I exposure.

Diagnostic ^{131}I

In a multicenter cohort [64] study of 35,074 patients, 50 thyroid cancers were observed through the Swedish Cancer Registry vs an expected number of 39.4 in the general population. This incidence was not significantly greater than expected and may have been influenced by the prevalence of underlying thyroid disease in this selected population. The mean age at first ^{131}I examination was about 44 years, with a mean total dose of 52 μCi and absorbed dose of 0.5 Gy. The mean follow-up was 20 year, with 527,056 person-years at risk, excluding the first 5 years after examination.

Therapeutic ^{131}I

Several studies of the effect of ^{131}I therapy for hyperthyroidism on subsequent malignancy have been performed. The largest of these [65] from the Cooperative Thyrotoxicosis Therapy Follow-up Study evaluated 35,593 patients, including 23,020 treated with ^{131}I. An elevated risk of thyroid cancer mortality following ^{131}I treatment was documented [65]; however, in absolute terms, the excess number of thyroid cancer deaths was small.

In a group of 4557 patients who received ^{131}I therapy for hyperthyroidism between 1951 and 1975 in Sweden, Holm [66] found no increased risk of thyroid cancer at doses estimated at 60–100 Gy. The mean age at treatment in this study was 56 years and an average follow-up time of only 9.5 years. An excess of thyroid cancer was found by Hoffman and associates [67] in a study of 1005 women treated with ^{131}I at the Mayo Clinic, but this excess was not statistically significant. In the study with the longest follow-up period (mean of 15 years for 85 % of recipient patients surviving), Holm and coworkers [68] found no increased risk of thyroid cancer in 3000 subjects treated for hyperthyroidism or cardiac disease, based on Swedish Cancer Registry data. Further mortality studies [69, 70] in women receiving ^{131}I therapy for hyperthyroidism have shown no excess thyroid cancer deaths.

At the Cleveland Clinic [71], 87 children and adolescents less than 18 years of age when they received ^{131}I treatment for hyperthyroidism were evaluated. The mean ^{131}I dose was 9.75 mCi. No thyroid cancers were detected in these patients or their offspring; the mean follow-up period was 12.3 years. Although ^{131}I in therapeutic doses may affect substantial cell killing and thereby mitigate any tumorigenic impact on the thyroid, long-term follow-up of exposed populations is needed to establish the effect of ^{131}I on subsequent thyroid cancer risk.

Fallout

Southwestern United States

People living in Nevada and Utah near the nuclear test site were exposed to radioactive fallout in the 1950s. At least 87 of the atmospheric tests between 1951 and 1958 resulted in offsite contamination [72]. Thyroid dose estimates range from 0.46 [73] to 25 Gy or more [72] with added uncertainty regarding the amount of consumption of contaminated milk. It is not known whether short-lived isotopes of iodine were involved. Thyroid examination 12–18 years later of 5179 children from the area of greatest exposure failed to disclose any increase in abnormalities [73]. However, an interview survey of a 1951 cohort of 4125 Mormons in this area disclosed an excess incidence of thyroid cancers from 1958 to 1980 [72]. This report was challenged by a subsequent mortality study of this region, which found no excess thyroid cancer deaths [74]. Owing to the lack of accurate dose information in this setting, no definite conclusions regarding the risk of fallout exposure are possible.

Continental United States

The National Cancer Institute published estimates of ^{131}I thyroid doses in the Continental United States from fallout exposure related to the Nevada tests of the 1950s [75]. An ecologic study of thyroid cancer death rates across the continental United States suggested an association with the thyroid dose received by children under 1 year of age but failed to demonstrate increased risk from doses received at ages 1–15 years [76]. This result may relate to biases inherent in an ecologic study design, especially limitations introduced by studying a mobile population. Based on the National Cancer Institute data, a committee of the US National Academy of Sciences Institute of Medicine and National Research Council [77] estimated that an excess of 11,300 thyroid cancer cases could be attributed to exposure from the Nevada atomic bomb testing. It was further calculated that 45 % of these cases had already occurred at the time of the report (1999).

Marshall Islands

In 1954, after detonation of a 15-megaton nuclear device at Bikini, an unanticipated wind shift caused exposure to fallout of at least 300 people on at least three of the atolls of the Marshall Islands [78–80]. Late effects of this exposure have been predominantly thyroid abnormalities from absorbed radioiodines (^{131}I, ^{132}I, ^{133}I, and ^{135}I), as well as penetrating whole-body γ radiation. Significant uncertainty exists regarding thyroid doses; rough estimates average 3.12 Gy in all exposed children. Although a significant increase in nodular thyroid disease and hypothyroidism has been shown throughout the northern atolls, few cancers have been documented, and the estimated risk only 1.9 times greater than unexposed Marshallese. The risk of thyroid cancer was lower in children under 10 year old at irradiation than in older populations, suggesting that dose estimates might be too low and that significant cell killing occurred in the younger group, which is reflected by their higher incidence of hypothyroidism. No thyroid cancer has been detected in the ten individuals exposed in utero, but two developed benign nodules.

Other Incidences

Wiklund and colleagues [81] studied a cohort of 2034 reindeer-breeding Lapps who had ingested large amounts of radioactive fallout products from nuclear weapons tests in the USSR. Exposure was through the lichen–reindeer–man food chain. From 1961 to 1984, an abundance in thyroid cancer incidence was not detected through the Swedish Cancer Registry.

^{131}I Risk in Children and Adolescents

Prior to the Chernobyl accident, data in the literature regarding ^{131}I exposures in individuals under age 20 are sparse [82]. Exposed populations were small, and only small numbers of thyroid cancer (23 cases) have been reported. Because of these factors, and the fact that some subjects were being investigated for thyroid diseases and others were administered ^{131}I doses in the cell-sterilization range, there is insufficient scientific information from earlier studies to make conclusions about the risk posed by ^{131}I in children and adolescents. However, analysis of post-Chernobyl thyroid cancer data has demonstrated conclusively that ^{131}I is a thyroid carcinogen in children and adolescents (see section on "The Chernobyl accident and thyroid cancer" below).

Analysis of Risk Assessment

Introduction

The association between radiation exposure and subsequent thyroid cancer has been conclusively demonstrated in epidemiological studies of children receiving head and neck irradiation and in survivors of the atomic bomb exposures in Japan. These studies indicate that radiation to the thyroid at high doses (>1 Gy) is highly linked with the subsequent development of cancer; the effect at lower doses is difficult to assess. Previous studies to assess doses of less than 0.10 Gy have produced no conclusive evidence of significant risk, but the requisite sample of greater than 100,000 exposed individuals and a similar control population have not been identified and analyzed.

Modifying Factors

Type and Duration of Exposure

External radiation is roughly four to five times as effective in causing thyroid cancer as is ^{131}I for each unit of absorbed dose [83], with other isotopes of iodine probably having an effect between that of ^{131}I and external radiation. Fractionation appears to provide an approx 30 % reduction in the tumorigenic effect on the thyroid [84]. However, X-ray technicians may have an increased risk over the general population [49, 50].

Age at Irradiation

The thyroid is more radiosensitive in children than in adolescents and similarly more so in adolescents than in adults. Tucker and colleagues [37] found that individuals treated at an early age and also after lower doses of radiation appeared to have a higher RR of thyroid cancer, suggesting some increased sensitivity to radiation. Shore [83] estimated that the geometric mean ERR of thyroid cancer following irradiation in adulthood was about 10 % of that in children. In the atomic bomb survivors, thyroid cancer in children had one of the highest ERR estimates among solid malignancies, whereas there was virtually no ERR for thyroid cancer in adults [20]. Large studies of women treated with radiation therapy for cervical cancer [39, 40] are among the few in adults that have demonstrated an excess risk for thyroid cancer, but the confidence intervals were very wide in each study.

Sex

The absolute risk in females is two to four times that of males, but the ERR/Gy is about the same in both sexes. In a study by Lundell and associates [25], most thyroid cancers occurred in females, but because of their higher background incidence rate, the sex-specific RR estimates were similar. Ron and associates [34] and Shore and coworkers [85] reported a greater excess number of cancers among females compared to males but no significant difference in the RR estimates. According to the report of the BEIR V Committee [86], females are about three times as susceptible to radiogenic and nonradiogenic thyroid cancer as males.

Race

The risk appears to be greater in individuals of Jewish ancestry. Thyroid cancer risks varied among different Jewish subgroups in the Israeli tinea study, with those born in Israel having one third the risk of those born in the Middle East or North Africa. Because the fathers of those born in Israel were themselves born in the Middle East or North Africa, environmental, rather than genetic, issues seem to be operative [86].

Iodine Deficiency

Iodine deficiency is a possible promoting factor, as decreased thyroid hormone results in increased stimulation of the thyroid epithelium by thyrotropin (TSH). However, at least two human studies indicate the opposite effect, and thyroid cancer is associated with a high dietary iodine intake [83]. Prior to the Chernobyl experience, only a few reports exist on iodine deficiency's influence on the risk of radiation-induced thyroid cancer [87, 88]. Analysis of post-Chernobyl data in one case–control study has demonstrated that iodine deficiency is a promoting factor in individuals exposed to ^{131}I, although this was not confirmed in a large cohort study (see section on "The Chernobyl accident and thyroid cancer" below).

Parity

The observation that thyroid cancer among the exposed Marshall Island population occurred exclusively in multiparous women implied that parity might increase the chance of radiation-induced thyroid cancer. Shore and colleagues [33] demonstrated that older age at first childbirth significantly increased the risk of radiation-induced thyroid cancer in patients irradiated for thymic enlargement in infancy. A similar effect was found with older age at menarche. Other studies reveal that a history of miscarriage increased this risk, especially for younger women [83].

Latency Period

The interval between initial exposure to radiation and detection of thyroid cancer varies widely among human clinical studies, from 5 to 50 year after irradiation, largely reflecting the study's follow-up interval. The latency period may also increase with the individual's age at irradiation.

Effect of Screening

Based on an intensive screening program that started in 1974 in Chicago, Ron and colleagues [89] reported that adjusted incidence rates of secondary thyroid cancer were seven times greater during the screening period (1974–1979) than before.

Temporal Pattern

The temporal pattern of risk remains uncertain owing to the limited long-term follow-up data available. Schneider and colleagues [27] estimated that the increased risk of radiation-induced thyroid cancer probably lasts throughout life. Similarly, Thompson and colleagues [20] found no evidence for decreased risk with time after exposure. Ron and coworkers [34] reported a continued increase in risk over their entire study period of up to 38 years. Shore and collaborators [33] indicated that the risk ratio declined over time but remained highly elevated at least 45 years after irradiation. Excess risk began 5 years after exposure.

Shore and coworkers [33] found that the ERR decreased during the entire study period but that there was no significant change over time in excess absolute risk (EAR). Conversely, Ron and coworkers [34] demonstrated no significant change in ERR but a continuing increase in EAR during the entire study period (mean follow-up: 30 year). These somewhat contradictory results highlight the need for even longer follow-up periods to clarify the temporal pattern.

Dose–Response Relationship

A strong dose–response relationship between radiation and incidence of thyroid cancer has been documented in Japanese atomic bomb survivors [20] and in studies of children and adolescents [25, 27, 34, 85]. A pooled analysis [84] of seven major studies over a wide range of doses demonstrated an ERR of 7.7 per Gy (95 % confidence limits: 2.1–28.7). For those exposed to radiation before age 15 years, linearity best described the dose–response relationship, even at 0.10 Gy. Although risk estimates are generally those of the linear no-threshold model, at very high doses, these estimates might not be valid because of cell killing [15]. Regardless of possible threshold effects at high doses owing to cell killing, the greatest need is for an understanding of carcinogenic effects of low-dose radiation.

The Chernobyl Accident and Thyroid Cancer

Radioactivity Release

Without question, the Chernobyl accident was the worst technological disaster in the history of nuclear power generation. On April 26, 1986 at 1:23 AM, two explosions occurred (from steam and hydrogen) in reactor 4 of the Chernobyl nuclear power station, ejecting large amounts of radioactive material into the atmosphere. Subsequently, the graphite within the reactor ignited, and fuel elements in the core of the reactor melted, resulting in the release of volatile radioactive products over a 10-day period. The immediate cause of the accident was operator error, but the reactor design (which lacked a concrete containment vessel) has been implicated in the serious consequences of the accident. Initial estimates from officials in Moscow [90] indicated that approx 4 % of the total activity of the core escaped into the atmosphere, resulting in the release of some 50 million Ci (2×10^{18} Bq). However, other researchers concluded that the release was much greater [91, 92]. After 18 months of study at the reactor site, Sich [93, 94] estimated that the total release was actually in the range of 120–150 million Ci. Over 80 different isotopes were released [95]; the most abundant volatile isotopes were those of iodine (^{131}I, ^{132}I, ^{133}I, and ^{135}I), tellurium (^{132}Te), and cesium (^{134}Cs and ^{137}Cs). Some radioactive isotopes released during the accident naturally decayed to isotopes of iodine, e.g., ^{132}Te has a 3-day half-life and decays to ^{132}I.

Geographic Distribution of Volatile Radioactive Isotopes

The distribution of volatile radioactive isotopes to different geographic regions was governed by the prevailing meteorologic conditions [96–99]. The initial plume of volatile isotopes drifted over northern Ukraine and the Gomel oblast (region) of southern Belarus (Fig. 7.1). Contaminated air masses moved west and then northwest, sweeping across the Brest and Grodno oblasts of Belarus, causing the deposition of isotopes in Sweden on April 27. The wind direction changed to the northeast and to the east on April 29, and a large cloud of radioactivity drifted over southern Belarus and the southwestern corner of the Russian Federation. A substantial deposit of radioactivity in the Gomel and Mogilev oblasts of Belarus and the Bryansk oblast of Russia resulted from rainfall during April 28–30, which washed fallout from the cloud onto the ground. Another substantial deposit about 500 km from Chernobyl was formed when the same cloud drifted over the Kaluga-Tula-Orel oblasts of Russia. Rain during April 28–30 washed fallout to the ground in these regions. Winds changed to the south and then shifted to the southwest during the last few days of the accident, contaminating the Balkans and Alps. The World Health Organization (WHO) estimated that 4.9 million people lived in areas where ground surface contamination exceeded 1 Ci/km^2 [100]. About 2.3 million children lived in locations that were significantly contaminated at the time of the accident [101].

Cesium-137 Release

Approximately 2 million Ci (8×10^{16} Bq) of ^{137}Cs was released, causing widespread soil contamination [96, 102]. The distribution of ^{137}Cs, which has a half-life of approx 30 years, has been carefully mapped [89] and was deposited in the following manner: Belarus, 33.5 %; Russia, 24 %; Ukraine, 20 %; Sweden, 4.4 %; and Finland, 4.3 %. The areas with the highest ^{137}Cs contamination are shown in Fig. 7.1.

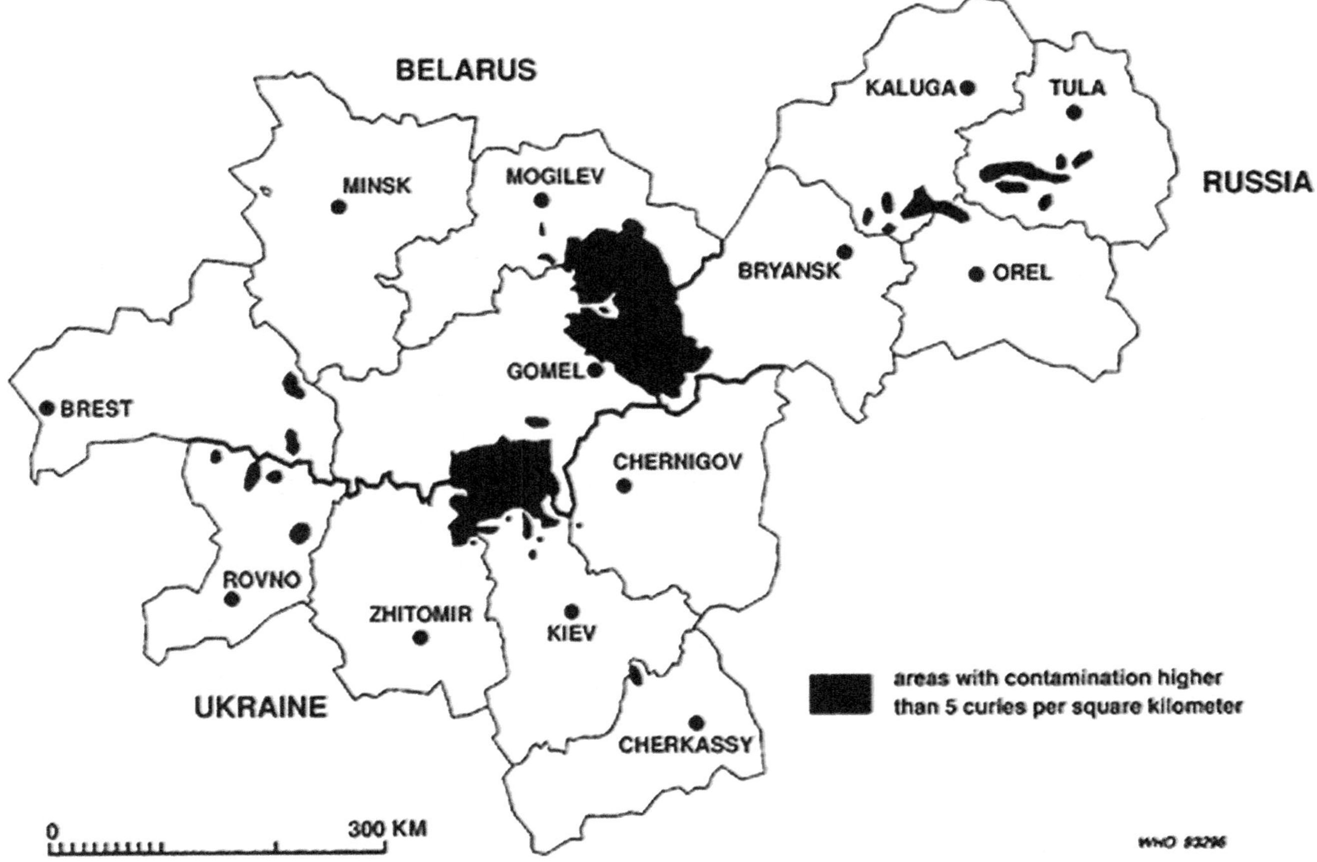

Fig. 7.1 Map showing the distribution of ^{137}Cs in Belarus, Ukraine, and Russia (From Ref. [100], courtesy of the World Health Organization)

Radioiodine Release

The heaviest initial exposure to the population resulted from isotopes of iodine. According to recent studies, the release of ^{131}I (half-life: 8.05 days) was 40–50 million Ci (approx 1.7×10^{18} Bq), representing about 50–60 % of the core inventory [102–105]. By comparison, the Three Mile Island accident released only 15–20 Ci of ^{131}I in the United States in 1979. During the first month following the Chernobyl accident, the major source of internal radiation exposure was ^{131}I, which was acquired by inhalation and ingestion of contaminated food. Deposits of ^{131}I on pasture lands and gardens in the rural agricultural areas surrounding the reactor introduced this radioisotope into the food chain. Ingestion of contaminated milk was the most important source of internal ^{131}I exposure in children [97]. Consumption of contaminated leafy vegetables was a secondary source of internal ^{131}I exposure.

Short-lived isotopes of iodine, such as ^{132}I (half-life: 2.3 h) and ^{133}I (half-life: 21 h), were also released from Chernobyl-4. Very few direct measurements of radioiodines were made in the initial days following the explosion. Therefore, data regarding ^{132}I and ^{133}I, which were important primarily in the first days after the accident, are scarce. Measurements made on April 28, 1986, in Warsaw, Poland, revealed that 28 % of the radioactivity in the air was from short-lived iodine isotopes [106]. Thus, populations near the reactor location were exposed to ^{132}I and ^{133}I via inhalation for at least 1 or 2 days.

Following the accident, a limited number of measurements of the ground deposition density of ^{131}I were conducted in Belarus by the Belarus Institute of Nuclear Physics (Minsk; [107]). A map (Fig. 7.2) of the ^{131}I deposition in Belarus [103] shows some obvious differences in the distribution of ^{131}I compared with the pattern of ^{137}Cs ground contamination (Fig. 7.1). Particularly, the Gomel and Mogilev oblasts were both heavily contaminated with ^{137}Cs, with relatively less contamination in the Brest oblast. In contrast, the ^{131}I contamination was highest in the Gomel oblast and lower but significant levels of deposition were seen in both the Mogilev and Brest oblasts. The contamination in the Brest oblast arose from the initial plume of radioactivity that passed over this area during the first day of the accident.

Reconstruction of Thyroid Doses

Ideally, to support careful epidemiological studies, accurate thyroid dose reconstructions are needed that separate out the contribution of (1) external radiation, (2) internal radiation owing to ^{131}I (from both inhalation and ingestion), and (3)

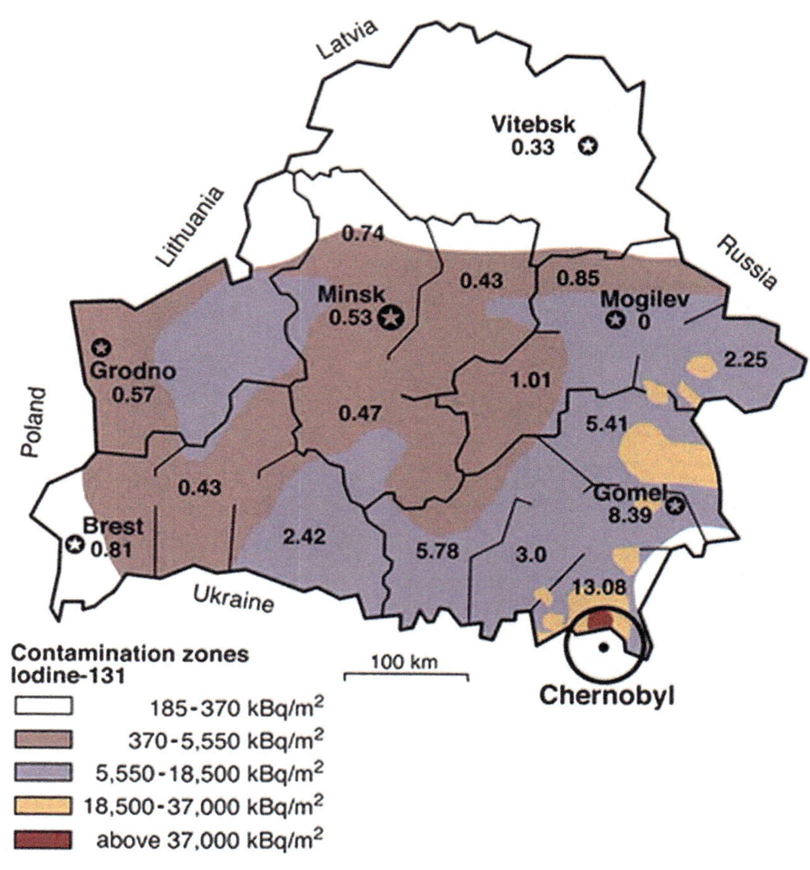

Fig. 7.2 Map showing the distribution of ^{131}I ground contamination in Belarus. Annual incidence rates of thyroid cancer in children in different geographic districts are shown per 100,000 children (Based on data in Ref. [135]. From Ref. [103] with permission of the American Association for the Advancement of Science. Color illustration is printed in insert following p. 198)

internal radiation from the short-lived iodine isotopes (^{132}I and ^{133}I), because these three components may have differing potential to cause thyroid cancer. For example, ^{132}I and ^{133}I, which decay more rapidly than ^{131}I, deliver their radiation dose over a shorter time interval and could theoretically have a carcinogenic effect on thyroid tissue similar to that of X-rays [108]. It has been suggested [101] that the majority of thyroid exposure (85 %) was from internally concentrated ^{131}I derived from ingestion. Approximately 15 % was estimated to have been derived from inhalation of short-lived iodine isotopes.

Following the accident, direct measurements of thyroid radioactive iodine content were made in Belarus, Russia, and Ukraine. From these, the exposure to ^{131}I can be extrapolated, but the measurements were made too late to provide useful information on ^{132}I and ^{133}I. Furthermore, the direct measurements were made on only a small proportion of the affected population. Thyroid dose reconstruction is required to determine the exposure for the rest of the population. Many factors may account for the variability in thyroid doses received by different individuals in the same geographic area. For example, many families grew their own vegetables and obtained milk from their own cows. Many individuals were outdoors most of the day at the time of the accident and slept with the windows open at night, thereby maximizing their exposure to ^{131}I by inhalation. The thyroid dose is known to be inversely related to thyroid mass. Thus, for a given uptake of ^{131}I, children achieve a higher thyroid dose than adults. The iodine level in the diet also influences the efficiency of uptake of ^{131}I. Southern Belarus suffers from mild iodine deficiency, with some relatively isolated pockets of severe iodine deficiency [109, 110]. Iodine supplementation measures had lapsed by 1985. The subsequent implications are that individuals living in iodine-deficient areas would have a greater thyroid uptake of radioiodine than those living in iodine-replete areas. An effective prophylaxis program utilizing potassium iodide, as was administered in Poland [99], could have limited radioiodine exposure. As exposed inhabitants were not immediately informed of the accident, and there was no immediate effort to systematically prophylax the population, potassium iodide was not administered early enough (if at all) in Belarus, Ukraine, and Russia to be effective.

Belarus

Direct measurements of thyroid ^{131}I content were made during May and June of 1986 in approx 300,000 individuals living in the contaminated areas of Belarus. About 200,000 records were verified and form the basis of a database for the calculation of individual thyroid doses of Belarussian residents [111–117]. Roughly 150,000 individuals in the database were interviewed regarding lifestyle and diet. Thyroid dose estimates have been completed for 130,000 residents of the Gomel and Mogilev oblasts and Minsk City who had direct thyroid measurements completed before June 6. Estimates were based on the direct measurements and information on lifestyle and diet (e.g., level of milk consumption). Calculations assumed ^{131}I intake by inhalation and ingestion of fresh milk after a single deposition of fallout on pasture grass [111]. Average thyroid doses have also been estimated for individuals living in 800 rural settlements without direct thyroid measurements. These reconstructions are calculated using the aforementioned database, considering the level of consumption of fresh cows' milk. A dose reconstruction study involving two cities and 2122 settlements in Belarus, as well as one city and 607 settlements in the Bryansk district of the Russian Federation, estimated an ERR of 23 per Gy [112].

Reported average thyroid doses of ^{131}I in Belarussian children living in different contaminated raions (administrative districts) of the Gomel and Mogilev oblasts ranged from 0.15 to 4.7 Gy [111–117]. Young children (age $\leq$7) in these districts generally received thyroid doses that were three- to fivefold higher than those recorded in adults living in the same district. Several hundred children in Belarus received doses of 10 Gy or more to the thyroid; the highest thyroid dose did not exceed 60 Gy.

Russian Federation

In addition to the 130,000 direct measurements in Belarus, 28,000 measurements were made in the Kaluga oblast, and 2000 measurements were made in the Bryansk oblast of Russia [118–120]. These oblasts also suffered from mild-to-moderate iodine deficiency [110]. The mean thyroid dose owing to iodine radionuclides in children in Bryansk was 0.5 Gy, but it was 2.2 Gy in the more heavily contaminated zones. In the Kaluga oblast, the mean dose in children was 0.25 Gy. In the more heavily contaminated areas, the mean dose was 0.5 Gy, and individual doses were as high as 10 Gy.

Ukraine

Direct measurements of thyroid ^{131}I content were made in 150,000 people in Ukraine in May to June of 1986, including 108,000 children and adolescents ages 0–18 years [121–125]. The measurements were conducted in four of the northern oblasts: Chernigov, Kiev, Zhitomir, and Vinnytsia. Large-scale thyroid dose reconstructions were carried out using the direct measurements in combination with environmental data and information on personal behavior and intake of milk and leafy vegetables. Empirical relations were developed between parameters of ^{131}I intake and the level of ^{137}Cs soil contamination and the distance and direction from the nuclear plant. These relations allowed estimation of thyroid ^{131}I content in territories without direct measurements, such as the Cherkassy and Rovno oblasts. In different administrative regions of northern Ukraine, average thyroid doses from ^{131}I in children and adolescents ranged from 0.03 to 1.6 Gy.

Thyroid Cancer Incidence in Children

Following the Chernobyl accident, Prisyazhiuk and colleagues [126] reported a small increase in thyroid cancer cases in children from three districts in the northern Ukraine within 80 km of the nuclear plant. Another report from Ukraine followed [127]. Local physicians had simultaneously detected a marked increase in the rate of childhood thyroid cancer in Belarus, starting in 1990 and primarily affecting the Gomel oblast [99, 128–131]. Whereas only 1 or 2 cases of thyroid cancer were seen annually in the Gomel oblast during 1986–1989, there were 14 cases in 1990 and 38 cases in 1991. Most cases from Belarus (128/131) were diagnosed as papillary carcinomas. The initial reports were met with some skepticism by the international scientific community. Therefore, a team of international scientists under the auspices of the WHO and Swiss government visited Belarus in July of 1992 to verify the accuracy of the histologic diagnoses of thyroid cancer. The international team studied the histologic specimens from 104 children diagnosed with thyroid cancer since 1989 and agreed with the diagnosis in 102 cases [132]. The team also reported a marked increase in the incidence of childhood cancer (age $\leq$14) in Gomel from 1990 onward, with 80 cancers per million children each year by 1992, compared with the usual background rate of around one case of cancer per million children each year.

Subsequent data [101] have shown a continued increase in thyroid cancer incidence in children from Belarus, northern Ukraine (Kiev, Chernigov, Cherkassy, Rovno, and Zhitomir oblasts), and southwestern Russia (Bryansk and Kaluga oblasts) since the accident (Table 7.3). As shown, rates are expressed as cases of pediatric (age $\leq$14) thyroid cancer per million children each year.

Belarus

The annual pediatric (age $\leq$14) thyroid cancer incidence rate in Belarus increased from 0.3 per million in 1981–1985 to 30.6 per million in 1991–1994, a 100-fold increase. A total of 333 cases of pediatric thyroid cancer were diagnosed in Belarus from 1986 to 1994 [101, 133, 134]. During 1995, 91 additional cases were diagnosed (57 in the first 7 months of the year). Yet, there were only seven pediatric cases in Belarus for 9 years preceding the accident (1977–1985). In the Gomel oblast, the incidence rate increased nearly 200-fold up to 96.4 per million.

Of the 390 pediatric cases reported in Belarus through mid-1995, 54.3 % were from the Gomel oblast, and 21.8 % were from the Brest oblast. Only 1.8 % of cases were from

Table 7.3 Incidence of thyroid cancer in children (under age 15 at diagnosis)

Location	Rate 1981–1985	1986–1990	1991–1994
Belarus	0.3	4	30.6
Gomel oblast	0.5	10.5	96.4
Ukraine	0.5	1.1	3.4
Kiev, Chernigov, Cherkassy, Rovno, and Zhitomir oblasts	0.1	2	11.5
Russia			
Bryansk and Kaluga oblasts	0	1.2	10

Data from Ref. [101]
Annual incidence rates per million children under age 15 are given

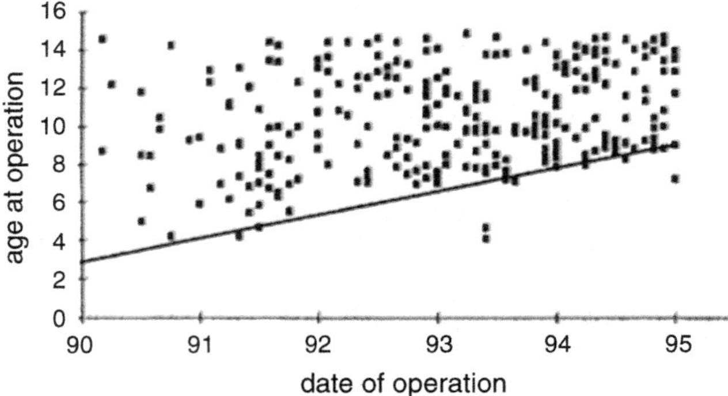

Fig. 7.3 Graph showing the age of Belarussian children at the time of thyroid surgery vs the date of surgery. The *bold line* corresponds to the age of a child born on November 26, 1986. Note that very few cases fall below the *bold line* (From Ref. [138], courtesy of the European Commission)

the Vitebsk oblast, which was not contaminated following the Chernobyl accident. Annual childhood thyroid cancer incidence rates for different geographic zones in Belarus are shown in Fig. 7.2 (in cases per 100,000 children/year for 1990–1991). There is a strong correlation between these incidence rates and soil ^{131}I contamination levels (Fig. 7.2), as documented by the study of Abelin and colleagues [135–137]. As noted by those authors, the higher incidence rates occurred along the two paths taken by the initial clouds of volatile radioisotopes: one pathway to the west and the other to the northeast. The highest annual incidence rate (130.8/million) was found in the southern part of the Gomel oblast, adjacent to Chernobyl, where the ^{131}I contamination level was highest. The association between childhood thyroid cancer incidence and ^{131}I deposition suggests that radioactive isotopes of iodine had an etiological role in the pathogenesis of the thyroid cancers.

The ratio of affected girls to boys in Belarus was 1.5: 1.0. Most affected children (386/390) were born either before the accident or near the time of the accident; only four of the children were born after 1986. The rate of thyroid cancer in children born after 1986 is low and approximates baseline levels before the accident. Figure 7.3 shows data from 298 children diagnosed with thyroid cancer at the Pathology Institute in Minsk from 1990 to 1994 [138]. Note that there is a sharp cutoff age (Fig. 7.3, bold line) below which few young children have presented with thyroid cancer, and the cutoff age increases with time. The bold line in Fig. 7.3 represents children who were born on November 26, 1986. Children born on this date would have been approx 10-weeks gestational age at the time of the Chernobyl accident. Because the fetal thyroid gland can concentrate iodine by 12 weeks, these children could have theoretically sustained significant thyroid exposure to ^{131}I in utero during the first month following the accident. These data strongly suggest that intrathyroidal accumulation of radioactive iodine isotopes—either in utero or after birth—was an important factor in the pathogenesis of the pediatric thyroid cancers in Belarus.

An analysis of thyroid cancer cases in Belarus by cohorts, defined according to the patient's date of birth, is shown in Fig. 7.4 [136, 139]. Clearly, increasing numbers of cases have occurred in each cohort at least until 1993. The largest number of new thyroid cancer cases has occurred in individuals who were age 4 and younger at the time of the accident (birth date: 1982–1986), followed by those who were ages 5–9 (birth date: 1977–1981); however, individuals as old as 19 at the time of the accident were still at risk. These data suggest that younger children are most susceptible to the carcinogenic effects of radioactive iodine isotopes.

The peak incidence of childhood papillary thyroid carcinoma (in patients up to age 14) occurred in Belarus in 1995 at 40 cases per million. Subsequently, a gradually decreasing frequency of papillary carcinoma has been observed in this age group. There were 84 cases observed in 1996, 66 cases in 1997, 54 cases in 1998, 49 cases in 1999, and 31 cases in 2000 [140]. This represents a total of 708 childhood cases presenting in Belarus from 1986 to 2000. After the latter half of 2001, only sporadic thyroid cancers were found in Belarussian children. The decrease is readily explained because over time, exposed individuals will reach age 15 or older and will no longer be reported in the data for children (up to age 14). In keeping with this analysis, since 1997, the incidence of thyroid cancer has increased in Belarussian adolescents ages 15–18 years old at the time of diagnosis or surgery. In 2001, the incidence was 112 per million in this patient cohort [141].

Russian Federation

In the contaminated oblasts of the Russian Federation, an increased incidence of thyroid cancer in children and adolescents has been registered [101, 119, 142, 143]. The annual

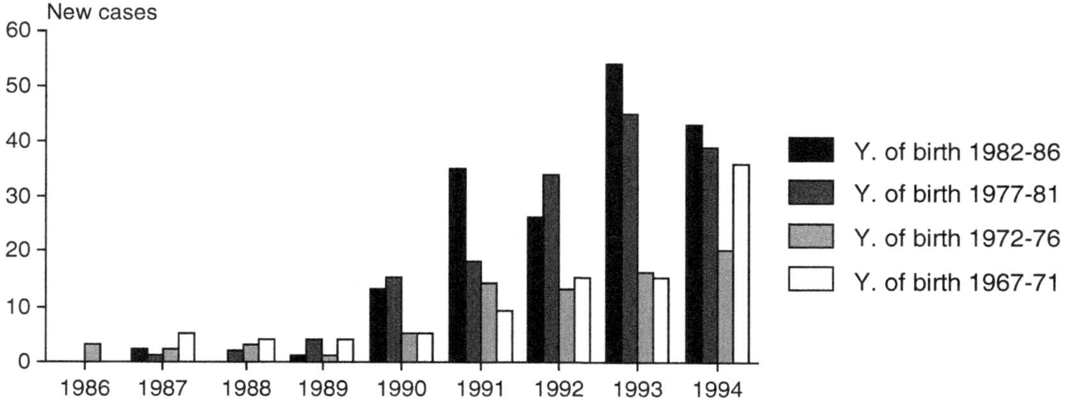

Fig. 7.4 Graph showing the number of new thyroid cancer cases during each year from 1986 to 1994 in cohorts of Belarussian children defined by year of birth (From Ref. [139], courtesy of the European Commission)

prevalence in children (age ≤14) in the Bryansk and Kaluga oblasts has increased from background to ten per million. The major increase occurred in the Bryansk oblast, with 21 cases reported between 1986 and 1994.

Ukraine

Between 1986 and 1994, 211 children (age ≤14) underwent surgery for thyroid cancer in Ukraine [101, 121, 122, 144, 145]. The incidence in children increased from 0.4 to 0.6 per million pre-Chernobyl to 4 per million by 1992–1994. The ratio of girls to boys was 1.4: 1.0. In the five most northern oblasts (Kiev, Chernigov, Zhitomir, Cherkassy, and Rovno) that were heavily contaminated by the Chernobyl accident, the incidence was much higher: 11.5 per million children. About 60 % of the cases in Ukraine originated from these 5 oblasts out of 25 oblasts in the country. Only two children presenting with thyroid cancer were born after 1986, equivalent to an incidence of less than one per million each year in children born after 1986. In Pripyat, located 3.5 km from the Chernobyl plant, the incidence in children and adolescents who were ages 0–18 years old at the time of the accident was 137 per million by 1990–1992. Throughout Ukraine, there was a 30-fold gradient in thyroid cancer incidence rates in individuals ages 0–18 at the time of the accident, directly corresponding to the gradient in thyroid doses from ^{131}I exposure [122]. This relationship between cancer incidence and thyroid ^{131}I dose strongly supports a role for radioactive iodine isotopes in the pathogenesis of the cancers.

Pathological and Biologic Features of the Pediatric Thyroid Cancers

The pathological features of the thyroid cancers presenting after the Chernobyl accident in children from Belarus, Ukraine, and Russia have been well characterized [146–155]. With few exceptions, all the cases have been papillary carcinomas. Several histological subtypes have been noted [146–149]: classical papillary architecture, often with mixed papillary/follicular elements (approx 11 %); a mixture of solid and follicular structures (73 %); and the diffuse sclerosing type (8 %). Primary tumors were 1 cm or larger in diameter in the vast majority of cases (79–88.5 % in three series; [133, 150, 151]).

Thyroid tumors that arise in children are typically more aggressive than those that arise in adults [156–161]. This phenomenon was also true in the Chernobyl-related cases. The tumors were often widely invasive within the thyroid gland (33 % in one series [151]; 59 % of cases in another series [146]). There was direct invasion of extrathyroidal tissue (T4 stage) in a high proportion of cases (48–63 %; [133, 134, 144, 146, 150, 154]). Lymphatic invasion was present in 77 % of cases and blood vessel invasion in 15–32 % [146, 150, 151]. Regional lymph node metastases (N1 stage) were present in 59–88 % of cases [133, 144, 150, 151, 154]. Distant metastases (M1 stage, usually to lung) were present in 5–9 % of cases [133, 150, 154].

Only a few cases showed features of "occult" or microcarcinoma. Taken together, these pathological and biological features argue strongly against the cancers being incidental findings [162–164]. In nearly all cases, the cancers represented clinically significant disease; only 9 % of the children in one series from Belarus were staged at T1 N0 M0 [150].

Molecular Characterization of Chernobyl-Associated Papillary Thyroid Carcinomas

Ret Oncogene

Activation of the *ret* oncogene by chromosomal rearrangement was initially reported in four of seven Chernobyl-associated pediatric cases by Ito and coworkers [165] and is the most characteristic type of molecular alteration in post-

Table 7.4 Studies of *Ret* rearrangements in post-Chernobyl papillary thyroid cancers

Authors (Ref.)	*N*	Dates of diagnosis	*Ret*/PTC1	*Ret*/PTC2	*Ret*/PTC3
A. Latency period[a]≤10 years (April 26, 1986, through April 26, 1996)					
Fugazzola et al. [166]	6	1991–1992	0 (0 %)	1 (17 %)	3 (50 %)
Nikiforov et al. [167]	38	1991–1992	6 (16 %)	1 (3 %)	22 (58 %)
Klugbauer et al. [168]	12	1993–1995	2 (17 %)	0 (0 %)	6 (50 %)
Smida et al. [182]	37	1993–4/16/1996	8 (22 %)	0 (0 %)	11 (29 %)
Rabes et al. [177, 178]	61	1993–4/26/1996	9 (15 %)	0 (0 %)	24 (39 %)
Pisarchik et al. [179]	4	2/1996	1 (25 %)	NT	NT
Pisarchik et al. [180]	3	2/1996	NT	NT	1 (33 %)
Pooled data			26 (16 %)	2 (1.3 %)	67 (43 %)
B. Latency period >10 years (after April 26, 1996)					
Pisarchik et al. [179]	27	10/1996–12/1996	8 (30 %)	NT	NT
Pisarchik et al. [180]	12	10/1996–12/1996	NT	NT	0 (0 %)
Pisarchik et al. [181]	37	1998	8 (22 %)	NT	5 (14 %)
Smida et al. [182]	14	5/1996–1997	4 (29 %)	0 (0 %)	2 (14 %)
Rabes et al. [177, 178]	130	5/1996–1998	39 (30 %)	0 (0 %)	14 (11 %)
Pooled data			59 (28 %)	0 (0 %)	21 (11 %)

NT not tested

[a]Interval between exposure and diagnosis/surgery

Chernobyl papillary thyroid carcinomas [165–186]. An analysis of pooled data regarding *ret* rearrangements from eight published studies [166–168, 177–182] is presented in Table 7.4. For purposes of this analysis, those cases diagnosed or undergoing surgery on or before April 26, 1996, are reported in part A; those presenting after April 26, 1996, are reported in part B. The original published case series have been segregated into two groups according to this criterion. For example, the first 37 cases of Smida et al. [182] underwent surgery from April 21, 1993, to April 16, 1996, and are recorded in part A. The remaining 14 from this series underwent surgery from May 3, 1996, to February 14, 1997, and are recorded in part B. The 191 cases of Rabes et al. [177, 178] were divided into groups of 61 and 130 by the original authors using the same criterion. Case numbers 3, 4, 5, and 6 as published by Pisarchik et al. [179, 180] underwent surgery in February 1996 and are included in part A. Cases numbered 7–39 underwent surgery from October 2, 1996, to December 27, 1996, and are reported in part B. All individuals reported in this analysis were under age 20 at the moment of the accident (April 26, 1986).

As demonstrated in Table 7.4, part A, *ret*/PTC3 is the most prevalent form of *ret* rearrangement in post-Chernobyl papillary carcinomas diagnosed during the first decade following the accident (until April 26, 1996). The overall prevalence of *ret*/PTC3 in these cases is 43 %, whereas the prevalence of *ret*/PTC1 is 16 % and that of *ret*/PTC2 is only 1.3 %.

In contrast with the earlier case series, Pisarchik and colleagues [179] found a higher prevalence of *ret*/PTC1 rearrangements (29 %) in 31 post-Chernobyl papillary thyroid carcinomas presenting in 1996. However, the prevalence of *ret*/PTC3 was found to be quite low (7 %) in a subset of these cases [180]. Pisarchik and colleagues [180] suggested that there was a switch in the ratio of *ret*/PTC3 to *ret*/PTC1 rearrangements in late (1996) vs early (1991–1992) post-Chernobyl papillary thyroid cancers. Smida and colleagues [182] independently arrived at a similar conclusion after studying 51 Chernobyl-related cases. These authors [182] suggested that *ret*/PTC3 may be typical for radiation-associated childhood papillary thyroid carcinomas with a short latency period, whereas *ret*/PTC1 may be a marker for carcinomas appearing after a longer latency period. These observations are confirmed by the pooled analysis in Table 7.4, part B. The overall prevalence of *ret*/PTC3 in these later cases is significantly lower at 11 %, whereas the prevalence of *ret*/PTC1 is higher at 28 %.

In addition to influencing the latency period, the type of *ret* rearrangement correlates strongly with morphological variants of papillary thyroid carcinoma. Nikiforov and colleagues [167] first reported that post-Chernobyl papillary thyroid carcinomas with a solid differentiation pattern are associated with *ret*/PTC3, and the classic papillary differentiation pattern is related to the *ret*/PTC1 rearrangement. This finding has been confirmed by Rabes and colleagues [177, 178], as well as Thomas and colleagues [183–185], and similar results have been obtained in transgenic mice [187–189].

The results regarding *ret* rearrangements are particularly interesting in view of the recent demonstration that X-irradiation (50–100 Gy) in vitro can induce *ret* oncogene rearrangements in undifferentiated human thyroid carcinoma cells [190]. Furthermore, Bounacer and colleagues [191] reported a high frequency of *ret* rearrangements (primarily *ret*/PTC1) in papillary thyroid carcinomas originating from

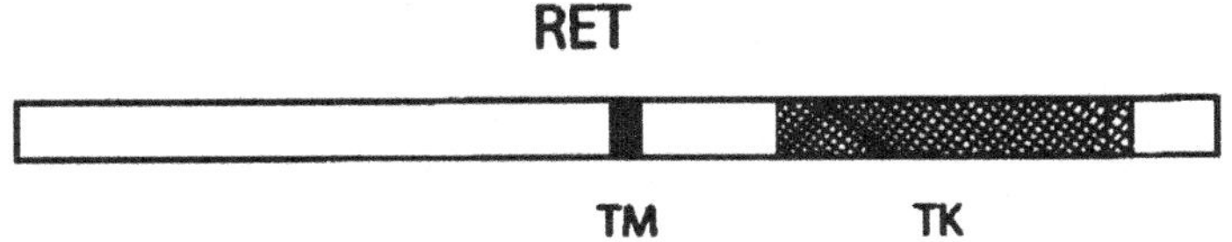

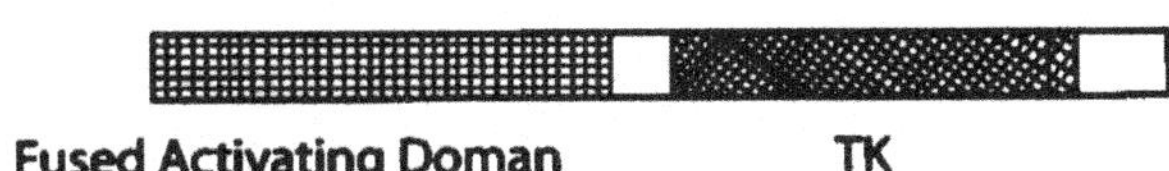

Rearrangement	Fused Activating Gene	Function	Chromosome
RET/PTC1	*H4*	Unknown	10q21
RET/PTC2	*RI α*	Regulatory subunit of cAMP-dependent protein Kinase A	17q23-24
RET/PTC3 } RET/PTC4	*ELE1 (ARA 70)*	Androgen receptor-associated protein (co-transcription factor)	10q11.2
RET/PTC5	*GOLGA5 (RFG5)*	Gogli integral membrane protein	14q
RET/PTC6	*hTIF1 α*	Transcription intermediary factor	7q32-34
RET/PTC7	*hTIF1 γ (RFG7)*	Transcription intermediary factor	1p13
RET/PTC8	*Kinectin*	Vesicle membrane anchored protein	14q22.1
RET/PTC9	*RFG9*	Putative intracellular transport protein	18q21-22
RET/PCM1	*PCM1*	Centrosomal protein	8p22-21.3
ELKS/RET	*ELKS*	Unknown	12p13

Fig. 7.5 Patterns of RET oncogene rearrangement found in papillary carcinomas

patients with a history of external radiation. Similar results using immunohistochemistry were reported by Collins and colleagues [192]. Taken together, they suggest that *ret* rearrangements are important in the pathogenesis of radiation-induced papillary thyroid carcinomas, and the specific type of molecular rearrangement (*ret*/PTC1 vs *ret*/PTC3) may influence the biology of the cancer (e.g., the latency period and morphological variant).

Following the Chernobyl accident, rare types of *ret*/PTC rearrangements were also described (Fig. 7.5). These include a variant of *ret*/PTC1 [193], *ret*/PTC4 [172], and other variants of *ret*/PTC3 [170, 171], *ret*/PTC5 [173], *ret*/PTC6 [174], *ret*/PTC7 [174], *ret*/PTC8 [175], and *ret*/PTC9 [176]. Three other rearrangements—*ret*/*PCM1* [194], *ELKS*/*RET* [195], and *ret*/*PTC1L* (another variant of *ret*/PTC1) [196]—were recently described.

Other Genetic Loci

Other genetic loci have been investigated [138, 146, 197–205] including *NTRK1*, *TP53*, the TSH receptor, the three *ras* genes (*H-RAS*, *K-RAS*, and *N-RAS*), and *BRAF*. Chromosomal rearrangements associated with the *NTRK1* gene [197] have been identified infrequently in post-Chernobyl papillary thyroid carcinomas [177, 178, 198]. Missense, silent, and nonsense mutations involving the *TP53* gene have been identified in a small number of Chernobyl-associated papillary thyroid carcinomas [199–204]. Alterations of the TSH receptor and *RAS* genes are very rare, suggesting that point mutations in these genes do not have a significant role in the pathogenesis of Chernobyl-associated thyroid cancers. A novel *AKAP9-BRAF* fusion resulting from an internal rearrangement of chromosome 7 has been described in a subset of post-Chernobyl papillary thyroid carcinomas [205]. In contrast, activating point mutations of *BRAF* are absent [205].

Summary Molecular Model

The available molecular data, taken together, suggest that the mechanism of Chernobyl radiation-induced papillary thyroid cancer pathogenesis is primarily related to double-stranded DNA breaks leading to chromosomal translocations and/or inversions and gene rearrangements (e.g., involving *ret*, *NTRK1*, and *BRAF* genes). The resulting hybrid gene products are expressed within thyroid follicular cells and exhibit ligand-independent activation. These hybrid proteins then constitutively activate the MAPK pathway. This is in contrast to sporadic papillary thyroid cancers where activating point mutations within elements of the MAPK pathway are more common.

Epidemiological Considerations

Following the initial reports of thyroid cancer cases in the regions surrounding Chernobyl, there were many questions about whether the cases were related to the accident or simply represented increased ascertainment [89, 206, 207]. The data reviewed in this chapter support the contention that nearly all the cancer cases were correctly diagnosed, and the majority represented clinically important disease, not incidental cases found by screening. Some oblasts that received little radiation (Vitebsk) were subjected to intensive screening but yielded very few cases. Thus, increased ascertainment cannot explain the dramatic and sustained increase in incidence that has been documented. The large number of cases and latency period support an association with the accident [108]. In addition, data reviewed previously suggest that radioiodine isotopes are implicated in the pathogenesis of the cancers. A small case–control epidemiological study has provided some further evidence for this point by demonstrating a dose–response relationship at the level of the individual thyroid dose [208, 209]. A study by Jacob et al. [210] showed a linear dose–response relationship between the thyroid dose, resulting from internal ^{131}I exposure and the risk of thyroid cancer. A recent analysis by Shibata et al. [211] further supports the concept that direct external or internal exposure to ^{131}I and short-lived radioiodine isotopes was a causative factor in the pediatric thyroid cancers. An analysis of children who lived within a 150-km radius from Chernobyl revealed that cancer frequently developed in children born in 1983–1986; however, no cases were seen in children born in 1987–1989 [211]. This is most likely explained by natural degradation of ^{131}I and short-lived radioiodine isotopes, as well as erosion of these isotopes from the contaminated territory by wind and rain. A large case–control study has definitively established a relationship between childhood radioiodine dose following the Chernobyl accident and the subsequent risk of thyroid cancer [212]. Risk is modified by iodine status; children living in iodine-deficient areas have greater risk of developing thyroid cancer following ^{131}I exposure [212]. Another case–control study by Davis and colleagues [213] demonstrated a dose-dependent relationship of thyroid cancer risk in the Bryansk oblast of the Russian Federation. Finally, a large-scale prospective cohort study involving 32,385 individuals under age 18 living in contaminated areas of Ukraine demonstrated an ERR of 5.25 per Gy during the first screening in 1998–2000 [214]. A linear dose–response relationship between individual ^{131}I dose and thyroid cancer risk persisted in this cohort for two decades following the Chernobyl accident, although at a somewhat lower ERR of 1.91 per Gy [215] based on screenings in 2001 through 2007. A major strength of this study was availability of individual ^{131}I dose estimates derived from radioactivity measurements taken within 2 months after the accident [214, 215]. This cohort study did not confirm a modifying effect of iodine status on ^{131}I- related risk of thyroid cancer [215].

References

1. Hanson GA, Komorowski RA, Cerletty JM, Wilson SD. Thyroid gland morphology in young adults: normal subjects versus those with prior low-dose neck irradiation in childhood. Surgery. 1983;94:984–8.
2. Spitalnik PF, Straus FH. Patterns of human thyroid parenchymal reaction following low-dose childhood irradiation. Cancer. 1978;41:1098–105.
3. Freedberg AS, Kurland GS, Blumgart HL. The pathologic effects of I-131 on the normal thyroid gland of man. J Clin Endocrinol. 1952;12:1315–48.
4. Carr RF, LiVolsi VA. Morphologic changes in the thyroid after irradiation for Hodgkin's and non-Hodgkin's lymphoma. Cancer. 1989;64:825–9.
5. Quimby EH, Werner SC. Late radiation effects in roentgen therapy for hyperthyroidism. JAMA. 1949;140:1046–7.

6. Winship T, Rosvoll RV. Thyroid carcinoma in childhood: final report on a 20 year study. Clin Proc Child Hosp Washington DC. 1970;26:327–49.
7. Roudebush CP, Asteris GT, DeGroot LJ. Natural history of radiation-associated thyroid cancer. Arch Intern Med. 1978;138:1631–4.
8. Samaan NA, Schultz PN, Ordonez NG, Hickey RC, Johnston DA. A comparison of thyroid carcinoma in those who have and have not had head and neck irradiation in childhood. J Clin Endocrinol Metab. 1987;64:219–23.
9. Mehta MP, Goetowski PG, Kinsella TJ. Radiation induced thyroid neoplasms 1920 to 1987: a vanishing problem? Int J Radial Oncol Biol Phys. 1989;16:1471–5.
10. Akslen LA, Haldorsen T, Thoresen SO, Glattre E. Incidence pattern of thyroid cancer in Norway: influence of birth cohort and time period. Int J Cancer. 1993;53:183–7.
11. Harach HR, Franssila KO, Wasenius V-M. Occult papillary carcinoma of the thyroid: a "normal" finding in Finland—a systematic autopsy study. Cancer. 1985;56:531–8.
12. Sampson RJ, Woolner LB, Bahn RC, Kurland LT. Occult thyroid carcinoma in Olmsted County, Minnesota: prevalence at autopsy compared with that in Hiroshima and Nagasaki, Japan. Cancer. 1974;34:2072–6.
13. Wilson SD, Komorowski R, Cerletty J, Majewski JT, Hooper M. Radiation-associated thyroid tumors: extent of operation and pathology technique influence the apparent incidence of carcinoma. Surgery. 1983;94:663–7.
14. Robbins J. Thyroid cancer: a lethal endocrine neoplasm—NIH conference. Ann Intern Med. 1991;115:133–47.
15. Mettler FA, Upton AC. Carcinogenesis at specific sites. In: Medical effects of ionizing radiation. Philadelphia: WB Saunders; 1995. p. 130–9.
16. Aldinger KA, Samaan NA, Ibanez M, Hill CS. Anaplastic carcinoma of the thyroid: a review of 84 cases of spindle and giant cell carcinoma of the thyroid. Cancer. 1978;41:2267–75.
17. Duffy BJ, Fitzgerald PJ. Cancer of the thyroid in children: a report of 28 cases. J Clin Endocrinol Metab. 1950;10:1296–308.
18. Simpson CL, Hempelmann LH. The association of tumors and roentgen-ray treatment of the thorax in infancy. Cancer. 1957;10:42–56.
19. Saenger EL, Silverman FN, Sterling TD, Turner ME. Neoplasia following therapeutic irradiation for benign conditions in childhood. Radiology. 1960;74:889–904.
20. Thompson DE, Mabuchi K, Ron E, Soda M, Tokunaga M, Ochikubo S, et al. Cancer incidence in atomic bomb survivors. Part II: solid tumors, 1958–1987. Radiat Res. 1994;137:817–67.
21. Parker LN, Belsky JL, Yamamoto T, Kawamoto S, Keehn RJ. Thyroid carcinoma after exposure to atomic radiation: a continuing survey of a fixed population, Hiroshima and Nagasaki, 1958–1971. Ann Intern Med. 1974;80:600–4.
22. Schull WJ. Atomic bomb survivors: patterns of cancer risk. Prog Cancer Res Ther. 1984;26:21–36.
23. Fjalling M, Tisell L-E, Carlsson S, Hansson G, Lundberg L-M, Oden A. Benign and malignant thyroid nodules after neck irradiation. Cancer. 1986;58:1219–24.
24. Furst CJ, Lundell M, Holm LE, Silfversward C. Cancer incidence after radiotherapy for skin hemangioma: a retrospective cohort study in Sweden. J Natl Cancer Inst. 1988;80:1387–92.
25. Lundell M, Hakulinen T, Holm L-E. Thyroid cancer after radiotherapy for skin hemangioma in infancy. Radiat Res. 1994;140:334–9.
26. Lindberg S, Karlsson P, Arvidsson B, Holmberg E, Lundberg LM, Wallgren A. Cancer incidence after radiotherapy for skin haemangioma during infancy. Acta Oncol. 1995;34:735–40.
27. Schneider AB, Ron E, Lubin J, Slovall M, Gierlowski TC. Dose-response relationships for radiation-induced thyroid cancer and nodules: evidence for the prolonged effects of radiation on the thyroid. J Clin Endocrinol Metab. 1993;77:362–9.
28. Schneider AB, Recant W, Pinsky SM, Ryo UY, Bekerman C, Shore-Freedman E. Radiation-induced thyroid carcinoma: clinical course and results of therapy in 296 patients. Ann Intern Med. 1986;105:405–12.
29. Viswanathan K, Gierlowski TC, Schneider AB. Childhood thyroid cancer: characteristics and long-term outcome in children irradiated for benign conditions of the head and neck. Arch Pediatr Adolesc Med. 1994;148:260–5.
30. Schneider AB, Shore-Freedman E, Weinstein RA. Radiation-induced thyroid and other head and neck tumors: occurrence of multiple tumors and analysis of risk factors. J Clin Endocrinol Metab. 1986;63:107–12.
31. Paloyan E, Lawrence AM. Thyroid neoplasms after radiation therapy for adolescent acne vulgaris. Arch Dermatol. 1978;114:53–5.
32. Hempelmann LH, Hall WJ, Phillips M, Cooper RA, Ames WR. Neoplasms in persons treated with x-rays in infancy: fourth survey in 20 years. J Natl Cancer Inst. 1975;55:519–30.
33. Shore RE, Hildreth N, Dvoretsky P, Andresen E, Moseson M, Pasternack B. Thyroid cancer among persons given x-ray treatment in infancy for an enlarged thymus gland. Am J Epidemiol. 1993;137:1068–80.
34. Ron E, Modan B, Preston D, Alfandary E, Stovall M, Boice JD. Thyroid neoplasia following low-dose radiation in childhood. Radiat Res. 1989;120:516–31.
35. Shore RE, Albert RE, Pasternack BS. Follow-up study of patients treated by x-ray epilation for tinea capitis: resurvey of post-treatment illness and mortality experience. Arch Environ Health. 1976;31:17–24.
36. Ron E, Modan B. Thyroid and other neoplasms following childhood scalp irradiation. Prog Cancer Res Ther. 1984;26:139–51.
37. Tucker MA, Morris Jones PH, Boice JD, Robison LL, Stone BJ, Stovall M, et al. Therapeutic radiation at a young age is linked to secondary thyroid cancer. Cancer Res. 1991;51:2885–8.
38. Hancock SL, Cox RS, McDougall IR. Thyroid diseases after treatment of Hodgkin's disease. N Engl J Med. 1991;325:599–605.
39. Boice JD, Day NE, Andersen A, Brinton LA, Brown R, Choi NW, et al. Second cancers following radiation treatment for cervical cancer: an international collaboration among cancer registries. J Natl Cancer Inst. 1985;74:955–75.
40. Boice JD, Engholm G, Klienerman RA, Blettner M, Stovall M, Lisco H, et al. Radiation dose and second cancer risk in patients treated for cancer of the cervix. Radiat Res. 1988;116:3–55.
41. Arai T, Nakano T, Fukuhisa K, Kasamatsu T, Tsunematsu R, Masubuchi K, et al. Second cancer after radiation therapy for cancer of the uterine cervix. Cancer. 1991;67:398–405.
42. Hay JH, Duncan W, Kerr GR. Subsequent malignancies in patients irradiated for testicular tumours. Br J Radiol. 1984;57:597–602.
43. Fossa SD, Langmark F, Aass N, Andersen A, Lothe R, Borrasen AL. Second non-germ cell malignancies after radiotherapy of testicular cancer with or without chemotherapy. Br J Cancer. 1990;61:639–43.
44. Kendall GM, Muirhead CR, MacGibbon BH, O'Hagan JA, Conquest AJ, Goodill AA, et al. Mortality and occupational exposure to radiation: first analysis of the National Registry for Radiation Workers. BMJ. 1992;304:220–5.
45. Beral V, Inskip H, Fraser P, Booth M, Coleman D, Rose G. Mortality of employees of the United Kingdom Atomic Energy Authority, 19461979. BMJ. 1985;291:440–7.
46. Wilkinson GS, Tietjen GL, Wiggs LD, Galke WA, Acquavella JF, Reyes M, et al. Mortality among plutonium and other radiation workers at a plutonium weapons facility. Am J Epidemiol. 1987;125:231–50.
47. Checkoway H, Pearce N, Crawford-Brown DJ, Cragle DL. Radiation doses and cause-specific mortality among workers

at a nuclear materials fabrication plant. Am J Epidemiol. 1988;127:255–66.

48. Wing S, Shy CM, Wood JL, Wolf S, Cragle DL, Frame EL. Mortality among workers at Oak Ridge Nationaal Laboratory: evidence of radiation effects in follow-up through 1984. JAMA. 1991;265:1397–402.
49. Wang J-X, Boice JD, Li B-X, Zhang J-Y, Fraumeni JF. Cancer among medical diagnostic x-ray workers in China. J Natl Cancer Inst. 1988;80:344–50.
50. Boice JD, Mandel JS, Doody MM, Yoder RC, McGowan R. A health survey of radiologic technologists. Cancer. 1992;69:586–98.
51. Smith PG, Doll R. Mortality from cancer and all causes among British radiologists. Br J Radiol. 1981;54:187–94.
52. Mátanosla GM, Seltser R, Sartwell PE, Diamond EL, Elliott EA. The current mortality rates of radiologists and other physician specialists: specific causes of death. Am J Epidemiol. 1975;101:199–210.
53. Stewart A, Kneale GW. Radiation dose effects in relation to obstetric x-rays and childhood cancers. Lancet. 1970;1:1185–8.
54. Mole RH. Childhood cancer after prenatal exposure to diagnostic x-ray examinations in Britain. Br J Cancer. 1990;62:152–68.
55. Oppenheim BE, Griem ML, Meier P. Effects of low-dose prenatal irradiation in humans: analysis of Chicago Lying-in data and comparison with other studies. Radiat Res. 1974;57:508–44.
56. Harvey EB, Boice JD, Honeyman M, Flannery JT. Prenatal x-ray exposure and childhood cancer in twins. N Engl J Med. 1985;312:541–5.
57. Rodvall Y, Pershagen G, Hrubec Z, Ahlbom A, Pedersen NL, Boice JD. Prenatal x-ray exposure and childhood cancer in Swedish twins. Int J Cancer. 1990;46:362–5.
58. Yoshimoto Y, Kato H, Schull WJ. Risk of cancer among children exposed in útero to A-bomb radiations, 1950–1984. Lancet. 1988;2:665–9.
59. Lee W, Chiacchierini RP, Shleien B, Telles NC. Thyroid tumors following I-131 or localized X irradiation to the thyroid and pituitary glands in rats. Radiat Res. 1982;92:307–19.
60. Forman D, Cook-Mozaffari P, Darby S, Davey G, Sratton I, Doll R, Pike M. Cancer near nuclear installations. Nature. 1987;329:499–505.
61. Jablon S, Urubec Z, Boice JD. Cancer in populations living near nuclear facilities: a survey of mortality nationwide and incidence in two states. JAMA. 1991;265:1403–8.
62. Davis S, Kopecky KJ, Hamilton T. Hanford thyroid disease final report. Seattle: Fred Hutchinson Cancer Research Center; 2002.
63. Committee on an Assessment of Centers for Disease Control and Prevention Radiation Studies from DOE Contractor Sites: Subcommittee to Review the Hanford Thyroid Disease Study Final Results and Report, National Academy of Sciences. Review of the Hanford thyroid disease study draft final report. Washington, DC: National Academies Press; 2000.
64. Holm L-E, Wiklund KE, Lundell GE, Bergman NA, Bjelkengren G, Cederquist ES, et al. Thyroid cancer after diagnostic doses of iodine 131: a retrospective cohort study. J Natl Cancer Inst. 1988;80:1132–8.
65. Ron E, Doody MM, Becker DV, Brill AB, Curtis RE, Goldman MB, et al. Cancer mortality following treatment for adult hyperthyroidism. JAMA. 1998;280:347–55.
66. Holm L-E. Malignant disease following iodine-131 therapy in Sweden. Prog Cancer Res Ther. 1984;26:263–71.
67. Hoffman DA, McConahey WM, Fraumeni JF, Kurland LT. Cancer incidence following treatment of hyperthyroidism. Int J Epidemiol. 1982;11:218–24.
68. Holm L-E, Dahlqvist I, Israelsson A, Lundell G. Malignant thyroid tumors after iodine-131 therapy: a retrospective cohort study. N Engl J Med. 1980;303:188–91.
69. Hoffman DA, McConahey WM, Diamond EL, Kurland LT. Mortality in women treated for hyperthyroidism. Am J Epidemiol. 1982;115:243–54.
70. Goldman MB, Maloof F, Monson RR, Aschengrau A, Cooper DS, Ridgway EC. Radioactive iodine therapy and breast cancer: a follow-up study of hyperthyroid women. Am J Epidemiol. 1988;127:969–80.
71. Safa AM, Schumacher OP, Rodriguez-Antunez A. Long-term follow-up results in children and adolescents treated with radioactive iodine (I-131) for hyperthyroidism. N Engl J Med. 1975;292:167–71.
72. Johnson CJ. Cancer incidence in an area of radioactive fallout downwind from the Nevada test site. JAMA. 1984;251:230–6.
73. Rallison ML, Dobyns BM, Keating PR, Rail JE, Tyler FH. Thyroid disease in children: a survey of subjects potentially exposed to fallout radiation. Am J Med. 1974;56:457–63.
74. Machado SG, Land CE, McKay FW. Cancer mortality and radioactive fallout in southwestern Utah. Am J Epidemiol. 1987;125:44–61.
75. National Cancer Institute. Estimated exposures and thyroid doses received by the American People from Iodine-131 in fallout following Nevada atmospheric nuclear bomb tests: a report from the National Cancer Institute. Washington, DC: U.S. Department of Health and Human Services; 1997.
76. Gilbert ES, Tarone R, Bouville A, Ron E. Thyroid cancer rates and 131-I doses from Nevada atmospheric nuclear bomb tests. J Natl Cancer Inst. 1998;90:1654–60.
77. Committee on Thyroid Screening Related to I-131 Exposure, Institute of Medicine, and Committee on Exposure of the American People to I-131 from the Nevada Atomic Bomb Tests, National Research Council. Exposure of the American people to Iodine-131 from Nevada nuclear-bomb tests: review of the National Cancer Institute Report and Public Health Implications. Washington, DC: National Academies Press; 1999.
78. Conard RA, Paglia DE, Larsen PR, Sutow WW, Dobyns BM, Robbins J, et al. Review of medical findings in a Marshallese population twenty-six years after accidental exposure to radioactive fallout. Brookhaven National Laboratory Report 1980; BNL 51261.
79. Conard RA. Late radiation effects in Marshall Islanders exposed to fallout 28 years ago. Prog Cancer Res Ther. 1984;26:57–71.
80. Hamilton TE, van Belle G, LoGerfo JP. Thyroid neoplasia in Marshall Islanders exposed to nuclear fallout. JAMA. 1987;258:629–36.
81. Wiklund K, Holm L-E, Eklund G. Cancer risks in Swedish Lapps who breed reindeer. Am J Epidemiol. 1990;132:1078–82.
82. Shore RE. Human thyroid cancer induction by ionizing radiation: summary of studies based on external irradiation and radioactive iodines. In: Karaoglou A, Desmet G, Kelly GN, Menzel HG, editors. The radiological consequences of the Chernobyl Accident. Brussels: European Commission; 1996. p. 669–75.
83. Shore RE. Issues and epidemiological evidence regarding radiation-induced thyroid cancer. Radiat Res. 1992;131:98–111.
84. Ron E, Lubin JH, Shore RE, Mabuchi K, Modan B, Pottern LM, et al. Thyroid cancer after exposure to external radiation: a pooled analysis of seven studies. Radiat Res. 1995;141:259–77.
85. Shore RE, Woodard E, Hildreth N, Dvoretsky P, Hempelmann L, Pasternack B. Thyroid tumors following thymus irradiation. J Natl Cancer Inst. 1985;74:1177–84.
86. National Academy of Sciences. Committee on the biological effects of ionizing radiations: health effects of exposure to low level of ionizing radiation (BEIR V). Washington, DC: National Academy Press; 1990.
87. Shakhtarin VV, Tsyb AF, Stepanenko VF, Orlov MY, Kopecky KJ, Davis S. Iodine deficiency, radiation dose, and the risk of thyroid cancer among children and adolescents in the Bryansk region of

Russia following the Chernobyl power station accident. Int J Epidemiol. 2003;32:584–91.
88. Niedziela M, Korman E, Breborowicz D, et al. A prospective study of thyroid nodular disease in children and adolescents in western Poland from 1996 to 2000 and the incidence of thyroid carcinoma relative to iodine deficiency and the Chernobyl disaster. Pediatr Blood Cancer. 2004;42:84–92.
89. Ron E, Lubin J, Schneider AB. Thyroid cancer incidence. Nature. 1992;360:113.
90. USSR State Committee on the Utilization of Atomic Energy. The accident at the Chernobyl nuclear power plant and its consequences. Information compiled for the International Atomic Energy Agency Experts Meeting, August 25–29, 1986, Vienna. Moscow: USSR State Committee on the Utilization of Atomic Energy; 1986.
91. Travis J. Chernobyl explosion. Inside look confirms more radiation. Science. 1994;263:750.
92. Warman EA. Paper presented at the New York Chapter Health Physics Society symposium on the effects of the nuclear reactor accident at Chernobyl. Upton: Brookhaven National Laboratory; 1987.
93. Sich AR. Chernobyl thesis. Science. 1994;266:1627–8.
94. Stone R. The explosions that shook the world. Science. 1996;272:352–4.
95. Sobotovich E, Bondarenko G, Petriaev E. Geochemistry of Chernobyl radionuclides. In: Karaoglou A, Desmet G, Kelly GN, Menzel HG, editors. The radiological consequences of the Chernobyl accident. Brussels: European Commission; 1996. p. 477–83.
96. Izrael YA, De Cort M, Jones AR, et al. The atlas of caesium-137 contamination of Europe after the Chernobyl accident. In: Karaoglou A, Desmet G, Kelly GN, Menzel HG, editors. The radiological consequences of the Chernobyl accident. Brussels: European Commission; 1996. p. 1–10.
97. Balonov M, Jacob P, Likhtarev I, Minenko V. Pathways, levels and trends of population exposure after the Chernobyl accident. In: Karaoglou A, Desmet G, Kelly GN, Menzel HG, editors. The radiological consequences of the Chernobyl accident. Brussels: European Commission; 1996. p. 235–49.
98. Tsaturov YS, De Cort M, Dubois G, Izrael YA, Stukin ED, Fridman SD, et al. The need for standardization in the analysis, sampling and measurement of deposited radionuclides. In: Karaoglou A, Desmet G, Kelly GN, Menzel HG, editors. The radiological consequences of the Chernobyl accident. Brussels: European Commission; 1996. p. 425–33.
99. Kazakov VS, Demidchik EP, Astakhova LN. Thyroid cancer after Chernobyl. Nature. 1992;359:21.
100. World Health Organization. International programme on the health effects of the Chernobyl accident. Geneva: World Health Organization; 1993.
101. Stsjazhko VA, Tsyb AF, Tronko ND, Souchkevitch G, Baverstock KF. Childhood thyroid cancer since accident at Chernobyl. BMJ. 1995;310:801.
102. Williams N, Balter M. Chernobyl research becomes international growth industry. Science. 1996;272:355–6.
103. Balter M. Children become the first victims of fallout. Science. 1996;272:357–60.
104. Goldman M, Catlin R, Anspaugh L. Health and environmental consequences of the Chernobyl nuclear power plant accident. Washington, DC: U.S. Department of Energy Report DOE/ER 0332; 1987.
105. Lange R, Dickerson MH, Gudiksen PH. Dose estimates from the Chernobyl accident. Nucl Technol. 1988;82:311–23.
106. Nauman J, Wolff J. Iodine prophylaxis in Poland after the Chernobyl reactor accident: benefits and risks. Am J Med. 1993;94:524–32.
107. Dubina YV, Schekin YK, Guskina LN. Systematisation and verification of the spectrometrical analysis data of soil, grass, milk and milk products samples with results of 131-iodine measurements. Minsk Belarus Institute of Nuclear Physics; 1990, In Russian.
108. Becker DV, Robbins J, Beebe GW, Bouville AC, Wachholz BW. Childhood thyroid cancer following the Chernobyl accident. Endocrinol Metab Clin North Am. 1996;25:197–211.
109. Mityukova T, Astakhova L, Asenchyk L, Orlov M, Van Middlesworth L. Urinary iodine excretion in Belarus children. Eur J Endocrinol. 1995;133:216–7.
110. Gerasimov G, Alexandrova G, Arbuzova M, Butrova S, Kenzhibaeva M, Kotova G, et al. Iodine deficiency disorders (IDD) in regions of Russia affected by Chernobyl. In: Karaoglou A, Desmet G, Kelly GN, Menzel HG, editors. The radiological consequences of the Chernobyl accident. Brussels: European Commission; 1996. p. 813–5.
111. Gavrilin Y, Khrouch V, Shinkarev S, Drozdovitch V, Minenko V, Shemyakina E, et al. Estimation of thyroid doses received by the population of Belarus as a result of the Chernobyl accident. In: Karaoglou A, Desmet G, Kelly GN, Menzel HG, editors. The radiological consequences of the Chernobyl accident. Brussels: European Commission; 1996. p. 1011–20.
112. Jacob P, Kenigsberg Y, Zvonova I, Goulko G, Buglova E, Heidenreich WF, et al. Childhood exposure due to the Chernobyl accident and thyroid cancer risk in contaminated areas of Belarus and Russia. Br J Cancer. 1999;80:1461–9.
113. Gavrilin YI, Gordeev KI, Ivanov VK, Ilyin LA, Kondrusev AI, Margulis UY, et al. The process and results of the reconstruction of internal thyroid doses for the population of contaminated areas of the Republic of Belarus. Vestn Acad Med Sci. 1992;2:35–43. In Russian.
114. Ilyin LA, Balonov MI, Buldakov LA, et al. Radiocontamination patterns and possible health consequences of the accident at the Chernobyl nuclear power station. J Radiol Prot. 1990;10:13–29.
115. Gavrilin YI, Gordeev KI, Ilyin LA, et al. Results of thyroid dose assessment for contaminated territories of Belarussia. Bull Acad Med Sci USSR. 1991;8:35. In Russian.
116. Gavrilin YI, Khrouch VT, Shinkarev SM. Internal thyroid exposure of the residents in several contaminated areas of Belarus. J Med Radiol. 1993;6:15–20. In Russian.
117. Khrouch VT, Gavrilin YI, Shinkarev SM, et al. Generalization of results of individual thyroid dose reconstruction: determination of connections between parameters of contamination of people residences and levels of irradiation on thyroid glands. (In Russian) Minsk: Final Report of Institute of Biophysics, Moscow Contract N 7-17/93 with the Ministry of Public Health; 1994.
118. Stepanenko V, Gavrilin Y, Khrousch V, et al. The reconstruction of thyroid dose following Chernobyl. In: Karaoglou A, Desmet G, Kelly GN, Menzel HG, editors. The radiological consequences of the Chernobyl accident. Brussels: European Commission; 1996. p. 937–48.
119. Tsyb AF, Parshkov EM, Shakhtarin VV, Stepanenko VF, Skvortsov VF, Chebotareva IV. Thyroid cancer in children and adolescents of Bryansk and Kaluga regions. In: Karaoglou A, Desmet G, Kelly GN, Menzel HG, editors. The radiological consequences of the Chernobyl accident. Brussels: European Commission; 1996. p. 691–7.
120. Zvonova I, Balonov MI. Radioiodine dosimetry and prediction of thyroid effects on inhabitants of Russia following the Chernobyl accident. In: Merwin SE, Balonov MI, editors. The Chernobyl papers, vol. I: doses to the Soviet population and early health effects studies. Richland: Research Enterprises; 1993. p. 71–126.
121. Sobolev B, Likhtarev I, Kairo I, Tronko N, Oleynik V, Bogdanova T. Radiation risk assessment of the thyroid cancer in Ukrainian children exposed due to Chernobyl. In: Karaoglou A, Desmet G, Kelly GN, Menzel HG, editors. The radiological consequences of

the Chernobyl accident. Brussels: European Commission; 1996. p. 741–8.
122. Likhtarev IA, Sobolev BG, Kairo IA, Tronko ND, Bogdanova TI, Oleinic VA, et al. Thyroid cancer in the Ukraine. Nature. 1995;375:365.
123. Likhtarev IA, Shandala NK, Gulko GM, Kairo IA, Chepurny NI. Ukrainian thyroid doses after the Chernobyl accident. Health Phys. 1993;64:594–9.
124. Likhtarev I, Sobolev B, Kairo I, et al. Results of large scale thyroid dose reconstruction in Ukraine. In: Karaoglou A, Desmet G, Kelly GN, Menzel HG, editors. The radiological consequences of the Chernobyl accident. Brussels: European Commission; 1996. p. 1021–34.
125. Likhtarev IA, Gulko GM, Sobolev BG, et al. Thyroid dose assessment for the Chernigov region (Ukraine): estimation based on 131I thyroid measurements and extrapolation of the results to districts without monitoring. Radiat Environ Biophys. 1994;33:149–66.
126. Prisyazhiuk A, Pjatak OA, Buzanov VA, Reeves GK, Beral V. Cancer in the Ukraine, post-Chernobyl. Lancet. 1991;338:1334–5.
127. Oleynic VA, Cheban AK. Thyroid cancer in children of Ukraine from 1981 to 1992. In: Robbins J, editor. Treatment of thyroid cancer in childhood. Proceedings of a workshop on September 10–11, 1992, at the National Institutes of Health. Publication No. DOE/EH-0406; 1992. p. 35.
128. Astakhova LN. Condition of the thyroid system and peculiarity of forming its pathology in the BSSR population under influence of the iodine-radionuclides in connection with Chernobyl nuclear accident. Zdravoohranenie Belorussi. 1990;6:11–5. In Russian.
129. Astakhova LN, Demidchuk EP, Davydova EV, et al. Health status of Byelorussian children and adolescents exposed to radiation as consequence of the Chernobyl atomic energy station accident. Vestn Akad Med Nauk USSR. 1991;11:25–7. In Russian.
130. Okeanov AE, Averkin YI. Analysis of malignant neoplasms in population of the Republic of Belarus before and after the Chernobyl accident. In: Matyukhin VA, Astakhova LN, Konigsberg YE, Nalivko SN, editors. Catastrophe at the Chernobyl atomic energy station and estimation of health state of population of the Republic of Belarus. Minsk: Research Institute of Radiation Medicine; 1991. p. 25–33.
131. Astakhova LN, Vorontsova TV, Drozd VM. Thyroid nodule pathology in children of Belarus following the Chernobyl accident. In: Robbins J, editor. Treatment of thyroid cancer in childhood. Proceedings of a workshop on September 10–11, 1992, at the National Institutes of Health. Publication No. DOE/EH-0406; 1992. p. 35.
132. Baverstock K, Egloff B, Finchera A, Ruchti C, Williams D. Thyroid cancer after Chernobyl. Nature. 1992;359:21–2.
133. Demidchik EP, Kazakov VS, Astakhova LN, et al. Thyroid cancer in children after the Chernobyl accident: clinical and epidemiological evaluation of 251 cases in the Republic of Belarus. In: Nagataki S, editor. Nagasaki symposium on Chernobyl: update and future. Amsterdam: Elsevier; 1994. p. 21.
134. Demidchik EP, Drobyshevskaya IM, Cherstvoy ED, et al. Thyroid cancer in children in Belarus. In: Karaoglou A, Desmet G, Kelly GN, Menzel HG, editors. The radiological consequences of the Chernobyl accident. Brussels: European Commission; 1996. p. 677–82.
135. Abelin T, Averkin JI, Egger M, et al. Thyroid cancer in Belarus post-Chernobyl: improved detection or increased incidence? Soz Praventivmed. 1994;39:189–97.
136. Averkin JI, Abelin T, Bleuer JP. Thyroid cancer in children in Belarus: ascertainment bias? Lancet. 1995;346:1223–4.
137. Abelin T, Egger M, Ruchti C. Belarus increase was probably caused by Chernobyl. BMJ. 1994;309:1298.
138. Williams ED, Cherstvoy E, Egloff B, et al. Interaction of pathology and molecular characterization of thyroid cancers. In: Karaoglou A, Desmet G, Kelly GN, Menzel HG, editors. The radiological consequences of the Chernobyl accident. Brussels: European Commission; 1996. p. 699–714.
139. Abelin T, Averkin JI, Okeanov AE, Bleuer JP. Thyroid cancer in Belarus: the epidemiologic situation. In: Karaoglou A, Desmet G, Kelly GN, Menzel HG, editors. The radiological consequences of the Chernobyl accident. Brussels: European Commission; 1996. p. 727–30.
140. Malko M. Chernobyl radiation induced thyroid cancers in Belarus. Joint Institute of Power and Nuclear Research, National Academy of Science of Belarus, pp. 240–55. Available on: http://www.rri.kyoto-u.ac.jp/NSRG/reports/kr79/kr79pdf/Malko2.pdf. Retrieved on 15 Jan 2012.
141. Demidchik YE, Demidchik EP. Thyroid carcinomas in Belarus 16 years after the Chernobyl disaster. In: Proceedings of symposium of Chernobyl-related health effects. Tokyo: Radiation Effects Association; 2002.
142. Tsyb AF, Parshkov EM, Ivanov VK, Stepanenko VF, Matveenko EG, Skoropad YD. Disease indices of thyroid and their dose dependence in children and adolescents affected as a result of the Chernobyl accident. In: Nagataki S, editor. Amsterdam: Elsevier Science; 1994. p. 9–19.
143. Remennik LV, Starinsky VV, Mokina VD, et al. Malignant neoplasms on the territories of Russia damaged owing to the Chernobyl accident. In: Karaoglou A, Desmet G, Kelly GN, Menzel HG, editors. The radiological consequences of the Chernobyl accident. Brussels: European Commission; 1996. p. 825–8.
144. Tronko N, Bogdanova T, Komissarenko I, et al. Thyroid cancer in children and adolescents in Ukraine after the Chernobyl accident. In: Karaoglou A, Desmet G, Kelly GN, Menzel HG, editors. The radiological consequences of the Chernobyl accident. Brussels: European Commission; 1996. p. 683–90.
145. Tronko N, Epstein Y, Oleinik V, et al. Thyroid gland in children after the Chernobyl accident (yesterday and today). In: Nagataki S, editor. Nagasaki symposium on Chernobyl: update and future. Amsterdam: Elsevier; 1994. p. 31–46.
146. Williams ED, Tronko ND. Molecular, cellular, biological characterization of childhood thyroid cancer. Brussels: European Commission; 1996.
147. Cherstvoy E, Pozcharskaya V, Harach HR, Thomas GA, Williams ED. The pathology of childhood thyroid carcinoma in Belarus. In: Karaoglou A, Desmet G, Kelly GN, Menzel HG, editors. The radiological consequences of the Chernobyl accident. Brussels: European Commission; 1996. p. 779–84.
148. Bogdanova T, Bragarnik M, Tronko ND, Harach HR, Thomas GA, William ED. The pathology of thyroid cancer in Ukraine post Chernobyl. In: Karaoglou A, Desmet G, Kelly GN, Menzel HG, editors. The radiological consequences of the Chernobyl accident. Brussels: European Commission; 1996. p. 785–9.
149. Abrosimov AY, Lushnikov EF, Tsyb AF, Harach HR, Thomas GA, Williams ED. The pathology of childhood thyroid tumours in the Russian Federation after Chernobyl. In: Karaoglou A, Desmet G, Kelly GN, Menzel HG, editors. The radiological consequences of the Chernobyl accident. Brussels: European Commission; 1996. p. 791–3.
150. Furmanchuk AW, Averkin JI, Egloff B, et al. Pathomorphological findings in thyroid cancers of children from the Republic of Belarus: a study of 86 cases occurring between 1986 ("post-Chernobyl") and 1991. Histopathology. 1992;21:401–8.
151. Nikiforov Y, Gnepp DR. Pediatric thyroid cancer after the Chernobyl disaster. Cancer. 1994;74:748–66.
152. Williams ED. Thyroid cancer in United Kingdom children and in children exposed to fallout from Chernobyl. In: Nagataki S, editor.

Nagasaki symposium on Chernobyl: update and future. Tokyo: Elsevier; 1994.
153. Nikiforov Y, Gnepp DR, Fagin JA. Thyroid lesions in children and adolescents after the Chernobyl disaster: implications for the study of radiation tumorigenesis. J Clin Endocrinol Metab. 1996;81:9–14.
154. Pacini F, Vorontsova T, Demidchik EP, et al. Diagnosis, surgical treatment and follow-up of thyroid cancers. In: Karaoglou A, Desmet G, Kelly GN, Menzel HG, editors. The radiological consequences of the Chernobyl accident. Brussels: European Commission; 1996. p. 755–63.
155. Nikiforov YE, Heffess CS, Korzenko AV, Fagin JA, Gnepp DR. Characteristics of follicular tumors and nonneoplastic thyroid lesions in children and adolescents exposed to radiation as a result of the Chernobyl disaster. Cancer. 1995;76:900–9.
156. Sierk AE, Askin FB, Reddick RL, Thomas CG. Pediatric thyroid cancer. Pediatr Pathol. 1990;10:877–93.
157. Harness JK, Thompson NW, Nishiyama RH. Childhood thyroid carcinoma. Arch Surg. 1971;102:278–84.
158. Richardson JE, Beaugie JM, Brown CL, Doniach I. Thyroid cancer in young patients in Great Britain. Br J Surg. 1974;61:85–9.
159. Tallroth E, Backdahl M, Einhorn J, Lundell G, Lowhagen T, Silfversward C. Thyroid carcinoma in children and adolescents. Cancer. 1986;58:2329–32.
160. Mizukami Y, Michigishi T, Nonomura A, et al. Carcinoma of the thyroid at young age: a review of 23 patients. Histopathology. 1992;20:63–6.
161. Robbins J. Characteristics of spontaneous and radiation induced thyroid cancers in children. In: Nagataki S, editor. Nagasaki symposium on Chernobyl: update and future. Amsterdam: Elsevier; 1994. p. 81.
162. Williams ED. Radiation-induced thyroid cancer. Histopathology. 1993;23:387–9.
163. Willams ED. Chernobyl, eight years on. Nature. 1994;371:556.
164. Williams D. Thyroid cancer and the Chernobyl accident. J Clin Endocrinol Metab. 1996;81:6–8.
165. Ito T, Seyama T, Iwamoto KS, Mizuno T, Tronko ND, Komissarenko IV, et al. Activated RET oncogene in thyroid cancers of children from areas contaminated by Chernobyl accident. Lancet. 1994;344:259.
166. Fugazzola L, Pilotti S, Pinchera A, et al. Oncogenic rearrangements of the RET proto-oncogene in papillary thyroid carcinomas from children exposed to the Chernobyl nuclear accident. Cancer Res. 1995;55:5617–20.
167. Nikiforov YE, Rowland JM, Bove KE, Monforte-Munoz H, Fagin JA. Distinct pattern of ret oncogene rearrangements in morphological variants of radiation-induced and sporadic thyroid papillary carcinomas in children. Cancer Res. 1997;57:1690–4.
168. Klugbauer S, Lengfelder E, Demidchik EP, Rabes HM. High prevalence of RET rearrangement in thyroid tumors of children from Belarus after the Chernobyl reactor accident. Oncogene. 1995;11:2459–67.
169. Rabes HM, Klugbauer S. Radiation-induced thyroid carcinomas in children: high prevalence of RET rearrangement. Verh Dtsch Ges Pathol. 1997;81:139–44. German.
170. Klugbauer S, Lengfelder E, Demidchik EP, Rabes HM. A new form of RET rearrangement in thyroid carcinomas of children after the Chernobyl reactor accident. Oncogene. 1996;13:1099–102.
171. Klugbauer S, Demidchik EP, Lengfelder E, Rabes HM. Molecular analysis of new subtypes of ELE/RET rearrangements, their reciprocal transcripts and breakpoints in papillary thyroid carcinomas of children after Chernobyl. Oncogene. 1998;16:671–5.
172. Fugazzola L, Pierotti M, Vigano E, Pacini F, Verontsova T, Bongarzone I. Molecular and biochemical analysis of RET/PTC4, a novel oncogeneic rearrangement between RET and ELE1 genes, in a post-Chernobyl papillary thyroid cancer. Oncogene. 1996;13:1093–7.
173. Klugbauer S, Demidchik EP, Lengfelder E, Rabes HM. Detection of a novel type of RET rearrangement (PTC5) in thyroid carcinomas after Chernobyl and analysis of the involved RET-fused gene RFG5. Cancer Res. 1998;58:198–203.
174. Klugbauer S, Rabes HM. The transcription coactivator HTIF1 and a related protein are fused to the RET receptor tyrosine kinase in childhood papillary thyroid carcinomas. Oncogene. 1999;18:4388–93.
175. Salassidis K, Bruch J, Zitzelsberger H, Lengfelder E, Kellerer AM, Bauchinger M. Translocation t(10;14)(q11.2:q22.1) fusing the kinectin to the RET gene creates a novel rearranged form (PTC8) of the RET proto-oncogene in radiation-induced childhood papillary thyroid carcinoma. Cancer Res. 2000;60:2786–9.
176. Klugbauer S, Jauch A, Lengfelder E, Demidchik E, Rabes HM. A novel type of RET rearrangement (PTC8) in childhood papillary thyroid carcinomas and characterization of the involved gene (RFG8). Cancer Res. 2000;60:7028–32.
177. Rabes HM, Demidchik EP, Sidorow JD, et al. Pattern of radiation-induced RET and NTRK1 rearrangements in 191 post-Chernobyl papillary thyroid carcinomas: biological, phenotypic, and clinical implications. Clin Cancer Res. 2000;6:1093–103.
178. Rabes HM. Gene rearrangements in radiation-induced thyroid carcinogenesis. Med Pediatr Oncol. 2001;36:574–82.
179. Pisarchik AV, Ermak G, Fomicheva V, Kartel NA, Figge J. The ret/PTC1 rearrangement is a common feature of Chernobyl-associated papillary thyroid carcinomas from Belarus. Thyroid. 1998;8:133–9.
180. Pisarchik AV, Ermak G, Demidchik EP, Mikhalevich LS, Kartel NA, Figge J. Low prevalence of the ret/PTC3r1 rearrangement in a series of papillary thyroid carcinomas presenting in Belarus ten year post-Chernobyl. Thyroid. 1998;8:1003–8.
181. Pisarchik AV, Yarmolinskii DG, Demidchik YE, Ermak GZ, Kartel NA, Figge J. ret/PTC1 and ret/PTC3r1 rearrangement in thyroid cancer cells, arising in residents of Belarus in the period after the accident at the Chernobyl nuclear power plant. Genetika. 2000;36:959–64. In Russian.
182. Smida J, Salassidis K, Hieber L, et al. Distinct frequency of ret rearrangements in papillary thyroid carcinomas of children and adults from Belarus. Int J Cancer. 1999;80:32–8.
183. Thomas GA, Bunnell H, Cook HA, et al. High prevalence of RET/PTC rearrangements in Ukrainian and Belarussian post-Chernobyl thyroid papillary carcinomas: a strong correlation between RET/PTC3 and the solid-follicular variant. J Clin Endocrinol Metab. 1999;84:4232–8.
184. Santoro M, Thomas GA, Vecchio G, et al. Gene rearrangement and Chernobyl related thyroid cancers. Br J Cancer. 2000;82:315–22.
185. Williams ED, Abrosimov A, Bogdanova T, et al. Thyroid carcinoma after Chernobyl latent period, morphology and aggressiveness. Br J Cancer. 2004;90:2219–24.
186. Elisei R, Romei C, Vorontsova T, et al. RET/PTC rearrangements in thyroid nodules: studies in irradiated and not irradiated, malignant and benign thyroid lesions in children and adults. J Clin Endocrinol Metab. 2001;86:3211–6.
187. Jhiang SM, Sagartz JE, Tong Q, et al. Targeted expression of the RET/PTC1 oncogene induces papillary thyroid carcinomas. Endocrinology. 1996;137:375–8.
188. Santoro M, Chiappetta G, Cerrato A, et al. Development of thyroid papillary carcinomas secondary to tissue-specific expression of the RET/PTC1 oncogene in transgenic mice. Oncogene. 1996;12:1821–6.
189. Powell Jr DJ, Russell J, Nibu K, et al. The RET/PTC3 oncogene: metastatic solid-type papillary carcinomas in murine thyroids. Cancer Res. 1998;58:5523–8.

190. Ito T, Seyama T, Iwamoto KS, et al. In vitro irradiation is able to cause RET oncogene rearrangement. Cancer Res. 1993;53:2940–3.
191. Bounacer A, Wicker R, Caillou B, et al. High prevalence of activating ret proto-oncogene rearrangements, in thyroid tumors from patients who had received external radiation. Oncogene. 1997;15:1263–73.
192. Collins BJ, Chiappetta G, Schneider AB, et al. RET expression in papillary thyroid cancer from patients irradiated in childhood for benign conditions. J Clin Endocrinol Metab. 2002;87:3941–6.
193. Elisei R, Romei C, Soldatenko PP, Cosci B, Vorontsova T, Vivaldi A, et al. New breakpoints in both the H4 and RET genes create a variant of PTC-1 in a post-Chernobyl papillary thyroid carcinoma. Clin Endocrinol. 2000;53:131–6.
194. Corvi R, Berger N, Balczon R, Romeo G. RET/PCM-1: a novel fusion gene in papillary thyroid carcinoma. Oncogene. 2000;19: 4236–42.
195. Nakata T, Kitamura Y, Shimizu K, Tanaka S, Fujimori M, Yokoyama S, Ito K, Emi M. Fusion of a novel gene, ELKS, to RET due to translocation t(10;12)(q11;p13) in a papillary thyroid carcinoma. Genes Chromosomes Cancer. 1999;25:97–103.
196. Giannini R, Salvatore G, Monaco C, Sferratore F, Pollina L, Pacini F, et al. Identification of a novel subtype of H4-RET rearrangement in a thyroid papillary carcinoma and lymph node metastasis. Int J Oncol. 2000;16:485–9.
197. Butti MG, Bongarzone I, Ferraresi G, Mondellini P, Borrello MG, Pierotti MA. A sequence analysis of the genomic regions involved in the rearrangements between TPM3 and NTRK1 genes producing TRK oncogenes in papillary thyroid carcinomas. Genomics. 1995;28:15–24.
198. Beimfohr C, Klugbauer S, Demidchik EP, Lengfelder E, Rabes HM. NTRK1 re-arrangement in papillary thyroid carcinomas of children after the Chernobyl reactor accident. Int J Cancer. 1999;80:842–7.
199. Nikiforov YE, Nikiforova MN, Gnepp DR, Fagin JA. Prevalence of mutations of ras and p53 in benign and malignant thyroid tumors from children exposed to radiation after the Chernobyl nuclear accident. Oncogene. 1996;13:687–93.
200. Hillebrandt S, Streffer C, Reiners C, Demidchik E. Mutations in the p53 tumor suppressor gene in thyroid tumors of children from areas contaminated by the Chernobyl accident. Int J Radial Biol. 1996;69:39–45.
201. Hillebrandt S, Streffer C, Demidchik EP, Biko J, Reiners C. Polymorphisms in the p53 gene in thyroid tumors and blood samples of children from areas in Belarus. Mutat Res. 1997;381:201–7.
202. Smida J, Zitzelsberger H, Kellerer AM, et al. P53 mutations in childhood thyroid tumors from Belarus and in thyroid tumors without radiation history. Int J Cancer. 1997;73:802–7.
203. Suchy B, Waldmann V, Klugbauer S, Rabes HM. Absence of RAS and p53 mutations in thyroid carcinomas of children after Chernobyl in contrast to adult thyroid tumors. Br J Cancer. 1998;77:952–5.
204. Pisarchik AV, Ermak G, Kartel NA, Figge J. Molecular alterations involving p53 codons 167 and 183 in papillary thyroid carcinomas from Chernobyl-contaminated regions of Belarus. Thyroid. 2000;10:25–30.
205. Ciampi R, Knauf JA, Kerler R, Gandhi M, Zhu Z, Nikiforova MN, Rabes HM, Fagin JA, Nikiforov YE. Oncogenic AKAP9-BRAF fusion is a novel mechanism of MAPK pathway activation in thyroid cancer. J Clin Invest. 2005;115(1):94–101.
206. Beral V, Reeves G. Childhood thyroid cancer in Belarus. Nature. 1992;359:680–1.
207. Shigematsu I, Thiessen JW. Childhood thyroid cancer in Belarus. Nature. 1992;359:681.
208. Beebe GW. Epidemiologic studies of thyroid cancer in the CIS. In: Karaoglou A, Desmet G, Kelly GN, Menzel HG, editors. The radiological consequences of the Chernobyl accident. Brussels: European Commission; 1996. p. 731–40.
209. Astakhova LN, Anspaugh LR, Beebe GW, Bouville A, Drozdovitch VV, Garber V, et al. Chernobyl-related thyroid cancer in children of Belarus: a case-control study. Radiat Res. 1998;150:349–56.
210. Jacob P, Goulko G, Heidenreich WF, et al. Thyroid cancer risk to children calculated. Nature. 1998;392:31–2.
211. Shibata Y, Yamashita S, Masyakin VB, Panasyuk GD, Nagataki S. 15 years after Chernobyl: new evidence of thyroid cancer. Lancet. 2001;358:1965–6.
212. Cardis E, Kesminiene A, Ivanov V, Malakhova I, Shibata Y, Khrouch V, Drozdovitch V, Maceika E, Zvonova I, Vlassov O, Bouville A, Goulko G, Hoshi M, Abrosimov A, Anoshko J, Astakhova L, Chekin S, Demidchik E, Galanti R, Ito M, Korobova E, Lushnikov E, Maksioutov M, Masyakin V, Nerovnia A, Parshin V, Parshkov E, Piliptsevich N, Pinchera A, Polyakov S, Shabeka N, Suonio E, Tenet V, Tsyb A, Yamashita S, Williams D. Risk of thyroid cancer after exposure to 131I in childhood. J Natl Cancer Inst. 2005;97(10):724–32.
213. Davis S, Stepanenko V, Rivkind N, Kopecky KJ, Voillequé P, Shakhtarin V, Parshkov E, Kulikov S, Lushnikov E, Abrosimov A, Troshin V, Romanova G, Doroschenko V, Proshin A, Tsyb A. Risk of thyroid cancer in the Bryansk oblast of the Russian Federation after the Chernobyl power station accident. Radiat Res. 2004;162(3):241–8.
214. Tronko MD, Howe GR, Bogdanova TI, Bouville AC, Epstein OV, Brill AB, Likhtarev IA, Fink DJ, Markov VV, Greenebaum E, Olijnyk VA, Masnyk IJ, Shpak VM, McConnell RJ, Tereshchenko VP, Robbins J, Zvinchuk OV, Zablotska LB, Hatch M, Luckyanov NK, Ron E, Thomas TL, Voillequé PG, Beebe GW. A cohort study of thyroid cancer and other thyroid diseases after the Chornobyl accident: thyroid cancer in Ukraine detected during first screening. J Natl Cancer Inst. 2006;98:897–903.
215. Brenner AV, Tronko MD, Hatch M, Bogdanova TI, Oliynik VA, Lubin JH, Zablotska LB, Tereschenko VP, McConnell RJ, Zamotaeva GA, O'Kane P, Bouville AC, Chaykovskaya LV, Greenebaum E, Paster IP, Shpak VM, Ron E. I-131 dose response for incident thyroid cancers in Ukraine related to the Chornobyl accident. Environ Health Perspect. 2011;119(7):933–9. Epub 2011 Mar 14.

Classification of Thyroid Malignancies

8

Virginia A. LiVolsi and Zubair W. Baloch

Pathologic Assessment and Classification of Thyroid Tumors

Many thyroid tumors arise in essentially normal thyroid tissue; however, one must be aware of the fact that definition of normal thyroid tissue in the era of ultrasound is subjective since approximately 60 % of the US population has one or more thyroid nodules. Thyroid neoplasms demonstrate a variety of morphologic patterns, which complicate their pathological interpretation [1]. All neoplasms that arise either from follicular or C cells may have some functional capacities. They may respond to TSH and may even produce excessive amounts of thyroid hormones or, if medullary carcinoma, release abnormal quantities of calcitonin and/or other hormones [2]. Localization of thyroid transcription factor (TTF-1) and thyroglobulin or calcitonin by immunohistochemistry aids in the classification of unusual thyroidal tumors and in providing definite identification of metastatic thyroid carcinomas [3]. Most thyroid cancers grow slowly and are amenable to appropriate treatment. The majority are papillary cancers, especially in those areas of the world in which adequate iodides are present in the diet and environment.

Proper pathologic assessment of the thyroid specimens is necessary for accurate diagnosis. Incomplete fixation of any thyroid tissue may produce loss of cellular details and pale nuclei in the sections (thus, a superficial resemblance to the nuclei of papillary carcinoma). The pathologic assessment of the thyroid lesions includes fine-needle aspiration and diagnosis, intraoperative evaluation, gross pathologic examination, and histopathologic reporting.

V.A. LiVolsi, MD • Z.W. Baloch, MD, PhD (✉)
Department of Pathology and Laboratory Medicine, University of Pennsylvania Medical Center, Perelman School of Medicine, 6 Founders Pavilion, 3400 Spruce Street, Philadelphia, PA 19104, USA
e-mail: linus@mail.med.upenn.edu; baloch@mail.med.upenn.edu

Fine-Needle Aspiration (FNA) of Thyroid Lesions

Fine-needle aspiration (FNA) of the thyroid has now been established as reliable and safe and has become an integral part in the management of thyroid nodules. Based on the examination of few groups of cells, it can effectively triage cases requiring clinical or surgical follow-up (for further discussion on FNA technique and specimen processing, please refer to Chap. 19). Thyroid FNA specimens are usually classified by employing a tiered system. Several classification schemes have been proposed by various authors based on personal/institutional experiences. In 2007, a six-tiered classification scheme for classifying thyroid FNAs known as Bethesda classification for thyroid FNA specimen was proposed (Table 8.1). In this scheme each diagnostic category is assigned a risk of malignancy based on literature review along with recommendations for management. It is also recommended that for some of the diagnostic categories, some degree of subcategorization can be informative and is often appropriate. Additional descriptive comments (beyond such subcategorization) are optional and left to the discretion of the cytopathologist [4, 7].

The brief description of the diagnostic categories in the Bethesda classification is as follows:

I. *Nondiagnostic or unsatisfactory*:
   (a) This diagnostic category applies to specimen which are nondiagnostic due to limited cellularity, no follicular cells, and adequate specimen which are uninterpretable due to poor fixation and preservation, i.e., obliteration of cellular details.
   (b) In some cases of solid nodules, it may be prudent to process and examine the entire specimen.

L. Wartofsky, D. Van Nostrand (eds.), *Thyroid Cancer*, DOI 10.1007/978-1-4939-3314-3_8

Table 8.1 The Bethesda system for reporting thyroid cytopathology: implied risk of malignancy and recommended clinical management [4–6]

Diagnostic category	Risk of malignancy (%)	Usual management
Nondiagnostic or unsatisfactory		Repeat FNA with ultrasound guidance
Benign	0–3 %	Clinical follow-up
Atypia of undetermined significance or follicular lesion of undetermined significance	~5–15 %	Repeat FNA
Follicular neoplasm or suspicious for a follicular neoplasm	15–30 %	Surgical lobectomy
Suspicious for malignancy	60–75 %	Near-total thyroidectomy or surgical lobectomy
Malignant	97–99 %	Near-total thyroidectomy

(c) It is recommended that solid nodules with repeat nondiagnostic FNA results should be excised because malignancy is eventually diagnosed in about 9 % of such cases.

II. *Benign*:

(a) The reported rate of malignancy for this diagnostic category is 0–3 %.

(b) The diagnostic terms in this category include but are not limited to nodular goiter, hyperplastic/adenomatoid nodule in goiter, chronic lymphocytic thyroiditis, and subacute thyroiditis.

(c) A thyroid nodule with a benign diagnosis should be followed periodically by US examination; a repeat FNA may be considered if the nodule increases in size (as per ATA guidelines the increase should be in 20 % in two dimensions of the nodule and that of solid component in case of cystic nodules) [8].

III. *Atypia of undetermined significance/follicular lesion of undetermined significance (AUS/FLUS)*:

(a) The literature review of the large cases series published after Bethesda classification scheme shows that this represents a heterogeneous diagnostic category (a true gray zone). The reported malignancy risk for cases diagnosed as such in these studies ranges from 6 to 48 % [9–11].

(b) It is recommended that the number of cases diagnosed as such should be kept to minimum, 7 % of the total diagnoses. The question arises what can serve as a guide for keeping the AUS/FLUS diagnosis in an acceptable range. One obvious answer is to use the AUS/FLUS to malignant diagnoses ratio similar to atypical squamous cell of undetermined significance to squamous intraepithelial lesion (ASCUS:SIL) ratio in cervical cytology; however, this needs to be proven by independent studies from multiple institutions.

(c) It is optional to describe the reason(s) for AUS/FLUS diagnosis. Some authors have shown that subclassifying this diagnosis further stratifies the risk of malignancy for this diagnostic category.

(d) It has been shown that repeat FNA is effective in arriving at definite management-based diagnosis in thyroid nodules initially diagnosed as indeterminate. Therefore, repeat FNA should be recommended in cases diagnosed as AUS/FLUS. These studies are clearly evident that RFNA has a definite role in the management of patients with thyroid nodules diagnosed as FLUS/AUS.

IV. *Follicular/follicular neoplasm with oncocytic features (AKA Hurthle cell) neoplasm or suspicious for follicular or follicular neoplasm with oncocytic features (AKA Hurthle cell) neoplasm*:

(a) These diagnostic terms encompass both benign and malignant tumors, i.e., follicular adenoma and carcinoma and oncocytic follicular adenoma and carcinoma. The cytologic diagnosis of "neoplasm" reflects the limitations of thyroid cytology, since the diagnosis of follicular carcinoma is only based on the demonstration of capsular and/or vascular invasion. Several authors have shown that, at most, only 20–30 % of cases diagnosed as "follicular neoplasm" are diagnosed as malignant on histological examination and the rest are either follicular adenomas or cellular adenomatoid nodules, i.e., benign. Interestingly, half or more of the malignant cases diagnosed as follicular neoplasm or suspicious for follicular neoplasm (FON/SFON) are found to be follicular variant of papillary thyroid carcinoma (FVPC) on surgical excision.

V. *Suspicious for malignancy*:

(a) This term includes suspicious for papillary carcinoma (malignancy risk 60–75 %), medullary carcinoma, other malignancies, lymphoma (flow cytometry can be recommended with repeat FNA), metastatic carcinoma/secondary tumor, and carcinoma (includes poorly differentiated and anaplastic carcinoma).

VI. *Malignant*:

(a) The thyroid FNA cases diagnosed as such carry a 97–100 % risk of malignancy.

The malignant tumors of the thyroid diagnosed on FNA include papillary carcinoma and variants, medullary carcinoma, poorly differentiated carcinoma, anaplastic carcinoma, metastatic carcinoma (with immunohistochemistry), and lymphoma (combined with flow cytometry).

Intraoperative Assessment/Frozen Section Examination of Thyroid Tumors

It has been shown that although frozen section diagnosis of thyroid tumors may be specific (90–97 %), it is not sensitive (60 %). In addition, deferred diagnoses at frozen section do nothing to alter the operative procedure or guide the surgeon [12]. In lieu of frozen sections, the initial approach to diagnose a thyroid nodule should be an aspiration biopsy (fine-needle aspiration (FNA)) [12–14]. For thyroid nodules which are unequivocally diagnosed as malignant, the surgeon should proceed with the appropriate surgery for that malignant diagnosis. In cases where the FNA diagnosis is suspicious for malignancy and that suspected lesion is papillary carcinoma or a variant thereof, intraoperative frozen section may be useful since the diagnosis relies on the nuclear morphology and not the finding of invasion. If the FNA diagnosis is "neoplasm/suspicious for neoplasm," frozen section will not provide a definitive diagnosis and therefore should not be requested [3, 15–17], since the limited sampling at the time of frozen section may not detect a random microscopic focus of capsular or vascular invasion required for the diagnosis of follicular carcinoma.

Gross Examination of Thyroid Specimens

As part of the macroscopic assessment of thyroid resection specimens, pertinent clinical and historical data should be provided to the pathologist. This includes age and sex of the patient, relevant clinical history (previous history of fine-needle aspiration biopsy and diagnosis, treatment, history of head and neck radiation, and family history of thyroid disease), and identification of the procedure type (lobectomy, near-total or total thyroidectomy). Radiologic, functional, and laboratory data should also be included. A detailed gross examination of a thyroid should be performed on the fresh specimen received and tumor size and appearance be documented before sections are taken for frozen section or other studies. The specimen should be oriented spatially by the surgeon. A detailed gross examination of the specimen should include weight and measurement (in three dimensions) of the specimen and description of the external surface and the cut surface (color, consistency); location, size, and physical characteristics (encapsulation, color, hemorrhage, FNA tracks, solid, cystic, calcified, necrosis) of the nodule(s) should be described. The surgical margins should be highlighted with ink, and the presence of gross extra-thyroidal extension should be noted. If the specimen contains regional lymph nodes, description of levels and characteristics of any grossly involved nodes should be given. The presence of parathyroid gland(s) should be documented. The gross examination determines the number of sections to be taken for histopathologic evaluation. Diffuse lesions of the thyroid such as thyroiditis or Graves' disease without any obvious nodules, up to three sections, should be submitted from each lobe and one from the isthmus. In the case of a solitary or dominant encapsulated nodule, it is recommended that the entire circumference of the nodule be sectioned. Each section should include tumor capsule and main tumor mass with a margin of normal surrounding parenchyma if present. For a nonencapsulated nodule, it is recommended that one section per 0.5 cm should be submitted.

Histopathologic Reporting of Thyroid Tumors

The final histopathologic report should be comprehensive and include all of the known prognostic parameters. The tumor description should include histologic type (Table 8.2) [18], number/multicentricity, size, encapsulation, the presence of tumor capsule and vascular invasion, perineural invasion, and extra-thyroidal invasion. If lymph node sampling or dissection was performed, the presence of lymph node metastases, by number and size, should be recorded. The identification of extra-nodal extension into the soft tissues should be mentioned. The number of parathyroid glands removed during

Table 8.2 Histologic classification of thyroid tumors [18]

Primary malignant tumors	1. *Malignant tumors of follicular cells*
	(a) Papillary carcinoma
	(b) Follicular carcinoma
	(c) Poorly differentiated carcinoma
	(d) Undifferentiated (anaplastic) carcinoma
	2. *Malignant tumor of C cells*
	(a) Medullary carcinoma
	3. *Malignant tumors of mixed follicular and C cells*
	4. *Miscellaneous epithelial tumors*
	(a) Squamous cell carcinoma
	(b) Mucoepidermoid carcinoma
	(c) Mucin-producing carcinoma
	(d) Spindle epithelial tumor with thymus-like differentiation (SETTLE)
	(e) Carcinoma showing thymus-like differentiation (CASTLE)
	(f) Hyalinizing trabecular neoplasms (predominantly adenomas)
	(g) Neoplasms associated with familial intestinal adenomatous
Thyroid adenoma and related tumors	1. Follicular adenoma
	2. Hyalinizing trabecular neoplasm
Malignant non-epithelial tumors	1. Lymphoma
	2. Sarcoma
Secondary tumors	Metastatic malignant tumors

surgery if any should be documented and their location given if possible. Additional pathologic findings in the thyroid such as nodular goiter, thyroiditis, and benign tumors should be described. Additional (optional) areas to include in the report are correlation with FNA findings (especially in discrepant cases) and correlation with intraoperative diagnosis and clinical information. The tumor stage should also be added according to the current AJCC staging system [19]. The results of special studies, special stains (Congo red for amyloid, elastic stain for vessels), immunostains (calcitonin, thyroglobulin, endothelial markers for vascular invasion), molecular studies, and flow cytometry, should be added as appropriate.

References

1. LiVolsi VA, Feind CR. Parathyroid adenoma and nonmedullary thyroid carcinoma. Cancer. 1976;38:1391–3.
2. LiVolsi VA. Surgical pathology of the thyroid. Philadelphia: WB. Saunders; 1990.
3. Baloch Z, LiVolsi VA. Pathology of the thyroid gland. Philadelphia: Churchill Livingston; 2002.
4. Cibas ES, Ali SZ. The Bethesda system for reporting thyroid cytopathology. Thyroid. 2009;19:1159–65.
5. Ali SZ. Thyroid cytopathology: Bethesda and beyond. Acta Cytol. 2011;55:4–12.
6. Baloch ZW, Cibas ES, Clark DP, Layfield LJ, Ljung BM, Pitman MB, Abati A. The National Cancer Institute Thyroid fine needle aspiration state of the science conference: a summation. Cytojournal. 2008;5:6.
7. Baloch ZW, LiVolsi VA, Asa SL, Rosai J, Merino MJ, Randolph G, Vielh P, DeMay RM, Sidawy MK, Frable WJ. Diagnostic terminology and morphologic criteria for cytologic diagnosis of thyroid lesions: a synopsis of the National Cancer Institute Thyroid Fine-Needle Aspiration State of the Science Conference. Diagn Cytopathol. 2008;36:425–37.
8. Cooper DS, Doherty GM, Haugen BR, Kloos RT, Lee SL, Mandel SJ, Mazzaferri EL, McIver B, Pacini F, Schlumberger M, Sherman SI, Steward DL, Tuttle RM. Revised American Thyroid Association management guidelines for patients with thyroid nodules and differentiated thyroid cancer. Thyroid. 2009;19:1167–214.
9. Faquin WC, Baloch ZW. Fine-needle aspiration of follicular patterned lesions of the thyroid: diagnosis, management, and follow-up according to National Cancer Institute (NCI) recommendations. Diagn Cytopathol. 2010;38:731–9.
10. Layfield LJ, Morton MJ, Cramer HM, Hirschowitz S. Implications of the proposed thyroid fine-needle aspiration category of "follicular lesion of undetermined significance": a five-year multi-institutional analysis. Diagn Cytopathol. 2009;37:710–4.
11. Nayar R, Ivanovic M. The indeterminate thyroid fine-needle aspiration: experience from an academic center using terminology similar to that proposed in the 2007 National Cancer Institute Thyroid Fine Needle Aspiration State of the Science Conference. Cancer Cytopathol. 2009;117:195–202.
12. Udelsman R, Westra WH, Donovan PI, Sohn TA, Cameron JL. Randomized prospective evaluation of frozen-section analysis for follicular neoplasms of the thyroid. Ann Surg. 2001;233:716–22.
13. Shaha AR, DiMaio T, Webber C, Jaffe BM. Intraoperative decision making during thyroid surgery based on the results of preoperative needle biopsy and frozen section. Surgery. 1990;108:964–7; discussion 970–1.
14. Shaha A, Gleich L, Di Maio T, Jaffe BM. Accuracy and pitfalls of frozen section during thyroid surgery. J Surg Oncol. 1990;44:84–92.
15. Basolo F, Baloch ZW, Baldanzi A, Miccoli P, LiVolsi VA. Usefulness of Ultrafast Papanicolaou-stained scrape preparations in intraoperative management of thyroid lesions. Mod Pathol. 1999;12:653–7.
16. Baloch ZW, Gupta PK, Yu GH, Sack MJ, LiVolsi VA. Follicular variant of papillary carcinoma. Cytologic and histologic correlation. Am J Clin Pathol. 1999;111:216–22.
17. Baloch ZW, Livolsi VA. Follicular-patterned lesions of the thyroid: the bane of the pathologist. Am J Clin Pathol. 2002;117:143–50.
18. DeLellis RA, Lloyd RD, Heitz PU, Eng C, editors. WHO: pathology and genetics. Tumours of endocrine organs. Lyon: IARC Press; 2004.
19. Wada N, Nakayama H, Suganuma N, Masudo Y, Rino Y, Masuda M, Imada T. Prognostic value of the sixth edition AJCC/UICC TNM classification for differentiated thyroid carcinoma with extrathyroid extension. J Clin Endocrinol Metab. 2007;92:215–8.

Staging of Thyroid Cancer

9

Leonard Wartofsky

Introduction

In general, the "stage" of a cancer refers to a phase in the course of the tumor when it has reached some defined level of extent. The extent of the tumor is a measure of its size and whether it has spread elsewhere. As thyroid cancers grow, they are first confined to the thyroid gland and then may extend in variable degrees to the subcutaneous tissues and lymph nodes of the neck and finally, potentially to distant sites of the body. Staging a tumor allows a more accurate description of the extent of disease in a given patient in objective and standardized terms. Stagingpermits communication between patients and physicians about their prognosis.

Definition and Utility of Staging

In general, the "stage" of a cancer refers to a phase in the course of the tumor when it has reached some defined level of extent. The extent of the tumor is a measure of its size and whether it has spread elsewhere. As thyroid cancers grow, they are first confined to the thyroid gland and then may extend in variable degrees to the subcutaneous tissues and lymph nodes of the neck and finally, potentially to distant sites of the body. Staging a tumor allows a more accurate description of the extent of disease in a given patient in objective and standardized terms. Staging permits communication between patients and physicians about their prognosis. This is facilitated by the fact that clinical investigators analyze and report their experience with various therapeutic approaches and express their results based on the staging of their patient population. Then therapeutic approaches may be selected for the patient based on these published studies on treatment results in comparably staged patients. A standardized staging vocabulary also allows more precise communication among physicians about the degree of disease present.

Thus, examining the thyroid cancer literature enables a better perspective of the potential outcome for our patients according to the results seen in hundreds or thousands of other patients at the same stage of disease. Prediction of outcome relates to prognosis of the various thyroid cancers and is discussed by Burch in several chapters below related to specific tumors. Prognosis may be expressed as life expectancy or the likelihood of achieving a full cure; remission; possible residual, but non-life-threatening, persistent disease; or in the worst case scenario, death. Tumors classified as stage 1 or 2 are typically considered to be "low-risk" tumors with excellent-to-good prognosis, whereas stage 3 or 4 tumors are often described as being "high risk," implying a greater chance of residual disease after initial treatment, recurrence, or death. The overwhelming majority of thyroid cancer patients will fall into stages 1 and 2 and have excellent prognosis with little risk for recurrence or death from their disease. In one large Mayo Clinic review of over 1400 patients with papillary thyroid cancer (PTC) [1], there was a remarkable 25-year survival of 97 % in patients who had complete surgical resection of their apparent disease. Thirty-year survival rates of 75–85 % are not unusual for such patients with low death rates. Stage 2 and 3 patients may have recurrences that require additional therapy but may still be at relatively low risk of death. A worse prognosis is associated with extensive local invasion at presentation and even more so with distant metastases, especially those to bone. Once distant metastases develop, the likelihood of subsequent presentation with bone metastases is extremely high [2]. Improved survival with bone metastases is associated

L. Wartofsky, MD, MACP (✉)
Department of Medicine, MedStar Washington Hospital Center, Georgetown University School of Medicine, 110 Irving Street, N.W., Washington, DC 20010-2975, USA
e-mail: leonard.wartofsky@medstar.net

L. Wartofsky, D. Van Nostrand (eds.), *Thyroid Cancer*, DOI 10.1007/978-1-4939-3314-3_9

with early detection and treatment by local resection of the bony lesion(s) followed by radioactive iodine therapy [3].

Outcome in patients with papillary cancer may vary widely because some of these tumors may be very small (<1.0 cm) or so-called microcarcinomas, and these tumors usually show little evidence of invasion and can have an excellent outcome [4–7] (see Chap. 30). Alternatively, other PTCs may grow rapidly, invade tissues aggressively, metastasize widely, and ultimately cause death. Staging of PTC is based on the patient characteristics that have been shown to impact prognosis. Many clinical and pathologic characteristics have been evaluated as predictors of tumor behavior and ultimate patient prognosis. For example, both the extent of disease and age of the patient at presentation are important determinants of outcome [8, 9]. The extent of disease could refer to invasion of the tumor into extrathyroidal soft tissues of the neck, spread to regional lymph nodes, or metastases to more distant sites. The extent of disease may be determined by clinical, radiological, and pathological examinations to include biopsy of suspicious lymph nodes. The most universally employed and useful imaging modality for the early determination of stage is ultrasonography of the neck. Indeed, even preoperative neck ultrasound has become commonplace at most major medical centers to facilitate the optimal surgical approach [10, 11]. Identification of pathologic lymph nodes is important because one component of stage assessment is the presence of lymph nodes involved with tumor, and ultrasound is the most sensitive technique available for determination of cervical lymphadenopathy. The characteristics of lymph nodes that suggest metastatic disease are described by Hegedus and colleaguesin Chap. 40. Once suspicious nodes are identified, the presence of tumor can be confirmed by fine-needle aspiration (FNA) cytology as well as by measurement of thyroglobulin (Tg) in the aspirate. Alternative imaging techniques such as MRI or PET/CT are not generally recommended at this early point in disease staging. Issues related to the possible benefit of central compartment (Level VI) lymph node dissection at the time of surgery are discussed in the chapter on surgical management.

Another important component of staging is whether there may be distant metastases present, and awareness of distant metastases may be suggested by the finding of high levels of serum Tg postoperatively. On the other hand, low postoperative levels of Tg in low-risk and intermediate-risk patients often herald a cure and allow follow-up without radioiodine ablation [12]. Identification of the extent and location of distant metastases usually awaits performance of post-ablation total-body radioisotopic survey scanning [13]. Thus, the latter sources of information in addition to details of the surgical pathologic findings form the basis for the postoperative assessment of tumor stage that provides useful information regarding both risk stratification that will influence future management and patient prognosis. In spite of the overall utility of the staging systems described below, they all fail to reliably predict prognosis to a high degree of certainty. They fail to do so because of the numerous other factors that may influence recurrence and response to therapy such as the histologic type of tumor (classic papillary vs. tall-cell variant, columnar variant, insular variant, Hurthle cell variant, etc.), as well as molecular characteristics (BRAF, RAS mutations, etc.), radioiodine resistance, and the location and extent of distant metastases, etc. Perhaps future staging systems will take these factors into account as we better understand the prognostic implications of each of these parameters.

Staging Scoring Systems

AMES System

A large number of staging systems currently exist that have been developed at various medical centers over the past several decades. Most systems include the key prognostic factors of patient age, tumor size, and extent of disease but may add other characteristics thought to lend greater specificity to the staging. According to preference, bias, or experience, different staging systems may be favored by various endocrinologists or may be more popular at certain specific medical centers. One such system is known as the AMES system, where the AMES letters refer to age (A), metastases (M), extent of tumor (E), and tumor size (S). This system classifies patients as either low or high risk [6]. Low-risk patients would include tumor size less than 5 cm, papillary cancer without evidence of extrathyroidal invasion, follicular carcinoma without major vascular or capsular invasion, and tumors in men less than 40 years old or women under 50 years old without evidence of metastatic disease. Any tumor that does not meet these criteria would be classified as high risk. Cady and Rossi [14] reported that 89 % of 310 patients were low-risk patients who were noted to have a recurrence rate of 5 %, whereas the remaining high-risk patients had a recurrence rate of 55 %. The same group reported the 20-year survival statistics on a subsequent larger series of 1019 patients, of whom the low-risk patients had a recurrence rate of 5 % and a survival of 98 % compared to 50 % recurrence rate in the high-risk group [15]. Moreover, recurrence in the high-risk patients was associated with a mortality rate of 75 %. They concluded that the AMES criteria were valid predictors of risk.

TNM System

Some differences pertain to staging systems used by clinicians compared to those used by pathologists. One of the most popular staging systems is called the "TNM" classification system, developed by the American Joint Commission

Table 9.1 TNM staging system

Tumor size	
TX	TX primary tumor cannot be assessed
T0	No evidence of primary tumor
T1	Tumor ≤2 cm in greatest dimension limited to thyroid
T2	Tumor >2 cm but <4 cm in greatest dimension and limited to the thyroid
T3	Tumor >4 cm in greatest dimension limited to the thyroid or tumor of any size with minimal extrathyroid extension (e.g., to sternothyroid muscle or perithyroid soft tissues)
T4a	Tumor of any size extending beyond the thyroid capsule and invading the local soft tissues, larynx, trachea, esophagus, or recurrent laryngeal nerve
T4b	Tumor invading prevertebral fascia and mediastinal vessels or encasing carotid artery in the neck
Nodes	
NX	Regional nodes cannot be assessed
N0	No metastases to regional nodes
N1	Metastases to regional nodes are present
N1A	To level 6 (pretracheal, paratracheal, prelaryngeal, and Delphian lymph nodes)
N1B	In other unilateral, bilateral, or contralateral cervical or mediastinal lymph nodes
Metastases	
Mx	Presence of distant metastases cannot be assessed
M0	No distant metastases
M1	Distant metastases are present

on Cancer (AJCC), and it is used by pathologists for most malignancies including thyroid cancer (Table 9.1). TNM refers to tumor size (T), involvement of lymph nodes (N), and the presence of distant metastases (M). Based on the tumor characteristics, the disease stage is described by assigning a numerical score to each of the characteristics reflecting the extent of disease present. The AJCC system was developed in 1959 and was derived from an earlier European system initiated by the International Union Against Cancer (Union Internationale Contre le Cancer (UICC; [16])). Updated versions of the AJCC manual for staging are published every few years; the most recent is the 7th edition published in 2009 and in effect since 2010 [9] with a newly revised version being currently under development in 2015. In 2007, Ito et al. [17] published an assessment of the validity of the UICC/AJCC classification based upon their analysis of outcomes in 1740 patients with PTC and found that age, clinical N1b node involvement, and both clinical and pathological tumor size T4a were independent predictors of both disease-free survival and cause-specific survival. Yang et al. developed a nomogram incorporating features of the TNM staging into prognostic estimates of future risk of mortality [18]. As described below, a key parameter affecting disease-free survival is the degree of extrathyroidal extension, with those patients with minimal invasiveness doing as well as those without extension beyond the thyroid.

Tumor Size

For tumor size, designations of T-0 to T-4 reflect a range of tumor sizes and whether local invasion was seen. For example, a small tumor of less than 2 cm confined to the thyroid is classified as T1; a very large tumor or one invading local tissues would be a T4, with intermediate levels designated as T2 or T3. When there is more than one tumor in the thyroid gland, i.e., multifocality, tumor size refers to the original single malignant nodule or the largest nodule in the gland. As can be seen in Table 9.2, it is only in patients over age 45 that tumor size influences the "T" score in the TNM system and ultimately the designated stage of disease. This is so because virtually all patients under age 45 fall into the category of low risk (stages 1 or 2), and by definition, there are no young patients classified as stage 3 or stage 4. The impact of tumor size on prognosis can be recognized by examining outcomes in a large series of patients with PTC seen at the Mayo Clinic [25]. Cancer-specific mortality was directly related to increasing tumor size with a 20-year mortality of 0.8 % for patients with tumors less than 2.0 cm in diameter, 6 % for tumors 2.0–3.9 cm, 16 % for tumors 4.0–6.9 cm, and 50 % for tumors greater than 7 cm. When the tumor was confined to the thyroid, the death rate was 1.9 %, whereas those patients whose tumor extended through the thyroid capsule into the surrounding tissues of the neck had a 20-year mortality of 28 %. Outcomes were the most poor in those patients with distant metastases at presentation who experienced a 10-year mortality rate of 69 %, compared to 3 % in patients with tumors confined to the neck.

Multifocality

In the majority (~70 %) of patients with thyroid cancer, the tumor is confined to one lobe or one side of the thyroid gland; in about 20–40 % of patients, the tumor is found in the contralateral lobe as well. Some studies have suggested that multifo-

Table 9.2 Impact of age on TNM staging

	Less than 45 years of age	45 years or older
Stage 1	Any T, any N, M0	T1, N0, M0
Stage 2	Any T, any N, M1	T2, N0, M0
Stage 3	N/A	T3, N0, M0 or T1–T3, N1A, M0
Stage 4A	N/A	T1–T3, N1B, M0
		T4a, N0–N1, M0
4B		T4b, Nx, M0
4C		Tx, Nx, M1

The staging for PTC is designated as stage 1, 2, 3, or 4 based on the TNM status and age of patient
N/A

cal tumors may have a worse prognosis [24], but this notion is controversial. Multifocality of cancer may relate to "seeding" of the tumor throughout the gland via intrathyroidal lymphatics or direct extension, but molecular typing also has demonstrated that many arise de novo. Multifocal tumors are also seen when there is a history of some carcinogenic environmental factor, such as exposure to external or internal radiation as seen after the Chernobyl nuclear plant accident in the Soviet Union in April 1986. Multifocal tumors are more likely to have regional lymph node involvement [19]. In one series of 2148 patients with PTC and FTC including 325 recurrences, multifocality, tumor size, and TNM stage were independent predictors of recurrence and early recurrences predicted a poor outcome [20]. Notwithstanding these earlier studies, the guidelines of the American Thyroid Association [21, 22] have modified the recommendation for management of the multifocal microcarcinoma. Previously, ablation was recommended for patients with multifocal microcarcinomas, presumably because of the possibility that another microscopic tumor could be present postoperatively in thyroid remnant tissue. Although a recent study indicates recurrence is more frequent in patients with multifocal microcarcinomas than in unifocal disease, radioiodine therapy was not associated with fewer recurrences [23]. Consequently, the most current guidelines [22] do not recommend routine ablation given that there may be no benefit of radioiodine administration. Ablation is also not recommended for a single tumor <1 cm unless there are worrisome aspects for higher risk such as lymph node metastases or a histologic variant such as tall-cell or insular tumors that are associated with higher recurrence rates and worse outcome.

Lymph Node Involvement

The "N" designation describes the extent of lymph nodes involved. Regional lymph nodes are defined as bilateral cervical and upper mediastinal nodes. Several staging systems include subcategories designated "A" or "B" to describe whether the involved lymph nodes were on the side of the neck of the original cancer or on the opposite side. About 35–40 % of patients presenting with papillary thyroid cancer have involvement of either cervical or mediastinal lymph nodes or both. When a papillary cancer is more aggressive, as evidenced by widespread involvement throughout the thyroid gland, the likelihood of lymph node metastases approaches 75 % [24]. In addition to the staging of lymph node involvement based on the surgical findings, the extent of lymph node involvement can be determined by ultrasound examinations of the neck or by computed tomography (CT) or magnetic resonance imaging (MRI) scans of the neck and mediastinum. The significance of lymph node metastases in the neck on prognosis and ultimate outcome has been debated. Different perspectives from different authors or medical centers may be owed to application of varying staging criteria to thyroid cancers of different pathologic type and grade. Based upon a large series of patients from the Mayo Clinic [25], it was concluded that the presence of tumor in lymph nodes had no adverse impact on either recurrence or survival. However, another series of patients reported by Mazzaferri and Jiang [24], which differed from the latter two series by the inclusion of the effect of routine radioiodine ablation on outcome, did demonstrate that lymph node metastases in the neck were an important independent predictive factor for both recurrence and survival. Most workers in the field of thyroid cancer now accept the importance of neck node metastases, and this is reflected in the various staging systems described. Beasley et al. [26] reviewed their experience with 347 patients with stage 1 disease and another 118 patients with stage 2 disease. Patients with multifocal intrathyroidal disease were more likely to have neck node metastases, and those patients with positive neck nodes had higher rates of recurrence and lower rates of disease-free survival, as well as reduced overall survival.

Those patients who presented with disease in lymph nodes outside of the central compartment of the neck (e.g., in the lateral compartments of the neck or in the mediastinum) were seen to have a greater than sixfold relative risk of recurrence. Because of this greater risk, it may be argued that larger ablative doses of radioiodine should be employed in such patients and a more frequent or greater degree of tumor surveillance should be exercised.

Certain risk factors for metastases to the cervical nodes have been identified for papillary microcarcinoma [27] and for the follicular variant of papillary thyroid carcinoma [28, 29] and include multifocality, angiolymphatic invasiveness, absence of tumor capsule, and extrathyroidal extension. Certain patterns of tumor spread from the thyroid to cervical lymph nodes have been identified and can serve as guides for the surgeon for node dissection [30]. The clinical importance and prognostic significance of positive lymph nodes will vary greatly, however, based upon their number, size, location, and the presence of extranodal extension [31]. Indeed, a recent study of patients with small nodes suspicious for metastasis demonstrated stability without progression, and the results argue for conservative management by monitoring without aggressive interventional measures [32, 33].

Distant Metastases

Distant metastases are scored as either present (M1) or absent (M0). Loh and coworkers [8] found the TNM system of staging to be a useful method in regard to correlation with observed outcomes based on a retrospective analysis of 700 patients over a 25-year period. CT, PET/CT, and MRI imaging are likely to be the most useful to determine if there are distant metastases. Because of their propensity to invade blood vessels, follicular carcinomas are more likely than papillary thyroid cancers to spread to distant sites in the lung or bone. The presence of silent distant metastases to the lung or bone is typically discovered on the first postoperative and post-radioiodine therapy nuclear scan. For lesions in the bone, radioactive iodine is generally more useful to detect metastases than technetium pyrophosphate. In one recent series, the follicular variant of papillary thyroid carcinoma had a relatively low propensity for distant metastases [34].

Impact of Age on Staging

In the AJCC system, two patients ages 25 and 45, with comparable tumor size and distant metastases, could be quite differently staged. The first would be classified as stage 2, and the older patient would be stage 4 because the AJCC system puts a great deal of weight on patient age (see Table 9.2). Indeed, age at diagnosis appears to be the most important factor in terms of having an impact on prognosis, with clearly more aggressive tumor behavior likely after age 40–45. In one large retrospective review of 15,698 cases of thyroid cancer, age was a stronger predictor of survival for patients with follicular carcinoma than for papillary carcinoma [35]. On the other hand, in a series of 261 patients with follicular (FTC) or Hurthle cell cancer reported by Besic et al. [36], tumor size and distant metastases were found to be independent prognostic variables, but age or lymph node metastases were not. Their data underscores the fact that some patients younger than age 45 who have T4 disease or distant metastases may have a poor prognosis even though they have only stage 2 disease. However, the observations of Sugino et al. [37] allow us to modify this conclusion somewhat. These workers followed 134 patients with FTC and not surprisingly found the best survival in the patients with $T<4$ cm, absence of distant metastases, age <45, and minimally invasive tumors. Age >45 and the presence of distant metastases were independent variables predicting poor outcome, and $T>4$ cm and age >45 were independent risk factors for distant metastasis. It would appear that age is more likely to be a negative factor with invasive tumors.

With papillary thyroid cancer, however, the impact of age on prognosis can be seen in the outcomes of a large series of patients seen at the Mayo Clinic over a 40-year period [25]. Cancer-specific mortality rates at 20 years were 0.8 % for patients below 50 years of age, 7 % for patients 50–59 years of age, 20 % for patients 60–69 years of age, and 47 % for patients ages 70 or older. Although not as important as age, the size of the original tumor is also important; tumors less than 1.5 cm have the best prognosis, and those more than 4 cm have the worst prognosis. Finally, a worse prognosis is also associated with extensive local invasion and even more so with distant metastases, especially those to bone. Some investigators have also incorporated the histologic grade of the tumor into the prognostic score [1, 38].

Histologic Variants of Papillary Cancer

Most patients with stage 1 or 2 PTC present with disease that is readily amenable to treatment, i.e., low-risk tumor. Not infrequently, pathologists see many follicular elements interspersed within the usual papillary cancer, and these tumors are designated as "follicular" variants of PTC. In their biological and clinical course, these tumors tend to behave like papillary cancers, rather than like follicular cancers. However, some subtypes of PTC typically behave somewhat more aggressively and, consequently, tend to have a worse prognosis than either the classic form or the follicular variant of papillary thyroid cancer. These subtypes are known by the pathologic terms used to describe the microscopic appearance of the cells and include tumors designated as the "tall-cell" variant, the "columnar" variant, and the "insular" variant of papillary thyroid cancer [39]. Because these variant tumors are relatively more rare, inferences regarding prognosis from small published series may not be accurate. Sywak et al. [40] collated all the cases in the published literature and analyzed 209 cases of the tall-cell variant, concluding that it was a more aggressive tumor that was associated with distant metastases in 22 % of patients and had a tumor-related mortality of 16 %. Similar outcomes with the tall-cell variant were observed by Prindiville et al. [41]. When encapsulated, the columnar cell variant had an excellent prognosis but was associated with an even higher mortality rate of 32 % when not encapsulated (41 reported cases). The insular variant (213 cases) was also seen to be more aggressive, with a 64 %

likelihood of recurrence or distant metastases and a 32 % mortality rate. Although these variants may behave more aggressively and may be associated with higher risk, the staging is not done differently from that of typical papillary carcinoma.

TNM Updates

It is the AJCC/UICC TNM staging system that was felt to have the greatest utility by the American Thyroid Association Guidelines [21, 22]. Periodic updated versions of the AJCC or UICC staging systems may revise assigned scoring, thereby impacting comparisons of outcomes to those reported in the literature that were based upon earlier and different criteria. In this regard, Dobert et al. [42] examined the influence of the differences between the recent UICC 5th and 6th editions by retrospectively applying the two scoring systems to a group of 169 patients. Comparing the two versions indicated that 32 % of the patients would have been stage 1 by the 5th edition, whereas the 6th edition placed 49 % as stage 1. As a result, 5th edition-scored T1 tumors had a 1-year relapse-free interval of 100 % compared to 96.8 % of T1 tumors scored by the 6th edition. Although the latter difference constitutes a slightly worse prognostic determination, Dobert et al. concluded that the differences did not appear to be sufficient enough to alter management strategies. In a comparison and evaluation of six different staging systems, Brierley et al. [43] concluded that no system provided any advantage over the TNM system and advocated its universal use to facilitate communication between medical centers worldwide.

ATA Risk of Recurrence Staging System

While the AJCC/UICC staging system has a good application to predicting the risk of mortality, a number of studies had shown some lack of utility or application of that system to predicting the risk of cancer recurrence [44, 45]. Knowing the potential risk of recurrence allows the clinician to differentially risk stratify and tailor therapeutic management accordingly. Risk stratifying for recurrence led to the suggestions proposed in the ATA Guidelines [21, 22] for a stratification system for risk of recurrence that classified patients based upon their postoperative status as either "low risk," "intermediate risk," or "high risk" for recurrence. The system was validated subsequently with at least short-term outcome data [46–48]. In brief, "low-risk" patients are defined as having had surgical removal of all visible tumor, lack of local tumor invasion, no positive lymph node or distant metastases, and not having one of the histologies associated with aggressive clinical behavior (tall-cell, insular, or columnar variants). In addition, although radioiodine (RAI) ablation is not routinely recommended for low-risk patients, in the event RAI was given for whatever reason, one would expect to see no evidence of extrathyroidal uptake on a post-treatment scan. On the contrary, an *intermediate-risk* patient would be one who did have positive lymph node metastases, vascular invasion or one of the aggressive histologies, evidence of local invasion into perithyroidal soft tissues, and finally uptake seen external to the thyroid bed on a post-therapy isotope scan. Finally, patients at *high risk* for recurrence are those with evidence of macroscopic tumor left behind by the surgeon, distant metastases, or the likelihood of more extensive or widespread disease on the basis of very elevated serum levels of thyroglobulin. Systems for risk stratification for recurrence recently proposed by the Latin American Thyroid Society (LATS) and the European Thyroid Association (ETA) are very similar to the ATA stratification system and differ primarily only in having a "very low risk" as well as a "low risk" for recurrence category. The ATA risk of recurrence system suffers the same deficiencies as mortality staging systems in not accounting for molecular mutational differences, degrees or extent of metastases, histologic variants, etc., and these variables will result in a range of values for actual risk of recurrence. These other factors can be taken into account on an individual or personalized risk estimate that would be applied to a given patient by their physician. The most recent ATA Guidelines [22] emphasize that risk stratification should be dynamic and that recurrence risk can get better or worse with time, and it is helpful, therefore, to periodically reassess and redefine the risk category and modulate any monitoring, diagnostic, or therapeutic interventions accordingly.

Periodic ultrasonography of the neck will be important for dynamic risk stratification [22, 49, 50], but the frequent periodic performance of diagnostic whole-body isotope scan has been largely abandoned. Other important parameters for assessment of recurrence risk include the serum levels of thyroglobulin (Tg) and anti-Tg antibodies (see Chap. 38) and the mutational status of the tumor, specifically if it was BRAF V600E positive or not (see Chap. 22).

Thyroglobulin and Thyroglobulin Antibodies: Tg autoantibodies have a twofold importance in that their presence can serve as an independent marker of tumor presence or recurrence, and because their presence can interfere with the usual measurements of Tg by radioimmunoassay, and cause falsely low serum Tg values [51]. Patients who had underlying Hashimoto thyroiditis are likely to have anti-Tg antibodies as well as anti-thyroperoxidase (TPO) antibodies. Because Tg antibody levels can serve as valuable a tumor marker for recurrence as Tg assay itself [52, 53], it is important to measure Tg antibody every time a Tg measurement is ordered [54, 55]. And should Tg antibody be negative or normal in a patient with Hashimoto thyroiditis, it would be wise to confirm that finding in an independent RIA for Tg antibody. Precise measurements of both Tg and Tg antibodies can be problematic, but when antibodies are present, the measurement of Tg by RIA may be most useful [56–58]. Risk of recurrence or even prognosis can be often predicted by the level of Tg measured postoperatively at the time of remnant ablation [59, 60]. TSH-stimulated levels of Tg, either by thyroxine withdrawal or rhTSH stimulation, provide a more sensitive estimate of recurrence than suppressed Tg levels especially in the presence of small or microscopic tumor remnants [61, 62]. However, it may not be necessary to obtain TSH-stimulated Tg levels if Tg is being measured with an ultrasensitive Tg assay system with a functional sensitivity of 0.1 ng/ml or less [63, 64]. Non-stimulated or suppressed undetectable Tg levels can misleadingly indicate cure [65–67] but when as low as <0.2 ng/ml, are likely to be associated with negative isotopic scans in ATA low- or intermediate-risk patients. When baseline-suppressed Tg is <1 ng/ml, there is little likelihood of a rise in Tg after TSH stimulation [68], while a TSH-stimulated Tg level >2 ng/ml is likely to be associated with discovery of underlying or latent disease. Just as calcitonin doubling time has utility in the management of medullary thyroid carcinoma, it has been proposed that Tg doubling time can serve to predict recurrence of differentiated thyroid cancer [69, 70].

BRAF V600E Mutational Status: Although still controversial, in assessing risk of recurrence in the ATA system, positive BRAF V600E status confers a greater risk of more aggressive disease with higher frequency of recurrence than does the wild-type BRAF, at least in some [71, 72], if not all, reports [73–75]. It remains uncertain whether knowledge of the BRAF status will significantly impact management. For example, it should not for intermediate- or high-risk patients who will be managed relatively aggressively irrespective of presence of the mutation. The data reflecting the impact of BRAF are mixed and inconclusive in low-risk patients, and other associated factors may play a larger role. For example, BRAF-positive multifocal tumors have a higher recurrence rate than BRAF-positive unifocal tumors [76]. Because BRAF-positive tumors are more likely to present with lymph node metastases, preoperative BRAF analysis of the thyroid tumor has been found to potentially be useful for determining the extent of surgical node resection [77].

Ohio State Scoring System

Although it has not been applied widely, Mazzaferri and colleagues proposed a variant on staging that is referred to as the Ohio State University Staging system [24]. Their system was based on a retrospective multivariate analysis of 1355 patients. Stage 1 patients had tumors less than 1.5 cm in size; stage 2 patients had tumors greater than 1.5 but less than 4.5 cm or lymph node metastases or greater than 3 multifocal tumors; patients were considered as stage 3 if their tumors were greater than 4.5 cm or if they had extra-thyroidal extension of tumor; and patients with distant metastases were classified as stage 4. As seen in Table 9.3, there was a clear correlation between mortality and stage of disease.

Table 9.3 The Ohio State University experience

Stage	% of patients	Disease-specific mortality (%)
1	13	0
2	70	6
3	15	14
4	2	65

AGES System

Physicians at the Mayo Clinic described and applied a staging system known as AGES (A, age; G, histologic grade; E, extent; and S, tumor size; [78]). Low-risk stage 1 patients were seen to have an excellent prognosis with a 1 % 20-year disease-specific death rate compared to 20 %, 67 %, and 87 % mortality for stages 2, 3, and 4, respectively. The AGES schema likely never became popular because it requires knowledge of tumor grade that is rarely reported by pathologists. Members of the same Mayo Clinic group subsequently modified AGES by devising the MACIS grading system, which eliminates the need to know tumor grade [78]. The Mayo group incorporated all the other factors into their MACIS scoring system (see below), which can reliably predict outcome based on data at initial presentation.

MACIS System

The MACIS scoring system is defined as metastases (M), age (A), completeness of resection (C), invasion (I), and tumor size (S) [79]. Hay [1] and others identified three varieties of presentation that reflected a different prognostic category regarding tumor recurrence. The three most important factors were the presence of postoperative local metastatic nodes, postoperative distant metastases, and local recurrence in the thyroid bed or adjacent tissue other than lymph nodes. They believe that this scoring system can more reliably predict outcome based on data at initial presentation than the TNM system, which is limited to fewer characteristics. Using the MACIS system, they described 20-year disease-specific mortality rates that directly correlated with the magnitude of scores (see Tables 9.4 and 9.5).

Table 9.4 The MACIS scoring system

Metastases	Absent	0
	Present	3
Patient age	<40	3.1
	>40	0.08 × age
Resection	Complete	0
	Incomplete	1
Invasion	Absent	0
	Present	1
Tumor size		0.3 × size in cm

Table 9.5 Correlation of MACIS score with mortality

Score	Stage	Mortality rates (%)
<6	1	1
6–6.99	2	11
7–7.99	3	44
>8	4	76

NTCTCS System

The most recently developed staging system was proposed by Sherman et al. [80] from the empirical development of a classification that considered patient data in a registry derived from 14 different medical centers, known as the National Thyroid Cancer Treatment Cooperative Study (NTCTCS). Prospective information on 1607 patients was analyzed and validated on the basis of initial follow-up. A comparison of the NTCTCS system to the other systems was performed for prediction of the disease-free state. The NTCTCS system provided somewhat better correlation than the AMES or Ohio State systems but did not appear to provide any advantage over the TNM system. The system was criticized as unnecessary and potentially flawed by Cady [81] and Sherman countered with a lively rebuttal [82].

Follicular Thyroid Cancer

Staging for follicular thyroid cancer (FTC) is done exactly the same as for PTC. Stage 1 follicular tumors, like papillary tumors, tend to have an excellent prognosis. The key underlying difference between these two cancer types is that the follicular cancers tend to be more invasive, invading blood vessels in the thyroid gland that can then lead to hematogenous metastases to the bone and lung. Several studies have attempted to determine which features or characteristics of a follicular tumor might be associated with a more negative prognosis. In one analysis [80], age at diagnosis, tumor size, poor differentiation, and extracervical metastases were the most important staging factors. These more "negative" features appear to be similar to those for papillary tumors and include age greater than 45 years, tumor size more than 4 cm, invasion of tumor into blood vessels or the capsule of the thyroid, extension of the cancer beyond the thyroid gland, and metastases to distant sites (e.g., bones and lungs). In a retrospective review of 504 patients with FTC, Simpson et al. [83] identified age at diagnosis, extrathyroidal invasion, primary tumor size, distant metastases, nodal involvement, and postoperative status as independently important prognostic factors. In another retrospective review of 214 patients with FTC [84], recurrence rates were less in those patients given radioiodine ablation, and no deaths occurred during a mean follow-up of 8.8 years, except in those with distant metastases at the time of presentation. Brennan et al. reported a retrospective analysis of 100 patients with FTC followed for up to 32 years (mean 17 years) who had an overall cancer-related mortality of 19 % [85]. Multivariate analysis suggested a "multiplier" effect with patients illustrating several negative prognostic features doing more poorly than those with only one negative indicator. High-risk patients with two or more negative risk predictors had a 5-year survival rate of 47 % and a 20-year survival rate of 8 %. Follicular thyroid carcinoma is relatively rare in children, and its behavior tends to parallel that in adults with vascular invasion being a poor prognostic factor [86].

Medullary Thyroid Cancer

Management and outcomes for medullary thyroid cancer (MTC) differ greatly from those for follicular cell-derived thyroid cancers [87, 88]. As may be seen in all of the various staging systems described in later chapters for MTC, patient age is not considered. Because the etiology and natural history of MTC differs broadly from that of follicular cell cancers, there may be some rationale for the development and use of a more specific analysis of staging and prognosis based on distinctions between familial and sporadic MTC and for the various described somatic and germline ret mutations. Boostrom et al. had assessed the utility of the 2002 TNM system in 173 patients with MTC and found them inadequate, for stage 4 disease in particular [89]. A poor outcome was not necessarily associated with elevated calcitonin levels as long as the levels were stable and that patients with lymph node metastases without other distant metastases were best classified as stage 3 rather than stage 4 and tend to have intermediate survival.

Anaplastic Carcinoma of the Thyroid

Because papillary thyroid cancer and FTC together account for about 95 % of thyroid cancers, this chapter primarily relates to these well-differentiated cancers. Prognostic issues related to anaplastic thyroid cancer and MTC are discussed in Chaps. 79 and 100. With very few exceptions, anaplastic cancer always has a poor prognosis and is automatically staged as stage 4, regardless of tumor size, patient age, or the presence of distant metastases [90, 91]. The current practice in staging anaplastic tumors is only to break the category down into stage 4A (surgically removable), 4B (not surgically removable), or 4C (with distant metastases). Ito et al. [92] found that prognosis with anaplastic cancer did correlate with whether the tumor was 4A, 4B, or 4C and that given the dismal prognosis, therapeutic initiatives should be tailored to the substage.

Relation of Staging to Prognosis

Prognosis of the different types of thyroid cancer is discussed by Burch in specific chapters below, and the topic is only briefly addressed here for well-differentiated follicular cancer in the context of staging. When analyzing reports or retrospective analyses of outcomes based on stage from different centers, it is important to note whether the patients' routine initial management (e.g., total thyroidectomy and radioiodine ablation) was comparable. Following thyroidectomy for papillary lesions more than 1.5 cm in the past, most workers employed radioiodine in doses of 30–150 mCi to ablate residual tissue and facilitate follow-up monitoring [13] as discussed in Chaps. 35 and 74. Early patient series have indicated that ^{131}I ablation of thyroid remnants was followed by a significantly lower recurrence rate [25, 93–95], but the conviction that such management is absolutely necessary in all patients and actually improves prognosis had been disputed by some experts earlier [1, 96] and much more so in recent years [97, 98]. For example, Hay et al. retrospectively reviewed 2444 PTC patients at the Mayo Clinic over a 60-year period and compared outcomes in the low-risk patients treated in the early decades without radioiodine ablation to those treated in the later decades with ablation [96]. They observed no difference in the rates of tumor recurrence or mortality rates from thyroid cancer, thereby implying that ablation did not improve outcomes and was not necessary in low-risk tumors. Alternatively, Simpson and coworkers [83, 99] in a series of 321 patients found that fewer recurrences occurred in those patients who underwent ablation, and 20-year survival was greater (90 % vs 40 %). Similarly, another retrospective analysis of 700 patients suggested that patients not treated with radioiodine ablation had a 2.1-fold greater risk of recurrence of their malignancy (p=0.0001) but no difference in death rates [8]. A careful meta-analysis of the literature concluded that ablation would reduce recurrence rates and improve outcome in high-risk patients, but definitive proof of necessity for ablation of low-risk tumors remains marginally convincing [100]. The reasons are not clear for the different outcomes in those studies supporting ablative therapy vs those that do not, and the issue for low-risk tumors remains controversial. Several authors have cited the need for a randomized, controlled clinical trial to address this question [101, 102]. Notwithstanding the earlier salutary effect of RAI ablation reported by Simpson et al. and Mazzaferri, the clear recent trend seen in well-controlled studies is away from the need for ablation in low-risk patients [97, 98]. As a reflection of the trend away from empiric radioiodine ablation, the ATA Guidelines both in 2009 [21] and 2015-2016 [22] have recommendations for ablation to large tumors or those with aggressive features with intermediate or high risk for recurrence.

Finally, the importance of age should be emphasized as a prognostic factor and can be appreciated by noting that all patients less than 45 years old without distant metastases are classified as stage 1, and those with distant metastases are not classified any higher than stage 2. The overwhelming majority of patients will fall into stages 1 and 2, with excellent prognosis and little risk for recurrence or death from their disease. There was a remarkable 25-year survival (97 %) in 1408 patients reviewed by Hay [1] who had complete surgical resection of their apparent disease. For such patients, 30-year survival rates of 75–85 % are not unusual. Stage 2 and 3 patients may have recurrences that require additional therapy but remain at relatively low risk for death [1, 24, 93, 94]. Numerous other factors have been assessed relating to prognosis, such as thyroglobulin levels [103, 104] and large lymph node metastases [105]. Most analyses tend to conclude that the most important staging factors influencing prognosis are patient age at diagnosis and the presence of distant metastases. A significant negative subsequent factor is a persistently elevated thyroglobulin level at 1 year post operation [106]. Blood vessel invasiveness has been cited by some authors as a correlate of tumor aggressiveness and prognosis. In a review of 358 patients with differentiated thyroid cancer, Furlan et al. [107] concluded that this was not necessarily the case regarding outcome for the short term of PTC and long term of FTC. Employing any one of the MACIS, TNM, or AMES criteria, angioinvasive PTC did have a worse prognosis, but the latter tumors were larger than nonangioinvasive tumors, raising the question of whether tumor size is the relevant parameter.

In the final analysis, it may not make a great difference which staging system is used; virtually all consider the most important factors, but it would obviously be optimal if we all used the same system to facilitate communication. In one comparison analysis [108], the TNM, AMES, AGES, and MACIS systems all provided comparably useful information correlating with prognosis. In another study [109] comparing MACIS, TNM, and AMES, the TNM system fared better in predicting disease-related mortality likely because it was the only system to include nodal metastases. Nine different staging systems were compared at two separate medical centers by Lang et al. [110] with the TNM system again being considered the most useful and the most consistent. The same conclusion was reached by Verburg et al. [111] after a comparison of 15 different prognostic classification systems in 1225 patients with PTC and FTC.

Although staging does allow more accuracy in predicting outcomes, true prognosis will be better defined as the course of the disease observed over months to years. This is because clinical staging typically is done early in the course of the disease, i.e., before any definitive treatment and on the basis of physical examination, imaging studies, and biopsy. Pathologic staging can be done shortly after thyroidectomy with the examination of the surgical specimen for precise tumor size and presence of involved lymph nodes or after the first administration of radioiodine. Data derived from correlations of stage and prognosis from large series of patients are, of course, average data. The stage designation may not accurately predict the outcome in a single given patient who may do better or worse than predicted. Those who have a worse outcome do because their tumors may become more aggressive with time than the average rate of progression anticipated for a given stage of tumor. One major clinical difficulty for both patients and their physicians is dealing with the indolent nature of these tumors. Thyroid cancer cells are usually slow growing; while this is favorable for recurrence and death rates, it also implies the absolute necessity for long-term meticulous follow-up because there can be recurrences in patients believed to be disease-free as late as 15–20 years after their original presentation.

Staging in Children

Thyroid cancer in children and adolescents is generally managed like that in adults [112, 113], with the same approaches: near total thyroidectomy, radioiodine ablation, radioiodine therapy for recurrence, and long-term monitoring with serum thyroglobulin measurements. Staging is done in a similar manner. The MACIS system has been used in the pediatric age group with excellent negative predictive value for persistent disease [114]. Other workers have found the TNM system to be inadequate for the classification of thyroid cancer in children [115], especially those with small tumors <2 cm who still may have lymph node metastases. Because of the importance of age as a prognostic factor and the obvious fact that these patients are young by definition, the prognosis tends to be excellent in children even with extensive local spread of disease. Indeed, in contrast to adults, the majority of children with thyroid cancer will already have local tumor spread in the neck to the lymph nodes at the time of initial diagnosis. Moreover, as many as 10–20 % of children and adolescents will have distant metastases at diagnosis, such as tumor in the lung, compared to only 5 % in adults [116]. Despite this apparently more aggressive appearance of these cancer tumors in children, the prognosis for cure remains good with therapy, with less than 10 % of children dying from their disease—a prognosis that is significantly better than mortality rates seen in adults. An exception to this general experience occurs in young children under 8 years of age, who may have more aggressive disease for unknown reasons. However, because of the usual excellent results with therapy, some physicians question whether aggressive approaches to therapy with large-dose radioiodine are necessary in children as it may be in adults, given the long-term radiation side effects that may ensue for these children. No clear-cut studies answer this question yet, but some physicians treating children with thyroid cancer will reserve aggressive radioiodine therapy for those with disease that has spread to the outside of the thyroid gland. Thus, as with adults, a reasonable approach is to individualize therapy rather than adopt an arbitrary standard approach, and long-term follow-up and monitoring is essential, owing to the slow-growing nature of thyroid cancer [117].

References

1. Hay ID. Papillary thyroid carcinoma. Endocrinol Metab Clin N Am. 1990;19:545–76.
2. Farooki A, Leung V, Tala H, Tuttle RM. Skeletal-related events due to bone metastases from differentiated thyroid cancer. J Clin Endocrinol Metab. 2012;97:2433–9.
3. Orita Y, Sugitani I, Matsuura M, et al. Prognostic factors and the therapeutic strategy for patients with bone metastasis from differentiated thyroid carcinoma. Surgery. 2010;147:424–31.
4. Pacini F. Management of papillary microcarcinoma: primum non nocere! J Clin Endocrinol Metab. 2013;98:1391–3.
5. Wartofsky L. Management of papillary microcarcinoma: primum non nocere? J Clin Endocrinol Metab. 2012;97:1169–72.
6. Durante C, Attard M, Torlontano M, Ronga G, Monzani F, Costante G, et al. Identification and optimal postsurgical follow-up of patients with very low risk papillary thyroid microcarcinoma. J Clin Endocrinol Metab. 2010;95:4882–8.
7. Wartofsky L. Should patients with papillary microcarcinoma undergo radioiodine ablation? Endocrine. 2013. doi:10.1007/s12020-013-0010-3.
8. Loh K-C, Greenspan FS, Gee L, et al. Pathological tumor-node metastasis (pTNM) staging for papillary and follicular thyroid carcinomas: a retrospective analysis of 700 patients. J Clin Endocrinol Metab. 1997;82:3553–62.
9. Sobin LH, Gospodarowicz MK, Wittekind C, editors. TNM classification of malignant tumors. 7th ed. Oxford: Wiley-Blackwell; 2009.
10. Marshall CL, Lee JE, Xing Y, et al. Routine pre-operative ultrasonography for papillary thyroid cancer: effects on cervical recurrence. Surgery. 2009;146:1063–72.
11. O'Connell K, Yen TW, Quiroz F, Evans DB, Wang TS. The utility of routine preoperative cervical ultrasonography in patients undergoing thyroidectomy for differentiated thyroid cancer. Surgery. 2013;154:697–730.
12. Ibrahimpasic T, Nixon IJ, Palmer FL, Whitcher MM, Tuttle RM, Shaha A, et al. Undetectable thyroglobulin after total thyroidectomy in patients with low- or intermediate-risk papillary thyroid cancer—is there a need for radioactive iodine therapy? Surgery. 2012;152:1096–105.

13. Van Nostrand D, Wartofsky L. Radioiodine for the treatment of thyroid cancer. Endocrinol Metab Clin N Am. 2007;36:807–22.
14. Cady B, Rossi R. An expanded view of risk-group definition in differentiated thyroid carcinoma. Surgery. 1988;104:947–53.
15. Sanders LE, Cady B. Differentiated thyroid cancer: reexamination of risk groups and outcome of treatment. Archives Surg. 1998;7. UICC 2002. Sobin LH, Wittekind C, editors. TNM classification of malignant tumors. 6th ed. New York: Wiley-Liss; 2002. p. 52–6.
16. UICC 2002, Sobin LH, Wittekind C. TNM classification of malignant tumors. 6th ed. New York: Wiley-Liss; 2002. p. 52–6.
17. Ito Y, Miyauchi A, Jikuzono T, et al. Risk factors contributing to a poor prognosis of papillary thyroid carcinoma: validity of UICC/AJCC TNM classification and stage grouping. World J Surg. 2007;31:838–48.
18. Yang L, Shen W, Sakamoto N. Population-based study evaluating and predicting the probability of death resulting from thyroid cancer and other causes among patients with thyroid cancer. J Clin Oncol. 2013;31:468–74.
19. Shah JP, Loree TR, Dharker D, et al. Prognostic factors in differentiated carcinoma of the thyroid gland. Am J Surg. 1992; 164:658–61.
20. Lin J-D, Hsueh C, Chao T-C. Early recurrence of papillary and follicular thyroid carcinoma predicts a worse outcome. Thyroid. 2009;19:1053–9.
21. Cooper DS, Doherty GM, Haugen BR, et al. Revised American Thyroid Association management guidelines for patients with thyroid nodules and differentiated thyroid cancer. Thyroid. 2009;19:1167–214.
22. Haugen BR, Alexander EK, Bible KC, Doherty GM, Mandel SJ, Nikiforov Y, et al. 2015 American Thyroid Association Management Guidelines for patients with thyroid nodules and differentiated thyroid cancer. Thyroid Available online at DOI:10.1089/thy.2015.0020; print version in Thyroid 26:2016.
23. Ross DS, Litofsky D, Ain KB, et al. Recurrence after treatment of micropapillary thyroid cancer. Thyroid. 2009;19:1043–8.
24. Mazzaferri EL, Jhiang SM. Long-term impact of initial surgical and medical therapy on papillary and follicular thyroid cancer. Am J Med. 1994;97:418–28.
25. McConahey W, Hay ID, Woolner LB, et al. Papillary thyroid cancer treated at the Mayo Clinic, 1946 through 1970: initial manifestations, pathologic findings, therapy, and outcome. Mayo Clin Proc. 1986;61:978–96.
26. Beasley NJP, Lee J, Eski S, et al. Impact of nodal metastases on prognosis in patients with well-differentiated thyroid cancer. Arch Otolaryngol Head Neck Surg. 2002;128:825–8.
27. Zhang L, Wei W-j, Ji Q-h, Zhu Y-x, Wang A-y, Wang Y, et al. Risk factors for neck nodal metastasis in papillary thyroid microcarcinoma: a study of 1066 patients. J Clin Endocrinol Metab. 2012;97:1250–7.
28. Blanchard C, Brient C, Volteau C, Sebag F, Roy M, Drui D, et al. Factors predictive of lymph node metastasis in the follicular variant of papillary thyroid carcinoma. Br J Surg. 2013;100:1312–7.
29. Yu X-M, Schneider DF, Leverson G, Chen H, Sippel RS. Follicular variant of papillary thyroid carcinoma is a unique clinical entity: a population-based study of 10,740 cases. Thyroid. 2013;23: 1263–8.
30. Eskander A, Merdad M, Freeman JL, Witterick IJ. Pattern of spread to the lateral neck in metastatic well-differentiated thyroid cancer: a systematic review and meta-analysis. Thyroid. 2013; 23:583–92.
31. Randolph GW, Duh Q-Y, Heller KS, LiVolsi VA, Mandel SJ, Steward DL, et al. The prognostic significance of nodal metastases from papillary thyroid carcinoma can be stratified based on the size and number of metastatic lymph nodes, as well as the presence of extranodal extension. Thyroid. 2012;22:1144–52.
32. Robenshtok E, Fish S, Bach A, Dominguez JM, Shaha A, Tuttle RM. Suspicious cervical lymph nodes detected after thyroidectomy for papillary thyroid cancer usually remain stable over years in properly selected patients. J Clin Endocrinol Metab. 2012; 97:2706–13.
33. Burman KD. Treatment of recurrent or persistent cervical node metastases in differentiated thyroid cancer: deceptively simple options (editorial). J Clin Endocrinol Metab. 2012;97:2623–5.
34. Vivero M, Kraft S, Barletta JA. Risk stratification of follicular variant of papillary thyroid carcinoma. Thyroid. 2013;23:273–9.
35. Gilliland FD, Hunt WC, Morris DM, Key CR. Prognostic factors for thyroid carcinoma: a population based study of 15698 cases from the surveillance, epidemiology and end results (SEER) program 19731991. Cancer. 1997;79:564–73.
36. Besic N, Zgajnar J, Hocevar M, Frkovic-Grazio S. Is patient's age a prognostic factor for follicular thyroid carcinoma in the TNM classification system? Thyroid. 2005;15:439–48.
37. Sugino K, Ito K, Nagahama M, et al. Prognosis and prognostic factors for distant metastases and tumor mortality in follicular thyroid carcinoma. Thyroid. 2011;21:751–7.
38. Samaan NA, Schultz PN, Hickey RC, et al. Well differentiated thyroid carcinoma and the results of various modalities of treatment: a retrospective review of 1599 cases. J Clin Endocrinol Metab. 1992;75:714–20.
39. Burman KD, Ringel MD, Wartofsky L. Unusual types of thyroid neoplasms. Endocrinol Metab Clin N Am. 1996;25:49–68.
40. Sywak M, Pasieka JL, Ogilvie T. A review of thyroid cancer with intermediate differentiation. J Surg Oncol. 2004;86:44–54.
41. Prendiville S, Burman KD, Ringel MD, et al. Tall cell variant: an aggressive form of papillary thyroid carcinoma. Otolaryngol Head Neck Surg. 2000;122:352–7.
42. Dobert N, Menzel C, Oeschger S, Grunwald F. Differentiated thyroid carcinoma: the new UICC 6th edition TNM classification system in a retrospective analysis of 169 patients. Thyroid. 2004; 14:65–70.
43. Brierley JD, Panzarella T, Tsang RW, et al. A comparison of different staging systems predictability of patient outcome. Thyroid carcinoma as an example. Cancer. 1997;79:2414–23.
44. Tuttle RM, Tala H, Shah J, Leboeuf R, Ghossein R, Gonen M, et al. Estimating risk of recurrence in differentiated thyroid cancer after total thyroidectomy and radioactive iodine remnant ablation using response to therapy variables to modify the initial risk estimates predicted by the new American Thyroid Association staging system. Thyroid. 2010;20:1341–9.
45. Vaisman F, Shaha A, Fish S, Tuttle R. Initial therapy with either thyroid lobectomy or total thyroidectomy without radioactive iodine remnant ablation is associated with very low rates of structural disease recurrence in properly selected patients with differentiated thyroid cancer. Clin Endocrinol 2011. doi:10.1111/j.1365-2265.2011.04002.
46. Vaisman F, Momesso D, Bulzico DA, Pessoa CH, Dias F, Corbo R, et al. Spontaneous remission in thyroid cancer patients after biochemical incomplete response to initial therapy. Clin Endocrinol. 2012;77:132–8.
47. Pitoia F, Bueno F, Urciuoli C, Abellerira E, Cross G, Tuttle RM. Outcomes of patients with differentiated thyroid cancer risk-stratified according to American thyroid association and Latin American thyroid society risk of recurrence classification systems. Thyroid. 2013;23:1401–7.
48. Nixon IJ, Ganly I, Patel SG, Palmer FL, Di Lorenzo MM, Grewal RK, et al. The results of selective use of radioactive iodine on survival and on recurrence in the management of papillary thyroid cancer, based on Memorial Sloan-Kettering Cancer Center Risk Group Stratification. Thyroid. 2013;23:683–94.
49. Durante C, Filetti S. Management of papillary thyroid cancer patients in absence of postoperative radioiodine remnant ablation:

tailoring follow-up by neck sonography. J Clin Endocrinol Metab. 2011;96:3059–61.
50. Moreno MA, Edeiken-Monroe BS, Siegel ER, Sherman SI, Clayman GL. In papillary thyroid cancer, preoperative central neck ultrasound detects only macroscopic surgical disease, but negative findings predict excellent long-term regional control and survival. Thyroid. 2012;22:347–55.
51. Spencer CA. Clinical utility of thyroglobulin antibody (TgAb) measurements for patients with differentiated thyroid cancers (DTC). J Clin Endocrinol Metab. 2011;96:3615–27.
52. Spencer CA, Fatemi S. Thyroglobulin antibody (TgAb) methods: strengths, pitfalls, and clinical utility for monitoring TgAb-positive patients with differentiated thyroid cancer. Best Pract Res Clin Endocrinol Metab. 2013;27:701–12.
53. Kim WG, Yoon JH, Kim WB, Kim TY, Kim EY, Kim JM, Ryu JS, Gong G, Hong SJ, Shong YK. Change in serum antithyroglobulin antibody levels is useful for prediction of clinical recurrence in thyroglobulin-negative patients with differentiated thyroid carcinoma. J Clin Endocrinol Metab. 2008;93:4683–9.
54. Verburg FA, Luster M, Cupini C, Chiovato L, Duntas L, Elisei R, et al. Implications of thyroglobulin antibody positivity in patients with differentiated thyroid cancer: a clinical position statement. Thyroid. 2013;23:1211–25.
55. Spencer CA. Commentary on: implications of thyroglobulin antibody positivity in patients with differentiated thyroid cancer: a clinical position statement. Thyroid. 2013;23:1190–2.
56. Giovanella L, Ceriani L. Comparison of thyroglobulin antibody interference in first- and second-generation thyroglobulin immunoassays. Clin Chem Lab Med. 2011;49:1025–7.
57. Stanojevic M, Savin S, Cvejic D, Djukic A, Jeremic M, Zivancevic SS. Comparison of the influence of thyroglobulin antibodies on serum thyroglobulin values from two different immunoassays in post surgical differentiated thyroid cancer patients. J Clin Lab Anal. 2009;23:341–6.
58. Stanojevic M, Savin S, Cvejic D, Djukic A, Zivancevic SS. Correlation of thyroglobulin concentrations measured by radioassay and immunometric assay and the influence of thyroglobulin antibody. J Immunoass Immunochem. 2009;30:197–207.
59. Webb RC, Howard RS, Stojadinovic A, Gaitonde DY, Wallace MK, Ahmed J, Burch HB. The utility of serum thyroglobulin measurement at the time of remnant ablation for predicting disease-free status in patients with differentiated thyroid cancer: a meta-analysis involving 3947 patients. J Clin Endocrinol Metab. 2012;97:2754–63.
60. Lee JI, Chong YJ, Cho BY, Chong SM, Seok JW, Park SJ. Postoperative-stimulated serum thyroglobulin measured at the time of 131-I ablation is useful for the prediction of disease status in patients with differentiated thyroid carcinoma. Surgery. 2013;153:828–35.
61. Cherk MH, Francis P, Topliss DJ, Bailey M, Kalff V. Incidence and implications of negative serum thyroglobulin but positive I-131 whole-body scans in patients with well-differentiated thyroid cancer prepared with rhTSH or thyroid hormone withdrawal. Clin Endocrinol (Oxf). 2012;76:734–40.
62. Giovanella L, Suriano S, Ceriani L, Verburg FA. Undetectable thyroglobulin in patients with differentiated thyroid carcinoma and residual radioiodine uptake on a postablation whole-body scan. Clin Nucl Med. 2011;36:109–12.
63. Trimboli P, La Torre D, Ceriani L, Condorelli E, Laurenti O, Romanelli F, et al. High sensitive thyroglobulin assay on thyroxine therapy: can it avoid stimulation test in low and high risk differentiated thyroid carcinoma patients ? Horm Metab Res. 2013;45:664–8.
64. Giovanella L, Treglia G, Sadeghi R, Trimboli P, Ceriani L, Verburg FA. Unstimulated high-sensitive thyroglobulin in follow-up of differentiated thyroid cancer patients: a meta-analysis. J Clin Endocrinol Metab. 2013. doi:10.1210/jc.2013-3156.
65. Robenshtok E, Grewal RK, Fish S, Sabra M, Tuttle RM. A low postoperative nonstimulated serum thyroglobulin level does not exclude the presence of radioactive iodine avid metastatic foci in intermediate-risk differentiated thyroid cancer patients. Thyroid. 2013;23:436–42.
66. Rosario PW, Xavier AC, Calsolari MR. Value of post-operative thyroglobulin and ultrasonography for the indication of ablation and (131)I activity in patients with thyroid cancer and low risk of recurrence. Thyroid. 2011;21:49–53.
67. Phan HT, Jager PL, van der Wal JE, Sluiter WJ, Plukker JT, Dierckx RA, Wolffenbuttel BH, Links TP. The follow-up of patients with differentiated thyroid cancer and undetectable thyroglobulin (Tg) and Tg antibodies during ablation. Eur J Endocrinol. 2008;158:77–83.
68. Spencer C, Fatemi S, Singer P, Nicoloff J, LoPresti J. Serum basal thyroglobulin measured by a second-generation assay correlates with the recombinant human thyrotropin-stimulated thyroglobulin response in patients treated for differentiated thyroid cancer. Thyroid. 2010;20:587–95.
69. Pacini F, Sabra M, Tuttle RM. Clinical relevance of thyroglobulin doubling time in the management of patients with differentiated thyroid cancer. Thyroid. 2011;21:691–2.
70. Miyauchi A, Kudo T, Miya A, Kobayashi K, Ito Y, Takamura Y, et al. Prognostic impact of serum thyroglobulin doubling-time under thyrotropin suppression in patients with papillary thyroid carcinoma who underwent total thyroidectomy. Thyroid. 2011; 21:707–16.
71. Elisei R, Viola D, Torregrossa L, Giannini R, Romei C, Ugolini C, et al. The BRAF V600E mutation is an independent poor prognostic factor for the outcome of patients with low-risk intrathyroid papillary thyroid carcinoma: single-institution results from a large cohort study. J Clin Endocrinol Metab. 2012;97:4390–8.
72. Lim JY, Hong SW, Lee YS, Kim B-W, Park CS, Chang H-S, Cho JY. Clinicopathologic implications of the GRAF V600E mutation in papillary thyroid cancer: a subgroup analysis of 3130 cases in a single center. Thyroid. 2013;23:1423–30.
73. Gandolfi G, Sancissi V, Torricelli F, Ragazzi M, Frasoldati A, Piana S, Ciarrocchi A. Allele percentage of the BRAF V600E mutation in papillary thyroid carcinomas and corresponding lymph node metastases: no evidence for a role in tumor progression. J Clin Endocrinol Metab. 2013;98:E934–42.
74. Li C, Lee KC, Schneider EB, Zeiger MA. BRAF V600E mutation and its association with clinicopathological features of papillary thyroid cancer: a meta-analysis. J Clin Endocrinol Metab. 2012;97:4559–70.
75. Li C, Han A, Lee KC, Lee LC, Fox AC, Beninato T, et al. Does BRAF V600E mutation predict aggressive features in papillary thyroid cancer? Results from four endocrine surgery centers. J Clin Endocrinol Metab. 2013;98:3702–12.
76. Neimeier LA, Kuffner AH, Song C, Carty SE, Hodak SP, Yip L. A combined molecular-pathologic score improves risk stratification of thyroid papillary microcarcinoma. Cancer. 2012;118:2069–77.
77. Joo J-Y, Park J-Y, Yoon Y-H, Choi B, Kim J-M, Jo YS, et al. Prediction of occult central lymph node metastasis in papillary thyroid carcinoma by preoperative BRAF analysis using fine-needle aspiration biopsy: a prospective study. J Clin Endocrinol Metab. 2012;97:3996–4003.
78. Hay ID, Grant CS, van Heerden JA, et al. Papillary thyroid microcarcinoma: a study of 535 cases observed in a 50-year period. Surgery. 1987;102:1088–95.
79. Hay ID, Bergstralh EJ, Goellner JR, et al. Predicting outcome in papillary thyroid carcinoma: development of a reliable prognostic scoring system in a cohort of 1779 patients surgically treated in one institution during 1940 through 1989. Surgery. 1993;114:1050–8.
80. Sherman SI, Brierley JD, Sperling M, et al. Prospective multicenter study of thyroid carcinoma treatment: initial analysis of

staging and outcome. National Thyroid Cancer Treatment Cooperative Study Registry Group. Cancer. 1998;83:1012–21.
81. Cady B. Staging in thyroid carcinoma. Cancer. 1998;83:844–7.
82. Sherman SI. Staging of thyroid carcinoma—reply. Cancer. 1998;83:848–50.
83. Simpson WJ, McKinney SE, Carruthers JS, et al. Papillary and follicular thyroid cancer: prognostic factors in 1,578 patients. Am J Med. 1987;83:479–88.
84. Young RL, Mazzaferri EL, Rahe AJ, Dorfman SG. Pure follicular thyroid carcinoma: impact of therapy in 214 patients. J Nucl Med. 1980;21:733–7.
85. Brennan MD, Bergstralh EJ, van Heerden JA, McConahey WM. Follicular thyroid cancer treated at the Mayo Clinic, 1946 through 1970: initial manifestations, pathologic findings, therapy, and outcome. Mayo Clin Proc. 1991;66:11–22.
86. Enomoto K, Enomoto Y, Uchino S, Yamashita H, Noguchi S. Follicular thyroid cancer in children and adolescents: clinicopathologic features, long-term survival, and risk factors for recurrence. Endocr J. 2013;60:629–35.
87. Massoll N, Mazzaferri EL. Diagnosis and management of medullary thyroid carcinoma. Clin Lab Med. 2004;24:49–83.
88. Boostrom SY, Grant CS, Thompson GB, et al. Need for a revised staging consensus in medullary thyroid carcinoma. Arch Surg. 2009;144:663–9.
89. Dottorini ME, Assi A, Sironi M, et al. Multivariate analysis of patients with medullary thyroid carcinoma. Prognostic significance and impact on treatment of clinical and pathologic variables. Cancer. 1996;77:1556–65.
90. McIver B, Hay ID, Giuffrida DF, et al. Anaplastic thyroid carcinoma: a 50-year experience at a single institution. Surgery. 2001;130:1028–34.
91. Smallridge RC, Ain KB, Asa SL, Bible KC, Brierley JD, Burman KD, et al. American Thyroid Association guidelines for management of patients with anaplastic thyroid cancer. Thyroid. 2012; 22:1104–39.
92. Ito Y, Higashiyama T, Hirokawa M, et al. Investigation of the validity of UICC stage grouping of anaplastic carcinoma of the thyroid. Asian J Surg. 2009;32:47–50.
93. Mazzaferri EL, Young RL, Oertel JE, et al. Papillary thyroid carcinoma: the impact of therapy in 576 patients. Medicine. 1977;56:171–96.
94. Mazzaferri EL, Young RL. Papillary thyroid carcinoma: a 10 year follow-up report of the impact of therapy in 576 patients. Am J Med. 1981;70:511–8.
95. Schlumberger M, Hay ID. Use of radioactive iodine in patients with papillary and follicular thyroid cancer: towards a selective approach. J Clin Endocrinol Metab. 1998;83:4201–3.
96. Hay ID, Thompson GB, Grant CS, et al. Papillary thyroid carcinoma managed at the Mayo Clinic during six decades (1940–1999): temporal trends in initial therapy and long-term outcome in 2444 consecutively treated patients. World J Surg. 2002;26: 879–85.
97. Ito Y, Masuoka H, Fukushima M, Inoue H, Kihara M, Tomoda C, et al. Excellent prognosis of patients with solitary T1N0M0 papillary thyroid carcinoma who underwent thyroidectomy and elective node dissection without radioiodine therapy. World J Surg. 2010;34:1285–90.
98. Schvartz C, Bonnetain F, Dabakuyo S, Gauthier M, Cueff A, Fieffe S, et al. Impact on overall survival of radioactive iodine in low-risk differentiated thyroid cancer patients. J Clin Endocrinol Metab. 2012;97:1526–35.
99. Simpson WJ, Panzarella T, Carruthers JS, et al. Papillary and follicular thyroid cancer: impact of treatment in 1578 patients. Int J Radiat Oncol Biol Phys. 1988;14:1063–75.
100. Sawka AM, Thephamongkhol K, Brouwers, et al. A systematic review and metaanalysis of the effectiveness of radioactive iodine remnant ablation for well-differentiated thyroid cancer. J Clin Endocrinol Metab. 2004;89:3668–76.
101. Haugen BR. Editorial: patients with differentiated thyroid carcinoma benefit from radioiodine remnant ablation. J Clin Endocrinol Metab. 2004;89:3665–7.
102. Mazzaferri EL. Editorial: a randomized trial of remnant ablation—in search of an impossible dream? J Clin Endocrinol Metab. 2004;89:3662–4.
103. Tubeau M, Touzery C, Arveux P, et al. Predictive value for disease progression of serum thyroglobulin levels measured in the postoperative period and after (131)I ablation therapy in patients with differentiated thyroid cancer. J Nucl Med. 2004;45:988–94.
104. Torre EM, Carballo MTL, Erdozan RMR, et al. Prognostic value of thyroglobulin serum levels and 131-I whole-body scan after initial treatment of low-risk differentiated thyroid cancer. Thyroid. 2004;14:301–6.
105. Sugitani I, Kasai N, Fujimoto Y, Yanagisawa A. A novel classification system for patients with PTC: addition of the new variables of large (3 cm or greater) nodal metastases and reclassification during the follow-up period. Surgery. 2004;135:139–48.
106. Eichhorn W, Tabler H, Lippold R, et al. Prognostic factors determining long-term survival in well-differentiated thyroid cancer: an analysis of 484 patients undergoing therapy and aftercare at the same institution. Thyroid. 2003;13:949–58.
107. Furlan JC, Bedard YC, Rosen IB. Clinicopathologic significance of histologic vascular invasion in papillary and follicular thyroid carcinomas. J Am Coll Surg. 2004;198:341–8.
108. D'Avanzo A, Ituarte P, Treseler P, et al. Prognostic scoring systems in patients with follicular thyroid cancer: a comparison of different staging systems in predicting the patient outcome. Thyroid. 2004;14:453–8.
109. Voutilainen PE, Siironen P, Franssila KO, et al. AMES, MACIS, and TNM prognostic classifications in papillary thyroid carcinoma. Anticancer Res. 2003;23:4283–8.
110. Lang BH-H, Chow S-M, Lo C-Y, et al. Staging systems for papillary thyroid carcinoma: a study of two tertiary referral centers. Ann Surg. 2007;246:114–21.
111. Verburg FA, Mader U, Kruitwagen CLJJ, Luster M, Reiners C. A comparison of prognostic classification systems for differentiated thyroid carcinoma. Clin Endocrinol. 2010;72:830–8.
112. Poorten VV, Hens G, Delaere P. Thyroid cancer in children and adolescents. Curr Opin Otolaryngol Head Neck Surg. 2013;21:135–42.
113. Rivkees SA, Mazzaferri EL, Verburg FA, Reiners C, Luster M, Breuer CK, et al. The treatment of differentiated thyroid cancer in children: emphasis on surgical approach and radioactive iodine therapy. Endocr Rev. 2011;32:798–826.
114. Powers PA, Dinauer CA, Tuttle RM, Francis GL. The MACIS score predicts the clinical course of papillary thyroid carcinoma in children and adolescents. J Pediatr Endocrinol. 2004;17:339–43.
115. Oommen PT, Romahn A, Linden T, Fruhwald MC, Bucsky P. UICC-2002 TNM classification is not suitable for differentiated thyroid cancer in children and adolescents. Pediatr Blood Cancer. 2008;50:1159–62.
116. LaQuaglia M, Black T, Holcomb G, et al. Differentiated thyroid cancer: clinical characteristics, treatment, and outcome in patients under 21 years of age who present with distant metastases. A report from the Surgical Discipline Committee of the Children's Cancer Group. J Pediatr Surg. 2000;35:955–9.
117. Powers PA, Dinauer CA, Tuttle RM, Francis GL. Treatment of recurrent papillary thyroid carcinoma in children and adolescents. J Pediatr Endocrinol. 2003;16:1033–40.

Recombinant Human Thyrotropin

10

Matthew D. Ringel and Stephen J. Burgun

Initial management of patients with thyroid cancer often includes total thyroidectomy, long-term treatment with L-thyroxine often at doses sufficient for suppression of pituitary production of thyrotropin (TSH), and eradication of iodine-avid tissue (benign or malignant) with radioactive iodine in selected cases [1]. Residual thyroid cancer will be present, or disease will recur, in ~15–20 % of patients, thereby leading to recommendations for long-term monitoring. In addition to careful interval patient history and physical examination, measurement of circulating levels of thyroglobulin and radiographic imaging are employed. Measurement of serum thyroglobulin, functional imaging with radioiodine, and structural imaging are used to monitor thyroid cancer patients [1]. Of these, thyroglobulin measurement and radioiodine scans are relatively thyroid specific, providing high degrees of specificity. However, the sensitivities of iodine scanning and, in some cases, thyroglobulin measurement are limited by the small relative amount of thyroid tissue present in patients treated by thyroidectomy and dedifferentiation of tumor cells compared to normal thyrocytes. Therefore, radioiodine imaging and therapy require stimulation of thyroid tissue by elevated levels of TSH, and thyroglobulin measurement is also enhanced by TSH stimulation.

To attain the elevated serum TSH concentrations, protocols have been designed to stimulate endogenous pituitary TSH production and secretion for radioiodine scanning and therapy. Most commonly, L-thyroxine is withdrawn ~4 weeks to achieve a TSH >30 mU/l which is felt to be adequate for radioiodine scanning and therapy. The precise level for highest sensitivity thyroglobulin levels has not been reported but has been assumed to be similar. In an effort to limit the duration of symptomatic hypothyroidism, some clinicians treat patients with triiodothyronine (T_3), an agent with a shorter circulating half-life than L-thyroxine, for 2 weeks following discontinuation of thyroxine, although the efficacy of this maneuver has been questioned [2]. Several days after scanning and/or therapy, one or both types of thyroid hormone are restarted. Using this paradigm, patients are clinically hypothyroid for approximately 4 weeks, which can result in symptomatic hypothyroidism and limit the ability to work [3–5]. Moreover, elevated TSH levels for extended periods of time have been associated with growth of metastatic tumor tissue that has potential to cause compromise, particularly patients with central nervous system metastases [6, 7]. For these reasons, effective alternative methods for thyroid cell stimulation that limit the degree of thyroid hormone withdrawal [8, 9] or do not require thyroid hormone withdrawal at all have been sought for decades [10]. In this chapter, the history and current use of exogenous thyroid-stimulating agents are reviewed with particular emphasis on recombinant human TSH (rhTSH) that is currently approved for clinical use.

Exogenous Thyrotropin-Releasing Hormone

Exogenous thyrotropin-releasing hormone (TRH) using intramuscular (IM), intravenous (IV), and oral preparations has been used to stimulate endogenous production of pituitary TSH release either alone or in conjunction with thyroxine withdrawal. When administered IV, TRH is rapidly inactivated, with a half-life of 4–5 min. TSH peaks approximately 20–30 min following administration of TRH in normal individuals, but this response is blunted in patients with hyperthyroidism or on thyroxine suppression [11–13]. Repeated doses and infusions have been shown to enhance

M.D. Ringel, MD (✉)
Department of Internal Medicine, Division of Endocrinology, Diabetes and Metabolism, Wexner Medical Center, The Ohio State University, 565 McCampbell Hall, 1581 Dodd Drive, Columbus, OH 43210, USA
e-mail: matthew.ringel@osumc.edu

S.J. Burgun, MD
Department of Medicine, University Hospitals, Case Western Reserve University, Chardon, OH, USA
e-mail: stephen.burgun@uhhospitals.org

L. Wartofsky, D. Van Nostrand (eds.), *Thyroid Cancer*, DOI 10.1007/978-1-4939-3314-3_10

the TSH response to TRH, but this agent has proven cumbersome for clinical use, and it is not currently available in the United States [14]. Several groups evaluated oral TRH as an adjunct to standard thyroxine withdrawal or as a method to elevate the serum TSH concentration while patients remain on their L-thyroxine therapy [14, 15]. Longer periods of TSH elevation were observed with oral TRH, compared to IV or IM TRH administration, particularly when used to augment thyroxine withdrawal. However, TRH administration alone was less effective in stimulating iodine uptake than standard thyroid hormone withdrawal [14, 15], and its addition to thyroxine withdrawal did not enhance the iodine uptake [16].

One possible reason for the lack of efficacy relates to differences in TSH glycosylation that occur after acute vs. chronic TRH stimulation [17]. Human TSH contains three asparagine-linked oligosaccharide chains that terminate either with sialic acid linked to galactose, or with sulfate attached to N-acetylgalactosamine. Two of these oligosaccharide chains are attached to the α-subunit and one is attached to the β-subunit. Laboratory experiments report that different forms exert different cellular effects, are metabolized differently, and have specific affinities for the α-subunit [18–24]. Therefore, it is possible that the forms of TSH released following TRH stimulation may not have equivalent biological activity to those present with a more gradual development of hypothyroidism following thyroxine withdrawal, and this may account for the lack of efficacy of TRH in patients.

Bovine Thyrotropin

Seidlin and colleagues [25] and Stanley and Astwood [26] reported administration of bovine TSH to stimulate radioiodine uptake in humans. The administration of bovine TSH during thyroxine therapy as an alternative to thyroid hormone withdrawal in preparation for radioiodine scanning was first reported in 1953 by Sturgeon et al. [27] and by Catz et al. in 1959 [28]. These reports suggested that bovine TSH administration may be an acceptable alternative to thyroid hormone withdrawal. In addition, similar binding and activity were seen for human and bovine TSH in the laboratory [29]. Schneider and coworkers [30] subsequently showed similar enhancement of thyroid iodine uptake in normal subjects following injection of either bovine or human pituitary TSH. These data provided the rationale for clinical studies designed to evaluate the efficacy of bovine TSH-stimulated radioiodine scanning and treatment in patients with thyroid cancer during thyroid hormone therapy and after a period of thyroxine withdrawal. Pharmacokinetic studies showed a peak serum TSH concentration 4 h after IM administration of bovine TSH, and that by 10 h, serum concentrations had decreased by 50 % [31]. Initial results in thyroid cancer patients suggested that administration of bovine TSH was effective, although it was not as effective in stimulating iodine uptake as thyroid hormone withdrawal [31–33].

Unfortunately, local and systemic adverse events were associated with bovine TSH [34]. These were particular evident in patients treated multiple times [33]. It was determined that detectable circulating neutralizing antibodies developed in the majority of patients who received multiple doses of bovine TSH [35–37]. These anti-bovine TSH antibodies also interfered with measurement of endogenous TSH, hindering the ability to monitor patients for efficacy of thyroid hormone suppression therapy [35, 38, 39]. Due to the combination of relative ineffectiveness with multiple dosing, concerns regarding side effects, and the development of antibodies, bovine TSH use subsequently diminished.

Human Thyrotropin

Human Pituitary TSH

Human pituitary TSH was proposed to be useful in preparing patients for radioiodine scanning. Studies reporting kinetics in humans show effective stimulation of thyroid hormone production and iodine uptake [40–43]. In the early 1980s, several cases of Creutzfeld-Jakob syndrome were reported in patients treated with human pituitary growth hormone [44]. In addition, the purity of the human TSH preparation was questioned. Thus, human pituitary TSH is unlikely to be clinically utilized.

Recombinant Human TSH

Preclinical Studies

The cloning of the gene encoding the human TSH-β subunit [45–47] raised the possibility of producing recombinant human TSH using molecular techniques. Bioactive recombinant human TSH was subsequently manufactured by cotransfecting mammalian cells with complementary DNAs encoding both the common human α subunit and the human TSH-β subunit [46, 48–50]. Because bacterial cells do not possess the enzymes necessary for protein glycosylation, mammalian gene expression systems were required. In vitro activity and the chemical structure of rhTSH were compared to the international human pituitary TSH standards utilized in clinical assays. Binding studies revealed that rhTSH had high affinity for human TSH receptors expressed endogenously on human fetal thyroid cells [51] and for human TSH receptors expressed on Chinese hamster ovary cells transfected with TSH receptor cDNA [23, 24, 47–50]. Moreover, rhTSH binding was not species specific, displaying relatively high affinities for both endogenous rat and mouse TSH receptors.

These in vitro studies led to studies in mice and rats [52–54] and primates [55] that confirmed bioactivity by documenting enhanced radioiodine uptake following administration of rhTSH. In those studies, it became apparent that there was a poor correlation between in vitro and in vivo activity and that differences in the glycosylation patterns of the batches were responsible. The in vivo bioactivity of the sialylated form of rhTSH was greater than sulfated form, presumably related to its longer serum half-life. The sulfated form is excreted in the kidneys and has a relatively short half-life, while the sialylated form is hepatically metabolized, resulting in a longer serum half-life [18, 21–24, 53]. Magner and colleagues [17] identified sialylated TSH as the predominant circulating TSH glycoprotein in humans. Therefore, in addition to its greater in vivo activity, sialylated rhTSH may be more similar to circulating endogenous TSH than sulfated rhTSH.

Clinical Studies

Studies in Normal Subjects

Based on the experience in preclinical models, rhTSH was then studied in normal subjects for activity. Ramirez et al. [56] evaluated six euthyroid subjects with no prior history of thyroid disease, normal thyroid physical examinations, and no biochemical evidence of thyroid disease. The subjects received 0.1 mg of recombinant human TSH intramuscularly on three consecutive days. Serum TSH, T_4, T_3, free thyroxine index, and thyroglobulin were monitored every 4 h for the first 12 h, at 24, 72, and 96 h, and 7 days after administration of the dose. The development of antibodies against human TSH following the injections was also assessed. Serum TSH rose from a baseline of 1.3 U/ml to a mean of 40 U/ml in 4 h and peaked after 24 h. It decreased to below baseline 7 days after the injection. Serum T_3 and T_4 concentrations showed similar patterns except the peak occurred after 48 h with continued elevation (still within the normal range) after 1 week. Serum thyroglobulin also rose following recombinant TSH administration, but the maximal rise did not occur until 48–72 h after the dose. The medication was well tolerated and no patients developed anti-TSH antibodies. Radioiodine uptake was not measured in this study of normal subjects. In a follow-up study, no further increase in normal thyroid uptake was seen following administration of 0.3 and 0.9 mg doses of recombinant human TSH in normal subjects [57].

Studies in Patients with Thyroid Cancer for Diagnostic Use

Many studies and case reports of use of rhTSH in patients with thyroid cancer have been published in the literature. The focus of this initial section is on the initial phases I, II, and III clinical trials that address rhTSH administration for diagnostic scans and measurements of serum thyroglobulin which led to its FDA approval in the United States. In each of these studies, patients were prepared first by recombinant human TSH during thyroid hormone therapy and second by thyroid hormone withdrawal. Randomization of scan order would subject some patients to a second period of hypothyroidism in preparation for radioiodine therapy. However, the possibility of reduced sensitivity of the withdrawal scan secondary to "stunning" by the first scanning dose must be considered as a potential confounding factor [1].

Meier and coworkers [58] performed a phase I/II clinical trial to compare the efficacy and pharmacokinetics of various dosing regimens of rhTSH administration on iodine uptake and serum thyroglobulin concentrations in patients with thyroid cancer. In addition, they also compared the efficacy of the various rhTSH preparation regimens with standard thyroid hormone withdrawal. They evaluated 19 patients with differentiated thyroid cancer. All patients were treated with triiodothyronine (T_3) for an average of 37 days before receiving recombinant human TSH. Suppressed serum TSH concentrations were documented in these patients, and they were randomized to receive a single intramuscular injection of recombinant TSH (10, 20, 30, or 40 units) or multiple doses (2 or 3) of 10 units or 2 doses of 20 units at 24-h intervals while they remained on T_3. The 10-unit dose was equivalent to 1 mg based on an international TSH reference standard. Laboratory evaluation included serum concentrations of TSH, thyroglobulin, free T_4, total T_3, and antithyroglobulin antibodies. Diagnostic whole-body radioiodine scans using 1–2 mCi of ^{131}I were performed 48 h after the last rhTSH injection. After the ^{131}I scan, patients were withdrawn from T_3 for an average of 29 days until the serum TSH concentration was above 30 U/ml. Patients then received a second diagnostic whole-body ^{131}I scan. Patients were treated as clinically indicated based upon the results of the scans and serum thyroglobulin concentrations. Diagnostic scans using the two preparations were compared by independent, blinded nuclear medicine physicians, and then later as paired samples in which the reviewers were blinded to the order and dates of the two scans. The pharmacokinetic study revealed that serum TSH concentrations were maximally elevated with higher doses of recombinant human TSH, but that the 10-unit dose resulted in mean serum TSH concentrations similar to withdrawal (127 U/ml versus 77 mU/l, respectively) after one dose with a greater peak after the second dose (mean value: 220 mU/l). The TSH elevation was maintained for a longer period of time with a multiple injection schedule. In the blinded review of scans, radioiodine scans were read as equivalent in 17 of 19 (89 %) patients. In two patients, the withdrawal scans were considered superior. In the paired evaluation, scans were of equivalent quality in only 12 of 19 cases; in four cases, the rhTSH scan was superior, and in three cases, the withdrawal scan was superior. The iodine uptake was lower in the rhTSH scans compared to withdrawal preparation in 72 % of patients regardless of dosing regimen. The uptake was similar in the group prepared with one or two doses of 10 units and one dose of 20 units. There was no correlation between degree of TSH elevation and the percentage uptake between the rhTSH groups. Retention of the ^{131}I dose in the neck was measured in seven patients. A twofold greater dose retention was demonstrated after thyroid hormone withdrawal than after rhTSH administration. This difference was corrected by controlling for whole-body retention. The likely cause of the longer retention time in the thyroid hormone withdrawal scans was thought to be reduced metabolism and clearance of iodine in the hypothyroid subjects.

Serum thyroglobulin concentrations also increased in response to the recombinant human TSH. Maximal serum concentrations in the thyroid cancer patients occurred 48 and 72 h after rhTSH administration. Serum thyroglobulin concentration increased more than twofold in 79 % of patients after thyroid hormone withdrawal compared to 58 % of patients after rhTSH. No data are provided about the frequency of lesser elevations of thyroglobulin or the correlation between withdrawal and rhTSH-induced elevations; 4 of 19 patients with circulating antithyroglobulin antibodies were not included in the analysis of thyroglobulin levels.

None of the patients in the study showed detectable levels of circulating antibodies against human TSH. Quality of life assessment using both the Billewicz Scale [3] to assess hypothyroid symptoms and the Profile of Mood State Comparison [59] to assess changes in mood and other psychological symptoms revealed more frequent abnormal scores during thyroid hormone withdrawal. This phase I/II study showed that, while in most patients rhTSH preparation for diagnostic whole-body scans led to similar scan results versus withdrawal, rhTSH preparation resulted in lower neck uptake, lower retention of isotope, and lower rises in serum thyroglobulin. Patients tolerated the rhTSH well and had fewer symptoms compared to withdrawal preparation. The two-injection 10-unit regimen produced similar rises in TSH to higher dose regimens and was well tolerated.

Based upon the results of this phase I/II trial, a phase III trial was initiated to further compare the diagnostic utility of rhTSH with standard withdrawal scanning in a larger group of patients. Ladenson and colleagues [5] reported the results of a similarly designed study of 152 patients with thyroid cancer who received rhTSH, 0. 9 mg intramuscularly, on two consecutive days during thyroid hormone suppression therapy with either/or L-T_4 and T_3, followed by a thyroid hormone withdrawal scan 4–6 weeks later. Thyroxine suppression was confirmed by serum TSH concentrations. Patients received 2- to 4-mCi doses of radioiodine 1 day after the second dose of rhTSH and were scanned 2 days later (Fig. 10.1). Serum concentrations of TSH and urinary iodine were measured. In 35 patients, serum thyroglobulin and antithyroglobulin antibodies were also measured. Whole-body

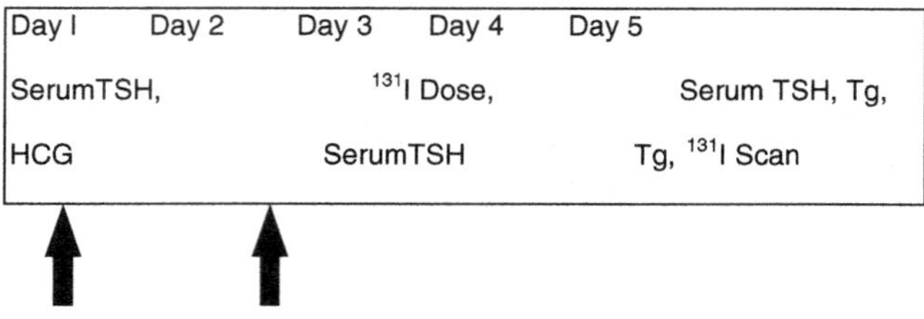

Fig. 10.1 Recommended dosing regimen for rhTSH: 0.9 mg of rhTSH (bioequivalence is 10 U/mg protein, Second World Health Organization International Reference Preparation, thyrotropin-pin, human, for bioassay) is administered on two consecutive days. Based on prior studies, the maximal rise in serum TSH occurs 24 and 48 h after the last dose of rhTSH, and the maximal rise in serum thyroglobulin (*Tg*) concentrations occurs 72 h after the last dose. Pregnancy tests (serum HCG) should be obtained from all women of childbearing age before rhTSH administration

radioiodine scans were interpreted by three independent reviewers in a blinded manner, and the results were compared. Hypothyroid symptoms and mood alterations were again measured by the Billewicz Scale [3] and the Profiles of Mood States Comparison [59], respectively. Of the initial 152 patients enrolled, 127 were included in the study evaluation. The majority of patients not included in the analysis were excluded for undefined protocol violations.

Mean serum TSH concentrations were 132 mU/l 24 h after the second rhTSH dose and 101 mU/l following thyroid hormone withdrawal. In 51 % of patients, scans revealed no uptake in both the withdrawal and rhTSH prepared scans. Among the 62 patients with uptake identified on one or both scans, 45 had thyroid bed uptake, 10 had cervical metastases, and 7 had distant metastases. Scans were considered discordant if additional areas of uptake were seen on one scan compared to the other, even if no change in tumor stage occurred. RhTSH and withdrawal scans were concordant in 66 % of the patients with positive scans. The rhTSH scan was superior in 5 %, and the withdrawal scan was superior in 29 %. Tumor stage was altered by the scan discordance in 6 of 17 patients with metastases. Including the concordant negative scans, the overall concordance rate for the 127 patients was 83 %. rhTSH scans were superior in 3 % of cases and withdrawal scans were superior in 14 % of cases.

Similar to the phase I/II study, local neck uptake was lower after rhTSH preparation, but when normalized for the differences in whole-body retention of ^{131}I, no difference was noted. Symptoms of hypothyroidism were significantly less common at the time of the rhTSH administration than after thyroid hormone withdrawal. Serum cholesterol, triglyceride, uric acid, and creatinine concentrations were also lower at the time of rhTSH stimulation than following withdrawal of thyroid hormone. Serum thyroglobulin concentrations were measured in only 35 of the patients. After rhTSH administration, thyroglobulin values were highest 72–96 h after the first dose. Thyroglobulin rose to a value greater

Table 10.1 Diagnostic accuracy of rhTSH monitoring compared to thyroid hormone withdrawal

Scans	2 injections (%)	3 injections (%)
A. Concordance between rhTSH-stimulated scans and thyroid	Hormone withdrawal scans are compared[a]	
Whole-body scan	$N=240$	$N=107$
Concordance	207 (86)	94 (88)
Discordance	33 (14)	13 (12)
Positive whole-body scan	$N=110$	$N=60$
Concordance	77 (70)	47 (78)
Discordance	33 (30)	13 (22)
rhTSH scan superior	6 (5)	5 (8)
Withdrawal scan superior (% of positive scans)	27 (24)	8 (13)
B. Accuracy of combined rhTSH scans and thyroglobulin concentrations are compared to a "Gold Standard" of positive withdrawal scan and/or an elevated withdrawal of thyroglobulin concentration		
Withdrawal scan and/or Tg >10 ng/ml[b]	$N=77$	$N=86$
rhTSH scan + or Tg >10 ng/ml		
Sensitivity (%)	94	97
Specificity (%)	93	81
Metastases on withdrawal scan	$N=9$	$N=23$
rhTSH scan + or Tg ≥3 ng/ml *N* (%)	9 (100)	23 (100)

[a]Data for the two injection regimen are combined from the two phase III trials. Overall concordance rates and concordance rates for those patients in whom at least one scan displayed uptake are shown. The definition of discordance differed in the two phase III studies (see text)

[b]Data are from the second phase III study only. Analysis of all subjects using 5 ng/ml as a positive rhTSH value yielded similar results to the 10 ng/ml value. Using the presence of uptake on rhTSH scanning or a rhTSH-stimulated thyroglobulin greater than 3 ng/ml identified recurrence in 32 of 32 patients with cervical and/or extracervical metastases

than 5 ng/ml in 13 patients after rhTSH and in 14 patients after withdrawal. No patients developed anti-TSH antibodies, including seven patients who previously received rhTSH in the phase I/II study. Adverse events were noted in 48 of 152 subjects. The most frequent adverse effect was nausea, which occurred in 25 patients and was generally mild and self-limited.

This phase III trial using a two-dose regimen demonstrated that among patients with recurrent or residual thyroid tissue, rhTSH preparation of patients for radioiodine scanning resulted in inferior scans in 29 % of cases. This frequency of inferior scans was concerning and several of these patients were treated differently based upon the discordant scan. However, measurement of a rhTSH-stimulated thyroglobulin appeared to be frequently concordant with thyroid hormone withdrawal-stimulated thyroglobulin. Unfortunately, this laboratory test was obtained from only 35 of the 127 patients in this study as this was not a primary endpoint. Most patients tolerated the rhTSH well, and symptoms of hypothyroidism were dramatically reduced with the use of rhTSH. Several reasons could account for the greater sensitivity of withdrawal compared to rhTSH scans, among these: (1) reduced clearance of the ^{131}I in hypothyroidism present after withdrawal results in a higher bioavailability for the iodine-avid tissue, (2) the longer duration of the elevated TSH levels after withdrawal may be important for maximally stimulating iodine uptake, and (3) the potentially higher total body iodine stores due to continuing L-thyroxine therapy [9].

To further define a potential role for rhTSH as a monitoring agent including thyroglobulin measurement in a larger group of patients, and to reevaluate the dosing regimen, a second phase III clinical trial comparing the two-injection regimen to a three-injection regimen in 226 patients was performed [60]. The protocol was designed in a similar manner to the study of Ladenson and coworkers [5] except that patients were randomized to receive either two or three 0. 9-mg doses of rhTSH intramuscularly. Patients received ^{131}I 24 h after the last dose of rhTSH, were scanned using 2–4 mCi ^{131}I 2 days later, and serum thyroglobulin concentrations were measured 48 and 72 h after the last dose of rhTSH. Following this scan, patients were withdrawn from thyroid hormone for diagnostic scans, serum thyroglobulin measurements, and treatment as needed.

In this study, scan discordance was defined as uptake on one scan that altered the stage of disease. Using this definition, the overall concordance rate between rhTSH and withdrawal ^{131}I whole-body scans was 89 %. Of the discordant studies, withdrawal whole-body scans were interpreted as superior in 8 % of cases, and rhTSH-stimulated scans were superior in 4 % of cases. No statistically significant difference was reported between the accuracy of rhTSH-stimulated scans and withdrawal scans using this definition. No statistical differences were seen between the two rhTSH preparation regimens. Combined data from the two phase III trials comparing the utility of the two- and three-injection regimens for radioiodine scanning versus withdrawal scanning are summarized in Table 10.1A.

Serum thyroglobulin measurements were measured 48 and 72 h after the last dose of rhTSH and following thyroid hormone withdrawal. Serial samples from individual patients were measured on the same assay. Analysis using different values of thyroglobulin to identify disease presence (detectable iodine-avid tissue on diagnostic and/or posttherapy scan) was performed for both basal and stimulated values. The lowest concentration that provided greatest accuracy for stimulated thyroglobulin concentrations using rhTSH or thyroid hormone withdrawal was determined to be 3 ng/ml. At values of 3 ng/ml or greater, the sensitivity and specificity were 72 and 95 % for rhTSH-stimulated thyroglobulin and 71 and 100 % for the withdrawal-stimulated thyroglobulin. Patients with circulating antithyroglobulin antibodies were excluded from this analysis. In general, serum thyroglobulin rose to similar levels following rhTSH stimulation and thyroid hormone withdrawal. The interpretation of these thyroglobulin data is dependent on the reproducibility of the thyroglobulin assay at lower values, a factor that varies greatly between different commercial laboratories. Using a TSH-stimulated value of 5 or 10 ng/ml as a "positive value," the combination of rhTSH-stimulated thyroglobulin and scan was 94 % sensitive and 93 % specific in predicting iodine-avid tissue on subsequent withdrawal and/or post-therapy scan. When a stimulated thyroglobulin value ≥3 ng/ml was used in combination with scanning, rhTSH stimulation identified all 32 patients with cervical or distant metastases. The study does not include neck ultrasound and newer more sensitive thyroglobulin assays were not available. Data from the second phase III study evaluating the accuracy of combining rhTSH scan and thyroglobulin measurement to identify metastases are summarized in Table 10.1B.

Studies Refining the Use of rhTSH in Thyroid Cancer Monitoring

Several investigators noted frequent discordant results between TSH-stimulated thyroglobulin and whole-body scanning, indicating greater sensitivity and less false-negative results with the TSH-stimulated thyroglobulin over whole-body scintigraphy [61–63]. Callieux and associates evaluated the accuracies of levothyroxine withdrawal thyroglobulin and ^{131}I whole-body scanning in 256 patients treated with thyroidectomy and 100 mCi of I-131 [62]. Six to 12 months after the radioiodine therapy, 46 of the 256 patients had a stimulated thyroglobulin of at least 1.0 ng/ml after L-thyroxine withdrawal. By contrast, diagnostic ^{131}I scintigraphy showed uptake in only 20 of the patients. Of the 210 patients with hypothyroid thyroglobulin concentration less than 1.0 ng/ml, only two had recurrent disease in 3 years of follow-up. Of the 15 patients with hypothyroid thyroglobulin concentrations of 10 ng/ml or more, only 3 had detectable thyroid bed uptake on scintigraphy, but 5 demonstrated persistent disease using other modalities. Thirty-seven patients from this cohort with hypothyroid concentrations greater than 1.0 ng/ml were followed further; nine developed evidence of disease between 3 and 117 months after initial surgery. Of these nine recurrences, only one was detected on diagnostic ^{131}I [61]. Thus, in this study, following L-thyroxine withdrawal, TSH-stimulated thyroglobulin was more sensitive than radioiodine whole-body scanning.

These observations were subsequently extended to rhTSH-stimulated Tg measurement. A retrospective review of 107 patients with differentiated thyroid cancer, without thyroglobulin antibodies, compared the results of rhTSH-stimulated thyroglobulin and whole-body 4 mCi (3.8–5.1 mCi) ^{131}I diagnostic whole-body scintigraphy [64]. Persistent disease was found in 11 patients. Using a rhTSH-stimulated thyroglobulin concentration of 2.0 ng/ml or more as the cut point, there was 100 % sensitivity and 100 % negative predictive value. By contrast, the diagnostic scan had a 73 % false-negative rate. The use of rhTSH-stimulated thyroglobulin alone was then studied prospectively in a multicenter trial of 300 patients with differentiated thyroid cancer and negative thyroglobulin antibody testing [65]. Serum thyroglobulin increased by at least 2 ng/ml in 53 patients (18 %) after rhTSH. Of 267 patients with thyroxine-suppressed thyroglobulin less than 1 ng/ml, 26 (10 %) had stimulated thyroglobulin of at least 2 ng/ml. Of the 53 patients with net increases in thyroglobulin of at least 2 ng/ml, 33 (62 %) had a history of negative ^{131}I whole-body scans.

An expert summary advocated the use of TSH-stimulated thyroglobulin alone instead of in combination with ^{131}I scanning as the preferred method of surveillance for patients with differentiated thyroid cancer at low risk for metastasis [66]. This consensus recommendation was limited to patients clinically at low risk for persistent or recurrent disease or cancer death and without thyroglobulin antibodies. The use of sensitive immunometric thyroglobulin assays was advocated, with simultaneous immunoassay for thyroglobulin antibody. A TSH-stimulated thyroglobulin concentration of 2.0 ng/ml was set as the threshold for further intervention. While hypothyroid- and rhTSH-stimulated thyroglobulin measurements were considered comparable for disease detection, the authors opined that rhTSH was preferable to L-thyroxine withdrawal due to the likelihood of hypothyroid symptoms and potential loss of productivity after withdrawal. This must be balanced against the cost of rhTSH, and the potential that shorter durations of thyroxine withdrawal or partial withdrawal (i.e., dose-reducing levothyroxine without discontinuation) have also been reported that might also reduce side effects [67].

The frequency or need for continued TSH-stimulated Tg monitoring over time, particularly with the increasing sensitivity of Tg assays and greater experience with neck ultrasound has been studied by several groups. Castagna et al. [68] investigated the role of rhTSH-stimulated thyroglobulin testing and neck ultrasound in patients felt to be free of disease after initial therapy. The series included 85 patients with differentiated thyroid cancer treated with total thyroidectomy and ^{131}I therapy that had thyroglobulin concentrations on levothyroxine below 1.0 ng/ml. At initial rhTSH-thyroglobulin testing within 1 year of the initial therapy, 68 had concentrations below 1.0 ng/ml, one of which had persistent disease identified on ultrasound and fine-needle aspiration. The other 67 had repeat rhTSH-stimulated thyroglobulin testing in 2–3 years. Of these, one had rhTSH-stimulated thyroglobulin concentration over 1 ng/ml, with disease also evident on ultrasound examination. The other 66 (98.5 %) had rhTSH-stimulated thyroglobulin concentrations below 1 ng/ml and negative ultrasound examinations. Thus, in this series of low-risk patients, neck ultrasound and rhTSH were highly sensitive in detecting recurrent thyroid cancer, and the combination was proposed to be particularly accurate. Importantly, the data suggest that in this group of patients, an undetectable TSH-stimulated thyroglobulin level after initial therapy predicted a 98.5 % likelihood of a similar result 3 years later suggesting that the frequency of continued TSH-stimulation testing might be able to be lengthened for many patients.

A retrospective series of 107 patients treated with initial thyroidectomy and remnant ablation were stratified by risk into three groups based on their follow-up posttherapy rhTSH-stimulated thyroglobulin concentration [69]. Patients were included if they were free of clinically apparent disease, had no thyroglobulin antibodies, and thyroglobulin concentration 1 ng/ml or lower on levothyroxine therapy. In those with rhTSH-stimulated thyroglobulin 0.5 ng/ml or less, the 7-year incidence of recurrence was 3 % – 2 of 62 patients. Those with rhTSH-stimulated thyroglobulin concentration greater than 2 ng/ml had an 80 % incidence of recurrence in 4.1 years. Of the intermediate group, with rhTSH-stimulated thyroglobulin 0.6–2 ng/ml followed for 8.1 years, 63 % had rhTSH-stimulated thyroglobulin concentration below 0.5 ng/ml on subsequent follow-up testing, and 11 % had recurrence after subsequent rhTSH-thyroglobulin concentration over 2 ng/ml. The implication of this longer-term series was that patients with low-risk disease and rhTSH-stimulated highly sensitive thyroglobulin concentration 0.5 ng/ml or below during follow-up may not require routine repeat rhTSH-stimulated thyroglobulin testing, but may be followed with thyroglobulin testing on levothyroxine and periodic neck ultrasound if they have papillary thyroid cancer. Serial testing of rhTSH-stimulated thyroglobulin concentration and thyroglobulin may be indicated for those with an initial concentration 1–2 ng/ml as a percentage will regress over time to a lower-risk category.

A third retrospective study in 278 patients treated with total thyroidectomy and ^{131}I was recently published [70]. Similar to prior studies, during a mean follow-up of 6.3 years (range 3–12), 96 % of the patients with undetectable rhTSH-stimulated thyroglobulin 1 year after initial therapy had undetectable results at the end of the study. Of the ten patients with an undetectable rhTSH-stimulated thyroglobulin 1 year after initial therapy who subsequently developed a detectable result, nine were detected by performing one subsequent rhTSH-stimulated thyroglobulin. However, only four had evidence of disease detected during follow-up. All of these patients had stimulated Tg levels >1.0 ng/ml and all but one were detected on neck ultrasound. One patient had a recurrence identified on neck ultrasound with an undetectable rhTSH-thyroglobulin level. The authors propose that performing a second round of rhTSH-thyroglobulin testing after an initial negative result allows for better refinement of further testing for patients with thyroid cancer and may define a group that does not require additional TSH-stimulation testing. In this study, however, the relative value of measuring even one repeat TSH-stimulated thyroglobulin beyond neck ultrasound was not assessed.

New generations of even more sensitive thyroglobulin assays that can accurately measure to levels below 0.1 ng/ml have been developed for thyroid cancer monitoring (Spencer). Using these assays, Spencer et al. [71] separated individuals into groups based on thyroglobulin levels on levothyroxine. Individuals with a thyroglobulin <0.1 ng/ml on TSH suppression rarely, if ever, have a rhTSH-stimulated thyroglobulin >2 ng/ml while those with Tg levels >0.2 frequently have elevated values. Thus, only the 22 % of individuals that had a thyroglobulin on levothyroxine between 0.1 and 0.2 ng/ml appear to benefit from rhTSH-stimulation. Moreover, the height of TSH stimulation correlated with the basal thyroglobulin level and was consistent in patients with multiple stimulated values over time as long as the basal levels were stable. Thus, if the results are confirmed, with use of this assay, it seems likely that most patients, especially those at low risk, will be able to be monitored using neck ultrasound and thyroglobulin levels on levothyroxine and only a minority will benefit from TSH-stimulation testing.

Whether or not this strategy of limited TSH-stimulated thyroglobulin tests and radiographic imaging using neck ultrasound is applicable to patients with non-papillary thyroid cancer or for patients with higher-risk tumors remains uncertain. For patients with follicular thyroid cancer, it seems unlikely that neck ultrasound would be highly sensitive, and further studies are needed to establish if radioiodine scanning adds to the accuracy of monitoring in this group of patients. The strategies and data described above also exclude individuals with anti-thyroglobulin antibodies. An approach to these patients is described elsewhere in the book. Finally, if strategies for monitoring rely on neck ultrasound, it presumes that a skilled neck ultrasound is available for patients. That is not the case in all locations; thus, strategies used in clinical practice may vary in order to provide optimal care for patients.

rhTSH Administration in Preparation for Radioiodine Therapy

The use of rhTSH as an alternative to thyroid hormone withdrawal preparation for the first radioiodine therapy after initial surgery for patients without known metastatic disease or residual cancer tissue is approved for use in the United States and some other countries. The use of rhTSH for remnant ablation was reported in a retrospective, non-randomized, single-center series [72]. In this series, 45 patients received rhTSH 0.9 mg IM on two consecutive days while continuing levothyroxine, and 42 patients had traditional hypothyroid preparation. The administered mean doses of radioiodine were 90.7 and 72.2 mCi for the rhTSH and hypothyroid groups, respectively. Follow-up diagnostic 131-iodine whole body scans performed approximately 11 months after therapy indicated a similar rate of complete ablation, 84.4 % with rhTSH, and 80.9 % with hypothyroidism. Thyroglobulin levels were also similar between the two groups at the time of the follow-up evaluation.

A prospective randomized study was performed to compare the efficacy and safety of rhTSH preparation with hypothyroid preparation for initial remnant ablation at a fixed ^{131}I dose of 100 mCi [73]. Sixty-three patients were randomized post-thyroidectomy either to two doses of intramuscular rhTSH 0.9 mg on consecutive days followed by ^{131}I administration the third day, versus withholding postoperative levothyroxine to achieve a serum TSH concentration greater than 25 mU/l. Efficacy was determined by posttherapy scan and also by diagnostic rhTSH-stimulated radioiodine uptake and whole-body scan 8 months after the treatment. The area of thyroid bed uptake was comparable on posttherapy scan, and all patients in both randomized groups had no visible uptake or uptake <0.1 % at 8 months. The radioiodine dose to the blood was lower in the rhTSH-stimulated euthyroid group than the hypothyroid group. As with the use of rhTSH in diagnostic testing, quality of life scores were favorable for euthyroid rhTSH over hypothyroidism at the time of ablation and at 4 weeks after ablation.

A subsequent single-center study then compared the efficacy of 100 and 50 mCi for initial therapy with euthyroid rhTSH preparation [74]. Successful ablation at 6–8 months determined by euthyroid rhTSH-stimulated diagnostic whole-body scan was the same at 88.9 % in both groups. The proportion achieving undetectable rhTSH-stimulated thyroglobulin concentrations at follow-up in the absence of anti-thyroglobulin antibody was also not significantly different between the two doses.

Comparison of clinical outcomes after rhTSH-stimulated versus hypothyroid first ^{131}I therapy was reported from a single center [75]. In this non-randomized series, 394 patients with differentiated thyroid cancer had postoperative radioiodine remnant ablation: 320 with rhTSH preparation and 74 with hypothyroid preparation. Radioiodine activity was selected based on clinical characteristics and ranged from 75 to over 150 mCi. The median ^{131}I activities were 109 and 103 mCi in the rhTSH-stimulated and hypothyroid groups, respectively. The primary outcome was considered no clinical evidence of disease, defined as a negative rhTSH-stimulated whole-body scan 12–18 months after therapy, all thyroid hormone-suppressed thyroglobulin concentrations less than 2 ng/ml, rhTSH-stimulated thyroglobulin less than 10 ng/ml, and no clinically evident recurrence. Median follow-up of 29 months indicated 76 % of the rhTSH group, and 62 % of the hypothyroid group met these criteria, which was not a significant difference. There was no significant difference in the rates of clinical disease recurrence, 4 % with rhTSH and 7 % with hypothyroid preparation. Because this is a non-randomized experience, there may have been selection biases in the two groups of patients that were not able to be quantified in the study.

Current product labeling in the United States indicates rhTSH for use with remnant ablation after total or near-total thyroidectomy for patients with no known residual thyroid cancer or metastatic disease. The recommended dosing is 0.9 mg by intramuscular injection to the buttock for two consecutive days, with ^{131}I administration on the third day. The protocol in the outcome study above employed a four-dose strategy, with 0.9 mg on days 1 and 2 followed by a diagnostic ^{131}I dose on day 3, with 0.9 mg on days 8 and 9 followed by the therapeutic ^{131}I dose on day 10 [75]. Therapeutic protocols with and without diagnostic scanning vary at other institutions.

Long-term outcomes after rhTSH-stimulated remnant ablation regarding survival and cancer recurrence are not yet known and may be difficult to discern in patients with low-risk disease who have an excellent prognosis. It also is not known whether the decreased radiation exposure to the blood seen with rhTSH relative to hypothyroid therapy will result in a reduced incidence of any secondary malignancy or other radioiodine off-target side effects such as sialadenitis or lacrimal duct stenosis.

Radioiodine therapy with rhTSH preparation for known metastatic thyroid cancer is not currently FDA approved. Clinical experience with rhTSH preparation in therapy for distant metastases from several centers has been reported. One retrospective study of 175 patients with radioiodine-avid distant metastases treated multiple times either with rhTSH preparation ($n=58$), thyroxine withdrawal ($n=35$), or the first dose with thyroxine withdrawal, and subsequent doses with rhTSH preparation ($n=82$) reported no differences in survival over 5.5 years between the groups [76]. On multivariate analysis, only patient age predicted outcome, not initial tumor stage or mode of preparation. In a retrospective second study from a different institution, outcomes of 15 patients with ^{131}I-avid distant metastases from differentiated thyroid cancer treated with rhTSH preparation were compared with 41 patients prepared with thyroid hormone withdrawal [77]. Doses were determined by treating clinicians. Sites of distant metastases were similar between the two groups. Rates of stable disease, partial remission, disease progression, and side effects were similar between the two groups over a mean follow-up time of 6 years. Although both studies suggest comparable responses between the treatment preparation options, they are retrospective and small with relatively short durations of follow-up. There may be important selection biases and dose differences in the treatments not able to be accounted for in the models. Thus, further studies are needed to better determine if rhTSH preparation is appropriate for patients with known metastatic thyroid cancer.

Summary of Recombinant Human TSH in Thyroid Cancer

For monitoring patients with previously treated thyroid cancer, it appears that rhTSH preparation is similar to thyroid hormone withdrawal in the detection of recurrent or residual thyroid cancer when thyroglobulin is included in the monitoring paradigm. There appears to be no significant advantage of the three-injection regimen as compared to the two-injection regimen. However, it is important to recognize that rhTSH ^{131}I scanning appears to be less sensitive than thyroid hormone withdrawal, although this type of monitoring is losing favor for papillary thyroid cancer monitoring due to its relatively low sensitivity. In all studies, euthyroid rhTSH preparation avoids the transient hypothyroidism that occurs with thyroid hormone withdrawal thereby improving quality of life. The advantage of avoiding hypothyroid symptoms must be balanced against cost for individual patients. Alternative strategies that reduce the severity of hypothyroidism, such as partial thyroid hormone withdrawal or shorter-term periods of hypothyroidism for thyroglobulin measurement, may also be considered. Finally, with the advent of more sensitive thyroglobulin assays, improved access to skilled neck ultrasound, and enhanced ability to predict long-term behavior of thyroid cancers based, repeated TSH-stimulated thyroglobulin measurement may not be necessary for many or most patients with thyroid cancer. Over time, refinement of these paradigms is expected to occur. Larger and prospective clinical studies are needed to adequately address several questions regarding the clinical use of rhTSH such as the following: (1) What is the sensitivity of rhTSH in patients with poorly differentiated tumors? (2) Is there a role for rhTSH stimulation for ^{131}I treatment in selected individuals with known residual or recurrent thyroid cancer? Finally, several groups are developing TSH receptor superagonists with enhanced effects on iodide uptake that have not yet been tested in clinical trials but may result in further refinement of thyroid cancer therapy and monitoring paradigms in the future [22, 78, 79].

References

1. Haugen BR, Alexander EK, Bible KC, Doherty GM, Mandel SJ, Nikiforov Y, Pacini F, Randolph G, Sawka A, Shepard D, Sosa J, Tuttle RM, Wartofsky L. 2015 American Thyroid Association Management Guidelines for adult patients with thyroid nodules and differentiated thyroid cancer. Available online at Thyroid 25: DOI:10.1089/thy.2015.0020; print version in Thyroid 26:2016.
2. Lee J, Yun MJ, Nam KH, Chung WY, Soh EY, Park CS. Quality of life and effectiveness comparisons of thyroxine withdrawal, triiodothyronine withdrawal, and recombinant thyroid-stimulating hormone administration for low-dose radioiodine remnant ablation of differentiated thyroid carcinoma. Thyroid. 2010;20(2):173–9.
3. Billewicz WZ, Chapman RS, Crooks J, Day ME, Gossage J, Wayne E, Young JA. Statistical methods applied to the diagnosis of hypothyroidism. Q J Med. 1969;38(150):255–66.
4. Dow KH, Ferrell BR, Anello C. Quality-of-life changes in patients with thyroid cancer after withdrawal of thyroid hormone therapy. Thyroid. 1997;7(4):613–9.
5. Ladenson PW, Braverman LE, Mazzaferri EL, Brucker-Davis F, Cooper DS, Garber JR, Wondisford FE, Davies TF, DeGroot LJ, Daniels GH, Ross DS, Weintraub BD. Comparison of administration of recombinant human thyrotropin with withdrawal of thyroid hormone for radioactive iodine scanning in patients with thyroid carcinoma. N Engl J Med. 1997;337(13):888–96.
6. Goldberg LD, Ditchek NT. Thyroid carcinoma with spinal cord compression. JAMA. 1981;245(9):953–4.
7. Sfakianakis GN, Skillman TG, George JM. Thyroxine withdrawal in thyroid cancer. Ohio State Med J. 1975;71(2):79–82.
8. Guimaraes V, DeGroot LJ. Moderate hypothyroidism in preparation for whole body 131I scintiscans and thyroglobulin testing. Thyroid. 1996;6(2):69–73.
9. Maxon HR. Detection of residual and recurrent thyroid cancer by radionuclide imaging. Thyroid. 1999;9(5):443–6.
10. Robbins J. Pharmacology of bovine and human thyrotropin: an historical perspective. Thyroid. 1999;9(5):451–3.
11. Sawin CT, Hershman JM. The TSH response to thyrotropin-releasing hormone (TRH) in young adult men: intra-individual variation and relation to basal serum TSH and thyroid hormones. J Clin Endocrinol Metab. 1976;42(5):809–16.
12. Spencer CA, Schwarzbein D, Guttler RB, LoPresti JS, Nicoloff JT. Thyrotropin (TSH)-releasing hormone stimulation test responses employing third and fourth generation TSH assays. J Clin Endocrinol Metab. 1993;76(2):494–8.
13. Wide L, Dahlberg PA. Quality requirements of basal S-TSH assays in prediction an S-TSH response to TRH. Scand J Clin Lab Invest Suppl. 1980;155:101–10.
14. Fairclough PD, Cryer RJ, McAllister J, Hawkins L, Jones AE, McKendrick M, Hall R, Besser GM. Serum TSH responses to intravenously and orally administered TRH in man after thyroidectomy for carcinoma of the thyroid. Clin Endocrinol (Oxf). 1973;2(4):351–9.
15. Wenzel KW, Meinhold H, Bogner U, Adlkofer F, Schleusener H. Serum TSH levels in thyroidectomized patients after withdrawal of thyroid hormone therapy or oral administration of TRH. Acta Endocrinol (Copenh). 1973;173(Suppl):15.
16. Ang ES, Teh HS, Sundram FX, Lee KO. Effect of lithium and oral thyrotrophin-releasing hormone (TRH) on serum thyrotrophin (TSH) and radioiodine uptake in patients with well differentiated thyroid carcinoma. Singapore Med J. 1995;36(6):606–8.
17. Magner JA, Kane J, Chou ET. Intravenous thyrotropin (TSH)-releasing hormone releases human TSH that is structurally different from basal TSH. J Clin Endocrinol Metab. 1992;74(6): 1306–11.
18. Canonne C, Papandreou MJ, Medri G, Verrier B, Ronin C. Biological and immunochemical characterization of recombinant human thyrotrophin. Glycobiology. 1995;5(5):473–81.

19. Matzuk MM, Kornmeier CM, Whitfield GK, Kourides IA, Boime I. The glycoprotein alpha-subunit is critical for secretion and stability of the human thyrotropin beta-subunit. Mol Endocrinol. 1988; 2(2):95–100.
20. Schaaf L, Leiprecht A, Saji M, Hubner U, Usadel KH, Kohn LD. Glycosylation variants of human TSH selectively activate signal transduction pathways. Mol Cell Endocrinol. 1997;132(1–2): 185–94.
21. Szkudlinski MW, Thotakura NR, Bucci I, Joshi LR, Tsai A, East-Palmer J, Shiloach J, Weintraub BD. Purification and characterization of recombinant human thyrotropin (TSH) isoforms produced by Chinese hamster ovary cells: the role of sialylation and sulfation in TSH bioactivity. Endocrinology. 1993;133(4):1490–503.
22. Szkudlinski MW, Thotakura NR, Weintraub BD. Subunit-specific functions of N-linked oligosaccharides in human thyrotropin: role of terminal residues of alpha- and beta-subunit oligosaccharides in metabolic clearance and bioactivity. Proc Natl Acad Sci U S A. 1995;92(20):9062–6.
23. Thotakura NR, Desai RK, Bates LG, Cole ES, Pratt BM, Weintraub BD. Biological activity and metabolic clearance of a recombinant human thyrotropin produced in Chinese hamster ovary cells. Endocrinology. 1991;128(1):341–8.
24. Thotakura NR, Szkudlinski MW, Weintraub BD. Structure-function studies of oligosaccharides of recombinant human thyrotrophin by sequential deglycosylation and resialylation. Glycobiology. 1994; 4(4):525–33.
25. Seidlin SM, Oshry E, Yalow AA. Spontaneous and experimentally induced uptake of radioactive iodine in metastases from thyroid carcinoma; a preliminary report. J Clin Endocrinol Metab. 1948;8(6):423–32.
26. Stanley MM, Astwood EB. The accumulation of radioactive iodide by the thyroid gland in normal and thyrotoxic subjects and the effect of thiocyanate on its discharge. Endocrinology. 1948;42(2):107–23.
27. Sturgeon CT, Davis FE, Catz B, Petit D, Starr P. Treatment of thyroid cancer metastases with TSH and I131 during thyroid hormone medication. J Clin Endocrinol Metab. 1953;13(11):1391–407.
28. Catz B, Petit DW, Schwartz H, Davis F, Mc CC, Starr P. Treatment of cancer of the thyroid postoperatively with suppressive thyroid medication, radioactive iodine, and thyroid-stimulating hormone. Cancer. 1959;12(2):371–83.
29. Reichert Jr LE. On the relationship between human thyrotrophin research standard A, the United States Pharmacopeia thyrotrophin standard (Bovine) and the International Standard for thyrotrophin (Bovine). J Clin Endocrinol Metab. 1970;31(3):331–3.
30. Schneider PB, Robbins J, Condliffe PG. Thyroid response to human thyrotropin in man. J Clin Endocrinol Metab. 1965;25:514–7.
31. Hershman JM, Edwards CL. Serum thyrotropin (TSH) levels after thyroid ablation compared with TSH levels after exogenous bovine TSH: implications for 131-I treatment of thyroid carcinoma. J Clin Endocrinol Metab. 1972;34(5):814–8.
32. Hays MT, Solomon DH, Pierce JG, Carstein ME. The effect of purified bovine thyroid-stimulating hormone in man. I. Dose-response characteristics studied with I-132. J Clin Endocrinol Metab. 1961;21:1469–74.
33. Hays MT, Solomon DH, Werner SC. The effect of purified bovine thyroid-stimulating hormone in men. II. Loss of effectiveness with prolonged administration. J Clin Endocrinol Metab. 1961;21: 1475–82.
34. Krishnamurthy GT. Human reaction to bovine TSH: concise communication. J Nucl Med. 1978;19(3):284–6.
35. Greenspan FS, Lew W, Okerlund MD, Lowenstein JM. Falsely positive bovine TSH radioimmunoassay responses in sera from patients with thyroid cancer. J Clin Endocrinol Metab. 1974;38(6):1121–2.
36. Greenspan FS, Lowenstein JM, West MN, Okerlund MD. Immunoreactive material to bovine TSH in plasma from patients with thyroid cancer. J Clin Endocrinol Metab. 1972;35(6):795–8.
37. Hays MT, Solomon DH, Beall GN. Suppression of human thyroid function by antibodies to bovine thyrotropin. J Clin Endocrinol Metab. 1967;27(11):1540–9.
38. Chaussain JL, Binet E, Job JC. Antibodies to human thyreotrophin in the serum of certain hypopituitary dwarfs. Rev Eur Etud Clin Biol. 1972;17(1):95–9.
39. Sain A, Sham R, Singh A, Silver L. Erroneous thyroid-stimulating hormone radioimmunoassay results due to interfering antibovine thyroid-stimulating hormone antibodies. Am J Clin Pathol. 1979;71(5):540–2.
40. Kuku SF, Harsoulis P, Young JL, Fraser TR. Concentrations of immunoreactive thyrotrophic hormone in urine of normal subjects, patients with thyroid disorders and hypopituitarism, and after infusion of human thyrotrophic hormone. J Endocrinol. 1974;62(3):645–55.
41. Law A, Jack GW, Tellez M, Edmonds CJ. In-vivo studies of a human-thyrotrophin preparation. J Endocrinol. 1986;110(2):375–8.
42. Ridgway EC, Weintraub BD, Maloof F. Metabolic clearance and production rates of human thyrotropin. J Clin Invest. 1974; 53(3):895–903.
43. Uller RP, Van Herle AJ, Chopra IJ. Comparison of alterations in circulating thyroglobulin, triiodothyronine and thyroxine in response to exogenous (bovine) and endogenous (human) thyrotropin. J Clin Endocrinol Metab. 1973;37(5):741–5.
44. Brown P, Gajdusek DC, Gibbs Jr CJ, Asher DM. Potential epidemic of Creutzfeldt-Jakob disease from human growth hormone therapy. N Engl J Med. 1985;313(12):728–31.
45. Hayashizaki Y, Miyai K, Kato K, Matsubara K. Molecular cloning of the human thyrotropin-beta subunit gene. FEBS Lett. 1985; 188(2):394–400.
46. Wondisford FE, Radovick S, Moates JM, Usala SJ, Weintraub BD. Isolation and characterization of the human thyrotropin beta-subunit gene. Differences in gene structure and promoter function from murine species. J Biol Chem. 1988;263(25):12538–42.
47. Wondisford FE, Usala SJ, DeCherney GS, Castren M, Radovick S, Gyves PW, Trempe JP, Kerfoot BP, Nikodem VM, Carter BJ, et al. Cloning of the human thyrotropin beta-subunit gene and transient expression of biologically active human thyrotropin after gene transfection. Mol Endocrinol. 1988;2(1):32–9.
48. Cole ES, Lee K, Lauziere K, Kelton C, Chappel S, Weintraub B, Ferrara D, Peterson P, Bernasconi R, Edmunds T, et al. Recombinant human thyroid stimulating hormone: development of a biotechnology product for detection of metastatic lesions of thyroid carcinoma. Biotechnology (N Y). 1993;11(9):1014–24.
49. Hussain A, Zimmerman CA, Boose JA, Froehlich J, Richardson A, Horowitz RS, Collins MT, Lash RW. Large scale synthesis of recombinant human thyrotropin using methotrexate amplification: chromatographic, immunological, and biological characterization. J Clin Endocrinol Metab. 1996;81(3):1184–8.
50. Watanabe S, Hayashizaki Y, Endo Y, Hirono M, Takimoto N, Tamaki M, Teraoka H, Miyai K, Matsubara K. Production of human thyroid-stimulating hormone in Chinese hamster ovary cells. Biochem Biophys Res Commun. 1987;149(3):1149–55.
51. Huber GK, Fong P, Concepcion ES, Davies TF. Recombinant human thyroid-stimulating hormone: initial bioactivity assessment using human fetal thyroid cells. J Clin Endocrinol Metab. 1991;72(6):1328–31.
52. Colzani RM, Alex S, Fang SL, Braverman LE, Emerson CH. The effect of recombinant human thyrotropin (rhTSH) on thyroid function in mice and rats. Thyroid. 1998;8(9):797–801.
53. East-Palmer J, Szkudlinski MW, Lee J, Thotakura NR, Weintraub BD. A novel, nonradioactive in vivo bioassay of thyrotropin (TSH). Thyroid. 1995;5(1):55–9.
54. Leitolf H, Szkudlinski MW, Hoang-Vu C, Thotakura NR, Brabant G, Weintraub BD, Muhlen A von zur. Effects of continuous and pulsatile administration of pituitary rat thyrotropin and recombinant human thyrotropin in a chronically cannulated rat. Horm Metab Res. 1995;27(4):173–8.

55. Braverman LE, Pratt BM, Ebner S, Longcope C. Recombinant human thyrotropin stimulates thyroid function and radioactive iodine uptake in the rhesus monkey. J Clin Endocrinol Metab. 1992;74(5):1135–9.
56. Ramirez L, Braverman LE, White B, Emerson CH. Recombinant human thyrotropin is a potent stimulator of thyroid function in normal subjects. J Clin Endocrinol Metab. 1997;82(9):2836–9.
57. Torres MS, Ramirez L, Simkin PH, Braverman LE, Emerson CH. Effect of various doses of recombinant human thyrotropin on the thyroid radioactive iodine uptake and serum levels of thyroid hormones and thyroglobulin in normal subjects. J Clin Endocrinol Metab. 2001;86(4):1660–4.
58. Meier CA, Braverman LE, Ebner SA, Veronikis I, Daniels GH, Ross DS, Deraska DJ, Davies TF, Valentine M, DeGroot LJ, et al. Diagnostic use of recombinant human thyrotropin in patients with thyroid carcinoma (phase I/II study). J Clin Endocrinol Metab. 1994;78(1):188–96.
59. Albrecht RR, Ewing SJ. Standardizing the administration of the Profile of Mood States (POMS): development of alternative word lists. J Pers Assess. 1989;53(1):31–9.
60. Haugen BR, Pacini F, Reiners C, Schlumberger M, Ladenson PW, Sherman SI, Cooper DS, Graham KE, Braverman LE, Skarulis MC, Davies TF, DeGroot LJ, Mazzaferri EL, Daniels GH, Ross DS, Luster M, Samuels MH, Becker DV, Maxon 3rd HR, Cavalieri RR, Spencer CA, McEllin K, Weintraub BD, Ridgway EC. A comparison of recombinant human thyrotropin and thyroid hormone withdrawal for the detection of thyroid remnant or cancer. J Clin Endocrinol Metab. 1999;84(11):3877–85.
61. Baudin E, Do Cao C, Cailleux AF, Leboulleux S, Travagli JP, Schlumberger M. Positive predictive value of serum thyroglobulin levels, measured during the first year of follow-up after thyroid hormone withdrawal, in thyroid cancer patients. J Clin Endocrinol Metab. 2003;88(3):1107–11.
62. Cailleux AF, Baudin E, Travagli JP, Ricard M, Schlumberger M. Is diagnostic iodine-131 scanning useful after total thyroid ablation for differentiated thyroid cancer? J Clin Endocrinol Metab. 2000;85(1):175–8.
63. Robbins RJ, Chon JT, Fleisher M, Larson SM, Tuttle RM. Is the serum thyroglobulin response to recombinant human thyrotropin sufficient, by itself, to monitor for residual thyroid carcinoma? J Clin Endocrinol Metab. 2002;87(7):3242–7.
64. Mazzaferri EL, Kloos RT. Is diagnostic iodine-131 scanning with recombinant human TSH useful in the follow-up of differentiated thyroid cancer after thyroid ablation? J Clin Endocrinol Metab. 2002;87(4):1490–8.
65. Wartofsky L. Management of low-risk well-differentiated thyroid cancer based only on thyroglobulin measurement after recombinant human thyrotropin. Thyroid. 2002;12(7):583–90.
66. Mazzaferri EL, Robbins RJ, Spencer CA, Braverman LE, Pacini F, Wartofsky L, Haugen BR, Sherman SI, Cooper DS, Braunstein GD, Lee S, Davies TF, Arafah BM, Ladenson PW, Pinchera A. A consensus report of the role of serum thyroglobulin as a monitoring method for low-risk patients with papillary thyroid carcinoma. J Clin Endocrinol Metab. 2003;88(4):1433–41.
67. Soroushyari A, Do D, Langton J, Hershman JM. Partial withdrawal of levothyroxine to stimulate serum thyroglobulin for thyroid cancer monitoring. Thyroid. 2004;14(12):1105–7.
68. Castagna MG, Brilli L, Pilli T, Montanaro A, Cipri C, Fioravanti C, Sestini F, Capezzone M, Pacini F. Limited value of repeat recombinant human thyrotropin (rhTSH)-stimulated thyroglobulin testing in differentiated thyroid carcinoma patients with previous negative rhTSH-stimulated thyroglobulin and undetectable basal serum thyroglobulin levels. J Clin Endocrinol Metab. 2008;93(1):76–81.
69. Kloos RT. Thyroid cancer recurrence in patients clinically free of disease with undetectable or very low serum thyroglobulin values. J Clin Endocrinol Metab. 2010;95(12):5241–8.
70. Klubo-Gwiezdzinska J, Burman KD, Van Nostrand D, Wartofsky L. Does an undetectable rhTSH-stimulated Tg level 12 months after initial treatment of thyroid cancer indicate remission? Clin Endocrinol (Oxf). 2011;74(1):111–7.
71. Spencer C, Fatemi S, Singer P, Nicoloff J, Lopresti J. Serum basal thyroglobulin measured by a second-generation assay correlates with the recombinant human thyrotropin-stimulated thyroglobulin response in patients treated for differentiated thyroid cancer. Thyroid. 2011;20(6):587–95.
72. Robbins RJ, Larson SM, Sinha N, Shaha A, Divgi C, Pentlow KS, Ghossein R, Tuttle RM. A retrospective review of the effectiveness of recombinant human TSH as a preparation for radioiodine thyroid remnant ablation. J Nucl Med. 2002;43(11): 1482–8.
73. Pacini F, Ladenson PW, Schlumberger M, Driedger A, Luster M, Kloos RT, Sherman S, Haugen B, Corone C, Molinaro E, Elisei R, Ceccarelli C, Pinchera A, Wahl RL, Leboulleux S, Ricard M, Yoo J, Busaidy NL, Delpassand E, Hanscheid H, Felbinger R, Lassmann M, Reiners C. Radioiodine ablation of thyroid remnants after preparation with recombinant human thyrotropin in differentiated thyroid carcinoma: results of an international, randomized, controlled study. J Clin Endocrinol Metab. 2006;91(3): 926–32.
74. Pilli T, Brianzoni E, Capoccetti F, Castagna MG, Fattori S, Poggiu A, Rossi G, Ferretti F, Guarino E, Burroni L, Vattimo A, Cipri C, Pacini F. A comparison of 1850 (50 mCi) and 3700 MBq (100 mCi) 131-iodine administered doses for recombinant thyrotropin-stimulated postoperative thyroid remnant ablation in differentiated thyroid cancer. J Clin Endocrinol Metab. 2007;92(9):3542–6.
75. Tuttle RM, Brokhin M, Omry G, Martorella AJ, Larson SM, Grewal RK, Fleisher M, Robbins RJ. Recombinant human TSH-assisted radioactive iodine remnant ablation achieves short-term clinical recurrence rates similar to those of traditional thyroid hormone withdrawal. J Nucl Med. 2008;49(5):764–70.
76. Tala H, Robbins R, Fagin JA, Larson SM, Tuttle RM. Five-year survival is similar in thyroid cancer patients with distant metastases prepared for radioactive iodine therapy with either thyroid hormone withdrawal or recombinant human TSH. J Clin Endocrinol Metab. 2011;96(7):2105–11.
77. Klubo-Gwiezdzinska J, Burman KD, Van Nostrand D, Mete M, Jonklaas J, Wartofsky L. Radioiodine treatment of metastatic thyroid cancer: Relative efficacy and side effect profile after preparation by thyroid hormone withdrawal vs. recombinant human TSH. Thyroid. 2012;22:310–317.
78. Szkudlinski MW. Past, presence and future of thyroid-stimulating hormone (TSH) superactive analogs. Cancer Treat Res. 2004;122:345–56.
79. Grossmann M, Leitolf H, Weintraub BD, Szkudlinski MW. A rational design strategy for protein hormone superagonists. Nat Biotechnol. 1998;16(9):871–5.

Part II

General Considerations II: Nuclear Medicine

11 Radioiodine Whole-Body Imaging

Frank B. Atkins and Douglas Van Nostrand

Introduction

Radioiodine imaging is an important diagnostic modality for the evaluation of differentiated thyroid carcinoma. A basic understanding of the physics, radioisotopes, equipment, and imaging techniques will help the physician fully comprehend the logistics, interpretation, strengths, and weaknesses of this diagnostic tool. This chapter presents a primer of the subjects noted in Table 11.1.

Overview of Atoms and Isotopes

An atom is made up of a central core (nucleus) and electrons, which circle around the nucleus in nearly the same way as satellites orbit the earth. A particular atom is designated by one or two letters, such as "I" for iodine, and is a distinct chemical element. The nucleus is composed of two types of particles, namely, protons and neutrons. The total number of protons and neutrons equals the mass number, which is labeled as "A." The number of protons is called the "atomic number" and is labeled as "Z." These qualifying labels are usually placed above and below the letter or letters used to designate the chemical element as noted in Fig. 11.1.

F.B. Atkins, PhD
Division of Nuclear Medicine, MedStar Washington Hospital Center, Georgetown University School of Medicine, Washington, DC, USA
e-mail: atkinsfb@gmail.com

D. Van Nostrand, MD, FACP, FACNM (✉)
Nuclear Medicine Research, MedStar Research Institute and Washington Hospital Center, Georgetown University School of Medicine, Washington Hospital Center, 110 Irving Street, N.W., Suite GB 60F, Washington, DC 20010, USA
e-mail: douglasvannostrand@gmail.com

This label is often shortened to include only the mass number (e.g., ^{131}I). In this case, the "I" identifies the element (iodine), and the "131" indicates the total number of protons and neutrons in the atom.

Although a given chemical element must always have the same number of protons, the number of neutrons may vary. In other words, the atomic number (*Z*) must always be the same, but the mass number (*A*) will change as the number of neutrons in the nucleus changes. When only the number of neutrons differs, those atoms of the same element are called isotopes. ^{131}I, ^{123}I, ^{124}I, and ^{127}I are all isotopes of the same chemical element, iodine, and are different because of the different number of neutrons in the nucleus. While all have 53 protons, ^{131}I has 78 neutrons, ^{123}I has 70 neutrons, ^{124}I has 71 neutrons, and ^{127}I has 74 neutrons. The number of neutrons affects the isotope's physical characteristics, which include the half-life and decay (see below), but the neutrons have no effect on its chemical behavior. Two isotopes—^{131}I and ^{123}I—are used routinely, and a third, namely, ^{124}I, has recently become available and is being evaluated for the diagnosis of thyroid carcinoma.

An important and distinct characteristic of the various isotopes of radioiodine is how that particular radioiodine releases its energy as it transforms from one iodine to another more stable element. This release of energy is called "decay," but this terminology is misleading. Although decay suggests deterioration, nothing is being destroyed. The element is only changing to another form with the release of energy.

The several types of decay have been discussed in "Radiation and Radioactivity" (see Chap. 55). One method involves releasing a wave. These waves are similar to light but cannot be seen by the human eye and can pass through tissue. These "waves of energy" are γ (gamma) *waves* or *rays* and can be seen only by special devices: γ *cameras*. Just as there are different types of light, there are different types of γ waves. The γ cameras used by the nuclear medicine physician or nuclear radiologist not only have the ability to see the γ waves but also have the ability to identify the types of γ wave.

L. Wartofsky, D. Van Nostrand (eds.), *Thyroid Cancer*, DOI 10.1007/978-1-4939-3314-3_11

Table 11.1 Overview of Topics in This Chapter

Overview of atoms and isotopes
Advantages and disadvantages of radioiodine isotopes
Overview of the γ camera
Nuclear medicine imaging techniques and systems
Types of whole-body scintigraphy
Selection of radioisotope and prescribed activity
Utility of whole-body scanning

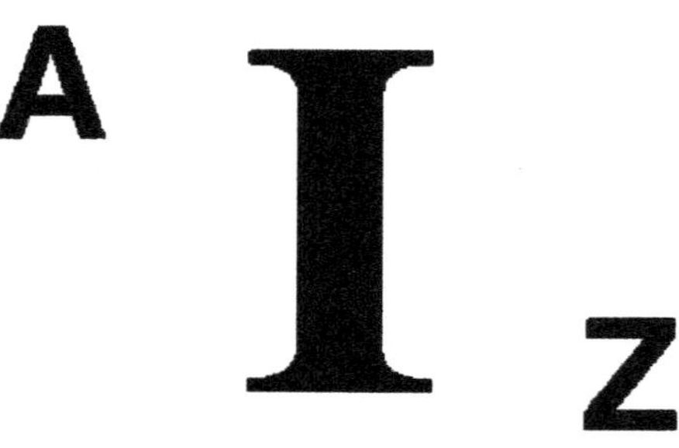

Fig. 11.1 Notation of an element. "I" represents the element. The superscript "A" represents the atomic weight, which is the total number of protons and neutrons. The subscript "Z"is the atomic number, which is the number of protons and determines the element iodine. Alternative forms might be written without the superscripts and subscripts, such as 131-I or I-131

Another way of releasing energy is in the form of a particle, which is similar to those particles that comprise the current that flows to and through a light bulb. The particle could be negatively or positively charged and is referred to as a β particle. The negatively charged β particles are identical to *electrons*, whereas the positively charged particles are called *positrons*. With this form of radioactive decay, energy is released by the nucleus as it "throws off" an electron or positron.

The methods of energy release are shown schematically in Fig. 11.2 (^{131}I) and Fig. 11.3 (^{123}I). The decay of ^{124}I is complex and beyond the scope of this chapter; however, a simplified decay scheme is shown in Fig. 11.4. When ^{123}I decays, it releases γ waves. When ^{131}I decays, it releases several types of γ waves, as well as a β particle. When ^{124}I decays, it releases energy in many different ways; the diagnostically important method is by the release of a positron. This positron collides with an electron, and both the positron and electron disintegrate or annihilate each other with the conversion of mass into two γ waves of the same energy which are released 180° apart.

Another important characteristic of any radionuclide is its half-life, which is the time it takes for half of the atoms to decay. The half-life could be seconds, minutes, hours, or days, but it is the same for all atoms of a given isotope. For example, for 100 atoms of ^{131}I, it would take 8.06 days for 50 of the atoms to transform into the element, xenon. For 100 atoms of ^{123}I, this same process would take 11.3 h for 50 atoms to transform into tellurium, and for ^{124}I, it would take 4.2 days. A summary of the decay mode, half-life, γ energy, production method, and typical prescribed activity is noted in Table 11.2.

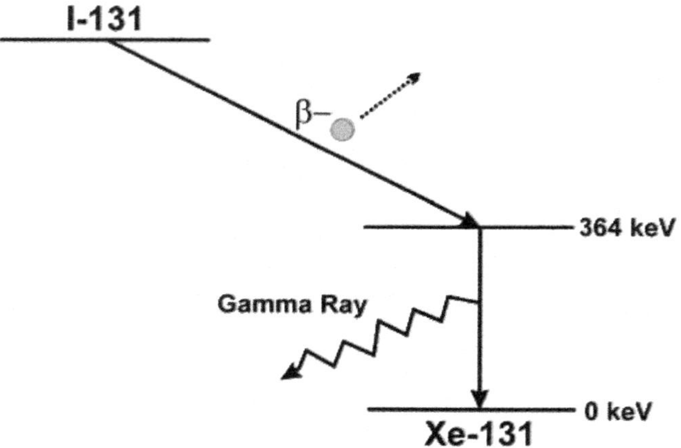

Fig. 11.2 β-decay for ^{131}I. This is a very simplified visual representation of the decay of ^{131}I, which does so by a process known as β-emission. β-emission is a mode of radioactive decay by which an unstable nucleus, one containing too few positively charged particles or protons, can become more stable. In this case, one of the neutral particles in the nucleus, i.e., the neutron, transforms into a proton. As this particle was originally neutral before changing to a positively charged particle, it must then also form a negatively charged particle so that the two charges cancel each other. The negatively charged particle produced is identical to the electrons that are the constituents of matter. However, because the electron does not belong within the confines of the nucleus, it is forcefully ejected during the transformation process. To identify this particle as having originated from within the nucleus, "β,"is used—β particle. Following the emission of the β particle, the nucleus usually emits a γ ray, in this case one that carries 364 keV of energy

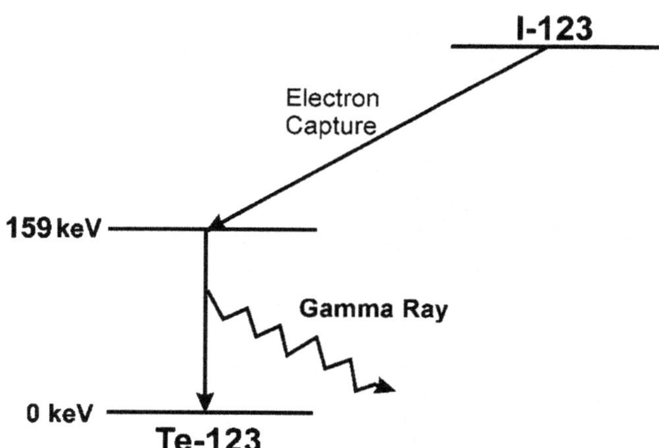

Fig. 11.3 Electron capture decay for ^{123}I. This is a simplified visual representation of the decay of ^{123}I, which does so by a process known as electron capture. In an unstable nucleus that contains too many positively charged particles or protons, electron capture is a mode of radioactive decay in which one of the protons in the nucleus captures one of the atom's orbital electrons. These two particles combine in such a way that the negative charge of the electron and positive charge of the proton effectively cancel each other out to produce a neutral particle, a neutron, which remains in the nucleus. Following the capture, the nucleus usually emits a γ ray

Advantages and Disadvantages of Radioiodine Isotopes of ^{123}I, ^{131}I, and ^{124}I

Some advantages and disadvantages of ^{123}I, ^{131}I, and ^{124}I are summarized in Table 11.3. The contents of this table are likely to change over time as a result of fluctuations in the cost of these isotopes or as new information becomes available.

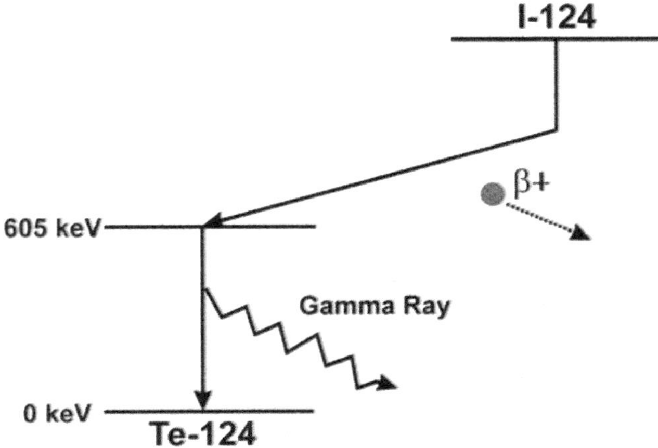

Fig. 11.4 Positron emission (β+) decay for ^{124}I. This is a simplified visual representation of the decay of ^{124}I, which does so by a process known as positron emission. Positron emission, like electron capture, is a mode of radioactive decay for an unstable nucleus that contains too many protons. In this case, to get rid of the excess positive charge, the proton transforms into a neutron and ejects a particle, which has the same mass as an electron except that it is positively charged. This positively charged electron is a positron or a β+ particle. Particles of this type are referred to as antiparticles. The ultimate fate of the positron is that after it loses most of its energy traveling through several millimeters of surrounding matter, the positron will combine with an electron. The two particles will annihilate each other with the subsequent production of two γ rays each with 511 keV of energy that travel in nearly opposite directions from the site of annihilation. It is these annihilation γ rays that are imaged using a PET scanner, which also exploits their simultaneous production and directionality of the two γ rays to form the image

Overview of the γ Camera

As noted above, the basic instrument used in nuclear medicine to form an image of the radionuclide distribution within a patient is the γ camera. This terminology is derived from the fact that it generates a two-dimensional (2D) image of an object (like a photographic camera) by detecting γ radiation, a particular type of radiation that is emitted from the tracer within the patient. Although there are numerous designs and configurations of γ cameras, most have one important component in common: the type of radiation detector used to measure the γ radiation. The device is a *scintillation detector*, as it is based on measuring a small burst of light that is produced by the γ radiation as it passes through the detector. For this reason, a γ camera is also frequently referred to as a *scintillation camera*. The technology is not new; in fact, the γ camera has been used in medical imaging since its invention by Hal Anger in the early 1960s. Since the γ camera was introduced, its design and performance have evolved considerably into the sophisticated device that is in widespread use today. Although there are numerous commercial versions of γ cameras currently available on the market, four components are common to virtually all of them: a collimator, scintillation crystal, photomultiplier tubes, and the electronics/computers to process and display the image. These components are shown in Fig. 11.5.

Collimator

The γ rays produced by the radioiodine within a patient are emitted randomly in all directions. However, to form an image requires knowledge or information about the direction that the γ rays are traveling. Because it is not possible to determine this directly, a collimator is used instead. The

Table 11.2 Radioiodines used for imaging of thyroid diseases

	Decay mode	Half-life	Gamma energy (keV)	Production method	Typical prescribed activity MBq (mCi)
^{123}I	Electron capture	13.6 h	159	Cyclotron methods. One method, referred to as a (p,5n), produces ^{123}I with no ^{124}I contamination and little ^{125}I The other approach, referred to as (p,2n), has a number of impurities that have high-energy γ's and long half-lives. These contaminations reduce image quality and increase the radiation exposure of the patient	15–148.8 (0.4–4.0)
^{124}I	Positron emission	4.2 days	511	Cyclotron	74–148 (2–4)
^{125}I	Electron capture	60.2 days	35	Cyclotron. Not used for imaging because the γ energy is too low. Also, the long half-life results in a significant radiation burden to the patient. This has primarily been used for radioimmunoassays and other in vitro laboratory tests	Not used for imaging owing to long half-life and low energy of γ ray
^{127}I	Stable	–	–	Naturally occurring	N/A
^{131}I	β-decay	8.02 days	364	Reactor produced either from direct bombardment of a target by neutrons or from the reprocessing of spent fuel rods from a nuclear power plant	Uptakes: 0.185 (0.005) Imaging: 37–185 (1–5) Treatment :1.07–37 GBq (29–1,000)

Table 11.3 Comparison of ^{123}I, ^{124}I, and ^{131}I

	^{123}I	^{124}I	^{131}I
Expense	$$	$$$	$
Readily available	Y (In some countries)	Just becoming available	Y
Reimbursed by insurance	Y	N	Y
Useful in the treatment of differentiated thyroid carcinoma	N	Y[a]	Y
Useful for dosimetry (blood/bone marrow)	Possibly	Y	Y
Useful for dosimetry (lesion)	Limited	Y	Limited
Stunning	No	Possibly	Possibly
Risk to personnel handling patient and radionuclide	Low	Medium	Medium
Necessity of radiation safety precautions for patient and public	N	Y	Y
Image quality	Good	Excellent	Fair
Delayed imaging (>48 h)	N[b]	Y	Y
PET scanner required	N	Y	N
Tomographic images (routinely)	N[c]	Y	N[c]
Image fusion with other modalities	N[c]	Y	N[c]

[a]The energy of the positron and half-life of ^{124}I would make it technically feasible for this radioiodine to be used for the treatment of differentiated thyroid carcinoma. However, even if sufficient quantities could be produced in today's market, the cost would be prohibitive

[b]Multiple studies have demonstrated the ability to obtain images at 48 h after administration of ^{123}I, and with higher prescribed activity, further delayed imaging may be possible

[c]With the development of single photon emission tomography (SPECT) tomographic images that can be fused with images obtained from other imaging modalities can be performed. However, this is not available at all facilities, and even if available, SPECT images of the whole body are not routinely performed because of significant increased time and expense

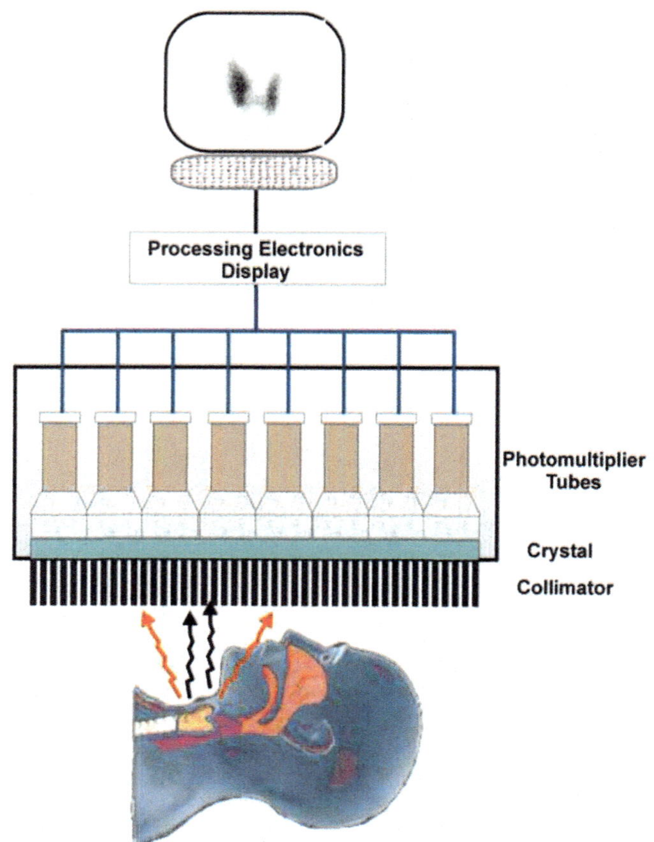

Fig. 11.5 Components of a γ camera. See text for discussion

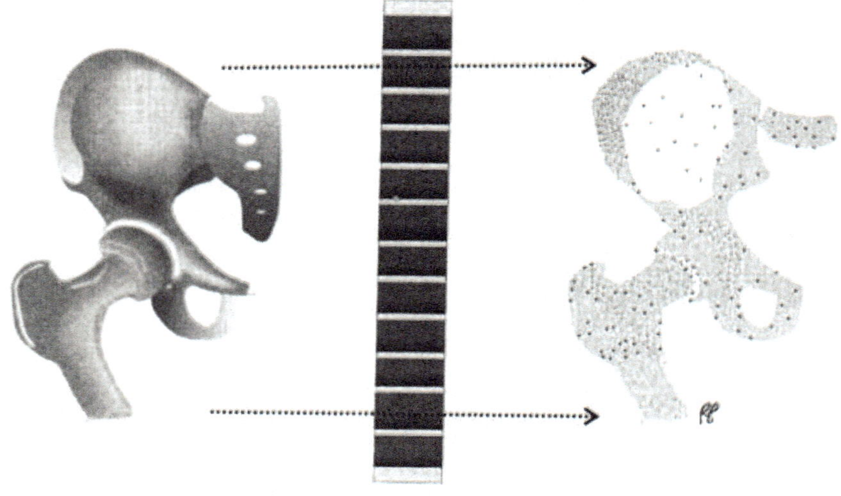

Fig. 11.6 Parallel-hole collimator. The collimator is an essential component of the γ camera. One type shown in this figure is a parallel-hole collimator because each channel through which the γ rays must pass before they can be recorded in the image is parallel to all of the other channels or holes. See text for more discussion (Reproduced with permission from Essentials of Nuclear Medicine Physics, Blackwell Publishers, Inc)

most common design of a γ camera collimator is shown in Fig. 11.6. It usually consists of a set of holes or channels (typically several thousand) in a block of lead, each of which is parallel to all the others. Hence, it is referred to as a *parallel-hole* collimator. γ rays that are traveling in a direction that pass through the channel will make it to the opposite side and enter the detector. Most γ rays that would cross from one channel to another will be absorbed in the lead that separates the holes and will not be recorded in the image. As a result, the γ rays that pass through the collimator form a distribution on its exit side, which is a representation of the radionuclide's spatial distribution within the patient.

To form an accurate representation of the distribution of radioiodine within the patient, it is important that as few γ rays as possible that have crossed between channels reach the detector. The γ rays that do are referred to as *penetration radiation*. Because of the nature of the passage of γ rays through material, it is not possible to completely stop all penetration, but it can be minimized through appropriate design and construction.

Several variables could be used to characterize the design of such a collimator and will have an impact on the quality of the image formed. These variables include the diameter of the hole, thickness of the collimator, and spacing between holes. By making the channel or hole wider, more γ rays will pass through the collimator and will be recorded in the image. Therefore, the statistical noise* in the image will be reduced. The importance of counts on the overall image quality is illustrated in Fig. 11.7.

However, the larger hole is less selective about the direction that the γ ray is traveling; therefore, the uncertainty about where the γ ray originated from within the patient is greater. Thus, larger channels will produce images with less statistical noise but also less sharpness or detail, i.e., greater blurring of images. The thickness of the material that separates one channel from an adjacent channel affects the amount of radiation that "penetrates" the collimator. Increasing this thickness reduces the penetration but also reduces the number of γ rays recorded in the image. Once again, the statistical noise can become a limiting factor. Furthermore, if it is too thick (>3 mm), the pattern of the holes or channels in the collimator can be visualized as it is superimposed on the patient's image. To compensate for this effect, the collimators can be increased in total height to maintain the spacing between channels at acceptable values.

Another important characteristic of γ rays is that the higher the energy of the photon, the more difficult it is to stop or absorb that radiation. This factor has a major impact on collimator design. Consequently, collimators are designed specifically for certain energy ranges. A typical and important rule followed in collimator design is that the number of γ rays that penetrate the collimator septa should be less than approx 5 % of the total number that pass through the collimator. Because ^{131}I emits a relatively high-energy γ ray (364 keV), it is important to use a collimator that has been designed for

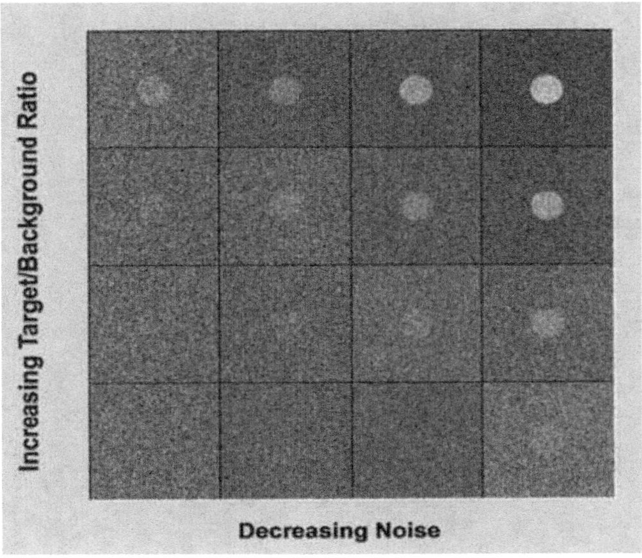

Fig. 11.7 Relationships of spatial resolution and detected events. This figure illustrates the importance of both counts (the number of γ rays recorded in the image) and the contrast (the relative ability of the tissue to concentrate the radionuclide compared to its surrounding tissues) on the ability to "detect" a lesion. The lesion in this case is a circular area in a uniform background. Along each row of this grid, the contrast is a constant value but increases progressively from the *bottom* to the *top*. Likewise, the statistical variations in the image (called "noise") are the same along a given column but decrease progressively from *left* to *right*. The *box* at the *lower left* has the lowest lesion contrast and the greatest noise level, whereas the *box* in the *upper right* corner has the highest lesion contrast and the least noise level. If you examine the bottom row, you will probably only be confident that the lesion is present in the *last box*. However, the lesion is present in every *box*; it is just obscured by the noise. For the second row from the *bottom*, the lesion is probably just detectable in the next to the *last box*. Similarly, for the next row up, the lesion is detectable in the last three *boxes*. This illustrates that as the contrast increases, the lesion can be detected in the presence of greater noise levels. The contrast depends on a number of physiological parameters that affect the ability of the metastatic thyroid tissue to concentrate the radioiodine relative to surrounding background tissues. One common way for the nuclear medicine physician to try and increase the lesion contrast is to delay the time of imaging an additional 24 h or longer. This takes advantage of the fact that non-protein-bound iodine is generally cleared or eliminated from normal tissues faster than it is from functioning thyroid metastasis. As a result, the contrast may increase over time, which would be equivalent to moving to a higher row in this image. What can also be observed in this figure is that even low-contrast lesions can be "seen" if the statistical noise is small enough. Noise can be reduced by recording more γ rays in the image. There are a variety of ways in which the number of detected γ rays can be increased. The simplest is to increase the imaging time. Another option might be to increase the administered prescribed activity. However, in the case of ^{131}I, this might increase the risk of stunning. The patient could be imaged sooner after the administration of the radioiodine while there is more activity in the patient, but this would result in a smaller lesion contrast as noted above

high-energy imaging. Usually, the penetration radiation is spread out diffusely over the entire patient image, but if there is a small intense area of ^{131}I concentration in the patient, it will be manifested as a star-like artifact, with rays projecting outward from the center like the points on a star. The number of points and shape of this artifact depend on the layout of the

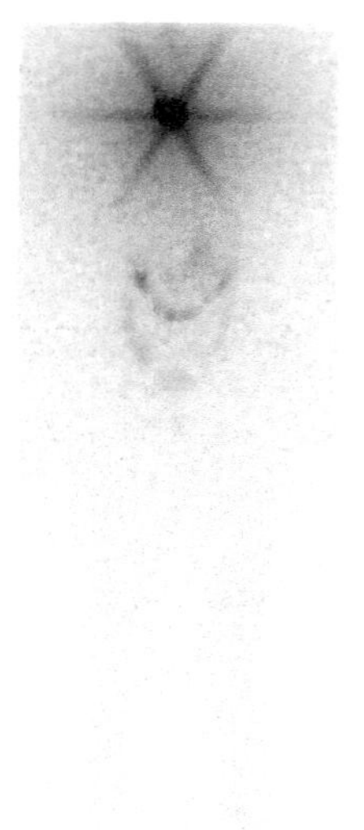

Fig. 11.8 Star artifact on radioiodine whole-body scan. See text and Chap. 12 for discussion

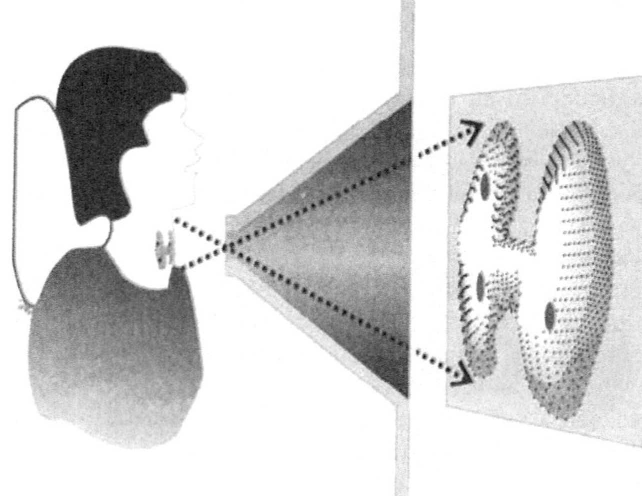

Fig. 11.9 Pinhole collimator. See text for discussion (Reproduced with permission from Essentials of Nuclear Medicine Physics, Blackwell Publishers, Inc)

channels and shape of the hole in the collimator. Basically, the projections are along paths where the material that separates one hole from its neighbor is the thinnest. An example is shown in Fig. 11.8.

The parallel-hole collimator is the most widely used type in nuclear medicine, but the pinhole collimator is another particularly useful design in imaging small organs like the thyroid gland.

The pinhole collimator is much simpler than the parallel-hole collimator in terms of its design and construction. The bulk of this collimator consists of a large lead conical shell with the tip cut off. The base of the cone will cover a large portion of the γ camera crystal. The purpose of this shell is to shield the detector from the γ rays that do not pass through the collimator itself. As implied by the name, the pinhole collimator itself consists of a single small hole (often referred to as an *aperture*) in the truncated tip of the cone. The diameter of this aperture is typically several millimeters. Ideally, the only γ rays that can reach the detector and contribute to the image are those that are emitted from the patient, pass through the pinhole, and strike the crystal. As γ rays travel along a straight line, each point on the crystal would then correspond to a small volume within the patient. This is illustrated in Fig. 11.9.

How well defined the patient's image is depends partly on how large the pinhole is. If it is too large, then γ rays from a broader region of the organ being imaged can pass through the aperture and strike the same location on the crystal. As a result, the image is not sharp. Alternatively, if the aperture is too small, then very few γ rays will pass through the opening, and the image (although sharp) will be of poor quality because of statistical limitations of low counts. For this reason, pinhole collimators are usually designed so that the aperture is changeable to accommodate different imaging conditions and requirements. A typical set of pinholes might include a diameter range of 2, 4, 6, and 8 mm. Generally, for lower-energy γ and higher administered activities (e.g., ^{99m}Tc pertechnetate), the smaller 2–4-mm pinhole is used; for higher energies (e.g., ^{131}I), a larger 6–8-mm pinhole is used.

Just as for parallel-hole collimators, penetration of the collimator by γ waves is also a problem for pinhole collimators. For this reason, the insert assembly is often manufactured using Tungsten, which is a strong metal that can be machined and is about 1.5 times more than the density of lead. Consequently, it is even more effective than lead at reducing the penetration radiation. Another advantage is its strength. Lead is a soft metal and can be easily damaged. For some research applications, an even denser metal has been used, i.e., *depleted uranium*. Naturally occurring uranium consists of a mixture by weight of three radionuclides of uranium: ^{238}U (99.27 %), ^{235}U (0.72 %), and ^{234}U (0.0054 %). The uranium used in nuclear power plants requires an "enriched" form in which the fraction of ^{235}U has been increased from 0.72 % to about 1.5–3 %. Depleted uranium is the uranium remaining after the enrichment process and contains only about 0.2 % of the fissionable ^{235}U. This material is even denser than tungsten and is about two times greater than the density of lead.

There are a number of important differences between pinhole and parallel-hole collimators. One is the *field of view* (FOV), which is how large an area of the patient the γ camera can image. For the parallel-hole collimator, the size of the FOV is essentially the physical size of the detector itself (aside from dead space around the periphery). However, for pinhole collimators, the area of an organ that can be imaged depends on how far the organ is from the pinhole. For objects only about 5 cm from the pinhole, the FOV is about one fourth to one third of the dimensions of the detector. As the object moves closer to the pinhole, the FOV decreases. In addition, as objects move away from the pinhole collimator, the number of γ rays that can pass through the pinhole falls off rapidly. Consequently, pinhole collimators are used to image small organs, such as the thyroid gland and neck bed, which can be positioned close to the collimator.

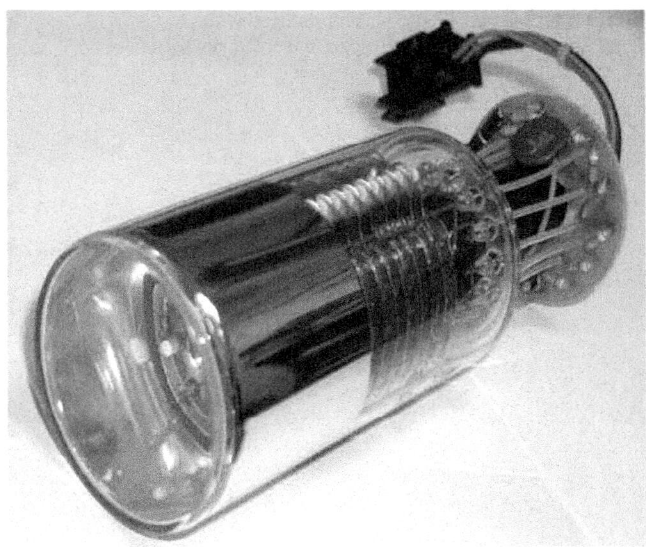

Fig. 11.10 Photomultiplier tube. The left end of the tube is coupled to the crystal. See text for discussion

Scintillation Crystal

Once the γ ray passes through the collimator, it must then be detected. This involves the use of a special type of material that will produce a brief flash of light (*scintillation*) when a γ ray interacts. This flash itself only lasts less than a 1/1,000,000 of a second. Although not all materials possess this capability, many that do are in a physical form, which we refer to as a "crystal," i.e., the atoms are lined up in a regular periodic structure. There are many different scintillation crystals, but the most commonly used for γ cameras is sodium iodide (NaI). The primary reasons for using NaI are the natural abundance of the raw materials and relative ease of growing the large crystals needed for this application. Both of these factors contribute to a relatively low cost for this component of the imaging system. The usual representation of the sodium iodide crystal is NaI(Tl). This indicates that a small amount (~0.1 %) of thallium (Tl) has been intentionally included in the growth of this scintillation crystal. A small amount of this impurity has been found to significantly increase the amount of light produced in the crystal by the radiation. When a γ ray interacts in the crystal, two important features help in the imaging process: (1) the light emanates from the point at which the γ interacts, and (2) the intensity of the light is proportional to the energy of the γ ray. The first factor allows an image of the location of the γ ray to be generated (i.e., where it came from in the patient), and the second factor allows the discrimination of γ rays of different energies, which then allows the discrimination of different radionuclides and γ wave scatter within the patient. Most γ cameras use a single, rectangular, large-area scintillation crystal that is capable of imaging a substantial portion of the patient at one time. Typical FOV are 20 in. wide by 15 in. in length.

Photomultiplier Tubes (PMT)

These electronic devices are designed for a single purpose—to detect and measure small amounts of light in a short period of time. The γ camera consists of an array of photomultipliers (PMTs) (see Fig. 11.10), which cover the surface of the scintillation crystal. Generally 2–3-in. diameter PMTs are used so that 50–100 of these devices are required. Each time a scintillation event occurs in the crystal (a γ ray is detected), some resultant light is detected by the PMT, and an electrical signal is produced. The more light that is "seen" by a PMT, the greater the signal it produces. Although "photomultiplier" implies the multiplication of photos (see Fig. 11.11), the PMT multiplies the electrical signal.

Processing Electronics and Image Display

The last component in the γ camera imaging chain is associated with the processing of the electrical signals from the PMTs and conversion of this information into an image. The closer a PMT is to the source of the light (i.e., the point in the crystal where the γ ray was absorbed), the more light it sees. Hence, the greater the electrical signal, the closer the PMT is to the scintillation event. By examining the signal distribution from a cluster of PMTs surrounding the interaction site, it is possible to determine the location of the γ interaction in the crystal itself with some degree of precision. In fact, despite the PMTs fairly large size (typically about 75 mm in diameter), this approach for localization can determine the site with a precision of about ±2.0 mm. Finally, the information from each detected event is stored in a 2D array, and each element of the array (called a pixel for picture element) contains the

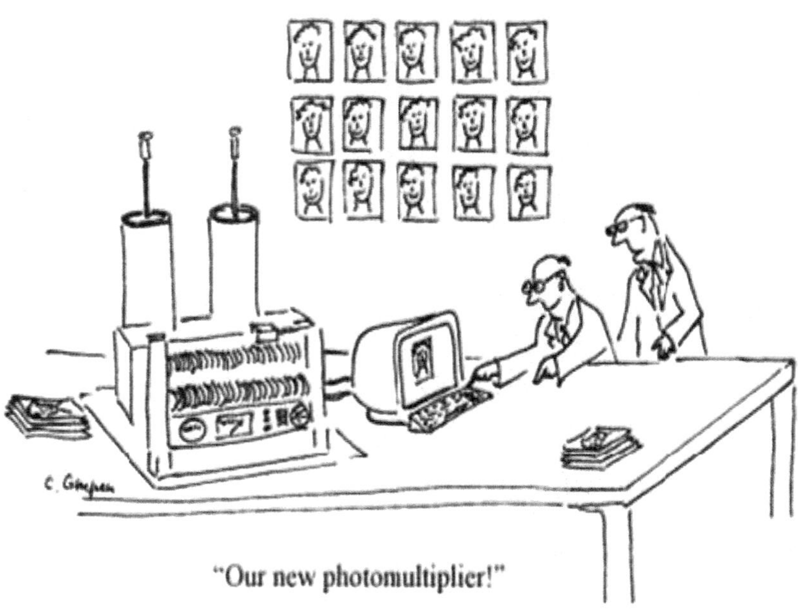

Fig. 11.11 See text (Photo was reproduced with permission of the Dr. Claus Grupen, the creator)

total number of γ rays that were detected at that location in the crystal during the entire acquisition period. The image displayed on the computer is a representation of the radioactivity distribution in the patient. Usually, the image is displayed in black and white, with the scale or darkness proportional to the number of λ rays that came from that region of the patient.

Nuclear Medicine Imaging Techniques and Systems

Several techniques can be used to image thyroid tissue and differentiated thyroid cancer using the γ camera and other systems.

Static Planar Imaging

The operating principles of the γ camera were described in the previous section. As indicated, this device consists of a large-area crystal to detect the γ rays and a collimator to select the γ rays on the basis of their direction of travel. Usually, the collimator is a parallel-hole design, which means that the γ rays recorded in the image are only those that are traveling (more or less) in a direction that is perpendicular to the crystal. If the detector has a dimension, e.g., of 15 by 20 in., then the area of the patient that would be examined is also approximately the same size. If the area of interest was much smaller than the camera area, such as the thyroid bed, then the detector would not be utilized efficiently. In this case, a different type of collimator might be used instead, i.e., a pinhole collimator, which has improved spatial resolution. Conversely, the FOV of the γ camera may not be large enough to cover all the areas of the patient that needs to be examined. In this instance, a series of images are acquired with the patient repositioned in front of the γ camera. Each image is often referred to as a "static" image or "spot" image since the patient and the γ camera are stationary during the imaging process, which may take 10–20 min.

Whole-Body Imaging (Metastatic Survey)

The whole-body or metastatic survey is a routinely performed imaging procedure to detect the metastatic spread of differentiated thyroid carcinoma. As thyroid cancer can metastasize to regions well outside the thyroid bed, it is necessary to image or *survey* a large portion of the patient's body. Hence, it is often referred to as *whole-body* scanning (WBS). In practice, however, the area scanned usually extends from the head to the knee or just below the knee because thyroid cancer rarely metastasizes more distally than this. The radionuclide used for this purpose is one of the radioisotopes of iodine. In the past, this has been generally ^{131}I; but more recently, ^{123}I has had increased usage, and the positron-emitter ^{124}I may have an important role in the not-too-distant future.

For either ^{123}I or ^{131}I, the device used is the γ camera to generate a 2D image of the radionuclide distribution within the patient, who is really a 3D object. Because some radiation is absorbed within the patient's body, the resulting image will be influenced to a greater extent by the radioiodine that is located closer to the patient's surface on the side that the γ camera is positioned. Thus, concentrations of activity (metastases) that are located posteriorly within the patient

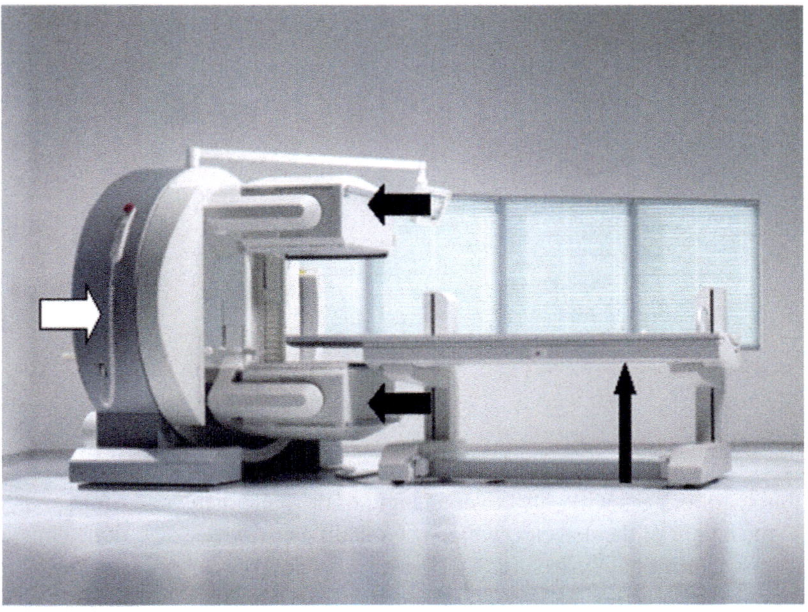

Fig. 11.12 Dual-head nuclear medicine γ camera. The *thick arrows* represent the dual γ camera heads. The *thin vertical arrow* represents the patient table, and the *white arrow* represents the camera gantry (Photo courtesy of Siemens Medical Solutions USA, Inc)

might not be visualized when viewed anteriorly and vice versa. Images are therefore obtained routinely from both the anterior and posterior projections.

To reduce imaging time, most systems currently employ two γ cameras that are mounted on a gantry, allowing the detectors to be positioned directly opposite each other, with the patient located between them (see Fig. 11.12). In this case, the anterior and posterior images can be acquired simultaneously. Furthermore, because the FOV along the length of the patient is typically only approx 15 in., multiple sets of images need to be acquired to cover or survey the patient's whole body. Although this could be accomplished by imaging each section of the patient individually, with some slight overlap between sections, this is a time-consuming approach for the patient and the technologist. Ultimately, the nuclear medicine physician must deal with assembling these images from all the different sections into the proper presentation. To facilitate the imaging of a substantial length of the patient, most imaging systems also have the capability of continuously scanning over the length of the patient as the data are collected. This scanning can either involve the patient's bed moving between the detectors or the camera gantry traversing along a track. In either case, the imaging system has been designed to incorporate the relative position of the γ cameras and table to generate a single image from each detector over the entire length that was scanned.

SPECT Imaging

One limitation of the imaging methods discussed so far is that these techniques all produce a 2D projection (image) of the radioiodine distribution within the patient, much like that of a conventional X-ray. As a result, the depth of a focal region of uptake cannot be determined from a single image. Since γ rays are absorbed or attenuated as they pass through tissue, the difference in the intensity of an area of interest between the anterior and posterior images, or any opposing views, can provide a clue as to whether the structure is closer to one surface or another, but this is not very precise. Static images from other orientations, such as a lateral projection, could provide more details. Regardless, the fact that each location in the image is a reflection of the superposition of the activity along a line through the patient, then overlying and/or underlying normal physiologic structures might obscure an abnormal area of radioiodine uptake. One approach to this limitation is that of SPECT (single photon emission computed tomography). This involves collecting a number of 2D images using the same γ camera described in this chapter over a set of angles that completely encircles the patient. Typically this set of images is acquired every 3–6° around the patient. Each of these images provides a different perspective of the internal distribution of the radioactivity within the patient. Using computer processing similar to that employed in conventional X-ray CT scanners, it is possible to construct a set of 2D transaxial sections of the activity within the patient. If we stack all of these slices up, we now have the 3D representation of the activity within the patient. Depth and overlying normal physiologic structures are no longer a problem. Clinical applications of SPECT imaging are discussed in Chap. 14. Although SPECT images may provide more information than whole-body or static images, there are several drawbacks. In order to produce high-quality, statistically useful SPECT studies, more γ rays need to be detected. However, this results in relatively longer imaging times (typically 30–45 min for a complete 360° set of images). In addition,

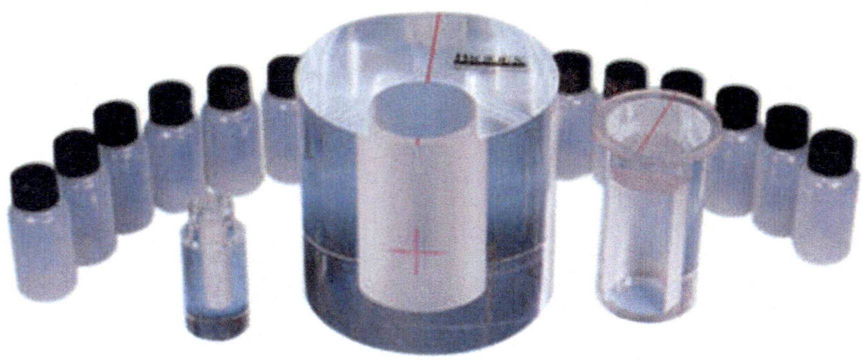

Fig. 11.13 Thyroid phantom. See text for discussion

this set of images will only cover a length of the patient equal to the height of the detector, which is typically in the order of 40 cm. Unfortunately, to survey the entire length of the patient would typically not be practical. Hence, the use of SPECT imaging in this setting might be to better evaluate areas of known metastatic disease or suspicious areas identified on the whole-body or static images. While SPECT imaging can improve lesion detectability and provide 3D localization, there are still farther limitations. Since γ rays are absorbed as they pass through tissue (for ^{131}I about 50 % for every 6 cm of tissue), there can be artifacts due to this attenuation as well as quantitative inaccuracies. Furthermore, there may be ambiguities in the anatomical localization of focal areas of uptake. To address these issues, the SPECT system may actually be a hybrid device that incorporates a CT scanner (or similar device) that can provide both the anatomical information and the necessary corrections to account for attenuation.

Radioiodine Uptake

An important factor often used to help select the prescribed activity for ablation or treatment of well-differentiated thyroid cancer with radioiodine is the *uptake*. Uptake is a measure of the fraction (usually expressed as a percentage) of the administered radioiodine present in some specific tissue at the time of measurement—usually 24 h after dosing. The tissue in question could be the thyroid gland, thyroid remnant left after near-total thyroidectomy, or metastatic thyroid carcinoma. The uptake is a significant parameter because it will directly impact the radiation dose that can be delivered to the tissue targeted for treatment and, hence, the potential effectiveness of the radioiodine therapy. The calculation itself is relatively simple:

$$\text{Uptake }(\%) = \text{radio activity in tissue} \times 100 / \text{administered activity}$$

Although the radioactivity in the tissue is measured at a specific time after the administration, the value used in this equation is what it would have been at the time of administration. Thus, this value is corrected for the decay of the radionuclide between the time of administration and measurement. If ^{123}I is being used for this measurement, then this amounts to a correction factor of about 3.4 for a 24-h period.

At issue is how to determine the activity in the tissue. There are basically two approaches to measure the uptake and use different instrumentation: an uptake probe and a γ camera. As the radiation detectors count γ rays while the patient is given an amount of radioiodine measured in units of *activity*, i.e., mega-Becquerel (MBq) or millicuries (mCi), then some conversion of the counts into radioactivity would be needed. In addition, because the thyroid gland is at some depth, albeit small, within the patient's neck, some loss of γ rays is from their absorption within the patient. Consequently, a separate measurement of a known amount of radioactivity (calibration source) of the radioiodine used for the uptake is also measured using the same device. In this case, the calibration source is (1) placed inside a phantom designed to mimic a typical neck size and tissue depth, and (2) the phantom is positioned in front of the uptake probe or the γ camera in the same manner as the patient would be. In order to achieve some measure of consistency, the neck phantom has been standardized by the International Atomic Energy Agency and is shown in Fig. 11.13.

A solid plastic cylinder simulates the neck of a patient approximately 5 in. in diameter by 5 in. in height with a cylindrical hole that extends partially through the phantom and is offset toward the "anterior" surface. If capsules containing the standard radioiodine are used, they are placed inside the plastic insert shown just to the left of the neck phantom. This insert is then placed inside the holder to the right of the neck, and the assembly is inserted into the hole in the phantom. If liquids are used instead of capsules, then one of the vials is filled with the radioiodine and placed into the insert. Frequently, the same capsule(s) to be administered to the patient are used for the calibration. The denominator in the equation above is simply the counts recorded using this measurement; no additional corrections are required.

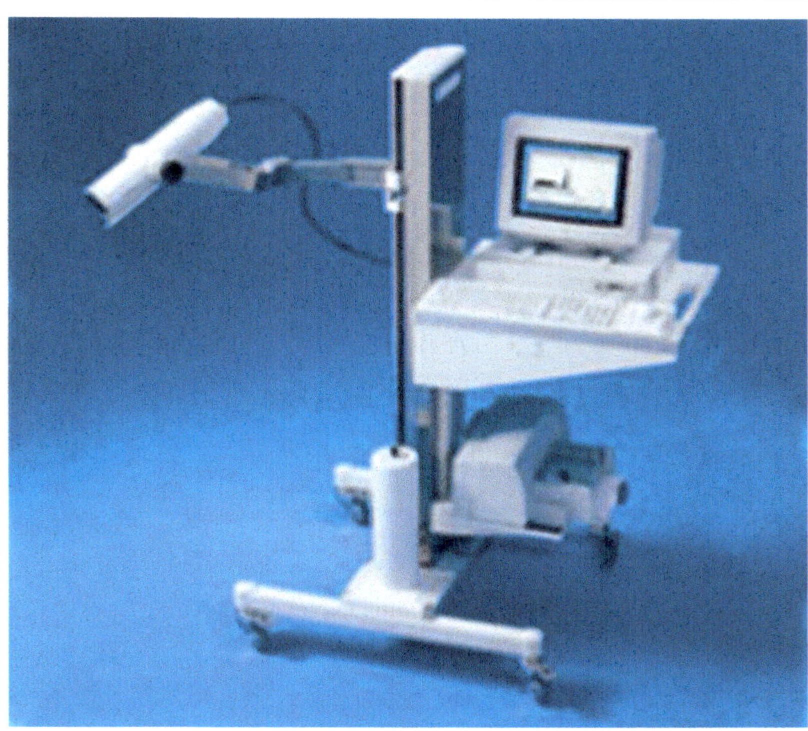

Fig. 11.14 Thyroid uptake probe. See text for discussion

Uptake Probe

The uptake probe typically uses a single small NaI (Tl) radiation detector that is mounted onto an articulating arm. The diameter of this detector is generally between 1 and 2 in. A collimator is in front of the detector and is a slightly tapered, cylindrical, lead-based shell of about 5 in. in length that blocks γ rays from striking the detector, unless they originate from a reasonably small volume at the end of the collimator. Because γ rays travel along straight lines, the size of the sensitive volume gradually increases with distance from the detector. Systems specifically designed as thyroid uptake probes are commercially available, and an example is shown in Fig. 11.14.

The arm holding the probe can move vertically along the counterbalanced stand to allow easy positioning over the anterior surface of the thyroid bed of the seated patient. The γ radiation emanating from the patient is then counted for about 1–5 min. As the number of γ rays that would strike the detector depends strongly on the distance of the source from the probe, there is also a movable device mounted on the side of the probe that allows the patient to be positioned at a consistent and reproducible distance about 3 in. from the collimator.

Acquisition Parameters and Technique

Scintigraphic protocols for imaging differentiated thyroid cancer depend on which radioiodine was administered and the mode of operation of the γ camera. To evaluate the patient for metastatic spread of the thyroid cancer, a large portion of the body must be imaged from the head to the knees. Although this can be accomplished in different ways, the most common technique is a whole-body scan, which was discussed earlier in this chapter. Today, most scintillation cameras are mounted on a gantry that enables either the patient bed to continuously translate the patient through the imaging field or the gantry and camera to "scan" along the length of the patient. In either case, a single image can be produced in which the width is equal to the camera's active width, whereas the height of the image corresponds to the distance that was scanned. Typically, the maximum length that can be scanned is approximately 200 cm. Furthermore, many scintillation camera systems currently have two detectors, such that anterior and posterior projections can be acquired simultaneously, thereby reducing the overall imaging time. If the imaging system is not capable of whole-body scanning, then separate overlapping images that span the appropriate length of the patient can be used. The whole-body scan or survey is an indispensable diagnostic tool; nevertheless, the image quality is not quite as good as that obtained from a static or "spot" view of a particular area of the patient. Table 11.4 lists typical acquisition parameters that might be used to acquire each image for the different modes of operation (whole-body scanning, static images, and pinhole images) for ^{123}I and ^{131}I. For some parameters, the values listed are guidelines and might differ somewhat between facilities. Additional information is also available from the Society of Nuclear Medicine [1].

Table 11.4 Typical acquisition parameters

Whole-body scanning					
Radionuclide	*Collimator*	*Peak (keV)*	*Window*	*Speed*	*Matrix*
^{123}I	Low energy	159	15–20 %	4–6 cm/min	512 × 1024
^{131}I	High energy	362	15–20 %	4–6 cm/min	512 × 1024
Static imaging					
Radionuclide	*Collimator*	*Peak (keV)*	*Window*	*Time/view*	*Matrix*
^{123}I	Low energy	159	15–20 %	10–20 min	256 × 256
^{131}I	High energy	362	15–20 %	10–20 min	256 × 256
Pinhole imaging					
Radionuclide	*Pinhole insert*	*Peak (keV)*	*Window*	*Time*	*Matrix*
^{123}I	4 mm	159	15–20 %	10–20 min	256 × 256
^{131}I	6 mm	362	15–20 %	10–20 min	256 × 256

Positron Emission Tomography (PET) Scanner

Because ^{124}I is a position-emitting radionuclide, a different device is required to image this radioiodine, the PET scanner, which is discussed further in Chap. 103.

Types of Whole-Body Scintigraphy

Understanding the different types of radioiodine whole-body scanning can be confusing because a whole-body scan can be performed many different ways, and the terminology varies between imaging facilities and also within the same facility. To aid the understanding and communication of the many different types of radioiodine whole-body scans, three factors are typically included in the name (see Table 11.5).

Table 11.5 Factors for describing radioiodine whole-body scan

The point in time during the patient's medical care when the scan is performed
The type of thyroid stimulation used in preparation for the scan
The specific radioiodine used

Time Points of Scanning

Scans may be typically performed at five time points during the patient's medical care.

Time Point 1: Pre-ablation Scan

The first scan is performed typically 4–6 weeks after the patient's initial thyroid surgery and before the first radioiodine ablation, hence, the terms *pre-ablation scan*, *first diagnostic scan*, or *postoperative* scan.

The objectives of this scan are:

1. To visually assess the extent and distribution of normal thyroid tissue still remaining after the thyroidectomy
2. To qualitatively demonstrate and quantitatively measure (uptake probe) the amount of radioiodine in the thyroid bed, which could affect the empiric, ablative prescribed activity of ^{131}I
3. To evaluate the presence of metastasis (e.g., cervical lymph nodes, bones, lungs, or brain) that may alter the immediate management of the patient

Although a large portion of facilities perform these pre-ablation scans, many facilities have eliminated them [2, 3]. These facilities typically use a single empiric prescribed activity of ^{131}I for all initial ablations in adults regardless of the results from the initial pre-ablation scan. The controversy of performing or not performing radioiodine scans before ^{131}I ablation is discussed further in Chaps. 14, 15, and 19. However, this author (dvn) believes that these scans are valuable for the reasons noted above and in Table 11.6. For the minor inconvenience to the patient and a cost equivalent to about one computed tomography (CT) scan, the information obtained is useful and could alter the physician's management of the patient.

Time Point 2: Follow-Up as a Screen for Recurrent Cancer (Surveillance Scan)

As part of the follow-up and screening for recurrent well-differentiated thyroid cancer in patients who have had a thyroidectomy and radioiodine ablation, a radioiodine whole-body scan may be used, and this is frequently called a *surveillance scan*. These scans may be performed as soon as 6 months or possibly as long as 2 years after the patient's initial ablation. Most surveillance scans are performed at approx 6 months to 1 year after remnant ablation or adjuvant treatment. However, with the availability of both thyroglobulin blood levels that can be used as a tumor marker and ultrasound, many facilities have stopped performing routine surveillance scans as part of the patient's routine follow-up

Table 11.6 Utility of the pre-ablation scan

Demonstration of the pattern and percent uptake of iodine in the thyroid bed or neck area that could, in turn, alter the patient's management, the amount of therapeutic ^{131}I prescribed activity, or both. Examples include:
1. A single area of significant uptake, such as 5–30 %, which suggests considering additional surgery or modifying the empiric prescribed activity of ^{131}I
2. A single area of low uptake such as <1 %, which suggests modifying the empiric prescribed activity of ^{131}I[a]
3. A pattern of radioiodine uptake consistent with cervical metastasis that may suggest (1) further evaluation with ultrasound or MR; (2) additional fine-needle aspiration, surgery, or both; and/or (3) the use of a larger empiric prescribed activity of ^{131}I
Demonstration of distant metastasis that may alter the evaluation and/or the management of the patient prior to ^{131}I therapy. Examples include:
1. Focal or diffuse uptake in lung that may warrant further evaluation with CT, pulmonary function tests, and dosimetry to determine the maximum tolerated prescribed activity without exceeding 48-h retained whole-body. The latter may increase or decrease prescribed activity relative to an empiric prescribed activity and may help minimize the potential for acute radiation pneumonitis and pulmonary fibrosis
2. Focal area suggesting bone metastasis that may need further evaluation with CT, larger empiric prescribed activity, dosimetry, and/or coordination of other treatment modalities such as metastasectomy, subsequent external radiotherapy, or radiofrequency ablation, to name a few
3. Focal uptake in the head that may warrant an MR exam of the brain. If the focal area is a brain metastasis, then consideration of surgery, external radiation therapy (i.e., gamma knife), reduction of the empiric prescribed activity, and/or treatment with steroids, glycerol, and/or mannitol prior to treatment with ^{131}I

[a]Various reports suggest that the prescribed activity for residual thyroid tissue in the thyroid bed be increased or decreased based upon the radioiodine uptake (see Chap. 58, Refs. [32–36])

and monitoring [4–7]. Nevertheless, surveillance scans may be of value in selected patients. Surveillance scans and follow-up baseline scans are discussed further in Chap. 41.

Time Point 3: Follow-Up Baseline

A scan may be performed 6–18 months after initial131I therapy in order to establish a new baseline scan, and this scan can be usedfor comparison should a subsequent scan be performed for evaluation ofpossible recurrence (See Chap. 41).

Time Point 4: When Metastasis Is Suspected

A scan may also be performed when recurrence of thyroid cancer is already known to be present or is suggested based on an elevated or rising thyroglobulin blood level, positive cytology obtained by fine-needle aspiration of a lymph node, a new mass on physical exam, and/or findings suggesting recurrence on CT, ultrasound, magnetic resonance (MR), or positron emission tomography (PET). Although some facilities also refer to this as a surveillance scan, the objective of this scan is no longer for surveillance. Rather, the objective of this scan depends on the patient's clinical situation. For example, if the patient's serum thyroglobulin level is rising, the objective of the scan may be to try to localize the site of the recurrent cancer for possible surgery, to determine whether the thyroid cancer has radioiodine uptake and could benefit from ^{131}I treatment or both. However, if a new mass is present, and its cytology by fine-needle aspiration is positive, the objective of the scan may be to determine whether it can be potentially treated with ^{131}I and/or if there are other sites of metastasis, which may alter management.

Time Point 5: Post-therapy Scan

This scan is typically performed between 3 and 7 days after the patient's ^{131}I ablation or treatment. Post-therapy scans have a particular advantage over the other scans discussed because of the much higher prescribed activity of ^{131}I used for the patient's ablation or treatment. As a result, these scans may demonstrate thyroid tissue or metastases that could not be detected on the postoperative or preablation scans. Although the information provided by the post-therapy scan typically does not alter the patient's immediate management, it could have an impact on subsequent follow-up and evaluation. This is discussed in more detail later in this chapter.

Method of Thyroid Stimulation

Patients may be prepared either by withdrawing their thyroid hormone to elevate their endogenous thyrotropin (TSH) level or by administering recombinant TSH. In regard to withdrawal, Hilt et al. [8] evaluated serial TSH levels after T3 withdrawal or thyroidectomy. After T3 was substituted for levothyroxine and then the T3 discontinued 4 weeks later, Hilt et al. reported a doubling time of 2 days until at least a TSH level of 40 uIU/ml was reached with a maximum at 20 days. The mean time required to reach a level of 50 uIU/ml was 11 days, and they suggested 11 days for TSH determination before I-131 imaging. After total thyroidectomy the dou-

Table 11.7 Terminology of radioiodine whole-body scanning

^{123}I postoperative withdrawal scan
^{123}I postoperative rhTSH scan
^{123}I pre-ablation withdrawal scan
^{123}I pre-ablation rhTSH scan
^{123}I first-time withdrawal scan
^{123}I first-time rhTSH scan
^{131}I postoperative withdrawal scan
^{131}I postoperative rhTSH scan
^{131}I pre-ablation withdrawal scan
^{131}I pre-ablation rhTSH scan
^{131}I first-time withdrawal scan
^{131}I first-time rhTSH scan
^{123}I surveillance or baseline withdrawal scan
^{123}I surveillance or baseline rhTSH scan
^{131}I surveillance or baseline withdrawal scan
^{131}I surveillance or baseline rhTSH scan
^{131}I withdrawal scan and dosimetry
^{131}I rhTSH scan and dosimetry
Post-therapy scan

Reproduced with permission from Van Nostrand et al.

bling time was more variable with a mean doubling time of 7.6 days. The use of thyroid hormone withdrawal and administration of rhTSH injections for preparation prior to ^{131}I therapy are discussed in further detail in Chaps. 34, 57, and 60.

Type of Radioiodine

As already discussed earlier in this chapter, the whole-body scan is performed with ^{123}I, ^{131}I, or ^{124}I.

Thus, by knowing these previous three factors, e.g., time, preparation, and type of radioiodine, the physician has a better understanding of the wide spectrum of terms that are used, types of whole-body scans available, and which whole-body scan may have been performed for their patients. Examples of terminology are shown in Table 11.7.

Selection of Radioisotope

As already noted in the Introduction, radioiodine whole-body scintigraphy is a valuable diagnostic tool in the assessment of patients with thyroid cancer. Two of the most controversial areas of radioiodine whole-body scanning involve the (1) selection of the radioisotope and (2) the prescribed activity to administer. The choices of radioiodine isotopes are ^{131}I, ^{123}I, and ^{124}I, and the physical characteristics of each have already been discussed earlier in this chapter. This section presents an overview of the choices of ^{131}I, ^{123}I, and ^{124}I. Further discussion regarding thyroid hormone withdrawal vs recombinant human (rh) TSH injections can be found in Chaps. 34, 57, and 60. Additional information regarding ^{124}I is also available in Chap. 103.

^{131}I

The most frequently used radiopharmaceutical to date is ^{131}I [9, 10]. Its major advantages are its long historical use, availability, reasonable cost, and half-life. ^{131}I has been used for clinical imaging for over 50 year, is readily available, and is relatively inexpensive for a diagnostic radiopharmaceutical. The half-life is approx 8 days, which allows additional delayed imaging to be performed as long as 3 or 4 days, and possibly even longer after administering ^{131}I. The value of delayed scanning is to allow significantly more time for the patient's background radioactivity to clear. Although the radioactivity of the normal or abnormal thyroid tissue may also have clearance over time, this decrease in radioactivity within the thyroid tissue or metastasis is typically less than the reduction of the whole-body background radioactivity. This causes increasing thyroid tissue-to-background ratios of radioactivity, thereby increasing the detection of functioning normal and abnormal thyroid tissue. The long half-life of ^{131}I also allows dosimetry to be performed, including whole-body counting, blood specimens, and urine specimens to be obtained and measured 5 days and even longer after radioiodine administration.

The major disadvantage of ^{131}I is the potential of "stunning." The concept and arguments for and against "stunning" are discussed in Chaps. 16, 17, and 18. In brief, stunning is the short-term reduction of radioiodine uptake after diagnostic amounts of prescribed activities of ^{131}I secondary to the radiation dose to the tissue. Again, as discussed elsewhere, this can potentially reduce the therapeutic effect of an ^{131}I treatment when administered shortly after a diagnostic ^{131}I study.

^{123}I

As an alternative to ^{131}I, ^{123}I has been used, and its advantages and disadvantages have been previously noted in Table 11.3. No documented stunning has been reported using ^{123}I, and given the relatively small estimated radiation doses from diagnostic amounts of ^{123}I, thyroid stunning of any significant degree is highly unlikely. Although frequently Hilditch et al.'s study [11] has been referenced as possibly indicating some stunning with ^{123}I, the authors suggest that the reduction of uptake after a therapeutic administration of ^{131}I is unlikely to be stunning from ^{123}I but rather a therapeutic effect from the therapeutic ^{131}I. ^{123}I also has better imaging characteristics than ^{131}I, resulting in high-quality images, and ^{123}I does not require a high- or medium-energy collimator. This allows great flexibility for obtaining images by various γ cameras within a nuclear medicine facility. Although the availability and cost for ^{123}I were previously problematic, ^{123}I has becoming more widely available in more countries, and the cost of ^{123}I has decreased as its use has increased.

Studies Involving ^{123}I

In evaluating (1) the prescribed activity of ^{123}I, (2) the time of imaging after dosing ^{123}I, and (3) the detection of thyroid tissue and thyroid cancer metastasis with ^{123}I relative to ^{131}I, multiple studies have been reported [12–17, 19–24].

Naddaf [13] compared 13 ^{123}I scans in 10 patients with post-therapy ^{131}I scans. The ^{123}I scans were performed 4, 24, and 48 h after the oral administration of 370 MBq (10 mCi) of ^{123}I. Anterior and posterior whole-body images were obtained for 60 min. The post-therapy scans were performed 5–7 days after 2.78–8 GBq (75–217 mCi) of ^{131}I. Of functioning thyroid tissue, 27 sites were identified on the post-therapy ^{131}I scans, and 24 of the 27 sites were identified on the ^{123}I scan. No comment was made regarding the relative utility of imaging ^{123}I at 4, 24, and 48 h.

Mandel et al. [10] evaluated 14 patients in whom the ^{123}I scans were obtained 5 h after administration of 48–56 MBq (1.3–1.5 mCi) ^{123}I. The ^{131}I scans were obtained at 48 h after the administration of 111 MBq (3 mCi) of ^{131}I. These scans were then compared with post-therapy scans performed 7 days after ^{131}I therapy. There were 35 foci identified, and ^{123}I images demonstrated that all 35 foci were in the thyroid bed and neck, whereas only 32 of 35 foci (91 %) were seen on the pre-therapy ^{131}I scan. Mandel et al. concluded that ^{123}I resulted in improved quality of images relative to ^{131}I in patients undergoing thyroid remnant ablation.

Berbano [14] reported that 15 of 16 patients had concordant findings on the ^{123}I scans relative to the ^{131}I scans. Only one patient had an additional site identified on the ^{131}I scan, which was not identified on the ^{123}I scan, and this was a patient with metastatic disease. The prescribed activity of ^{123}I was 370 MBq (10 mCi). The ^{131}I scans were performed after radioiodine therapy, with prescribed activities ranging from 75 to 2.8–7.4 GBq (200 mCi). Berbano [14] also evaluated ^{123}I scans at 24 and 48 h after dosing. He reported no advantage for imaging at 48 h in comparison to 24 h.

Maxon [15] evaluated 13 administrations of ^{123}I in 11 patients. The average prescribed activity of ^{123}I was 743 MBq (20.1 mCi); the ^{123}I scans were compared with scans performed 2–3 days after ^{131}I therapy. He reported no false-negative ^{123}I scans when those scans were imaged at 18–24 h after administration of ^{123}I. Scans performed 2 h after ^{123}I administration had a false-negative rate of 38 % (5/13). Pre-therapy scans with ^{131}I were performed with 74 MBq (2 mCi) of ^{131}I, and the results of analyzing the ^{123}I scans with ^{131}I scans were not reported.

Yaakob [16] examined 13 patients with ^{123}I with prescribed activities of 30–37 MBq (0.8–1.0 mCi). Images were obtained 24 h after ^{123}I administration and compared with scans performed 7–10 day after ^{131}I therapy. There were 11 ^{123}I scans that correlated with the post-therapy scan. One patient had an additional area detected on the ^{131}I post-therapy scan that was not detected on ^{123}I scan, and one patient had an additional area detected on the ^{123}I scan that was not seen on the ^{131}I post-therapy scan. The latter was attributed to physiologic esophageal activity.

Shankar [17] compared ^{123}I and ^{131}I scans in 26 patients. The ^{123}I scans were performed 4 h after the administration of 55.5 MBq (1.5 mCi) of ^{123}I, and the ^{131}I scans were performed 48 h after the administration of 111 MBq (3 mCi) of ^{131}I. ^{123}I scans identified 56 foci of activity, whereas the ^{131}I scan demonstrated only 44 of the 56 foci seen on the ^{123}I scan. All 56 foci of activity were seen on the post-therapy ^{131}I scan, and the post-therapy ^{131}I scan showed one additional area not seen on the ^{123}I scan. Of the 56 foci, 54 foci were in the neck and thyroid bed, with one focus each in the mediastinum and lung. In a separate report, Shankar et al. [18] demonstrated that the imaging with ^{123}I was superior at 24 h relative to 5 h after administration of the ^{123}I.

In a comparison of ^{123}I scans with post-therapy ^{131}I scans, Gerard et al. [19] identified 37 sites on post-therapy scan; 26 were identified with ^{123}I for a sensitivity of 70 %. Of the 11 sites missed by ^{123}I, 7 were seen on the post-therapy scan relative to the early scan. A total of ten patients had 48-h ^{123}I scans, and eight were of good quality. Lesion detection was improved on the 48-h scans. ^{123}I scans after withdrawal of thyroid hormone were performed with 3–5 mCi 111–185 MBq (3–5 mCi) of ^{123}I at 6, 24, and 48 h.

Alzahrani et al. [20] had 238 pairs of pre-therapy ^{123}I scans and post-therapy ^{131}I scans with a concordance rate of 94 %. Siddiqi [21] compared ^{123}I whole-body scans to post-therapy ^{131}I scans in 12 patients who had elevated serum thyroglobulin levels and previous negative ^{131}I whole-body scans. On subsequent evaluations, the ^{123}I dose was 185 MBq (5 mCi), and images were obtained at 2 and 24 h after administration of ^{123}I. The post-therapy scans were performed 4–7 days after the therapy with 150 mCi 5.55 GBq (150 mCi). The ^{123}I scans were concordant with the ^{131}I post-therapy scan in 11 of 12 patients.

Sarkar et al. [22] compared ^{123}I and ^{131}I in 12 patients, and both revealed residual disease in nine patients. ^{131}I detected metastases in five studies of four patients. In four of the five studies, ^{123}I missed metastases shown by ^{131}I in eight body regions including the neck, mediastinum, lungs, and bone and detected three other sites of metastasis only in retrospect. No lesion was better seen with ^{123}I than ^{131}I. Although ^{123}I is adequate for imaging residual disease, it appears to be less sensitive than ^{131}I for minimal thyroid cancer metastasis.

Khan et al. [23] compared ^{123}I scans with prescribed activity of 5.55–111 MBq (1.5–3.0 mCi) with post-therapy ^{131}I in

183 patients, showing a similar number of lesions in similar locations in 91 %, but the time of imaging was not noted. Nine patients (4.5 %) had more lesions detected in the ^{123}I scan when compared to the 7-day post-therapy ^{131}I scan. Likewise, nine patients had more lesions detected on the 7-day post-therapy scan. Post-therapy scans were obtained 7 days after 2.22–7.4 GBq (60–200 mCi). It is assumed that some of these lesions were included in earlier reports from the same institution [10, 17].

Anderson et al. [24] evaluated 101 consecutive ^{123}I and 101 consecutive ^{131}I scans after preparation with rhTSH injections. There were 96 patients in the ^{131}I group and 98 patients in the ^{123}I group who had received previous ^{131}I ablations or treatments. They used 111 MBq (3 mCi) of ^{123}I and 148 MBq (4 mCi) of ^{131}I, and images were obtained 24 h after ^{123}I and 48 h after ^{131}I. The rhTSH-stimulated ^{123}I scans and thyroglobulin levels were concordant in 90 % (91/101) of patients; the results of rhTSH-stimulated ^{131}I scans and thyroglobulin levels were concordant in 84 % (85/101) of patients. ^{123}I whole-body scans detected nine foci of disease in six patients, and ^{131}I whole-body scans detected ten foci of disease in nine patients. Anderson proposed that rhTSH-stimulated ^{123}I scans might prove to be as sensitive as rhTSH-stimulated ^{131}I scans for the detection of metastatic disease.

^{124}I

^{124}Is a positron-emitting radioisotope and has recently become commercially available for research studies. The advantages and disadvantages of ^{124}I have been previously noted in Table 11.3 and include superior image quality, tomographic images, bone marrow and metastatic lesion dosimetry, and the ability to fuse the tomographic images with CT, MR, or both. The physical half-life of ^{124}I is approx 4 days, which is sufficiently long enough to allow delayed imaging and dosimetry. The major disadvantages of ^{124}I are its availability (production sites are limited), cost, and requirement for a PET imaging system, and it is not approved by the FDA. Another potential disadvantage of ^{124}I is stunning, as the radiation-absorbed dose is about half that of a comparable prescribed activity of ^{131}I. A few studies have already been reported using ^{124}I [25, 26], and ^{124}I has been discussed further in Chap. 103.

^{99m}Tc Pertechnetate

Multiple studies have been published evaluating ^{99m}Tc pertechnetate (^{99m}Tc04) as an alternative radioisotope to evaluation patients with differentiated thyroid cancer postoperatively and pre-^{131}I therapy [27–30]. ^{99m}Tc04 would avoid the issue of stunning from ^{131}I. However, because of higher background radioactivity, the negative predictive value of ^{99m}Tc04 does not appear as good as radioisotopes of iodine [28].

Table 11.8 Factors that affect scanning and radioisotope selection

Factors
Time of the whole-body scintigraphy
First scan, which is performed after initial diagnosis, thyroidectomy, and prior to radioiodine remnant ablation or adjuvant treatment
Surveillance scan[a]
Follow-up baseline scan
Pretreatment scan[a]
Patient preparation
Thyroid hormone withdrawal
rhTSH injections
Whether thyroglobulin levels are obtained before or simultaneously with radioiodine scan
Presence or absence of increased thyroglobulin blood levels when suppressed or stimulated prior to whole-body scanning
Physician's belief in the potential for stunning
Physician's approach to the selection of prescribed activities for first-radioiodine remnant ablation or adjuvant treatment (e.g., fixed or variable empiric prescribed activity or dosimetrically determined prescribed activity)
Physician's approach to subsequent selection of prescribed activities for treatment (e.g., recurrence and/or distant metastases) of differentiated metastatic thyroid carcinoma (e.g., "blind treatment," empiric vs dosimetrically determined prescribed activity for treatments)

[a]Defined in text

Utility of Whole-Body Scanning: Pre-ablation, Surveillance, Pre-treatment, and Post-therapy

So, should one scan or not, and if one scans, what isotope of radioiodine does one use? The choice depends on multiple factors, such as those shown in Table 11.8, as well as the factor(s) that the physician and/or patients consider the most important. Four of the more common situations are discussed briefly below and the reader is referred to the chapters that discuss these situations in more detail.

Pre-ablation Scan

For those facilities that administer a standard empiric prescribed activity for remnant ablation or adjuvant treatment and would not alter their ^{131}I therapy based on any radioiodine scan finding, a scan is obviously unnecessary. For those facilities that believe that a radioiodine scan offers useful information prior to the first therapy, the use of ^{123}I is an excellent choice. Not only does this author believe that pre-therapy scans are useful (as already discussed above, in Table 11.6, and in Chap. 19), but this author also believes that if ^{123}I is available, it is the radioisotope of choice. At the time of this publication, ^{123}I is a reasonably cost-effective isotope that can demonstrate both the pattern and percent uptake of radioiodine activity in the thyroid bed. In addition, its sensitivity is as good or at least comparable to ^{131}I to show functioning metastasis that would result in altering management of anticipated initial ^{131}I therapy. Although ^{123}I may arguably miss a small focus with low uptake in residual thyroid disease or metastasis, the failure to detect these small or low-uptake foci will be infrequent. In addition, regardless of whether or not ^{131}I may cause significant stunning, ^{123}I virtually eliminates the possibility and consideration of stunning (see Chaps. 16, 17, and 18). In regard to ^{124}I, this radioisotope is not approved for use within the United States (see Chap. 103).

Surveillance Scan (to Be Distinguished from a Follow-Up Baseline Scan or Pre-treatment Scan)

The term, "surveillance scan," has been used in a number of contexts, which has been discussed earlier and in more detail in Chap. 41. In brief, a surveillance scan is a radioiodine scan performed at some routine interval, which is typically every year beginning 6 months to 1–2 years after ablation or treatment. The objective of this scan is to *screen* for recurrent and/or metastatic functioning differentiated thyroid cancer in patients who are in otherwise clinical remission. Clinical remission is defined here as no evidence of disease on physical exam, undetectable serum thyroglobulin levels on thyroid hormone suppression or stimulation, and no evidence by any other imaging modalities such as ultrasound that has been performed.

As defined above, a surveillance scan should be differentiated from a "pre-therapy scan," which is a radioiodine scan performed in "anticipation" of ^{131}I therapy in patients in whom the physician is suspicious of recurrent local thyroid cancer or metastases or patients who have documented recurrence or metastatic disease. A surveillance scan should also be differentiated from a follow-up "baseline scan." A baseline scan is performed after an ^{131}I therapy such as remnant ablation, adjuvant treatment, or treatment for locoregional and/or distant metastases in order to establish a new baseline scan to be used for any future comparison (see Chap. 41).

Although surveillance scans in the past have been frequently performed every 6 months to 1 or 2 years after the initial therapy of residual thyroid tissue or adjuvant treatment, the utility and cost-effectiveness of such a surveillance scan in patients who are in a low-risk group or clinical remission is no longer warranted [4–7]. This fact is especially true when the patient must undergo a prolonged period of hypothyroidism during thyroid hormone withdrawal. Again, surveillance scans are discussed further with proposed recommendations from various organization groups and societies in Chap. 41.

However, if a physician believes a surveillance scan is still valuable for his or her patients, then which isotope should be used? Again, either ^{123}I or ^{131}I may be used when the patient is prepared with thyroid hormone withdrawal. For those patients who are prepared with injection of rhTSH, many facilities use ^{131}I because ^{131}I was the radioisotope used in the initial studies with rhTSH. However, ^{123}I may also be used. To our knowledge, no prospective study is available comparing ^{123}I and ^{131}I scans after rhTSH preparation for surveillance scanning.

Pre-treatment Scan

(A) *Before therapy when an empiric prescribed activity of ^{131}I is planned for adjuvant treatment of suspected residual cancer or treatment of known recurrent or metastatic disease*:
The *preferred* radioiodine isotope in the opinion of this author is ^{123}I if the patient has known or highly suspected recurrent or metastatic disease and the physician anticipates treating with an empiric prescribed activity of ^{131}I. This choice is again based on the objective of the scan, namely, identification of findings that would potentially alter management. The findings are similar to some already noted in Table 11.4.

B) *Before therapy when dosimetrically determined prescribed activity of ^{131}I is planned in suspected or known recurrent or metastatic disease*:
The preferred radioiodine isotope is ^{131}I. Although the prescribed activity used in different facilities may vary from 37 to 148 MBq (1–4 mCi), this author recommend the lowest prescribed activity that still allows the performance of dosimetry while attempting to minimize the likelihood of stunning. In the author's facility, this ranges from 37 to 74 MBq (1–2 mCi). For ^{123}I, high-prescribed activities up to 740 MBq] (20 mCi) have been used [15], and further study is warranted using high diagnostic prescribed activity of ^{123}I for dosimetry. Initial studies have already demonstrated the potential of ^{124}I for dosimetry [25, 26], but additional research is needed regarding its potential for stunning. Table 11.9 summarizes several proposed recommendation for the use of first-time pre-ablation scans, surveillance scans, and pre-therapy scans.

Post-therapy Scans

Post-therapy scans image the ^{131}I administered for the radiotherapy, and this scan is performed between 3 and 7 days after radioiodine remnant ablation or adjuvant treatment and has been shown to be useful and is routinely performed [3, 31–37]. Fatourechi et al. [35] reported that 13 % of (17/117) post-therapy scans demonstrated an abnormal foci of ^{131}I that was originally undetected on the pre-therapy scan. The areas of newly detected abnormal uptake were located in the neck (5), lung (5), mediastinum (4), bone (2), and adrenal (1). The prescribed activity of the pre-therapy scan was 111 MBq (3 mCi) of ^{131}I, and post-therapy images were obtained between 1 and 5 days after therapy. The likelihood of detecting new

Table 11.9

First-time pre-remnant ablation or adjuvant treatment scan	
After thyroid hormone withdrawal After rhTSH injection	• ^{123}I using 74–148 MBq (2–4 mCi) with imaging at 24 h • Consider ^{123}I using 74–148 MBq (2–4 mCi) with injection after the second injection of rhTSH with imaging at 24 h followed by ^{131}I therapy later that day
Surveillance scan[a]	
After thyroid hormone withdrawal After rhTSH injections	• ^{123}I using 74–148 MBq (2–4 mCi) with imaging at 24 h • ^{131}I with 148 MBq (4 mCi) and imaging at 48 h • Consider ^{123}I using 74–148 MBq (2–4 mCi) with injection after the second injection of rhTSH with imaging at 24 h
Pre-therapy scan[a] with the intent to treat with an empiric prescribed activity of ^{131}I for recurrent and/or metastatic differentiated thyroid cancer	• ^{123}I using 74–148 MBq (2–4 mCi) with imaging at 24 h
Pre-therapy scan[a] with the intent to treat with dosimetrically determined prescribed activity of ^{131}I for recurrent and/or differentiated thyroid cancer	• ^{131}I using the lowest prescribed activity possible to perform dosimetry and to minimizing potential of stunning (typically 37–74 MBq [1–2 mCi])

[a]Defined in text and see Chap. 41

Table 11.10 Post-therapy radioiodine scans

Reference	Patients	Pair scans	Days on which scans were performed	Recommend scanning time
Bourgeois [39]	43	49	3 vs 6	Early and late
Chong [42]	52	52	3 vs 7	Late
Hung [41]	239	717	3–4 vs 5–6 vs 10–11	Early
Khan [38]	18	18	2 vs 7	Late
Lee [43]	81	81	3 vs 10	Early
Oliveira [40]	164	164	2 vs 7	Low risk: early
				High risk: early and late
Salvatori [45]	134	134	3 vs 7	Early
Wakabayisha[44]	42	42	3 vs 7	Early SPECT-CT

uptake on the post-therapy scans decreases after each successive therapy. Sherman et al. [33] reported that 22 % (31/143) new lesions were detected on the post-therapy scan that were not seen on the pre-therapy scan. They used 74–185 MBq (2–5 mCi) for the pre-therapy scan, and the post-therapy scan was performed between 5 and 12 days after therapy. In regard to the effects of post-therapy scans on management strategies, Fatourechi et al. [35] reported that 9 % of scans affected management (e.g., future decisions about plans for diagnostic scanning or ^{131}I therapy) or changed the patient's risk-group category. Post-therapy scans are widely performed and accepted as useful.

However, when post-therapy scans should be performed is more controversial, and multiple authors have evaluated this issue [38–45] (see Table 11.10). Hung et al. [41] evaluated 239 patients evaluating three sequential radioiodine whole-body scans at 3–4 days, 5–6 days, and 10–11 days after ^{131}I therapy. For remnants, imaging at 3–4 days, 5–6 days, and 10–11 days missed 1.1 % (2/170), 1.8 % (3/170), and 5.4 % (9/170) foci, respectively. For metastases, imaging at 3–4 days, 5–6 days, and 10–11 days missed 6.3 % (7/112), 2.5 % (3/112), and 25 % (28/112) areas, respectively. The trend was that earlier imaging was better than later imaging in order to identify remnant thyroid tissue and metastases.

Salvatori et al. [39] evaluated 124 patients that were performed on the third (early) and seventh (late) day. The early and late scans were concordant in 80.5 % (108/134) of patients. However, 7.5 % (10/134) of the early scans demonstrated lymph nodes (seven patients) and distant metastatic uptake (three patients) that were not seen on the late scan. In addition, in 12 % (16/134) of the patients, the late scan showed thyroid remnants (4), lymph nodes (7), and distant metastases (5) that were not seen on the early scan. Bourgeois et al. [38] suggested considering performing both scans, whereas Oliveira et al. [39] suggested early scanning for low-risk patients and early and late scans for high-risk patients. Salvatori et al. proposed that performing the early scan yields highly accurate results while saving the expense of a second scan and avoiding an additional visit to the imaging facility for the patient. However, in this case, one could miss up to 12.5 % of other foci.

Based on my interpretation of Salvatori et al.'s data, the early and late scans were either completely concordant, positive on the early scan and negative on the late scan, or negative on the early scan and positive on the late scan. No patient showed some lesions on the early and different lesions on the late scan. If correct, then I would propose that one may wish to consider performing an early scan at 3–4 days, and if that scan is negative, then consider performing a late scan at 7 days. This would result in only 12.5 % of the patients requiring a second scan.

In closing this section, two caveats are appropriate. First, if one is performing only an early 3-day scan or only a late 7-day scan and that scan is negative, then that does not necessarily mean that the patient's differentiated thyroid cancer no longer takes up radioiodine. Based on Salvatori et al.'s data, one would miscategorize that patient as radioiodine-negative in 7.5–12.5 % of the patients. Salvatori et al.'s paper also provokes an interesting question regarding stunning. Although Salvatori et al. did not report performing pre-ablation scans, if a focus of radioiodine uptake was observed on a pre-ablation scan but not observed on the post-therapy scan, that is not in of itself indicative of stunning. It may indicate that only a 3-day or only a 7-day scan was performed and missed the foci and that the foci were not stunned. Clearly, further study is warranted.

Summary

Radioiodine whole-body scans are important diagnostic tools in the evaluation of patients with differentiated thyroid carcinoma. With a basic understanding of such factors as radioelements, scientific notation, decay, physical half-life, γ cameras, and protocols, the physician will have a better understanding of how the radioiodine whole-body scans are performed, as well as their utility and controversial aspects. The next chapter presents a primer and atlas for the basic interpretation of radioiodine whole-body scans.

References

1. Silberstein EB, Alavi A, Balon HR, Becker D, Charkes ND, Clarke SEM, Divgi CR, Donohoe KJ, Delbeke D, Goldsmith SJ, Meier DA, Sarkar SD, Waxman AD, Society of Nuclear Medicine procedure guideline for scintigraphy for differentiated papillary and follicular thyroid cancer http://snmmi.files.cms-plus.com/docs/Scintigraphy%20for%20Differentiated%20Thyroid%20Cancer%20V3%200%20(9-25-06).pdf
2. Schlumberger M, Tubiana M, De Vathaire F, et al. Long term results of treatment of 283 patients with lung bone and metastases from differentiated thyroid carcinoma. J Clin Endocrinol Metab. 1998;63:960–7.
3. Pacini F, Lippi F, Formica N, et al. Therapeutic doses of iodine-131 reveal undiagnosed metastases in thyroid cancer patients with detectable serum thyroglobulin levels. J Nucl Med. 1987;28:1888–91.
4. Cailleux AF, Baudin E, Travagli JP, Schlumberger RM. Is diagnostic iodine-131 scanning useful after total thyroid ablation for differentiated thyroid cancer? J Clin Endocrinol Metab. 2000; 85:175–8.
5. Wartofsky L. Clinical utility of rh-TSH-stimulated thyroglobulin testing without scan in the follow-up of differentiated thyroid cancer. Denver: Program of the 83rd Annual Meeting of the Endocrine Society; 2000:P2–P535.
6. Mazzaferri EL, Kloos RT. Is diagnostic iodine-131 scanning with recombinant human TSH useful in the follow-up of differentiated thyroid cancer after thyroid ablation? J Clin Endocrinol Metab. 2002;87:1490–8.
7. Wartofsky L. Using baseline and recombinant human TSH-stimulated Tg measurements to manage thyroid cancer without diagnostic I-131 scanning. J Clin Endocrinol Metab. 2002;87: 1486–9.
8. Hilt SV, Hellman D, Anderson J, Woolfenden J, Van Antwerp J, Serial PD, TSH. Determination after T3 withdrawal or thyroidectomy in the Therapy of Thyroid Carcinoma. J Nucl Med. 1979;20:928–32.
9. Maxon HR, Smith HR. Radioiodine-131 in the diagnosis and treatment of metastatic well-differentiated thyroid cancer. Endocrinol Metab Clin North Am. 1990;19:685–718.
10. Mandel SJ, Shankar LK, Benard F, et al. Superiority of iodine-123 compared with iodine-131 scanning for thyroid remnants in patients with differentiated thyroid cancer. Clin Nucl Med. 2001;26:6–9.
11. Hilditch TE, Dempsey MF, Bolster AA, McMenemin RM, Reed RS. Self-stunning in thyroid ablation: evidence from comparative studies of diagnostic ^{131}I and ^{123}I. Eur J Nucl Med. 2002;29: 783–8.
12. Jeevanram RK, Shah DH, Shama M, et al. Influence of initial large dose on subsequent uptake of therapeutic radioiodine in thyroid cancer patient. Nucl Med Biol. 1986;13:277.
13. Naddaf S, Young I, Rapun R, et al. Comparison between iodine-123 (I-123) and iodine-^{131}I sodium iodide total body scanning in thyroid cancer patients. J Nucl Med. 1996;37:251P.
14. Berbano B, Naddaf S, Echemendia, et al. Use of iodine-123 as a diagnostic tracer for neck and whole body scanning in patients with well-differentiated thyroid cancer. Endocr Pract. 1998;4:11–6.
15. Maxon JR, Thomas SR, Washburn LC, et al. High-activity ^{123}I for the diagnostic evaluations of patients with thyroid cancer. J Nucl Med. 1993;34:42P.
16. Yaakob W, Gordon L, Spicer KM, Nitke SJ. The usefulness of iodine-123 whole-body scans in evaluating thyroid carcinoma and metastases. J Nucl Med Technol. 1999;27:279–81.
17. Shankar LK, Mandel S, Benard F. The promising role of ^{123}I Scintigraphy in the management of differentiated thyroid cancer. J Nucl Med. 2002;43:526.
18. Shankar LK, Yamamoto AJ, Alavi A, et al. Comparison of I-123 scintigraphy at 5 and 24 hours in patients with differentiated thyroid cancer. J Nucl Med. 2002;43:72–6.
19. Gerard SK, Cavalieri RR. ^{123}I diagnostic thyroid tumor whole-body scanning with imaging at 6, 24, and 48 hours. Clin Nucl Med. 2002;27:1–8.
20. Alzahrani AS, Bakheet S, Mandil MAL, et al. ^{123}I isotope as a diagnostic agent in the follow-up of patients with differentiated thyroid cancer: comparison with post ^{131}I therapy whole body scanning. J Clin Endocrinol Metab. 2001;86:5294–300.
21. Siddiqi A, Foley RR, Britton KE, et al. The role of ^{123}I diagnostic imaging in the follow-up of patients with differentiated thyroid carcinoma as compared to ^{131}I scanning; avoidance of negative therapeutic uptake due to stunning. Clin Endocrinol. 2001;55:515–21.
22. Sarkar SD, Kalapparambath TP, Palestro CJ. Comparison of ^{123}I and ^{131}I for whole body imaging in thyroid cancer. J Nucl Med. 2002;43:632–4.
23. Khan J, Hickeson M, Zhuang HM, et al. Diagnostic scanning by ^{123}I vs ^{131}I in thyroid remnant following surgery for differentiated thyroid cancer. J Nucl Med. 2002;43:129P.
24. Anderson GS, Fish S, Nakhoda K, et al. Comparison of ^{123}I and ^{131}I for whole body imaging after stimulation by recombinant human thyrotropin: a preliminary report. Clin Nucl Med. 2003;28:93–6.
25. Eschmann SM, Reischl G, Bilger K, et al. Evaluation of dosimetry of radioiodine therapy in benign and malignant thyroid disorders by means of iodine-124 and PET. Euro J Nucl Med. 2002;29:760–7.

26. Sgouros G, Kolbert KS, Sheikh A, et al. Patient-specific dosimetry for I-131 thyroid cancer therapy using I-124 PET and 3-dimensionalinternal dosimetry (3D-ID) software. J Nucl Med. 2004;45:1366–72.
27. Nadig MR, Pant GS, Bal C. Usefulness of ^{99m}Tc-pertechnetate single-photon emission computed tomography in remnant mass estimation of postsurgical patients of differentiated thyroid cancer during internal dosimetry. Nucl Med Commun. 2008;29:809–14.
28. Kueh SSH, Roach PJ, Schembri GP. Role of Tc-99m pertechnetate for remnant scintigraphy post-thyroidectomy. Clin Nucl Med. 2010;35:671–4.
29. Markovic V, Eterovic D, Punda A, et al. Preoperative Tc-99m-pertechnetate scan visualization of gross neck metastases from microcarcinoma papillare and another papillary carcinoma of tall cell variant scintigraphically presented like small warm nodule in Graves Disease Patient. Clin Nucl Med. 2010;35:858–61.
30. Giovanella L, Suriano S, Ricci R, et al. Postsurgical thyroid remnant estimation by (99m) Tc-pertechnetate scintigraphy predicts radioiodine ablation effectiveness in patients with differentiated thyroid carcinoma. Head Neck. 2011;33:552–6.
31. Nemec J, Rohling S, Zamarazil V, Pohunkova D. Comparison of the distribution of diagnostic and thyroablative I-131 in the evaluation of differentiated thyroid cancers. J Nucl Med. 1997; 20:92–7.
32. Balachandran S, Sayle BA. Value of thyroid carcinoma imaging after therapeutic doses of radioiodine. Clin Nucl Med. 1981;6:162–7.
33. Sherman SI, Tielens ET, Sostre S, et al. Clinical utility of post treatment radioiodine scans in the management of patients with thyroid carcinoma. J Clin Endocrinol Metab. 1994;78:629–34.
34. Spies WG, Wojtowicz CH, Spies SM, et al. Value of post-therapy whole-body I-131 imaging in the evaluation of patients with thyroid carcinoma having undergone high-dose I-131 therapy. Clin Nucl Med. 1989;14:793–800.
35. Fatourechi V, Hay ID, Mullan BP, et al. Are post therapy radioiodine scans informative and do they influence subsequent therapy of patients with differentiated thyroid cancer? Thyroid. 2000;10:573–7.
36. Pineda JD, Lee T, Ain K, et al. Iodine-131 therapy for thyroid cancer patients with elevated thyroglobulin and negative diagnostic scan. J Clin Endocrinol Metab. 1995;80:1488–92.
37. Rosario PWSD, Barroso AL, Rezende LL, et al. Post I-131 therapy scanning in patients with thyroid carcinoma metastases; an unnecessary cost or a relevant contribution? Clin Nucl Med. 2004;29:795–8.
38. Khan S, Waxman A, Magarj N, Braunstein G. Optimization of post ablative I-131 scintigraphy: comparison of 2 day vs 7 day post therapy study in patients with differentiated thyroid cancer (DTC). J Nucl Med. 1994;35:15P.
39. Bourgeois P, Bordet J. Imaging the patients 3 and/or 7 days after treatment with 131-I for differentiated thyroid cancer (DTC)? Eur J Nucl Med Mol Imaging. 2005;32:S240.
40. Oliveira C, Neto J, Barros C, Ferreira P, Almeida A, Curvo-Semedo A, et al. Post-therapy whole-body scan: what is the best time to do? Eur J Nucl Med Mol Imaging. 2008;35:S266.
41. Hung BT, Huang SH, Huagn YE, Wang PW. Appropriate time for post-therapeutic I-131 whole body scan. Clin Nucl Med. 2009; 34:339–42.
42. Chong A, Song HC, Min JJ, Jeong SY, Ha JM, Kim JA, et al. Improved detection of lung or bone metastases with an I-131 whole body scan on the 7th day after high-dose I-131 therapy in patients with thyroid cancer. Nucl Med Mol Imaging. 2010;44:273–81.
43. Lee JW, Lee SM, Koh GP, Lee DH. The comparison of (131)I whole-body scans on the third and tenth day after (131) therapy in patients with well-differentiated thyroid cancer: preliminary report. Ann Nucl Med. 2011;15:439–46.
44. Wakabayashi H, Nakajima K, Fukuoka M, Inaki A, Nakamura A, Kayano D, et al. Double-phase ^{131}I whole body scan nad ^{131}I SPECT-CT images in patients with differentiated thyroid cancer: their effectiveness for accurate identification. Ann Nucl Med. 2011;25:609–15.
45. Salvatori M, Peotti G, Villani MF, Mazza R, Maussier ML, Indovina L, Sigismondi A, Dottorini ME, Giodano A. Determining the appropriate time of execution of an I-131 post-therapy whole-body scan: comparison between early and late imaging. Nucl Med Commun. 2013;34:900–8.

12 Primer and Atlas for the Interpretation of Radioiodine Whole Body Scintigraphy

Douglas Van Nostrand and Frank B. Atkins

Introduction

Radioiodine whole body scintigraphy remains an important diagnostic modality in the evaluation of patients with differentiated thyroid carcinoma. The advantages and disadvantages of the various radioiodine isotopes, and how the images are obtained, are discussed in Chap. 11. This chapter presents a primer and atlas for the interpretation of radioiodine whole body scintigraphy. The objective of the primer is to present a simple, consistent, and reliable approach to the evaluation and interpretation of radioiodine whole body scans. The objectives of the atlas are to demonstrate (1) a spectrum of thyroid tissue uptake, residual activity in the thyroid bed and elsewhere, (2) a spectrum of non-thyroidal physiological uptake, (3) various patterns of metastatic disease, (4) examples of false-positives and artifacts, and (5) several techniques to help the interpreter differentiate metastatic disease from physiological uptake, false-positives, and artifacts. Although all patterns of physiological uptake, false-positive uptake, and artifacts cannot be presented, a comprehensive review of the literature of thyroidal uptake, non-thyroidal uptake, false-positives, and artifacts of radioiodine uptake is presented in Chap. 13).

D. Van Nostrand, MD, FACP, FACNM (✉)
Nuclear Medicine Research, MedStar Research Institute and Washington Hospital Center, Georgetown University School of Medicine, Washington Hospital Center, 110 Irving Street, N.W., Suite GB 60F, Washington, DC 20010, USA
e-mail: douglasvannostrand@gmail.com

F.B. Atkins, PhD
Division of Nuclear Medicine, MedStar Washington Hospital Center, Georgetown University School of Medicine, 110 Irving Street NW, Washington, DC 20010, USA
e-mail: fbatkins@gmail.com

Primer

A Systematic Approach for the Evaluation and Interpretation of Radioiodine Whole Body Scans

When a medical student or physician in-training sees a radioiodine whole body scan for the first time, the initial response is frequently either "it's easy—just look for the hot spots" or "the findings are so nonspecific." However, both responses are incorrect. The interpretation of radioiodine whole body scans is not easy, and the findings can be very specific.

Like most nuclear medicine scans, the process of interpreting radioiodine whole body scans can be divided into three simple but important steps: (1) ensuring adequate quality of the imaging technique, (2) observation, and (3) interpretation.

The first step is to review the scan in terms of the quality of the imaging technique. Ensuring that adequate quality of the scan has been achieved is not difficult but is frequently taken for granted. Failure to ensure that the scan is performed according to the facility's procedural guidelines can be without exaggeration, disastrous. The physician must ensure quality by:

1. Interviewing the patient before beginning the scan to ascertain his or her compliance with thyroid hormone withdrawal, thyrotropin injections, and/or low-iodine diet
2. Reviewing β human choriogonadotropin (hCG) levels when warranted, thyrotropin (TSH) blood levels, images, and the placement of markers
3. When necessary, questioning the technologist regarding window settings, exposure intensity, duration of imaging, counts, scanning speed, collimator, and other factors that may affect the acquisition of the images

This is only a partial list. However, without first ensuring adequate quality of preparation and technique, the remaining steps may have reduced or no value.

L. Wartofsky, D. Van Nostrand (eds.), *Thyroid Cancer*, DOI 10.1007/978-1-4939-3314-3_12

The second step is simply to observe and describe all areas of increased radioactivity on the whole body scan or camera views. The physician who states that the radioiodine whole body scan is easy typically performs only this step.

The third step of interpretation involves the evaluation of each area of increased radioactivity noted on the previous step for etiology. The physician who claims that the radioiodine whole body scans are nonspecific, albeit at times correct, usually does not use the five databases noted in Table 12.1, SPECT-CT (see Chaps. 14 and 15), and the many tools noted in Table 12.2 to markedly improve the specificity of radioiodine uptake. SPECT-CT is the most important tool in improving specificity, and its value in altering management, thereby potentially altering outcomes, is well documented in the literature. Although most of the tools fall into the category of "common sense," they are not commonly considered. The physician who follows these guidelines will discover that the radioiodine whole body scans are neither easy nor nonspecific.

Atlas

Atlas of Radioiodine Whole Body Scans

The atlas is divided into six sections:

1. A spectrum of thyroid tissue uptake (Figs. 12.1 to 12.5)
2. A spectrum of non-thyroidal physiological uptake (Figs. 12.6 to 12.14)
3. Several patterns of metastatic disease (Figs. 12.15 to 12.25)
4. Examples of false-positive uptake and artifacts (Figs. 12.26 to 12.29)
5. Several tools to help differentiate metastases from non-thyroidal physiological uptake, false-positives, and artifacts (Figs. 12.31 to 12.34)
6. Miscellaneous (Fig. 12.35)

For each scan, only the teaching point for the figure is typically noted and discussed in the legend.

Table 12.1 Five databases

Patient's detailed history for specific scan findings
Normal physiological distribution and patterns of radioiodine at various times after dosing
Normal variants
Artifacts
Tools to distinguish all of the above from metastasis

Table 12.2 Tools to help distinguish metastases from non-thyroidal physiological uptake, false-positives, and artifacts

Obtain "uptake-specific" history, such as:
• Recent surgery
• Colostomies
• Prostheses
• Dentures
• Contact lens, artificial eye, and so on
Examine the patient regarding:
• Colostomies
• Ureterostomies
• Nephrostomies
• Skin lesions
Localize the area of radioiodine accumulation within the patient with:
• SPECT-CT, but when SPECT-CT is not available, then consider using:
• Marker images with external radioactive sources placed on the patient to provide anatomical reference points on the scan, e.g., to help establish that the region of uptake corresponds to the submandibular gland or a palpable mass
• Marker image to help localize area of radioactivity on scan or patient, which, in turn, may help facilitate the evaluation of the area on CT, MRI, or ultrasound
• Lateral views to localize the radioiodine as deep or superficial, such as helping to differentiate the rib from lung, sternum from mediastinum, gastrointestinal tract from bone, and brain from bone
Improve resolution:
• Pinhole images
Manipulate the radioactivity:
• Decontamination
• Additional views 1 or 2 d later
• Administration of water
• Administration of sialogogues (lemon)
• Administration of laxatives
Compare:
• With previous study
Perform additional diagnostic studies, such as:
• Chest X-ray
• Plain films
• Ultrasound (US)
• Computer tomography (CT)
• Magnetic resonance imaging (MR)
• Positron emission tomography scan (PET)
• Bone scan
• Renal scan

Part 1: A Spectrum of Thyroid Tissue Uptake

Preoperative Thyroid Scan with Hypofunctioning Area

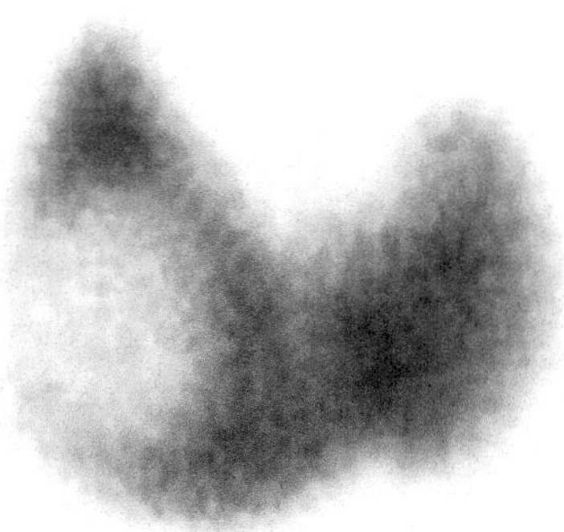

Fig. 12.1 This is a preoperative pinhole collimator image of the thyroid performed 24 h after the administration of ^{123}I. A large hypofunctioning area is noted in the right lobe, which corresponded to a palpable nodule. The patient subsequently had fine-needle aspiration with cytology that demonstrated differentiated papillary thyroid carcinoma. The patient had a near-total thyroidectomy (Reproduced with permission from Keystone Press, Inc [1]). Preoperative thyroid scanning is not routinely performed unless thyroid function blood levels suggest a functioning adenoma, the latter having increased uptake on thyroid scan (see Chap. 24)

Comment Why does thyroid cancer appear "cold" on thyroid scans and "hot" on radioiodine whole body scans? Although the primary site or metastases of differentiated thyroid cancer can take up radioiodine, the degree of this uptake is generally much less than the surrounding normal functioning thyroid tissue and, as a result, appears "cold" on a preoperative thyroid scan. However, after most of the thyroid gland has been surgically removed and the residual thyroid tissue ablated with radioiodine, metastases will then frequently appear "hot" and functioning relative to background activity. Over time, a metastasis of differentiated thyroid cancer may lose its function (dedifferentiated) and no longer take up radioiodine.

Minimal Postoperative Residual Thyroid Tissue (Thyroid Remnant)

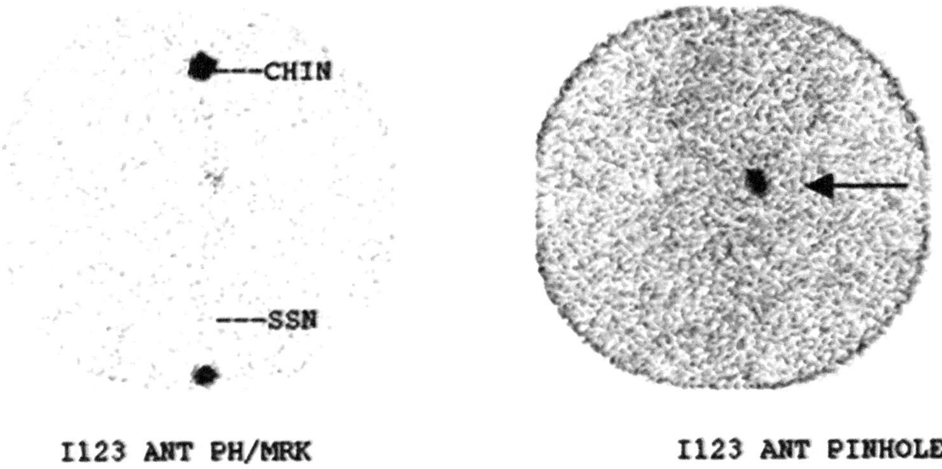

Fig. 12.2 The pinhole collimator image on the *left* represents a marker image, in which the chin and suprasternal notch (SSN) are marked by placing radioactive sources on the patient. After the markers are removed and without moving the patient, a second pinhole collimator image is performed for a significantly longer interval of time. The resulting image on the *right* demonstrates a single well-defined focal area of modest radioiodine uptake in the upper aspect of the thyroid bed. The patient received radioiodine to ablate this minimal residual thyroid tissue. (The label for the SSN is slightly higher than the actual marker.)

Comment The surgeon typically leaves behind some normal residual thyroid tissue in order to avoid injury to the laryngeal nerves and to preserve some parathyroid gland tissue. However, the volume and the number of individual foci of thyroid tissue left by the surgeon vary not only between surgeons but also among patients operated on by the same surgeon.

A question frequently asked is whether or not this focus of uptake could represent a focus of metastatic thyroid carcinoma. It is possible but not likely. Again, the surgeon seeks to remove any areas of metastatic thyroid carcinoma while leaving normal thyroid tissue to spare the recurrent laryngeal nerve and to leave functioning parathyroid gland tissue. Although it is possible to remove all thyroid tissue while leaving only distant metastatic thyroid carcinoma within the thyroid bed, it is less likely.

Could thyroid carcinoma still be present in the remaining normal residual thyroid tissue? Yes, and this is one of the objectives of ^{131}I adjuvant treatment (i.e., the destruction of any additional area of thyroid cancer) (see Chap. 33).

Large Postoperative Residual Thyroid Tissue

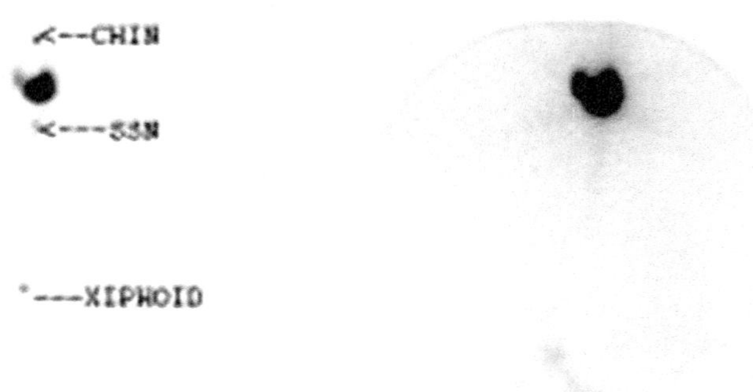

Fig. 12.3 Using a parallel collimator (see Chap. 11), the image on the *left* represents a marker image in which the chin, suprasternal notch (SSN), and xiphoid are all marked. After the markers are removed, and without moving the patient, a second parallel-hole collimator image is performed for a significantly longer time. The resulting image on the *right* demonstrates a large focus of significant increased radioiodine uptake. This figure, together with the previous figure, illustrates the two extremes of residual thyroid activity after a near-total thyroidectomy

Comment Because of the significant amount of thyroid tissue remaining in the thyroid bed after the initial surgery, additional surgery may have to be considered. However, whether more surgery is warranted is beyond the scope of this chapter.

If the facility administers a fixed empiric prescribed activity of ^{131}I for remnant ablation, regardless of the result of these postoperative scans, then these scans would obviously not need to be performed. However, many facilities use these scans along with uptakes to modify the therapy approach such as modification of the empiric prescribed activity (see Chaps. 19 and 33).

Functioning Thyroid Tissue in the Thyroglossal Tract

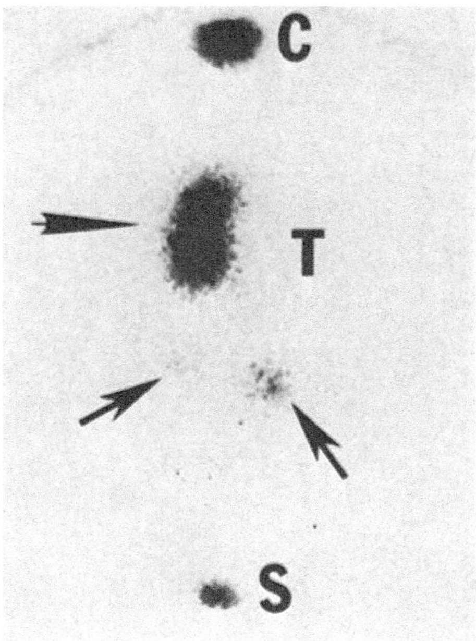

Fig. 12.4 An ^{131}I image of the neck bed was performed using a pinhole collimator. An elongated area of radioactivity is present in the midline at the level of the thyroid cartilage (*T*) and is consistent with the functioning thyroid tissue within the thyroglossal duct remnant (*arrowhead*). Two small foci of residual radioactivity are also noted in the thyroid bed (*arrows*). The location of the chin (*C*) and suprasternal notch (*S*) are marked using cobalt sources (Reproduced with permission from Lippincott, Williams, and Wilkins [2])

Comment The thyroid gland embryologically develops from the foramen cecum at the junction of the anterior two thirds and posterior one third of the tongue. It then descends and bifurcates in the neck. During thyroid development and migration, various embryologic maldevelopments may occur, including functioning thyroid tissue in the thyroglossal tract (as noted above), lingual thyroid, and aberrant thyroid tissue (see Table 13.1) entitled "False positives and artifacts of radioiodine imaging").

The diagnosis of thyroglossal duct remnant is suggested by the midline location and the linear-oval distribution of radioactivity. Although one can help exclude esophageal activity with techniques such as clearing the esophageal activity by drinking water and repeating the scan (see Table 12.2 and Fig. 12.9 in this chapter), one may not be able to differentiate thyroglossal duct remnant from local lymph node metastasis. However, based on the combination of the intensity, location, and presence of the radioactivity on the presurgical scan, thyroglossal duct remnant would be most likely. SPECT-CT may also be valuable.

Struma Ovarii

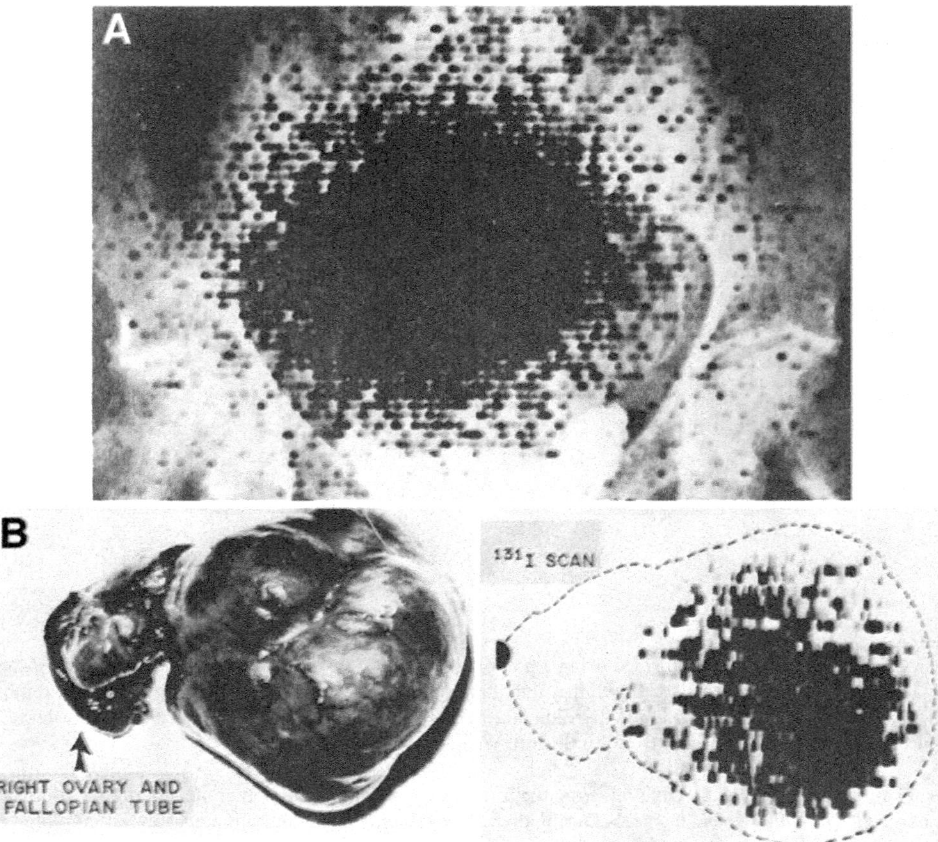

Fig. 12.5 Part (**A**) is an overlay of the patient's ^{131}I rectilinear scan onto her pelvic radiograph, and this combined image demonstrates ^{131}I uptake in the pelvic region. This uptake corresponded to a 10-cm pelvic mass, which was an infarcted teratoma composed mostly of active thyroid tissue (struma ovarii). With the bladder catheterized, the 24-h ^{131}I uptake over the mass was 17 %. The image on the *left* in part (**B**) is the gross surgical specimen; the image on the *right* is the corresponding in vitro ^{131}I image of the specimen. The ^{131}I had been administered 9 days prior to surgery (This figure was originally published in *JNM*. Yeh et al. [6]. © by the Society of Nuclear Medicine and Molecular Imaging, Inc.)

Comment Although struma ovarii itself is very rare, the likelihood of the simultaneous occurrence with thyroid carcinoma is even more remote [3–5]. Pelvic or abdominal ^{131}I uptake in struma ovarii could be mistaken for metastatic thyroid carcinoma [6, 7].

Part 2: A Spectrum of Non-thyroidal Physiological Uptake

"Facial" Radioactivity

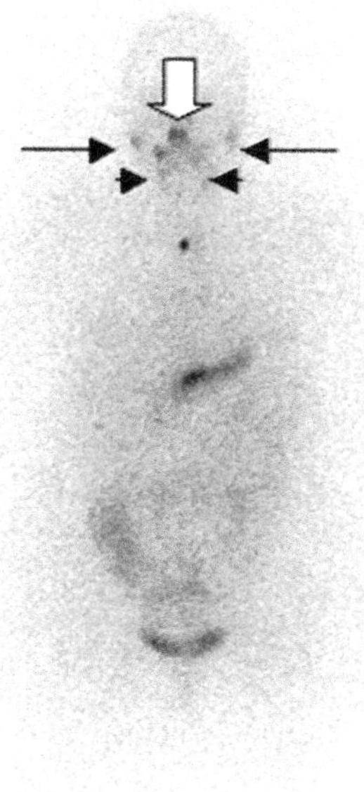

Fig. 12.6 The above radioiodine whole body image was performed 48 h after the ^{131}I administration. Physiological uptake is present in the facial area. Modest uptake is found in the parotid glands (*long, black, thin arrows*), and less intense radioactivity is noted in the submandibular glands (*short, black, thin arrows*). Slightly more intense activity is indicated in the midline (*white arrow*), which is most likely nasal uptake (see Figs. 12.7 and 12.8), and a small asymmetric area (no *arrow*) is noted slightly inferior to the nasal area and medial to the right parotid (no *arrow*), consistent with asymmetric oropharyngeal activity

Comment Radioiodine normally concentrates in the salivary glands, including the parotid, submandibular, and sublingual glands, and is secreted into the oral pharynx. Uptake may also be present in the nasal area, which is discussed further below.

"Facial" Radioiodine Accumulation

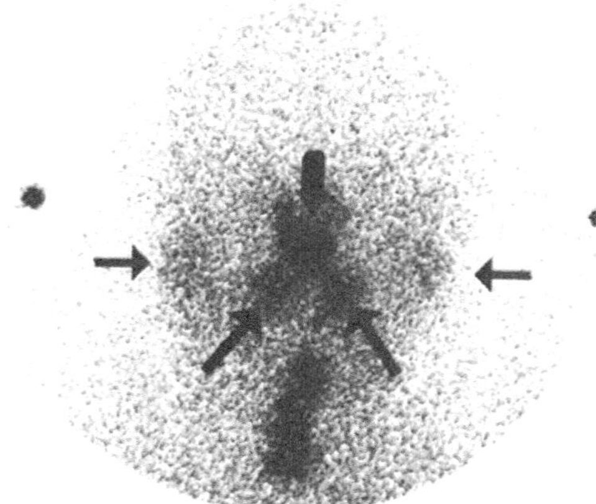

Fig. 12.7 Using a parallel-hole collimator of the head, face, and neck, this anterior image demonstrates typical areas of facial uptake and the variability of radioactivity in more detail than Fig. 12.6. Normal radioiodine uptake is noted in the parotid (*short arrows*) with slightly greater activity in the right parotid relative to the *left*. More intense radioactivity is found in the mouth and/or sublingual salivary gland area (*long arrows*). On this anterior image, no definitive radioiodine accumulation is noted in the submandibular glands. The radioactivity in the midline (*thick arrow*) represents nasal activity. The faint radioactivity that outlines the head is secondary to residual radioactivity in the blood pool. (The radioactivity in the midline below the two long arrows was discussed in the legend to Fig. 12.4) (Reproduced with permission from Lippincott, Williams, and Wilkins [2])

Comment Uptake in the facial area can be variable. Although the radioactivity in each group of salivary glands is usually symmetrical, this is not always the case (as noted here). Asymmetric uptake may be caused by disease of the salivary gland, asymmetric development of the salivary glands, previous ^{131}I treatment that resulted in asymmetric sialoadenitis, or even a slight rotation of the head during imaging.

Kulkarni et al. [8] have suggested that assessment of salivary gland uptake on the postoperative preablation/therapy scan may help predict sialoadenitis. If this is confirmed, the scan may help identify patients for whom the management should be altered, such as a reduced ablative or therapeutic prescribed activity and/or additional medications administered prophylactically to try to reduce the radiation exposure to the salivary glands from the treatment.

"Facial Uptake"

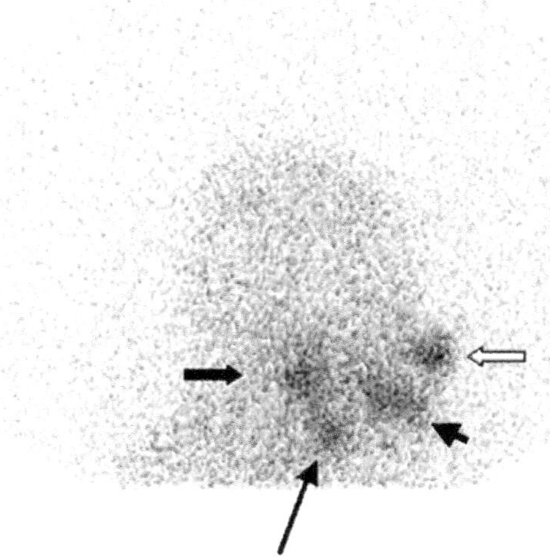

Fig. 12.8 This right lateral view of the head was obtained approx 72 h after the administration of ^{131}I. It demonstrates radioiodine accumulation in the nose (*open arrow*), parotid gland (*medium-length arrow*), submandibular gland (*long arrow*), and oral pharyngeal area (*short arrow*)

Comment Uptake in the nose is a common finding. Norby et al. [9] reported that 95 % (20/21) of patients had nasal radioactivity greater than background on whole body scans performed 72 h after the administration of 18.5 MBq (5 mCi) of ^{131}I. The intensity of radioiodine accumulation was 1+ (greater than background but less than parotid gland and/or mouth activity) in 33 % (6/20), 2+ (equal to parotid and/or mouth) in 33 % (6/20), and 3+ (greater than parotid and/or mouth) in 40 % (8/20). The pattern was ovoid in 75 % (15/20) of patients but could also be linear.

The mechanism of radioiodine accumulation in the nose is not known. However, mucous glands are present in the tip of the nose and may be responsible. Focal uptake in the tip of the nose should not be considered a bone metastasis. Nasal pain and epistaxis have been reported after large therapeutic prescribed activities (7.4–14.8 GBq [200–400 mCi]) of ^{131}I, and they are hypothesized to be the result of significant radiation absorbed dose to the tip of the nose [10]. Assessment of the radioiodine whole body scan may help identify patients who may be at risk for these nasal side effects and who may warrant a change in management, such as reduced prescribed activity and/or medication(s) to reduce the nasal uptake.

Esophagus: Swallowed Radioactivity or Aberrant Thyroid Tissue?

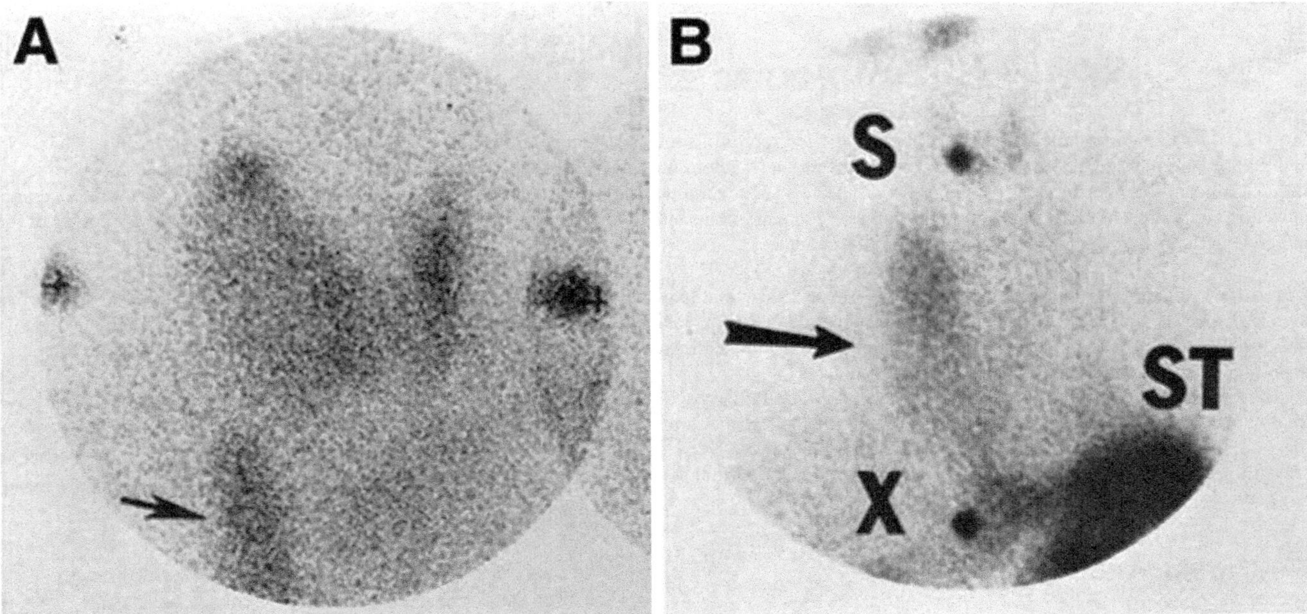

Fig. 12.9 Although these preoperative thyroid images were performed using $^{99m}TcO_4$, they illustrate the potential pitfall of esophageal radioactivity. The anterior image of the thyroid performed using a pinhole collimator (**A**) demonstrates a large linear area of radioactivity inferior to the right lobe of the thyroid (*arrow*). Image (**B**) was obtained with a parallel-hole collimator and shows that the radioactivity extends to the xiphoid region (*large arrow*). After the patient drank several glasses of water, the radioactivity cleared. The patient had achalasia, and the area of radioactivity most likely represented persistent radioactivity in the dilated esophagus, which had been secreted by the salivary glands and swallowed (*X* xiphoid, *S* suprasternal notch, *ST* stomach) (Reproduced with permission from Lippincott, Williams, and Wilkins [2])

Comment ^{131}I, like $^{99m}TcO_4$, may end up in the esophagus via several mechanisms. First, the ^{131}I that concentrates in the salivary glands may be secreted into the oropharynx and subsequently swallowed into the esophagus. Second, ^{131}I that is secreted by the gastric mucosa into the stomach may reflux into the esophagus. Third, ectopic gastric mucosa in the esophagus, such as a Barrett's esophagus, may secrete ^{131}I. Although the esophageal radioactivity from any of these mechanisms should clear rapidly, stasis may occur with Zenker's diverticulum or achalasia. To help differentiate physiological radioactivity from metastases, further manipulations may be necessary.

Thymus

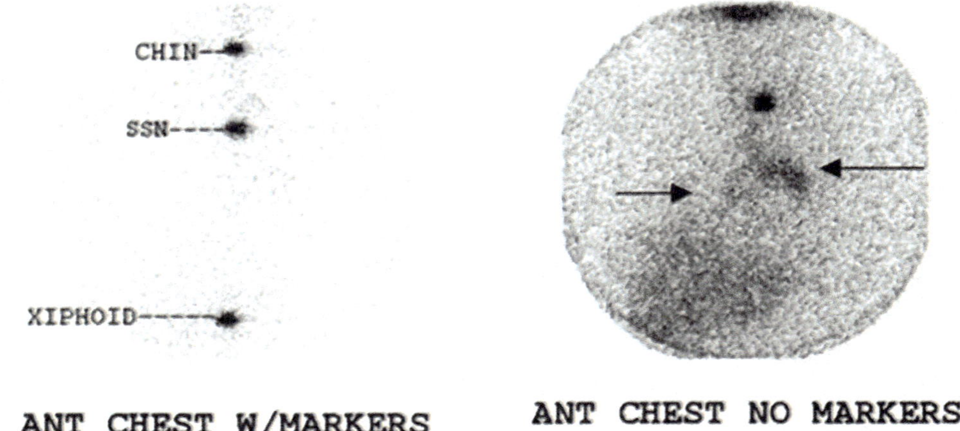

Fig. 12.10 The parallel-hole collimator image on the *left* represents a marker image, in which the location of the chin, suprasternal notch (*SSN*), and xiphoid are marked. After the markers are removed, and without moving the patient, a second parallel-hole collimator image was performed for a significantly longer time. These images were performed several days after ^{131}I ablation. The image on the *right* demonstrates a bilobed area of radioactivity present in the mediastinum (*arrows*) secondary to normal thymic uptake. The modest radioactivity noted in the lower corner of the image is in the liver, which is discussed later in this chapter.

Comment Radioiodine uptake in thymus has been reported by multiple authors, and the uptake has been observed in both hyperplastic and normal thymic tissue [11–13, 18, 19]. Wilson et al. has also reported $^{99m}TcO_4$ uptake in a thymoma [12]. The mechanism of radioiodine accumulation in the thymus is not known, but Vermiglio et al. [13] have suggested that the radioiodine localizes in cystic Hassall's bodies. Although thymic uptake is more frequently observed in children, it can also be seen in adults [11].

In a group of 175 patients, Davidson [18] reported radioiodine accumulation in thymus in four of 325 diagnostic scans and three of 200 post-treatment scans. Michigishi [19] has suggested that the mediastinal uptake may become more prominent after successive ^{131}I therapies. Uptake in the thymus should not be mistaken for mediastinal metastasis. SPECT-CT or computed tomography (CT) without contrast may be helpful in confirming the presence of thymic tissue or confirming an abnormal mass or nodes that suggest metastases.

Cardiac Blood Pool

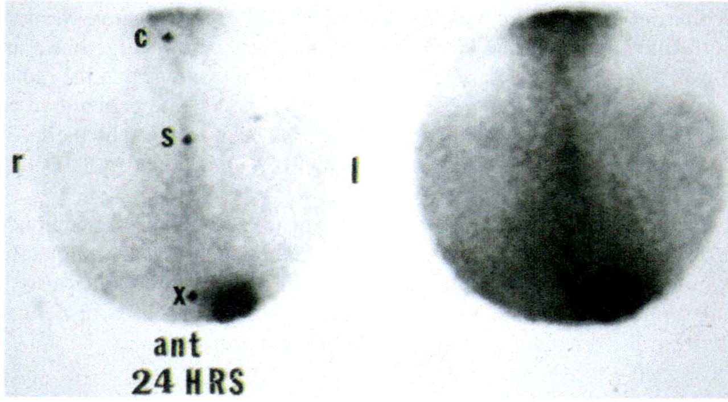

Fig. 12.11 This anterior neck and chest image was obtained 24 h after the administration of 37 MBq (1.0 mCi) of ^{131}I orally. Increased ^{131}I activity is noted in the cardiac region and represents normal cardiac blood pool activity at this time point. This area cleared on the 72-h image (not shown). The chin (C), suprasternal notch (S), and xiphoid (X) are noted using cobalt markers. The right (r) and left (l) side of the patient are also marked (Reproduced with permission from Lippincott, Williams, and Wilkins [2])

Comment The physician should be alert for and recognize blood pool activity, which may be more frequent on 24-h images with either ^{131}I or ^{123}I. It is normal and should not be mistaken for diffuse metastasis. Blood pool radioactivity may mask metastasis in both the lower lung and possibly the lower hilar regions. Delayed views on subsequent days may be needed to allow further clearance of the blood pool (background) activity.

Diffuse Liver Radioactivity

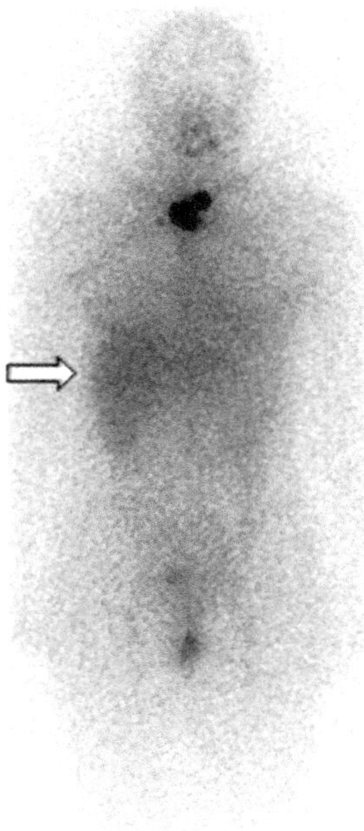

Fig. 12.12 This post-therapy ^{131}I whole body scan was performed approx 12 days after ablation with ^{131}I and demonstrates diffuse radioactivity in the liver (*arrow*) (Reproduced with permission from Keystone Press, Inc. [20])

Comment Ziessman [14] reported that liver uptake is commonly seen in 44 % (12/27) of patients and 35 % (21/60) of scans and can be present on post-therapy scans, as well as on diagnostic scans. Of 19 post-therapy scans performed following 1.11–7.4 GBq (30-200 mCi) of ^{131}I, liver radioactivity was present on a subjective scale of 3+ in six, 2+ in four, 1+ in four, and 0 in five. In contrast, of 41 patients receiving 74–370 MBq (2–10 mCi) of ^{131}I, liver radioactivity was present on the same scale with 3+ in one, 2+ in two, 1+ in six, and 0 in 32. The post-therapy scans were performed 3–7 days after the therapy, and the diagnostic scans were performed 48 h after administration of the diagnostic prescribed activity.

Chung et al. [15] reported that 60 % of 399 patients and 36 % of 1,115 radioiodine whole body scans had diffuse hepatic uptake more than grade 2, which was defined as definite but faint liver activity. In the diagnostic scans, 12 % showed uptake in the liver, whereas the frequency of liver uptake on post-therapy scans increased based on the therapy dose. Liver uptake was present in 39 % of scans performed after treatment with 1.11 GBq (30 mCi), 62 % after 2.775–3.7 GBq (75–100 mCi), and 71.3 % after 5.55 ^{131}I –7.4 GBq (150–200 mCi). Similarly, as the uptake in residual thyroid tissue increased visually, the liver intensity also increased. However, 15 patients showed diffuse liver uptake without uptake in the thyroid or metastases. Chung et al. [15] also showed a relationship of the degree of hepatic uptake to release of ^{131}I-labeled thyroglobulin.

Ziessman [14] also reported that the presence of liver uptake correlated with both the administered prescribed activity of ^{131}I and the absolute thyroid uptake (actual number of becquerels [millicuries] of ^{131}I in the thyroid) but not with the percent uptake. With few exceptions, patients with liver visualization had an absolute thyroid uptake of more than 37 MBq (1 mCi), and most without liver visualization had thyroid uptake of less than 37 MBq (1 mCi). He also suggested that the longer the time interval between administration of the radioiodine and the time to imaging, the greater the frequency would be as well as the degree of increased uptake of liver radioactivity.

Radiolabeled thyroxine localizes in the liver within hours after injection [16], and the liver deiodinates 40 % of the whole body T-4 and 70 % of the T-3 production [17].

Gastrointestinal Radioactivity

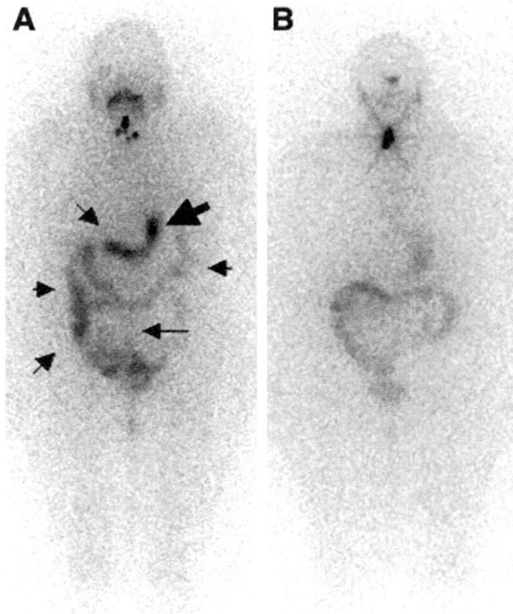

Fig. 12.13 (Part **A**) demonstrates normal physiological radioactivity in the stomach (*large arrow*) and gastrointestinal system (*small arrowheads*). The patterns of gastrointestinal radioactivity are variable (part **B**)

Comment Radioiodine in the stomach and gastrointestinal tract may be secondary to a combination of at least three mechanisms: swallowed radioactive saliva, radioactivity secreted by the gastric mucosa, and deiodinated thyroid hormone in the liver excreted through the biliary tree.

Because it is highly unusual for well-differentiated thyroid carcinoma to metastasize to the gastrointestinal system, differentiating physiological gastrointestinal uptake from a gastrointestinal metastasis is typically not a diagnostic problem. Rather, the problem is differentiating physiological gastrointestinal uptake from a metastasis in bone. This is usually facilitated by SPECT-CT (see Chap. 14) and the pattern, localization, and use of multiple tools as listed in Table 12.2. Gastrointestinal radioactivity is typically indicated by an area of radioactive that has a tubular rather than a focal pattern of activity, localizes on lateral views to the abdomen, does not localize to the bone, and changes configuration on delayed views with or without laxatives.

In addition to the above, delayed and lateral views may help assess the bones that are obscured by overlying gastrointestinal radioactivity. Identification of significant gastrointestinal radioactivity on a diagnostic scan may also help encourage the physician to manage more aggressively a patient with stool softeners and/or laxatives after remnant ablation or treatment. This may reduce the residence time and amount of the radioactivity in the intestine, thereby reducing the radiation absorbed dose to the gastrointestinal tract.

Urinary Bladder

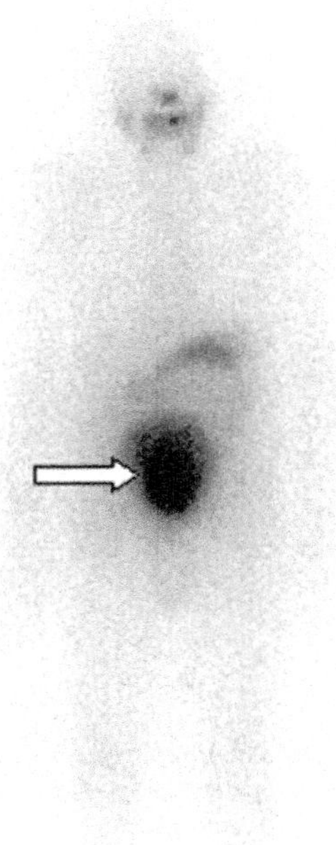

Fig. 12.14 A large area of radioactivity is noted in the pelvis, extending into the lower abdomen (*white arrow*), which is a distended urinary bladder. Gastrointestinal activity is also noted slightly cephalad

Comment The kidneys are the principal means by which the radioiodine is cleared from the body; accordingly, radioiodine will accumulate in the urinary bladder. The importance of urinary bladder radioactivity is that:

1. It is variable in intensity, size, and sometimes configuration.
2. It should not be mistaken for bony metastasis.
3. It can obscure the assessment of the underlying or even overlying pelvic bones for bony metastases.
4. The patient should be encouraged to void before beginning the scan.
5. Hydration and frequent voiding after ^{131}I therapy will help reduce the radiation absorbed dose to the urinary bladder wall, adjacent bowel, colon, ovaries, and testes.
6. Distended bladders, such as this patient's bladder, may need to be catheterized when the patient is unable to void a significant amount of urine in order to minimize the radiation absorbed dose to the urinary bladder wall after radioactivity ablation or treatment.

Part 3: Patterns of Metastatic Disease

Regional Lymph Node Metastasis

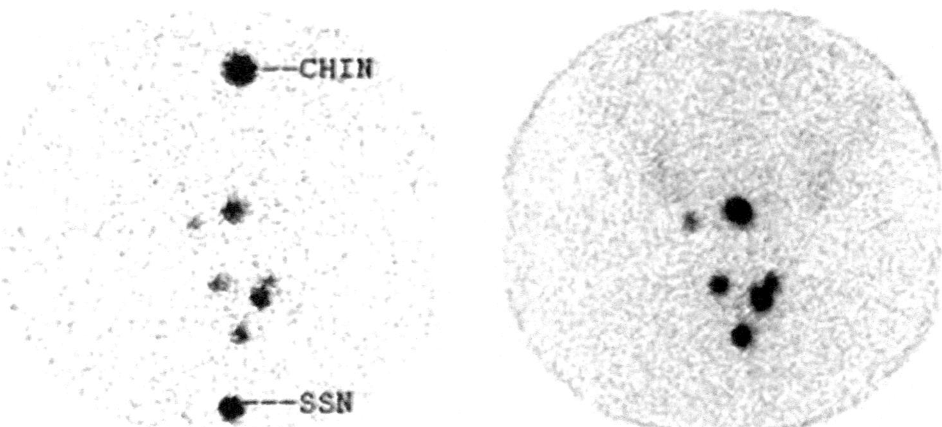

Fig. 12.15 The pinhole collimator image on the *left* represents a marker image in which the locations of the chin and suprasternal notch (*SSN*) are marked. After the markers are removed, and without moving the patient, a second pinhole collimator image is performed for a significantly longer time. The resulting image on the *right* demonstrates six areas of focal radioactivity. Several of these were confirmed as cervical lymph nodes with metastatic disease

Comment One author (dvn) proposes that as the number of focal areas of radioactivity increases, the likelihood of lymph node metastases increases, and the likelihood of normal post-operative residual tissue decreases. Although we are unaware of any study that has confirmed this relationship, Chennupati et al. have evaluated the relationship of the number of foci remaining after near-total or total thyroidectomy for three surgeons at Medstar Washington Hospital Center in patients who had a very low a priori likelihood of locoregional metastases [21]. If >5 foci observed on a ^{123}I 24-h image using a pinhole collimator imaging was the threshold for suggesting further evaluation for locoregional disease, then the combined false-positive rate would have been 3 % (3/87) for the three surgeons.

If metastatic disease is confirmed in the lymph nodes using fine-needle aspiration, then additional surgery may need to be considered prior to performing ^{131}I remnant ablation or therapy.

Although some facilities will give a fixed empiric prescribed activity for ^{131}I remnant ablation or therapy in this patient, other facilities will consider increasing the empiric prescribed activity of ^{131}I or will perform lesional dosimetry [22, 23].

Mediastinal Metastasis

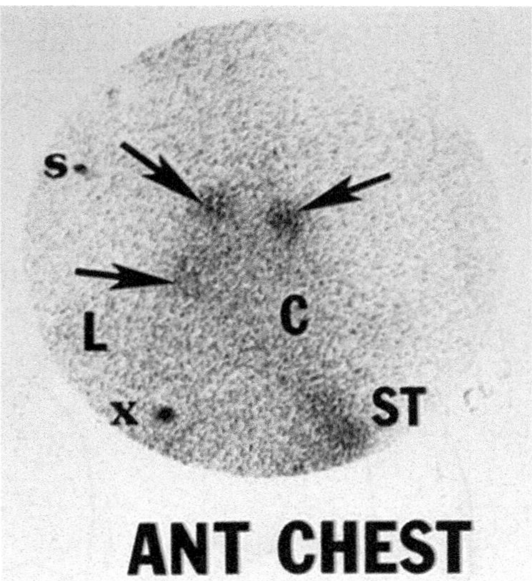

Fig. 12.16 This parallel-hole collimator image of the chest demonstrates three areas of metastastic thyroid cancer in the mediastinum (*black arrows*). "s" represents the level of the suprasternal notch, but the marker was placed to the right side of the patient. "x" designates the xiphoid, and again this marker is also placed to the right of the midline. "L" represents the lower lung area. "C" represents cardiac areas, and "ST" represents the stomach (Reproduced with permission from Lippincott, Williams, and Wilkins [2])

Comment This is an example of metastasis to the mediastinal lymph nodes, which is a frequent location of metastasis from differentiated thyroid carcinoma. The determination of the prescribed radioactivity to treat this patient is problematic. The prescribed activity could range from an empiric fixed prescribed activity of 3.7 GBq (100 mCi) to 11.1 GBq (300 mCi). Lesional dosimetry, blood (bone marrow) dosimetry, or both have also been performed to help determine an appropriate prescribed amount of radioactivity for treatment.

Pulmonary Metastasis: Patterns

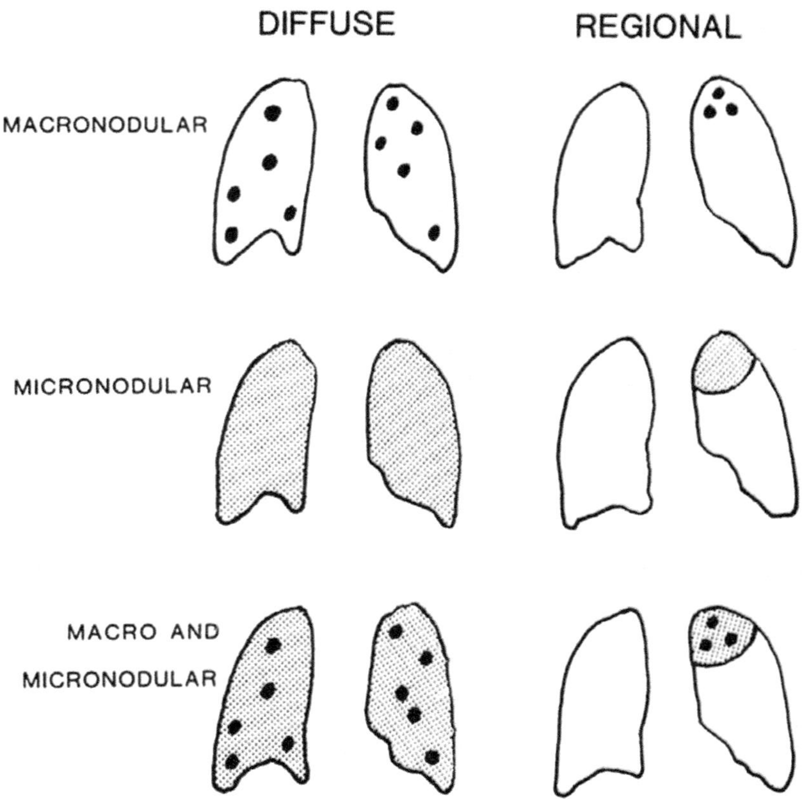

Fig. 12.17 The above drawings demonstrate three potential patterns of radioactive uptake secondary to metastastic thyroid cancer to the lungs. These patterns are macronodular (*upper*), micronodular (*middle*), and mixed (*lower*) and may also be diffuse or regional (Reproduced with permission from Lippincott, Williams, and Wilkins [2])

Comment The terms "micronodular" and "macronodular" may be used to describe the pattern of pulmonary metastases on either radioiodine scan or radiographs, albeit most authors use the terms to describe radiograph findings. Although no precise measurement differentiates macronodular from micronodular metastases, 1 cm or greater has been used by Schlumberger as the threshold for macronodular and less than 1 cm as micronodular [24]. Casara et al. [41] have used the threshold of more than 5 mm as macronodular and less than 5 mm as micronodular.

Pulmonary metastasis may present in a wide spectrum of patterns from a diffuse miliary pattern of micrometastases throughout both lungs with good radioiodine uptake and normal chest X-ray to a pattern of a single large focal macronodular metastasis on chest X-ray with no radioiodine uptake.

Although the association of the pattern of pulmonary metastasis to either prognosis or the frequency and severity of side effects of radioiodine treatment has not been well characterized (see Chaps. 48 and 79 regarding prognosis, Chap. 56 regarding ^{131}I treatment of distant metastases, and Chap. 62 for side effects), several potential relationships have been suggested. First, good uptake of radioiodine in a diffuse miliary pattern may be associated with a better prognosis than multiple focal macronodular metastases with poor radioiodine uptake [24–28]. In addition, when the chest X-ray/CT is negative for evidence of pulmonary metastasis, Hindié et al. [29] observed that the prognosis may be even better. Schlumberger et al. [26] observed complete remission in 83 % of lesions that were not visible on chest X-ray, in 53 % of micronodular (<1 cm) metastases, and in only 14 % of macronodular (>1 cm) metastases. However, the pattern of diffuse functioning micronodular metastases may be more likely to be associated with diffuse acute radiation pneumonitis, pulmonary fibrosis, or both, rather than the latter pattern (see Chap. 56).

Pulmonary Metastasis: Diffuse Miliary (Micronodular) Metastases

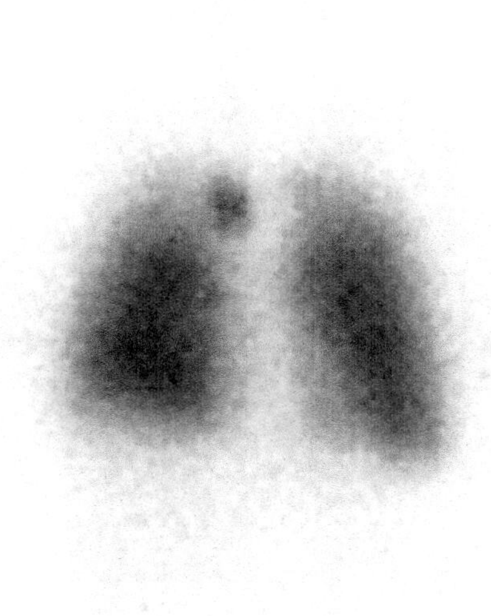

Fig. 12.18 This is a whole body anterior image performed 72 h after the administration of ^{131}I. Marked diffuse radioactivity is noted throughout both lung fields, which is typical for a miliary pattern of pulmonary metastasis. The radiograph demonstrates a miliary pattern throughout both lungs. Although the scan suggests a focal area of radioactivity in the upper medial aspect of the right lung, the radiographs showed only a similar miliary pattern. Histopathologic examination confirmed papillary follicular differentiated thyroid carcinoma. Owing to the intense uptake in both lungs, the outline of the patient's body is not readily visualized at the brightness and contrast settings used in this image (Reproduced with permission from Keystone Press, Inc. [20])

Comment Several authors have reported that this pattern is associated with a good prognosis. However, this patient may be more susceptible to acute radiation pneumonitis, fibrosis, or both after ^{131}I therapy. As previously discussed, the selection of an appropriate prescribed activity of ^{131}I for treatment is problematic. In the adult patient, the prescribed activity has ranged between an empiric fixed prescribed activity of 3.7 GBq (100 mCi) and 11.1 GBq (300 mCi). This author suggests that bone marrow (blood) dosimetry, as described by Benua and Leeper, has value in determining the maximum allowable prescribed activity and has a long history of successful usage, with little or no acute radiation pneumonitis and/or pulmonary fibrosis when appropriate restrictions are followed. (See Chap. 58 entitled "Dosimetrially-Determined Prescribed Activity of ^{131}I for the Treatment of Metastatic Differentiated Thyroid Cancer" and Chap. 62 entitled "Side Effects of ^{131}I for Therapy of Differentiated Thyroid Carcinoma.")

Pulmonary Metastasis: Macronodular

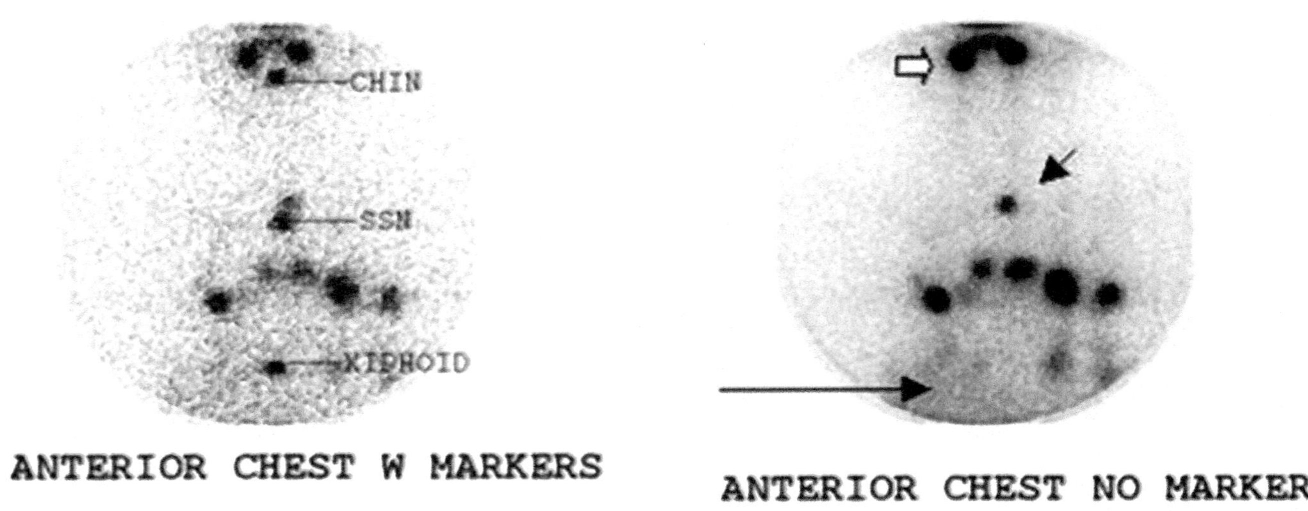

Fig. 12.19 The parallel-hole collimator image on the *left* represents a marker image in which the location of the chin, SSN, and xiphoid are marked. After the markers are removed, and without moving the patient, a second parallel-hole collimator image was performed for a significantly longer time. The resulting image on the *right* demonstrates multifocal macronodular metastases in the lung and possibly mediastinum (*short arrow*). The activity designated by the *long arrow* was physiological liver activity

Comment Again, the selection of an appropriate prescribed activity of ^{131}I for treatment is problematic and discussed above. Unlike the previous figure, this pattern of pulmonary metastases may be associated with a lower likelihood of diffuse acute radiation pneumonitis and/or pulmonary fibrosis. In addition, if either one or both occur, the diffuse acute radiation pneumonitis or fibrosis should be more localized to the area around the macronodules. However, as reported in the external radiation therapy literature, abscopal effects may occur, which are pulmonary changes outside the radiation port [27–30].

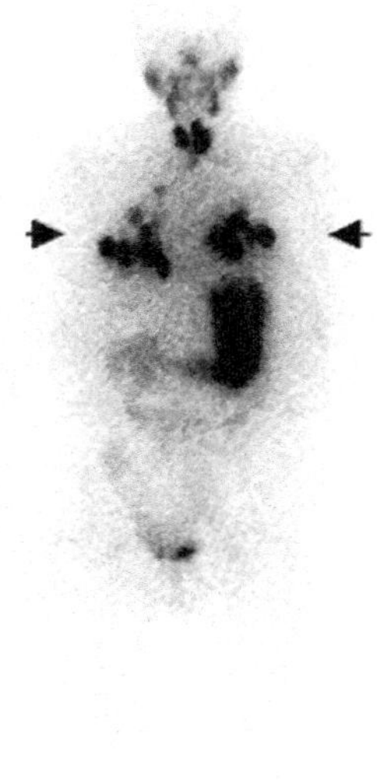

Fig. 12.20 This whole body image performed 48 h after radioiodine administration again demonstrates predominantly macronodules more localized to the mid- and lower lung fields (*arrow heads*)

Pulmonary Metastasis: Macro- and Micronodular

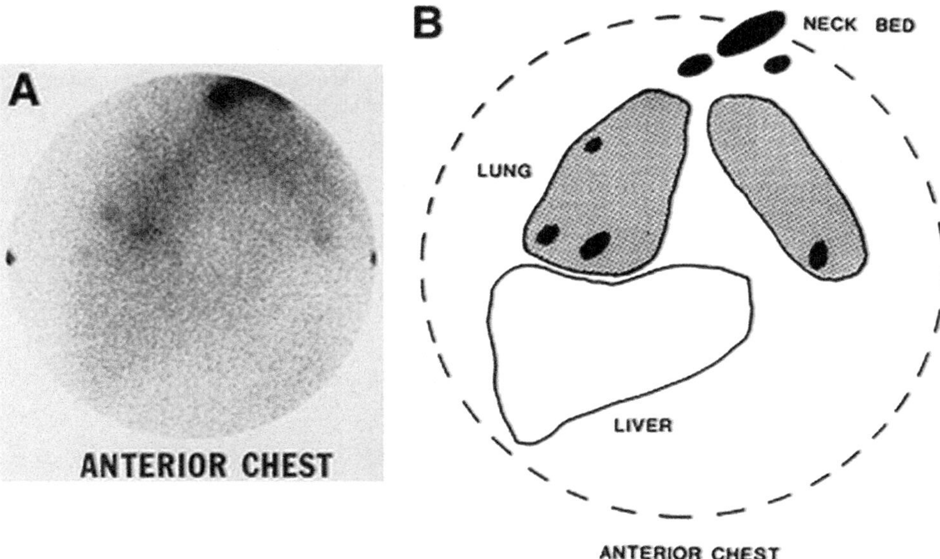

Fig. 12.21 The patient was shifted slightly to his *left* for this anterior chest and abdominal image (**A**), and the accompanying diagram (**B**) should aid in identification of the findings. This image demonstrates increased radioiodine in the thyroid bed, diffuse moderately increased radioiodine throughout most of both lungs (which is indicative of micronodular metastases), and faint but definite focal areas of increased radioiodine in the mid- to lower lung fields. The focal areas of radioactivity were attributed to pulmonary macronodular metastases. The CT of the chest confirmed both micronodular and macronodular pattern in the lung without any changes in the bones to account for bony metastasis. Trace amount of radioactivity is noted in the liver and is normal. This case demonstrates that both pulmonary patterns of macronodular and micronodular disease may occur together (Reproduced with permission from Lippincott, Williams, and Wilkins [2])

Liver Metastases

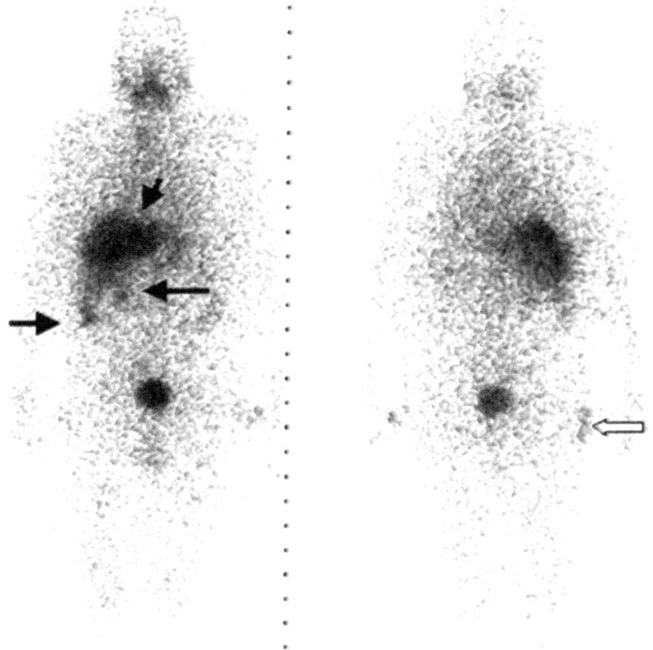

Fig. 12.22 These whole body images demonstrate inhomogeneous accumulation of ^{131}I in the liver (*black arrows*) secondary to confirmed multiple liver metastases. The patient had a total thyroidectomy, and the images were performed prior to ^{131}I treatment. The *left* and *right* panels are the anterior and posterior whole body images, respectively. A radioactivity-contaminated handkerchief (*white arrow*) is seen in the posterior view in the right pocket. These images were contributed by Milton G. Gross, MD, University of Michigan Medical School, and Ann Arbor, MI

Comment Metastasis to the liver is rare but does occur. Physiological radioiodine uptake in the liver can be distinguished from metastatic disease by assessment of the pattern of uptake (diffuse vs focal), distribution of uptake (homogeneous versus inhomogeneous), and possibly intensity (low vs high). Physiological uptake would be typically more diffuse and more homogeneous, have lower intensity, and be associated with significant uptake of radioactivity in the thyroid bed or in other functioning metastases [14]. (See Fig. 12.12 of physiological liver uptake above.) Metastases would be more focal, inhomogeneous, and not necessarily associated with significant uptake of radioactivity elsewhere. Of course, further diagnostic imaging, such as with CT, magnetic resonance imaging (MRI), ultrasound, and/or SPECT should be useful.

No significant data are available regarding how the presence of liver metastases would influence the prescribed activity of ^{131}I or the side effects of ^{131}I in patients with liver metastases. A hyperfunctioning liver metastasis has been reported [31].

Bone Metastases

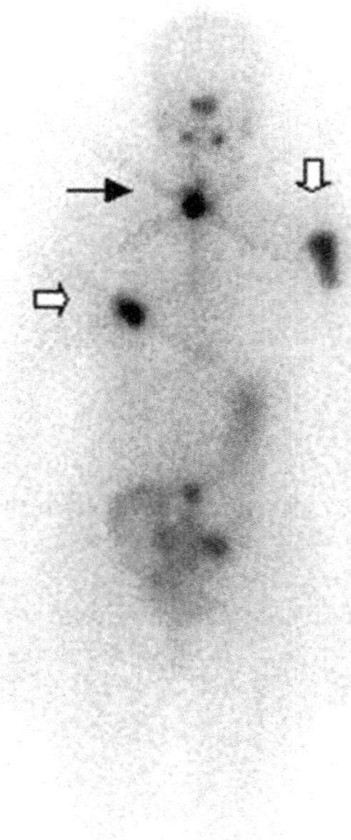

Fig. 12.23 This pretherapy whole body scan performed 72 h after administration of ^{131}I demonstrates abnormal radioiodine uptake in the proximal left humerus and one of the anterior right ribs (*white arrows*). The abnormality in the left humerus was confirmed histopathologically to be metastatic differentiated thyroid carcinoma, and a CT of right anterior ribs confirmed changes consistent with bone metastasis. Significant residual radioactivity is noted in the thyroid bed consistent with postoperative residual thyroid tissue after a near-total thyroidectomy (*black arrow*). Note the starburst-pattern artifact of radioactivity in the area of uptake in the thyroid bed and possibly the right rib (see Fig. 12.28)

Comment Focal uptake that appears to be in the bone on anterior and/or posterior views should be confirmed with SPECT-CT or lateral or oblique planar views. Bone uptake should not be taken as prima facie evidence for metastatic bone disease. Plain radiographs, CT without contrast, and/or MRI should be performed to help confirm the presence of metastases or to identify other etiologies for the bony uptake. If a metastasis to the bone is confirmed, consider (1) increasing the empiric prescribed activity for ^{131}I treatment, (2) determining the maximal prescribed activity for ^{131}I treatment by dosimetry, and/or (3) treating with external beam radiotherapy. Radiofrequency ablation has also been used with success (see Chaps. 65 and 67).

Brain Metastasis

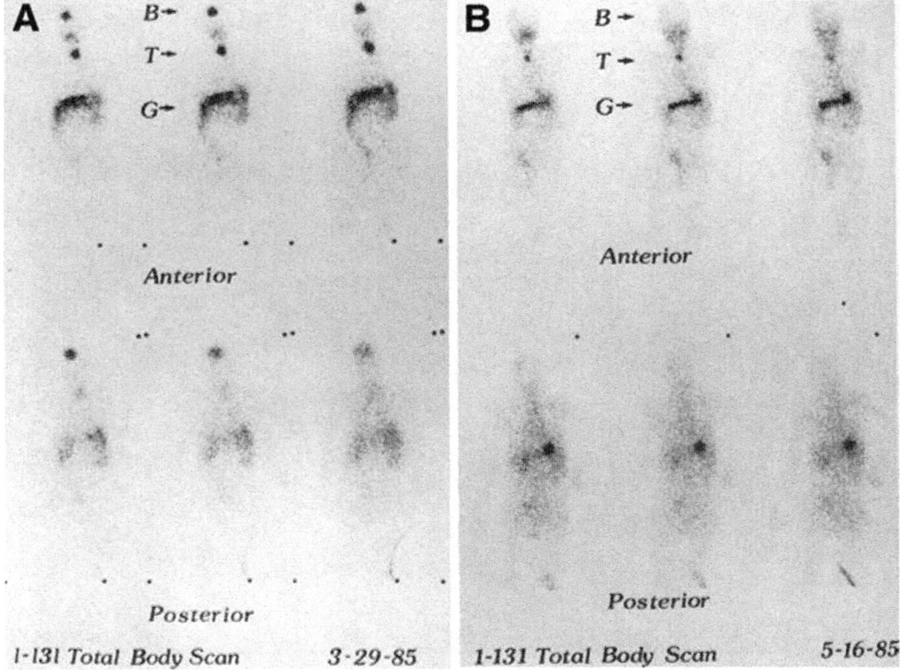

Fig. 12.24 Parts (**A, B**) are coronal tomographic whole body ^{131}I images. Proceeding from *left* to *right* and *top* to *bottom*, the coronal slices progress from anterior to posterior. Part (**A**) demonstrates abnormal radioiodine accumulation in the head (*B*), which was confirmed as an intracerebral metastasis. Activity is present in the thyroid bed (*T*) and gastrointestinal areas (*G*). After the intracerebral metastasis was resected, repeat images approx 48 days after administration (part **B**) illustrate resolution of the abnormal uptake in the intracerebral metastasis with residual faint background activity. The latter was attributed to postoperative blood pool (Reproduced with permission of the American Medical Association [32])

Comment Focal uptake that appears to be in the brain on anterior and/or posterior views should be confirmed with SPECT-CT or with lateral or oblique planar views. An MR is also warranted. Intracerebral metastases are infrequent (see Chap. 56). Misaki et al. [32] report intracerebral metastasis in 5.4 % of 167 patients who had lung or bone metastases. In this group, none of the brain lesions had significant uptake of radioiodine despite accumulation in most of the extracerebral metastases.

Management includes surgical resection, stereotactic radiosurgery, external beam irradiation, and/or radioiodine. If ^{131}I is to be administered for the treatment of intracerebral metastasis, pretreatment of the patient on steroids, glycerol, or mannitol should be considered.

Renal Metastasis

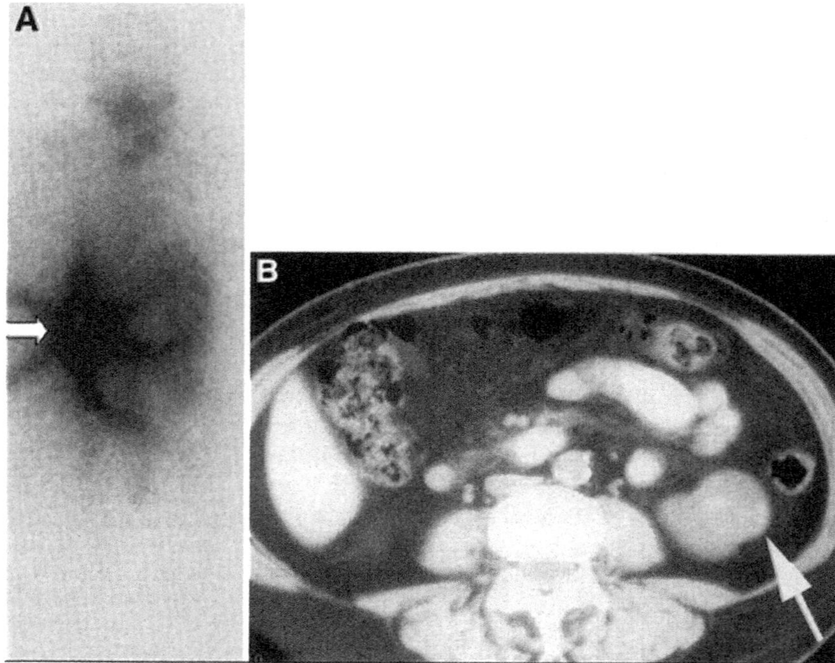

Fig. 12.25 Part (**A**) is a post-therapy posterior ^{131}I whole body scan that demonstrates a prominent "star" artifact (*white arrow*) in the upper left quadrant of the abdomen, which was secondary to a renal metastasis from well-differentiated thyroid cancer. The "star" artifact is discussed in Fig. 12.28. Part (**B**) is the transverse CT image of the abdomen, demonstrating (*white arrow*) the metastasis in the inferolateral aspect of the kidney. Metastatic well-differentiated thyroid cancer was confirmed in the renal mass by histopathology (Reproduced with permission of Mary Ann Liebert, Inc. [33])

Comment Renal metastasis from well-differentiated thyroid carcinoma has been reported but is rare [31, 32]. Radioiodine is excreted by the kidneys, and radioiodine accumulation in the kidney secondary to radioiodine retention in the renal collecting system should not be mistaken for a renal metastasis [35].

Part 4: Examples of False-Positive Uptake and Artifacts

Ovarian Cystadenoma

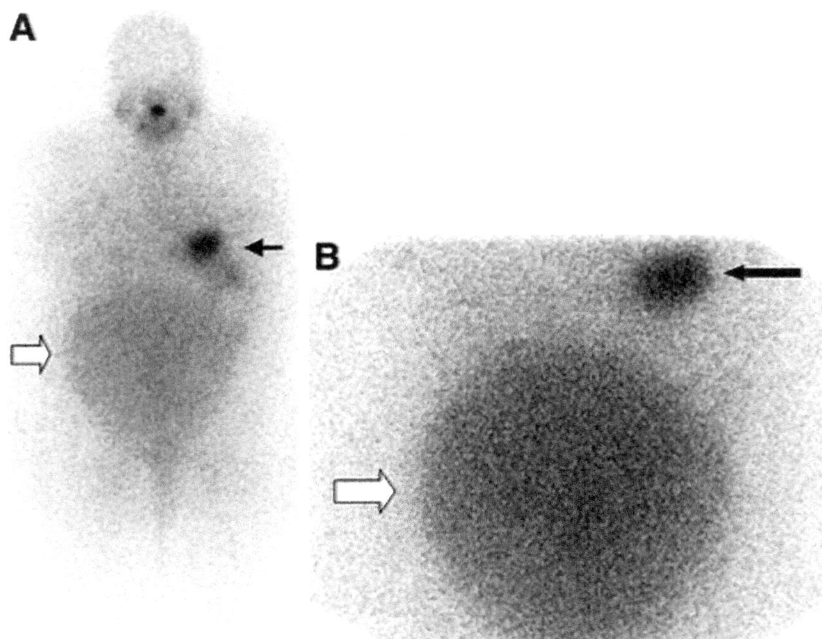

Fig. 12.26 The whole body scan (**A**) was performed 24 h after the administration of 37 MBq (1 mCi) of ^{123}I and demonstrates a large circular area of modest radioiodine accumulation (*white arrow*). (**B**) is a static image of the abdominal-pelvic area showing the same finding (*white arrow*). Surgery confirmed a large ovarian cystadenoma. The more intense radioiodine accumulation in the left upper quadrant of the abdomen (*black arrows*) was attributed to physiological activity in the stomach

Comment Radioiodine accumulation in an ovarian cystadenoma has been reported [37]. The mechanism of radioiodine accumulation in the ovarian cyst is unknown.

Dentures

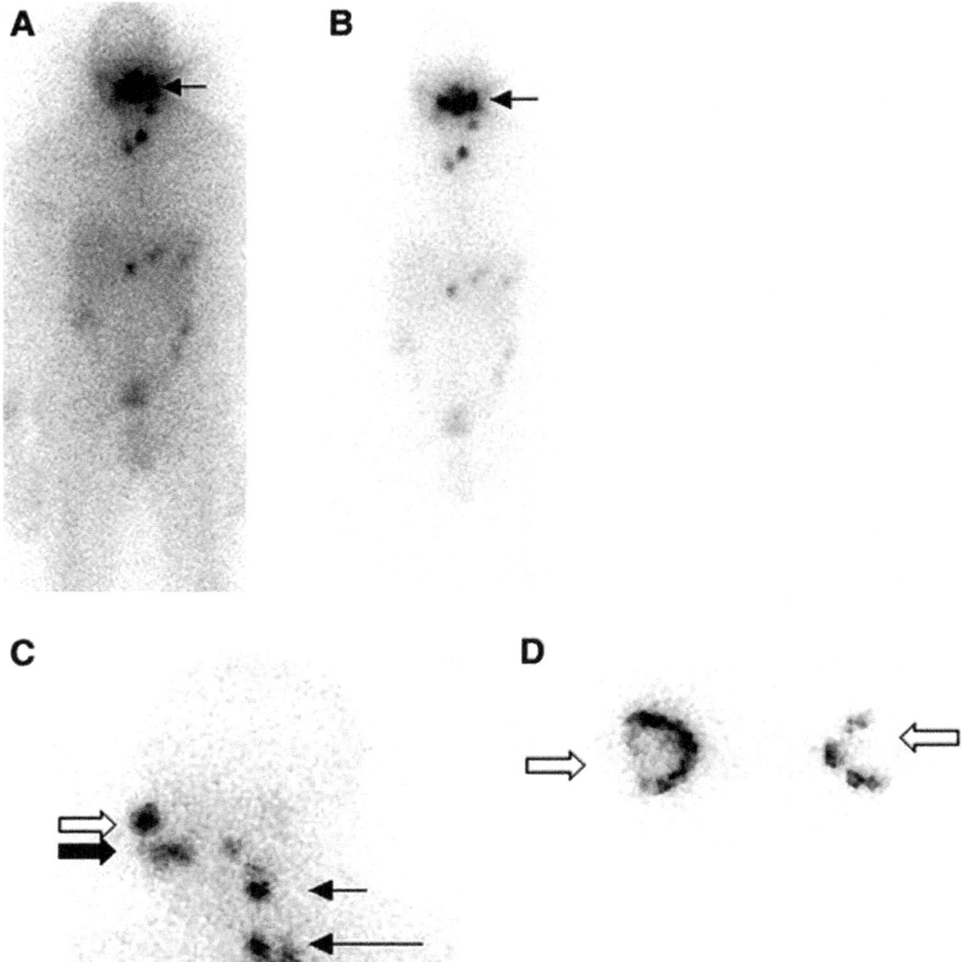

Fig. 12.27 The whole body radioiodine image (**A**) demonstrates uptake in the neck and face; however, the radioactivity in the mouth area is more prominent than usual (*arrow* in high intensity image in **A** and low-intensity image in **B**). Upon further history and after removal of the patient's dentures, the patient was reimaged, and the radioactivity in the mouth region was normal (**C**) (*large white arrow* nose; *large black arrow* oral area; *thin black arrow* salivary gland or metastases; *long thin arrow* thyroid tissue). Separate images of the *upper* and *lower* dentures illustrated the significant radioactivity around the dentures (**D**) (*white arrows*)

Comment The etiologies of false-positive areas of radioiodine accumulation are extensive and discussed in detail in Chap. 13. Uptake from poor dental hygiene has been reported [38].

Septal Penetration

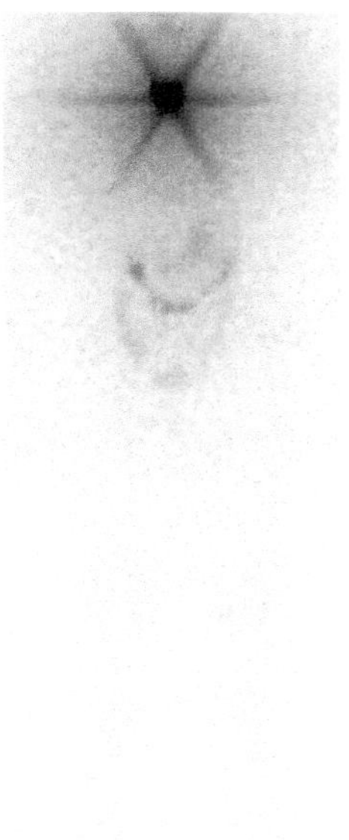

Fig. 12.28 This whole body scan was performed 48 h after the oral administration of 148 MBq (4 mCi) of ^{131}I and demonstrates significant uptake in the thyroid bed, which is not a radioactive marker. Radioactivity is noted, projecting outward in six symmetrical linear "rays" from the intense focal area of radioactivity in the thyroid bed. Owing to the configuration of this pattern, this area has been described as a "star" artifact

Comment For a full discussion, see Chap. 11. This is truly an "artifact" because the events being recorded in the image along those projections did not originate at those locations within the patient but instead are malpositioned events that come from the thyroid bed uptake. This phenomenon occurs throughout the image, but it is only apparent around areas of intense radioiodine concentration.

In brief, the γ waves from the ^{131}I have penetrated the thinnest portion of the lead septa of the parallel-hole collimator and are thus visualized. The thinnest portion may depend on the shape and construction of the collimator. In this example, the collimator hole is a hexagon, and the thinnest portion is that portion of the septa between each junction.

This artifact may limit the ability of the scan to show nearby functioning metastases. In addition, because of the intense radioiodine uptake in the thyroid bed, the pattern of radioactivity in that area cannot be demonstrated. As pointed out in the previous figure, this may be important for comparison with subsequent scans. A pinhole collimator does not produce this artifact and will resolve this dilemma.

Off-Peak Artifacts

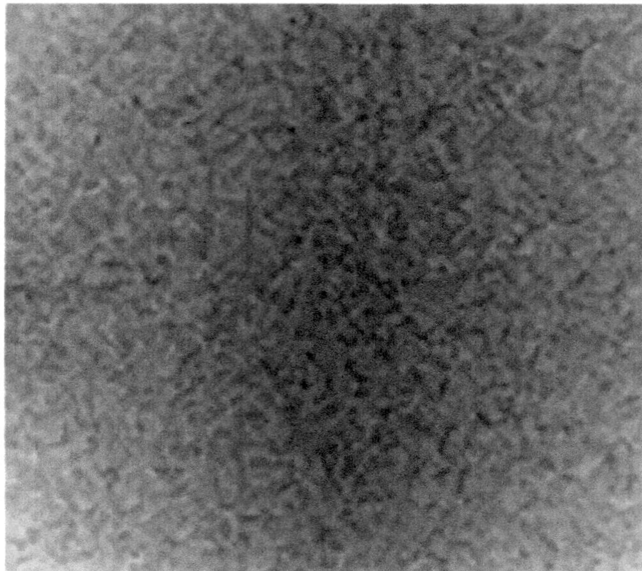

Fig. 12.29 The above image is a whole body scan obtained 48-h post-administration of ^{131}I. No identifiable uptake, structure, or outline of the body is noted. The technologist was using an incorrect energy peak for ^{131}I

Comment As noted at the beginning of the chapter, the physician must ensure that the images are obtained according to the facility's protocol and are of diagnostic quality. Although the newer cameras help minimize the various setup and acquisition errors and the nuclear medicine technologist should be able to identify and correct these errors, errors may still occur. The interpreting physician must still have a good working knowledge of technical artifacts to be able to identify and troubleshoot them. This figure is an example of one of the many technical artifacts.

Low Counts

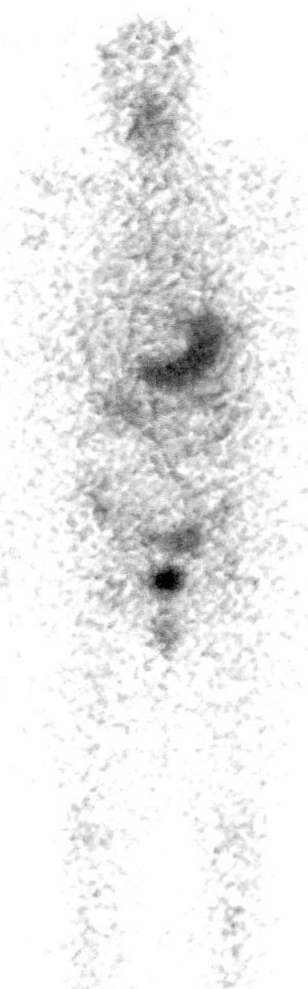

Fig. 12.30 This whole body scan was performed 48 h after the administration of ^{131}I. The image appears "grainy," which is a result of low counts

Comment Low counts in the image may be the result of such factors as (1) low diagnostic prescribed activity administered, (2) partially infiltrated dose, (3) delayed imaging in a patient with fast clearance, and/or (4) shortened acquisition time of the study.

When there are insufficient counts in a whole body scan, the sensitivity of the scan for the detection of functioning metastases is reduced. The higher the counts are, the more likely that significant accumulation of radioiodine can be differentiated from background and noise.

Part 5: Tools Other than SPECT-CT to Help Differentiate Metastases from Non-thyroidal Physiological Uptake, False-Positives, and Artifact

The Value of "Uptake-Specific" History and Patient Examination

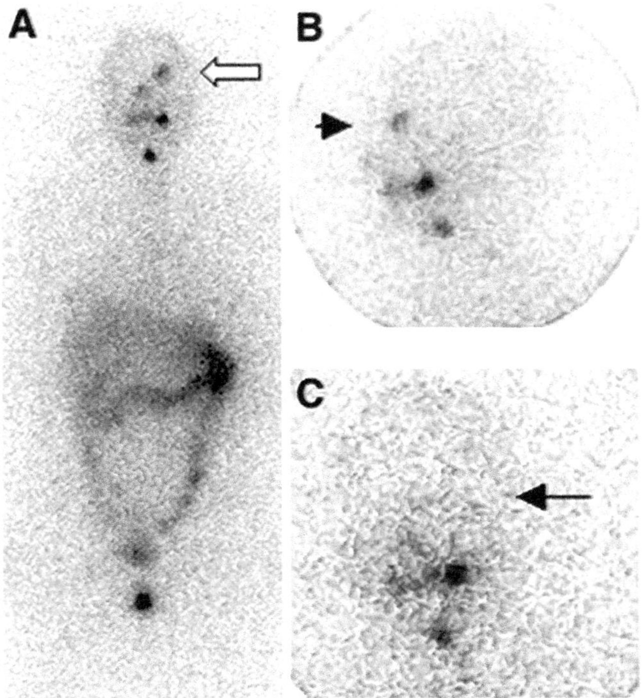

Fig. 12.31 This whole body scan (**A**) was performed 24 h after the administration of low prescribed activity of ^{123}I (18.5 MBq [500 uCi]) and demonstrated several asymmetric areas of uptake in the neck and face. The area of interest is the accumulation of radioactivity in the left eye or skull region (*arrow*). The lateral view (**B**) suggests that the uptake was either in the left eye or adjacent bone, raising the possibility of a bone metastasis (*arrow*). With additional "uptake-specific" history and examination, it was determined that the patient had an artificial eyeball prosthesis on this side. After removing the artificial eyeball and re-imaging the face, the foci of radioactivity disappeared (**C**) (*arrow*)

Comment "Uptake-specific" history (i.e., questions directed specifically at areas of suspicious uptake seen on the scan) and examination of the patient can frequently resolve the etiology of an area of radioactivity uptake and improve the specificity of the whole body radioiodine scan. Although this teaching point should be self-evident, knowledge of an adequate history and a thorough physical examination in the area of interest are not universal performed. Uptake secondary to an artificial eyeball [39] should not be interpreted as bone or brain metastasis.

This is only one example of the wide spectrum of false-positive or artifactual radioiodine accumulation (see Chap. 13).

Utility of Pinhole Collimator Images

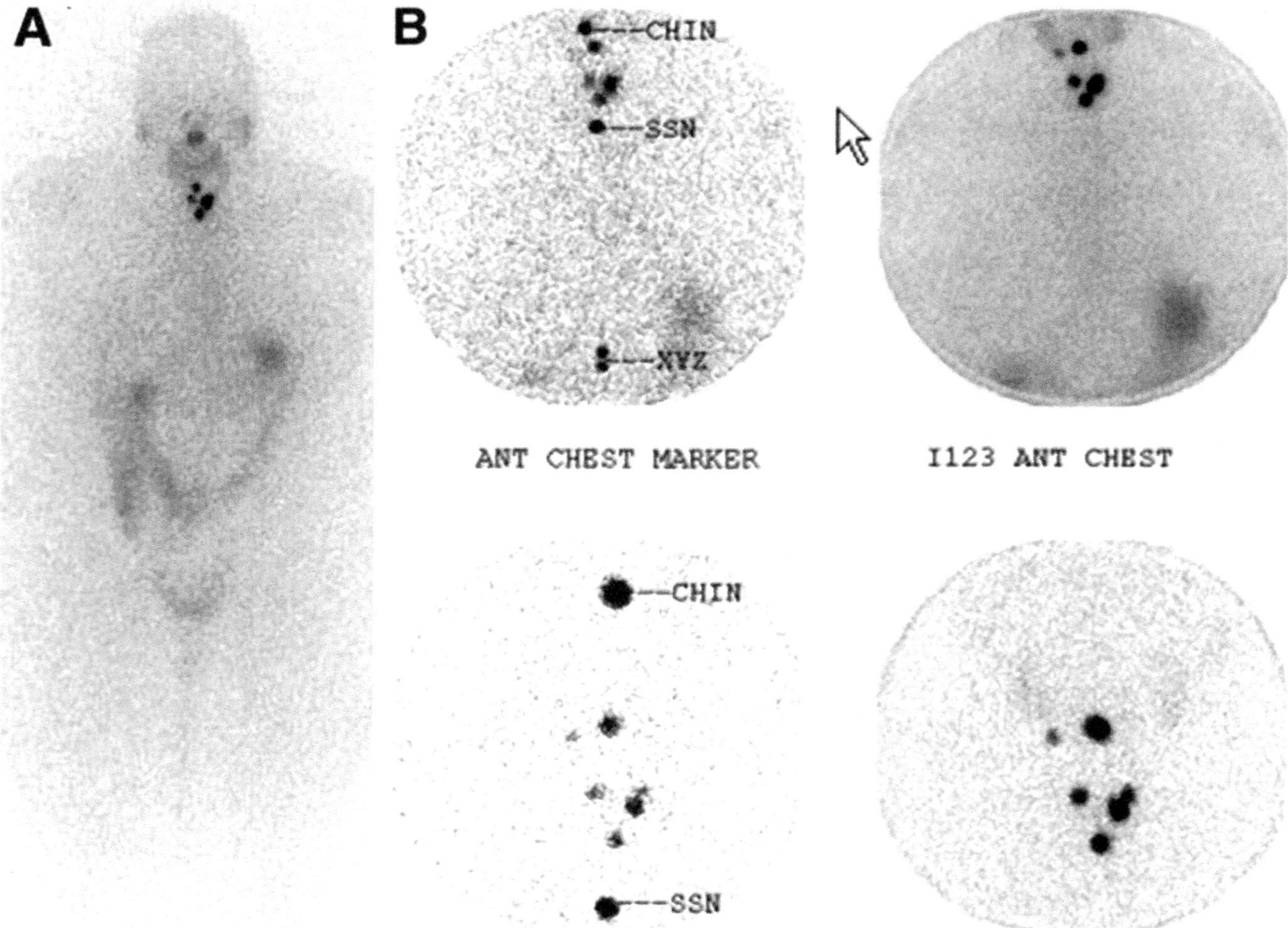

Fig. 12.32 This figure demonstrates the utility of pinhole collimator images, which are discussed in more detail in Chap. 11). (**A**) is the whole body image that shows four distinct areas of uptake in the thyroid bed consistent with normal residual tissue remaining after a near-total thyroidectomy. In imaging (**B**), the *upper left* image was obtained using a parallel-hole collimator, and external markers were placed over the chin, suprasternal notch (*SSN*), and xiphoid (*XYZ*) to "mark" these anatomical locations on the image. After the markers are removed, and without moving the patient, a second image was performed for a significantly longer time. The resulting image on the *upper right* demonstrates five areas of thyroid tissue. The lower set of images of (**B**) was obtained using a pinhole collimator with the "marker" image on the *left*. The image on the *lower right*, which has no markers, illustrates six distinct foci of radioiodine accumulation with several outside the thyroid bed.

Comment Pinhole collimator images have higher resolution than "spot-camera" or whole body camera images performed with a parallel-hole collimator for small targeted areas, e.g., the thyroid bed. In this patient, the differentiation of six, rather than four, foci of radioiodine accumulation and location suggest a higher likelihood of cervical lymph node metastases. Kulkarni et al. have reported on the value of pinhole images vs individual or whole body images obtained with a parallel-hole collimator [36].

For those facilities that administer a fixed empiric prescribed activity of ^{131}I for ablation without first performing a scan or regardless of the scan findings, the additional findings seen on the pinhole collimator images would not be of value. However, for those facilities that will either reconsider additional imaging, fine-needle aspiration, additional surgery, and/or an increase in the prescribed activity of ^{131}I for adjuvant therapy rather than remnant ablation, then pinhole collimator images are valuable.

The pinhole images also provide a superior baseline study for future comparison. If the patient has persistent elevation of serum thyroglobulin levels or develops evidence of some other recurrence, a previous baseline pinhole collimator image helps differentiate whether the radioactivity on a new scan is a new region or one of the previous areas that was not completely ablated.

Value of Lateral Views

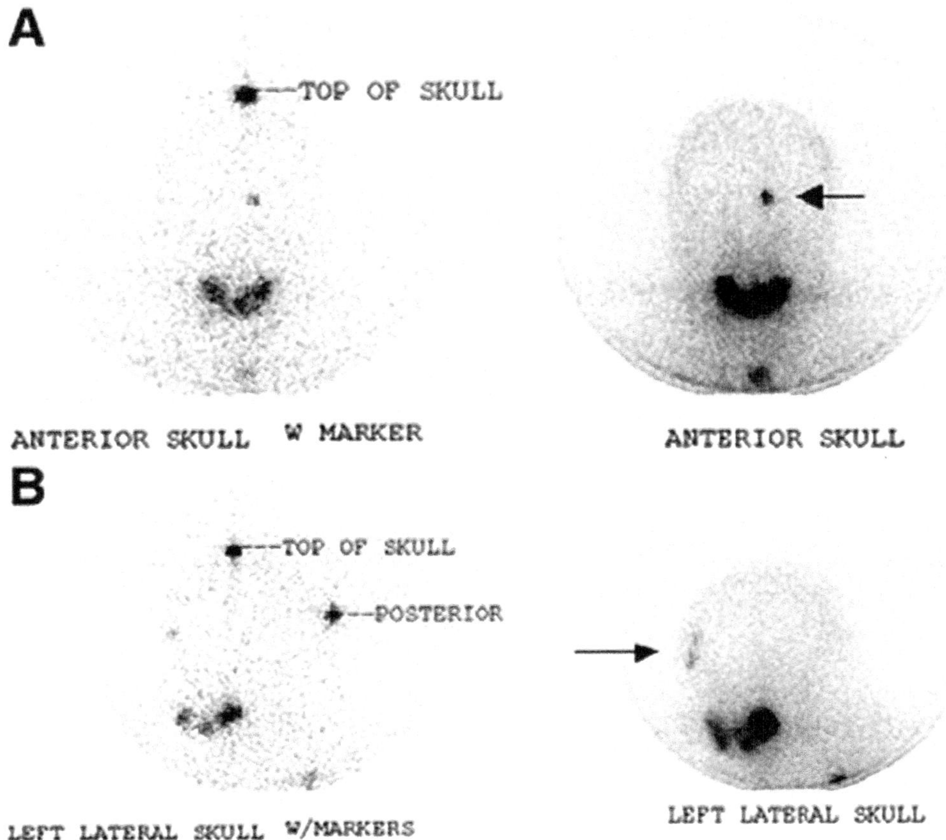

Fig. 12.33 The image on the *upper left* of (**A**) was obtained using a parallel-hole collimator camera, taken of the head in the anterior view with a marker on the *top* of the calvarium (a "spot-camera" view). The acquisition time was only long enough to allow the marker to be clearly visualized. The marker was then removed, and without moving the patient, an image was performed for a significantly longer duration. This latter image, which is shown on the *upper right*, demonstrates a focus of intense radioactivity in the midline (*arrow*). The radioactivity immediately inferior to this represents physiological oropharyngeal-nasal radioiodine accumulation. The lateral view with markers (*left image* in **B**) and without markers (*right image* in **B**) suggests that the radioactivity is in the bone, not the brain, which a non-contrast CT confirmed

Comment When a SPECT-CT is not available, lateral views can be useful to further localize radioactivity and are frequently helpful to improve the specificity of radioiodine accumulation. Although the lateral view may not always localize conclusively the radioiodine accumulation, it may still be useful either (1) as a guide for CT and MRI evaluation or (2) for comparison with future scans.

Further confirmation is always warranted such as with a non-contrast CT or MRI.

Value of Patient Markers

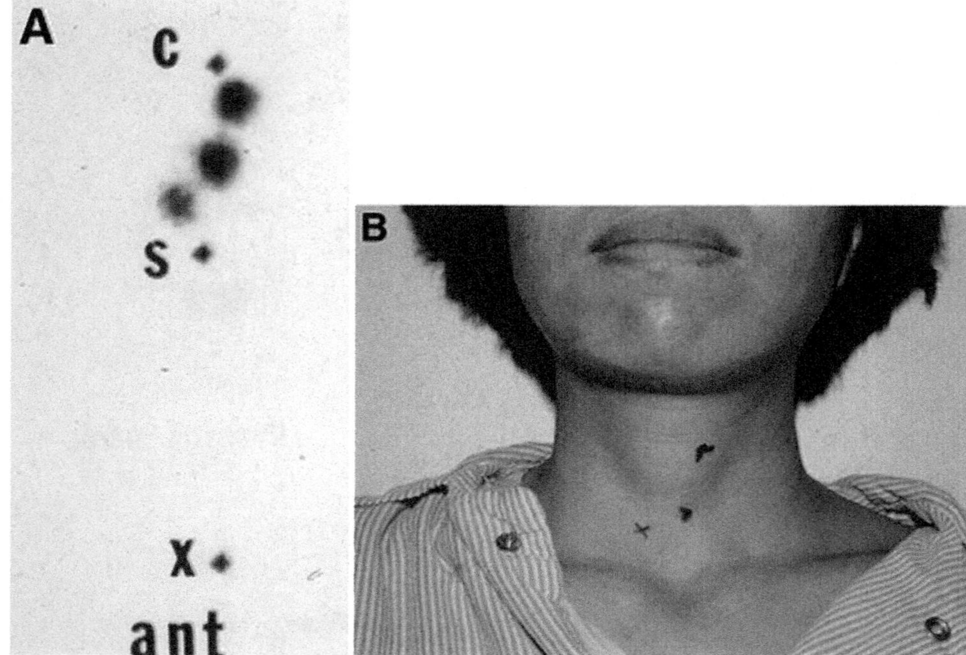

Fig. 12.34 Part (**A**) is an anterior (*ant*) parallel-hole collimator image obtained 48 h after ^{131}I administration. Radioactive markers are placed at the chin (*c*), suprasternal notch (*s*), and xiphoid (*x*). Three focal areas of radioiodine uptake are noted in the thyroid bed. With the use of a radioactive marker, these areas were localized to the patient's skin (**B**)

Comment As already noted in many earlier figures, radioactive markers can be useful to denote anatomical landmarks and are frequently so indispensable that they are virtually mandatory. Marking the patient's skin can also be valuable by demonstrating that an area of radioiodine accumulation localizes to a palpable mass, lymph node, or salivary gland. Subsequently, these anatomical markers may guide ultrasound evaluation. Of note, radioactive markers should not be positioned in such a way that the uptake is obscured under the marker, except when used to localize the region within the patient. Also, when a pinhole collimator is used, the pinhole may distort the location of a marker relative to a deeper structure. This is beyond the scope of this atlas, but when marking a focal area of activity with a pinhole collimator, always place the focal area of activity in the center of the field of view of the pinhole collimator before marking the skin surface.

Part 6: Miscellaneous

^{124}I PET

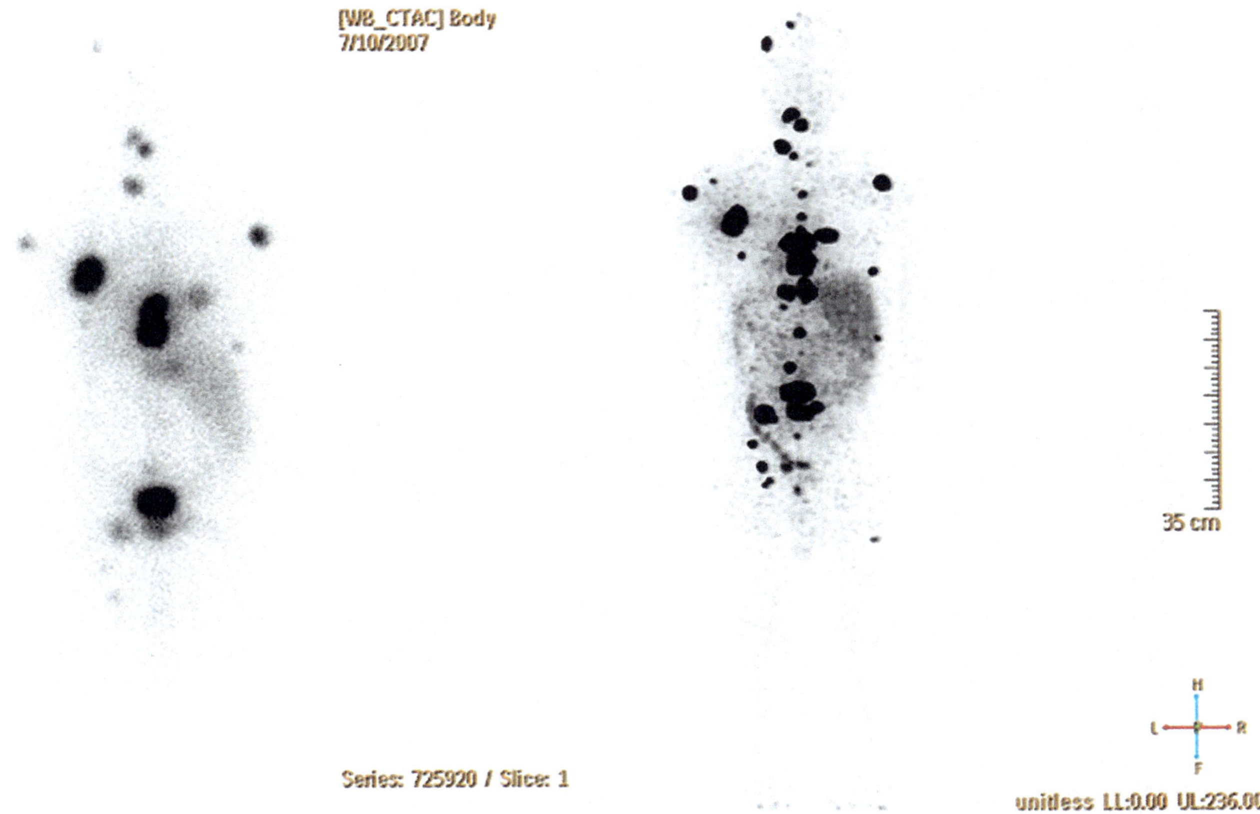

Fig. 12.35 Both of the above images were obtained in the same patient. The image on the *left* is a pretherapy anterior planar ^{131}I whole body image demonstrating approximately 18 foci of ^{131}I uptake indicative of metastatic differentiated thyroid cancer. The image on the *right* is the anterior ^{124}I PET image from the maximum intensity projection (MIPS) demonstrating multiple additional foci of ^{124}I uptake suggesting metastatic differentiated thyroid cancer that were not detected on the ^{131}I images (This figure was originally published in Van Nostrand et al. [42]. Reproduced with permission from Mary Ann Liebert, Inc. Publishers)

Comment The potential advantages and disadvantages of ^{124}I PET have already been discussed in detail in Chap. 103. The advantages include:

- Higher spatial and contrast resolution
- Tomographic images
- A half-life that permits delayed imaging
- The ability to perform lesional, blood (bone marrow), and other organ dosimetries
- The ability to fuse and thereby coregister the PET images with CT and/or MRI for more precise anatomical localization and improved specificity of the ^{124}I foci of radioactivity

The present disadvantages are availability, cost, and the potential for stunning (Reproduced with permission from Mary Ann Liebert, Inc.) [42].

References

1. Wartofsky L. Thyroid nodules. In: Van Nostrand D, Bloom G, Wartofsky L, editors. Thyroid cancer: a guide for patients. Baltimore: Keystone Press; 2004. p. 15–31.
2. Manier S, Van Nostrand D, Atkins F, Wu SY. I-131 neck and chest scintigraphy. In: Van Nostrand D, Baum S, editors. Primers and atlases of clinical nuclear medicine. Philadelphia: J.B. Lippincott Co.; 1988.
3. Makani S, Kim W, Gaba AR. Struma ovarii with a focus of papillary thyroid cancer: a case report and review of the literature. Gynecol Oncol. 2004;94:835–9.
4. Griffiths AN, Jain B, Vine SJ. Papillary thyroid carcinoma of struma ovarii. J Obstet Gynaecol. 2004;24:92–3.
5. DeSimone CP, Lele SM, Modesitt SC. Malignant struma ovarii: a case report and analysis of cases reported in the literature with focus on survival and I-131 therapy. Gynecol Oncol. 2003;89:543–8.
6. Yeh E, Mead RC, Ruetz PP. Radionuclide study of struma ovarii. J Nucl Med. 1973;14:118–24.
7. Salvatori M, Rufini V, Daidone MS, et al. Occasional detection of "struma ovarii" in a patient with thyroid cancer. La Radiologia Med. 1991;81:744–7.
8. Kulkarni K, Kim SM, Intenzo C. Can salivary gland uptakes on a diagnostic I-131 scan predict acute salivary gland dysfunction in patients receiving radioiodine therapy for thyroid cancer? J Nucl Med. 2004;5S:291P.
9. Norby EH, Neutze J, Van Nostrand D, et al. Nasal radioiodine activity; a prospective study of frequency, intensity, and pattern. J Nucl Med. 1990;31:52–4.
10. Van Nostrand D, Neutze J, Atkins F. Side effects of "rational dose" iodine-131 therapy for metastatic well differentiated thyroid carcinoma. J Nucl Med. 1986;27:1519–27.
11. Jackson GL, Flickinger FW, Graham WP, Kennedy TJ. Thymus accumulation of radioactive iodine. Penn Med. 1979;11:37–8.
12. Wilson RL, Cowan R. Tc-99m pertechnetate uptake in a thymoma: case report. Clin Nucl Med. 1982;7:149–50.
13. Vermiglio F, Baudin E, Travagli P, et al. Iodine concentration by the thymus in thyroid carcinoma. J Nucl Med. 1996;37:1830–1.
14. Ziessman HA, Bahar H, Fahey FH, Dubiansky V. Hepatic visualization of iodine-131 whole body thyroid cancer scans. J Nucl Med. 1987;28:1408–11.
15. Chung JK, Lee YJ, Jeong YM, et al. Clinical significance of hepatic visualization on iodine-131 whole body scan in patients with thyroid carcinoma. J Nucl Med. 1997;38:1191–5.
16. Oppenheimer JH. Thyroid hormones in liver. Mayo Clin Proc. 1972;47:854–63.
17. Hillier AP. Deiodination of thyroid hormones by the perfused rat liver. J Physiol. 1972;222:475–85.
18. Davidson J, McDougall IR. How frequently is the thymus seen on whole body iodine-131 diagnostic and post-treatment scans? Eur J Nucl Med. 2000;27:425–30.
19. Michigishi T, Mizukami Y, Shuke N, et al. Visualization of the thymus with therapeutic doses of radioiodine in patients with thyroid cancer. Eur J Nucl Med. 1993;20:75–9.
20. Van Nostrand. Radioiodine whole body scanning: overview and the different types of scans for well-differentiated thyroid cancer. In: Van Nostrand D, Bloom G, Wartofsky L, editors. Thyroid cancer: a guide for patients. Baltimore: Keystone Press; 2004. p. 111–23.
21. Chennupati S, Van Nostrand D, Kharazi P, et al. Determination of the Number of Foci of Normal Thyroid Tissue Remaining After Thyroidectomy in Patients with Differentiated Thyroid Cancer: The Washington Hospital Center Experience. J Nucl Med 2011; 52(Suppl):1300.
22. Thomas SR, Maxon HR, Kereiakes JG. In vivo quantitation of lesion radioactivity using external counting methods. Med Phys. 1976;3:253–5.
23. Thomas SR, Maxon HR, Kereiakes JG, Saenger EL. Quantitative external counting techniques enabling improved diagnostic and therapeutic decisions in patients with well-differentiated thyroid cancer. Radiology. 1997;122:731–7.
24. Schlumberge M, Challeton C, De Vathaire F, et al. Radioactive iodine treatment and external radiotherapy for lung and bone metastases from thyroid carcinoma. J Nucl Med. 1996;l37:598–605.
25. Nemec J, Zamrazil V, Pohunkova D, Roohling S. Radioiodide treatment of pulmonary metastases of differentiated thyroid cancer. Results and prognostic factors. Nuklearmedizin. 1979; 18:86–90.
26. Schlumberger M, Tubiana M, De Vathaire F, et al. Long-term results of treatment of 283 patients with lung and bone metastases from differentiated thyroid cancer. J Clin Endocrinol Metab. 1986;63:960–7.
27. Bennett DE, Million RR, Ackerman IV. Bilateral radiation pneumonitis. A complication of the radiotherapy of bronchogenic carcinoma. Cancer. 1969;23:1001–18.
28. Fulkerson WJ, McLendon RE, Prosnitz LR. Adult respiratory distress syndrome after limited radiotherapy. Cancer. 1986;57: 1941–6.
29. Hindié E, Melliere D, Lange F, et al. Functioning pulmonary metastases of thyroid cancer: does radioiodine influence the prognosis? J Nucl Med. 2003;30:974–81.
30. Monson JM, Start P, Reilly JJ, et al. Clinical radiation pneumonitis and radiographic changes after thoracic radiation therapy for lung carcinoma. Cancer. 1998;82:842–50.
31. Guglielmi R, Pacella CM, Dottorini ME, et al. Severe thyrotoxicosis due to hyperfunctioning liver metastasis from follicular carcinoma: treatment with (131)I and interstitial laser ablation. Thyroid. 1999;9:173–7.
32. Misaki T, Iwata M, Kasagi K, Konishi J. Brain metastasis from differentiated thyroid cancer in patients treated with radioiodine for bone and lung lesions. Ann Nucl Med. 2000;14:111–4.
33. Parker LN, Wu SY, Kim DD, et al. Recurrence of papillary thyroid carcinoma presenting as a focal neurologic deficit. Arch Int Med. 1986;146:1985–7.
34. Smallridge RC, Castro MR, Morris JC, et al. Renal metastases from thyroid papillary carcinoma: study of sodium iodide symporter expression. Thyroid. 2001;11:795–804.
35. Bakheet SM, Hammami MM, Powe J. False-positive radioiodine uptake in the abdomen and the pelvis: radioiodine retention in the kidneys and review of the literature. Clin Nucl Med. 1996;21: 932–7.
36. Kulkarni K, Van Nostrand D, Young-Rok S, Aiken M, Mete M, Burman K, Wartofsky L. Detectability of foci of radioiodine uptake in the thyroid bed and neck comparing pin-hole with parallel-hole collimators. Nucl Med Commun. 2011;32:369–74.
37. Kim EE, Pjura G, Gobuty A, et al. 131-I uptake in a benign serous cystadenoma of the ovary. Eur J Nucl Med. 1984;9:433–5.
38. Morgan R, Cote M. Abnormal uptake of I-131 mimicking salivary gland uptake in a patient with diffuse dental disease. Clin Nucl Med. 2000;25:314–5.
39. Howarth DM, Forstrom LA, O'Connor MK, et al. Patient-related pitfalls and artifacts in nuclear medicine imaging. Semin Nucl Med. 1996;26:295–307.
40. Sgouros G, Kolbert KS, Sheikh A, et al. Patient-specific dosimetry for ^{131}I thyroid cancer therapy using 124-I PET and 3-dimensional internal dosimetry (3D-ID) software. J Nucl Med. 2004;45: 1366–72.
41. Casara D, Rubello D, Saladini G, et al. Different features of pulmonary metastases in differentiated thyroid cancer: natural history and multivariate statistical analysis of prognostic variables. J Nucl Med. 1993;34:1626–31.
42. Van Nostrand D, Moreau S, Bandaru VV, Atkins A, Chennupati S, Mete M, Burman K, Wartofsky L. ^{124}I positron emission tomography versus ^{131}I planar imaging in the identification of residual thyroid tissue and/or metastasis in patients who have well-differentiated thyroid cancer. Thyroid. 2010;20:879–83.

False-Positive Radioiodine Scans in Thyroid Cancer

13

Brahm Shapiro, Vittoria Rufini, Ayman Jarwan, Onelio Geatti, Kimberlee J. Kearfott, Lorraine M. Fig, Ian David Kirkwood, John E. Freitas, Anca M. Avram, Ka Kit Wong, and Milton D. Gross

Introduction

Whole-body radioiodine imaging of patients with thyroid cancer after thyroidectomy is widely accepted as a critical component necessary for appropriate decision-making in the treatment of this disease for over six decades [1–14]. The value of the technique lies in the identification and functional localization of foci of normal thyroid tissues, residual tumor, and locoregional and distant metastatic spread which is virtually undetectable by any other imaging modality [6, 8–10]. Furthermore, uptake of radioiodine on diagnostic imaging facilitates selection of patients for subsequent radioiodine therapy [6, 8, 9].

It is the singularly unique property of thyroid tissue(s) to concentrate, organify, and retain radioiodine that makes the modality so valuable in the diagnosis and treatment of thyroid cancer where foci of uptake on postthyroidectomy scans are highly specific for the presence of thyroid tissue, be it a residual remnant of normal thyroid or malignancy in the neck or in distant metastases [2, 7–9, 11–19]. Unfortunately, the otherwise high specificity of radioiodine for tissues of thyroid origin is confounded by uptake in other tissues with the ability to concentrate, but not organify radioiodine (Fig. 13.1). These tissues include the choroid plexus, salivary glands, nasopharynx, stomach, and other organs that participate in iodine metabolism and excretion such as the kidney, liver, gut, and bladder [2, 6–9, 11, 16–18]. The literature is replete with an increasing collection of reports of radioiodine accumulation in

B. Shapiro, MBChB, PhD
Radiology (Nuclear Medicine), Formerly, University of Michigan Health System, Ann Arbor, MI, USA

Division of Nuclear Medicine, Department of Radiology, University of Michigan Medical School, Ann Arbor, MI, USA

Nuclear Medicine and Radiation Safety Service, Department of Veterans Affairs Health Systems, Washington, DC (field based) and Ann Arbor, MI, USA
e-mail: lfig@umich.edu

V. Rufini, MD
Institute of Nuclear Medicine, Agostino Gemelli University Polyclinic, Rome, Italy
e-mail: v.rufini@rm.unicatt.it

A. Jarwan, MD • K.J. Kearfott, ScD
Department of Nuclear Engineering and Radiological Sciences, University of Michigan, Ann Arbor, MI, USA
e-mail: kearfott@umich.edu

O. Geatti, MD
Servizio di Medicina Nucleare, Ospedale Maggiore, Trieste, Italy

L.M. Fig, MBChB, MPH
Department of Nuclear Medicine, University of Michigan, Ann Arbor, MI, USA
e-mail: lfig@umich.edu

I.D. Kirkwood, MBBS
Department of Nuclear Medicine, Royal Adelaide Hospital, Adelaide, SA, Australia
e-mail: ian.kirkwood@health.sa.gov.au

J.E. Freitas, MD
Department of Radiology, St. Joseph Mercy Health System, Ypsilanti, MI, USA
e-mail: freitasj@trinity-health.org

A.M. Avram, MD
Division of Nuclear Medicine, Department of Radiology, University of Michigan, 1500 E. Medical Center Drive, Ann Arbor, MI 48109, USA

BIG505G University Hospital, Ann Arbor, MI 48109, USA
e-mail: ancaa@umich.edu

K.K. Wong, MBBS, FRACP (✉)
Division of Nuclear Medicine, Department of Radiology, University of Michigan Health System, Ann Arbor, MI, USA
e-mail: kakit@med.umich.edu

M.D. Gross, MD
Division of Nuclear Medicine, Department of Radiology, University of Michigan Medical School, Ann Arbor, MI, USA

Nuclear Medicine and Radiation Safety Service, Department of Veterans Affairs Health Systems, Washington, DC (field based) and Ann Arbor, MI, USA

L. Wartofsky, D. Van Nostrand (eds.), *Thyroid Cancer*, DOI 10.1007/978-1-4939-3314-3_13

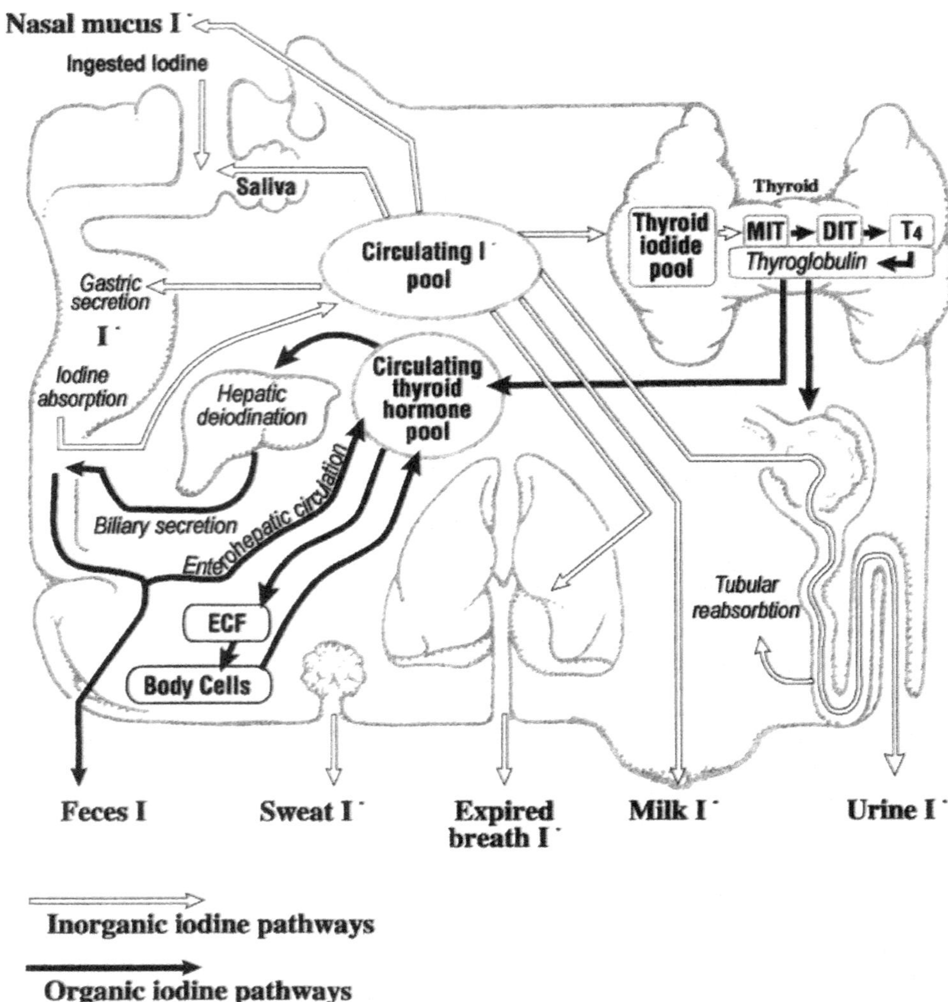

Fig. 13.1 A schematic representation of iodine metabolism (From Shapiro et al. [275] with permission from Elsevier)

these organs and tissues and in associated diseases and other related pathological processes [1, 4, 6, 8, 12–16, 20–23].

Accurate interpretation of postthyroidectomy whole-body radioiodine images requires a thorough knowledge and understanding of all these potential confounding phenomena [1, 2, 4, 6–9, 13, 21–23]. Imaging after the therapeutic administration of large doses of radioiodine permits verification of the biodistribution of radioiodine and has been used to depict a greater extent of disease than that seen on prior diagnostic imaging [6, 9]. The same problem of interpretation applies in this post-therapeutic situation as in the diagnostic images, regardless of whether recombinant human TSH or thyroid hormone withdrawal is used to produce the necessary TSH stimulation of radioiodine uptake. Unfortunately, the literature that describes nonthyroid radioiodine imaging is scattered and consists primarily of isolated case reports and small case series or is hidden within larger reports as anecdotal descriptions [1, 3, 4, 6, 8, 12, 16, 21–27]. We have sought to clarify this literature by utilizing a detailed and updated review based upon underlying physiological principles governing the biodistribution of radioactive iodine. By this approach, we can create a logical classification and pathophysiological interpretation of this disparate literature concerning artifacts, anatomical and physiological variants, and nonthyroidal diseases that are responsible for false-positive radioiodine scans in thyroid cancer. The administration of large activities of radioiodine for the treatment of residual or metastatic well-differentiated thyroid cancer is a uniquely effective systemic therapy when applied to appropriate patients [3–9, 11]. Correct interpretation of post-therapy images will prevent misinterpretation and inappropriate use of radioiodine therapy.

Since the prior edition, there is a growing body of literature describing the incremental value of SPECT-CT over planar and SPECT only imaging. The value of functional SPECT and anatomic CT as a combination useful for problem-solving has been reported [28–34]. SPECT-CT reduces equivocal findings on planar imaging and can be used to distinguish typical patterns of normal remnant thyroid tissue(s) after surgery from regional nodal disease [35–37]. Judicious use of SPECT-CT has been shown to clarify and confirm the vast majority of benign mimics of disease improving anatomic localization and diagnostic interpretation [38–40]. Regardless of the inherent value of SPECT-CT, it should not be used to replace standard practice of clinical history, additional views, delayed imaging or other maneuvers such as swallowing water to discern esophageal radioiodine accumulation or removing surface contamination by washing or removing clothing as part of the imaging process when necessary [38].

Artifacts Related to Ectopic Normal Thyroid Tissue

The embryological origin of the thyroid gland from the foramen cecum at the junction between the anterior two thirds and the posterior one third of the tongue, with its subsequent descent and bifurcaton in the neck, gives rise to a wide variety of abnormalities owing to embryological maldevelopment (Table 13.1) [4, 20, 41–75]. Thus, complete failure to migrate leads to a lingual thyroid (Fig. 13.2) and incomplete migration leads to a high cervical thyroid, whereas excessive migration causes a superior mediastinal thyroid or even a paracardiac gland [4, 20, 41–58]. Foci of functioning tissue may remain anywhere along the embryological thyroglossal duct tract [4, 41–43, 47, 57–59]. Abnormal migration results in widely divergent ectopic foci (e.g., esophageal, intratracheal, and intrahepatic) [4, 41–43, 49, 50, 60, 61, 75–76]. The so-called lateral aberrant thyroid tissue is highly controversial, and many believe that it is, in fact, well-differentiated thyroid cancer metastatic to and completely replacing cervical lymph nodes, with the primary thyroid tumor being occult [4, 42, 43, 71, 73–76]. Finally, normally differentiated

Table 13.1 Ectopic normal thyroid tissue

Ectopic normal thyroid tissue sites	Mechanism for radioiodine uptake	Embryonic thyroid migration/development
Lingual thyroid [4, 42–44, 58, 250]	Normal thyroid radioiodine uptake/organification	Failure to migrate (descend)
High cervical thyroid [4, 15, 20, 42, 43, 46, 48, 49, 58]	Same as above	Incomplete migration
Thoracic superior mediastinal thyroid [4, 15, 16, 28, 51–55]	Same as above	Excessive migration
Paracardiac thyroid [4, 42, 51, 52, 55, 56]	Same as above	Same as above
Intracardiac (struma cordis)	Same as above	Same as above
Pericardial Thyroglossal tract [4, 38, 42, 43, 47, 57, 58, 77]	Same as above	Foci of functioning thyroid tissue along the route of migration, may be stimulated by ↑ TSH postthyroidectomy
Esophageal thyroid [4, 42, 43, 50, 58, 61]	Same as above	Abnormal migration
Intratracheal thyroid [4, 42, 50, 60]	Same as above	Same as above
Ovarian thyroid (struma ovarii) [4, 28, 42, 43, 63–68]	Same as above	Differentiation of thyroid tissue in a benign ovarian teratoma/malignant with metastases
Lateral aberrant thyroid [4, 16, 42, 43, 73–74]	Same as above	Many/all are metastases to cervical lymph nodes
Intrahepatic thyroid tissue [4, 42, 43, 49, 75, 76]	Same as above	Must be distinguished from biliary cyst(s)

From Shapiro et al. [275] with permission from Elsevier
SPECT-CT may be expected to assist with diagnostic interpretation of these entities

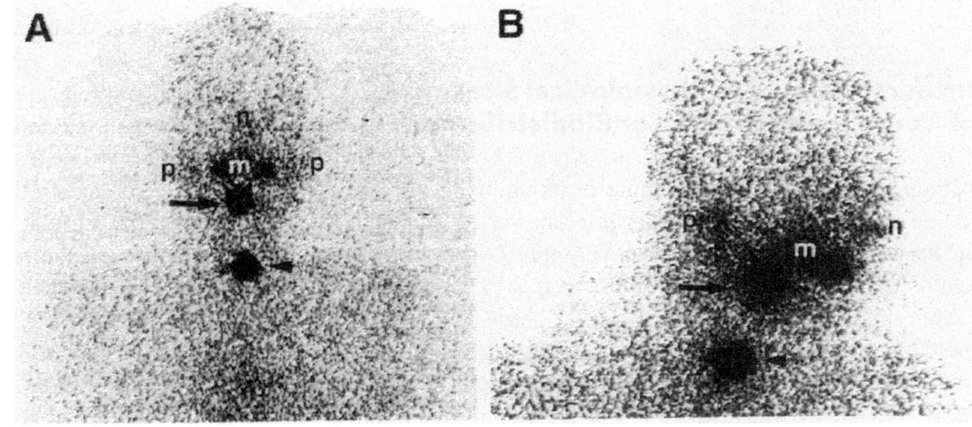

Fig. 13.2 (**a**) Anterior and (**b**) lateral views of the head, neck, and upper chest 24 h after 2 mCi (74 MBq) of radioiodine following a total thyroidectomy for papillary thyroid cancer. There was a small thyroid bed remnant (*arrowhead*) and normal uptake of radioiodine in the nose (*n*), mouth (*m*), and parotid glands (*p*). The intense midline focus of uptake below the floor of the mouth was a lingual thyroid remnant in the base of the tongue (*arrow*) (From Shapiro et al. [275] with permission from Elsevier)

Table 13.2 Physiological sites of nonthyroidal uptake or biodistribution

Physiological sites of nonthyroidal uptake/ distribution	Mechanism for radioiodine uptake	Comments regarding normal biodistribution
Normal cardiac blood pool displaced by pectus excavatum [4, 122]	Radioiodine transported from site of absorption via circulation	Activity fades as blood pool clears with time (not to be confused with lung lesions)
Carotid ectasia [4, 21, 88, 123]	Same as above	Activity fades as blood pool clears with time (not to be confused with tumor spread to cervical lymph nodes)
Salivary gland uptake [4, 6, 18, 20, 38, 79, 90, 246, 257]	Site of active radioiodine transport	Knowledge of normal biodistribution required for image interpretation
Gastric mucosal uptake [4, 18, 88]	Same as above	Same as above
Nasal mucosal uptake [4, 38, 88]	Same as above	Same as above
Thymic uptake [38, 131–142]	Site of active radioiodine transport previously unexplained	May be associated with a mediastinal mass at CT scan owing to thymic hyperplasia
Gut activity	Translocation of activity secreted by gastric mucosa	Same as above
Urinary tract excretion [4, 24, 110, 111]	Major route of clearance	Same as above
Choroid plexus uptake	Site of active radioiodine transport	Not to be confused with brain or skull metastases
Persistent uptake in cardiac and great vessel blood pool or dilated veins [2, 4, 89, 112, 113, 120, 258]	Slow renal clearance in renal disease or absent renal clearance in renal failure and on dialysis	Slow or absent renal clearance from blood pool owing to kidney disease
Nonlactating breast uptake [4, 18, 38, 86, 99, 101, 102, 103, 266]	Site of active radioiodine transport	Usually faint but intensity may be quite variable (not to be confused with lung metastases)
Lactating breast uptake (see Fig. 13.3) [4, 10, 15, 18, 80, 83–88, 96–98, 101, 103]	Site of active radioiodine transport	Uptake may be intense; breastfeeding must stop before scintigraphy as significant radioiodine may be transferred to the infant
Liver uptake [4, 92, 117, 118, 121, 261]	Diffuse hepatic uptake of radioiodine-labeled thyroid hormones synthesized by functioning normal or neoplastic thyroid tissue	The uptake by normal residual thyroid tissue or functioning thyroid cancer deposits is usually focal and very obvious
Gallbladder uptake [4, 92, 110, 121, 244]	Enterohepatic excretion of radioiodine thyroid hormone and metabolites	Unusual cause for focal uptake in right upper quadrant, may be discharged into gut by gallbladder contraction
Swallowed saliva in pharynx and esophagus [4, 81]	Activity migrates from site of secretion in salivary glands	Knowledge of normal bio-distribution required for image interpretation, restudy after swallow of water
Lacrimal gland [4, 106, 241, 267]	Site of active radioiodine transport	Secretion in tears
Menstruating uterus [29, 30]	Radioiodine within blood pool	
Hematocolpos [256]	Radioiodine within blood pool	

From Shapiro et al. [275] with permission from Elsevier

thyroid tissue may occur in the ovary (struma ovarii) as the thyroidal component of a teratoma or as a solitary tissue focus in isolation [4, 42, 43, 62–71].

Artifacts Related to Physiological Sites of Nonthyroidal Uptake or Biodistribution

Although thyroid tissue is unique in its ability to organify iodide and synthesize thyroid hormones, a variety of glandular tissues share the ability to actively transport radioiodine against a chemical gradient of up to a 20:1 uptake ratio (Table 13.2) [2, 18, 78]. Tissues that share this property include gastric mucosa, nasal mucosa, salivary glands, lacrimal glands, and the lactating or nonlactating breast (Fig. 13.3) [2, 4, 15, 18, 79–109]. The choroid plexus, although not a glandular epithelium, is nevertheless a site of secretory function for the formation of cerebrospinal fluid (CSF) and also shows radioiodine uptake [4].

As a small ion, iodide is readily cleared by glomerular filtration and is subject to a balance between tubular secretion and reabsorption such that the urine is the principal route of radioiodine excretion [2, 4, 24, 110–112]. Clearance of radioiodine is delayed in patients on dialysis [111–115]. Urinary iodide concentration or excretion rates are a good index of the state of iodine nutrition.

Thyroid hormones undergo metabolic degradation and excretion in conjugated form into the gut [4, 88]. Hence, radioiodine uptake by the liver several days after radioiodine administration is an index of the amount of functioning (hormone synthesizing) tissue present [4, 88, 92, 110, 116–121]. The gallbladder may occasionally be depicted when biliary

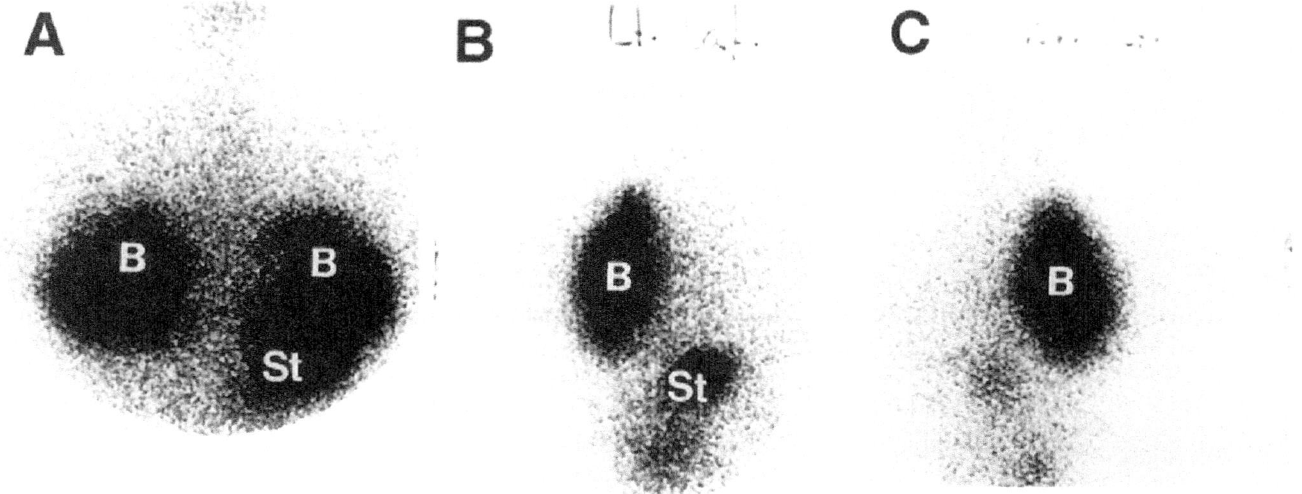

Fig. 13.3 A diagnostic 2-mCi (74 MBq) radioiodine scan was performed 1 week after cessation of breastfeeding. The patient has been breastfeeding for 18 months. Some milk could still be expressed from the breast. (panel **a**) Anterior, (panel **b**) left lateral, and (panel **c**) right lateral images of the neck and chest, showing (*B*) intense bilateral breast uptake and normal gastric uptake (*S*). This clearly demonstrates that a delay of longer than 1 week after weaning is required for resolution of breast uptake of radioiodine (From Shapiro et al. [275] with permission from Elsevier)

excretion is extensive [4, 92, 110, 121]. The majority of the various iodine-containing compounds excreted via the liver undergo further metabolism and reabsorption with reutilization in the enterohepatic circulation [4, 92, 110, 117–121].

After the prompt and efficient absorption of radioiodine in the upper gastrointestinal tract, the anion is carried to all tissues of the body via the circulation, and, particularly at earlier imaging time points, radioiodine within the vascular compartment may be visualized [4, 122123]. Examples of artifactual cardiovascular uptake include the heart and great vessels, particularly in the presence of pectus excavatum and carotid ectasia [2, 4, 21, 87]. In the presence of renal insufficiency, clearance from the vascular compartment will be delayed.

The main function of the thyroid gland is to concentrate iodine up to 20 to 40 times that of plasma concentration [124–126]. Iodine uptake is mediated by an intrinsic membrane glycoprotein in the thyrocyte, the sodium-iodide symporter (NIS) driven by an electrochemical sodium gradient from Na+/K+ –ATPase [124–128]. The human NIS gene was cloned in 1996 and is located on chromosome 9p12 13.2 [129]. NIS is expressed in the thyroid, salivary glands, gastric mucosa, and the lactating mammary gland [127]. It is also detected in the lacrimal glands, choroid plexus, ciliary body of the eye, skin, placenta, and thymus [124–130]. Lower levels are detected in the prostate, ovary, adrenal gland, lung, and heart [125–127]. In the lactating breast, NIS concentrates iodine into milk for the neonate, under hormonal control of prolactin, estrogen, and oxytocin. NIS has not been found in colon, orbital fibroblasts, or nasopharyngeal mucosa. Distributions of radioiodine on scintigraphy in humans have informed researchers of which sites to evaluate for NIS expression. Conversely, the identification of NIS expression in tissues such as thymus provides a mechanism to explain thymic uptake, previously classified as unexplained but now understood to be related to NIS expression [32, 131–142].

Artifacts Related to Contamination by Physiological Secretions

A wide variety of potentially misleading artifacts can arise from contamination by physiological or pathological secretions derived from those organs that are capable of uptake and excretion of radioiodine (Table 13.3). These include urine, saliva, nasal secretions, other respiratory tract secretions, sweat, vomit, and breast milk (Figs. 13.4 and 13.5) [1, 10, 22, 80, 82–84, 87–89, 91–94, 96, 98, 101, 106, 107, 109, 111, 143–162]. Although NIS expression is found in 6 % of nonlactating breasts [128] particularly in young women, it appears to peak in the mammary gland at gestation and lactation [125]. Any focus of radioiodine uptake for which there is not an obvious physiological or pathological explanation must be suspected as arising from contamination by secretions. Patients should always be imaged in clean gowns, and, if necessary, they should be replaced after an attempt is made to wash away any unexplained foci of radioiodine [111, 120, 145, 163–166].

Irritants or foreign bodies such as tracheostomy tubes, bronchitis, nose rings, ocular prosthesis, chewing gum, or chewing tobacco may exaggerate this phenomenon [11, 152, 153, 157, 158]. Unless sweating is excessive due to fever or high ambient temperature, this route of iodide excretion is seldom prominent but may be increased in cystic fibrosis [145–147].

Table 13.3 Contaminationby physiological secretions

Sources of contamination by physiological secretions	Mechanism for radioiodine uptake (consequence of normal physiological concentration or route of excretion)	Comments regarding normal radioiodine biodistribution
Urine [22, 111, 144–154]	Major route of radioiodine excretion	Clothing must be changed just before scanning; attempts to wash away unexplained foci should always be made if there is any suspicion of contamination (not to be confused with pathological uptake)
Saliva [4, 79, 94, 152–156, 239]	Active radioiodine transport into saliva	Typically onto the hair, skin, clothing; may be seen on neurosurgical immobilization frame
Nasal secretions [38, 82, 89, 92, 93, 101, 109, 149, 150, 152–154]	Active radioiodine transport by mucus glands	Same as above
Nasal secretions on nose ring [149]	Active radioiodine transport by mucus glands and drying on the ring	Same as above
Respiratory secretions (especially with tracheostomy) [38, 151, 156, 157, 274]	Active radioiodine transport by mucus glands	Same as above
Sweat [143, 146, 147, 151, 158]	Active radioiodine transport into sweat	Sweat iodide excretion may be greater in cystic fibrosis
Vomit [87, 151]	Active radioiodine transport into gastric secretions	Vomiting may occur as a side effect of radioiodine therapy
Breast milk [1, 79, 83, 84, 86, 90, 95, 105, 107, 159–161]	Active radioiodine transport into milk (iodine is an essential micronutrient for the infant)	Activity may be transmitted to infant
Lacrimal, on artificial eye [106, 108, 155, 251]	Active radioiodine transport into tears	Could be washed off prosthesis
Chewing gum and chewing tobacco [150]	Stimulate salivation with transport of radioiodine saliva	Gum, tobacco quid, and expectorated saliva may cause extensive contamination
External contamination (source unknown) [115, 144, 151, 162–165]	Origin of skin or clothing contamination not always obvious	Contamination above the waist usually saliva/nasal, below waist often urine
Laryngocele [269]	Active radioiodine transport into saliva	

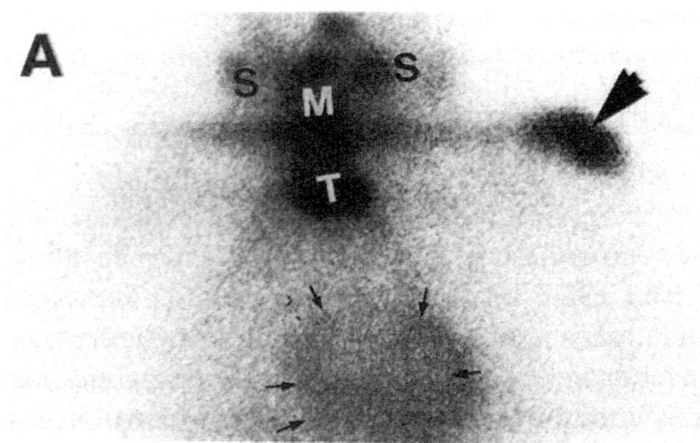

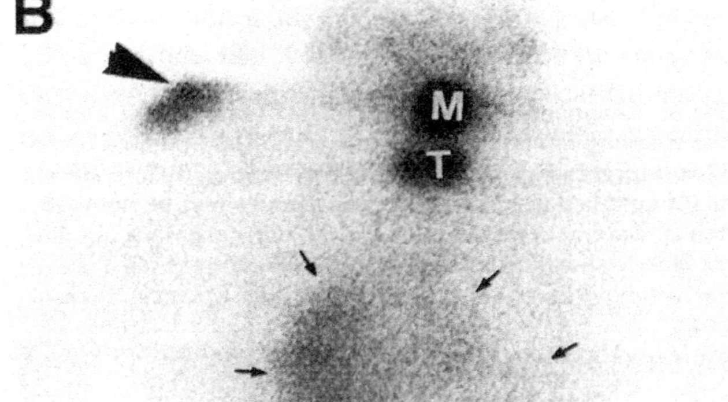

Fig. 13.4 (**a**) Anterior and (**b**) posterior views of the neck and chest in a patient 6 weeks after a near-total thyroidectomy for papillary thyroid cancer obtained 24 h after a 2-mCi (74 MBq) radioiodine tracer dose shows (s) normal salivary gland uptake and (m) mouth activity. There was extensive salivary contamination of the shirt over the patient's shoulder (*arrowhead*) and a prominent halo around the heart from a pericardial effusion secondary to hypothyroidism (*small arrows*) (From Shapiro et al. [275] with permission from Elsevier)

Artifacts Related to Ectopic Gastric Mucosa

The ability of gastric mucosa to concentrate radioiodine is a prominent feature on whole-body radioiodine scintigraphy, and this property is retained by ectopic gastric mucosa (Table 13.4) [4, 18, 21, 88, 166–179]. Ectopic gastric mucosa may arise de novo as an abnormality of embryological development in diverticuli (e.g., Meckel's diverticulum), or in duplication cysts almost anywhere along the foregut and midgut, or as a component of ovarian or other teratomas [59, 167–169]. Chronic inflammatory changes may cause metaplastic transformation of gastrointestinal epithelium of various types of gastric mucosa (e.g., squamous to gastric mucosa in Barrett's esophagus and gastric metaplasia in chronic colitis) [180]. Finally, normal

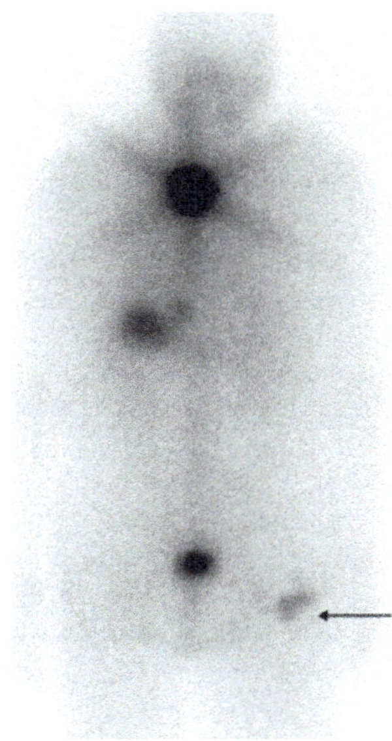

Fig. 13.5 Anterior whole-body scan of a patient with significant thyroid remnant activity in the neck. A focus of radioiodine in the region of the hip (*arrow*) is a handkerchief in the patient's left pocket

gastric mucosa may be anatomically displaced to abnormal anatomic sites. Mechanisms for this phenomenon include hiatal hernia (Fig. 13.6) and surgical procedures such as gastric pull-through [4, 18, 21, 169–173, 175–177].

Artifacts Related to Abnormalities of Gastrointestinal Uptake Other than Ectopic Gastric Mucosa

A variety of pathophysiological processes other than active gastric transport of radioiodine may result in altered radioiodine biodistribution (Table 13.5). These include active concentration by salivary glands with secretion into saliva and subsequent abnormal transfer of the radioactivity into upper gastrointestinal diverticuli, delay by mechanical esophageal stricture or dysmotility [4, 16, 18, 46, 81, 88, 99, 105, 152, 153, 166, 180–183]. Poorly dissolved radioiodine capsules may be retained in the esophagus under these circumstances [184]. Asymmetric depiction of the salivary glands themselves may follow ductal obstruction owing to stone (Fig. 13.7), stricture, or tumor [4, 6,

Table 13.4 Uptake by ectopic gastric mucosa

Sites of uptake by ectopic gastric mucosa	Mechanism for radioiodine uptake	Comments regarding normal function of gastric mucosal
Meckel's diverticulum [4, 38, 166]	Owing to normal active radioiodine transport into gastric secretions	Gastric mucosa at abnormal site[a]
Gastric duplication cysts (may occur in esophagus, duodenum, small bowel) [4, 104, 168]	Same as above	Gastric mucosa at abnormal site[a]
Normal stomach in abnormal locations (hiatus hernia, gastric pull-through) [4, 18, 21, 38, 104, 174, 176]	Same as above	Displacement of stomach from normal site[a]
Barrett's esophagus [177]	Same as above	Gastric mucosa present at abnormal site in esophagus[a]

[a]From Shapiro et al. [275] with permission from Elsevier
SPECT-CT may assist diagnostic interpretation of these entities

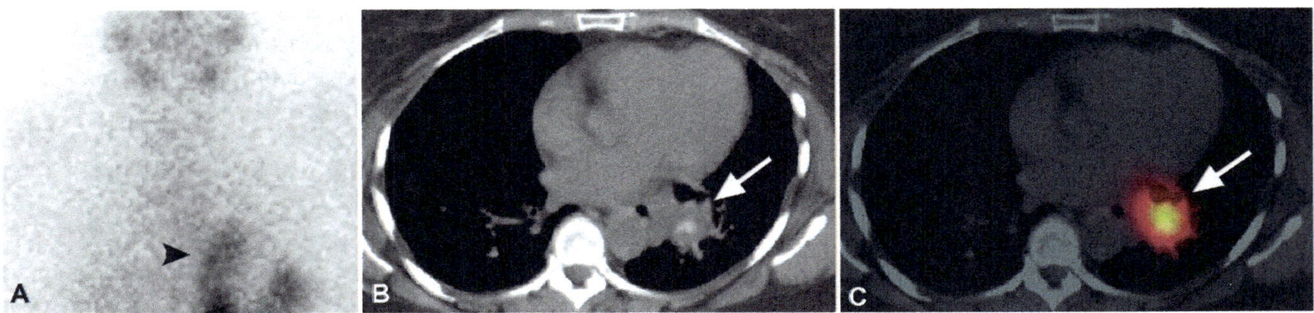

Fig. 13.6 Physiologic uptake in a hiatal hernia mimicking thoracic disease on radioiodine imaging in a 63-year-old woman, postoperative Tg 89 ng/ml (TSH 63mIU/L). (**a**) Planar image shows activity over the left medial anterior chest wall (*arrowhead*) (**b**, **c**) Axial CT and fused SPECT-CT localizes this activity to a hiatal hernia (*arrows*) consistent with physiologic activity in gastric mucosa (With permission Wong et al. [37])

Table 13.5 Abnormalities of gastrointestinal uptake other than ectopic gastric mucosa

Sites of other abnormalities of gastrointestinal uptake	Mechanism for radioiodine uptake (owing to normal active radioiodine transport into secretions)	Comments regarding abnormal motility or structure
Zenker's diverticulum [178, 180, 265]	Active radioiodine transport into saliva	Owing to retention of activity in swallowed saliva in diverticulum[a]
Stricture of esophagus [98, 181]	Same as above	Retention of saliva above stricture
Achalasia/esophageal dysmotility [46, 80, 165, 178, 182, 187, 188]	Same as above	Delayed clearance from esophagus
Poorly dissolved radioiodine capsule [184]	Lack of absorption and retention in the esophagus	Often combined with retention of saliva above stricture and delayed clearance from esophagus
Colonic bypass of esophagus [170, 176]	Active radioiodine transport into saliva and gastric secretions	Delayed clearance and reflux from stomach
Gastroesophageal reflux [1, 16, 87, 104, 174]	Active radioiodine transport into gastric secretions	Reflux of gastric activity into esophagus is very common; always rescan after drink of water if mediastinal activity is present
Abnormal location of bowel with normal radioiodine content (e.g., diaphragmatic or other hernias) [38, 87, 167, 172, 243, 260]	Active radioiodine secreted into the lumen in patients	Luminal radioiodine activity observed at abnormal location[a]
Constipation [190]	Active radioiodine transport into gastric secretions and translocation by luminal transport to small bowel and colon	Delayed transport of luminal radioiodine activity owing to abnormal colonic motility (may be a result of hypothyroidism)
Parotid gland uptake [188]	Active radioiodine secreted into the lumen in patients with ectasia	Pooling of activity in dilated duct as distinct from diffuse uptake in gland
Asymmetrical salivary glands [186]	Active radioiodine transport into saliva	Owing to obstruction of salivary duct by stone, stricture, or tumor (or absence of normal gland owing to prior surgical removal or injury by radiation therapy)

SPECT-CT may assist diagnostic interpretation of these entities
[a]From Shapiro et al. [275] with permission from Elsevier]

8, 16, 18, 46, 79, 84, 88, 184–189]. Prior surgery or radiotherapy may reduce salivary gland radioiodine uptake and this may be asymmetric. Intraluminal radioiodine within the upper gastrointestinal tract is derived from swallowed saliva or active gastric secretion and can be refluxed into the esophagus (Fig. 13.8) [4, 18, 81, 88, 99, 105, 167, 183, 186, 187]. This phenomenon is extremely common, and to distinguish esophageal reflux activity from mediastinal nodal metastases, studies must be performed after a drink of water or more stubborn cases may require upright imaging [3, 4, 6, 8, 16, 105, 109].

Radioiodine secreted by the stomach and radioiodine-labeled metabolites of thyroxine metabolism excreted into the bile will often result in depiction of the colon and may mask metastases elsewhere as well as increase radiation exposure to the colon [1, 3, 4, 7, 8, 16, 110, 116–118, 120, 189–190]. Decreased colonic motility that accompanies hypothyroidism previously required for whole-body radioiodine imaging is likely a major contributing factor that can be mitigated with laxatives or obviated with the use of human recombinant TSH.

Artifacts Related to Urinary Tract Abnormalities

The urinary tract is the principal route of iodide excretion after glomerular filtration of the small anion and a balance between tubular secretion and reabsorption (Table 13.6) [2–4, 17, 19, 24, 105]. Thus, the urine within the bladder is often the most intense radioactive focus on a whole-body radioiodine scan, particularly at 24 and 48 h post-administration [2, 3, 6–8, 16, 21, 24, 105, 155], and as a consequence, all dilations, diverticuli, and fistulae of the kidney, ureter, and bladder may show focal radioiodine retention [3, 4, 6–8, 16, 24, 43, 105, 155]. The same is also true of ectopic, horseshoe, and transplanted kidneys [24]. Renal cysts may show radioiodine uptake if they communicate with the urinary tract or if the epithelium which lines them has the capacity to concentrate and secrete iodide [24, 191]. When suspected, the simultaneous depiction of the urinary tract with a suitable renal imaging agent such as ^{99m}Tc-DTPA or ^{99m}Tc-MAG3 may be useful in characterizing the etiology of these urinary tract abnormalities.

Artifacts Related to Mammary Variations and Abnormalities

The glandular epithelium of the breast during lactation is capable of actively transporting the essential micronutrient iodide from plasma into milk with an efficiency of approximately 20 to 1 under systemic hormonal influence including priming by estrogens, secretory stimulation by prolactin, and milk ejection by oxytocin, which acts on both breasts (Table 13.7) [17, 18, 80, 83, 84, 87, 88, 91, 96, 97, 106, 107, 160–162, 192–199]. As a result, the lactating

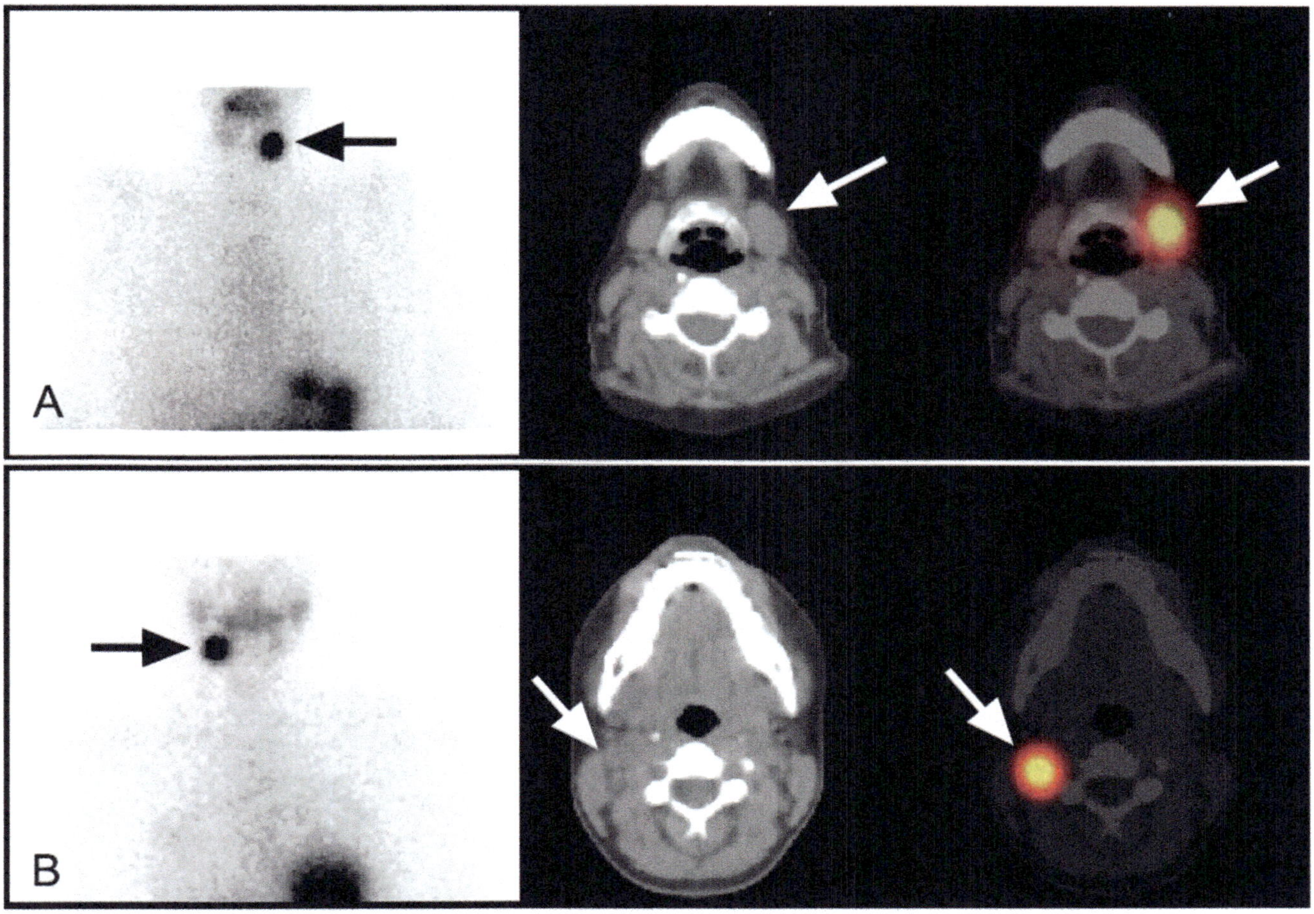

Fig. 13.7 (**a**) Benign focal uptake related to asymmetric radioactivity in the salivary glands after total thyroidectomy in a 49-year-old woman with papillary thyroid cancer. Planar anterior image obtained 24 h after oral administration of 37 MBq of radioiodine shows focal radiotracer uptake in the left side of the neck (*arrow*). SPECT/CT localizes focal radioiodine uptake to the normal left submandibular gland, representing asymmetric physiologic uptake in an otherwise normal gland (*arrows*). Transient or permanent narrowing or obstruction of the salivary duct may cause this pattern and is most commonly associated with previous radioiodine therapy. (**b**) Patient with papillary thyroid cancer status postthyroidectomy underwent diagnostic radioiodine SPECT/CT with 37 MBq. There is a focus of uptake in the right submandibular region on planar images suspicious for nodal disease (*arrow*). SPECT/CT demonstrates focal radioiodine uptake corresponds to a pathologically enlarged, right, level II lymph node (*arrows*) compatible with N1 disease (With permission Glazer et al. [276])

breast often shows intense radioiodine uptake [4, 13, 18, 79, 82–84, 86, 87, 90, 95–98, 100, 102, 108]. Local reflex secretory stimulation that is asymmetrical, or unilateral suckling can result in persistent asymmetric radioiodine uptake for weeks or even months after cessation of lactation. Faint to moderate radioiodine uptake is also seen in nonlactating breast tissue related to NIS expression [4, 18, 85, 99, 101, 102]. This phenomenon may be symmetric or asymmetric and may be seen in unilateral mammary hypertrophy, supernumerary breasts, and lactational duct cysts (Figs. 13.9 and 13.10) [99, 101, 107, 192–195].

Artifacts Related to Uptake in Serous Cavities and Cysts

The epithelia lining of the pleura, peritoneum, and pericardium do not actively transport radioiodine but may be permeable to passive diffusion even in the absence of inflammation (Table 13.8). This leads to the accumulation of radioiodine in pleural, peritoneal and pericardial effusions, scrotal hydroceles, and pleuropericardial cysts [22, 200–208]. Similar processes appear to operate in ovarian cysts and lymphoepithelial cysts [204, 205].

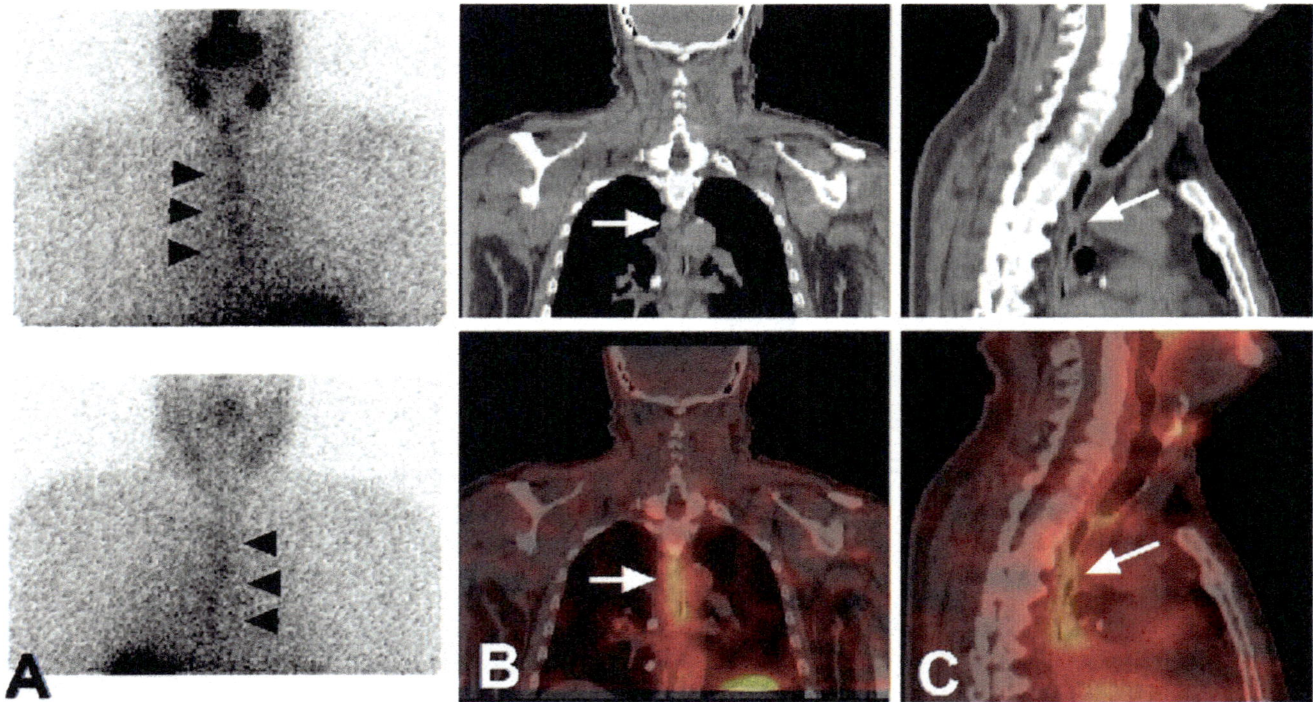

Fig. 13.8 Physiologic uptake due to retained esophageal secretions on radioiodine scan in a patient with papillary thyroid cancer following total thyroidectomy. (**a**) Planar image *Top*; anterior, *Bottom*; posterior shows linear activity in the midline of the thorax (*arrowheads*). (**b**) Coronal and (**c**) Sagittal, *Top*; CT, *Bottom*; fused SPECT-CT localizes this activity to the esophagus (*arrows*)

Table 13.6 Urinary tract abnormalities

Sites of urinary tract abnormalities	Mechanism for radioiodine uptake	Comments regarding slow clearance from urinary tract or abnormal structures in communication with urinary tract[a]
Hydronephrosis, extrarenal pelvis, and caliectasis [3, 4, 6, 8, 21, 23, 43]	Renal clearance of radioiodine into the urine as the major route of excretion	Slow clearance from dilated and/or obstructed renal collecting system
Renal cysts [24, 38, 191]	Same as above	Cyst communicates with urinary tract or nephrons[b]
Urinary tract diverticuli (e.g., affecting renal pelvis, ureter, and bladder) [4, 6, 8, 18, 23, 24, 43]	Same as above	Delayed clearance from diverticuli[b]
Urinary tract fistulae [4, 6, 8, 24, 108]	Same as above	Radioiodine in urine transferred to abnormal locations by fistulous communications[b]
Atonic or dilated bladder [4, 6, 8, 21, 24, 43]	Same as above	Delayed clearance from bladder owing to obstruction or abnormal motility
Ectopic kidney or transplanted kidney [1, 4, 8, 24, 43, 108, 238]	Same as above	Normal renal handling of radioiodine at abnormal location[b]

From Shapiro et al. [275] with permission from Elsevier

[a]Simultaneous imaging of urinary tract with suitable radiopharmaceutical (e.g., Tc-99m-DTPA or Tc-99mMAG3) may be helpful

[b]SPECT-CT may assist with diagnostic interpretation

Artifacts Related to Uptake in Sites of Inflammation or Infection

Inflammation, whether it be sterile (autoimmune, traumatic, postsurgical or ischemic) or due to infection, results in increased blood flow from vasodilation, and increased capillary permeability owing to the complex interplay of various inflammatory cells, immune mediators, lymphokines, and other systemic and paracrine factors (Table 13.9). This results in the accumulation of radioiodine at the sites of a wide variety of inflammatory and infectious processes in which increased blood flow delivers increased levels of radioiodine which then diffuses through the permeable capillaries accumulating in extracellular water spaces (e.g., edema fluid) (Fig. 13.11) [1, 6, 12, 22, 23, 108, 155, 186, 203, 204, 206–220]. These processes seem to be independent of the active iodide transport seen in thyroid, gastric, salivary, and other specialized epithelia [18].

Table 13.7 Mammary abnormalities

Sites of mammary abnormalities	Mechanism for radioiodine uptake (breast duct epithelium actively transports radioiodine into the lumen)	Comments regarding related abnormalities of location or structure
Unilateral mammary hypertrophy [99, 101, 192, 193, 249, 270]	Site of active radioiodine transport	Asymmetrical exaggeration of normal breast uptake
Supernumerary breast [107]	Same as above	Additional foci of breast tissue may be found from axilla to groin
Asymmetrical lactation [107, 192–194]	Same as above	Asymmetrical suckling may stimulate radioiodine uptake into breast with greatest milk secretion
Lactational duct cyst [195]	Same as above	Cyst may be lined with epithelium able to transport radioiodine into cyst lumen

From Shapiro et al. [275] with permission from Elsevier

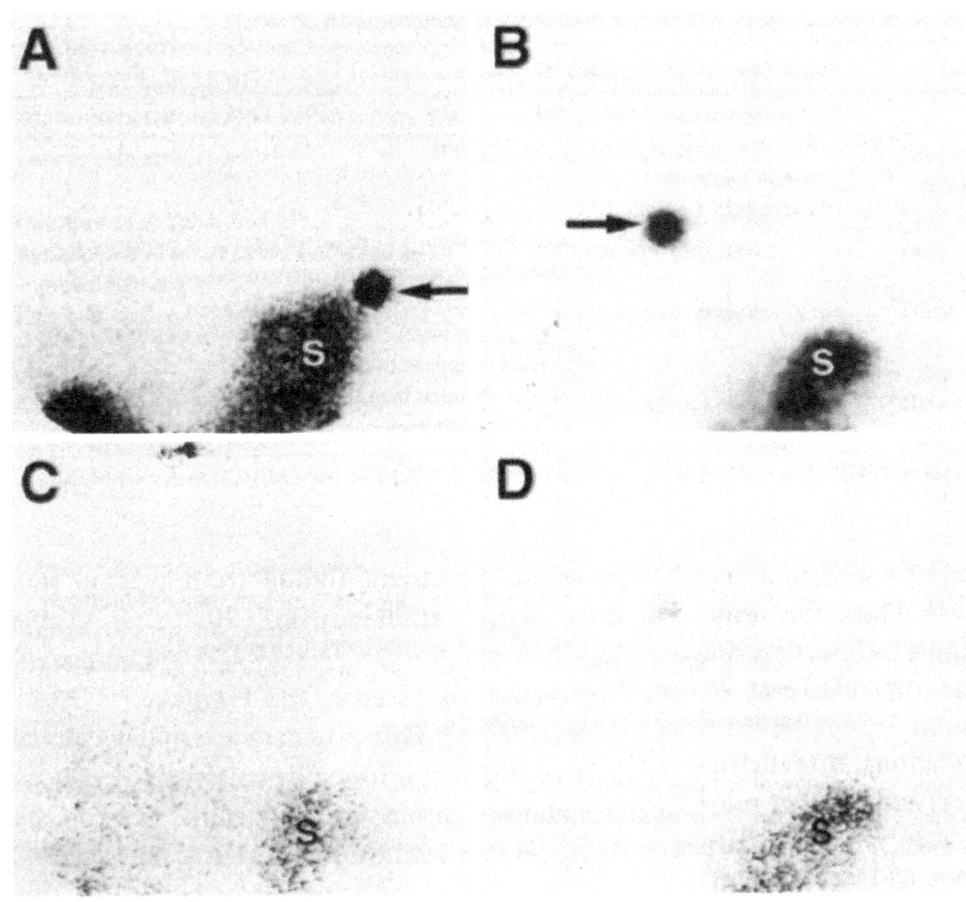

Fig. 13.9 Diagnostic radioiodine scans of the chest performed 24 h after a 2-mCi (74 MBq) tracer dose in a patient with a previously resected papillary thyroid carcinoma (anterior **a**, left lateral **b**). A small intense focus of activity corresponded to a palpable breast cyst (arrow). After aspiration of the cyst fluid contents, the radioiodine uptake virtually disappeared as shown in **c** (anterior) and **d** (left lateral), which are images obtained for lesser total counts. This indicates that the vast majority of the radioiodine activity was in the cyst fluid. Normal gastric uptake (S) (From Shapiro et al. [275] with permission from Elsevier)

Artifacts Related to Uptake by Nonthyroidal Neoplasms

A wide variety of nonthyroidal neoplasms have been reported to demonstrate radioiodine uptake (Table 13.10) [62–68, 71, 82, 85, 204, 205, 221–236]. The mechanisms for this uptake are diverse and include increased vascularity and capillary permeability similar to that seen in inflammation and infection (these include meningiomas, ovarian adenocarcinoma and cystadenoma, uterine fibroma (Fig. 13.12), and neurilemmoma [85, 205, 224, 232, 235, 236]), and many of the tumors are derived from epithelia that show normal physiological iodide transport [18]. These include gastric adenocarcinoma, bronchial adenocarcinoma, salivary adenocarcinoma, and ovarian and other teratomas containing gastric, salivary, thyroid, and similar tissues [59–68, 71, 83, 121, 131–234].

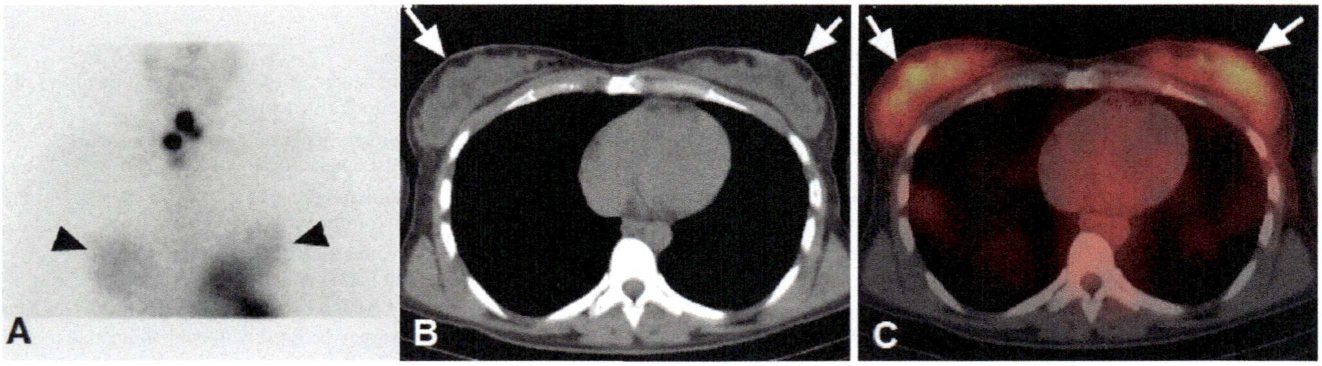

Fig. 13.10 Physiologic uptake in bilateral nonlactating breast tissue. Radioiodine scan in a female patient with papillary thyroid cancer following total thyroidectomy. (**a**) Planar image shows bilateral activity projected over the anterior chest wall (*arrowheads*). There is also focal uptake in the neck compatible with remnant thyroid tissue and cervical nodal metastases (**b**, **c**) Axial CT and fused SPECT-CT localizes this activity to a bilateral breast tissue (*arrows*) consistent with physiologic activity in nonlactating breast tissue presumed due to NIS expression

Table 13.8 Uptake in serous cavities and cysts

Sites of uptake in serous cavities or cysts	Mechanism for radioiodine uptake	Comments regarding diverse locations and factors that may be involved
Pericardial effusion (not associated with inflammation; also see Table 13.9) [22, 202, 203]	Cysts are lined by epithelia not able to actively transport	May be associated with hypothyroidism[a]
Scrotal hydrocele	Radioiodine; passive diffusion into cyst fluid with subsequent slow clearance	Must be distinguished from urinary contamination
Lymphoepithelial cysts	Same as above	
Ovarian cysts [199, 205, 275]	Same as above	This does not include lesions (teratomas) with ectopic gastric, salivary gland, or thyroid epithelium[a]
Pleuropericardial cysts [207]	Same as above	
Bronchogenic cyst [27]	Same as above	

[a]SPECT-CT may assist with diagnostic interpretation

Table 13.9 Uptake in sites of inflammation or infection

Uptake in sites of inflammation/infection	Mechanism for radioiodine uptake	Comments regarding diverse locations possible (inflammatory process need not be infectious in cause)
Pulmonary (e.g., rheumatoid lung, bronchiectasis, fungal infection, or acute respiratory tract infection) 23, 108, 200, 209–211, 247, 255, 259]	Inflammation results in increased perfusion, vasodilation, and capillary permeability	Increased production of mucus may be an additional factor[a]
Pericarditis [22, 155, 203, 204]	Same as above	Frequently autoimmune in cause[a]
Skin burns, superficial abrasions [201]	Same as above	Need not be infected to show radioiodine uptake
Dental disease/periodontal surgery [12, 212–213]	Same as above	May not be clinically evident[a]
Arthritis (e.g., rheumatoid) [214]	Same as above	Usually noninfected inflammatory lesion
Chronic sinusitis [1, 108, 215]	Same as above	Increased production of mucus may be an additional factor[a]
Dacryocystitis [1, 108]	Same as above	Increased uptake in gland beyond that owing to concentration in tears
Psoriatic plaques [6]	Same as above	Noninfected inflammatory lesion
Acute or chronic cholecystitis [216]	Same as above	Biliary excretion may also occur[a]
Scalp folliculitis [217]	Same as above	Same as above
Sialoadenitis [186]	Same as above	Same as above
Recent myocardial infarct [218]	Increased capillary permeability and inflammation in region of infarcted myocardium implies coronary redistribution	Should not be confused with normal gastric uptake of radioiodine or activity in a hiatus hernia[a]
Infected sebaceous cyst [216, 219]	Inflammation results in increased perfusion, vasodilation, and capillary permeability	Sebaceous glands may also concentrate radioiodine

(continued)

Table 13.9 (continued)

Uptake in sites of inflammation/infection	Mechanism for radioiodine uptake	Comments regarding diverse locations possible (inflammatory process need not be infectious in cause)
Frontal sinus mucocele [215]	Sinus mucosa capable of iodide transport	To be distinguished from acute or chronic sinusitis[a]
Sinusitis [206]	Sinus mucosa capable of iodide transport	Same as above
Site of needle biopsy [220]	Inflammation at site of trauma	Uninfected inflammation
Intestinal scar [271]	Inflammation at site of surgery	Uninfected inflammation
Appendix after surgery [240]	Inflammation at site of surgery	Uninfected inflammation
Hepatic hydatid cyst [262]	Infected cyst	Uninfected inflammation

From Shapiro et al. [275] with permission from Elsevier
[a]SPECT-CT may assist diagnostic interpretation

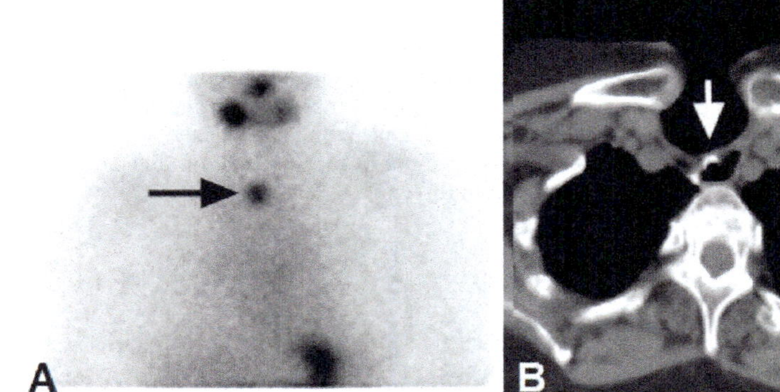

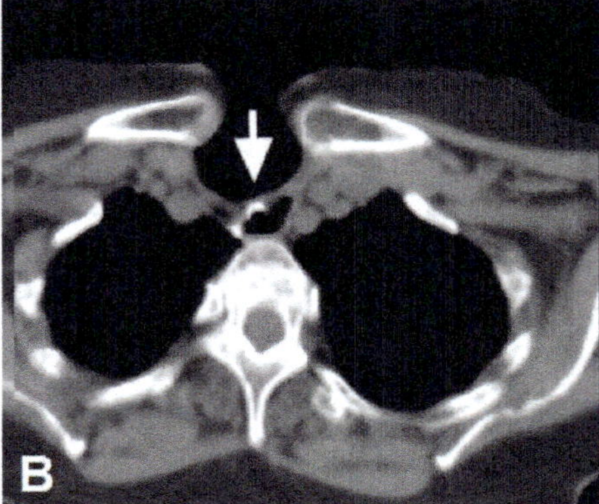

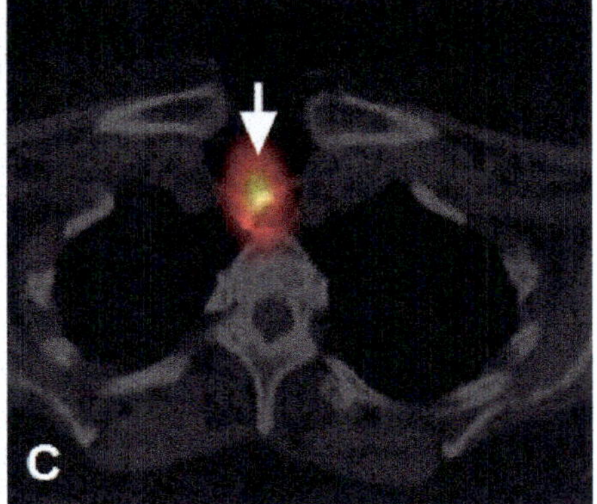

Fig. 13.11 Physiologic uptake due to retained secretions at a tracheostomy site. Radioiodine scan in a woman with invasive papillary thyroid cancer following total thyroidectomy and tracheostomy tube placement. (**a**) Planar image shows intense focal uptake in the central neck (*arrow*). (**b**, **c**) Axial CT and fused SPECT-CT localizes this activity to the patient's tracheostomy site (*arrows*) compatible with benign retained secretions within the stoma

Table 13.10 Uptake by nonthyroidal neoplasms

Sites of nonthyroidal neoplasms	Mechanism for radioiodine uptake[a]	Comments regarding both primary and metastatic tumors
Gastric adenocarcinoma [85, 221, 222]	Gastric mucosa actively transports radioiodine	Probably owing to preservation of normal gastric mucosal active iodide
Meningioma [223, 224]	Mechanism unclear (highly vascular)	
Lung cancer (adenocarcinoma, oat cell carcinoma, squamous cell carcinoma, and bronchoalveolar) [204, 215, 225–228, 254]	Bronchial mucus glands actively transport radioiodine	This would explain uptake in adenocarcinoma but not squamous or oat cell cancers
Salivary adenocarcinoma (Warthin's tumor) [229, 242]	Salivary glands actively transport radioiodine	Other salivary tumors are less likely to show radioiodine uptake; must be distinguished from uptake owing to ductal obstruction
Ovarian adenocarcinoma and ovarian cystadenoma [205, 264, 272]	Mechanism unclear	Mechanism differs from that in ovarian teratomas[b]
Ovarian teratoma (benign/malignant) [29, 62–69, 230–233, 245, 253]	Owing to uptake of radioiodine into salivary gland, gastric mucosa, or thyroid gland tissue present in tumor	Tissues that normally take up radioiodine may differentiate in such tumors[b]
Teratomas at other sites (benign or malignant) [234]	Owing to uptake of radioiodine into salivary gland, gastric mucosa, or thyroid gland tissue present	Tissues that normally take up radioiodine may differentiate in such tumors[b]
Uterine fibromyoma [248]	Mechanism unclear	May be difficult to separate from bladder and bowel activity[b]
Abdominal neurilemmoma [85, 235]	Mechanism unclear	May be difficult to separate from bladder and bowel activity[b]
Vertebral hemangioma [165]	Mechanism unclear	Possible pooling of radioiodine activity in endocapillary structure

[a]Some, by no means all, of these tumors are derived from tissues that can normally concentrate radioiodine
[b]SPECT-CT may assist diagnostic interpretation

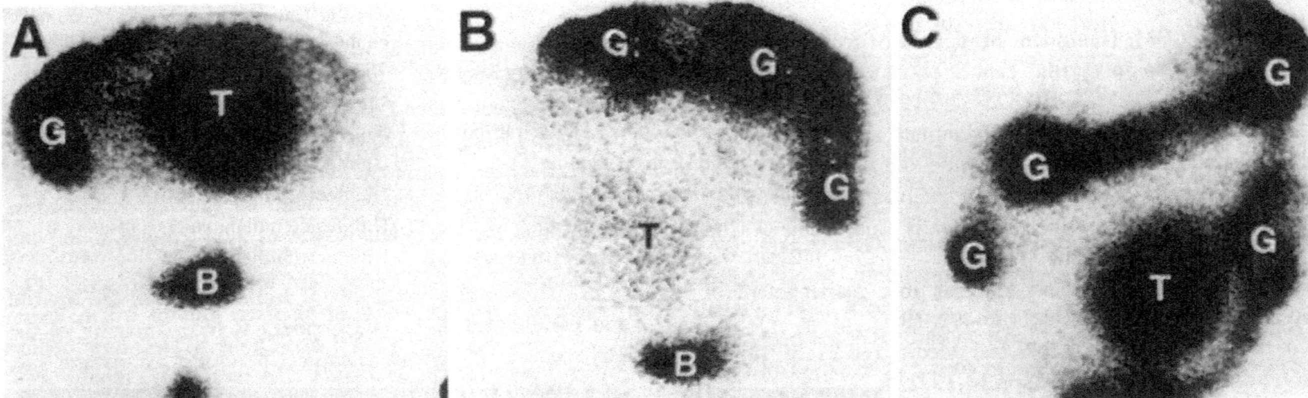

Fig. 13.12 Diagnostic studies performed 24 h after a dose of 2 mCi (74 MBq) of radioiodine as part of a metastatic survey after a total thyroidectomy for papillary cancer. There was intense and extensive gut radioactivity (*G*) owing constipation caused by hypothyroidism required for preparation for imaging. There was normal urinary excretion of radioiodine in the bladder (*B*) and urinary contamination of the vulva. A large abnormal focus of radioiodine uptake in the anterior pelvis (*T*), separate from the gut and bladder was best depicted on the (panel **a**) anterior and (panel **c**) right anterior oblique projections. On the (panel **b**) posterior projection, the focus was much fainter, indicating a relatively anterior location. The abnormal radioiodine uptake was in a large fibroid uterus, which extended out of the pelvis (From Shapiro et al. [275] with permission from Elsevier)

Table 13.11 Currently unexplained sites of uptake

Other sites and causes	Mechanisms for radioiodine uptake	Factors to be considered in otherwise unexplained thoracic radioiodine
Uptake related to metal dental fillings [237]	Currently unexplained	May represent a reaction between metal cations found in filling material, Ag+, Hg+, with I-
Unexplained mediastinal uptake (? normal variant) [135, 136]	Same as above	To be considered in otherwise unexplained thoracic radioiodine
Unexplained uptake of porencephaly [140]	Same as above	Trauma occurred 25 years earlier
Posttraumatic cerebral malacia [139]	Possible chronic inflammation of cerebral or overlying tissues	Prior surgery for cerebral abscess 25 years earlier
Subdural hematoma [263]	Currently unexplained	Possible radioiodine activity from blood pool retained in hematoma

From Shapiro et al. [275] with permission from Elsevier

Currently Unexplained Sites of Artifactual Uptake

There remain a few reports of focal radioiodine uptake in postthyroidectomy patients for which there remains no obvious physiological or pathophysiological explanation (Table 13.11). Focal uptake in the mouth has been attributed to the iodide anion reacting with metallic cations within dental metal filling materials [38, 237], while focal uptake of radioiodine at sites of porencephaly and cerebral malacia occurring up to 25 years after the original cerebral injury remains unexplained but likely relate to ongoing low level, chronic inflammation [139, 140].

Conclusions

This classification and organization of artifacts, anatomical and physiological variants, and nonthyroidal diseases causing false-positive whole-body radioiodine scans in thyroid cancer patients aids in the correct interpretation of both diagnostic and post-therapeutic radioiodine studies. This update of our previous chapter provides a single compendium reference of the available English language literature on the subject with ongoing publication of reports of benign etiologies of radioiodine uptake indicating continued interest in this topic [29, 209, 238–275]. The organizational schema is offered as a means to interpret and clarify additional future observations in this area that will undoubtedly change with the use of human recombinant TSH that facilitates imaging without induction of hypothyroidism and the introduction of the new hybrid imaging technology of SPECT-CT.

References

1. Bakheet SM, Hammami MM, et al. False positive radioiodine whole-body scan in thyroid cancer patients due to unrelated pathology. Clin Nucl Med. 1994;19:325–9.
2. Berson SA, Yallow RS, et al. Quantitative aspects of iodine metabolism: the exchangeable organic iodine pool and the rates of

thyroid secretion, peripheral degradation and fecal excretion of endogenously synthesized organically bound iodine. J Clin Invest. 1954;33:1533–52.
3. Cavalieri RR, et al. Nuclear imaging in the management of thyroid carcinoma. Thyroid. 1996;6:485–92.
4. Datz FL, et al. Gamuts in nuclear medicine. 3rd ed. St. Louis: Mosby-Yearbook; 1995. p. 14–5, 27–34.
5. Echenique R, Kasi L, Haynie TP, et al. Critical evaluation of serum thyroglobulin levels and I-131 scans in post-therapy patients with differentiated thyroid carcinoma: concise communication. J Nucl Med. 1982;23:235–40.
6. Fogelman I, Maisey MN, et al. The thyroid scan in the management of thyroid disease. In: Freeman LM, Weissmann HS, editors. Nuclear medicine annual. New York: Raven Press; 1989. p. 1.
7. Freitas JE, Gross MD, Ripley S, et al. Radionuclide diagnosis and therapy of thyroid cancer: current status report. Semin Nucl Med. 1985;15:106–31.
8. Johnson PM, et al. Thyroid and whole-body scanning. In: Werner SC, Ingbar SH, editors. The thyroid, a fundamental and clinical text. 4th ed. Hagerston: Harper & Row; 1978. p. 247–97.
9. Maxon RH, Smith HS, et al. Radioiodine-131 in the diagnosis and treatment of metastatic well differentiated thyroid cancer. Endocrinol Metab Clin North Am. 1990;19:685–718.
10. Ramanna L, Waxman AD, Brachman MB, et al. Correlation of thyroglobulin measurements and radioiodine scans in the follow-up of patients with differentiated thyroid cancer. Cancer. 1985;55:1525–9.
11. Riggs DS, et al. Quantitative aspects of iodine metabolism in man. Pharmacol Rev. 1952;4:283–93.
12. Sutter CW, Masilungan BG, Stadalnik RC, et al. False-positive results of I-131 whole-body scans in patients with thyroid cancer. Semin Nucl Med. 1995;25:279–82.
13. Carlisle MR, Lu C, McDougall IR. The interpretation of ^{131}I scans in the evaluation of thyroid cancer, with an emphasis on false positive findings. Nucl Med Commun. 2003;24:715–35.
14. Mitchell G, Pratt BE, Vini L, et al. False positive ^{131}I whole body scans in thyroid cancer. Br J Radiol. 2000;73:627–35.
15. Zalis ED, Ellison RB, Captain MC, et al. A diagnostic pitfall with radioiodine scanning. Am J Roentgenol. 1965;94:837–8.
16. Wu S, Brown T, Milne N, et al. Iodine-131 total body scan: extrathyroidal uptake of radioiodine. Semin Nucl Med. 1986;16:82–4.
17. Wolff J, et al. Iodide concentrating mechanisms. In: Tall JE, Kopin IJ, Berson SA, editors. The thyroid and biogenic amines: methods in investigative and diagnostic endocrinology, vol. 1. Amsterdam: North-Holland Publishing Co; 1972. p. 115–203.
18. Spitzweg C, Joba W, Eisenmenger W, et al. Analysis of human sodium iodide symporter gene expression in extrathyroidal tissues and cloning of its complementary deoxyribonucleic acids from salivary gland, mammary gland, and gastric mucosa. J Clin Endocrinol Metab. 1998;83:1746–51.
19. Wayne EJ, Koutras DA, Alexander WD, editors. Clinical aspects of iodine metabolism. Philadelphia: Davis Company; 1964. p. 1–303.
20. Coover LR. False positive result of a total body scan caused by benign thyroidal tissue after ^{131}I ablation. Clin Nucl Med. 1999;24:182–3.
21. Greenler DP, Klein HA, et al. The scope of false-positive iodine-131 images for thyroid carcinoma. Clin Nucl Med. 1989;14:111–7.
22. Geatti O, Shapiro B, Orsolon PG, et al. An unusual false positive scan in a patient with pericardial effusion. Clin Nucl Med. 1994;19:678–82.
23. Bakheet S, Powe J, Hammami M, et al. Radioiodine uptake in the chest. J Nucl Med. 1997;38:984–6.
24. Bakheet S, Hammami M, Powe J, et al. False-positive radioiodine uptake in the abdomen and the pelvis: radioiodine retention in the kidneys and review of the literature. Clin Nucl Med. 1996;21: 932–7.
25. Haveman JW, Phan HT, Links TP, Jager PL, Plukker JT. Implications of mediastinal uptake of 131I with regard to surgery in patients with differentiated thyroid carcinoma. Cancer. 2005;103:59–67.
26. Leitha T, Staudenherz A. Frequency of diagnostic dilemmas in ^{131}I whole body scanning. Nuklearmedizin. 2003;42:55–62.
27. Agriantonis DJ, Hall L, Wilson MA. Pitfalls of I-131 whole body scan interpretation: bronchogenic cyst and mucinous cystadenoma. Clin Nucl Med. 2008;33:325–7.
28. Dumcke CW, Madsen JL. Usefulness of SPECT/CT in the diagnosis of intrathoracic goiter versus metastases from cancer of the breast. Clin Nucl Med. 2007;32(2):156–9.
29. Macdonald W, Armstrong J. Benign struma ovarii in a patient with invasive papillary thyroid cancer: detection with I-131 SPECT-CT. Clin Nucl Med. 2007;32:380–2.
30. Rachinsky I, Driedger A. Iodine-131 uptake in a menstruating uterus: value of SPECT/CT in distinguishing benign and metastatic iodine-positive lesions. Thyroid. 2007;17:901–2.
31. Thust S, Fernando R, Barwick T, Mohan H, Clarke SE. SPECT/CT identification of post-radioactive iodine treatment false-positive uptake in a simple renal cyst. Thyroid. 2009;19:75–6.
32. Wong KK, Avram AM. Posttherapy I-131 thymic uptake demonstrated with SPECT/CT in a young girl with papillary thyroid carcinoma. Thyroid. 2008;18:919–20.
33. Avram AM, Fig LM, Frey KA, Gross MD, Wong KK. Preablation ^{131}I scans with SPECT/CT in postoperative thyroid cancer patients: what is the impact on staging? J Clin Endocrinol Metab. 2013;98:1163–71.
34. Xue YL, Qiu ZL, Song HJ, Luo QY. Value of ^{131}I SPECT/CT for the evaluation of differentiated thyroid cancer: a systematic review of the literature. Eur J Nucl Med Mol Imaging. 2013;40:768–78.
35. Wong KK, Zarzhevsky N, Cahill JM, Frey KA, Avram AM. Incremental value of diagnostic ^{131}I SPECT/CT fusion imaging in the evaluation of differentiated thyroid carcinoma. AJR Am J Roentgenol. 2008;191:1785–94.
36. Wong KK, Sisson JC, Koral KF, Frey KA, Avram AM. Staging of differentiated thyroid carcinoma using diagnostic ^{131}I SPECT-CT. AJR Am J Roentgenol. 2010;195:730-6.
37. Wong KK, Zarzhevsky N, Cahill JM, Frey KA, Avram AM. Hybrid SPECT-CT and PET-CT imaging of differentiated thyroid carcinoma. Br J Radiol. 2009;82:860–76.
38. Glazer DI, Brown RK, Wong KK, Savas H, Gross MD, Avram AM. SPECT/CT evaluation of unusual physiologic radioiodine biodistributions: pearls and pitfalls in image interpretation. Radiographics. 2013;33:397–418.
39. Oh JR, Ahn BC. False-positive uptake on radioiodine whole-body scintigraphy: physiologic and pathologic variants unrelated to thyroid cancer. Am J Nucl Med Mol Imaging. 2012;2:362–85.
40. Blum M, Tiu S, Chu M, Goel S, Friedman K. I-131 SPECT/CT elucidates cryptic findings on planar whole-body scans and can reduce needless therapy with I-131 in post-thyroidectomy thyroid cancer patients. Thyroid. 2011;21:1235–47.
41. Turlington B, et al. Embryology and anatomy of the thyroid and parathyroid glands. In: Eisenberg B, editor. Imaging of the thyroid and parathyroid glands. New York: Churchill Livingstone; 1991. p. 1–8.
42. Larochelle D, Arcand P, Belzile M, et al. Ectopic thyroid tissue: a review of the literature. J Otolaryngol. 1979;8:523–30.
43. Sloan LW, Feind CR, et al. Clinical aspects of anomalous development. In: Werner SC, Ingbar SH, editors. The thyroid. New York: Harper & Row; 1971. p. 317–33.
44. Weider DJ, Parker W, et al. Lingual thyroid. Ann Otol Rhinol Laryngol. 1977;86:841–8.
45. Strain J, Oates E, Nejad A, et al. Unusual appearance of lingual thyroid in congenital hypothyroidism. Clin Nucl Med. 1998;23:460.
46. Lin DS, et al. Thyroid imaging-mediastinal uptake in thyroid imaging. Semin Nucl Med. 1983;13:395–6.

47. Leung AKC, Wong AL, Robson WLM, et al. Ectopic thyroid gland simulating a thyroglossal duct cyst: a case report. Can J Surg. 1995;38:87–9.
48. Sironi M, Assi A, Andruccioli M, et al. Submandibular ectopic thyroid gland. Clin Nucl Med. 1996;21:585.
49. Touliopoulos P, Oates E, et al. Autonomously functioning thyroid rests following total thyroidectomy for Graves' disease. Clin Nucl Med. 1993;18:914.
50. Dowling EA, Johnson IM, Collier FCD, et al. Intratracheal goiter: a clinico-pathologic review. Ann Surg. 1962;156:258–67.
51. Dundas P, et al. Intrathoracic aberrant goiter. Acta Chir Scand. 1964;128:729–36.
52. Fogelfeld L, Rubinstein U, Bar-On J, et al. Severe thyrotoxicosis caused by an ectopic intrathoracic goiter. Clin Nucl Med. 1986;11:20–2.
53. Salvatore M, Gallo A, et al. Accessory thyroid in the anterior mediastinum: case report. J Nucl Med. 1975;16:1135–6.
54. Salvatore M, Rufini V, Corsellow SM, et al. Thyrotoxicosis due to ectopic retrotracheal adenoma treated with radioiodine. J Nucl Biol Med. 1993;37:69–72.
55. Thakore K, Vansant J, et al. Hyperthyroidism due to toxic, intrathoracic thyroid tissue with absent cervical thyroid gland. Clin Nucl Med. 1993;18:535–6.
56. Rieser GD, Ober KP, Cowan RJ, et al. Radioiodine imaging of struma cordis. Clin Nucl Med. 1988;13:421–2.
57. Aldasouqi S, Edmondson J, Prince M, et al. Carcinoma of thyroglossal duct remnants: report of three cases and a review of the literature. Endocrinologist. 1996;6:238–44.
58. Gaby M, et al. The role of thyroid dysgenesis and maldescent in the etiology of sporadic cretinism. J Pediatr. 1962;60:830–5.
59. Gorbman A, Dickhoff WW, Vigna SR, et al. The thyroid gland. In: Gorbman A, editor. Comparative endocrinology. New York: Wiley; 1983. p. 185–202.
60. Myers EN, Pantangco IP, et al. Intratracheal thyroid. Laryngoscope. 1975;85:1833–40.
61. Postlethwait RN, Detmer DE, et al. Ectopic thyroid nodule in the esophagus. Ann Thorac Surg. 1975;19:98–100.
62. Braun WW, Shetty KR, Rosenfeld PS, et al. Hyperthyroidism due to struma ovarii: demonstration by radioiodine scan. Acta Endocrinol. 1973;73:266–72.
63. Falsetti L, Schivardi MR, Maira G, et al. Riscontro di struma ovarii in una paziente in trattamento per cacinoma tiroideo. Ann Ost Gin Med Perin. 1985;106:290–3.
64. March DE, Desai AG, Park CH, et al. Struma ovarii: hyperthyroidism in a postmenopausal woman. J Nucl Med. 1988;29:263–5.
65. Salvatore M, Rufini V, Daudone MS, et al. Occasional detection of "struma ovarii" in a patient with thyroid cancer. Radiol Med (Torino). 1991;81:744–67.
66. Thomas RD, Batty VB, et al. Metastatic malignant struma ovarii: two case reports. Clin Nucl Med. 1992;17:577–8.
67. Yeh E-L, Meade RC, Reutz PP, et al. Radionuclide study of struma ovarii. J Nucl Med. 1973;14:118–21.
68. Zwas ST, Heyman Z, Lieberman LM, et al. ^{131}I ovarian uptake in a whole-body scan for thyroid carcinoma. Semin Nucl Med. 1989;19:340–2.
69. Konez O, Hanelin LG, Jenison EL, Goyal M, Randolph W. Functioning liver metastases on a whole-body scan: a case of malignant struma ovarii. Clin Nucl Med. 2000;25:465–6.
70. Ziessman HA, Bahar H, Fahey FH, et al. Hepatic visualization on iodine-131 whole-body thyroid cancer scans. J Nucl Med. 1987;28:1408–11.
71. Joja I, Asakawa T, Mitsumori A, et al. I-123 uptake in nonfunctional struma ovarii. Clin Nucl Med. 1998;23:10–2.
72. Moses DC, Thompson NW, Nishiyama RH, et al. Ectopic thyroid tissue in the neck, benign or malignant? Cancer. 1976;38: 361–5.
73. Ryo UY, Stachura ME, Schneider AB, et al. Significance of extrathyroidal uptake of Tc-99m and I-123 in the thyroid scan: concise communication. J Nucl Med. 1981;22:1039–42.
74. Sud AM, Gross MD, et al. Radioiodine uptake following thyroidectomy for thyroid cancer: recurrence or ectopic tissue? Clin Nucl Med. 1991;16:894–7.
75. Todino V, Pacella CM, Crescenzi A, et al. Ectopic thyroid tissue in the liver: case report. Eur J Nucl Med. 1996;23:1055 (abstract).
76. Bakheet S, Powe J, Hammami MM, et al. Isolated porta hepatis metastasis of papillary thyroid cancer. J Nucl Med. 1996;37:993–4.
77. Feuerstein IM, Harbert JC, et al. Hypertrophied thyroid tissue in a thyroglossal duct remnant. Clin Nucl Med. 1986;11:135.
78. Freinkel KA, Ingbar SH, et al. Concentration gradients for inorganic iiodide I-131 and chloride in mixed human saliva. J Clin Invest. 1953;32:1077–84.
79. Ahlgren L, Ivarsson S, Johansson L, et al. Excretion of radionuclides in human breast milk after the administration of radiopharmaceuticals. J Nucl Med. 1985;26:1085–90.
80. Bakheet S, Hammami MM, et al. False positive thyroid cancer metastasis on whole body radioiodine scanning due to retained radioactivity in the oesophagus. Eur J Nucl Med. 1993;20:415–9.
81. Boxen I, Zhang M, et al. Nasal secretion of iodine-131. Clin Nucl Med. 1990;15:610–1.
82. Coakley AJ, Mountford PJ, et al. Nuclear medicine and the nursing mother. Br Med J. 1985;291:159–60.
83. Clode WH, Sobral JMV, Lima-Basto E, et al. Elective uptake of radioiodine by cancer of the stomach. Surgery. 1961;50:725–7.
84. Duong RB, Fernandez-Ulloa M, Planitz MK, et al. ^{123}I breast uptake in a young primipara with postpartum transient thyrotoxicosis. Clin Nucl Med. 1983;8:35.
85. Ganatra RD, Atmaram SH, Sharma SM, et al. An unusual site of radioiodine concentration in a patient with thyroid cancer (letter). J Nucl Med. 1972;13:777.
86. Hedrick WR, DiSimone RN, Keen RL, et al. Radiation dosimetry from breast milk excretion of radioiodine and pertechnetate. J Nucl Med. 1986;27:1569–71.
87. Honour AJ, Myant NB, Rowlands EN, et al. Secretion of redioiodine in digestive juices and milk in man. Clin Sci (Colch). 1952;11:447–62.
88. Lopez OL, Maisano ER, et al. Vascular retention of Tc-99m pertechnetate simulating ectopic or metastatic thyroid tissue. Clin Nucl Med. 1983;8:503–4.
89. Malpani BL, Samuel AM, Ray S, et al. Deferential kinetics of parotid and submandibular gland function as demonstrated by scintigraphic means and its possible implications. Nucl Med Commun. 1995;16:706–9.
90. Mountford PJ, Coakley AJ, et al. A review of the secretion of radioactivity in human breast milk: data, quantitative analysis and recommendations. Nucl Med Commun. 1989;10:15–27.
91. Neutze JA, Norby EH, VanNostrand D, et al. Nasal radioiodine uptake: a prospective study of frequency, degree, and pattern. Presented at the 34th Annual Meeting. J Nucl Med. 1987;28:686, (Abstract 542).
92. Norby EH, Neutze J, Van Nostrand D, et al. Nasal radioiodine activity: a prospective study of frequency, intensity and pattern. J Nucl Med. 1990;31:52–4.
93. Park HM, Tarver RD, Schauwecker DS, et al. Spurious thyroid cancer metastasis: saliva contamination artifact in high dose iodine-131 metastases survey. J Nucl Med. 1986;27:634–6.
94. Riccabona G, et al. Differentiated thyroid carcinoma. In: Murray IPC, Ell PJ, editors. Nuclear medicine in clinical diagnosis and treatment. Churchill Livingstone; 1998. p. 941–57.
95. Romney B, Nicholoff EF, Esser PD, et al. Excretion of radioiodine in breast milk. J Nucl Med. 1989;30:124–6.
96. Romney BM, Nicholoff EL, et al. Diagnostic nuclear medicine and the nursing mother. Appl Radiol. 1987;16:51–6.

97. Romney BM, Nickoloff EL, Esser PD, et al. Radionuclide administration to nursing mothers: mathematically derived guidelines. Radiology. 1986;160:549–54.
98. Schuster DM, Alazraki N, et al. Esophageal scarring causing false-positive uptake on I-131 whole-body imaging. Clin Nucl Med. 1998;23:334.
99. Hammami MM, Bakheet S, et al. Radioiodine breast uptake in non-breast feeding women. Clinical and scintigraphic characteristics. J Nucl Med. 1996;37:26–31.
100. Park HM, Wellman H, et al. Hot nose after I-131 sodium iodide thyroablation therapy. Clin Nucl Med. 1992;17:130–1.
101. Allen T, Wiest P, Vela S, et al. I-131 uptake in the breast for thyroid cancer surveillance with biopsy-proven benign tissue. Clin Nucl Med. 1998;23:585–7.
102. Baemler GR, Joo KG, et al. Radioactive iodine uptake by breasts (letter). J Nucl Med. 1986;27:149–51.
103. Watanabe N, Matsumoto M, Ohtake H, et al. Bilateral breast uptake of T1-201 chloride in a nursing woman. Clin Nucl Med. 1996;21:818–9.
104. McDougall IR, et al. Whole body scintigraphy with radioiodine-131: a comprehensive list of false-positives with some examples. Clin Nucl Med. 1995;20:869–75.
105. Robinson PS, Barker P, Campbell A, et al. Iodine-131 in breast milk following therapy for thyroid carcinoma. J Nucl Med. 1994;35:1797–801.
106. Bakheet S, Hammami M, Hemidan A, et al. Radioiodine secretion in tears. J Nucl Med. 1998;39:1452–4.
107. Bakheet SM, Hammami MM, et al. Patterns of radioiodine uptake by the lactating breast. Eur J Nucl Med. 1994;21:604–8.
108. Howarth DV, Forstrom LA, O'Connor MK, et al. Patient-related and pitfalls artifacts in nuclear medicine imaging. Semin Nucl Med. 1996;26:295–307.
109. Achong DM, Oates E, Lee SL, et al. Gallbladder visualization during post-therapy iodine-131 imaging of thyroid carcinoma. J Nucl Med. 1991;32:2275–7.
110. Nishizawa K, Ohara K, Ohshima M, et al. Monitoring of iodine excretions and used materials of patients treated with ^{131}I. Health Phys. 1980;38:467–81.
111. Daumerie C, Vynckier S, Caussin J, et al. Radioiodine treatment of thyroid carcinoma in patients on maintenance hemodialysis. Thyroid. 1996;6:301–4.
112. Howard N, Glasser M, et al. Iodine-131 ablation therapy for a patient on maintenance haemodialysis. Br J Radiol. 1981;54:259–61.
113. Mello AM, Isaacs R, Petersen J, et al. Management of thyroid papillary carcinoma with radioiodine in a patient with end-stage renal disease on hemodialysis. Clin Nucl Med. 1994;19:776–81.
114. Morris DW, Filipow JL, McEwan AJ, et al. ^{131}I treatment of thyroid papillary carcinoma in a patient with renal failure. Cancer. 1990;66:2509–13.
115. Nibhanupudy JR, Hamilton W, Sridhar R, et al. Iodine-131 treatment of hyperthyroidism in a patient on dialysis for chronic renal failure. Am J Nephrol. 1993;13:214–7.
116. Rosenbaum RC, Johnston GS, Valente WA, et al. Frequency of hepatic visualization during 131I imaging for metastatic thyroid carcinoma. Clin Nucl Med. 1988;13:657–60.
117. Schober B, Cohen P, Lyster D, et al. Diffuse liver uptake of ^{131}I (letter). J Nucl Med. 1990;31:1575–6.
118. Nodine JH, Maldia G, et al. Pseudostruma ovarii. Obstet Gynecol. 1961;17:460–3.
119. You DL, Tzen KY, Chen JF, et al. False-positive whole-body iodine-131 scan due to intrahepatic duct dilatation. J Nucl Med. 1997;38:1977–9.
120. Varoglu E, Yildirim M, Bayrakdar R, Kantarci M, Uslu H. Radioiodine pooling in dilated greater saphenous vein mimicking contamination. Clin Nucl Med. 2003;28:866–8.
121. Chung JK, Lee YJ, Jeong JM, et al. Clinical significance of hepatic visualization on I-131 whole-body scan in patients with thyroid carcinoma. J Nucl Med. 1997;38:1191–5.
122. Muherji S, Ziessman HA, Earll JM, et al. False-positive iodine-131 whole-body scan due to pectus excavatum. Clin Nucl Med. 1988;13:207–8.
123. Giuffrida D, Garofalo MR, Cacciaguerra G, et al. False positive I-131 total body scan due to an ectasia of the common carotids. J Endocrinol Invest. 1993;16:207–11.
124. Carvalho DP, Ferreira AC. The importance of sodium/iodide symporter (NIS) for thyroid cancer management. Arq Bras Endocrinol Metabol. 2007;51:672–82.
125. Chung JK. Sodium iodide symporter: its role in nuclear medicine. J Nucl Med. 2002;43:1188–200.
126. Filetti S, Bidart JM, Arturi F, Caillou B, Russo D, Schlumberger M. Sodium/iodide symporter: a key transport system in thyroid cancer cell metabolism. Eur J Endocrinol. 1999;141:443–57.
127. Bizhanova A, Kopp P. Minireview: the sodium-iodide symporter NIS and pendrin in iodide homeostasis of the thyroid. Endocrinology. 2009;150:1084–90.
128. Shen DH, Kloos RT, Mazzaferri EL, Jhian SM. Sodium iodide symporter in health and disease. Thyroid. 2001;11:415–25.
129. Dai G, Levy O, Carrasco N. Cloning and characterization of the thyroid iodide transporter. Nature. 1996;379:458–60.
130. Dohan O, De la Vieja A, Paroder V, et al. The sodium/iodide symporter (NIS): characterization, regulation, and medical significance. Endocr Rev. 2003;24:48–77.
131. Bestagno M, Pagliavni R, Maira G, et al. Mediastinal uptake of ^{131}I in patients with thyroid cancer: may it be referred to normal thymus? Eur J Nucl Med. 1993;20:648 (abstr).
132. Goldman M, Bauer SR, et al. A comparative study of iodine uptake by thyroid and thymus glands of male and female Sprague-Dawley rats of different ages. Acta Endocrinol. 1977;85:64–70.
133. Jackson GL, Graham WP, Flickinger FW, et al. Thymus accumulation of radioactive iodine. Pa Med. 1979;82:37–8.
134. Michigishi T, Mizukami Y, Shuke N, et al. Visualization of the thymus with therapeutic doses of radioiodine in patients with thyroid cancer. Eur J Nucl Med. 1993;20:75–9.
135. Veronikis IE, Simkin P, Braverman LE, et al. Thymic uptake of iodine-131 in the anterior mediastinum. J Nucl Med. 1996;37:991–2.
136. Vermiglio F, Baudin E, Travagli JP, et al. Iodine concentration by the thymus in thyroid carcinoma. J Nucl Med. 1996;37:1830–1.
137. Wilson L, Barrington SF, Kettle AG, et al. Physiological uptake occurs in the thymus of young patients treated with radioiodine for thyroid carcinoma. J Nucl Med. 1998;38:152P (abstr).
138. Wilson LM, Barrington SF, Morrison ID, et al. Therapeutic implications of thymic uptake of radioiodine in thyroid carcinoma. Eur J Nucl Med. 1998;25:622–8.
139. Salvatore M, Saletmich I, Rufini V, et al. Unusual false-positive radioiodine whole-body scans in patients with differentiated thyroid carcinoma. Clin Nucl Med. 1997;22:380–4.
140. Andreas J, Bruhl K, Eissmer D, et al. False-positive I-131 whole body imaging after I-131 therapy for a follicular carcinoma. Clin Nucl Med. 1997;22:123–4.
141. Davidson J, McDougall IR. How frequently is the thymus seen on whole-body iodine-131 diagnostic and post-treatment scans. Eur J Nucl Med. 2000;27:425–30.
142. Mello ME, Flamini RC, Corbo R, Mamede M. Radioiodine concentration by the thymus in differentiated thyroid carcinoma: report of five cases. Arq Bras Endocrinol Metabol. 2009;53:874–9.
143. Abdel-Dayem HM, Halker K, El Sayed M, et al. The radioactive wig in iodine-131 whole-body imaging. Clin Nucl Med. 1984;9:454–5.
144. Bakheet SM, Hammami MM, et al. Spurious thyroid cancer bone metastases on radioiodine scan due to external contamination. Eur J Radiol. 1993;16:239–42.

145. Bakheet S, Hammami MM, et al. Spurious lung metastases on radioiodine thyroid and whole body imaging. Clin Nucl Med. 1993;18:307–12.
146. Brodkey JS, Gibbs GE, et al. Sweat iodide excretion in patients with cystic fibrosis of the pancreas. J Appl Physiol. 1960;15:501–2.
147. Camponovo EJ, Goyer PF, Silverman ED, et al. Axillary iodine-131 accumulation due to perspiration. Clin Nucl Med. 1989;14:762–3.
148. Chandramouly BS, Scagnelli T, Burgess CK, et al. Artifact on iodine-131 whole body scan due to contaminated handkerchief. Clin Nucl Med. 1989;14:762–3.
149. Dick C, Mudun A, Alazraki NP, et al. False-positive images mimicking thyroid cancer metastasis: the nose ring sign. Clin Nucl Med. 1995;20:876–7.
150. Gritters LS, Wissing J, Gross MD, et al. Extensive salivary contamination due to concurrent use of chewing tobacco during I-131 radioablative therapy. Clin Nucl Med. 1993;18:115–7.
151. Ibis E, Wilson CR, Collier BD, et al. Iodine-131 contamination from thyroid cancer patients. J Nucl Med. 1992;33:2110–5.
152. Pochis WT, Krasnow AZ, Isitman AT, et al. The radioactive handkerchief sign: a contamination artifact in I-131 imaging for metastatic thyroid carcinoma. Clin Nucl Med. 1990;15:491–4.
153. Carey JE, Kumpuris TM, Wrobel MC, et al. Release of patients containing therapeutic dosages of iodine-131 from hospitals. J Nucl Med Technol. 1995;23:144–9.
154. Ryo UY, Alavi A, Colllier BD et al., editors. The thyroid. In: Atlas of nuclear medicine artifacts and variants. Chicago: Yearbook Medical Publishers; 1995. p. 23–33.
155. Silva F, Negron JA, et al. Unusual contamination after a therapeutic dose of iodine-131. J Nucl Med. 1996;37:75.
156. Ain KB, Shih WJ, et al. False-positive I-131 uptake at a tracheostomy site: discernment with T1-201 imaging. Clin Nucl Med. 1994;19:619–21.
157. Kirk GA, Schulz EE, et al. Post-laryngectomy localization of I-131 at tracheostomy site on a total body scan. Clin Nucl Med. 1984;9:409–11.
158. Joyce WT, Cowan RJ, et al. A potential false-positive post-therapy radioiodine scan secondary to I-131 excretion in perspiration. Clin Nucl Med. 1995;20:368–9.
159. Lawes SC, et al. ^{123}I excretion in breast milk-additional data. Nucl Med Commun. 1992;13:570–2.
160. Weaver JC, Kamm ML, Dobson RL, et al. Excretion of radioiodine in human milk. JAMA. 1960;173:872–5.
161. Spencer RP, Spitznagle LA, Karimeddini MK, et al. Breast milk content of ^{131}I in a hypothyroid patient. Nucl Med Biol. 1986;13:585.
162. Wiseman J, et al. Bony metastasis from thyroid carcinoma or contamination? Clin Nucl Med. 1984;9:363.
163. Bruno R, Giannasio P, Ronga G, et al. Sodium iodide symporter expression and radioiodine distribution in extrathyroidal tissues. J Endocrinol Invest. 2004;27:1010–4.
164. Schechter D, Krausz Y, Moshe S, et al. Radioiodine hot hand sign. Clin Nucl Med. 1998;23:378–9.
165. Barzel US, Chun KJ, et al. Artifact of I-131 whole-body scan with thoracic vertebral uptake in a patient with papillary thyroid carcinoma. Clin Nucl Med. 1997;22:855.
166. Caplan RH, Gundersen GA, Abellera M, et al. Uptake of iodine-131 by a Meckel's diverticulum mimicking metastatic thyroid cancer. Clin Nucl Med. 1987;12:760–2.
167. Ho Y, Hicks R, et al. Hiatus hernia: a potential cause of false-positive iodine-131 scan in thyroid carcinoma. Clin Nucl Med. 1998;23:621–2.
168. Kamoi I, Nishitani H, Oshiumi Y, et al. Intrathoracic gastric cyst demonstrated by Tc-99m pertechnetate scintigraphy. AJR Am J Roentgenol. 1980;134:1080–1.
169. McNamara M, Tsang H, et al. Hiatal hernia with reflux resulting in false positive I-131 scan. Clin Nucl Med. 1998;23:178–9.
170. Misaki T, Iida Y, Kasayi K, et al. First impressions: unusual extrathyroidal uptake. J Nucl Med. 1998;39:1650.
171. Schneider JA, Divgi CR, Scott AM, et al. Hiatal hernia on whole-body radioiodine survey mimicking metastatic thyroid cancer. Clin Nucl Med. 1993;18:751–3.
172. Unal S, Oguz H, Alagol F, et al. Misinterpretation of I-131 scintigraphy because of diaphragmatic hernia. Clin Nucl Med. 1996;21:151–2.
173. White JE, Flickinger FW, Morgan ME, et al. ^{131}I accumulation in gastric pull-up simulating pulmonary metastases on total-body scan for thyroid cancer. Clin Nucl Med. 1990;15:809–10.
174. Willis LL, Cowan RJ, et al. Mediastinal uptake of I-131 in a hiatal hernia mimicking recurrence of papillary thyroid carcinoma. Clin Nucl Med. 1993;18:961–3.
175. Bekis R, Durak H, et al. Intrathoracic stomach causing a pitfall on thyroid imaging. Clin Nucl Med. 1998;23:848–9.
176. Ceccarelli C, Pancini F, Lippi F, et al. An unusual case of a false-positive iodine-131 whole-body scan in a patient with papillary thyroid cancer. Clin Nucl Med. 1987;3:192–3.
177. Berquist TH, Nolan NG, Stephens DM, et al. Radioisotope scintigraphy in diagnosis of Barrett's esophagus. AJR Am J Roentgenol. 1971;123:401–11.
178. Nair N, Basu S, Pakhale H. Unusual uptake of radioiodine in the chest in a patient with thyroid carcinoma. Br J Radiol. 2004;77:63–7.
179. Boulahdour H, Meignan M, Melliere D, et al. False-positive I-131 scan induced by Zenker's diverticulum. Clin Nucl Med. 1992;17:243–4.
180. Dhawan VM, Kaess KR, Spencer RP, et al. False positive thyroid scan due to zenker's diverticulum. J Nucl Med. 1978;19:1231–2.
181. Kistler AM, Yudt WM, Bakalar RS, et al. Retained esophageal activity on iodine-131 survey in patient with benign esophageal stricture. Clin Nucl Med. 1993;18:908–9.
182. Ozdemir A, Gungor F, Ozugur S, et al. Abnormal iodine-131 uptake in the mediastinum caused by achalasia. Clin Nucl Med. 1998;23:706–7.
183. Grossman M, et al. Gastroesophageal reflux: a potential source of confusion in technetium thyroid scanning: case report. J Nucl Med. 1977;18:548–9.
184. Robertson JS, Verhasseet M, Wahnet HW, et al. Use of ^{123}I for thyroid uptake measurements and depression of radioiodine thyroid uptake by incomplete dissolution of capsule filler. J Nucl Med. 1974;15:770–4.
185. Kipper MS, Krohn LD, et al. Increased submandibular gland uptake on thyroid scintigraphy due to Wharton's duct stone. Clin Nucl Med. 1996;21:881–2.
186. Kolla IS, Alazraki NP, Watts NB, et al. Sialadenitis mimicking metastatic thyroid carcinoma. Clin Nucl Med. 1989;14:564–6.
187. Tyson JW, Wilkinson RH, Witherspoon LR, et al. False-positive I-131 total body scans. J Nucl Med. 1974;15:1052–3.
188. Wolff H, Breda DJ, DaSilva N, et al. False-positive I-131 deposition in a parotid gland duct ectasia. Clin Nucl Med. 1998;23:257–9.
189. Carlisle M, Cortes A, McDougall IR, et al. Uptake of I-131 in the biliary tract: a potential cause of a false-positive result of scintiscan. Clin Nucl Med. 1998;23:524–7.
190. Schall GL, Temple R, et al. Importance of proper bowel cleansing before I-131 whole body scan or retention study. J Nucl Med. 1972;13:181–2.
191. Brachman MB, Rothman BJ, Ramanna L, et al. False-positive iodine-131 body scan caused by a large renal cyst. Clin Nucl Med. 1988;13:416–8.
192. Bakheet MS, Powe J, Hammami MM, et al. Unilateral radioiodine breast uptake. Clin Nucl Med. 1998;23:170–1.

193. Robinson PS, Surveyor I, et al. Response to letter: unilateral iodine-131 uptake in the lactating breast. J Nucl Med. 1995;36:1725.
194. Grunwald F, Palmedo H, Biersack HJ, et al. Unilateral iodine-131 uptake in the lactating breast. J Nucl Med. 1995;36:1724–5.
195. Serafini A, Sfakianakis G, Georgiou M, et al. Breast cyst simulating metastases of iodine-131 imaging in thyroid carcinoma. J Nucl Med. 1998;39:1910–2.
196. Blue PW, Dydek GJ, Ghaed N, et al. Radiation dosimetry from breast milk excretion of iodine-123. J Nucl Med. 1987;28:544–5.
197. Nurnberger CE, Lipscomb A, et al. Transmission of radioiodine (I-131) to infants through human maternal milk. JAMA. 1952;150:1398–400.
198. Rubow S, Klopper J, et al. Excretion of radioiodine in human milk following a therapeutic dose of 131I. Eur J Nucl Med. 1988;14:632–3.
199. Lungo M, Tenenbaum F, Chaumerliac P, Vons C, Mirat A, Beuzen F, Luton JP, Richard B. Ann Endocrinol. 2000;61:147–50.
200. Bakheet SM, Hammami MM, Powe J, Bazarbashi M, Al Subaibani H. Radioiodine in inactive tuberculosis. Eur J Nucl Med. 1999;26:659–62.
201. Regalbuto C, Buscema M, Arena S, Vigneri R, Squatrito S, Pezzino V. False-positive findings on ^{131}I whole-body scans because of posttraumatic superficial scabs. J Nucl Med. 2002;43:207–9.
202. Maslack MM, Wilson CA, et al. Iodine-131 accumulation in a pericardial effusion (letter). J Nucl Med. 1987;28:133.
203. Silva F, Garcia L, Flores C, et al. Pericardial effusion: unusual complication in thyroid cancer. Clin Nucl Med. 1996;21:218–20.
204. Haubold-Reuter BG, Landolt U, Schulthess GKV, et al. Bronchogenic carcinoma mimicking metastatic thyroid carcinoma. J Nucl Med. 1993;34:809–11.
205. Kim EE, Pjura G, Gobuty A, et al. radioiodine uptake in a benign serous cystadenoma of the ovary. Eur J Nucl Med. 1984;9:433–5.
206. Bakheet SM, Hammami MM, Pove J, Larrson S. Radioiodine in the head and neck. Endocr Pract. 2000;6:37–41.
207. Francese C, Schlumberger M, Travagli JP, et al. Iodine-131 uptake in a pleuropericardial cyst: case report of a false-positive radioiodine total body scan result in a patient with a thyroid cancer. Eur J Nucl Med. 1991;18:779–80.
208. Duque JJ, Begona Miguel M, Ruiz E, et al. False-positive ^{131}I whole-body scan in follicular thyroid carcinoma caused by frontal sinus mucocele. Clin Nucl Med. 2000;25:137–8.
209. Bakheet SM, Hammami MM, Powe J, et al. Radioiodine bronchogram in acute respiratory tract infection. Clin Nucl Med. 1997;22:308–9.
210. Bakheet SM, Hammami MM, Powe J, et al. Radioiodine uptake in rheumatoid arthritis-associated lung disease mimicking thyroid cancer metastases. Clin Nucl Med. 1988;23:319–20.
211. Hoschl R, Choy DHL, Grandevia B, et al. Iodine-131 uptake in inflammatory lung disease: a potential pitfall in treatment of thyroid carcinoma. J Nucl Med. 1988;29:701–6.
212. Herzog G, Kisling G, Bekerman C, et al. Diagnostic significance of dental history in the clinical evaluation of patients with thyroid carcinoma: periodontal surgery mimicking a metastasis on I-131 whole-body survey. Clin Nucl Med. 1992;17:589–90.
213. Wadhwa SS, Mansberg R, et al. Benign oral disease as a cause of false-positive iodine-131 scans. Clin Nucl Med. 1998;23:747–9.
214. Otsuka N, Fukunaga M, Morita K, et al. 131I uptake in patient with thyroid cancer and rheumatoid arthritis during acupuncture treatment. Clin Nucl Med. 1990;15:29–31.
215. Matheja P, Lerch H, Schmid K, et al. Frontal sinus mucocele mimicking a metastasis of papillary thyroid carcinoma. J Nucl Med. 1997;38:1022–4.
216. Brucker-Davis F, Reynolds JC, Skarulis MC, et al. False-positive iodine-131 whole-body scans due to cholecystitis and sebaceous cyst. J Nucl Med. 1996;37:1690–3.
217. Kinuya S, Yokoyama K, Michigishi T, et al. I-131 accumulation in folliculitis of the scalp. Clin Nucl Med. 1996;21:807–8.
218. Froncova K, et al. Uptake of radioiodine by myocardium following infarction. Cas Lek Cesk 103:64, (1964), quoted by Brucer, M., In: Nuclear cardiology-coronary and myocardial phase. Vignettes in Nuclear Medicine No. 89. St. Louis: Mallinkrodt; 1978. p. 9.
219. Turoglu HT, Naddaf S, Young I, et al. Infected sebaceous cyst: a cause for false-positive total-body I-123 metastatic survey for thyroid cancer. Clin Nucl Med. 1996;23:887.
220. Naddaf S, Akisik MF, Omar WS, et al. I-123 uptake in the chest wall after needle biopsy of a pulmonary nodule. Clin Nucl Med. 1997;22:572–3.
221. Langsteger W, Koltringer P, Meister E, et al. False-positive scans in papillary thyroid carcinoma (letter). J Nucl Med. 1993;34:2280.
222. Wu S, Kollin J, Coodley E, et al. I-131 total body scan: Localization of disseminated gastric adenocarcinoma. Case report and survey of the literature. J Nucl Med. 1984;25:1204–9.
223. Berding, Forsting M, Georgi P, et al. Unspezifische speichergung in J-131-Ganzkorperszintigramm bei de Nachsorgeeines metasterierienden papillaren. Schilddrusencarcinoms bedingt durch ein meningeom. Nucl Compact. 1990;21:163–4.
224. Priesman RA, Halpern SE, Shishido R, et al. Uptake of radioiodine by a papillary meningioma. AJR Am J Roentgenol. 1977;128:349–50.
225. Acosta J, Chitkara R, Kahn F, et al. Radioactive iodine uptake by a large cell-undifferentiated bronchogenic carcinoma. Clin Nucl Med. 1982;7:368–9.
226. Fernandez-Ulloa M, Maxon HR, Mehta S, et al. Iodine-131 uptake by primary lung adenocarcinoma, misinterpretation of ^{131}I scan. JAMA. 1976;236:857–8.
227. Langsteger W, Lind P, Koltringer P, et al. Misinterpretation of iodine uptake in papillary thyroid carcinoma and primary lung adenocarcinoma. J Cancer Res Clin Oncol. 1990;116:8–12.
228. Misaki T, Takeuchi R, Miyamoto S, et al. Radioiodine uptake by squamous-cell carcinoma of the lung. J Nucl Med. 1994;35:474–5.
229. Burt RW, et al. Accumulation of ^{123}I in a Warthin's tumor. Clin Nucl Med. 1978;3:155–6.
230. Harbert JC, et al. Radio iodine therapy of differentiated thyroid carcinoma. In: Harbert JC, Robertson JS, Held KD, editors. Nuclear medicine therapy. New York: Thieme Medical Publishers; 1987. p. 37–89.
231. Wynne HMN, McCartney JC, McClendon JF, et al. Struma ovarii. Am J Obstet Gynecol. 1940;39:263–75.
232. Willemse PHB, Oosterhuis JW, Aalders JG, et al. Malignant struma ovarii treated by ovariectomy, thyroidectomy and I-131 administration. Cancer. 1987;60:178–82.
233. Brenner W, Bohuslavizki KH, Wolf H, et al. Radiotherapy with iodine-131 in recurrent malignant struma ovarii. Eur J Nucl Med. 1996;23:91–4.
234. Lakshmanan M, Reynolds JC, DelVecchio S, et al. Pelvic radioiodine uptake in a rectal wall teratoma after thyroidectomy for papillary carcinoma. J Nucl Med. 1992;33:1848–50.
235. Wang PW, Chen HY, Li CH, et al. Uptake of I-131 by an abdominal neurilemoma mimicking metastatic thyroid carcinoma. Clin Nucl Med. 1993;18:964–6.
236. Wilson RL, Cowan RJ, et al. Tc-99m pertechnetate uptake in a thymoma: case report. Clin Nucl Med. 1982;7:149–50.
237. Savas H, Wong KK, et al. SPECT/CT characterization of oral activity on radioiodine scintigraphy. J Clin Endocrinol Metab. 2013;98:4410–6.
238. Attard M, Marozzi P, Gambino L, et al. False-positive results of an iodine-131 whole-body scan caused by an ectopic kidney. Clin Nucl Med. 2001;26:271–3.
239. Bhargava P, Choi WS. Artifactual I-131 activity in the hairs after thyroid remnant ablation. Thyroid. 2006;16:1187–9.

240. Borkar S, Grewal R, Schoder H. I-131 uptake demonstrated in the appendix on a posttreatment scan in a patient with thyroid cancer. Clin Nucl Med. 2008;33:551–2.
241. Brockmann H, Wilhelm K, Joe A, Palmedo H, Biersack HJ. Nasolacrimal drainage obstruction after radioiodine therapy: case report and a review of the literature. Clin Nucl Med. 2005;30:543–5.
242. Caglar M, Tuncel M, Usubutun A. Increased uptake on I-131 whole-body scintigraphy in Warthin tumor despite false-negative Tc-99m pertechnetate salivary gland scintigraphy. Clin Nucl Med. 2003;28:945–6.
243. Ceylan GE, Erdogan A. Mediastinal radioiodine uptake due to hiatal hernia: a false-positive reason in 131I scan. Rev Esp Med Nucl. 2010;29:95.
244. De la Riva Perez PA, Castro Montano J, Iglesias Jerez R, Lopez Munoz N, Gil Martinez EM, Rodriguez de Quesada B. Atypical uptake of gallbladder as cause of false-positive iodine-131 in post-surgical removal scanning of thyroid remains. Rev Esp Med Nucl. 2007;26:52–3.
245. Deandreis D, Lumbroso J, Al Ghuzlan A, Baudin E, Schlumberger M, Leboulleux S. Abnormal pelvic uptake on post-therapeutic radioiodine (^{131}I) whole-body scan. Eur J Nucl Med Mol Imaging. 2011;38:1957.
246. Frew J, Mallick U, Perros P. A patient with asymmetric parotid uptake on a diagnostic iodine-131 scan during thyroid cancer follow-up. Thyroid. 2007;17:801–2.
247. Garcia Alonso MP, Balsa Breton MA, Paniagua Correa C, et al. Iodine uptake in the chest in the follow-up of well-differentiated thyroid cancer. Rev Esp Med Nucl. 2011;30:24–8.
248. Hirata K, Shiga T, Kubota KC, Okamoto S, Kamibayashi T, Tamaki N. Radioiodine therapy for thyroid cancer depicted uterine leiomyoma. Clin Nucl Med. 2009;34:180–1.
249. Hsiao E, Huynh T, Mansberg R, Bautovich G, Roach P. Diagnostic I-123 scintigraphy to assess potential breast uptake of I-131 before radioiodine therapy in a postpartum woman with thyroid cancer. Clin Nucl Med. 2004;29:498–501.
250. Iglesias P, Olmos-Garcia R, Riva B, Diez JJ. Iodine 131 and lingual thyroid. J Clin Endocrinol Metab. 2008;93:4198–9.
251. Karyagar S, Uyanik E, Karyagar SS, Uslu R. False-positive orbital uptake on (131)I scintigraphy due to ocular prothesis. Hell J Nucl Med. 2008;11:193.
252. Khan S, Dunn J, Strickland N, Al-Nahhas A. Iodine-123 uptake in vertebral haemangiomas in a patient with papillary thyroid carcinoma. Nucl Med Rev Cent East Eur. 2008;11:30–3.
253. Lim ST, Jeong HJ, Chung MJ, Yim CY, Sohn MH. Malignant struma ovarii demonstrated on post-therapy radioiodine scan after total thyroidectomy for papillary thyroid cancer. Clin Nucl Med. 2008;33:429–31.
254. Malhotra G, Nair N, Menon H, et al. Bronchoalveolar carcinoma of lung masquerading as iodine avid metastasis in a patient with minimally invasive follicular carcinoma of thyroid. Clin Nucl Med. 2008;33:26–9.
255. Manka-Waluch A, Palmedo H, Tasci S, Biersack HJ, Bucerius J. False-positive ^{131}I whole-body scan and shrinkage of a pulmonary aspergilloma under ^{131}I therapy in a patient with thyroid cancer. Thyroid. 2006;16:197–8.
256. Mattern M, Staab E. I-131 localization in hematocolpos: a differential diagnosis consideration for pelvic I-131 uptake. Clin Nucl Med. 2007;32:659–60.
257. Meltzer DE, Gebara NV, Goel SR, Ghesani M, Kuriloff DB, Shatzkes DR. Asymmetric I-131 uptake in the submandibular gland in the setting of thyroid carcinoma. Clin Nucl Med. 2008;33:638–40.
258. Mena Bares LM, Vallejo Casas JA, Moreno Ortega E, del Real Nunez R, Maza Muret FR, Latre Romero JM. I-131 visualization of thoracic aortic aneurysm after radioiodine administration for thyroid carcinoma. Clin Nucl Med. 2008;33:553–4.
259. Modoni S, Crocetti U, Torlontano M, Urbano N. Abnormal lung iodine-131 uptake in a patient with cystic fibrosis and papillary thyroid carcinoma. Thyroid. 2005;15:89–90.
260. Nguyen BD, Roarke MC. Epiphrenic diverticulum: potential pitfall in thyroid cancer iodine-131 scintigraphy. Clin Nucl Med. 2005;30:631–2.
261. Omur O, Akgun A, Ozcan Z, Sen C, Ozkilic H. Clinical implications of diffuse hepatic uptake observed in postablative and post-therapeutic I-131 scans. Clin Nucl Med. 2009;34:11–4.
262. Omur O, Ozbek SS, Akgun A, Yazici B, Mutlukoca N, Ozcan Z. False-positive I-131 accumulation in a hepatic hydatid cyst. Clin Nucl Med. 2007;32:930–2.
263. Ong SC, Eng DN, Sundram FX, Chan LL. A novel case of false-positive I-131 whole-body scan in thyroid carcinoma caused by subdural hematoma. Clin Nucl Med. 2004;29:164–6.
264. Qiu ZL, Xu YH, Song HJ, Luo QY. Unusual ^{131}I uptake in a benign mucinous cystadenoma of the ovary in a patient with papillary thyroid cancer. Clin Nucl Med. 2010;35:965–6.
265. Rashid K, Johns W, Chasse K, Walker M, Gupta SM. Esophageal diverticulum presenting as metastatic thyroid mass on iodine-131 scintigraphy. Clin Nucl Med. 2006;31:405–8.
266. Ronga G, Bruno R, Puxeddu E, et al. Radioiodine uptake in non-lactating mammary glands: evidence for a causative role of hyperprolactinemia. Thyroid. 2007;17:363–6.
267. Sakahara H, Yamashita S, Suzuki K, Imai M, Kosugi T. Visualization of nasolacrimal drainage system after radioiodine therapy in patients with thyroid cancer. Ann Nucl Med. 2007;21:525–7.
268. Schlosser J, Paliou M, Bravo-Vera R, Sheikh A, Gouller A. False positive uptake in post-treatment iodine-131 whole-body scans secondary to contamination. Thyroid. 2007;17:81–2.
269. Schmidt M, Dietlein M, Schroder U, Schicha H. False-positive uptake of I-131 in a laryngocele mimicking thyroid remnant after thyroidectomy for papillary thyroid carcinoma. Clin Nucl Med. 2006;31:716–7.
270. Sinha A, Bradley KM, Steatham J, Weaver A. Asymmetric breast uptake of radioiodine in a patient with thyroid malignancy: metastases or not? J R Soc Med. 2008;101:319–20.
271. Sioka C, Dimakopoulos N, Kouraklis G, Kotsalou I, Zouboulidis A. False-positive whole-body scan after I-131 therapy in a patient with intestinal scar. Clin Nucl Med. 2006;31:232–3.
272. Turker O, Dogan I, Kumanlioglu K. Radioiodine accumulation in a large adnexal cystadenofibroma. Thyroid. 2010;20:561–2.
273. Utamakul C, Sritara C, Kositwattanarerk A, Balachandra T, Chotipanich C, Chokesuwattanaskul P. I-131 uptake in bilateral ovarian endometrial cysts. Clin Nucl Med. 2009;34:537–8.
274. Vallejo Casas JA, Mena Bares ML, Galvez Moreno MA, Latre Romero JM. Tracheostomy cannula as a cause of false positive in the body scan with (131)I in the follow-up of differentiated thyroid cancer. Rev Esp Med Nucl. 2011.
275. Shapiro B, Rufini V, Jarwan A, et al. Semin Nucl Med. 2000;30:115–32.
276. Glazer D, Brown RKJ, Wong KK, Savas H, Gross MD, Avram AM. Radiographics. 2013;33:375–96.

The Utility of SPECT-CT in Differentiated Thyroid Cancer

14

Kanchan Kulkarni, Frank B. Atkins, and Douglas Van Nostrand

Introduction

For over 60 years, planar scintigraphy using ^{131}I has been an important part of the standard of care for imaging patients who have differentiated thyroid cancer (DTC), and more recent planar scintigraphy using ^{123}I has in part or in toto replaced ^{131}I in several countries. The range of sensitivities reported for detecting recurrent or metastatic disease with planar technique using these radioisotopes of iodine is 45–75 %, while the specificity ranges from 55 % to 100 % [1–8]. However, the limited contrast resolution of the planar images, the presence of physiological activity, and the lack of anatomical landmarks on the planar whole-body scan (WBS), "spot" camera images, or pinhole camera images make the interpretation of radioiodine scans frequently problematic. Single-photon emission computer tomography (SPECT) by its virtue of better contrast resolution and the presence of anatomical landmarks from computer tomography (CT) images overcomes several of these shortcomings, and therefore, SPECT-CT can be used for evaluation of equivocal results on planar imaging. As a result of SPECT-CT integrating the functional and anatomic information, it plays an increasingly important role in imaging of differentiated thyroid cancer.

This chapter will review radioiodine SPECT-CT imaging prior to ^{131}I therapy, immediately (i.e., 3–7 days) after ^{131}I therapy, and at follow-up with special emphasis on SPECT-CT's impact on altering staging, prognosis, and patient management.

K. Kulkarni, MD
Division of Nuclear Medicine, MedStar Washington Hospital Center, Washington, DC, USA
e-mail: Kanchan.kulkarni@medstar.net

F.B. Atkins, PhD
Division of Nuclear Medicine, MedStar Washington Hospital Center, Georgetown University School of Medicine, Washington, DC, USA
e-mail: Francis.B.Atkins@Medstar.net

D. Van Nostrand, MD, FACP, FACNM (✉)
Nuclear Medicine Research, MedStar Research Institute and Washington Hospital Center, Georgetown University School of Medicine, Washington Hospital Center, 110 Irving Street, N.W., Suite GB 60F, Washington, DC 20010, USA
e-mail: douglasvannostrand@gmail.com

Technical Aspect of SPECT-CT

SPECT is an acronym that describes a form of nuclear medicine imaging. The letters "SP" refer to the fact that the image data are collected using conventional gamma cameras in which a *single photon* at a time from the radionuclide decay is used in forming the image as opposed to those positron emitting radionuclides in which two photons resulting from the collision and annihilation of a positron with an electron must be detected simultaneously. "ECT" refers to *emission computer tomography*. In order to generate tomographic slices, it is necessary to view the patient from a large number of angles completely around the patient, typically every 3–6° over a full 360°. Therefore, SPECT imaging systems consist of one or more conventional gamma cameras that are mounted on a gantry that allows these detectors to be precisely and automatically rotated around the patient while collecting each of these images. The complexity of the mathematical processing (often referred to as *reconstruction*) has become feasible with the high speed and low cost of computers. The first research SPECT devices were made available in the 1960s and the commercial devices in the early 1980s.

On some planar radioisotope studies, one may identify anatomic structures that allow the anatomic localizaion of the radioisotope uptake. However, for thyroid radioisotope imaging anatomic structures for localization are typically not present. In addition, it can sometimes be difficult to distinguish normal physiologic distributions from regions of abnormal uptake without precise anatomical landmarks for

L. Wartofsky, D. Van Nostrand (eds.), *Thyroid Cancer*, DOI 10.1007/978-1-4939-3314-3_14

correlation. Relatively recent advances in imaging technology have resulted in hybrid devices that help to address this dilemma. One such device is the SPECT-CT system, which is a hybrid of a SPECT camera and a *computer tomography* (CT) scanner. This was pioneered by Lang et al. [9] and is now the configuration of the majority of systems sold by the major commercial SPECT vendors. These various hybrid devices all have a common feature – namely, the SPECT unit and the CT unit, sharing the same patient table so that the same transaxial slice through the patient can be identified on both modalities. Often these two sets of images are displayed superimposed on each other with the physician able to control the degree of blending (fusion) dynamically on the computer monitor.

Radiation Absorbed Dose

The radiation exposure from this imaging procedure is low, and it is not clear what adverse effect, if any, low-dose radiation might cause. Since the effect of these low radiation dose levels will likely never be scientifically established, the recommendations of the regulatory bodies are to adopt a conservative position and assume that the risk varies linearly with the radiation dose and to extrapolate this from observations obtained from high levels (e.g., derived largely from long-term follow-up of Japanese atomic bomb survivors) to the very low levels associated with medical imaging. However, these estimated values are not patient specific. For radiopharmaceuticals, the estimates are based only on stylized models of adults and children and assumptions about their biokinetic and multiple other factors like distribution of radiopharmaceutical in the body and radiosensitivities of the organs, to name two. Therefore, another approximate measure that has been introduced is called the *effective radiation dose* that applies different weighting factors (based on stochastic risk factors) to the radiation dose based on the organ that was exposed. These are then summed over all of the body parts that were exposed. The weighting factors typically used are based on the recommendations of the ICRP report 103 [10]. CT and other radiographic procedures only expose a portion of the body to the ionizing radiation. For CT imaging, the effective dose will depend upon the institution's imaging protocol and the body part examined (e.g., head, chest, and/or abdomen). Typical effective doses from several diagnostic radiographic [11] and nuclear medicine procedures [12] that a patient with thyroid cancer might undergo are shown in Fig. 14.1.

Advantages and Disadvantages

The advantages as well as disadvantages of SPECT-CT are multiple. One of the major advantages of SPECT imaging is that the images produced are 3-D in nature – the superposition of over- and underlying normal tissue is removed. Hence, SPECT imaging results in increased image contrast resolution and potentially improved lesion detection. In conventional imaging, two or more lesions with radioiodine accumulation positioned along a single plane would at best be seen as a single abnormal area. However, on the tomographic image, each abnormal focal area would typically be visualized separately, providing more information about the extent of disease and depth of the lesion(s) within the patient. Thus, SPECT-CT by virtue of improved contrast resolution results in improved sensitivity for the detection of foci of uptake of normal residual thyroid tissue and functioning metastatic differentiated thyroid cancer (DTC).

As the name implies, SPECT images are tomographic images, which allow review of individual cross-sectional images of the body rather than planar images. By combining the SPECT gamma camera with a CT, one may co-register the functional images with the anatomic images of the CT, which in turn improves significantly the specificity of the study [13–22]. This has significantly helped in differentiating physiological or artifactual radioiodine uptake from normal residual thyroid tissue and functioning metastatic DTC. SPECT-CT also offers the potential for lesional and whole-body dosimetry for treatment planning [23, 24].

However, SPECT-CT has some inherent disadvantages. The image reconstruction process itself tends to enhance statistical noise in the images, and the primary way of compensating for this degradation is to collect more counts in the images. Thus, a SPECT acquisition may take about 30–45 min to complete. However, this only covers an axial extent through the patient equal to the height of the detector, which is typically about 40 cm. This process would have to be repeated four to five times or more in order to cover the patient's entire axial extent, which would not be practical. Instead, SPECT studies would normally be a supplement to whole-body imaging and be limited to a suspicious anatomical region that requires more detailed investigation. Another disadvantage is that the cross-sectional tomographic images obtained both on the SPECT camera and the CT may be misregistered resulting in either a false-positive or false-negative study. Although dedicated SPECT-CT cameras minimize this problem, misregistration artifacts can still occur secondary to patient motion during imaging or even respiratory motion, especially when evaluating chest lesions [25]. To help reduce misregistration artifacts, various techniques are available to help, such as the use of external markers [22, 26]. Third, the patient receives additional radiation exposure from the CT, which may vary depending on whether the CT radiation exposure is from a nondiagnostic CT performed for attenuation correction and localization or from a regular diagnostic CT. Finally, SPECT imaging systems are frequently more expensive than conventional whole-body devices, and in any evaluation of the utility of imaging, cost analysis is important.

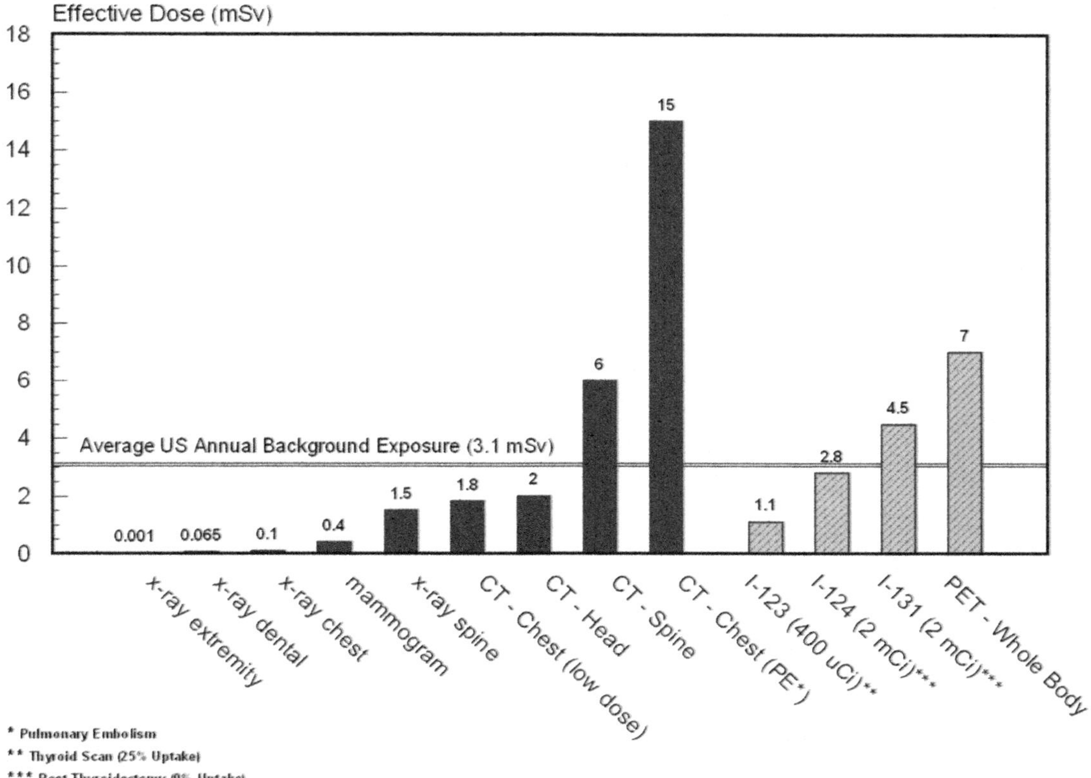

Fig. 14.1 Effective dose (mSv) for several radiographic and nuclear medicine studies [11, 12]. A reference line is also indicated at 3.1 mSv, which corresponds to the average annual radiation exposure each person in the United States receives from naturally occurring sources (e.g., cosmic, terrestrial, radon gas). The darker bars are for radiographic procedures and the lighter bars are for nuclear medicine studies for typical administered activities. The radiation-absorbed dose from the nuclear medicine study only depends on the radioactivity administered and not on the number of scans performed, imaging time, or equipment used. If a SPECT-CT study is also performed, then an additional radiation absorbed dose would be delivered from the CT scan. If a low-dose CT is performed for anatomical localization and attenuation correction, the additional effective dose would be added to the radioiodine study, but this would be less than the effective dose of a diagnostic CT

Utility of Pre-therapy SPECT Scanning

Pre-therapy scans are often used to evaluate the presence of thyroid remnant size and locoregional and distant metastases as well as to potentially guide the prescribed activity for the therapeutic ^{131}I (see Chapt. 19). Several publications investigating the utility of SPECT-CT prior to ^{131}I therapy have concluded that results were superior in comparison to planar scintigrams [13–15, 19]. In regard to specificity, SPECT-CT imaging is proven to be consistently superior to planar imaging because of the better localization offered by the CT (see Table 14.1).

The better localization offered by CT helps in distinguishing thyroid bed remnants from cervical nodes (see fig 14.2) or even physiological activity like the salivary glands or radioactivity in the lumen of the esophagus [17]. CT with SPECT may also help in characterizing normal variants of thyroid tissue like thyroglossal tract remnants. Within the chest, SPECT may improve sensitivity of detection of pulmonary nodules and mediastinal nodes and/or help distinguish nonmalignant conditions like bronchiectasis from distant metastases. Distant metastatic sites may be identified with more specificity. The accuracy offered by SPECT-CT imaging increases the confidence of interpretation of the radioiodine scan and may assist or change clinical management by more accurate staging of the disease, selection of additional surgery, altering the therapeutic prescribed activity of ^{131}I, or even avoidance of an unnecessary ^{131}I therapy [15, 19, 22, 27]. The incremental value of SPECT in these diagnostic scans is reported to be in the range of 47–85 %. Studies suggest that the postsurgical staging may change in as many as 21 % of the patients, and proposed therapeutic activity may be impacted in as many as 47–58 % of the patients [13–15]. In a recent study by Avram et al., routine SPECT-CT of the neck and chest changed staging in 4 % of younger patients and 25 % of the older patients [28].

Utility of Post-therapy Spect Scanning

Imaging with SPECT-CT at the time of post-therapy scanning is also valuable given the higher administered prescribed activities for therapy and a better target to background ratio

Table 14.1 Utility of SPECT-CT prior to ^{131}I therapy

Author	Patients	Body area imaged	Incremental value	Comments
Wong [13]	53 patients with 56 scans. 52 diagnostic scans and 4 post-therapy scans.	Selected areas based on findings on planar images.	SPECT-CT had incremental value for 70/147 (47.6 %) foci, and this included 53 of 130 foci in the neck and 17 of 17 distant foci.	
Chen [14]	66 pre-therapy scans with subsequent thyroidectomy.	Selected areas based on inconclusive planar findings.	Precise localization and characterization were achieved in 69/81 (85.2 %) and 67/81 (82.7 %) foci, respectively. Therapeutic strategy was changed in 8 (47 %) of 17 patients.	Uncommon metastatic lesions found in 9/66 (13.6 %) patients with SPECT-CT. Unusual locations of uptake (e.g., subcutaneous, erector spinae muscle, parotid gland, and femoral metastases) identified by SPECT-CT.
Wong [15]	48 patients before first ^{131}I therapy Retrospective.	Neck and upper thorax in 45 patients. Head, abdomen, and proximal lower extremities in 3 patients.	SPECT-CT changed planar scan interpretation in 19/48 (40 %) patients, detecting regional nodal metastases in four patients and clarifying equivocal focal neck uptake in 15 patients. SPECT in combination with chest radiographs and planar images changed postsurgical staging in 10/48 (21 %) of patients. SPECT-CT changed the proposed ^{131}I therapeutic dosage in 28/48 (58 %) patients.	The improved interpretation led to changes in staging and prescribed activity of therapeutic ^{131}I.
Blum [27]	Retrospective analysis of 184 scans. 40 scans had indeterminate findings. 15/40 scans performed before therapy. 25/40 scans performed post-therapy.	Head, neck, chest, abdomen, and pelvis depending on location of cryptic findings.	In 15 pre-therapy patients, the SPECT-CT was important in determining if ablative I-131 therapy was to be performed. In 25 post-therapy patients, SPECT-CT helped distinguish thyroid cancer mets or remnants.	Reduces needless therapies by resolving cryptic findings.
Avram [28]	320 scans post thyroidectomy 138 <45 years old, and 182 >45 years old	Routine SPECT-CT from skull base to diaphragm and all other foci of abnormal activity on planar images.	In young patients (<45 years), pre-therapy scans detected distant metastases (4 %) and nodal mets in 61/138 (44 %) including 24/62 (38 %) originally assigned pN0 and pNx. In older patients, distant metastases detected in 18/182 (10 %) and nodal metastases in 51/182 (28 %) including unsuspected nodal metastases in 26/108 (24 %) originally assigned pN0 and pNx.	I-131 SPECT-CT detected regional metastases in 35 % and distant metastases in 8 % of patients leading to upstaging in 4 % of the younger and 35 % of the older patients.

secondary to the longer interval between the ^{131}I therapy and the post-therapy scan [29].

Multiple publications demonstrating the superior results of post-therapy scanning of selected locations with SPECT-CT relative to planar scintigraphy have been published (see Table 14.2) [17–20, 26, 27, 29–32]. These studies demonstrate the superior utility of SPECT-CT relative to planar scintigraphy in the diagnosis of additional sites of metastases and clarification of equivocal foci in as many as 28–88 %.

Within the neck, cervical nodal metastases at times may be masked by the intense activity in thyroid remnants on the post-therapy scans; SPECT-CT can be helpful by distinguishing thyroid remnant tissue and nodal metastases (see Fig. 14.2). Neck SPECT-CT can also better localize radioactivity to physiological structures like salivary glands, dental caries, oral cavity, etc. [15]. The nodal staging is reported to change in as many as 22–36 % [17, 20, 21, 33]. Thoracic SPECT-CT can help distinguish rib cage involvement from peripheral soft tissue metastases, lung metastases, or bronchial metastases (see Fig. 14.3) [22]. Additional distant metastatic sites were identified in 10–25 % of patients [20, 31]. The accurate staging may lead to an alteration in patient management in as many as 11–41 % [18–20].

In addition to the value of identification of the true extent of disease and altering management, surveillance SPECT-CT may have added utility in regard to evaluating prognosis. Aide et al. [16] demonstrated that post-therapy SPECT-CT

Table 14.2 Utility of SPECT-CT immediately after (i.e., 3–7 days) ^{131}I therapy

Author	Patients	Body area imaged	Incremental value	Comments
Aide [16]	55 patients. Prospective study. Median follow-up 21 months.	Neck and thorax	SPECT-CT enabled more accurate diagnosis than whole-body scans (WBS) and reduced the number of indeterminate interpretations from 29 % on whole-body scans to 7 % with SPECT-CT.	Neck node involvement was accurately localized to central or lateral compartments.
Schmidt [17]	57 patients	Neck	Altered nodal staging in 20/57 (35 %) patients by upstaging in 8 patients or down staging in 12 patients. Change in nodal stage resulted in new risk stratification in 14/57 (25 %) patients.	Authors proposed routine use of SPECT-CT since it can identify lymph node mets in patients who are on stage N0.
Ruf [18]	25 patients. Prospective.	Inconclusive foci on planar images.	Additional use of SPECT-CT allowed improved interpretation of inconclusive ^{131}I findings in planar scans. Impacted management in ~25 % of patients.	
Yamamato [26]	17 patients		SPECT-CT fusion imaging was considered to be of benefit in 15/17 (88 %) of patients.	Fusion images using external markers, which were considered simple and practical.
Grewal [29]	148 patients. Retrospective.	Neck and upper chest, abdomen, and pelvis, as needed.	SPECT-CT reduced the need for additional cross-sectional imaging studies in 29/148 (20 %) patients and changed the initial risk of recurrence (ATA classification) in 6.4 %.	This was first study of its kind to assess risk stratification per the 2009 ATA guidelines as well as the cost-effective value of SPECT-CT.
Ciappuccini [30]	170 patients. Prospective. Median follow-up of 29 months.	Neck and thorax – routine. Abdomen and pelvis selectively.	SPECT was shown to be the sole independent prognostic variable for disease-free survival. Combining WBS and SPECT-CT identified previously unknown distant metastases in 10 patients and clearly showed lymph node involvement in 12 patients.	Assessed the prognostic value of SPECT-CT in recurrent or persistent metastatic DTC compared to standard clinical, biological, and pathological predictive factors. Only WBS with SPECT-CT was associated with an increased risk of persistent/recurrent disease.
Tharp [19]	71 patients of which 17 pre-therapy scans and 54 post-therapy scans were performed. Retrospective.	Inconclusive foci on planar images.	SPECT-CT had an incremental diagnostic value compared to planar imaging in 41/71 (57 %) patients. Changed therapeutic approach in 7/17 (41 %) of the patients.	Image fusion particularly useful for structures in the neck.
Kohlfuerest [20]	41 patients	Inconclusive findings on planar images.	Changed nodal staging in 12/33 (36.4 %) of patients Direct impact on 8/33 (63.6 %) patients who underwent surgery. Upstaged M stage in 4/19 (21.1 %) of patients with distant metastases Direct impact on 2/19 (10.5 %) patients who had external radiation therapy.	SPECT-CT provided valuable additional information for neck lesions by precise localization.
Wang [31]	94 patients. Retrospective.	Patients with abnormal uptake on planar imaging.	Provided additional clinical data in 7/94 patients. Identified 10 (11 %) new metastases missed by WBS. Caused physicians to reconsider the ^{131}I therapeutic prescribed activity in 22/94 (23 %) patients based on altered staging relative to prior staging. Upstaged in 7 patients. Downstaged 15 patients.	
Mustafa [21]	151 patients. Prospective.	Head and neck on all patients.	Changed nodal staging in 24.5 % of patients with microcarcinomas.	Authors suggested use of SPECT-CT as a routine tool in all T1 papillary thyroid cancer patients in whom lymph node dissection was not performed.
Qiu [32]	561 patients. Prospective.	Neck	SPECT-CT identified parapharyngeal metastases in 14/561 patients (2.5 %).	Parapharyngeal mets were associated with regional and/or distant metastases.
Maruoka [33]	Retrospective. 147 patients.	Routine from skull base to diaphragm and additional SPECT-CT depending on the planar scan findings	Interpretation of 24/108 (22.2 %) foci for lymph node metastases was changed with SPECT-CT. SPECT-CT helped changed clinical staging in 9/147 (6.1 %) patients and therapeutic planning in 3/147 (2.0 %).	Post-therapy SPECT-CT improved localization, detection of lymph node and distant metastases

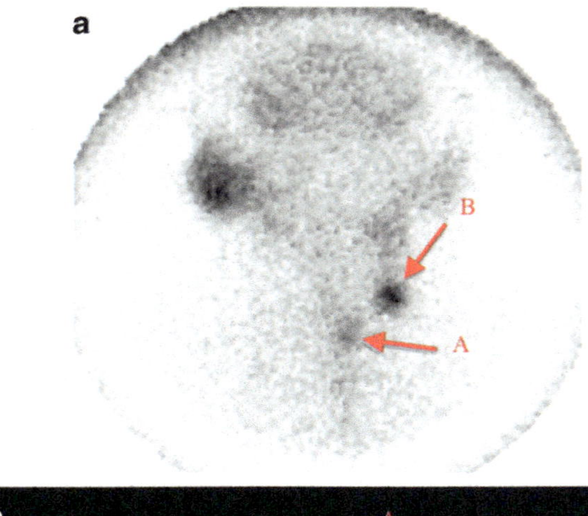

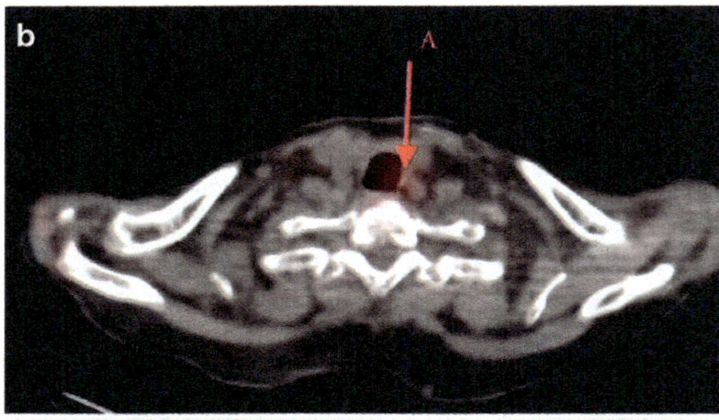

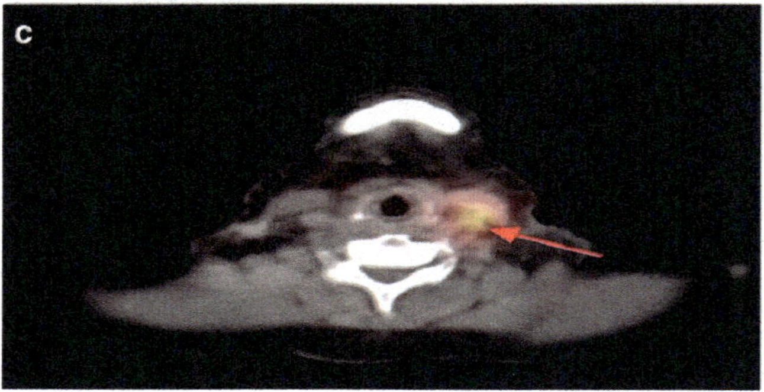

Fig. 14.2 A 71-year-old female, status post-near-total thyroidectomy. After near-total thyroidectomy, the pathology of a nodule within the thyroid demonstrated unifocal papillary thyroid cancer measuring 2.2 cm in its greatest dimension. Two perithyroidal lymph nodes were removed and were negative for metastases. The patient was referred for ^{123}I postoperative scan and remnant ablation with ^{131}I. (**a**) A pinhole image in the anterior projection of the neck performed after the administration of 74 MBq (2 mCi) of ^{123}I demonstrated two focal areas of radioactivity on the *left side* – one in the lower neck (*A*) and the other more superiorly (*B*) (see *arrows* in Fig. **a**). SPECT-CT was performed to characterize these two foci. The inferior focus (*A*) is localized in the left thyroid bed (Fig. **b**), while the left superior cervical focus is confirmed to be a left lymph node (Fig. **c**). The patient's thyroid cancer was upstaged and the ^{131}I therapy prescribed activity was increased

scans predicted treatment failure at 2 years better than planar WBS. Similarly, in a prospective study with a median follow-up of 29 months, Ciapuccini et al. [30] demonstrated that only a positive post-therapy WBS with SPECT-CT was an independent variable of disease-free survival. Positive scans were related to an increased risk of persistent or recurrent disease (HR = 65.21, 95 % CI: 26.03–163.39; $p < 0.001$) and suggested a post-therapy scan including a WBS and neck-thorax SPECT-CT may be used in combination. SPECT-CT by virtue of the increased specificity and timely diagnosis may be precluding additional imaging [29]. In selecting which patients may benefit from a SPECT-CT post-ablation, Ciapuccini et al. [30] suggested that patients with stimulated thyroglobulin level of >29 ng/ml may particularly benefit from SPECT-CT, and a threshold stimulated thyroglobulin level of 30 ng/ml may be appropriate for selection of patients to perform SPECT-CT.

Utility of SPECT-CT in Surveillance Scanning

The utility of SPECT-CT for diagnosis of recurrent disease during follow-up on surveillance imaging is validated by several authors (see Table 14.3) [22, 34–36]. The precise localization offered by SPECT-CT helps in accurate detection of the recurrent disease sites and may lead to altered and more appropriate treatment of these patients, or save additional imaging procedures (see Fig. 14.4). SPECT-CT was reported to be of incremental value in 42–67.8 % of patients.

Utility of SPECT-CT Compared to PET-CT Imaging

^{18}F fluorodeoxyglucose positron emission tomography-computerized tomography (^{18}F-FDG PET-CT) is often used for detection of non-iodine avid metastases in thyroid cancer [37, 38], and ^{18}F-FDG PET-CT has been discussed in more detail in multiple other chapters (see Chapt. 43, 76, 87, 93, and 97). Oh et al. [39] compared the diagnostic accuracy of ^{131}I SPECT-CT with ^{131}I WBS and ^{18}F-FDG PET-CT. SPECT-CT was accurate in patients with one ^{131}I therapy while ^{18}F-FDG PET-CT presented higher diagnostic performance in patients with multiple therapies. The authors attributed the difference between SPECT-CT and PET-CT to possible dedifferentiation of tumors in patient with multiple ^{131}I therapies, and ^{18}F fluorodeoxyglucose PET-CT identifies dedifferentiated tumors better than imaging with radioiodine.

Summary

The consensus of the literature is that SPECT-CT consistently has superior specificity of imaging compared to planar imaging. The advantages of SPECT-CT with particular reference to its incremental role in better anatomical localization and characterization of areas of radioiodine uptake over planar

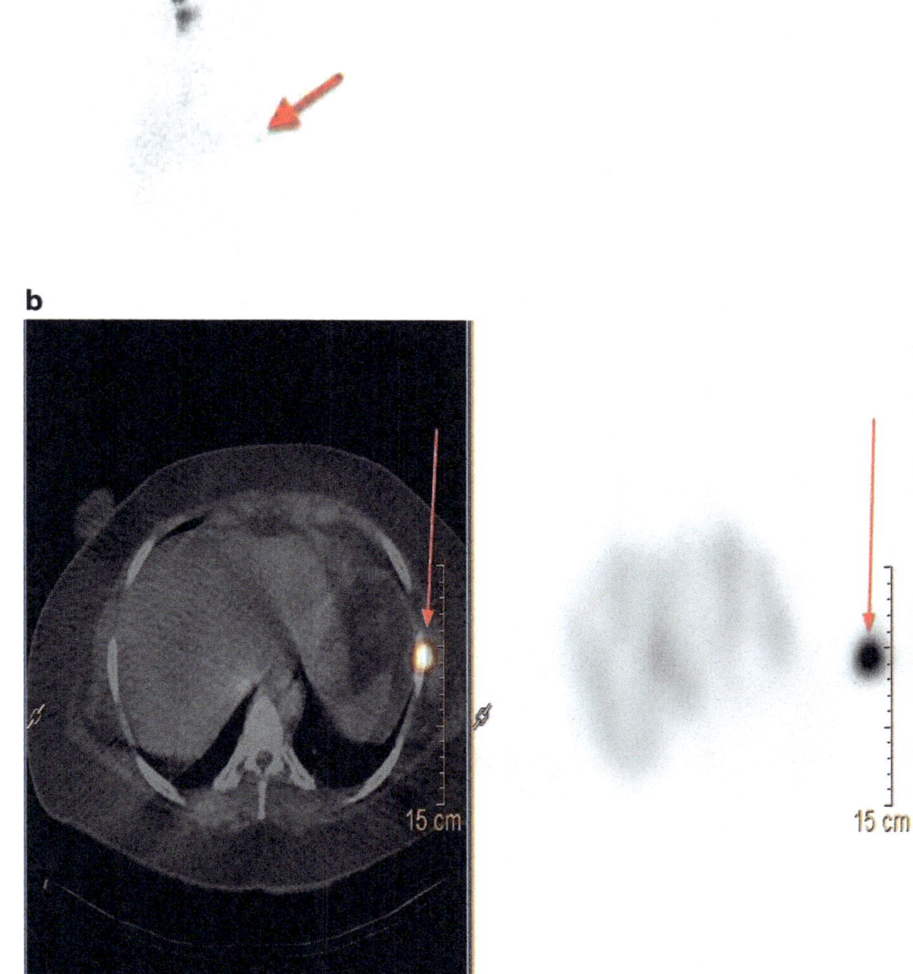

Fig. 14.3 A 31-year-old female with history of 1.1 cm follicular carcinoma of the thyroid. Postoperative ^{123}I scan demonstrated only thyroid bed remnant tissue, and the patient received 3.7 GBq (100 mCi) of ^{131}I for ablation. The post-therapy scan (shown below) was performed 7 days after administration of ^{131}I and showed a focus of radioactivity in the left lateral thorax (*arrow*) on the planar "spot" camera views (see **a**), and SPECT-CT (**b**) localized the focus to a rib indicative of skeletal metastases. SPECT-CT helped accurately localize this focus of skeletal metastases in this patient confirmed by a CT-guided biopsy

Table 14.3 Utility of SPECT-CT for follow-up surveillance scanning

Author	Patients	Body areas imaged	Incremental value	Comments
Schmidt [34]	61 patients with one radioablation. Retrospective.	Neck	All patients (61) without SPECT-CT evidence of lymph node metastases post-ablation had no uptake in the follow-up scan 5 months later.	SPECT-CT has a negative predictive value with regard to occurrence of radioiodine-positive lymph node metastases 5 months after therapy. Most of the positive lymph node metastases disappeared within 5 months.
Geerlings [36]	87 patients. Retrospective.	Neck and thorax	SPECT added additional sensitivity to the planar scan. 6/22 patients had uptake identified only on SPECT within the head and neck area. 9 patients had lesions outside the head and neck areas on SPECT.	SPECT-CT was highly recommended to improve detection rate of recurrent disease as a complimentary technique to planar imaging for head and neck as well as chest areas.

(continued)

Table 14.3 (continued)

Author	Patients	Body areas imaged	Incremental value	Comments
Spanu [22]	117 total patients. 99 surveillance scans. 8 diagnostic pre-therapy scans. 9 post-therapy scans. Prospective Fusion software used.	Routine neck and chest. Additional areas questionable by planar imaging.	Improved interpretation by precise localization in 67.8 % of patients. Resulted in more appropriate therapeutic treatment in 35.6 % of patients with positive findings. Identified occult lesions in 17 patients.	Authors highly recommended SPECT-CT in follow-up of thyroidectomized DTC patients when planar imaging was inconclusive.
Barwick [35]	79 patients. Follow-up ^{123}I scans at 6 months post-ablation. Retrospective.	Neck and thorax	Provided additional diagnostic information in 42 % of the cases.	Included patients with non-radioiodine avid disease. Because SPECT characterized focal uptake better and enabled more accurate localization, authors suggested patients may be spared further imaging procedures or even unnecessary ^{131}I therapy.

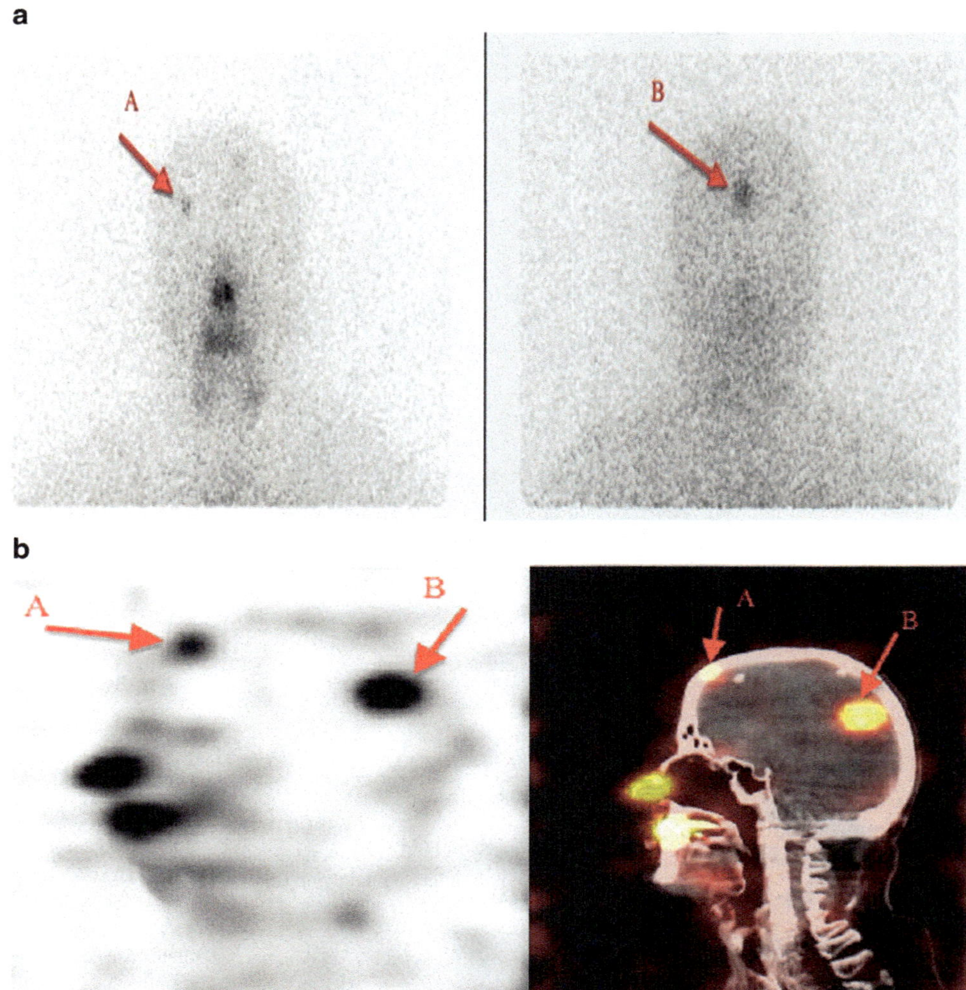

Fig. 14.4 A 62-year-old patient with metastatic papillary thyroid cancer with known metastases to the lungs and skull. This patient was referred for dosimetry to help determine his prescribed activity for an anticipated ^{131}I therapy. The diagnostic images were performed approximately 48 h after administration of 74 MBq (2 mCi) of ^{131}I, and planar images demonstrated two lesions (*A* and *B*) in the area of the head (see Fig. **a**). The anteriorly located lesion (*A*) correlated to the skull metastases seen on a recent bone scan. SPECT-CT performed for further evaluation of the additional posterior lesion (*B*) demonstrated that the activity was a brain metastase (see Fig. **b**). (Of note, the two calcifications are dural calcifications and are nonspecific chronic changes.) Because we generally perform at our facility either surgical resection or gamma knife irradiation initially for single brain metastases, the ^{131}I therapy was canceled and a gamma knife treatment of the brain metastase was performed. This was then followed by a dosimetric-determined prescribed activity of ^{131}I for therapy

imaging has significantly added to the diagnostic accuracy of radioiodine imaging. The potential incremental value of SPECT relative to planar imaging is reported to range from 35 % to 74 % and may potentially change management in 10–64 % of patients. However, given that we believe it is unlikely that SPECT-CT can replace the traditional planar WBS because of time and cost, SPECT-CT will be complementary and used to clarify equivocal areas of radioiodine uptake on WBS or other imaging modalities. SPECT-CT may also be used for better evaluation of the stage and prognosis. Further prospective studies with larger number of patients would be valuable to assess whether altered management results in altered patient outcomes.

References

1. Spies WJ, Wojtowicz CH, Spies SM, et al. Value of post-therapy whole body ^{131}I imaging in the evaluation of patients with thyroid carcinoma having undergone high-dose ^{131}I therapy. Clin Nucl Med. 1989;14:892–00.
2. Simpson WJ, Panzarella T, Carruthers JS, et al. Papillary and follicular thyroid cancer: impact of treatment in 1578 patients. Int J Radiat Oncol Biol Phys. 1998;14:1063–75.
3. van Sorge-van Boxtel RA, van Eck-Smit BL, Goslings BM. Comparison of serum thyroglobulin, ^{131}I and ^{201}Tl scintigraphy in the prospective follow-up of differentiated thyroid cancer. Nucl Med Commun. 1993;14:365–72.
4. Lubin E, Mechlis-Frisch S, Zatz S, et al. Serum thyroglobulin and iodine-131 whole body scan in the diagnosis and assessment of treatment for metastatic differentiated thyroid carcinoma. J Nucl Med. 1994;35:257–62.
5. Sutter CW, Masilungan B, Stadalnik RC. False-positive results of ^{131}I whole body scans in patients with thyroid cancer. Semin Nucl Med. 1995;25:279–82.
6. Franceschi M, Kusic Z, Franceschi D, et al. Thyroglobulin determination, neck ultrasonography and iodine-131 whole-body scintigraphy in differentiated thyroid carcinoma. J Nucl Med. 1996;37:446–51.
7. Filesi M, Signore A, Ventroni G, et al. Role of initial iodine-131whole-body scan and serum thyroglobulin in differentiated thyroid carcinoma metastases. J Nucl Med. 1998;39:1542–6.
8. Lind P, Kohlufurest S. Respective roles of thyroglobulin, radioiodine imaging, and positron emission tomography in assessment of thyroid cancer. Semin Nucl Med. 2006;36:194–205.
9. Lang T, Hasagawa B, Liew S, et al. Description of a prototype emission-transmission computed tomography imaging system. J Nucl Med. 1992;33:1881–7.
10. The 2007 Recommendations of the International Commission on Radiological Protection, ICRP publication 103. Ann ICRP. 2007; 37:1–332.
11. Mettler F, Huda W, Yoshizumi TT, et al. Effective doses in radiology and diagnostic nuclear medicine: a catalog. Radiology. 2008;248:254–63.
12. MIRD Dose Estimate Report No. 5 (data gathered in human subjects). J Nucl Med 1975;16:857–60 (25% thyroid uptake).
13. Wong KK, Zarzhevsky N, Cahill JM, Frey KA, Avram AM. Incremental value of diagnostic ^{131}I SPECT-CT fusion imaging in the evaluation of differentiated thyroid carcinoma. Nucl Med Mol Imaging. 2008;191:1785–94.
14. Chen L, Luo Q, Shen Y, et al. Incremental value of ^{131}I SPECT-CT in the management of patients with differentiated thyroid carcinoma. J Nucl Med. 2008;49:1952–7.
15. Wong KK, Sisson JC, Koral KF, et al. Staging of differentiated thyroid carcinoma using diagnostic ^{131}I SPECT/CT. Nucl Med Mol Imaging. 2010;195:730–6.
16. Aide N, Heutte N, Rame JP, et al. Clinical relevance of SPECT-CT of the neck and thorax in postablation ^{131}I scintigraphy for thyroid cancer. J Clin Endocrinol Metab. 2009;94:2075–84.
17. Schmidt D, Szikszai A, Linke R, Bautz W, et al. Impact of ^{131}I SPECT-spiral CT on nodal staging of differentiated thyroid carcinoma at the first radioablation. J Nucl Med. 2009;50:18–23.
18. Ruf J, Lehmkuhl L, Bertram H, et al. Impact of SPECT and integrated low-dose CT after radioiodine therapy on the management of patients with thyroid carcinoma. Nucl Med Commun. 2004; 25:1177–82.
19. Tharp K, Israel O, Hausmann J, et al. Impact of ^{131}I-SPECT/CT images obtained with an integrated system in the follow-up of patients with thyroid carcinoma. Eur J Nucl Med Mol Imaging. 2004;31:1435–42.
20. Kohlfuerst S, Igerc I, Lobnig M, et al. Post-therapeutic ^{131}I SPECT-CT offers high diagnostic accuracy when the findings on conventional planar imaging are inconclusive and allows a tailored patient treatment regimen. Eur J Nucl Med Mol Imaging. 2009;36:886–93.
21. Mustafa M, Kuwert T, Weber K, et al. Regional lymph node involvement in T1 papillary thyroid carcinoma: a bicentric prospective SPECT/CT study. Eur J Nucl Med Mol Imaging. 2010;37:1462–6.
22. Spanu A, Solinas ME, Chessa, et al. ^{131}I SPECT/CT in the follow-up of differentiated thyroid carcinoma: incremental value versus planar imaging. J Nucl Med. 2009;50:184–90.
23. Sgouros G, Frey E, Wahl R, et al. Three dimensional imaging-based radiobiological dosimetry. Semin Nucl Med. 2008;38:321–34.
24. Prideaux AR, Song H, Hobbs RF, et al. Three-dimensional radiobiologic dosimetry: application of radiobiologic modeling to patient-specific-3dimensional imaging-based internal dosimetry. J Nucl Med. 2007;48:1008–16.
25. Bennewitz C, Kuwert T, Han J, et al. Computer-aided evaluation of the anatomical accuracy of hybrid SPECT/spiral-CT imaging of lesions localized in the neck and upper abdomen. Nucl Med Commun. 2012;33:1153–9.
26. Yamamoto Y, Nishiyama Y, Monden T, et al. Clinical usefulness of fusion of ^{131}I SPECT and CT images in patient with differentiated thyroid carcinoma. J Nucl Med. 2003;44:1905–10.
27. Blum M, Tiu S, Chu M, Goel S, Friedman K. I-131 SPECT/CT elucidates cryptic findings on planar whole-body scans and can reduce needless therapy with iodine-131 in post-thyroidectomy thyroid cancer patients. Thyroid. 2011;21:1235–47.
28. Avram AM, Fig LM, Frey KA, Gross MD, Wong KK. Preablation 131-I scans with SPECT/CT in postoperative thyroid cancer patients: what is the impact on staging? J Clin Endocrinol Metab. 2013;98:1163–71.
29. Grewal RK, Tuttle RM, Fox J, et al. The effect of post-therapy ^{131}I SPECT/CT on risk classification and management of patients with differentiated thyroid cancer. J Nucl Med. 2010;51:1361–7.
30. Ciappuccini R, Heutte N, Trzepla G, et al. Postablation ^{131}I scintigraphy with neck and thorax SPECT/CT and stimulated serum thyroglobulin level predict the outcome of patients with differentiated thyroid cancer. Eur J Endocrinol. 2011;164:961–9.
31. Wang H, Fu HL, Li JN, et al. The role of single-photon emission computed tomography/computed tomography for precise localization of metastases in patients with differentiated thyroid cancer. Clin Imaging. 2009;33:49–54.
32. Qiu ZL, Xu YH, Song HJ, et al. Localization and identification of parapharyngeal metastases from differentiated thyroid carcinoma by ^{131}I-SPECT/CT. Head Neck. 2011;33:171–7.
33. Maruoka Y, Abe K, Baba S, Isoda T, Sawamoto H, Tanabe Y, Sasaki M, Honda H. Incremental diagnostic value of SPECT/CT

with ^{131}I scintigraphy after radioiodine therapy in patients with well-differentiated thyroid carcinoma. Radiology. 2012;265: 902–9.
34. Schmidt D, Linke R, Uder M. Five months follow-up of patients with and without iodine-positive lymph node metastases of thyroid carcinoma as disclosed by ^{131}I-SPECT/CT at the first radioablation. Eur J Nucl Med Mol Imaging. 2010;37:699–705.
35. Barwick T, Murray I, Megadmi H, et al. SPECT/CT using ^{123}I in patients with differentiated thyroid cancer: additional value over whole body planar imaging and SPECT. Eur J Endocrinol. 2010;162:1131–9.
36. Geerlings JAC, van Zuijlen A, Lohmann EM, et al. The value of ^{131}I SPECT in the detection of recurrent differentiated thyroid cancer. Nucl Med Commun. 2010;31:417–22.
37. Alnafisi NS, Driedger AA, Coates G, et al. FDG PET of recurrent or metastatic ^{131}I-negative papillary thyroid carcinoma. J Nucl Med. 2000;41:1010–5.
38. Fletcher JW, Djubegocuc, Soares HP, et al. Recommendations on the use of ^{18}F-FDG PET in oncology. J Nucl Med. 2008;49:480–508.
39. Oh JR, Byun BH, Hong SP, et al. Comparison of ^{131}I whole body imaging, ^{131}I-SPECT/CT, and ^{18}F-FDG PET/CT in the detection of metastatic thyroid cancer. Eur J Nucl Med Mol Imaging. 2011;38:1459–68.

Radioiodine Scintigraphy with SPECT/CT: An Important Diagnostic Tool for Staging and Risk Stratification

15

Anca M. Avram

The concept of managing thyroid cancer patients according to risk stratification based on clinical-pathological criteria (i.e., age of patient and the results of surgical pathology) has been established by the current ATA guidelines: ^{131}I ablation is recommended for patients with distant metastases, grossly invasive or >4 cm primary tumor, and in selected patients with 1–4 cm tumors confined to the thyroid, who have documented node metastases or other high-risk features; ^{131}I ablation is not recommended in low-risk patients [1]. A clinically important question remains: what is the role of radioiodine imaging (^{131}I; ^{123}I and/or ^{124}I) in risk stratification of patients with thyroid cancer and what contribution does it bring to completion of staging and to the decision to omit or proceed with ^{131}I therapy?

Staging and risk stratification are used for determining if patients would benefit (and should be referred for) ^{131}I ablative therapy, with new ATA guidelines recommending against ^{131}I ablation in patients with unifocal or mutifocal tumors <1 cm (microcarcinomas) without high-risk features [1]. However, when the ^{131}I therapy is omitted, staging without post-therapy ^{131}I whole-body scan (WBS) and stimulated thyroglobulin (Tg) level has the potential to underestimate the recurrence risk in non-ablated patients, and in a slowly growing malignancy such as differentiated thyroid cancer (DTC), this risk may become apparent only after long-term follow-up [2].

The most commonly occurring papillary thyroid cancer in the USA is now a microcarcinoma: 45 % of tumors in older (≥45 years) and 34 % of tumors in younger (<45 years) patients are microcarcinomas [3]. Although the long-term outcome of papillary microcarcinoma is excellent, it frequently spreads to cervical lymph nodes, as documented in 40.9 % of cases in a series of 445 patients [4] and may occasionally metastasize to distant sites [5–8]. The cumulative risk of developing lymph node metastases increases continuously with primary tumor diameter ≥5 mm; therefore, the concept of "very low-risk" papillary thyroid cancer (PTC) based on tumor size alone becomes questionable [9].

Performing postoperative diagnostic radioiodine scans provides the opportunity of identifying patients with unsuspected regional and distant metastases, defines the target of ^{131}I therapy, and is essential for dosimetry calculations if high-dose ^{131}I therapy is necessary. For making a rational decision regarding the prescribed therapeutic ^{131}I activity, the primary goal of ^{131}I therapy should be determined prior to ^{131}I dose administration and must take into account clinical and histopathologic information and the findings on preablation radioiodine scintigraphy for each individual patient. An understanding of the purpose of therapeutic ^{131}I administration is essential: remnant ablation, defined as the use of ^{131}I for elimination of normal residual functional thyroid tissue (thyroid remnant) for facilitating long-term follow-up and to maximize the therapeutic effect of any subsequent ^{131}I treatment; adjuvant ^{131}I therapy, defined as the use of ^{131}I for elimination of suspected but unproven metastatic disease; or targeted ^{131}I therapy, defined as the use of ^{131}I for treatment of known local-regional and distant metastases [10].

We consider that the patients' risk stratification should not be solely based on clinical and histopathologic criteria, but should include specific thyroid cancer imaging to evaluate for the presence of regional and distant metastases. Diagnostic ^{131}I scintigraphy (planar studies with or without SPECT/CT imaging) can detect metastases in normal-size cervical lymph nodes (that would not be visible on postoperative neck ultrasonography), can identify pulmonary micrometastases (which are too small to be detected on routine chest x-ray and may remain undetected on computer tomography), and can diagnose bone metastases at an early

A.M. Avram, MD (✉)
Division of Nuclear Medicine, Department of Radiology, University of Michigan, 1500 E. Medical Center Drive, Ann Arbor, MI 48109, USA

BIG505G University Hospital, Ann Arbor, MI 48109, USA
e-mail: ancaa@umich.edu

L. Wartofsky, D. Van Nostrand (eds.), *Thyroid Cancer*, DOI 10.1007/978-1-4939-3314-3_15

stage before cortical disruption is visible on bone x-rays. Since thyroid cancer osseous metastases are predominantly osteolytic, bone scans with 99m-Tc MDP and/or 18-F fluoride may not portray the full extent of skeletal metastatic disease and are most often positive only in larger lesions and advanced-stage disease. More importantly, since ^{131}I therapy is most effective for smaller metastatic deposits, early identification of regional and distant metastases is crucial for successful therapy [11, 12].

Several studies bring evidence that pre-ablation scans impact the staging of patients with thyroid cancer, and the information obtained with pre-ablation scintigraphy changes management decisions (such as whether to proceed or omit therapeutic ^{131}I administration, refer the patient for surgical debulking prior to ^{131}I therapy, or perform additional imaging studies when non-iodine avid disease is demonstrated by negative radioiodine scans but elevated thyroglobulin). The findings on pre-ablation scans may also alter the prescribed ^{131}I activity for thyroid cancer patients, either by adjusting empiric ^{131}I doses, or performing dosimetry calculations for maximizing therapeutic ^{131}I activity for treatment of distant metastatic disease. In a study based on the review of 355 diagnostic iodine scans (after administration of 1–4 mCi of either ^{123}I or ^{131}I), Van Nostrand and colleagues demonstrated that in 53 % of cases, the findings on pre-ablation scans may alter the patients' management plan [13]. Similar conclusions have been reached by other investigators who demonstrated in a group of 48 patients studied with pre-ablation scans that the information obtained from diagnostic ^{131}I scans (planar and SPECT/CT studies) changed the prescribed ^{131}I activity in 58 % cases [14].

Diagnostic ^{131}I scans are essential when high-dose ^{131}I therapy is considered for treatment of metastatic thyroid cancer: dosimetry calculations based on % whole-body retentions at 48 h identify those patients in whom prescribed ^{131}I activity may be increased, or should be decreased in order to not exceed the maximum tolerated activity [15, 16].

Radioiodine scintigraphy when combined with SPECT/CT has become a powerful diagnostic tool for identification of regional and distant metastases in thyroid cancer. The synergistic combination of functional and anatomical information provided by SPECT/CT has been found to have many advantages over traditional planar imaging in different clinical settings. Optimal co-registration of tomographic volumes of data obtained by gamma cameras with inline computer tomography (CT), with the patient in the same bed position, allows precise anatomic localization of radioactivity foci. Additional benefits include CT-based attenuation correction and morphological information from a non-contrast CT with reduced mAs and kV. The advantages of SPECT/CT have been outlined in several excellent reviews on the clinical applications of hybrid imaging [17–21].

The initial reports on the use of SPECT/CT in thyroid cancer described the advantages of SPECT/CT applied to post-therapy ^{131}I scintigraphy: in a study evaluating co-registration of separately acquired SPECT and CT data with the aid of external fiducial markers, combined SPECT/CT improved diagnostic evaluation compared to SPECT alone in 15/17 (88 %) patients [22]. Similarly, in a series of 25 patients with post-therapy ^{131}I scans, SPECT/CT improved diagnostic interpretation compared to planar images in 44 % of radioactivity foci, resulting in change to management in 25 % patients [23]. In a study of 71 patients, of whom 54 had post-therapy and 17 had diagnostic I-131 imaging, Tharp and colleagues reported incremental diagnostic value of SPECT/CT over planar imaging in 57 % of patients; when considering only the group of 17 patients who underwent diagnostic ^{131}I studies, the findings on SPECT/CT changed the therapeutic approach for 41 % of these patients [24].

Aide and colleagues reported that in 55 patients studied with post-therapy ^{131}I scans, there were 29 % indeterminate results on planar imaging and only 7 % with SPECT/CT. Of the 16 patients with indeterminate planar scans, reclassification with SPECT/CT as positive or negative for disease correlated with success or failure of radioiodine treatment at follow-up [25].

One clear advantage of SPECT/CT is to substantially reduce the number of equivocal foci seen on planar imaging alone: Chen and colleagues reported that SPECT/CT accurately characterized 85 % of foci considered inconclusive on planar imaging, resulting in altered management for 47 % patients [26]. Kohlfuerst et al. reported on the impact of post-therapy SPECT/CT in a group of 41 patients: in 33 patients with neck lesions, SPECT/CT changed N status in 12/33 patients (36.4 %) and led to a treatment change in 8/33 patients (24.2 %); in 19 patients with lesions distant from the neck, SPECT/CT changed M status in 4/19 patients (21.1 %) and led to a treatment change in 2/19 patients (10.5 %); for the entire group of 41 patients, SPECT/CT led to a treatment change in 10/41 patients (24.4 %) [27].

Schmidt and colleagues reported on nodal staging in 57 patients who underwent planar and SPECT/CT after first radioablation, and they concluded that SPECT/CT determines lymph nodal status more accurately than planar imaging: 6 of 11 lesions considered nodal metastases on planar were reclassified as benign on SPECT/CT, and 11 of 15 lesions considered indeterminate on planar were reclassified as nodal metastases on SPECT/CT; SPECT/CT provided information which clarified nodal status in 20/57 patients (35 %), which resulted in a change in risk stratification in 25 % of patients [28]. Furthermore, the same group determined that the information obtained with ^{131}I SPECT/CT performed at the first radioablation can predict the occurrence and/or persistence of iodine avid cervical nodal metastases in subsequent follow-up: 94 % of nodal metastatic deposits smaller than 0.9 ml were eliminated after radioablation, while nodal metastases exceeding this size were less likely to completely resolve with ^{131}I therapy [12]. Consequently, the size information obtained on CT data from the SPECT/CT study can be used for guiding patient selection for further surgery for excision of large metastatic deposits.

SPECT/CT improved anatomic localization of activity foci seen on planar post-therapy ^{131}I imaging in 21 % of cases, as demonstrated by Wang and colleagues in a study of 94 patients; in addition, SPECT/CT identified new metastatic foci unsuspected on planar imaging in 7 % of patients. Most importantly, the additional information obtained with SPECT/CT resulted in reconsideration of therapeutic approach in 22/94 (23 %) of patients [29].

The use of post-therapy SPECT/CT at first radioablation has also extended our knowledge regarding the incidence of nodal metastases in patients with T1 tumors (≤2 cm, limited to the thyroid). In a large, bicentric study of 151 patients, by using a combination of nodal staging based on histopathology (pN1) information (in 46 % patients who underwent surgical neck dissection) and imaging information (SPECT/CT in 54 % patients who did not undergo neck dissection), Mustafa et al. reported that nodal metastases occurred in 26 % of T1 tumors and in 22 % of microcarcinomas (T1a tumors, ≤1.0 cm). Regarding nodal staging, SPECT/CT was more accurate than planar imaging in 24.5 % of patients [30].

The use of SPECT/CT technology permitted identification of parapharyngeal metastases 14/561 (2.5 %) patients; in these patients, parapharyngeal metastases were also associated with regional and/or distant metastases [31].

The effect of post-therapy ^{131}I SPECT/CT on ATA risk classification was assessed by Grewal et al. in a group of 148 intermediate- and high-risk patients (as initially assessed on clinical and histopathology criteria): 74 % of patients underwent first radioablation, while 26 % patients received ^{131}I therapy for treatment of recurrent or metastatic disease with rising thyroglobulin levels. SPECT/CT changed nodal status in 15 % postsurgical patients and 21 % patients with suspected disease recurrence or persistence. Based on SPECT/CT findings, ATA risk classification changed in 7/109 (6.4 %) patients. Importantly, review of CT data of SPECT/CT study identified non-iodine avid metastases in 32/148 (22 %) patients and demonstrated that the size of nodal metastases can be measured on CT component of SPECT/CT; additional imaging studies were avoided in 48 % patients [32].

Ciappucinni and colleagues demonstrated that post-ablation scintigraphy (planar and SPECT/CT imaging) has prognostic value for predicting therapeutic outcome of patients with thyroid cancer after total thyroidectomy and first radioablation. The study group comprised 170 patients followed for median of 29 months (range 1.5–4.5 years) after initial ^{131}I ablative therapy: 32 (19 %) patients presented with persistent or recurrent disease in subsequent follow-up: 18 patients with nodal metastases, 8 patients with distant metastases, and 6 patients with both nodal and distant metastases. In all patients free of disease at follow-up evaluations, initial post-ablative SPECT/CT was negative or equivocal for disease. However, SPECT/CT was positive for disease in 78 % patients identified with persistent/recurrent disease at follow-up; the fact that post-therapy scintigraphy was negative in 22 % patients with persistent/recurrent disease during follow-up points to the presence of non-iodine metastases, also reported by other groups in 20–30 % of patients [32, 33], The authors conclude that post-ablation scintigraphy (planar WBS and SPECT/CT) has 78 % sensitivity and 100 % specificity for predicting recurrent/persistent disease, and it is the sole independent prognostic variable for disease-free survival [34].

SPECT/CT also improved dual phase (3 days and 7 days) post-therapy ^{131}I planar WBS scan interpretation in a group of 42 patients regarding characterization of focal radioiodine accumulations as benign or malignant [35]. Table 15.1 summarizes the results of studies reporting on the use of post-therapy ^{131}I scintigraphy with SPECT/CT for accurate lesion localization and characterization.

Unusual patterns of radioiodine biodistribution that could mimic metastatic disease are well recognized and are known to raise a diagnostic dilemma on planar scintigraphy interpretation [36, 37]. SPECT/CT is an excellent diagnostic tool for rapid evaluation of suspected physiological mimics and can accurately localize radioiodine distribution to the salivary glands, dental fillings, retrosternal goiter, esophageal and/or airway secretions, hiatal hernias, bowel diverticuli, breast, skin contamination, and benign uptake related to radioiodine retention in cysts, bronchiectasis, thymus, benign struma ovarii, or menstruating uterus [38–44]. Several reports outline the usefulness of SPECT/CT for solving difficult diagnostic interpretations and revealing unusual metastatic lesions in the liver, kidney, central nervous system, erector spinae, and rectus abdominis muscles [45–49].

SPECT/CT technology has also been used in conjunction with diagnostic pre-ablation ^{123}I or ^{131}I scans and demonstrated incremental diagnostic information resulting in increased specificity as compared to classic planar scintigraphy. Barwick et al. demonstrated in a group of 79 consecutive patients studied with ^{123}I planar, SPECT, and SPECT/CT imaging that SPECT/CT provided additional diagnostic information in 42 % patients and provided further characterization in 70 % of foci seen on planar images. The authors calculated the diagnostic performance of SPECT/CT compared to planar scans and SPECT alone: planar studies demonstrated a sensitivity of 41 %, specificity of 68 %, and accuracy of 61 %; SPECT studies demonstrated a sensitivity of 45 %, specificity of 89 %, and accuracy of 78 %; SPECT/CT provided significant improvement in specificity, with a

Table 15.1 Studies reporting utility of post-Rx. ^{131}I SPECT/CT for evaluation of differentiated thyroid cancer

Author Journal	No. pts/scans Design	Setting Indication	Scan type Activity	Camera CT settings	Site of radioactivity foci Findings/comments
Ciappuccini R et al. (2011) *EJE* [34]	170/170 Pros	First RA Routine	Post-Rx I-131 0.9–4.8 GBq	Symbia T2	Neck/distant; Follow-up: median, 29 months, range 1.5–4.5 years Prognostic value of post-ablation SPECT/CT for recurrence was assessed in follow-up evaluation: 32 (19 %) pts. had persistent/recurrent ds: 18 with nodal mets, 8 with distant mets and 6 with both SPECT/CT was negative or equivocal in all patients free of disease at follow-up SPECT/CT was positive in 78 % and negative in 22 % pts with persistent or recurrent disease Post-ablation scintigraphy has 78 % sensitivity and 100 % specificity for predicting recurrent disease
Qiu Z et al. (2010) *Head and neck* [47]	561/ Pros	First RA RAI Rx for mets Selected	Post-Rx I-131 3.7–7.4 GBq	Millennium Hawkeye 140 kV, 2.5 mAs	Neck SPECT/CT identified parapharyngeal metastases in 14/561 (2.5 %) pts Parapharyngeal mets were associated with regional and/or distant mets
Grewal et al. (2010) *JNM* [32]	148/148 Retro	First RA (74 %) Recurrent or metastatic ds (26 %) Routine	Post-Rx I-131 1.7–8 GBq	Philips Precedence 120 kV, adjusted mAs/kg	Neck/distant SPECT/CT changed N in 15 % postsurgical pts. and in 21 % recurrence pts SPECT/CT changed ATA risk classification in 7/109 (6.4 %) pts SPECT/CT identified non-iodine avid metastases in 32/148 (22 %) pts Size of nodal mets was measured on CT component of SPECT/CT SPECT/CT avoided additional imaging in 48 % pts
Mustafa et al. (2010) *EJNMMI* [30]	151/151 Pros	First RA Routine	Post-Rx I-131 1.8–5.3 GBq	Symbia T2, T6 140 kV, 20–40 mAs	Neck Accuracy SPECT/CT > planar in 24.5 % pts SPECT/CT revised N score in 24.5 % pts LNM occurs in 26 % pts with T1 and 22 % pts with microcarcinoma (≤1 cm)
Schmidt et al. (2010) *EJNMMI* [12]	81/81 Retro	First RA Routine	Post-Rx I-131 1.5–5.3 GBq	Symbia T2, T6 140 kV, 40 mAs	Neck 60/61 pts with negative SPECT/CT were disease-free at 5 months 17/20 pts with positive SPECT/CT were disease-free at 5 months Metastasis size <0.9 ml predicted treatment success
Aide et al. (2009) *JCEM* [25]	55/55 Pros	First RA Routine	Post-Rx I-131 2.9–4.0 GBq	Symbia T2 ?kV, 60 mAs	Neck SPECT/CT clarified diagnosis in16 pts with indeterminate planar scans: 9/9 pts without disease had negative SPECT/CT 4/5 pts with disease had positive SPECT/CT
Kohlfuerst et al. (2009) *EJNMMI* [27]	41/53 Pros	First RA (23 pts) FU (18 pts) Selected	Post-Rx I-131 2.9–7.5 GBq	Symbia T 130 kV, 25 mAs	Neck/distant SPECT/CT impact 21/33 (63.6 %) pts, changed N score 12/33 (36.4 %) SPECT/CT impact 14/19 (73.7 %) pts, change M score 4/19 (21.1 %) Changed treatment in 10/41 (24.4 %) pts 8/33 (24.2 %) changed treatment due to N score 2/19 (10.5 %) changed treatment due to M score
Wang et al. (2009) *Clin Imag* [29]	94/94 Retro	First RA Routine	Post-Rx I-131 3.7–7.4 GBq	Infinia Hawkeye 140 kV, 2.5 mAs	Neck/distant Accuracy SPECT/CT > planar in 20/94 (21 %) pts Changed treatment in 22/94 (23 %) pts SPECT/CT identified unsuspected metastases in 7/94 (7 %) pts

Schmidt et al. (2009) *EJNMMI* [28]	57/57 Retro	First RA Routine	Post-Rx I-131 1.5–5.3 GBq	Symbia T2, T6 140 kV, 40 mAs	Neck SPECT/CT completes N staging SPECT/CT changed N score in 20/57 (35 %) pts SPECT/CT changed risk stratification in 14/57 (25 %) pts
Chen et al. (2008) *JNM* [26]	23/37 Pros	First RA Selected	Post-Rx I-131 3.7–7.4 GBq	Millennium Hawkeye 140 kV, 2.5 mAs	Neck/distant Incremental diagnostic value SPECT/CT > planar in 17/23 (74 %) pts SPECT/CT clarified 69/81 (85 %) inconclusive planar foci Changed treatment in 8/17 (47 %) pts
Tharp et al. (2004) *EJNMMI* [24]	71/71 Retro	First RA (28/54) FU (26/54) Selected	Post-Rx I-131 1.4–9.7 GBq (54 pts) Diagn. I-131 143– 187 MBq (17pts)	Millennium VG Hawkeye 140 kV, 2.5 mAs	Neck/distant Incremental diagnostic value SPECT/CT > planar in 41/71 (57 %) pts Diagnostic SPECT/CT changed treatment in 7/17 (41 %) pts
Ruf et al. (2004) *NMC* [23]	25/25 Pros	First RA Selected	Post-Rx I-131 3.7 GBq	Millennium Hawkeye 140 kV, 2.5 mAs	Neck/distant SPECT/CT impact in 17/39 (44 %) foci Changed treatment in 6/24 (25 %) pts
Yamamoto et al. (2003) *JNM* [22]	17/17 Retro	First RA Routine	Post-Rx I-131 3.7–7.4 GBq	Aquilon CT Picker Prism	Neck/distant Accuracy SPECT/CT > SPECT 15/17 (88 %) pts Co-registration with external fiducial markers feasible

Pts. patients, *ds.* disease, *Retro* retrospective, *Pros* prospective, *First RA* postsurgery at time of first radioablation with I-131, *FU* follow-up from postsurgery 6 months onward, *Routine* SPECT/CT performed on consecutive pts, *Selected* SPECT/CT performed on selected pt group, *Post-Rx* post-therapy scan, *LNM* lymph node metastases, *Sen* sensitivity, *Spec* specificity calculated sensitivity of 50 %, specificity of 100 %, and accuracy of 87 % (the study group included 11 patients with non-iodine avid disease demonstrated on anatomic imaging and elevated Tg levels) [50].

The incremental value of SPECT/CT as compared with planar whole-body scan (WBS) results from better identification and interpretation of focal uptake, correct anatomic localization and characterization of activity foci, and precise differentiation between metastatic lesions and physiologic uptake. In a group of 117 patients studied with planar WBS and SPECT/CT (of whom 108 patients underwent diagnostic ^{123}I and 9 patients underwent post-therapy ^{131}I scans), Spanu et al. demonstrated that SPECT/CT has incremental value over planar scan in 67.8 % patients, SPECT/CT identified more foci of pathologic activity (158 foci on SPECT/CT compared to only 116 foci on planar), and SPECT/CT changed treatment approach in 35.6 % patients with disease and led to avoidance of unnecessary I-131 therapy in 20 % patients without disease [51].

Similarly, Wong et al. demonstrated incremental diagnostic value of SPECT/CT over planar imaging for interpretation of 47.6 % of foci seen on WBS in a group of 53 patients studied with ^{131}I planar and SPECT/CT protocol (the group comprised of 47 patients studied with diagnostic pre-ablation scans and 6 patients studied with post-therapy scans): SPECT/CT provided incremental information for interpretation of 53/130 (41 %) neck activity foci and 17/17 (100 %) distant foci by providing clear anatomic lesion localization and lesion size measurement for predicting the likelihood for response to ^{131}I therapy and assessing therapeutic response in subsequent follow-up. Rapid exclusion of physiologic activity or contamination resulted in elimination of equivocal interpretations on planar scans. Reader confidence increased for interpretation of 104/147 (71 %) of foci seen on planar images after the review of SPECT/CT [52].

In a group of 48 patients studied with diagnostic pre-ablation ^{131}I scans (planar and SPECT/CT protocol), Wong and colleagues demonstrated that SPECT/CT using low diagnostic activities (37 MBq ^{131}I) is feasible and can be used in addition to histopathologic information to complete staging and risk stratification prior to radioablation [14]. Although long-standing controversy regarding radioablation continues (regarding the indications, patient selection, and prescribed ^{131}I activity), there is agreement, however, that accurate staging is important for treatment decisions and subsequent follow-up. In this study, staging of patients was done according to TNM system using three levels of sequential information: histopathology and chest radiograph, planar WBS, and SPECT/CT. The patients were restaged according to the findings on ^{131}I scintigraphy (planar, and then planar, and SPECT/CT information). Compared to histopathologic analysis, planar and SPECT/CT changed postsurgical DTC stage for 21 % of patients. Identification of unsuspected nodal and distant metastases resulted in prescription of higher therapeutic activities (e.g., 5.5 GBq for regional metastatic disease; 7.4–14.8 GBq or dosimetry calculations for distant metastatic disease), while demonstration of only residual functional thyroid tissue in the surgical bed (i.e., thyroid remnant) in the absence of high-risk histopathologic features resulted in prescription of low ^{131}I activity (e.g., 1.1 GBq). Information obtained with diagnostic pre-ablation planar WBS and SPECT/CT scans changed prescribed radioactivity in 58 % patients as compared to initially proposed therapy based on histopathologic risk stratification alone [14]. In a larger cohort of 320 patients studied with pre-ablation ^{131}I scans, diagnostic pre-ablation ^{131}I planar and SPECT/CT scintigraphy detected regional-nodal metastases in 22 % and distant metastases in 8 % of patients, leading to upstaging of 4 % young (<45 years old) patients and 25 % older (≥45 years old) patients, as compared to pTNM staging based on surgical pathology alone [53].

Table 15.2 summarizes the results of studies reporting on the use of diagnostic pre-ablation ^{123}I or ^{131}I scintigraphy with SPECT/CT for accurate lesion localization and characterization.

The use of radioiodine SPECT/CT has been reported to change clinical management in significant numbers of patients, both when utilized routinely on all consecutive patients, or on selected patients with inconclusive planar images. Proposed changes in management include the decision to give or withhold radioiodine treatment, indicating and guiding the extent of surgery, selecting patients for external beam radiation therapy, and indicating the need for alternative imaging strategies such as FDG PET. Depending on patients' clinical context, timing of radioiodine scan (pre-ablation or post-therapy), and therapeutic protocols at each institution, change in management has been reported in 11 % [50], 23 % [29], 24 % [27], 25 % [23], 36 % [51], 41 % [24], 47 % [26], and 58 % of patients [54].

The use of SPECT/CT technology in the setting of diagnostic pre-ablation radioiodine scintigraphy allows recommended staging and risk stratification for patients with thyroid cancer [1] prior to management decisions. The advantages are the prescription of appropriately higher activities delivered at first ^{131}I therapy for high-risk patients, when the iodine-concentrating ability of the tumor is presumably highest, and reduction of activity prescribed for, or omission of, radioablation for thyroid remnants. In fact, particularly the patients in whom ablation is omitted may benefit from a postoperative diagnostic scan to exclude the presence of regional and/or distant metastases and afford the opportunity of obtaining a baseline stimulated thyroglobulin measurement.

The information obtained with diagnostic radioiodine scans has the potential to impact staging and risk stratification,

Table 15.2 Studies reporting utility of diagnostic pre-ablation ^{123}I/^{131}I SPECT/CT for evaluation of differentiated thyroid cancer

Author Journal	No. pts/scans Design	Setting Indication	Scan type Activity	Camera CT settings	Site of radioactivity foci Findings/comments
Wong et al. (2010) *AJR* [54]	48/48 Retro	First RA Selected	Diagn. I-131 37 MBq	Symbia T6 140 kV, 100 mAs	Neck/distant SPECT/CT changed TNM stage in 10/48 (21 %) pts SPECT/CT changed proposed I-131 dose selection in 28/48 (58 %) pts SPECT/CT identified unsuspected metastases in 4/8 pts with M1
Barwick et al. (2010) *EJE* [50]	79/85 Retro	FU Routine	Diagn. I-123 350–400 MBq	Millennium Hawkeye 140 kV, 2.5 mAs	Neck/distant Planar: Sen 41 % Spec 68 % Accuracy 61 % SPECT: Sen 45 % Spec 89 % Accuracy 78 % SPECT/CT: Sen 50 % Spec 100 % Accuracy 87 % SPECT/CT provided additional information in 42 % pts and 70 % foci
Spanu et al. (2009) *JNM* [51]	117/117 Pros	First RA (8 %) FU (92 %) Routine	Diagn. I-123 185 MBq (108 pts) Infinia Hawkeye 4 Post-Rx I-131 3.7 GBq (9 pts)	Millennium Hawkeye 140 kV, 2.5 mAs	Neck/distant SPECT/CT has incremental value over planar scan in 67.8 % pts SPECT/CT changed treatment in 35.6 % pts with disease SPECT/CT led to avoidance of I-131 therapy in 20 % pts without disease SPECT/CT identified 158 foci compared to only 116 foci on planar
Wong et al. (2008) *AJR* [52]	53/56 Retro	First RA (47 pts) FU (6 pts) Selected	Diagn. I-131 37 MBq (47 pts) 150 MBq (6 pts)	Symbia T6 140 kV, 100 mAs	Neck/distant Diagnostic value SPECT/CT > planar in 53/130 (41 %) neck foci Diagnostic value SPECT/CT > planar in 17/17 (100 %) distant foci SPECT/CT using diagnostic I-131 activities feasible Allows adjustment of prescribed radioiodine activity

Pts., patients, *Retro* retrospective, *Pros* prospective, *First RA* postsurgery at time of first radioablation with I-131, *FU* follow-up after surgery and initial radioablation, 6 months onward, *Routine* SPECT/CT performed on consecutive pts, *Selected* SPECT/CT performed on selected pt group, *Diagn.* diagnostic pre-ablation scan, *Post-Rx* post-therapy scan, *LNM* lymph node metastases, *Sen* sensitivity, *Spec* specificity

the decision to proceed or omit ^{131}I therapy, and also determines the long-term follow-up strategy. The initial ^{131}I treatment should be targeted at destroying residual and/or metastatic carcinoma, with the absorbed dose of radiation in the tumor as the best predictor of success for ^{131}I therapy. Future directions for the use of hybrid radioiodine imaging involve the use of SPECT/CT to perform lesion-specific dosimetry. Lesion radioiodine uptake and retention can be quantified on SPECT, and tumor volume can be measured on the CT component of SPECT/CT study, permitting calculation of radiation absorbed dose to tumor. Follow-up with SPECT/CT can be used to determine therapeutic responses and assess for tumor shrinkage. An example of this approach has been reported in a patient with a large skull metastasis causing infringement on the brain [55]. Sgourous and colleagues demonstrated the feasibility of patient-specific three-dimensional (3D) dosimetry using multiple SPECT/CT images, in which the patient's own anatomy and spatial distribution of radioactivity over time are factored into the calculation of radiation absorbed dose to tumor (lesion dosimetry) or to an organ of interest (organ dosimetry): the CT images of SPECT/CT studies are used to provide the density and composition of each voxel for use in a Monte Carlo calculation and also to define organs or regions of interest for computing spatially averaged doses; the longitudinal series of SPECT images are used to perform time integration of activity in each voxel and to obtain the cumulated activity per voxel [56, 57]. The goal of patient-specific voxel-based absorbed dose calculations is better prediction of biologic effects of radionuclide therapy.

In summary, SPECT/CT is a powerful diagnostic tool that allows accurate anatomic localization and characterization of radioiodine foci. The interpretation of radioiodine scintigraphy has been substantially improved by the addition of SPECT/CT: due to CT-based attenuation correction, SPECT/CT can reveal more foci of pathologic activity as compared to planar studies, and anatomic co-registration allows more precise differentiation between malignant and benign radioactivity distributions. SPECT/CT contributes to completion of staging for patients with thyroid cancer by improved characterization of N and M scores. The information obtained with planar and SPECT/CT imaging impacts management in a significant number of patients.

The new technology of SPECT/CT has changed the field and should lead to reassessment of current management protocols and guidelines in thyroid cancer. When applied in the setting of pre-ablation scintigraphy, SPECT/CT brings us closer to our goal of radioiodine therapy in a way that planar scintigraphy could not: avoiding excessive prescribed activity in low-risk patients and optimizing the prescribed ^{131}I activity for targeting locoregional and distant metastases at first therapy.

References

1. Haugen BR, Alexander EK, Bible KC, Doherty GM, Mandel SJ, Nikiforov YE, Pacini F, Randolph GW, Sawka AM, Schlumberger M, Schuff KG, Sherman SI, Sosa JA, Steward DL, Tuttle RM, Wartofsky L. 2015 American Thyroid Association Management Guidelines for Adult Patients with Thyroid Nodules and Differentiated Thyroid Cancer: American Thyroid Association Guidelines Task Force on Thyroid Nodules and Differentiated Thyroid Cancer. Thyroid. 2016;26:1–133.
2. Dietlein M, Verburg FA, Luster M, Reiners C, Pitoia F, Schicha H. One should not just read what one believes: the nearly irresolvable issue of producing truly objective, evidence-based guidelines for the management of differentiated thyroid cancer. Eur J Nucl Med Mol Imaging. 2011;38:793–8.
3. Hughes DT, Haymart MR, Miller BS, Gauger PG, Doherty GM. The most commonly occurring papillary thyroid cancer in the United States is now a microcarcinoma in a patient older than 45 years. Thyroid. 2011;21:231–6.
4. Mercante G, Frasoldati A, Pedroni C, Formisano D, Renna L, Piana S, Gardini G, Valcavi R, Barbieri V. Prognostic factors affecting neck lymph node recurrence and distant metastasis in papillary microcarcinoma of the thyroid: results of a study in 445 patients. Thyroid. 2009;19:707–16.
5. Hay ID, Grant CS, van Heerden JA, Goellner JR, Ebersold JR, Bergstralh EJ. Papillary thyroid microcarcinoma: a study of 535 cases observed in a 50-year period. Surgery. 1992;112:1139–46; discussion 46–7.
6. Hay ID, Hutchinson ME, Gonzalez-Losada T, McIver B, Reinalda ME, Grant CS, Thompson GB, Sebo TJ, Goellner JR. Papillary thyroid microcarcinoma: a study of 900 cases observed in a 60-year period. Surgery. 2008;144:980–7; discussion 87–8.
7. Strate SM, Lee EL, Childers JH. Occult papillary carcinoma of the thyroid with distant metastases. Cancer. 1984;54:1093–100.
8. Ross DS, Litofsky D, Ain KB, Bigos T, Brierley JD, Cooper DS, Haugen BR, Jonklaas J, Ladenson PW, Magner J, Robbins J, Skarulis MC, Steward DL, Maxon HR, Sherman SI. Recurrence after treatment of micropapillary thyroid cancer. Thyroid. 2009;19:1043–8.
9. Machens A, Holzhausen HJ, Dralle H. The prognostic value of primary tumor size in papillary and follicular thyroid carcinoma. Cancer. 2005;103:2269–73.
10. Van Nostrand D. The benefits and risks of I-131 therapy in patients with well-differentiated thyroid cancer. Thyroid. 2009;19:1381–91.
11. Durante C, Haddy N, Baudin E, Leboulleux S, Hartl D, Travagli JP, Caillou B, Ricard M, Lumbroso JD, De Vathaire F, Schlumberger M. Long-term outcome of 444 patients with distant metastases from papillary and follicular thyroid carcinoma: benefits and limits of radioiodine therapy. J Clin Endocrinol Metab. 2006;91:2892–9.
12. Schmidt D, Linke R, Uder M, Kuwert T. Five months' follow-up of patients with and without iodine-positive lymph node metastases of thyroid carcinoma as disclosed by (131)I-SPECT/CT at the first radioablation. Eur J Nucl Med Mol Imaging. 2010;37:699–705.
13. Van Nostrand D, Aiken M, Atkins F, Moreau S, Garcia C, Acio E, Burman K, Wartofsky L. The utility of radioiodine scans prior to iodine 131 ablation in patients with well-differentiated thyroid cancer. Thyroid. 2009;19:849–55.
14. Wong KK, Sisson JC, Koral KF, Frey KA, Avram AM. Staging of differentiated thyroid carcinoma using diagnostic ^{131}I SPECT/CT. AJR Am J Roentgenol. 2010;195:730–6.
15. Van Nostrand D, Atkins F, Moreau S, Aiken M, Kulkarni K, Wu JS, Burman KD, Wartofsky L. Utility of the radioiodine whole-body retention at 48 hours for modifying empiric activity of 131-iodine for the treatment of metastatic well-differentiated thyroid carcinoma. Thyroid. 2009;19:1093–8.
16. Sisson JC, Shulkin BL, Lawson S. Increasing efficacy and safety of treatments of patients with well-differentiated thyroid carcinoma by measuring body retentions of ^{131}I. J Nucl Med. 2003;44:898–903.
17. Bockisch A, Freudenberg LS, Schmidt D, Kuwert T. Hybrid imaging by SPECT/CT and PET/CT: proven outcomes in cancer imaging. Semin Nucl Med. 2009;39:276–89.
18. Buck AK, Herrmann K, Stargardt T, Dechow T, Krause BJ, Schreyogg J. Economic evaluation of PET and PET/CT in oncology: evidence and methodologic approaches. Journal of Nuclear Medicine. 2010;51:401–12.
19. Delbeke D, Schoder H, Martin WH, Wahl RL. Hybrid imaging (SPECT/CT and PET/CT): improving therapeutic decisions. Semin Nucl Med. 2009;39:308–40.
20. Even-Sapir E, Keidar Z, Bar-Shalom R. Hybrid imaging (SPECT/CT and PET/CT) – improving the diagnostic accuracy of functional/metabolic and anatomic imaging. Semin Nucl Med. 2009;39:264–75.
21. Mariani G, Bruselli L, Kuwert T, Kim EE, Flotats A, Israel O, Dondi M, Watanabe N. A review on the clinical uses of SPECT/CT. Eur J Nucl Med Mol Imaging. 2010;37:1959–85.
22. Yamamoto Y, Nishiyama Y, Monden T, Matsumura Y, Satoh K, Ohkawa M. Clinical usefulness of fusion of ^{131}I SPECT and CT images in patients with differentiated thyroid carcinoma. J Nucl Med. 2003;44:1905–10.
23. Ruf J, Lehmkuhl L, Bertram H, Sandrock D, Amthauer H, Humplik B, Ludwig Munz D, Felix R. Impact of SPECT and integrated low-dose CT after radioiodine therapy on the management of patients with thyroid carcinoma. Nucl Med Commun. 2004;25:1177–82.
24. Tharp K, Israel O, Hausmann J, Bettman L, Martin WH, Daitzchman M, Sandler MP, Delbeke D. Impact of ^{131}I-SPECT/CT images obtained with an integrated system in the follow-up of patients with thyroid carcinoma. Eur J Nucl Med Mol Imaging. 2004;31:1435–42.
25. Aide N, Heutte N, Rame JP, Rousseau E, Loiseau C, Henry-Amar M, Bardet S. Clinical relevance of single-photon emission computed tomography/computed tomography of the neck and thorax in postablation (131)I scintigraphy for thyroid cancer. J Clin Endocrinol Metab. 2009;94:2075–84.
26. Chen L, Luo Q, Shen Y, Yu Y, Yuan Z, Lu H, Zhu R. Incremental value of ^{131}I SPECT/CT in the management of patients with differentiated thyroid carcinoma. J Nucl Med. 2008;49:1952–7.
27. Kohlfuerst S, Igerc I, Lobnig M, Gallowitsch HJ, Gomez-Segovia I, Matschnig S, Mayr J, Mikosch P, Beheshti M, Lind P. Posttherapeutic

(131)I SPECT/CT offers high diagnostic accuracy when the findings on conventional planar imaging are inconclusive and allows a tailored patient treatment regimen. Eur J Nucl Med Mol Imaging. 2009;36:886–93.

28. Schmidt D, Szikszai A, Linke R, Bautz W, Kuwert T. Impact of ^{131}I SPECT/spiral CT on nodal staging of differentiated thyroid carcinoma at the first radioablation. J Nucl Med. 2009;50:18–23.
29. Wang H, Fu HL, Li JN, Zou RJ, Gu ZH, Wu JC. The role of single-photon emission computed tomography/computed tomography for precise localization of metastases in patients with differentiated thyroid cancer. Clin Imaging. 2009;33:49–54.
30. Mustafa M, Kuwert T, Weber K, Knesewitsch P, Negele T, Haug A, Linke R, Bartenstein P, Schmidt D. Regional lymph node involvement in T1 papillary thyroid carcinoma: a bicentric prospective SPECT/CT study. Eur J Nucl Med Mol Imaging. 2010;37:1462–6.
31. Qiu ZL, Xu YH, Song HJ, Luo QY. Localization and identification of parapharyngeal metastases from differentiated thyroid carcinoma by ^{131}I-SPECT/CT. Head Neck. 2011;33:171–7.
32. Grewal RK, Tuttle RM, Fox J, Borkar S, Chou JF, Gonen M, Strauss HW, Larson SM, Schoder H. The effect of posttherapy 131I SPECT/CT on risk classification and management of patients with differentiated thyroid cancer. J Nucl Med. 2010;51:1361–7.
33. Mian C, Barollo S, Pennelli G, Pavan N, Rugge M, Pelizzo MR, Mazzarotto R, Casara D, Nacamulli D, Mantero F, Opocher G, Busnardo B, Girelli ME. Molecular characteristics in papillary thyroid cancers (PTCs) with no ^{131}I uptake. Clin Endocrinol (Oxf). 2008;68:108–16.
34. Ciappuccini R, Heutte N, Trzepla G, Rame JP, Vaur D, Aide N, Bardet S. Postablation (131)I scintigraphy with neck and thorax SPECT/CT and stimulated serum thyroglobulin level predict the outcome of patients with differentiated thyroid cancer. Eur J Endocrinol. 2011;164:961–9.
35. Wakabayashi H, Nakajima K, Fukuoka M, Inaki A, Nakamura A, Kayano D, Kinuya S. Double-phase (131)I whole body scan and (131)I SPECT/CT images in patients with differentiated thyroid cancer: their effectiveness for accurate identification. Ann Nucl Med. 2011;25:609–15.
36. Shapiro B, Rufini V, Jarwan A, Geatti O, Kearfott KJ, Fig LM, Kirkwood ID, Gross MD. Artifacts, anatomical and physiological variants, and unrelated diseases that might cause false-positive whole-body ^{131}I scans in patients with thyroid cancer. Semin Nucl Med. 2000;30:115–32.
37. Mitchell G, Pratt BE, Vini L, McCready VR, Harmer CL. False positive ^{131}I whole body scans in thyroid cancer. Br J Radiol. 2000;73:627–35.
38. Wong KK, Zarzhevsky N, Cahill JM, Frey KA, Avram AM. Hybrid SPECT/CT and PET-CT imaging of differentiated thyroid carcinoma. Br J Radiol. 2009;82:860–76.
39. Wong KK, Avram AM. Posttherapy I-131 thymic uptake demonstrated with SPECT/CT in a young girl with papillary thyroid carcinoma. Thyroid. 2008;18:919–20.
40. Dumcke CW, Madsen JL. Usefulness of SPECT/CT in the diagnosis of intrathoracic goiter versus metastases from cancer of the breast. Clin Nucl Med. 2007;32:156–9.
41. Macdonald W, Armstrong J. Benign struma ovarii in a patient with invasive papillary thyroid cancer: detection with I-131 SPECT/CT. Clin Nucl Med. 2007;32:380–2.
42. Thust S, Fernando R, Barwick T, Mohan H, Clarke SE. SPECT/CT identification of post-radioactive iodine treatment false-positive uptake in a simple renal cyst. Thyroid. 2009;19:75–6.
43. Rachinsky I, Driedger A. Iodine-131 uptake in a menstruating uterus: value of SPECT/CT in distinguishing benign and metastatic iodine-positive lesions. Thyroid. 2007;17:901–2.
44. Jong I, Taubman K, Schlicht S. Bronchiectasis simulating pulmonary metastases on iodine-131 scintigraphy in well-differentiated thyroid carcinoma. Clin Nucl Med. 2005;30:688–9.
45. Agriantonis DJ, Hall L, Wilson MA. Utility of SPECT/CT as an adjunct to planar whole body I-131 imaging: liver metastasis from papillary thyroid cancer. Clin Nucl Med. 2009;34:247–8.
46. Aide N, Lehembre E, Gervais R, Bardet S. Unusual intratracheal metastasis of differentiated thyroid cancer accurately depicted by SPECT/CT acquisition after radioiodine ablation. Thyroid. 2007;17:1305–6.
47. Qiu ZL, Luo QY. Erector spinae metastases from differentiated thyroid cancer identified by I-131 SPECT/CT. Clin Nucl Med. 2009;34:137–40.
48. von Falck C, Beer G, Gratz KF, Galanski M. Renal metastases from follicular thyroid cancer on SPECT/CT. Clin Nucl Med. 2007; 32:751–2.
49. Zhao LX, Li L, Li FL, Zhao Z. Rectus abdominis muscle metastasis from papillary thyroid cancer identified by I-131 SPECT/CT. Clin Nucl Med. 2010;35:360–1.
50. Barwick T, Murray I, Megadmi H, Drake WM, Plowman PN, Akker SA, Chew SL, Grossman AB, Avril N. Single photon emission computed tomography (SPECT)/computed tomography using Iodine-123 in patients with differentiated thyroid cancer: additional value over whole body planar imaging and SPECT. Eur J Endocrinol. 2010;162:1131–9.
51. Spanu A, Solinas ME, Chessa F, Sanna D, Nuvoli S, Madeddu G. ^{131}I SPECT/CT in the follow-up of differentiated thyroid carcinoma: incremental value versus planar imaging. J Nucl Med. 2009;50: 184–90.
52. Wong KK, Zarzhevsky N, Cahill JM, Frey KA, Avram AM. Incremental value of diagnostic ^{131}I SPECT/CT fusion imaging in the evaluation of differentiated thyroid carcinoma. AJR Am J Roentgenol. 2008;191:1785–94.
53. Avram AM, Doherty GM, Fig LM, Wong KK. Diagnostic ^{131}I fusion SPECT/CT Imaging in postoperative thyroid cancer patients: what is the impact on staging? Thyroid. 2011;21:193.
54. Wong KK, Sisson JC, Koral KF, Frey KA, Avram AM. Staging of differentiated thyroid carcinoma using diagnostic ^{131}I SPECT/CT. AJR Am J Roentgenol. 2010;195:730–6.
55. Sisson JC, Dewaraja YK, Wizauer EJ, Giordano TJ, Avram AM. Thyroid carcinoma metastasis to skull with infringement of brain: treatment with radioiodine. Thyroid. 2009;19:297–303.
56. Song H, He B, Prideaux A, Du Y, Frey E, Kasecamp W, Ladenson PW, Wahl RL, Sgouros G. Lung dosimetry for radioiodine treatment planning in the case of diffuse lung metastases. J Nucl Med. 2006;47:1985–94.
57. Prideaux AR, Song H, Hobbs RF, He B, Frey EC, Ladenson PW, Wahl RL, Sgouros G. Three-dimensional radiobiologic dosimetry: application of radiobiologic modeling to patient-specific 3-dimensional imaging-based internal dosimetry. J Nucl Med. 2007;48:1008–16.

Stunning by ^{131}I Scanning: Untoward Effect of ^{131}I Thyroid Imaging Prior to Radioablation Therapy

16

Hee-Myung Park and Stephen K. Gerard

Introduction

Thyroid stunning is a radiobiological phenomenon. It may be defined as a temporary suppression of iodine-trapping function of the thyrocytes and thyroid cancer cells as a result of the radiation given off by the scanning (or first) dose of ^{131}I. The tissue-absorbed radiation dose from the scanning is often sufficient to cause hypofunction but usually not enough to destroy the target cells. The stunned cells may not be able to take up the ensuing therapeutic ^{131}I to the degree of their original unaffected capacity. It may lead to an incomplete ablation of the thyroid remnant or metastatic lesion. Stunning is radiation dose dependent, i.e., the higher the radiation-absorbed dose to the target tissue, the greater the stunning effect. Stunning is a matter of quantity, not quality, and certainly is not an "all or none" phenomenon; there is a spectrum of severity. When severe, there is often a visually apparent reduction in uptake of the therapy dose of ^{131}I in the target lesion when the diagnostic and post-therapy scans are compared. When mild, it may be noticeable only when the thyroid iodide uptake function is measured. However, the visual evidence of decreased radioiodine uptake caused by stunning could be confounded by one or more uncontrolled differences in technical and/or physiologic constraints between the diagnostic and post-therapy scans. Such differences might relate to the post-dose imaging time, differential radioiodine washout, nonlinear camera response between low and high doses of radioiodine, the thyrotropin (TSH) level, and extent of iodine depletion at the time of dose administration.

Moreover, calculating the "thyroid uptake" a second time using ^{131}I is not an easy task because of the presence of high residual ^{131}I activity in the thyroid tissue. This difficulty is especially apparent after a large scanning dose or after the first portion in a fractionated treatment regimen is administered. Nevertheless, several investigators have succeeded in measuring the thyroid uptake using various methods, proving that the radiation from the diagnostic dose of ^{131}I indeed suppressed the iodide uptake of the target tissues.

To avoid stunning, another isotope of iodine can be used. With all factors considered, ^{123}I seems to be the ideal scanning agent among the 24 possible isotopes of iodine [1].

Park et al. first noticed this phenomenon many years ago when liberal amounts (up to 370 MBq [10 mCi]) of ^{131}I were commonly used as a scanning dose. When treatable lesions were found, the patients were admitted to the hospital and received ^{131}I therapy (3.7–5.55 GBq [100–150 mCi]). Post-therapy whole-body scans were obtained initially at 24–48 h, which was when the retained ^{131}I activity fell below 1.1 GBq (30 mCi) but before the patient was discharged from the hospital. Those images often unexpectedly showed little or no apparent uptake of the therapy dose of ^{131}I in the remnant that had been iodine-avid on diagnostic scans. Systematic review revealed the stunning effect [2]. The evidence indicating that stunning was radiation induced was especially convincing when they noticed the effect was dose dependent. The frequency of visually apparent stunning was 40 %, 67 %, and 89 % after 111, 185, and 370 MBq (3, 5, and 10 mCi) doses of ^{131}I, respectively [3]. A few illustrative cases of thyroid stunning are shown in Figs. 16.1, 16.2, 16.3, and 16.4.

The time of recovery from stunning is not known and is difficult to determine because it requires repetitive whole-body scanning with necessary patient preparation, which can be quite burdensome to patients. In a few patients who underwent repeat diagnostic scanning, the thyroid showed no uptake and thus no evidence of recovery after 2 weeks, 27 days, 40 days, and even 7 months [4]. A diagnostic dose may be lethal if the absorbed tissue dose is sufficient.

H.-M. Park, MD
Department of Radiology, Indiana University Hospital, Indianapolis, IN, USA

S.K. Gerard, MD, PhD (✉)
Department of Nuclear Medicine, Department of Pathology, Seton Medical Center, 1900 Sullivan Avenue, Daly City, CA 94015, USA
e-mail: stephengerard@dochs.org

L. Wartofsky, D. Van Nostrand (eds.), *Thyroid Cancer*, DOI 10.1007/978-1-4939-3314-3_16

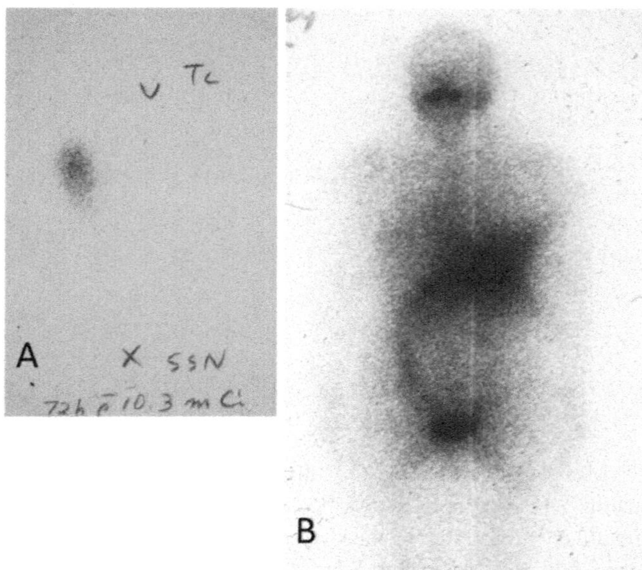

Fig. 16.1 Stunning due to 370 MBq (10 mCi) ^{131}I scanning. A follow-up scan with 370 MBq (10 mCi) ^{131}I 1 year after an ablation therapy in a 37-year-old female shows a persistent remnant in the *right upper pole* (**a**). Due to the patient's family situation, the patient received 3.7 GBq (100 mCi) ^{131}I therapy (her second) 6 weeks later. The 24 h whole-body scan shows no discernible uptake of the therapy dose in the remnant (**b**). The target tissue was undoubtedly stunned by the scanning dose and lost iodide-trapping function. Radioiodine is distributed physiologically in the stomach, GI tract, and bladder

Physical Properties of ^{131}I and Thyroid Radiation-Absorbed Dose

^{131}I emits β particles and has a half-life of 8 days. The radiation-absorbed dose to the thyroid tissue increases daily until the ^{131}I loses all of its radioactivity. The ultimate absorbed tissue dose is reached at 8–10 weeks. Most of the radiation-absorbed dose, however, is absorbed during the first few days.

How much radiation would thyroid tissue receive from a scanning dose of ^{131}I? How does it compare with that from the ^{131}I therapy given for hyperthyroidism? When 1 uCi of ^{131}I is deposited in 1 g of thyroid tissue and is allowed to decay completely, the tissue would have received approximately 100 cGy (rad). It is believed that approximately 10,000 rad (100 Gy; or 100 uCi of ^{131}I/g) is needed to treat Graves' disease. In a postoperative thyroid cancer patient, if the weight of a thyroid remnant is 1 g and the iodine uptake is 1 %, a 370 MBq (10 mCi) scanning dose of ^{131}I would have delivered 3.7 MBq (100 uCi) to the thyroid tissue. The remnant would have received approximately 10,000 cGy (rad) – a therapeutic dose for Graves' disease. Therefore, it becomes obvious why such irradiated thyroid tissue may not function normally and cannot fully trap the ensuing therapeutic dose.

The threshold radiation dose, below which no functional changes would occur, is not clearly known. In terms of administered quantity of ^{131}I, a 7.4 MBq (2 mCi) diagnostic dose, according to McDougall, did not cause visually apparent stunning except in 2 of 147 cases [5]. However, Medvedec

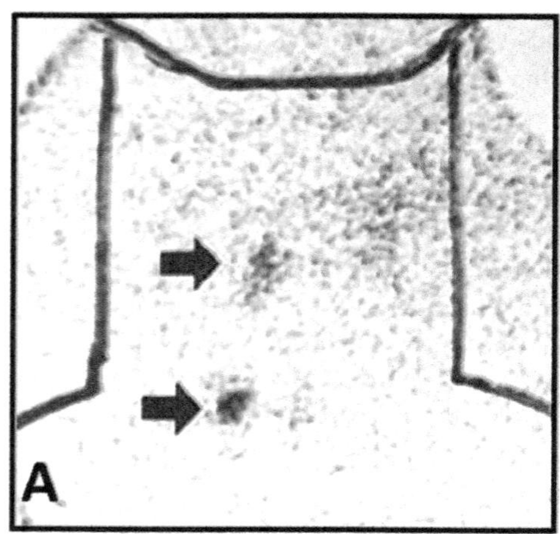

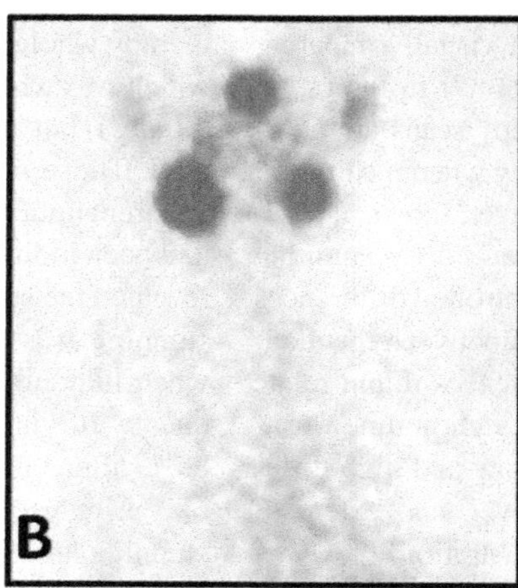

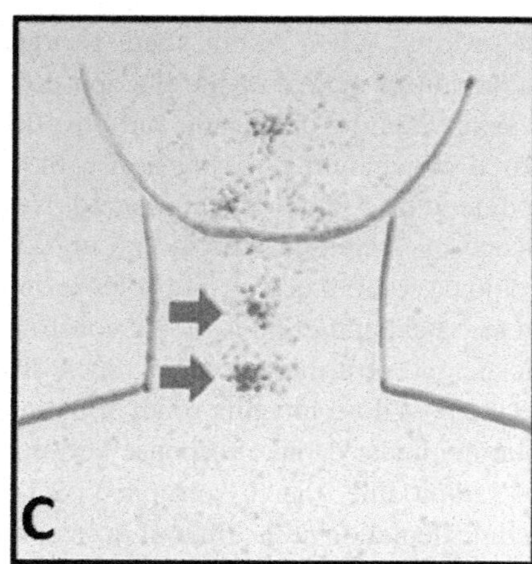

185 MBq (5 mCi) ^{131}I **3.7 GBq (100 mCi) ^{131}I** **185 MBq (5 mCi) ^{131}I (1 y f/u)**

Fig. 16.2 Stunning due to 185 MBq (5 mCi) ^{131}I scanning. After a total thyroidectomy in a 53-year-old male with papillary cancer, two foci of thyroid remnant were identified in a 72-h diagnostic scan with 185 MBq (5 mCi) ^{131}I (**a**) (*arrows*). Four weeks later, a 3.7 GBq (100 mCi) ^{131}I ablation therapy dose was given, and a 72-h post-therapy scan was obtained, which shows no evidence of uptake of the therapy dose by the severely stunned remnant tissues (**a**). A 1-year follow-up scan at 72 h following a 185 MBq (5 mCi) ^{131}I diagnostic dose again shows the same remnant tissue present in the same locations (**c**). The therapy dose was evidently wasted and obviously failed to ablate the target tissues

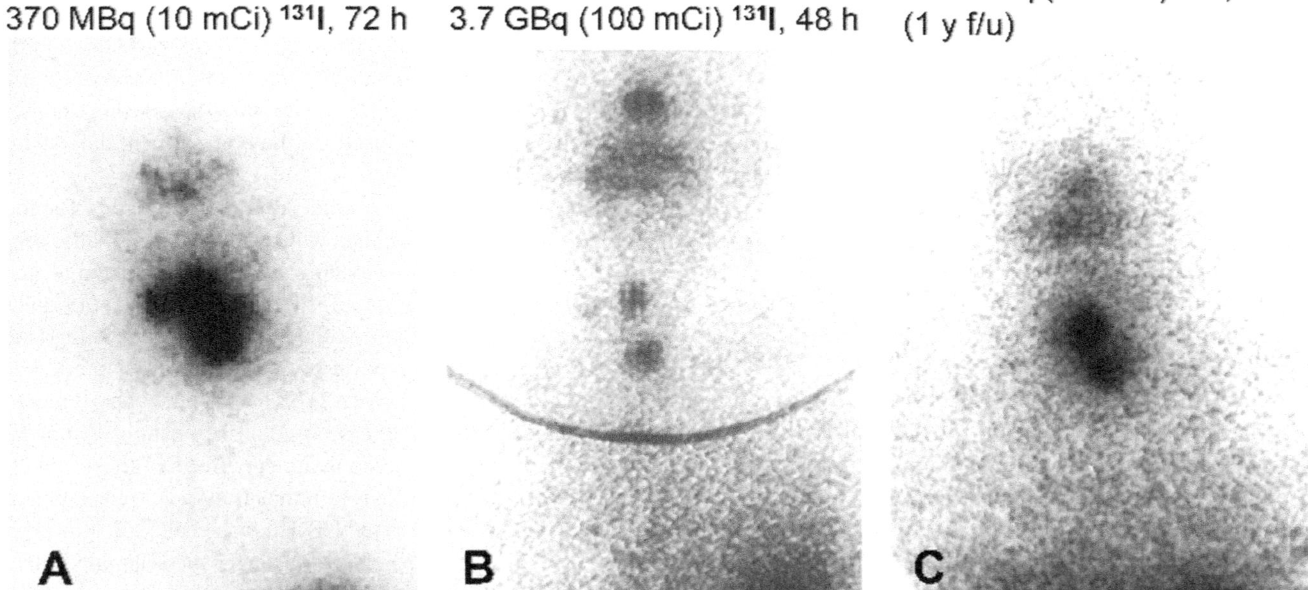

Fig. 16.3 Stunning due to 370 MBq (10 mCi) ^{131}I scanning. Postoperative iodine-avid thyroid remnants are shown by radioiodine scanning 72 h after the 370 MBq (10 mCi) ^{131}I scanning dose was given to a 44-years-old male with papillary thyroid cancer (**a**). The patient received a 3.7 GBq (100 mCi) ablative dose of ^{131}I on the day of diagnostic scanning, and a post-therapy scan obtained 48 h later shows unexpectedly low ^{131}I activity in the remnants. Certainly not much of the therapy dose was taken up by these relatively mildly stunned tissues (**b**). A 1-year follow-up scan shows evidence of failure of ablation (**c**)

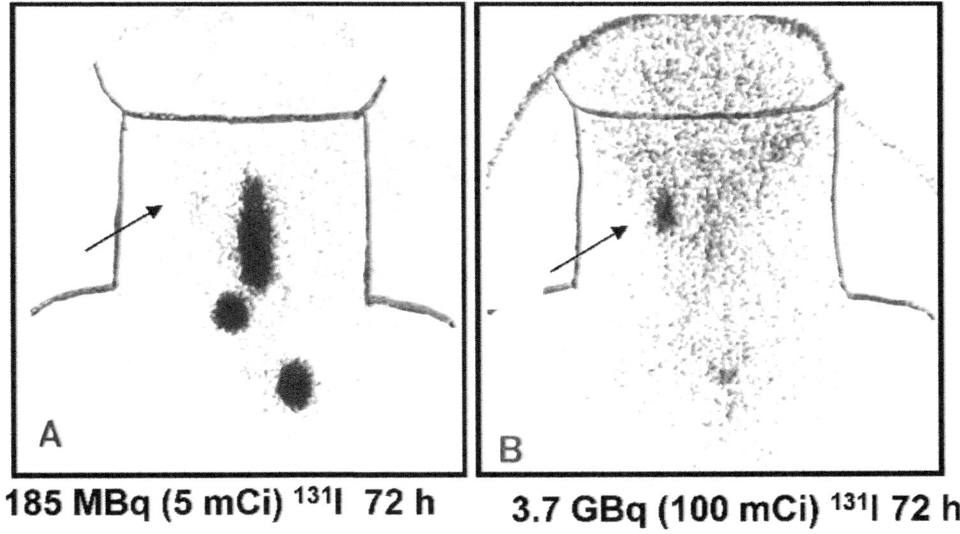

Fig. 16.4 The greater the uptake, the more the stunning. Postoperative thyroid scan using 185 MBq (5 mCi) dose of ^{131}I shows several foci of remnant, including the vertical pyramidal lobe. There are different degrees of uptake. The *arrow points* to a probable nodal metastasis with minimal uptake (**a**). The 72-h post-therapy scan after the 3.7 GBq (100 mCi) therapy dose shows more uptake in the node (*arrow*) than the other radioiodine-avid remnant tissues, the latter obviously being stunned to a higher degree (**b**)

et al. measured the changes in uptake values and found that 7.4 MBq (2 mCi) of ^{131}I lowered the uptake by 40 % [6, 7]. Moreover, McMenemin et al. showed that a potentially significant decrease caused by stunning may not be visually apparent in the post-therapy images [8]. For three thyroid cancer patients treated with ^{131}I, a reduction in post-therapy uptake to 86 %, 59 %, and 40 % of the pretreatment value was not seen by visual comparison of the scans. Therefore, qualitative comparison of diagnostic and post-therapy scans may be an insensitive indicator of stunning.

Evidence of Stunning

Numerous studies have documented proof of stunning. Quantitative studies more consistently identify the stunning effect [6, 9–14] than qualitative visual assessment reports [5, 15, 16], which are likely to be less sensitive. Sabri et al. studied the effect of the first half of a therapy dose to the thyroid uptake function [12]. In 171 patients with benign thyroid conditions (toxic diffuse goiter and toxic multinodular goiter), they found that the first dose (432.9±247.9 MBq [11.7±6.2 mCi] with a range of 244.2–1,209.9 MBq [6.6–32.7 mCi]) reduced thyroid uptake by 31.7 % (on average) when measured 4 days later. They also found that the stunning effect was dependent on the radiation-absorbed tissue dose. Postgard et al. performed an elegant in vitro study using a monolayer of porcine thyrocytes in a culture medium [11]. When the cells were irradiated with ^{131}I that was added to the medium and the cells received 300 rad (3 Gy), their iodide transport function was reduced by 50 % with a precipitous dose-response curve for higher exposures. In a clinical situation, 300 cGy (rads) would be equivalent to the absorbed tissue dose received by 1 g of thyroid tissue trapping 0.1 % of a 111 MBq (3 mCi) scanning dose of ^{131}I. Using a similar in vitro experimental model, Lundh et al. reported similar but more severe inhibitory effects of pretreatment by ^{131}I on iodide transport by cultured porcine thyrocytes [17]. A 50 % reduction in transport was observed following a dose of 1.5 Gy (150 rad) caused by exposure to ^{131}I. More recent studies from this group using the same experimental model found that the administered radiation doses to the cultured cells resulted in decreased expression of the sodium iodide symporter (NIS), identified by measurement of the NIS mRNA [18, 19]. This suggests a possible underlying molecular mechanism for the stunning phenomenon.

Hilditch et al. described an apparent stunning effect caused by the ^{131}I treatment dose itself [20]. Two groups of patients underwent radioiodine treatment following thyroidectomy for differentiated thyroid cancer. There were 26 patients in group 1 who underwent prior diagnostic whole-body scanning with 120 MBq (3.2 mCi) of ^{131}I 3–38 days prior to the therapeutic administration (median delay = 14 days). The 16 patients in group 2 had diagnostic whole-body scanning with ^{123}I followed by ^{131}I treatment 5–47 days later (median delay = 19 days). The percent uptake of the diagnostic and therapeutic doses for each patient was estimated from the geometric mean of anterior and posterior thyroid counts with appropriate use of high-count mode for post-therapy scanning. The measured thyroid counts were calibrated against those measured in a neck phantom containing a known quantity of the same radioiodine tracer that was imaged and counted in the identical manner. The mean therapeutic/diagnostic uptake ratio was 32.8 % for group 1 (^{131}I diagnostic scan) vs 58.8 % for group 2 (^{123}I diagnostic scan; $p<0.001$). At first glance, the reader might be tempted to conclude that ^{123}I also caused stunning in the group 2 patients, given that there was a 41.2 % average reduction of therapeutic ^{131}I uptake compared to the percentage of prior diagnostic ^{123}I uptake for these patients. However, as noted by the authors, this decreased therapeutic ^{131}I uptake among those in the group scanned with ^{123}I was more likely caused by the early radiation treatment effects of the absorbed ^{131}I in the thyroid remnant. Another possible contributor to the apparent posttreatment dose decrement could be a nonlinear count response by the gamma camera for the posttreatment scans, despite the use of high-count mode to avoid this liability. However, even in that event, one would not expect such a systematic error to behave differently based on whether I-123 or I-131 had been used for the pretreatment diagnostic whole-body scan.

It is noteworthy in this study that the use of ^{123}I for the diagnostic scan was associated with a significantly smaller decrement of subsequent therapeutic ^{131}I uptake compared to that seen among patients for whom ^{131}I was used for the prior diagnostic scan. Similar evidence of reduced therapeutic ^{131}I uptake compared to that measured in prior diagnostic ^{131}I scans was also described by Sisson et al. [21]. There is little opportunity to mitigate the potential decrease in total therapeutic ^{131}I uptake caused by the early radiation treatment effects of the ^{131}I treatment dose itself on the thyroid remnant tissue, a phenomenon that was suggested in the study by Hilditch et al. [20]. However, the choice of ^{123}I instead of ^{131}I for diagnostic scanning in this study was correlated with a larger subsequent fractional uptake of the ^{131}I treatment dose, which is clearly in the interest of optimal therapeutic outcome.

Kao and Yen reviewed diagnostic and posttreatment ^{131}I scans of 468 patients that were treated for differentiated thyroid cancer [22]. Diagnostic scanning was performed 3 days after administration of 111 MBq (3 mCi) ^{131}I. A therapeutic dose of 3.7–7.4 GBq (100–200 mCi) ^{131}I was administered 1 week to 1 month following the diagnostic scan with posttreatment scanning at 10 days post dose. Of the total patients treated, 344 (73.5 %) had some degree of reduced ^{131}I uptake in the posttreatment scans compared to that seen in the prior diagnostic scans, and 50 patients (10.7 %) had no uptake at sites of differentiated thyroid tissue, which was considered "stunning." The authors recommended using ^{123}I in lieu of ^{131}I for diagnostic scanning to avoid compromising uptake of the therapeutic dose.

A study by Lassman et al. quantified the stunning effect of a repeat 7.4 MBq (2 mCi) ^{131}I diagnostic dose in six patients approximately 5 weeks following the initial diagnostic dose [13]. The average reductions in both uptake and half-life for the second ^{131}I administration were 44 % and 51 %, respectively ($p<0.001$ for both). Decreased fractional uptake and biological half-life would both contribute to decreases in the absorbed tissue dose in the interval between the first and second diagnostic scans in this study. These intervals were longer than those typical in clinical practice in the United States. This greater "lag time" between the two doses may amplify the stunning effect, from the longer residence time of the first dose prior to the administration of the second dose. Particularly, some have advocated that keeping this dose interval as short as possible will avoid the effects of stunning [5, 15]. However, Medvedec et al. reported no difference in the degree of stunning by decreasing this dose interval from a mean of 8.5 days to a mean of 4.3 days [14]. These data suggest that most of the damage is already done at 4.3 days, and although reducing the dose interval should be helpful to decrease further stunning, it may not avoid it completely. Apparently, the waiting period after administration of the scanning dose should be shortened to reduce the stunning. The usual waiting period of 72 h would allow the β particles to bombard the thyroid tissue for just as many hours. The thyroid tissue would have received 72.7 % of the ultimate total radiation dose at 72 h when the total effective half-life is 2 days or 54.1 % when the total effective half-life is 4 days [4]. Thyroid tissue receives much less radiation if the scan is done at 24 h instead.

Stunning Effect on the Outcome of Ablation Therapy

The outcome-based evidence for stunning is perhaps most compelling as it may not be a function of technical variables that confound comparisons of diagnostic and post-therapy scans. Park et al. reported that there was a lower success rate of ablation after ^{131}I scans than after ^{123}I scans (56 % vs 72 %) in 47 and 43 patients, respectively [23].

Muratet et al. examined 229 patients and found that successful outcome was significantly less frequent after a scanning dose of 111 MBq (3 mCi) than after 37 MBq (1 mCi) of ^{131}I (50 % vs 76 %, p<0.001). Even 37 MBq (1 mCi) of ^{131}I caused stunning in a few cases [24].

Chmielowiec et al. [25] evaluated the efficacy of ^{131}I treatments among post-thyroidectomy patients without evidence of metastatic disease. The total cumulative ^{131}I dose and total number of ^{131}I treatments required to achieve complete remnant ablation in the post-therapy scan was determined for patients who had pretreatment diagnostic scans with either a low dose (LD) or a high dose (HD) of ^{131}I. There were 126 patients who had received 200 MBq (5.4 mCi) ^{131}I in the HD group and 105 patients in the LD group, for whom the ^{131}I diagnostic dose was 50 MBq (1.35 mCi). They found that on average, significantly less total cumulative ^{131}I was required to completely ablate patients in the LD group vs those in the HD group (5.126±2.9 GBq [138.5±78.4 mCi] vs 7.45±4.64 GBq [201.5±125.4 mCi], respectively, $p<0.01$). Similarly, fewer total ^{131}I treatments on average were required for the LD group vs the HD group (1.51±0.75, vs 1.83±1.13, respectively, $p<0.01$). The significantly larger mean total cumulative dose and significantly greater mean number of ^{131}I treatments required to achieve complete remnant ablation for patients in the HD group reflects the stunning effect of the larger ^{131}I dose used in the pretreatment diagnostic scans.

Lees et al. reported a 47 % ablation success rate in the ^{131}I (185 MBq [5 mCi]) scan group vs 86 % in the ^{123}I (740 MBq [20 mCi]) scan group divided equally among 72 patients ($p<0.005$) [26].

Morris et al. reported no difference in the success rates between an ^{131}I-scanned group and the non-scanned group when the success was based on follow-up scans obtained at 4–42 months [27].

Similarly, Silberstein found no significant difference in the efficacy of ^{131}I remnant ablation for two groups of patients following thyroidectomy for differentiated thyroid cancer, differing only in the choice of either ^{123}I or ^{131}I for pretreatment diagnostic scanning [28]. In group 1, for whom 14.8 MBq (400 uCi) ^{123}I was used for the diagnostic scan, 81 % (21/26) of patients had effective ablation based on post-therapy thyroglobulin levels and radioiodine scanning. This was compared to a treatment efficacy of 74 % (17/23) of group 2 patients who had pretreatment diagnostic scans with 74 MBq (2 mCi) ^{131}I.

Conversely, Verburg et al. reported a significant reduction in the efficacy of radioiodine ablation depending upon whether or not pretreatment diagnostic scanning with just 40 MBq (1.1 mCi) ^{131}I had been performed [29]. All patients (48) from one hospital had pretreatment ^{131}I diagnostic scans and were compared to treatment outcomes with a group of 51 patients from another hospital treated with ^{131}I without prior diagnostic scanning. Based on non-detectible thyroglobulin levels and the results of post-therapy radioiodine scanning, ^{131}I ablation was successful in 33 % (17/51) of patients who had first undergone diagnostic scanning with ^{131}I compared to 65 % (31/48) of patients without prior ^{131}I diagnostic scanning ($p=0.002$). Some uncertainty is likely introduced by comparing outcomes between groups of patients from two different hospitals. However, the two treatment protocols were described as being identical with the only exception being the use of the pretreatment scan.

Hu et al. evaluated the efficacy of remnant ablation with and without prior diagnostic scanning with 185 MBq (5 mCi) ^{131}I 4–11 days prior to ^{131}I treatment [30]. Of the 126 cases who had a prior diagnostic ^{131}I scan, 56 (44.4 %) had effective remnant ablation vs 86/119 (72.2 %) of those without a prior diagnostic scan ($p<0.001$). Paradoxically, only 13/126 (10.3 %) of the patients who had a prior diagnostic scan with ^{131}I had visible evidence of stunning in the post-therapy scan despite a much larger proportion of those with unsuccessful remnant ablation. Therefore, visually detectable stunning in this study proved to be an insensitive marker for therapeutic compromise.

Dam et al. described a similar lack of correlation between stunning in post-therapy ^{131}I scans and therapeutic efficacy [16]. Pre- and post-therapy ^{131}I scans were compared among patients with follow-up who underwent ^{131}I treatment and prior post-thyroidectomy diagnostic scanning with 185 MBq (5 mCi) ^{131}I. For the patients without visible evidence of stunning, 48/55 had effective remnant ablation (87 %) vs 10/11 (91 %) of those with evidence of stunning on the post-therapy scan. A similar noncorrelation between stunning and treatment efficacy was found for metastatic lesions, which were primarily lymph nodes. However, as noted by Gerard [31], technical issues may have compromised the validity of this evaluation. There were substantial differences in the post-dose scanning times for the diagnostic and post-therapy imaging (2 days vs 7 days). Pre- and post-therapy scans with a 20–40-fold difference in the administered ^{131}I dose were only compared qualitatively. Medium energy rather than high-energy collimation was used for ^{131}I imaging, which is contrary to published procedure guidelines [32]. In addition, the criteria for therapeutic efficacy were based only on the post-therapy scan without the use of thyroglobulin measurement.

The discrepancy between these conflicting results may arise from the lack of uniform protocols for ^{131}I scanning and treatment, the lack of uniform criteria for successful ablation between the reporting institutions, uncontrolled differences between study cohorts within a given study, and inherent differences between patient populations being studied across multiple institutions. More data using the same protocol with a larger patient population is needed to show significant differences. Also, it is likely that at least 12 months should elapse before an attempt is made to determine the outcome. Stunned lesions with no uptake on earlier scans may have uptake on the later scans after recovery. Therapeutic effect depends on the amount of radiation absorbed by the thyroid tissue from any ^{131}I dose. In a few patients, we have observed that the scanning dose of ^{131}I was later found to be actually lethal to the target tissue [4].

Considerations in Fractionated ^{131}I Therapy

Similar to the situation in the United States until 1997, nuclear regulations in many countries still limit the amount of ^{131}I that can be given to outpatients. In certain areas, hospitals are required to have a specifically designed stainless steel septic tank large enough to hold ^{131}I waste from the patients to allow near-complete decay of ^{131}I.

Understandably, fractionated dosing is a common practice to manage therapies within such strict nuclear regulations. The longer the interval between the divided doses in fractionated ^{131}I treatment, the greater the absorbed radiation dose would be from the first dose, and the lower the uptake would be from the subsequent ^{131}I doses. The therapeutic contribution of the second or third dose must be lower than the first dose because the amount of ^{131}I taken up by the stunned thyroid tissue from the first dose should be smaller, decreasing the cumulative radiation-absorbed dose. "Satisfactory" results were indicated with fractionated therapy in treating benign thyroid conditions and thyroid cancer. Such an inhibitory effect by the first ^{131}I dose fraction on the second ^{131}I dose fraction was in fact shown by Wu et al. [33] when treating patients with thyroid cancer and by Krohn et al. [34] for the treatment of patients with benign thyroid disease.

However, a paucity of reports analyzed the therapeutic effect of the first dose and subsequent doses separately because at least in part the full effect of the first dose may not become evident for up to 12 months. Such a study would not be justifiable in patients with thyroid cancer because the consequence of probable incomplete treatment may be harmful.

The Use of ^{123}I vs ^{131}I as a Scanning Agent

^{123}I emits γ rays but not β particles and has a half-life of 13 h. The radiation-absorbed tissue dose from pure ^{123}I is only 1 % of that from ^{131}I [35]. No stunning has been observed after the use of pure ^{123}I (Fig. 16.5). Notably, depending on the production methods, some ^{123}I preparations contain ^{124}I as contaminant, which will raise the absorbed tissue dose.

In nuclear imaging studies, it is generally known that a higher scanning dose provides better image quality. Waxman showed that higher ^{131}I doses gave greater sensitivity [36]. The ^{131}I scans using 3.7 GBq (100 mCi) therapy dose that are obtained 7 days later when the background is low may be considered as the "gold standard" provided no pretreatment diagnostic ^{131}I was used. The accuracy of diagnostic scans may be compared to this standard. Gerard and Cavalieri have shown that the sensitivity of ^{123}I (111–185 MBq [3–5 mCi]) compared with the early post-therapy scans was 86.7 % and that good-quality images can be obtained up to 48 h after administration [37]. Gulzar et al. showed that ^{123}I scans (185 MBq [5 mCi]) had a 92.6 % concordance rate between 24-h ^{123}I scan and post-therapy ^{131}I scan. The quality of 24-h ^{123}I scans was found to be slightly better than 4-h ^{123}I images [38].

Comparing diagnostic scans using either ^{123}I or ^{131}I, Mandel et al. reported that ^{123}I (44.4–55.5 MBq [1.2–1.5 mCi]) 5-h scans were slightly superior to ^{131}I (111 MBq [3 mCi]) 48-h scans for whole-body imaging. ^{123}I scans showed 35 foci, whereas ^{131}I scans showed 32 foci [39].

Ali et al. evaluated ^{123}I for diagnostic scanning using doses of 185–270 MBq (5–7.3 mCi; 40). A negative diagnostic whole-body ^{123}I scan in 125 patients provided the basis for deferring ^{131}I treatment. In 50 patients with positive diagnostic ^{123}I scans, 49 were confirmed as "true positive" in the subsequent post-therapy ^{131}I scans. These investigators thereby identified high specificity of diagnostic ^{123}I scanning for the identification of differentiated thyroid tissue. They acknowledged that ^{123}I avoids stunning and is the tracer of choice for diagnostic scanning of thyroid cancer patients.

Owing to the relatively short half-life, ^{123}I scans are commonly done at 24 h, whereas the ^{131}I scans are obtained at

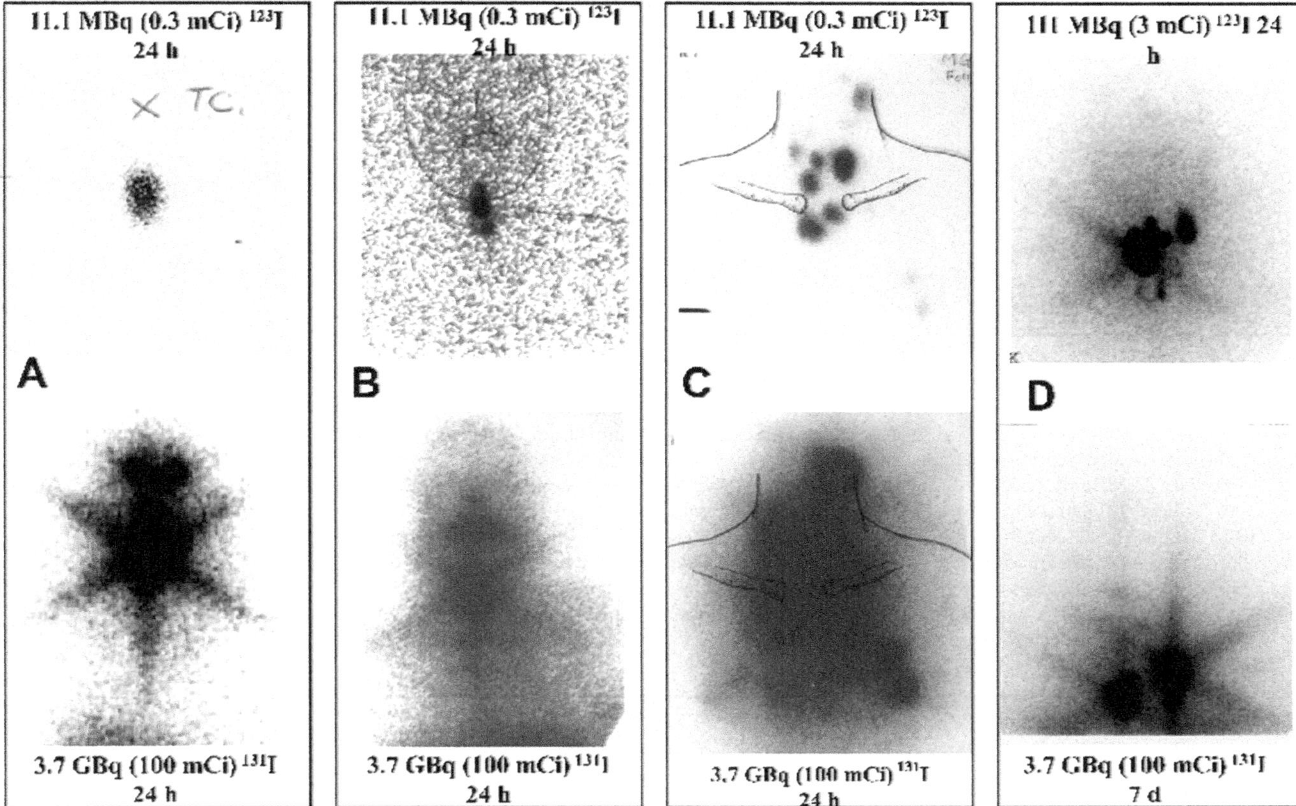

Fig. 16.5 Excellent uptake of therapeutic ^{131}I by not-stunned thyroid. Four different postoperative cases where ^{123}I was used to scan prior to ^{131}I therapy (**a–d** *top row*). In each case, the post-therapy scan shows markedly increased uptake of the therapy dose in the target tissues (**a–d** *bottom row*). The star artifact is caused by penetration of the collimator on the gamma camera by the gamma rays from the highly concentrated ^{131}I activity in the target tissues

48–72 h. Some slow-functioning lesions may be identified only on the scans obtained much later. Sarkar et al. reported four cases in which 24-h ^{123}I scans (74–129.5 MBq [2–3.5 mCi]) missed metastases that were seen on the 72–96-h ^{131}I scans (111–185 MBq [3–5 mCi]; 41). In one patient, both the 24-h ^{123}I and 24-h ^{131}I scans missed some of the metastases that were seen on the 96-h ^{131}I scan. This result emphasized the benefit of delayed imaging and washout of background activity to raise the target-to-background ratios. However, the 24-h ^{123}I images showed all of the postoperative remnants present in nine patients. Alternatively, Bautovich et al. reported superior detection of metastases from diagnostic scans using a large ^{123}I dose (1 GBq [27 mCi]) and 48-h imaging in eight of ten previously ablated patients compared to that with 185 MBq (5 mCi) ^{131}I [42]. The ^{131}I diagnostic scans missed 13 more foci than were seen with ^{123}I in comparison to the post-therapy scans as the gold standard. Admittedly, routine use of such large doses could be cost-prohibitive. However, ^{123}I used in large enough doses sufficient to permit 48-h delayed imaging may afford competitive or superior sensitivity without the associated risks of stunning with diagnostic ^{131}I scanning.

On a dose-for-dose basis, ^{123}I scans seem to offer equal or higher sensitivity in diagnostic scanning as do ^{131}I scans for the detection of thyroid remnant [39, 43]. Gerard and Cavalieri have shown that ^{123}I scans obtained at 48 h are good quality when doses of at least 185 MBq (5 mCi) are used [37], which has also been shown by others (26, 42, 44, 45; Figs. 16.6, 16.7, and 16.8). Others have reported competitive sensitivity of ^{123}I for diagnostic scanning when compared to the post-therapy ^{131}I scans, even when used in doses of 37–111 MBq (1–3 mCi) [46, 47].

Thus, a growing body of literature indicates that ^{123}I is preferred for whole-body imaging in thyroid cancer metastasis screening [45, 48, 49].

The disadvantages of ^{123}I include limited availability, the higher cost necessitated by production at a cyclotron facility, as well as its short half-life, which is problematic for long-distance shipping and quantitative dosimetry. The cost of a 185 MBq (5-mCi) dose can be reduced by ordering the tracer directly from the manufacturer and administering it orally as a liquid [37, 50]. We believe that the additional cost of ^{123}I is justified to avoid a suboptimal therapeutic outcome. One caveat in ^{123}I imaging is to recognize that salivary activity is

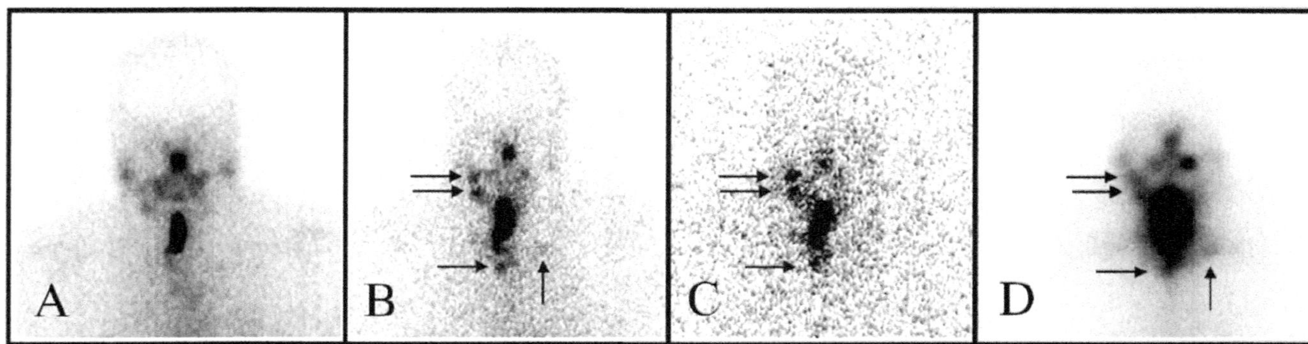

Fig. 16.6 Increasing target-to-background activity in 6-, 24-, and 48-h ^{123}I images. A 40-year-old female post-thyroidectomy for multifocal papillary thyroid cancer had invasion into sternocleidomastoid muscle on the right with positive resection margins. Diagnostic scanning was performed with 181 MBq (4.9 mCi) ^{123}I. The anterior view is shown at 6 h in (**a**), 24 h in (**b**), and 48 h in (**c**). The patient was treated with 7.44 GBq (201 mCi) ^{131}I. The 3-day posttreatment anterior image is shown in (**d**). The *horizontal arrows* in (**b–d**) identify two *upper right* cervical lymph nodes (two *upper adjacent arrows*) and two sites of thyroid tissue below the larger vertical midline neck accumulation (*lower single arrow*). These images show a progressive increase in ^{123}I target-to-background activity ratio from 6 to 24 h and again from 24 to 48 h in the thyroid tissue sites delineated by the *horizontal arrows*. Relatively symmetric parotid salivary gland activity most evident in the 6-h ^{123}I image, lateral to the lymph node uptake, also becomes relatively less conspicuous at 24 h and 48 h in this case. The *vertical arrow* in (**d**) identifies a more weakly avid site of posttreatment ^{131}I accumulation, either lymph node or soft tissue metastasis. This focus was identified only in hindsight in the 24-h image (*vertical arrow* in **b**) and for which the counts were too low to visualize in the 48-h image (**c**). Note the superior resolution of the ^{123}I images in (**a–c**) vs the ^{131}I image in (**d**)

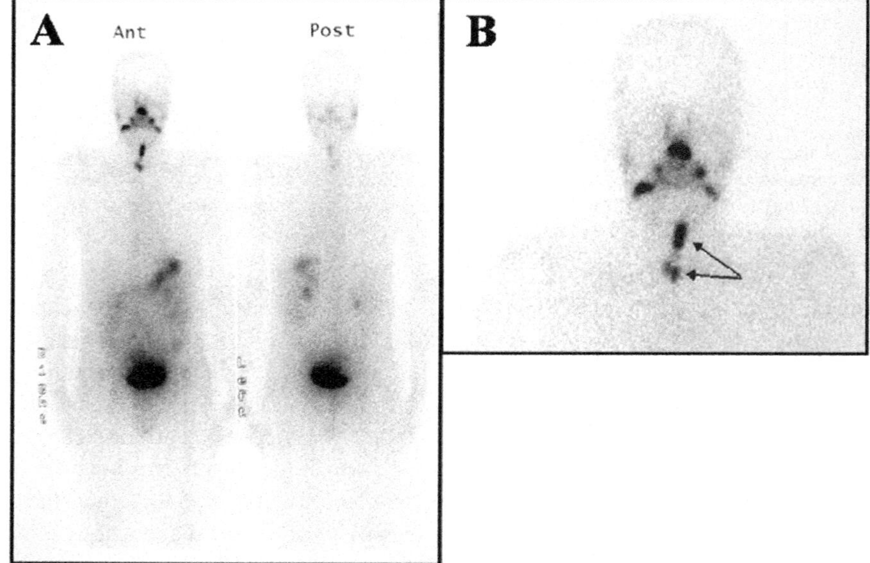

Fig. 16.7 ^{123}I 24-h whole-body imaging with rhTSH. A 51-year-old male patient following total thyroidectomy for papillary thyroid cancer underwent whole-body imaging with 281 MBq (7.6 mCi) ^{123}I with rhTSH. The 24-h images are shown in (**a**), and an enlargement of the anterior head and neck image is shown in (**b**). The *arrows* in (**b**) show two or three foci in the lower neck and a higher midline focus, representing pyramidal lobe remnant. These sites were confirmed in the post-^{131}I therapy scan (not shown). Of interest in this case, the patient's thyroglobulin measured 72 h following the second intramuscular rhTSH injection was only 0.8 ng/mL with a TSH level of 69 μU/mL on the day of ^{123}I dose administration. The thyroglobulin level following full withdrawal preparation for therapy, including 2 weeks off of T3, was similarly only 1.7 ng/mL with TSH level of 35 μU/mL at the time of treatment. Importantly, antithyroid antibodies were negative in this patient. This case represents an example of the complementary sensitivity of ^{123}I diagnostic imaging and thyroglobulin measurement for detection of residual differentiated thyroid tissue. Had the practice been only to do the latter, a decision to defer radioiodine ablation might have been inappropriate

present in the esophagus at 24 h. Repeat scanning after allowing the patient to drink a glass of water clears this activity.

Experience with ^{123}I for diagnostic scanning with recombinant human TSH (rhTSH) suggests comparable sensitivity to that achieved with ^{131}I under the same conditions [51–53]. ^{131}I therapy with rhTSH for thyroid remnant ablation appears to be as effective as therapy performed following thyroid hormone withdrawal [54–60]. Therefore, the option to avoid

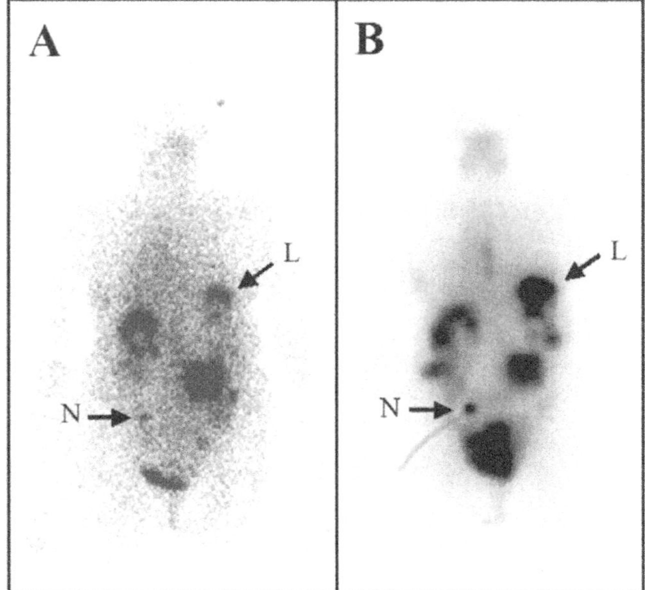

Fig. 16.8 ^{123}I diagnostic scan and early ^{131}I post-therapy scan with rhTSH. An 82-year-old female patient with history of metastatic follicular thyroid cancer was assessed with ^{123}I diagnostic scanning with rhTSH, followed by ^{131}I treatment also with rhTSH (second dose 1 week later). The patient had a known history of metastasis to the liver, a high tumor burden with thyroglobulin levels >30,000, for whom thyroid hormone withdrawal did not result in adequate TSH elevation. (**a**) The posterior whole-body diagnostic scan at 24 h following an ^{123}I dose of 233 MBq (6.3 mCi). (**b**) Posterior whole-body posttreatment scan at 3 days following an ^{131}I dose of 5.59 GBq (151 mCi). In both images, the sites of liver metastasis and retroperitoneal lymph node metastasis are labeled with an "L" arrow and an "N" arrow, respectively. Intensely labeled kidneys in both images are seen in the lower right and upper left of the abdomen. The post-therapy scan also shows some midline esophageal activity in the lower thorax. Both sites of metastatic involvement were also confirmed in the 8-day post-therapy image (not shown) (the spot of activity in the diagnostic scan on the right side of the head is surface contamination at the site of the patient's hair clip)

the morbidity of severe hypothyroidism could be applied more routinely to both diagnostic scanning and therapy. This opportunity emphasizes the need to further validate rhTSH diagnostic scanning using ^{123}I to avoid stunning by ^{131}I. Some evidence shows that thyroidal iodine residence time with rhTSH may be longer compared to that in the withdrawal setting [61], which could potentiate the stunning effect.

Examples of rhTSH ^{123}I whole-body scans are shown in Figs. 16.7 and 16.8.

Using Low Dose of ^{131}I When ^{123}I Is Not Available

In places where ^{123}I is not available, the only choice may be to use ^{131}I as the imaging agent. Relevant to this option, Medvedec reviewed studies with evaluable ^{131}I dosimetric data from which he estimated a threshold absorbed dose for stunning of the thyroid of only 4–5 Gy [62]. This radiation absorbed dose would be achieved in a normal euthyroid patient with intact thyroid gland from just 11.8 MBq (317 uCi) ^{131}I or alternatively from 1.173 GBq (31.7 mCi) of ^{123}I [63]. It is physiologically challenging to translate these absorbed dose estimates for the euthyroid patient with intact thyroid gland to the post-thyroidectomy patient with variable amounts of residual remnant with high TSH levels, as is the case for those patients undergoing diagnostic whole-body radioiodine scanning prior to ^{131}I therapy. Nonetheless, Medvedec's suggestion that "… there is no scintigraphically sufficient diagnostic amount of ^{131}I that can be given prior to ^{131}I therapy for a thyroid cancer that does not cause thyroid stunning…" seems in the least possible and perhaps likely [62].

Therefore, it would be prudent to lower the administered dose as much as possible to prevent stunning prior to a planned ^{131}I therapy. However, other measures may also help reduce stunning: (1) to scan early (e.g., at 24 h instead of at 72 h, to decrease the interval between diagnostic dose and time of scanning) and (2) to administer the ^{131}I treatment dose soon after scanning, preferably on the same day, considering that the stunning effect increases over time. The 72-h scans may have slightly higher sensitivity, but a clinical decision to treat can often be made on the 24-h scans. If the 24-h scan shows no thyroid tissue uptake, further delayed scans should be obtained.

Discussion

Generally, to successfully ablate the target tissues, a sufficient dose of ^{131}I should be administered at once to "hit them hard the first time." As early as 1951, Rawson et al. warned against giving a "noncancericidal" dose of ^{131}I, which results in inadequate therapy for differentiated thyroid cancers [64]. Efforts are continuously made to improve the radioiodine uptake by the target cells to their maximum capacity before radioablation therapy. Most physicians involved with ^{131}I therapy prepare the patients with T4 withdrawal or rhTSH injection to raise the serum TSH level. Patients are placed on a low-iodine diet to decrease the body iodide pool as low as possible to allow the target cells to take up as much administered ^{131}I as possible [65]. Some suggest the use of lithium to increase the resident time of ^{131}I in the thyroid tissue; others are developing methods to increase sodium iodide symporter (NIS) gene expression in the thyroid cancer cells. In line with these efforts, stunning of the thyroid target cells should be avoided or minimized. Stunning the thyroid cells, or making them temporarily nonfunctional or less functional prior to the intended radioablation therapy, will work against most of our other efforts to improve the radioiodine uptake with the thyroid remnant or metastatic thyroid cancer cells.

To avoid thyroid stunning altogether or to increase patient convenience, some suggest administering ^{131}I therapy blindly to all postoperative patients without conducting a diagnostic survey scan. Unfortunately, this practice may end up giving a large amount of ^{131}I to a few patients without treatable lesions. Moreover, diagnostic whole-body radioiodine scanning for thyroid cancer, although not perfect, is one of the best imaging tests for staging the extent of disease prior to treatment. These data are often included in the treatment algorithm for determination of the ^{131}I dose [66].

^{123}I is available or may soon become available in many parts of the world. Using it for scanning will alleviate the problem of stunning, and a lower therapeutic dose may be needed to treat lesions that are not stunned. Then, if the current therapy dose of ^{131}I is lowered, can the same ablation success rate still be achieved? What other factors are required to achieve the success rate of 100 %? These are some questions that need to be answered by future research.

Summary

Thyroid stunning is a predictable, verifiable radiobiological suppressive phenomenon that occurs when a scanning dose of ^{131}I deposits a sufficient radiation dose to the target tissue to temporarily reduce its iodide-trapping function. The stunned cells are unable to take up the ensuing therapeutic dose of ^{131}I to the degree of their prior unaffected maximal capacity, and the intended ablation may become incomplete. There must be factors other than stunning that account for some ^{131}I ablation failures. Nevertheless, stunning is one of the known causes of reduced ^{131}I uptake by the target cells and may negate all other efforts to increase the ^{131}I uptake before radioablation therapy.

^{123}I has many desirable characteristics as a thyroid imaging agent and does not stun the target cells. Wherever available, it would be prudent to utilize ^{123}I for scanning purposes before ^{131}I therapy in the management of well-differentiated thyroid cancers. It is not known if there exists a safe but effective scanning dose of ^{131}I [62]. However, in places where ^{123}I is not available, thereby requiring the use of ^{131}I for pretreatment diagnostic scanning, efforts should be made to minimize the stunning effect by administering a minimum dose of 74 mBq (2 mCi) or less and by keeping the time between the diagnostic and treatment doses as short as possible.

Acknowledgments The authors are grateful to Drs. Richard Schnute, Christine Park, and Trudy Lionel for reviewing this article and rendering helpful suggestions and to Dr. S. Bae of Koshin University, Korea, for providing images for Figs. 16.2 and 16.4.

References

1. Park HM. ^{123}I: almost a designer radioiodine for thyroid scanning. J Nucl Med. 2002;43:77–8.
2. Park HM. Potential adverse effect of high survey dose of ^{131}I administered prior to ^{131}I therapy in the management of differentiated thyroid cancers. In: Schmidt H, Van Der Schoot JB, editors. Nuclear medicine: the state of the art of nuclear medicine in Europe. Stuttgart: Schattauer; 1991. p. 340–2.
3. Park HM, Perkins OW, Edmondson JW, Shnute RB, Manatunga A. Influence of diagnostic radioiodines on the uptake of ablative dose of ^{131}I. Thyroid. 1994;4:49–54.
4. Park HM. The stunning effect in radioiodine therapy of thyroid cancer. Nucl Med Ann. 2001: 49–67.
5. McDougall IR. 74 MBq ^{131}I does not prevent uptake of therapeutic doses of ^{131}I in differentiated thyroid cancer. Nucl Med Commun. 1997;18:505–12.
6. Huic D, Medvedec M, Dodig D, Popovic S, Ivancevic D, Pavlinovic Z, Zuvic M. Radioiodine uptake in thyroid cancer patients after diagnostic application of low-dose ^{131}I. Nucl Med Commun. 1996;17:839–42.
7. Medvedec M, Pavlinovic Z, Dodig D. 74 MBq radioiodine ^{131}I does prevent uptake of therapeutic activity of ^{131}I in residual thyroid tissue. Eur J Nucl Med. 1999;26:1013.
8. McMenemin RM, Hilditch TE, Dempsey MF, Reed NS. Thyroid stunning after ^{131}I diagnostic whole-body scanning. J Nucl Med. 2001;42:986–7.
9. Jeevanram RK, Shah DH, Sharma SM, Ganatra RD. Influence of initial large dose on subsequent uptake of therapeutic radioiodine in thyroid cancer patients. Nucl Med Biol. 1986;13:277–9.
10. Leger FA, Izembart M, Dagousset F, et al. Decreased uptake of therapeutic doses of ^{131}I after 185 mBq ^{131}I diagnostic imaging for thyroid remnants in differentiated thyroid carcinoma. Eur J Nucl Med. 1998;25:242–6.
11. Postgard P, Himmelman J, Lindencrona L, Bhogal N, Wiberg D, Berg G, Jansson S, Nystrom E, Forssell-Aronsson E, Nilsson M. Stunning of iodide transport by ^{131}I irradiation in cultured thyroid epithelial cells. J Nucl Med. 2002;43:828–34.
12. Sabri O, Zimny M, Schreckenberger M, Meyer-Oelmann A, Reinartz P, Buell U. Does thyroid stunning exist? A model with benign thyroid disease. Eur J Nucl Med. 2000;27:1591–7.
13. Lassmann M, Luster M, Hänscheid H, Reiners C. Impact of ^{131}I diagnostic activities on the biokinetics of thyroid remnants. J Nucl Med. 2004;45:619–25.
14. Medvedec M, Grosev D, Loncaric S, Pavlinovic Z, Dodig D. As soon as possible is already too late. J Nucl Med. 2001;42:322P (abstract).
15. Cholewinski S, Yoo K, Klieger P, O'Mara R. Absence of thyroid stunning after diagnostic whole-body scanning with 185 MBq ^{131}I. J Nucl Med. 2000;41:1198–202.
16. Dam HQ, Kim SM, Lin HC, Intenzo CM. ^{131}I therapeutic efficacy is not influenced by stunning after diagnostic whole-body scanning. Radiology. 2004;232:527–33.
17. Lundh C, Norden MM, Nilsson M, Forssell-Aronsson E. Reduced iodide transport (stunning) and DNA synthesis in thyrocytes exposed to low absorbed doses from ^{131}I in vitro. J Nucl Med. 2007;48:481–6.
18. Norden MM, Larsson F, et al. Down-regulation of the sodium/iodide symporter explains ^{131}I-induced thyroid stunning. Cancer Res. 2007;67:7512–7.
19. Lundh C, Lindencrona U, et al. Radiation-induced thyroid stunning: differential effects of ^{123}I, ^{131}I, ^{99m}Tc, and ^{111}at on iodide transport and NIS mRNA expression in cultured thyroid cells. J Nucl Med. 2009;50:1161–7.
20. Hilditch TE, Dempsey MF, et al. Self-stunning in thyroid ablation: evidence from comparative studies of diagnostic ^{131}I and ^{123}I. Eur J Nucl Med. 2002;29:783–8.
21. Sisson JC, Avram AM, et al. The so-called stunning of thyroid tissue. J Nucl Med. 2006;47:1406–12.
22. Kao CH, Yen TC. Stunning effects after a diagnostic dose of ^{131}I. Nuklearmedizin. 1998;37:23–5.
23. Park H, Park Y, Zhou X. Detection of thyroid remnant/metastasis without stunning: an ongoing dilemma. Thyroid. 1997;7:277–80.
24. Muratet J, Daver A, Minier J, Larra F. Influence of scanning doses of ^{131}I on subsequent first ablative treatment outcome in patients

operated on for differentiated thyroid carcinoma. J Nucl Med. 1998;39:1546–50.
25. Chmielowiec C, Logus JW, et al. The effect of thyroid gland stunning by ^{131}I sodium iodide diagnostic scans on subsequent patient ablation doses – a 25 year retrospective study. Eur J Nucl Med. 2000;27:1154.
26. Lees W, Mansberg R, Roberts J, Towson J, Chua E, Turtle J. The clinical effects of thyroid stunning after diagnostic whole-body scanning with 185 MBq ^{131}I. Eur J Nucl Med. 2002;29:1421–7.
27. Morris LF, Waxman AD, Braunstein GD. J Clin Endocrinol Metab. 2001;86:3507–11.
28. Silberstein EB. Comparison of outcomes after ^{123}I versus ^{131}I preablation imaging before radioiodine ablation in differentiated thyroid carcinoma. J Nucl Med. 2007;48:1043–6.
29. Verburg FA, Verkooijen RB, Stokkel MP, van Isselt JW. The success of ^{131}I ablation in thyroid cancer patients is significantly reduced after a diagnostic activity of 40 MBq ^{131}I. Nuklearmedizin. 2009;48:138–42.
30. Hu Y, Wang P, Wang S, et al. Influence of ^{131}I diagnostic dose on subsequent ablation in patients with differentiated thyroid carcinoma: discrepancy between the presence of visually apparent stunning and the impairment of successful ablation. Nucl Med Commun. 2004;25:793–7.
31. Gerard SK. Stunning with ^{131}I diagnostic whole body imaging of patients with thyroid cancer. Radiology. 2005;234:972–3.
32. Becker D, Charkes ND, Dworkin H, et al. Procedure guideline for extended scintigraphy for differentiated thyroid cancer: 1.0. Society of nuclear medicine. J Nucl Med. 1996;37:1269–71.
33. Wu H, Hseu H, et al. Decreased uptake after fractionated ablative doses of iodine-131. Eur J Nucl Med Mol Imaging. 2005;32:167–73.
34. Krohn T, Meyer PT, Ocklenburg C, et al. Stunning in radioiodine therapy of benign thyroid disease. Quantification and therapeutic relevance. Nuklearmedizin. 2008;47:248–54.
35. Berman M, Braverman LE, Burke J, et al. MIRD (Medical Internal Radiation Dose) Committee Report # 5 Summary of current radiation dose estimates to humans from ^{123}I, ^{124}I, ^{125}I, ^{126}I, ^{130}I, ^{131}I, and ^{132}I as sodium iodide. J Nucl Med 1975; 16:857–860.
36. Waxman A, Ramanna L, Chapman N, et al. Significance of ^{131}I scan dose in patients with thyroid cancer: determination of ablation: concise communication. J Nucl Med. 1981;22:861–5.
37. Gerard SK, Cavalieri RR. ^{123}I diagnostic thyroid tumor whole body scanning with imaging at 6, 24, and 48 hours. Clin Nucl Med. 2002;27:1–8.
38. Gulzar Z, Jana S, Young I, et al. Neck and whole-body scanning with a 5 mCi dose of ^{123}I as diagnostic tracer in patients with well-differentiated thyroid cancer. Endocr Pract. 2001;7:244–9.
39. Mandel SJ, Shankar LK, Benard F, Yamamoto A, Alavi A. Superiority of iodine-123 compared with iodine-131 scanning for thyroid remnants in patients with differentiated thyroid cancer. Clin Nucl Med. 2001;26:6–9.
40. Ali N, Sebastian C, Foley R, et al. The management of differentiated thyroid cancer using ^{123}I for imaging to assess the need for ^{131}I therapy. Nucl Med Commun. 2006;27:165–9.
41. Sarkar SD, Kalapparambath TP, Palestro CJ. Comparison of ^{123}I and ^{131}I for whole-body imaging in thyroid cancer. J Nucl Med. 2002;43:632–4.
42. Bautovich GJ, Towson JE, Eberl S, Turtle J, Chua E, Rawdry R, MacKinnon I, McHarg D. Comparison of Iodine-123 and Iodine-131 as a scanning agent for the detection of metastatic thyroid cancer. J Nucl Med. 1997;38:150P–1 (abstract).
43. Shankar LK, Yamamoto AJ, Alavi A, Mandel SJ. Comparison of ^{123}I scintigraphy at 5 and 24 hours in patients with differentiated thyroid cancer. J Nucl Med. 2002;43:72–6.
44. De Geus-Oei LF, Pauwels EKJ, Stokkel MPM. A comparison between low and high dose ^{123}I WBS in the follow-up of thyroid cancer. Eur J Nucl Med. 2000;27:931.
45. Klein HA, DiSibio KJ, et al. ^{123}I whole body scanning: case report and discussion. Clin Nucl Med. 2005;30:312–6.
46. Urhan M, Dadparvar S, Mavi A, et al. Iodine-123 as a diagnostic imaging agent in differentiated thyroid carcinoma: a comparison with iodine-131 post-therapy scanning and serum thyroglobulin measurement. Eur J Nucl Med Mol Imaging. 2007;34:1012–7.
47. Thomas DL, Mendas Y, Bushnell D. A comparison between diagnostic ^{123}I and post-therapy ^{131}I scans in the detection of remnant and locoregional thyroid disease. Clin Nucl Med. 2009;34:745–8.
48. Kalinyak JE. ^{123}I as a diagnostic tracer in the management of thyroid cancer. Editorial. Nucl Med Commun. 2002;23:509–11.
49. McDougall IR, Iagaru A. Thyroid stunning: fact or fiction? Semin Nucl Med. 2011;41:105–12.
50. Berbano R, Naddaf S, Echemendia E, et al. Use of Iodine-123 as a diagnostic tracer for neck and whole body scanning in patients with well-differentiated thyroid cancer. Endocr Pract. 1998;4:11–6.
51. Anderson GS, Fish S, Nakhoda K, Zhuang H, Alavi A, Mandel S. Comparison of ^{123}I and ^{131}I for whole-body imaging after stimulation by recombinant human thyrotropin: a preliminary report. Clin Nucl Med. 2003;28:93–6.
52. Alzahrani AS, Alshaikh O, Tuli M, et al. Diagnostic value of recombinant human thyrotropin-stimulated ^{123}I whole-body scintigraphy in the follow-up of patients with differentiated thyroid cancer. Clin Nucl Med. 2012;37:229–34.
53. Kim HY, Gelfand MJ, Sharp SE. SPECT/CT imaging in children with papillary thyroid carcinoma. Pediatr Radiol. 2011;41:1008–12.
54. Berg G, Lindstedt G, Suurkula M, Jansson S. Radioiodine ablation and therapy in differentiated thyroid cancer under stimulation with recombinant human thyroid-stimulating hormone. J Endocrinol Invest. 2002;25:44–52.
55. Robbins RJ, Larson SM, Sinha N, et al. A retrospective review of the effectiveness of recombinant human TSH as a preparation for radioiodine thyroid remnant ablation. J Nucl Med. 2002;43:1482–8.
56. Jarzab B, Handkiewicz-Junak D, Roskosz J, et al. Recombinant human TSH-aided radioiodine treatment of advanced differentiated thyroid carcinoma: a single-centre study of 54 patients. Eur J Nucl Med Mol Imaging. 2003;30:1077–86.
57. Duntas LH, Cooper DS. Review on the occasion of a decade of recombinant human TSH: prospects and novel uses. Thyroid. 2008;18:509–16.
58. Middendorp M, Grünwald F. Update on recent developments in the therapy of differentiated thyroid cancer. Semin Nucl Med. 2010;40:145–52.
59. Schlumberger M, Catargi B, Borget I, et al. Strategies of radioiodine ablation in patients with low-risk thyroid cancer. N Eng J Med. 2012;366:1663–73.
60. Mallick U, Harmer C, Yap B, et al. Ablation with low-dose radioiodine and thyrotropin alfa in thyroid cancer. New Eng J Med. 2012;366:1674–85.
61. Luster M, Sherman SI, Skarulis MC, Reynolds JR, Lassman M, Hanscheid H, Reiners C. Comparison of radioiodine biokinetics following the administration of recombinant human thyroid stimulating hormone and after thyroid hormone withdrawal in thyroid carcinoma. Eur J Nucl Med Mol Imaging. 2003;30:1371–7.
62. Medvedec M. Thyroid stunning *in vivo* and *in vitro*. Nucl Med Commun. 2005;28:731–5.
63. Stabin MG, Stubbs JB, Toohey RE. Radiation dose estimates for radiopharmaceuticals. NUREG/CR-6345 Radiation Internal Dose Information Center. Oak Ridge: Oak Ridge Institute for Science and Education; 1996. 37831–0117, April.
64. Rawson RW, Rall JE, Peacock W. Limitations and indications in the treatment of cancer of the thyroid with radioactive iodine. J Clin Endocrinol Metab. 1951;11:1128–31.
65. Pluijmen MJHM, Eustatia-Rutten C, Goslings BM, et al. Effects of low-iodide diet on postsurgical radioiodide ablation therapy in patients with differentiated thyroid carcinoma. Clin Endocrinol. 2003;58:428–35.
66. Silberstein EB, Alavi A, Balon HR, Balon HR, et al. The SNM practice guideline for therapy of thyroid disease with ^{131}I 3.0. J Nucl Med. 2012;53:1–19.

Stunning Is Not a Problem

17

Iain Ross McDougall

Introduction

To stun has been defined in several ways. The Webster dictionary provides synonyms of "to make senseless," "to daze or stupefy," or "to shock deeply." The adjective form also means excellent or attractive. None of these accurately represent what is meant by "stunning" in relation to treatment of thyroid cancer. In this context, stunning means that a diagnostic prescribed activity of radioiodine (^{131}I) can do sufficient damage to the thyroid that the follicular cells are incapable of trapping therapeutic prescribed activities of ^{131}I [1, 2]. It is true that some of us were "stunned" when the concept was first presented. The early reports implied that there would be no uptake of the therapeutic ^{131}I. Thus, when a pretreatment diagnostic scan was compared to a post-therapy scan, the latter would show the absence of uptake at one or more sites previously seen on the pretreatment diagnostic scan. Subsequently, the term was expanded to cover the possibility that the percentage of uptake of the therapeutic prescribed activity would be less than that of the prior diagnostic scintiscan, i.e., a quantitatively different finding. Lastly, the term "stunning" was expanded to include a worse outcome after treatment than when there was no diagnostic activity administered [3–6]. Whether or not stunning actually occurs has divided opinions into two perspectives, generating considerable debate [7–17]. This section presents data arguing against the concept of stunning. However, it might be considered superfluous since many clinicians are treating patients with ^{131}I without a prior diagnostic scan (although this is not the author's recommendation), and those who obtain a diagnostic scan are more frequently employing ^{123}I that theoretically should not cause stunning. We always use this radionuclide for diagnostic whole-body scanning. The author also exhorts the reader to study carefully the details of published reports with attention to the quantity of ^{131}I administered for the diagnostic scan, the percentage of uptake in thyroid tissue identified on scan (this is seldom available), and the delay between the administration of the diagnostic and therapeutic radioiodine (this also is often omitted in articles). Our group treats patients with a specified quantity of ^{131}I that is determined from the diagnostic images, pathology, and Tg value and that specified quantity of ^{131}I is ordered and administered on the same day as the diagnostic scan information is obtained. In several countries, there can be a delay of weeks or months between testing and treatment, and this alters the radiobiological effects of the former greatly. In a recent publication from Japan where patients treated with ^{131}I for thyroid cancer have to be admitted to hospital and where there is a shortage of appropriate rooms, about one half of patients are not treated within 180 days of thyroidectomy [18].

One additional comment is necessary. ^{131}I can ablate thyroid tissue, which has been known for more than 60 years. It is the basis of radioiodine treatment of hyperthyroidism and functioning thyroid cancer. This treatment is very successful provided thyroid tissues absorb sufficient radiation. Less absorbed radiation might fail to cure the patient, yet reduce the function and/or volume of thyroid tissue. This leads to the semantic debate whether the latter should be considered treatment or stunning. I review the data arguing against stunning and how it can be avoided recognizing that at high extremes of absorbed radiation doses there could be a therapeutic effect that might be judged to be stunning.

The first argument opposing stunning is self-evident. Diagnostic whole-body scanning with ^{131}I has been employed for five decades, and yet the treatment of thyroid cancer with ^{131}I has been remarkably successful [19]. The second argument is that it has been an accepted practice to obtain diagnostic and

I.R. McDougall, MD, PhD, FRCP (✉)
Department of Radiology, Nuclear Medicine, Stanford University Hospital and Clinics, 300 Pasteur Drive, Stanford, CA 94305, USA
e-mail: RossMcDougall@Stanford.edu

L. Wartofsky, D. Van Nostrand (eds.), *Thyroid Cancer*, DOI 10.1007/978-1-4939-3314-3_17

post-therapy scans for more than 30 years. There are a number of publications that demonstrate post-therapy scans show more lesions than the corresponding diagnostic images—not less lesions. Nemec et al. were probably the first to report on this in 1979 [20]. It is true that these investigators used a small diagnostic prescribed activity of 18.5 MBq (0.5 mCi) of ^{131}I; however, the post-therapy scan made after 3.7 GBq (100 mCi) showed an additional 25 % of lesions. Waxman et al. compared therapeutic scans with diagnostic images obtained with 370 MBq (10 mCi) ^{131}I [21]. When 1.1 GBq (30 mCi) ^{131}I was administered for treatment, 5/9 patients showed more lesions, and when 3.7 GBq (100 mCi) ^{131}I was the therapy prescribed activity, 5/10 patients showed more abnormalities on the post-therapy scintiscans. A third report, published as an abstract, also found 40 % more lesions were identified on the post-therapy scan [22]. The post-therapy scan can show the site of thyroglobulin production when the diagnostic scan is faintly positive and in some cases negative [23–25]. None of these reports provide evidence of reduced or absent uptake of therapeutic ^{131}I as a result of the diagnostic prescribed activity of ^{131}I.

Many authors writing on the topic of stunning cite the 1951 publication by Rawson et al. as the first to recognize this phenomenon [26]. Rawson et al. pointed out that ^{131}I can reduce the efficacy of subsequent therapeutic ^{131}I. However, they are reporting on this finding after a prescription of 925 MBq (25 mCi) of ^{131}I that was administered for treatment. There is no discussion of diagnostic or post-therapy rectilinear or scintiscan, and the response to treatment was judged by the percentage of radioactive iodine excreted in the urine. This does not fit the essence of stunning defined earlier. If stunning is a true finding, then it is more likely to occur after absorption of a large dose of radiation, and the factors that lead to that are the administration of a significant quantity of ^{131}I and a delay between conducting the diagnostic procedure and administering treatment.

In those publications that directly compare the pre- and post-therapy scans, several show little or no effect of the diagnostic prescribed activity. These reports cover a range of diagnostic prescribed activities of ^{131}I.

Park and colleagues were, as far as I can determine, the first to use the term *stunning* [1]. This was based on their review of post-therapy scans in patients who had preliminary diagnostic scans with 111 MBq (3 mCi), 185 MBq (5 mCi), or 370 MBq (10 mCi) ^{131}I. The numbers of patients were small, but there was a linear relationship of stunning and the quantity of ^{131}I administered. It is of considerable interest that the same investigators in a later publication found there was no statistical difference in successful ablation after the first or second application of therapy whether or not the patients had a diagnostic scan using ^{123}I or ^{131}I [1, 2]. In particular these investigators found no evidence of stunning when the diagnostic prescribed activity of ^{131}I was 111 MBq (3 mCi) or less.

A total of 122 patients were treated by Cholewinski et al. [27]. The investigators prescribed a diagnostic activity of 185 MBq (5 mCi) and scanned after a delay of 72 h. The treatment-prescribed activities covered a range from 1.1 to 7.4 GBq (30–200 mCi). However, 85 % of the patients received 5.5 GBq (150 mCi), and the treatment was administered on the same day as the diagnostic scan. There were no areas of absent uptake on the posttreatment scintiscans that were also obtained after 72 h. The authors then evaluated the outcome of the ^{131}I therapy by follow-up scan. In this analysis they separated the patients into two groups, the first where the operation had been a total thyroidectomy and the second where a lobectomy was conducted. In the first group consisting of 92 patients, 84 % were successfully ablated. The authors conclude "diagnostic whole-body scanning can be performed effectively with a 185 MBq (5 mCi) of ^{131}I 72 h before radioiodine ablation without concern for thyroid stunning."

Investigators from the Mayo Clinic compared diagnostic and post-therapy scans in a study designed to determine whether or not the latter provided additional information [28]. The data also allowed the question of stunning to be assessed. Diagnostic prescribed activities of ^{131}I ranged from 37 to 111 MBq (1–3 mCi) with a mean of 96 MBq (2.6 mCi), and imaging was conducted after 48 h. The authors did not note when the therapy was administered, but posttreatment scans were obtained after 3–5 days. They found reduced uptake on 4 % (5 of 117) of the post-therapy scans. In four of these five cases, they identified an alternative reason to stunning to explain the reduced uptake. With regard to these five patients, they comment "a stunning effect might have been the cause although it appears unlikely." Of their patients' scans, 96 % definitely showed no evidence of stunning.

One publication that is used by some to strengthen the argument for stunning I find supports the opposite. In the report by Bajen et al., the post-therapy scan showed less uptake in 78 (21 %) of 373 patients [29]. A prescribed activity of 185 MBq (5 mCi) was administered for the diagnostic scan, and patients were treated 7–8 weeks later. The average therapeutic prescribed activity of ^{131}I was 4 GBq (108 mCi). Follow-up scans were conducted in 76 of these 78 patients and were negative in 68 (89 %). Thyroglobulin (Tg) was <3 ng/ml in 61 of the 68 patients. Of the remaining eight patients (76–68), seven had improvement on the follow-up scan and had low values of Tg. Thus, although it appears that stunning occurred in 21 % of the patients, 89 % of the so-called stunned group had no functioning thyroid on follow-up, and in 88 % of the remainder, there was evidence of benefit from ^{131}I therapy. These investigators concluded "our data suggests that a stunning effect does not exist for prescribed activity of 185 MBq (5 mCi) ^{131}I."

For several decades physicians at the Memorial Sloan Kettering Cancer Center have employed dosimetric measurements prior to treatment with ^{131}I. The aim is to ensure the bone marrow does not receive 2 Gy (200 rad) or more radiation-absorbed dose. The measurements require scans and blood measurements over 4 or 5 days, which can only be achieved with ^{131}I since the half-life of ^{123}I is too short. They used 1–5 mCi (37–185 MBq) of ^{131}I for diagnostic measurements. The researchers compared the uptake of the therapeutic prescribed activity to the diagnostic one and concluded "we did not observe a strong correlation between administered activity and the magnitude of stunning" [30].

This author has compared diagnostic and post-therapy scans in 305 patients. The diagnostic scans were usually obtained 66–72 h after 74 MBq (2 mCi) of ^{131}I (the patients received the test prescribed activity on a Friday and were scanned on the following Monday). Treatment was administered as soon as possible after the information from the diagnostic scan was reviewed. Forty percent were treated on the same day and a further 34 % by 24 h. Post-therapy scans were obtained after an average of 8 days. Reduced uptake was identified on ten (3.3 %) of these scans. Follow-up scan and Tg measurements were negative in eight of these ten patients. Earlier results from this investigation have been published [31].

Several years ago our group stopped using ^{131}I for diagnostic scanning in favor of ^{123}I. The change was not because of concern of stunning but the better quality of ^{123}I images and reduced total radiation to the patient. It was a surprise when we found post-therapy scans that showed reduced uptake in 4 (13 %) of 30 patients who were treated with ^{131}I shortly after the diagnostic scan [32]. It is not probable, and indeed it is not possible that the prescribed activity of 74 MBq (2 mCi) ^{123}I that was employed at that time could deliver sufficient radiation to cause stunning over 24 h. We have demonstrated that post-therapy scans can vary with less lesions being identified with the passage of time from administration of the diagnostic activity. Therapeutic ^{131}I can be released from various sites of uptake at different rates, so all lesions seen on an early image might not be seen after many days. This has been demonstrated in a publication by the author [33]. Lee et al. compared post-therapy scans conducted 3 and 10 days after therapy [34]. The lesion to background ratio fell from 10.8 + 7.6 to 5.4 + 5.2 ($p < 0.001$), and ratio in the thyroid remnant to background fell from 12.0 + 10.8 to 8.0 + 7.6 ($p < 0.02$). When a region shows absent or reduced uptake on delayed scan, this should not immediately be blamed on stunning. It has long been recognized that cancerous thyroid cells may trap and organify iodine less efficiently than normal thyroid and there may be more rapid turnover. This is a likely explanation for reports of stunning in some patients. Because of an increasing body of information that ^{123}I is a better radionuclide for whole-body scanning, our group and others now routinely use 148–185 MBq (4–5 mCi) of ^{123}I [3]. Van Nostrand et al. established the importance of the information obtained from the diagnostic scan on determining appropriate therapy [5].

Returning to the discussion of diagnostic whole-body scan and stunning, the articles discussed above demonstrate no evidence of stunning, and several also demonstrate no loss of therapeutic efficacy. One criticism of most of these publications is the lack of quantitative comparisons. In defense of this missing information, the question remains of the reliability of uptake measurement of large therapeutic prescribed activities and the relevance of a difference between a 24–72 h diagnostic result and a 7–8 day post-therapy result.

Because there has been a movement away from obtaining a diagnostic scan for fear of stunning, some physicians proceed directly to therapy [35]. The goal of this presentation is not only to argue against stunning but also to promote the value of technically high-quality diagnostic scan that aids the physician to select the most appropriate therapeutic prescribed activity of ^{131}I [5]. Morris et al. were able to compare the outcome in two well-matched groups of patients. One group had a diagnostic scan using prescribed activities of 111–185 MBq (3–5 mCi) ^{131}I and the other did not [36]. There was no difference in outcome with 65 % of the former group being ablated versus 67 % of the latter. Treatment was administered 2–5 days after the diagnostic scan.

Rosario et al. compared outcome after ^{131}I treatment in 145 patients who had a preliminary diagnostic scan using 185 MBq (5 mCi) ^{131}I [37]. Seventy-six patients were treated without a diagnostic scan. There was no difference in the rates of ablation whether the patients were treated for residual thyroid tissue or for pulmonary metastases. A similar investigation compared the therapeutic outcome in 20 patients who had a diagnostic scan with 185 MBq (5 mCi) ^{131}I versus 20 matched patients who had no scan. Follow-up whole-body scan, ultrasound, and Tg measurements were used to determine therapeutic success. There was no difference ($p = 0.6$) [38].

A retrospective multivariate analysis of factors that influence the success of ^{131}I ablation in 389 patients found the most important factor was the size of the therapeutic prescribed activities [39]. They concluded with the statement "higher diagnostic doses were not associated with higher rates of ablation failure."

In Vitro Data

Postgard et al. conducted an experiment using thyroid cells in culture in a chamber [40]. They incubated the cells with ^{131}I for 48 h and then 3 days later studied the ability of the cells to transport iodine. 3 Gy (300 rad) reduced transport by 50 % and 30 Gy (3,000 rad) by approximately 90 %. In a later study they demonstrated that provided there was no delay between testing and treatment, trapping actually increased over 72 h, thus supporting the benefit of treating soon after a diagnostic scan employing ^{131}I. Researchers from the same center also studied the effects of ^{131}I, ^{123}I, ^{99m}Tc, and ^{211}At [41]. Thyroid cells in culture were exposed to radiation for 48 h. They found that ^{131}I caused no reduction in mRNA NIS expression 24 h after radiation, but by 5 days it had fallen to 80 %. Paradoxically, ^{123}I produced a 55 % drop in NIS mRNA expression at 24 h, but this returned to normal by 5 days. The paradox is explained by the fact they used the same absorbed dose of radiation and the absorbed dose per unit of activity is about 100 times greater for ^{131}I than ^{123}I. Thus, the probability of stunning with 148–185 MBq (4–5 mCi) ^{123}I would be about 1/100th that of 148–185 MBq (4–5 mCi) of ^{131}I.

Another Possible Example of Stunning

In patients with negative radioiodine scans but measurable Tgs, there is a body of data supporting the use of ^{18}F fluorodeoxyglucose (^{18}F FDG) positron emission tomography/ computer tomography (PET/CT) scans to identify the site(s) of Tg production. A meta-analysis provides data on sensitivity and specificity and a comprehensive list of references, and this subject has been reviewed elsewhere in this book (see Chaps. 43, 47, and 76) [42]. In several non-thyroidal cancers, ^{18}F FDG PET/CT scans can be falsely negative after external radiation, i.e., a form of stunning. This raised concern that ^{131}I might cause stunning on ^{18}F FDG PET/CT scans. Hung et al. compared six patients who had PET/CT scans within 4 months of ^{131}I therapy to ten patients who had not been treated. The standardized uptake values (SUVs) were lower in the treated patients. However, the two groups were not equivalent with regard to age and TSH values. This area needs clarification.

Dosimetric evidence against stunning can be derived from knowledge of how much radiation is required to ablate thyroid tissue. Maxon et al. calculated that 300 Gy (30,000 rad) has to be delivered for reliable success [43, 44]. Some authorities suggest a similar dose could be required for 100 % success in treating hyperthyroidism caused by hyperfunctioning nodules [45]. Therefore, it seems reasonable that the prescribed activity required to cause stunning would be significant. Let us consider two reasonable examples. First, consider a patient with remnant tissue of 1 g who has an uptake of 1 % and is scanned 72 h after a prescribed activity of 74 MBq (2 mCi) of ^{131}I administered for diagnostic scanning and treatment performed shortly after the diagnostic scan. Assuming almost instantaneous uptake of the tracer, the absorbed radiation dose to the thyroid from the diagnostic prescribed activity would be approximately 6 Gy (600 rad). Second, a patient with a 1 g remnant tissue and uptake of 4 % receives a diagnostic prescribed activity of 370 MBq (10 mCi) ^{131}I and treatment delayed for 1 week. The thyroid could receive 160 Gy (16,000 rad) assuming an effective half-life of 100 h. The former's absorbed dose would not be enough to cause ablation but the latter could. These numbers make the obvious point that larger diagnostic amounts of prescribed activity and **longer** delays between diagnosis and therapy result in thyroid tissue receiving more radiation, in fact enough to cause ablation or certainly a significant reduction in function, and could be interpreted as stunning when a post-therapy scan made some time later shows reduced uptake. Therefore, when ^{131}I is used for a diagnostic whole-body scan, it is prudent to use 37–111 MBq (1–3 mCi) and be prepared to treat as soon as possible after the test. Although several studies indicate that prescribed activities of 185 MBq (5 mCi) of ^{131}I do not cause stunning, it would be more important that treatment should certainly not be delayed.

In summary, there are several studies involving large numbers of patients that do not support the concept of stunning whether this means absent uptake on the post-therapy scan or reduced efficacy of ^{131}I treatment. Is it possible to state stunning never occurs? No. When a large diagnostic prescribed activity of ^{131}I is administered and there is a significant delay before therapy is given, stunning can be anticipated. These facts argue in favor of diagnostic imaging with ^{123}I and treating as soon as possible with an administered prescribed activity determined by the clinical risk and scan and Tg findings.

References

1. Park H, Perkins OW, Edmondson JW, Schnute RB, Manatunga A. Influence of diagnostic radioiodines on the uptake of ablative dose of iodine-131. Thyroid. 1994;4:49–54.
2. Park H, Park YH, Zhou XH. Detection of thyroid remnant/ metastasis without stunning: an ongoing dilemma. Thyroid. 1997; 7:277–80.
3. Mandel SJ, Shankar LK, Benard F, Yamamoto A, Alavi A. Superiority of iodine-123 compared with iodine-131 scanning for thyroid remnants in patients with differentiated thyroid cancer. Clin Nucl Med. 2001;26:6–9.
4. Gerard SK. Whole-body thyroid tumor ^{123}I scintigraphy. J Nucl Med. 2003;44:852.
5. Van Nostrand D, et al. The utility of radioiodine scans prior to iodine 131 ablation in patients with well-differentiated thyroid cancer. Thyroid. 2009;19:849–55.
6. Urhan M, et al. Iodine-123 as a diagnostic imaging agent in differentiated thyroid carcinoma: a comparison with iodine-131 post-treatment scanning and serum thyroglobulin measurement. Eur J Nucl Med Mol Imaging. 2007;34:1012–7.
7. Allman KC. Thyroid stunning revisited. J Nucl Med. 2003;44:1194.
8. Coakley A. Thyroid stunning. Eur J Nucl Med. 1998;25:203–4.
9. Brenner W. Is thyroid stunning a real phenomenon or just fiction? J Nucl Med. 2002;43:835–6.
10. Hurley JR. Management of thyroid cancer: radioiodine ablation, "stunning," and treatment of thyroglobulin-positive, ^{131}I scan-negative patients. Endocr Pract. 2000;6:401–6.

11. Medvedec M. Thyroid stunning. J Nucl Med. 2001;42:1129–31.
12. Diehl M, Grunwald F. Stunning after tracer dosimetry. J Nucl Med. 2001;42:1129.
13. Kalinyak JE, McDougall IR. Whole-body scanning with radionuclides of iodine and the controversy of thyroid stunning. Nucl Med Commun. 2004;25:883–9.
14. McDougall IR, Iagaru A. Thyroid stunning: fact or fiction? Semin Nucl Med. 2011;41:105–12.
15. Sisson JC, et al. The so-called stunning of thyroid tissue. J Nucl Med. 2006;47:1406–12.
16. Filesi M, et al. Thyroid stunning in clinical practice: is it a real problem? Minerva Endocrinol. 2009;34:29–36.
17. Hilditch TE, et al. Re: the so-called stunning of thyroid tissue. J Nucl Med. 2007;48:675–6.
18. Higashi T, Nishii R, Yamada S, Nakamoto Y, Ishizu K, Kawase S, Togashi K, Itasaka S, Hiraoka M, Misaki T, Konishi J. Delayed initial radioactive iodine therapy resulted in poor survival in patients with metastatic differentiated thyroid carcinoma: a retrospective statistical analysis of 198 cases. J Nucl Med. 2011;52:683–9.
19. Mazzaferri E, Jhiang SM. Long-term impact of initial surgical and medical therapy on papillary and follicular thyroid cancer. Am J Med. 1994;97:418–28.
20. Nemec J, Röhling S, Zamrazil V, Pohunková D. Comparison of the distribution of diagnostic and thyroablative I-131 in the evaluation of differentiated thyroid cancers. J Nucl Med. 1979;20:92–7.
21. Waxman A, Ramana L, Chapman N, et al. The significance of I-131 scan dose in patients with thyroid cancer: determination of ablation: concise communication. J Nucl Med. 1981;22:61–865.
22. Spies W, Wojtowicz CH, Spies SH, Shah AY, Zimmer AM. Value of post-therapy whole-body I-131 imaging in the evaluation of patients with thyroid carcinoma having undergone high-dose I-131 therapy. Clin Nucl Med. 1989;14:793–800.
23. Pacini F, Lippi L, Formica M, et al. Therapeutic doses of iodine-131 reveal undiagnosed metastases in thyroid cancer patients with detectable serum-thyroglobulin levels. J Nucl Med. 1987;28:1888–91.
24. Schlumberger M, Mancusi F, Baudin E, Pacini F. ^{131}I therapy for elevated thyroglobulin levels. Thyroid. 1997;7:273–6.
25. Pineda J, Lee T, Ain K, Reynolds JC, Robbins J. Iodine-131 therapy for thyroid cancer patients with elevated thyroglobulin and negative diagnostic scan. J Clin Endocrinol Metab. 1995;80:1488–92.
26. Rawson R, Rall JE, Peacock W. Limitations and indications in the treatment of thyroid cancer with radioactive iodine. J Clin Endocrinol Metab. 1951;11:1128–42.
27. Cholewinski SP, Yoo KS, Klieger PS, O'Mara RE. Absence of thyroid stunning after diagnostic whole-body scanning with 185 MBq ^{131}I. J Nucl Med. 2000;41:1198–202.
28. Fatourechi V, Hay ID, Mullan BP, Wiseman GA, Eghbali-Fatourechi GZ, Thorson LM, Gorman CA. Are posttherapy radioiodine scans informative and do they influence subsequent therapy of patients with differentiated thyroid cancer? Thyroid. 2000; 10:573–7.
29. Bajen M, Mane S, Munoz A, Garcia JR. Effect of a diagnostic dose of 185 MBq ^{131}I on postsurgical thyroid remnants. J Nucl Med. 2000;41:2038–42.
30. Yeung H, Humm JL, Larson SM. Thyroid stunning. J Nucl Med. 2001;42:1130–1 (letter).
31. McDougall IR. 74 MBq radioiodine ^{131}I does not prevent uptake of therapeutic doses of 131I (i.e. it does not cause stunning) in differentiated thyroid cancer. Nucl Med Commun. 1997;18:505–12.
32. Cohen J, Kalinyak JE, McDougall IR. Clinical Implications of the differences between diagnostic 123I and post-therapy ^{131}I scans. Nucl Med Commun. 2004;25:129–34.
33. McDougall IR. Thyroid disease in clinical practice. New York: Oxford UP; 1992. p. 80.
34. Lee JW, et al. The comparison of ^{131}I whole-body scans on the third and tenth day after ^{131}I therapy in patients with well-differentiated thyroid cancer: preliminary report. Ann Nucl Med. 2011;25: 439–46.
35. Hu YH, et al. Influence of ^{131}I diagnostic dose on subsequent ablation in patients with differentiated thyroid carcinoma: discrepancy between the presence of visually apparent stunning and the impairment of successful ablation. Nucl Med Commun. 2004;25:793–7.
36. Morris LF, Waxman AD, Braunstein GD. The nonimpact of thyroid stunning: remnant ablation rates in ^{131}I-scanned and nonscanned individuals. J Clin Endocrinol Metab. 2001;86:3507–11.
37. Rosario PW, et al. 5 mCi pretreatment scanning does not cause stunning when the ablative dose is administered within 72 hours. Arq Bras Endocrinol Metabol. 2005;49:420–4.
38. Amin A, Amin M, Badwey A. Stunning phenomenon after a radioactive iodine- ^{131}I diagnostic whole-body scan: is it really a point of clinical consideration? Nucl Med Commun. 2013;34:771–6.
39. Karam M, Gianoukas A, Feustel PJ, Postal ES, Cooper JA. Influence of diagnostic and therapeutic doses on thyroid remnant ablation rates. Nucl Med Commun. 2003;24:489–95.
40. Postgard P, et al. Stunning of iodide transport by ^{131}I irradiation in cultured thyroid epithelial cells. J Nucl Med. 2002;43:828–34.
41. Lundh C, et al. Radiation-induced thyroid stunning: differential effects of ^{123}I, ^{131}I, ^{99m}Tc, and ^{211}At on iodide transport and NIS mRNA expression in cultured thyroid cells. J Nucl Med. 2009;50:1161–7.
42. Dong MJ, et al. Value of ^{18}F-FDG-PET/PET-CT in differentiated thyroid carcinoma with radioiodine-negative whole-body scan: a meta-analysis. Nucl Med Commun. 2009;30:639–50.
43. Maxon HR, Thomas SR, Hertzberg VS, Kereiakes JG, Chen IW, Sperling MI, Saenger EL. Relation between effective radiation dose and outcome of radioiodine therapy for thyroid cancer. N Engl J Med. 1983;309:937–41.
44. Maxon HR. Quantitative radioiodine therapy in the treatment of differentiated thyroid cancer. Q J Nucl Med. 1999;43:313–23.
45. Gorman CA, Robertson JS. Radiation dose in the selection of ^{131}I or surgical treatment for toxic thyroid adenoma. Ann Intern Med. 1978;89:85–90.

Stunning: Does It Exist? A Commentary

18

Douglas Van Nostrand

Do diagnostic prescribed activities (dosages) of ^{131}I cause stunning or not?

In the first part of this section, Drs. Park and Gerard present arguments supporting the presence of stunning secondary to the administration of diagnostic dosages of ^{131}I, and in the second section, Dr. McDougall presents arguments against the presence of stunning. In the end, many physicians may select the information that one believes makes the stronger arguments or best supports one's prior viewpoint. However, a third viewpoint exists to either a "yes" or "no" answer. It is a viewpoint that proposes that ". . . diagnostic prescribed activity (dosages) of ^{131}I results in a spectrum ranging from no stunning to significant stunning and even treatment."

I submit that the authors of the above two sections, as well as the authors of all of the references cited [1–4] and many more, are good physicians, observers, and researchers. Consequently, although one particular study may be flawed, it would be statistically unlikely that all the authors, their data, and their arguments on either the pro or con side of the argument are all wrong. Notably, all the authors appear to agree that the radiation-absorbed dose of ^{131}I to thyroid tissue and metastases as well as the documentation of stunning depends on many factors (see Table 18.1). Although the specific factors that may account for the discordant observations between the various articles cannot be identified, it is more likely that such uncontrolled factors as those listed again in Table 18.1 produced these discordant results, rather than that all the data on one or the other particular side of the argument were completed wrong. Accordingly, to answer the question, "Does stunning exist?" my response is: ". . . it is a spectrum ranging from no stunning to significant stunning and even treatment," and Drs. Parks, Gerard, and McDougall acknowledge this in their respective discussions.

Although it is not my intent to re-discuss here the arguments on either side of the controversy, in my opinion two interesting observations deserves emphasis. First, Hilditch et al. [5, 6] and Sisson et al. [7] have proposed that the radiation-absorbed dose from the ^{131}I therapy itself may in fact be causing the "stunning" – or as may be more appropriately referred to as the "treatment" – of the thyroid tissue resulting in reduced uptake on the post-^{131}I therapy scans rather than "stunning" from the diagnostic dosage of ^{131}I. This possibility certainly confounds the controversy. Second, Salvatori et al. [8] evaluated uptake on post-therapy scans performed early and late (i.e. 3 and 7 days after ^{131}I therapy, respectively) (see Chap. 11). The early scans demonstrated 7.5 % more information compared with the late scans and the late scans provided 12 % more information than the early scans. If one is only doing an early or late scan and one does not see the uptake on that scan that was originally observed on the pre-therapy scan, one might conclude that that is prima facie evidence of stunning. But stunning may not necessarily be occuring. In addition, if the pre-therapy scan was done at 1 or 2 days after dosing and if any radioiodine uptake on that scan was not seen on the 3 or 7 day post-therapy scan, this simply may be an issue of clearance and timing, possibly even the results of the treatment itself affecting the clearance—not stunning. Salvatori et al.'s article at a minimum raises the issue that stunning from diagnostic prescribed activities of ^{131}I and the relatively immediate effects of treatment from therapeutic prescribed activities of ^{131}I may be far more complex than we may think.

Nevertheless, some readers may still want to continue the debate by taking either one or the other extreme of the stunning issue. However, to do so provides no actions toward progress, and it will be more productive to redirect our

D. Van Nostrand, MD, FACP, FACNM (✉)
Nuclear Medicine Research, MedStar Research Institute and Washington Hospital Center, Georgetown University School of Medicine, Washington Hospital Center, 110 Irving Street, N.W., Suite GB 60F, Washington, DC 20010, USA
e-mail: douglasvannostrand@gmail.com

L. Wartofsky, D. Van Nostrand (eds.), *Thyroid Cancer*, DOI 10.1007/978-1-4939-3314-3_18

Table 18.1 Factors influencing the radiation-absorbed dose to thyroid tissue and/or the detection of stunning

Amount of diagnostic prescribed activity (dosage) of ^{131}I administered
Uptake of ^{131}I by the thyroid tissue or metastasis
Variability of residence time of ^{131}I in the thyroid tissue or thyroid metastasis
Volume of thyroid tissue or metastasis
Whether the tissue consists of normal thyroid cells or metastatic cells
Whether the metastatic cells are well-differentiated or more dedifferentiated
Interval of time from the diagnostic prescribed activity (dosage) to the time of ^{131}I treatment
Investigator compulsiveness in looking for "stunning"
Ability to differentiate whether or not decreased radioactivity in a foci on the post-therapy scan is due to the effects of initial treatment of the therapeutic dose of ^{131}I
Method to confirm or disprove stunning

Table 18.2 Alternative approaches to eliminate or minimize the effects of stunning

Use ^{123}I for scanning
If ^{131}I needs to be used because either ^{123}I is not available or ^{131}I must be used for dosimetry, then use the smallest amount of ^{131}I possible to achieve the desired objective
Administration of the ^{131}I therapeutic dose as soon as possible after the completion of the ^{131}I diagnostic scan in order to minimize any time for significant stunning to occur
Use $^{99m}TcO_4$ scanning
Use ^{99m}Tc sestamibi or tetrofosmin scanning
Use ^{201}thallium chloride scanning

energy – regardless of the frequency or severity of stunning or treatment – into alternatives to eliminate, or at least to minimize, the real or theoretical effects of stunning by diagnostic amounts of ^{131}I and/or to seek additional developments or research that would allow us to manage better any potential stunning. The alternatives and the ideas for further development or research are listed in Tables 18.2 and 18.3, respectively.

Finally, an additional option that some individuals may propose is not performing any pre-therapy diagnostic radioiodine scan at all. This is another controversial area, and the reader is referred to Chaps. 14, 15, and 19 for a more detailed discussion.

Table 18.3 Ideas for further development and research

Encourage commercial companies to increase the availability of ^{123}I at reasonable costs in areas that do not have access to ^{123}I
If stunning occurs, further evaluate the onset of stunning to help determine the time for administration of the therapeutic ^{131}I after a diagnostic dose of ^{131}I
Evaluate more extensively the use of $^{99m}TcO_4$ scanning
Evaluate the use of ^{99m}Tc sestamibi or tetrofosmin scanning
Encourage commercial companies to increase the radioactivity of ^{123}I available in a single dose at a reasonable cost for ^{123}I dosimetry
Evaluating the utility of ^{124}I and whether or not it results in stunning at acceptable diagnostic amounts of prescribed activity (dosages)

In summary, stunning is a controversial issue with many confounding factors at work. However, regardless of its presence or absence and, if present, regardless of its frequency and severity, many reasonable alternatives are available. In addition, these alternatives as well as the issue of stunning offer many opportunities for research that may have a potential immediate impact on clinical care of our patients with differentiated thyroid cancer. So, let's use our alternatives and let's get back to work.

References

1. Dam HQ, Kim SM, Lin HC, Intenzo CM. ^{131}I therapeutic efficacy is not influenced by stunning after diagnostic whole body scanning. Radiology. 2004;232:527–33.
2. Mf B, Mane S, Munoz A, Garcia JR. Effect of diagnostic dose of 185MBq ^{131}I on postsurgical thyroid remnants. J Nucl Med. 2000;41:2038–42.
3. Gerard SK. Stunning with ^{131}I diagnostic whole-body imaging of patients with thyroid cancer. Radiology. 2004;232:972–3.
4. Dam HQ. Stunning with ^{131}I diagnostic whole-body imaging of patients with thyroid cancer. Radiology. 2004;232:973–4.
5. Hilditch TE, Dempsey MF, Boslter AA, et al. Self-stunning in thyroid ablation: evidence from comparative studies of diagnostic ^{131}I and ^{123}I. Euro J Nucl Med and Molec Imaging. 2002;29:783–8..
6. Hilditch TE, Bolster AA, Dempsy MF, et al. Re: the so-called stunning of thyroid tissue. J Nucl Med. 2007;48:675–6.
7. Sisson JC, Avram AM, Lawson SA, Gauger PG, Doherty GM. The so-called stunning of thyroid tissue. J Nucl Med. 2006;47: 1406–12.8.
8. Salvatori M, Perotti G, Villani MF, Mazza R, Maussier ML, Indovina L, Sigismondi A, Dottorin ME, Giordano A. Determining the appropriate time of execution of an I-131 post-therapy whole. Nuclear medicine communications. 2013;34: 900–8.

To Perform or Not to Perform Radioiodine Scans Prior to ^{131}I Remnant Ablation? PRO

19

Douglas Van Nostrand

Introduction

A review of the recommendations for the use of radioiodine scan prior to ^{131}I remnant ablation of differentiated thyroid cancer by the American Thyroid Association (ATA) [1], European Consensus (EC) [2], National Cancer Center Network (NCCN) [3], British Thyroid Association (BTA) [4], and Society of Nuclear Medicine [5] is presented in Table 19.1, and the utility of radioiodine pre-remnant ablation scans remains controversial [1–15].

However, I believe that the controversy regarding whether or not a radioiodine scan should be performed prior to an ^{131}I remnant ablation revolves around five major arguments that are typically presented: (1) "no useful data are obtained from pre-remnant ablation radioiodine scans that will alter my management," (2) "everything I need to know is on the post-therapy scan," (3) "^{131}I may cause stunning," (4) "the benefits of pre-remnant ablation radioiodine scans do not warrant the cost, inconvenience, and radiation exposure," and (5) "until data are published demonstrating that the pre-^{131}I therapy scans alter patient outcomes, these scans should not be performed." These arguments will be individually discussed, and in addition, several rarely if ever discussed issues will be explored, issues that I believe may account for one of the more important reasons for the differences in opinions regarding the utility of pre-remnant ablation radioiodine scans.

D. Van Nostrand, MD, FACP, FACNM (✉)
Nuclear Medicine Research, MedStar Research Institute and Washington Hospital Center, Georgetown University School of Medicine, Washington Hospital Center, 110 Irving Street, N.W., Suite GB 60F, Washington, DC 20010, USA
e-mail: douglasvannostrand@gmail.com

No Useful Data Are Obtained From Pre-remnant Ablation Radioiodine Scans That Will Alter May Management

In the discussions regarding the utility of pre-ablation scans, a frequent comment is "*I don't find pre-remnant ablation radioiodine scans useful, because the information will not alter my management.*" Now, to determine whether or not you, the reader, would alter your management prior to your administration of ^{131}I for remnant ablation based on a pre-remnant ablation radioiodine scan, I suggest you perform the following exercise. For Cases 1 through 7 (see Figs. 19.1, 19.2, 19.3, 19.4, 19.5, 19.6, and 19.7), determine whether or not you would alter your management prior to ^{131}I remnant ablation.

If you answered that you would not alter your management based on any or all these scans, then our difference of our opinion is not regarding the utility of pre-ablation scans. The difference of our opinions is in regard to the *management of these patients* with these radioiodine pre-ablation scan findings. If you answered that you would alter your management to any or all of these images, then the next question becomes whether or not the findings for which you would alter your management occurred frequently enough to justify the cost, inconvenience, and radiation exposure of the pre-remnant ablation radioiodine scan.

These frequencies have been previously reported from our facility and are noted in Table 19.2 [6] as well as other reports such as Chen et al. [7]. It is also important to note that our population studied excluded patients who had (1) a known recent history of large iodine intake (e.g., radiographic contrast, kelp, amiodarone), (2) a spot urine iodine >300 mg/L, (3) thyrotropin (TSH) <25 mIU within 4 days prior to radioiodine administration in patients undergoing thyroid hormone withdrawal, (4) locoregional disease and/or distant metastases suspected or known prior to the radioiodine scan (e.g., physical exam, ultrasound, chest

L. Wartofsky, D. Van Nostrand (eds.), *Thyroid Cancer*, DOI 10.1007/978-1-4939-3314-3_19

Table 19.1 Recommendations proposed by various professional organizations

Organization	Recommendation number and/or section number	Guidelines	Recommendation grade and/or category
American Thyroid Association [1]	B35	"Post-operative diagnostic radioiodine whole-body scans may be useful when the extent of the thyroid remnant or residual disease cannot be accurately ascertained from the surgical report or neck ultrasonography, and when the results may alter the decision to treat, or the activity of RAI that is to be administered. Identification and localization of uptake foci may be enhanced by concomitant SPECT/CT. When performed, pretherapy diagnostic scans should utilize ^{123}I (1.5–3 mCi) or a low activity of ^{131}I (1–3 mCi), with the therapeutic activity optimally administered within 72 hours of the diagnostic activity"	Weak recommendation, low-quality evidence
European Consensus [2]	Page 792	"The value of a diagnostic scan before thyroid ablation has been questioned based on its low clinical utility, the possibility of a stunning effect on the subsequent therapeutic activity of ^{131}I, and the consideration that the post-therapy WBS performed 3–5 days after radioiodine administration is much more sensitive than the diagnostic WBS. Thus, this procedure may be avoided without loss of information. Centers may choose to perform pre-ablations in some circumstances such as uncertainty concerning the extent of thyroidectomy"	
National Compr-ehensive Cancer Network (NCCN) [3]	PAP-5	"Total body radioiodine imaging with adequate TSH stimulation"	2B = recommendation based on low level evidence and there is non-uniform NCCN consensus (but no major disagreement)
British Thyroid Association and Royal College of Physicians. Guidelines/ Statements the British Thyroid Association 2014 edition of the Thyroid Cancer Guidelines (Draft) [4]	9.2 page 5	"A pre-ablation scan is not indicated routinely if the patient has had optimal surgery. If there is any doubt over completeness of surgery or radiological evidence of a large remnant, further resection should be discussed before proceeding to RRA"	4 = expert opinion D = evidence level 3 or 4; or extrapolated evidence from studies rated as 2+
Society of Nuclear Medicine Guidelines [5]	Page 7	Routine pre-ablation planar scintigraphy can be useful in guiding ^{131}I therapy. (including a lengthy discussion of argument for and against)	

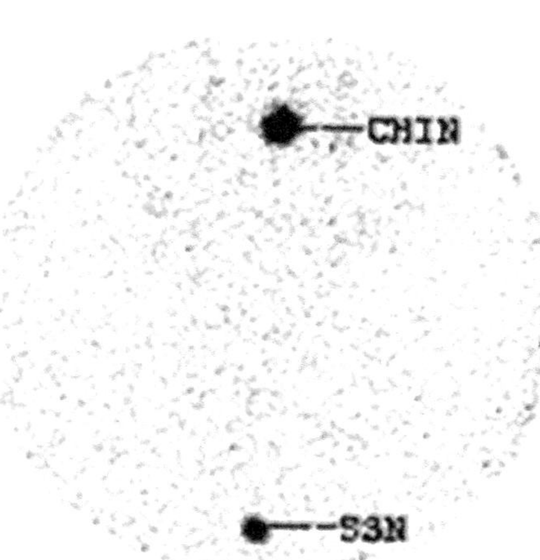

Fig. 19.1 This anterior pinhole collimator view of the thyroid bed and neck was performed 24 h after the administration of ^{123}I. No uptake is present. Would you continue with your planned ^{131}I ablation or would you alter your management such as evaluating further the camera technique, urine iodine level, TSH level, and/or eliminating radioiodine ablation (see Table 19.3)? (This figure was originally published in Kulkarni et al. [22]. Reproduced with permission by Wolter Kluwer)

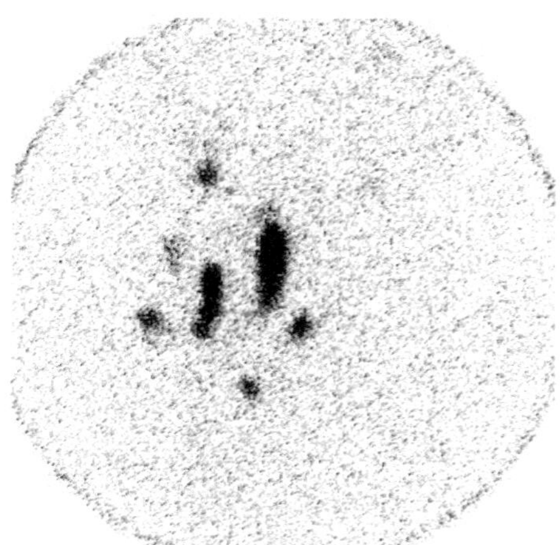

Fig. 19.2 This anterior pinhole collimator view of the thyroid bed/neck was performed 24 h after the administration of ^{123}I. Multiple foci are present in the thyroid bed and possibly outside the thyroid bed. Specifically, 8 foci were considered present. Would you continue with your planned empiric prescribed activity of ^{131}I for you remnant ablation or would you alter your management such as evaluating further with ultrasound, FNA, additional surgery, and/or increasing your prescribed activity of ^{131}I (see Table 19.3)? (Reproduced with permission from Mary Ann Liebert) [5]

x-ray, computer tomography [CT], positron emission computer tomography [PET], magnetic resonance imaging [MRI], etc.), (6) any history prior to the pre-remnant ablation scan that would likely result in altered physiologic radioiodine uptake in the breast such as recent cessation of breastfeeding, and/or (7) inadequate records to determine any of the above. All patients had negative ultrasounds of the neck.

I would submit that most readers would indeed have altered their management of their patient prior to ^{131}I remnant ablation for most, if not all, of the findings in Cases 1 through 7 and at least 1 through 6, and I would submit that the altered management would include one or more of those listed in Table 19.3. Depending on which or all images would alter one's management, one's management could be altered in as many as 29 % of patients [6].

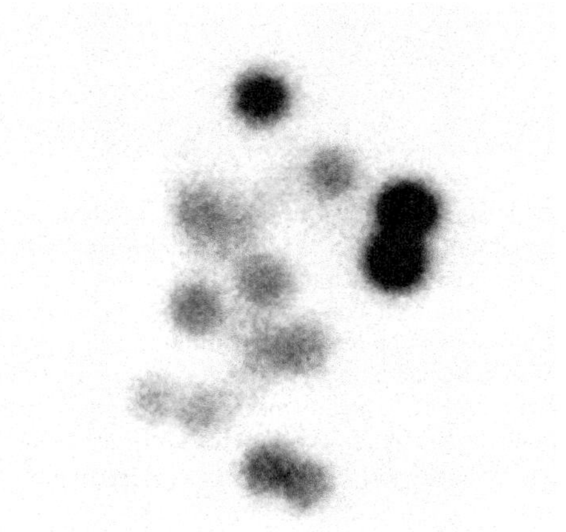

Fig. 19.3 This anterior pinhole collimator view of the thyroid bed and neck was performed 24 h after the administration of ^{123}I. Multiple foci are present in the thyroid bed and several were outside the thyroid bed. No radioactive markers are present in this image. Specifically, twelve foci were counted. Would you continue with your planned empiric prescribed activity of ^{131}I for remnant ablation or would you alter your management such as evaluating further with ultrasound, FNA, additional surgery, and/or increasing your prescribed activity of ^{131}I (see Table 19.3)? (Reproduced with permission from Mary Ann Liebert) [5]

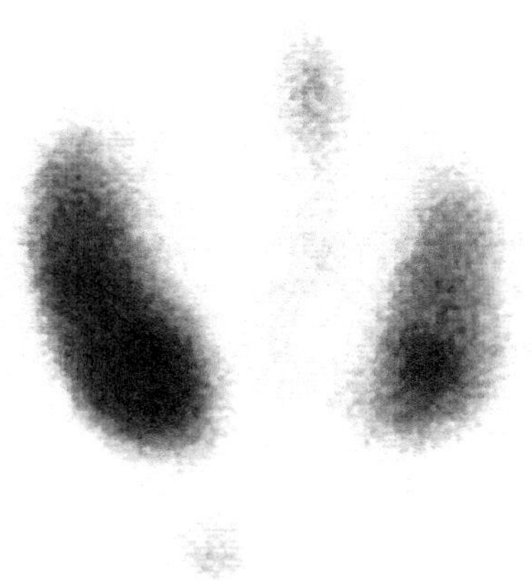

Fig. 19.5 This anterior pinhole collimator view of the thyroid bed and neck was performed 24 h after the administration of ^{123}I. Despite the report that the patient had a near-total thyroidectomy, significant residual tissue is suggested. Would you continue with your planned empiric prescribed activity of ^{131}I for remnant ablation or would you alter your management such as performing additional surgery and/or modifying your prescribed activity of ^{131}I (see Table 19.3)? (Reproduced with permission from Mary Ann Liebert) [5]

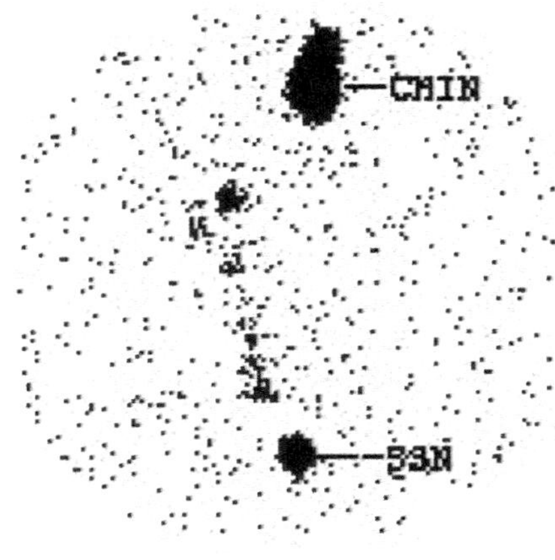

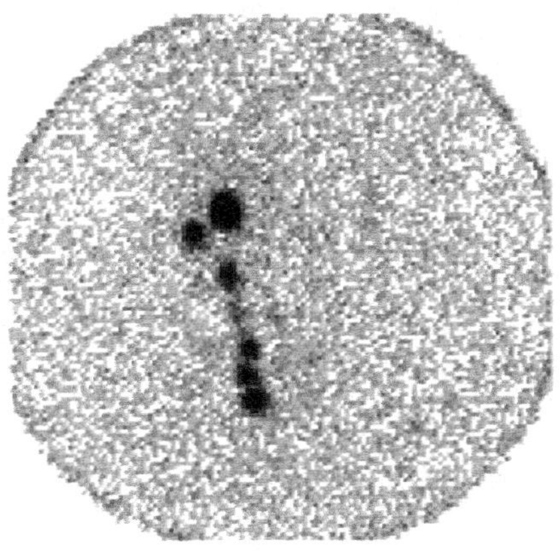

Fig. 19.4 These anterior pinhole collimator views of the thyroid bed and neck were performed 24 h after the oral administration of ^{123}I. The image on the *left* is the marker image with a marker on the chin and suprasternal notch (SSN). The image on the *right* was performed after removing the chin and SSN markers without repositioning the patient. Multiple foci are present outside the thyroid bed. Would you continue with your planned empiric prescribed activity of ^{131}I for remnant ablation or would you alter your management such as evaluating further with ultrasound, FNA, additional surgery, and/or increasing your prescribed activity of ^{131}I (see Table 19.3)? (Reproduced with permission from Mary Ann Liebert) [5]

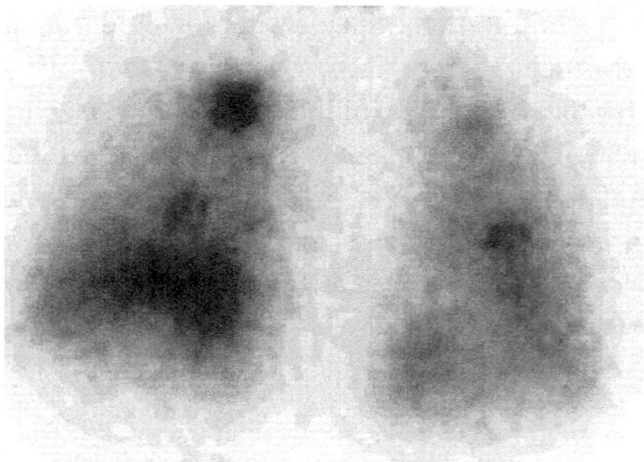

Fig. 19.6 This anterior parallel-hole collimator view of the chest was performed 24 h after the administration of ^{123}I. Diffuse micro and macronodular pattern of uptake is noted in the chest indicative of metastases to the lung, respectively. The chest radiograph was negative. Would you continue with your planned empiric prescribed activity of ^{131}I for remnant ablation or would you alter your management such as evaluating further with pulmonary function tests, additional imaging with CT without contrast for baseline study for future comparison, increasing your prescribed activity of ^{131}I, and/or performing dosimetry (see Table 19.3)? (Reproduced with permission from Mary Ann Liebert) [5]

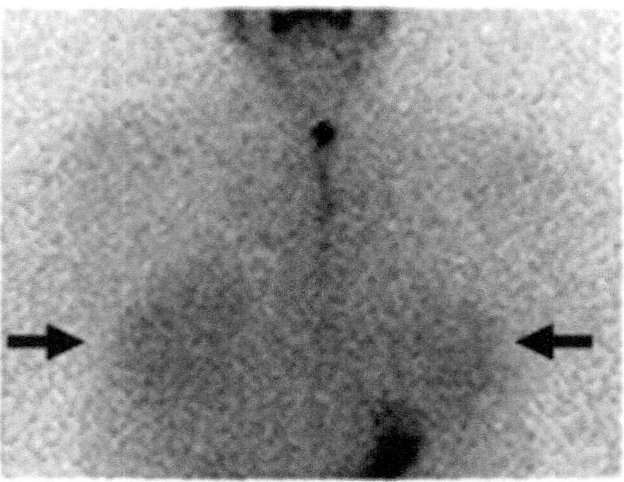

Fig. 19.7 This anterior parallel-hole view of the chest was performed 48 h after the administration of ^{131}I. Bilateral diffuse breast uptake was present (arrows). The patient was not lactating and had not been previous lactating. Would you continue with your planned empiric prescribed activity of ^{131}I for remnant ablation or would you alter your management such as evaluating the patient's history regarding galactorrhea, postponement of ^{131}I treatment, and/or treatment with carbergoline or bromocryptine (see Table 19.3)? (Reproduced with permission from Mary Ann Liebert) [5]

Table 19.2 Potential findings on radioiodine pre-remnant ablation scan

No uptake in the thyroid bed or neck	6 % (22)
Six or more foci in the thyroid bed or neck suggestive of regional metastases	12 % (44)
Foci located outside the thyroid bed strongly suggestive of regional metastases	14 % (48)
One or more foci uptake greater than or equal to the size of one lobe of a thyroid gland	1 % (4)
Uptake in the thyroid bed/neck >15 %	8 % (27)
Findings suggesting distant metastases	4 % (11)
Breast uptake	6 % (20)
Total patients with at least one of the above (some may have had more than one)	29 %

Of course, if none of these findings would have affected your management, then the statement "*I don't find pre-remnant ablation radioiodine scans useful, because the information will not alter my management*" appears circular and even tautological. For example, the statement that "*I don't find the internet useful because it does not alter what I do*" is not evidence that the Internet has *no value*. Rather the statement indicates that that particular individual making that statement chooses not to *use* the information from the Internet. If one is not going to alter one's management despite seeing no uptake on the scan, despite findings suggesting locoregional disease, and despite findings suggesting distant metastases, that is not evidence that the pre-ablation scans have no value but rather that that particular physician chooses not to *use* the information from the pre-ablation scan.

Table 19.3 Potential altered management based on findings in cases 1–7

Recheck camera technique (Case 1)
Recheck the patient's history for compliance with low iodine diet and/or thyroid hormone withdrawal (Case 2)
Recheck TSH level and urine iodine level (Case 1)
Postpone the radioiodine therapy (Case 1, 2, 3, 4, 6, and 7)
Perform additional imaging (e.g., ultrasound, MR) (Case 2, 3, 4, and 6)
Perform additional imaging of the chest (e.g., CT without contrast) (Case 6)
Perform additional FNA aspiration (Case 2, 3, and 4)
Perform additional surgery (Case 2, 3, 4, and 5)
Altered (higher or lower) empiric prescribed activity for ^{131}I therapy (Case 2, 3, 4, 5, and 6)
Determine dosimetrically prescribed activity for ^{131}I therapy (Case 2, 3, 4, and 6)
Perform pulmonary function tests (Case 6)
Obtain absolute neutrophil and platelet counts (Case 6)
Perform patient history/physical exam regarding breast disease and reconsideration of repeat ^{123}I image after an interval of time with or without intervention to reduce the breast uptake (Case 7)

Everything I Need to Know That Will Alter My Management of the Patient I Will Identify on the Post ^{131}I Therapy Scan

An additional statement that is also frequently heard is: "*Everything I need to know that will alter my management of the patient I will identify on the post131I therapy scan.*" Again, the same counter argument to the first statement of

"*I don't find pre-remnant ablation radioiodine scans useful, because the information will not alter my management*" applies equally as well to this statement. So, I ask the same question again as above: if any of the findings on the above seven cases are identified on the post ^{131}I therapy scan, will any or all of those findings alter your management? If you answered yes to any or all of these findings, then why would they alter your management after your ^{131}I therapy but not before your ^{131}I therapy scan? Again, this is not an issue of whether or not the pre ^{131}I therapy scan has value; it is an issue that the individual chooses to alter management only after the post ^{131}I therapy scan and chooses not to alter management after the pre ^{131}I therapy scan. In summary, significant useful information is obtained that may potentially alter the patient's management *before* the ^{131}I therapy is administered, and again, data addressing this issue have been published [6, 7].

^{131}I May Cause Stunning

A third argument for not performing pre-ablation radioiodine scans is the potential of stunning. The pro and con arguments for the existence of stunning have been discussed in detail in Chaps. 16, 17, and 18, and whether or not one believes in stunning or the degree of stunning, there are three reasonable alternatives that either eliminate stunning and/or significantly reduce the effects of stunning. In the first place, one may replace ^{131}I with ^{123}I. Two counter arguments to this option are non-availability of ^{123}I and ^{123}I could cause stunning. In regard to the first counter argument, one could use ^{99m}Tc04, ^{99m}Tc sestamibi, or ^{99m}Tc tetrofosmin. A discussion of these options is beyond the scope of this chapter, but these options are discussed further Chap. 44 on Alternative Imaging. In regard to ^{123}I causing stunning, a review of the literature helps put this into perspective. The ATA guidelines [1] state that ". . . stunning [of ^{123}I] may also occur though to a lesser degree than with ^{131}I." This is based on the article of Hilditch et al. [16], but as suggested in a letter to the editor by Gerard and Park [17], the ATA guidelines may be misleading. Although Hilditch et al. [16] demonstrated a reduction in the uptake of therapeutic ^{131}I after the administration of 200 MBq (5.4 mCi) of ^{123}I in 15 of 16 patients, Hilditch et al. noted that this reduction ". . . could not be explained by . . . the radiation dose delivered by the ^{123}I." They went on further to say that ". . . the resultant radiation dose to the thyroid remnant, as the therapeutic radioiodine is being taken up, may be sufficient to inhibit the uptake process, thus leading to a reduction in maximum uptake compared with that of a diagnostic activity of radioiodine." As Gerard and Park noted [17], "it is misleading to attribute this decrement in therapeutic ^{131}I uptake to potential stunning caused by the ^{123}I tracer dose since it is well known that the ^{123}I dosimetry to thyroid tissue is 100-fold less than that of ^{131}I." Although I believe that significant stunning is highly unlikely at the prescribed activity of 37–200 MBq (1–5 mCi) of ^{123}I [18], I also agree with Lundh et al. [19] that ". . . stunning by ^{123}I cannot be excluded in patients." However, neither can one say that ". . . stunning [of ^{123}I] may also occur though to a lesser degree than with ^{131}I." With all data presently available at the time that this book went to press, ^{123}I remains an excellent alternative to ^{131}I, and if ^{123}I is not available, typically ^{99m}Tc04 is available in most countries that have access to radioisotopes for imaging.

The second alternative to reducing significant potential for stunning is to lower the prescribed activity of ^{131}I for the diagnostic scans. Although the reduction of the prescribed diagnostic activity of ^{131}I from 128–370 MBq (4–10 mCi) to 64 MBq (2 mCi) or even 37 MBq (1 mCi) may reduce the utility of the ^{131}I pre-remnant ablation radioiodine scan, the frequency of the findings reported in our study on pre-ablation radioiodine scans [6] were all observed administering only 37–64 MBq (1–2 mCi) of ^{123}I with images performed at 24 h. I would submit that the frequency of detection of the above findings in the seven cases already shown herein would be as good, if not better, with 37–64 MBq (1–2 mCi) of ^{131}I with imaging performed at 48–72 h with little to no stunning.

The third alternative, which has been suggested by McDougal et al. [20], is administering the ^{131}I therapeutic prescribed activity within a short time (e.g., 24 h) after the administration of the diagnostic dosage of ^{131}I, and data from Hilditch support this as a potential option to avoid risk of stunning [16].

With either of the above three alternatives, stunning is more of a theoretical than a real problem.

The Benefits of Pre-remnant Ablation Radioiodine Scans Do Not Warrant the Cost, Inconvenience, and Radiation Exposure

Another justification for not performing pre-ablation radioiodine scans that one frequently hears is "*pre-ablation scanning is expensive, an inconvenience to the patient, and results in additional unnecessary radiation to the patient.*" In the United States, the cost of a scan varies not only from region to region but also depending upon whether the cost is borne by the patient or by the various third-party payers. As a result, it is difficult to gather precise and consistent costs. However, in an attempt to compare reimbursements and to allow at least a better sense of the relative costs, Table 19.4 lists the reimbursements by Medicare in the District of Columbia in the United States for radioiodine whole-body imaging, ^{131}I, ^{123}I, various other imaging studies, and recombinant human thyroid stimulating hormone (rhTSH) at the time this textbook went to print. In relative terms, the reimbursement for a ^{131}I whole-body scan was only modestly

Table 19.4 Reimbursements for various imaging studies, procedures, radiopharmaceuticals, and pharmaceuticals[a]

Ultrasound of the neck (76536)	$ 102
Thyroid mets uptake (78020)	$ 0[b]
^{131}I whole-body scan (78018)	$ 308
^{123}I whole-body scan (78018)	$ 308[c]
Ultrasound-guided fine-needle aspiration (just for the aspiration)	$ 175
SPECT-CT of the neck (78803)	$ 516
Diagnostic CT of the chest (71250)	$ 411
Abdomen and pelvis (74176)	$ 411
MRI of the neck (72141)	$ 726
PET-CT of the neck (78814)	$ 1,043
Two recombinant human thyrotropin injections (J3240)	$ 2,424

[a]As of 17 December 2013
[b]The cost of the uptake is included within the reimbursement of the radioiodine whole-body scan
[c]The cost of the ^{131}I and ^{123}I are included within the reimbursement of the radioiodine whole-body scan. However, ^{123}I does cost the imaging facility more

more than an ultrasound. ^{123}I added no increased costs for the patient but increased the expense to the facility as it is now included in the imaging charge. In comparison to the reimbursement for a radioiodine whole-body scans (WBS), a diagnostic CT was 2 ½ times greater for just a CT of the chest and much more for a diagnostic CT of the chest and abdomen-pelvis. A MRI of the neck or PET scan was ~3 times as much as a WBS. Two injections of rhTSH were over seven times as much as the reimbursement for radioiodine WBS. As already discussed, these ratios can vary from region to region and country to country, but these comparisons help put the cost of a radioiodine whole-body scan in perspective. The cost of a radioiodine whole-body scan is reasonable and approximately equally or significantly less than most other studies.

The second argument in this category is patient inconvenience. While we have to be sensitive to the convenience of the patient, convenience should not be sacrosanct. We have to weigh convenience versus potential benefit to the patient's health. The inconvenience of a visit to receive several capsules by mouth and a second visit that lasts typically less than the length of an average football game, movie, or a few afternoon television "soap-operas" does not seem, in my judgment, to be a major inconvenience in exchange for information that could potentially modify the patient's management.

Finally, the additional radiation absorbed dose to the patient from a diagnostic prescribed activity of ^{131}I is inconsequential relative to the prescribed activity of 1.11–3.7 GBq (30–50 mCi) for the patient's anticipated ^{131}I remnant ablation. In fact, at least within the United States, the prescribed activity of the delivered amount of ^{131}I to be administered for the ^{131}I remnant ablation may legally vary by ± 10 % of the prescribed activity. Thus, for a therapeutic prescribed activity of 1.11 GBq (30 mCi), the administered prescribed activity may vary by as much as 222 MBq (6 mCi). The radiation absorbed dose from a prescribed diagnostic activity of 1–2 mCi (37–64 MBq) of ^{131}I is inconsequential relative to even the accepted variability of the anticipated therapeutic prescribed activity let alone the larger therapeutic prescribed activity itself, and to my knowledge no one has raised concern about any increase in the radiation absorbed dose from the variable imprecision of the final therapeutic prescribed activity of ^{131}I. Moreover, the radiation absorbed dose from ^{123}I for radioiodine scanning is inconsequential. Thus, the potential benefit of a pre-ablation remnant scan far outweighs the expense, inconvenience to the patient, and additional radiation absorbed dose to the patient.

Until Data Are Published Demonstrating That the Pre-^{131}I Therapy Scans Alter Patient Outcomes, These Scans Should Not Be Performed

Evidence-based medicine is important in deciding what test, imaging scan, and/or treatment are valuable to perform or not to perform. However, in our desire to make our medical decisions "evidence based," I submit that many of us use the lack of evidence that a test, imaging scan, or treatment alters patient outcomes as our "argument of last resort" that that test, imaging scan, or treatment should not be performed. Certainly, a decision regarding whether or not a *new* imaging scan should be implemented should be based on good evidence that either the patients' outcomes or a surrogate for the patients' outcomes are altered. However, when that imaging scan has been used for 10, 20, 30, 40, or even 50 or more years with no definitive outcome data published but with many expert physicians supporting the value of that imaging scan based on their extensive empiric experience, should that imaging scan now not be performed because there is no evidence to demonstrate that the patients' outcomes are altered? I submit that the argument of a lack of "evidence-based" data is not an argument against the use of pre-ablation imaging scan. In testimony to this, I would also submit that that is not how most professional organizations' guidelines manage their recommendations. When there is no good evidence-based medicine that outcomes are altered by an imaging scan, neither the ATA, European Consensus, NCCN, the BTA, nor the SNM recommend that that imaging scan should no longer be performed until there are good studies demonstrating that the patients' outcomes or surrogates for the patients' outcomes are altered. Instead, they propose a recommendation based on "expert opinion," which of course is based on the empirical experience of the specific members of that committee. Accordingly, the fact that data have not been published demonstrating that pre-^{131}I therapy scans alter patients' outcomes should not be the reason that pre-^{131}I therapy scans should not be performed. Instead, it should be noted that the use of pre-^{131}I therapy scans is controversial and that in the absence of definitive data, expert opinions for and against the use of that imaging scan will differ.

But Are These the Only Factors for and Against Pre-ablation Scans?

In the blockbuster J.K. Rowling's Harry Potter series, the archenemy of Harry Potter is referred to as "He-Who-Must-Not-Be-Named," and everyone fears what may happen should one speaks "his name" – Lord Voldemort. In a discussion of why do reasonable, knowledgeable, and excellent clinicians and investigators have such extreme differences of opinions regarding the utility of pre-remnant ablation radioiodine scans, it appears to me that there are "Reasons-That-Must-Not-Be-Named." At the fear and risk of what may happen to me, I submit that there may be three important reasons, which to my knowledge have never been named or discussed.

One important potential reason for a significant difference in opinion relates to the equipment and technique for the performance of radioiodine scans. It is well known that equipment and technique can make a significant difference in the quality and utility of scans (see Chap.11). If one has any doubt about that, one's doubt should be assuaged by referring to Dr. Yong Whee Bhak's book. Although this book addresses pinhole imaging of the bones relative to whole-body scanning of the bones or even parallel-hole collimator images [21], the superiority and utility of pinhole imaging applies equally to thyroid cancer imaging of the thyroid bed and neck. In short, technique does make a difference. But perhaps this may not be as well appreciated regarding radioiodine imaging of the thyroid. In fact, a common failure to recognize these differences may be implicit in the common use of the expression referring to radioiodine imaging of patients with thyroid cancers as "*whole-body imaging.*" When one uses this term, I would suggest that for many there is an assumption, or at least a tacit implication, that all radioiodine "whole-body imaging" techniques are equivalent.

Radioiodine "whole-body imaging" techniques may be very different. Not only may the "whole-body imaging" quality vary because of factors such as type of whole-body scanners, whole-body table scanning speeds, times after dosing for imaging, and collimators, but "whole-body imaging" in one facility may only include the use of a whole-body scanner without additional individual "spot" parallel-hole collimator images of selected areas or even more importantly, individual "spot" pinhole collimator images of the thyroid bed and neck (see Chap.11). As one example of the differences in what one may detect using various techniques, Kulkarni et al. [22] compared the ability of images obtained with a whole-body scanner to images obtained with individual parallel-hole collimators and pinhole collimators used to detect individual foci of uptake in or adjacent to the thyroid bed. Kulkarni et al. demonstrated that individual pinhole collimator images distinguished significantly more foci of radioiodine uptake relative to images obtained with a whole-body scanner and even those obtained with individual parallel-hole collimator imaging. The number of foci detected in the thyroid bed and neck on whole-body scanner images, "spot" parallel-hole collimator images, and pinhole collimator images in the same patient group was 694, 916, and 1079, respectively (see Fig. 19.8 and Graph 19.1). If one is obtaining images with only a whole-body scanner or just with a "spot" parallel-hole collimator, one may be failing to identify patients with a significant number of foci either within or outside the thyroid bed area that may suggest regional disease. Of note, Kulkarni et al. [22] excluded patients with known or suspected locoregional disease. Although it may be argued that one does not know how many foci of tissue a specific surgeon may normally leave behind after near total or total thyroidectomy in order to know what numbers of foci would raise suspicious of locoregional disease, this can be easily determined for each surgeon at one's facility as reported by Chennupati et al. [23]. Nevertheless, the limitation of only performing images on a whole-body scanner or even a parallel-hole collimator is best demonstrated by a "star artifact," which has been well described (see Chap.12). A "star artifact" is an intense focal area of uptake such as in the thyroid bed with multiple streak-like areas radiating out form the intense focal area of uptake (Fig. 19.9). This is a result of significant uptake of radioiodine in the thyroid bed and/or neck with significant penetration of the septum of the collimator by the emitted gamma rays which result in the "star pattern" on the images. With a "star artifact," the interpreting physician loses essentially all or almost all of his/her ability to obtain any useful information of the thyroid bed or neck. Perhaps this is an important reason why one physician who only performs whole-body scanned images finds pre-^{131}I therapy images of little to no value.

Finally, in regard to equipment and technique, the above arguments do not even consider SPECT-CT imaging, and multiple publications have demonstrated additional, significant improvement in the utility of pre-ablation radioiodine scans (see Chaps. 14 and 15). This is a result of improved contrast resolution and anatomical localization with non-diagnostic or diagnostic computed tomography. As examples of some of the initial publications, Spanu et al. [14] evaluated the incremental value of SPECT-CT over planar imaging in 117 patients. Although nine of these SPECT-CT scans were post-therapy, the overwhelming majority of SPECT-CT scans were pre-therapy, and these authors demonstrated an incremental value over planar imaging of 67.8 % of patients,

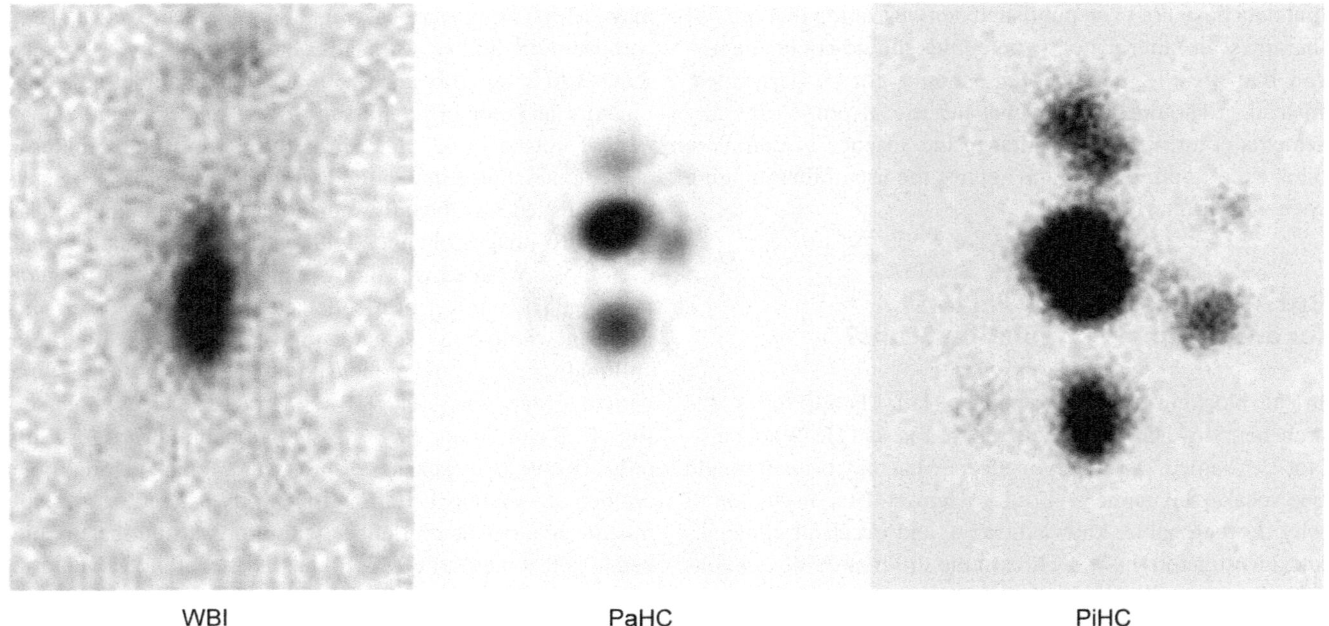

Fig. 19.8 These images demonstrate that technique makes a major difference. WBI is an image of the thyroid bed and neck performed by a whole-body scanner (WBI). PaHC is an image performed of the same area in the same patient using a parallel-hole collimator, and PiCH image is performed using a pinhole collimator of the same area in the same patient. The PiHC image delineates more foci of uptake in the thyroid bed and neck than either the PaHC image or the WBI. The PaHC image also delineated more foci of radioiodine uptake in the thyroid bed and neck than the WBI. The numbers of foci in each image were reported as 2 (WBI), 4 (PaHC), and 7 (PiHC). Based on the WBI and although we could not differentiate whether or not the activity on the WBI represented normal functioning remnant tissue with or without residual thyroid cancer, I would interpret the iHC image as strongly suggestive persistent locoregional thyroid cancer with residual functioning thyroid cancer, and this would alter my management. Altered management may include performing additional imaging (e.g., ultrasound or MRI), fine-needle aspiration, additional surgery, higher empiric prescribed activity of radioiodine, and/or dosimetrically-determined prescribed activity of radioiodine. Technique makes a difference (Reproduced with permission from Keystone Press, Inc.)

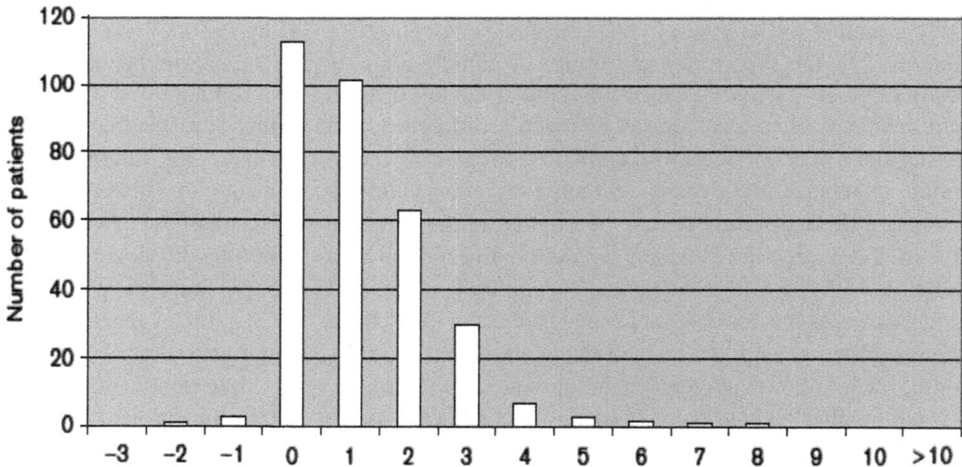

Graph 19.1 The difference in the number of foci detected. Number of *additional* foci detected on pinhole "spot" images vs whole-body images using a parallel-body collimator (This image was reproduced with permission from Kulkarni et al. [22])

modification of therapeutic management in 36 % of positive cases, and avoidance of unnecessary treatment in 20 % of patients. Tharp et al. [15] demonstrated an incremental value of pre-therapy SPECT-CT in 11/17 (65 %) of patients of which tumor was excluded in two patients, lymph node involvement was demonstrated in three patients, and distant metastasis were diagnosed and localized in six. SPECT-CT adds even greater value to pre-ablation scans, and again a more in-depth discussion of publications is noted in Chaps. 14 and 15. Accordingly, I submit that one of the major reasons that reasonable, knowledgeable, and excellent clinicians and investigators may have such extreme differences in opinions

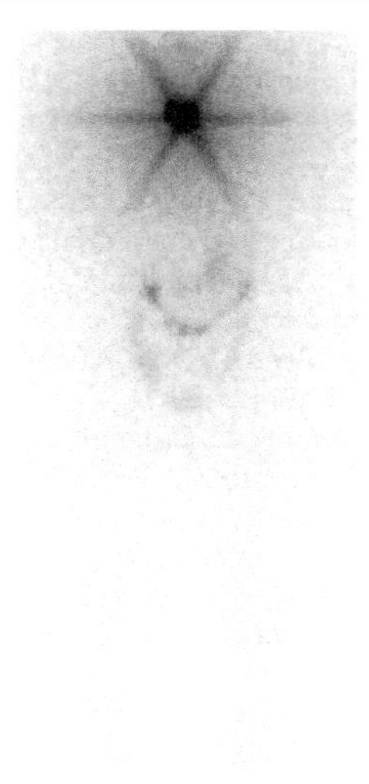

Fig. 19.9 This ^{131}I whole-body image obtained with a whole-body scanner demonstrates the "star artifact" resulting from penetration of the lead septum of the wall of the collimator by gamma rays from an area of intense uptake in the thyroid bed/neck. The intense uptake of the "star artifact" reduces the discrimination of the number of foci and location of the foci of uptake in or outside the thyroid bed and neck area

regarding the utility of pre-ablation radioiodine scans is the imaging equipment and parameters that they either have to use or choose to use.

The second "Reason-That-Must-Not-Be-Named" is *money*. One needs no reference to acknowledge that self-referral in a fee for service practice may increase utilization of a test, a scan, and/or a treatment for income. Of course, we believe we can easily identify this action within others and that we ourselves have "risen above" this self-interest. However, inappropriate self-referral may be so occult and even subconsciousness that it is not recognized within ourselves. Accordingly, I submit that money may be a factor in not only supporting the use of pre-^{131}I therapy scans but also in arguing against the use of pre-^{131}I therapy scans. Whether in a non-fee-for-service practice (i.e., salaried or contracted), a government-based practice, and/or a health maintenance organization, there can be subtle and even major financial incentives consciously or subconsciously to reduce the use of tests, imaging scans, and/or treatments, including but not limited to budget restrictions, staffing limitations, incentives, and bonuses, to name only few.

A third potential "Reason-That-Must-Not-Be-Named" is *work* involved. In the same non-fee-for-service practice, government-based practice, and/or health maintenance organization in which the physician is salaried, the approach that offers the *least amount of work* to the management of a patient for first-time ^{131}I ablation is to eliminate a pre-^{131}I therapy scan and administer a predetermined empiric prescribed amount of activity of ^{131}I. It is less complex, requires less thinking, requires no extra views, and requires less time dealing with the referring physician and the patient. Again, I am sure that all of us believe that none of the above applies to us, and that we have risen above this. But have we?

For the record, my staff and I receive fixed wages. We are not fee for service and receive no bonuses for volumes. When we discover findings that we believe should alter management – no uptake in the thyroid bed, five/six or more foci in the thyroid bed, uptake outside the thyroid bed, and/or focal distant uptake requiring a SPECT-CT or extra views – we receive no additional compensation; we just work harder.

In short, I submit that there may be reasons that are rarely discussed that could influence whether or not we support the use of pre-^{131}I therapy scans, and these reasons may fuel, at least in part, the controversy between reasonable, knowledgeable, and excellent clinicians and investigators.

References

1. Haugen B, Alexander E, Bible K, Doherty G, Mandel S, Nikiforov Y, Pacini F, Randolph G, Sawka A, Schlumberger M, Schuff K, Sherman S, Sosa J, Steward D, Tuttle, R, Wartofsky L. 2015 American Thyroid Association Management Guidelines for Adult Patients with Thyroid Nodules and Differentiated Thyroid Cancer. Thyroid. 2016;26:1–133.
2. Pacini F, Schlumberger M, Dralle H, Elisei R, Smit JWA, Wiersinga W, European Thyroid Cancer Taskforce. European consensus for the management of patients with differentiated thyroid carcinoma of the follicular epithelium. Eur J Endocrinol. 2006;154:787–803.
3. National Comprehensive Cancer Network (NCCN). Clinical practice guidelines in oncology. Thyroid carcinoma. Follicular thyroid carcinoma. V.2.2013.
4. British Thyroid Association and Royal College of Physicians. Guidelines/statements the British Thyroid Association 2014 edition of the Thyroid Cancer Guidelines (Draft). Available at: http://www.british-thyroid-association.org/Guidelines/.
5. Silberstein EB, Alvai A, Balon H, et al. The SNM pracice guideline for therapy of thyroid disease with ^{131}I, 3.0. J Nucl Med. 2012;53:1633–51.
6. Van Nostrand D, Aiken M, Atkins F, Moreau S, Garcia C, Acio E, Burman K, Wartofsky L. The utility of radioiodine scans prior to ^{131}I ablation in patients with well-differentiated thyroid cancer. Thyroid. 2009;19:849–55.
7. Chen MK, Yasrebi M, Samii J, Staib LH, Doddamane I, Cheng DW. The utility of I-123 pretherapy scan in I-131 radioiodine therapy for thyroid cancer. Thyroid. 2012;22:304–9.
8. McDougall IR. Differentiated thyroid cancer. In: McDougall IR, editor. Management of thyroid cancer and related nodular disease. London: Springer; 2006. p. 173.
9. Amdur RJ, Mazzaferri EL. The role of a diagnostic radioiodine whole body scan (DxSCAN). In: Amdur RJ, Mazzaferri E, editors. Essentials of thyroid cancer management. Springer: New York; 2005. p. 63.
10. Haq MS, Harmer C. Non-surgical management of thyroid cancer. In: Mazzaferri E, Harmer C, Mallick UK, Kendall-Taylor P, editors. Practical management of thyroid cancer. London: Springer; 2006. p. 174.
11. Schlumberger MJ, Leboulleux SM, Pacini F. Follow-up of patients with differentiated thyroid carcinoma. In: Mazzaferri EL, Harmer

C, Mallick UJ, Kendall-Taylor P, editors. Practical management of thyroid cancer. New York: Springer; 1996. p. 231.
12. Schlumberger MJ, Pacini F. The low utility of pretherapy scans in thyroid cancer patients. Thyroid. 2009;19:815–6.
13. McDougall IR. The case for obtaining a diagnostic whole-body scan prior to iodine 131 treatment of differentiated thyroid cancer. Thyroid. 2009;19:811–3.
14. Spanu A, Solinas ME, Chessa F, Sanna D, Nuvoli S, Madeddu S. ^{131}I SPECT-CT in the follow-up of differentiated thyroid carcinoma: incremental value versus planar imaging. J Nucl Med. 2009;50:184–90.
15. Tharp K, Israel O, Hausmann J, Bettman L, Martin WH, Daitzchman M, Sandler MP, Delbeke D. Impact of ^{131}I-SPECT/CT images obtained with an integrated system in the follow-up of patients with thyroid carcinoma. Eur J Nucl Med Mol Imaging. 2004;31:1435–42.
16. Hilditch TE, Dempsey MF, Bolster AA, McMenemin RM, Reed NS. Self-stunning in thyroid ablation: evidence from comparative studies of diagnostic ^{131}I and ^{123}I. Eur J Nucl Med Mol Imaging. 2002;29:783–8.
17. Gerard SK, Park HM. Stunning and I-123 use for diagnostic whole body scanning: letter to the editor. Thyroid. 2006;16:817.
18. MIRD (Medical Internal Radiation Dose) Committee 1975 Report #5. Summary of current radiation dose estimates to humans from ^{123}I, ^{124}I, ^{125}I, ^{126}I, ^{130}I, ^{131}I, and ^{132}I as sodium iodide. J Nucl Med. 1975; 16:857–60.
19. Lundh C, Lindencrona U, Postgard P, Carlsson T, Nilsson M, Forssell-Aronsson E. Radiation-induced thyroid stunning: differential effects of ^{123}I, ^{131} I, ^{99m}Tc, and ^{211}AT on iodide transport and NIS mRNA expression in cultured thyroid cells. J Nucl Med. 2009;50:116–1171.
20. McDougall IR, Iagaru A. Thyroid stunning: fact or fiction. Sem Nucl Med. 2011;41:105–12.
21. Bahk YW, editor. Combined scintigraphic and radiographic diagnosis of bone and joint diseases. 2nd ed. Berlin: Springer; 2000.
22. Kulkarni K, Van Nostrand D, Young-Rok S, Aiken M, Mete M, Burman K, Wartofsky L. Detectability of foci of radioiodine uptake in the thyroid bed and neck comparing pinhole with parallel-hole collimators. Nuc Med Comm. 2011;32:369–74.
23. Chennupati S, Van Nostrand D, Kharazi P, Khorjekar G. Determination of the number of foci of normal thyroid tissue remaining after thyroidectomy in patients with differentiated thyroid cancer: the Washington hospital center experience. J Nucl Med. 2011;52S:1300.

Part III

The Thyroid Nodule

The Thyroid Nodule: Evaluation, Risk of Malignancy, and Management

20

Leonard Wartofsky

Introduction

Palpable nodules of the thyroid are frequently encountered in clinical practice, and their evaluation requires the physician to be familiar with a growing number of diagnostic tools that can be employed to identify those nodules that may represent cancer and require surgical intervention. Until recently, what constituted optimal clinical management of a thyroid nodule varied from center to center and even between physicians at a given center. The routine management of thyroid nodules today is less controversial as our major professional organizations have published consensus guidelines for the diagnosis and management of thyroid nodules [1–7] that have been widely accepted. A discussion of the special circumstances surrounding thyroid nodules detected during pregnancy is discussed in Chap. 54 and in the guidelines of the American Thyroid Association on management of thyroid disease in pregnancy [8].

Prevalence

The detection of thyroid nodules has been increasing significantly related to the more widespread use of ultrasonography of the neck for various indications. It is controversial whether the actual incidence of thyroid cancer is increasing or whether we are seeing more cancers because of the increased detection of nodules. The latter argument has been made [9] because the increases in thyroid cancers that have been seen were largely microcarcinomata and because no parallel increase in mortality has been noted that might have been anticipated by an increased incidence of larger tumors with worse prognosis. In my view, the data extant are suggestive but not fully convincing that the etiology of the increasing incidence is due solely to improved detection and screening. Conceivably, enhanced risks of thyroid malignancy could be derived from interventions such as therapeutic and diagnostic radiation to the head and neck and nuclear fission with radiation fallout. Other potential contributing factors include autoimmune phenomena, genetic mutation, alterations in iodine intake, and potential environmental carcinogens, both known and unknown [10]. If the increase is simply due to improved detection, it is difficult to explain the observations that incidence appears to be increasing faster in developing countries (which can ill afford the expensive technology for detection) than in the West. Davies and Welch [9] argue that because cancer mortality has been stable over several decades implies that most of the carcinomas detected may be papillary microcarcinomata found early enough to have an excellent prognosis. On the other hand, it is possible that the mortality rates are stable in spite of increasing incidence because of improvement in diagnostic and therapeutic approaches. Moreover, analyses published subsequently have indicated that the incidence of thyroid cancer is indeed increasing with increases seen in tumors >2 cm as well as in microcarcinomata [11–13].

Solitary nodules of the thyroid gland are present in about 6.4 % of women and 1.5 % of men in the United States. The incidence noted in surveys in northeast England are comparable with 5.3 % of adult women and 0.8 % of adult men found to have nodules [14]. Most thyroid nodules in children are benign with an overall low prevalence in children of ~1.5 % but which increases linearly with age. Although nodules are less common in children than in adults, nodules in children are more likely to be malignant than in adults [15]. The risk of malignancy is highest below age 15 and over age 45. During a 15-years follow-up of the Framingham population, new nodules appeared in 0.1 % of patients per year

L. Wartofsky, MD, MACP (✉)
Department of Medicine, MedStar Washington Hospital Center, Georgetown University School of Medicine,
110 Irving Street, N.W., Washington, DC 20010-2975, USA
e-mail: leonard.wartofsky@medstar.net

L. Wartofsky, D. Van Nostrand (eds.), *Thyroid Cancer*, DOI 10.1007/978-1-4939-3314-3_20

[16]. Palpation will detect that approximately 4–8 % of the population will have a thyroid nodule. Many single palpable nodules thought to be solitary are actually in a multinodular thyroid gland. Although autopsy studies indicate thyroid nodules can be seen in as many as 50 % of consecutive necropsies, many may be small and clinically inapparent [1–3]. High-resolution ultrasound has identified nodules in 13–40 % of patients evaluated for nonthyroid problems [17–19]. Indeed, nodules may be detected by ultrasound in up to 70 % of adults but most will be quite small and of uncertain clinical importance. Thus, a discrepancy exists between the true prevalence of thyroid nodules and that detected on physical examination. Generally, nodules must approach a size of 1 cm in diameter to be recognized on palpation, and nodules greater than 1 cm in size are thought to have a greater risk of harboring malignancy. The significance of nonpalpable nodules incidentally found by ultrasound, or so-called incidentalomas, is discussed below, and these nonpalpable nodules generally are considered to have the same risk of malignancy as a palpable nodule of the same size. Thus, the clinical significance of thyroid nodules relates to the likelihood that a given nodule may be malignant or harbor a malignancy. Given that thyroid nodules are quite common, and given both the cost and risks of undergoing surgical thyroidectomy for a nodule, to operate on all nodules would not be medically prudent and would constitute an extraordinary burden on health care costs. With only approximately 5 % of nodules that will be malignant, the challenge to the physician is to follow a reasonably aggressive, yet cost-effective approach to sift through the numerous nodules in the population to determine whether a given nodule might represent thyroid cancer. Thyroidectomy would then be recommended for those nodules either shown to harbor malignancy or to be at sufficient risk of malignancy to warrant undergoing surgery.

Pathogenesis

While the cause of thyroid nodules is not known for the most part, possible relationships to nodule formation include iodine deficiency and indirectly, elevation in blood levels of thyrotropin (TSH). Nodules that do not take up radioactive iodine on scanning are referred to as "cold" nodules. Cold nodules occur about 2.5 times more often in areas of low naturally occurring iodine. In rats, iodine deficiency enhances TSH secretion and the development of thyroid nodules, some of which will be malignant [20]. The precise relationship to TSH is unclear, but the response of benign nodular thyroid enlargement to thyroxine-induced suppression of TSH [2, 21, 22], as well as the improved prognosis of patients with papillary thyroid cancer treated with thyroxine [23, 24], suggests a role of relative increases in serum TSH in human neoplasia. Not all lines of experimental evidence point to a role of TSH as a growth factor or mitogen for both benign and malignant thyroid tumors [25]. However, recent clinical studies indicate that the likelihood that a given nodule is malignant correlates directly to the level of serum TSH [26–28] and thyroid cancer patients with elevated TSH levels may be more likely to have more advanced disease or evidence of extrathyroidal extension [29] at time of presentation.

Radiation exposure can cause thyroid neoplasia, with a linear relationship between radiation doses up to 1,800 rad and the incidence of thyroid nodules and cancer. The increased risk of clinically significant thyroid cancer associated with prior radiotherapy to the head and neck given for thymic enlargement, tonsillitis, acne, and adenitis, is around 3 % [30–32]. The patient with thyroid cancer and a prior history of radiation exposure typically is a childhood cancer survivor in whom the thyroid was exposed to radiation therapy with inadequate or no shielding. Radiation exposure during childhood is more likely to produce thyroid neoplasia than similar exposure at a later age, possibly related to greater cellular mitotic activity at the earlier age of insult. Among individuals in the United States who received head and neck irradiation as children, palpable nodules are found in 16–29 % and carcinoma in one third of these nodules [32–35]. Most nodules tend to occur within 10–20 year of exposure, but the risk may exist for 40 years or more. The irradiated thyroid gland often presents with multiple nodules; at surgery, the lesion of initial concern may prove to be benign, whereas one or more carcinomas will be found elsewhere in the gland. Thus, those nodules associated with a radiation history do not demonstrate a reduced cancer risk when the thyroid contains multiple nodules. Early studies have indicated that one cannot predict malignancy following radiation exposure based upon either the size of a nodule or the radiation dose [36]. This has been confirmed by a study demonstrating that the risk of malignancy is not mitigated by multinodularity or the size of the nodule [37]. In the latter study, 31 % of patients with two or more nodules had a thyroid cancer, and a FNA of only the largest nodule would have missed almost 50 % of the cancers subsequently identified. While some other studies have ascribed a higher risk of malignancy to the multinodular gland [38], a recent meta-analysis indicated either no difference or a lower risk [39]. The ATA guideline recommendation [4] to perform FNA on nodules of less than 1 cm when there is a history of radiation is consistent with these reports. The dramatic increase in thyroid nodules and thyroid cancer occurring in Belarus after the 1986 Chernobyl nuclear disaster is discussed in detail in Chap. 7 by J. Figge and associates.

Exposure of the thyroid gland to higher doses of irradiation, e.g., that from external radiation therapy for Hodgkin's disease (>2,000 rad) or internal radiation from ^{131}I therapy for toxic goiter, does not appear to be related to subsequent development of thyroid carcinoma. In both cases, the high-dose exposure with attendant cell destruction and fibrosis often leads to hypothyroidism, and the reduced functioning tissue mass may serve to attenuate any carcinogenic effect that is seen with lesser degrees of radiation injury.

Differential Diagnosis

As indicated in Table 20.1, the differential diagnosis of apparent thyroid nodules covers a wide range of pathology [1–6]. Most true intrathyroidal nodules will represent colloid adenomas (27–60 %) or simple follicular adenomas (26–40 %). About 5 % of thyroid nodules are classified as hyperfunctioning and are "hot" on radionuclide scanning based on a relative increased ability to trap iodide. Most hot nodules are autonomously functioning and are associated with either subclinical or overt hyperthyroidism in more than half of patients over 60 year of age. Of nodules greater than 3 cm in diameter, 20 % are associated with hyperthyroidism [40] compared with 2 % of smaller lesions. Although most toxic autonomous nodules secrete both thyroxine (T4) and triiodothyronine (T3), elevations of either T3 or T4 alone occasionally may be seen. Moreover, even when T3 and T4 levels are "normal," a low or undetectable serum TSH by a sensitive assay may be commonly seen, suggesting supraphysiologic iodothyronine production or "subclinical" hyperthyroidism.

Table 20.1 Differential diagnosis of apparent thyroid nodules

Benign thyroid neoplasms
Follicular adenoma
Colloid
Simple
Fetal
Embryonal
Hurthle cell
Papillary adenoma
Teratoma
Lipoma
C-cell adenoma
Dermoid cyst
Malignant thyroid neoplasms
Papillary carcinoma
Follicular carcinoma
Medullary thyroid carcinoma
Anaplastic carcinoma
Metastatic carcinoma
Sarcoma
Lymphoma
Other thyroid abnormalities
Thyroiditis
Thyroid cyst
Hemiagenetic thyroid
Infectious granulomatous disease (e.g., sarcoidosis)
Nonthyroid lesions
Lymphadenopathy
Aneurysm
Thyroglossal duct cyst
Parathyroid cyst
Parathyroid adenoma
Laryngocele
Cystic hygroma

Cancers are found in 10–14 % of patients presenting with palpable thyroid nodules [1–6]. Papillary carcinomas account for about 80–85 % of all thyroid cancer in Americans, with follicular carcinoma as the next most common (10–12 %) and anaplastic and medullary thyroid carcinomas comprising the remaining 3–5 %. The thyroid gland has a rich blood supply, and a thyroid nodule occasionally may represent a secondary or metastatic neoplasm to the thyroid gland, commonly seen with cancers such as malignant melanoma, renal cell, breast, or bronchogenic carcinoma. In 2013, the American Cancer Society estimated that there will be approximately 60,220 new thyroid cancer cases diagnosed and 1,850 thyroid cancer-related deaths in the United States [41]. Thyroid cancer is estimated to be among the top leading causes of new cases of cancer in women. Autopsy studies have revealed occult thyroid cancer in 6 % of autopsies in North American series [42]. There is general agreement that these small, occult, and mostly papillary cancers are of little or no clinical significance, and their increased prevalence does not correlate with an increase in the death rate from thyroid carcinoma [43].

Diagnostic Evaluation

As the vast majority of thyroid nodule morbidity is related to those lesions representing carcinoma, the evaluation is focused on the identification of nodules that may be malignant.

History and Physical Examination

The single most important historical risk factor for cancer is exposure to radiation. It is important to determine the age at time of exposure, exact region of the body irradiated, and, if possible, the type and dose of radiation to the thyroid. Although women are more prone to thyroid nodules and thyroid cancer than men, the probability of cancer is higher among men with nodules, especially in those over age 70. The incidence of thyroid cancer increases with age, but a higher percentage of nodules in patients less than 20 years of age will be malignant. The presence of cervical lymphadenopathy can indicate the presence of thyroid cancer because most thyroid cancers are of the papillary type which typically spread to cervical lymph nodes. Thus, the features regarding history and physical examination that are more suggestive that a given nodule may be malignant include male sex, age less than 15 or greater than 60, history of irradiation of the head and neck, and associated cervical lymphadenopathy. Risk of malignancy in a given nodule may also be stratified based upon ultrasonographic characteristics of the nodule (see below) as a guide to which nodules require FNA for cytologic examination. This approach is recommended in the ATA guidelines [4, 7].

Thyroid lymphoma should be considered in patients with rapid thyroid enlargement and a previous diagnosis of Hashimoto's thyroiditis, especially in women over age 50. Such lesions may present as a dominant "cold" nodule, and there is often coincident diabetes mellitus. A family history of pheochromocytoma, hypercalcemia, mucosal abnormalities, or medullary thyroid carcinoma raises suspicion of the latter diagnosis as part of a multiple endocrine neoplasia (MEN) syndrome. Although family history of benign goiter may be reassuring, the rare Pendred's syndrome of familial goiter and deaf mutism is linked with a higher cancer risk [1, 3]. Other genetic entities in the family history that confer greater risk for thyroid cancer include multiple endocrine neoplasia (MEN2), familial polyposis, Werner syndrome, Carney complex, and Cowden's syndrome [44].

Most thyroid nodules are discovered incidentally in asymptomatic patients. Although only a single nodule may be detected on physical examination, as many as 50 % of glands will actually harbor multiple nodules [45]. As noted in Table 20.2, many symptoms or physical findings are believed to be more common in malignant than in benign nodules, but as few as 5–10 % of patients with malignancy actually present with symptoms. Patients with advanced disease may present with bulky lymphadenopathy, hard nodules, nodule growth while under observation, thyroid pain and tenderness, and vocal cord paralysis, all of which point to the likelihood of malignancy. A thyroid nodule that is very firm, or relatively fixed in the neck with little movement with swallowing, or associated with enlarged cervical lymph nodes or recurrent laryngeal nerve paralysis is highly likely to be malignant.

Table 20.2 Physical and historical factors increasing risk of carcinoma in a thyroid nodule

History	Physical exam
Radiation	Cervical lymphadenopathy
Family history of MEN	Firmness
Rapid growth	Documented growth
Hoarseness	Vocal cord paralysis
Pain	Fixation
Dysphagia	Horner's syndrome
Respiratory obstructive symptoms	
Growth with thyroxine medication	

Laboratory Tests

In regard to indicating the presence of malignancy, thyroid function tests are usually of little value. However, the first step in the evaluation of thyroid nodules should be a measurement of TSH. As indicated above, higher TSH levels can be associated with malignant nodules, and the presence of a high TSH is another indication for fine-needle aspiration of the nodule. On the contrary, a nodule associated with low or suppressed TSH levels will rarely be malignant. The finding of a suppressed TSH suggests that the nodule is likely to be a toxic (hyperfunctioning or autonomous) adenoma, and the recommended next step in evaluation would be a thyroid scan. Serum levels of thyroglobulin (Tg) levels may be elevated in patients with thyroid malignancy but preoperative blood levels do not differentiate malignant nodules from those associated with benign adenomas or thyroiditis and their measurement is not recommended preoperatively for diagnostic purposes [4, 7]. However, serum Tg is a critically useful measurement as a tumor marker for surveillance for residual or recurrent cancer in the routine follow-up of patients after they have undergone total thyroidectomy with or without radioiodine ablation [7, 46–48], and measurement of Tg in aspirates of lymph nodes confirms the presence of metastasis [49]. The measurement of serum antithyroglobulin and antimicrosomal (TPO, or antithyroid peroxidase) antibodies also has limited value in the initial phase of diagnosis of the nature of a thyroid nodule. However, once the diagnosis may have been made by fine-needle aspiration cytology, it will be of interest to know the antibody status of the patient. The presence of positive thyroid peroxidase (TPO) antibodies indicating underlying Hashimoto's thyroiditis has implications for prognosis and family screening, as well as indicating a greater likelihood of associated antithyroglobulin antibodies. Elevated antithyroglobulin antibodies have been said to represent an independent risk factor for thyroid malignancy [50, 51] possibly due to linkage to underlying Hashimoto's disease. The presence of the latter antibodies renders difficult the ability to obtain accurate measurements of Tg and it is very useful to know whether anti-Tg antibodies are present this early in the course of management. During subsequent periods of surveillance, the disappearance or reappearance of antithyroglobulin antibodies may herald cure or recurrence, respectively, of thyroid cancer [51, 52]. An assay utilizing mass spectrometry has been developed recently and if validated holds some promise to provide measurement of Tg in the presence of interfering Tg antibodies in the serum [53].

Of the several familial syndromes that can be associated with thyroid cancer, medullary thyroid cancer (MTC) is the most common. Special diagnostic studies are available for the detection of MTC, which may present as a dominant thyroid cold nodule per se or as part of a MEN syndrome [54–56].

MEN2A is characterized by MTC with pheochromocytoma and, in some cases, hyperparathyroidism. The familial MTC of MEN2A differs from sporadic MTC in being often preceded by C-cell hyperplasia, leading to multifocal tumors. MEN2B includes MTC, pheochromocytoma, and several phenotypic abnormalities, e.g., mucosal neuromata. The RET proto-oncogene is the gene responsible for MEN2A and 2B, and mutations in differing codons and exons of RET have been identified in sporadic MTC as well. It is possible to routinely identify RET in material obtained by fine-needle aspiration (FNA) of a thyroid nodule. Differentiation between the mutations known for sporadic vs. familial MTC provides information that helps to determine whether preoperative screening for pheochromocytoma is necessary prior to thyroidectomy.

MTC may secrete calcitonin, carcinoembryonic antigen (CEA), chromogranin, and other peptides [57–59]. As tumor markers (analogous to thyroglobulin for follicular thyroid cancer), these measurements are most useful for the detection of recurrence after initial thyroidectomy, rather than for initial diagnosis. Not all patients with proven MTC have elevated levels of calcitonin [60, 61]. Pentagastrin for provocative testing and stimulation of calcitonin secretion is no longer available in the United States. Generally, the measurement of basal plasma calcitonin or CEA or assessment for the RET proto-oncogene intended to identify whether a nodule represents MTC is not cost-effective in the initial evaluation of the nodular thyroid. However, this is controversial [62–69] and not universally held. Screening serum calcitonin was deemed to be worthwhile in one large series of patients [70], and the ostensibly earlier detection of MTC was associated with a better prognosis for the patients detected by screening. False-positive elevated calcitonin may be seen in Hashimoto's disease [71], in the presence of heterophile antibodies [72], with renal failure [73], with proton pump inhibitor drug therapy [74], or in pseudohypoparathyroidism [75]. False-positive rates may be reduced by employing an upper limit of normal of 15 ng/L rather than 10 ng/L [76]. In one screening study of 2,733 patients, only 43 patients were found to have an elevated calcitonin and 12/43 or less than 25 % turned out to have MTC [63]. Although the European consensus guidelines [77] recommend calcitonin measurement in the evaluation of thyroid nodules, the American Thyroid Association guidelines [4, 7] recommend neither for nor against screening with calcitonin measurements. Inability to provide a more specific recommendation is due in part to concern as to whether screening is cost-effective, as well as to the fact that pentagastrin for stimulation testing, which has proven useful for detection of MCT in Europe, is not available in the United States. "Normal" individuals usually have serum calcitonin levels of less than 10 pg/mL [65]. Calcitonin levels correlate with MTC tumor size and cost-effectiveness of calcitonin screening may depend upon the size of the nodule, as well as the dollar cost of the assay and the number of times that the measurement might have to be repeated in serial follow-up [78]. In patients with proven MTC, preoperative calcitonin levels have been shown to correlate with prognosis [79]. Measurement of calcitonin in washout fluid of aspirates of thyroid nodules or lymph nodes may be useful for diagnosis [80–82].

Fine-Needle Aspiration

The single best preoperative method to identify a malignant thyroid nodule is to obtain cells from the nodule for cytopathologic examination by a FNA technique [83–87]. FNA with a 22–25 gauge needle provides the highest rate of successful sampling and the lowest rate of complications while yielding diagnostic precision that is equal or superior to other methods [1, 5]. Both the collection technique and availability of a skilled cytopathologist are critical to the adequate collection and interpretation of a specimen. As a result, the best success is achieved when both the operator and pathologist have considerable, continuous experience; false-negatives should average only 1 % and false-positives 2 % or less. It should be emphasized that the material obtained by FNA constitutes only cells for cytologic examination and consequently does not represent a tissue biopsy. True core needle biopsy of thyroid nodules for tissue is still done in some centers with reportedly higher yields than FNA [88] but is likely to have significantly more morbidity.

Authoritative cytopathologists indicate that adequacy for cytologic interpretation of a FNA requires the presence of at least six groups of follicular cells, each group of which may have 10–15 cells. When insufficient material is obtained, several reports have indicated that to then perform FNA under ultrasound guidance will be associated with a higher yield of satisfactory specimens, thereby enabling improved diagnostic accuracy [89, 90], and this is consistent with ATA guidelines [7].

The greatest likelihood of malignancy is seen in older men with nodules >3–4 cm whereas young women with smaller nodules have a much lower risk. In general, approximately 5–10 % of aspirates may be clearly malignant, 65–70 % clearly benign, 10–20 % indeterminate, and 10–15 % inadequate for diagnosis and may require subsequent re-aspiration. A clearly benign aspirate does not require repeat FNA unless enlargement is noted during subsequent follow-up. The indeterminate group presents a special problem in management to the clinician. The varied cytologic diagnoses that may fall under the indeterminate group include designations such as follicular neoplasm, follicular tumor, atypia of unknown significance, or simply suspicious for malignancy. In the past, the decision has been either to repeat the FNA in 3–4 months if the nodule remains stable in size or to refer these nodules for thyroidectomy.

One risks the possible morbidity of surgical complications versus the failure to identify a malignancy that will be present in up to 50 % of these indeterminate nodules. Very large thyroid nodules of greater than 4 or 5 cm present an increased risk of sampling error by FNA leading to a false-negative diagnosis. Consequently, some authors have suggested that patients with these larger nodules be subjected to lobectomy or subtotal thyroidectomy to obtain more precise diagnosis [91]. However, this was not confirmed in a more recent study [92]. In another recent study, an increase in malignancy was seen in nodules starting at a size of 2 cm. While there was no greater frequency of papillary thyroid carcinoma in nodules >2 cm, the frequency of follicular carcinoma did so increase [93].

A serum TSH should be done prior to surgery to ensure that the TSH is not undetectable which could indicate a hyperfunctioning or autonomous adenoma, in which case the management may differ and a thyroid scan would be indicated. The difficulty inherent in the differential diagnosis between benign lesions like a cellular or follicular adenoma vs. follicular carcinoma or Hurthle cell adenoma vs. Hurthle cell carcinoma relates to the need to visualize capsular or vascular invasion to confirm malignancy, neither of which can be seen in FNA specimens. Prior to the recent availability of more specific molecular mutational analysis (see below) to indicate malignancy, NCCN guidelines [5] recommended thyroidectomy for the patient with a cytologic diagnosis of follicular neoplasm with normal or high serum TSH levels.

Most cytopathologists are currently adhering to guidelines proposed by the National Cancer Institute which have come to be known as the Bethesda Classification System [94–97]. This classification provides a standard nomenclature for indeterminate lesions and a correlation of the cytologic interpretation to the risk of malignancy. In accord with the now fairly universally accepted "Bethesda system" of reporting, the results of a FNA of a thyroid nodule are generally categorized as "nondiagnostic or unsatisfactory," "benign," "malignant," or "indeterminate" with "indeterminate" subdivided into "atypia of undetermined significance or follicular lesion of undetermined significance," "follicular neoplasm or suspicious for follicular neoplasm," and "suspicious for malignancy." The distinctions between these categories are discussed by Drs. Baloch and LiVolsi in the chapter devoted to cytology and pathology. While not fully clarifying the dilemma presented by the indeterminate nodule, the Bethesda guidelines are considered helpful in weighing risk of cancer and relative indication for surgical thyroidectomy. In one study of 197 patients with FNA cytology read as "follicular lesion of undetermined significance" who went to thyroidectomy, the overall incidence of malignancy was 16.2 % with 17 cases (8.6 %) that were follicular carcinoma, 6 cases (3.1 %) that were classic PTC, and 9 cases (4.6 %) that were follicular variant PTC [98].

FNA carries no significant risk, reported cases of tumor seeding in the needle track are exceedingly rare [99] and an infectious complication is also rare [100]. Should an attempt at FNA be unsuccessful, ATA guidelines recommend repeating the procedure under ultrasonographic guidance [4, 7]. Over the past decade, the use of FNA has had a clear salutary effect on the economics of nodule management by reducing the required frequency of surgical thyroidectomy by approximately 50 % and doubling the yield of cancer in those patients undergoing operation [101, 102]. FNA cytologic examination is also applied to the identification of thyroid carcinoma in lymph nodes, and measurement of thyroglobulin in the needle washout [103] or RT-PCR for TSH-receptor and thyroglobulin mRNA [104] may prove useful adjuncts to cytology. When a benign diagnosis is obtained on a nodule by FNA cytology, it is common practice to repeat the FNA in a year or two while monitoring the patient, but in expert hands the original diagnosis is almost always correct [105].

In summary, and consistent with the most recent American Thyroid Association guidelines [7], FNA is the diagnostic procedure of choice for thyroid nodules. The indication for FNA of a given nodule can be based on the ultrasonographic features of the nodule with FNA recommended for any nodule >1 cm with moderate to highly suspicious features and for nodules with minimally suspicious features that are >1.5 cm. Smaller nodules and purely cystic lesions do not require FNA. Having the indication based upon sonographic criteria indicates that the guidelines mandate an initial ultrasound for any patient with a known or suspected thyroid nodule. The guidelines also state that FNA cytology results are to be reported employing the Bethesda classification. Should the interpretation be of "atypia of uncertain significance" (AUS) or "follicular lesion of uncertain significance" (FLUS), the ATA recommendation would be to try to obtain a more specific diagnosis by repeating the FNA and doing mutational testing (see below) if the same AUS/FLUS reading is obtained or alternatively referring to a surgeon for thyroidectomy. Approximately 30–40 % of these FNA's will be AUS/FLUS on the repeat FNA. No immediate further workup is warranted when the FNA cytology is benign, whereas the patient whose cytology is interpreted as indicating malignancy will be referred for thyroidectomy.

Molecular Mutational Analysis

For quite some time, various workers have sought to use cytometric DNA analysis to improve the predictive value of FNA. Although the older methodology employed was not entirely successful in separating benign from malignant disease, it did correlate with the outcome and survival in patients with proven malignancy [106, 107]. Subsequently, a number of biochemical and cellular markers were identified and examined regarding their potential association with malignancy and their potential use to distinguish benign from malignant nodules [106]. These markers are described in greater detail below in Chap. 22 by Xing and in earlier reviews [107–111], and the hope has been that better understanding of the significance of molecular markers would avoid unnecessary surgeries and the attendant potential complications [112]. Perhaps the earliest potential marker studied was Galectin-3 [113], the measurement of which was not recommended for diagnostic purposes in the 2006 guidelines of the American Thyroid Association but was so recommended in the 2009 guidelines [4]. The 2014 guidelines [7] have expanded on the issue of molecular testing given the more recent advances in the field. It is recommended that clinical decisions be based only on molecular analyses performed in approved CLIA- or CAP-certified laboratories and that these tests should be considered when the FNA results are indeterminate (e.g., atypia of uncertain significance (AUS), follicular lesion of uncertain significance (FLUS), follicular neoplasm, suspicious for follicular neoplasm).

The presence of the BRAF V600E mutation of the BRAF gene was found to be linked to papillary thyroid carcinoma over 10 years ago [114] and innumerable studies since have linked this mutation with bilaterality, more aggressive tumor behavior, greater frequency of lymph nodes metastases, and poorer prognosis [115–119]. Nikiforov et al. performed a meta-analysis of 22 reports of 1,117 BRAF+ thyroid nodules indicating that over 99 % were malignant. Notwithstanding these implications of the mutation, one study concluded that surgical approaches to the tumor do not need to be any different [120].

The 2015–2016 ATA guidelines [7] have addressed two of the newest molecular profiling methods with promise to more clearly distinguish between benign and malignant neoplasms [121–129]. With one of these methods, a small portion of the FNA is tested for the common mutations known to be associated with thyroid cancer such as *BRAF* but in addition will also determine *RET/PTC*, *PAX8/PPARγ*, and *RAS*. When these mutations are found, there is a very high likelihood of malignancy, but other cancers can be missed when these specific markers are not present. Other approaches have employed mRNA expression analysis to classify risk in FNA's on a genomic basis or in proteomic analysis using microRNAs for diagnosis [130–135] or to predict progression or indicate therapy for a given tumor [136, 137].

As this volume goes to press, the two molecular analyses of fine-needle aspirates that are commercially available are the miRinform molecular mutational panel offered by Asuragen, Inc., and the Afirma gene expression classifier offered by Veracyte, Inc. A third, and arguably more comprehensive analysis is provided by the so-called ThyroSeq assay [138] that reports a panel analyzed for point mutations in 14 genes and 42 types of gene fusions known to occur in thyroid carcinoma. The Afirma method is a multigene expression classifier (GEP) performed on mRNA from cells in the aspirate that compares the sample to over 160 known genes reflecting benign cytologies and provides a report that can indicate that the nodule is considered benign with approximately 95 % negative predictive value (NPV), 38 % positive predictive value (PPV), and 92 % sensitivity given a frequency of carcinoma of about 25 % [139]. A test result for an AUS/FLUS lesion read as "negative" would reduce the likelihood of cancer from about 24 % to 5 % and implies that the patient could be followed without surgical intervention. The test has been validated in some preliminary subsequent trials [140, 141]. The high NPV implies that surgeries can now be avoided in those patients with indeterminate nodules on FNA who previously had to undergo thyroidectomy in order to obtain a definitive tissue diagnosis [140, 142]. Employing the mutational panel testing for BRAF, RET/PTC, RAS, etc., will indicate malignancy in 20–40 % of FNA samples with about an 85–90 % PPV, but there is still a remaining risk of cancer of 10–15 %. When positive, mutational testing on the FNA material is helpful to guide the surgical approach and indicate that a total rather than a lesser thyroidectomy should be performed. These tests are currently quite expensive but should be looked upon as potentially cost saving in terms of the avoidance of surgery or at least the avoidance of a two-stage thyroidectomy. For this reason, molecular testing with either mutational analysis [143] or with the gene expression classifier [125] has been declared cost-effective. When the nodule cytology is interpreted to be "suspicious," mutational analysis can help define the relative risk of malignancy and guide the choice for surgery. Thus, when the mutational analysis is negative, there is a 25–30 % risk of cancer and such nodules should be referred for thyroidectomy irrespective of the results of either mutational analysis or the gene expression classifier. The thyroidectomy could be either a subtotal or total, perhaps subtotal being acceptable with negative mutational analysis and/or based on strong patient preference and the absence of other risk factors.

RAS is another common mutation found in nodules with indeterminate cytology and one recent study found that such nodules have a high risk for cancer, typically lack suspicious ultrasonographic features, and are more likely to be low-grade follicular variants of papillary thyroid carcinoma [144]. The recent ATA guidelines [7] suggest that a test with high NPV and sensitivity might be employed best in those patients for whom we want to avoid surgery. Earlier, a working committee of the ATA had described the pros and cons as to which method to have performed on a given indeterminate FNA and urged caution in the use of these analyses until more evidence-based data are available [145]. It is highly likely that other molecular markers will be developed and the cost of these analyses should fall in the future. Another marker of peripheral serum RNA is the assay for TSH mRNA but with only limited data on its utility to date.

Thyroid Scanning

Specific aspects of radionuclide scanning are described in depth in various chapters (see Index), and this section serves only as an introduction to these procedures as they are applied to the initial evaluation of a thyroid nodule. Notably, scans reveal little about nodule size or shape and instead find their greatest utility in describing the functional state of a nodule. The majority of thyroid adenomas and carcinomas have defects in iodide accumulation and/or organification. Such defects can be demonstrated by images consistent with focal reduction in isotope accumulation (reduced trapping of radionuclide), leading to the designation of a "cold" nodule. On radionuclide scanning, about 5 % of nodules are found to be "hot" (hyperfunctioning), 10 % are "warm" (normal functioning), and 84 % are "cold" (nonfunctioning).

The Hyperfunctioning ("Hot") Thyroid Nodule

A thyroid scan is useful in identifying hyperfunctioning nodules in patients with symptoms of hyperthyroidism, suppressed TSH levels, or biopsy results suggestive of follicular neoplasm. Hot nodules rarely represent malignancy, warm nodules carry an intermediate risk of about 5 %, and cold nodules, although with the highest risk [1, 3, 99] of malignancy, still represent benign pathology in more than 80 % of cases. Therefore, radioisotopic scans are of low specificity despite their high sensitivity for nodules over 1 cm in diameter. Scanning is usually done with ^{123}I, ^{131}I, or ^{99}mTc pertechnetate (often referred to as "technetium scans"). Regardless of some limitations, the qualities of low-radiation dose, low cost, short-scanning interval, and reliability of hypofunctioning scans have led to the continued use of Tc at many centers. ^{123}I also delivers lower radiation than ^{131}I and is the preferred iodine-scanning agent but is not universally employed primarily because of its brief half-life (12 h) and the higher cost associated with its use. Although hyperfunctioning nodules are usually benign, caution had been suggested with the assumption that this is always the case in children [146]. In addition to functional information, scans may reveal evidence of multinodularity in up to one third of clinically palpable solitary lesions—a finding that has been thought to be associated with a decreased risk of malignancy, at least in the past. Some recent studies still support this perspective [147], but the majority of studies (particularly those that have utilized ultrasound to detect additional nodules) have demonstrated no difference in the frequency of malignancy in patients with single vs. multiple nodules [45, 148, 149] or in fact a greater likelihood of malignancy in multinodular glands [38].

With the finding of multiple nodules, the question arises as to which nodule or nodules to subject to FNA for cytologic examination. The 2014 and 2009 ATA guideline on this issue have not changed since the 2006 ATA guidelines and recommend FNA of any nodule with suspicious findings on ultrasonography, and if no suspicious characteristics are noted to, then do FNA on the largest of the nodules identified. Note, however, that thyroid cancer can arise in multiple foci within the gland as either independent tumors or on a monoclonal basis [150, 151].

A recent vogue in Europe, which is yet to gain wide popularity in the United States, is the percutaneous injection of 95 % ethanol into thyroid nodules and, in this case, specifically into a hyperfunctioning nodule [152, 153]. This therapeutic approach has also been applied to benign thyroid cysts after aspiration, as well as to cold nodules proven initially to be benign by FNA. The procedure can be painful for the patient and has been associated with transient increases in serum thyroglobulin and thyroid hormones with self-limited thyrotoxicosis. Fever, local pain and hematoma, and vocal cord paralysis are also possible complications with inexperienced physicians. Although it has been claimed that no serious side effects of ethanol ablation have occurred, there is one case reported of fairly dramatic toxic necrosis of the larynx and overlying skin [154, 155]. Ultrasound-guided laser photocoagulation has also been employed for ablation of both hyperfunctioning [156] and cold thyroid nodules [157], as well as for small nodules proven on FNA to be papillary carcinoma in patients who are not deemed candidates for surgical thyroidectomy [158].

The frequency of cancer within a hyperfunctioning nodule has been estimated to be 0.34 % based upon one series of 296 patients [157]. While this cancer occurrence rate is clearly low, one advantage of management of the hot nodule by surgical excision (usually lobectomy) is the acquisition of a definitive histopathologic diagnosis, which would be lacking with management by radioiodine therapy or ethanol injection. Nevertheless, surgery is infrequently recommended for hyperfunctioning nodules because of its associated risks, the low incidence of cancer, and the proven efficacy and low morbidity of radioiodine therapy. One exception may be those very large (>4 cm diameter) hot nodules for which the required ablative dose of radioiodine is so great that it increases the risk of subsequent radiation-induced neoplasia in the contralateral lobe.

The differential diagnosis for thyroid pain is quite short and includes thyroiditis, hemorrhage, and thyroid cancer. Hemorrhagic necrosis, heralded by pain, may occur during the natural history of a hyperfunctioning adenoma. With infarction of the hyperfunctioning nodule, the subsequent loss of the existing hyperfunction leads to reduced TSH suppression, return of TSH levels to normal with time, and resumption of function in the previously suppressed extranodular thyroid tissue. The previously hyperfunctioning nodule may then appear cold on scintiscanning, which taken together with the history of pain could be misinterpreted to represent a carcinoma. The functional state of a solitary autonomous nodule may not be sufficiently active to cause hyperthyroidism. Such patients will be euthyroid and have measurable levels of TSH and will appear as a hot nodule on the scan but with visible extranodular uptake of radionuclide. Hot nodules often enlarge with time, and there is a correlation of size with associated hyperthyroidism with approximately 4 % of patients per year developing thyrotoxicosis [159].

Other Scanning Modalities

Although no longer available at most centers, fluorescent thyroid scanning offers special advantages in childhood and pregnancy owing to minimal radiation exposure. The procedure has been reported as nearly 100 % sensitive but only 64 % specific when cold areas are taken to represent positive results. The procedure employs ^{241}Am, which has the ability to excite thyroid iodine, causing release of X-rays that quantitatively correlate with iodine content of the imaged tissue. The required equipment is not widely available, and accumulated data remain too limited to recommend standard use of this technique.

A variety of other scanning techniques, including ^{99}mTc-SestaMIBI [160], ^{201}Tl [161–165], ^{75}Sel, ^{67}Ga, and ^{131}Cs, have been investigated, and none have been proven to be reliable indicators of malignancy [166, 167]. ^{131}I metaiodobenzylguanidine has been used successfully to image medullary carcinoma of the thyroid [168]. Fluorodeoxyglucose-positron emission tomography (PET) scanning has an important role in the follow-up of patients with thyroid cancer and, although not routinely recommended, has also been used earlier in the preoperative evaluation of thyroid nodules [169]. The significance of PET positivity of a thyroid nodule is discussed below.

Ultrasonography

A full discussion of thyroid ultrasound appears in Chap. 40 by Hegedus, and the utility of this diagnostic modality to determine which thyroid nodules might be malignant has been well described [170–175]. With the refinement of equipment, low cost, absence of radiation exposure, and the more universal office-based application of ultrasound, it has become arguably the most useful and important imaging technique for disorders of the thyroid gland. Ultrasonographic characteristics suggestive of malignancy in a thyroid nodule include: hypoechogenicity, microcalcifications, a speculated nodule margin, and a taller than wide shape and absence of halo [176, 177]. The presence of these characteristics, especially microcalcifications, together with BRAF^{v600e} positivity can be highly suggestive of malignancy [177, 178]. Similarly, ultrasound characteristics suggestive of a benign process, such as isogenicity and a spongiform appearance, may allow deferral of fine-needle aspiration [179].

One putative problem with ultrasound is its increasing sensitivity, with the ability to delineate nodules as small as 1 mm [180]. This sensitivity raises the management problem of what to do with such little nodules, especially when found incidentally during an ultrasound study for some other purpose ("incidentalomas"), as discussed below. Although the field of view is characteristically small with conventional ultrasound, newer approaches have employed computerized modifications that allow panoramic images of the entire thyroid gland [181]. Elastography applied to ultrasound is a technique that has been around for some time but has only recently been enjoying increasing application to the determination of malignancy in thyroid nodules. The procedure consists of applying a probe with slight pressure on the nodule to gain a measure of the elasticity of the nodule. A color scale assigns red to greater elasticity which correlates with benignity, whereas nodules displaying the lowest elasticity are indicated as blue and are most likely to represent cancer [182–185]. The validity of the method in predicting malignancy is reduced by certain ultrasonographic features of a given nodule such as underlying Hashimoto's disease as well as operator variability. Some workers have employed a "strain index" as the ratio of measured nodule strain to the strain of the most normal or softest extranodular thyroid tissue. In skilled hands, the strain index can provide a negative predictive value indicative of a benign lesion that could preclude the likelihood of thyroid cancer and the need for fine-needle aspiration cytology [186].

In contrast to radioisotopic-scanning techniques, ultrasound enables guidance for FNA, thereby improving diagnos-

Table 20.3 Potential utility of ultrasonography of thyroid nodules

Differentiation of solid vs. cystic consistency
Detection of multinodularity
Detection of occult thyroid malignancy in cases of metastatic cervical lymphadenopathy from unknown primary
Monitoring nodule size, including response to suppressive therapy
Determination of solid vs. hemorrhagic expansion in thyroid lesions showing rapid increase in size
Guidance for needle aspiration cytology in selected difficult cases
Guidance for therapy with ethanol or laser photocoagulation
(?) Monitoring irradiated thyroids
(?) Monitoring for local recurrence of thyroid carcinoma

tic yield and accuracy [89, 90, 148, 149, 187–191] or guidance for therapeutic ablative therapy [156, 192, 193] (Table 20.3). Some workers have characterized the blood flow within nodules by color Doppler ultrasonography to distinguish between benign and malignant follicular neoplasms [194]. In the case of nodules that are purely cystic lesions, neither the ATA [4, 7] nor the NCCN guidelines [5] mandate FNA cytology in view of the low likelihood of malignancy of 5 % or less in these pure cysts. Some series of patients indicate that only 5 % of even partially cystic nodules may be malignant but advise that the presence of microcalcifications further increases the risk of cancer [195]. The ATA guidelines [7] recommend preoperative ultrasonography of the contralateral lobe and lateral node compartments for nodules positive or highly suspicious for carcinoma, as well as consideration for FNA of any suspicious-appearing lymph nodes seen on ultrasound. When there is suspicion of more advanced disease that could involve deeper structures in the neck, the guidelines recommend cross-sectional imaging with CT or MRI, but PET/CT is not recommended.

Thyroid Incidentaloma

Thyroid nodules discovered during routine imaging for other purposes have been termed "incidentalomas" if less than 1.5 cm in size. Because of the presumed rare occurrence of carcinoma in these small tumors, FNA with cytology has generally not been recommended for nodules of less than 1 cm; rather, it has been suggested that prudent follow-up by ultrasound examination was sufficient and more cost-effective [196]. However, opinions on this subject have since evolved [197] in view of recent literature describing early detection of malignancy in incidentalomas with PET scanning [198–202] and studies implying that the frequency of malignancy in small lesions is no different than that in nodules greater than 1.5 cm [174, 187, 199, 200]. High standardized uptake values (SUV) on the PET scan appear to correlate well with the likelihood of malignancy and may prove useful to guide management in the future, specifically to determine which incidentalomas to biopsy [199, 200]. Those tumors that are FDG-PET positive are likely to be more aggressive and consequently demand further investigation [203]. Other workers have found no significant difference in SUV values on FDG-PET scanning between benign and malignant nodules and suggest that this diagnostic modality is of limited value for differential diagnosis preoperatively [204]. FDG-PET uptake can be either diffuse or focal, the diffuse type suggesting underlying Hashimoto's disease and not thyroid cancer. Approximately a third of PET positive thyroid nodules will prove to be malignant [205]. The ATA guidelines [4, 7] do not recommend preoperative FDG-PET scanning as part of an initial evaluation. However, when the "incidentaloma" finding appeared on a PET scan done for another purpose, the guidelines suggest that nodules with SUV of 3 or less are likely benign, and greater concern would apply to those with SUV of >6. Hence, FNA is recommended in nodules confirmed on ultrasound that have significant PET positivity.

Based on ultrasonographic criteria, the features of greatest concern that indicate possible cancer are a solid or hypoechoic appearance, irregular or blurred margins, intranodular vascularity on Doppler, a taller than wide shape [206], and microcalcifications [174, 207]. The "spongiform" nodule on ultrasound is so-called because of the appearance on ultrasound of cystic or lacunar spaces over more than 50 % of the nodule. Such nodules are almost always benign, and the ATA guidelines [4, 7] indicate that FNA could be deferred with these findings, although the NCCN guidelines [5] recommend considering FNA when the spongiform nodule is >2 cm in size. Other features that would indicate further evaluation of an incidentaloma include a history of irradiation to the head and neck, the presence of cervical lymphadenopathy, or a history of thyroid cancer in a first-degree relative. Based on their review of the literature, Silver and Parangi [208] recommended FNA of all incidentalomas seen on ultrasound that measure between 8 and 15 mm, when at least one of the telltale ultrasound features is present. On the other hand, Mazzaferri and Sipos [209] did not recommend FNA of nodules smaller than 5 mm because of the likelihood of obtaining an inadequate sample and instead suggested monitoring for increase in size by periodic ultrasonography.

The finding of medullary thyroid cancer in an incidentaloma represents yet another unique clinical problem. Some of these patients have had only subtotal thyroidectomy, raising the question of whether complete thyroidectomy is necessary for a small medullary tumor. Fortunately, many of these patients may do well with conservative management and close follow-up [210]. The risk of malignancy in incidentalomas is discussed further in Chap. 29 on papillary thyroid cancer. The ATA guidelines [4, 7] largely dismiss the incidentalomas of <0.7 cm because of the low cost/benefit ratio of a full evaluation unless some of the suspicious characteristics that are associated with greater risk of cancer are present on ultrasonography.

Thyroid Hormone Suppression

Thyroid hormone had been used for many years to reduce the size of thyroid lesions thought to be dependent on TSH stimulation. As a diagnostic test, the assumption is that benign lesions will show preferential reduction in size while malignant nodules, being autonomous, will grow. Typically, patients were given a 3–6-month trial of L-thyroxine at a dose titrated to result in TSH suppression to, or slightly below, the lower limit of a normal in a sensitive TSH assay. The presumption is that growth of a nodule or lack of reduction in size during such therapy suggests malignancy. This notion has been significantly challenged by the observations that even benign nodules grow with time [211, 212]. A greater than 75 % reduction in size on L-thyroxine therapy likely occurs in only 5–10 % of cases, whereas a 50 % decline in size has been reported in an average of 30 % of cases [1, 5]. Generally, those nodules that shrink with thyroxine suppression tend to enlarge again if therapy is withdrawn [213, 214].

The controversy regarding whether to treat a nodule proven to be benign by FNA with thyroid hormone has been discussed [21, 22, 215–217]. Numerous trials of suppressive therapy have variably met with failure or success [215, 218–223] compared to placebo [224–226], and there may be certain nodule cytologic characteristics that predict responsiveness [227]. Overall, long-term benefits of suppressive therapy may not be significant [226]. Most clinical thyroidologists tend to no longer recommend suppressive therapy with levothyroxine and the ATA guidelines recommend against it [4, 7]. Others feel that more carefully controlled studies of large patient populations are required to clarify whether there might still be a role for suppression therapy of proven benign thyroid nodules. The increasing concern about the possible risk of osteopenia after long-term suppressive doses of thyroid hormone has been somewhat allayed by careful analyses of the data [228]. Use of prudent suppression doses of thyroxine has not been shown to contribute to osteopenia [229] and low-dose TSH suppression has been shown to have as comparable a salutary effect on nodule size as higher dose TSH suppression in some [230], but not all [226], studies.

A trial of thyroid hormone suppression is neither sensitive nor specific and, although not recommended, may have utility as an adjunct to other modalities of evaluation. In addition, suppressive therapy may have benefit in preventing the development of additional nodules. In a study examining recurrence rates for thyroid nodules after partial surgical thyroidectomy for benign disease in patients with a previous history of radiation, treatment with thyroid hormone postoperatively decreased the risk of benign recurrence from 36 % to 8.4 % [231].

Some patients given thyroxine may have concomitant underlying autoimmune thyroid disease and/or other hyperfunctioning nonsuppressible nodules, in addition to the cold nodule being treated. These patients may require less levothyroxine because of the presence of functioning tissue that complements the exogenously administered hormone. An approximate suppressive dosage is 1.7 μg/kg body weight per day [232], which usually results in a serum T4 at, or somewhat above, the upper limit of the normal range. The dose is incremented by 0.025 mg/day every 5–6 weeks with TSH monitoring until the desired degree of TSH suppression is observed. Nodules are assessed for change in size by physical examination every 6 weeks for the first 6 months (or less frequently by ultrasound if required). The follow-up intervals may be more prolonged when significant decreases in size are observed, eventually extending to annual follow-up. Because of its long half-life, levothyroxine is administered as a single daily dose. Although the serum T3 may be superior to the serum T4 as an indicator of the metabolic state in the patient receiving levothyroxine, the optimal dose is best determined by clinical criteria and measurement of serum TSH by an ultrasensitive assay. An elevated serum TSH indicates that treatment is insufficient, and an elevated serum T3 demonstrates that it is excessive. A decrease in dosage may be required with progressive emergence of autonomy and hyperfunction in a uninodular or multinodular goiter. In the setting of autonomous nodules, exposure to a high-iodine source may lead to clinical thyrotoxicosis. FNA biopsy should be repeated immediately when a "cold" nodule enlarges during suppressive therapy, and surgical exploration should be considered inevitable unless cystic fluid or hemorrhage with benign cytology is obtained. FNA should also be repeated when there is a failure to achieve a significant reduction in nodule size after 6–12 months of suppressive therapy. With failure of suppression to achieve size reduction, levothyroxine therapy should be discontinued.

Summary: Approach to the Thyroid Nodule

The majority of thyroid nodules will be follicular adenomas, which are benign tumors that may occur singly or in multiples and may mimic normal thyroid function, trapping iodide and producing thyroid hormones. On a radionuclide scan, they may be nonfunctional (cold), normally functional (warm), or hyperfunctioning (hot). Hot nodules are almost always benign. Hot nodules that cause hyperthyroidism are treated with radioiodine or surgery, whereas euthyroid patients with hot nodules may be followed without therapy, advised to avoid iodine excess, and monitored periodically with thyroid function tests. Other common benign nodules include colloid adenomas or cysts.

Concern should be raised that a thyroid nodule may be malignant in patients with a history of irradiation to the neck in childhood, associated cervical lymphadenopathy, a family history of thyroid cancer or pheochromocytoma, or recent or rapid nodule enlargement. Symptoms and signs that may be more suggestive of a malignant nodule include odynophagia, pain or pressure (compressive symptoms), vocal cord paralysis, or superior vena caval syndrome. Routine laboratory tests do not distinguish between benign and malignant nodules, and FNA for cytology is the initial procedure of choice [83–86, 233]. Molecular analytical techniques to improve diagnosis of carcinoma in suspicious aspirates have been developed, such as the detection of BRAF and other mutations in aspirates by polymerase chain reaction-restriction fragment length polymorphism analysis [234, 235] and detection of Galectin-3 [103] and other markers. In the near future, molecular analysis is certain to assume a routine role in management, specifically for clarifying the nature of nodules with indeterminate cytology, with the increasing availability and reduced cost and popularity of these assays. The Afirma test with its high NPV and sensitivity will be employed best in those patients for whom we want to avoid surgery, while the miRiform mutational analysis will prove most useful when there is higher suspicion for malignancy and the clinician and/or patient favors surgical intervention.

Ultrasound for sizing, detection of cystic components, and evaluation for characteristics suggestive of cancer is essential to the evaluation and likely to be beneficial, and a scintiscan to confirm a hyperfunctional state is useful when TSH is very low or undetectable. Thyroxine suppression therapy is rarely recommended today, although cysts or colloid adenomas demonstrated to be benign on FNA may have their size reduced with levothyroxine therapy by as much as 40–50 %. L-T4 treatment is not an alternative to appropriate diagnostic evaluation to include ultrasonography and fine-needle aspiration cytology and is contraindicated for autonomous hyperfunctioning adenomata.

The clinical challenge in thyroid nodule management is the formulation of the most accurate and cost-effective diagnostic protocol. Figure 20.1 suggests an algorithm that may be useful in a practice where FNA is frequently utilized with experienced cytopathology support. Use of radionuclide scans as the initial step may result in increased cost, as only 5–10 % of scans obviate the need for aspiration, whereas 60–80 % of FNAs eliminate scan requirements. Most investigators place a greater emphasis on the role of ultrasonography in the evaluation of patients with nodules [236], and a spherical shape of nodules has been shown to be highly associated with malignancy [237] as has a taller than wide shape [206]. Sonography also may permit identification of other nodules than the dominant nodule felt on palpation, as well as disclosing the presence of metastatic disease in lymph nodes preoperatively. The ATA guidelines [4, 7] recommend serial follow-up by ultrasound for nodules >1 cm that were proven benign by FNA cytology, with the frequency of repeat ultrasounds being reduced with each passing year assuming stability of nodule size. The 2014 guidelines recommend that long-term follow-up for benign nodules be based on ultrasonographic criteria. A repeat ultrasound with FNA is recommended in 6–12 months for those nodules >5 mm with a more suspicious initial appearance on ultrasound, while those nodules with a less suspicious appearance may wait 18–24 months for repeat ultrasound and FNA. Moreover, a 50 % increase in volume or a 20 % increase in two dimensions on a follow-up ultrasound would also warrant repeat FNA for cytology. Finally, routine sonographic follow-up in deemed unnecessary for nodules <5 mm and those >5 mm that have had no change in size documented over the course of 24-month follow-up with confirmation of negative cytology for malignancy. While real-time elastography was indicated in one study to be useful for decisions

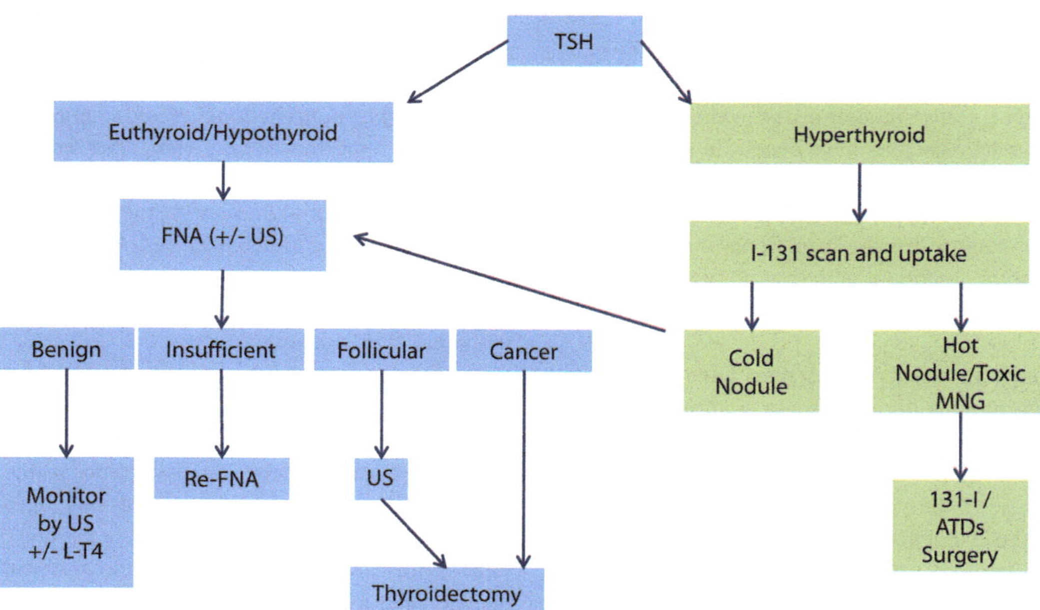

Fig. 20.1 Suggested algorithm for diagnosis and management of thyroid nodules, starting with serum TSH level

for operative intervention on the thyroid nodule with indeterminate cytology [181], this was not confirmed in a subsequent study [238].

For patients with proven benign nodules, a trial of levothyroxine suppressive therapy may be attempted but is not recommended by ATA guidelines or most clinicians. Adequate TSH suppression is usually achieved at a dose of approx 1.7 μg/kg. Patients may be started on lower doses based on age and potential underlying cardiovascular disease, with patient reevaluations within 6 weeks to monitor for symptoms of hyperthyroidism and to evaluate serum TSH levels. Starting from the initial dose, the dose is then incremented by 0.025 mg every 6 weeks until the desired degree of TSH is achieved, unless the patient has symptoms that require lowering the thyroxine dose. Nodules should be assessed for change in size every 2 months for the first 6 months. If the nodule significantly decreases in size, follow-up intervals may be gradually prolonged, with eventual annual follow-up. A strong argument against long-term suppressive thyroxine therapy relates to the risks of adverse effects on bone density and the heart. Thyroxine therapy is discontinued and FNA may be repeated when nodules fail to respond to thyroxine suppression after 6–12 months and sooner for any nodule that seems to be enlarging. Of repeat FNAs, 98 % confirm the original diagnosis [137].

Patients with a history of irradiation present a special situation. Historically, these patients have been immediately referred to surgery because of their higher likelihood of cancer. Some clinicians now advocate FNA in the management of these patients as well, but sufficient evidence for reliability of benign results is still lacking owing to the frequent coexistence of both benign and malignant nodules [239]. When surgical therapy is recommended, the choice of procedure will vary related to the clinical situation. While a total thyroidectomy will be preferred when there is a history of external radiation, an ipsilateral lobectomy and isthmusectomy is a common approach in the absence of a radiation history for single nodules where the preoperative diagnosis is uncertain (see Chap. 26). Frequently, intraoperative frozen-section histologic evaluation is inconclusive or unreliable, and final diagnosis requires careful examination of permanent sections [240]. Many papillary carcinomas have multicentric growth, with tumor foci in the contralateral lobe in 30–82 % of cases [241]. In questionable diagnostic cases, gene profiling of surgical thyroid tissue may distinguish benign follicular adenoma from carcinoma [107, 242]. Accordingly, when the ultimate diagnosis is carcinoma, it is customary to complete a near-total thyroidectomy within 1 week of the first surgery. Studies have not shown any differences in survival or recurrence rates between total and near-total thyroidectomy, as well as greater morbidity associated with total thyroidectomy [243]. Inspection of regional lymph nodes with excision of suspicious nodes should also be conducted in all cases of thyroid cancer. Near-total thyroidectomy is the initial preferred procedure in patients with thyroid nodules and a history of thyroid irradiation because of the high incidence (54–75 %) of bilateral disease [243]. Nonsurgical approaches to ablation of benign nodules have been employed in some medical centers [244–246].

References

1. Gharib H, Papini E. Thyroid nodules: clinical importance, assessment, and treatment. Endocrinol Metab Clin N Am. 2007;36:707–35.
2. Iyer NG, Shaha AR. Management of thyroid nodules and surgery for differentiated thyroid cancer. Clin Oncol. 2010;22:405–12.
3. Miller MC. The patient with a thyroid nodule. Med Clin N Am. 2010;94:1003–15.
4. Cooper DS, Doherty GM, Haugen BR, Kloos RT, Lee SL, Mandel SJ, Mazzaferri EL, et al. Revised American Thyroid Association Management Guidelines for patients with thyroid nodules and differentiated thyroid cancer. Thyroid. 2009;19:1167–214.
5. National Comprehensive Cancer Network (NCCN) Thyroid carcinoma: clinical practice guidelines 2011. J Natl Compr Cancer Netw; Version 3.2011.
6. Wartofsky L. Highlights of the American Thyroid Association Guidelines for patients with thyroid nodules or differentiated thyroid cancer. Thyroid. 2009;19:1139–43.
7. Haugen BR, Alexander EK, Bible KC, Doherty GM, Mandel SJ, Nikiforov Y, et al. American Thyroid Association Management Guidelines for patients with thyroid nodules and differentiated thyroid cancer. Thyroid 25: doi:10.1089/thy.2015.0020. Print version in Thyroid 26:2016. (in Press).
8. Stagnaro-Green A, Abalovich M, Alexander E, Azizi F, Mestman J, Negro R, et al. Guidelines of the American Thyroid Association for the diagnosis and management of thyroid disease during pregnancy and postpartum. Thyroid. 2011;21:1081–125.
9. Davies L, Welch HG. Increasing incidence of thyroid cancer in the United States, 1973–2002. JAMA. 2006;295:2164–7.
10. Ito Y, Nikiforov YE, Schlumberger M, Vigneri R. Increasing incidence of thyroid cancer: controversies explored. Nat Rev Endocrinol. 2013;9:178–84.
11. Chen AY, Jemal A, Ward EM. Increasing incidence of differentiated thyroid cancer in the United States, 1988–2005. Cancer. 2009;115:3801–7.
12. Erewold L, Zhu K, Ron E, et al. Rising thyroid cancer incidence in the United States by demographic and tumor characteristics, 1980–2005. Cancer Epidemiol Biomarkers Prev. 2009;18:784–91.
13. Cramer JD, Fu P, Harth KC, et al. Analysis of the rising incidence of thyroid cancer using the surveillance, epidemiology and end results national cancer data registry. Surgery. 2010;148:1147–52.
14. Tunbridge WMG, Evered DC, Hall R, et al. The spectrum of thyroid disease in a community: the Wickham survey. Clin Endocrinol. 1977;7:481–93.
15. Gupta A, Ly S, Castroneves LA, Frates MC, Benson CB, Feldman HA, et al. A standardized assessment of thyroid nodules in children confirms higher cancer prevalence than in adults. J Clin Endocrinol Metab. 2013;98:3238–45.
16. Vander JB, Gaston EA, Dawber TR. The significance of nontoxic thyroid nodules: final report of a 15-year study on the incidence of thyroid malignancy. Ann Intern Med. 1968;69:537–40.
17. Hopkins CR, Reading CC. Thyroid and parathyroid imaging. Semin Ultrasound CT MR. 1995;16:279–95.
18. Horlocker TT, Hay JE, James EM. Prevalence of incidental nodular thyroid disease detected during high resolution parathyroid

ultrasonography. In: Medeiros-Neto G, Gaitan E, editors. Frontiers in thyroidology, vol. 1. New York: Plenum Press; 1986. p. 1309–12.
19. Brander A, Viikinkoski P, Nickels J, Kivisaari L. Thyroid gland: ultrasound screening in a random adult population. Radiology. 1991;181:683–7.
20. Burrow GN. The thyroid: nodules and neoplasia. In: Felig P, Baxter JD, Broadus AE, Frohman LA, editors. Endocrinology and metabolism. New York: McGraw-Hill; 1987. p. 473–507.
21. Richter B, Neises G, Clar C. Pharmacotherapy for thyroid nodules: a systematic review and meta-analysis. Endocrinol Metab Clin N Am. 2002;31:699–722.
22. Hegedus L, Bonnema SJ, Bennedback FN. Management of simple nodular goiter: current status and future perspectives. Endocr Rev. 2003;24:102–32.
23. Mazzaferri EL, Young RL, Oertel JE, et al. Papillary thyroid carcinoma: the impact of therapy in 576 patients. Medicine. 1977;56:171–96.
24. Hovens GC, Stokkel MP, Kievit J, Corssmit EP, Pereira AM, Romijn JA, Smit JWA. Associations of serum thyrotropin concentrations with recurrence and death in differentiated thyroid cancer. J Clin Endocrinol Metab. 2007;92:2610–5.
25. Derwahl M, Broecker M, Kraiem Z. Thyrotropin may not be the dominant growth factor in benign and malignant thyroid nodules. J Clin Endocrinol Metab. 1999;84:829–34.
26. Boelaert K, Horacek J, Holder RL, Watkinson JC, Sheppard MC, Franklyn JA. Serum thyrotropin concentration as a novel predictor of malignancy in thyroid nodules investigated by fine-needle aspiration. J Clin Endocrinol Metab. 2006;91:4295–301.
27. Jin J, Machekano R, McHenry CR. The utility of preoperative serum thyroid-stimulating hormone level for predicting malignant nodular thyroid disease. Am J Surg. 2010;199:294–7.
28. Jonklaas J, Nsouli-Maktabi H, Soldin SJ. Endogenous thyrotropin and triiodothyronine concentrations in individuals with thyroid cancer. Thyroid. 2008;18:943–52.
29. Haymart MR, Repplinger DJ, Leverson GE, Elson DF, Sippel RS, Jaume JC, Chen H. Higher serum thyroid stimulating hormone level in thyroid nodule patients is associated with greater risks of differentiated thyroid cancer and advanced tumor stage. J Clin Endocrinol Metab. 2008;93:809–14.
30. Sarne D, Schneider AB. External radiation and thyroid neoplasia. Endocrinol Metab Clin N Am. 1996;25:181–96.
31. Ron E, Kleinerman RE, Boice Jr JD, et al. A population-based case-control study of thyroid cancer. J Natl Cancer Inst. 1987;79:1–12.
32. Favus MJ, Schneider AB, Stachura ME, et al. Thyroid cancer occurring as a late consequence of head-and-neck irradiation. N Engl J Med. 1976;294:1019–25.
33. DeGroot LJ, Reilly M, Pinnameneni K, Refetoff S. Retrospective and prospective study of radiation-induced thyroid disease. Am J Med. 1983;74:852–62.
34. Cardis R, Kesminiene A, Ivanov V, et al. Risk of thyroid cancer after exposure to 131-I in childhood. J Natl Cancer Inst. 2005;97:724–32.
35. Boice JD. Radiation-induced thyroid cancer—what's new? J Natl Cancer Inst. 2005;97:703–5.
36. Imaizumi M, Usa T, Tominaga T, et al. Long-term prognosis of thyroid nodule cases compared with nodule-free controls in atomic bomb survivors. J Clin Endocrinol Metab. 2005;90:5009–14.
37. Mihailescu DV, Schneider AB. Size, number, and distribution of thyroid nodules and the risk of malignancy in radiation-exposed patients who underwent surgery. J Clin Endocrinol Metab. 2008;93:2188–93.
38. Castro MR, Espiritu RP, Bahn RS, Henry MR, Gharib H, Caraballo PJ, Morris JC. Predictors of malignancy in patients with cytologically suspicious thyroid nodules. Thyroid. 2011;21:1191–8.
39. Brito JP, Yarur AJ, Prokop LJ, McIver B, Murad MH, Montori VM. Prevalence of thyroid cancer in multinodular goiter versus single nodule: a systematic review and meta-analysis. Thyroid. 2013;23:449–55.
40. Hamburger JI. The autonomously functioning thyroid nodule: Goetsch's disease. Endocr Rev. 1987;8:439–47.
41. Siegel R, Naishadham D, Jemal A. Cancer statistics, 2013. CA Cancer J Clin. 2013;63(1):11–30.
42. Sampson RJ, Woolner LB, Bahn RC. Occult thyroid carcinoma in Olmsted County, Minnesota. Prevalence at autopsy compared with that in Hiroshima and Nagasaki. Cancer. 1974;34:2070–6.
43. Sampson RJ. Prevalence and significance of occult thyroid cancer. In: DeGroot LJ, Frohman LA, Kaplan EL, Refetoff S, editors. Radiation-associated thyroid carcinoma. New York: Grune & Stratton; 1977. p. 137–43.
44. Richards ML. Familial syndromes associated with thyroid cancer in the era of personalized medicine. Thyroid. 2010;20:707–13.
45. McCall A, Jarosz H, Lawrence AM. The incidence of thyroid carcinoma in solitary cold nodules and in multinodular goiters. Surgery. 1986;100:1128–31.
46. Spencer CA, Wang C-C. Thyroglobulin measurement: techniques, clinical benefits, and pitfalls. Endocrin Metab Clin N Am. 1995;24:841–64.
47. Whitley RJ, Ain KB. Thyroglobulin: a specific serum marker for the management of thyroid carcinoma. Clin Lab Med. 2004;24:29–47.
48. Spencer CA, LoPresti JS, Fatemi S, Nicoloff JT. Detection of residual and recurrent differentiated thyroid carcinoma by serum thyroglobulin measurement. Thyroid. 1999;9:435–41.
49. Giovanella L, Bongiovanni M, Trimboli P. Diagnostic value of thyroglobulin assay in cervical lymph node fine-needle aspirations for metastatic differentiated thyroid cancer. Curr Opin Oncol. 2013;25:6–13.
50. Kim ES, Lim DJ, Baek KH, Lee JM, Kim MK, Kwon HS, et al. Thyroglobulin antibody is associated with increased cancer risk in thyroid nodules. Thyroid. 2010;20:885–91.
51. Verburg FA, Luster M, Cupini C, Chiovato L, Duntas D, Elisei R, et al. Implications of thyroglobulin antibody positivity in patients with differentiated thyroid cancer: a clinical position paper. Thyroid. 2013;23:1211–1225.
52. Spencer CA, Takeuchi M, Kazaroxyan M, et al. Serum thyroglobulin autoantibodies: prevalence, influence on serum thyroglobulin measurement, and prognostic significance in patients with differentiated thyroid carcinoma. J Clin Endocrinol Metab. 1998;83:1121–7.
53. Hoofnagle AN, Roth MY. Improving the measurement of serum thyroglobulin with mass spectrometry. J Clin Endocrinol Metab. 2013;98:1343–52.
54. Marsh DJ, Learoyd DL, Robinson BG. Medullary thyroid carcinoma: recent advances and management update. Thyroid. 1995;5:407–24.
55. Pacini F, Fontanelli M, Fugazzola L, et al. Routine measurement of serum calcitonin in nodular thyroid diseases allows the preoperative diagnosis of unsuspected sporadic medullary thyroid carcinoma. J Clin Endocrinol Metab. 1994;78:826–9.
56. Vitale G, Caraglia M, Ciccarelli A, et al. Current approaches and perspectives in the therapy of medullary thyroid carcinoma. Cancer. 2001;91:1797–808. 35.
57. Wells Jr SA, Dilley WG, Farndon JA, et al. Early diagnosis and treatment of medullary thyroid carcinoma. Arch Intern Med. 1985;145:1248–52.
58. Hanna FWF, Ardill JES, Johnston CF, et al. Regulatory peptides and other neuroendocrine markers in medullary carcinoma of the thyroid. J Endocrinol. 1997;152:275–81.
59. Franke WG, Pinkert J, Runge R, et al. Chromogranin A: an additional tumor marker for postoperative recurrence and metastases of medullary thyroid carcinomas? Anticancer Res. 2000;20:5257–60.

60. Redding AH, Levine SN, Fowler MR. Normal preoperative calcitonin levels do not always exclude medullary thyroid carcinoma in patients with large palpable thyroid masses. Thyroid. 2000;10:919–22.
61. Bockhorn M, Frilling A, Rewerk S, et al. Lack of elevated serum carcinoembryonic antigen and calcitonin in medullary thyroid carcinoma. Thyroid. 2004;6:468–70.
62. Hodak SP, Burman KD. Editorial: The calcitonin conundrum—is it time for routine measurement of serum calcitonin in patients with thyroid nodules? J Clin Endocrinol Metab. 2004;89:511–4.
63. Chambon G, Alovisetti C, Idoux-Louche C, Reynaud C, Rodier M, Guedj A-M, et al. The use of preoperative routine measurement of basal serum thyrocalcitonin in candidates for thyroidectomy due to nodular thyroid disorders: results from 2733 consecutive patients. J Clin Endocrinol Metab. 2011;96:75–81.
64. Vierhapper H, Raber W, Bieglmayer C, et al. Routine measurement of plasma calcitonin in nodular thyroid diseases. J Clin Endocrinol Metab. 1997;82:1589–93.
65. Hahm JR, Lee MS, Min YK, et al. Routine measurement of serum calcitonin is useful for early detection of medullary thyroid carcinoma in patients with nodular thyroid diseases. Thyroid. 2001;11:73–80.
66. Daniels GH. Screening for medullary thyroid carcinoma with serum calcitonin measurements in patients with thyroid nodules in the United States and Canada. Thyroid. 2011;21:1199–207.
67. Pacini F. Screening of thyroid nodules by serum calcitonin measurements: why not? Thyroid. 2012;22:103.
68. Borget GDP, Schlumberger M. Editorial: Calcitonin determination in patients with nodular thyroid disease. J Clin Endocrinol Metab. 2007;92:425–7.
69. Costante G, Meringolo D, Durante C, Bianchi D, Nocera M, Tumino S, et al. Predictive value of serum calcitonin levels for preoperative diagnosis of medullary thyroid carcinoma in a cohort of 5817 consecutive patients with thyroid nodules. J Clin Endocrinol Metab. 2007;92:450–5.
70. Elisei R, Bottici V, Luchetti F, et al. Impact of routine measurement of serum calcitonin on the diagnosis and outcome of medullary thyroid cancer: experience in 10,864 patients with nodular thyroid disorders. J Clin Endocrinol Metab. 2004;89:163–8.
71. Karanikas G, Moameni A, Poetzi C, et al. Frequency and relevance of elevated calcitonin levels in patients with neoplastic and nonneoplastic thyroid disease and in healthy subjects. J Clin Endocrinol Metab. 2004;89:515–9.
72. Tommasi M, Brocchi A, Cappellini A, et al. False high serum calcitonin levels using a non-competitive two-site IRMA. J Endocrinol Invest. 2001;24:356–60.
73. Kotzmann H, Schmidt A, Scheuba C, et al. Basal calcitonin levels and the response to pentagastrin stimulation in patients after kidney transplantation or on chronic hemodialysis as indicators of medullary carcinoma. Thyroid. 1999;9:943–7.
74. Erdogan MF, Gullu S, Baskal N, et al. Omeprazole: calcitonin stimulation test for the diagnosis, follow-up and family screening in medullary thyroid carcinoma. J Clin Endocrinol Metab. 1997;82:897–9.
75. Vlaeminck-Guillem V, D'Herbomez M, Pigny P, et al. Pseudohypoparathyroidism Ia and hypercalcitoninemia. J Clin Endocrinol Metab. 2001;86:3091–6.
76. Rink T, Truong P-N, Schroth H-J, Diener J, Zimny M, Grunwald F. Calculation and validation of a plasma calcitonin limit for early detection of medullary thyroid carcinoma in nodular thyroid disease. Thyroid. 2009;19:327–32.
77. Pacini F, Schlumberger M, Dralle H, Elisei R, Smit JW, Wiersinga W. European consensus for the management of patients with differentiated thyroid carcinoma of the follicular epithelium. Eur J Endocrinol. 2006;154:787–803.
78. Cheung K, Roman SA, Wang TS, Walker HD, Sosa JA. Calcitonin measurement in the evaluation of thyroid nodules in the United States: a cost effectiveness and decision analysis. J Clin Endocrinol Metab. 2008;93:2173–80.
79. Machens A, Schneyer U, Holzhausen H-J, Dralle H. Prospects of remission in medullary thyroid carcinoma according to basal calcitonin level. J Clin Endocrinol Metab. 2005;90:2029–34.
80. Abraham D, Gault PM, Hunt J, Bentz J. Calcitonin estimation in neck lymph node fine-needle aspirate fluid prevents misinterpretation of cytology in patients with metastatic medullary thyroid cancer. Thyroid. 2009;19:1015–6.
81. Boi F, Maurelli I, Pinna G, Atzeni F, Piga M, Lai ML, Mariotti S. Calcitonin measurement in wash-out fluid from fine needle aspiration of neck masses in patients with primary and metastatic medullary thyroid carcinoma. J Clin Endocrinol Metab. 2007;92:2115–8.
82. Giovanella L, Ceriani L, Bongiovanni M. Calcitonin measurement on fine needle washouts: preanalytical issues and normal reference values. Diagn Cytopathol. 2013;41:226–9.
83. Oertel YC. Fine needle aspiration and the diagnosis of thyroid cancer. Endocrin Metab Clin N Am. 1996;25:69–92.
84. Ravetto C, Colombo L, Dottorini ME. Usefulness of fine needle aspiration in the diagnosis of thyroid carcinoma: a retrospective study in 37,895 patients. Cancer. 2000;90:357–63.
85. Gharib H, Goellner JR. Fine needle aspiration biopsy of the thyroid: an appraisal. Ann Intern Med. 1993;118:282–9.
86. Ko HM, Jhu IK, Yang SH, et al. Clinicopathologic analysis of fine needle aspiration cytology of the thyroid. A review of 1613 cases and correlation with histopathologic diagnoses. Acta Cytol. 2003;47:727–32.
87. Layfield LJ, Cibas ES, Gharib H, Mandel SJ. Thyroid aspiration cytology: current status. CA Cancer J Clin. 2009;59:99–110.
88. Harvey JN, Parker D, De P, Shrimali RK, Otter M. Sonographically guided core biopsy in the assessment of thyroid nodules. J Clin Ultrasound. 2005;33:57–62.
89. Danese D, Sciacchitano S, Farsetti A, et al. Diagnostic accuracy of conventional versus sonography-guided fine-needle aspiration biopsy of thyroid nodules. Thyroid. 1998;8:15–21.
90. Hatada T, Okada K, Ishii H, et al. Evaluation of ultrasound-guided fine-needle aspiration biopsy for thyroid nodules. Am J Surg. 1998;175:133–6.
91. McCoy KL, Jabbour N, Ogilvie JB, Ohori NP, Carty SE, Yim JH. The incidence of cancer and rate of false-negative cytology in thyroid nodules greater than or equal to 4 cm in size. Surgery. 2007;142:837–44.
92. Burch HB, Shrestha M, Crothers BA. The impact of thyroid nodule size on the risk of malignancy and accuracy of fine needle aspiration: a ten-year study from a single institution. Thyroid. 2012;22:1251–6.
93. Kamran SC, Marqusee E, Kim MI, Frates MC, Ritner J, Peters H, et al. Thyroid nodule size and prediction of cancer. J Clin Endocrinol Metab. 2013;98:564–70.
94. Bongiovanni M, Spitale A, Faquin WC, Mazzucchelli L, Baloch ZW. The Bethesda system for reporting thyroid cytopathology: a meta-analysis. Acta Cytol. 2012;56:333–9.
95. Cibas E, Ali SZ. The Bethesda system for reporting thyroid cytopathology. Thyroid. 2009;19:1159–65. Am J Clin Path 2009; 132:658–665.
96. Theoharis CGA, Schofield KM, Hammers L, Udelsman R, Chhieng DC. The Bethesda thyroid fine-needle aspiration classification system: year 1 at an academic institution. Thyroid. 2009;19:1215–23.
97. Bose S, Walts AE. Thyroid fine needle aspirate: a post-Bethesda update. Adv Anat Pathol. 2012;19:160–9.
98. Teixeira GV, Chikota H, Teixeira T, Manfro G, Pal SI, Tufano RP. Incidence of malignancy in thyroid nodules determined to be follicular lesions of undetermined significance on fine-needle aspiration. World J Surg. 2012;36:69–74.

99. Ito Y, Asahi S, Matsuzuka F, Nakamura Y, Amino N, Miyauchi A. Needle tract implantation of follicular neoplasm after fine-needle aspiration biopsy: report of a case. Thyroid. 2006;16:1059–62.
100. Polyzos SA, Anastasilakis AD. Infectious thyroiditis as a complication of fine-needle biopsy: a systematic review. Expert Rev Endocrinol Metab. 2010;5:673–9.
101. Singer PA. Evaluation and management of the thyroid nodule. Otolaryngol Clin N Am. 1996;29:577–92.
102. Backdahl M, Wallin G, Lowhagen T, et al. Fine-needle biopsy cytology and DNA analysis: their place in the evaluation and treatment of patients with thyroid neoplasms. Surg Clin N Am. 1987;67:197–211.
103. Baskin HJ. Detection of recurrent papillary thyroid carcinoma by thyroglobulin assessment in the needle washout after fine-needle aspiration of suspicious lymph nodes. Thyroid. 2004;14:959–63.
104. Wagner K, Arciaga R, Siperstein A, et al. Thyrotropin receptor/thyroglobulin messenger ribonucleic acid in peripheral blood and fine-needle aspiration cytology: diagnostic synergy for detecting thyroid cancer. J Clin Endocrinol Metab. 2005;90:1921–4.
105. Oertel YC, Miyahara-Felipe L, Mendoza MG, Yu K. Value of repeated fine needle aspirations of the thyroid: an analysis of over ten thousand FNAs. Thyroid. 2007;17:1061–6.
106. Finley DJ, Arora N, Zhu B, et al. Molecular profiling distinguish papillary carcinoma from benign thyroid nodules. J Clin Endocrinol Metab. 2004;89:3214–23.
107. Finley DJ, Lubitz CC, Wei C, Zhu B, Fahey III TJ. Advancing the molecular diagnosis of thyroid nodules: defining benign lesions by molecular profiling. Thyroid. 2005;15:562–8.
108. Weber F, Eng C. Update on the molecular diagnosis of endocrine tumors: toward-omics-based personalized healthcare? J Clin Endocrinol Metab. 2008;93:1097–104.
109. Nikiforov Y, Nikiforova MN. Molecular genetics and diagnosis of thyroid cancer. Nat Rev Endocrinol. 2011;7:569–80.
110. Prasad NB, Kowalski J, Tsai H-L, Talbot K, Somervell H, Kouniavsky G, et al. Three-gene molecular diagnostic model for thyroid cancer. Thyroid. 2012;22:275–84. 88D, Nikiforova MN.
111. Nikiforov YE. Molecular diagnostics and predictors in thyroid cancer. Thyroid. 2009;19:1351–61.
112. Alexander EK. Approach to the patient with a cytologically indeterminate thyroid nodule. J Clin Endocrinol Metab. 2008;93:4175–82.
113. Chiu CG, Strugnell SS, Griffith OL, Jones SJM, Gown AM, Wlaker B, Nabi IR, Wiseman SM. Diagnostic utility of galectin-3 in thyroid cancer. Am J Pathol. 2010;176:2067–81.
114. Cohen Y, Xing M, Mambo E, Guo Z, Wu G, Trink B, et al. BRAF mutation in papillary thyroid carcinoma. J Natl Cancer Inst. 2003;95:625–7.
115. Rossi ED, Martini M, Capodimonti S, Lombardi CP, Pontecorvi A, Vellone VG, et al. BRAF (V600E) mutation analysis on liquid-based cytology-processed aspiration biopsies predicts bilaterality and lymph node involvement in papillary thyroid microcarcinoma. Cancer Cytopathol. 2013;121:291–7.
116. Colanta A, Lin O, Tafe L, Ghossein R, Nafa K, Mitchell T, et al. BRAF mutation analysis of fine-needle aspiration biopsies of papillary thyroid carcinoma: impact on diagnosis and prognosis. Acta Cytol. 2009;55:563–9.
117. Xing M. BRAF V600E mutation and papillary thyroid cancer: chicken or egg? J Clin Endocrinol Metab. 2012;97:2295–8.
118. Adeniran AJ, Hui P, Chhieng DC, Prasad ML, Scholfield K, Theoharis C. BRAF mutation testing of thyroid fine-needle aspiration specimens enhances the predictability of malignancy in thyroid follicular lesions of undetermined significance. Acta Cytol. 2011;55:570–5.
119. Lee S-T, Kim SW, Ki C-S, Jang J-H, Shin JH, Oh YL, et al. Clinical implication of highly sensitive detection of the BRAF V600E mutation in fine-needle aspirations of thyroid nodules: a comparative analysis of three molecular assays in 4585 consecutive cases in a BRAF V600E mutation-prevalent area. J Clin Endocrinol Metab. 2012;97:2299–306.
120. Kleiman DA, Sporn MJ, Beninato T, Crowley MJ, Nguyen A, Uccelli A, et al. Preoperative BRAF(V600E) mutation screening is unlikely to alter initial surgical treatment of patients with indeterminate thyroid nodules. Cancer. 2013;119:1495–502.
121. Ringel MD. Molecular markers of aggressiveness of thyroid cancer. Curr Opin Endocrinol Diabetes Obes. 2009;16:361–6.
122. Nikiforov YE, Steward DL, Robinson-Smith TM, Haugen BR, Klopper JP, Zhu A, Fagin JA, Falciglia M, Weber K, Nikiforova MN. Molecular testing for mutations in improving the fine-needle aspiration diagnosis of thyroid nodules. J Clin Endocrinol Metab. 2009;94:2092–9.
123. Moses W, Weng J, Sansano I, Peng M, Kanafshar E, Ljung B-M, Duh Q-Y, Clark OH, Kebebew E. Molecular testing for somatic mutations improves the accuracy of thyroid fine-needle aspiration biopsy. World J Surg. 2010;34:2589–94.
124. Kim SK, Hwang TS, Yoo YB, Han HS, Kim d-L, Song K-H, Lim SD, Kim WS, Paik NS. Surgical results of thyroid nodules according to a management guideline based on the BRAFV600E mutation status. J Clin Endocrinol Metab. 2011;96:658–64.
125. Li H, Robinson KA, Anton B, Saldanha IJ, Ladenson PW. Cost-effectiveness of a novel molecular test for cytologically indeterminate thyroid nodules. J Clin Endocrinol Metab. 2011;96:E1719–26.
126. Lassalle S, Hofman V, Ilie M, et al. Clinical impact of the detection of BRAF mutations in thyroid pathology: potential usefulness as diagnostic, prognostic and theragnostic applications. Curr Med Chem. 2010;17:1839–50.
127. Ferraz C, Eszlinger M, Paschke R. Current state and future perspective of molecular diagnosis of fine-needle aspiration biopsy of thyroid nodules. J Clin Endocrinol Metab. 2011;96:2016–26.
128. Duick DS. Overview of molecular biomarkers for enhancing the management of cytologically indeterminate thyroid nodules and thyroid cancer. Endocr Pract. 2012;18:611–5.
129. Chudova D, Wilde JI, Wang ET, Wang H, Rabbee N, Egidio CM, Reynolds J, et al. Molecular classification of thyroid nodules using high-dimensionality genomic data. J Clin Endocrinol Metab. 2010;95:5296–304.
130. Chen YT, Kitabayashi N, Zhou XK, Fahey TJ, Scognamiglio T. MicroRNA analysis as a potential diagnostic tool for papillary thyroid carcinoma. Mod Pathol. 2008;21:1139–46.
131. Nikiforova MN, Tseng GC, Steward D, et al. MicroRNA expression profiling of thyroid tumors: biological significance and diagnostic utility. J Clin Endocrinol Metab. 2008;93:1600–8.
132. Kitano M, Rahbari R, Patterson EE, Steinberg SM, Prasad NB, Wang Y, et al. Evaluation of candidate diagnostic microRNAs in thyroid fine-needle aspiration biopsy specimens. Thyroid. 2012;22:285–91.
133. Shen R, Liyanarachchi S, Li W, Wakely Jr PE, Saji M, Huang J, et al. MicroRNA signature in thyroid fine needle aspiration cytology applied to "atypia of undetermined significance" cases. Thyroid. 2012;22:9–16.
134. Yu S, Liu Y, Wang J, Guo Z, Zhang Q, Yu F, et al. Circulating microRNA profiles as potential biomarkers for diagnosis of papillary thyroid carcinoma. J Clin Endocrinol Metab. 2012;97:2084–92.
135. Vriens MR, Weng J, Suh I, Huynh N, Guerrero MA, Shen WT, et al. MicroRNA expression profiling is a potential diagnostic tool for thyroid cancer. Cancer. 2011;118:3426–32.
136. Menon MP, Khan A. Micro-RNAs in thyroid neoplasms: molecular, diagnostic and therapeutic implications. J Clin Pathol. 2009;62:978–85.
137. de la Chapelle A, Jazdzewski K. MicroRNAs in thyroid cancer. J Clin Endocrinol Metab. 2011;96:3326–36.
138. Nikiforov YE, Carty SE, Chiosea SI, Coyne C, Duvvuri U, Ferris RL, Gooding WE, et al. Impact of the multi-gene thyroseq nextgen-

eration sequencing assay on cancer diagnosis in thyroid nodules with atypia of undetermined significance/follicular lesion of undetermined significance cytology. Thyroid 2015;25:1217–1223.
139. Alexander EK, Kennedy GC, Baloch ZW, Cibas ES, Chudova D, Diggans J, et al. Preoperative diagnosis of benign thyroid nodules with indeterminate cytology. N Engl J Med. 2012;367:705–15.
140. Duick DS, Klopper JP, Diggnas JC, Friedman L, Kennedy GC, Lanman RB, McIver B. The impact of benign gene expression classifier test results on the endocrinologist-patient decision to operate on patients with thyroid nodules with indeterminate fine-needle aspiration cytopathology. Thyroid. 2012;22:996–1001.
141. Alexander EK, Schorr M, Klopper J, Kim C, Sipos J, Nabhan F, et al. Multicenter clinical experience with the Afirma gene expression classifier. J Clin Endocrinol Metab 2015;373:2347–2356.
142. Jameson JL. Minimizing unnecessary surgery for thyroid nodules. N Engl J Med. 2012;367:765–6.
143. Yip L, Farris C, Kabaker AS, Hodak SP, Nikiforova MN, McCoy KL, et al. Cost impact of molecular testing for indeterminate thyroid nodule fine-needle aspiration biopsies. J Clin Endocrinol Metab. 2012;97:1905–12.
144. Gupta N, Dasyam AK, Carty SE, Nikiforova MN, Ohori NP, Armstrong M, et al. RAS mutations in thyroid FNA specimens are highly predictive of predominantly low-risk follicular cancers. J Clin Endocrinol Metab. 2013;98:E914–22.
145. Hodak SP, Rosenthal DS. Information for clinicians: commercially available molecular diagnosis testing in the evaluation of thyroid nodule fine-needle aspiration specimens. Thyroid. 2013;23:131–4.
146. Tfayli HM, Teot LA, Indyk JA, Witchel SF. Papillary thyroid carcinoma in an autonomously hyperfunctioning thyroid nodule: case report and review of the literature. Thyroid. 2010;20:1029–32.
147. Kumar H, Daykin J, Holder R, et al. Gender, clinical findings, and serum thyrotropin measurements in the prediction of thyroid neoplasia in 1005 patients presenting with thyroid enlargement and investigated by fine-needle aspiration cytology. Thyroid. 1999;9:1105–9.
148. Tollin SR, Mery GM, Jelveh N, et al. The use of fine-needle aspiration biopsy under ultrasound guidance to assess the risk of malignancy in patients with a multinodular goiter. Thyroid. 2000;10:235–41.
149. Marqusee E, Benson CB, Frates MC, et al. Usefulness of ultrasonography in the management of nodular thyroid disease. Ann Intern Med. 2000;133:696–700.
150. Shattuck TM, Westra WH, Ladenson PW, Arnold A. Independent clonal origins of distinct tumor foci in multifocal papillary thyroid carcinoma. N Engl J Med. 2005;352:2406–12.
151. Utiger RD. The multiplicity of thyroid nodules and carcinomas. N Engl J Med. 2005;352:2376–8.
152. Bennedbaek FN, Hegedus L. Treatment of recurrent thyroid cysts with ethanol: a randomized double-blind controlled trial. J Clin Endocrinol Metab. 2003;88:5773–7.
153. Guglielmi R, Pacella CM, Bianchini A, et al. Percutaneous ethanol injection treatment in benign thyroid lesions: role and efficacy. Thyroid. 2004;14:125–31.
154. Mauz PS, Stiegler M, Holderried M, Brosch S. Complications of ultrasound guided percutaneous ethanol injection therapy of the thyroid and parathyroid glands. Ultraschall Med. 2005;26: 111142–5.
155. Mauz PS, Maassen MM, Braun B, Brosch S. How safe is percutaneous ethanol injection for treatment of thyroid nodules? Report of a case of severe toxic necrosis of the larynx and adjacent skin. Acta Otolaryngol. 2004;124:1226–30.
156. Dossing H, Bennedbaek FN, Hegedus L. Ultrasound-guided interstitial laser photocoagulation of an autonomous thyroid nodule: the introduction of a novel alternative. Thyroid. 2003;13:885–8.
157. Valcavi R, Riganti F, Bertani A, Formisano D, Pacella CM. Percutaneous laser ablation of cold benign thyroid nodules: a 3-year follow-up study in 122 patients. Thyroid. 2010;20:1253–61.
158. Papini E, Guglielmi R, Hosseim G, Misischi I, Graxiano F, et al. Ultrasound-guided laser ablation of incidental papillary thyroid microcarcinoma: a potential therapeutic approach in patients at surgical risk. Thyroid. 2011;21:917–20.
159. Corvilain B. The natural history of thyroid autonomy and hot nodules. Ann Endocrinol. 2003;64:17–22.
160. Boi F, Lai ML, Deias C, et al. The usefulness of 99mTC-SestaMIBI in the diagnostic evaluation of thyroid nodules with oncocytic cytology. Eur J Endocrinol. 2003;149:493–8.
161. Maki K, Okumura Y, Sato S, et al. Quantitative evaluation by TI-201 scintigraphy in the diagnosis of thyroid follicular nodules. Ann Nucl Med. 2003;17:91–8.
162. Chang CT, Liu FY, Tsai JJ, et al. The clinical usefulness of dual phase 201Tl thyroid scan for false-negative fine-needle aspiration cytological diagnoses in non-functioning cold thyroid nodules. Anticancer Res. 2003;23:2965–7.
163. Erdogan MF, Anil C, Ozer D, Kamel N, Erdogan G. Is it useful to routinely biopsy hot nodules in iodine deficient areas? J Endocrinol Invest. 2003;26:128–31.
164. Tamizu A, Okumura Y, Sato S, et al. The usefulness of serum thyroglobulin levels and Tl-201 scintigraphy in differentiating between benign and malignant thyroid follicular lesions. Ann Nucl Med. 2002;16:95–101.
165. Sinha PS, Beeby DI, Ryan P. An evaluation of thallium imaging for detection of carcinoma in clinically palpable solitary, nonfunctioning thyroid nodules. Thyroid. 2001;11:85–9.
166. Cases JA, Surks MI. The changing role of scintigraphy in the evaluation of thyroid nodules. Semin Nucl Med. 2000;30: 81–7.
167. Meller J, Becker W. The continuing importance of thyroid scintigraphy in the era of high-resolution ultrasound. Eur J Nucl Med Mol Imaging. 2002;29 Suppl 2:S425–38.
168. Asari AN, Siegel ME, DeQuattro V. Imaging of medullary thyroid carcinoma and hyperfunctioning adrenal medulla using iodine-131 metaiodobenzylguanidine. J Nucl Med. 1986;27:1858–60.
169. Kresnik E, Gallowitsch HH, Mikosch P, et al. Fluorine-18-fluorodeoxyglucose positron emission tomography in the preoperative assessment of thyroid nodules in an endemic goiter area. Surgery. 2003;133:294–9.
170. Fish SA, Langer JE, Mandel SJ. Sonographic imaging of thyroid nodules and cervical lymph nodes. Endocrinol Metab Clin N Am. 2008;37:401–17.
171. Sipos JA. Advances in ultrasound for the diagnosis and management of thyroid cancer. Thyroid. 2009;19:1363–72.
172. Moon W-J, Baek JH, Jung SL, Kim DW, Kim EK, Kim JY, Kwak JY. Ultrasonography and the ultrasound-based management of thyroid nodules: consensus statement and recommendations. Korean J Radiol. 2011;12:1–14.
173. Iared W, Shigueoka DC, Cristofoli JC, et al. Use of color Doppler ultrasonography for the prediction of malignancy in follicular thyroid neoplasms: systematic review and meta-analysis. J Ultrasound Med. 2010;29:419–25.
174. Henrichsen TL, Reading CC. Thyroid ultrasonography. Part 2: Nodules. Radiol Clin N Am. 2011;49:417–24.
175. Ito Y, Amino N, Yokozawa T, Ota H, Ohshita M, Murata N, Morita S, et al. Ultrasonographic evaluation of thyroid nodules in 900 patients: comparison among ultrasonographic, cytological, and histological findings. Thyroid. 2007;17:1269–76.
176. Moon W-J, Jung SL, Lee JH, Na DG, Baek J-H, Lee YH, et al. Benign and malignant thyroid nodules: US differentiation – multicenter retrospective study. Radiology. 2008;247: 762–70.

177. Rossi M, Buratto M, Bruni S, Filieri C, Tagliati F, Trasforini G, et al. Role of ultrasonographic/clinical profile, cytology, and BRAF V600E mutation evaluation in thyroid nodule screening for malignancy: a prospective study. J Clin Endocrinol Metab. 2012;97:2354–61.
178. Kabaker AS, Tublin E, Nikiforov YE, Armstrong MJ, Hodak SP, Stang MT, et al. Suspicious ultrasound characteristics predict BRAF^{V600e}-positive papillary thyroid carcinoma. Thyroid. 2012;22:585–9.
179. Smith-Bindman R, Lebda P, Feldstein VA, Goldstein RB, Brasic N, Jin C, Kornak J. Risk of thyroid cancer based on thyroid ultrasound imaging characteristics: results of a population-based study. JAMA Intern Med. 2013;173(19):1788–96.
180. Solbiati L, Charboneau JW, James EM, Hat ID. The thyroid gland. In: Rumack CM, Wilson SR, Charboneau JW, editors. Diagnostic ultrasound. 2nd ed. St Louis: Mosby-Yearbook; 1998. p. 703–29.
181. Shapiro RS. Panoramic ultrasound of the thyroid. Thyroid. 2003;13:177–81.
182. Rago T, Scutari M, Santini F, Loiacono V, Piaggi P, et al. Real-time elastosonography: useful tool for refining the presurgical diagnosis in thyroid nodules with indeterminate or nondiagnostic cytology. J Clin Endocrinol Metab. 2010;95:5274–80.
183. Sebag F, Vaillant-Lombard J, Berbis J, Griset V, Henry JF, Petit P, Oliver C. Shear wave elastography: a new ultrasound imaging mode for the differential diagnosis of benign and malignant thyroid nodules. J Clin Endocrinol Metab. 2010;95:5281–8.
184. Lippolis PV, Tognini S, Materazzi G, Polini A, Mancini R, Ambrosini CE, et al. Is elastography actually useful in the presurgical selection of thyroid nodules with indeterminate cytology? J Clin Endocrinol Metab. 2011;96:E1816–25.
185. Hegedus L. Can elastography stretch our understanding of thyroid histomorphology? J Clin Endocrinol Metab. 2010;95:5213–5.
186. Magri F, Chytiris S, Capelli V, Gaiti M, Zerbini F, Carrara R, et al. Comparison of elastographic strain index and thyroid fine-needle aspiration cytology in 631 thyroid nodules. J Clin Endocrinol Metab. 2013;98:4790–7.
187. Nam-Goong IS, Kim HY, Gong G, et al. Ultrasonography-guided fine-needle aspiration of thyroid incidentaloma: correlation with pathological findings. Clin Endocrinol. 2004;60:21–8.
188. Leenhardt L, Hejblum G, Franc B, et al. Indications and limits of ultrasound-guided cytology in the management of nonpalpable thyroid nodules. J Clin Endocrinol Metab. 1999;84:24–8.
189. Bellantone R, Lombardi CP, Raffaelli M, et al. Management of cystic or predominantly cystic thyroid nodules: the role of ultrasound-guided fine-needle aspiration biopsy. Thyroid. 2004;14:43–7.
190. Alexander EK, Heering JP, Benson CB, et al. Assessment of non-diagnostic ultrasound-guided fine needle aspirations of thyroid nodules. J Clin Endocrinol Metab. 2002;87:4924–7.
191. Braga M, Cavalcanti TC, Collaco LM, Graf H. Efficacy of ultrasound-guided fine-needle aspiration biopsy in the diagnosis of complex thyroid nodules. J Clin Endocrinol Metab. 2001;86:4089–91.
192. Dossing H, Bennedbaek FN, Karstrup S, Hegedus L. Benign solitary solid cold thyroid nodules: US-guided interstitial laser photocoagulation—initial experience. Radiology. 2002;225:53–7.
193. Pacini F. Role of percutaneous ethanol injection in management of nodular lesions of the thyroid gland. J Nucl Med. 2003;44:211–2.
194. Fukunari N, Nagahama M, Sugino K, Mimura T, Ito K, Ito K. Clinical evaluation of color Doppler imaging for the differential diagnosis of thyroid follicular lesions. World J Surg. 2004;28:1261–5.
195. Lee M-J, Kim E-K, Kwak JY, Kim MJ. Partially cystic thyroid nodules on ultrasound: probability of malignancy and sonographic differentiation. Thyroid. 2009;19:341–6.
196. Burguera B, Gharib H. Thyroid incidentalomas. Prevalence, diagnosis, significance, and management. Endocrinol Metab Clin N Am. 2000;29:187–203.
197. Bailey RH, Aron DC. The diagnostic dilemma of incidentalomas: working through uncertainty. Endocrinol Metab Clin N Am. 2000;29:91–105.
198. Van den Bruel A, Maes A, De Potter T, et al. Clinical relevance of thyroid fluorodeoxyglucose-whole body positron emission tomography incidentaloma. J Clin Endocrinol Metab. 2002;87:1517–20.
199. Cohen MS, Arslan N, Dehdashti F, et al. Risk of malignancy in thyroid incidentalomas identified by fluorodeoxyglucose-positron emission tomography. Surgery. 2001;130:941–6.
200. Kang HW, Kim S-K, Kang H-S, et al. Prevalence and risk of cancer of focal thyroid incidentaloma identified by 18F-fluorodeoxyglucose positron emission tomography for metastasis evaluation and cancer screening in healthy subjects. J Clin Endocrinol Metab. 2003;88:4100–4.
201. Stack Jr BC, Bodenner DL, Bartel TB, Boeckmann J. Focal thyroid uptake on 18F-fluorodeoxyglucose positron emission tomography: interpreting the data. Thyroid. 2013;23:636–7.
202. Bertagna F, Treglia G, Piccardo A, Giubbini R. Diagnostic and clinical significance of F-18-FDG-PET/CT thyroid incidentalomas. J Clin Endocrinol Metab. 2012;97:3866–75.
203. Are C, Hsu JF, Ghossein RA, Schoder H, Shah JP, Shaha AR. Histological aggressiveness of fluorodeoxyglucose positron-emission tomogram (FDG-PET)-detected incidental thyroid carcinomas. Ann Surg Oncol. 2007;14:3210–5.
204. Kim JM, Ryu JS, Kim TY, Kim WB, Kwon GY, Gong G, Moon DH, et al. 18F-fluorodeoxyglucose positron emission tomography does not predict malignancy in thyroid nodules cytologically diagnosed as follicular neoplasm. J Clin Endocrinol Metab. 2007;92:1630–4.
205. Soelberg KK, Bonnema SJ, Brix TH, Hegedus L. Risk of malignancy in thyroid incidentalomas detected by 18F-fluorodeoxyglucose positron emission tomography: a systematic review. Thyroid. 2013;22:918–25.
206. Moon HJ, Kwak JY, Kim E-K, Kim MJ. A taller than wide shape in thyroid nodules in transverse and longitudinal ultrasonographic planes and the prediction of malignancy. Thyroid. 2011;21:1249–53.
207. Kang HW, No JH, Chung JH, et al. Prevalence, clinical and ultrasonographic characteristics of thyroid incidentalomas. Thyroid. 2004;14:29–33.
208. Silver RJ, Parangi S. Management of thyroid incidentalomas. Surg Clin N Am. 2004;84:907–19.
209. Mazzaferri EL, Sipos J. Should all patients with subcentimeter thyroid nodules undergo fine-needle aspiration biopsy and preoperative neck ultrasonography to define the extent of tumor invasion? Thyroid. 2008;18:597–602.
210. Raffel A, Cupisti K, Krausch M, et al. Incidentally found medullary thyroid cancer: treatment rationale for small tumors. World J Surg. 2004;28:397–401.
211. Quadbeck B, Pruellage J, Roggenbuck U, et al. Long-term follow-up of thyroid nodule growth. Exp Clin Endocrinol Diabetes. 2002;110:348–54.
212. Alexander EK, Hurwitz S, Heering JP, et al. Natural history of benign solid and cystic thyroid nodules. Ann Intern Med. 2003;138:315–8.
213. Zelmanovitz R, Genro S, Gross JL. Suppressive therapy with levothyroxine for solitary thyroid nodules: a double-blind controlled clinical study and cumulative meta-analyses. J Clin Endocrinol Metab. 1998;83:3881–5.
214. Gharib H, Mazzaferri EL. Thyroxine suppressive therapy in patients with nodular thyroid disease. Ann Intern Med. 1998;128:386–94.

215. Castro MR, Caraballo PJ, Morris JC. Effectiveness of thyroid hormone suppressive therapy in benign solitary thyroid nodules: a metaanalysis. J Clin Endocrinol Metab. 2002;87:4154–9.
216. Ridgway EC. Medical treatment of benign thyroid nodules: have we defined a benefit? Ann Intern Med. 1998;128:403–5.
217. Hoermann R. Thyroid-hormone suppressive therapy in benign thyroid nodules—is it effective? Lancet. 2002;360:1899–900.
218. Cheung PSY, Lee JMH, Boey JH. Thyroxine suppressive therapy of benign solitary thyroid nodules: a prospective randomized study. World J Surg. 1989;13:818–22.
219. Celani MF, Mariani M, Mariani G. On the usefulness of levothyroxine suppressive therapy in the medical treatment of benign solitary, solid, or predominantly solid thyroid nodules. Acta Endocrinol. 1990;123:603–8.
220. Papini E, Bacci V, Panunzi C, et al. A prospective randomized trial of levothyroxine suppressive therapy for solitary thyroid nodules. Clin Endocrinol. 1993;38:507–13.
221. LaRosa GL, Lupo L, Giuffrida D, et al. Levothyroxine and potassium iodide are both effective in treating benign solitary solid cold nodules of the thyroid. Ann Intern Med. 1995;122:1–8.
222. Lima N, Knobel M, Cavaliere H, et al. Levothyroxine suppressive therapy is partially effective in treating patients with benign, solid thyroid nodules and multinodular goiters. Thyroid. 1997;7:691–7.
223. Wemeau JL, Caron P, Schvartz C, et al. Effects of TSH suppression with levothyroxine in reducing volume of solitary thyroid nodules and improving extranodular nonpalpable changes. J Clin Endocrinol Metab. 2002;87:4928–34.
224. Gharib H, James EM, Charboneau JW. Suppressive therapy with levothyroxine for solitary nodules. N Engl J Med. 1987;317:70–5.
225. Reverter JL, Lucas A, Salinas I, et al. Suppressive therapy with levothyroxine for solitary thyroid nodules. Clin Endocrinol. 1992;36:25–8.
226. Papini E, Petrucci L, Guglielmi R, et al. Long term changes in nodular goiter: a 5 year prospective randomized trial of levothyroxine suppressive therapy for benign cold thyroid nodules. J Clin Endocrinol Metab. 1998;83:780–3.
227. La Rosa GL, Ippolito AM, Lupo L, et al. Cold thyroid nodule reduction with L-thyroxine can be predicted by initial nodule volume and cytological characteristics. J Clin Endocrinol Metab. 1996;81:4385–7.
228. Stathatos N, Wartofsky L. Effects of thyroid hormone on bone. Clin Rev Bone Mineral Metab. 2004;2:135–50.
229. Marcocci C, Golia F, Bruno-Bossio G, et al. Carefully monitored levothyroxine suppressive therapy is not associated with bone loss in premenopausal women. J Clin Endocrinol Metab. 1994; 78:818–23.
230. Koc M, Ersoz HO, Akpinar I, et al. Effect of low-and high-dose levothyroxine on thyroid nodule volume: a crossover placebo-controlled trial. Clin Endocrinol. 2002;57:621–8.
231. Fogelfeld L, Wiviott MBT, Shore-Freedman E, et al. Recurrence of thyroid nodules after surgical removal in patients irradiated in childhood for benign conditions. N Engl J Med. 1989;320: 835–40.
232. Hennessey JV, Evaul JE, Tseng YL, et al. L-thyroxine dosage: a re-evaluation of therapy with contemporary preparations. Ann Intern Med. 1986;105:11–6.
233. Wartofsky L, Oertel Y. Fine needle aspiration biopsy of thyroid nodules. In: Van Nostrand D, editor. Nuclear medicine atlas. Philadelphia: J. B. Lippincott; 1987. p. 193–200.
234. Hayashida N, Namba H, Kumagai A, et al. A rapid and simple detection method for the BRAF T1796A mutation in fine needle aspirated thyroid carcinoma cells. Thyroid. 2004;14:910–5.
235. Xing M, Tufano RP, Tufaro AP, et al. Detection of BRAF mutation on fine needle aspiration biopsy specimens: a new diagnostic tool for papillary thyroid cancer. J Clin Endocrinol Metab. 2004; 89:2867–72.
236. Mandel SJ. A 64 year old woman with a thyroid nodule. JAMA. 2004;292:2632–42.
237. Alexander EK, Marqusee E, Orcutt J, et al. Thyroid nodule shape and prediction of malignancy. Thyroid. 2004;14:953–8.
238. Lippolis PV, Tognini S, Materazzi G, Polini A, Mancini R, Ambrosini CE, et al. Is elastography actually useful in the presurgical selection of thyroid nodules with indeterminate cytology? J Clin Endocrinol Metab. 2011;96:E1826–30.
239. Rosen IB, Palmer JA, Bain J, et al. Efficacy of needle biopsy in postradiation thyroid disease. Surgery. 1983;94:1002–7.
240. Duek DS, Goldenberg D, Linn S, et al. The role of fine-needle aspiration and intaoperative frozen section in the surgical management of solitary thyroid nodules. Surg Today. 2002;32:857–61.
241. Lennquist S. The thyroid nodule: diagnosis and surgical treatment. Surg Clin N Am. 1987;67:213–32.
242. Finley DJ, Zhu B, Barden CB, Fahey III TJ. Discrimination of benign and malignant thyroid nodules by molecular profiling. Ann Surg. 2004;240:425–37.
243. Norton JA, Doppman JL, Jensen RT. Cancer of the endocrine system. In: Devita Jr VT, Hellman L, Rosenberg SA, editors. Cancer: principles and practice of oncology. Philadelphia: J. B. Lippincott; 1989. p. 1269–87.
244. Faggiano A, Ramundo V, Assanti AP, et al. Thyroid nodules treated with percutaneous radiofrequency thermal ablation: a comparative study. J Clin Endocrinol Metab. 2012;97:4439–45.
245. Lim HK, Lee JH, Ha EJ, Sung JY, Kim JK, Baek JH. Radiofrequency ablation of benign non-functioning thyroid nodules: 4-year follow-up results for 111 patients. Eur Radiol. 2013;23:1044–9.
246. Gharib H, Hegedus L, Pacella CM, Baek JH, Papini E. Nonsurgical, image-guided, minimally invasive therapy for thyroid nodules. J Clin Endocrinol Metab. 2013;98:3949–57.

21 Fine-Needle Aspiration

Zubair W. Baloch and Virginia A. LiVolsi

Introduction

Fine-needle aspiration (FNA) is a quick, valuable, minimally invasive procedure to assess the nature of a thyroidal mass. It should not be confused with "needle biopsy," which requires a Tru-Cut or Vim-Silverman needle and yields tissue fragments for histologic diagnosis. Details of the FNA technique and the equipment required have been described. Of particular importance is the use of a syringe holder and needles with clear plastic hubs [1]. It is essential to use little or no suction when aspirating the lesions [2, 3].

Equipment

1. The syringe holder or handle is an indispensable item. The commonly used ones are the Cameco syringe pistol (Precision Dynamics Corporation, Burbank, CA) and a less expensive, plastic handle is the Aspir Gun (The Everest Company, Linden, NJ).
2. Plastic disposable syringes: 10 cc and, rarely, 20 cc.
3. Disposable needles: 25 or 27 gauge, preferably 1.5 in.
4. Plain glass slides, preferably with one frosted end.
5. Appropriate staining solutions (we prefer the Diff-Quik stain, a hematological stain similar to the May-Grünwald-Giemsa stain) if on-site evaluation is being performed.

Z.W. Baloch, MD, PhD (✉) • V.A. LiVolsi, MD
Department of Pathology and Laboratory Medicine, University of Pennsylvania Medical Center, Perelman School of Medicine, 6 Founders Pavilion, 3400 Spruce Street, Philadelphia, PA 19104, USA
e-mail: balocj@mail.med.upenn.edu; linus@mail.med.upenn.edu

Procedure

Thyroid FNA can be performed manually by palpation or employing ultrasound guidance. It is recommended that FNA is performed by a clinician, radiologist, or pathologist who is proficient/experienced in thyroid FNAB [4]. The use of ultrasound guidance ensures that the sample is obtained from the nodule in question and allows directing the needle into the solid portions of a complex solid and cystic nodule, thus improving the diagnostic yield [5]. The specimen should be obtained by using either a 25- or 27-gauge needle which can be either attached or not (non-aspiration technique) to a syringe; however, the former method is the most favored one. The correlation between the gauge of the needle and the cellularity of the specimen has been discussed in the literature [6]. A higher rate of specimen adequacy has been reported with a thinner gauge needle. Various studies have compared FNAB of thyroid by employing aspiration and non-aspiration (capillary action) techniques. Some authors have shown no difference between the two sampling techniques while others have reported a higher rate of adequacy with non-aspiration technique. In any event this is highly dependent upon the preference and experience of the operator with either technique [6–9]. Multiple passes in a thyroid nodule may not prove to be useful in acquiring adequate cellularity as thyroid nodules are inheritably vascular and lead to increased bleeding resulting in diluted specimen [7, 10]. Following FNA technique has been recommended by many authors.

1. Ask the patient if he or she knows the procedure. While you explain the procedure, ask the patient to hold an ice pack on the area to be aspirated. Oertel recommended the use of ice pack as a substitute for local anesthesia because it not only numbs the area but also reduces bleeding due to vasoconstriction [1]. Then have the patient lie down on the examining table and is instructed not to swallow or talk during the insertion of the needle and the specimen procurement (it is advisable to explain to the patient

L. Wartofsky, D. Van Nostrand (eds.), *Thyroid Cancer*, DOI 10.1007/978-1-4939-3314-3_21

that the thyroid gland moves during swallowing and talking). A local anesthetic may be used during the procedure, approximately 1–2 ml of 1 % lidocaine hydrochloride solution. Proceed in the following way:

2. Place the thyroid mass between the index and middle fingers of your non-dominant hand in a position suitable for needling. In case of ultrasound-guided FNA, the transducer (usually high-resolution linear array transducer) encased in a sterile cover is placed directly over the lesion for preaspiration scanning for lesion localization. Doppler mapping may also be used to find blood vessels in and around the nodule to avoid FNA-related bleeding [11].
3. Clean the skin with an alcohol swab. Dry the skin with a gauze sponge to avoid the stinging sensation caused by residual alcohol when inserting the needle. In ultrasound-guided FNA, it is important to clean ultrasound gel from the area of needle insertion. In our experience when mixed with blood and colloid, the ultrasound gel may hamper the cellular details in the slides prepared for on-site evaluation. As recommended by Oertel, we often ask patients if they need someone to hold their hand during the procedure (patients often mention how helpful and reassuring it is for someone to hold their hands) [2, 3].
4. Ask the patient to swallow. (If necessary, water can be provided through a bent straw.) After the patient has swallowed, hold down the lesion between your left index and middle fingers.
5. Pierce the needle through the skin, making sure that the syringe is in "the resting position" (plunger at the 0-cc mark). In case of ultrasound-guided FNA, the needle is placed just above the transducer and may be entered into the nodule parallel or perpendicular to the transducer. The needle tip should be monitored during the entire FNA procedure.
6. Once the needle has entered the nodule, move it back and forth in the same plane (do not vary the angle of the needle) *without applying any suction*. Perform this maneuver twice; if nothing appears in the clear plastic needle hub, then apply suction gradually and gently by pulling the plunger of the syringe.
7. While inserting the needle in the lesion, it is advisable to keep talking to the patient with encouraging words; such expressions are very helpful in calming the patient. As you apply suction, gradually push the needle deeper, with gentle movements back and forth in the lesion, maintaining the suction. Usually, when the plunger of the syringe is at the 2- or 3-cc mark, you should see material in the clear plastic needle hub. However, if the lesion is firm, and no material appears in the needle hub, keep applying suction until you reach the 10-cc mark. Again, move the needle back and forth with gentle jabbing movements. By now you should have hemorrhagic material in the needle hub. Release the plunger to stop the suction. Shift your fingers from the "trigger" to hold the outside of the handle.
8. Withdraw the needle.
9. Ask the patient to apply *firm* pressure at the site of the aspiration using cotton gauze. While the patient is still applying pressure, move quickly to prepare the smears (in case of on-site evaluation) or express the contents into a transport medium (Normosol®, Cytolyt®). Because the aspirate tends to clot promptly, we cannot emphasize enough that *rapid preparation of the smears is extremely important*. Once the smears have been prepared, the physician may help the patient sit up, and continue to apply pressure at the site of aspiration until the smear is ready for microscopic examination. Then tell the patient to apply pressure while the slides are examined under the microscope. The patient remains seated or propped up on the examining table until after the smears have been examined and decided which size needle to use in the next aspiration if more passes are needed to obtain adequate specimen. These simple precautions, i.e., sitting up between aspirates (to improve the venous drainage) and applying steady pressure at the puncture site, prevent the formation of post-FNA hematomas. However, if the patient feels dizzy and does not want to sit up, allow the patient to remain lying down. Also, if the patient cannot tolerate pressure on the neck (e.g., the lesion is over the trachea and pressure produces coughing), apply an ice pack to the site.
10. Once satisfied that you have sampled the lesion thoroughly, tell the patient that there are no restrictions and that he or she can go back to work or routine activities. (We seldom put a small adhesive bandage on the area that has been aspirated.)
11. *Technical hints* [1, 3, 12]: Obtaining an adequate and representative sample is crucial for a correct diagnosis. We reiterate that the technique is deceptively simple.
    (a) While applying suction and moving the needle into the lesion, look at the needle hub. If fluid appears, continue applying suction until the syringe is filled or until there is no more fluid aspirated. If blood appears in the needle hub, immediately stop applying suction, whether the plunger is at the 1- or 4-cc mark. If no blood appears, continue applying suction up to the 10-cc mark on the syringe.
    (b) Observe your patient's face. If you see grimacing or any signs of discomfort, state that you are almost done, that it will take a little longer, to bear with you, and so on. If you notice that the patient is about to swallow, release the plunger immediately, and pull out of the lesion. Sometimes, a patient will start swallowing and surprise you; then just move along, do not offer resistance, release the plunger, and pull out of the lesion as quickly as possible.

(c) *Do not forget to release the plunger*. When unexperienced, it is a common mistake to withdraw the needle from the nodule while still applying suction. This action will cause the aspirated material to flow into the syringe. To recover the material, rinse the syringe and prepare a filter specimen.
(d) After inserting the needle in the lesion, the needle should be moved up and down (if the patient is lying down) or back and forth (if the patient is sitting upright), with gentle jabbing movements and without applying any suction. There should *not* be any lateral movements. If bright red blood is seen immediately in the needle hub, the procedure should be stopped, and the needle should be withdrawn at once.
(e) The on-site smear(s) should be checked under the microscope. Depending on the microscopic findings, change the needle gauge or apply more suction in the next aspirate.

The FNA Specimen

It is well understood that the precise and management-based cytologic diagnosis is highly dependent upon an adequate specimen with well-preserved cellular details. Therefore, regardless of the cytologic preparation, i.e., smears, cytospins, monolayer preps, and cell block, an adequate and well-preserved thyroid FNA specimen is important for rendering cytologic interpretation [13–16]. Many experts have proposed various criteria for cell adequacy in thyroid FNAB specimens [17–20]; it is well understood that these criteria of adequacy apply to solid nodule and solid and cystic nodule and not to cystic nodules with no solid component on ultrasound evaluation. The most commonly used criterion for specimen adequacy is six to eight groups of follicular cells with 10–20 cells per groups on two different slides. Adequate cellularity of a thyroid FNA specimen reflects adequate and representative sampling of the nodule, granted this is highly operator dependent [20]. In our experience an adequate and representative thyroid FNAB specimen is acquired by using ultrasound guidance and making sure that the biopsy needle samples are multiple portions rather than one portion of the nodule.

On-Site Evaluation

The on-site evaluation of thyroid FNA specimens with performance of rapid stains leads to adequate specimens and lessens nondiagnostic rates; however, this may not be possible in all clinical settings. The clinical utility of the on-site assessment of thyroid FNA is similar to the interpretation of frozen sections in surgical pathology. A number of questions can be answered by on-site evaluation, which includes adequacy of specimen; classification of lesion, primary vs. metastatic; and if additional studies are needed (flow cytometry, serum calcitonin measurements to rule out medullary carcinoma and molecular studies) [10, 21, 22].

The number of on-site smears should be kept low, 2–3 smears/per pass; they can be air-dried for Romanowsky stain or fixed in 95 % alcohol or spray fixed for Papanicolaou stain. The Romanowsky staining method is one of the best available methods available for immediate evaluation of FNA specimens; however, some authors have proposed rapid Papanicolaou staining method. Papanicolaou stain is vital to the diagnosis of thyroid lesion. It effectively highlights the nuclear details and alterations (grooves and inclusions), which are crucial for the diagnosis of papillary thyroid carcinoma. It also is helpful in the diagnosis of Hurthle cell and C-cell lesions. If one is not providing on-site assessment than FNA, specimen can be placed into appropriate medium for monolayer preparation (ThinPrep®, SurePath®, etc.) or other concentration techniques and preparations [10].

It is well established now that molecular testing can serve to further refine the cytologic interpretation. Therefore, a portion or an entire thyroid FNA pass may be processed for molecular diagnosis. This is highly dependent upon the molecular test(s). In case of BRAF mutational analysis, DNA can be extracted from the FNA material in routinely air-dried smears or leftover needle rinse; however, mutational analysis for multiple genes will require a dedicated FNA pass stored at −80 °C [23].

Core Needle Biopsy

Although FNA is the most commonly employed method for obtaining diagnostic material from a thyroid nodule, in some cases it may not yield sufficient diagnostic material even with multiple passes and repeat procedures. It has been shown that core biopsy (18–20-gauge needle) can increase the diagnostic yield by 10 % as compared to fine-needle aspiration. The core biopsy does provide a large amount of histologic material to be examined for evaluation of cytologic as well as architectural features; however, the success of this procedure is highly dependent upon the operator well versed in this procedure as there is also an increased risk of complications such as hematoma formation [10, 24, 25].

References

1. Oertel YC. A pathologist's comments on diagnosis of thyroid nodules by fine needle aspiration. J Clin Endocrinol Metab. 1995; 80:1467–8.
2. Oertel YC. Who should perform fine-needle aspirations? Cytopathology. 1997;8:134–8.

3. Oertel YC. Emerging role of the interventional pathologist. Diagn Cytopathol. 2004;30:295–6.
4. American Thyroid Association Guidelines Task Force on Thyroid Nodules and Differentiated Thyroid Cancer. Haugen BR, Alexander EK, Bible KC, Doherty GM, Mandel SJ, Nikiforov YE, Pacini F, Randolph GW, Sawka AM, Schlumberger M, Schuff KG, Sherman SI, Sosa JA, Steward DL, Tuttle RM, Wartofsky L. 2015 American Thyroid Association Management Guidelines for Adult Patients with Thyroid Nodules and Differentiated Thyroid Cancer. Thyroid 2016; 26:1–133.
5. Moon HJ, Kwak JY, Kim EK, Kim MJ. Ultrasonographic characteristics predictive of nondiagnostic results for fine-needle aspiration biopsies of thyroid nodules. Ultrasound Med Biol. 2011;37:549–55.
6. Cappelli C; Pirola I; Gandossi E; De Martino E; Agosti B; Castellano M. Fine-needle aspiration cytology of thyroid nodule: does the needle matter? Southern Medical Journal. 2009;102:498–501.
7. Carpi A, Di Coscio G, Iervasi G, Antonelli A, Mechanick J, Sciacchitano S, Nicolini A. Thyroid fine needle aspiration: how to improve clinicians' confidence and performance with the technique. Cancer Lett. 2008;264:163–71.
8. Carpi A, Ferrari E, Sagripanti A, Nicolini A, Iervasi G, De Gaudio C, Romani R, Di Coscio G. Aspiration needle biopsy refines preoperative diagnosis of thyroid nodules defined at fine needle aspiration as microfollicular nodule. Biomed Pharmacother. 1996;50:325–8.
9. Carpi A, Ferrari E, Toni MG, Sagripanti A, Nicolini A, Di Coscio G. Needle aspiration techniques in preoperative selection of patients with thyroid nodules: a long-term study. J Clin Oncol. 1996;14:1704–12.
10. Pitman MB, Abele J, Ali SZ, Duick D, Elsheikh TM, Jeffrey RB, Powers CN, Randolph G, Renshaw A, Scoutt L. Techniques for thyroid FNA: a synopsis of the National Cancer Institute thyroid fine-needle aspiration state of the science conference. Diagn Cytopathol. 2008;36:407–24.
11. Kim MJ, Kim EK, Park SI, Kim BM, Kwak JY, Kim SJ, Youk JH, Park SH. US-guided fine-needle aspiration of thyroid nodules: indications, techniques, results. Radiographics. 2008;28:1869–86. discussion 1887.
12. Oertel YC. Fine-needle aspiration and the diagnosis of thyroid cancer. Endocrinol Metab Clin North Am. 1996;25:69–91.
13. Baloch ZW, LiVolsi VA. Fine-needle aspiration of the thyroid: today and tomorrow. Best Pract Res. 2008;22:929–39.
14. Baloch ZW, Tam D, Langer J, Mandel S, LiVolsi VA, Gupta PK. Ultrasound-guided fine-needle aspiration biopsy of the thyroid: role of on-site assessment and multiple cytologic preparations. Diagn Cytopathol. 2000;23:425–9.
15. Tulecke MA, Wang HH. ThinPrep for cytologic evaluation of follicular thyroid lesions: correlation with histologic findings. Diagn Cytopathol. 2004;30:7–13.
16. Malle D, Valeri RM, Pazaitou-Panajiotou K, Kiziridou A, Vainas I, Destouni C. Use of a thin-layer technique in thyroid fine needle aspiration. Acta Cytol. 2006;50:23–7.
17. Kini SR, Miller JM, Hamburger JI. Cytopathology of thyroid nodules. Henry Ford Hosp Med J. 1982;30:17–24.
18. Oertel YC, Burman K, Boyle L, Ringel M, Wartofsky L, Shmookler B, Yeganeh F, Van Nostrand D. Integrating fine-needle aspiration into a daily practice involving thyroid disorders: the Washington Hospital Center approach. Diagn Cytopathol. 2002;27:120–2.
19. Hamburger JI. Fine needle biopsy diagnosis of thyroid nodules. Perspective. Thyroidology. 1988;1:21–34.
20. Goellner JR, Gharib H, Grant CS, Johnson DA. Fine needle aspiration cytology of the thyroid. Acta Cytol. 1987;31:587–90.
21. Redman R, Zalaznick H, Mazzaferri EL, Massoll NA. The impact of assessing specimen adequacy and number of needle passes for fine-needle aspiration biopsy of thyroid nodules. Thyroid. 2006; 16:55–60.
22. Ghofrani M, Beckman D, Rimm DL. The value of onsite adequacy assessment of thyroid fine-needle aspirations is a function of operator experience. Cancer. 2006;108:110–3.
23. Ferraz C, Eszlinger M, Paschke R. Current state and future perspective of molecular diagnosis of fine-needle aspiration biopsy of thyroid nodules. J Clin Endocrinol Metab. 2011;96:2016–26.
24. Park KT, Ahn SH, Mo JH, Park YJ, do Park J, Choi SI, Park SY. Role of core needle biopsy and ultrasonographic finding in management of indeterminate thyroid nodules. Head Neck. 2011;33:160–5.
25. Zhang S, Ivanovic M, Nemcek Jr AA, Defrias DV, Lucas E, Nayar R. Thin core needle biopsy crush preparations in conjunction with fine-needle aspiration for the evaluation of thyroid nodules: a complementary approach. Cancer. 2008;114:512–8.

22 Diagnostic and Prognostic Molecular Markers in Thyroid Cancer

Mingzhao Xing

Introduction

Thyroid nodules are extremely common, which are present in approximately 5–10 % of adult people on physical examination and in 50–70 % of people over the age of 60 years on ultrasonography [25, 46]. About 5–8 % of thyroid nodules are malignant. A major effort in the clinical workup of a thyroid nodule is thus to determine whether it is cancer. A diagnostic mainstay for thyroid nodule has been fine-needle aspiration biopsy (FNAB) for the last several decades. Cytological classification of FNAB has been evolving and is currently based on the "Bethesda classification system" in the United States [3]. Five cytological categories are classified on this system, including benign, malignant, atypia of undetermined significance/follicular lesion of undetermined significance (AUS/FLUS), follicular neoplasm/suspicious for follicular neoplasm (FN/SFN), and suspicious for malignancy, which are associated with the malignancy rates of 0–1 %, 98–100 %, 5–10 %, 20–30 %, and 50–75 %, respectively. In the majority of cases, FNAB provides a nearly definitive diagnosis (malignant or benign) for thyroid nodules, which can reliably guide their clinical management (e.g., thyroidectomy or no thyroidectomy). In 20–30 % of cases, however, FNAB yields indeterminate cytological results, including AUS/FLUS, FN/SFN, and suspicious for malignancy. Surgery was classically recommended for such indeterminate nodules for their risk of malignancy, which, overall, is about 25 % when confirmed histopathologically upon thyroidectomy. As a result, about 75 % of patients with cytologically indeterminate thyroid nodules would undergo unnecessary thyroid surgeries for nodules that prove to be benign only after surgery. This historically represents a major dilemma in the diagnostic management of thyroid nodules, to which other conventional diagnostic modalities, such as ultrasonography, are also unable to provide definitive solution [14].

Accompanying the high prevalence of thyroid nodules is the worldwide rapidly rising incidence of diagnosed thyroid cancer in recent years [28, 31]. There will be 62,450 new cases of thyroid cancer and 1,950 deaths from thyroid cancer estimated for 2015 in the United States [28]. Aside from the diagnostic challenge of thyroid nodule, there is also the prognostic dilemma of thyroid cancer. This starts even at the preoperative stage when a nodule is diagnosed as cancer by FNAB; even though a diagnosis of malignancy is established, it is often uncertain what type of treatment is ideal given the sometimes uncertain prognosis of thyroid cancer. The use of conventional clinicopathological risk factors, which are often unavailable preoperatively, seems to have currently reached its limit in its efficiency in improving further the prognostication and treatment of thyroid cancer.

Molecular marker-based diagnostic and prognostic strategies have proven to be promising and, in fact, clinically useful in tackling these diagnostic and prognostic dilemmas [72]. Many molecular markers have been investigated in this context, among which several have demonstrated high diagnostic or prognostic values and drawn particular attention. This chapter is focused on the discussion of those molecular markers that have proven to be clinically useful or most promising for the diagnosis and prognostication of thyroid cancer.

Diagnostic Molecular Markers of Thyroid Cancer

There are many diagnostic molecular markers identified for thyroid cancer in recent years whose corresponding functional molecules play fundamental roles in thyroid tumori-

M. Xing, MD PhD (✉)
Department of Medicine/Endocrinology and Metabolism, Johns Hopkins Hospital, 1830 East Monument Street/Suite 333, Baltimore, MD 21287, USA
e-mail: mxing1@jhmi.edu

L. Wartofsky, D. Van Nostrand (eds.), *Thyroid Cancer*, DOI 10.1007/978-1-4939-3314-3_22

genesis, providing the biological basis for their value as biomarkers for thyroid cancer [72, 74]. As summarized in Table 22.1, these molecular markers include RNA-related markers [e.g., the gene expression classifier (GEC) system, human telomerase reverse transcriptase (hTERT) mRNA, thyroid-stimulating hormone (TSH) mRNA, galectin-3 mRNA, and microRNA], genetic alteration-related markers (e.g., *BRAF* and *RAS* mutations, *RET-PTC* and *PAX8-PPARγ* rearrangements), protein markers [e.g., galectin-3, CK-19, HBME-1, and thyroid peroxidase (TPO)], and epigenetic markers (e.g., aberrant gene hypermethylation markers). Most of these markers are tested on FNAB specimens and thyroid tumor tissues, and some can be tested in peripheral blood (e.g., thyrotropin [TSH] receptor mRNA [44, 49] and gene methylation markers [29]). Some of these biomarkers do not show sufficiently high diagnostic values and are therefore unlikely to be clinically useful. Others demonstrate high diagnostic values, making them clinically useful or highly clinically promising. Among these, three types stand out for their best diagnostic values on testing on FNAB specimens, including the gene expression classifier (GEC) system, genetic markers, and galectin-3. Blood-based diagnostic biomarker tests for thyroid nodules are also attractive although they are in their early development stage at this time. These categories of molecular markers for the diagnostic evaluation of thyroid nodules have drawn the widest attention and are each specifically discussed here.

Gene Expression Classifier (GEC)

The GEC is a RNA array system consisting of 142 mRNAs that was shown to have a high diagnostic value for the evaluation of thyroid nodules when applied to FNAB specimens [2].

Table 22.1 Summary of studies on diagnostic molecular markers for thyroid nodules with indeterminate cytology

Authors, year	n[a]	% malig[b]	Marker(s)	Prospective	Multicenter	Blinded	Sensitivity	NPV	Specificity	PPV
Faroux et al. 1997 [19]	69	13 %	A	?	No	?	89 %	97 %	58 %	24 %
Umbricht et al. 2004 [63]	100	48 %	B	No	Yes	?	90 %	87 %	65 %	70 %
Saggiorato et al. 2005 [56]	125	60 %	C	No	No	Yes	100 %	100 %	82 %	78 %
Bartolazzi et al. 2008 [5]	432	30 %	D	Yes	Yes	Yes	78 %	91 %	93 %	82 %
Franco et al. 2009 [21]	138	51 %	E	Yes	No	?	95 %	92 %	76 %	83 %
Nikiforov et al. 2009 [52]	52	40 %	F	Yes	Yes	Yes	71 %	84 %	100 %	100 %
Moses et al. 2010 [51]	137	31 %	F	Yes	No	Yes	48 %	80 %	94 %	78 %
Milas et al. 2010 [44]	61	75 %	G	No	No	No	59 %	80 %	90 %	39 %
Samija et al. 2011 [57]	142	20 %	H	Yes	No	Yes	79 %	91 %	53 %	28 %
Fadda et al. 2011 [18]	119	45 %	I	?	No	?	89 %	85 %	64 %	71 %
Nikiforov et al. 2011 [53]	513	24 %	J	Yes	No	No	61 %	89 %	98 %	89 %
Shen et al. 2012 [58]	68	65 %	K	No	No	Yes	89 %	79 %	79 %	89 %
Keutgen et al. 2012 [33]	72	31 %	L	Yes	Yes	Yes	100 %	100 %	86 %	73 %
Agretti et al. 2012 [1]	53	28 %	M	Yes	No	Yes	60 %	78 %	58 %	39 %
Rossi et al. 2012 [55]	123	36 %	N	Yes	No	?	32 %	73 %	100 %	100 %
Alexander et al. 2012 [2]	265	32 %	O	Yes	Yes	Yes	92 %	93 %	52 %	47 %
Hu et al. 2006 [29]	15	73 %	P	Yes	No	No	73 %	–	100 %	–

Adapted with modifications from Xing et al. [72]
[a]Number of indeterminate fine-needle aspiration biopsy (FNAB) with histopathology correlation
[b]Percent malignancy rate among indeterminate FNAB nodules
A – Thyroid peroxidase (*TPO*) immunocytochemistry (positive for malignancy <80 % cells)
B – hTERT (human telomerase) mRNA
C – Galectin-3 + CK-19 + HBME-1 immunocytochemistry
D – Galectin-3 immunohistochemistry
E – Galectin-3 + HBME-1 immunohistochemistry, either marker positive (>10 % cells staining)
F – BRAF and Ras mutations, Ret/PTC and Pax8-PPARγ rearrangements
G – Peripheral blood (nonserum, nonerythrocyte) thyrotropin/thyroid-stimulating hormone receptor mRNA (>1 ng/μg RNA is positive)
H – Galectin-3 mRNA RT-PCR (visual band on gel)
I – Galectin-3 and HBME-1 immunocytochemistry (>50 % cell staining, either marker positive)
J – BRAF and Ras mutations, Ret/PTC and Pax8-PPARγ rearrangements
K – Four microRNA set (miR-30d, miR-146b, miR-187, miR-221) linear discrimination analysis
L – Four microRNA set (miR-21, miR-197, miR-222, miR-328) support vector machine, radial basis kernel (SVM-RBF) model
M – Three microRNA set (miR-146b, miR-155, miR-221) decision-tree analysis
N – BRAFV600E mutation
O – Gene expression classifier (mRNA expression levels of 142 genes)
P– DNA methylation of five genes (CALCA, CDH1, TIMP3, DAPK, and RARβ2), detected in serum by methylation-specific real-time PCR
Other than G and P, which were peripheral blood-based tests, all were tested on fine-needle aspiration biopsy specimens

The test was established through a number of testing procedures, including iterative training and testing against known and unknown histopathology/cytopathology samples from multicenters. Unique gene expression patterns revealed in the GEC are used to distinguish benign from malignant thyroid tumors. There is a good overlap of such gene expression patterns between benign and malignant tumors. Consequently, the diagnostic specificity of the GEC for thyroid nodules with indeterminate cytology is low, which was only 52 %, with a positive predictive value of only 47 %. These values make GEC unreliable as a test to rule in a diagnosis of malignancy for the recommendation of thyroidectomy. On the bright side, however, GEC had high diagnostic sensitivities – 90 % for both AUS/FLUS and FN/SFN. Given their corresponding pretest probabilities of 24 % and 25 % in the study [2], the negative predictive values were 95 % and 94 % for AUS/FLUS and FN/SFN, respectively. This high negative predictive values make it reasonable to apply GEC to AUS/FLUS and FN/SFN to help identify patients with benign thyroid nodules for exclusion from thyroidectomy. Specifically, with a negative result on GEC test, the risk for malignancy in a thyroid nodule in the cytology category of AUS/FLUS or FN/SFN is dramatically decreased from 24–25 % to 5–6 %. Given the generally non-aggressive and indolent nature of thyroid cancer, with such GEC results, it is currently reasonable and acceptable to recommend conservative nonsurgical management of such thyroid nodules in appropriate clinical settings. Although the positive predictive value of GEC for AUS/FLUS or FN/SFN is relatively low at round 50 %, it is not negligible. With a positive (suspicious) GEC test result, thyroid nodules cytologically classified as AUS/FLUS or FN/SFN would be most reasonably considered for surgical treatments as would conventionally be recommended for cytologically indeterminate thyroid nodules. The cytological category of "suspicious for malignancy" has a high pretest probability, which was 62 % in the study [2]. Correspondingly, the negative predictive value of GEC for this category of thyroid nodule was relatively low at 85 %, which is too low to make GEC a reliable test in excluding patients from pursuing surgery. Therefore, GEC test adds limited diagnostic value to help the management of thyroid nodules in the cytological category of "suspicious for malignancy." Because the "suspicious for malignancy" cytology category is associated with a high enough risk for malignancy, it should be reasonable at the current time to recommend thyroid surgery without further diagnostic molecular testing, including GEC. This practice may be changed when more useful diagnostic molecular markers become available in the future. Thus, practically, the most applicable aspect of GEC is its usage, when the test is negative, with thyroid nodules in the cytological categories of AUS/PLUS and FN/SFN to favor nonsurgical conservative management. This approach in the management of thyroid nodules using GEC has been shown to be cost-effective as a large number of thyroid nodule patients with AUS/PLUS and FN/SFN can be spared from thyroid surgery [37]. Application of GEC to the management of thyroid nodules has become increasingly accepted and is likely to have a significant impact on the practice of thyroid tumor medicine. It should be noted, however, that the acceptance of the 5–6 % false-negative test rate of GEC applied to AUS/PLUS and FN/SFN is the result of overall consideration of all the aspects of thyroid nodules, such as the generally non-aggressive nature of thyroid cancer, cost, and potential complications of thyroid surgery, and the advertise affects associated with thyroid hormone replacements after thyroidectomy. However, this false-negative rate of GEC should be clearly discussed with the patient and accepted by the patient before pursuing GEC in the management of thyroid nodules. Also, the excellent negative predictive values with GEC were achieved based on the pretest probabilities of 24–25 % for AUS/PLUS and FN/SFN in the study [2]. In settings or institutions where the pretest probabilities are higher than 24–25 %, the false-negative rates of GEC when applied to AUS/PLUS and FN/SFN would be higher than 5–6 %, and, depending on the actual values, GEC could result in a high enough false-negative rate that may render the test unacceptable.

Perhaps new gene expression patterns can be identified to enhance the current GEC system in the future to further improve its diagnostic accuracy. It should also be noted that the GEC data and the recommendations based on them discussed above are solely from one study [2]. This study is not short of limitations. For example, among the 4,812 FNABs performed at 49 clinical sites in the study, only 577 (12 %) were cytologically indeterminate, representing a lower rate of this cytological category than generally seen [34, 72]. Among these, only 265 (46 %) were included in the final GEC testing after certain inclusion criteria were met. Thus, there seemed to be a selection bias, which could potentially call into question the generalization of this GEC test. In fact, a recent study at an academic center on a limited number of patients showed only a 16 % rate of histopathologically confirmed malignancy in GEC-positive (suspicious) nodules [47], which was much lower than the originally reported malignancy rate of around 50 % [2]. Thus, a large independent study that is more inclusive may be needed to more definitively evaluate the utility of this diagnostic approach for thyroid nodules.

Diagnostic Genetic Molecular Markers

Genetic molecular marker-based diagnostic approach to thyroid nodule has attracted wide interest and proven to be useful. Many genetic markers have been investigated, and the best known are *BRAF* mutation, *RAS* mutation, *RET-PTC* rearrangement, and *PAX8-PPARγ* rearrangement. *BRAF* V600E mutation is the most common genetic alteration in thyroid cancer that is present in about 45 % of papillary thyroid cancer (PTC) and 25 % of anaplastic thyroid cancer (ATC) on average [68]. Since its initial discovery in 2003 in thyroid cancer by a Johns Hopkins group [11], a work that won a United States patent, *BRAF* mutation has been extensively studied for its diagnostic value. Initial original studies demonstrated a 100 % diagnostic specificity of *BRAF* mutation for thyroid cancer when tested on thyroid FNAB specimens [12, 66]. The sensitivity of this diagnostic marker, however, is low, which was about 50 % in the initial original study [66], reflecting the similar prevalence of this mutation in PTC, which is the most common thyroid cancer and accounts for about 90 % of all thyroid malignancies [28, 31]. In the category of indeterminate thyroid cytological specimens, the cancer diagnostic sensitivity of *BRAF* mutation is even lower, which was, on average, only 8 % in an early meta-analysis [68]. This is because most of thyroid nodules with indeterminate cytology are benign nodules, which do not harbor *BRAF* mutation, and malignant thyroid nodules in the indeterminate cytology category are mostly follicular thyroid cancer (FTC) or follicular-variant papillary thyroid cancer (FVPTC), with the former harboring no *BRAF* mutation and the latter harboring the mutation only with a prevalence of 10–20 % [68, 75]. This low diagnostic sensitivity confers the testing of *BRAF* mutation alone limited diagnostic value in the evaluation of thyroid nodule. The diagnostic sensitivity of *BRAF* mutation, however, is dramatically increased in areas of the world, such as South Korea, where the *BRAF* mutation rate in PTC is up to 80–90 % and 95 % of all thyroid cancers are PTC [35, 36, 62, 69]. In such areas, *BRAF* mutation testing on FNAB specimens is a useful diagnostic approach to the evaluation of thyroid nodule.

Testing of *RET-PTC* on FNAB specimens for the diagnostic evaluation of thyroid nodule was initially performed more than 10 years ago, which was shown to be able to help refine the diagnosis of thyroid nodules [8]. *RAS* mutations and *PAX8-PPARγ* rearrangement have been also investigated for their diagnostic value for thyroid nodules. In general, these markers have an inferior specificity compared with *BRAF* mutation as they can occur, albeit relatively infrequently, in benign thyroid nodules [24, 43, 71, 74]. The combination use of these genetic markers has been shown to significantly improve the diagnostic sensitivity for cytologically indeterminate thyroid nodules [53]. In this later study, a panel of genetic markers were collectively tested, consisting of *BRAF* V600E, *N-RAS* codon 61, *HRAS* codon 61, and *KRAS* codons 12/13 point mutations and *RET-PTC1*, *RET-PTC3* , and *PAX8-PPARγ* rearrangements. In 479 patients who contributed 513 FNAB samples that were surgically confirmed for the final pathological diagnosis, the diagnostic sensitivities of these markers tested collectively for malignancy of thyroid nodules were 88 %, 87 %, and 95 % for cytological categories of AUS/PLUS, FN/SFN, and suspicious for malignancy, respectively. The false-negative values of this genetic testing for these cytological categories were correspondingly 6 %, 14 %, and 28 %, respectively. The authors concluded that this genetic molecular analysis has a significant diagnostic value for indeterminate cytology. Several institutions in the United States are currently applying the diagnostic approach using this panel of genetic markers to the evaluation of thyroid nodules and have found this approach to be helpful. It has been demonstrated that diagnostic use of this panel of genetic markers in assisting the decision making for the management of thyroid nodules would be cost-effective [78]. It should be noted, though, that the false-negative rate of this approach is relatively high, particularly in the cytological categories of FN/SFN and suspicious for malignancy. Very few cases positive for *RET-PTC* and *PAX8-PPARγ* were found, and they were exclusively found in malignant nodules in this study. Also, the RAS mutation rate in benign thyroid tumors was unusually low. These results are all somehow inconsistent with the relatively common findings of genetic rearrangement markers and *RAS* mutations in benign thyroid tumors [24, 43, 71, 74]. It seems to be ideal to have an independent large study to further evaluate and define the diagnostic values of this panel of genetic markers in the evaluation of thyroid nodules. Addition of new genetic markers recently discovered in thyroid cancer, such as *RASAL1* mutations [39] and *TERT* promoter mutations [41, 42, 76] (see below), may enhance the diagnostic sensitivity and specificity.

Diagnostic Protein Maker Galectin-3

Galectin-3 (Gal-3) is a 30-kDa protein that binds to beta-galactosidase residues on cell surface glycoproteins and has been well known to play an important role in cell proliferation, adhesion, differentiation, angiogenesis, and apoptosis in normal and pathologic tissues; it is also closely involved in tumor cell transformation, migration, invasion, and metastasis [60]. Consequently, it is not surprising that Gal-3 is commonly overexpressed in many human cancers, including thyroid cancer [10]. As such, Gal-3 has been extensively investigated as a protein biomarker for its diagnostic value in thyroid cancer [10, 79]. Gal-3 was first proposed as a marker for thyroid malignancy in 1995 [77]. Using the immunohistochemical (IHC) staining approach, this study demonstrated that both PTC and FTC were positive for Gal-3, but benign samples were negative. Many other studies have confirmed these results, albeit with varying values of sensitivity and specificity, using IHC and reverse transcription polymerase chain reaction [13, 15, 20, 26, 45, 54]. Many more recent studies continued to show a good diagnostic value of Gal-3 for thyroid nodules. The largest one among these was a study testing the diagnostic value of Gal-3 in thyroid nodules cytologically determined to be indeterminate [5]. In this study, HIC staining of FNAB specimens to detect Gal-3 expression was performed in 432 cytologically indeterminate cases that had final pathological diagnosis established after thyroidectomy. The overall sensitivity of this Gal-3 test for thyroid malignancy was 78 % (95 % CI 74–82), and the specificity was 93 % (95 % CI 90–95). Estimated positive predictive value was 82 % (79–86), and negative predictive value was 91 % (88–93). The preoperative diagnostic accuracy was 88 % (381/432). Although these diagnostic values of Gal-3 are slightly inferior to the GEC system and the genetic markers discussed above, Gal-3 testing is easier to perform and does not require sophisticated equipments [4]. Even currently without available data to assess the cost-effectiveness of Gal-3 testing, this test is expected to be less costly than the markers discussed above. Thus, in economically constrained settings, Gal-3 may be a better choice than the GEC system and the genetic markers for the diagnostic evaluation of thyroid nodule. It should be kept in mind, though, that, like any IHC examination of protein markers, observer's subjective bias in reading the IHC results could potentially complicate the diagnosis determination.

Peripheral Blood-Based Diagnostic Tests for Thyroid Nodules

Among several blood biomarkers that have been investigated in recent years is the thyrotropin/thyroid-stimulating hormone receptor (TSHR) mRNA in peripheral blood [9, 49]. In an analysis on 61 cases of patients with cytologically indeterminate thyroid nodule, preoperative test of TSHR mRNA by real-time PCR showed a diagnostic sensitivity of 59 % and specificity of 90 %, with a negative predictive value of 80 % and positive predictive value of 39 % [44]. Another blood marker is aberrant DNA methylation, which was first demonstrated in 2006 [29]. In this study, methylation-specific real-time PCR was used to detect aberrant hypermethylation of five tumor suppressor genes – *CALCA*, *CDH1*, *TIMP3*, *DAPK*, and *RARβ2* – on 57 serum DNA samples isolated preoperatively from patients undergoing for thyroidectomy for thyroid tumors. The results showed a diagnostic sensitivity of 68 % (26 of 38) for surgically confirmed thyroid cancer and a specificity of 95 % (18 of 19) for surgically confirmed benign thyroid tumors, with an overall preoperative diagnostic accuracy of 77 % and positive and negative predictive values of 96 % and 60 %, respectively. In a limited number of patients with cytologically indeterminate thyroid nodules, this serum DNA methylation testing revealed a diagnostic sensitivity of 73 % (8/11) and specificity of 100 % (4/4). Although the diagnostic values of these peripheral blood biomarkers are limited at the present time in these early studies, they are promising and the convenient nature of blood tests makes these diagnostic approaches for thyroid nodules attractive. Further studies are worth pursuing to improve these tests.

Prognostic Molecular Markers of Thyroid Cancer

BRAF V600E Mutation in the Recurrence of PTC

The *BRAF* V600E mutation causes constitutive activation of the MAP kinase pathway, which is the primary mechanism for the oncogenic role of this mutation in human cancers [16]. As this is the major oncogene in PTC [68], its prognostic potential for PTC has drawn considerable attention since its initial discovery. In 2005, *BRAF* V600E mutation was for the first time demonstrated to be associated with increased disease recurrence of PTC, along with other aggressive clinicopathological characteristics of PTC [67]. Numerous other studies were subsequently pursued to investigate the prognostic value of *BRAF* V600E in PTC [36, 62, 69]. Although the studies were not all consistent, most of them showed a significant association of *BRAF* V600E with poor clinicopathological outcomes, such as large tumor size, extrathyroidal invasion, lymph node metastasis, and disease recurrence of PTC. This association of *BRAF* mutation with PTC recurrence was lost in some studies upon multivariable adjustment for common pathological characteristics, such as lymph node metastasis and extrathyroidal invasion of the tumor. This is partially explained by the fact that these aggressive tumor behaviors are the main source of PTC recurrence, and *BRAF* mutation, through well-established molecular mechanisms [74], promotes PTC aggressiveness by aggravating these aggressive tumor behaviors. As such, in statistical multivariable models, the importance of *BRAF* mutation may be artificially diminished or even lost when adjustment is made for aggressive tumor behaviors. Also, many of the individual studies were relatively small and could not provide a large enough power to accurately address the prognostic value of *BRAF* mutation.

A recent large retrospective multicenter study on 2,099 cases of PTC demonstrated a strong association of *BRAF* mutation with PTC recurrence even after multivariable adjustment for conventional clinicopathological factors [75]. The 2,099 patients consisted of 1,615 females and 484 males, with a median age of 45 (interquartile range – IQR = 34–58) years and a median follow-up time of 36 (IQR = 14–75) months. The overall *BRAF* V600E mutation prevalence was 48.5 % (1,017/2,099). PTC recurrence was found in 20.9 % (213/1,017) of *BRAF* V600E mutation-positive and 11.6 % (125/1,082) of *BRAF* V600E mutation-negative patients.

Recurrence rates in terms of recurrences per 1,000 person-years were 47.71 (95 % CI=41.72–54.57) versus 26.03 (95 % CI=21.85–31.02) in *BRAF* mutation-positive versus mutation-negative patients ($P<0.001$) with a hazard ratio (HR)=1.82 (95 % CI=1.46–2.28). This HR remained significant after the multivariable adjustment for patient sex and age at diagnosis, medical center, tumor size, extrathyroidal invasion, and lymph node metastasis. Significant association between *BRAF* mutation and PTC recurrence was also found in patients with conventionally low-risk disease stage I and II and micro PTC and within various subtypes of PTC, including follicular-variant PTC (FVPTC). In *BRAF* mutation-positive versus mutation-negative FVPTC, recurrence was found in 21.3 % (19/89) and 7.0 % (24/342) of patients, with recurrence rates of 53.84 (95 % CI=34.34–84.40) versus 19.47 (95 % CI=13.05–29.04) recurrences per 1,000 person-years ($P<0.001$) and a HR=3.20 (95 % CI=1.46–7.02) after adjustment for clinicopathological factors. A poorer recurrence-free probability was found to be associated with *BRAF* mutation on Kaplan-Meier survival analyses in various clinicopathological categories. Thus, this large multicenter study established an independent prognostic value of *BRAF* V600E mutation for PTC recurrence in various clinicopathological categories. It is of interest that the prognostic power of *BRAF* mutation was highest in FVPTC. This result may be particularly useful as the prevalence of *BRAF* mutation in FVPTC is only 10–20 % [68, 75], making it practically possible to relatively focus on a small group of patients with FVPTC for relatively more aggressive treatment.

It is worth noting that *BRAF* mutation has a high negative predictive value for the absence of PTC recurrence. In a previous study on preoperative testing for *BRAF* mutation on FNAB specimens in 190 patients with PTC of mixed risks, the negative predictive values of preoperative testing for *BRAF* mutation to predict the absence of future recurrence of PTC were 88 % for patients with any PTC and 92 % for patients with conventional PTC (CPTC) [70]. In a subsequent study on 319 patients with stages I–II PTC (intrathyroid tumor and no metastases; T1–T2) and a mean follow-up time of 5.3±0.8 years, the negative predictive value for a negative test of *BRAF* mutation to predict the absence of PTC recurrence was 97 % [17]. This high negative predictive power of *BRAF* mutation should be particularly useful in helping appropriately minimize surgical extents and reduce overtreatments of PTC in many patients.

Testing of FNAB specimens for *BRAF* mutation may not only be helpful diagnostically as discussed above, but it may also be helpful prognostically. A 2009 study for the first time tested the preoperative predictive power of *BRAF* mutation on FNAB specimens for poor pathological characteristics of PTC and the risk of future recurrence [70]. This study demonstrated a strong association of *BRAF* mutation detected preoperatively with aggressive pathological characteristics of the tumor discovered postoperatively, including lymph node metastasis, extrathyroidal invasion, and advanced disease stages as well as future tumor recurrence. Several other studies subsequently also demonstrated a significant association of *BRAF* mutation detected preoperatively on FNAB specimens with postoperatively discovered aggressive clinicopathological outcomes of PTC, including a strong prediction of occult lymph node metastases by preoperative BRAF mutation testing [32, 38]. Thus, preoperative testing of *BRAF* mutation can provide useful prognostic information on PTC that conventional clinical and imaging evaluations may not be able to provide. Such preoperative information of *BRAF* mutation status may be useful in helping physicians define the surgical and medical treatments of PTC.

BRAF V600E Mutation in PTC-Related Patient Mortality

Thyroid cancer usually has an indolent clinical course with a very low mortality rate. Consequently, it is often not easy to achieve a large enough cohort of patients with clinical follow-up that is sufficiently long to investigate patient mortality. This has been also the case with the research of *BRAF* mutation. As a result, there were fewer studies that investigated the role of *BRAF* mutation in PTC-related patient mortality and most of the studies that did lacked sufficient power to reliably conclude on this role of *BRAF* mutation. A recent large retrospective multicenter study has been able to thoroughly explore the role of *BRAF* mutation in PTC-related patient mortality [73]. This study investigated the relationship between *BRAF* V600E mutation and PTC-related mortality in 1,849 patients (1,411 women and 438 men) with a median age of 46 years (interquartile range: 34–58 years) and an overall median follow-up time of 33 months (interquartile range: 13–67 months). Patient death was found in 5.3 % (45/845; 95 % CI, 3.9–7.1 %) and 1.1 % (11/1,004; 95 % CI, 0.5–2.0 %) in *BRAF* mutation-positive and mutation-negative patients, respectively, with death rates in terms of deaths per 1,000 person-years being 12.87 (95 % CI, 9.61–17.24) vs. 2.52 (95 % CI, 1.40–4.55) in the former versus the latter ($P<0.001$) and the hazard ratio [HR] being 2.66 (95 % CI, 1.30–5.43) after adjustment for age at diagnosis, sex, and medical center. When only focused on CPTC, deaths per 1,000 person-years were 11.80 (95 % CI, 8.39–16.60) vs. 2.25 (95 % CI, 1.01–5.00) in *BRAF* mutation-positive versus mutation-negative patients, with the adjusted HR being 3.53 (95 % CI, 1.25–9.98). A higher *BRAF* mutation-associated patient mortality was also observed within several clinicopathological subcategories. As an example, in patients with lymph node metastasis, deaths per 1,000 person-years were 26.26 (95 % CI, 19.18–35.94) vs. 5.93 (95 % CI, 2.96–11.86) in *BRAF* mutation-positive vs. mutation-negative groups

(HR 4.43; 95 % CI, 2.06–9.51), and in patients with distant tumor metastasis, deaths per 1,000 person-years were 87.72 (95 % CI, 62.68–122.77) vs. 32.28 (95 % CI, 16.14–64.55) in *BRAF* mutation-positive versus mutation-negative patients (HR 2.63, 95 % CI 1.21–5.72). These data thus demonstrated a significant association of *BRAF* V600E mutation with increased PTC-related patient mortality. When tumor behaviors, such as lymph node metastasis, extrathyroidal invasion, and distant metastasis, were included in the multivariable model, the association of *BRAF* mutation with PTC-related mortality was no longer significant with HR being crossing 1.0 although a strong trend was still present. This does not mean the lack of an important role of *BRAF* mutation in PTC-related mortality as were concerned by some authors [7]. All cancer-related patient deaths are a consequence of tumor aggressiveness, and thyroid cancer is no exception; PTC-related patient death would not occur if no aggressive tumor behavior is present, such as lymph node metastasis, extrathyroidal invasion, and distant metastasis. Mutations themselves do not directly cause patient death. This and any mutation alone cannot independently cause PTC-related patient death if none of the aggressive tumor behaviors exists. As such, the impact of *BRAF* mutation on patient death could be expectedly lost on the multivariable model adjusting for aggressive tumor behaviors. Theoretically, if given a long enough follow-up time for sufficient number of deaths to occur, including deaths that occur from recurrent diseases in patients without measurable initial classical aggressive tumor behaviors, one may be able to see an independent effect of BRAF mutation on PTC-related mortality. Oncogenes, such as mutated *BRAF* gene, can aggravate poor clinical outcomes, such as cancer-related patient death, but this is achieved by promoting aggressive pathological tumor behaviors. Therefore, as the JAMA study showed [73], *BRAF* mutation is strongly associated with PTC-related mortality, but this is not independent of aggressive tumor behaviors within the studied follow-up time. Given this mechanism, it is not surprising to see that, as the JAMA study demonstrated, *BRAF* mutation and some of the classical aggressive clinicopathological risk factors, such as old patient age, lymph node metastasis, and distant metastasis, synergistically aggravate PTC-related mortality rates. The synergy index was much larger than 1.0 for the interaction between *BRAF* mutation and these high-risk factors, suggesting a strong synergy of *BRAF* mutation with them. Thus, even patients with known classical high-risk factors can be separated into two groups by the *BRAF* mutation status; the *BRAF* mutation-positive group has a even higher risk of mortality than the risk conferred by the conventional clinicopathological risk factor alone, representing an incremental prognostic value of *BRAF* mutation for PTC-related mortality. For example [73], in patients <60 years old, death occurred in 0.6 % (5/819) of *BRAF* mutation-negative patients versus 2.3 % (14/617) of *BRAF* mutation-positive patients (P=0.009), implying that in 100 patients <60 years old the presence of *BRAF* mutation could only increase 1–2 patient death; in contrast, in patients ≥60 years old, patient death occurred in 3.2 % (6/185) of *BRAF* mutation-negative patients versus 13.6 % (31/228) of *BRAF* mutation-positive patients (P<0.001), implying that in 100 patients ≥60 years old, the presence of *BRAF* mutation could additionally cause 10 patient deaths. As another example [73], in the absence of distant metastasis, patient death occurred in 0.3 % (3/944) of *BRAF* mutation-negative patients versus 1.4 % (11/772) of *BRAF* mutation-positive patients (P=0.01), implying that in 100 patients without distant metastasis the presence of *BRAF* mutation could only increase one patient death; in contrast, in the presence of distant metastasis, patient death occurred in 18.2 % (8/44) of *BRAF* mutation-negative patients versus 51.5 % (34/66) of *BRAF* mutation-positive patients (P<0.001), implying that in 100 patients with distant metastasis the presence of *BRAF* mutation could additionally cause 33 patient deaths. Thus, from a practical perspective, the impact of *BRAF* mutation on patient deaths is profound in certain clinical settings, although this impact, from a mathematical perspective, would misleadingly disappear on the multivariable statistical model adjusting for the conventional risk factors. It is also interesting to see that in this study in patients with micro PTC (tumor ≤1.0 cm), death occurred in 0 % (0/267) *BRAF* mutation-negative patients versus 2.4 % (4/168) *BRAF* mutation-positive patients (P=0.02). Thus, although there were only few deaths in patients with micro PTC, they all occurred in the *BRAF* mutation-positive group, suggesting a high negative predictive value of *BRAF* mutation to predict the absence of PTC-related mortality, which was also seen in other clinicopathological settings [73]. This high negative predictive value of *BRAF* mutation for PTC-related mortality, together with its high negative predictive value for PTC recurrence discussed above, can be useful in assisting clinical decision making for less aggressive treatments of PTC patients in appropriate clinical settings.

Potential Prognostic Values of *RAS* Mutations and *RET-PTC* Rearrangement in Thyroid Cancer

RAS mutations, particularly *N-RAS* mutations, have been demonstrated to be associated with increased aggressiveness and poorer clinicopathological outcomes of thyroid cancer, particularly poorly differentiated thyroid cancer (PDTC) and FTC. For example, an early study demonstrated that *RAS* mutations were more commonly associated with PDTC or ATC than differentiated thyroid cancer [23]. In this study, 74.3 % (26/35) of patients positive for *RAS* mutation versus 31.9 % (23/72) patients negative for the mutation died as a result of thyroid cancer ($P<0.001$). When only differentiated thyroid cancer and PDTC were examined, 55.0 % (11/20) of patients positive for *RAS* mutation versus 15.5 % (9/58) of patients negative for the mutation died of thyroid cancer ($P=0.016$). A later study demonstrated a significant association of *N-RAS* mutation with poorer disease-specific survival of patients with PDTC [65]. A more recent study demonstrated a significant association of *N-RAS* mutation with distant metastasis of FTC and FTC-related patient mortality [22]. These studies suggest a potential prognostic role of *RAS* mutations in thyroid cancer, particularly PDTC and FTC. Further studies are needed to determine how testing for *RAS* mutations can assist decision making for the clinical management of these cancers.It should be noted that this aggressive role of RAS mutation may not necessarily represent the sole effect of RAS mutation itself. It is possible that its coexistence with other oncogenic genetic alterations, such as TERT promoter mutations, synergistically promotes tumor aggressiveness and poor prognosis while RAS mutation alone may not be a strong promoter. This is similar to the synergistic effect between BRAF mutation and TERT promoter mutations (see below). Further studies are needed to test this possibility.

In contrast, *RET-PTC* has been shown not to be associated with aggressive features of thyroid cancer, such as large tumor size, extrathyroidal invasion, and metastasis of thyroid cancer [61]. This is consistent with the only mild extent of aggressive molecular derangements associated with *RET-PTC* , such as loss of thyroid iodide-handling gene expression, in contrast with the profound extent of aggressive molecular derangements associated with the *BRAF* mutation in thyroid cancer [74]. Thus, unlike *BRAF* mutation, a positive test of *RET-PTC* predicts a good prognosis of thyroid cancer, which may be useful information in the management decision making to favor less aggressive treatments of thyroid cancer in appropriate clinical settings.

New Genetic Molecular Markers in Thyroid Cancer

RASAL1 Mutations and Hypermethylation in Thyroid Cancer

RASAL1 is a GTPase-activating protein that activates the intrinsic GTPase of RAS. The normal function of RASSAL1 is thus to promote the conversion of the active form of GTP-bound RAS to the inactive form of GDP-bound RAS, terminating the RAS signaling. A recent study for the first time established RASAL1 as a prominent tumor suppressor in thyroid cancer by demonstrating the tumor suppressor function of RASAL1 and its inactivation by mutations and hypermethylation of the *RASAL1* gene in thyroid cancer [39]. In this study, several mutations of the *RASAL1* gene were for the first time identified, which were found only in thyroid cancer, but not in benign thyroid tumors. Aberrant hypermethylation of the *RASAL1* gene was also commonly found in thyroid cancer, but not in benign thyroid tumors. *RASAL1* mutations and hypermethylation may thus be potentially novel diagnostic molecular markers for thyroid cancer. Interestingly, these genetic and epigenetic alterations of the *RASAL1* gene were more commonly found in aggressive type of thyroid cancer, such as ATC, suggesting a prognostic potential of these genetic and epigenetic molecular markers of *RASAL1* for thyroid cancer. Further studies are needed to define the diagnostic and prognostic values of these *RASAL1* markers.

TERT Promoter Mutations in Thyroid Cancer

The *TERT*gene encodes telomerase reverse transcriptase (TERT) which is the catalytic subunit of telomerase, a ribonucleoprotein complex that plays a primary role in maintaining telomere length at the end of chromosomes [50, 59]. TERT has long been known to play an important role in human cancers [6]. Early in 2013, two interesting somatic mutations, chr5:1,295,228 C>T and chr5:1,295,250 C>T (termed here as C228T and C250T, respectively), in the promoter of the *TERT* gene were identified in melanoma, which represent nucleotide changes of −124 C>T and −146 C>T from the ATG translation start site of the *TERT* gene, respectively [27, 30]. These mutations confer *TERT* increased transcriptional activities. The two *TERT* promoter mutations were soon discovered in thyroid cancer [41]. In this initial study on a large number of thyroid tumors, the C228T *TERT* mutation was found to be in about 12 % of PTC and FTC and 30–40 % of PDTC and ATC, but not in benign thyroid tumors, suggesting a potential diagnostic value for thyroid cancer in the evaluation of thyroid nodules. The preferential occurrence of *TERT* promoter mutations in aggressive types of thyroid cancer, such as PDTC and ATC, as well as *BRAF* V600E mutation-positive PTC, suggests a role of *TERT* promoter mutations in the development of aggressiveness of thyroid cancer. A subsequent study demonstrated a strong association of *TERT* promoter mutations with various aggressive pathological characteristics, and this association was particularly prominent when coexisting with *BRAF* mutation [41]. These findings were confirmed in several other studies [40, 48, 64]. A more recent large study demonstrated that coexistence of *TERT* promoter mutations with *BRAF* V600E mutation was associated with the highest recurrence and the most common aggressive features of PTC [76]. Coexistence of BRAF mutation and TERT promoter mutations has been recently also shown to be associated the worst PTC-related mortality. Thus, coexisting BRAF mutation and TERT promoter mutations provide a unique genetic background that defines the most aggressive PTC [80]. As such, *TERT* promoter mutation is a novel diagnostic and prognostic molecular marker for thyroid cancer. Inclusion of *TERT* promoter mutations will likely enhance the diagnostic sensitivity and specificity of the current panel of diagnostic genetic markers of thyroid cancer. *TERT* promoter mutations are also novel powerful prognostic makers for thyroid cancer, particularly for PTC when used in combination with *BRAF* V600E mutation.

Summary and Conclusions

Considerable progress has occurred in recent years in the identification and development of diagnostic and prognostic molecular markers for thyroid nodule and thyroid cancer. Several of these biomarkers have been proven to be clinically useful and are increasingly used as adjunct diagnostic molecular tests with FNAB for thyroid nodules. These include the GEC, the genetic panel of *BRAF* mutation, *RAS* mutations, *RET-PTC* and *PAX8-PPAR*γ, and the protein marker galectin-3. The best studied prognostic maker is *BRAF* V600E mutation, which has been proving to be useful in assisting the current risk stratification of PTC; this will now be enhanced by the recently discovered *TERT* promoter mutations. *RAS* mutations have a potential prognostic value in FTC and PDTC, which is worth further investigating; its sole prognostic role particularly needs to be determined. Several other molecular markers, such as the peripheral blood-based molecular markers, hold great promises as diagnostic and prognostic molecular markers for thyroid cancer and deserve to be further explored. It is expected that appropriate selection and application of the right molecular markers will significantly improve the current management of thyroid nodule and thyroid cancer. As more molecular markers are discovered and the current markers become better characterized to fit appropriate clinical settings, this biomarker-based approach will have an even more profound impact on the practice of thyroid tumor medicine.

References

1. Agretti P, Ferrarini E, Rago T, Candelieri A, De Marco G, Dimida A, Niccolai F, Molinaro A, Di Coscio G, Pinchera A, Vitti P, Tonacchera M. MicroRNA expression profile helps to distinguish benign nodules from papillary thyroid carcinomas starting from cells of fine-needle aspiration. Eur J Endocrinol. 2012;167: 393–400.
2. Alexander EK, Kennedy GC, Baloch ZW, Cibas ES, Chudova D, Diggans J, Friedman L, Kloos RT, LiVolsi VA, Mandel SJ, Raab SS, Rosai J, Steward DL, Walsh PS, Wilde JI, Zeiger MA, Lanman RB, Haugen BR. Preoperative diagnosis of benign thyroid nodules with indeterminate cytology. N Engl J Med. 2012;367:705–15.
3. Baloch ZW, LiVolsi VA, Asa SL, Rosai J, Merino MJ, Randolph G, Vielh P, DeMay RM, Sidawy MK, Frable WJ. Diagnostic terminology and morphologic criteria for cytologic diagnosis of thyroid lesions: a synopsis of the National Cancer Institute Thyroid Fine-Needle Aspiration State of the Science Conference. Diagn Cytopathol. 2008;36:425–37.
4. Bartolazzi A, Bellotti C, Sciacchitano S. Methodology and technical requirements of the galectin-3 test for the preoperative characterization of thyroid nodules. Appl Immunohistochem Mol Morphol. 2012;20:2–7.
5. Bartolazzi A, Orlandi F, Saggiorato E, Volante M, Arecco F, Rossetto R, Palestini N, Ghigo E, Papotti M, Bussolati G, Martegani MP, Pantellini F, Carpi A, Giovagnoli MR, Monti S, Toscano V, Sciacchitano S, Pennelli GM, Mian C, Pelizzo MR, Rugge M, Troncone G, Palombini L, Chiappetta G, Botti G, Vecchione A, Bellocco R, Italian Thyroid Cancer Study Group (ITCSG). Galectin-3-expression analysis in the surgical selection of follicular thyroid nodules with indeterminate fine-needle aspiration cytology: a prospective multicentre study. Lancet Oncol. 2008;9:543–9.
6. Blasco MA. Telomeres and human disease: ageing, cancer and beyond. Nat Rev Genet. 2005;6:611–22.
7. Cappola AR, Mandel SJ. Molecular testing in thyroid cancer: BRAF mutation status and mortality. JAMA. 2013;309:1529–30.
8. Cheung CC, Carydis B, Ezzat S, Bedard YC, Asa SL. Analysis of ret/PTC gene rearrangements refines the fine needle aspiration diagnosis of thyroid cancer. J Clin Endocrinol Metab. 2001;86: 2187–90.
9. Chia SY, Milas M, Reddy SK, Siperstein A, Skugor M, Brainard J, Gupta MK. Thyroid-stimulating hormone receptor messenger ribonucleic acid measurement in blood as a marker for circulating thyroid cancer cells and its role in the preoperative diagnosis of thyroid cancer. J Clin Endocrinol Metab. 2007;92:468–75.
10. Chiu CG, Strugnell SS, Griffith OL, Jones SJ, Gown AM, Walker B, Nabi IR, Wiseman SM. Diagnostic utility of galectin-3 in thyroid cancer. Am J Pathol. 2010;176:2067–81.
11. Cohen Y, Xing M, Mambo E, Guo Z, Wu G, Trink B, Beller U, Westra WH, Ladenson PW, Sidransky D. BRAF mutation in papillary thyroid carcinoma. J Natl Cancer Inst. 2003;95:625–7.
12. Cohen Y, Rosenbaum E, Clark DP, Zeiger MA, Umbricht CB, Tufano RP, Sidransky D, Westra WH. Mutational analysis of BRAF in fine needle aspiration biopsies of the thyroid: a potential application for the preoperative assessment of thyroid nodules. Clin Cancer Res. 2004;10:2761–5.
13. Coli A, Bigotti G, Zucchetti F, Negro F, Massi G. Galectin-3, a marker of well-differentiated thyroid carcinoma, is expressed in thyroid nodules with cytological atypia. Histopathology. 2002;40:80–7.
14. Haugen BR, Alexander EK, Bible KC, Doherty GM, Mandel SJ, Nikiforov Y, Pacini F, Randolph G, Sawka A, Shepard D, Sosa J, Tuttle RM, Wartofsky L. 2015 American Thyroid Association Management Guidelines for adult patients with thyroid nodules and differentiated thyroid cancer. Available online at Thyroid 25: DOI:10.1089/thy.2015.0020; print version in Thyroid 26:1–133, 2016.
15. Cvejic D, Savin S, Paunovic I, Tatic S, Havelka M, Sinadinovic J. Immunohistochemical localization of galectin-3 in malignant and benign human thyroid tissue. Anticancer Res. 1998;18:2637–41.
16. Davies H, Bignell GR, Cox C, Stephens P, Edkins S, Clegg S, Teague J, Woffendin H, Garnett MJ, Bottomley W, Davis N, Dicks E, Ewing R, Floyd Y, Gray K, Hall S, Hawes R, Hughes J, Kosmidou V, Menzies A, Mould C, Parker A, Stevens C, Watt S, Hooper S, Wilson R, Jayatilake H, Gusterson BA, Cooper C, Shipley J, Hargrave D, Pritchard-Jones K, Maitland N, Chenevix-Trench G, Riggins GJ, Bigner DD, Palmieri G, Cossu A, Flanagan A, Nicholson A, Ho JW, Leung SY, Yuen ST, Weber BL, Seigler HF, Darrow TL, Paterson H, Marais R, Marshall CJ, Wooster R, Stratton MR, Futreal PA. Mutations of the BRAF gene in human cancer. Nature. 2002;417:949–54.

17. Elisei R, Viola D, Torregrossa L, Giannini R, Romei C, Ugolini C, Molinaro E, Agate L, Biagini A, Lupi C, Valerio L, Materazzi G, Miccoli P, Piaggi P, Pinchera A, Vitti P, Basolo F. The BRAF(V600E) mutation is an independent, poor prognostic factor for the outcome of patients with low-risk intrathyroid papillary thyroid carcinoma: single-institution results from a large cohort study. J Clin Endocrinol Metab. 2012;97:4390–8.
18. Fadda G, Rossi ED, Raffaelli M, Pontecorvi A, Sioletic S, Morassi F, Lombardi CP, Zannoni GF, Rindi G. Follicular thyroid neoplasms can be classified as low- and high-risk according to HBME-1 and Galectin-3 expression on liquid-based fine-needle cytology. Eur J Endocrinol. 2011;165:447–53.
19. Faroux MJ, Theobald S, Pluot M, Patey M, Menzies D. Evaluation of the monoclonal antibody antithyroperoxidase MoAb47 in the diagnostic decision of cold thyroid nodules by fine-needle aspiration. Pathol Res Pract. 1997;193:705–12.
20. Fernández PL, Merino MJ, Gómez M, Campo E, Medina T, Castronovo V, Sanjuán X, Cardesa A, Liu FT, Sobel ME. Galectin-3 and laminin expression in neoplastic and non-neoplastic thyroid tissue. J Pathol. 1997;181:80–6.
21. Franco C, Martínez V, Allamand JP, Medina F, Glasinovic A, Osorio M, Schachter D. Molecular markers in thyroid fine-needle aspiration biopsy: a prospective study. Appl Immunohistochem Mol Morphol. 2009;17:211–5.
22. Fukahori M, Yoshida A, Hayashi H, Yoshihara M, Matsukuma S, Sakuma Y, Koizume S, Okamoto N, Kondo T, Masuda M, Miyagi Y. The associations between RAS mutations and clinical characteristics in follicular thyroid tumors: new insights from a single center and a large patient cohort. Thyroid. 2012;22:683–9.
23. Garcia-Rostan G, Zhao H, Camp RL, Pollan M, Herrero A, Pardo J, Wu R, Carcangiu ML, Costa J, Tallini G. Ras mutations are associated with aggressive tumor phenotypes and poor prognosis in thyroid cancer. J Clin Oncol. 2003;21:3226–35.
24. Guerra A, Carrano M, Angrisani E, Puzziello A, Izzo G, Di Crescenzo V, Vatrella A, Vitale M. Detection of RAS mutation by pyrosequencing in thyroid cytology samples. Int J Surg. 2014;12:S91–4. pii: S1743-9191(14)00144-7.
25. Guth S, Theune U, Aberle J, Galach A, Bamberger CM. Very high prevalence of thyroid nodules detected by high frequency (13 MHz) ultrasound examination. Eur J Clin Invest. 2009;39:699–706.
26. Herrmann ME, LiVolsi VA, Pasha TL, Roberts SA, Wojcik EM, Baloch ZW. Immunohistochemical expression of galectin-3 in benign and malignant thyroid lesions. Arch Pathol Lab Med. 2002;126:710–3.
27. Horn S, Figl A, Rachakonda PS, Fischer C, Sucker A, Gast A, Kadel S, Moll I, Nagore E, Hemminki K, Schadendorf D, Kumar R. TERT promoter mutations in familial and sporadic melanoma. Science. 2013;339:959–61.
28. Howlader N, Noone AM, Krapcho M, Garshell J, Miller D, Altekruse SF, et al. 2015 SEER Cancer Statistics Review, 1975-2012, National Cancer Institute. Bethesda, MD, http://seer.cancer.gov/csr/1975-2012/, based on November 2014 SEER data submission, posted to the SEER web site, April 2015. Accessed on June 10, 2015.
29. Hu S, Ewertz M, Tufano RP, Brait M, Carvalho AL, Liu D, Tufaro AP, Basaria S, Cooper DS, Sidransky D, Ladenson PW, Xing M. Detection of serum deoxyribonucleic acid methylation markers: a novel diagnostic tool for thyroid cancer. J Clin Endocrinol Metab. 2006;91:98–104.
30. Huang FW, Hodis E, Xu MJ, Kryukov GV, Chin L, Garraway LA. Highly recurrent TERT promoter mutations in human melanoma. Science. 2013;339:957–9.
31. Jemal A, Bray F, Center MM, Ferlay J, Ward E, Forman D. Global cancer statistics. CA Cancer J Clin. 2011;61:69–90.
32. Joo JY, Park JY, Yoon YH, Choi B, Kim JM, Jo YS, Shong M, Koo BS. Prediction of occult central lymph node metastasis in papillary thyroid carcinoma by preoperative BRAF analysis using fine-needle aspiration biopsy: a prospective study. J Clin Endocrinol Metab. 2012;97:3996–4003.
33. Keutgen XM, Filicori F, Crowley MJ, Wang Y, Scognamiglio T, Hoda R, Buitrago D, Cooper D, Zeiger MA, Zarnegar R, Elemento O, Fahey 3rd TJ. A panel of four miRNAs accurately differentiates malignant from benign indeterminate thyroid lesions on fine needle aspiration. Clin Cancer Res. 2012;18:2032–8.
34. Keutgen XM, Filicori F, Fahey 3rd TJ. Molecular diagnosis for indeterminate thyroid nodules on fine needle aspiration: advances and limitations. Expert Rev Mol Diagn. 2013;13:613–23.
35. Kim KH, Kang DW, Kim SH, Seong IO, Kang DY. Mutations of the BRAF gene in papillary thyroid carcinoma in a Korean population. Yonsei Med J. 2004;45:818–21.
36. Kim TH, Park YJ, Lim JA, Ahn HY, Lee EK, Lee YJ, Kim KW, Hahn SK, Youn YK, Kim KH, Cho BY, do Park J. The association of the BRAF(V600E) mutation with prognostic factors and poor clinical outcome in papillary thyroid cancer: a meta-analysis. Cancer. 2012;118:1764–73.
37. Li H, Robinson KA, Anton B, Saldanha IJ, Ladenson PW. Cost-effectiveness of a novel molecular test for cytologically indeterminate thyroid nodules. J Clin Endocrinol Metab. 2011;96: E1719–26.
38. Lin KL, Wang OC, Zhang XH, Dai XX, Hu XQ, Qu JM. The BRAF mutation is predictive of aggressive clinicopathological characteristics in papillary thyroid microcarcinoma. Ann Surg Oncol. 2010;17:3294–300.
39. Liu D, Yang C, Bojdani E, Murugan AK, Xing M. Identification of RASAL1 as a major tumor suppressor gene in thyroid cancer. J Natl Cancer Inst. 2013;105:1617–27.
40. Liu T, Wang N, Cao J, Sofiadis A, Dinets A, Zedenius J, Larsson C, Xu D. The age- and shorter telomere-dependent TERT promoter mutation in follicular thyroid cell-derived carcinomas. Oncogene. 2013. doi:10.1038/onc.2013.446 [Epub ahead of print].
41. Liu X, Bishop J, Shan Y, Pai S, Liu D, Murugan AK, Sun H, El-Naggar AK, Xing M. Highly prevalent TERT promoter mutations in aggressive thyroid cancers. Endocr Relat Cancer. 2013;20:603–10.
42. Liu X, Qu S, Liu R, Sheng C, Shi X, Zhu G, Murugan AK, Guan H, Yu H, Wang Y, Sun H, Shan Z, Teng W, Xing M. TERT promoter mutations and their association with BRAF V600E mutation and aggressive clinicopathological characteristics of thyroid cancer. J Clin Endocrinol Metab. 2014;99:E1130–6.
43. Marotta V, Guerra A, Sapio MR, Vitale M. RET/PTC rearrangement in benign and malignant thyroid diseases: a clinical standpoint. Eur J Endocrinol. 2011;165:499–507.
44. Milas M, Shin J, Gupta M, Novosel T, Nasr C, Brainard J, Mitchell J, Berber E, Siperstein A. Circulating thyrotropin receptor mRNA as a novel marker of thyroid cancer: clinical applications learned from 1758 samples. Ann Surg. 2010;252:643–51.
45. Martins L, Matsuo SE, Ebina KN, Kulcsar MA, Friguglietti CU, Kimura ET. Galectin-3 messenger ribonucleic acid and protein are expressed in benign thyroid tumors. J Clin Endocrinol Metab. 2002;87:4806–10.
46. Mazzaferri EL. Management of a solitary thyroid nodule. N Engl J Med. 1993;328:553–9.
47. McIver B, Castro MR, Morris JC, Bernet V, Smallridge R, Henry M, Kosok L, Reddi H. An independent study of a gene expression classifier (afirma™) in the evaluation of cytologically indeterminate thyroid nodules. J Clin Endocrinol Metab. 2014;99:4069–77 [Epub ahead of print].
48. Melo M, da Rocha AG, Vinagre J, Batista R, Peixoto J, Tavares C, Celestino R, Almeida A, Salgado C, Eloy C, Castro P, Prazeres H,

Lima J, Amaro T, Lobo C, Martins MJ, Moura M, Cavaco B, Leite V, Cameselle-Teijeiro JM, Carrilho F, Carvalheiro M, Máximo V, Sobrinho-Simões M, Soares P. TERT promoter mutations are a major indicator of poor outcome in differentiated thyroidcarcinomas. J Clin Endocrinol Metab. 2014;99:E754–65.

49. Milas M, Mazzaglia P, Chia SY, Skugor M, Berber E, Reddy S, Gupta M, Siperstein A. The utility of peripheral thyrotropin mRNA in the diagnosis of follicular neoplasms and surveillance of thyroid cancers. Surgery. 2007;141:137–46.
50. Mocellin S, Pooley KA, Nitti D. Telomerase and the search for the end of cancer. Trends Mol Med. 2013;19:125–33.
51. Moses W, Weng J, Sansano I, Peng M, Khanafshar E, Ljung BM, Duh QY, Clark OH, Kebebew E. Molecular testing for somatic mutations improves the accuracy of thyroid fine-needle aspiration biopsy. World J Surg. 2010;34:2589–94.
52. Nikiforov YE, Steward DL, Robinson-Smith TM, Haugen BR, Klopper JP, Zhu Z, Fagin JA, Falciglia M, Weber K, Nikiforova MN. Molecular testing for mutations in improving the fine-needle aspiration diagnosis of thyroid nodules. J Clin Endocrinol Metab. 2009;94:2092–8.
53. Nikiforov YE, Ohori NP, Hodak SP, Carty SE, LeBeau SO, Ferris RL, Yip L, Seethala RR, Tublin ME, Stang MT, Coyne C, Johnson JT, Stewart AF, Nikiforova MN. Impact of mutational testing on the diagnosis and management of patients with cytologically indeterminate thyroid nodules: a prospective analysis of 1056 FNA samples. J Clin Endocrinol Metab. 2011;96:3390–7.
54. Nucera C, Mazzon E, Caillou B, Violi MA, Moleti M, Priolo C, Sturniolo G, Puzzolo D, Cavallari V, Trimarchi F, Vermiglio F. Human galectin-3 immunoexpression in thyroid follicular adenomas with cell atypia. J Endocrinol Invest. 2005;28:106–12.
55. Rossi M, Buratto M, Bruni S, Filieri C, Tagliati F, Trasforini G, Rossi R, Beccati MD, Degli Uberti EC, Zatelli MC. Role of ultrasonographic/clinical profile, cytology, and BRAF V600E mutation evaluation in thyroid nodule screening for malignancy: a prospective study. J Clin Endocrinol Metab. 2012;97:2354–61.
56. Saggiorato E, De Pompa R, Volante M, Cappia S, Arecco F, Dei Tos AP, Orlandi F, Papotti M. Characterization of thyroid 'follicular neoplasms' in fine-needle aspiration cytological specimens using a panel of immunohistochemical markers: a proposal for clinical application. Endocr Relat Cancer. 2005;12:305–17.
57. Samija I, Matea N, Lukac J, Kusic Z. Galectin-3 and CD44v6 as markers for preoperative diagnosis of thyroid cancer by RT-PCR. Diagn Mol Pathol. 2011;20:233–41.
58. Shen R, Liyanarachchi S, Li W, Wakely Jr PE, Saji M, Huang J, Nagy R, Farrell T, Ringel MD, de la Chapelle A, Kloos RT, He H. MicroRNA signature in thyroid fine needle aspiration cytology applied to "atypia of undetermined significance" cases. Thyroid. 2012;22:9–16.
59. Smekalova EM, Shubernetskaya OS, Zvereva MI, Gromenko EV, Rubtsova MP, Dontsova OA. Telomerase RNA biosynthesis and processing. Biochemistry (Mosc). 2012;77:1120–8.
60. Song L, Tang JW, Owusu L, Sun MZ, Wu J, Zhang J. Galectin-3 in cancer. Clin Chim Acta. 2014;431:185–91.
61. Tallini G, Santoro M, Helie M, Carlomagno F, Salvatore G, Chiappetta G, Carcangiu ML, Fusco A. RET/PTC oncogene activation defines a subset of papillary thyroid carcinomas lacking evidence of progression to poorly differentiated or undifferentiated tumor phenotypes. Clin Cancer Res. 1998;4:287–94.
62. Tufano RP, Teixeira GV, Bishop J, Carson KA, Xing M. BRAF mutation in papillary thyroid cancer and its value in tailoring initial treatment: a systematic review and meta-analysis. Medicine (Baltimore). 2012;91:274–86.
63. Umbricht CB, Conrad GT, Clark DP, Westra WH, Smith DC, Zahurak M, Saji M, Smallridge RC, Goodman S, Zeiger MA. Human telomerase reverse transcriptase gene expression and the surgical management of suspicious thyroid tumors. Clin Cancer Res. 2004;10:5762–8.
64. Vinagre J, Almeida A, Pópulo H, Batista R, Lyra J, Pinto V, Coelho R, Celestino R, Prazeres H, Lima L, Melo M, da Rocha AG, Preto A, Castro P, Castro L, Pardal F, Lopes JM, Santos LL, Reis RM, Cameselle-Teijeiro J, Sobrinho-Simões M, Lima J, Máximo V, Soares P. Frequency of TERT promoter mutations in human cancers. Nat Commun. 2013;4:2185.
65. Volante M, Rapa I, Gandhi M, Bussolati G, Giachino D, Papotti M, Nikiforov YE. RAS mutations are the predominant molecular alteration in poorly differentiated thyroid carcinomas and bear prognostic impact. J Clin Endocrinol Metab. 2009;94:4735–41.
66. Xing M, Tufano RP, Tufaro AP, Basaria S, Ewertz M, Rosenbaum E, Byrne PJ, Wang J, Sidransky D, Ladenson PW. Detection of BRAF mutation on fine needle aspiration biopsy specimens: a new diagnostic tool for papillary thyroid cancer. J Clin Endocrinol Metab. 2004;89:2867–72.
67. Xing M, Westra WH, Tufano RP, Cohen Y, Rosenbaum E, Rhoden KJ, Carson KA, Vasko V, Larin A, Tallini G, Tolaney S, Holt EH, Hui P, Umbricht CB, Basaria S, Ewertz M, Tufaro AP, Califano JA, Ringel MD, Zeiger MA, Sidransky D, Ladenson PW. BRAF mutation predicts a poorer clinical prognosis for papillary thyroid cancer. J Clin Endocrinol Metab. 2005;90:6373–9.
68. Xing M. BRAF mutation in thyroid cancer. Endocr Relat Cancer. 2005;12:245–62.
69. Xing M. BRAF mutation in papillary thyroid cancer: pathogenic role, molecular bases, and clinical implications. Endocr Rev. 2007;28:742–62.
70. Xing M, Clark D, Guan H, Ji M, Dackiw A, Carson KA, Kim M, Tufaro A, Ladenson P, Zeiger M, Tufano R. BRAF mutation testing of thyroid fine-needle aspiration biopsy specimens for preoperative risk stratification in papillary thyroid cancer. J Clin Oncol. 2009;27:2977–82.
71. Xing M. Genetic alterations in the phosphatidylinositol-3 kinase/Akt pathway in thyroid cancer. Thyroid. 2010;20:697–706.
72. Xing M, Haugen BR, Schlumberger M. Progress in molecular-based management of differentiated thyroid cancer. Lancet. 2013;381:1058–69.
73. Xing M, Alzahrani AS, Carson KA, Viola D, Elisei R, Bendlova B, Yip L, Mian C, Vianello F, Tuttle RM, Robenshtok E, Fagin JA, Puxeddu E, Fugazzola L, Czarniecka A, Jarzab B, O'Neill CJ, Sywak MS, Lam AK, Riesco-Eizaguirre G, Santisteban P, Nakayama H, Tufano RP, Pai SI, Zeiger MA, Westra WH, Clark DP, Clifton-Bligh R, Sidransky D, Ladenson PW, Sykorova V. Association between BRAF V600E mutation and mortality in patients with papillary thyroid cancer. JAMA. 2013;309:1493–501.
74. Xing M. Molecular pathogenesis and mechanisms of thyroid cancer. Nat Rev Cancer. 2013;13:184–99.
75. Xing M, Alzahrani AS, Carson KA, Shong YK, Kim TY, Viola D, Elisei R, Bendlová B, Yip L, Mian C, Vianello F, Tuttle RM, Robenshtok E, Fagin JA, Puxeddu E, Fugazzola L, Czarniecka A, Jarzab B, O'Neill CJ, Sywak MS, Lam AK, Riesco-Eizaguirre G, Santisteban P, Nakayama H, Clifton-Bligh R, Tallini G, Holt EH, and Sýkorová V. Association between *BRAF* V600E mutation and recurrence of papillary thyroid cancer. J Clin Oncol. 2015 Jan 1;33(1):42-50
76. Xing M, Liu R, Liu X, Murugan AK, Zhu G, Zeiger MA, Pai S, Bishop J. BRAF V600E and TERT promoter mutations cooperatively identify the most aggressive papillary thyroid cancer with highest recurrence. J Clin Oncol. 2014;32:2718–26. pii: J Clin Oncol. 2014.55.5094. [Epub ahead of print].
77. Xu XC, el-Naggar AK, Lotan R. Differential expression of galectin-1 and galectin-3 in thyroid tumors. Potential diagnostic implications. Am J Pathol. 1995;147:815–22.

78. Yip L, Farris C, Kabaker AS, Hodak SP, Nikiforova MN, McCoy KL, Stang MT, Smith KJ, Nikiforov YE, Carty SE. Cost impact of molecular testing for indeterminate thyroid nodule fine-needle aspiration biopsies. J Clin Endocrinol Metab. 2012; 97:1905–12.
79. Yip L. Molecular diagnostic testing and the indeterminate thyroid nodule. Curr Opin Oncol. 2014;26:8–13.
80. Xing M, Liu R, Bishop J. TERT promoter and BRAF mutations cooperatively promote papillary thyroid cancer-related mortality. Thyroid. 2014b; 24: A–131.

Ultrasonic Imaging of the Thyroid Gland

23

Enrico Papini, Claudio Maurizio Pacella, Andrea Frasoldati, and Laszlo Hegedüs

Diagnostic Ultrasonography

Basic Concepts of B-Mode US

Medical ultrasonography (US) is performed by using a pulse-echo approach. A short, spatially located pulse of ultrasound is produced by a device (*transducer*) and is transmitted into target tissue. US echoes directed back toward the transducer are produced as the pulse travels along a straight path (*ultrasound beam*) through the tissues. As the pulse travels deeper into the tissues, there is a long train of echoes en route back toward the transducer, where they are detected. The different reflectivities of various structures encountered by the pulse cause a corresponding variation of the strength of the echo detection. The detected echo signals are processed and translated into luminance, resulting in a *brightness mode* or B-mode image display. In B-mode images, more reflective structures appear brighter than less reflective ones (*gray-scale resolution*[1]). A complete image is obtained by repeating this pulse-echo cycle for coplanar paths (or *beam lines*). After the echoes from a beam line have been detected by the transducer, further pulses are transmitted for subsequent beam lines. After all the echoes from all the beam lines have been detected and processed, all signals are mapped to the proper locations in the image pixel matrix, and the complete B-mode image is displayed. The entire process is immediately repeated to obtain echoes for the next image frame, generally at rates of 20–40 frames per second (*temporal resolution*[2]).

E. Papini, MD, FACE
Endocrinology Unit, Regina Apostolorum Hospital,
Rome, Albano Laziale, Italy
e-mail: enrico.papini@fastwebnet.it

C.M. Pacella, MD
Department of Diagnostic Imaging and Interventional Radiology,
Regina Apostolorum Hospital, Via S, Francesco, 50,
Rome, Albano Laziale 00041, Italy
e-mail: claudiomauriziopacella@gmail.com;
claudiomaurizio.pacella@fastwebnet.it

A. Frasoldati, MD, PhD
Endocrinology Unit, Arcispedale S. Maria Nuova - IRCCS,
Reggio Emilia, Italy
e-mail: frasoldati.andrea@asmn.re.it

L. Hegedüs, MD, DMSc (✉)
Department of Endocrinology and Metabolism,
Odense University Hospital and University of Southern Denmark,
Kloevervaenget 6, 6th floor, Odense, Funen 5000 C, Denmark
e-mail: laszlo.hegedus@ouh.rsyd.dk

Basic Ultrasound Physics

Ultrasound consists of mechanical waves with frequency above the upper auditory limit of 20 kHz. Mechanical waves must travel through some physical medium like air, water, or tissue. An ultrasound acoustic wave is a *longitudinal* compressional wave consisting of a series of compressions and rarefactions. The term longitudinal refers to waves that cause oscillatory motion of the medium in the same direction as the direction of wave propagation. The pressure wave moves through the medium at a characteristic propagation velocity for each tissue and depends on the elastic modules and density of the tissue medium. A good average value of velocity of sound in tissue is nominally 1,540 m/s. The sound wave also has a characteristic frequency (number of pressure peaks per second) and wavelength (distance between pressure peaks), both of which depend on the transducer design. Because the velocity is constant, the wavelength (λ) must decrease as the frequency of the sound wave increases. For clinical purposes, it is useful to image with the highest possible frequency because as the wavelength decreases, the axial resolution increases. Medical US devices commonly use longitudinal waves with a frequency range between 2 and 15 MHz.

[1] *Gray-scale resolution* is the maximum number of gray shades available in a system, broken into steps from white to black.

[2] *Temporal resolution* is the number of times per second the ultrasound system scans. This is displayed as frames per second.

L. Wartofsky, D. Van Nostrand (eds.), *Thyroid Cancer*, DOI 10.1007/978-1-4939-3314-3_23

Interaction of Ultrasound with Tissue

As ultrasound pulses and echoes travel through tissue, their intensity is reduced (*attenuated*). In general, the amount of *attenuation* increases with the distance from the transducer and with the frequency of ultrasound waves. Thus, imaging of superficial structures (e.g., thyroid or parathyroid glands) demands higher frequencies than deeper lying structures (e.g., liver, kidney, and pancreas). As long as the acoustic characteristics of the tissue in the sound field are constant, the wave will continue to propagate away from the transducer. When tissue with different characteristics is encountered, some of the sound energy will be reflected back to the transducer. The relative amount of energy reflected back depends on the differences between the two tissues. Therefore, echo generation results from the interaction between the incident ultrasound pulse with structures in the tissue medium. Of the different and specific types of interaction, the most important is a tissue property called the *acoustic impedance*. This quantity is correlated with the density of the tissue and velocity of sound in the tissue. Hence, the intensity of the reflected echo increases with increasing impedance difference between tissues. It follows that when the tissues have identical impedance, the result is no echoes. In contrast, all the energy will be reflected when there is a strong difference of acoustic impedance between the tissues (e.g., tissue-air). Interfaces between tissues (excluding the lung and bone) generally produce very-low-intensity echoes. For normal (or 90°) angle of incidence, this type of interaction is called *specular reflection*. If the angle of incidence is not 90°, the echo will not travel directly back toward the transducer but rather will be reflected at an angle equal to the angle of incidence. If the interface between the tissues is rough, the echo will be *diffusely reflected* through a wide range of angles. If the ultrasound pulse encounters reflectors whose dimensions are smaller than the ultrasound wavelength, *scattering* occurs. This results in echoes that are reflected echo intensity through a wide range of angles. On US images most biologic tissue appears as though it is filled with tiny scattering structures. The speckle signal that provides the visible texture in organs like the thyroid gland is the result of interference between multiple scattered echoes. While most of the signal visible in US images results from scatter interactions, the amount and type of reflection depend also on the relationship between the size of the interface and the wavelength. *Reflection* from a large area interface, such as between the liver and the diaphragm (where λ is much less than the object size), is *specular*, like a mirror (the echo travels directly back toward the transducer). Intermediate-size interface (where λ is about the same size as the object) *diffracts* the beam, while small objects, such as blood cells (where λ is much larger than the object size), *scatter* the acoustic wave in all directions. Finally, attenuation is due not only to reflection and scattering but also to friction-like losses resulting from the induced oscillatory tissue motion produced by the pulse, which causes conversion of energy from the original mechanical form to heat. This energy loss is referred to as *absorption* and is the most important component of ultrasound attenuation.

Ultrasound Pulse Formation and Scanning the Ultrasound Beam

A *transducer*, or probe as it is commonly called, is any device that converts energy from one form to another. An ultrasound transducer converts electrical energy to mechanical energy (ultrasound waves). The most important components of ultrasound transducers are piezoelectric elements. The application of electrical waveforms to the piezoelectric elements induces their vibration and the emission of ultrasounds. On the other hand, when sound waves reach the piezoelectric element, they induce vibrations that are converted by the piezoelectric material into electric signals. Thus, an electric current applied across a crystal would result in a vibration that generates sound waves, and, in turn, sound waves striking a crystal would produce an electric voltage. Composite piezoelectric elements commonly consist of tiny rods of lead zirconate titanate ceramic embedded in a matrix of epoxy. Ultrasound pulses that are short in duration and in extent produce US images with the greatest sharpness in the axial direction (axial resolution[3]). Similarly, ultrasound pulses that are narrow in lateral direction produce images with greatest sharpness in that direction (lateral resolution[4]) [1–6].

Most modern US imagers automatically scan the ultrasound beam using transducers consisting of an array of many narrow piezoelectric elements. The array may consist of as many as 128–196 elements [7]. In linear-array transducers, frequently used for US examination of the thyroid gland, the ultrasound beam is created by electrically exciting only a subset of these elements. The ultrasound pulse is emitted perpendicular to the element array and is centered over the element subset. Successive beams are obtained by shifting the subset of excited elements across the face of the array, slightly shifting the beam line laterally. A larger subset of elements is used to receive the returning echoes. The ultrasound beam can be electronically swept across an entire rectangular field in 1/10 s. or faster. The timing is adjusted so that the elements are not all excited simultaneously.

[3] *Axial resolution* defines the ability of the ultrasound transducer to detect two closely spaced reflectors along the direction of sound travel and is directly proportional to the pulse length. The distribution of frequencies present in a beam varies with pulse length: the frequency distribution broadens as the pulse gets shorter. The axial resolution of the imaging system depends on the pulse length: the shorter the pulse length, the better the axial resolution. Short pulses have the broadest frequency distribution but the best axial resolution.

[4] *Lateral resolution* defines the ability of the ultrasound transducer to discern two points perpendicular to the direction of propagation.

Array transducer fields of view (FOVs) are smaller than those produced by past static B-mode scanners, but this disadvantage is compensated for by a more rapid, real-time scanning (*motion mode* or M-mode) that is devoid of motion artifacts.

Echo Detection and Signal Processing

The US image is processed to optimize the appearance on the display. All echo signals are uniformly preamplified after detection by the transducer, and uniform user-controllable *gain* is applied. Equally reflective structures are displayed in the B-mode image with the same brightness, regardless of their depth. The *dynamic range* of the echo signals is also compressed to reduce the gain for larger signal magnitudes and increase the gain for smaller signal magnitudes. These signals are also demodulated to remove oscillations at the ultrasound frequency, and very small signals are removed in order to reduce image noise and clutter. Other steps are designed to obtain sharper edges and improved contrast. Among recent innovations in B-mode US, a mode called *spatial compound imaging* is a new approach to smooth the speckle in order to make the images look less grainy. Spatial compound images smooth the speckle, noise, clutter, and refractive shadows and improve contrast and margin definition [8].

Color and Power Doppler US

The differences in amplitude of backscattered ultrasound produce a gray-scale image, and precise timing allows determination of the depth from which the echo originates. Thus, these differences are related to strength of the interface reflecting the incident sound and are not related to the movement of the target. Rapidly moving targets, such as red blood cells within the bloodstream, produce echoes of such low amplitude that they are not commonly displayed. Nevertheless, the backscattered signal varies from the transmitted signal in frequency as well as amplitude, if the target is moving relative to the transducer. These frequency changes are related to velocity of the moving target by the Doppler equation and are evaluated in the Doppler mode of US signal processing. The Doppler shift is a change in frequency that occurs when sound is emitted from, or bounced off of, a moving object. Movement toward the transducer produces a positive frequency shift, while movement away from the transducer produces a negative frequency shift. The Doppler effect is used to make quantitative measurements of absolute blood velocity and to map blood flow over a large FOV in a semiquantitative manner. Color Doppler (CD) US measurements may be used to determine the presence of flow, determine the direction of flow, identify time-varying velocity characteristics, and detect velocity disturbances. State-of-the-art instrumentation uses intensity and color coding to display complex physiologic and anatomic data to the clinician in a format that can easily be comprehended. The color and intensity represent the direction and magnitude of the velocities present in the image. Analysis of the color flow image gives a graphic illustration of the direction and speed of blood flow within soft tissue. In contrast, power Doppler (PW) considers all frequency shifts to be equivalent, integrating the total amount of motion detected. The assigned color represents the total amount of flow present, independent of the velocity. PW ultrasound is a technique that encodes the power in the Doppler signal in color. This parameter is fundamentally different from the mean frequency shift encoded with CD. The frequency is determined by the velocity of the red blood cells, while the power depends on the amount of blood present. PW has shown several key advantages over CD, including higher sensitivity to flow, better edge definition, and depiction of continuity of flow. The higher sensitivity to slow flow, which is poorly imaged with conventional CD and the improved detailing of the course of tortuous and irregular vessels, has made PW a technique for imaging intratumoral vessels and to improve the accuracy of CD in predicting the likelihood of benign versus malignant nodules. In addition, PD has been used to identify the decreased flow that is characteristic of areas of ischemia, to demonstrate the inflammatory hyperemia, and to assess vascular changes related to therapy [9–14].

Equipment

Accurate ultrasound examination of the superficial structures requires high-frequency broadband transducers, sophisticated electronic focusing, and computing facilities. These instruments provide high-quality B-mode imaging and sensitive Doppler analysis. Broadband technology is useful for systems offering both Doppler analysis and B-mode imaging. The low-frequency component optimizes flow evaluation, while the higher-frequency component allows the study of morphology and structure through gray-scale imaging. High-frequency real-time handheld-specific transducers ranging from at least 7.5 MHz to 15 MHz or more, and focused in the near field, provide enough resolution to discern very subtle differences of acoustic impedance among soft tissues. High-frequency probes can enhance both *spatial resolution* (axial and lateral) and *contrast resolution*[5]. Superficial structures make it possible to increase the frequency of the Doppler signal which is used for both spectrum analysis and color flow mapping (CFM) and to improve the *resolution of vascular structures*[6] [15, 16]. Modern full-size US scanners are relatively portable and inexpensive,

[5] *Contrast resolution* defines the ability to discriminate the differences of acoustic impedance among tissues. It is affected by echo amplitude and tissue attenuation.

[6] *Vascular resolution* describes sensitivity for the detection of very low Doppler signal intensities and Doppler frequency shifts.

especially compared with imaging units for modalities such as MR imaging and CT. Hardware miniaturization and the use of integrated circuitry allow smaller and less expensive US scanners which greatly extends the role of US in the diagnosis and follow-up of thyroid tumors.

How to Perform Thyroid US

The patient is typically scanned in the supine position with the neck slightly hyperextended over a small pillow or a foam wedge. The US machine is usually positioned at the right side of the examining table while the operator is to the right of the patient. For the right-handed operator, the ultrasound equipment is set up such that the right hand does the scanning and the left hand adjusts the scanning features of the machine at the beginning and during the examination. The thyroid gland is initially scanned in both the longitudinal and the transverse planes for a general overview. Next, the entire region is systematically explored in the longitudinal plane starting in the midline to explore the isthmus and then laterally on each side to view the medial, central, and lateral aspects of each lobe as well as the region peripheral to the gland. Each longitudinal scan is performed from the sternal notch to the hyoid region. The common carotid artery and the jugular vein are the useful vascular landmarks that help to define the most lateral or outer border of the thyroid. Still in the longitudinal plane, scanning superiorly beyond the level of the thyroid cartilage depicts cranial structures such as the pyramidal lobe or thyroglossal duct cysts. Next, the entire gland is systematically studied in the transverse plane in the upper, middle, and lower regions of each lobe. Representative images are taken in regions where pathology has been found.

When to Perform Thyroid US

In patients without a palpable nodule, US evaluation of the thyroid gland should be performed when a thyroid disorder is suspected on clinical grounds, when a suspicious cervical adenopathy is revealed by neck palpation, or if risk factors for malignancy (previous head and neck irradiation or a family history of medullary carcinoma, MEN 2A, or papillary thyroid carcinoma in first-degree relatives) are present [17–20]. When a focal lesion of the thyroid gland is revealed by imaging techniques (CT, MRI, PET-CT, or isotope scan), performed for other clinical reasons, a focused US evaluation should be performed to assess the risk of malignancy and the indication for FNA [18–20].

Thyroid US should be performed in all patients with palpable thyroid nodules or goiter to detect US features suggestive of malignancy and to prioritize nodules for FNA. Importantly, US examination additionally provides a reliable measure of the volume of nodules (and the goiter) for follow-up, reveals coexistent thyroid lesions, and aids in the evaluation of differential diagnostic conditions mimicking a thyroid nodule, such as chronic lymphocytic thyroiditis or asymmetrical gland enlargement [21].

A careful US neck examination should always be performed before surgery or radioiodine treatment for a thyroid disorder. US staging provides relevant information about the size of a biopsy-proven malignant nodule, its extracapsular growth, its possible multifocality, and the coexistence of a secondary adenopathy [22, 23].

Thyroid US Reporting

The US report should provide all the information useful for clinical management of thyroid lesions and enable the reader to evaluate the described lesions as for relative risk of malignancy. Qualitative features of thyroid lesions, such as content, type of calcification, border, shape, echotexture, and vascularity – when evaluated in combination – can provide information about the risk of malignancy and should be documented [24, 25]. The following US features of nodules must be reported accurately: (*1*) nodule size, (*2*) internal content, (*3*) nodule shape, (*4*) nodule margins, (*5*) echogenicity, (*6*) calcifications, (*7*) extracapsular invasion, and (*8*) vascularity. While the echotexture of a nodule may be homogeneous or heterogeneous, this feature seems of little help in distinguishing malignant from benign nodules due to low sensitivity and specificity [23, 26].

The nodule *size* should be measured in all three dimensions, but, for minor lesions, usually only the maximal diameter of the nodule can be measured and documented. It is suggested to place the calipers at the outer margin of the halo, when present [27].

The *internal content* of a nodule is generally categorized in terms of the ratio of the cystic portion to the solid component of the nodule: solid (fluid component ≤10 %), predominantly solid (>10 % up to ≤50 %), predominantly cystic (>50 % up to ≥90 %), and cystic (fluid component >90 %) [26]. The nodule may be classified as spongiform when it appears as an aggregation of multiple microcystic components affecting more than 50 % of its volume [26]. The presence of vascularity (Fig. 23.1) or microcalcifications in the solid component should be well documented and stressed in the US imaging report [28–31].

The *shape* of a nodule may be classified as ovoid to round (the anteroposterior diameter of the nodule is equal to or less than its axial diameter on a transverse or longitudinal plane), taller than wide (the anteroposterior diameter of the nodule is longer than its axial diameter on a transverse or longitudinal plane), or irregular, when a nodule is neither ovoid to round nor taller than wide but with a completely uneven shape (Fig. 23.2) [32].

The *margin* of a nodule may be smooth, spiculated (irregular), or ill defined [26, 31–33]. With high-frequency transducer US techniques, previously described ill-defined margins may well be spiculated and jagged edge borders with sharp boundaries (Figs. 23.3 and 23.4).

The *echogenicity* of the solid component of the nodule may be categorized as follows: *marked hypoechoic* when it

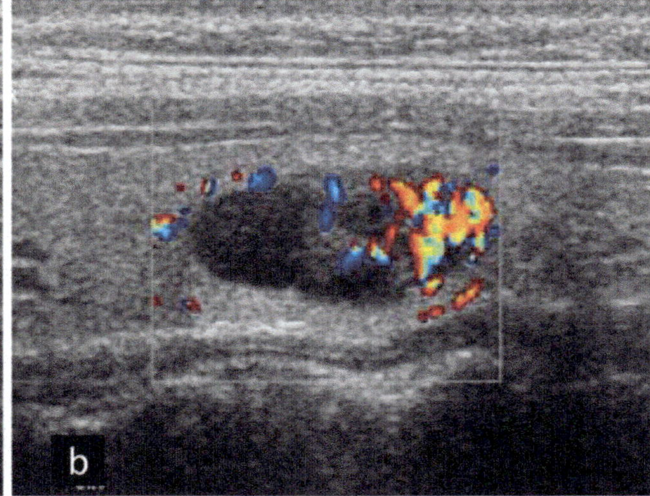

Fig. 23.1 Role of color Doppler US. Sagittal US image of predominantly cystic thyroid nodule with a solid component containing flow. (**a**) Sagittal gray-scale image shows predominantly cystic nodule with solid-appearing mural component. (**b**) Addition of color Doppler mode shows vascularity within the solid mural component, indicating increased likelihood that it is tissue and not debris. US-guided FNA, directed into this zone, showed that it was a papillary carcinoma

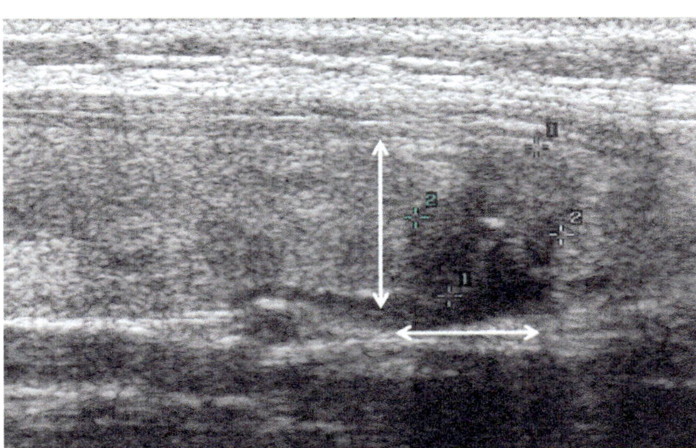

Fig. 23.2 Gray-scale image of a nodule with taller-than-wide shape. US image shows a lesion (*calipers*) with anteroposterior diameter longer than its axial diameter (*arrows*) on sagittal plane. This was a papillary carcinoma

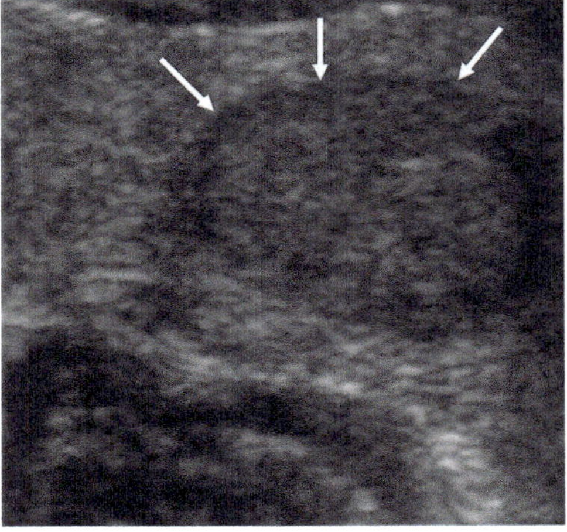

Fig. 23.3 Poorly defined margins of a thyroid nodule. Sagittal US gray-scale image shows blurred and ill-defined margins in the superior part of the nodule (*arrows*). This feature is highly suggestive of malignancy. FNA and surgery confirmed papillary carcinoma. Note also the hypoechogenicity of the lesion

has an echogenicity lower than that of the adjacent strap muscle (Fig. 23.5), *hypoechoic* when the echogenicity of the nodule is comparatively inferior to the surrounding thyroid parenchyma, *isoechoic* when the nodule has the same echogenicity as that of the thyroid parenchyma, and *hyperechoic* when the nodule appears echogenic relative to the surrounding thyroid parenchyma. The latter finding may be present in patients with chronic autoimmune thyroiditis [26].

Calcifications are classified as *microcalcifications* when there are tiny, punctuate echogenic foci of 1 mm or less either with or without posterior shadowing (Fig. 23.6) or as *macrocalcifications* when echogenic foci are larger than 1 mm in size with definite posterior shadowing and as *rim calcifications* when a nodule has peripheral curvilinear or eggshell calcification (Fig. 23.7) [25, 26, 32–37].

As regards the *extracapsular invasion*, the operator should observe carefully at US examination whether nodule margins merge into surrounding thyroid tissue or crosses the thyroid capsule or invades the adjacent structures (usually the perithyroid tissue or, in some cases, the trachea, esophagus, or thyroid cartilage) (Fig. 23.8) [33].

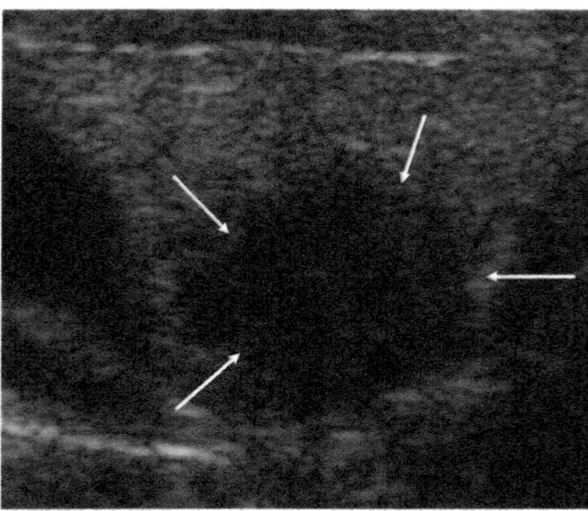

Fig. 23.4 Irregular margins in a thyroid nodule. Sagittal US gray-scale image shows spiculated and jagged margins (*arrows*) of the nodule. In addition, the nodule appears markedly hypoechoic. FNA and surgery confirmed that it was a papillary carcinoma

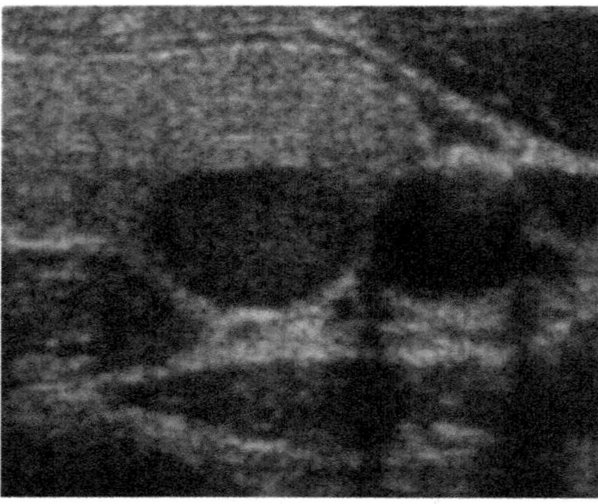

Fig. 23.5 Marked hypoechogenicity of a thyroid nodule. Transverse gray-scale US image shows a nodule with regular margins but marked hypoechogenicity. This was a papillary carcinoma both at cytology examination and at surgery

CD US and PW US are well suited for the evaluation of the intralesional *vascularity* of thyroid nodules (Fig. 23.9) [38, 39].

If US evaluation reveals the presence of multiple nodules, a short general description of the thyroid size and structure and of the number and size of the nodules is suggested. However, the report should be specifically focused on the nodule(s) with US features associated with risk of malignancy and on the presence/absence of suspicious lymph nodes or signs suggestive of extracapsular growth [23].

US Criteria of Malignancy

US Features Suggestive of Malignancy

The risk of malignancy, at the individual level, is independent of whether the patient has a single or multiple palpable thyroid nodules [33], but the challenge of diagnosing it in the latter may be pronounced [17, 40]. One of the major reasons for the increasing use of diagnostic imaging, and imaging-guided FNA, is the wish to offer nonsurgical therapeutical alternatives to the vast majority of patients (>95 %) who are in need of therapy but do not have thyroid malignancy [17–19]. Unfortunately, there is a significant overlap of the US features between benign and malignant thyroid lesions. On the basis of several retrospective and prospective reports [27, 32, 33, 35, 36, 41–43] and two recent South Korean studies [26, 44], the *features predictive of malignancy* in thyroid nodules can be categorized as follows [17]:

- Taller-than-wide shape (sensitivity 40–64 % and specificity 91–100 %).
- The presence of margin abnormalities (microlobulated or spiculated margins) (sensitivity 48–69 % and specificity 92–98 %).
- Marked hypoechogenicity (sensitivity 41–64 % and specificity 92–98 %).
- The presence of microcalcifications (sensitivity 40–44 % and specificity 91–98 %).
- Evidence of aggressive growth (extension of the lesion beyond the thyroid capsule, invasion of the strap muscles, or infiltration of the tracheal cartilage). This is infrequent, but with nearly 100 % specificity for malignancy.
- Coexistence of suspicious lymphadenopathy (enlarged neck lymph nodes with no hilum, cystic changes, and/or microcalcifications) (sensitivity 18 % and specificity 100 %). Lymph nodes with a rounded hypoechoic appearance and hypervascularity are a more frequent but less specific finding [45].

US findings *suggestive of a benign thyroid lesion*:

- Spongiform appearance (sensitivity 10 % and specificity 100 %)
- Isoechoic US appearance (sensitivity 57 % and specificity 88 %)
- Well-defined smooth and regular margins (sensitivity 61 % and specificity 74 %)
- Purely cystic lesion (specificity 100 %).

Borderline features that are associated with thyroid carcinoma but with a low diagnostic accuracy are:

- Hypoechogenicity (sensitivity 11 % and specificity 78 %)
- Macrocalcifications (intranodular macrocalcifications and interrupted eggshell calcifications) (sensitivity 10 % and specificity 86 %)
- Predominant central vascularization (sensitivity 6 % and specificity 89 %)

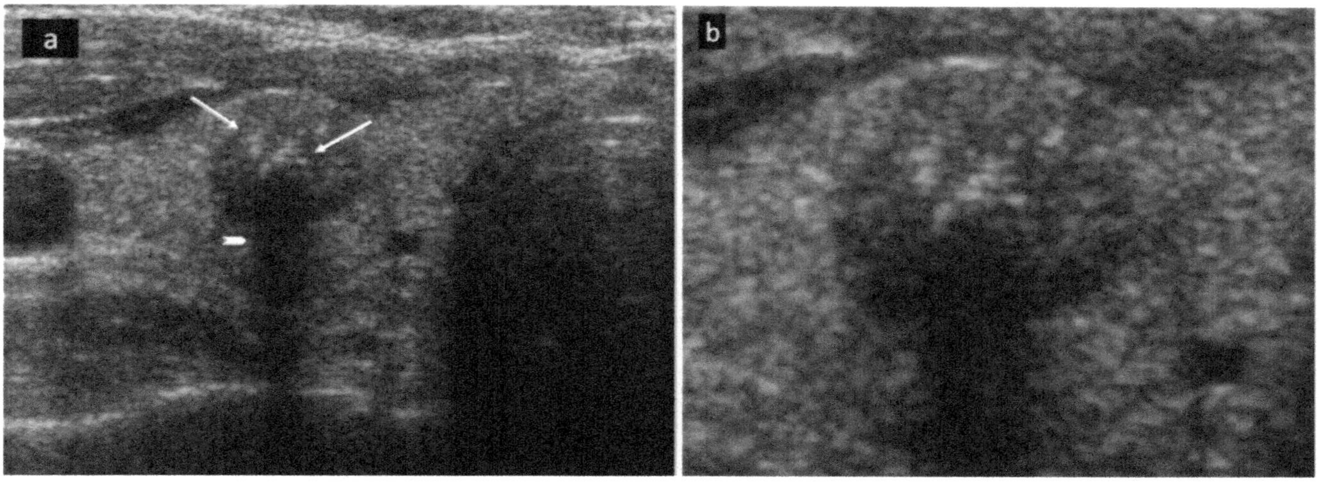

Fig. 23.6 Postsurgical neuroma in a patient previously treated by thyroidectomy and lateral neck dissection. The lesion is superficially located and appears as an oval, slightly inhomogeneous lump, with a hyperechoic posterior margin (Panel **a**). At one pole, the hypoechoic and almost avascular structure continues in an elongated tail (Panel **b**)

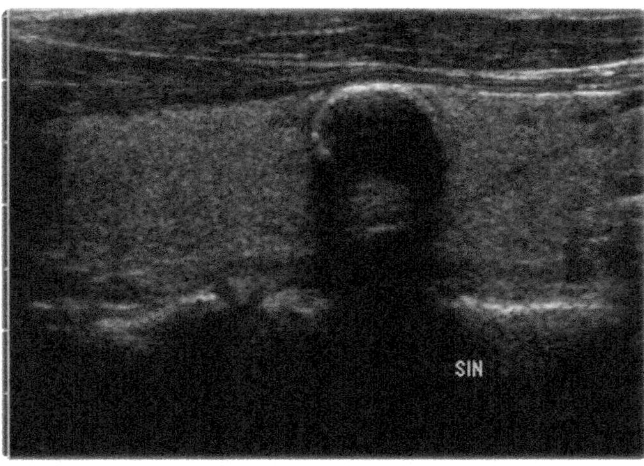

Fig. 23.7 Peripheral curvilinear or eggshell calcification in a thyroid nodule. Sagittal gray-scale US image shows peripheral partial curvilinear calcification in the superior part of the lesion with evident posterior shadow. This US finding is suggestive of a benign thyroid lesion

A taller-than-wide shape is highly predictive of malignancy because it is the expression of a centrifugal growth of the nodule across the tissue plane, while benign lesions usually enlarge along a direction that is parallel to the tissue plane. Unfortunately, an ovoid to round shape is only partially suggestive of a benign nodule because papillary microcarcinomas may appear as well-defined round hypoechoic lesions.

The finding of irregular margins is strongly predictive of malignancy, because it is the expression of an infiltrative growth. Ill-defined or poorly defined margins may be seen in both benign and malignant nodules. Benign thyroid nodules, indeed, are known to be incompletely encapsulated and poorly marginated, and they can merge with normal tissue [46].

Hypoechogenicity is a marker of risk of malignancy, since most thyroid carcinomas are characterized by a hypoechoic US appearance. However, many benign nodules are hypoechoic as well, and only marked hypoechogenicity is strongly predictive of malignancy.

The presence of intranodular microcalcifications, due to psammoma bodies (laminar calcific deposits within the tumor papillae), is highly predictive of papillary thyroid carcinoma. Unfortunately, the high specificity of this finding is associated with a rather low sensitivity [46]. Macrocalcifications are frequently encountered in medullary thyroid carcinomas and in anaplastic carcinomas, but they are more often seen as a consequence of tissue necrosis in benign long-standing nodular goiters.

The vascularity pattern, using CD or PW US, is of little help in differentiating benign from malignant nodules [47, 48]. Intratumoral hypervascularity is frequently detected in thyroid carcinomas, but the presence of intranodular vascular signals is a highly nonspecific finding. Perinodular flow is mainly a characteristic of benign nodules, but it is detected in a nonnegligible number of malignant nodules as well. Probably only a few qualitative features, like the presence of a marked chaotic intranodular vascularization or of large penetrating "swordlike" vessels, may be of use in selected malignant lesions [49].

The size of the nodule and the rate of growth in most cases do not distinguish a benign from a malignant nodule [21, 33]. Many benign nodules are characterized by a slow but progressive volume increase during long-term follow-up, and only aggressive tumors (poorly differentiated and anaplastic carcinomas, thyroid lymphomas, and sarcomas) demonstrate a rapid growth over a period of weeks or months [50].

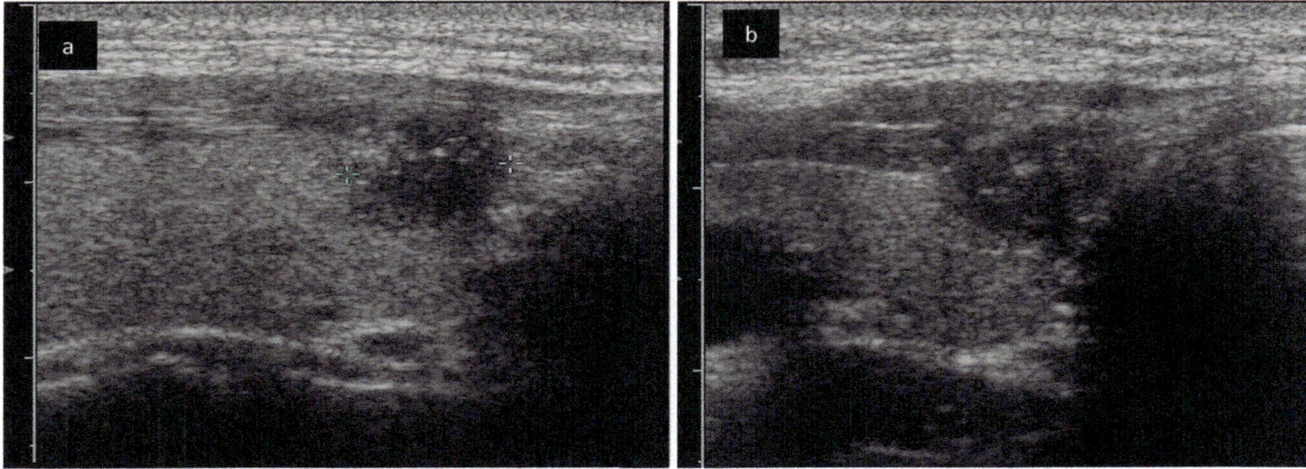

Fig. 23.8 Representative cases of nodules with evidence of aggressive growth. (**a**) Transverse US B-mode image shows a hypoechoic nodule (*calipers*) with irregular margins and intralesional microcalcifications that cross the thyroid capsule and invade the adjacent perithyroid structures. (**b**) Transverse US image shows a nodule with intralesional microcalcifications that invade perithyroid tissue and the contiguous tracheal wall. Cytology and surgery confirmed papillary carcinoma in both cases

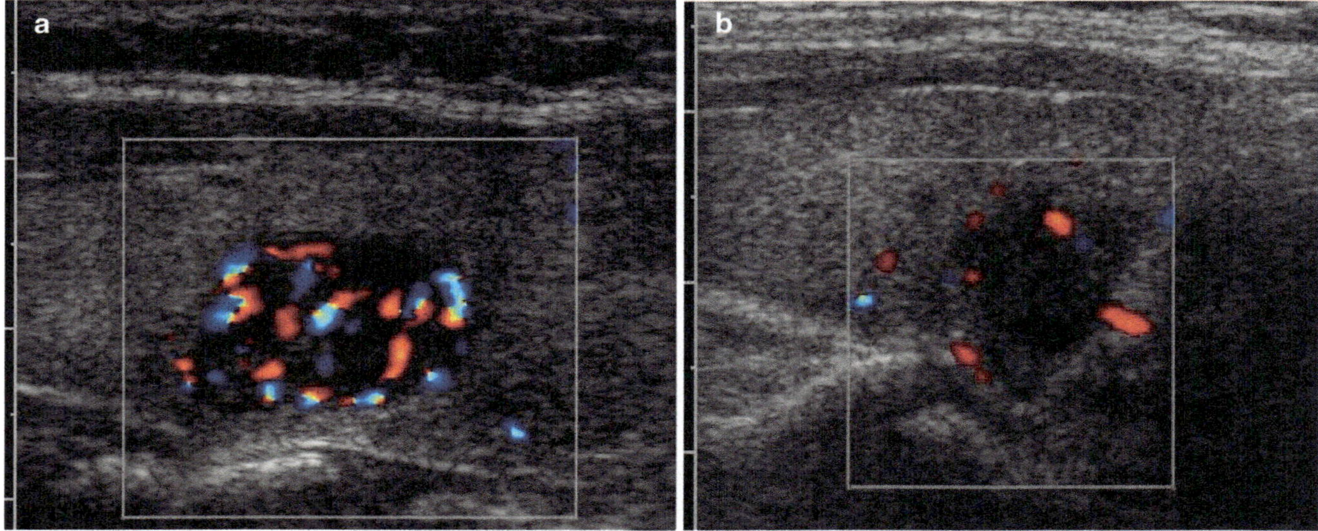

Fig. 23.9 Role of color Doppler US. (**a**) Color Doppler mode shows marked internal vascularity, indicating increased likelihood that the nodule is malignant. (**b**) Color Doppler mode shows little internal vascularity in a markedly hypoechoic nodule with irregular margins. Cytology and surgery confirmed papillary carcinoma, in both cases

Pure cysts are invariably benign, but partially cystic thyroid lesions are reported as malignant in 5–26 % of cases [30]. US evidence of a relevant solid component with marked vascular signals or microcalcifications should raise suspicion of a partially cystic carcinoma.

When to Perform US-Guided Thyroid Biopsy

FNA biopsy should be performed:

- In patients with a history of neck irradiation or family history of papillary thyroid carcinoma, medullary thyroid carcinoma, or multiple endocrine neoplasia type II. This should be performed independent of nodule size, if technically feasible.
- In patients with US findings suggestive of extracapsular growth or with metastatic cervical lymph nodes. This should be performed independent of nodule size, if technically feasible.
- In patients without a high-risk history and with nodules smaller than 10 mm, only in the presence of at least one suspicious US finding.
- In patients without a high-risk history and with nodules greater than 10 mm but smaller than 20 mm, only in the presence of at least one borderline US finding.

- In all patients with nodules greater than 20 mm or with progressive growth.
- In patients with thyroid incidentalomas detected by PET-CT with ^{18}F-fluorodeoxyglucose or with Tc99m sestamibi scan.

Interventional Ultrasonography

US-Assisted Thyroid Biopsy

FNA is the pivotal procedure for the assessment of malignancy risk of thyroid nodules and cervical lymph nodes. US guidance of FNA is necessary for cytological sampling of nonpalpable nodules and of lesions in anatomically difficult sites. Routine use of US-guided FNA is strongly recommended in palpable thyroid nodules as well, due to the increased diagnostic accuracy and the decreased risk of complications [19]. A team comprising an operator and a trained nurse can reliably perform US-guided FNA. The US machine should be equipped with a linear transducer with a 3.5–4.0 cm footprint and multiple frequency settings ranging between 7.5 and 14 MHz and CD/PW capability. Small curvilinear transducers may be useful for imaging otherwise inaccessible locations, especially in the lower neck The clinical usefulness of an elastosonography software is still under evaluation and debated [51, 52].

The operator is situated on the left side of the patient, and the assistant, or the nurse, stands on the right side. The US equipment is placed on the right side of the patient at the level of her head. The assistant is required to handle the US machine switches, such as freeze, depth, gain, color, and power color adjustments. The operator holds the transducer with the left hand and watches images on the monitor in front of her, aims the guide to the target, and inserts the needle with the right hand. If the procedure is carried out by two physicians, the operator can perform the biopsy maneuver while the assistant holds the transducer and supervises the needle track. The monitor should be placed in front of the operator, allowing a straight comfortable field of vision. A setup tray should include the material for topical cleansing, transducer sterile covers, sterile coupling gel, syringes (from 5 to 20 ml), and hypodermic needles of different gauges (G) and lengths. FNA is usually performed with 25–27G needles, but the sampling of dense, fibrotic lesions is better accomplished with 22–23G needles. The drainage of sticky colloid collections may require even larger needles up to 19–20G. Spinal or stylet-type needles are more expensive than ordinary needles, but in selected cases, they are of use since they avoid the uploading into the needle lumen of gel, blood, or follicular cells from normal thyroid parenchyma while advancing the needle toward the lesion of interest. Needles of variable length are required. Spinal needles inserted through the needle guide should be 75–90 mm long, while shorter needles are used for US-assisted procedures in cases where a guide attachment is not required.

Pistol grip holders allow the operator to use the left hand to hold the transducer for direct control of the target view and the right hand to fit and move the needle. This procedure allows continuous real-time vision of the target. A detachable needle guide, adapted for the transducer, may permit the operator to act on his own, with the assistance of a nurse. When using syringe holders, the operator should carefully avoid to apply an excessive aspiration pressure, especially on highly vascularized thyroid lesions. In these cases, the optimal sampling is obtained without any or with very little suction.

A worktable prepared with glass slides and fixing materials (95 % alcohol solution bottles for slide glass immersion or isofix spray) should be available for immediate smearing and fixation. If the physician has no or limited experience in the sampling maneuver and slide smearing, the entire procedure is at risk of failure. The expression of the sampled material into transport media, for subsequent liquid-based cytology or cell block preparation, is preferable in such situations.

Waste boxes to dispose needles and biologic material should be at hand. Two 4 ml tubes, containing normal saline solution 1 ml, should be available for the analysis of relevant biochemical markers in the needle washout (thyroglobulin, calcitonin, parathyroid hormone, and other markers).

An extended field of view of the thyroid gland should be obtained before the biopsy procedure. A careful preliminary US evaluation allows the operator to choose the most relevant lesion(s), the best percutaneous approach, and the length and type of needle. A Doppler imaging assessment of the gland rules out the presence of large intrathyroid vessels along the supposed path of the needle and provides information about the lesion's vascularity.

The transducer is enclosed in a plastic cover or Parafilm to avoid contact of the probe with the patient's blood. The skin of the neck is cleaned with antiseptic solution. Local anesthesia with subcutaneous injection of 2 % lidocaine, or with an anesthetic spray, is usually unnecessary for FNA performed with 25–22G needles. When warranted, lidocaine should be injected from the subcutaneous tissue down to the strap muscles and the thyroid capsule.

The US-guided FNA procedure can, basically, be performed with a "parallel" or a "perpendicular" approach [53]. According to the parallel approach, the needle is inserted at either of the short sides of the probe, and it is angled down toward the nodule. The parallel approach has the advantage to show nearly completely the track of the needle from its insertion into the skin until its penetration into the target lesion. This approach is best suited for procedures performed with a guiding device because the path of the needle must be continuously maintained in the scan plane of the transducer while the tip advances toward the lesion.

The perpendicular approach requires two experienced operators because the tip of the needle is visualized only in the final phase of the procedure. Both the point of needle insertion into the skin and the nodule to be aspirated must be carefully centered at the midpoint of the long axis of the probe. The needle must be inserted with the precise angle of descent (usually a 30–40° angle with the vertically placed transducer) to allow placing the needle tip into the nodule. As the initial part of the needle course is not visualized, the operator should be able to predict the needle path in order to avoid an excessively cranial or caudal placement of the needle bevel [54].

US-guided FNA may obtain material from a nodule by means of "aspiration" (or closed suction) or by "nonaspiration" (or needle-only) techniques [55, 56]. According to the aspiration technique, a 22–25G needle attached to a 10–20 ml syringe is inserted into the lesion and only after the correct placement of its tip is a gentle aspiration performed, withdrawing the plunger of the syringe for a 1–5 ml volume. The needle is rapidly moved back and forth within the lesion for 5–10 s, then the syringe plunger is completely released, and the needle is quickly withdrawn from the neck. The needle is disconnected, 5 ml of air is aspirated into the syringe, the needle is reinserted, and the aspirated material is expressed onto a glass slide for smear or into a transport medium for liquid-based cytology. This technique is rapid and effective for most solid thyroid nodules and especially for the nonpalpable or deeply located lesions.

The nonaspiration technique is of use for highly vascularized nodules and for complex lesions with a component of degeneration and/or fluid. The hub of a 25–27G needle is held by the operator with her fingertips in a pencillike way and is inserted within the lesion while performing rapid back and forth movements according to the aforementioned procedure. After about 5 s, a fingertip is placed over the needle hub to close it, the needle is withdrawn, and it is attached to a syringe with an already retracted plunge. This procedure leads to a capillary-driven uploading of material into the needle. The absence of any aspiration avoids the dilution of the cellular material with colloid fluid or blood. In deeply located lesions, the procedure can be performed with a spinal needle that is attached to a 10–20 ml syringe with its plunge partially retracted or removed.

The recommended biopsy sites are as follows [40]:

- In large nodules, the peripheral part of the lesion rather than the central area, in order to escape sampling degenerative changes and fluid collections which may hamper sample adequacy.
- In entirely cystic areas, the center of the lesion should be reached in order to drain the fluid content completely. Cyst fluid should be submitted to the laboratory within the syringe for evaluation after centrifugation. Most colloid fluids are clear yellow with minimal blood staining. Clear-colorless fluid suggests the sampling from a parathyroid gland and parathyroid hormone should be measured. Bloody liquid is usually drained from hemorrhagic pseudocysts, and this finding may represent a malignant lesion, although most often it is not.
- In mixed thyroid nodules, before the drainage of the fluid component, a careful sampling should be performed from the solid pedicles growing into the cystic lumen. The needle tip should be aimed at hubs that are vascularized at PW examination or at their basis, because the extremities of the pedicles usually contain mostly necrotic debris and degenerative changes. After a complete drainage of the fluid, both the solid areas and the peripheral borders of the lesion should be sampled.

Ideally, the request form for the cytopathology laboratory should provide the following clinical data: location and size of the nodule, suspicious US findings, thyroid function including the presence of autoimmunity and calcitonin level – if available, current medical treatment, history of neck irradiation, and personal or family history of thyroid malignancy. Suspicion of malignancy, whether clinical or based on the US findings, should always be expressed.

US-Guided Core Biopsy

The role of FNA in the initial evaluation of thyroid nodules is widely accepted. However, inadequate or suboptimal specimens constitute major limitations. Inadequate specimens are obtained in up to 15–25 % of FNA procedures, and suboptimal samples, due to insufficient cellularity or blood contamination, are even more frequent. Core needle biopsy (CNB) is an US-guided biopsy aimed at obtaining a small size tissue sample for histological evaluation by means of a 22–20G cutting needle. The procedure is usually performed with disposable spring-activated devices widely available on the market. These needles are small enough to precisely sample thyroid lesions in the 8–20 mm range with a very low risk of local bleeding or of damage to the cervical structures [40].

CNB should be performed under US guidance and by experienced operators only. After skin cleansing with an antiseptic solution, a careful local anesthesia with the injection of 2 % lidocaine from the subcutaneous tissue down to the muscle layers of the neck and the thyroid capsule is required to reduce local pain.

For a safe procedure, the longitudinal (craniocaudal) approach is recommended, because this needle track is not directed toward vital structures of the neck (large vessels or trachea). The needle is inserted into the lesion under US monitoring, and the absence of local bleeding should be ensured during the insertion through US images in different planes. The needle tip should never break outside the lesion before needle firing. After careful placing of the needle and instructing the patient not to swallow or speak, the needle is triggered and rapidly extracted [57, 58].

Material may be traditionally processed by fixation of the tissue in formalin for hematoxylin and eosin examination and/or gently crushed between two slides to prepare an air-dried sample for cytological examination [59]. Pressure and ice pack should immediately be placed on the biopsy site to prevent local bleeding, pain, and discomfort. An oral analgesic effectively controls pain, if present. An US control after 30 min, mainly to rule out hemorrhage, is suggested before patient discharge.

The rate of unsatisfactory thyroid nodule sampling with CNB has been reported as low as 3.4 % and importantly without significant procedure complications [59]. Thin-needle CNB provided an impressive 98.3 % adequacy rate in a series of 258 patients with a previous unsatisfactory FNA sampling [60].

CNB is a safe technique, when performed by experienced operators, and may be recommended in solid thyroid nodules which despite repeated (usually two) FNAs has yielded unsatisfactory samples. CNB may be performed simultaneously with FNA when one or two aspiration samplings have yielded insufficient or suboptimal material from fibrous nodules or lesions with a rubbery consistence (such as chronic lymphocytic thyroiditis). CNB may be the first-choice procedure in case of unusual thyroid lesions that are suspicious for metastatic tumors, lymphoma, sarcoma, or undifferentiated thyroid carcinoma. In all these cases, CNB may provide some architectural definition as well as a quantity of material enabling immunohistochemical or molecular biology evaluations.

US-Assisted Mini-invasive Procedures for Thyroid Malignancy and Neck Recurrence

Most differentiated thyroid carcinomas are cured by the initial surgical treatment, which is usually followed by radioiodine ablation. However, some patients with thyroid carcinoma are found to have neck lymph node metastases during their long-term clinical and US follow-up. The recurrence rate within a 30-year follow-up is reported to be as high as 9–20 % in patients with differentiated thyroid carcinoma and up to 25 % in patients with medullary thyroid carcinoma. In some of these cases, radioiodine treatment is not effective in eradicating nodal metastases due to their scanty or absent 131-I uptake. In such situations, current US techniques make it possible to identify subcentimetric and clinically occult cervical metastases, which can rapidly be confirmed by US-guided FNA but which may be beyond surgical reach. Additionally, a few of these patients have previously undergone repeated neck explorations, and when further metastases are revealed, their resection is cumbersome and confer a high risk of surgical complications due to the extensive neck scarring. Based on these considerations, and on the commonly indolent course of neck metastases from thyroid carcinomas, the use of nonsurgical ablation techniques has been proposed and is currently under evaluation for the treatment of cases at high surgical risk of complications [61].

Percutaneous Ethanol Injection

Percutaneous ethanol injection (PEI) was first used for the chemical ablation of small hepatocellular carcinomas [62]. Ethanol induces coagulation necrosis of the lesion as a result of cellular dehydration, protein denaturation, and chemical occlusion of small lesion vessels. PEI has also been proposed as a nonsurgical treatment of secondary/tertiary hyperparathyroidism [63] to ablate parathyroid tissue [64, 65]. Subsequently, PEI has been employed to treat both hyperfunctioning nodules and benign cold nodules of the thyroid gland [66, 67]. Due to technical limitations, short- and long-term complications – mainly caused by ethanol seepage along the needle tract – as well as recurrences due to incomplete ablation, the therapy has been abandoned by all the centers that initiated the therapy in the first place [68]. At present, the only remaining indication for PEI is treatment of cysts or predominantly cystic lesions [21, 69–71].

In 1999, PEI was first proposed as a palliative treatment in a case of inoperable thyroid carcinoma [72]. Subsequently, PEI has been evaluated as a possible treatment for thyroid cancer metastases in cervical lymph nodes in patients who were not candidates for surgical resection or radioiodine therapy [73]. In a series of 14 patients with 29 neck nodal metastases (NNM) from papillary thyroid cancer (PTC), US follow-up after PEI showed a mean volume decrease from 492 mm^3 at baseline, to 76 mm^3 after 12 months, to 20 mm^3 after 24 months [73, 74]. In a second series of 20 patients with 23 nodal metastases, six lesions disappeared completely after PEI, while seven lymph nodes required a second treatment. A complete control was reported in 15 patients with an average injection of only 0.7 ml of ethanol [75]. In a third trial, six patients with biopsy-proven neck recurrences of well-differentiated thyroid cancer were treated with PEI and had 18.7 months' clinical and US follow-up. Four patients showed a rapid reduction of the volume of their metastatic lymph nodes, while two of them needed repeated treatments. No neck disease persistence was reported, and serum thyroglobulin levels dropped from a mean pretreatment value of 6.1–2.0 ng/ml [76].

Lim et al. [77] used US-guided PEI on 24 recurrent lesions (eight in thyroid beds and 16 in neck nodes) of 16 papillary thyroid carcinoma patients. Ethanol was injected at 3-month intervals under US guidance. The median diameter of the lesions was significantly reduced, from 9.9 mm (range 5.5–25.0 mm) to 5.3 mm (range 0.0–17.0 mm) by PEI. Four recurrent lesions disappeared sonographically. Kim et al. [78] treated 27 patients with 47 cervical metastases by PEI with a mean follow-up of 28.2 (14–38 months). Ethanol (99 %) was repeatedly injected with adjusting needle position until the entire lymph node was ablated. All metastases significantly decreased in volume (range 30–100 %; mean 93.6 %). The mean number of sessions, the total volume of ethanol per NNM-PTC, and the mean volume of ethanol per session per NNM-PTC were 2.1 sessions (range 1–6), 2.4 ml (range 0.3–10.1), and 1.1 ml/session (range 0.3–3.0), respectively. More recently, Heilo et al. [79] described their experience in 69 patients with 109 neck metastases of papillary thyroid carcinoma. A total of 101 of the 109 (93 %) metastatic lymph nodes responded to PEI treatment, 92 (84 %) completely, and 9 incompletely. Two did not respond, and four progressed. Two lymph nodes previously considered successfully treated showed evidence of malignancy during follow-up. Serum TG values were available from 62 patients before PEI and from 60 at the end of follow-up. Of 51 patients without TG antibodies, 13 had undetectable serum TG levels (<0.2 μg/l) before PEI, despite biopsy-proven metastatic disease. Of the 38 patients with elevated serum TG values before PEI, 30 patients had undetectable values after PEI treatment.

Although the procedure has proven to be quite safe, and few complications have been reported [76–79], PEI treatment of neck lesions devoid of a capsule is usually characterized by a transient but sharp pain radiating to the jaw and the chest, likely related to the leakage of ethanol into surrounding cervical soft tissue. Potential complications to PEI include damage to the recurrent laryngeal nerves or the parathyroid glands. In addition, a posttreatment local fibrosis is frequent. A relevant limitation of PEI, for ablation of cancer recurrences, is the difficulty of achieving – with a single treatment – a definite area of coagulative necrosis with certainty associated with complete ablation of the target tissue. Ethanol diffusion is unpredictable, and there is no precise correlation between the amount of ethanol injected into the lesion and the size of the coagulative zone [69]. While the aforementioned data look convincing, it is important to recognize that there is ongoing discussion of whether PEI should be employed for this purpose. Most centers do not and there are no data on cost-effectiveness and whether the procedure influences quality of life or the prognosis of the patients.

Radiofrequency Ablation

The goal of radiofrequency (RF) ablation is to induce thermal injury to the tissue through electromagnetic energy deposition. In the more popular monopolar mode, the patient is part of a closed-loop circuit that includes a radiofrequency generator, an electrode needle, and a large dispersive electrode (ground pads). An alternating electric field is created within the tissue of the patient. Because of the relatively high electrical resistance of tissue in comparison with the metal electrodes, there is marked agitation of the ions present in the target tissue that surrounds the electrode. This is due to the tissue ions attempting to follow the changes in direction of alternating electric current. The agitation results in frictional heat around the electrode. The discrepancy between the small surface area of the needle electrode and the large area of the ground pads causes the generated heat to be focused and concentrated around the needle electrode. Several electrode types are available for clinical RF ablation, including internally cooled electrodes and multiple-tined expandable electrodes with or without perfusion [80, 81].

RF was first applied to a group of eight patients with locally recurrent well-differentiated thyroid carcinoma (WTC) [82]. The mean diameter of the lesions was 2.4 cm, and the treatment was performed under US guidance and using intravenous conscious sedation. The RF electrode was inserted into the site of the recurrent lesion and treated with the maximum allowable current for between 2 and 12 min. All patients were treated as outpatients. A minor skin burn and one case of vocal cord paralysis occurred. With a mean follow-up of 10 months, no recurrent disease at the treatment site was detected [82]. Subsequent histological examination showed no evidence of a tumor in the treated lymph nodes in six patients [82]. The same center reported a second series (not specified if in part coincident) [76] of 12 patients who underwent RF treatment of biopsy-proven recurrent thyroid carcinoma in the neck. No recurrent disease was detected at the treatment site in over 80 % of the patients after a mean follow-up of 41 months. A minor skin burn and one permanent vocal cord paralysis occurred after RF treatment. Thus, RF ablation shows promise as an alternative to surgical treatment of recurrent differentiated thyroid carcinoma in patients at surgical risk. Clearly, adequately controlled long-term studies are necessary to determine the possible role of RF in the treatment of recurrent malignant thyroid tumors.

Laser Ablation

The term "laser ablation" should be used for ablation with laser light energy applied via fibers directly inserted into the tissue. A great variety in laser sources and wavelengths are available. In addition, different types of laser fibers, modified tips, and applicators can be used. A spherical volume of coagulative necrosis up to 2 cm in diameter can be produced from a single, bare 300–400 μm laser fiber. Two methods have been developed for producing larger volumes of necrosis. One utilizes firing multiple bare fibers arrayed at 1.5–1.8 cm spacing throughout a target lesion [80, 81, 83–86]. The other employs cooled-tip diffuser fibers that can deposit up to 30 W over a large surface area, thus diminishing local overheating [80, 87–89].

Laser ablation (LA) has been tested in undifferentiated thyroid carcinomas. The first reported case was a 75-year-old woman with a rapidly progressive anaplastic thyroid carcinoma [90]. After achieving the ablation of a large proportion of the tumor, an external beam radiation therapy was performed. The volume of the tumor and local symptoms (dysphagia and cervical pain) were markedly reduced and stabilized during the following 4 months. A similar, albeit transient, improvement was reported in another inoperable anaplastic carcinoma patient with an aggressive course [91].

Recently, with a 1,064 nm Nd:YAG laser source operating in continuous wave mode, using 300 μm plane-cut optic fibers inserted through the sheath of two 21 gauge spinal needles and a total energy of 3,600 J, an incidental solitary papillary microcarcinoma (PTMC) of 8 mm in maximum diameter, confined to the thyroid gland, was completely ablated in an elderly patient at high surgical risk. US-guided FNA and a core-needle biopsy performed at 1 and 12 months after the procedure showed necrotic material and absence of viable neoplastic tissue. A contrast-enhanced US (CEUS) scan performed after 24 months showed that the neoplastic lesion was completely replaced by a large avascular hypoechoic area [92].

Solbiati et al. [93] used the same technique [83, 94] to treat 23 metastatic nodes (mean size 1.2 cm; range 0.6–2.6 cm) from papillary cancer of the thyroid gland in 19 patients who had previously (13–54 months earlier) undergone thyroidectomy and central and laterocervical lymph node dissection. All cases were negative at ^{131}I whole-body scan but had marked uptake at 18F-FDG PET and elevated serum levels of TG. Lymph nodes were treated with one or two [6] fiber insertions, each one with a power of 3 W for 400–600 s (total energy applied 1,200–1,800 J). After withdrawing the fiber, CEUS was performed to assess the lack of enhancement in the treated lesion. All cases were followed at 3 and 6 months with B-mode US, CEUS, 18F-FDG PET, and assessment of serum levels of TG. In 21 of 23 (91.3 %) cases, complete ablation (disruption of the parenchymal structure at B-mode US, lack of enhancement at CEUS, no uptake at 18F-FDG PET with normalization of peak standard uptake value (SUV) (Fig. 23.10), and >90 % decrease of TG serum levels) was achieved. In two cases, residual uptake at 18F-FDG PET with abnormal SUV was found, and laser ablation was repeated and subsequent normalization of all parameters was achieved.

LA treatment of four cases of local recurrence of poorly differentiated thyroid carcinoma has been described [95, 96]. All patients were elderly and had previously had total thyroidectomy followed by cervical lymphadenectomy and external beam radiation therapy for repeated cervical recurrences. Neck metastases were not iodine avid and symptoms of local invasion (cervical pain, dysphagia, and dysphonia) were present and progressive. In all cases, from two to five LA treatments were performed during a mean period of 20 months, which induced a marked tumor shrinkage and a clinically significant improvement of local symptoms. LA was combined with a further cycle of external beam irradiation in two patients and with a bronchoscopic laser treatment for control of tracheal invasion in one case. Laser procedures were well tolerated and only caused mild cervical pain, which was controlled by betamethasone and ketoprofen given for 24 h. No major complications were recorded [95, 96].

Despite the limited number of cases, percutaneous US-guided LA is a promising therapeutic tool for PTMC ablation in fragile patients at high surgical risk and for neck metastases from differentiated thyroid carcinoma in patients already treated with repeated lymphadenectomy. Thermal ablation may be used for local recurrences of poorly differentiated or medullary thyroid carcinomas that are not amenable to traditional surgical treatment, for improving local compressive symptoms, and for inducing a decrease of the volume of neoplastic tissue prior to external radiation therapy or target therapy [61].

Although not the focus of this chapter, we have to stress the important outcomes achieved by these hyperthermic techniques when treating, percutaneously, benign thyroid lesions. US-guided thermal techniques result in a satisfactory long-term clinical response with improvement in pressure symptoms and cosmetic complaints in the majority of the patients with a benign solitary solid thyroid nodule [97–102].

High-intensity focused ultrasound (HIFU), a technique which delivers US-guided thermal destruction without penetration of the skin, has recently shown promise in the therapy of small benign nodules in the thyroid [103, 104]. In principle, this technique holds promise also for ablating malignant thyroid tissue.

Perspectives

Ultrasound Elastography of the Thyroid

Principles

Thyroid nodules that are hard and fixed at physical examination are well recognized as clinically suspicious [40]. The B-mode US examination of the thyroid offers a valuable guide for assessing the risk of malignancy of thyroid lesions, but it does not provide any information about its hardness. Hence, the hardness of nonpalpable thyroid nodules cannot be evaluated by either US or palpation. US elastography (sonoelastography) is a noninvasive imaging technique that can be used to map relative tissue stiffness or displacement (strain) in response to an imparted force [105, 106]. Stiff tissue deforms less and exhibits less strain than does compliant tissue, in response to the same applied force. Thus, the basis of elastography is analogous to manual palpation [106]. This novel

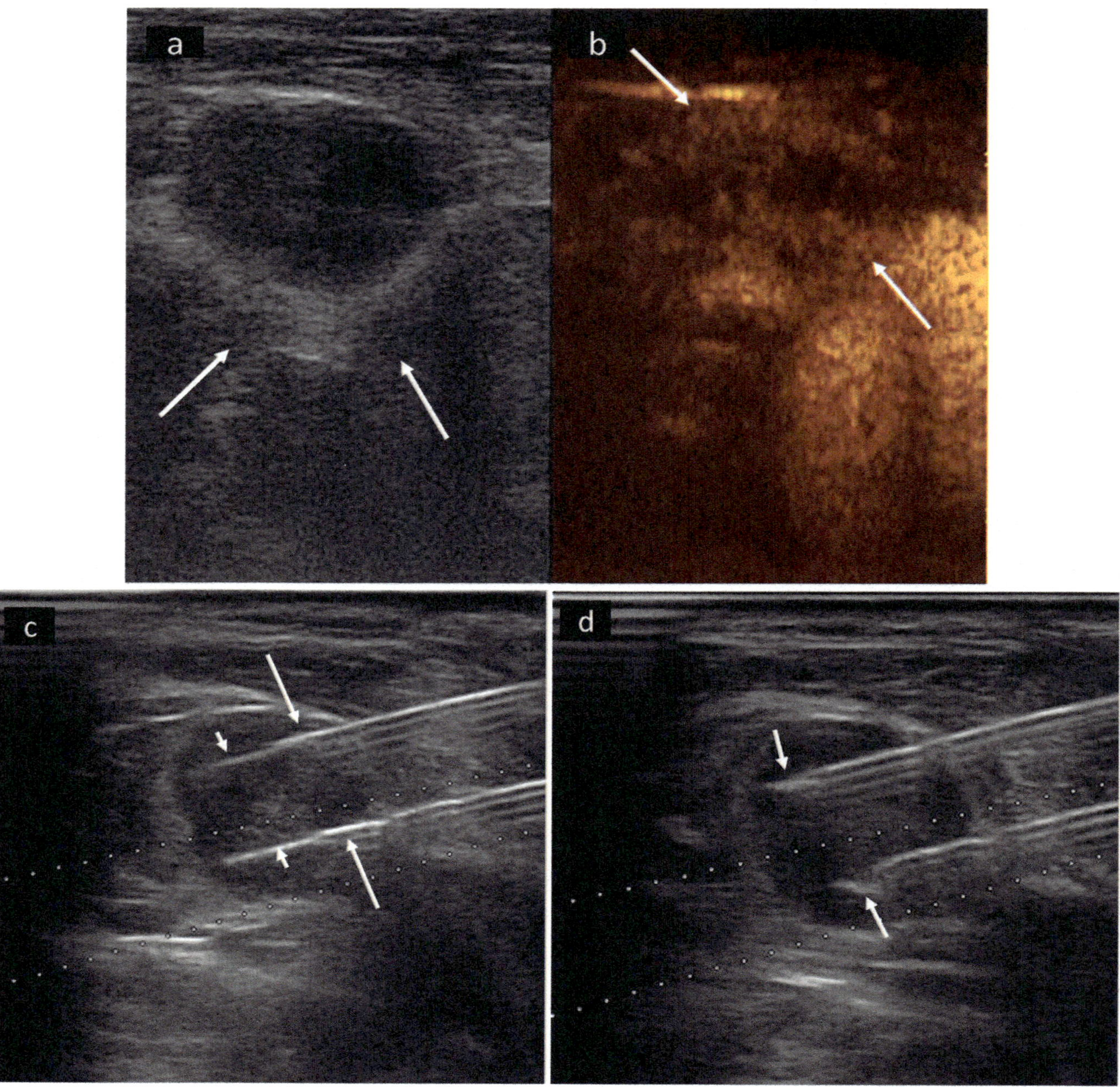

Fig. 23.10 Laser ablation (LA) for the percutaneous treatment of neck nodal metastases (NNM) from papillary thyroid cancer (PTC). (**a**) Transverse B-US image shows a metastatic neck lymph node of 2.0 cm in diameter (*arrows*), before contrast-enhanced ultrasound (CEUS). (**b**) CEUS performed before the LA procedure shows evident enhancement of the lymph node (*arrows*). (**c**) Longitudinal B-US image shows two 21G fine needles (*arrows*) and two plane-cut fibers (*arrowheads*) with interneedle spacing of 1.0 cm into the lesion at the beginning of an LA session. (**d**) Longitudinal B-US image shows the needles and the fibers during the treatment. Vapor is clearly visible (*arrow*) as small hyperechoic foci close to the tips of the fibers. (**e**) Transverse gray-scale image shows the lymph node as a hypoechoic area (*arrows*), close to the carotid artery, at the end of the LA session. (**f**) CEUS, performed after LA treatment, shows the absence of enhancement due to complete ablation of the metastatic neoplastic tissue. (**h**) 18F-FDG PET image shows marked uptake (*arrow*). (**i**) No uptake with 18F-FDG PET is visible 3 months after an LA procedure

modality, first proposed for breast lesions [107], utilizes US to evaluate the stiffness of thyroid nodules [51]. This parameter is assessed by determining the grade of distortion that occurs in a target lesion under external pressure [108]. The most common technique is to apply an external pressure on the thyroid gland using the US probe. The transducer is placed vertically over the region of interest, and a small pressure is rhythmically applied with the probe. A dedicated software compares the

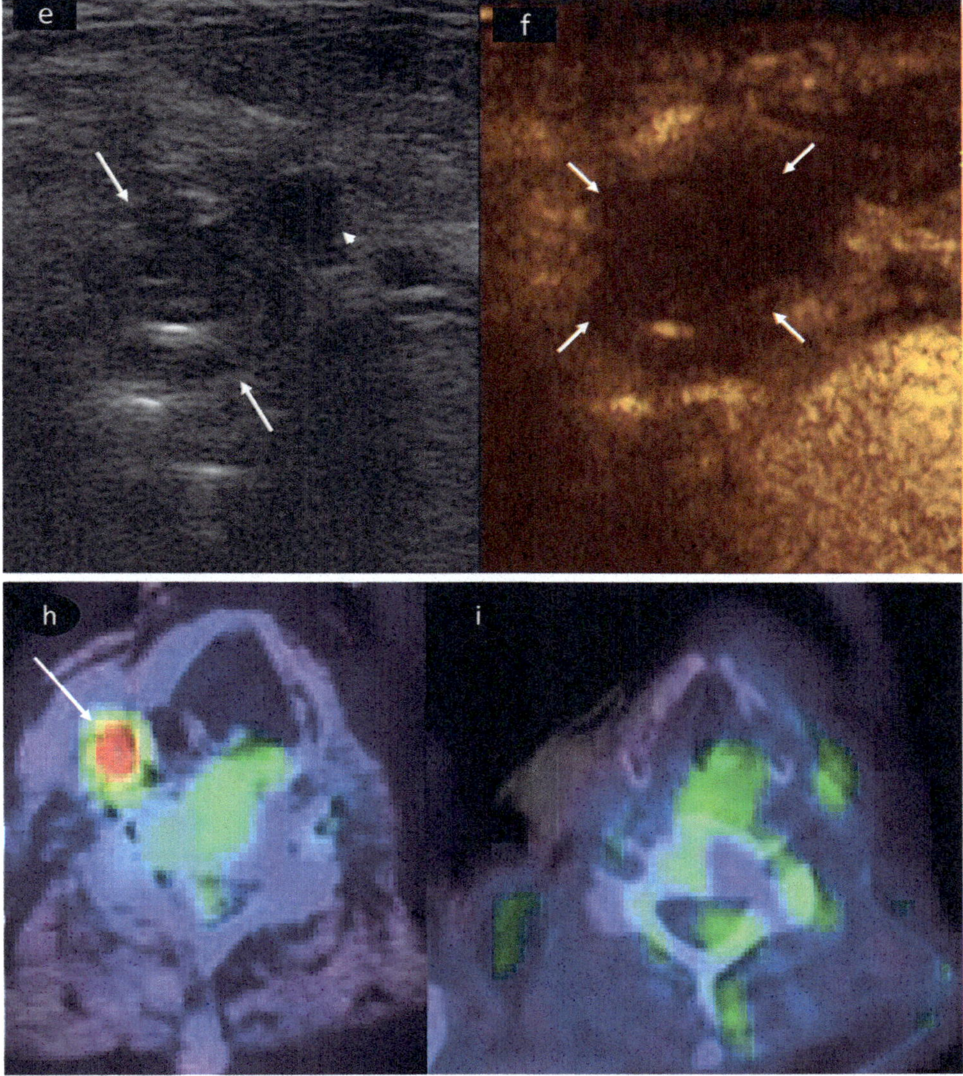

Fig. 23.10 (continued)

deformation of the lesion under evaluation to that of the surrounding parenchyma, and the relative stiffness of the lesion is illustrated by both a quantitative measure (or "strain index") and a qualitative color representation superimposed on the B-mode US image [109]. Other techniques, like the use of carotid pulsation as a compression source, are less widely used due to the frequent presence of artifacts [110].

Predictive Value of Malignancy

Thyroid Nodules

Rago et al. [111] evaluated, by real-time elastography, 96 solitary thyroid nodules that were undergoing surgery due to suspicious cytology or local pressure symptoms. Results were expressed according to a five-class qualitative score that was obtained by a subjective analysis of elastographic color images. Scores 1 and 2 were observed only in benign lesions, score 3 was observed mostly in benign nodules, and scores 4 and 5 were associated with thyroid carcinoma only. The predictive value of elastography was remarkably high. Thus, sensitivity for malignancy of scores 4–5 was 97 % with a specificity of 100 % (Fig. 23.11).

Lymph Nodes

Lyshchik et al. [112] examined 141 lymph nodes in 43 patients undergoing surgery for suspected head and neck malignancies. A strain index, calculated on the basis of lymph node versus cervical muscle stiffness, was highly predictive of malignancy. A cutoff of 1.5 was associated with a 98 % sensitivity and a 85 % specificity for malignancy. While the two [111, 112] studies demonstrated an impressively high positive predictive value of elastography in the diagnosis of malignancy, both were characterized by a num-

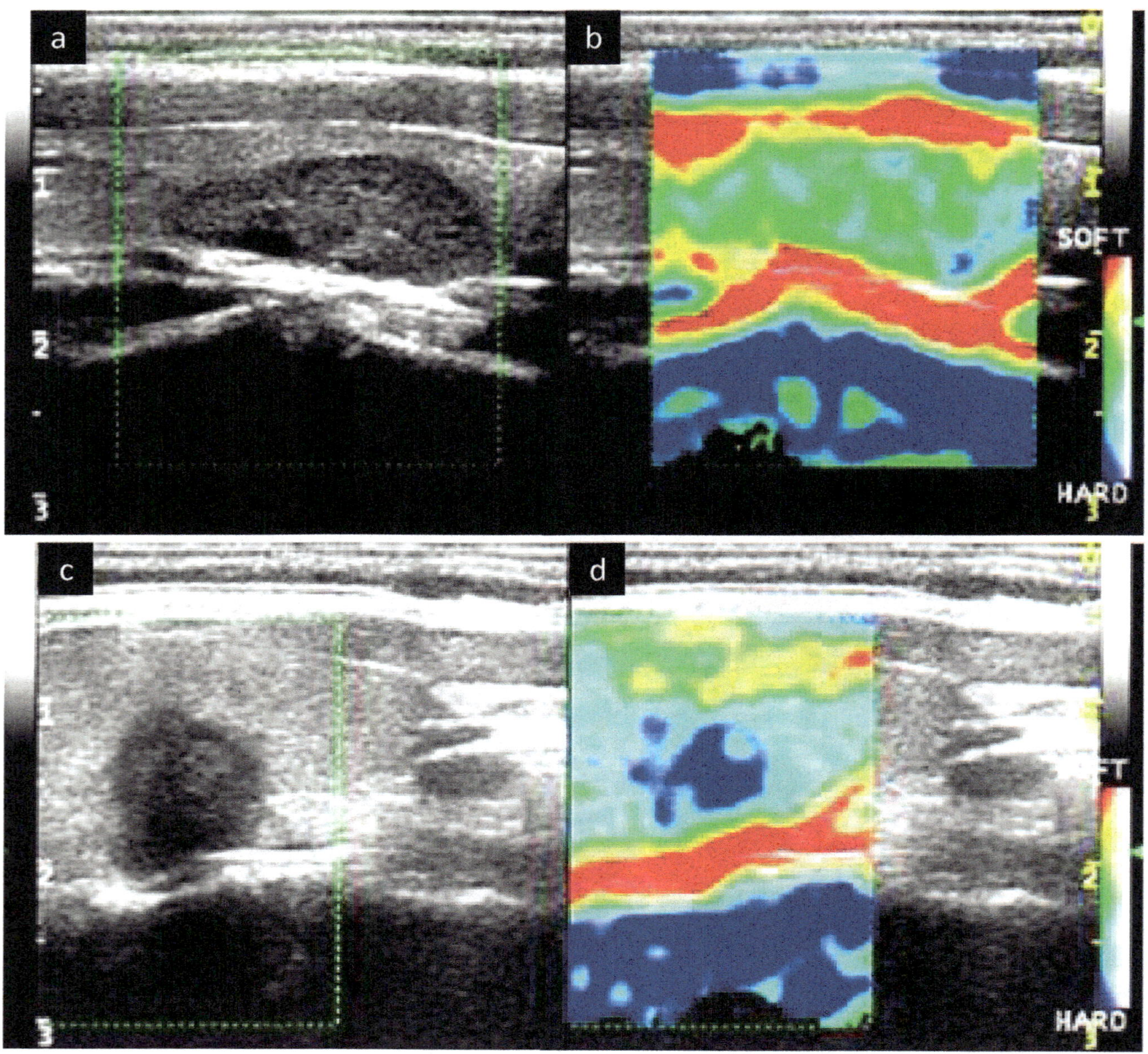

Fig. 23.11 Role of US elastography. (**a**) Sagittal conventional gray-scale image shows a thyroid nodule with US findings suggestive of a benign thyroid lesion . (**b**) US elastography image shows the nodule with elasticity score of 1. US-guided FNA confirmed the benign nature of the nodule. (**c**) Sagittal conventional B-mode US shows a marked hypoechoic nodule with irregular margins. (**d**) US elastography shows that the nodule presents an elasticity score of 5. This lesion was cytologically a papillary carcinoma

ber of shortcomings, most importantly selection bias with a very high prevalence of malignancy. Based on this, the value of elastography in a broader range of patients with nodular thyroid disease needs further evaluation [52].

Technical Limits

Elastography cannot be performed on nodules with peripheral rim calcification or intranodular macrocalcifications, due to the inability of the US beam to penetrate this hard material. Mixed nodules with a cystic component provide unreliable results because the elasticity is markedly influenced by the elasticity of the fluid component. Large size, certain localizations of the nodule(s), and abnormalities of the thyroid parenchyma (as in chronic autoimmune thyroiditis) also influence the evaluations and the value of elastography examinations [52, 109].

Clinical Use

The diagnostic accuracy of elastography for thyroid malignancy, its inter- and intraobserver reproducibility, and its cost-effectiveness, when compared with the traditional US information, are not yet clearly established. Controlled prospective trials in larger numbers of unselected patients are needed. Hence, the use of elastography in routine clinical practice is still of limited value and remains an ancillary technique in most thyroid centers. Elastography, however, may provide rather useful information in selected clinical settings. Thus, small thyroid nodules that show nonsuspicious or indeterminate US features are usually followed up clinically without FNA. In such cases, evidence of low elasticity should strengthen the indication for FNA. A similar approach may be used for the management of cervical lymphadenopathy of uncertain significance revealed by US neck examination during follow-up of patients with thyroid carcinoma.

Contrast-Enhanced Ultrasound

Introduction

Vascularization plays a primary role in the characterization of pathologic tissue by imaging techniques. The limitations of CT and MRI in detecting density or signal differences in pathologic tissues lead to the use of iodinated contrast agents for CT and that of paramagnetic contrast agents for MRI. Similar considerations have been applied to US imaging.

The first-generation contrast medium was a simple isotonic saline solution containing air microbubbles. Second- and third-generation contrast media contain microbubbles of a gas characterized by low solubility in biologic fluids and is enclosed in lipidic or proteinous shells. These involucres increase the resistance to external pressure and provide a protracted half-life (more than 5 min for third-generation media). Contrast media are employed with US equipment and software that detect the harmonic components of the US that are scattered by microbubbles. Incident ultrasound, with a frequency close to the resonant frequency of microbubbles, starts an oscillatory motion which generates ultrasound with a dominant second harmonic component. When the receiver is tuned to this frequency, contributes from contrast media are clearly discriminated from those from solid tissues [113]. Microbubbles are small enough to pass through capillaries, and their diameter influences the resonance frequency. When a microbubble resonates, it absorbs a great quantity of the colliding energy. The microbubble becomes a scattering body which generates US waves that are spherically dispersed. If the energy is high, generated US waves are a distorted copy of the colliding ones, with a dominant frequency which is twofold that of the incident signals. The ability of microbubbles to scatter a distorted copy of the colliding energy is defined as nonlinear, or harmonic, property. Wideband transducers that can detect the harmonic response of microbubbles transmit a fundamental frequency equal to the resonance frequency of microbubbles (i.e., 2 MHz) and receive the second harmonic scattered back by the microbubbles (4 MHz). The harmonic response of contrast media is usually revealed firing sequential ultrasound impulses (typically two or three), one the inverse of the other, and then subtracting the received signals. Only the nonlinear (harmonic) component is detected. The limitations of this technique are a reduced time resolution (reduced frame rate of US scan), an increase in the transmitted energy that causes the destruction of the injected microbubbles, and the possibility of movement artifacts. The introduction of coded-pulse techniques has reduced the potential drawbacks, and currently, US equipments produce high-quality contrast-enhanced images. The usefulness of CEUS in the examination of the abdomen is established, but its use for small part examinations is still under investigation [114].

Procedure

A preliminary US evaluation of the thyroid gland should be performed, and vascular signals of the lesion should be evaluated with CD, performed with a pulse repetition frequency of 1,200, and PW, to detect slow flows. The amplifier gain should be raised until random color noise appears and then slightly lowered. The wall filter should be set low (100 Hz), and once set, the parameters should remain unchanged during the whole CEUS examination. CEUS can be performed with commercially available US scanners equipped with an electronically focused near-field linear array transducer with a 7.0–15.0 MHz bandwidth and a pulse inversion imaging software. The field of interest should be carefully selected. When possible, the area should include the carotid artery or some other major arterial vessels, the whole lesion, and a part of the surrounding normal thyroid parenchyma. The patient should be instructed not to speak or breathe deeply during the examination, and after the bolus injection, swallowing should be avoided for 2 min. After selection of the area of interest, the transducer should remain stable without modifications in its position on the neck, avoiding changes of inclination, vibrations, or involuntary movements. A precontrast clip lasting 10 s should be obtained and digitally stored in a PC-based workstation connected with or built into the US unit. A 22G peripheral intravenous needle is placed into the brachial vein, and US contrast agent is injected as a bolus in 15 s, followed by rapid flushing with 5 ml of 0.9 % saline solution. A low frame rate (5 Hz) and a very low mechanical index (MI=0.05–0.08) should be used with the US focus placed at a lower level than the nodule under examination, in order to minimize microbubble destruction. A postcontrast clip lasting 2 min should be acquired and digitally stored for subsequent editing.

The contrast-enhancement pattern can be evaluated on the basis of:

(a) US changes at visual appearance

(b) Time-intensity curves
(c) Three-dimensional reconstruction.

Visual Appearance

Contrast enhancement may be classified as absent (no difference in enhancement between the lesion and the surrounding tissue after contrast injection), dotted (tiny scattered spots of enhancement throughout the lesion), or diffuse (homogeneous enhancement of the whole lesion). Assessment of the changes in time-intensity curves is performed at the level of regions of interest (ROI) within the nodule, the surrounding thyroid parenchyma, and the common carotid artery. Calculations of the signal intensity curves are performed using a linear scale, and results are transformed into a logarithmic scale to reduce the range of variation in the intensity values. Second-generation contrast media are devoid of human or animal substances, but a few side effects, or even rare fatal complications, have been described. The use of contrast agents is currently off label for thyroid gland visualization, and it is suggested that an informed written consent is signed by the patients. A study, performed in 2001, with a first-generation galactose-based US contrast agent claimed that the analysis of time-intensity curves was able to differentiate benign from malignant lesions [115]. A subsequent well-controlled study in 18 patients with a solitary thyroid nodule could not confirm these findings. Signal-intensity values, after the injection of a second-generation contrast medium, showed a diffuse pattern of contrast enhancement in nodules with intranodular vascular signals at baseline Doppler assessment unrelated to histological diagnoses [116]. We recently performed a blinded US study of 28 hypofunctioning solid thyroid nodules with benign, indeterminate, or malignant cytology before surgery [96]. Contrast-enhanced evaluation did not add any information to the precontrast data for the prediction of malignancy. Therefore, in our view, only future large-scale studies with surgical confirmation can clarify whether contrast-enhanced US improves the sensitivity and specificity in the selection of thyroid nodules at highest risk of harboring malignancy and whether using this technology improves the prognosis of the patients.

Clinical Use

(a) Evaluation of thyroid nodules with contrast-enhanced US (CEUS):
- Differentiation of benign from malignant lesions: visual appearance offers no advantage over conventional CD and PW.
- Time to peak, wash-in, and washout curves give no relevant information. Blood volume is reduced in small malignant lesions, but diagnostic accuracy is low and the technique is cumbersome.
- 3-D reconstruction improves visual assessment of blood volume differences and may be of aid in evaluating the risk of malignancy.

(b) Assessment of ablation treatment with CEUS seems useful for the evaluation of the extension of the coagulation zone induced by hyperthermic ablation (Fig. 23.12).

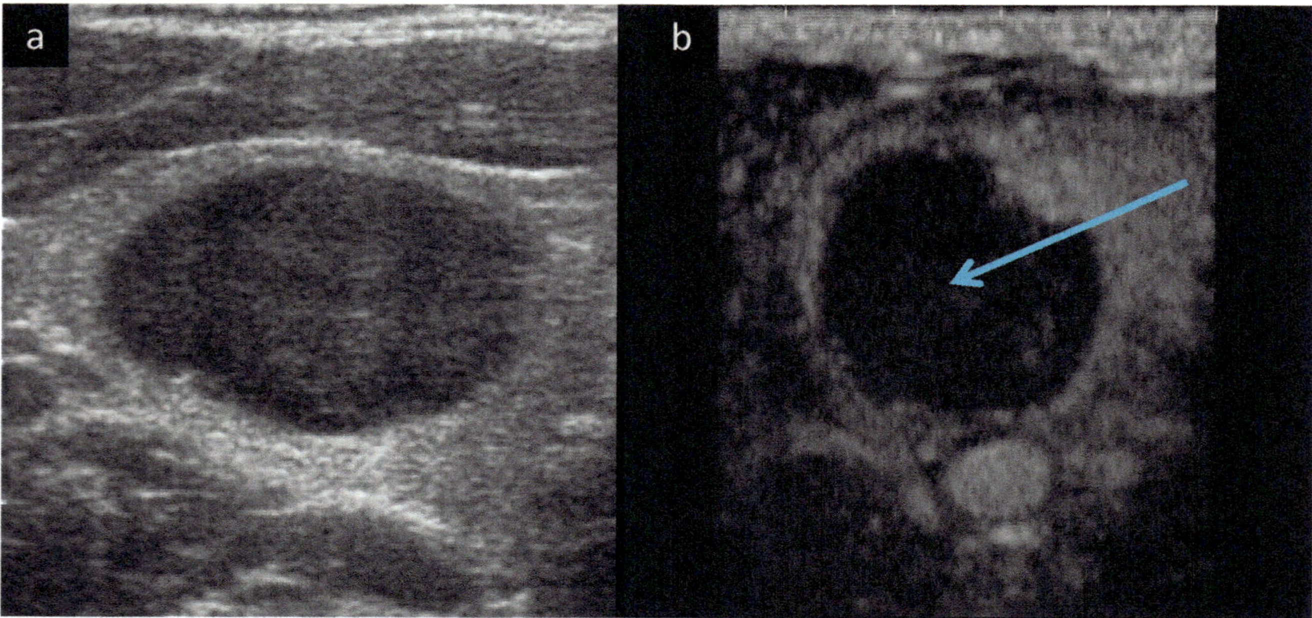

Fig. 23.12 US contrast media for the assessment of LA-induced thyroid tissue coagulation. (**a**) Transverse gray-scale image shows a solid benign nodule before LA treatment. (**b**) CEUS, 6 h after an LA session, shows a large area of coagulation (*blue arrow*) due to hyperthermic ablation

CEUS evaluation should be performed 6 h after thermal ablation to avoid the artifacts due to the presence of microbubbles of gas within the thyroid tissue. B-mode US does not provide a correct evaluation of the area of necrosis until 24 h posttherapy. Information obtained by CEUS is similar to findings by CT examination with contrast injection. However, CT is more expensive and time-consuming and requires the intravenous injection of an iodinated contrast agent.

Conclusions

First- and second-generation contrast agents seem to provide only ancillary data for the diagnosis of malignant nodules. Preliminary data using third-generation contrast media demonstrate their utility in obtaining early and valid evidence of the extent of thyroid tissue destruction induced by mini-invasive ablation procedures (laser and radiofrequency treatment) [96]. Currently, variation in time-intensity curves, during transit time of the injected microbubbles, offers only a modest improvement over prediction of malignancy provided by CD or PW evaluations [96].

References

1. Foley WD. Physical principles and instrumentation. In: Foley WD, editor. Color Doppler flow imaging. Boston: Andover Medical Publishers; 1991. p. 3–13.
2. Zagzebski J. Essentials of ultrasound physics. St Louis: Mosby; 1996.
3. Kremkau FW. Diagnostic ultrasound. Philadelphia: Saunders; 1998.
4. Goldstein A, Powis RL. Medical ultrasonic diagnostics. Phys Acoust. 1999;23:43–191.
5. Carson P. Ultrasound tissue interactions. In: Goldman L, Fowlkes J, editors. Categorical course in diagnostic radiology physics: CT and US cross-sectional imaging. Oak Brook: Radiological Society of North America; 2000. p. 9–20.
6. Bushberg J, Seibert J, Leidholdt E, Boone J. The essential physics of medical imaging. Philadelphia: Lippincott Williams & Wilkins; 2002. p. 469–553.
7. Thomenius K. Instrumentation for B-mode imaging. In: Goldman LW, Fowlles JB, editors. Categorical course in diagnostic radiology physics: CT and US cross-sectional imaging. Oak Brook: Radiological Society of North America; 2000. p. 21–32.
8. Jespersen SK, Wilhjelm JE, Sillesen H. Multi-angle compound imaging. Ultrason Imaging. 1998;20(2):81–102.
9. Burns PN. The physical principles of Doppler and spectral analysis. J Clin Ultrasound. 1987;15(9):567–90.
10. Nelson TR, Pretorius DH. The Doppler signal: where does it come from and what does it mean? AJR Am J Roentgenol. 1988;151(3):439–47.
11. Rubin JM, Bude RO, Carson PL, Bree RL, Adler RS. Power Doppler US: a potentially useful alternative to mean frequency-based color Doppler US. Radiology. 1994;190(3):853–6.
12. Stavros AT, Rapp CL, Thickman D. Sonography of inflammatory condition. Ultrasound Q. 1995;13:1–26.
13. Bude RO, Rubin JM. Power Doppler sonography. Radiology. 1996;200(1):21–3.
14. Raza S, Baum JK. Solid breast lesions: evaluation with power Doppler US. Radiology. 1997;203(1):164–8.
15. Holland SK, Orphanoudakis SC, Jaffe CC. Frequency-dependent attenuation effects in pulsed Doppler ultrasound: experimental results. IEEE Trans Biomed Eng. 1984;31(9):626–31.
16. Rizzatto G. Ultrasound transducers. Eur J Radiol. 1998;27 Suppl 2:S188–95.
17. Hegedus L, Bonnema SJ, Bennedbaek FN. Management of simple nodular goiter: current status and future perspectives. Endocr Rev. 2003;24(1):102–32.
18. Hegedus L. Clinical practice. The thyroid nodule. N Engl J Med. 2004;351(17):1764–71.
19. Hegedus L. Therapy: a new nonsurgical therapy option for benign thyroid nodules? Nat Rev Endocrinol. 2009;5(9):476–8.
20. Gharib H, Papini E, Paschke R, et al. American Association of Clinical Endocrinologists, Associazione Medici Endocrinologi, and European Thyroid Association medical guidelines for clinical practice for the diagnosis and management of thyroid nodules. J Endocrinol Invest. 2010;33(5 Suppl):1–50.
21. Gharib H, Papini E. Thyroid nodules: clinical importance, assessment, and treatment. Endocrinol Metab Clin North Am. 2007;36(3):707–35, vi.
22. American Thyroid Association Guidelines Task Force on Thyroid Nodules and Differentiated Thyroid Cancer. Haugen BR, Alexander EK, Bible KC, Doherty GM, Mandel SJ, Nikiforov YE, Pacini F, Randolph GW, Sawka AM, Schlumberger M, Schuff KG, Sherman SI, Sosa JA, Steward DL, Tuttle RM, Wartofsky L. 2015 American Thyroid Association Management Guidelines for Adult Patients with Thyroid Nodules and Differentiated Thyroid Cancer. Thyroid 2016; 26:1–133.
23. Paschke R, Hegedus L, Alexander E, Valcavi R, Papini E, Gharib H. Thyroid nodule guidelines: agreement, disagreement and need for future research. Nat Rev Endocrinol. 2011;7(6):354–61.
24. Solbiati L, Osti V, Cova L, Tonolini M. Ultrasound of thyroid, parathyroid glands and neck lymph nodes. Eur Radiol. 2001; 11(12):2411–24.
25. Kwak JY, Han KH, Yoon JH, et al. Thyroid imaging reporting and data system for US features of nodules: a step in establishing better stratification of cancer risk. Radiology. 2011;260(3):892–9.
26. Moon WJ, Jung SL, Lee JH, et al. Benign and malignant thyroid nodules: US differentiation – multicenter retrospective study. Radiology. 2008;247(3):762–70.
27. Frates MC, Benson CB, Charboneau JW, et al. Management of thyroid nodules detected at US: Society of Radiologists in Ultrasound consensus conference statement. Radiology. 2005; 237(3):794–800.
28. Hatabu H, Kasagi K, Yamamoto K, et al. Cystic papillary carcinoma of the thyroid gland: a new sonographic sign. Clin Radiol. 1991;43(2):121–4.
29. Watters DA, Ahuja AT, Evans RM, et al. Role of ultrasound in the management of thyroid nodules. Am J Surg. 1992;164(6):654–7.
30. Chan BK, Desser TS, McDougall IR, Weigel RJ, Jeffrey Jr RB. Common and uncommon sonographic features of papillary thyroid carcinoma. J Ultrasound Med. 2003;22(10):1083–90.
31. Hoang JK, Lee WK, Lee M, Johnson D, Farrell S. US features of thyroid malignancy: pearls and pitfalls. Radiographics. 2007;27(3):847–60; discussion 861–845.
32. Kim EK, Park CS, Chung WY, et al. New sonographic criteria for recommending fine-needle aspiration biopsy of nonpalpable solid nodules of the thyroid. AJR Am J Roentgenol. 2002;178(3):687–91.
33. Papini E, Guglielmi R, Bianchini A, et al. Risk of malignancy in nonpalpable thyroid nodules: predictive value of ultrasound and color-Doppler features. J Clin Endocrinol Metab. 2002; 87(5):1941–6.
34. Yoon DY, Lee JW, Chang SK, et al. Peripheral calcification in thyroid nodules: ultrasonographic features and prediction of malignancy. J Ultrasound Med. 2007;26(10):1349–55; quiz 1356–1347.

35. Khoo ML, Asa SL, Witterick IJ, Freeman JL. Thyroid calcification and its association with thyroid carcinoma. Head Neck. 2002;24(7):651–5.
36. Peccin S, de Castsro JA, Furlanetto TW, Furtado AP, Brasil BA, Czepielewski MA. Ultrasonography: is it useful in the diagnosis of cancer in thyroid nodules? J Endocrinol Invest. 2002;25(1):39–43.
37. Kim BM, Kim MJ, Kim EK, et al. Sonographic differentiation of thyroid nodules with eggshell calcifications. J Ultrasound Med. 2008;27(10):1425–30.
38. Martinoli C, Pretolesi F, Crespi G, et al. Power Doppler sonography: clinical applications. Eur J Radiol. 1998;27 Suppl 2:S133–40.
39. Frates MC, Benson CB, Doubilet PM, Cibas ES, Marqusee E. Can color Doppler sonography aid in the prediction of malignancy of thyroid nodules? J Ultrasound Med. 2003;22(2):127–31; quiz 132–124.
40. Gharib H, Papini E, Paschke R, et al. American Association of Clinical Endocrinologists, Associazione Medici Endocrinologi, and European Thyroid Association medical guidelines for clinical practice for the diagnosis and management of thyroid nodules: executive summary of recommendations. J Endocrinol Invest. 2010;33(5 Suppl):51–6.
41. Nam-Goong IS, Kim HY, Gong G, et al. Ultrasonography-guided fine-needle aspiration of thyroid incidentaloma: correlation with pathological findings. Clin Endocrinol (Oxf). 2004;60(1):21–8.
42. Alexander EK, Marqusee E, Orcutt J, et al. Thyroid nodule shape and prediction of malignancy. Thyroid. 2004;14(11):953–8.
43. Wienke JR, Chong WK, Fielding JR, Zou KH, Mittelstaedt CA. Sonographic features of benign thyroid nodules: interobserver reliability and overlap with malignancy. J Ultrasound Med. 2003;22(10):1027–31.
44. Lee YH, Kim DW, In HS, et al. Differentiation between benign and malignant solid thyroid nodules using an US classification system. Korean J Radiol. 2011;12(5):559–67.
45. Leenhardt L, Hejblum G, Franc B, et al. Indications and limits of ultrasound-guided cytology in the management of nonpalpable thyroid nodules. J Clin Endocrinol Metab. 1999;84(1):24–8.
46. Reading CC, Charboneau JW, Hay ID, Sebo TJ. Sonography of thyroid nodules: a "classic pattern" diagnostic approach. Ultrasound Q. 2005;21(3):157–65.
47. Tamsel S, Demirpolat G, Erdogan M, et al. Power Doppler US patterns of vascularity and spectral Doppler US parameters in predicting malignancy in thyroid nodules. Clin Radiol. 2007; 62(3):245–51.
48. Moon HJ, Kwak JY, Kim MJ, Son EJ, Kim EK. Can vascularity at power Doppler US help predict thyroid malignancy? Radiology. 2010;255(1):260–9.
49. Lacout A, Marcy PY, Thariat J. RE: role of Duplex Doppler US for thyroid nodules: looking for the "sword" sign. Korean J Radiol. 2011;12(3):400–1.
50. Alexander EK, Hurwitz S, Heering JP, et al. Natural history of benign solid and cystic thyroid nodules. Ann Intern Med. 2003;138(4):315–8.
51. Lyshchik A, Higashi T, Asato R, et al. Thyroid gland tumor diagnosis at US elastography. Radiology. 2005;237(1):202–11.
52. Hegedus L. Can elastography stretch our understanding of thyroid histomorphology? J Clin Endocrinol Metab. 2010;95(12): 5213–5.
53. Duick S, Mandel S. Ultrasound-guided aspiration of thyroid nodules. In: Baskin JH, Duick DS, Levine RA, editors. Thyroid ultrasound and ultrasound-guided FNA. 2nd ed. New York: Springer Science; 2008. p. 97–110.
54. Gao J, Kazam JK, Kazam E. Imaging and biopsy guidance in the perioperative management of thyroid carcinoma. In: Carpi A, Mechanick JI, editors. Thyroid cancer: from emergent biotechnologies to clinical practice guidelines. New York: CRC Press; 2011. p. 117–32.
55. Gobien RP. Aspiration biopsy of the solitary thyroid nodule. Radiol Clin North Am. 1979;17(3):543–54.
56. Gharib H. Diagnosis of thyroid nodules by fine-needle aspiration biopsy. Curr Opin Endocrinol Diabetes. 1996;3:433–8.
57. Silverman JF, West RL, Finley JL, et al. Fine-needle aspiration versus large-needle biopsy or cutting biopsy in evaluation of thyroid nodules. Diagn Cytopathol. 1986;2(1):25–30.
58. Screaton NJ, Berman LH, Grant JW. US-guided core-needle biopsy of the thyroid gland. Radiology. 2003;226(3):827–32.
59. Zhang S, Ivanovic M, Nemecek AA, De Frias DVS, Lucas E, Nayar R. Thin core needle biopsy crush preparation in conjunction with fine-needle aspiration for the evaluation of thyroid nodules. A complementary approach. Cancer Cytopathol. 2008; 114:512–8.
60. Park KT, Ahn SH, Mo JH, et al. Role of core needle biopsy and ultrasonographic finding in management of indeterminate thyroid nodules. Head Neck. 2011;33(2):160–5.
61. Papini E, Bianchini A, Guglielmi R, et al. Image-guided mini-invasive ablation of thyroid tumors and distant metastases. In: Carpi A, Mechanick JI, editors. Thyroid cancer: from emergent biotechnologies to clinical practice guidelines. New York: CRC Press; 2011. p. 213–30.
62. Livraghi T, Giorgio A, Marin G, et al. Hepatocellular carcinoma and cirrhosis in 746 patients: long-term results of percutaneous ethanol injection. Radiology. 1995;197(1):101–8.
63. Solbiati L, Giangrande A, De Pra L, Bellotti E, Cantu P, Ravetto C. Percutaneous ethanol injection of parathyroid tumors under US guidance: treatment for secondary hyperparathyroidism. Radiology. 1985;155(3):607–10.
64. Charbonneau JW, Hay ID, van Heerden JA. Persistent primary hyperparathyroidism: successful ultrasound-guided percutaneous ethanol ablation of an occult adenoma. Mayo Clin Proc. 1988;63:913–7.
65. Karstrup S, Holm HH, Glenthoj A, Hegedus L. Nonsurgical treatment of primary hyperparathyroidism with sonographically guided percutaneous injection of ethanol: results in a selected series of patients. AJR Am J Roentgenol. 1990;154(5):1087–90.
66. Livraghi T, Paracchi A, Ferrari C, et al. Treatment of autonomous thyroid nodules with percutaneous ethanol injection: preliminary results. Work in progress. Radiology. 1990;175(3):827–9.
67. Bennedbaek FN, Nielsen LK, Hegedus L. Effect of percutaneous ethanol injection therapy versus suppressive doses of L-thyroxine on benign solitary solid cold thyroid nodules: a randomized trial. J Clin Endocrinol Metab. 1998;83(3):830–5.
68. Bennedbaek FN, Karstrup S, Hegedus L. Percutaneous ethanol injection therapy in the treatment of thyroid and parathyroid diseases. Eur J Endocrinol. 1997;136(3):240–50.
69. Papini E, Pacella C. Percutaneous ethanol injection of benign thyroid nodules and cysts using ultrasound. In: Baskin HJ, editor. Thyroid ultrasound and ultrasound-guided FNA biopsy. 1st ed. Boston: Kluwer Academic Publishers; 2000. p. 169–213.
70. Valcavi R, Frasoldati A. Ultrasound-guided percutaneous ethanol injection therapy in thyroid cystic nodules. Endocr Pract. 2004;10(3):269–75.
71. Guglielmi R, Pacella CM, Bianchini A, et al. Percutaneous ethanol injection treatment in benign thyroid lesions: role and efficacy. Thyroid. 2004;14(2):125–31.
72. Goletti O, Lenziardi M, De Negri F, et al. Inoperable thyroid carcinoma: palliation with percutaneous injection of ethanol. Eur J Surg. 1993;159(11–12):639–41.
73. Hay ID, Charboneau JW. The coming of age of ultrasound-guided percutaneous ethanol ablation of selected neck nodal metastases in well-differentiated thyroid carcinoma. J Clin Endocrinol Metab. 2011;96(9):2717–20.
74. Lewis BD, Hay ID, Charboneau JW, McIver B, Reading CC, Goellner JR. Percutaneous ethanol injection for treatment of cer-

vical lymph node metastases in patients with papillary thyroid carcinoma. AJR Am J Roentgenol. 2002;178(3):699–704.
75. Hay ID, Charbonneau JW, Lewis BD, et al. Successful ultrasound-guided percutaneous ethanol ablation of neck metastases in 20 patients with postoperative TNM stage I papillary thyroid carcinoma resistant to conventional therapy. (abstract). In: 74th Meeting ATA. Los Angeles; 2002. p. 176.
76. Monchik JM, Donatini G, Iannuccilli J, Dupuy DE. Radiofrequency ablation and percutaneous ethanol injection treatment for recurrent local and distant well-differentiated thyroid carcinoma. Ann Surg. 2006;244(2):296–304.
77. Lim CY, Yun JS, Lee J, Nam KH, Chung WY, Park CS. Percutaneous ethanol injection therapy for locally recurrent papillary thyroid carcinoma. Thyroid. 2007;17(4):347–50.
78. Kim BM, Kim MJ, Kim EK, Park SI, Park CS, Chung WY. Controlling recurrent papillary thyroid carcinoma in the neck by ultrasonography-guided percutaneous ethanol injection. Eur Radiol. 2008;18(4):835–42.
79. Heilo A, Sigstad E, Fagerlid KH, et al. Efficacy of ultrasound-guided percutaneous ethanol injection treatment in patients with a limited number of metastatic cervical lymph nodes from papillary thyroid carcinoma. J Clin Endocrinol Metab. 2011;96(9): 2750–5.
80. Tranberg KG. Percutaneous ablation of liver tumours. Best Pract Res Clin Gastroenterol. 2004;18(1):125–45.
81. Lencioni R. Loco-regional treatment of hepatocellular carcinoma. Hepatology. 2010;52(2):762–73.
82. Dupuy DE, Monchik JM, Decrea C, Pisharodi L. Radiofrequency ablation of regional recurrence from well-differentiated thyroid malignancy. Surgery. 2001;130(6):971–7.
83. Pacella CM, Bizzarri G, Francica G, et al. Percutaneous laser ablation in the treatment of hepatocellular carcinoma with small tumors: analysis of factors affecting the achievement of tumor necrosis. J Vasc Interv Radiol. 2005;16(11):1447–57.
84. Gough-Palmer AL, Gedroyc WM. Laser ablation of hepatocellular carcinoma – a review. World J Gastroenterol. 2008;14(47):7170–4.
85. Walser EM. Percutaneous laser ablation in the treatment of hepatocellular carcinoma with a tumor size of 4 cm or smaller: analysis of factors affecting the achievement of tumor necrosis. J Vasc Interv Radiol. 2005;16(11):1427–9.
86. Pacella CM, Francica G, Di Lascio FM, et al. Long-term outcome of cirrhotic patients with early hepatocellular carcinoma treated with ultrasound-guided percutaneous laser ablation: a retrospective analysis. J Clin Oncol. 2009;27(16):2615–21.
87. Vogl TJ, Eichler K, Straub R, et al. Laser-induced thermotherapy of malignant liver tumors: general principals, equipment(s), procedure(s) – side effects, complications and results. Eur J Ultrasound. 2001;13(2):117–27.
88. Stafford RJ, Fuentes D, Elliott AA, Weinberg JS, Ahrar K. Laser-induced thermal therapy for tumor ablation. Crit Rev Biomed Eng. 2010;38(1):79–100.
89. Ahrar K, Gowda A, Javadi S, et al. Preclinical assessment of a 980-nm diode laser ablation system in a large animal tumor model. J Vasc Interv Radiol. 2010;21(4):555–61.
90. Pacella CM, Bizzarri G, Spiezia S, et al. Thyroid tissue: US-guided percutaneous laser thermal ablation. Radiology. 2004;232(1): 272–80.
91. Cakir B, Topaloglu O, Gul K, et al. Ultrasound-guided percutaneous laser ablation treatment in inoperable aggressive course anaplastic thyroid carcinoma: the introduction of a novel alternative palliative therapy – second experience in the literature. J Endocrinol Invest. 2007;30(7):624–5.
92. Papini E, Guglielmi R, Hosseim G, et al. Ultrasound-guided laser ablation of incidental papillary thyroid microcarcinoma: a potential therapeutic approach in patients at surgical risk. Thyroid. 2011;21(8):917–20.
93. Solbiati L, Cova L, Ierace T, Pacella CM, Baroli A, Lomuscio G. Percutaneous US-guided interstitial laser ablation of new metastatic lymph nodes in the neck from papillary thyroid carcinoma following thyroidectomy and lymphadenectomy (abstract). In: RSNA, (ed.) 97th Scientific assembly and annual meeting. Chicago; 2011.
94. Ritz JP, Lehmann KS, Zurbuchen U, et al. Ex vivo and in vivo evaluation of laser-induced thermotherapy for nodular thyroid disease. Lasers Surg Med. 2009;41(7):479–86.
95. Pacella CM, Bizzarri G, Bianchini A, Guglielmi R, Pacella S, Papini E. US-guided laser thermal ablation of benign and malignant thyroid lesions (abstract). In: RSNA, (ed.) 84th scientific assembly and annual meeting November 30–December 5. Chicago; 2003. p. 1974.
96. Papini E, Bizzarri G, Bianchini A, et al. Contrast-enhanced ultrasound in the management of thyroid nodules. In: Baskin HJ, Duick DS, Levine RA, editors. Thyroid ultrasound and ultrasound-guided FNA. New York: Springer; 2008. p. 151–71.
97. Baek JH, Kim YS, Lee D, Huh JY, Lee JH. Benign predominantly solid thyroid nodules: prospective study of efficacy of sonographically guided radiofrequency ablation versus control condition. AJR Am J Roentgenol. 2010;194(4):1137–42.
98. Pacella CM, Bizzarri G, Guglielmi R, et al. Thyroid tissue: US-guided percutaneous interstitial laser ablation-a feasibility study. Radiology. 2000;217(3):673–7.
99. Dossing H, Bennedbaek FN, Hegedus L. Ultrasound-guided interstitial laser photocoagulation of an autonomous thyroid nodule: the introduction of a novel alternative. Thyroid. 2003;13(9):885–8.
100. Dossing H, Bennedbaek FN, Hegedus L. Effect of ultrasound-guided interstitial laser photocoagulation on benign solitary solid cold thyroid nodules – a randomised study. Eur J Endocrinol. 2005;152(3):341–5.
101. Papini E, Guglielmi R, Bizzarri G, et al. Treatment of benign cold thyroid nodules: a randomized clinical trial of percutaneous laser ablation versus levothyroxine therapy or follow-up. Thyroid. 2007;17(3):229–35.
102. Dossing H, Bennedbaek FN, Hegedus L. Long-term outcome following interstitial laser photocoagulation of benign cold thyroid nodules. Eur J Endocrinol. 2011;165(1):123–8.
103. Esnault O, Franc B, Menegaux F, et al. High-intensity focused ultrasound ablation of thyroid nodules: first human feasibility study. Thyroid. 2011;21(9):965–73.
104. Kovatcheva RD, Vlahov JD, Shinkov AD, et al. High-intensity focused ultrasound to treat primary hyperparathyroidism: a feasibility study in four patients. AJR Am J Roentgenol. 2010; 195(4):830–5.
105. Lerner RM, Huang SR, Parker KJ. "Sonoelasticity" images derived from ultrasound signals in mechanically vibrated tissues. Ultrasound Med Biol. 1990;16(3):231–9.
106. Konofagou EE. Quo vadis elasticity imaging? Ultrasonics. 2004;42(1–9):331–6.
107. Itoh A, Ueno E, Tohno E, et al. Breast disease: clinical application of US elastography for diagnosis. Radiology. 2006;239(2):341–50.
108. Lyshchik A, Higashi T, Asato R, et al. Elastic moduli of thyroid tissues under compression. Ultrason Imaging. 2005;27(2): 101–10.
109. Levine RA. Ultrasound elastography of the thyroid. In: Baskin J, Duick D, Levine R, editors. Thyroid ultrasound and ultrasound-guided FNA. 2nd ed. New York: Springer Science; 2008. p. 237–43.
110. Bae U, Dighe M, Dubinsky T, Minoshima S, Shamdasani V, Kim Y. Ultrasound thyroid elastography using carotid artery pulsation: preliminary study. J Ultrasound Med. 2007;26(6):797–805.
111. Rago T, Santini F, Scutari M, Pinchera A, Vitti P. Elastography: new developments in ultrasound for predicting malignancy in thyroid nodules. J Clin Endocrinol Metab. 2007;92(8): 2917–22.

112. Lyshchik A, Higashi T, Asato R, et al. Cervical lymph node metastases: diagnosis at sonoelastography – initial experience. Radiology. 2007;243(1):258–67.
113. Wilson SR, Burns PN. Microbubble contrast for radiological imaging: 2. Applications. Ultrasound Q. 2006;22(1):15–8.
114. Huang-Wei C, Bleuzen A, Bourlier P, et al. Differential diagnosis of focal nodular hyperplasia with quantitative parametric analysis in contrast-enhanced sonography. Invest Radiol. 2006;41(3):363–8.
115. Spiezia S, Farina R, Cerbone G, et al. Analysis of color Doppler signal intensity variation after levovist injection: a new approach to the diagnosis of thyroid nodules. J Ultrasound Med. 2001;20(3):223–31; quiz 233.
116. Bartolotta TV, Midiri M, Galia M, et al. Qualitative and quantitative evaluation of solitary thyroid nodules with contrast-enhanced ultrasound: initial results. Eur Radiol. 2006;16(10):2234–41.

Radionuclide Imaging of Thyroid Nodules

24

Douglas Van Nostrand, Mark Schneider, and Elmo R. Acio

Introduction

Thyroid scintigraphy has been used for many years to evaluate thyroid nodules. The clinical value of thyroid scintigraphy has been established based on the knowledge that (1) functioning nodules have not only increased radioiodine uptake relative to normal functioning thyroid tissue but also have a low probability of malignancy and (2) thyroid cancers have no or very low radioiodine accumulation relative to normal thyroid tissue. This chapter presents an overview of thyroid scintigraphy in the evaluation of thyroid nodules (see Table 24.1).

Radiopharmaceuticals and Mechanisms

The most frequently used radiopharmaceuticals for thyroid scintigraphy have been ^{131}I, $^{99m}TcO_4$, and ^{123}I. The physical characteristics of the various radiopharmaceuticals are shown in Table 24.2; their respective advantages and disadvantages are listed in Table 24.3. Because of the significant radiation-absorbed dose to normal functioning thyroid tissue, ^{131}I is no longer routinely used for scanning when $^{99m}TcO_4$ and ^{123}I are available, and the latter are widely available in the United States and many other countries. Although ^{123}I is more expensive than $^{99m}TcO_4$, the cost of ^{123}I has decreased significantly over the last several years. Both $^{99m}TcO_4$ and ^{123}I result in good images; ^{123}I is slightly better, and as an isotope of iodine, ^{123}I is both trapped and organified, whereas $^{99m}TcO_4$ only reflects trapping.

D. Van Nostrand, MD, FACP, FACNM (✉)
Nuclear Medicine Research, MedStar Research Institute and Washington Hospital Center, Georgetown University School of Medicine, Washington Hospital Center, 110 Irving Street, N.W., Suite GB 60F, Washington, DC 20010, USA
e-mail: douglasvannostrand@gmail.com

M. Schneider, MD
Cardiovascular/Metabolic, Boehringer Ingelheim, Chicago, IL, USA
e-mail: abschnei@uic.edu

E.R. Acio, MD
Division of Nuclear Medicine, Department of Medicine, MedStar Washington Hospital Center, Washington, DC, USA

Imaging Procedure

The Society of Nuclear Medicine has published guidelines for thyroid scintigraphy [1]. For thyroid scintigraphy, the prescribed activity of ^{123}I ranges typically between 7.4 and 14.8 MBq (200 and 400 uCi) with images performed 6–24 h later. The prescribed activity of $^{99m}TcO_4$ is approximately 370 MBq (10 mCi), and images are performed 20–30 min later. Images are obtained on γ-camera with a pinhole collimator in the anterior, left anterior oblique (LAO), and right anterior oblique (RAO) positions. Markers may be placed on various landmarks such as the suprasternal notch and chin.

After completion of the standard images, the thyroid gland should be examined and additional images—with or without radioactive markers placed on nodules or anatomical landmarks—may need to be performed. The radioactive markers on the palpable nodule(s) help determine whether the nodule is *cold*, *hot*, *warm*, *indeterminate*, *normofunctioning*, *or hyperfunctioning*, and these terms are defined later in this chapter. However, when using a pinhole collimator, caution should be taken when using markers to correlate the nodule to the findings in the pinhole collimator image. As discussed in greater detail in Chap. 11 entitled "Radioiodine Whole Body Imaging," pinhole collimators have the best resolution, but they may distort the location of the anatomy—a phenomenon that has been called "parallax" [2]. Structures or markers located close to the face of the pinhole collimator are recorded on the final image farther toward the edge of the field of view than deeper structures. Thus, a marker placed on the skin surface near the face of the pinhole collimator, precisely over a deep, underlying nodule

L. Wartofsky, D. Van Nostrand (eds.), *Thyroid Cancer*, DOI 10.1007/978-1-4939-3314-3_24

Table 24.1 Topics

Radiopharmaceuticals and mechanisms
Imaging procedure
Radiation dosimetry
Terminology for describing the function of nodules assessed on thyroid scintigraphy and the frequency of thyroid cancer
Hyperfunctioning nodules and association with thyroid cancer
Discordance of ^{123}I and $^{99m}TcO_4$ pertechnetate scans
Utility of thyroid scintigraphy
Summary

Table 24.2 Radiopharmaceuticals used for thyroid scintigraphy

Typical prescribed					
Decay mode		Half-life	γ-energy (keV)	Production method	Activity MBq (mCi)
^{123}I	Electron capture	13.6 h	159	Cyclotron methods; one method referred to as a (p,5n) produces ^{123}I with no ^{124}I contamination and little ^{125}I. The other approach referred to as (p,2n) has a number of impurities that have high-energy γ and long half-lives. These contaminations reduce image quality and increase the radiation exposure of the patient	1.5–3.0 (0.2–0.4)
^{99m}Tc	Isomeric transition	6.02 h	140	Molybdenum 99 generator	7.4–370 (2–10)
^{131}I	β-decay	8.02 days	364	Reactor produced either from direct bombardment of a target by neutrons or from the reprocessing of spent fuel rods from a nuclear power plant	0.185 (0.005) for uptakes
					37–185 (1–5) for imaging
					1.07–37 (29–1000) for therapy

Table 24.3 Comparison of ^{123}I, ^{99m}Tc, and ^{131}I

Advantages/disadvantages			
Characteristics	^{123}I	$^{99m}TcO_4$	^{131}I
Expense	$$	$	$
Readily available	Y	Y	Y
Reimbursed by insurance	Y	Y	Y
Image quality	Excellent	Excellent but not as good when trapping is low because of higher background	Good
Mechanism of accumulation of radioactivity in the thyroid	Organification	Trapping	Organification
Esophageal or vascular radioactivity	Unlikely	Possibly	Unlikely
Patient convenience	Requires longer time between administration and imaging (6–24 h)	More rapid exam: imaging within 30 min of administration	Imaging typically 24 h after administration
Radiation dose to thyroid	Depends on method of production[a]	Low	Significant
Ability to obtain 24-h uptake	Y	N (can obtain a 20-min trapping)	Y
Risk to personnel handling patients and radionuclides	Very low	Very low	Low

[a]Although the radiation-absorbed dose to the thyroid from ^{123}I is low, the presence of contaminants of ^{124}I and ^{125}I in the preparation of ^{123}I can result in higher radiation-absorbed doses to the thyroid, and the presence of contaminants depends on the method of ^{123}I production. ^{123}I produced by the (p,5n) cyclotron method has no contaminants of ^{124}I and little contaminants of ^{125}I. ^{123}I produced by the (p,2n) cyclotron method can have significant contaminants of ^{124}I and ^{125}I

may appear on the images to be lateral to the cold or hot area. The only location in the field of view of a pinhole collimator where it can be determined that all the structures line up on the image, regardless of their depth, is at the center. Standard and marker images can usually be completed within 30–60 min.

Radiation Dosimetry

Estimates of radiation-absorbed dose for adults for ^{123}I, ^{99m}TcO$_4$, and ^{131}I are noted in Table 24.4. For standard prescribed activity for imaging, ^{131}I delivers the highest radiation-absorbed dose to the thyroid, but all three radioisotopes have reasonably low whole-body radiation-absorbed doses. As noted above and because of the radiation-absorbed dose to the thyroid, ^{131}I is infrequently used when ^{123}I or ^{99m}TcO$_4$ is available.

Terminology for Nodule Function Assessed on Thyroid Scintigraphy

The terminology for describing the function of nodules on thyroid scans can be confusing. "Cold," "hypofunctioning," and "nonfunctioning" nodules have reduced radioiodine uptake relative to adjacent normal or abnormal tissue (see Fig. 24.1). Of note, an important adjective of this definition is the use of the word "radioiodine." Hypofunctioning nodules on radioiodine scans may not be hypofunctioning on ^{99m}TcO$_4$ scans, which is discussed further in the "Discordance of ^{123}I and ^{99m}TcO$_4$ Scans" section of this chapter. Nevertheless, in a study of 2237 patients, Borner et al. [3] reported a 21 % frequency of cold nodules in patients ages 15 and 16 and a 44 % frequency in patients over age 65. Thyroid cancer was present in 11 % of cold nodules in patients ages 45–65 and evident in 25 % of patients over age 65. In a review of the literature, Ashcraft and Van Herle [4] reported that 16–21 % of cold nodules harbored a malignancy.

The designation of "indeterminate" means that there is no abnormality on scan and/or the function of a palpable nodule cannot be determined. Small hypofunctioning nodules located posteriorly in the thyroid may be obscured by radioiodine uptake in normal thyroid tissue that anteriorly overlies the small thyroid nodule. Similarly, a small hypofunctioning nodule located anteriorly in the thyroid may not be apparent if it does not significantly attenuate the radioactivity coming from the normal underlying thyroid tissue. The half value for attenuation by tissues of ^{123}I is approximately 6 cm (i.e., it would require as large as a 6-cm nodule overlying normal thyroid tissue to attenuate 50 % of the radioactivity from the underlying normal thyroid tissue). The half value for attenuation of ^{99m}TcO$_4$ is approximately 5 cm. Thus, although a nodule may be truly hypofunctioning relative to normal thyroid tissue, its "cold" appearance on the scan may not be seen at all. In this case, it would be called "indeterminate." Ashcraft and Van Herle [4] reported that 9 % of intermediate nodules harbored malignancy. Sandler et al. [5] have stated that indeterminate nodules have equivalent significance as a hypofunctioning nodule.

The terms "normo-functioning," "isofunctioning," or "warm" are more problematic because the interpreter of the thyroid scan may be using the terms in either one or two ways. The terms are frequently used interchangeably with "indeterminate"; the interpreter is stating that in the region of the palpable nodule, the function appears to be "normo-functioning," "isofunctioning," or "warm." But as already discussed above, they may in fact be hypofunctioning, and again these nodules have the equivalent clinical significance as a hypofunctioning nodule [5]. However, these terms have also been used when the interpreter can in fact determine that the nodule does have function approximately equal to normal adjacent thyroid tissue and thus has a very low likelihood of malignancy as further discussed below.

Table 24.4 Absorbed radiation dose in adults for ^{123}I, ^{99m}Tc, and ^{131}I

	^{123}I	^{99m}TcO$_4$	^{131}I
Activity administered	0.2–0.6 mCi	1–10 mCi	0.05–0.2 mCi
	(7.4–25 MBq)	(37–370 MBq)	(1.85–7.4 MBq)
Organ receiving the largest radiation-absorbed dose	Thyroid	Upper large intestine	Thyroid
Thyroid	7.7 rad/0.4 mCi[a]	0.390 rad/3 mCi	78 rad/0.1 mCi[a]
	(77 mGy/14.8 MBq)	(3.9 mGy/111 MBq)	(780 mGy/3.7 MBq)
Total body	0.014 rad/0.4 mCi[a]	0.042 rad/3 mCi	0.047 rad/0.1 mCi[a]
	(0.14 mGy/14.8 MBq)	(0.42 mGy/111 MBq)	(0.47 mGy/3.7 MBq)

[a]Thyroid uptake of 15 %

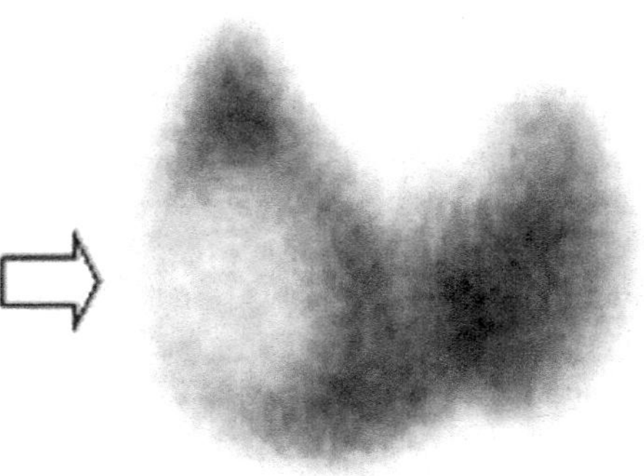

Fig. 24.1 A prominent, "cold," or hypofunctioning area in the mid-aspect of the right lobe (*white arrow*) is demonstrated (Reproduced with permission from Keystone Press, Inc. [49])

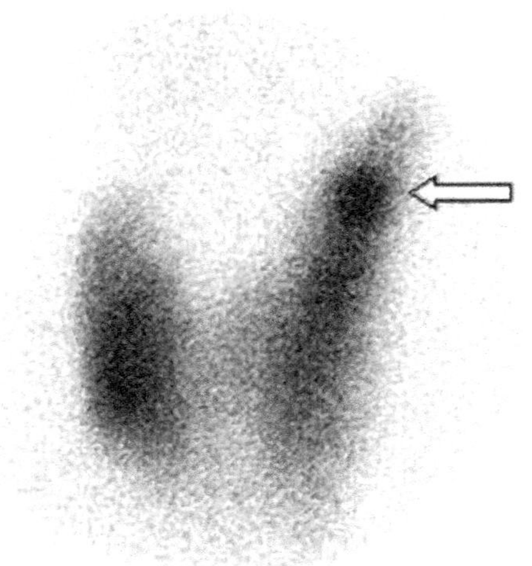

Fig. 24.2 A small area of increased activity ("warm" or hyperfunctioning) in the upper pole of the left lobe of the thyroid (*white arrow*) is demonstrated. No significant suppression of the remaining thyroid is apparent. This finding is most consistent with a hypertrophic area, which is not necessarily autonomous (not under the regulation of TSH), toxic, or suppressing the remainder of the thyroid tissue. However, the scan cannot exclude the less likely possibility that the small hyperfunctioning area is autonomous but is not yet toxic or producing enough thyroid hormone to suppress the patient's TSH and the remainder of his thyroid tissue (Reproduced with permission from Keystone Press, Inc. [49])

"Hot" or "hyperfunctioning" nodules indicate having increased radioiodine uptake relative to normal thyroid tissue with or without suppression of the remaining thyroid tissue (see Figs. 24.2, 24.3, and 24.4). "Warm" has also been used to describe the latter, which is appropriate when an area on the scan has slightly increased radioiodine uptake in association with adjacent normal thyroid tissue. Although "hot" or "hyperfunctioning" tacitly may imply that the nodules are

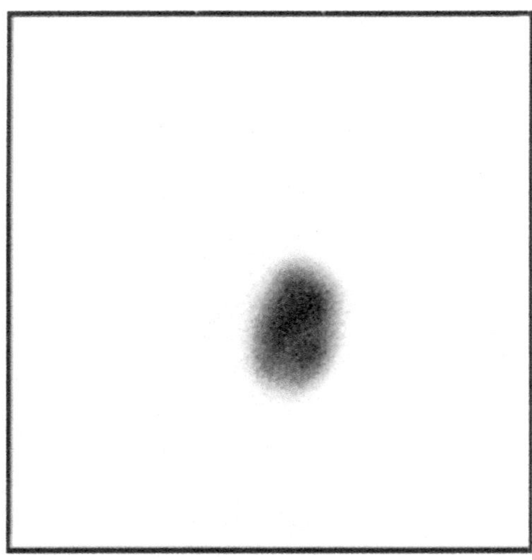

Fig. 24.3 A single, prominent "hot" or hyperfunctioning area with no visualization of the remaining thyroid. This is consistent with an autonomous and toxic hyperfunctioning thyroid nodule with suppression of the TSH and the remainder of the thyroid tissue is not visualized

autonomous, the nodule may not necessarily be autonomous. A "hot" or "hyperfunctioning" nodule may either be "hypertrophic" and under the regulation of thyrotropin (TSH) or "autonomous" and not under the regulation of TSH, and the lack of suppression of the remainder of the thyroid tissue does not necessarily differentiate whether that nodule is autonomous or not. Of course, if the rest of the thyroid tissue is suppressed, then the "hot" or "hyperfunctioning" nodule must be an "autonomous" nodule, and this situation also implies that the patient is hyperthyroid.

Hyperfunctioning Nodules and Association with Thyroid Cancer

Relative to the frequency of thyroid cancer in cold thyroid nodules, only a limited number of cases report the presence of malignancy associated with a hyperfunctioning nodule [6–40], and Schneider et al. [41] have previously reviewed the literature (see Table 24.5). Lupi et al. [31] have also described four scenarios regarding the coexistence of thyroid carcinoma and hyperfunctioning tissue, which is graphically displayed in Fig. 24.4. The thyroid cancer may be (1) in a different location than the hyperfunctioning nodule, the hyperfunctioning nodule itself being benign; (2) within a portion of the hyperfunctioning benign adenoma; (3) a true hyperfunctioning thyroid carcinoma; or (4) a large cancer mass, which despite having less radioactivity per gram of tissue than normal functioning thyroid tissue, the volume of the large cancer results in the appearance of greater "function" than the normal thyroid tissue [31]. Of course, SPECT-CT would help resolve the latter.

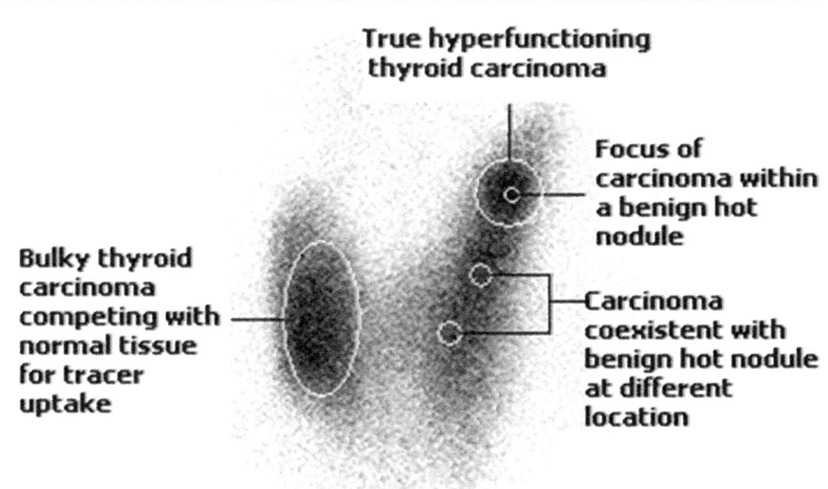

Fig. 24.4 Four scenarios regarding the coexistence of thyroid carcinoma and hyperfunctioning tissue. The thyroid cancer may be (1) in a different location than the hyperfunctioning nodule, the hyperfunctioning nodule itself being benign; (2) within a portion of the hyperfunctioning benign adenoma; (3) a true hyperfunctioning thyroid carcinoma; or (4) a large cancer mass, which despite having less radioactivity per gram of tissue than normal functioning thyroid tissue, the volume of the large cancer results in the appearance of greater "function" than the normal thyroid tissue

Lupi et al. [31] further suggested that the coexistence of carcinoma and focally hyperfunctioning tissue in the same gland in different locations is not uncommon and may approximate the incidence of thyroid carcinoma that exists in the absence of a hyperfunctioning thyroid nodule. Thyroid carcinoma coexisting and adjacent to a hyperfunctioning adenoma is reflected in the majority of reports [10, 13, 17, 18], and documented true hyperfunctioning thyroid carcinomas are extremely rare [6–8, 11–13, 15, 16, 19–21, 24, 26, 31, 33, 35, 36, 40]. Ghose et al. [11] confirmed high radioiodine uptake in a thyroid carcinoma by autoradiography, and Sandler et al. [5] showed low in vitro iodine content by X-ray fluorescence. Regarding Lupi's fourth possibility above, Lupi acknowledged that this is unlikely.

Finally, the descriptive phrase, "owl's eye," has been used to denote a cold area within an autonomous hyperfunctioning area [5]. The cold area often represents cystic degeneration and/or hemorrhage in an autonomously functioning thyroid nodule. Although sudden onset of a nodule and/or cold area may favor hemorrhage, further evaluation with ultrasound and possible fine-needle aspiration may be warranted.

Discordance of ^{123}I and $^{99m}TcO_4$ Scans

As discussed above, radioiodine scans demonstrate organification of the iodine, and $^{99m}TcO_4$ scans show only trapping of the $^{99m}TcO_4$ because $^{99m}TcO_4$ is not organified by the thyroid tissue. As a result, discordant findings on ^{123}I and $^{99m}TcO_4$ scans may be observed. Kusic et al. [42] found six different discordant ^{123}I and $^{99m}TcO_4$ patterns, and the overall incidence of discordance was 5–8 %. These patterns were: ^{99m}Tc hot/^{123}I normal, ^{99m}Tc hot/^{123}I cold, ^{99m}Tc normal/^{123}I cold, ^{99m}Tc normal/^{123}I hot, ^{99m}Tc cold/^{123}I normal, and ^{99m}Tc cold/^{123}I hot. Although Kusic reported thyroid cancer in 4 % (12 of 16) of patients, none of the patients with thyroid cancer had a discordant pattern. Ryo et al. [43] reported a discordance of 33 % (40 of 122) of patients, many of whom had a functioning or "warm" nodule on $^{99m}TcO_4$ scanning and a hypofunctioning nodule on ^{123}I scanning. Erjaec et al. [44] reported disparate results in 31 % (18 of 58) of patients; of the 18 patients, 78 % (14 of 18) had cancer. Turner and Spencer [14] reviewed the literature to approximately 1976 and determined that a discordant pattern of ^{123}I and $^{99m}TcO_4$ scanning was associated with cancer in approximately 1 of 30 studies.

Consequently, should thyroid scans be performed only with radioiodine? Or if $^{99m}TcO_4$ is used, does a radioiodine scan need to be performed in those patients with hyperfunctioning or warm nodules on the $^{99m}TcO_4$ scan? Certainly, arguments may be presented that support the recommendation that only ^{123}I scans should be performed in order to obtain the slightly superior quality of ^{123}I images, to eliminate the potential discordance of a "hot" nodule on ^{99m}Tc scan/cold nodule on subsequent ^{123}I scan, and/or to obtain a 6- or 24-h uptake.

However, counterarguments also exist for performing only a $^{99m}TcO_4$ scan or performing a $^{99m}TcO_4$ scan as the first scan, and if the nodule is "hot," then performing a subsequent ^{123}I scan [45]. $^{99m}TcO_4$ is inexpensive, provides good images, and allows imaging within 15–30 min rather than the 6–24 h required after administration of ^{123}I. With a theoretical example, the cost and convenience of using $^{99m}TcO_4$ with subsequent ^{123}I scans for further evaluation of "hot" nodules on $^{99m}TcO_4$ scans (group A) can be compared with ^{123}I scans performed in all patients (group B). If 100 ^{99m}Tc scans are performed and 5 % of these scans have "hot" nodules, then group A would have had 100 scans performed with $^{99m}TcO_4$ along with five scans performed with ^{123}I scans. Group B would have 100 scans performed with ^{123}I only. Assuming that the cost of the scans for either radioisotope are equal and assuming that the cost for the

Table 24.5 Review of the literatue of reported thyroid cancers in or adjacent to hyperfunctioning thyroid nodules

Author	Ref. #	# of cases	Age	Isotope	Dominant size (cm)	Location of cancer	Unifocal vs. multifocal tumor	Presence of (+) lymph nodes
Mulnar	[6]	1	28	^{131}I	0.5 and 0.2	Within	Multifocal	NS[a]
Becker	[7]	2	21 and 23	^{131}I	2.5 × 3.0 1.0	Both within	Both unifocal	Both no
Dische	[8]	1	NS	^{131}I	6	Within	Unifocal	NS
McLaughlin	[9]	1	56	^{131}I	4	NS	Unifocal	NS, but mets[b] to humerus
Meier	[10]	1	34	^{131}I	NS	Outside	Unifocal	NS
Ghose	[11]	1	68	^{131}I	3	Within	Unifocal	NS, but skull mets
Fujimoto	[12]	1	27	No info	2 to <3	Within	Unifocal	Yes
Hamburger	[13]	3	NS	NS	NS	1 within 2 Outside	1 unifocal 2 multifocal	NS
Turner	[14]	1	24	$^{99m}TcO_4$ and ^{131}I	NS	NS	Unifocal	NS
Livadas	[15]	2	50 and 67	Both ^{131}I	NS	1 within with vessel 1 outside	Both unifocal	NS
Raikar	[16]	1	19	^{131}I	4 × 3.5 × 4	Within	NS	No
Wolfstein	[17]	1	41	^{131}I	1.7	Outside	Multifocal	NS
Blizer	[18]	1	36	^{131}I	1.5	Outside	Unifocal	Yes
Khan	[19]	1	44	^{131}I	Micro <1	Within	Unifocal	No
Hoving	[20]	1	29	^{131}I	1 to <2	Within	Unifocal	Yes
Sander	[21]	1	67	NS	3	Within	Unifocal	Yes
Rubenfeld	[22]	1	35	^{123}I	Micro <1	Within	Unifocal	NS
De Rosa	[23]	1	25	^{131}I	1 to <2	NS	Multifocal	NS
Castelli	[24]	1	59	^{131}I	Micro <1	Within	Unifocal	NS
Das	[25]	1	NS	NS	NS	NS	NS	No
Sato	[26]	1	67	^{123}I	0.7 × 0.7 × 0.7	Within	Unifocal	Yes
Cirillo	[27]	1	17	$^{99m}TcO_4$ & ^{123}I	2 to <3	NS	Multifocal	Yes
Appetecchia	[28]	1	23	^{131}I	3 to <4	NS	Multifocal	NS
Valenti	[29]	1	34	^{131}I	1 to <2	NS	Unifocal	No info
Mircescu	[30]	1	11	$^{99m}TcO_4$ and ^{131}I	>4	NS	Unifocal	No info
Lupi	[31]	2	Case 1:46 Case 2: 55	Case 1: $^{99m}TcO_4$ Case 2: $^{99m}TcO_4$	Case 1: 4.5 Case 2: no Info	Case 1: within Case 2: within	Case 1: unifocal Case 2: unifocal	Case 1: no Case 2: no info
Logani	[32]	1	36	NS	NS	NS	Unifocal	NS
Yaturu	[33]	1	39	NS	NS	Within	Unifocal	No
Dell Erba	[34]	1	61	$^{99m}TcO_4$ and ^{131}I	3 to <4	NS	Multifocal	Yes
Pucci	[35]	1	77	^{131}I 3.7GBq	3.5	Within	Unifocal	No
Nishida	[36]	1	62	NS	NS	Within	Multifocal	No
Tfayli	[37]	1	11	NS	1 to <2	NS	Unifocal	NS
Bommireddipalli	[38]	1	63	^{123}I	3 to <4	NS	Unifocal	No
Azevedo	[39]	1	47	^{131}I	3 to <4	NS	Unifocal	NS
Hernan-Martinez	[40]	1	31	^{131}I	Micro <1	Within	Multifocal	NS

[a]*NS* not specified
[b]*Mets* metastasis

^{123}I is $150 and the cost of the $^{99m}TcO_4$ is $10, then group A would have spent $1750 (100 doses of $^{99m}TcO_4$ plus five doses of ^{123}I) vs. $15,000 (100 doses of ^{123}I) for group B. Additionally, patients in group B would have had to come to the imaging facility 200 times (e.g., for each patient, the patient would come for one visit for the oral administration of the radioiodine and one visit for imaging), whereas patients in group A would have had to come to the imaging facility for 110 visits (100 for the injection of $^{99m}TcO_4$ scan and 2 visits each for the additional five ^{123}I dosages and scans). In addition, those that argue for only a $^{99m}TcO_4$ scan might propose the following question. If only $^{99m}TcO_4$ scans are performed with no subsequent ^{123}I scan to evaluate "hot" nodules on the $^{99m}TcO_4$ scan, how many cancers would be missed? Again, a theoretical example helps put this into perspective. If (1) 1000 $^{99m}TcO_4$ scans are performed, (2) 5 % of these scans have "hot" nod-

Table 24.6 Organizational recommendations

Organization	Recommendation	Rating
NCCN [46] (page: THYR-1)	If a thyroid nodule has a low TSH, then perform radioiodine imaging. If cold, then FNA, and if hot, then evaluate and treat for thyrotoxicosis as indicated. Malignancy is rare	Category 2A (recommendation based on a low level of evidence and there is uniform NCCN consensus)
NCCN (page: THYR-2)	If FNA of a nodule shows follicular or Hürthle cell neoplasm or follicular lesion of undetermined significance (including terms of *atypia of undetermined significance*, *rule out neoplasm*, *atypical follicular lesion*, and *cellular follicular lesion*) and the TSH is low, then perform radioiodine imaging. If cold, repeat FNA, and consider surgery based on clinical grounds, concerning growth, or suspicious sonographic findings. If hot, then evaluate and treat for thyrotoxicosis as indicated. Again, malignancy is rare	Category 2A (recommendation based on a low level of evidence and there is uniform NCCN consensus)
ATA [47] (page: 1171)	If the serum TSH is subnormal, a radionuclide thyroid scan should be obtained to document whether the nodule is hyperfunctioning (i.e., tracer uptake is greater than the surrounding normal thyroid), isofunctioning or "warm" (i.e., tracer uptake is equal to the surrounding thyroid), or nonfunctioning (i.e., has uptake less than the surrounding thyroid tissue). Since hyperfunctioning nodules rarely harbor malignancy, if one is found that corresponds to the nodule in question, no cytologic evaluation is necessary	Rating A (the recommendation is based on good evidence that the service or intervention can improve important health outcomes. Evidence includes consistent results from well-designed, well-conducted studies in representative populations that directly assess effects on health outcomes)
	Measure serum TSH in the initial evaluation of a patient with a thyroid nodule. If the serum TSH is subnormal, a radionuclide thyroid scan should be performed using either ^{99m}Tc pertechnetate or ^{123}I	
European Consensus [48] (page 154)	Although the advent of thyroid US has limited the use of the thyroid scan, this test is still useful to confirm the functioning nature of a nodule when the serum thyrotropin (TSH) is low or undetectable and in patients with multinodular goiter, because it frequently demonstrates the presence of autonomous functioning nodules	

ules, (3) 10 % of these "hot nodules" are truly "cold" on ^{123}I scans, and (4) 20 % of these "cold" nodules on ^{123}I scans harbor cancer, then one thyroid cancer would be missed out of 1000 patients if only $^{99m}TcO_4$ scans had been performed initially. However, this estimate is different if one is using a $^{99m}Tc0_4$ scan when the TSH is suppressed. In this theoretical situation in which 1000 $^{99m}TcO_4$ scans are performed in *patients with suppressed TSH* and assuming (1) that 50 % (arbitrary selection) of these scans have "hot" nodules, (2) that 10 % of these "hot nodules" are truly "cold" on ^{123}I scans, and (3) that 20 % of these "cold" nodules on ^{123}I scans harbor cancer, then thyroid cancer would be missed in 10 out of 1000 (1 %) patients with suppressed TSH if only $^{99m}TcO_4$ scans had been performed initially. In summary, because of the radiation-absorbed dose to the thyroid from ^{131}I, this isotope of radioiodine is not recommended when ^{123}I and $^{99m}TcO_4$ are available. However, if thyroid scintigraphy is to be performed, then both $^{99m}TcO_4$ and ^{123}I are reasonable alternatives, each with their own strengths and weaknesses.

Utility of Thyroid Scintigraphy

Presently, the major role(s) of thyroid scintigraphy as noted by the various societies and other organizations are noted in Table 24.6, and the primary indication for thyroid scintigraphy is the evaluation of a thyroid nodule when the patient has a concomitant low TSH blood level.

Summary

Historically, thyroid scintigraphy has been a valuable imaging modality in the evaluation and characterization of the function of thyroid nodules. ^{123}I and $^{99m}TcO_4$ are the preferred radioisotopes, and the thyroid scintigraphic procedure is simple to perform. However, despite the historical utility of thyroid scintigraphy, its role in the evaluation of thyroid nodules has been significantly altered with the refinement of ultrasound (see Chap. 23) and the ease, safety, and reliability of fine-needle aspiration (see Chaps. 20 and 21). A thyroid scan may still be useful in selected patients with signs or symptoms of hyperthyroidism or suppressed TSH. Nevertheless, it is time to look for "smarter" radiolabeled molecular tracers that will help differentiate benign from malignant nodules.

References

1. Society of Nuclear Medicine Procedure Guideline for Thyroid Scintigraphy, version 2.0, approved February 7, 1999. Procedure Guidelines Manual, Society of Nuclear Medicine, 2003:29–32.
2. McKitrick WL, Park HM, Kosegi JE. Parallax error in pinhole thyroid scintigraphy: a critical consideration in the evaluation of substernal goiters. J Nucl Med. 1985;26:418–20.
3. Borner W, Lautsch M, et al. Die diagnostiche bedeutung des "kalten Knotens" im schilddrusenszintigramm. Med Welt. 1965;17:892–7.
4. Ashcraft MW, Van Herle AJ. Management of thyroid nodules. II. Scanning techniques, thyroid suppressive therapy, and fine needle aspiration. Head Neck Surg. 1981;3:296–322.

5. Sandler MP, Coleman RE, Patton JA, et al. Diagnostic nuclear medicine. 4th ed. Philadelphia: Lippincott Williams & Wilkins; 2003.
6. Mulnar GD, Childs DS, Wollner LB. Histologic evidence of malignancy in a thyroid gland bearing a "hot" nodule. J Clin Endocrinol Metab. 1958;18:1132–4.
7. Becker FO, Economou PH, Schwartz TB. The occurrence of carcinoma in "hot" thyroid nodules: report of two cases. Ann Intern Med. 1963;58:877–82.
8. Dische S. The radioisotope scan applied to the detection of carcinoma in the thyroid swellings. Cancer. 1963;17:473–9.
9. McLaughlin RP, Scholz DA, McConahey WM, et al. Metastatic thyroid carcinoma with hyperthyroidism: two cases with functioning metastatic follicular thyroid carcinoma. Mayo Clin Proc. 1970;45:328–35.
10. Meier DA, Hamburger JI. An autonomously functioning thyroid nodule, cancer, and prior radiation. Arch Surg. 1971;12:759–61.
11. Ghose MK, Genuth SM, Abellera RM, et al. Functioning primary thyroid carcinoma and metastases producing hyperthyroidism. J Clin Endocrinol Metab. 1971;33:639–46.
12. Fujimoto Y, Oka A, Nagataki S. Occurrence of papillary carcinoma in hyperfunctioning thyroid nodule report of a case. Endocrinol Japanonica. 1972;19:371–4.
13. Hamburger JI. Solitary autonomously functioning thyroid lesions. Am J Med. 1975;58:740–9.
14. Turner JW, Spencer RP. Thyroid carcinoma presenting as a pertechnetate "hot" nodule, but without I131 uptake; case report. J Nucl Med. 1976;17:22–3.
15. Livada DP, Kotoulad OB, Bouropoulos V, Sfonouris J, et al. The coexistence of thyroid malignancy with autonomous hot nodules of the thyroid. Clin Nucl Med. 1977;2:350–4.
16. Raikar UR, Ganatra RD, Raghunath B. Thyroid carcinoma in an autonomously functioning nodule. J Nucl Med. 1977;18:1001–2.
17. Wolfstein RS. Enigma of the "hyperfunctioning" thyroid carcinoma resolved? J Nucl Med. 1978;19:441–2.
18. Blitzer A. Thyroid carcinoma in a patient with a coexisting functional adenoma. Otolaryngol Head and Neck Surg. 1979;87:768–74.
19. Khan O, Ell PJ, Maclennan KA, Kurtz A, et al. Thyroid carcinoma in an autonomously hyperfunctioning thyroid nodule. Postgrad Med J. 1981;57:172–5.
20. Hoving J, Piers DA, Vermey A, et al. Carcinoma in hyperfunctioning thyroid nodule in recurrent hyperthyroidism. Eur J Nucl Med. 1981;6:131–2.
21. Sandler MP, Fellmeth B, Salhany KE, et al. Thyroid carcinoma masquerading as a solitary benign hyperfunctioning nodule. Clin Nucl Med. 1988;13:410–5.
22. Rubenfeld S, Wheeler TM. Thyroid cancer presenting as a hot thyroid nodule: report of a case and review of the literature. Thyroidology. 1988;1:63–8.
23. DeRosa G, Testa A, Maurizi M, et al. Thyroid carcinoma mimicking a toxic adenoma. Eur J Nucl Med. 1990;17:179–84.
24. Castelli V, Moscogiuri D, Taviani AP, et al. Occurrence of papillary carcinoma in a hyperfunctioning thyroid nodule: report of a case and diagnostic considerations. Thyroidol Clin Exp. 1994;6:69–72.
25. Das AB, Alam MN, Haq SA, et al. Solitary thyroid nodule: a study of 100 cases. Bangladesh Med Res Clin Bull. 1996;22:12–8.
26. Sato Y, Sakurai A, Miyamoto T, Hiramatsu K, et al. Hyperfunctioning thyroid adenoma concomitant with papillary thyroid carcinoma, follicular thyroid adenoma and primary hyperparathyroidism. Endocr J. 1998;45:61–7.
27. Cirillo Jr RL, Pozderac RV, Caniano DA, et al. Metastatic pure papillary thyroid carcinoma presenting as a toxic hot nodule. Clin Nucl Med. 1998;23:345–9.
28. Appetecchia M, Ducci M. Hyperfunctioning differentiated thyroid carcinoma. J Endocrinol Invest. 1998;21:189–92.
29. Valenti TM, Macchia E, Pisa R, et al. Toxic adenoma and papillary thyroid carcinoma in a patient with Graves disease. J Endocrinol Invest. 1999;22:701–4.
30. Mircescu H, Parma J, Huot C, et al. Hyperfunctioning malignant thyroid nodule in an 11-y.o. J Pediatr. 2000;137:585–7.
31. Lupi A, Orsolon P, Cerisara D, Migliorati Deantoni G, Dri VA. "Hot" carcinoma of the thyroid. Minerva Endocrinol. 2002;27:53–6.
32. Logani S, Osei SY, LiVolsi VA, et al. Fine-needle aspiration of follicular variant of papillary carcinoma in a hyperfunctioning thyroid nodule. Diagn Cytopathology. 2001;25:80–1.
33. Yaturu S, Fowler MR. Differentiated thyroid carcinoma with functional autonomy. Endocr Pract. 2002;8:36–9.
34. Dell'Erba L, Gerundini P, Caputo M, et al. Association of hyperfunctioning thyroid adenoma with thyroid cancer resenting as "trapping only" nodule at 99mTcO4 – scintigraphy. J Endocr Invest. 2003;26:1124–7.
35. Pucci A, Suppo M, Lucchesi G, et al. Papillary thyroid carcinoma presenting as a solitary soft tissue arm metastasis in an elderly hyperthyroid patient. Case report and review of the literature. Virchows Arch. 2006;448:857–61.
36. Nishida A, Hirano S, Asato R, et al. Multifocal hyper functioning thyroid carcinoma without metastases. Auris Nasus Larynx. 2008;35:432–6.
37. Tfayli HM, Teot LA, Indyk JA, et al. Papillary thyroid carcinoma in an autonomous hyperfunctioning thyroid nodule: case report and review of the literature. Thyroid. 2010;20:1029–32.
38. Bommireddipalli S, Goel S, Gadiraju R, et al. Follicular variant of papillary thyroid carcinoma presenting as a toxic nodule by I-123 scintigraphy. Clin Nucl Med. 2010;35:770–5.
39. Azevedo MF, Casulari LA. Hyperfunctioning thyroid cancer: a 5 yr follow up. Arq Bras Endocrinol Metab. 2010;54:78–80.
40. Hernan-Martinez J, Uzcategui M, Corder E, et al. Hyperthyroidism, hyperfunctioning thyroid nodule, and thyroid cancer in a young female: a rare and unusual coexistence. P R Health Sci J. 2010;29:78–82.
41. Schneider MT, Glister O, Hall JP, Acio E, Kulkarni KP, Tran AT, Van Nostrand D. Thyroid cancer in functioning thyroid nodules. Presented at the 2012 ACNM Mid-Winter meeting.
42. Kusic Z, Becker DV, Saenger EL, et al. Comparison of technetium99m and iodine-123 imaging of thyroid nodules: correlation with pathologic findings. J Nucl Med. 1990;31:393–9.
43. Ryo UY, Vaidya PV, Schneider AB, et al. Thyroid imaging agents: a comparison of I-123 and Tc-99m pertechnetate. Radiology. 1983;148:819–22.
44. Erjavec M, Movrin T, Auersperg M, Golough R. Comparative accumulation of ^{99m}Tc and ^{131}I in thyroid nodules: case report. J Nucl Med. 1977;18:346–7.
45. Dos Remedios LV, Weber PM, Jasko IA. Thyroid scintiphotography in 1,000 patients: rational use of 99mTC and 131-I compounds. J Nucl Med. 1971;12:673–7.
46. Comprehensive Cancer Network (NCCN). Clinical practice guidelines in oncology. Thyroid carcinoma. Follicular Thyroid Carcinoma. V.1.2010.
47. Cooper DS, Doherty GM, Haugen BR, Kloos RT, Lee SL, Mandel SJ, Mazzaferri EL, McIver B, Pacini F, Schlumberger M, Sherman SI, Steward DL, Tuttle RM. Revised American thyroid association management guidelines for patients with thyroid nodules and differentiated thyroid cancer. Thyroid. 2009;19:1167–214.
48. Pacini F, Schlumberger M, Dralle H, Elisei R, Smit JWA, Wiersinga W, the European Thyroid Cancer Taskforce. European consensus for the management of patients with differentiated thyroid carcinoma of the follicular epithelium. Eur J Endocrinol. 2006;154:787–803.
49. Wartofsky L, Van Nostrand D, Bloom G. Thyroid cancer: a guide for patients. Baltimore: Keystone Press; 2004. p. 15–31.

^{18}F Fluorodeoxyglucose PET and Thyroid Nodules

25

Carlos Alberto Garcia

Introduction

Fluorine-18 fluorodeoxyglucose (^{18}F-FDG) positron emission tomography (PET) scan is a valuable tool in the management of patients with cancer of many different organs, and the usage is increasing. The basis of this increased usage lies within its ability to detect varying degrees of metabolic activity (glucose consumption) by different cell types, benign and malignant. The first studies to clearly demonstrate increased glucose consumption by neoplastic tumors in general were those of Warburg et al. in 1933 [1]. Adler and Bloom were the first to study thyroid nodules with ^{18}F-FDG-PET scans [2]. In 1987, Joensuu and Ahonen were the first to report ^{18}F-FDG localization of metastatic thyroid cancer [3].

Subsequently, multiple reports have documented incidentally detected thyroid lesions (ITL) on ^{18}F-FDG-PET scans in patients with no known prior history of thyroid disease [3–6]. These ITLs have also been called "incidentalomas," defined as unpalpable "nodules" detected serendipitously during a radiological investigation, and these incidentalomas may be found in up to 50 % of patients [4, 7–9]. When detected by ^{18}F-FDG-PET, these incidentalomas are a combination of metabolic and anatomic information and warrant a higher degree of suspicion than lesions detected by sonogram or CT [10–13]. The clinical meaning of the thyroid ^{18}F-FDG-PET incidentaloma may be more significant than initially assumed in the interpretation of ^{18}F-FDG-PET scans [5, 7, 14, 15]. It is hypothesized that incidental thyroid carcinomas (ITC) detected by ^{18}F-FDG-PET-CT may have more aggressive histological features than those detected by other means. Previous studies have shown that primary nonincidental carcinomas, as well as their metastases detected by ^{18}F-FDG-PET computer tomography (CT), tended to be less well differentiated, possessed more aggressive histological features, and behaved more aggressively. Again, these adverse prognostic features and aggressive histotypes may be present in the majority of patients regardless of size [16]. The objective of this chapter is to review the ^{18}F-FDG-PET and PET-CT detection of incidental uptake in the thyroid, the patterns of ^{18}F-FDG-PET uptake, the significance of the standard uptake value (SUV), and the management of ^{18}F-FDG-PET incidental thyroid lesions.

Background

In the United States, 4–7 % of adults have a palpable thyroid nodule [10], and their prevalence increases with age. At age 55, as many as 45 % of women and 32 % of men may harbor one or more thyroid nodules, many detectable by palpation, and some only detectable by ultrasonography [7]. The risk of finding cancer in a thyroid nodule identified on physical examination alone is approximately 7.6 %, and the frequency of cancer in the resulting surgically excised nodules ranges from 8 % to 17 % [17, 18]. The age-adjusted annual incidence rate of thyroid malignancy in the United States is 4.5 per 100,000 according to the Surveillance, Epidemiology, and End Results (SEER) data from 1986 to 1990 [17, 18].

Multiple imaging modalities employed in the evaluation of the thyroid gland are available such as ultrasound, CT, magnetic resonance (MR), and ^{18}F-FDG-PET scanning, and further reading is available in Chaps. 23, 43, and 45.

Incidental abnormalities of the thyroid gland are commonly encountered at a rate of 16 % on cross-sectional imaging, 27 % on ultrasonography, and in 9.4 % of carotid duplex scans [11, 19]. The role of these imaging modalities in characterizing thyroid lesions is limited, providing only

C.A. Garcia, MD (✉)
Division of Nuclear Medicine, Department of Medicine, MedStar Washington Hospital Center/Georgetown University, 110 Irving Street, NW, Suite GB-01, Washington, DC 20010, USA
e-mail: carlos.garcia@medstar.net

L. Wartofsky, D. Van Nostrand (eds.), *Thyroid Cancer*, DOI 10.1007/978-1-4939-3314-3_25

morphologic features, but inadequate information to assess the risk for containing malignancy [20]. Ultrasonography is excellent for detection and characterizations of thyroid nodule features such as microcalcifications, solid structure, hypoechogenicity, irregular margins, and/or central vascular flow, which may help determine the risk of malignancy, but there may be significant overlap in the appearance of benign and malignant lesions [21, 22]. CT scanning may also detect and demonstrate thyroid nodules, but CT detects 40 % less thyroid nodules than ultrasound examination with no reliable CT-specific features that help distinguish between benign and malignant nodules [22]. The sensitivity, specificity, and negative and positive predictive values of these modalities appear to vary greatly between institutions reflecting operator dependence [23]. In all institutions, nodule size is consistently not predictive of malignancy, and the feature with the highest sensitivity for cancer—solid composition (69–70 %)—has a positive predictive value of only 15.6–27 % [6, 24].

Unlike sonography and CT imaging, ^{18}F-FDG-PET provides information about tumor location, biologic activity, and potential for aggressive behavior in patients with thyroid incidentalomas. A hypermetabolic thyroid lesion detected by ^{18}F-FDG-PET is both a biologic and anatomic abnormality, and in most cases incidentalomas detected by CT or ultrasonography are purely physical or radiographic findings [14, 16, 22].

Patterns of ^{18}F-FDG-PET and PET-CT Uptake in the Thyroid

The normal thyroid gland typically has very low-grade or no uptake on an ^{18}F-FDG-PET scan (see Fig. 25.1), and when low-grade uptake (> background activity but <2.5 SUV) is seen, it is typically diffuse in nature. Thyroid gland activity is considered abnormal on an ^{18}F-FDG-PET when significant uptake (SUV >2.5) is seen, whether it is diffuse or focal.

Abnormal bilateral, diffuse ^{18}F-FDG activity in the thyroid (see Fig. 25.2) has been previously reported to be associated with chronic thyroiditis, nodular goiter, Graves' disease, or a normal variant. Kang et al. [22] reported that the risk of malignancy is extremely low in patients with diffuse or bilateral uptake (1.4 %). In their series of 1330 patients, 8 patients were documented to have diffuse thyroid uptake of whom 7 were noted to have chronic thyroiditis. Are et al. [14] reported that only 2 out of 162 patients with diffuse thyroid uptake harbored malignancy at a rate of 1.4 %. Chen et al. [5] described two rare cases of diffuse ^{18}F-FDG uptake in the thyroid incidentally found on ^{18}F-FDG-PET that were related to malignancy; one case harbored a papillary carcinoma associated with Hashimoto's thyroiditis, and the other case was a metastasis from lung cancer. Although the rate of malignancy is very low in a diffuse goiter, one must always consider that a diffuse ^{18}F-FDG uptake such as secondary to

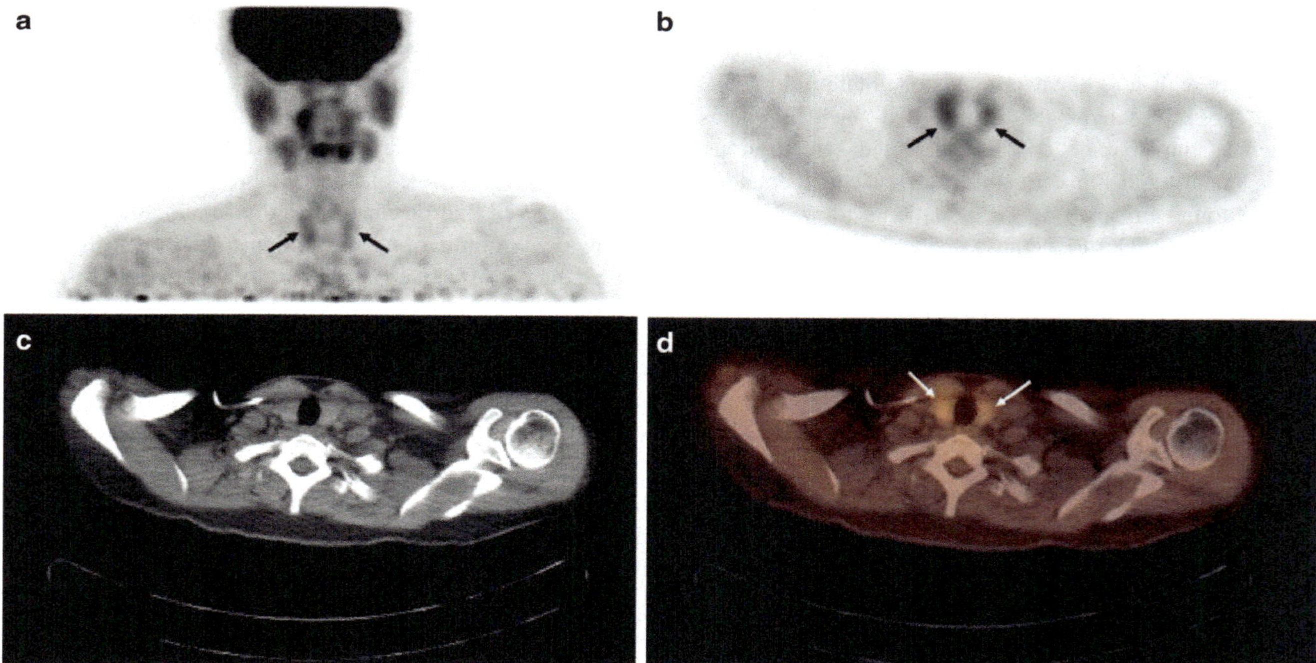

Fig. 25.1 Normal thyroid ^{18}F-FDG uptake. Faintly visualized activity may be seen throughout both thyroid lobes (arrows) with no regions of abnormal focal increased metabolic activity. (**a**) Coronal ^{18}F-FDG-PET scan. (**b**) Axial ^{18}F-FDG-PET projection. (**c**) Axial CT projection. (**d**) Fused PET-CT axial projection.

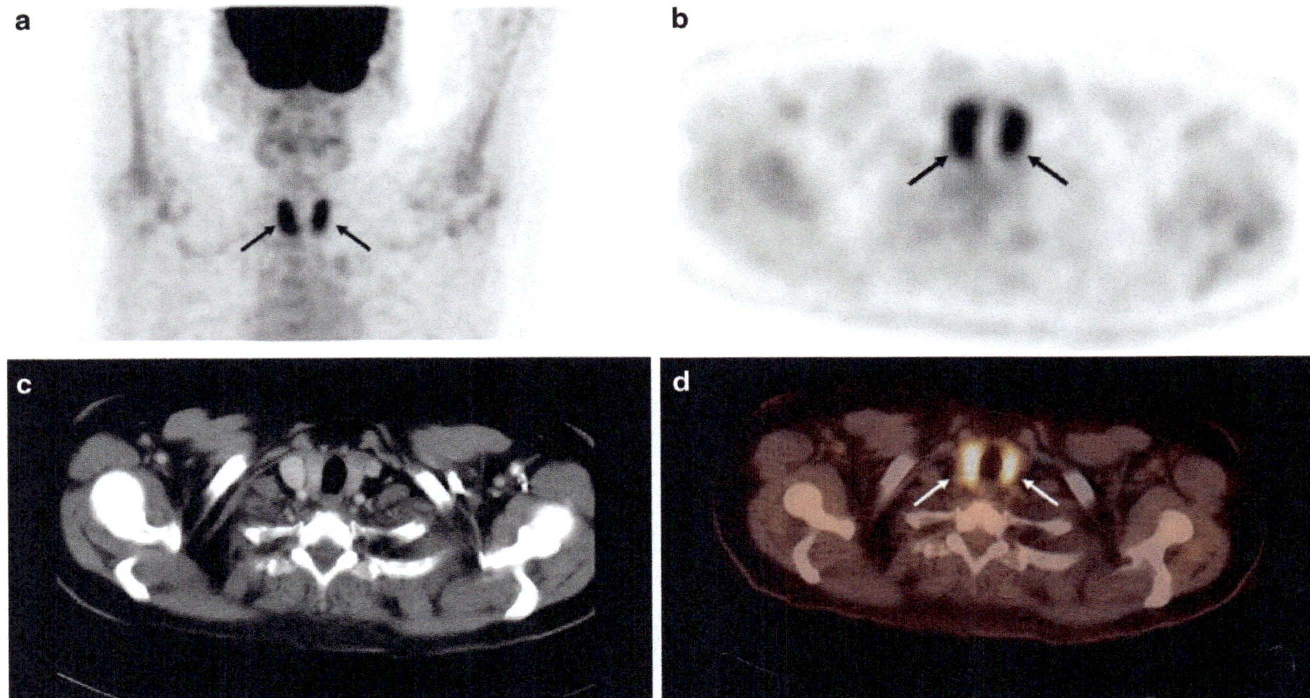

Fig. 25.2 Diffuse thyroid ^{18}F-FDG-PET uptake. Diffuse intense hypermetabolic activity seen throughout both thyroid lobes with no focal lesions (arrows). (**a**) Coronal ^{18}F-FDG-PET scan. (**b**) Axial ^{18}F-FDG-PET projection. (**c**) Axial CT projection. (**d**) Fused ^{18}F-FDG-PET-CT axial projection. This intense diffuse activity is suggestive of a thyroiditis

chronic thyroiditis could still obscure a thyroid nodule with focal ^{18}F-FDG uptake [15].

Focal thyroidal ^{18}F-FDG uptake is not likely to be misinterpreted as adjacent nodal uptake or physiological activity when concurrent CT images are used. Published reports have suggested an improvement in lesion localization, characterization of the uptake, and overall diagnostic confidence of ^{18}F-FDG-PET-CT compared with ^{18}F-FDG-PET alone (see Fig. 25.3) [25, 26].

Frequency of Cancer in ^{18}F-FDG Incidentalomas

Abnormal focal uptake of ^{18}F-FDG in the thyroid on PET or PET-CT has been reported in multiple series (see Table 25.1). From seven publications, 84,113 ^{18}F-FDG-PET scans were reviewed, and focal ^{18}F-FDG uptake was identified in the thyroid in 1514 patients, a prevalence of 1.8 %. Of the 1514 patients, 462 (31 %) patients had tissue obtained, and of these patients, 135 (29 %) had a malignancy with a range in the individual reports of 14–54 % [25–27, 30]. These numbers reflect a pattern seen throughout the literature of a low prevalence of ^{18}F-FDG-PET-positive focal lesions but a high prevalence of malignancy in patients with a histological diagnosis [14, 16, 29, 31, 32].

Of the types of malignancies found, not all focal ^{18}F-FDG uptakes found within the thyroid gland are related to a primary thyroid malignancy. This is particularly true in patients with an antecedent malignancy, such as metastatic renal cell carcinoma, squamous cell carcinoma, lymphoma, and melanoma of which have all been described presenting as incidental PET finding involving the thyroid (see Table 25.2) [28, 33]. Cancer metastasis to the thyroid gland is rare, accounting for 1.4–3 % of thyroid malignancies in most clinical series involving surgical resection or fine-needle aspiration biopsy of the thyroid. Renal cell carcinoma accounts for 48.1 % of these metastases, as demonstrated by Chung et al. in an extensive literature review of the last decade [34]. The frequency of thyroid metastases identified at autopsy is greater, ranging between 2 % and 26 %, which probably depends on the thoroughness of the pathologic examination [10, 34]. Data from autopsy series show that most metastatic disease in the thyroid originates from breast, melanoma, and lung cancers, with lung neoplasms accounting for up to 43 % of thyroid metastases [34]. This review also demonstrated that metastases of non-thyroid malignancies to the thyroid are more common in women than men and also in nodular glands. In many patients, the thyroid metastases are present when the primary cancer is initially diagnosed and can be the initial presentation of a primary malignancy [19, 21, 30, 35].

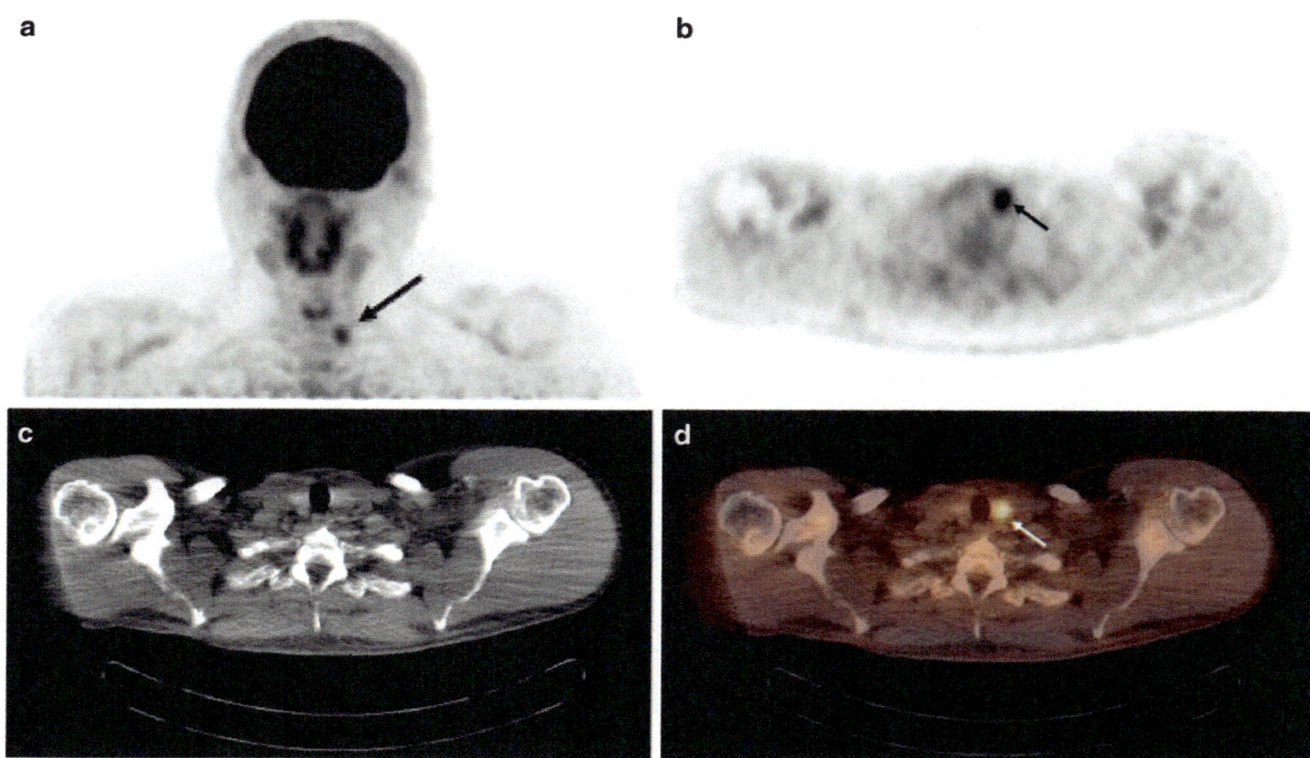

Fig. 25.3 Focal thyroid ^{18}F-FDG-PET uptake. Thyroid incidentaloma located in the mid-portion of the left thyroid lobe. (**a**) Coronal ^{18}F-FDG-PET scan (*arrow* indicates solitary nodule). (**b**) Axial FDG-PET projection. (**c**) Axial CT projection. (**d**) Fused PET-CT axial projection

Table 25.1 Incidence of malignancy in incidental thyroid lesions detected by ^{18}F-FDG-PET imaging

		Focal PET-positive findings			Biopsy-proven malignancy	
Author	Total patients	Patients	Prevalence (%)	Histological examination	Patients	Percent
Are [14]	8800	263	2.9	57	24	42
Bertagna [27]	49,519	729	1.4	211	72	34
Bogsrud [28]	7347	79	1.1	48	15	31
Chen [5]	4803	60	1.2	50	7	14
Cohen [23]	4525	102	2.3	15	7	47
Ishimori [29]	1912	29	1.5	11	6	54
Kang [22]	1330	29	2.2	15	4	27

Table 25.2 Primary tumor in incidental thyroid lesions detected by ^{18}F-FDG-PET imaging

PET-CT initial cancer indication	No. of patients	No. of patients with ^{18}F-FDG (+) ITL	^{18}F-FDG (+) ITL histology-proven thyroid cancer
Healthy subject screening	666	58	5 (8.6 %)
Breast	893	97	7 (7.2 %)
Head and neck	428	17	0
GI tract	311	25	4 (16 %)
Pulmonary	306	21	2 (9.5 %)
Gynecologic	297	31	3 (9.6 %)
Lymphoma	163	19	1 (5.2 %)
Liver and biliary tract	159	8	1 (12.5 %)
Other primary tumors	132	6	0
Unknown cancer site	24	3	0

ITL incidental thyroid lesions, *FDG* fluorodeoxyglucose

The Role of SUV in Incidental Thyroid Lesions

It is unclear whether the SUV level correlates with the likelihood of malignancy in a thyroid incidentaloma. Several authors report that elevated SUVs are associated with increased likelihood of thyroid malignancy (Table 25.3) [2]. Others suggest that the degree of ^{18}F-FDG uptake is not predictive of incidental thyroid lesion malignancy [14, 36].

Although it is not entirely clear why there are discrepancies in the literature concerning the association of SUV levels with incidental thyroid lesion malignancy, several issues may contribute to these disparate findings. The first is a variable level of mitochondrial activity causing overlap between benign and malignant lesions—the higher level of activity and higher level of ^{18}F-FDG uptake does not neces-

Table 25.3 Correlation of SUV and incidental thyroid lesions detected by ^{18}F-FDG-PET imaging

	Benign lesion SUV_{max}	Malignant lesion SUV_{max}	p-value
Adler [2]	3.0–4.3	10.8	<0.05
Kang [22]	6.5	14.2	<0.05
Mitchell [4]	1.1–3.3	6.5	<0.05
Choi [36]	6.7	10.7	<0.05
Are [14]	8.2	9.2	0.07
Bogsrud [28]	5.6	6.4	0.12
Kim [15]	3.6	3.4	0.83
Eloy [37]	3.4 ± 2.6	2.9 ± 1.6	0.63
Bae [26]	6.64 ± 4.12	3.35 ± 1.69	0.001
Shiea [17]	6.8 ± 4.6	4.6 ± 2.1	0.001
Ho [32]	8.2 ± 4.5	5.6 ± 3.2	0.048

SUVmax maximal standard uptake value

sarily imply malignancy as certain benign adenomas such as Hürthle cell adenomas may have high levels of mitochondrial activity with reported average SUVs greater than 5 [38]. A second reason for variable SUV values in benign and malignant disease may be a result of partial volume effects underestimating SUV levels as seen in some papillary thyroid carcinomas. Kresnick et al. demonstrated that 6 out of 12 patients with papillary thyroid cancer in his series had SUVs less than 5.3 [38]. Third, thyroid-stimulating hormone (TSH) stimulates ^{18}F-FDG uptake by differentiated thyroid carcinoma with resulting increase in SUV values and tumor to background ratios. Petrich et al. in a series of 30 patients demonstrated that ^{18}F-FDG-PET is more accurate under rhTSH than under suppression in both number of lesions detected and tumor/background contrast [39].

Regardless of the degree of correlation between SUV levels and the risk of thyroid carcinoma, it is clear that the presence of any ^{18}F-FDG uptake on PET scan seems to be more important in terms of clinical decision making than the actual SUV level. Considering uptake alone, it would be the pattern of activity—diffuse or focal, in the thyroid gland, which would be the most useful predictive factor in determining the likelihood of malignancy. However, as previously noted, a histological diagnosis cannot be replaced or excluded to establish the true benign or malignant nature of a thyroid lesion.

Management of ^{18}F-FDG-PET-CT Incidental Thyroid Lesions

Although numerous guidelines exist that indicate the appropriate management of palpable thyroid nodules [40, 41], there are no accepted guidelines for the increasingly common incidental PET thyroid lesion (incidentaloma) [7, 37, 42]. Some factors, such as the extent of disease of the primary malignancy and other comorbidities, may prevent further workup of these incidental abnormalities, despite their high prevalence of malignancy once tissue diagnosis has been established [14]. The literature suggests that patients with incidental thyroid abnormalities should be subjected to further investigation leading to possible operative intervention. Eloy et al. [37] proposed a multidisciplinary treatment algorithm in the absence of a consensus for these thyroid lesions, differing from the revised American Thyroid Association (ATA) Guidelines [40] and from the National Comprehensive Cancer Network (NCCN) Guidelines [41], in the management of benign or atypical cell results from thyroid nodule fine-needle aspirations (FNA) (Fig. 25.4). The ATA and NCCN guidelines suggest observation and follow-up for benign FNA results, and if nodule growth is observed, repeat FNA or consideration of surgical intervention is recommended. In this same subgroup of patients, Eloy et al. [37] suggested a hemithyroidectomy with intraoperative frozen section and completion thyroidectomy if malignant results were observed. This recommendation was based on his findings of a five-time greater risk of malignancy (27.8 % rate), within lesions incidentally found on ^{18}F-FDG-PET when compared to other nodules.

The revised ATA guidelines also state that in microcarcinomas (<1 cm), a total thyroidectomy may not be necessary. Eloy et al. articulated that if this recommendation were to be followed, three of nine PET-positive unilateral incidental thyroid carcinomas described by Law et al. [43], which in fact harbored contralateral tumors, could have possibly undergone hemithyroidectomy instead of a total thyroidectomy. The contralateral tumor foci in these patients were not detected by ^{18}F-FDG-PET or ultrasound examination, and a tumor focus would have been left behind in the contralateral lobe. Although the long-term outcome of leaving small contralateral tumor foci after hemithyroidectomy remains poorly understood, the possibility of locoregional recurrence remains.

It is important to note that not all incidental thyroid carcinomas behave in the same benign manner and that some should be managed in much the same way as clinically significant carcinomas. The true management of incidental thyroid carcinomas, particularly subcentimeter nodules, remains controversial with some investigators even advocating observation with regular ultrasound surveillance as primary treatment, even though most would perform surgical resection [44].

Summary

The current widespread usage of whole-body ^{18}F-FDG-PET and ^{18}F-FDG-PET-CT studies as a screening tool for evaluation of malignant tumors has resulted in an increase in the detection of incidentally found thyroid lesions. Multiple studies have demonstrated that the prevalence of focal

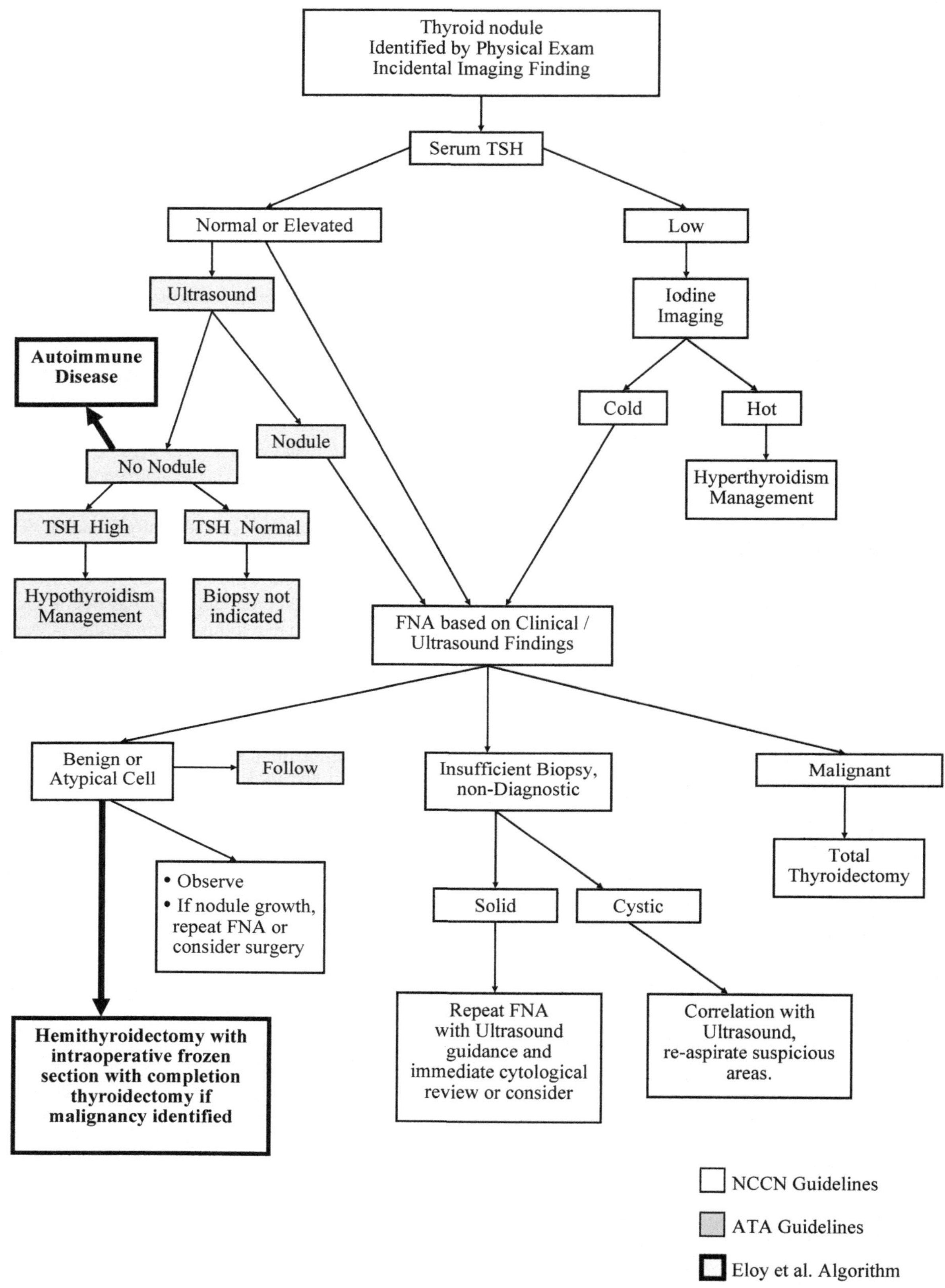

Fig. 25.4 Combined incidental thyroid nodule management algorithm. Proposed treatment algorithm for PET incidentalomas by Eloy et al. (*light gray*), Revised American Thyroid Association (ATA) Guidelines (*dark gray*), and the National Comprehensive Cancer Network (NCCN) Guidelines (*white*)

thyroid lesions incidentally found on ^{18}F-FDG-PET-CT ranges from 2.2 % to 2.9 % and that when tissue is obtained, cancer is identified from 14 % to 54 %.

When focal uptake of ^{18}F-FDG in the thyroid gland is demonstrated to be cancer, it is overwhelming thyroid cancer, but a small percentage of cancers may be secondary to metastatic lesions to the thyroid. Diffuse thyroid uptake in most instances is considered benign, but thyroiditis is possible. The role of SUV in determining malignancy is variable because papillary carcinoma may present with lower SUV levels and several benign thyroid lesions, such as Hürthle cell adenomas, may present with elevated SUV. Nevertheless, the consensus among most investigators is that histological analysis of a thyroid nodule with focal ^{18}F-FDG uptake is importance to determine benign versus malignant etiologies of thyroid incidentalomas.

References

1. Warburg O, Wind F, Neglers E. On the metabolism of tumors in the body. In: Warburg O, editor. Metabolism of tumors. London: Constable; 1930. p. 254–70.
2. Adler LP, Bloom AD. Positron emission tomography of thyroid masses. Thyroid. 1993;3:195–200.
3. Joensuu H, Ahonen A. Imaging of metastases of thyroid carcinoma with fluorine-18 fluorodeoxyglucose. J Nucl Med. 1987;28:910–4.
4. Mitchell J, Parangi S. The thyroid incidentaloma: an increasingly frequent consequence of radiologic imaging. Semin Ultrasound CT MR. 2005;26:37–46. Review.
5. Chen W, Parsons M, Torigian DA, Zhuang H, Alavi A. Evaluation of thyroid FDG uptake incidentally identified on FDG-PET/CT imaging. Nucl Med Commun. 2009;30:240–4.
6. Vriens D, de Wilt JH, van der Wilt GJ, Netea-Maier RT, Oyen WJ, de Geus-Oei LF. The role of [(18)F]-2-fluoro-2-deoxy-d-glucose-positron emission tomography in thyroid nodules with indeterminate fine-needle aspiration biopsy: systematic review and meta-analysis of the literature. Cancer. 2011;117:4582–94.
7. Gough J, Scott-Coombes D, Palazzo FF. Thyroid incidentaloma: an evidence-based assessment of management strategy. World J Surg. 2008;32:1264–8.
8. Van Den Bruel A, Maes A, De Potter T, Mortelmans L, Drijkoningen M, Van Damme B, Delaere P, Bouillon R. Clinical relevance of thyroid fluorodeoxyglucose-whole body positron emission tomography incidentaloma. J Clin Endocrinol Metab. 2002;87:1517–20.
9. Tan GH, Gharib H. Thyroid incidentalomas: management approaches to nonpalpable nodules discovered incidentally on thyroid imaging. Ann Intern Med. 1997;126:226–31.
10. Brander A, Viikinkoski P, Nickels J, Kivisaari L. Thyroid gland: US screening in a random adult population. Radiology. 1991;181:683–7.
11. Youserm DM, Huang T, Loevner LA, Langlotz CP. Clinical and economic impact of incidental thyroid lesions found with CT and MR. Am J Neuroradiol. 1997;18:1423–8.
12. Nishimori H, Tabah R, Hickeson M, How J. Incidental thyroid "PETomas": clinical significance and novel description of the self-resolving variant of focal thyroid uptake. Can J Surg. 2011;54:83–8.
13. Pak K, Kim SJ, Kim IJ, et al. The role of 18F-fluorodeoxyglucose positron emission tomography in differentiated thyroid cancer before surgery. Endocr Relat Cancer. 2013;20:R203–13.
14. Are C, Hsu JF, Schoder H, et al. FDG-PET detected thyroid incidentalomas: need for further investigation? Ann Surg Oncol. 2007;14:239–47.
15. Kim TY, Kim WB, Ryu JS, Gong G, Hong SJ, Shong YK. 18F-fluorodeoxyglucose uptake in thyroid from positron emission tomogram (PET) for evaluation in cancer patients: high prevalence of malignancy in thyroid PET incidentaloma. Laryngoscope. 2005;115:1074–8.
16. Are C, Hsu JF, Ghossein RA, et al. Histological aggressiveness of fluorodeoxyglucose positron-emission tomogram (FDG-PET)-detected incidental thyroid carcinomas. Ann Surg Oncol. 2007;14:3210–5.
17. Shiea P, Cardarellib R, Sprawlsb K, Fuldab KG, Taur A. Systematic review: prevalence of malignant incidental thyroid nodules identified on fluorine-18 fluorodeoxyglucose positron emission tomography. Nucl Med Commun. 2009;30:742–8.
18. Mazzaferri EL. Current concepts: management of a solitary thyroid nodule. N Engl J Med. 1993;328:553–9.
19. Steele SR, Martin MJ, Mullenix PS, et al. The significance of incidental thyroid abnormalities identified during carotid duplex ultrasonography. Arch Surg. 2005;140:981–5.
20. Shetty SK, Maher MM, Hahn PF, et al. Significance of incidental thyroid lesions detected on CT: correlation among CT, sonography, and pathology. AJR. 2006;187:1349–56.
21. Yi JG, Marom EM, Munden RF, Truong MT, Macapinlac HA, Gladish GW, Sabloff BS, Podoloff DA. Focal uptake of fluorodeoxyglucose by the thyroid in patients undergoing initial disease staging with combined PET/CT for non–small cell lung cancer. Radiology. 2005;236:271–5.
22. Kang KW, Kim SK, Kang HS, et al. Prevalence and risk of cancer of focal thyroid incidentalomas identified by 18F-Fluorodeoxyglucose positron emission tomography for metastasis evaluation and cancer screening in healthy subjects. J Clin Endocrinol Metab. 2003;88:4100–4.
23. Cohen MS, Arslan N, Dehdashti F, Doherty G, Lairmore TC, Brunt M, Moley JF. Risk of malignancy in thyroid incidentalomas identified by fluorodeoxyglucose-positron emission tomography. Surgery. 2001;130:941–6.
24. Frates MC, Benson CB, Charboneau JW, et al. Management of thyroid nodules detected at US, Society of Radiologists in Ultrasound consensus conference statement. Ultrasound Q. 2006;22:231–8.
25. Even-Sapir E, Lerman H, Gutman M, Lievshitz G, Zuriel L, Polliack A, et al. The presentation of malignant tumours and premalignant lesions incidentally found on PET-CT. Eur J Nucl Med Mol Imaging. 2006;33:541–52.
26. Bae JS, Chae BJ, Park WC, Kim JS, Kim SH, Jung SS, Song BJ. Incidental thyroid lesions detected by FDG-PET/CT: prevalence and risk of thyroid cancer. World J Surg Oncol. 2009;7:63.
27. Bertagna F, Treglia G, Piccardo A, et al. F18-FDG-PET/CT thyroid incidentalomas: a wide retrospective analysis in three Italian centres on the significance of focal uptake and SUV value. Endocrine. 2013;43:678–85.
28. Bogsrud TV, Karantanis D, Nathan MA, et al. The value of quantifying 18F-FDG uptake in thyroid nodules found incidentally on whole-body PET-CT. Nucl Med Commun. 2007;28:373–81.
29. Ishimori T, Patel PV, Wahl RL. Detection of unexpected additional primary malignancies with PET/CT. J Nucl Med. 2005; 46:752–7.
30. Nakhjavani MK, Gharib H, Goellner JR, van Heerden JA. Metastasis to the thyroid gland: a report of 43 cases. Cancer. 1997;79:574–8.
31. Katz SC, Shaha A. PET-associated incidental neoplasms of the thyroid. J Am Coll Surg. 2008;207:259–64.
32. Ho TY, Liou MJ, Lin KJ, Yen TC. Prevalence and significance of thyroid uptake detected by (18)F-FDG PET. Endocrine. 2011;40:297–302.

33. Basu S, Alavi A. Metastatic malignant melanoma to the thyroid gland detected by FDG-PET imaging. Clin Nucl Med. 2007;32:388–9.
34. Chung AY, Tran TB, Brumund KT, Weisman RA, Bouvet M. Metastases to the thyroid: a review of the literature from the last decade. Thyroid. 2012;22:258–68.
35. Singh R, Lehl SS, Sachdev A, Handa U, D'Cruz S, Bhalla A. Metastasis to thyroid from lung carcinoma. Indian J Chest Dis Allied Sci. 2003;45:203–4.
36. Choi JY, Lee KS, Kwon OJ, et al. Improved detection of second primary cancer using integrated [18F] fluorodeoxyglucose positron emission tomography and computed tomography for initial tumor staging. J Clin Oncol. 2005;23:7654–9.
37. Eloy JA, Brett EM, Fatterpekar GM, Kostakoglu L, Som PM, Desai SC, Genden EM. The significance and management of incidental [18F]fluorodeoxyglucose–positron-emission tomography uptake in the thyroid gland in patients with cancer. AJNR Am J Neuroradiol. 2009;30:1431–4.
38. Kresnik E, Gallowitsch HJ, Mikosch P, et al. Fluorine-18-fluorodeoxyglusocse positron emission tomography in the preoperative assessment of thyroid nodules in an endemic goiter area. Surgery. 2003;133:294–9.
39. Petrich T, Borner AR, Otto D, et al. Influence of rhTSH on [(18)F] fluorodeoxyglucose uptake by differentiated thyroid carcinoma. Eur J Nucl Med Mol Imaging. 2002;29:641–7.
40. Cooper DS, Doherty GM, Haugen BR, Kloos RT, Lee SL, Mandel SJ, Mazzaferri EL, McIver B, Pacini F, Schlumberger M, Sherman SI, Steward DL, Tuttle RM, The American Thyroid Association (ATA) Guidelines Taskforce on Thyroid Nodules and Differentiated Thyroid Cancer. Revised American Thyroid Association management guidelines for patients with thyroid nodules and differentiated thyroid cancer. Thyroid. 2009;19(11):1167.
41. National Comprehensive Cancer Network (NCCN) Guidelines in oncology. Thyroid Carcinoma. Version 3.2013.
42. Deandreis D, Al Ghuzlan A, Auperin A, Vielh P, Caillou B, Chami L. Is 18F-fluorodeoxyglucose-PET/CT useful for presurgical characterization of thyroid nodules with indeterminate fine needle aspiration cytology? Thyroid. 2012;22:165–72.
43. Law TT, Hung-Hin Lang B. Incidental thyroid carcinoma by FDG-PET/CT: a study of clinicopathological characteristics. Ann Surg Oncol. 2011;18:472–8.
44. Ito Y, Miyauchi A, Inoue H, et al. An observational trial for papillary thyroid microcarcinoma in Japanese patients. World J Surg. 2010;34:28–35.

Thyroid Nodules and Cancer Risk: Surgical Management

26

Gerard M. Doherty

Risk of a Nodule Being Thyroid Cancer

Thyroid nodules are common, and most are not cancer. About 5 % of women and 1 % of men have palpable thyroid nodules, and smaller nodules detectable on ultrasound are far more common in the population affecting as many as 50 % or more depending on age, gender, and geography. Only about 5 % of all nodules are malignant, and so the challenge is to efficiently identify those patients with malignant nodules, and to treat them appropriately, while minimizing unnecessary intervention in the remainder [1]. Important factors that increase the risk that a thyroid nodule is malignant are listed in Table 26.1.

Management of a patient with a nodule and decision-making regarding operation requires individual assessment of risks based on history, physical examination, and the results of clinical evaluation. Most people with thyroid cancer have no risk factors based on the history, and no obvious advanced disease on examination, and so the evaluation largely depends upon the imaging and cytology results. These results and the implied risk of malignancy must then be judged through the lens of the individual patient's risk tolerance. Patient preferences after thorough counseling may include operation for low-risk lesions rather than facing a possible delay in treatment of a small cancer or an interval surveillance plan for a similar lesion in a different patient to whom the importance of the operative risk is greater [1–4].

The minority of patients who have significant risk factors in their history need special consideration. A family history of thyroid cancer is infrequent in patients with follicular cell-derived thyroid lesions; conversely, about 5 % of patients with papillary and Hürthle cell cancer have familial thyroid cancer, while follicular thyroid cancer is rarely familial. Patients with autosomal dominant disorders that cause disseminated gastrointestinal polyposis or Gardner syndrome (large and small bowel tumors, desmoid tumors, lipomas, and epidermoid cysts) and Cowden syndrome (multiple hamartomas, breast cancer, colon cancer, and nodular goiter) have an increased risk of their nodules being thyroid cancer [5, 6].

The probability of medullary thyroid cancer in a patient from a *Ret*-proto-oncogene kindred (especially if they are known to be a mutation carrier) who has a thyroid nodule is high. This familial disease occurs in three forms, all associated with specific *Ret*-proto-oncogene abnormalities:

1. Familial MTC without other endocrinopathy.
2. Familial medullary cancer with multiple endocrine neoplasia, type IIA (MENIIA), which can include MTC, hyperparathyroidism, and pheochromocytoma.
3. Familial MTC with MENIIB, which can include pheochromocytoma, marfanoid habitus, mucosal neuromas, and ganglioneuromatosis.

Direct genetic testing for RET germ line point mutations can now identify the specific genetic abnormality, which can reveal the risk of cancer as well as the likelihood of the development of some of the other features of the syndromes [7–9].

Exposure to low or moderate doses of therapeutic radiation also increases the risk that an individual nodule is thyroid cancer. There does not appear to be a threshold dose, as exposure to as little as 6 cGy of radiation appears to increase the patient's risk of thyroid cancer sixfold. An almost linear increase in cancer frequency occurs as the dose of radiation increases from 6 to 2,000 cGy. Higher doses of radiation, such as 5,000–6,000 cGy, can cause hypothyroidism, but thyroid cancer occurrence does not appear to increase appreciably, likely because the thyroid cells are destroyed [10, 11]. Age at exposure, as well as time since exposure, is important. Younger children are especially vulnerable to the

G.M. Doherty, MD, FACS (✉)
Department of Surgery, Boston Medical Center,
Boston University, 88 East Newton Street, Collamore Building
Suite 500, Boston, MA 02118, USA
e-mail: dohertyg@bu.edu

L. Wartofsky, D. Van Nostrand (eds.), *Thyroid Cancer*, DOI 10.1007/978-1-4939-3314-3_26

Table 26.1 Increased risk of thyroid cancer

Increased risk of thyroid cancer
History
Family history of thyroid cancer
Known membership in MEN-2/ret-proto-oncogene kindred
Cowden syndrome
Familial polyposis (Gardner syndrome)
Exposure to low- or moderate-dose therapeutic radiation
Repeated external radiation exposure
Nuclear fallout exposure
New thyroid nodule in young person (<20 year) or older person (>60 year)
Physical examination
Hard thyroid nodule
Thyroid nodule with adjacent lymphadenopathy
Hoarseness with vocal cord paralysis
Evaluation
Elevated TSH
Suspicious or definitive result on multimodal evaluation
Fine-needle aspiration cytology
Ultrasound
Fluorodeoxyglucose positron emission tomography

Table 26.2 Thyroid cytopathology diagnostic categories and associated risk of malignancy

Diagnostic categories	Alternate category terms	Risk of malignancy
Benign		<1 %
Follicular lesion of undetermined significance	Atypia of undetermined significance	5–10 %
	R/O neoplasm	
	Atypical follicular lesion	
	Cellular follicular lesion	
Neoplasm	Suspicious for neoplasm	20–30 %
Follicular neoplasm	Suspicious for follicular neoplasm	
Hürthle cell neoplasm	Suspicious for Hürthle cell neoplasm	
Suspicious for malignancy		50–75 %
Malignant		100 %
Nondiagnostic	Unsatisfactory	

From: Baloch et al. [15]

cancer-inducing effect of radiation exposure. In addition, there appears to be hereditary influence on the effect of exposure to low-dose therapeutic radiation or radiation fallout on the frequency of thyroid cancer [12–14].

Finally, thyroid nodules that develop in people younger than 20 or over 60 years of age are more likely to be cancerous. All of these features of the history must be considered when counseling patients regarding the optimal management of their nodule(s) and their cancer risk.

Physical examination features that can affect operative management of nodules are mainly signs of local invasion or advanced disease. Nodules associated with vocal cord paralysis and hoarseness, rapidly growing nodules, hard solitary nodules, fixed nodules, or nodules associated with palpable ipsilateral lymphadenopathy all merit operation management, regardless of the results of other evaluations.

Cytologic Diagnosis

Fine-needle aspiration (FNA) for cytological examination helps to determine the nature of a nodule. FNA requires a trained cytopathologist to interpret the aspirate. Cytological examination can help establish the risk that a thyroid nodule is thyroid cancer. The cytologic diagnosis should be reported in one of six categories, and individual institutions should ensure that their cytology assessments are consistent with this system (Table 26.2) [15]. The clinician and patient then synthesize the overall clinical situation including history and physical exam findings as well as the imaging results and cytology category to make a management plan. When there is no concordance among these findings, then resection is an appropriate option to avoid diagnostic delay, even in the setting of a benign FNA result.

Operative Approach

The minimal thyroid operation that should be done for a thyroid nodule that might be malignant is an ipsilateral total thyroid lobectomy and isthmusectomy [1]. If further operation is necessary, it is less likely to be in the area of prior resection; thus, there should be no appreciable increased risk of complications, such as hypoparathyroidism or recurrent laryngeal nerve injury. It is more difficult to completely remove the remaining thyroid gland after partial thyroid lobectomy because the remaining thyroid tissue is often adherent to the surrounding tissue.

The easiest time to conduct a total thyroidectomy is during the initial operation. Therefore, if it can be known that there is thyroid cancer present during the diagnostic procedure for a thyroid nodule, then the optimal operation for thyroid cancer generally should be completed. This must be agreed upon with the patient preoperatively, so that the various contingencies can be anticipated (should a central neck dissection be included? What are the additional risks imposed by the suggested operation?). Some patients may opt to have only the diagnostic lobectomy performed at the initial anesthetic, no matter what information is available intraoperatively, so that they can more actively participate in the decision-making.

Before thyroidectomy, ultrasonography of the neck is recommended to evaluate both the thyroid and cervical lymph nodes [1]. During the initial thyroid operation, the surgeon should also carefully identify and palpate the lymph nodes adjacent to the thyroid tumor and medial to the carotid sheath. If there are abnormal lymph nodes, then intraoperative pathology assessment may demonstrate thyroid cancer, allowing for the definitive operation. The preoperative ultrasound may provide targets for intraoperative assessment or for preoperative cytology sampling.

Intraoperative pathology assessment of the primary thyroid lesion by frozen section examination is unfortunately not very effective in differentiating between benign or malignant follicular and Hürthle cell neoplasms [16]. Since these are also the most difficult to definitively assess by preoperative cytology, they represent a continuing challenge. Intraoperative frozen section evaluation of the thyroid nodule may be used on a routine or selective basis, or not at all in various institutions, but for any of these strategies, it is imperfect.

New approaches using molecular assessment of fine-needle aspiration samples promise to clarify these situations for at least some patients with follicular lesions, allowing either definitive operation for molecularly diagnosed cancer or deferral of operation for lesions highly likely to be benign based upon the molecular profile. Development of optimal strategies for using this information is ongoing, but the promise of decreasing the number of diagnostic thyroid operations necessary seems excellent.

References

1. Haugen BR, Alexander EK, Bible KC, Doherty GM, Mandel SJ, Nikiforov Y, Pacini F, Randolph G, Sawka A, Shepard D, Sosa J, Tuttle RM, Wartofsky L. 2015 American Thyroid Association Management Guidelines for adult patients with thyroid nodules and differentiated thyroid cancer. Available online at Thyroid 25: DOI:10.1089/thy.2015.0020; print version in Thyroid 26:1–133, 2016.
2. Alexander EK, Heering JP, Benson CB, et al. Assessment of nondiagnostic ultrasound-guided fine needle aspirations of thyroid nodules. J Clin Endocrinol Metab. 2002;87(11):4924–7.
3. Haymart MR, Repplinger DJ, Leverson GE, et al. Higher serum thyroid stimulating hormone level in thyroid nodule patients is associated with greater risks of differentiated thyroid cancer and advanced tumor stage. J Clin Endocrinol Metab. 2008;93(3):809–14.
4. Rago T, Di Coscio G, Basolo F, et al. Combined clinical, thyroid ultrasound and cytological features help to predict thyroid malignancy in follicular and Hupsilonrthle cell thyroid lesions: results from a series of 505 consecutive patients. Clin Endocrinol (Oxf). 2007;66(1):13–20.
5. Vriens MR, Suh I, Moses W, Kebebew E. Clinical features and genetic predisposition to hereditary nonmedullary thyroid cancer. Thyroid. 2009;19(12):1343–9.
6. Khan A, Smellie J, Nutting C, Harrington K, Newbold K. Familial nonmedullary thyroid cancer: a review of the genetics. Thyroid. 2010;20(7):795–801.
7. Fialkowski EA, Moley JF, Fialkowski EA, Moley JF. Current approaches to medullary thyroid carcinoma, sporadic and familial. J Surg Oncol. 2006;94(8):737–47.
8. Yip L, Cote GJ, Shapiro SE, et al. Multiple endocrine neoplasia type 2: evaluation of the genotype-phenotype relationship. Arch Surg. 2003;138(4):409–16. discussion 416.
9. Kloos RT, Eng C, Evans DB, et al. Medullary thyroid cancer: management guidelines of the American Thyroid Association. Thyroid. 2009;19(6):565–612.
10. Williams D. Radiation carcinogenesis: lessons from Chernobyl. Oncogene. 2008;27 Suppl 2:S9–18.
11. Hundahl SA. Perspective: National Cancer Institute summary report about estimated exposures and thyroid doses received from iodine 131 in fallout after Nevada atmospheric nuclear bomb tests. CA Cancer J Clin. 1998;48(5):285–98.
12. Sinnott B, Ron E, Schneider AB. Exposing the thyroid to radiation: a review of its current extent, risks, and implications. Endocr Rev. 2010;31(5):756–73.
13. Naing S, Collins BJ, Schneider AB. Clinical behavior of radiation-induced thyroid cancer: factors related to recurrence. Thyroid. 2009;19(5):479–85.
14. Mihailescu DV, Schneider AB. Size, number, and distribution of thyroid nodules and the risk of malignancy in radiation-exposed patients who underwent surgery. J Clin Endocrinol Metab. 2008;93(6):2188–93.
15. Baloch ZW, LiVolsi VA, Asa SL, et al. Diagnostic terminology and morphologic criteria for cytologic diagnosis of thyroid lesions: a synopsis of the National Cancer Institute Thyroid Fine-Needle Aspiration State of the Science Conference. Diagn Cytopathol. 2008;36(6):425–37.
16. Udelsman R, Westra WH, Donovan PI, Sohn TA, Cameron JL. Randomized prospective evaluation of frozen-section analysis for follicular neoplasms of the thyroid. Ann Surg. 2001;233(5):716–22.

27 Thyroid Nodules in Children and Cancer Risk

Andrew J. Bauer

Introduction

Thyroid nodules are diagnosed less frequently in children and adolescents when compared to adults. However, similar to adults, the incidence of both thyroid nodules and thyroid cancer in pediatric patients has increased over the last several decades. The reason for the increase is not entirely clear but is likely related to a combination of several factors, to include an increase in incidentally discovered thyroid nodules found during non-thyroid-related head and neck imaging (ultrasound (US), CT, and MRI), increased use of radiological surveillance for children at risk of developing thyroid malignancy (i.e., survivors of primary malignancy exposed to radiation therapy), and variety of additional factors with unknown but confounding impact such as the presence of autoimmune thyroid disease, the degree of iodine sufficiency, and exposure to medical and environmental ionizing radiation. In adult patients, there is controversy whether the increasing incidence of thyroid cancer is related to the identification of subclinical disease [1–3]. This same concern is relevant to the pediatric age as well, however, because of a fivefold risk of malignancy for a nodule discovered in a child or adolescent when compared to an adult patient (25 % vs 5 %, respectively) [4, 5]. Thorough evaluation of the nodule found in a child or adolescent should be based on individual risk factors and ultrasound features rather than on the method of discovery.

These considerations highlight the importance of establishing appropriate clinical expertise and resources in order to perform accurate evaluation and management.

A.J. Bauer, MD (✉)
Division of Endocrinology and Diabetes, Department of Pediatrics, The Children's Hospital of Philadelphia, The Perelman School of Medicine, The University of Pennsylvania, 34th Street and Civic Center Boulevard Suite 11 NW 30, Philadelphia, PA 19014, USA
e-mail: bauera@chop.edu

Prevalence and Presentation of Thyroid Nodules

Estimates suggest that approximately 1.5 % of pediatric-aged patients have a thyroid nodule(s) discoverable by routine physical exam [6, 7] and up to 18 % of pediatric-aged patients may have a thyroid lesion found by radiological exam [8]. In general, these observations follow the same pattern as in adults, with a higher prevalence based on the method of discovery and advancing age. In adults, by age 25–30 years, up to 20 % of patients can be found to have a thyroid lesion by US, and by 70 years of age, up to 50 % [9]. The data in children are less robust, but current estimates predict that for every 1 year of advancing age, there may be as high as a 9 % increased risk of finding a thyroid abnormality by radiological exam. Risk factors associated with a higher incidence of thyroid nodules include female gender, postpubertal age, personal or family history of thyroid disease, and history of exposure to radiation.

There is considerable debate, and variation in practice, in regard to the routine use of ultrasound screening for patients at increased risk of developing thyroid nodules and thyroid cancer. The most notable patient groups include survivors of non-thyroid malignancy, patients with autoimmune thyroid disease (Hashimoto's and Graves' disease) [10, 11], and patients with genetic syndromes with increased predisposition to developing thyroid disease (see "Pathogenesis") [12–18]. Those in favor of routine screening base their decision on the increased risk of thyroid malignancy within these subpopulations [10, 19, 20]. Those against routine screening raise concern over the potential increased number of procedures that will be performed for the detection of a small number of clinically significant thyroid malignancies [21]. For patients with autoimmune thyroid disease, the risk of developing a thyroid malignancy appears to be generally low and the heterogeneous echotexture on US suggests that routine screening will result in an excess of procedures for a low yield of finding a malignancy. In contrast, US surveillance

L. Wartofsky, D. Van Nostrand (eds.), *Thyroid Cancer*, DOI 10.1007/978-1-4939-3314-3_27

may be appropriate for patients with a history of radiation exposure, the most important known predisposing risk factor for developing differentiated thyroid cancer. This is most evident in survivors of non-thyroid childhood malignancies exposed to therapeutic radiation therapy who show a 27-fold increase in the likelihood of developing thyroid nodules and a 10–18-fold increased incidence of developing thyroid carcinoma [20]. For this latter group, the causal inference between radiation exposure, the increased prevalence of developing thyroid nodules, and the increased risk of subsequently developing differentiated thyroid cancer suggests that routine screening within this population is warranted.

Table 27.1 Risk factors for the development of thyroid nodules and/or thyroid cancer in children and adolescents

Exposure to radiation
Adolescent female
Family history of thyroid nodules or thyroid cancer (isolated or syndrome)
Personal history of thyroid disease
Iodine deficiency

Pathogenesis

Multiple factors are associated with an increased risk of developing a nodule and/or thyroid cancer in pediatric-aged patients (Table 27.1): iodine deficiency [22]; selenium deficiency [23]; a family history of thyroid nodules and thyroid cancer [24–33]; a personal history of thyroid disease, both congenital and acquired [10, 11]; genetic syndromes, i.e., PTEN hamartoma tumor syndrome [34], DICER1 syndrome [35], familial adenomatous polyposis [36–38]; Cowden [14, 39, 40], McCune-Albright [17], and Carney complex syndromes [15]; and previous history of exposure to radiation, either related to medical evaluation [41], treatment (i.e., Hodgkin's lymphoma) [19, 20, 42–53] or environmental exposure [54–59].

Alterations of thyrotropin (TSH) levels and the TSH-receptor pathway are additional etiologies of thyroid nodular disease. Hyperthyrotropinemia is positively correlated with iodine deficiency [60] and may be a contributor to altered thyrocyte growth and goiter, nodule formation, and, potentially, thyroid tumorigenesis [61]. The mechanism of goitrogenesis and nodulogenesis is complex, and multiple confounding variables are likely associated with the clinical course, to include genetic predisposition [62]; obesity and insulin resistance [63]; exposure to dietary or environmental goitrogens, such as hydrogen cyanide from tobacco smoke or dietary sources such as cassava root [64, 65]; the relationship between micronutrient deficiencies and autoimmunity (i.e., zinc) [66]; and exposure to ionizing radiation [67]. Somatic mutations in the TSH receptor (*TSHR*) and *GNAS* genes are also associated with the formation of functional ("hot") thyroid nodules which can be associated with subclinical or overt hyperthyroidism [68].

While all of these factors may increase the likelihood of developing a nodule, the reason for the increased risk that a nodule may harbor malignancy within the pediatric population is not fully understood. Activation of the *RAS-RAF-MEK-ERK* signaling pathway is commonly found and appears to play a critical role, in thyroid tumorigenesis in adults as well as children [4, 5, 69–71]. In contrast to adults, however, where a mutation in *BRAF* is the most common identifiable genetic abnormality, and is associated with invasive and non-RAI avid disease, BRAF mutations are similarly common, but they do not appear to predict more aggressive disease [72, 73, 74–77]. In early reports, *BRAF* mutations were detected in less than 5 % of the pediatric tumors [70, 78]; however, in more recent reports up to 30–35 % of pediatric PTC harbor a *BRAF* mutation [72, 73]. *RET/PTC* rearrangements are also common in pediatrics, do correlated with tumor invasiveness [79], and *RET/PTC* has been identified in nonmalignant as well as malignant thyroid tumors [80, 81]. Additional thyroid oncogenes and gene fusions have also been found in pediatric thyroid cancer and it is conceivable that the presence of these molecular alterations in the growth-promoting microenvironment of childhood may result in increased susceptibility for malignant transformation and, ultimately, the increased incidence of malignancy that is observed in thyroid nodules in pediatric-aged patients. This potential explanation, while unproven, is supported by reports showing increased expression of insulin-like growth factor-1 (IGF-1), it's receptor IGF-1-R [82], and nuclear Ki-67, a marker of cell proliferation, in thyroid tumors from pediatric-aged patients [83].

The higher thyroid cell proliferation index [83] as well as an increased expression of the sodium-iodide symporter (NIS) [84] may explain why children are at increased risk of developing thyroid nodules and thyroid cancer after exposure to either radiation from medical evaluation and/or treatment or environmental radioiodine [41]. Survivors of childhood cancer who received head and neck irradiation during treatment of Hodgkin's or non-Hodgkin's lymphoma, as well CNS tumors, have the greatest risk of developing thyroid nodules and thyroid cancer [85, 86]. The risk of radiation-induced thyroid cancer is linear between 0.1 and 15 Gray (Gy), with an estimated relative risk of 1.3 per Gy over this range and a peak relative risk of approximately 14.6-fold (95 % CI, 6.8–31.5) after exposure to a maximum of 20 Gy [51, 85]. The risk decreases as the dose exceeds 20 Gy as higher doses induce a killing and sclerosing effect [51, 85, 87]. Age at the time of exposure, female gender, and time since exposure increase the excess absolute risk [85], and the younger the age at the time of exposure, the shorter the latency to develop a thyroid malignancy [87]. Within the pediatric oncology community, radiation-sparing protocols have been implemented, but there are a significant number of patients previously treated who require lifelong surveillance as the latency to develop thyroid cancer spans over three to four decades of life [51, 85, 87].

The Chernobyl accident provides the most powerful reminder of the interaction of iodine deficiency and the increased incidence of thyroid malignancy when persons are exposed to internal ionizing radiation [88, 89] (see Chap. 7). Perhaps the most notable lesson to remember from this unfortunate accident is that the thoughtful and purposeful public distribution plan of cold iodine to a population exposed to internal ionizing radiation can effectively prevent the risk of developing radiation-induced thyroid malignancy [90].

Differential Diagnosis

The differential diagnosis of an anterior, midline, and/or thyroid neck mass in a child or adolescent is listed in Table 27.2. For lesions that are extrathyroidal, the differential is similar to adults; however, the prevalence of congenital, nonmalignant malformations is greater in the pediatric-aged group [91, 92]. The most common extrathyroidal lesions include thyroglossal duct cysts [93] and cervical thymic tissue [91]. Branchial cleft cysts are typically located in the lateral neck, although, with abscess formation, they may extend medially and even extend into the thyroid [92].

For intrathyroidal lesions, the differential is divided between benign and malignant lesions. While there is a fivefold increased risk that a thyroid nodule will be malignant when found in a child or adolescent compared to an adult, the majority of lesions will be benign, either a colloid cyst or a follicular adenoma [5, 94]. Hyperfunctioning or autonomously functioning nodules occur within the pediatric age, with symptoms ranging from subacute to overt hyperthyroidism [95]. In the adolescent age group, there is often a discrepancy between symptoms and the degree of thyroid function abnormalities with patients complaining of fairly disruptive symptoms, such as anxiousness, difficulty concentrating, and difficulty sleeping, despite having only high normal to mildly elevated T4 and T3. In these cases, TSH may be suppressed or be in the low-normal range. US imaging typically reveals increased intranodular flow and radionucleotide uptake and scan showing increased uptake within the nodule.

Table 27.2 Differential diagnosis of a thyroid nodule in the pediatric-aged group

Anterior-midline
Thyroglossal duct cyst
Cervical thymic tissue
Cervical lymphadenopathy
Intrathyroidal
Benign thyroid nodules (follicular adenoma, colloid or simple cyst, others)
Differentiated thyroid cancer
Medullary thyroid cancer
Pseudonodule associated with autoimmune thyroid disease
Intrathyroidal thymic remnant
Intrathyroidal parathyroid gland
Venous malformation
Teratoma

Ectopic intrathyroidal thymic inclusions are benign lesions that are typically limited to presentation within pediatrics. Patients typically present with an asymptomatic nodule found incidentally during head and neck radiographic imaging or during thyroid US performed for the evaluation of congenital hypothyroidism or autoimmune thyroid disease. On US, the lesions are hypoechoic, with punctuate, bright internal echoes ("spiculated"), features that may mistakenly be interpreted for microcalcifications [8, 96]. If fine needle aspiration is performed, small, round monotonous lymphoid cells will be found in the absence of thyroid follicular cells [97]. Flow cytometry of the FNA aspirate will confirm lymphoid cell lineage [97]. Because these characteristics raise concern over a thyroid malignancy or lymphoid neoplasm and surgical resection is frequently pursued, careful US interrogation of the thyroid will often reveal an unusual shape to the lesion with extension to and often beyond the edge of the thyroid gland. The extension is often in a caudal direction toward adjacent cervical thymic tissue (Fig. 27.1). On occasion, the lesions may be bilateral. These US characteristics are pathognomonic and if identified should allay the need for biopsy or surgical intervention. One must remember that the size of the thymus gland peaks during adolescence prior to undergoing involution. Close US surveillance should be pursued to ensure stability of characteristics. While the maximum length of follow-up in the literature is 34 months [98], the rarity of the lesion in adult series suggests that the ectopic, intrathyroidal thymic tissue follows an expectant timeline of involution.

The differential diagnosis of malignant lesions in the thyroid is mostly confined to primary thyroid malignancy. More than 90 % of malignant lesions are papillary thyroid cancer (PTC) and the remaining follicular thyroid cancer (FTC) [4, 5, 99–101]. Sporadic medullary thyroid cancer and dedifferentiated and anaplastic thyroid cancer are nearly exclusive to the adult population. The only exception is MEN 2B where sporadic disease is common. MEN 2B is associated with specific signs, including alacrima (inability to produce tears) and constipation (secondary to ganglioneuromatosis) as well as specific physical exam features, most notably long-narrow facies, marfanoid body habitus, and mucosal neuromas of the lips, tongue, conjunctiva, and urinary and gastrointestinal tract [102]. Thyroid nodules are typically located in the mid-lateral portion of the gland and are associated with the presence of micro- or macrocalcifications, although there do not appear to be any US features that definitively help distinguish MTC from PTC [103]. A high index of suspicion and

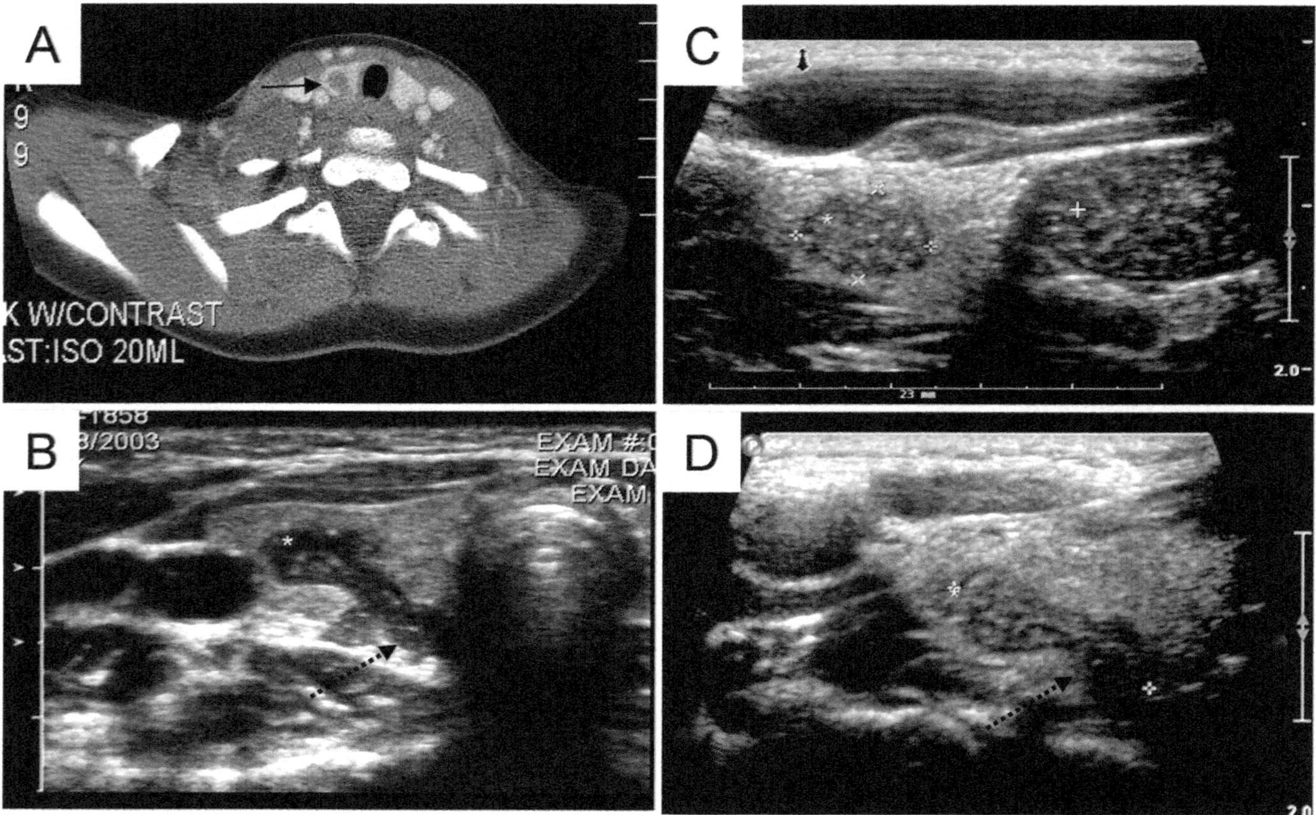

Fig. 27.1 Intrathyroidal thymic remnant. An intrathyroidal thymic remnant (*) noted on CT scan during evaluation of a 2-year-old with seizures (**a** – *arrow*). The same lesion on ultrasound showing classic features of an unusual shape: speckled intranodular echogenicity and extension beyond the edge of the thyroid (**b** – *dashed arrow*). (**c**) and (**d**) show a similar lesion in a different child with ectopic, cervical thymic tissue abutting against the thyroid (**c**) and similar classic features (**d**)

timely investigation are warranted in patients with any of the above features. Unfortunately, a great number of these patients are diagnosed late, during adolescents, and are found to have metastasis at the time of diagnosis [102, 104]. Lastly, intrathyroidal thymomas (spindle epithelial tumor with thymus-like differentiation = SETTLE tumors [105]) and teratomas [106] have been reported in the pediatric-aged group, and rarely, the thyroid gland may be a target for metastasis from non-thyroid malignancy.

Diagnostic Evaluation

History and PE

The majority of pediatric patients are asymptomatic at the time of diagnosis with the thyroid mass discovered incidentally by the patient, parent, or health-care provider. With the more frequent use of radiological imaging, there have been an increased number of patients referred for the evaluation of incidentally discovered thyroid nodules found during ultrasound, CT, or MR imaging of the head and/or neck [8]. While a significant number of these referrals are often for low-risk lesions (purely cystic), there is no evidence in the pediatric literature to suggest that an incidentally discovered thyroid nodule is associated with a lower likelihood of malignancy. However, several factors are associated with an increased risk of developing a nodule and thyroid malignancy (Table 27.1), the single greatest risk being exposure to radiation [20, 51, 85, 90]. Additional risk factors and features associated with an increased risk of malignancy include female gender starting in adolescence [107] and evidence of abnormal cervical adenopathy, particularly in cervical regions II, III, IV, and VI, noted during physical exam or US imaging [108]. In keeping with this, no matter the method of discovery, the risk of malignancy is more likely related to the patient's risk factors rather than the method of discovery and a thorough investigation to include thyroid and neck US followed by fine needle aspiration biopsy (FNA) of lesions with suspicious US features (Table 27.3) should be pursued in the majority of pediatric patients with a thyroid nodule.

Table 27.3 Ultrasound features consistent with benign or malignant thyroid nodules

Characteristics suggestive of benign lesions
Hyperechoic pattern
Completely cystic composition
Translucent halo
Homogenous internal consistency
Eggshell calcifications
Smooth, well-defined margin
Characteristics suggestive of malignant lesions
Hypoechoic pattern
Calcifications
Poorly defined, infiltrative or microlobulated margins
Increased intranodular blood flow
Solid
Taller than wide in transverse view
Abnormal cervical lymph nodes[a]

[a]See Table 27.4

Laboratory Tests

There are limited preoperative laboratory tests that will help discern the risk of malignancy in a thyroid nodule. A suppressed thyroid-stimulating hormone (TSH) may be the exception, suggestive of an autonomous functioning thyroid nodule (AFTN). These lesions are typically associated with a lower risk of malignancy; however, due to exposure of the unaffected thyroid tissue to radioiodine, and the potential risk of radiation-induced thyroid malignancy over a child's lifetime, the majority of pediatric patients with an AFTN are referred for surgical resection [109]. In adults, preoperative thyroglobulin (Tg) levels are generally viewed as unhelpful in estimating the malignancy risk; however, levels above 300–400 ng/ml may help distinguish between follicular adenoma and carcinoma [110, 111]. Similar data has not been examined in the pediatric population.

There are conflicting recommendations in regard to obtaining serum calcitonin (CT) levels in patients with sporadic thyroid nodules. The European Thyroid Cancer Taskforce recommends routine screening of serum CT [112]; however, the American Thyroid Association guidelines do not support this recommendation [113]. A baseline serum CT should be obtained in a child and adolescent with a thyroid nodule and a family history of, or consistent with, multiple endocrine neoplasia type 2 (MEN 2) [102, 104]. This is particularly important for families that carry a MEN 2A diagnosis in which the child presents for evaluation beyond the recommended age of prophylactic thyroidectomy based on the specific RET proto-oncogene mutation or for a child with a thyroid nodule and physical exam features suggestive of MEN 2B (marfanoid body habitus, mucosal neuromas) [102, 104, 113]. RET proto-oncogene mutation analysis should accompany the CT measurement if not previously obtained. For all other pediatric patients with a thyroid nodule, a random serum Ct measurement is very unlikely to be of diagnostic utility due to the low incidence of sporadic MTC. There are limited data on the normal range for basal CT levels in children [114], and, while stimulated CT levels may be of greater utility, pentagastrin is not available in the United States and calcium-stimulated levels in children have not been validated.

Radiological Imaging

There are an increasing number of radiological technologies available to perform anatomic imaging of the thyroid and neck, but when performed and read by members of a skilled radiology department, thyroid ultrasound (US) provides the most accurate information with the least cost and no exposure to radiating energy. Ultrasound can detect lesions as small as 2–3 mm in size and provides information on the size, location, echogenicity, blood flow, multiplicity, and potential involvement of regional lymph nodes which may be helpful in steering which nodules should undergo FNA [115]. There are several US features that suggest the malignant potential of a thyroid nodule (Table 27.3) but few that are specific enough to provide definitive diagnosis. The two exceptions are small, purely cystic lesions, which are almost without exception benign, and lesions with microcalcifications which carry a high correlation with malignancy (both PTC and MTC) [103, 108, 116, 117]. Combining two or more US features appears to increase the diagnostic accuracy of predicting malignancy [116, 117]. In children, the size of the nodule does not appear to be predictive of malignancy [108] and must be interpreted in relation to the age and height of the patient as the thyroid does not reach adult size until mid to late puberty [94].

A complete evaluation of a thyroid nodule includes US interrogation of the most common sites for thyroid cancer metastasis, levels VI (central neck), III, IV, and II, in decreasing order of frequency [118]. This data is extremely important, aiding in diagnosis [108] and ultimately serving as preoperative staging for patients diagnosed with thyroid cancer. Up to 70–80 % of pediatric patients with PTC will have metastasis to the regional lymph nodes at the time of presentation [119–124]. Discovery of cervical lymph nodes with features suggestive of metastatic disease (Table 27.4) increases the likelihood of malignancy for the primary thyroid lesion [108, 125].

While US is arguably the most reliable and sensitive radiological technique to inspect the thyroid and cervical region, there are several limitations worthy of mention. The first limitation is reduced sensitivity of US to identify metastasis to level VI (central neck) lymph nodes due to the thyroid gland obstructing the central neck prior to surgical resection [126].

Table 27.4 US features of lymph nodes suggestive of malignancy

Round shape
Presence of peripheral vascularity
Loss of echogenic hilum
Cystic changes
Presence of microcalcifications

While a discussion on prophylactic central neck dissection is beyond the scope of this chapter, if there is evidence of metastatic disease in the lateral neck on preoperative US, central neck dissection should be pursued. CT (without contrast) or MRI of the neck may also increase the sensitivity of identifying level VI disease preoperatively [127]. The second limitation of US is not unique to pediatrics but may be more common, the ability of US to discern reactive lymph nodes from lymph nodes harboring metastatic disease. If the US features of the lymph nodes are nondiagnostic, fine needle aspiration biopsy (FNA) should be considered prior to extending surgical dissection, especially into the lateral neck. The addition of FNA washout for the measurement of thyroglobulin (Tg) from a lymph node sample may increase the accuracy of diagnosis if cytology is equivocal [128].

The use of these additional radiological modalities, to include radionuclide scanning, positron-emission tomography (PET), and others, is rarely helpful in diagnosing thyroid malignancy, exposes the patient to additional radiation, and should be avoided. The only exception is in patients with a thyroid nodule and suppressed TSH where radionuclide scanning should be pursued to confirm the presence of an autonomously functioning thyroid nodule.

FNA

Once a nodule has been identified, the next step in the evaluation is fine needle aspiration biopsy (FNA). Conscious sedation for younger children and anxiolytics for adolescents is appropriate and recommended but must be performed in a setting with fully qualified and credentialed pediatric providers. The use of ultrasound guided FNA [129], and having cytological confirmation of sample adequacy at the bedside, decreases the rate of insufficient sampling.

In the setting of providers with experience and regular practice in performing and interpreting the FNA results, the clinical utility of FNA in pediatrics is similar to adults. A meta-analysis which included 12 studies and 475 FNAs reported a sensitivity of 94 % (95 % confidence interval [CI], 86–100 %) and specificity of 81 % (95 % CI, 72–91 %) [130]. Assuming a 20 % rate of malignancy for a nodule, the accuracy was 83.6 %, positive predictive value (PPV) 55.3 %, and negative predictive value 98.2 %. Reduced specificity and PPV were secondary to including specimens with a cytological diagnosis of follicular neoplasm (FN) as a false positive if the histological diagnosis was confirmed to be a follicular adenoma.

There are multiple classification schemes to describe the cytological results from FNA, the most basic having four categories: inadequate, benign (0–3 % risk of malignancy), indeterminate, and malignant (97–99 % risk of malignancy). The most descriptive is the Bethesda classification scheme in which the indeterminate category is divided into subcategories of malignancy risk: follicular lesion of undetermined significance (FLUS; 5–15 % risk of malignancy), follicular or Hürthle cell neoplasm (FN or HN; 15–50 % risk), or suspicious for malignancy (60–75 % risk) [131].

The indeterminate category poses the greatest clinical challenge among all age groups. Great strides have been made to identify molecular markers that reliably increase the specificity, PPV, and NPV of FNA. Unfortunately, there are exceedingly few reports which have included pediatric-aged patients in the sample population. While there are differences in the oncogene profile between children and adults with differentiated thyroid cancer (DTC) [70, 74, 77, 78], preliminary reports of oncogene analysis for pediatric patients with nodules displaying indeterminate cytology have also show improved preoperative prediction for malignancy [73, 132].

With a lack of consensus on how to incorporate the molecular markers to more accurately identify benign from malignant disease in the indeterminate classification category, in a pediatric patient with FLUS or FN, most clinicians advocate for lobectomy/isthmusectomy or total thyroidectomy (TT) based on clinical criteria such as age of the patient, nodule size and distribution (unilateral vs bilateral), ultrasound criteria, family history, and/or history of radiation exposure (environmental or medical). This approach is not ideal leading to a significant number of patients either referred for completion thyroidectomy when DTC is found on histological examination or placed at undue surgical risk when final histology reveals benign disease.

In patients with multinodular disease, FNA should be performed on as many nodules as possible [133]. At a minimum, in patients with multiple nodules, FNA should be directed toward nodules with different US features. Criteria based on the size of the nodule must be used cautiously, with size interpreted based on the age and size of the patient as well as the potential for gland atrophy from previous exposure to ionizing radiation. The lower prevalence of nodules, and the higher incidence of malignancy in a pediatric patient with a nodule, should lead to increased consideration for performing FNA. The only exception is purely cystic nodules where the likelihood of achieving an adequate sample and the risk of malignancy are both low.

Thyroid Hormone Suppression for the Treatment of Benign Thyroid Nodules

There is very little data on the use of thyroid hormone replacement or suppressive therapy in the management of thyroid nodules in children and adolescents. Data from the adult literature suggests that a L-thyroxine-induced decrease in nodule size is not predictive of benign histology; however, an increase in size while on L-thyroxine therapy warrants repeat FNA and/or resection [134–136].

There are many limitations to using L-thyroxine in the pediatric patients, most notably the difficulty in defining "low risk" for a population that in general has a fivefold increased risk of malignancy when a nodule is detected. In addition, even if one could be assured that a nodule in a child or adolescent was benign, there are no data to define the dose of L-thyroxine therapy, replacement vs suppressive dosing, or the duration of treatment. In considering a dose, one must balance the potential negative consequences of suppressive L-thyroxine therapy on cognition, behavior, and cardiovascular and bone health with the potential benefits associated with reducing the size of the nodule.

In a strictly selected population, defined by a negative history of a previous non-thyroid cancer, no history of radiation exposure, and no history of congenital thyroid disease, US features that were reassuring for a benign nodule (Table 27.3) and benign FNA, one could consider the use of L-thyroxine replacement therapy to reduce the size of the nodule for cosmetic reasons or if there were any complaints of compressive symptoms [137]. Even in this very select group of patients, there is no data to know the required length of therapy, the potential non-thyroid-related consequences of long-term therapy, or the potential change in nodule characteristics if or when L-thyroxine therapy is stopped.

The limited data on the best course of action for pediatric patients with a benign thyroid nodule is complicated by a lack of data on the natural history of disease in this age group. This is a significant shortfall in data when one considers that up to 70 % of nodules in pediatric patients are benign. In addition, the impact of surveillance, to include physical exam, serial US exams, and the potential need for repeat FNA, is unknown but of significant concern. Oftentimes, when patients and families are faced with the option of lifelong surveillance or surgical resection, they opt for surgery. Taken together, these gaps in knowledge highlight the need to collect data on the natural history of disease, the impact on quality of life imposed by surveillance compared to surgical resection, and the potential role for L-thyroxine therapy or other techniques, such as thermal or percutaneous laser ablation in an effort to change disease course in pediatric patients with benign nodules [138].

Summary: Approach to the Thyroid Nodule

Over the last two decades, the incidence of pediatric thyroid cancer has steadily increased. Thyroid cancer is now the eighth most common cancer diagnosed in 15–19-year-olds and the second most common cancer diagnosed in Caucasian girls in this same age group (see Chap. 4 for review of pediatric thyroid cancer) [139]. Concomitant with this increased rate of thyroid malignancy, there are increased numbers of children and adolescents referred for the evaluation of thyroid nodules.

Irrespective of the method of discovery, the evaluation of a thyroid nodule in a pediatric patient starts with a history and physical exam focused on review of risk factors (Table 27.1) and detection of abnormal physical exam features, to include thyroid exam, assessment for abnormal cervical adenopathy, and evidence of syndromic features: MEN 2B (marfanoid habitus, mucosal neuromas), PTEN hamartoma tumor syndrome, Carney Complex (lentigines), and others. Laboratory testing can be limited to TSH, T4, and specific genetic testing based on suspicion of a related tumor syndrome. If not completed, a thyroid US is essential, the US characteristics affording some assessment for the risk of malignancy and, more importantly, allowing for selection of which nodules should undergo FNA. US imaging of the lateral neck will aid in the ability to predict the malignant potential of the thyroid nodule and serve for preoperative staging if malignancy is found. With a lack of consensus on defining "low risk" in the pediatric-aged group, FNA of a nodule with any solid component should be considered. In patients with multiple nodules, at a minimum, all nodules with different US features should undergo FNA. The size of the nodule must be interpreted in the context of patient age and risk factors. Performing FNA in a center with expertise in pediatric sedation, thyroid FNA, and in interpretation of the cytology is critical. Figure 27.2 outlines a suggested course of action based on results within the context of the Bethesda classification scheme.

While the incidence and prevalence of thyroid nodules in pediatric patients is less than the adult population, there are significant challenges in evaluating a pediatric-aged patient discovered to have a thyroid nodule. These challenges are exaggerated by limited resources for routine and thorough evaluation as well as a lack of data and consensus for appropriate determination of risk and stratification of evaluation and treatment. Despite following a well-established adult paradigm for evaluation, many children and adolescents with indeterminate or biopsy-proven benign nodules are ultimately referred for surgical resection due to concerns over potential malignancy and the unknown impact of long-term surveillance on quality of life. This lack of reliance on preoperative screening is reflected by a 1.5-fold likelihood of an

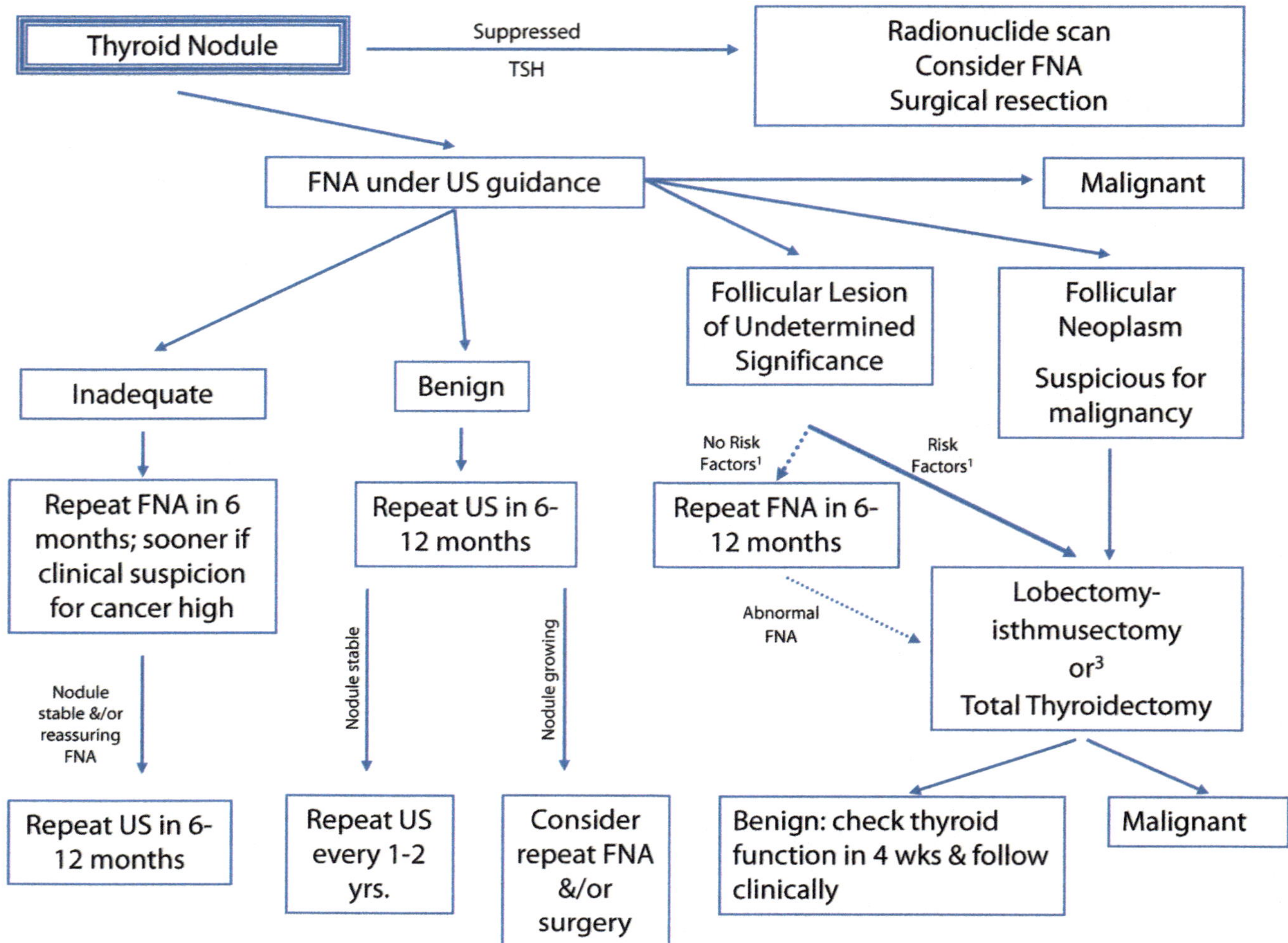

Fig. 27.2 Outline of a suggested course of action based on results within the context of the Bethesda classification scheme

adult patient being diagnosed with a thyroid malignancy after surgical resection compared to a pediatric-aged patient [5, 140, 141]. These observations emphasize the need for improved collaboration and data collection in order to more clearly define the natural history of benign nodules and to find and validate methods for assessing the risk of malignancy in indeterminate lesions within the categories of FLUS and FN [113].

References

1. Davies L, Welch HG. Increasing incidence of thyroid cancer in the United States, 1973–2002. JAMA. 2006;295:2164–7.
2. Morris LG, Myssiorek D. Improved detection does not fully explain the rising incidence of well-differentiated thyroid cancer: a population-based analysis. Am J Surg. 2010;200:454–61.
3. Wartofsky L. Increasing world incidence of thyroid cancer: increased detection or higher radiation exposure? Hormones (Athens). 2011;9:103–8.
4. Jarzab B, Handkiewicz-Junak D. Differentiated thyroid cancer in children and adults: same or distinct disease? Hormones (Athens). 2007;6:200–9.
5. Niedziela M. Pathogenesis, diagnosis and management of thyroid nodules in children. Endocr Relat Cancer. 2006;13:427–53.
6. Rallison ML, Dobyns BM, Keating Jr FR, Rall JE, Tyler FH. Thyroid nodularity in children. JAMA. 1975;233:1069–72.
7. Chiesa F, Tradati N, Calabrese L, Gibelli B, Giugliano G, Paganelli G, De Cicco C, Grana C, Tosi G, DeFiori E, Cammarano G, Cusati A, Zurrida S. Thyroid disease in northern Italian children born around the time of the Chernobyl nuclear accident. Ann Oncol. 2004;15:1842–6.
8. Avula S, Daneman A, Navarro OM, Moineddin R, Urbach S, Daneman D. Incidental thyroid abnormalities identified on neck US for non-thyroid disorders. Pediatr Radiol. 2010;40:1774–80.
9. Mazzaferri EL. Management of a solitary thyroid nodule. N Engl J Med. 1993;328:553–9.
10. Corrias A, Cassio A, Weber G, Mussa A, Wasniewska M, Rapa A, Gastaldi R, Einaudi S, Baronio F, Vigone MC, Messina MF, Bal M, Bona G, de Sanctis C. Thyroid nodules and cancer in children and adolescents affected by autoimmune thyroiditis. Arch Pediatr Adolesc Med. 2008;162:526–31.

11. Niedziela M, Korman E. Thyroid carcinoma in a fourteen-year-old boy with Graves disease. Med Pediatr Oncol. 2002;38:290–1.
12. Cetta F, Montalto G, Gori M, Curia MC, Cama A, Olschwang S. Germline mutations of the APC gene in patients with familial adenomatous polyposis-associated thyroid carcinoma: results from a European cooperative study. J Clin Endocrinol Metab. 2000;85:286–92.
13. Herraiz M, Barbesino G, Faquin W, Chan-Smutko G, Patel D, Shannon KM, Daniels GH, Chung DC. Prevalence of thyroid cancer in familial adenomatous polyposis syndrome and the role of screening ultrasound examinations. Clin Gastroenterol Hepatol. 2007;5:367–73.
14. Ngeow J, Mester J, Rybicki LA, Ni Y, Milas M, Eng C. Incidence and clinical characteristics of thyroid cancer in prospective series of individuals with Cowden and Cowden-like syndrome characterized by germline PTEN, SDH, or KLLN alterations. J Clin Endocrinol Metab. 2011;96:E2063.
15. Sandrini F, Matyakhina L, Sarlis NJ, Kirschner LS, Farmakidis C, Gimm O, Stratakis CA. Regulatory subunit type I-alpha of protein kinase A (PRKAR1A): a tumor-suppressor gene for sporadic thyroid cancer. Genes Chromosomes Cancer. 2002;35:182–92.
16. Uchino S, Noguchi S, Yamashita H, Watanabe S, Ogawa T, Tsuno A, Murakami A, Miyauchi A. Mutational analysis of the APC gene in cribriform-morula variant of papillary thyroid carcinoma. World J Surg. 2006;30:775–9.
17. Congedo V, Celi FS. Thyroid disease in patients with McCune-Albright syndrome. Pediatr Endocrinol Rev. 2007;4 Suppl 4:429–33.
18. Ishikawa Y, Sugano H, Matsumoto T, Furuichi Y, Miller RW, Goto M. Unusual features of thyroid carcinomas in Japanese patients with Werner syndrome and possible genotype-phenotype relations to cell type and race. Cancer. 1999;85:1345–52.
19. Chow EJ, Friedman DL, Stovall M, Yasui Y, Whitton JA, Robison LL, Sklar CA. Risk of thyroid dysfunction and subsequent thyroid cancer among survivors of acute lymphoblastic leukemia: a report from the Childhood Cancer Survivor Study. Pediatr Blood Cancer. 2009;53:432–7.
20. Sklar C, Whitton J, Mertens A, Stovall M, Green D, Marina N, Greffe B, Wolden S, Robison L. Abnormalities of the thyroid in survivors of Hodgkin's disease: data from the Childhood Cancer Survivor Study. J Clin Endocrinol Metab. 2000;85:3227–32.
21. Eden K, Mahon S, Helfand M. Screening high-risk populations for thyroid cancer. Med Pediatr Oncol. 2001;36:583–91.
22. Paschke R. Nodulogenesis and goitrogenesis. Ann Endocrinol. 2011;72:117–9.
23. Rasmussen LB, Schomburg L, Kohrle J, Pedersen IB, Hollenbach B, Hog A, Ovesen L, Perrild H, Laurberg P. Selenium status, thyroid volume, and multiple nodule formation in an area with mild iodine deficiency. Eur J Endocrinol. 2011;164:585–90.
24. Alsanea O, Wada N, Ain K, Wong M, Taylor K, Ituarte PH, Treseler PA, Weier HU, Freimer N, Siperstein AE, Duh QY, Takami H, Clark OH, Department of Surgery UoCSF USA. Is familial non-medullary thyroid carcinoma more aggressive than sporadic thyroid cancer? A multicenter series. Surgery. 2000;128(6):1043–51.
25. Capezzone M, Marchisotta S, Cantara S, Busonero G, Brilli L, Pazaitou-Panayiotou K, Carli AF, Caruso G, Toti P, Capitani S, Pammolli A, Pacini F. Familial non-medullary thyroid carcinoma displays the features of clinical anticipation suggestive of a distinct biological entity. Endocr Relat Cancer. 2008;15:1075–81.
26. Eng C. Familial papillary thyroid cancer – many syndromes, too many genes? J Clin Endocrinol Metab. 2000;85:1755–7.
27. Hemminki K, Eng C, Chen B. Familial risks for nonmedullary thyroid cancer. J Clin Endocrinol Metab. 2005;90:5747–53.
28. Musholt TJ, Musholt PB, Petrich T, Oetting G, Knapp WH, Klempnauer J. Familial papillary thyroid carcinoma: genetics, criteria for diagnosis, clinical features, and surgical treatment. World J Surg. 2000;24:1409–17.
29. Nose V. Familial non-medullary thyroid carcinoma: an update. Endocr Pathol. 2008;19:226–40.
30. Prazeres H, Torres J, Soares P, Sobrinho-Simoes M. The familial counterparts of follicular cell – derived thyroid tumors. Int J Surg Pathol. 2010;18:233–42.
31. Sturgeon C, Clark OH. Familial nonmedullary thyroid cancer. Thyroid. 2005;15:588–93.
32. Takami H, Ozaki O, Ito K. Familial nonmedullary thyroid cancer: an emerging entity that warrants aggressive treatment. Arch Surg. 1996;131:676.
33. Zivaljevic V, Paunovic I, Diklic A, Krgovic K, Kalezic N, Kazic M, Tatic S, Savic D, Stojanovic D, Perunovic R. The incidence of familial nonmedullary thyroid cancer in a large case series. Acta Chir Belg. 2008;108:328–32.
34. Doros D, Schultz KA, Stewart DR, et al. DICER1 related disorders. In: Pagon RA, Adam MP, Ardinger HH, et al., editors. GeneReviews® [Internet]. Seattle: University of Washington, Seattle; 1993–2016. 24 Apr 2014. http://www.ncbi.nlm.nih.gov/books/NBK196157/.
35. Eng C. PTEN hamartoma tumor syndrome (PHTS). In: Pagon RA, Adam MP, Ardinger HH, et al., editors. GeneReviews® [Internet]. Seattle: University of Washington, Seattle; 1993–2016. 29 Nov 2001 [updated 23 Jan 2014]. http://www.ncbi.nlm.nih.gov/books/NBK1488/.
36. Brasseur B, Dahan K, Beauloye V, Bletard N, Chantrain C, Dupont S, Guarin JL, Vermylen C, Brichard B. Multiple neoplasia in a 15-year-old girl with familial adenomatous polyposis. J Pediatr Hematol Oncol. 2009;31:530–2.
37. Cameselle-Teijeiro J, Menasce LP, Yap BK, Colaco RJ, Castro P, Celestino R, Ruiz-Ponte C, Soares P, Sobrinho-Simoes M. Cribriform-morular variant of papillary thyroid carcinoma: molecular characterization of a case with neuroendocrine differentiation and aggressive behavior. Am J Clin Pathol. 2009;131:134–42.
38. Harach HR, Williams GT, Williams ED. Familial adenomatous polyposis associated thyroid carcinoma: a distinct type of follicular cell neoplasm. Histopathology. 1994;25:549–61.
39. Yeager N, Klein-Szanto A, Kimura S, Di Cristofano A. Pten loss in the mouse thyroid causes goiter and follicular adenomas: insights into thyroid function and Cowden disease pathogenesis. Cancer Res. 2007;67:959–66.
40. Smith JR, Marqusee E, Webb S, Nose V, Fishman SJ, Shamberger RC, Frates MC, Huang SA. Thyroid nodules and cancer in children with PTEN hamartoma tumor syndrome. J Clin Endocrinol Metab. 2011;96:34–7.
41. Sinnott B, Ron E, Schneider AB. Exposing the thyroid to radiation: a review of its current extent, risks, and implications. Endocr Rev. 2010;31:756–73.
42. Favus MJ, Schneider AB, Stachura ME, Arnold JE, Ryo UY, Pinsky SM, Colman M, Arnold MJ, Frohman LA. Thyroid cancer occurring as a late consequence of head-and-neck irradiation. Evaluation of 1056 patients. N Engl J Med. 1976;294:1019–25.
43. von der Weid NX. Adult life after surviving lymphoma in childhood. Support Care Cancer. 2008;16:339–45.
44. Cohen A, Rovelli A, Merlo DF, van Lint MT, Lanino E, Bresters D, Ceppi M, Bocchini V, Tichelli A, Socie G. Risk for secondary thyroid carcinoma after hematopoietic stem-cell transplantation: an EBMT Late Effects Working Party Study. J Clin Oncol. 2007;25:2449–54.
45. Mazonakis M, Damilakis J, Varveris H, Fasoulaki M, Gourtsoyiannis N. Risk estimation of radiation-induced thyroid cancer from treatment of brain tumors in adults and children. Int J Oncol. 2003;22:221–5.
46. Tucker MA, Jones PH, Boice Jr JD, Robison LL, Stone BJ, Stovall M, Jenkin RD, Lubin JH, Baum ES, Siegel SE, et al. Therapeutic

radiation at a young age is linked to secondary thyroid cancer. The Late Effects Study Group. Cancer Res. 1991;51:2885–8.
47. Mehta MP, Goetowski PG, Kinsella TJ. Radiation induced thyroid neoplasms 1920 to 1987: a vanishing problem? Int J Radiat Oncol Biol Phys. 1989;16:1471–5.
48. Acharya S, Sarafoglou K, LaQuaglia M, Lindsley S, Gerald W, Wollner N, Tan C, Sklar C. Thyroid neoplasms after therapeutic radiation for malignancies during childhood or adolescence. Cancer. 2003;97:2397–403.
49. Laughton SJ, Merchant TE, Sklar CA, Kun LE, Fouladi M, Broniscer A, Morris EB, Sanders RP, Krasin MJ, Shelso J, Xiong Z, Wallace D, Gajjar A. Endocrine outcomes for children with embryonal brain tumors after risk-adapted craniospinal and conformal primary-site irradiation and high-dose chemotherapy with stem-cell rescue on the SJMB-96 trial. J Clin Oncol. 2008;26:1112–8.
50. Oberfield SE, Sklar CA. Endocrine sequelae in survivors of childhood cancer. Adolesc Med. 2002;13:161–9, viii.
51. Ronckers CM, Sigurdson AJ, Stovall M, Smith SA, Mertens AC, Liu Y, Hammond S, Land CE, Neglia JP, Donaldson SS, Meadows AT, Sklar CA, Robison LL, Inskip PD. Thyroid cancer in childhood cancer survivors: a detailed evaluation of radiation dose response and its modifiers. Radiat Res. 2006;166:618–28.
52. Sigurdson AJ, Ronckers CM, Mertens AC, Stovall M, Smith SA, Liu Y, Berkow RL, Hammond S, Neglia JP, Meadows AT, Sklar CA, Robison LL, Inskip PD. Primary thyroid cancer after a first tumour in childhood (the Childhood Cancer Survivor Study): a nested case-control study. Lancet. 2005;365:2014–23.
53. Sadetzki S, Chetrit A, Lubina A, Stovall M, Novikov I. Risk of thyroid cancer after childhood exposure to ionizing radiation for tinea capitis. J Clin Endocrinol Metab. 2006;91:4798–804.
54. Williams ED, Abrosimov A, Bogdanova T, Demidchik EP, Ito M, LiVolsi V, Lushnikov E, Rosai J, Tronko MD, Tsyb AF, Vowler SL, Thomas GA. Morphologic characteristics of Chernobyl-related childhood papillary thyroid carcinomas are independent of radiation exposure but vary with iodine intake. Thyroid. 2008;18:847–52.
55. Reiners C, Demidchik YE, Drozd VM, Biko J. Thyroid cancer in infants and adolescents after Chernobyl. Minerva Endocrinol. 2008;33:381–95.
56. Demidchik YE, Saenko VA, Yamashita S. Childhood thyroid cancer in Belarus, Russia, and Ukraine after Chernobyl and at present. Arq Bras Endocrinol Metabol. 2007;51:748–62.
57. Baverstock K. The recognition of childhood thyroid cancer as a consequence of the Chernobyl accident: an allegorical tale of our time? J R Soc Med. 2007;100:407–9.
58. Nikiforov YE. Radiation-induced thyroid cancer: what we have learned from chernobyl. Endocr Pathol. 2006;17:307–17.
59. Gilbert ES, Huang L, Bouville A, Berg CD, Ron E. Thyroid cancer rates and 131I doses from nevada atmospheric nuclear bomb tests: an update. Radiat Res. 2010;173:659–64.
60. Oberlin O, Plantin-Carrenard E, Rigal O, Wilkinson C. Goitre and iodine deficiency in Afghanistan: a case-control study. Br J Nutr. 2006;95:196–203.
61. Fiore E, Rago T, Provenzale MA, Scutari M, Ugolini C, Basolo F, Di Coscio G, Berti P, Grasso L, Elisei R, Pinchera A, Vitti P. Lower levels of TSH are associated with a lower risk of papillary thyroid cancer in patients with thyroid nodular disease: thyroid autonomy may play a protective role. Endocr Relat Cancer. 2009;16:1251–60.
62. Singer J, Eszlinger M, Wicht J, Paschke R. Evidence for a more pronounced effect of genetic predisposition than environmental factors on goitrogenesis by a case control study in an area with low normal iodine supply. Horm Metab Res. 2011;43:349–54.
63. Radetti G, Longhi S, Baiocchi M, Cassar W, Buzi F. Changes in life style improve body composition, thyroid function and structure in obese children. J Endocrinol Invest. 2011.
64. Knudsen N, Bulow I, Laurberg P, Perrild H, Ovesen L, Jorgensen T. High occurrence of thyroid multinodularity and low occurrence of subclinical hypothyroidism among tobacco smokers in a large population study. J Endocrinol. 2002;175:571–6.
65. Knudsen N, Laurberg P, Perrild H, Bulow I, Ovesen L, Jorgensen T. Risk factors for goiter and thyroid nodules. Thyroid. 2002;12:879–88.
66. Ertek S, Cicero AF, Caglar O, Erdogan G. Relationship between serum zinc levels, thyroid hormones and thyroid volume following successful iodine supplementation. Hormones (Athens). 2010;9:263–8.
67. Ron E, Brenner A. Non-malignant thyroid diseases after a wide range of radiation exposures. Radiat Res. 2010;174:877–88.
68. Lania AG, Mantovani G, Spada A. Mechanisms of disease: mutations of G proteins and G-protein-coupled receptors in endocrine diseases. Nat Clin Pract Endocrinol Metab. 2006;2:681–93.
69. Vasko V, Bauer AJ, Tuttle RM, Francis GL. Papillary and follicular thyroid cancers in children. Endocr Dev. 2007;10:140–72.
70. Penko K, Livezey J, Fenton C, Patel A, Nicholson D, Flora M, Oakley K, Tuttle RM, Francis G. BRAF mutations are uncommon in papillary thyroid cancer of young patients. Thyroid. 2005; 15:320–5.
71. Yamashita S, Saenko V. Mechanisms of disease: molecular genetics of childhood thyroid cancers. Nat Clin Pract Endocrinol Metab. 2007;3:422–9.
72. Henke LE, Perkins SM, Pfeifer JD, et al. BRAF V600E mutational status in pediatric thyroid cancer. Pediatr Blood Cancer. 2014;61(7):1168–72.
73. Prasad ML, Vyas M, Horne MJ, et al. NTRK fusion oncogenes in pediatric papillary thyroid carcinoma in northeast United States. Cancer. 2016;122(7):1097–107.
74. Smida J, Salassidis K, Hieber L, Zitzelsberger H, Kellerer AM, Demidchik EP, Negele T, Spelsberg F, Lengfelder E, Werner M, Bauchinger M. Distinct frequency of ret rearrangements in papillary thyroid carcinomas of children and adults from Belarus. Int J Cancer. 1999;80:32–8.
75. Pisarchik AV, Iarmolinskii DG, Demidchik Iu E, Ermak GZ, Kartel NA, Figge J. ret/PtC1 and ret/PTC3r1 rearrangement in thyroid cancer cells, arising in residents of Belorus in the period after the accident at the Chernobyl nuclear power plant. Genetika. 2000;36:959–64.
76. Rabes HM, Klugbauer S. Molecular genetics of childhood papillary thyroid carcinomas after irradiation: high prevalence of RET rearrangement. Recent Results Cancer Res. 1998;154:248–64.
77. Fenton CL, Lukes Y, Nicholson D, Dinauer CA, Francis GL, Tuttle RM. The ret/PTC mutations are common in sporadic papillary thyroid carcinoma of children and young adults. J Clin Endocrinol Metab. 2000;85:1170–5.
78. Kumagai A, Namba H, Saenko VA, Ashizawa K, Ohtsuru A, Ito M, Ishikawa N, Sugino K, Ito K, Jeremiah S, Thomas GA, Bogdanova TI, Tronko MD, Nagayasu T, Shibata Y, Yamashita S. Low frequency of BRAFT1796A mutations in childhood thyroid carcinomas. J Clin Endocrinol Metab. 2004;89:4280–4.
79. Basolo F, Molinaro E, Agate L, Pinchera A, Pollina L, Chiappetta G, Monaco C, Santoro M, Fusco A, Miccoli P, Elisei R, Capezzone M, Pacini F. RET protein expression has no prognostic impact on the long-term outcome of papillary thyroid carcinoma. Eur J Endocrinol. 2001;145:599–604.
80. Sadetzki S, Calderon-Margalit R, Modan B, Srivastava S, Tuttle RM. Ret/PTC activation in benign and malignant thyroid tumors arising in a population exposed to low-dose external-beam irradiation in childhood. J Clin Endocrinol Metab. 2004;89:2281–9.
81. Elisei R, Romei C, Vorontsova T, Cosci B, Veremeychik V, Kuchinskaya E, Basolo F, Demidchik EP, Miccoli P, Pinchera A, Pacini F. RET/PTC rearrangements in thyroid nodules: studies in irradiated and not irradiated, malignant and benign thyroid lesions in children and adults. J Clin Endocrinol Metab. 2001;86:3211–6.

82. Gydee H, O'Neill JT, Patel A, Bauer AJ, Tuttle RM, Francis GL. Differentiated thyroid carcinomas from children and adolescents express IGF-I and the IGF-I receptor (IGF-I-R). Cancers with the most intense IGF-I-R expression may be more aggressive. Pediatr Res. 2004;55:709–15.
83. Saad AG, Kumar S, Ron E, Lubin JH, Stanek J, Bove KE, Nikiforov YE. Proliferative activity of human thyroid cells in various age groups and its correlation with the risk of thyroid cancer after radiation exposure. J Clin Endocrinol Metab. 2006;91:2672–7.
84. Faggiano A, Coulot J, Bellon N, Talbot M, Caillou B, Ricard M, Bidart JM, Schlumberger M. Age-dependent variation of follicular size and expression of iodine transporters in human thyroid tissue. J Nucl Med. 2004;45:232–7.
85. Bhatti P, Veiga LH, Ronckers CM, Sigurdson AJ, Stovall M, Smith SA, Weathers R, Leisenring W, Mertens AC, Hammond S, Friedman DL, Neglia JP, Meadows AT, Donaldson SS, Sklar CA, Robison LL, Inskip PD. Risk of second primary thyroid cancer after radiotherapy for a childhood cancer in a large cohort study: an update from the childhood cancer survivor study. Radiat Res. 2010;174:741–52.
86. Friedman DL, Whitton J, Leisenring W, Mertens AC, Hammond S, Stovall M, Donaldson SS, Meadows AT, Robison LL, Neglia JP. Subsequent neoplasms in 5-year survivors of childhood cancer: the Childhood Cancer Survivor Study. J Natl Cancer Inst. 2010;102:1083–95.
87. Ron E, Lubin JH, Shore RE, Mabuchi K, Modan B, Pottern LM, Schneider AB, Tucker MA, Boice Jr JD. Thyroid cancer after exposure to external radiation: a pooled analysis of seven studies. Radiat Res. 1995;141:259–77.
88. Nesterenko AV, Nesterenko VB. 14. Protective measures for activities in Chernobyl's radioactively contaminated territories. Ann N Y Acad Sci. 2009;1181:311–7.
89. Nesterenko AV, Nesterenko VB, Yablokov AV. Introduction: the difficult truth about Chernobyl. Ann N Y Acad Sci. 2009;1181:1–3.
90. Cardis E, Kesminiene A, Ivanov V, Malakhova I, Shibata Y, Khrouch V, Drozdovitch V, Maceika E, Zvonova I, Vlassov O, Bouville A, Goulko G, Hoshi M, Abrosimov A, Anoshko J, Astakhova L, Chekin S, Demidchik E, Galanti R, Ito M, Korobova E, Lushnikov E, Maksioutov M, Masyakin V, Nerovnia A, Parshin V, Parshkov E, Piliptsevich N, Pinchera A, Polyakov S, Shabeka N, Suonio E, Tenet V, Tsyb A, Yamashita S, Williams D. Risk of thyroid cancer after exposure to 131I in childhood. J Natl Cancer Inst. 2005;97:724–32.
91. Cigliano B, Baltogiannis N, De Marco M, Faviou E, Antoniou D, De Luca U, Soutis M, Settimi A. Cervical thymic cysts. Pediatr Surg Int. 2007;23:1219–25.
92. Friedman ER, John SD. Imaging of pediatric neck masses. Radiol Clin North Am. 2011;49:617–32, v.
93. Acierno SP, Waldhausen JH. Congenital cervical cysts, sinuses and fistulae. Otolaryngol Clin North Am. 2007;40:161–76, vii–viii.
94. Babcock DS. Thyroid disease in the pediatric patient: emphasizing imaging with sonography. Pediatr Radiol. 2006;36:299–308; quiz 372–293.
95. Niedziela M, Breborowicz D, Trejster E, Korman E. Hot nodules in children and adolescents in western Poland from 1996 to 2000: clinical analysis of 31 patients. J Pediatr Endocrinol Metab. 2002;15:823–30.
96. Megremis S, Stiakaki E, Tritou I, Bonapart IE, Tsilimigaki A. Ectopic intrathyroidal thymus misdiagnosed as a thyroid nodule: sonographic appearance. J Clin Ultrasound. 2008;36:443–7.
97. Aguayo-Figueroa L, Golightly MG, Hu Y, Cohen HL, Wilson TA. Cytology and flow cytometry to identify ectopic thymic tissue masquerading as a thyroid nodule in two children. Thyroid. 2009;19:403–6.
98. Segni M, di Nardo R, Pucarelli I, Biffoni M. Ectopic intrathyroidal thymus in children: a long-term follow-up study. Horm Res Paediatr. 2010;75:258–63.
99. Handkiewicz-Junak D, Wloch J, Czarniecka A, Roskosz J, Prokurat A, Pomorski L, Krajewska J, Kropinska A, Kukulska A, Jarzab B. Completion total thyroidectomy in children with differentiated thyroid cancer. Endokrynol Pol. 2006;57:356–61.
100. Harness JK, Thompson NW, McLeod MK, Pasieka JL, Fukuuchi A. Differentiated thyroid carcinoma in children and adolescents. World J Surg. 1992;16:547–53; discussion 553–44.
101. Schlumberger M, Travagli JP, Lemerle J, Parmentier C. Differentiated thyroid carcinoma in childhood. Experience at Institute Gustave-Roussy, Villejuif. Acta Otorhinolaryngol Belg. 1987;41:804–8.
102. Waguespack SG, Rich TA, Perrier ND, Jimenez C, Cote GJ. Management of medullary thyroid carcinoma and MEN2 syndromes in childhood. Nat Rev Endocrinol. 2011;7:596–607.
103. Lee S, Shin JH, Han BK, Ko EY. Medullary thyroid carcinoma: comparison with papillary thyroid carcinoma and application of current sonographic criteria. AJR. 2010;194:1090–4.
104. Kloos RT, Eng C, Evans DB, Francis GL, Gagel RF, Gharib H, Moley JF, Pacini F, Ringel MD, Schlumberger M, Wells Jr SA. Medullary thyroid cancer: management guidelines of the American Thyroid Association. Thyroid. 2009;19:565–612.
105. Casco F, Illanes Moreno M, Gonzalez Campora R, Moreno A, Galera Ruiz H. Spindle epithelial tumor with thymuslike differentiation in a 2-year-old boy: a case report. Anal Quant Cytol Histol/ Int Acad Cytol Am Soc Cytol. 2010;32:53–7.
106. Martino F, Avila LF, Encinas JL, Luis AL, Olivares P, Lassaletta L, Nistal M, Tovar JA. Teratomas of the neck and mediastinum in children. Pediatr Surg Int. 2006;22:627–34.
107. Wu X, Groves FD, McLaughlin CC, Jemal A, Martin J, Chen VW. Cancer incidence patterns among adolescents and young adults in the United States. Cancer Causes Control. 2005;16:309–20.
108. Corrias A, Mussa A, Baronio F, Arrigo T, Salerno M, Segni M, Vigone MC, Gastaldi R, Zirilli G, Tuli G, Beccaria L, Iughetti L, Einaudi S, Weber G, De Luca F, Cassio A. Diagnostic features of thyroid nodules in pediatrics. Arch Pediatr Adolesc Med. 2010;164:714–9.
109. Tfayli HM, Teot LA, Indyk JA, Witchel SF. Papillary thyroid carcinoma in an autonomous hyperfunctioning thyroid nodule: case report and review of the literature. Thyroid. 2010;20:1029–32.
110. Besic N, Sesek M, Peric B, Zgajnar J, Hocevar M. Predictive factors of carcinoma in 327 patients with follicular neoplasm of the thyroid. Med Sci Monit. 2008;14:CR459–67.
111. Petric R, Perhavec A, Gazic B, Besic N. Preoperative serum thyroglobulin concentration is an independent predictive factor of malignancy in follicular neoplasms of the thyroid gland. J Surg Oncol. 2011.
112. Pacini F, Schlumberger M, Dralle H, Elisei R, Smit JW, Wiersinga W. European consensus for the management of patients with differentiated thyroid carcinoma of the follicular epithelium. Eur J Endocrinol. 2006;154:787–803.
113. Francis GL, Waguespack SG, Bauer AJ, et al. Management guidelines for children with thyroid nodules and differentiated thyroid cancer: American Thyroid Association Guidelines Task Force. Thyroid. 2015;25(7):716–59.
114. Verga U, Morpurgo PS, Vaghi I, Radetti G, Beck-Peccoz P. Normal range of calcitonin in children measured by a chemiluminescent two-site immunometric assay. Horm Res. 2006;66:17–20.
115. Ahn SS, Kim EK, Kang DR, Lim SK, Kwak JY, Kim MJ. Biopsy of thyroid nodules: comparison of three sets of guidelines. AJR. 2010;194:31–7.
116. Lyshchik A, Drozd V, Demidchik Y, Reiners C. Diagnosis of thyroid cancer in children: value of gray-scale and power doppler US. Radiology. 2005;235:604–13.

117. Saavedra J, Deladoey J, Saint-Vil D, Boivin Y, Alos N, Deal C, Van Vliet G, Huot C. Is ultrasonography useful in predicting thyroid cancer in children with thyroid nodules and apparently benign cytopathologic features? Horm Res Paediatr. 2011;75:269–75.
118. Carty SE, Cooper DS, Doherty GM, Duh QY, Kloos RT, Mandel SJ, Randolph GW, Stack Jr BC, Steward DL, Terris DJ, Thompson GB, Tufano RP, Tuttle RM, Udelsman R. Consensus statement on the terminology and classification of central neck dissection for thyroid cancer. Thyroid. 2009;19:1153–8.
119. Demidchik YE, Demidchik EP, Reiners C, Biko J, Mine M, Saenko VA, Yamashita S. Comprehensive clinical assessment of 740 cases of surgically treated thyroid cancer in children of Belarus. Ann Surg. 2006;243:525–32.
120. Handkiewicz-Junak D, Wloch J, Roskosz J, Krajewska J, Kropinska A, Pomorski L, Kukulska A, Prokurat A, Wygoda Z, Jarzab B. Total thyroidectomy and adjuvant radioiodine treatment independently decrease locoregional recurrence risk in childhood and adolescent differentiated thyroid cancer. J Nucl Med. 2007;48:879–88.
121. Hay ID, Gonzalez-Losada T, Reinalda MS, Honetschlager JA, Richards ML, Thompson GB. Long-term outcome in 215 children and adolescents with papillary thyroid cancer treated during 1940 through 2008. World J Surg. 2010;34:1192–202.
122. Jarzab B, Handkiewicz Junak D, Wloch J, Kalemba B, Roskosz J, Kukulska A, Puch Z. Multivariate analysis of prognostic factors for differentiated thyroid carcinoma in children. Eur J Nucl Med. 2000;27:833–41.
123. O'Gorman CS, Hamilton J, Rachmiel M, Gupta A, Ngan BY, Daneman D. Thyroid cancer in childhood: a retrospective review of childhood course. Thyroid. 2010;20:375–80.
124. Spinelli C, Bertocchini A, Antonelli A, Miccoli P. Surgical therapy of the thyroid papillary carcinoma in children: experience with 56 patients < or =16 years old. J Pediatr Surg. 2004;39:1500–5.
125. Frates MC, Benson CB, Charboneau JW, Cibas ES, Clark OH, Coleman BG, Cronan JJ, Doubilet PM, Evans DB, Goellner JR, Hay ID, Hertzberg BS, Intenzo CM, Jeffrey RB, Langer JE, Larsen PR, Mandel SJ, Middleton WD, Reading CC, Sherman SI, Tessler FN. Management of thyroid nodules detected at US: Society of Radiologists in Ultrasound consensus conference statement. Ultrasound Q. 2006;22:231–8; discussion 239–40.
126. Park JS, Son KR, Na DG, Kim E, Kim S. Performance of preoperative sonographic staging of papillary thyroid carcinoma based on the sixth edition of the AJCC/UICC TNM classification system. AJR. 2009;192:66–72.
127. Choi JS, Kim J, Kwak JY, Kim MJ, Chang HS, Kim EK. Preoperative staging of papillary thyroid carcinoma: comparison of ultrasound imaging and CT. AJR. 2009;193:871–8.
128. Bournaud C, Charrie A, Nozieres C, Chikh K, Lapras V, Denier ML, Paulin C, Decaussin-Petrucci M, Peix JL, Lifante JC, Cornu C, Giraud C, Orgiazzi J, Borson-Chazot F. Thyroglobulin measurement in fine-needle aspirates of lymph nodes in patients with differentiated thyroid cancer: a simple definition of the threshold value, with emphasis on potential pitfalls of the method. Clin Chem Lab Med. 2010;48:1171–7.
129. Izquierdo R, Shankar R, Kort K, Khurana K. Ultrasound-guided fine-needle aspiration in the management of thyroid nodules in children and adolescents. Thyroid. 2009;19:703.
130. Stevens C, Lee JK, Sadatsafavi M, Blair GK. Pediatric thyroid fine-needle aspiration cytology: a meta-analysis. J Pediatr Surg. 2009;44:2184–91.
131. Cibas ES, Ali SZ. The Bethesda system for reporting thyroid cytopathology. Am J Clin Pathol. 2009;132:658–65.
132. Ballester LY, Sarabia SF, Sayeed H, et al. Integrating molecular testing in the diagnosis and management of children with thyroid lesions. Pediatr Dev Pathol. 2016;19(2):94–100.
133. Frates MC, Benson CB, Doubilet PM, Kunreuther E, Contreras M, Cibas ES, Orcutt J, Moore Jr FD, Larsen PR, Marqusee E, Alexander EK. Prevalence and distribution of carcinoma in patients with solitary and multiple thyroid nodules on sonography. J Clin Endocrinol Metab. 2006;91:3411–7.
134. Castro MR, Caraballo PJ, Morris JC. Effectiveness of thyroid hormone suppressive therapy in benign solitary thyroid nodules: a meta-analysis. J Clin Endocrinol Metab. 2002;87:4154–9.
135. Richter B, Neises G, Clar C. Pharmacotherapy for thyroid nodules. A systematic review and meta-analysis. Endocrinol Metab Clin N Am. 2002;31:699–722.
136. Ridgway EC. Medical treatment of benign thyroid nodules: have we defined a benefit? Ann Intern Med. 1998;128:403–5.
137. Corrias A, Mussa A, Wasniewska M, Segni M, Cassio A, Salerno M, Gastaldi R, Vigone MC, Bal M, Matarazzo P, Weber G, De Luca F. Levothyroxine treatment in pediatric benign thyroid nodules. Horm Res Paediatr. 2011;75:246–51.
138. Hegedus L. Therapy: a new nonsurgical therapy option for benign thyroid nodules? Nat Rev Endocrinol. 2009;5:476–8.
139. Raval MV, Bentrem DJ, Stewart AK, Ko CY, Reynolds M. Utilization of total thyroidectomy for differentiated thyroid cancer in children. Ann Surg Oncol. 2010;17:2545–53.
140. Oertel YC, Miyahara-Felipe L, Mendoza MG, Yu K. Value of repeated fine needle aspirations of the thyroid: an analysis of over ten thousand FNAs. Thyroid. 2007;17:1061–6.
141. Yang J, Schnadig V, Logrono R, Wasserman PG. Fine-needle aspiration of thyroid nodules: a study of 4703 patients with histologic and clinical correlations. Cancer. 2007;111:306–15.

28 Management of the Thyroid Nodule: A Comparison of Published International Guidelines

Joanna Klubo-Gwiezdzinska

In the past couple of years, several society-sponsored guidelines on thyroid nodules and thyroid cancer management have been published, including those by the European Thyroid Association (ETA) in 2006 [1], the British Thyroid Association (BTA) in 2007 [2], the National Cancer Institute (NCI) in 2008 [3], the American Thyroid Association (ATA) in 2009 [4], the Latin American Thyroid Society (LATS) in 2009 [5], the French Thyroid Association (FTA) in 2011 [6], and the National Comprehensive Cancer Network Guidelines in 2011 [7]. There were also attempts to standardize the guidelines in order to make them practically applicable for wider populations of patients. These efforts resulted in the publication of a joint statement of three large societies: American Association of Clinical Endocrinologist (AACE), Italian Association of Clinical Endocrinologists (AME), and the ETA in 2010 [8]. The Japanese Thyroid Association (JTA) guidelines for the diagnosis and management of thyroid nodules are now under preparation and will include classification and prevalence of thyroid nodules, recommendations for diagnosis and management of thyroid nodules, clinical data for the Japanese population, and comparison with the other guidelines.

All of the respective societies have attempted to use the best available published evidence as well as incorporating the expertise of multidisciplinary expert panels into their final recommendations. Interestingly, despite agreement on many issues, notable differences in management do exist. This variable interpretation of the available data may be due to the different practice patterns and geographic differences in the prevalence of thyroid diseases or on the availability of economic resources and health priorities [9]. The aim of this chapter is to summarize the available recommendations and to compare and contrast guidelines for management of thyroid nodules.

In general, the methodology employed for guideline development began with a survey and search of peer-reviewed journals for studies focused on diagnosis and management of thyroid nodules. The quality of the available data was critically assessed, with the highest rank given to prospective, randomized trials. When not available, retrospective and observational data were utilized as well as expert opinions. Consensus was achieved following review of all available data and discussion in the task force. Therefore, for all guidelines with the exception of the NCI and LATS guidelines, the recommendations acknowledge the level of evidence upon which recommendations were made [9].

Recommended Workup for Patients with Thyroid Nodules

Laboratory Studies

All guidelines are unequivocal in recommending evaluation of TSH levels as a screening thyroid function test in patients diagnosed with a thyroid nodule [1–8]. Clinically relevant thyroid nodules are defined by most of the guidelines as being >1 cm in any diameter or, as indicated by the ATA [4], characterized by positive FDG-PET uptake (Table 28.1). Additional testing is recommended when the TSH level is abnormal. The AACE/AME/ETA [8] and the FTA [6] point out specifically what additional laboratory data should be obtained. If the TSH level is decreased, a free thyroxine (FT4) and total or free triiodothyronine (T3) should be measured, while if TSH level is increased, FT4 and thyroperoxidase antibody (TPOAb) levels should be assessed.

The experts are not unanimous in the establishment of the role of routine CT measurement in patients with thyroid nodules. The combined AACE, AME, and ETA task force [8]

J. Klubo-Gwiezdzinska, MD, PhD (✉)
Combined Divisions of Endocrinology, National Institutes of Health, Bethesda, MD, USA
e-mail: joanna.klubo-gwiezdzinska@nih.gov

L. Wartofsky, D. Van Nostrand (eds.), *Thyroid Cancer*, DOI 10.1007/978-1-4939-3314-3_28

Table 28.1 Comparison of the guidelines on diagnosis and management of thyroid nodules

Laboratory tests recommended in patients with thyroid nodules	
Areas of general agreement	Areas of disagreement
TSH measurement for patients with clinically relevant thyroid nodules	**CT measurement**: ATA – cannot recommend for or against BTS and LATS – for suspicion of MTC or family history of MTC FTA – MTC, flushing, motility-related diarrhea, in cases suspicious for malignancy, before any intervention for goiter or nodule AACE, AME, and ETA – might be useful as a routine in patient with thyroid nodules
Imaging studies	
Neck ultrasound should be performed in all patients with known or suspected thyroid nodules Exemption – BTA guidelines for low-risk patients (no recommendation for or against) US features should be used as a tool for the malignancy risk stratification MRI, CT, PET-CT – should not be performed routinely. They may be useful in specific clinical situations: large goiters extending to the mediastinum and airway obstructions	**Indications for the radioisotope scanning**: ATA and BTA – radioisotope scan for the patients with decreased TSH levels FTA – scintigraphy may be useful as a second-line investigation in multinodular goiters (nodules >10 mm), regardless of the TSH level, when the anatomical conditions do not enable a precise analysis of the entire gland LATS, AACE, AME, ETA – toxic and nontoxic nodular goiters
FNAB	
Indications	
Hot nodules on scintigraphy do not require FNAB The threshold for FNAB of the solid nodule is 1 cm or lower for nodules characterized by high-risk clinical features Exemptions: BTA – no recommendation on US analysis of thyroid nodules FTA – FNAB for all nodules with high-risk clinical features and at least 2 suspicious US findings	**Diagnostic FNAB for purely cystic nodules**: ATA, NCCN, FTA, and NCI – purely cystic nodules do not require FNAB LATS, AACE, AME, ETA – not addressed the management of purely cystic nodules **Diagnostic FNAB for nodules without high-risk US or clinical features**: ATA, NCCN, FTA – the threshold warranting FNAB is 2 cm LATS, AACE, AME, ETA – not addressed the indications for FNAB for mixed cystic-solid nodules and spongiform nodules
Technique	
The gauge of the needle, the number of passes, and the need for a negative suction depend on the nodule composition and clinical situation. The 25–27 gauge needles for initial biopsies and increasing needle size up to 20 gauges in cases of drainage of viscous cyst content are advocated. Three to four needle passes generally constitute an effective FNA cytology test Samples can be processed via a direct smear on a glass slide or by liquid-based preparations Recommendation against initial core biopsy	**Palpation vs. US-guided FNAB**: BTA – does not recommend the routine use of US guidance ATA, FTA, NCI, and NCCN – recommend US guidance for nonpalpable, predominantly cystic, or located posteriorly nodules AACE, EMA, and ETA – favor US for its ability to reduce the rate of nondiagnostic and false-negative aspirates Detailed description of immunocytochemical staining placed only in the FTA guidelines
Classification of FNABs	
5 categories of FNAB samples: 1. Nondiagnostic/inadequate/unsatisfactory 2. Benign/nonneoplastic 3. Follicular lesion (AACE, AME, ETA, BTA) or indeterminate lesion (ATA). The NCI and FTA guidelines subdivide this category into three classes 4. Suspicious 5. Malignant	**The subdivision of the indeterminate FNABs**: NCI and FTA – subdivision of indeterminate nodules into three classes: follicular lesion of undetermined significance, follicular neoplasm, and suspicious for malignancy AACE, AME, ETA, BTA – one category of follicular lesion ATA – one category of indeterminate FNAB

Management of thyroid nodules in function of FNAB classification	
Category 1 – requires repeated US-guided FNAB. Partially cystic nodules with repeated nondiagnostic aspirates need close observation or surgical excision. Surgery should be more considered if the cytological nondiagnostic nodule is solid Category 2 – conservative approach for benign/nonneoplastic thyroid nodules unless nodule size increases progressively or shows suspicious clinical or US findings Indications for the surgery (addressed in LATS, AACE, AME, ETA, and FTA guidelines): neck pressure, dysphagia, a choking sensation, respiratory abnormalities (especially when supine), dyspnea on exertion, hoarseness, or pain Categories 4 and 5 – surgery for suspicious and malignant thyroid nodules	**Category 3**: ATA, NCCN, LATS – surgery is recommended for most "follicular lesions"/"indeterminate lesions" BTA, AACE, AME, ETA, NCI, and FTA – "follicular lesions" with favorable clinical, cytology, and ultrasound characteristics and "atypical cells of an undetermined significance" might be considered for the a clinical follow-up without immediate surgery and repeat FNAB

indicates that measurement of basal serum CT level may be useful in the initial evaluation of thyroid nodules. They recommend consideration of measurement of non-stimulated serum CT level before thyroid surgery for nodular goiter. They also indicate the subsequent follow-up strategy when the basal CT level is elevated. The panel advocates that a CT measurement should be repeated and, if an abnormal finding is confirmed in the absence of modifiers, a pentagastrin or calcium stimulation test may be performed to increase the diagnostic accuracy. The authors also point out that the measurement of CT is mandatory in patients with a family history or clinical suspicion of medullary thyroid cancer (MTC) or multiple endocrine neoplasia (MEN2). A narrower application of CT measurement is proposed by the FTA [6], BTA [2], and LATS [5]. The FTA states that CT should be measured when there is a known genetic background of MTC, flushing, motility-related diarrhea, in cases of suspicion for malignancy, and as a rule before any intervention for goiter or nodule. The BTA recommends its use only in case of suspicion of MTC, while LATS would measure CT if the family history suggests MTC. On the other hand, the ATA panel [4] concluded that they could neither recommend for nor against the routine measurement of serum CT (Table 28.1). The NCCN guidelines [7] underscored controversy surrounding cost-effectiveness of this practice in the United States, especially in the absence of a confirmatory pentagastrin test.

These equivocal recommendations from different societies suggest variable interpretation of existing literature focused on the utility of CT measurement in the management of patients with thyroid nodules. There are several reasons underlying this controversy. Advocates of routine CT measurement point out that several prospective studies found serum CT measurements as a highly sensitive screening tool for diagnosis of occult MTC in patients with thyroid nodules [10–16]. Moreover, Elisei et al. [13] found an improved outcome in MTC diagnosed by serum CT screening as compared with MTC patients diagnosed based upon cytology or pathology without prior screening. These authors found a 10-year survival rate of 86.8 % in MTC-screened patients compared with a 43.7 % 10-year survival rate in non-screened patients. Similar results were obtained by Karga et al. who observed that MTC tumors were smaller and the 15-year disease-specific survival rate was higher in screened patients (85 %) compared with non-screened ones (35 %) [17].

The epidemiological data strongly suggest a relatively high prevalence of occult MTC (approximately 0.39 %) in patients with thyroid nodules [18]. The prevalence of MTC in autopsy studies varies from 0.1 % to 3.4 % with a median of around 0.3 % [18]. Consequently, there is presumably a large reservoir of medullary microcarcinomas which might be detected by screening. However, the malignant potential of these micro-tumors is uncertain, so there is a risk that detection of minimally elevated serum CT levels may lead to unnecessary surgery and an increase in the patient's anxiety level.

Some of the arguments against universal screening refer to the specificity of basal serum CT measurements. There are several conditions other than MTC causing elevated basal CT levels including pernicious anemia, drugs inhibiting gastric acid secretion, or gastrinomas [18]. d'Herbomez et al. [19] evaluated 375 clinically euthyroid individuals with five different CT assays and found that 2.5–9.8 % of patients presented with elevated CT levels, despite the lack of apparent C-cell disease. There was an association between the increased CT concentration and male sex and smoking. The diagnostic accuracy of this test may be increased by performing stimulation tests with pentagastrin or calcium. Unfortunately, pentagastrin is not available widely in all countries, including the Untied States, and there is limited data regarding the interpretation of calcium stimulation test [18].

Imaging Studies

Neck Ultrasound

The majority of the guidelines uniformly recommend that neck ultrasound (US) should be performed in all patients with known or suspected thyroid nodules [1–8]. Some societies (FTA, AACE, AME, and ETA) also provide a detailed description of the standards for neck ultrasound examination, documentation, reporting, equipment, and methods of assessment of thyroid nodules. The one and only exception is the BTA consensus [2] which lacked a formal recommendation for or against routine use of neck US in low-risk patients with thyroid nodules. The reason for that relates to the health-care system in the United Kingdom, where low-risk patients are managed by general practitioners without subspecialty referral (Table 28.1). The guidelines uniformly imply that US should be used as one of the tools for malignancy risk stratification. Suspicious nodules are described as taller than wider, hypoechoic, with microcalcifications, infiltrative margins, increased nodular vascularity, and accompanied by enlarged or suspicious cervical lymph nodes [1–8]. Additionally, some societies comment on the utility of additional US modalities. LATS [5] states that "*nodular characteristics on color Doppler alone, including vascular pattern, resistive index and maximal systolic velocity values, are not useful parameters for distinguishing malignant from benign thyroid nodules*". Furthermore, ATA [4] and FTA [6] guidelines comment on the applicability of elastography. Both societies point out that despite the fact that elastography has proven very useful in several studies, its wider use requires further investigation [20–22].

Radioisotope Scans

There is a minor disagreement in terms of the indications for nuclear scintigraphy. All guidelines recommend radioisotope scanning when a patient with thyroid nodule has a decreased TSH level. Additionally, the AACE, AME, and ETA [8] as well as LATS guidelines [5] recommend scintigraphy in patients with multinodular goiters irrespective of the TSH levels. The rationale for this is the high prevalence of hyperthyroidism due to a solitary or multiple hot nodules in iodine-deficient areas [23], as well as the fact that hot nodules can also be found in patients with nontoxic goiters who have been shown to develop hyperthyroidism at an annual rate of 5 % [24]. Another indication for scintigraphy pointed out by the FTA guidelines [6] is its usage as a second-line investigation in multinodular goiters, regardless of the TSH level, when the anatomical conditions do not enable a precise analysis of the entire gland.

MRI, CT, and PET-CT

The published guidelines do not recommend routine use of MRI, CT, or PET-CT in patients with thyroid nodules [1–8]. Instead, they specify clinical situations in which these techniques might be used such as for goiters extending into upper mediastinum or compressing the airways. Additionally, the ATA [4], NCCN [7], and combined AACE, AME, and ETA [8] guidelines point out that thyroid incidentalomas discovered by FDG-PET-CT are characterized by an increased risk of malignancy.

Fine-Needle Aspiration Biopsy (FNAB)

Indications

All guidelines recommend appropriate risk stratification based on clinical and US features of the thyroid nodules [1–8]. This approach is intended to limit unnecessary intervention in low malignancy risk disease. Therefore, diagnostic FNAB is not indicated for hot nodules detected with radionuclide scan as recommended by all guidelines and for purely cystic nodules as suggested by ATA [4], NCCN [7], FTA [6], and NCI [3]. There are minor discrepancies related to the specific thyroid nodule features warranting further cytological diagnosis. ATA recommends FNAB for any nodules accompanied by cervical lymph node enlargement and for nodules larger than 5 mm when there is a family history of thyroid cancer, history of external beam radiation or ionizing radiation in childhood or adolescence, prior surgery for thyroid cancer, FDG avidity on PET scanning, MEN2/FMTC-associated RET protooncogene mutation, or CT >100 pg/ml. For the patients without high clinical risk of thyroid cancer, the threshold warranting FNAB is 1 cm, for solid nodules; 1.5 cm, for mixed cystic-solid nodules with any suspicious US features; and 2 cm, for the remaining types of nodules. The majority of remaining societies agree with the threshold of 1 cm for FNAB of solid nodules and below that threshold when there are high-risk clinical features. They however do not comment on the size of mixed cystic-solid or spongiform nodules warranting FNAB. At a little variance is the latest FTA guidelines [6] recommending FNAB for any nodules characterized by high-risk clinical feature and for any nodules with at least two suspicious US criteria and propose a threshold of 2 cm for the remaining types of nodules. Finally, the BTA guidelines [2] make no recommendation on US analysis of thyroid nodules.

FNAB Technique

The NCI [3], FTA [6], and combined AACE, EMA, and ETA [8] documents provide a detailed description of the appropriate FNAB technique. The gauge of the needle, the number of passes, and the need for a negative suction depend on the nodule composition and clinical situation. The guidelines recommend the use of 25–27 gauge needles for initial biopsies and increasing needle size up to 20 gauge in cases of drainage of viscous cyst content. Three to four needle passes generally constitute an effective sampling for FNA cytology. FNA cytology samples can be processed via a direct smear on a glass slide or by liquid-based preparations.

All guidelines recommend against initial core biopsy with exception of specific situations, such as suspicion of thyroid lymphoma, anaplastic carcinoma, or pathologic lymph nodes when it might be used as an alternative [25].

The guidelines are equivocal in terms of FNAB based on palpation vs. US guidance. BTA does not recommend the routine use of ultrasound guidance procedures [1]. ATA [4], FTA [6], NCI [3], and NCCN [7] recommend ultrasound guidance for those nodules that are nonpalpable, predominantly cystic, or located posteriorly in the thyroid. Combined AACE, EMA, and ETA [8] guidelines favor US for its ability to reduce the rate of nondiagnostic and false-negative aspirates [26]. Ultrasound guidance is of particular relevance for FNA of suspicious lymph nodes. ATA [4], FTA [6], NCI [3], and AACE, EMA, and ETA [8] recommend the measurement of Tg (or CT) in the needle washout to increase the diagnostic accuracy of cytological sampling. The recent FTA guidelines are the only one to address the role of immunocytochemical studies as an aid for establishing the appropriate diagnosis. The indications for immunocytochemistry in thyroid cytology are as follows:

- Suspicion of medullary carcinoma: if the morphology is not clear, the fine-needle aspiration product can be investigated for expression of CT and/or chromogranin, carcinoembryonic antigen, and possibly thyroglobulin. A serum measurement of CT is indicated.

- Suspicion of anaplastic carcinoma: pan-cytokeratin staining can be performed.
- Suspicion of secondary tumor: perform immunocytochemistry of TTF1. If negative, diversify the range of antibodies according to the standard morphology and the clinical context.
- Suspicion of lymphoma: the expression of T and B lymphocytic markers can be investigated with immunocytochemistry. Some teams perform this phenotypic characterization using the flow cytometry technique.
- Suspicion of parathyroid lesion: perform immunocytochemistry of the parathyroid hormone, TTF1, and chromogranin. A parathyroid hormone measurement on the fine-needle aspiration product complements the immunocytochemistry study

The Classification of FNABs

All guidelines recommend classification of FNAB samples into five categories:

1. Nondiagnostic (AACE, AME, ETA, BTA), nondiagnostic or inadequate (ATA), unsatisfactory (NCI, FTA).
2. Benign or "nonneoplastic" (ATA).
3. Follicular lesion (AACE, AME, ETA, BTA) or indeterminate (ATA). The NCI and FTA guidelines subdivide this category into three classes: follicular lesion of undetermined significance, follicular neoplasm, and suspicious for malignancy.
4. Suspicious.
5. Malignant.

Obviously, the major disagreement between the guidelines refers to the division of "indeterminate" cytology into three different subcategories to better define cancer risk. This classification recommended by NCI and FTA is accurate in defining the risk of malignancy, though at the expense of increased complexity and more detailed cytological differentiation.

Although there is some variability in terms of labeling of the category 1 cytology samples, the majority of guidelines state that a satisfactory FNAB of solid nodules consists of a minimum five to six groups with a least ten cells, preferably on a single slide [1–8]. There are exceptions of this rule which include cystic lesions and inflammatory processes.

Management of Thyroid Nodules

FNAB Category 1

The majority of the guidelines agree that the US guidance should be used when repeating the FNA procedure for a nodule with an initial nondiagnostic cytology result [1–8]. Despite good initial technique and repeated biopsy, still 5–30 % of nodules remain nondiagnostic because of factors inherent to the lesion [27]. In nondiagnostic specimens, the reported malignancy rate varies from 2 % to 12 % [27]. Partially cystic nodules that repeatedly yield nondiagnostic aspirates need close observation or surgical excision. Surgery should be more strongly considered if the cytological nondiagnostic nodule is solid [4].

FNAB Category 2

The guidelines are uniform in recommending a conservative approach for benign/nonneoplastic thyroid nodules unless nodule size increases progressively or shows suspicious clinical or US findings. The majority of the guidelines recommend routine clinical and US evaluation of the nodules at 6–18 month intervals and, if stable, at progressively longer intervals of 2, 5, and 10 years. The BTA [1] makes no recommendation for the time interval of the follow-up. The majority of the guidelines recommend repeated FNAB in the presence of suspicious clinical signs (hard nodule, adherent, presence of adenopathy, etc.), of rapid and significant increase in size (increase of diameter greater than 20 % or of 2 mm in two dimensions) of a non-cystic nodule, or when there is suspicious modification of ultrasound data. On the contrary, the FTA guidelines [6] indicate that "during monitoring of cytologically benign nodules, a repeated fine-needle aspiration is to be carried out".

All guidelines recommend against routine use of levothyroxine as the therapeutic options for benign thyroid nodules in iodine-sufficient populations [1–8]. The FTA guidelines [6] however point out that particularly in regions of relative iodine deficiency, suppressive treatment with levothyroxine may lead to a decrease in the volume of thyroid nodules, especially when the nodules are small, recent, and colloid [28]. The French panel states that levothyroxine treatment may be indicated in patients living in iodine-deficient areas presenting with a recent colloid thyroid nodule that is stable or progressive and in young patients with nodular thyroid dystrophy, particularly in women before pregnancy [8].

Surprisingly, not all the guidelines cover in detail the surgical options for benign nodules (Table 28.1). Indications for surgery include neck pressure, dysphagia, a choking sensation, respiratory abnormalities (especially when supine), dyspnea on exertion, hoarseness, or pain. Surgery may also occasionally be reasonable for cosmetic reasons or if severe growth is noted. In the case of surgery, the preferred extent is lobectomy plus isthmectomy for uninodular and total or near total thyroidectomy for multinodular goiter, irrespective of whether the patient is euthyroid or hyperthyroid.

The majority of the guidelines support radioactive iodine (RAI) treatment for autonomously functioning nodules [1–8]. However, only the combined AACE, AME, ETA [8], and LATS [5] guidelines analyze the indications for RAI therapy in detail. Their expert panels indicate that RAI therapy reduces the nodule size by 35–45 % over the subsequent 12–24 months.

In multinodular goiter, indications for RAI treatment are hyperfunctioning and/or symptomatic goiter, previous thyroid surgery, or comorbidities causing a high surgical risk. Based on relatively few adverse effects and a 40–50 % goiter size reduction within 1–2 years, RAI is an effective alternative to surgery for the treatment of large goiters, whether the patient is euthyroid or hyperthyroid. The panels underscore the usefulness of recombinant human TSH (rhTSH) as an adjunct to RAI therapy of goiters characterized by low RAI uptake. rhTSH has been shown to increase the uptake two- to fourfold at the expense of a higher risk of early posttreatment thyrotoxicosis [29–31].

Alternative methods to ablate thyroid nodules such as percutaneous ethanol injection, percutaneous laser ablation, and radiofrequency ablation are addressed as potential therapeutic options in detail by the AACE, AME, ETA, and LATS guidelines. Moreover, the LATS guidelines [5] also suggest some experimental therapies such as the use of metformin to reduce nodule size in patients with insulin resistance [32].

FNAB Category 3

This category of FNAB reading is associated with the most vivid discussion between the experts forming the recommendation panels. The lack of the uniform statement is partially due to different and often confusing nomenclature as well as a wide range for the risk of malignancy within this group of thyroid lesions. The latter fact formed the rationale for the NCI and FTA to subdivide this category into the previously mentioned three subgroups of indeterminate nodules (follicular lesion of undetermined significance, follicular neoplasm, and suspicious for malignancy), characterized by different malignancy risk. Nevertheless, surgery is recommended for most "follicular lesions" or "indeterminate lesions." A minority opinion by the BTA [2] and combined AACE, AME, and ETA [8] statement indicates that "follicular lesions" with favorable clinical, cytology, and ultrasound characteristics and NCI "atypical cells of an undetermined significance" might be considered for the clinical follow-up without immediate surgery and repeat FNAB.

Since the risk of overtreatment and referrals for unnecessary surgery is particularly high in this indeterminate diagnostic category, several attempts have been made to improve stratification of malignancy risk using molecular biology techniques. The ATA [4] and NCCN [7] guidelines suggest consideration of the use of molecular markers like *BRAF*, *RAS*, *RET/PTC*, *PAX8-PPARγ*, or galectin-3 for patients with indeterminate cytology on FNA. If detectable, these markers can help guide thyroid nodule management. The combined AACE, AME, and ETA [8] guidelines reserve the use of molecular markers for selected cases and do not recommend their application for routine clinical use. The BTA [2] and LATS [5] guidelines do not comment on usage of molecular markers, while the FTA [6] points out that the application of molecular techniques for the management of thyroid nodules is still an area of clinical research.

FNAB Categories 4 and 5

All societies are concordant in recommending surgery for suspicious and malignant thyroid nodules. The extent of the surgery and further management is summarized in detail in subsequent chapters on the management of thyroid cancer. All societies comment relatively briefly on the management of the thyroid nodules in children. The consensus is to apply similar strategies as described above for adults [1–8]. All guidelines are also unequivocal in terms of the management of thyroid nodules during pregnancy. The evaluation is the same as for a nonpregnant patient, with the exception that a radionuclide scan is contraindicated. In addition, for patients with nodules diagnosed as thyroid cancer by FNAB during pregnancy, delaying surgery until after delivery does not affect the outcome [33]. When the decision for surgery has been made, it should be done in the second trimester before 24 weeks gestation in order to minimize the risk of miscarriage [34].

To summarize, there is consensus regarding the majority of diagnostic and therapeutic procedures for patients with thyroid nodules. There are few areas of disagreement, such as indications for scintigraphy or CT screening. They probably could be resolved by generating data from well-designed clinical studies covering those topics. Finally, there are clinically relevant areas of uncertainty such as the routine application of molecular biology tools for the risk stratification of indeterminate nodules, which remains to be addressed by further research and clinical experience.

As we go to press with this volume, the draft-revised ATA 2015 guidelines have been submitted for publication. In brief, review of the draft reveals only minor changes that relate to the threshold for FNAB of the thyroid nodules with high-risk sonographic features. Only nodules of 1 cm or larger should be biopsied – in contrast to ATA 2009 guidelines where the size cutoff for high-risk nodules was 5 mm. This recommendation was based on increasing incidence of thyroid microcarcinomas characterized by the indolent course, not warranting aggressive therapy. Current guidelines also point that focal FDG-PET uptake within a sonographically confirmed thyroid nodule conveys an increased risk of thyroid cancer (30 %), and fine-needle aspiration is recommended.

If molecular testing is being considered, patients should be counseled regarding the potential benefits and limitations of testing and about the possible uncertainties in the therapeutic and long-term clinical implications of results. If intended for clinical use, molecular testing should be performed in CLIA-/CAP-certified molecular laboratories, as reported quality assurance practices may be superior compared to other settings [35].

References

1. Pacini F, Schlumberger M, Dralle H, Elisei R, Smit JW, Wiersinga W, European Thyroid Cancer Taskforce. European consensus for the management of patients with differentiated thyroid carcinoma of the follicular epithelium. Eur J Endocrinol. 2006;154(6): 787–803.
2. Guidelines for the management of thyroid cancer. British Thyroid Association. 2007; http://www.british-thyroid-association.org/news/Docs/Thyroid_cancer_guidelines_2007.pdf.
3. Pitman MB, Abele J, Ali SZ, Duick D, Elsheikh TM, Jeffrey RB, Powers CN, Randolph G, Renshaw A, Scoutt L. Techniques for thyroid FNA: a synopsis of the national cancer institute thyroid fine-needle aspiration state of the science conference. Diagn Cytopathol. 2008;36(6):407–24.
4. American Thyroid Association (ATA) Guidelines Taskforce on Thyroid Nodules and Differentiated Thyroid Cancer, Cooper DS, Doherty GM, Haugen BR, Kloos RT, Lee SL, Mandel SJ, Mazzaferri EL, McIver B, Pacini F, Schlumberger M, Sherman SI, Steward DL, Tuttle RM. Revised American Thyroid Association management guidelines for patients with thyroid nodules and differentiated thyroid cancer. Thyroid. 2009;19(11):1167–214.
5. Camargo R, Corigliano S, Friguglietti C, Gauna A, Harach R, Munizaga F, Niepomniszcze H, Pitoia F, Pretell E, Vaisman M, Ward LS, Wohllk N, Tomimori E, Latin American thyroid society. Latin American thyroid society recommendations for the management of thyroid nodules. Arq Bras Endocrinol Metabol. 2009;53(9):1167–75.
6. Wémeau JL, Sadoul JL, d'Herbomez M, Monpeyssen H, Tramalloni J, Leteurtre E, Borson-Chazot F, Caron P, Carnaille B, Léger J, Do C, Klein M, Raingeard I, Desailloud R, Leenhardt L. Guidelines of the French society of endocrinology for the management of thyroid nodules. Ann Endocrinol. 2011;72:251–81.
7. Tuttle RM, Ball DW, Byrd D, Dilawari RA, Doherty GM, Duh QY, Ehya H, Farrar WB, Haddad RI, Hunt JP, Kandeel F, Kloos RT, Kopp P, Lamonica DM, Loree TR, Lydiatt WM, McCaffrey J, Moley JF, Olson JA, Parks L, Ridge JA, Shah JP, Sherman SI, Sturgeon C, Waguespack SG, Wang TN, Wirth LJ. NCCN clinical practice guidelines in oncology: thyroid carcinoma version 3. 2011. http://www.nccn.org.
8. Gharib H, Papini E, Paschke R, Duick DS, Valcavi R, Hegedüs L, Vitti P, AACE/AME/ETA Task Force on Thyroid Nodules. American Association of Clinical Endocrinologists, Associazione Medici Endocrinologi, and European Thyroid Association medical guidelines for clinical practice for the diagnosis and management of thyroid nodules. J Endocrinol Invest. 2010;33(5 Suppl):1–50.
9. Paschke R, Hegedüs L, Alexander E, Valcavi R, Papini E, Gharib H. Thyroid nodule guidelines: agreement, disagreement and need for future research. Nat Rev Endocrinol. 2011;7(6):354–61.
10. Herrmann BL, Schmid KW, Goerges R, Kemen M, Mann K. CT screening and pentagastrin testing: predictive value for the diagnosis of medullary carcinoma in nodular thyroid disease. Eur J Endocrinol. 2010;162:1141–5.
11. Rink T, Truong PN, Schroth HJ, Diener J, Zimny M, Grunwald F. Calculation and validation of a plasma CT limit for early detection of medullary thyroid carcinoma in nodular thyroid disease. Thyroid. 2009;19:327–32.
12. Costante G, Meringolo D, Durante C, Bianchi D, Nocera M, Tumino S, Crocetti U, Attard M, Maranghi M, Torlontano M, Filetti S. Predictive value of serum CT levels for preoperative diagnosis of medullary thyroid carcinoma in a cohort of 5817 consecutive patients with thyroid nodules. J Clin Endocrinol Metab. 2007;92:450–5.
13. Elisei R, Bottici V, Luchetti F, Di Coscio G, Romei C, Grasso L, Miccoli P, Iacconi P, Basolo F, Pinchera A, Pacini F. Impact of routine measurement of serum CT on the diagnosis and outcome of medullary thyroid cancer: experience in 10,864 patients with nodular thyroid disorders. J Clin Endocrinol Metab. 2004;89:163–8.
14. Karanikas G, Moameni A, Poetzi C, Zettinig G, Kaserer K, Bieglmayer C, Niederle B, Dudczak R, Pirich C. Frequency and relevance of elevated CT levels in patients with neoplastic and non-neoplastic thyroid disease and in healthy subjects. J Clin Endocrinol Metab. 2004;89:515–9.
15. Iacobone M, Niccoli-Sire P, Sebag F, De Micco C, Henry JF. Can sporadic medullary thyroid carcinoma be biochemically predicted? Prospective analysis of 66 operated patients with elevated serum CT levels. World J Surg. 2002;26:886–90.
16. Vierhapper H, Niederle B, Bieglmayer C, Kaserer K, Baumgartner-Parzer S. Early diagnosis and curative therapy of medullary thyroid carcinoma by routine measurement of serum CT in patients with thyroid disorders. Thyroid. 2005;15:1267–72.
17. Karga H, Giagourta I, Papaioannou G, Doumouchtsis K, Polymeris A, Thanou S, Papamichael K, Zerva C. Changes in risk factors and tumor node metastasis stage of sporadic medullary thyroid carcinoma over 41 years, before and after the routine measurements of serum CT. Metabolism. 2011;60:604–8.
18. Daniels GH. Screening for medullary thyroid carcinoma with serum CT measurements in patients with thyroid nodules in the United States and Canada. Thyroid. 2011;21(11):1199–207.
19. d'Herbomez M, Caron P, Bauters C, Cao CD, Schlienger JL, Sapin R, Baldet L, Carnaille B, We'meau JL, French Group GTE (Groupe des Tumeurs Endocrines). Reference range of serum CT levels in humans: influence of CT assays, sex, age, and cigarette smoking. Eur J Endocrinol. 2007;157:749–55.
20. Lyshchik A, Higashi T, Asato R, Tanaka S, Ito J, Mai JJ, Pellot-Barakat C, Insana MF, Brill AB, Saga T, Hiraoka M, Togashi K. Thyroid gland tumor diagnosis at US elastography. Radiology. 2005;237:202–11.
21. Rago T, Santini F, Scutari M, Pinchera A, Vitti P. Elastography: new developments in ultrasound for predicting malignancy in thyroid nodules. J Clin Endocrinol Metab. 2007;92:2917–22.
22. Tranquart F, Bleuzen A, Pierre-Renoult P, Chabrolle C, Sam Giao M, Lecomte P. Élastographie ultrasonore des lésions thyroïdiennes. J Radiol. 2008;89:35–9.
23. Laurberg P, Pedersen KM, Vestergaard H, Sigurdsson G. High incidence of multinodular toxic goitre in the elderly population in a low iodine intake area vs. high incidence of Graves' disease in the young in a high iodine intake area: comparative surveys of thyrotoxicosis epidemiology in East-Jutland Denmark and Iceland. J Intern Med. 1991;229:415–20.
24. Sandrock D, Olbricht T, Emrich D, Benker G, Reinwein D. Long-term follow-up in patients with autonomous thyroid adenoma. Acta Endocrinol (Copenh). 1993;128:51–5.
25. Zhang S, Ivanovic M, Nemcek Jr AA, Defrias DV, Lucas E, Nayar R. Thin core needle biopsy crush preparations in conjunction with fine-needle aspiration for the evaluation of thyroid nodules: a complementary approach. Cancer. 2008;114:512–8.
26. Danese D, Sciacchitano S, Farsetti A, Andreoli M, Pontecorvi A. Diagnostic accuracy of conventional versus sonography-guided fine-needle aspiration biopsy of thyroid nodules. Thyroid. 1998;8:15–21.
27. Kini SR. Specimen adequacy and assessment, reporting system. In: Thyroid cytopathology: an atlas and text. Philadelphia: Lippincott Williams & Wilkins; 2008. p. 17–26.
28. Wémeau JL, Caron P, Schvartz C, Schlienger JL, Orgiazzi J, Cousty C, Vlaeminck-Guillem V. Effects of thyroid-stimulating hormone suppression with levothyroxine in reducing the volume of solitary thyroid nodules and improving extranodular nonpalpable changes: a randomized, double-blind, placebo controlled trial by the French thyroid research group. J Clin Endocrinol Metab. 2002;87:4928–34.
29. Bonnema SJ, Nielsen VE, Boel-Jørgensen H, Grupe P, Andersen PB, Bastholt L, Hegedüs L. Improvement of goiter volume reduc-

tion after 0.3 mg recombinant human thyrotropin-stimulated radioiodine therapy in patients with a very large goiter: a double-blinded, randomized trial. J Clin Endocrinol Metab. 2007;92: 3424–8.
30. Bonnema SJ, Nielsen VE, Hegedüs L. Radioiodine therapy in non-toxic multinodular goitre. The possibility of effect-amplification with recombinant human TSH (rhTSH). Acta Oncol. 2006;45(8):1051–8.
31. Nielsen VE, Bonnema SJ, Jørgensen HB, Grupe P, Hegedüs L. Stimulation with 0,3 mg recombinant human thyrotropin (rhTSH) increases the effect of 131I therapy in patients with non-toxic nodular goiter. A prospective, randomized, double-blind trial – secondary publication. Ugeskr Laeger. 2006;168:4098–101.
32. Rezzónico J, Rezzónico M, Pusiol E, Pitoia F, Niepomniszcze H. Metformin treatment for small benign thyroid nodules in patients with insulin resistance. Metab Syndr Relat Disord. 2011;9(1): 69–75.
33. Moosa M, Mazzaferri EL. Outcome of differentiated thyroid cancer diagnosed in pregnant women. J Clin Endocrinol Metab. 1997;82:2862–6.
34. Mestman JH, Goodwin TM, Montoro MM. Thyroid disorders of pregnancy. Endocrinol Metab Clin North Am. 1995;24: 41–71.
35. Haugen BR, Alexander EK, Bible KC, Doherty GM, Mandel SJ, Nikiforov Y, Pacini F, Randolph G, Sawka A, Shepard D, Sosa J, Tuttle RM, Wartofsky L. 2015 American Thyroid Association Management Guidelines for adult patients with thyroid nodules and differentiated thyroid cancer. Available online at Thyroid 25: DOI:10.1089/thy.2015.0020; print version in Thyroid 26:1–133, 2016.

Part IV

Well-Differentiated Thyroid Cancer: Papillary Carcinoma – Presentation

Papillary Carcinoma: Clinical Aspects

29

Leonard Wartofsky

Introduction

Papillary thyroid carcinoma (PTC) is a cancer of the thyroid follicular epithelium; like follicular carcinoma, it is the more highly differentiated of all of the classes of thyroid malignancy. The biological behavior of PTC varies widely, from small (<1.0 cm) tumors found at autopsy with surprisingly high frequency that show little evidence of invasion to rapidly growing, locally invasive tumors that may be resistant to radioiodine therapy, eventually metastasizing and can cause death. To date, it has not been possible in a given patient to predict which course the tumor may take until several years, or even decades, of follow-up have elapsed. Fortunately, the overwhelming majority of tumors less than 1.5 cm in diameter tend to behave in a more biologically benign manner and can be completely cured with definitive therapy. This reflects the importance of age and tumor size on prognosis and risk of recurrence or death [1]. Although PTC tends to affect women more often than men (~2:1), the risk of cancer in thyroid nodules in men is equally, if not more, significant because of the much lower frequency of any type of thyroid disease in men.

This chapter deals with several clinical aspects of these tumors, and descriptions of pathology and management appear in the immediate chapters that follow. In general, the discussion applies to all papillary cancers although there is a histologic basis to distinguish between classic papillary thyroid carcinoma and follicular variant papillary carcinoma. Moreover, both of the latter subtypes can be further classified into encapsulated or nonencapsulated papillary cancers as described in Chap. 32 on pathology by Baloch and LiVolsi. The importance of the distinction may relate to a clinical correlation in that encapsulated follicular variant papillary cancers may behave more like follicular carcinomas with a greater tendency to vascular invasion and distant metastases rather than local invasion with lymph node metastases [2], although in one recent series, the follicular variant of papillary thyroid carcinoma had a relatively low propensity for distant metastases [3].

Epidemiology

According to 2013 data from the American Cancer Society, thyroid cancer is the most rapidly increasing cancer in frequency in the USA in women, representing 5 % of all cancers in women, about 1 % in men, and approx 1.4 % of all cancers in children. They estimate 49,020 new cases of thyroid cancer in 2011 (11,470 in men; 36,550 in women), with an estimated 1,740 deaths from thyroid cancer [4]. Approximately 80 % of these tumors are papillary carcinomas. Because most patients with thyroid cancer are followed for a long time, it is estimated that there are approximately 350,000 patients alive with the disease in the USA. The frequency of thyroid cancer has been increasing each year of the past decade and represents a significant economic and clinical burden on world health [5]. The reasons for this rise are not clear and may relate to earlier diagnosis owing to the ever-increasing use of ultrasound and fine-needle aspiration (FNA), but many believe that it is because of exposure to ionizing radiation, such as from the nuclear tests of the 1950s and 1960s [6].

Thyroid cancer is the most common malignancy of the endocrine system, and papillary carcinoma (PTC) is the most common type of thyroid malignancy, accounting for ~80 % of all thyroid cancers [7, 8]. The frequency of papillary cancer appears to be increasing relative to the incidence of follicular thyroid cancer, which has been attributed to the higher iodine content of the American diet. Incidence of follicular cancer has not declined in geographic areas with

L. Wartofsky, MD, MACP (✉)
Department of Medicine, MedStar Washington Hospital Center, Georgetown University School of Medicine, 110 Irving Street, N.W., Washington, DC 20010-2975, USA
e-mail: leonard.wartofsky@medstar.net

L. Wartofsky, D. Van Nostrand (eds.), *Thyroid Cancer*, DOI 10.1007/978-1-4939-3314-3_29

relative iodine deficiency. High iodine intake was also found to be associated with a higher frequency of the BRAF mutation in one epidemiologic study [9]. PTC tends to occur in younger patients, most commonly in the third and fourth decades of life, and has the best prognosis of all the varieties of thyroid malignancy. There is a weak association with breast cancer in that White (but not Black) women with a history of thyroid cancer have a somewhat greater risk (relative risk [RR] = 1.42) of developing breast cancer, but women with breast cancer do not have a greater risk of developing thyroid cancer [10]. Difference between the presentation of PTC in adults and that in children or adolescents has been described [11–14] and is discussed in Chap. 51.

A number of clinical and pathological characteristics have been evaluated as predictors of tumor behavior and ultimate patient prognosis. The more useful of these parameters are described in the chapter on staging and prognosis. Exposure to radiation is a risk factor for PTC, where the risk of malignancy in a thyroid nodule rises from 5–10 % to 30–50 % [15]. This chapter discusses general aspects of typical papillary carcinoma, but the discussion also largely applies to the follicular variant of papillary carcinoma (FVPTC) although some differences have been noted [16, 17]. FNA cytology may not be sufficiently sensitive to distinguish between PTC and FVPTC preoperatively [18, 19]. Some studies have indicated that the FVPTC may be less invasive and associated with a lower frequency of neck node metastases [18, 20], but it may present with larger original tumor size and higher tumor stage [20]. Experts have proposed that clear-cut histopathologic features should be present to make the diagnosis of FVPTC [21]. Other variants of papillary carcinoma, such as the tall cell variant, columnar variant, and insular variant, may behave in a more aggressive or invasive manner [22–28] and are discussed in Chaps. 80 and 81.

Annual incidence rates for well-differentiated thyroid cancer range from 1 to 10 cases per 100,000 population, and a detailed description of the epidemiology of these tumors appears in Chap. 4. One of the largest cohorts of patients with PTC was followed at the Mayo Clinic and reviewed by Hay [29]. Of 1,500 patients, two thirds were women (2:1 ratio), and age at diagnosis ranged widely from only 5 to 93 years of age. Most patients presented between ages 30 and 60. There are major differences in frequencies of PTC in other ethnic groups. For example, the female-to-male ratio among Japanese has been reported as high as 13:1 [30].

Clinical Presentation

In most patients, the first clinical presentation of PTC is that of a thyroid nodule, discovered during routine physical examination by a physician or noted as a lump in the neck by a friend or relative. As recommended by the guidelines of the American Thyroid Association [31], the diagnostic evaluation of the nodule should always include ultrasonography [32, 33] and FNA cytology, which can demonstrate the tumor's pathognomonic cytologic features. The tumors are almost always solid and anechoic on ultrasound examination and may contain microcalcifications. Although purely cystic nodules rarely contain malignancy, large, mixed cystic/solid nodules pose a greater risk that demand closer management with subsequent reaspiration if not excised. Other imaging techniques, such as CT or MRI (Chap. 45), are rarely required but can demonstrate the extent of metastatic lymphadenopathy either before or after surgery and are recommended for more advanced disease [31]. It is common for a patient to present for evaluation of a thyroid mass found incidentally because a CT scan or MRI was performed for another unrelated problem.

Fine needle aspiration cytology clearly indicating carcinoma mandates thyroidectomy. In more indeterminate cytologies, the use of new molecular biologic techniques may distinguish benign from malignant cytologies and are under intensive study [34]. One of the molecular mutations that has been most studied is BRAF, in particular the V600E point mutation of BRAF that when present in papillary thyroid cancer is often [35–38] but not always [39, 40] associated with a greater likelihood for extrathyroidal invasiveness, cervical lymph node metastases [41], and higher stage disease. BRAF positivity occurs in 30–80 % of tumors [42–45] and is associated to a greater degree with male gender and larger tumors, but not with Hashimoto thyroiditis [36]. BRAF positivity may lead clinicians to manage a given tumor more aggressively, e.g., electing central compartment (Level VI) node dissection at the time of thyroidectomy as well as postoperative radioiodine ablation. Many other variables in a given patient determine the recommendation for the extent of surgery (total or subtotal thyroidectomy, lymph node dissection, etc.) and whether postoperative radioiodine ablation is warranted. These issues are covered in the guidelines for evaluation, diagnosis, and long-term management of thyroid cancer that have been published by several authoritative sources [31, 46, 47].

As much as one third of patients with a PTC will have some underlying thyroid disease, such as Hashimoto's disease or multinodular or adenomatoid goiter. In one series of 596 PTC patients from the Mayo Clinic [29], 40 % had other benign thyroid disease, 33 % had coexistent thyroid nodules, and 20 % had Hashimoto's thyroiditis. Although a link of PTC to Hashimoto's disease has been questioned [48], other workers find that underlying Hashimoto's disease appears to be a favorable prognostic factor for both reduced rates of recurrence and increased survival [49]. This may relate to a lymphocyte-mediated immune response against the cancer [50]. Some familial papillary cancers occur in association with Hashimoto's thyroiditis [51, 52], and a family history of thyroid cancer could be highly relevant at presentation, either indicating a possible medullary carcinoma or a familial type of PTC [53]. Indeed, in one study, the relative risk of thyroid cancer was ten times higher in relatives of thyroid cancer patients than in controls [54].

In some of the cancer literature, papillary tumors have been classified as occult, intrathyroidal, or extrathyroidal. An occult tumor has been defined as typically less than 1.0 cm in size, an intrathyroidal tumor is more than 1.0 cm in size but confined to the thyroid gland, and an extrathyroidal tumor demonstrates extension to the soft tissues or lymph nodes of the neck. An initial presentation to a physician of PTC as cervical lymphadenopathy is fairly common, and this evaluation then leads to detection of the primary thyroid tumor [55]. The lymphadenopathy is from local metastases of the tumor, and the most frequent presentation is to nodes on the ipsilateral side of the tumor's neck, as well as down into the superior mediastinum. Metastases to the contralateral cervical chains of nodes occur with either more advanced or more aggressive disease. This may be related to initial intrathyroidal seeding via the thyroidal lymphatic system because microscopic to macroscopic foci of papillary carcinoma are often found in the contralateral thyroid lobe. Certain risk factors for metastases to the cervical nodes have been identified for papillary microcarcinoma [56] and for the follicular variant of papillary thyroid carcinoma [16, 17] and include multifocality, angiolymphatic invasiveness, absence of tumor capsule, and extrathyroidal extension. Patterns of tumor spread from the thyroid to cervical lymph nodes have been identified and serve as guides for node dissection [57]. The clinical importance and prognostic significance of any lymph nodes involved with tumor will vary based upon their number, size, location, and the presence of extranodal extension [58]. Indeed, a recent study of patients with small nodes suspicious for metastasis demonstrated stability without progression and argued for conservative management by monitoring without aggressive interventional measures [59].

In the Mayo series [29] of 1,500 patients, the primary tumor was confined to one lobe in 71 %, bilateral in 19 %, and with multicentric lesions in 26 %. Cervical lymph node involvement was diagnosed in 38 % (573 of 1,500; median number of nodes = 4), and 2 % (32 of 500) had distant metastases at time of initial diagnosis. These findings are comparable to the series reported by Mazzaferri and Jhiang [60] in which 32 % of the tumors were multicentric and 43 % had nodal involvement. When the papillary cancer is more aggressive, as evident by vascular invasion [61] or widespread involvement throughout the thyroid gland, the likelihood of lymph node metastases is approx 75 %. This was seen frequently in the series of 129 patients reported by DeJong and associates [55] in whom 34 % had metastases to the ipsilateral jugular nodes, 41 % had bilateral jugular nodes, and 81 % had metastasis in the central compartment. In their total series of 243 patients with PTC, DeJong's group found that 21 % actually presented with lateral cervical nodes and no palpable thyroid nodule(s).

Patients presenting with palpable cervical lymph nodes at varying intervals after their original thyroidectomy should be evaluated for metastatic disease to the neck. The extent of the lymphadenopathy can be assessed easiest and usually best by ultrasonography [62], but computed tomography (CT) or magnetic resonance imaging (MRI) scans of the neck and mediastinum may also be useful. Such recurrent disease is usually suggested by rising levels of serum thyroglobulin (Tg) either basally or after recombinant human thyrotropin (rhTSH) administration [63–65] and in some cases can be predicted by the presence of positive preoperative BRAF analysis of the FNA material [66, 67] or the number of lymph node metastases or extranodal tumor extension [67]. The most specific diagnostic maneuver is an FNA aspirate of suspicious lymph nodes [68], and enlarged palpable lymph nodes can be readily aspirated with or without ultrasound guidance for cytological examination and Tg measurement of the aspirate.

Because these tumors are so frequently detected incidentally, it is obvious that most are asymptomatic. Symptoms arise only from increasing size and/or invasion. Symptoms commonly include a sense of fullness or pressure in the neck, as well as cough, dysphagia, or odynophagia. Occasionally, patients complain of an aching in the area of the involved lobe. The differential diagnosis of pain in the thyroid gland is not extensive, consisting of only three entities: invasive thyroid cancer, subacute thyroiditis, and hemorrhage within a nodule, tumor, or cyst.

Young (≤17 years old) patients may have metastases of PTC to the lungs [12, 69, 70], although the frequency appears to be decreasing. Patients with lung metastases may present with hemoptysis or dyspnea at rest or upon exertion. Pulmonary metastases were confirmed in one report by cytological examination after bronchoalveolar lavage [71]. Although PTC can metastasize to the lungs, follicular thyroid carcinoma is more likely to invade blood vessels and appear in distant sites, such as the bone and lung [72], and present with symptoms of local bone pain [73–75] and dyspnea, respectively. While pulmonary micrometastases may respond to radioiodine therapy, pulmonary macrometastases of PTC are typically difficult to completely eradicate with radioiodine therapy [76–78], and the best results were seen in younger patients with positive radioiodine uptake on scan (see Chap. 41). More rare sites for metastasis of PTC include the eyes and skin [79], and other rare sites for metastasis are described in Chap. 66. Initial presentation with distant metastasis heralds a very poor ultimate outcome with half of such patients dying of their disease within 5 years [78].

Patients with PTC only rarely present with local thyroid or cervical pain, in contrast to the patients with less differentiated more aggressive thyroid cancers. Involvement of the recurrent laryngeal nerve results in palsy of the ipsilateral vocal cord and hoarseness. The texture or consistency of a malignant thyroid nodule may be no different from that of a benign follicular adenoma; the classic, firm-to-hard consistency of a nodule of papillary cancer may be related to the nodule's content of calcium (psammoma bodies). Medullary cancers (in which calcifications are frequent) and anaplastic carcinoma are much harder on palpation than are well-differentiated tumors.

Management

Pacini and Castagna have provided a concise summary of the issues involved with the management of PTC [80], and McLeod et al. have written an excellent analysis of the controversies underlying management [81]. Virtually all patients with PTC presenting as a thyroid nodule are euthyroid; hence there is little need for routine thyroid function tests. Occasional patients with underlying Hashimoto's disease may have associated hypothyroidism, which is coincidental and not related to the tumor per se, as it is only the more aggressive anaplastic forms of cancer that replace so much normally functioning thyroid parenchyma to cause thyroid hypofunction. In patients undergoing thyroidectomy for either a benign cause or malignancy, there may be some advantage in knowing the preoperative levels of serum TSH and free thyroxine to have target levels for subsequent levothyroxine replacement therapy. However, such information is rarely pragmatic for the very early postoperative management of patients with malignant disease. This is so because both in the early management of thyroid cancer and more long-term in patients with persistent disease, the dosage of thyroxine therapy is selected to be suppressive, rather than for replacement, and thus the preoperative hormone levels are irrelevant. Interestingly, the likelihood that a given nodule is malignant correlates directly to the level of serum TSH [82–84], and thyroid cancer patients with elevated TSH levels may be more likely to have more advanced disease or evidence of extrathyroidal extension [85] at time of presentation.

Once the diagnosis is established, surgical thyroidectomy is the next step, which is usually a near-total to total thyroidectomy with or without central compartment (Level 6) ipsilateral dissection and exploration for enlarged lymph nodes, especially on the side ipsilateral to the nodule, as described in Chaps. 49 and 50 and in recent reviews [86–88]. A case may be made for lobectomy or subtotal thyroidectomy in certain circumstances [31, 89]. Central neck compartment dissection may be considered either as prophylactic or therapeutic depending on the aim of the surgery. Whether or not to do prophylactic Level 6 dissection as part of the initial thyroidectomy remains controversial [90–92] particularly because of the potential complications [90] especially in less skilled hands. On the other hand, the indications for a therapeutic or comprehensive Level 6 node dissection relate to persistent or recurrent disease [93]. Total thyroidectomy is associated with greater risk of complications (recurrent laryngeal nerve trauma with subsequent hoarseness or temporary to permanent hypoparathyroidism) but is more likely to result in a lower rate of recurrence, presumably from the removal of bilateral or multifocal foci of tumor. In earlier series, patients who underwent only lobectomy or subtotal thyroidectomy were said to have a 2.5-fold risk of death compared with those undergoing total thyroidectomy [94]. Prior attempts at modeling for life expectancy and quality-adjusted life years indicated that total thyroidectomy was the preferred procedure in both low- and high-risk patients with PTC [95], but current surgical guidelines have become more selective and individualized [31, 86, 87]. Dackiw and Zeiger [96] summarized the benefits of total thyroidectomy as:

- Radioiodine may be used to find and treat residual tissue or metastases.
- Serum Tg measurements can be used more effectively with all normal thyroid tissue excised.
- There is a 50–85 % chance of microscopic cancer in the contralateral lobe.
- Residual tumor could dedifferentiate into anaplastic cancer.
- Frequency of recurrence is reduced.
- Without total thyroidectomy, recurrence occurs in 7 % of patients, and 50 % of patients with recurrence may die from their disease.
- Improved survival statistics.
- Later surgery for recurrence is associated with more complications.

Clearly, there are compelling arguments for total thyroidectomy. However, patients with tumors of 1.5 cm diameter or less usually have an excellent prognosis after only a lobectomy with isthmusectomy, without postoperative radioiodine ablation of the residual contralateral thyroid lobe [31, 46, 47]. This includes the so-called incidental "microcarcinomas" (discussed below) that may be found in a thyroid gland resected for some other indication, such as Graves' disease or nodular goiter, and that tend to have an excellent prognosis. These tumors are often found in the thyroid at postmortem examination. Based on the findings at surgery, tentative staging may be considered, but the full assignment of stage is based on both the extent of disease, as determined by clinical, radiological, and pathological examinations, and patient age at presentation [97]. Appropriate staging is critical to optimal patient management. Staging of papillary cancer is discussed in Chap. 9. Whether or not to perform radioiodine ablation may be based upon the level of thyroglobulin postoperatively together with the findings on ultrasonography of the neck [31, 98].

The use of radioactive iodine for ablation postoperatively has been decreasing in recent years and with current practices being increasingly based on risk stratification [99]. Following thyroidectomy for papillary lesions that are greater than 2.0 cm, many physicians employ radioiodine in doses of 30–100 mCi to ablate residual tissue and facilitate follow-up monitoring [100, 101]. The degree of success with ablation depends on the dose of radioiodine administered [102]. Data from the early series of patients receiving 131I ablation of thyroid remnants indicated a subsequent significantly lower recurrence rate [103, 104]. However, the belief that such management is necessary and actually improves prognosis has been disputed [29] and remains a matter of some controversy [105–107]. A review of 2,638 patients by Ito et al. [108] demonstrated excellent outcomes for 10-year disease-free survival after thyroidectomy and elective node dissection alone without radioiodine ablation. When comparing differing results from studies, it is important to ask whether the patient populations were truly matched. Another retrospective analysis of 700 patients suggested that patients that were not treated with radioiodine ablation had a 2.1-fold greater risk of recurrence of their malignancy ($p=0.0001$) but no difference in death rates [94]. Several studies have been done that assessed the efficacy of radioiodine ablation after preparation with recombinant human TSH (rhTSH; Thyrogen®) rather than ablation during traditional thyroid hormone withdrawal and hypothyroidism ([109, 110]; see Chap. 27) and have been found to be just as effective for ablation [111–114] and associated with comparable long-term outcomes [98, 115]. Standard ablation doses as low as 30 mCi have been found to be perfectly adequate for ablation [112–114]. In earlier studies employing rhTSH for ablation, it was thought that higher doses were required because of the more rapid renal clearance of isotope in the euthyroid patient receiving rhTSH in comparison with the slowed renal clearance in hypothyroidism [110, 111]. rhTSH stimulation can be employed with dosimetric therapies with higher 131-I dosage activities [116], but it is not possible to achieve the same degree of iodide depletion in these patients because of the contribution to dietary iodine of the iodine in their levothyroxine or L-triiodothyronine medications. Notwithstanding the difference in biokinetics of radioiodine, dose selection with rhTSH preparation for ablation does not differ significantly from that administered after withdrawal [116, 117]. Minor but important differences in the surgical and radioiodine treatment approaches in children have been well summarized by Rivkees et al. [70] and in Chap. 42.

The postoperative follow-up of patients regarding thyroxine suppressive therapy and monitoring with periodic radioisotopic scans and serum Tg measurement is discussed in Chaps. 46 and 47 [118, 119]. Increasingly sensitive assays for Tg have revolutionized the approach to monitoring these patients [120]. Highly predictive insights into the risk of residual or recurrent tumors are provided by assays for Tg postoperatively and at 6–12 months subsequently [118, 121]. Measurement of serum Tg is not always feasible, however, because of the high prevalence of interfering anti-Tg antibodies in serum [122, 123]. When basal Tg levels are undetectable on levothyroxine suppressive therapy, 18–26 % of patients may still have occult tumor, which may be uncovered by Tg measurement after rhTSH stimulation [124]. Because papillary thyroid cancer may grow very slowly, patients may be mistakenly presumed to be free of disease when thyroglobulin levels are very low or even undetectable [125]. Establishing that a true cure has occurred is often only possible after several sequential rhTSH-stimulation tests [63]. Indeed, rhTSH-stimulated Tg is sufficiently sensitive that abandonment of diagnostic scanning has been advocated by some [126, 127] but not all centers and is especially useful when coupled with ultrasound of the neck [128, 129].

Another problematic area for clinicians is the therapeutic approach to documented residual or recurrent disease in the neck. With papillary thyroid cancer, this often will have been detected with the finding of enlarged, abnormal-appearing lymph nodes in the neck with tumor confirmed by ultrasound-guided FNA cytology. The prognosis of such patients has been shown to depend upon the age at recurrence, histology (e.g., tall cell variant), and the size and location of the recurrence [130]. Assuming that all patients had an initial total thyroidectomy and radioiodine ablation, whether or not a second surgical intervention for lymph node dissection is deemed successful may depend upon the definition of "cure," i.e., what level of thyroglobulin is achieved, suppressed, or stimulated. With lymph node reoperations, Al-Saif et al. [131] achieved a biochemically complete response in only 27 % of patients and then after several surgeries in some patients. Yim et al. [132] were more successful, achieving biochemical remission in 51 % after the first reoperation defined as a TSH-stimulated Tg of <1 ng/ml. The failures tended to have the highest preoperative Tg levels. While reoperation provides greater risk of adverse outcome to the recurrent laryngeal nerve or parathyroid glands, it has been pointed out that the alternative therapeutic approach of radioiodine also has significant side effects with repeated doses [133].

Detection of significantly measurable serum Tg or residual uptake with isotopic imaging generally leads to a search to better delineate the presence of tumors, e.g., additional imaging, to determine whether additional therapy is needed and the appropriate approach to further therapy. Because residual or recurrent papillary carcinoma presents most often in the neck, ultrasound examination of the neck has become the first choice for surveillance monitoring in both adults [32, 62, 98] and children [134]. Detection of residual or recurrent tumor prompts consideration for additional therapy. The choice of therapy will depend upon many factors including whether the disease is localized (and might be amenable to surgical excision) or is more diffuse and could be best treated with radioactive iodine (see Chaps. 33 and 34) When the choice is for radioiodine therapy, most centers employ relatively standard or empiric dosage of radioiodine, whereas a few more highly specialized thyroid cancer treatment centers also employ 131I dosage dosimetrically determined with either 131I [135–137] or 124I [138]. Dosimetric approaches have also been modified for children [139] and characterized in association with rhTSH administration [136, 140].

Unfortunately too often, tumor is identified but found not to trap tracer radioiodine, thereby likely excluding the possibility of therapy with radioiodine, although empiric therapy with radioiodine may be attempted [141, 142]. The clue to the presence of disease in such cases may be detectable or rising levels of serum thyroglobulin, and the management of the "radioisotope scan-negative but thyroglobulin-positive" patient is discussed in Chap. 47. The negative scans and loss of iodine uptake in these patients are presumed to be the result of dedifferentiation and loss of the sodium iodide symporter (NIS). An active area of research involved attempts to restore NIS and thus enable therapy in these patients. Very limited success has been achieved with various approaches to this "redifferentiation therapy" resulting in less enthusiasm for this approach that had been hoped earlier [143]. External radiation therapy [144] has been used with variable success for tumors that do not trap radioiodine or are resistant to such therapy. Targeted chemotherapy is another alternative in such patients [145–147].

Further discussion of aspects of follow-up and prognosis of papillary thyroid cancer follow in the chapters by Burch. The availability of rhTSH (Thyrogen®) [65, 148] has radically altered routine follow-up evaluations for residual or recurrent disease of patients after their initial management by thyroidectomy and radioiodine ablation. Although rhTSH is FDA approved for radioiodine ablation only and not therapy, studies have indicated comparable efficacy of preparation with rhTSH to withdrawal for treatment of patients with metastatic disease [149–151]. A full discussion of the application of rhTSH to management is in Chap. 10.

Malignant Thyroid Incidentaloma and Microcarcinoma

With the increasing use of imaging procedures of the head and neck, such as ultrasound, CT, or MRI, a large number of small thyroid nodules are being detected. These so-called incidentalomas (because of their incidental discovery during an imaging procedure) may be benign nodules but if malignant are most likely to be papillary thyroid microcarcinomas. These tumors may also be found during thyroidectomy performed for an indication other than tumor and can range in size from 2 mm to 1.5 cm in diameter and are usually nonencapsulated [152, 153]. These small tumors have been thought to have a clearly different natural history than larger lesions, appearing to remain biologically silent in most cases with minimal morbidity. This impression was supported by studies such as that by Hay and colleagues [153], representing a review of 900 microcarcinoma cases, of which the median tumor size was 7 mm and 98 % were histologically grade 1 tumors with no local invasion apparent in 98 % of the patients. However, three patients (0.3 %) had distant metastases at presentation, and an average of 30 % had positive nodes at presentation that correlated with higher risk of recurrence. The prognosis was nevertheless excellent after near-total thyroidectomy alone, irrespective of whether radioiodine remnant ablation was done, and only three patients died of thyroid cancer. The low frequency of malignancy in incidentally discovered small thyroid nodules and the excellent prognosis even if malignant, as implied by the experience of Hay et al., lead to some complacency and the development of fairly nonaggressive guidelines for management of incidental nodules [31, 46, 47]. Indeed, one long-term observational trial concluded that such small tumors could be safely followed without intervention unless there were signs of progression [154]. Based on the experience of other groups, these guidelines may prove to be too conservative to apply to all patients with microcarcinoma. For example, Hughes et al. [155] noted that although the most common tumor in patients >45 years of age is a microcarcinoma, a significant number are found to be Stage III or Stage IV with an associated worse prognosis. And Ross et al. [156] observed that recurrence rates were not unusual in microcarcinoma patients, particularly those presenting with lymph node metastases irrespective of whether radioiodine had been administered. Sometimes the microcarcinoma discovered may be one of the more aggressive variants, like the diffuse sclerosing type or tall cell variant. In such cases, the tumors are often associated with lymph node metastases and extrathyroidal extension even though the tumor is "only" a microcarcinoma [157]. Management strategies may need to differ based upon potentially three different types of presentation of papillary microcarcinoma [158].

Identification of malignancy within a small thyroid nodule may be facilitated with positron emission tomography (PET) [159]. PET scanning with 18F-fluoro-deoxyglucose (see Chap. 25) also has proven to be a useful procedure for the detection of residual or recurrent malignancy [160] and is based on the presence of an increased number of Glut transporters in cancer cells. With the increasing use of PET scans, incidental thyroid cancers are being detected at a greater frequency [161, 162]. A recent retrospective review of 299 patients with microcarcinoma [163] confirms that these small tumors should not routinely be considered to follow a benign natural history. In a series of 292 patients, persistent disease was found during follow-up in 77 (26 %), 68 patients had locoregional metastases, and ten had distant metastases. Fortunately, no patients died of their disease during follow-up, and tumor size was not predictive of relapse. Although the management of cancers less than 1.5 cm has often been either subtotal thyroidectomy or near-total thyroidectomy but without radioiodine ablation, the authors and those of an accompanying editorial [164] make a good case for total thyroidectomy followed by radioiodine ablation. Based on their experience, ablation would be warranted in those patients who were more likely to have recurrent or residual disease after thyroidectomy and included those with multicentric tumors, positive lymph node metastases, or vascular or capsular invasion. Notably, multifocality is no longer an indication for radioiodine ablation in the revised ATA guidelines, however [31]. Also instructive in this regard is a study from Japan in which 162 patients with papillary microcarcinoma on FNA elected to be conservatively followed without surgery, and 70 % had stable tumors during a follow-up period of just under 4 years [165]. Thus, the clinician is faced with conflicting data bearing on the potential management of the papillary microcarcinoma, and risk stratification is required to determine when more aggressive management is warranted [166]. Unfortunately, optimal management strategies that take all relevant factors into account (including costs of evaluation and therapy vs benefits of earlier cancer diagnosis) are not available, and properly controlled randomized studies are needed.

Current management trends for patients with papillary thyroid microcarcinoma (PTMC) of <1 cm are based upon a predicted excellent outcome without radioiodine ablation. Guidelines suggest that postsurgical ablation is not necessary for such small tumors and rather that the patients may be followed by monitoring serum thyroglobulin and performing periodic neck ultrasonography [31]. In this regard, Gallicchio et al. [167] report on a retrospective 14-month follow-up of 85 pT1 patients with PTMC who received ablation of whom 35 % were shown subsequently to have lymph node metastases on SPECT/CT. They suggest that perhaps we may have abandoned ablative therapy either prematurely or too broadly and that the criteria for or against ablation of these PTMC patients need to be reexamined. Similar caution was raised recently by Malandrino et al. [168] from a survey of two cancer registries, one in Sicily and one in the USA, from which the same proportion, i.e., 35 % of patients, were noted to have two or more risk factors for recurrence that included lymph nodes, multifocality, younger age, and extrathyroidal extension. The significance of lymph node metastases lies in their association with future recurrence. This issue was recognized in the most recent ATA guidelines [31] which, while not advocating radioiodine ablation for small tumors or even for multifocality, did leave the door open for ablation of those tumors with higher-risk features such as lymph node metastases, local invasiveness, or aggressive histologies such as tall cell, insular, or columnar variants of PTC.

It is conceivable that the selected cutoff size of 1 cm may be too arbitrary and can be further refined with better discrimination in regard to which PTMCs might be associated with lymph node metastases or subsequent recurrence. Thus, Lee et al. [169] proposed a tumor size of 7 mm as the cutoff point for PTMC having noted that tumors <7 mm were less likely to have aggressive features such as lymph node metastases (30.6 %) compared with larger tumors of 7–10 mm of which 47.8 % had central compartment lymph node metastases. Experience has taught us that the TNM pathologic classification of risk status is suboptimal or poorly applicable to many patients with thyroid cancer. Other recommendations for risk stratification that establish risk of recurrence or establish subsequent risk based on responses to initial therapy are becoming more useful [170, 171] and could be considered in the postoperative decision for or against radioiodine ablation. Even when the preoperative diagnosis is uncomplicated PTMC, a decision might be made to recommend radioiodine ablation postoperatively on the basis of either the operative findings (e.g., incomplete tumor resection, aggressive histologic type, etc.) or a higher than expected serum thyroglobulin. Such patients would be restratified from "low risk" to "intermediate risk" for whom RAI ablation serves to facilitate disease surveillance and offers some benefit in improving overall survival or reducing the risk of local relapse of disease.

What criteria or characteristics of PTMC might be useful as risk factors for recurrence? Male gender and lateral cervical node metastases were found by Kim et al. [172] to be associated with recurrence, and Zhang et al. [56] identified multifocality, male gender, tumor size >6 mm, and extrathyroidal extension as risk factors for lymph node metastasis. Their presence in patients with PTMC might warrant central neck lymph node dissection as well as subsequent radioiodine ablation. In the very near future, it is likely that we will be looking to some aspect of molecular mutational analysis of these tumors to determine which mutations in a microcarcinoma are associated with extrathyroidal extension, multifocality, or lateral neck lymph node metastases [173]. The group of Nikiforov et al. proposed risk stratification of patients with PTMC based upon their BRAF status [174], and as mentioned above, some studies [43, 44] but not all [40, 175] associate the presence of BRAF with more aggressive biological behavior. While the analysis of Gallicchio et al. implies some benefit of radioiodine ablation for PTMC, we should remain mindful that too aggressive therapy has pitfalls inherent in the potential adverse effects of radioisotope therapy [133, 173] and a balanced approach is required.

References

1. Toniato A, Boschin I, Casara D, et al. Papillary thyroid carcinoma: factors influencing prognosis. Ann Surg Oncol. 2008;15:1518–22.
2. Rivera M, Tuttle RM, Patel S, et al. Encapsulated papillary thyroid carcinoma: a clinico-pathologic study of 106 cases with emphasis on it morphologic subtypes (histologic growth pattern). Thyroid. 2009;19:119–27.
3. Vivero M, Kraft S, Barletta JA. Risk stratification of follicular variant of papillary thyroid carcinoma. Thyroid. 2013;23:273–9.
4. Siegel R, Naishadham D, Jemal A. Cancer statistics, 2013. CA Cancer J Clin. 2013;63:11–30.
5. Aschebrook-Kilfoy B, Schechter RB, Shih Y-C, Kaplan EL, Chiu BC-H, Angelos P, Grogan RH. The clinical and economic burden of a sustained increase in thyroid cancer incidence. Cancer Epidemiol Biomarkers Prev. 2013. doi:10.1158/1055-9965.EPI-13-0242.
6. Wartofsky L. Rising world incidence of thyroid cancer: increased detection or higher radiation exposure? Hormones. 2010;9:103–8.
7. Ain KB. Papillary thyroid carcinoma: etiology, assessment, and therapy. Endocrinol Metab Clin N Am. 1995;24:711–60.
8. Schlumberger MJ. Papillary and follicular thyroid carcinoma. N Engl J Med. 1998;338:297–306.
9. Guan H, Ji M, Bao R, Yu H, Wang Y, Hou P, et al. Association of high iodine intake with the T1799A BRAF mutation in papillary thyroid cancer. J Clin Endocrinol Metab. 2009;94:1612–7.
10. Chen AY, Levy L, Goepfert H, et al. The development of breast carcinoma in women with thyroid carcinoma. Cancer. 2001; 92:225–31.
11. Enomoto K, Enomoto Y, Uchino S, Yamashita H, Noguchi S. Follicular thyroid cancer in children and adolescents: clinicopathologic features, long-term survival, and risk factors for recurrence. Endocr J. 2013;60:629–35.
12. Hay I, Gonzalez-Losada T, Reinalda MS, Honetschlager JA, Richards ML, Thompson GB. Long-term outcome in 215 children and adolescents with papillary thyroid cancer treated during 1940 through 2008. World J Surg. 2010;34:1192–202.
13. Wada N, Sugino K, Mimura T, Nagahama M, Kitagawa W, Shibuya H, et al. Pediatric differentiated thyroid carcinoma in stage I: risk factor analysis for disease free survival. BMC Cancer. 2009;9:306.
14. Vriens MR, Moses W, Weng J, Peng M, Griffin A, Bleyer A, et al. Clinical and molecular features of papillary thyroid cancer in adolescents and young adults. Cancer. 2011;117:259–67.
15. Robbins J, Merino MJ, Boice JD, et al. Thyroid cancer: a lethal endocrine neoplasm. Ann Intern Med. 1991;115:133–47.
16. Blanchard C, Brient C, Volteau C, Sebag F, Roy M, Drui D, et al. Factors predictive of lymph node metastasis in the follicular variant of papillary thyroid carcinoma. Br J Surg. 2013;100:1312–7.
17. Yu X-M, Schneider DF, Leverson G, Chen H, Sippel RS. Follicular variant of papillary thyroid carcinoma is a unique clinical entity: a population-based study of 10,740 cases. Thyroid. 2013;23:1263–8.
18. Jain M, Khan A, Patwardhan N, et al. Follicular variant of papillary thyroid carcinoma: a comparative study of histopathologic features and cytology results in 141 patients. Endocr Pract. 2001;7:79–84.
19. Kesmodel SB, Terhune KP, Canter RJ, et al. The diagnostic dilemma of follicular variant of papillary thyroid carcinoma. Surgery. 2003;134:1005–12.
20. Burningham AR, Krishnan J, Davidson BJ, Ringel MD, Burman KD. Papillary and follicular variant of papillary carcinoma of the thyroid: initial presentation and response to therapy. Otolaryngol – Head Neck Surg. 2005;132(6):840–4.
21. Lloyd RV, Erickson LA, Casey MB, et al. Observer variation in the diagnosis of follicular variant of papillary thyroid carcinoma. Am J Surg Pathol. 2004;28:1336–40.
22. Morris LGT, Shaha AR, Tuttle RM, Sikora AG, Ganly I. Tall-cell variant of papillary thyroid carcinoma: a matched-pair analysis of survival. Thyroid. 2010;20:153–8.
23. Regalbuto C, Malandrino P, Frasca F, Pellegriti G, LeMoli R, Vigneri R, Pezzino V. The tall cell variant of papillary thyroid carcinoma: clinical and pathological features and outcomes. J Endocrinol Invest. 2013;36:249–54.
24. Roman S, Sosa JA. Aggressive variants of papillary thyroid cancer. Curr Opin Oncol. 2013;25:33–8.
25. van den Brekel MWM, Hekkenberg RJ, Asa SL, et al. Prognostic features in tall cell papillary carcinoma and insular thyroid carcinoma. Laryngoscope. 1997;107:254–9.
26. Prendiville S, Burman KD, Ringel MD, et al. Tall cell variant: an aggressive form of papillary thyroid carcinoma. Otolaryngol Head Neck Surg. 2000;122:352–7.
27. Volante M, Landolfi S, Chiusa L, et al. Poorly differentiated carcinomas of the thyroid with trabecular, insular, and solid patterns: a clinicopathologic study of 183 patients. Cancer. 2004;100:950–7.
28. Chao T-C, Lin J-D, Chen M-F. Insular carcinoma: infrequent subtype of thyroid cancer with aggressive clinical course. World J Surg. 2004;28:393–6.
29. Hay ID. Papillary thyroid carcinoma. Endocrinol Metab Clin North Am. 1990;19:545–76.
30. Ito J, Noguchi S, Murakami T, et al. Factors affecting the prognosis of patients with carcinoma of the thyroid. Surg Gynecol Obstet. 1980;150:539.
31. Haugen BR, Alexander EK, Bible KC, Doherty GM, Mandel SJ, Nikiforov YE, Pacini F, Randolph GW, Sawka AM, Schlumberger M, Schuff KG, Sherman SI, Sosa JA, Steward DL, Tuttle RM, Wartofsky L. 2015 American Thyroid Association Management Guidelines for Adult Patients with Thyroid Nodules and Differentiated Thyroid Cancer: American Thyroid Association Guidelines Task Force on Thyroid Nodules and Differentiated Thyroid Cancer. Thyroid. 2016;26:1–133.
32. Ito Y, Amino N, Miyauchi A. Thyroid ultrasonography. World J Surg. 2010;34:1171–80.
33. O'Connell K, Yen TW, Quiroz FF, Evans DB, Wang TS. The utility of routine preoperative cervical ultrasonography in patients undergoing thyroidectomy for differentiated thyroid cancer. Surgery. 2013;154:697–730.
34. Nikiforov YE, Yip L, Nikiforova MN. New strategies in diagnosing cancer in thyroid nodules: impact of molecular markers. Clin Cancer Res. 2013;19:2283–8.
35. Park YJ, Kim YA, Lee YJ, et al. Papillary microcarcinoma in comparison with larger papillary thyroid carcinoma in BRAF(V600E) mutation, clinicopathological features, and immunohistochemical findings. Head Neck. 2010;32:38–45.
36. Lim JY, Hong SW, Lee YS, Kim B-W, Park CS, Chang H-S, Cho JY. Clinicopathologic implications of the BRAF V600E mutation in papillary thyroid cancer: a subgroup analysis of f3130 cases in a single center. Thyroid. 2013;23:1423–30.
37. Elisei R, Viola D, Torregrossa L, Giannini R, Romei C, Ugolini C, et al. The BRAF V600E mutation is an independent poor prognostic factor for the outcome of patients with low-risk intrathyroid papillary thyroid carcinoma: single-institution results from a large cohort study. J Clin Endocrinol Metab. 2012;97:4390–8.
38. Guerra A, Fugazzola L, Marotta V, Cirillo M, Rossi S, Cirello V, et al. A high percentage of BRAF V600E alleles in papillary thyroid carcinoma predicts a poorer outcome. J Clin Endocrinol Metab. 2012;97:2333–40.
39. Kebebew E, Weng J, Bauer J, et al. The prevalence and prognostic value of BRAF mutation in thyroid cancer. Ann Surg. 2007;246:466–70.
40. Gandolfi G, Sancissi V, Torricelli F, Ragazzi M, Frasoldati A, Piana S, Ciarrocchi A. Allele percentage of the BRAF V600E mutation in papillary thyroid carcinomas and corresponding

lymph node metastases: no evidence for a role in tumor progression. J Clin Endocrinol Metab. 2013;98:E934–42.

41. Alzahrani AS, Xing M. Impact of lymph node metastases identified on central neck dissection (CND) on the recurrence of papillary thyroid cancer: potential role of BRAFV600E mutation in defining CND. Endocr Relat Cancer. 2013;20:13–22.
42. Li C, Lee KC, Schneider EB, Zeiger MA. BRAF V600E mutation and its association with clinicopathological features of papillary thyroid cancer: a meta-analysis. J Clin Endocrinol Metab. 2012;97:4559–70.
43. Li C, Han A, Lee KC, Lee LC, Fox AC, Beninato T, et al. Does BRAF V600E mutation predict aggressive features in papillary thyroid cancer? Results from four endocrine surgery centers. J Clin Endocrinol Metab. 2013;98:3702–12.
44. Xing M, Alzahrani AS, Carson KA, Viola D, Elisei R, Bendlova B, et al. Association between BRAF V600E mutation and mortality in patients with papillary thyroid cancer. JAMA. 2013;309: 1493–501.
45. Xing M, Haugen BR, Schlumberger M. Progress in molecular based management of differentiated thyroid cancer. Lancet. 2013;381:1058–69.
46. National Comprehensive Cancer Network (NCCN) Thyroid Carcinoma: clinical practice guidelines 2011. J Natl Compr Cancer Netw; Version 3.2011;5:568–621.
47. British Thyroid Association. Guidelines for the management of differentiated thyroid cancer in adults. Available at: www.british-thyroidassociation.org/guidelines.htm. 2nd ed. 2007.
48. Jankovic B, Le KT, Hershman JM. Hashimoto's thyroiditis and papillary thyroid carcinoma: is there a correlation? J Clin Endocrinol Metab. 2013;98:474–82.
49. Dvorkin S, Robenshtok E, Hirsch D, Strenov Y, Shimon I, Benbassat CA. Differentiated thyroid cancer is associated with less aggressive disease and better outcome in patients with coexisting Hashimotos thyroiditis. J Clin Endocrinol Metab. 2013;98:2409–14.
50. Modi J, Patel A, Terrell R, et al. Papillary thyroid carcinomas from young adults and children contain a mixture of lymphocytes. J Clin Endocrinol Metab. 2003;88:4418–25.
51. Mechler C, Bounacer A, Suarez H, et al. Papillary thyroid carcinoma: 6 cases from 2 families with associated lymphocytic thyroiditis harbouring RET/PTC rearrangements. Br J Cancer. 2001;85:1831–7.
52. Uchino S, Noguchi S, Kawamoto H, et al. Familial nonmedullary thyroid carcinoma characterized by multifocality and a high recurrence rate in a large study population. World J Surg. 2002;26: 897–902.
53. Alsanea O, Clark OH. Familial thyroid cancer. Curr Opin Oncol. 2001;13:44–51.
54. Pal T, Vogl FD, Chappuis PO, et al. Increased risk for nonmedullary thyroid cancer in the first degree relatives of prevalent cases of non-medullary thyroid cancer: a hospital-based study. J Clin Endocrinol Metab. 2001;86:5307–12.
55. DeJong S, Demeter J, Jarosz H, et al. Primary papillary thyroid carcinoma presenting as cervical lymphadenopathy. Am Surg. 1993;59:172–7.
56. Zhang L, Wei W-j, Q-h J, Zhu Y-x, Wang A-y, Wang y, et al. Risk factors for neck nodal metastasis in papillary thyroid microcarcinoma: a study of 1066 patients. J Clin Endocrinol Metab. 2012;97:1250–7.
57. Eskander A, Merdad M, Freeman JL, Witterick IJ. Pattern of spread to the lateral neck in metastatic well-differentiated thyroid cancer: a systematic review and meta-analysis. Thyroid. 2013;23:583–92.
58. Randolph GW, Duh Q-Y, Heller KS, LiVolsi VA, Mandel SJ, Steward DL, et al. The prognostic significance of nodal metastases from papillary thyroid carcinoma can be stratified based on the size and number of metastatic lymph nodes, as well as the presence of extranodal extension. Thyroid. 2012;22:1144–52.
59. Robenshtok E, Fish S, Bach A, Dominguez JM, Shaha A, Tuttle RM. Suspicious cervical lymph nodes detected after thyroidectomy for papillary thyroid cancer usually remain stable over years in properly selected patients. J Clin Endocrinol Metab. 2012;97: 2706–13.
60. Mazzaferri EL, Jhiang SM. Long-term impact of initial surgical and medical therapy on papillary and follicular thyroid cancer. Am J Med. 1994;97:418–28.
61. Falvo L, Catania A, D'Andrea V, et al. Prognostic importance of histologic vascular invasion in papillary thyroid carcinoma. Ann Surg. 2005;241:640–6.
62. Durante C, Filetti S. Management of papillary thyroid cancer patients in absence of postoperative radioiodine remnant ablation: tailoring follow-up by neck sonography. J Clin Endocrinol Metab. 2011;96:3059–61.
63. Klubo-Gwiezdzinska J, Burman KD, Van Nostrand D, Wartofsky L. Does an undetectable rhTSH-stimulated Tg level 12 months after initial treatment of thyroid cancer indicate remission? Clin Endocrinol. 2011;74:111–7.
64. Robbins RJ, Srivastava S, Shaha A, et al. Factors influencing the basal and recombinant human thyrotropin-stimulated serum thyroglobulin in patients with metastatic thyroid carcinoma. J Clin Endocrinol Metab. 2004;89:6010–6.
65. Klubo-Gwiezdzinska J, Burman KD, Van Nostrand D, Wartofsky L. Diagnostic and therapeutic use of human recombinant thyrotropin (rhTSH) (Thyrogen®) in well differentiated thyroid cancer – current indications and future perspectives. Curr Pharm Anal. 2010;6:1–14.
66. Joo J-Y, Park J-Y, Yoon Y-H, Choi B, Kim J-M, Jo YS, et al. Prediction of occult central lymph node metastasis in papillary thyroid carcinoma by preoperative BRAF analysis using fine-needle aspiration biopsy: a prospective study. J Clin Endocrinol Metab. 2012;97:3996–4003.
67. Ricarte-Filho J, Ganly I, Rivera M, Katabi N, Fu W, Shaha A, et al. Papillary thyroid carcinomas with cervical lymph node metastases can be stratified into clinically relevant prognostic categories using oncogenic BRAF, the number of nodal metastases, and extranodal extension. Thyroid. 2012;22:575–84.
68. Baskin HJ. Detection of recurrent papillary thyroid carcinoma by thyroglobulin assessment in the needle washout after fine-needle aspiration of suspicious lymph nodes. Thyroid. 2004;14:959–63.
69. Poorten VV, Hens G, Delaere P. Thyroid cancer in children and adolescents. Curr Opin Otolaryngol Head Neck Surg. 2013;21:135–42.
70. Rivkees SA, Mazzaferri EL, Verburg FA, Reiners C, Luster M, Breuer CK, et al. The treatment of differentiated thyroid cancer in children: emphasis on surgical approach and radioactive iodine therapy. Endocr Rev. 2011;32:798–826.
71. Mello CJ, Veronikis I, Fraire AE, et al. Metastatic papillary thyroid carcinoma to lung diagnosed by bronchoalveolar lavage. J Clin Endocrinol Metab. 1996;81:406–10.
72. Haugen BR, Kane MA. Approach to the thyroid cancer patient with extracervical metastases. J Clin Endocrinol Metab. 2010;95:987–93.
73. Farooki A, Leung V, Tala H, Tuttle RM. Skeletal-related events due to bone metastases from differentiated thyroid cancer. J Clin Endocrinol Metab. 2012;97:2433–9.
74. Wexler JA. Approach to the thyroid cancer patient with bone metastases. J Clin Endocrinol Metab. 2011;96:2296–307.
75. Muresan MM, Olivier P, Leclere J, Sirveaux F, Brunaud L, Klein M, et al. Bone metastases from differentiated thyroid carcinoma. Endocr Relat Cancer. 2008;15:37–49.
76. Sisson JC, Jamadar DA, Kazerooni EA, et al. Treatment of micronodular lung metastases of papillary thyroid cancer: are the

tumors too small for effective irradiation from radioiodine? Thyroid. 1998;8:215–21.
77. Ronga G, Filesi M, Montesano T, et al. Lung metastases from differentiated thyroid carcinoma: a 40 years' experience. Q J Nucl Med. 2004;48:12–9.
78. Nixon IJ, Whitcher MM, Palmer FL, Tuttle RM, Shaha AR, Shah JP, et al. The impact of distant metastases at presentation on prognosis in patients with differentiated carcinoma of the thyroid gland. Thyroid. 2012;22:884–9.
79. Avram AM, Gielczyk R, Su L, et al. Choroidal and skin metastases from papillary thyroid cancer: case and a review of the literature. J Clin Endocrinol Metab. 2004;89:5303–7.
80. Pacini F, Castagna MG. Approach to the treatment of differentiated thyroid carcinoma. Med Clin N Am. 2012;96:369–83.
81. McLeod DS, Sawka AM, Cooper DS. Controversies in primary treatment of low-risk thyroid cancer. Lancet. 2013;381:1046–57.
82. Boelaert K, Horacek J, Holder RL, Watkinson JC, Sheppard MC, Franklyn JA. Serum thyrotropin concentration as a novel predictor of malignancy in thyroid nodules investigated by fine-needle aspiration. J Clin Endocrinol Metab. 2006;91:4295–301.
83. Jin J, Machekano R, McHenry CR. The utility of preoperative serum thyroid-stimulating hormone level for predicting malignant nodular thyroid disease. Am J Surg. 2010;199:294–7.
84. Jonklaas J, Nsouli-Maktabi H, Soldin SJ. Endogenous thyrotropin and triiodothyronine concentrations in individuals with thyroid cancer. Thyroid. 2008;18:943–52.
85. Haymart MR, Repplinger DJ, Leverson GE, Elson DF, Sippel RS, Jaume JC, Chen H. Higher serum thyroid stimulating hormone level in thyroid nodule patients is associated with greater risks of differentiated thyroid cancer and advanced tumor stage. J Clin Endocrinol Metab. 2008;93:809–14.
86. Mazeh H, Chen H. Advances in surgical therapy for thyroid cancer. Nat Rev Endocrinol. 2011;7:581–8.
87. Dralle H, Machens A. Primary surgery for differentiated thyroid cancer in the new millennium. J Endocrinol Invest. 2012; 35:10–5.
88. Liao S, Shindo M. Management of well-differentiated thyroid cancer. Otolaryngol Clin N Am. 2012;45:1163–79.
89. Nixon IJ, Ganly I, Patel SG, Palmer FL, Whitcher MM, Tuttle RM, Shaha A, Shah JP. Thyroid lobectomy for treatment of well differentiated intrathyroid malignancy. Surgery. 2012;151:571–9.
90. Giordano D, Valcavi R, Thompson GB, Pedroni C, Renna L, Gradoni P, Barbieri V. Complications of central neck dissection in patients with papillary thyroid carcinoma: results of a study on 1087 patients and review of the literature. Thyroid. 2012; 22:911–7.
91. Mazzaferri EL, Doherty GM, Steward DL. The pros and cons of prophylactic central compartment lymph node dissection for papillary thyroid carcinoma. Thyroid. 2009;19:683–9.
92. Carling T, Carty SE, Ciarleglio MM, Cooper DS, Doherty GM, Kim LT, et al. American Thyroid Association design and feasibility of a prospective randomized controlled trial of prophylactic central lymph node dissection for papillary thyroid carcinoma. Thyroid. 2012;22:237–44.
93. Clayman GL, Agarwal G, Edeiken BS, Waguespack SG, Roberts DB, Sherman SI. Long-term outcome of comprehensive central compartment dissection in patients with recurrent/persistent papillary thyroid carcinoma. Thyroid. 2011;21:1309–16.
94. Loh K-C, Greenspan FS, Gee L, et al. Pathological tumor-node-metastasis (pTNM) staging for papillary and follicular thyroid carcinomas: a retrospective analysis of 700 patients. J Clin Endocrinol Metab. 1997;82:3553–62.
95. Esnaola NF, Cantor SB, Sherman SI, et al. Optimal treatment strategy in patients with papillary thyroid cancer: a decision analysis. Surgery. 2001;130:921–30.
96. Dackiw APB, Zeiger M. Extent of surgery for differentiated thyroid cancer. Surg Clin N Am. 2004;84:817–32.
97. American Joint Committee on Cancer. The thyroid gland. In: AJCC cancer staging manual. 6th ed. New York: Springer; 2002. p. 77–87.
98. Rosario PW, Xavier ACM, Calsolari MR. Value of postoperative thyroglobulin and ultrasonography for the indication of ablation and 131-I activity in patients with thyroid cancer and low risk of recurrence. Thyroid. 2011;21:49–53.
99. Wartofsky L, Van Nostrand D. Radioiodine treatment of well-differentiated thyroid cancer. Endocrine. 2012;42:506–13.
100. Heufelder AE, Gorman CA. Radioiodine therapy in the treatment of differentiated thyroid cancer: guidelines and considerations. Endocrinologist. 1991;1:273–80.
101. Bal CS, Kumar A, Pant GS. Radioiodine dose for remnant ablation in differentiated thyroid carcinoma: a randomized clinical trial in 509 patients. J Clin Endocrinol Metab. 2004;89:1666–73.
102. Van Nostrand D. The benefits and risks of I-131 therapy in patients with well-differentiated thyroid cancer. Thyroid. 2009;19: 1381–91.
103. Sacks W, Fung CH, Chang JT, Waxman A, Braunstein GD. The effectiveness of radioactive iodine for treatment of low-risk thyroid cancer: a systematic analysis of the peer-reviewed literature from 1966 to April 2008. Thyroid. 2010;20:1235–45.
104. Mazzaferri EL. Thyroid remnant 131-I ablation for papillary and follicular thyroid carcinoma. Thyroid. 1997;7:265–71.
105. Sawka AM, Thephamongkhol K, Brouwers M, et al. A systematic review and metaanalysis of the effectiveness of radioactive iodine remnant ablation for well differentiated thyroid cancer. J Clin Endocrinol Metab. 2004;89:3668–76.
106. Mazzaferri E. Editorial: a randomized trial of remnant ablation—in search of an impossible dream? J Clin Endocrinol Metab. 2004;89:3662–4.
107. Haugen BR. Editorial: patients with differentiated thyroid carcinoma benefit from radioiodine remnant ablation. J Clin Endocrinol Metab. 2004;89:3665–7.
108. Ito Y, Masuoka H, Fukushima M, et al. Excellent prognosis of patients with solitary T1N0M0 papillary thyroid carcinoma who underwent thyroidectomy and elective lymph node dissection without radioiodine therapy. World J Surg. 2010;34:1285–90.
109. Luster M, Lippi F, Jarzab B, et al. rhTSH-aided radioiodine ablation and treatment of differentiated thyroid carcinoma: a comprehensive review. Endocr Relat Cancer. 2005;12:49–64.
110. Robbins RJ, Tuttle RM, Sonenberg M, et al. Radioiodine ablation of thyroid remnants after preparation with recombinant human thyrotropin. Thyroid. 2001;11:865–9.
111. Robbins RJ, Larson SM, Sinha N, et al. A retrospective review of the effectiveness of recombinant human TSH as a preparation for radioiodine thyroid remnant ablation. J Nucl Med. 2002;43: 1482–8.
112. Schlumberger M, Catargi B, Borget I, Deandreis D, Zerdoud S, Bridji B, et al. Strategies of radioiodine ablation in patients with low-risk thyroid cancer. N Engl J Med. 2013;366:1663–73.
113. Mallick U, Harmer C, Yap B, Wadsley J, Clarke S, Moss L, et al. Ablation with low-dose radioiodine and thyrotropin alfa in thyroid cancer. N Engl J Med. 2013;366:1674–85.
114. Barbaro D, Boni G, Meucci G, et al. Radioiodine treatment with 30 mCi after recombinant human thyrotropin stimulation in thyroid cancer: effectiveness for postsurgical remnants ablation and possible role of iodine content in L-thyroxine in the outcome of ablation. J Clin Endocrinol Metab. 2003;88:4110–5.
115. Tuttle RM, Brokhin M, Omry G, et al. Recombinant human TSH-assisted radioactive iodine remnant ablation achieves short-term clinical recurrence rates similar to those of traditional thyroid hormone withdrawal. J Nucl Med. 2008;49:764–70.

116. Hänscheid H, Lassmann M, Luster M, et al. Iodine biokinetics and dosimetry in radioiodine therapy of thyroid cancer: procedures and results of a prospective international controlled study of ablation after rhTSH or hormone withdrawal. J Nucl Med. 2006;47:648–54.
117. Remy H, Borget I, Leboulleux S, Guilabert N, Lavielle F, Garsi J, Bournaud C, Gupta S, Schlumberger M, Ricard M. 131I effective half-life and dosimetry in thyroid cancer patients. J Nucl Med. 2008;49:1445–50.
118. Malandrino P, Latina A, Marescalco S, et al. Risk-adapted management of differentiated thyroid cancer assessed by a sensitive measurement of basal serum thyroglobulin. J Clin Endocrinol Metab. 2011;96:1703–9.
119. Zucchelli G, Iervasi A, Ferdeghini M, Iervasi G. Serum thyroglobulin measurement in the follow-up of patients treated for differentiated thyroid cancer. Q J Nucl Med Mol Imaging. 2009;53:482–9.
120. Smallridge RC, Meek SE, Morgan MA, et al. Monitoring thyroglobulin in a sensitive immunoassay has comparable sensitivity to recombinant human TSH-stimulated thyroglobulin in follow-up of thyroid cancer patients. J Clin Endocrinol Metab. 2007;92:82–7.
121. Toubeau M, Touzery C, Arveux P, et al. Predictive value for disease progression of serum thyroglobulin levels measured in the postoperative period and after (131)I ablation therapy in patients with differentiated thyroid cancer. J Nucl Med. 2004;45:988–94.
122. Spencer CA. Clinical utility of thyroglobulin antibody (TgAb) measurements for patients with differentiated thyroid cancers (DTC). J Clin Endocrinol Metab. 2011;96:3615–27.
123. Spencer CA, Petrovic I, Fatemi S. Current thyroglobulin autoantibody (TgAb) assays often fail to detect interfering TgAb that ca result in the reporting of falsely low/undetectable serum Tg IMA values for patients with differentiated thyroid cancer. J Clin Endocrinol Metab. 2011;96:1283–91.
124. Mazzaferri EL, Robbins RJ, Spencer CA, et al. A consensus report of the role of serum thyroglobulin as a monitoring method for low-risk patients with papillary thyroid carcinoma. J Clin Endocrinol Metab. 2003;88:1433–41.
125. Kloos RT. Thyroid cancer recurrence in patients clinically free of disease with undetectable or very low serum thyroglobulin values. J Clin Endocrinol Metab. 2010;95:5241–8.
126. Mazzaferri EL, Kloos RT. Is diagnostic iodine-131 scanning with recombinant human TSH useful in the follow-up of differentiated thyroid cancer after thyroid ablation? J Clin Endocrinol Metab. 2002;87:1490–8.
127. Robbins RJ, Chon JT, Fleisher M, et al. Is the serum thyroglobulin response to recombinant human thyrotropin sufficient, by itself, to monitor for residual thyroid carcinoma? J Clin Endocrinol Metab. 2002;87:3242–7.
128. Pacini F, Molinaro E, Castagna MG, et al. Recombinant human thyrotropin-stimulated serum thyroglobulin combined with neck ultrasonography has the highest sensitivity in monitoring differentiated thyroid carcinoma. J Clin Endocrinol Metab. 2003;88: 3668–73.
129. Antonelli A, Miccoli P, Fallahi P, et al. Role of neck ultrasonography in the follow-up of children operated on for thyroid papillary cancer. Thyroid. 2003;13:479–84.
130. Ito Y, Higashiyama T, Takamura Y, Kobayashi K, Miya A, Miyauchi A. Prognosis of patients with papillary thyroid carcinoma showing postoperative recurrence to the central neck. World J Surg. 2011;35:767–72.
131. Al-Saif O, Farrar WB, Bloomston M, Porter K, Ringel MD, Kloos RT. Long-term efficacy of lymph node reoperation for persistent papillary thyroid cancer. J Clin Endocrinol Metab. 2010;95:2187–94.
132. Yim JH, Kim WB, Kim EY, Kim WG, Kim TY, Ryu J-S, et al. The outcomes of first reoperation for locoregionally recurrent/persistent papillary thyroid carcinoma in patients who initially underwent total thyroidectomy and remnant ablation. J Clin Endocrinol Metab. 2011;96:2049–56.
133. Schuff KG. Management of recurrent/persistent papillary thyroid carcinoma: efficacy of the surgical option. J Clin Endocrinol Metab. 2011;96:2038–9.
134. Brignardello E, Corrias A, Isolato G, et al. Ultrasound screening for thyroid carcinoma in childhood cancer survivors: a case series. J Clin Endocrinol Metab. 2008;93:4840–3.
135. Van Nostrand D, Atkins F, Yeganeh F, et al. Dosimetrically determined doses of radioiodine for the treatment of metastatic thyroid carcinoma. Thyroid. 2002;12:121–34.
136. Klubo-Gwiezdzinska J, Van Nostrand D, Atkins FB, et al. Efficacy of dosimetric versus empirically determined prescribed activity of 131-I for therapy of differentiated thyroid cancer. J Clin Endocrinol Metab. 2011;96:3217–25. doi:10.1210/jc.2011-0494. jc 2011-0494.
137. Lassman M, Hanscheid H, Verburg FA, Luster M. The use of dosimetry in the treatment of differentiated thyroid cancer. Q J Nucl Med Mol Imaging. 2011;55:107–15.
138. Sgouros G, Hobbs RF, Atkins FB, et al. Three-dimensional radiobiological dosimetry (3D-RD) with 124-I PET for 131-I therapy of thyroid cancer. Eur J Nucl Med Mol Imaging. 2011;38 Suppl 1:541–7.
139. Verburg FA, Reiners C, Hanscheid H. Approach to the patient: role of dosimetric RAI Rx in children with DTC. J Clin Endocrinol Metab. 2013;98:3912–9.
140. de Keizer B, Hoekstra A, Konijnenberg MW, et al. Bone marrow dosimetry and safety of high 131-I activities given after recombinant human thyroid-stimulating hormone to treat metastatic differentiated thyroid cancer. J Nucl Med. 2004;45:1549–54.
141. Mazzaferri EL. Empirically treating high serum thyroglobulin levels. J Nucl Med. 2005;46:1079–88.
142. Ma C, Xie J, Kuang A. Is empiric 131-I therapy justified for patients with positive thyroglobulin and negative 131-K whole-body scanning results? J Nucl Med. 2005;46:1164–70.
143. Park J-W, Clark OH. Redifferentiation therapy for thyroid cancer. Surg Clin N Am. 2004;84:921–43.
144. Brierley JD. Update on external beam radiation therapy in thyroid cancer. J Clin Endocrinol Metab. 2011;96:2289–95.
145. Brilli L, Pacini F. Targeted therapy in refractory thyroid cancer: current achievements and limitations. Future Oncol. 2011;7:657–68.
146. de la Fouchardiere C, Droz JP. Targeted therapies and thyroid cancer: an update. Anticancer Drugs. 2011;22:688–99.
147. Takami HE. Current status of molecularly targeted drugs for the treatment of advanced thyroid cancer. Endocr J. 2011;58:151–3.
148. Duntas LH, Cooper DS. Review on the occasion of a decade of recombinant human TSH: prospects and novel uses. Thyroid. 2008;18:509–16.
149. Klubo-Gwiezdzinska J, Burman KD, Van Nostrand D, Mete M, Jonklaas J, Wartofsky L. Radioiodine treatment of metastatic thyroid cancer: relative efficacy and side effect profile after preparation by thyroid hormone withdrawal vs. recombinant human TSH. Accepted for publication. Thyroid. 2012;22:310–7.
150. Van Nostrand D, Khorjekar G, O'Neil J, Moreau S, Atkins F, Kharazi P, et al. Recombinant human thyroid stimulating hormone versus thyroid hormone withdrawal in the identification of metastasis in differentiated thyroid cancer with 131I planar whole body and 124I PET. J Nucl Med. 2012;53:359–62.
151. Klubo-Gwiezdzinska J, Burman KD, Van Nostrand D, Mete M, Jonklaas J, Wartofsky L. Potential use of recombinant human thyrotropin in the treatment of distant metastases in patients with differentiated thyroid cancer. Endocr Pract. 2013;19:139–48.
152. Burguera B, Gharib H. Thyroid incidentalomas. Prevalence, diagnosis, significance, and management. Endocrinol Metab Clin N Am. 2000;29:187–203.

153. Hay ID, Hutchinson ME, Gonzalez-Losada T, et al. Papillary thyroid micro-carcinoma: a study of 900 cases observed in a 60-year period. Surgery. 2008;144:980–8.
154. Ito Y, Miyauchi A, Inoue H, et al. An observational trial for papillary thyroid microcarcinoma in Japanese patients. World J Surg. 2010;34:28–35.
155. Hughes DT, Haymart MR, Miller BS, Gauger PG, Doherty GM. The most commonly occurring papillary thyroid cancer in the United States is now a microcarcinoma in a patient older than 45 years. Thyroid. 2011;21:231–6.
156. Ross DS, Litofsky D, Ain KB, et al. Recurrence after treatment of micropapillary thyroid cancer. Thyroid. 2009;19:1–6.
157. Kuo EJ, Goffredo P, Sosa JA, Roman SA. Aggressive variants of papillary thyroid microcarcinoma are associated with extrathyroidal spread and lymph-node metastases: a population-level analysis. Thyroid. 2013;23:1305–11.
158. Sugitani I, Toda K, Yamada K, et al. Three distinctly different kinds of papillary thyroid microcarcinoma should be recognized: our treatment strategies and outcomes. World J Surg. 2010; 34:1222–31.
159. Nilsson I-L, Arnberg F, Zedenius J, Sundin A. Thyroid incidentaloma detected by fluorodeoxyglucose positron emission tomography/computed tomography: practical management algorithm. World J Surg. 2011;35:2691–7.
160. Nahas Z, Goldenberg D, Fakhry C, et al. The role of positron emission tomography/computed tomography in the management of recurrent papillary thyroid carcinoma. Laryngoscope. 2005; 115:237–43.
161. Yun M, Noh T-W, Cho A, et al. Visually discernible [18F] Fluorodeoxyglucose uptake in papillary thyroid microcarcinoma: a potential new risk factor. J Clin Endocrinol Metab. 2010;95: 3182–8.
162. Kang HW, Kim S-K, Kang H-S, et al. Prevalence and risk of cancer of focal thyroid incidentaloma identified by 18F-fluorodeoxyglucose positron emission tomography for metastasis evaluation and cancer screening in healthy subjects. J Clin Endocrinol Metab. 2003;88:4100–4.
163. Pellegriti G, Scollo C, Lumera G, et al. Clinical behavior and outcome of papillary thyroid cancers smaller than 1.5 cm in diameter: study of 299 cases. J Clin Endocrinol Metab. 2004;89:3713–20.
164. Pearce EN, Braverman LE. Editorial: papillary thyroid microcarcinoma outcomes and implications for treatment. J Clin Endocrinol Metab. 2004;89:3710–2.
165. Ito Y, Uruno T, Nakano K, et al. An observation trial without surgical treatment in patients with papillary microcarcinoma of the thyroid. Thyroid. 2003;13:381–7.
166. Durante C, Attard M, Torlontano M, et al. Identification and optimal postsurgical follow-up of patients with very low-risk papillary thyroid microcarcinomas. J Clin Endocrinol Metab. 2010;95:4882–8.
167. Gallicchio R, Giacomobono S, Capacchione D, Nardelli A, Barbato F, Nappi A, et al. Should patients with remnants from thyroid microcarcinoma really not be treated with iodine-131 ablation? Endocrine. 2013;44:426–33.
168. Malandrino P, Pellegriti G, Attard M, Violi MA, Giordano C, Sciacca L, et al. Papillary thyroid microcarcinomas: a comparative study of the characteristics and risk factors at presentation in two cancer registries. J Clin Endocrinol Metab. 2013;98:1427–34.
169. Lee KJ, Cho YJ, Kim SJ, Lee SC, Kim JG, Ahn CJ, Lee DH. Analysis of the clinicopathologic features of papillary thyroid microcarcinoma based on 7-mm tumor size. World J Surg. 2011;35:318–23.
170. Tuttle RM, Rondeau G, Lee NY. A risk-adapted approach to the use of radioactive iodine and external beam radiation in the treatment of well-differentiated thyroid cancer. Cancer Control. 2011;18:89–95.
171. Castagna MG, Maino F, Cipri C, Belardini V, Theodoropoulou A, Cevenini G, Pacini F. Delayed risk stratification to include the response to initial treatment (surgery and radioiodine ablation) has better outcome predictivity in differentiated thyroid cancer patients. Eur J Endocrinol. 2011;165:441–6.
172. Kim TY, Hong SJ, Kim JM, Kim WG, Gong G, Ryu JS, et al. Prognostic parameters for recurrence of papillary thyroid microcarcinoma. BMC Cancer. 2008;8:296. doi:10.1186/1471-2407-8-296.
173. Wartofsky L. Management of papillary microcarcinoma: primum non nocere? J Clin Endocrinol Metab. 2012;97:1169–72.
174. Niemeier LA, Kuffner AH, Song C, Carty SE, Hodak SP, Yip L, et al. A combined molecular-pathologic score improves risk stratification of thyroid papillary microcarcinoma. Cancer. 2011; 118:2069–77.
175. Lee ST, Kim SW, Ki CS, Jang JH, Shin JH, Oh YL, et al. Clinical implications of highly sensitive detection of the BRAF V600E mutation in fine needle aspirations of thyroid nodules: a comparative analysis of three molecular assays in 4585 consecutive cases in a BRAF V600E mutation-prevalent area. J Clin Endocrinol Metab. 2012;97:2299–306.

30 Papillary Microcarcinoma

Victor J. Bernet

This chapter is focused on issues particularly germane to the management of patients with papillary microcarcinoma (PMC). The reader is referred to other chapters within this book as to issues related to papillary thyroid cancer in general.

The occurrence of PMC is frequently faced in the clinical care of patients with thyroid cancer. Data derived from the SEER database reveals a 2.4-fold rise in the incidence of thyroid cancer between 1973 and 2002 [1]. While the incidence of all variants of thyroid cancer appears to be increasing, new cases of papillary thyroid cancer account for the largest proportion in this rise [2]. World Health Organization guidelines define thyroid microcarcinoma as a malignancy less than 1 cm in size [3]. Reports indicate that the incidence of PMC has also risen from 19 % between 1945 and 1955 up to 35 % between 1995 and 2004 [4]. A more recent increase of 49 % (95 % CI, 47–51 %) in PMC rate has been noted for the time span between 1988 and 2002 [1]. Another report indicates that PMC in a patient older than 45 years has become the most common form of PTC in the United States [5]. Additionally, autopsy reports indicate that 6–36 % cases examined are found to have evidence for the presence of papillary microcarcinoma [6–8].

Similar for thyroid cancers >1 cm, the growing frequency of thyroid microcarcinoma cases is at least partly attributable to an enhanced detection related to the widespread use of thyroid ultrasound and other sensitive imaging modalities. However, as papillary thyroid cancers >2 cm in size are also more commonly diagnosed, increased detection alone does not appear to completely explain the upsurge in thyroid cancer cases. Papillary thyroid microcarcinoma may present in an "occult" or "incidental" manner. Unanticipated micro-foci of papillary thyroid cancer are commonly found during inspection of the thyroid gland following thyroidectomy. These foci of PMC are sometimes found in tissue outside the initial nodule of interest which may or may not have harbored a malignancy.

As cases of PMC are frequently encountered in clinical practice and as they are associated with a relatively benign course in comparison to larger papillary carcinomas, it is imperative to be familiar with the recommended management of PMC so as to ensure proper therapy while avoiding unnecessary and cost-ineffective interventions.

As previously stated, by definition, papillary microcarcinomas do not exceed 1 cm. The average size of these foci is reported to be about 6 mm [4]. Mutlifocality is discovered in about 30–40 % of cases and bilateral thyroid involvement is found in approximately 20 % of patients [9, 10]. Those patients >45 years of age may be at increased risk for development of bilateral disease [11]. Available data indicate that these multiple cancer foci may represent intraglandular metastasis or be independent foci of separate clonal origin [12]. Cervical lymphadenopathy is detected in between 25 % and 43 % of patients with PMC. The minute size of PMC tumors does not exclude the potential of extra-glandular disease. Extrathyroidal extension, typically microscopic, not gross invasion, is noted in about 15–21 %. Furthermore, it is reported that about 3.5 % of PMC cases are found to have vascular invasion, while distant metastases are relatively uncommon at a rate of 1.0–2.8 % [4, 9, 10].

As with papillary thyroid cancer tumors >1 cm, surgery plays an integral role in the management of PMC. Data indicate that the amount of thyroid resection required for an optimal outcome differs based of the presenting tumor burden. As all treatment modalities for thyroid cancer should be optimized as to improve outcome while minimizing risk, deciding on the appropriate extent of surgical excision is essential. In general, total thyroidectomy is associated with some increased risk for perioperative complications such as

V.J. Bernet, MD (✉)
Division of Endocrinology, Mayo Clinic,
4500 San Pablo Road, Jacksonville, FL 32224, USA
e-mail: Bernet.Victor@mayo.edu

L. Wartofsky, D. Van Nostrand (eds.), *Thyroid Cancer*, DOI 10.1007/978-1-4939-3314-3_30

hypoparathyroidism or recurrent laryngeal nerve injury in comparison to lesser degrees of thyroid resection. Therefore, it is imperative that a defined benefit, either in decreased morbidity or mortality, be proven to justify pursuing a total/completion thyroidectomy over a lesser extent of thyroid surgery such as lobectomy. The circumstances surrounding the discovery of the microcarcinoma will impact this decision process as well. For example, in cases where a PMC is discovered following a hemi-lobectomy +/− isthmusectomy, one must consider the benefits and risks associated with proceeding to a completion thyroidectomy in comparison to no further surgery. In patients with a residual thyroid lobe, there is concern for potential disease in the remaining thyroid tissue. Studies have revealed as high as a 20 % rate of contralateral lobe involvement even in instances when only a lone focus of PTC was evident by preoperative evaluation [9].

One must also weigh the impact that additional factors should have on surgical decision-making. The presence or absence of unifocal or multi-focal disease, cervical lymphadenopathy, distant metastasis, local invasion, extranodal invasion, aggressive subtypes of PTC (e.g., tall cell, columnar, insular, poorly differentiated, diffuse sclerosing, etc.); older age, gender, and family history of PTC and the existence of underlying Graves' disease should all be considered [13–17]. The existence of any of these abovementioned factors may provide varying levels of justification for proceeding with a more complete excision of thyroid tissue.

Available data strongly indicate that death related to papillary microcarcinoma is exceedingly rare being <1 %. Thus, with expected survival being excellent for PMC patients overall, proof of benefit for treatment interventions instead shifts toward achieving a reduction in morbidity. The results from studies addressing this issue yield somewhat conflicting results. The initial data from a report on 535 PMC cases found a reduction in recurrence rates with "bilobar resections" in comparison to unilateral procedures [18]. However, a later reanalysis of this same cohort as it reached 900 patients and a 60-year period of observation did not find any difference in recurrence rates related to the extent of surgery [4]. Another somewhat smaller study concurred with these findings as well [10]. Conversely, a study of 281 cases of papillary microcarcinoma monitored for 7.3 years discovered a noteworthy reduction in recurrence from 70 % in those patients who underwent less than a total thyroidectomy to 30 % after a total thyroidectomy [9]. The 20 2015 American Thyroid Association thyroid cancer guidelines recommend that patients with <1 cm micro-tumors need not undergo completion thyroidectomy especially when the tumor(s) is found to be intrathyroidal and unifocal and is without any lymph node involvement or metastasis [19].

Multifocality is of special interest as it appears to be associated with an increased risk for recurrent disease. Results from one study revealed that whereas only 1.2 % of patients with unifocal PTC developed recurrent disease, 8.6 % suffered recurrence when multifocal disease was present [9]. As multifocality appears to be associated with increased recurrence rates, it is important to understand if any management interventions can reduce this rate. The degree of thyroid resection has been assessed as a potential factor. Recurrence rates for patients with multifocality have been found to be only 2.3–5 % with total thyroidectomy, while the rates rose to between 8.2 % and 25 % in the case of lobectomy and/or isthmusectomy [9, 10]. However, patients with unifocal tumors undergoing lobectomy and isthmusectomy had only a 3–4 % recurrence rate [9, 20]. Data from the National Thyroid Cancer Treatment Cooperative Study Group Registry which included 611 patients with PMC revealed 6.2 % of patients having recurrent disease [20]. In those patients having a near-total thyroidectomy, recurrence rates were higher in the face of multifocality in comparison to unifocal disease. A trend of fewer recurrences with multifocal disease was found in patients undergoing total or near-total thyroidectomy than in those undergoing less extensive resection (6 % vs 18 %, $p=0.058$). Multifocality has been associated with an increased risk for locoregional lymph node involvement with up to a 5.6-fold increase in rate by at least one report [10]. Furthermore, while distant metastases are infrequent in PMC patients, multifocal disease tends to be present in the cases when it does occur [9].

In summary, multifocality is associated with a higher rate of recurrence. While the evidence is not definitive, total or near-total thyroidectomy appears to reduce the risk of recurrence in comparison to patients receiving less aggressive resection. AT A guidelines refer to multifocal PMC as low risk disease potentially manageable with lobectomy alone with pursuit of a total or completion thyroidectomy limited to selected cases. [19].

As previously mentioned, cervical lymph node involvement may be encountered in patients with PMC. The occurrence of lymph node distribution within the neck has been reported to be as follows: central neck (40.3 %), lateral neck (4.2 %), ispsilateral/paratracheal (37.5 %), pretracheal (11.1 %), superior mediastinal (5.6 %), and contralateral paratracheal (1.4 %) [21]. Cervical lymphadenopathy detected at presentation is associated with a lymph node recurrence rate of about 11–22 % in comparison to 0.8–6 % in node-negative patients [4, 20]. Patients with palpable cervical lymphadenopathy have been shown to have a recurrence rate of 16 % after therapeutic node dissection in comparison to only 0.43 % in those having undergone a prophylactic lymph node dissection instead [20]. Data from additional studies indicate around an 11-fold rise in risk for distant metastasis with the presence of cervical lymphadenopathy [10]. The degree of lymph node involvement may modify the risk for recurrence in PMC cases as well. Available data suggest that macroscopic lymph node involvement and/or the presence of extracapsular extension, tumor penetrating the lymph node capsule, holds a greater risk for recurrence than lymph node involvement noted microscopically alone [22]. PMC patients with ultrasonographically documented abnormal lymph nodes have been reported to have improved recurrence-free survival after modified radical neck dissection [23]. Patients found to have abnormal cervical lymph nodes preoperatively should undergo therapeutic central lymph node dissection, and if evidence of lateral lymph node disease is found, then dissection on the involved side should occur [19].

While Graves' disease has been associated with more aggressive disease in patients with tumors >1 cm, this trend is not apparent in cases of microcarcinomas [24]. Graves' disease patients with incidental PMC have been found to do somewhat better than controls with a respective 99 % versus 93 % disease-free follow-up over 20 years. Of note, these results are tempered by the fact that the Graves' patients underwent near-total thyroidectomy while lobectomy predominated in the controls. As far as cases of PMC, it is unclear that Graves' disease is actually associated with any significant negative impact on prognosis.

Radioactive iodine (RAI) ablation can be utilized to destroy any residual thyroid bed thyroid tissue following surgery, typically total or near-total thyroidectomy. RAI can also be used for its potential tumoricidal effect on persistent thyroid cancer cells within the thyroid bed or cervical lymph nodes. Destruction of any residual thyroid tissue by means of RAI simplifies thyroid cancer surveillance by improving the specificity of iodine whole-body scans and thyroglobulin levels. Nevertheless, an amassing body of data does not reveal RAI to improve disease specific survival or lower tumor recurrence for cases of low-stage, minimal-risk PTC. Furthermore, available studies appear to indicate that RAI may not hold any particular benefit until PTC tumors are >1.5 cm in size. The 2015 ATA and NCCN guidelines specify that patients with stage I disease (specifically those with tumors ≤1 cm which are intrathyroidal or microscopic and unifocal) should not receive RAI unless other high-risk features are identified [25]. The vast majority of PMC cases fall within this low-risk classification. The guidelines do stipulate that RAI can be considered in patients with additional risk factors such as multifocality, lymphadenopathy, local extension, or distant metastasis. However, two studies evaluating the efficacy of RAI in cases of PMC with multiple foci have not revealed any improvement in outcome [4, 20] So while patients with multifocal disease exhibit a greater rate of recurrence, ablation therapy with RAI has not been shown to reduce such recurrences. One large retrospective study actually reported a higher recurrence rate in patients having received RAI. However, the retrospective nature of this study leaves open the possibility of an undetermined selection bias for use of RAI possibly associated with a higher risk for recurrence independent of RAI.

In summary, without any clearly defined benefit, the use of RAI ablation for patients with PMC is generally not recommended especially in uncomplicated stage I–II patients. While guidelines leave open the use of RAI for cases of multifocality and/or cervical lymphadenopathy, data do not reveal any improvement in disease-free survival. Patients >45 years of age with T3/T4 disease related to locoregional extra-thyroidal extension should be considered for use of RAI. The presence of distant metastasis or frank local invasion indicating aggressive tumor behavior also is a valid reason to pursue RAI ablation/therapy.

TSH suppression by means of levothyroxine therapy has been a mainstay in the management of thyroid cancer patients for many decades. While data from a meta-analysis support that TSH suppression is associated with a reduction in PTC tumor recurrence in general [26], the benefit for PMC patients, especially for those with stage 1 disease, has not been shown. Data from the National Thyroid Cancer Treatment Cooperative Study Group report in 2006 did not show an overall survival benefit with TSH suppression in cases of stage I PTC. However, keeping TSH at the subnormal to undetectable range did show a benefit in stage II patients, and higher-risk patients had improved overall survival when TSH levels were suppressed to the undetectable range. Therefore, the degree of TSH suppression indicated in a particular case should be based on the documented stage of disease [24]. In targeting a TSH goal in PMC patients, a low-normal TSH of 0.5–1.0 mU/L appears reasonable for uncomplicated stage I patients, while a TSH goal of 0.1–0.5 mU/L is appropriate for stage II patients, and more aggressive TSH suppression to <0.1 mU/L should be considered in patients with stage III or IV disease [27]. When considering the use of TSH suppression, one must balance the potential benefits with the risks associated with prolonged TSH suppression on bone and cardiac health [28]. Those risks can be minimized by lowering thyroxine dosing and allowing the TSH goal to rise the longer the patient exhibits a disease-free state.

Patients with PMC tend to have excellent overall rates for both survival and disease-free state. The mortality rate reported with PMC is very low, averaging around 0.4–1.0 % [29]. Data from Chow et al. indicate an expected 10-year survival of 100 %, a locoregional failure-free survival of 92 %, and a distant metastasis-free survival of 97 % [10]. The size of the PMC primary foci may play a role in prognosis. At least one report indicates a higher recurrence rate when the primary lesions are >5 mm [30]. However, this association is not a consistent finding [9, 20]. The preliminary results from a meta-analysis of nine studies of PMC patients found that when the total size of all involved PTC micro-foci are >1 cm, then the risk of recurrence doubles in comparison to patients with unifocal lesions <1 cm in size [31]. The studies in this meta-analysis included mainly subjects from Asian populations, so further confirmation in other populations groups is necessary. Interestingly, incidentally discovered PMC tumors may have a lower rate of multifocality, extrathyroidal extension, lymph node involvement, and improved disease-free survival in comparison to those identified prior to surgery [32, 33]. This finding may partially be related to PMC tumor foci size.

Age >45 years, stage of disease pT3 and higher, and presentation with clinically apparent lymph nodes and gross extrathyroidal extension have all been associated with increased risk of recurrence [34]. Based on results from three reports, the distant metastasis rate appears to be very low in PMC patients ranging between 0.2 % and 2.85 % [9, 10, 20, 35]. PTC patients with distant metastasis, PMC cases included, have a significantly worse prognosis than those without evidence of extrathyroidal disease. Patients with PMC and distant metastasis should be treated with more aggressive intervention to include extent of surgery, use of RAI ablation/treatment, and the degree of TSH suppression.

Much promise is held for the potential use of molecular markers to determine prognosis in thyroid cancer. The BRAF V600E (valine to glutamate) point mutation has a prevalence of about 45 % in conventional PTC, and growing data suggest that BRAF-positive lesions tend to be more aggressive, although this is not universally the case [36]. The BRAF mutation has been reported to occur in PMC anywhere between 30 % and 65 % of cases [37]. At this time, some reports suggest that the BRAF mutation may be associated with a higher likelihood of cervical lymph node metastasis, extrathyroidal extension, and overall higher stage of disease, while some other studies have not confirmed these findings [38, 37]. One group has found that PMC patients can be separated into high, moderate, and low risk for extrathyroidal spread and recurrence by means of BRAF status in addition to the presence of three histopathologic characteristics: tumor fibrosis, superficial tumor location within the gland, and intraglandular spread/multifocality [39]. This promising discovery requires confirmation at present. Naturally, even more helpful would be a preoperative marker prognostic for long-term disease recurrence risk and which could be used to guide extent of surgery and additional management interventions. While much promise exists for such a tool, one has yet to be clinically applied and proven useful.

As previously mentioned, the majority of patients with thyroid microcarcinoma tend to do extremely well long term with low rates of recurrence. As a consequence, surveillance testing should be tailored to correlate with the extent of disease with the most aggressive follow-up regimens occurring in patients at higher risk for persistent/recurrent disease. When considering cancer surveillance in cases of microcarcinoma, one must account for the fact that the efficacy of various testing can be impacted by the extent of thyroid gland resection and whether or not post-thyroidectomy RAI has been utilized. As means of monitoring for recurrence, both serum thyroglobulin levels and radioiodine WBS are less specific in the presence of residual thyroid tissue. Many patients with PMC do not meet the recommended criteria for proceeding with ablation therapy, and some patients can be properly managed with lobectomy alone. Following a total/near-total thyroidectomy, slightly more than 50 % of the patients will have serum TG levels of <1 ng/ml, while the remainder will have TG levels >1 ng/ml with some rising up to 25 ng/ml after TSH stimulation [40]. Secondary to the aforementioned limitations with WBS and TG testing, the use of neck ultrasound, which is very effective in detecting local PTC recurrence, has become a valuable surveillance tool in patients with PMC. Ultrasound imaging can be used to detect locoregional disease within the cervical lymph nodes which is known as the most common area of recurrence in PTC. In low-risk patients, the combination of stimulated serum TG and neck ultrasound has been found to have a sensitivity of 96.3 % as well as a negative predictive value of 99.5 % [41]. Patients found to have suspicious-appearing cervical lymph nodes (enlarged and rounded in shape, with loss of the hyperechoic hilar signal and/or vascular flow in the lymph node periphery) should undergo further evaluation [42]. Fine-needle aspiration of suspicious lymph nodes can be performed as to assess for presence of cancer. Measurement of TG in aspirate washings can enhance the sensitivity for cancer as well [43]. However, ultrasound imaging has become more and more sensitive and incidental nonpathologic lymph nodes are commonly noted during surveillance imaging as well. Guidelines recommend fine-needle aspiration for lymph nodes with concerning ultrasound characteristics indicative for metastasis and a size greater than 5–8 mm in the shortest diameter [19].

After the initial diagnosis, more frequent monitoring should occur for the first 6–12 months and then testing can be spread out to longer intervals if the patient remains disease-free. The scope of testing should be based on the probability of disease being present. The National Comprehensive Cancer Network Practice Guidelines indicate that in select low-risk patients, surveillance ultrasound need only be done "if there is a reasonable suspicion for recurrence" [25]. Nevertheless, as recurrences in PMC can occur many years after initial management, some form of regular interval monitoring should continue long term.

In summary, patients with PMC as a group have an excellent prognosis with a very low disease-specific mortality. Age >45 years, multifocal disease, locoregional lymph node metastasis, gross extrathyroidal invasion, and distant metastasis are associated with an increased risk of recurrence. Lobectomy appears adequate for unifocal low-risk tumors, whereas total thyroidectomy should be considered in patients with presence of worrisome features. To date, RAI ablation has not been proven beneficial in uncomplicated cases of PMC and has not been shown to lessen recurrence in patients with multifocal disease. RAI can be considered in patients with stage II or higher disease and particularly in any PMC patients with higher-risk features. In uncomplicated cases of PMC, the TSH goal should be initially a level of 0.1–0.5 mU/L and can gradually be allowed to rise to 0.3–2.0 mU/L if the patient remains cancer-free. More aggressive TSH suppression is indicated in patients with persistent disease, other aggressive features, or distant metastases. Neck ultrasound and non-TSH-stimulated TG levels are effective surveillance tools, while stimulated TG levels and WBS should be reserved for patients having received RAI. Prognostic markers, such as BRAF tumor status, are likely to be further developed to permit separation of low-risk from high-risk cases and allow for more targeted treatment intervention in the later group of patients.

References

1. Davies L, Welch HG. Increasing incidence of thyroid cancer in the United States, 1973–2002. JAMA. 2006;295:2164–7.
2. SEER stat fact sheets: thyroid cancer, surveillance, epidemiology, and end results (SEER) program of the National Cancer Institute. 2013. Available at: http://seer.cancer.gov/statfacts/html/thyro.html. Last accessed 21 Nov 2013.
3. Hedinger C, Williams ED, Sobin LH. Histological typing of thyroid tumours. Second edition. No. 11 in: International Histological Classification of Tumours, World Health Organization. Berlin, Heidelberg, New York, London, Paris, Tokyo, Hong Kong: Springer-Verlag, 1988.
4. Hay ID, Hutchinson ME, Gonzalez-Losada T, McIver B, Reinalda ME, Grant CS, Thompson GB, Sebo TJ, Goellner JR. Papillary thyroid microcarcinoma: a study of 900 cases observed in a 60-year period. Surgery. 2008;144(6):980–7.
5. Hughes DT, Haymart MR, Miller BS, Gauger PG, Doherty GM. The most commonly occurring papillary thyroid cancer in the United States is now a microcarcinoma in a patient older than 45 years. Thyroid. 2011;21(3):231–6.
6. Sampson RJ, Key CR, Buncher CR, Iijima S. Thyroid carcinoma in Hiroshima and Nagasaki: prevalence of thyroid carcinoma at autopsy. JAMA. 1969;209(1):65–70.
7. Harach HR, Franssila KO, Wasenius VM. Occult papillary carcinoma of the thyroid. A "normal" finding in Finland. A systematic autopsy study. Cancer. 1985;56(3):531–8.
8. Lang W, Borrusch H, Bauer L. Occult carcinomas of the thyroid. Evaluation of 1,020 sequential autopsies. Am J Clin Pathol. 1988;90(1):72–6.
9. Baudin E, Travagli JP, Ropers J, Mancusi F, Bruno-Bossio G, Caillou B, Cailleux AF, Lumbroso JD, Parmentier C, Schlumberger M. Microcarcinoma of the thyroid gland: the Gustave-Roussy Institute experience. Cancer. 1998;83(3):553–9.
10. Chow SM, Law SC, Chan JK, Au SK, Yau S, Lau WH. Papillary microcarcinoma of the thyroid-prognostic significance of lymph node metastasis and multifocality. Cancer. 2003;98(1):31–40.
11. Ricci JA, Alfonso AE. Multifocal micropapillary thyroid cancer: a new indication for total thyroidectomy? Am Surg. 2012;78(11):1211–4.
12. Shattuck TM, Westra WH, Ladenson PW, Arnold A. Independent clonal origins of distinct tumor foci in multifocal papillary thyroid carcinoma. N Engl J Med. 2005;352(23):2406–12.
13. Mazzaferri EL. Management of low-risk differentiated thyroid cancer. Endocr Pract. 2007;13(5):498–512.
14. Lupoli G, Vitale G, Caraglia M, Fittipaldi MR, Abbruzzese A, Tagliaferri P, Bianco AR. Familial papillary thyroid microcarcinoma: a new clinical entity. Lancet. 1999;353(9153):637–9.
15. Stocker DJ, Burch HB. Thyroid cancer yield in patients with Graves' disease. Minerva Endocrinol. 2003;28(3):205–12.
16. Sanders LE, Rossi RL. Occult well differentiated thyroid carcinoma presenting as cervical node disease. World J Surg. 1995;19(4):642–6; 646–7.
17. Volante M, Landolfi S, Chiusa L, Palestini N, Motta M, Codegone A, Torchio B, Papotti MG. Poorly differentiated carcinomas of the thyroid with trabecular, insular, and solid patterns: a clinicopathologic study of 183 patients. Cancer. 2004;100:950–7.
18. Hay ID, Grant CS, van Heerden JA, Goellner JR, Ebersold JR, Bergstralh EJ. Papillary thyroid microcarcinoma: a study of 535 cases observed in a 50-year period. Surgery. 1992;112(6): 1139–46.
19. Haugen BR, Alexander EK, Bible KC, Doherty G, Mandel SJ, Nikiforov Y, Pacini F, Randolph G, Sawka A, Schlumberger M, Schuff K, Sherman SI, Sosa JA, Steward D, Tuttle RM, Wartofsky L. American Thyroid Association Management Guidelines for Adult Patients with Thyroid Nodules and Differentiated Thyroid Cancer. Thyroid. Ahead of print. doi:10.1089/thy.2015.0020 print version in Thyroid 26:1–133, 2016.
20. Ross DS, Litofsky D, Ain KB, Bigos T, Brierley JD, Cooper DS, Haugen BR, Jonklaas J, Ladenson PW, Magner J, Robbins J, Skarulis MC, Steward DL, Maxon HR, Sherman SI. Recurrence after treatment of micropapillary thyroid cancer. Thyroid. 2009;19(10):1043–8.
21. Roh JL, Kim JM, Park CI. Central lymph node metastasis of unilateral papillary thyroid carcinoma: patterns and factors predictive of nodal metastasis, morbidity, and recurrence. Ann Surg Oncol. 2011;18(8):2245–50.
22. Yamashita H, Noguchi S, Murakami N, Toda M, Uchino S, Watanabe S, Kawamoto H. Extracapsular invasion of lymph node metastasis. A good indicator of disease recurrence and poor prognosis in patients with thyroid microcarcinoma. Cancer. 1999;86(5):842–9.
23. Ito Y, Tomoda C, Uruno T, Takamura Y, Miya A, Kobayashi K, Matsuzuka F, Kuma K, Miyauchi A. Preoperative ultrasonographic examination for lymph node metastasis: usefulness when designing lymph node dissection for papillary microcarcinoma of the thyroid. World J Surg. 2004;28(5):498–501.
24. Kasuga Y, Sugenoya A, Kobayashi S, Masuda H, Iida F. The outcome of patients with thyroid carcinoma and Graves' disease. Surg Today. 1993;23(1):9–12.
25. National Comprehensive Cancer Network. Thyroid carcinoma. 2009. www.nccn.org/Professionals/physician_gls/PDF/thyroid.pdf. Accessed 1 Mar 2010.
26. McGriff NJ, Csako G, Gourgiotis L, Lori CG, Pucino F, Sarlis NJ. Effects of thyroid hormone suppression therapy on adverse clinical outcomes in thyroid cancer. Ann Med. 2002;34:554–64.
27. Pacini F, Schlumberger M, Dralle H, Elisei R, Smit JW, Wiersinga W. European Thyroid Cancer Taskforce. European consensus for the management of patients with differentiated thyroid carcinoma of the follicular epithelium. Eur J Endocrinol. 2006;154(6): 787–803.
28. Biondi B, Cooper DS. Benefits of thyrotropin suppression versus the risks of adverse effects in differentiated thyroid cancer. Thyroid. 2010;20(2):135–46.
29. Neuhold N, Schultheis A, Hermann M, Krotla G, Koperek O, Birner P. Incidental papillary microcarcinoma of the thyroid-further evidence of a very low malignant potential: a retrospective clinicopathological study with up to 30 years of follow-up. Ann Surg Oncol. 2011;18(12):3430–6.
30. Noguchi S, Yamashita H, Uchino S, Watanabe S. Papillary microcarcinoma. World J Surg. 2008;32(5):747–53.

31. Zhao Q, Ming J, Liu C, Shi L, Nie X, Huang T. What role does multifocality play in papillary thyroid microcarcinoma(PTMC)? Thyroid. 2011;21(S1):Abstract 92:42.
32. Pellegriti G, Scollo C, Lumera G, Regalbuto C, Vigneri R, Belfiore A. Clinical behavior and outcome of papillary thyroid cancers smaller than 1.5 cm in diameter: study of 299 cases. J Clin Endocrinol Metab. 2004;89(8):3713–20.
33. Ito Y, Higashiyama T, Takamura Y, Miya A, Kobayashi K, Matsuzuka F, Kuma K, Miyauchi A. Prognosis of patients with benign thyroid diseases accompanied by incidental papillary carcinoma undetectable on preoperative imaging tests. World J Surg. 2007;31(8):1672–6.
34. Cho JK, Kim JY, Jeong CY, Jung EJ, Park ST, Jeong SH, Ju YT, Lee YJ, Hong SC, Ha WS, Choi SK. Clinical features and prognostic factors in papillary thyroid microcarcinoma depends on age. J Korean Surg Soc. 2012;82(5):281–7.
35. Lin HW, Bhattacharyya N. Survival impact of treatment options for papillary microcarcinoma of the thyroid. Laryngoscope. 2009;119(10):1983–7.
36. Kebebew E, Weng J, Bauer J, Ranvier G, Clark OH, Duh QY, Shibru D, Bastian B, Griffin A. The prevalence and prognostic value of BRAF mutation in thyroid cancer. Ann Surg. 2007;246(3):466–70.
37. Xing M. BRAF mutation in papillary thyroid cancer: pathogenic role, molecular bases, and clinical implications. Endocr Rev. 2007;28(7):742–62.
38. Park YJ, Kim YA, Lee YJ, Kim SH, Park SY, Kim KW, Chung JK, Youn YK, Kim KH, do Park J, Cho BY. Papillary microcarcinoma in comparison with larger papillary thyroid carcinoma in BRAF(V600E) mutation, clinicopathological features, and immunohistochemical findings. Head Neck. 2010;32(1):38–45.
39. Niemeier LA, Kuffner Akatsu H, Song C, Carty SE, Hodak SP, Yip L, Ferris RL, Tseng GC, Seethala RR, Lebeau SO, Stang MT, Coyne C, Johnson JT, Stewart AF, Nikiforov YE. A combined molecular-pathologic score improves risk stratification of thyroid papillary microcarcinoma. Cancer. 2012 Apr 15;118(8):2069–77.
40. Torlontano M, Crocetti U, Augello G, D'Aloiso L, Bonfitto N, Varraso A, Dicembrino F, Modoni S, Frusciante V, Di Giorgio A, Bruno R, Filetti S, Trischitta V. Comparative evaluation of recombinant human thyrotropin-stimulated thyroglobulin levels, 131I whole-body scintigraphy, and neck ultrasonography in the follow-up of patients with papillary thyroid microcarcinoma who have not undergone radioiodine therapy. J Clin Endocrinol Metab. 2006;91:60–3.
41. Pacini F, Molinaro E, Castagna MG, Agate L, Elisei R, Ceccarelli C, Lippi F, Taddei D, Grasso L, Pinchera A. Recombinant human thyrotropin-stimulated serum thyroglobulin combined with neck ultrasonography has the highest sensitivity in monitoring differentiated thyroid carcinoma. J Clin Endocrinol Metab. 2003;88(8): 3668–73.
42. Sipos JA. Advances in ultrasound for the diagnosis and management of thyroid cancer. Thyroid. 2009;19(12):1363–72.
43. Pacini F, Fugazzola L, Lippi F, Ceccarelli C, Centoni R, Miccoli P, Elisei R, Pinchera A. Detection of thyroglobulin in fine needle aspirates of nonthyroidal neck masses: a clue to the diagnosis of metastatic differentiated thyroid cancer. J Clin Endocrinol Metab. 1992;74:1401–4.

Surgical Approach to Papillary Thyroid Cancer

31

Gerard M. Doherty

Papillary thyroid cancer has an excellent prognosis, with few deaths from disease compared to most solid tumors. The measures of quality intervention depend more upon outcomes other than survival, disease-free survival, quality of life, complications from therapy, and the need for ongoing surveillance or treatment, which are all interrelated. To be most effective by these measures, operative treatment for papillary thyroid cancer should be thorough without morbidity and tailored to the specific patient situation [1].

The goals of initial therapy for differentiated thyroid cancer as delineated by the American Thyroid Association are [1]:

1. To remove the primary tumor, disease that has extended beyond the thyroid capsule, and involved cervical lymph nodes
2. To minimize treatment-related morbidity
3. To permit accurate staging of the disease
4. To facilitate postoperative treatment with radioactive iodine, where appropriate
5. To permit accurate long-term surveillance for disease recurrence
6. To minimize the risk of disease recurrence and metastatic spread

Preoperative cervical ultrasound to evaluate the central and lateral cervical lymph node compartments is required prior to operation for thyroid carcinoma. This is necessary in order to identify involved lymph node compartments so that a thorough initial operation can be planned [2]. If there is imageable lymphadenopathy in the lateral compartment, then fine-needle aspiration of a lateral neck node with thyroglobulin measurement of the aspirate can determine the need for therapeutic neck dissection in that basin. Selective neck dissection based upon the levels of the involved lymph nodes should include any compartment involved.

For those with the very best prognosis (tumor <10 mm, normal lymph nodes, age <45 years), thyroid lobectomy is clearly adequate therapy. Patients with large (>4 cm) or metastatic tumors should have an initial operation that includes removal of the entire thyroid gland [3]. Patients with intermediate-sized tumors (1–4 cm) may be selected for therapy with either total thyroidectomy or thyroid lobectomy, depending upon risk factors for recurrence and plans for adjuvant radioiodine therapy. In addition, any lymph nodes involved by cancer based on preoperative or intraoperative assessment should be removed by complete compartmental dissection. The utility of prophylactic level 6 lymph node dissection for those patients with apparently uninvolved lymph nodes is controversial but may provide important prognostic information and may affect use of adjuvant therapy [4, 5]. The therapeutic benefit of prophylactic level 6 neck dissection is not clear.

Surgical Approach

The extent of the planned operation is dictated by the locations of disease. Known disease should be removed. A part of the controversy regarding management of the level 6 lymph nodes stems from the fact that they are difficult to image by ultrasound when the thyroid gland is in place. This compartment is opened during the operation (as the thyroid gland is also in the central neck); if there is no plan to remove the central neck nodes prophylactically, then they must be actively assessed intraoperatively to ensure a thorough operation. The value of total thyroidectomy includes removal of potential multifocal disease in the thyroid gland and preparation for postoperative radioiodine therapy. If a thyroid lobectomy alone is used to manage a thyroid carcinoma, then

G.M. Doherty, MD, FACS (✉)
Department of Surgery, Boston Medical Center, Boston University, 88 East Newton Street, Collamore Building Suite 500, Boston, MA 02118, USA
e-mail: dohertyg@bu.edu

L. Wartofsky, D. Van Nostrand (eds.), *Thyroid Cancer*, DOI 10.1007/978-1-4939-3314-3_31

radioiodine generally cannot be utilized. Similarly, the value of postoperative surveillance with thyroglobulin levels as a tumor marker is enhanced by total thyroidectomy.

This operation is best done under general anesthesia. Though many thyroid operations can be done using local anesthesia and sedation, the inclusion of central and lateral neck dissection makes this quite difficult. The key steps of the operation are listed in Table 31.1 and principles of safety in Table 31.2. Thyroidectomy can be complicated by infection, bleeding, and anesthetic reactions though these are quite unlikely. The more worrisome complications of thyroidectomy are nerve injury and hypoparathyroidism, both because they are more common and because they can cause permanent functional deficits for the patient.

The use of nerve stimulators and laryngeal muscle action potential monitors has been investigated as a tool to try to limit or avoid nerve injuries. The data do not currently support the mandatory use of these devices; however, many experienced surgeons now routinely use a nerve monitoring system intraoperatively [6].

Table 31.1 Key technical steps and potential pitfalls of total thyroidectomy

Key technical steps:
1. Low collar incision within or parallel to natural skin lines
2. Raise subplatysmal flaps
3. Separate the strap muscles in the midline exposing the thyroid gland
4. If using an intraoperative nerve monitoring system, expose the vagus nerve in the carotid sheath and confirm function of the monitor by stimulating the vagus nerve prior to exposure of the recurrent laryngeal nerve
5. Separate the lateral border of the thyroid gland from the strap muscles and carotid sheath; enter the avascular plane medial to the upper pole without damaging the cricothyroid muscle fascia; isolate and divide the upper pole vessels
6. Rotate the thyroid lobe anteriorly and identify the recurrent laryngeal nerve in the tracheoesophageal groove using the nerve monitoring system if available; dissect craniad along the nerve, separating from the thyroid, up to the cricothyroid muscle
7. Divide the ligament of Berry anterior to the passage of the nerve into the larynx
8. Separate the thyroid posterior surface from the trachea
9. Identify and inspect the parathyroid glands; re-implant them if their vascularity is in question
10. If using the nerve monitor, confirm unchanged function of the vagus nerve-recurrent laryngeal nerve-vocalis muscle system by stimulating the vagus nerve
Potential intraoperative pitfalls:
1. Injury to the recurrent laryngeal or superior laryngeal nerves
2. Injury to the parathyroid glands
3. Tumor invasion into surrounding structures, such as the larynx, trachea, esophagus, carotid sheath, or strap muscles

Table 31.2 Principles of safe thyroid dissection

(1)	Avoid dividing any structures in the tracheoesophageal groove until the nerve is definitively identified. Small branches of the inferior thyroid artery may seem like they can clearly be safely transected; however, the distortion of tumor, retraction, or previous scar may lead the surgeon to mistakenly divide a branch of the RLN
(2)	Identify the nerve low in the neck, well below the inferior thyroid artery, at the level of the lower pole of the thyroid gland, or below. This allows dissection of the nerve at a site where it is not tethered by its attachments to the larynx or its relation to the inferior thyroid artery
(3)	Keep the nerve in view during the subsequent dissection of the thyroid gland from the larynx
(4)	Minimize the use of powered dissection posterior to the thyroid gland
(5)	Treat each parathyroid gland as though it were the last one
(6)	Autograft any parathyroid glands that have questionable viability

Management of Complications

Nerve Injury

The main nerves adjacent to the thyroid gland that can be deliberately or inadvertently affected include the recurrent laryngeal nerve (RLN) immediately adjacent to the thyroid and the external branch of the superior laryngeal nerve. Damage to the RLN causes unilateral paralysis of the muscles that controls the ipsilateral vocal cord. Unilateral RLN injury changes the voice substantially in most patients and also significantly affects swallowing. Bilateral RLN injury causes paralysis of both cords and usually results in a very limited airway lumen at the cords. These patients usually have a normal-sounding speaking voice but severe limitations on inhalation velocity because of upper airway obstruction.

RLN paresis is usually temporary and resolves over days to months. If a unilateral paresis proves to be permanent, then palliation of the cord immobility and voice changes can be achieved with vocal cord injection or laryngoplasty. These procedures stiffen and medialize the paralyzed cord, in order to allow the contralateral cord to appose the paralyzed cord during speech. If both cords are affected, then the palliative procedures are more limited and involve creating an adequate airway for ventilation; improvements in voice quality are not likely, as there is no muscular control of the cord function.

About 10 % of patients have some evidence of RLN paresis after thyroidectomy; however, this resolves in most patients. About 1 % or fewer patients have permanent nerve injury when total thyroidectomy is performed by experienced surgeons [5].

The external branch of the superior laryngeal nerve (EBSLN) courses adjacent to the superior pole vessels of the thyroid gland, before separating to penetrate the cricopharyngeus muscle fascia at its supero-posterior aspect. The nerve supplies motor innervation of the inferior constrictor muscles of the larynx. Damage to this nerve changes the ability of the larynx to control high-pressure phonation, such as high-pitched singing or yelling.

To avoid damaging this nerve, the dissection of the upper pole vessels should proceed from a space where the nerve is safely sequestered under the cricopharyngeal fascia, to the superior vessels themselves, thus safely separating the nerve from the tissue to be divided.

Parathyroid Gland Injury

The parathyroid glands are small, delicate structures that share a blood supply with the thyroid gland. Their size and fragility expose them to damage during thyroidectomy. Avoidance of permanent hypoparathyroidism is far more desirable than treatment of it. This can be accomplished by preservation of the parathyroid glands on their native blood supply or autografting of parathyroid tissue to a muscular bed [7]. If the parathyroid glands cannot be preserved on their native blood supply, then transfer of the gland to a convenient grafting site can maintain function. For normal parathyroid glands, transfer to the sternocleidomastoid muscle provides a convenient vascular bed for autograft. The parathyroid gland must be reduced to pieces that can survive on the diffusion of nutrients temporarily, while neovascular ingrowth occurs over several weeks.

The symptoms of hypoparathyroidism are those of severe hypocalcemia. Patients have numbness and tingling in the distal extremities and around the mouth or tongue in the earliest phases. For mild hypocalcemia with tingling, oral calcium supplements (calcium carbonate, 500–1500 mg p.o., two to four times daily) are often sufficient to resolve the hypocalcemia. If supplementation beyond this level is necessary (as it is for most patients with severe hypocalcemia), then the addition of supplemental vitamin D (calcitriol 0.25–1.0 mcg daily) increases the gastrointestinal absorption of calcium. Hypocalcemia not controlled by oral supplements, or accompanied by severe symptoms such as muscle cramping, is best managed by intravenous calcium administration. Intravenous calcium gluconate is the only option for intravenous calcium supplementation (calcium chloride should never be used).

Permanent hypoparathyroidism requires lifelong support with calcium supplements and vitamin D analogues. Missing doses of the supplements will usually produce symptoms, of varying severity, and which, while manageable, are often quite bothersome for patients.

References

1. Haugen BR, Alexander EK, Bible KC, Doherty GM, Mandel SJ, Nikiforov Y, Pacini F, Randolph G, Sawka A, Shepard D, Sosa J, Tuttle RM, Wartofsky L. 2015 American Thyroid Association Management Guidelines for adult patients with thyroid nodules and differentiated thyroid cancer. Available online at Thyroid 25: DOI:10.1089/thy.2015.0020; print version in Thyroid 26:1–133, 2016.
2. Kouvaraki MA, Lee JE, Shapiro SE, Sherman SI, Evans DB. Preventable reoperations for persistent and recurrent papillary thyroid carcinoma. Surgery. 2004;136(6):1183–91.
3. Bilimoria KY, Bentrem DJ, Ko CY, et al. Extent of surgery affects survival for papillary thyroid cancer [see comment]. Ann Surg. 2007;246(3):375–81; discussion 381–374.
4. Doherty GM. Prophylactic central lymph node dissection: continued controversy [comment]. Oncology. 2010;23(7):603, 608.
5. Hughes DT, White ML, Miller BS, Gauger PG, Burney RE, Doherty GM. Influence of prophylactic central lymph node dissection on postoperative thyroglobulin levels and radioiodine treatment in papillary thyroid cancer. Surgery. 2010;148(6):1100–6; discussion 1006–1107.
6. Dralle H, Sekulla C, Lorenz K, Brauckhoff M, Machens A, German ISG. Intraoperative monitoring of the recurrent laryngeal nerve in thyroid surgery. World J Surg. 2008;32(7):1358–66.
7. Olson Jr JA, DeBenedetti MK, Baumann DS, Wells Jr SA. Parathyroid autotransplantation during thyroidectomy. Results of long-term follow-up [see comment]. Ann Surg. 1996;223(5):472–8; discussion 478–80.

Papillary Carcinoma: Cytology and Pathology

32

Zubair W. Baloch and Virginia A. LiVolsi

Introduction

Papillary thyroid carcinoma (PTC) is the most common thyroid cancer and endocrine malignancy, constituting 75–85 % of the malignant thyroid lesions in regions where iodine-deficient goiter is no longer present [1, 2]. It represents most of the thyroid cancers that occur in children and young adults, whether idiopathic or related to radiation. A small proportion is familial [3]. Generally, PTCs grow slowly and therefore behave in an indolent fashion and spread mostly by lymphatic vessels to regional lymph nodes. Vascular invasion is rare in papillary thyroid carcinoma and metastases outside the confines of neck are rare [4]. Both gross and microscopic features are varied, depending on cellularity, amount and type of stroma, architectural features, and the presence or absence of cystic degeneration. Cytologic and pathologic features of the more common variants of PTC are described in this chapter and in Chap. 80, 82, and 66 with clinical descriptions in Chap. 81.

Classic Variant

The *classic variant of papillary carcinoma* predominantly consists of true papillae, i.e., fingerlike projections with core-containing vessel(s) and connective tissue surrounded by tumor cells (Fig. 32.1). Few follicles intermixed with papillae are a common finding in this variant [1]. Minor cystic changes are common. The gross appearance is a firm opaque mass, usually poorly defined and with a granular or finely nodular-cut surface. Irregular scarring is typical, and foci of calcification can be found frequently. If part of the tumor is rich in colloid, this is translucent and gelatinous and has some resemblance to goitrous thyroid tissue or a colloid nodule. If there are numerous psammoma bodies, the tissue feels gritty, and it should be decalcified before paraffin embedding [2, 5].

In histological sections, the cells are larger than normal follicular cells and are cuboidal to low columnar (Fig. 32.2). The cytoplasm is typically amphophilic to slightly eosinophilic. Nuclei are relatively large (but vary somewhat in size), ovoid, and subtly irregular in shape and in their positions in the cells. Nuclear indentations/grooves and round intranuclear inclusions of cytoplasm are common, but these vary in number and degree in different tumors and in different parts of the same tumor. Nucleoli are usually small and situated close to the nuclear membranes (eccentric), along with the heterochromatin, thereby causing the nuclear membrane to seem "thick" and much of the interior of the nucleus to be "pale," "empty," "clear," or "ground glass" in appearance. Follicles may be colloid filled or empty and occur as micro- or macrofollicles. Many are abnormally shaped and may be elongated (almost tubular; Fig. 32.3). Papillae differ greatly in size and complexity (Fig. 32.1). Each papilla consists of a fibrovascular core that is covered by a single layer of cuboidal to low columnar cells. The longer papillae are typically twisted and slightly irregular [2].

Nearly all PTCs show positive immunoreactions for thyroglobulin (cytoplasmic) thyroid transcription factor (TTF-1) and cytokeratins (membranous and cytoplasmic). Psammoma bodies occur in about 40 % [5] and are lamellated round to oval calcified structures that represent the "ghosts" of dead papillae (Fig. 32.8). These are usually seen

Z.W. Baloch, MD, PhD (✉)
Department of Pathology & Laboratory Medicine, University of Pennsylvania Medical Center, Perelman School of Medicine, 6 Founders Pavilion 3400 Spruce Street, Philadelphia, PA 19104, USA
e-mail: balocj@mail.med.upenn.edu

V.A. LiVolsi, MD
Department of Pathology & Laboratory Medicine, University of Pennsylvania/Perelman School of Medicine, Philadelphia, PA, USA
e-mail: linus@mail.med.upenn.edu

L. Wartofsky, D. Van Nostrand (eds.), *Thyroid Cancer*, DOI 10.1007/978-1-4939-3314-3_32

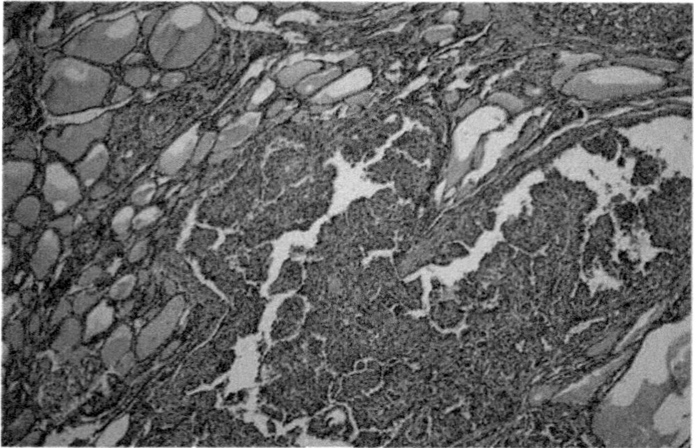

Fig. 32.1 Papillary carcinoma (classic pattern) invades the normal gland (H&E stain)

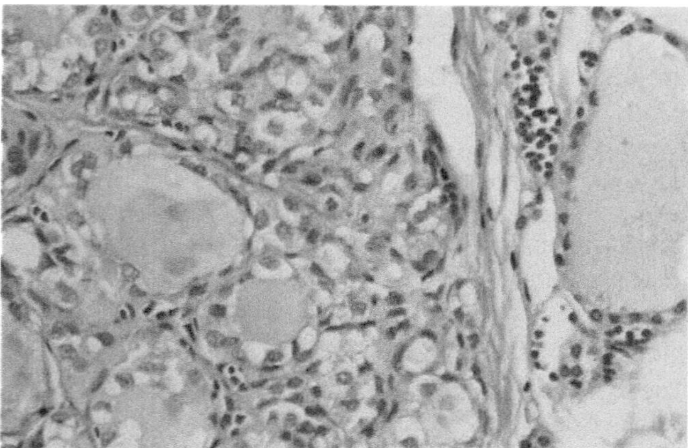

Fig. 32.2 Normal thyroid tissue lies to the right in the figure. Note that the cells of the cancer are much larger than the normal follicular epithelial cells (H&E stain)

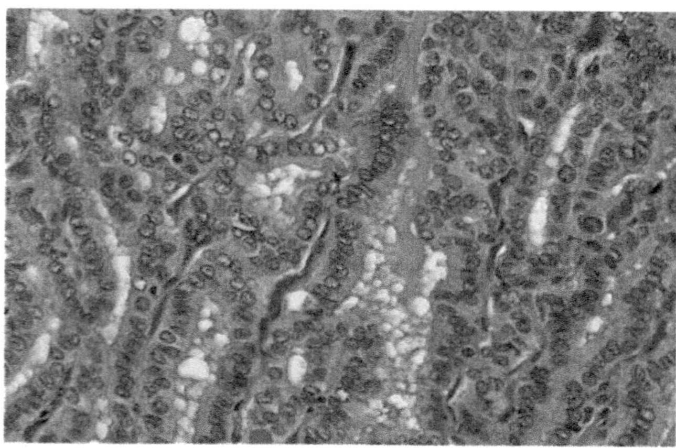

Fig. 32.3 Small papillae of the papillary carcinoma are crowded together, and follicular spaces are elongated (H&E stain)

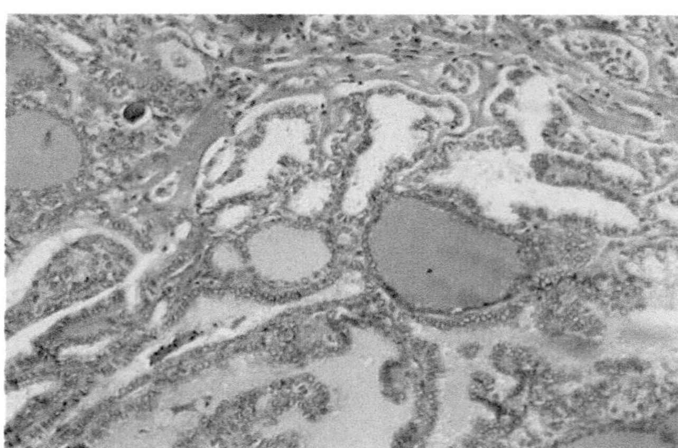

Fig. 32.4 A psammoma body lies in the upper left of the figure (H&E stain)

within the cores of papillae or in the tumor stroma of PTC; however, they can also be seen in intrathyroidal lymphatics representing intraglandular spread. Rarely psammoma bodies are found in benign conditions of the thyroid gland [6, 7]. The finding of psammoma bodies in a cervical lymph node is a strong indicator of a PTC in the thyroid [8]. Foci of irregular calcification (even ossification with rare cases showing bone marrow elements) are moderately common. The colloid may be dense or thin; dense colloid often appears "stringy" or globular. Fibrosis occurs in an erratic pattern, often as trabeculae or nodules of dense collagenous tissue [9]. A latticework of dense fibrous tissue often is present.

There may be many chronic inflammatory cells, mostly lymphocytes, within and around a PTC. The papillae may be filled with lymphocytes and/or histiocytes, often foamy histiocytes. Presumably, this inflammatory response is a reflection of the high incidence of the deposition of immunoglobulin G and complement factors on the cells of papillary carcinoma [10]. Histiocytes in the tumor may contain lipofuscin and/or hemosiderin, particularly when hemorrhage and/or cystic change is present. Foreign-body-type giant cells (multinucleated histiocytes) are moderately frequent in the classic papillary carcinomas. Some may be closely associated with psammoma bodies (Fig. 32.4).

Papillary carcinoma can also present as multifocal tumors within the same gland [2]. It has been shown that papillary carcinomas are clonal proliferations. Recent RET/PTC and LOH studies have shown that multifocal papillary microcarcinomas can represent separate primary cancers instead of intraglandular spread from one tumor source [11, 12]. Venous invasion can be identified in up to 7 % of papillary cancers [13]. Regional lymph node metastases are extremely common (50 % of more) at initial presentation of usual papillary cancer [14]. The histology of the nodal metastases in papillary can-

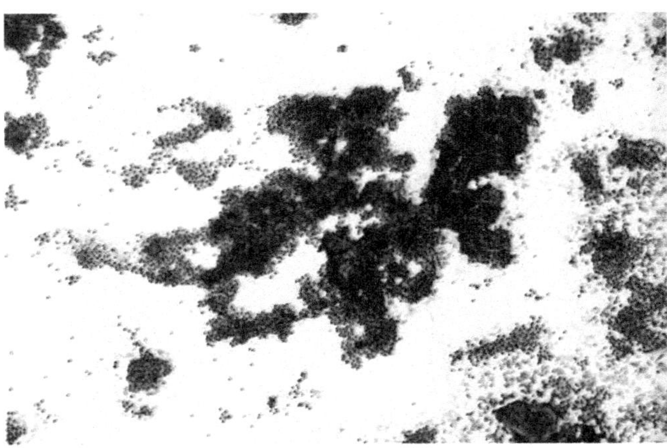

Fig. 32.5 Aspirate showing papillary tissue fragments of the papillary carcinoma (Diff-Quik stain)

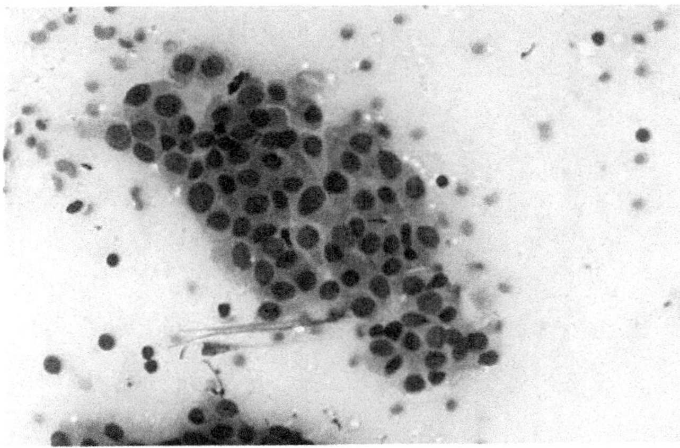

Fig. 32.6 Aspirate of a papillary carcinoma showing neoplastic cells with variation in nuclear sizes (Diff-Quik stain)

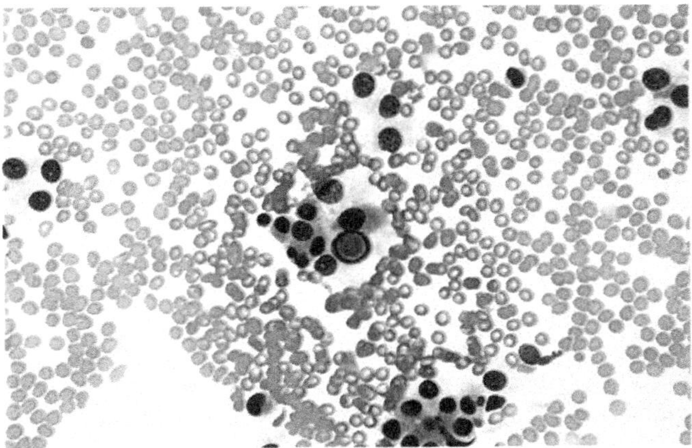

Fig. 32.7 Aspirate of a papillary carcinoma showing "intranuclear cytoplasmic pseudoinclusion" in large nucleus in the center of the field (Diff-Quik stain, low magnification)

cer may appear papillary, mixed, or follicular. This feature does not adversely affect long-term prognosis [2, 15]. Tumor grading is of no use in PTC since over 95 % of these tumors are grade 1 [16]. It has been recommended that adverse histological features such as numerous mitotic figures, abnormal mitoses, and tumor necrosis in a tumor that demonstrates a papillary growth pattern should warrant a diagnosis of a high-grade or poorly differentiated papillary carcinoma [16]. In some tumors, either in the primary site or in recurrences, transformation to poorly differentiated carcinoma can occur. This change is characterized by solid growth of tumor and mitotic activity, and cytologic atypia can be found. Such lesions have a much more guarded prognosis [17]. Anaplastic transformation in a papillary cancer can occur, although it is uncommon [18]. Distant metastases of papillary carcinoma to the lungs, bones, and brain occur in 5–7 % of cases [19].

By immunohistochemistry PTCs express thyroglobulin and TTF1 and not calcitonin [20]. From an extensive list of these immunohistochemical markers, the ones that have shown some promise include cytokeratin19, HBME1, and Glacetin3 [21–26]. However, none of these have proven to be specific since all can be expressed in some benign lesions of thyroid. Multiple foci of cancer cells are common in the thyroid, both as spread through the lymphatic vessels and as several simultaneous primary sites. Cervical lymph nodes are the most typical sites of metastatic foci.

The cytologic preparations of PTC contain large numbers of cells ("tumor cellularity"). Tight clusters of neoplastic cells—some in a papillary arrangement (Fig. 32.5)—and single cells are observed. The cell groups may show a typical concentric arrangements of lesional cells described as "cellular swirls." These tumor cells have enlarged and oval nuclei (at least twice the size of red blood cells; Fig. 32.6), dense chromatin, distinct nuclear borders on occasion showing nuclear membrane irregularities, and variable shapes (round, ovoid, and triangular). Nucleoli are seldom seen. Nuclear "grooves" are rarely evident in smears stained with Diff-Quik and Papanicolaou-stained preparations. Intranuclear cytoplasmic inclusions are seen frequently (Figs. 32.7 and 32.8); these usually appear as sharply demarcated punched out holes in the nucleus. The cytoplasm is usually dense and well demarcated. Colloid may range from scarce to abundant, appearing as thick strands ("ropy" or "bubblegum" colloid) (Figs. 32.9 and 32.10), irregular masses, or dense balls that stain bright pink (Fig. 32.10) to lavender. Psammoma bodies often are seen (Fig. 32.11). Multinucleated histiocytes are commonly a conspicuous feature ([27]; Fig. 32.12).

Follicular Variant

A diagnosis of the follicular variant of papillary carcinoma (FVPTC) may be made when more than 90 % of the histological pattern is composed of neoplastic follicles lined by

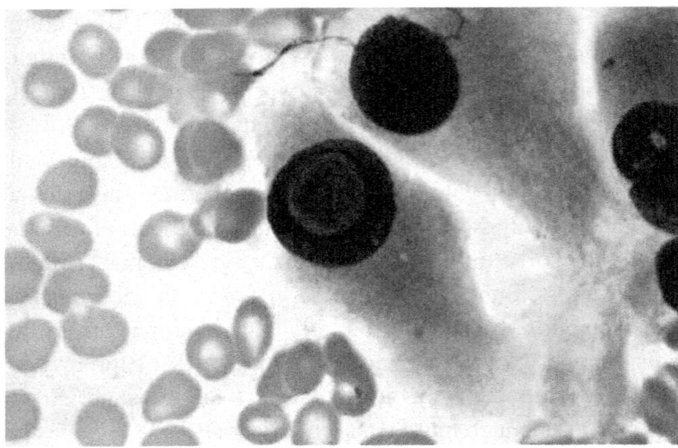

Fig. 32.8 Aspirate of a papillary carcinoma showing "intranuclear cytoplasmic pseudoinclusion" (Diff-Quik stain, high magnification)

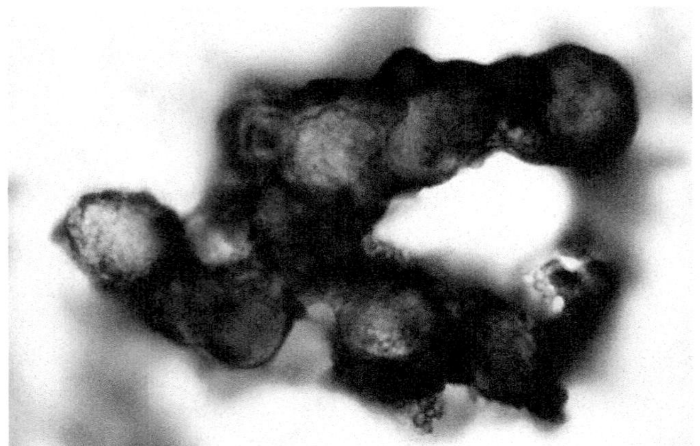

Fig. 32.11 Papillary carcinoma aspirate showing psammoma bodies (Diff-Quik stain)

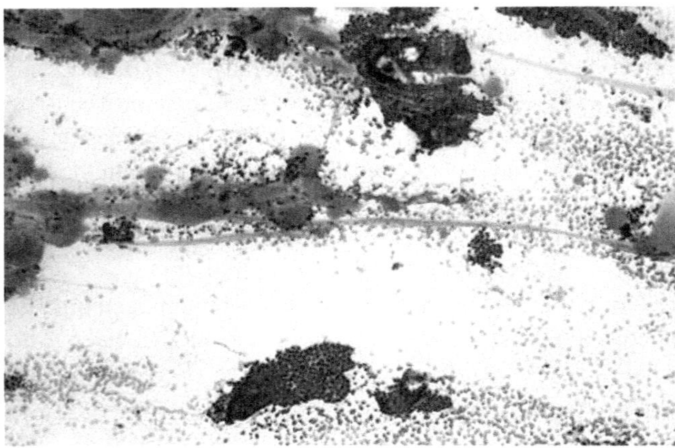

Fig. 32.9 Aspirate of a papillary carcinoma showing bubble gum (chewing gum or ropy) colloid (Diff-Quik stain)

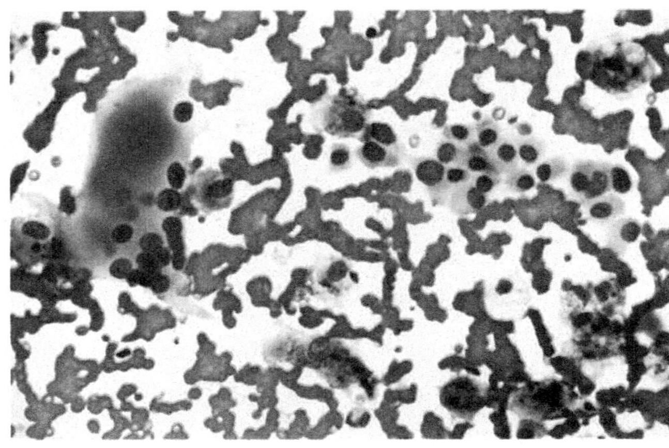

Fig. 32.12 Multinucleated histiocyte (on the *left*) and neoplastic cells of a papillary carcinoma. Many erythrocytes lie in the background of the smear (Diff-Quik stain)

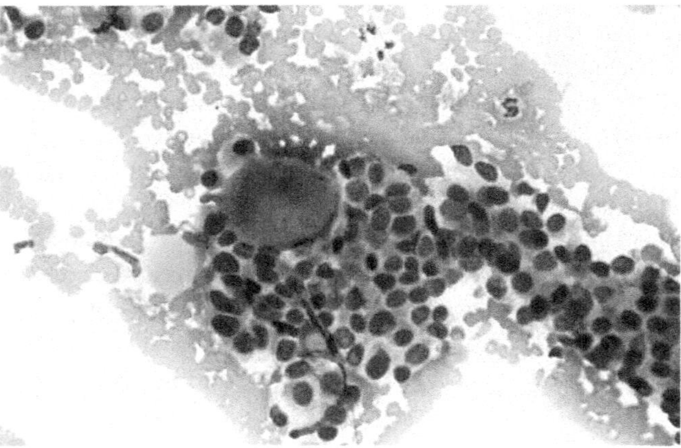

Fig. 32.10 Papillary carcinoma. Aspirate showing neoplastic cells surrounding colloid, which appears as a "pink ball" (Diff-Quik stain)

cells demonstrating diagnostic nuclear morphology of PTC (Fig. 32.13). Three distinct types of follicular variant include the infiltrative type, the diffuse follicular variant, and the encapsulated follicular variant. In the infiltrative type, the tumor which is a solitary mass or nodule is unencapsulated and invades the surrounding thyroid gland. Lymphatic invasion, nodal metastases, and extraglandular extension are common (almost as common as classic papillary carcinoma). In the diffuse follicular variant, the gland is diffusely replaced by tumor [28, 29]. Lymph node and distant metastases are common in these patients. The prognosis appears to be poor in these patients, although only a handful of cases have been described [29, 30]. If follicles in a FVPTC are small and contain little colloid, and if papillae are tiny and scarce, the tumor will appear fleshy and opaque on gross examination; it

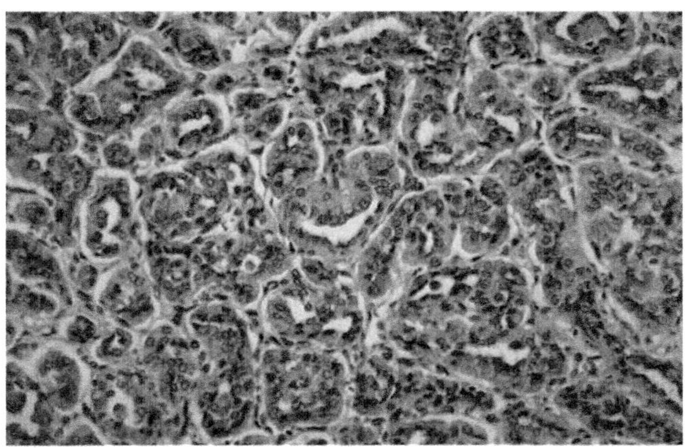

Fig. 32.13 Papillary carcinoma, follicular pattern. The nuclei are irregular in shape, size, and in their position in the cells. Follicles are tiny and generally appear empty (H&E stain)

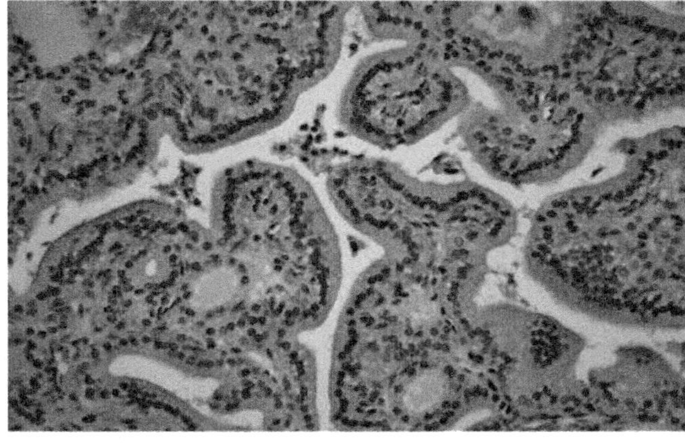

Fig. 32.15 Benign adenomatoid nodule with papillae. Compare these regular nuclei with those of papillary carcinoma in the other figures (H&E stain)

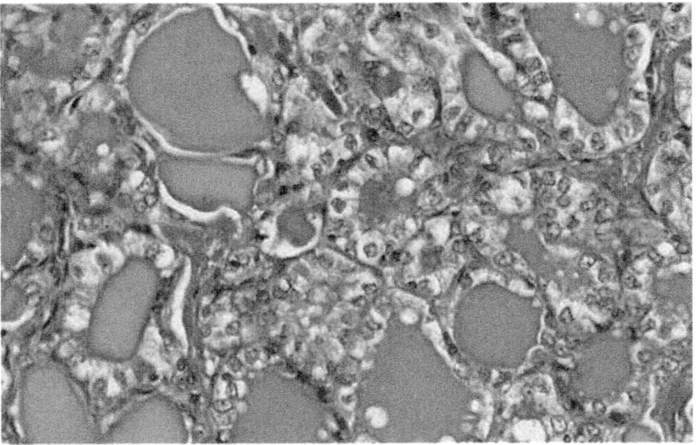

Fig. 32.14 Papillary carcinoma, follicular pattern. Much colloid is present, and the irregularity of the nuclei readily apparent (H&E stain)

may be misclassified as a follicular adenoma or follicular carcinoma on microscopic examination. If most follicles are medium to large sized, and there is abundant colloid (Fig. 32.14), then the tumor resembles an adenomatoid nodule or macrofollicular adenoma (macrofollicular variant), both grossly and microscopically; it may be mistaken for an adenomatoid nodule (Fig. 32.15).

The encapsulated follicular variant is characterized by the presence of a capsule around the lesion [31, 32]. Encapsulated FVPTCs are associated with an excellent prognosis [28]. In some cases, the diagnosis of this particular variant of papillary carcinoma can be difficult due to presence of multifocal rather than diffuse distribution of nuclear features of papillary thyroid carcinoma. Because of this peculiar morphologic presentation, these tumors can be misdiagnosed as adenomatoid nodule or follicular adenoma [28, 33]. Some authors have suggested that these tumors be classified as "tumors of undetermined malignant potential" due to excellent prognosis [34]; however, others have shown that some cases belonging in this category can lead to distant metastasis [32].

It is now well documented that FVPTC does share some morphologic and clinical features with follicular carcinoma. This has also been confirmed by gene expression profiling studies and comparative genomic hybridization analysis; RAS gene mutation, an abnormality seen in follicular adenoma and carcinoma, is exclusively seen in FVPTC and not in classic PTC [35, 36] in the papillary carcinoma group; similarly RET gene translocations and BRAF mutations which are common in classic PTC are rare in cases of FVPTC [35–37]. Therefore, in view of morphologic features, clinical behavior, and molecular analysis, encapsulated FVPTC most likely is a hybrid of papillary carcinoma and follicular adenoma or carcinoma. Thus a well-sampled tumor without any capsular and vascular invasion will behave more as a follicular adenoma and the ones with capsular and vascular invasion as follicular carcinoma [32].

Cytologic preparations from fine-needle aspiration (FNA) of FVPTC can be markedly cellular. The enlarged neoplastic cells form small follicles with well-demarcated lumina (Fig. 32.16) or lie in clusters, forming rosettes and tubules. Occasionally, papillary tissue fragments may be seen. The background may contain variable amount of thick and thin colloid depending upon the presence of micro- and macrofollicles within the tumor. Pink-staining thick colloid appears inside follicles (Fig. 32.17) or as balls and masses of variable shapes in close proximity to the neoplastic cells. The nuclei are dark staining, have smooth contours, and differ in size and shape; a few are triangular, resembling arrowheads. Intranuclear cytoplasmic inclusions, psammoma bodies, and multinucleated histiocytes are less frequent than in the classic type of papillary carcinoma [38]. Therefore, a good proportion of FVPTCs are diagnosed as suspicious for papillary carcinoma on cytology.

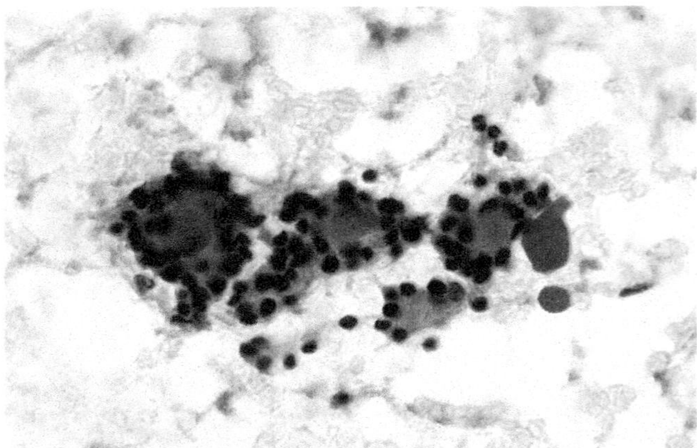

Fig. 32.16 Papillary carcinoma, follicular variant. Aspirate showing multiple microfollicles with inspissated luminal colloid (Papanicolaou stain)

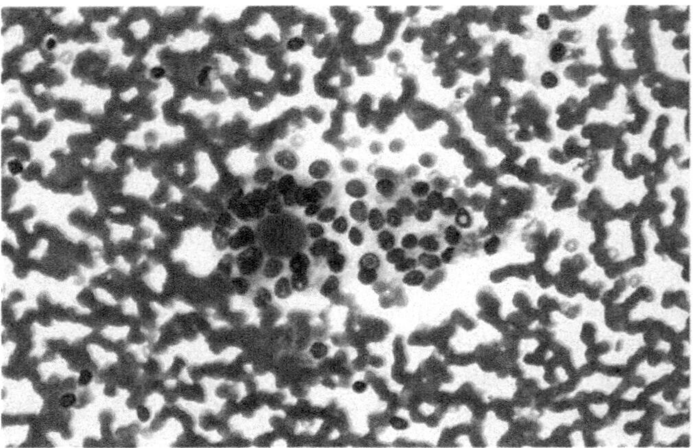

Fig. 32.17 Papillary carcinoma, follicular variant. Aspirate showing a rosette (on the *right*) and a microfollicle with "pink colloid" in its lumen (Diff-Quik stain)

Encapsulated Variant

About 10–20 % of the clinical papillary cancers are encapsulated variants. Some are cystic and encapsulated; thus, the gross appearance is extremely varied. Capsules range from delicate to thick. These neoplasms have a lower incidence of nodal metastases than the other types, but careful search of the periphery of such a tumor usually reveals microscopic evidence of penetration of its capsule or foci of neoplastic cells in the thyroid tissue just outside the tumor's capsule. Therefore, gross evidence of invasion is often absent, but microscopic evidence of aggressiveness is usually present [39].

Many papillary carcinomas have irregular and dense fibrous tissue that accompanies their infiltrating cells, producing a "pseudocapsule" around part of the neoplasm. This should be differentiated from the well-organized, continuous, real capsule just described. Cytologic smears are diagnosed as papillary carcinoma on FNA.

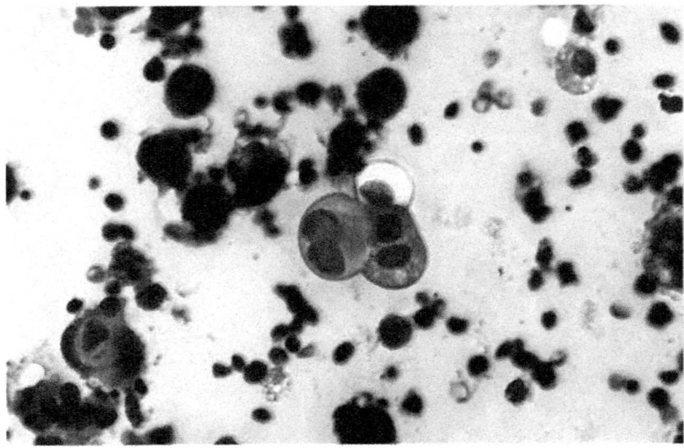

Fig. 32.18 Papillary carcinoma with cystic change. Aspirate showing neoplastic cells with dense well-demarcated cytoplasm and one with pale cytoplasm (Diff-Quik stain)

Cystic Carcinoma

Small cystic foci are fairly common in PTC, but in some cases the cystic component may occupy most of the lesion. The fluid often contains bits of tissue and flecks of calcific material, and papillary fronds may be visible on gross examination. Sometimes, there is so little epithelium that the tumor appears as a fluid-filled sac [40]. These cancers are often encapsulated, suggesting a reduced risk of metastases [41]. Aspiration yields at least 1.0 mL of fluid, often a larger amount, typically thin and pale yellow, greenish, brown, or thick and brown. The fluid may re-accumulate rapidly. If a residual mass can be detected after fluid evacuation and collapse of the cyst, this should be aspirated. It is important to remember that most cystic thyroid masses are benign.

Direct smears and smears from sediment after centrifugation of the fluid should be prepared; monolayer preparations are often helpful in these cases [42]. Large numbers of hemosiderin-laden histiocytes and considerable cellular debris are present. Sheets of intact follicular cells may be seen, which resemble those from cellular adenomatoid nodules [43]; however, these will demonstrate nuclear cytology suspicious or diagnostic of PTC. In a benign cystic lesion, such epithelial cells should be shrunken and degenerate, and the presence of apparently well-preserved cells is therefore a warning of a possible neoplasm. These cells are slightly larger than normal follicular cells, their cytoplasm is denser, they lack paravacuolar granules, and their nuclei are larger than normal nuclei and are not pyknotic. Some groups of larger cells with clear cytoplasm and dense, convex cellular borders also are seen. The edges of these cellular clusters have a scalloped appearance [44] (Fig. 32.18). In other cases, the predominant cell type resembles a histiocyte with clear cytoplasm and an enlarged atypical nucleus; these are presumably partly degenerated neoplastic epithelial cells [45, 46].

Squamous metaplasia have been reported in cases of cystic PTCs. Dense globules of pink-staining colloid ("pink balls") may be present.

Microcarcinoma

Papillary microcarcinoma is defined as tumor measuring 1.0 cm or less. In the literature some authors have labeled these as "occult carcinomas"; however, this term should only be reserved for tumors that are not easily identifiable by physical or radiologic examination. Papillary microcarcinoma is a common incidental finding at autopsy or in thyroidectomy specimens for benign disease or removed during resection of carcinomas involving neighboring structures. Histologically, the tumors may be either completely follicular patterned or show papillary architecture as well. Sclerosis may be prominent; the lesions can be encapsulated or infiltrate the surrounding thyroid [5]. Lymph node metastases from papillary microcarcinoma can occur; metastases from lesions less than 0.5 cm have been reported [47, 48]. Distant metastases, although very rare, are also documented [49]. A familial form of papillary microcarcinoma has been described which is associated with aggressive clinical course.

PTC with Nodular Fasciitis-Like Stroma

Extensively fibrotic tumors are rare and typically infiltrative. Little epithelium is present, and the stroma may be dense, myxomatous, or fasciitis-like. The gross appearance depends on the amount and density of the stroma. Due to these features these tumors may be mistaken for anaplastic carcinoma; however, these tumors strongly express thyroglobulin and TTF-1. Few case reports of these tumors have been reported in cytology literature [50].

Diffuse Sclerosis Variant

In diffuse papillary carcinoma, most of a lobe or the entire thyroid gland is involved, and the tissue is firm, pale, and opaque. Usually, no discrete mass can be found. The lymphatic vessels of the gland are permeated by the cancer, and typical chronic lymphocytic thyroiditis is often present. Frequently, there is diffuse fibrosis throughout (Fig. 32.19) but not always. Psammoma bodies and foci of squamous metaplasia in the cancer are common. Adjacent lymph nodes often are involved, and metastatic spread to the lungs is common, but these features do not necessarily portend short survival, as many of the patients are young women [51, 52]. Cytologic preparations show papillary carcinoma with solid growth pattern and numerous psammoma bodies.

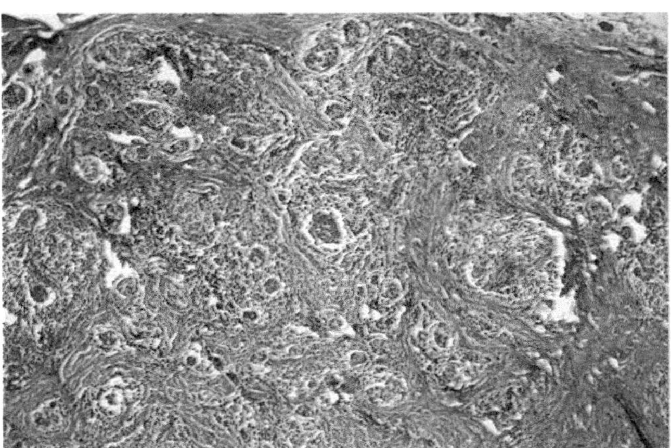

Fig. 32.19 Papillary carcinoma of the diffuse sclerosing type (H&E stain)

Oxyphilic Papillary Carcinoma

Only a small number of papillary carcinomas with oxyphilic cells occur; only a few have been studied, and they may be infiltrative or encapsulated. Some pathologists believe this variant is considerably more aggressive than the usual papillary carcinoma. Others have not been able to detect any clear differences, allowing for the other prognostic factors also present [53]. Aspirates may be misdiagnosed as follicular neoplasms of the Hürthle cell type because of the cytoplasmic characteristics. In the oxyphilic papillary carcinoma, nucleoli are rarely visible, intranuclear cytoplasmic inclusions are common, and multinucleated histiocytes are seen frequently [54].

Warthin-Like Variant

By light microscopy these tumors resemble "Warthin's tumor" of the salivary gland. These tumors usually arise in a background of lymphocytic thyroiditis and show papillary architecture. The clinical course of this variant is similar to conventional papillary carcinoma [55, 56]. Cytologic preparations of this tumor demonstrate oncocytic tumor cells with nuclear features of papillary carcinoma and an infiltrate of lymphocytes and plasma cells within the tissue fragments of tumor cells.

Clear-Cell Papillary Carcinoma

A few cells with clear cytoplasm are present in a modest proportion of papillary carcinomas. Only a few cancers have many or most of their cells with clear cytoplasm. This feature does not have any known prognostic significance [57, 58].

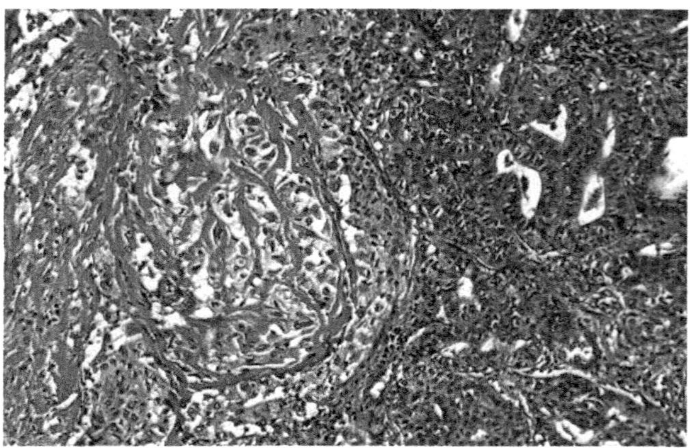

Fig. 32.20 Less well-differentiated papillary carcinoma. Relatively tall and irregular cells are on the *left*; a trabecular pattern with tall cells is on the *right*. Almost no colloid is visible (H&E stain)

However, it is of utmost importance to exclude metastases from a clear-cell renal cell carcinoma by performing immunostains for thyroglobulin and TTF-1 before making a diagnosis of clear-cell variant of papillary thyroid carcinoma.

Tall-Cell Variant

The tall-cell variant of papillary carcinoma is uncommon and has a poor prognosis, with a greater tendency to recur or metastasize. The neoplastic cell has a height three times as great as its width. Cytoplasm is usually eosinophilic [59, 60]. Dedifferentiation to anaplastic carcinoma with spindle and squamous cell features has been described in tall-cell variant of PTC [61, 62]. The FNA specimens of these tumors demonstrate characteristics features: larger cells with abundant oxyphilic cytoplasm, more frequent intranuclear cytoplasmic inclusions, and fewer psammoma bodies than in classic papillary carcinoma [63].

Papillary Carcinomas with Less Well-Differentiated Growth Pattern

Papillary cancers with less well-differentiated architecture are classified as grades 2 and 3 by the Mayo Clinic Broders' classification and are described as "moderately differentiated papillary carcinoma" [64], i.e., papillary carcinoma with marked atypia (multilayered epithelium, notable variations in size and shape of the cells and nuclei, and nuclei with hyperchromatism and abnormal chromatin distribution [65]. Other investigators include the tall-cell and columnar-cell cancers as less well-differentiated papillary carcinomas ([66]; Fig. 32.20.

An extensive trabecular pattern of growth has been stated to indicate a worse prognosis [67], but such cases may overlap with the tall-cell variant [68]. Patterns of solid growth might not be significant, especially in young persons [69]. Focal necrosis and invasion of blood vessels may also indicate a higher grade of malignancy [16].

When follicles are empty and closed, or when papillae or trabeculae are pressed together, a neoplasm may appear solid, without actually having a solid diffuse pattern of growth. True solid regions are moderately typical in papillary carcinoma but are usually only a minor component. Sometimes the solid foci are the result of focal squamous metaplasia; this is often not a significant feature. The solid variant of is most commonly seen in children and has been reported in greater than 30 % of patients with papillary carcinoma following the Chernobyl nuclear accident [70, 71].

The entire neoplasm is only solid or predominantly solid in a few instances. Aspirates may show malignant features without specifically resembling a papillary thyroid carcinoma. We have diagnosed a few of these cases as "carcinoma, cannot further classify."

Columnar-Cell Carcinoma

Columnar-cell papillary carcinoma is rare, occurring in adults of all ages. It is usually a solid, nodular, light-colored mass, either encapsulated or infiltrative, and contains tall, slender, columnar cells arranged in patterns that are papillary or trabecular. Solid regions may present with small polygonal and/or spindled cells. Follicles of multiple sizes may be present. An alveolar pattern is sometimes suggested. Cytoplasm is usually clear, sometimes eosinophilic or amphophilic, and is scanty. Nuclei are hyperchromatic, rarely pale, and elongated in the tall cylindrical cells and may contain longitudinal grooves; intranuclear cytoplasmic inclusions are rare. These elongated nuclei differ sufficiently in their positions in the cells to produce a stratified or pseudostratified appearance. Nucleoli are inconspicuous, and there are many mitotic figures [72, 73]. The cells contain glycogen, thyroglobulin, and sometimes keratin. A few psammoma bodies may be found.

Neoplasms have been reported where the columnar-cell pattern was mixed with tall-cell papillary carcinoma [74, 75], as well as with solid regions of typical papillary carcinoma [75]. Reports suggest that the locally infiltrative tumors are usually fatal [72, 76], but those that are encapsulated may be resected successfully. The FNA specimens of this tumor demonstrate papillary fragments composed of pseudostratified columnar cells crowded together. The neoplastic cells had oval to elongated nuclei and resembled respiratory epithelial cells. The background of the smears was devoid of colloid [77–79].

Rare Variants of Papillary Carcinoma

Other rare variants of PTC which have been described include the spindle-cell variant [80], papillary carcinoma with lipomatous stroma [81, 82], papillary carcinoma with fasciitis-like stroma [50], and cribriform variant [83, 84]. The last of these is often seen in patients with familial adenomatous polyposis although it may occur as a sporadic tumor. Recently, an aggressive form of PTC known as "hobnail" variant has been described [85].

References

1. Rosai J, Carcangui ML, DeLellis RA. Tumors of the thyroid gland. Washington, DC: Armed Forces Institute of Pathology; 1992.
2. Carcangiu ML, Zampi G, Rosai J. Papillary thyroid carcinoma: a study of its many morphologic expressions and clinical correlates. Pathol Annu. 1985;20(Pt 1):1–44.
3. Moses W, Weng J, Kebebew E. Prevalence, clinicopathologic features, and somatic genetic mutation profile in familial versus sporadic nonmedullary thyroid cancer. Thyroid. 2011;21:367–71.
4. Mazzaferri EL. Papillary thyroid carcinoma: factors influencing prognosis and current therapy. Semin Oncol. 1987;14:315–32.
5. LiVolsi VA. Surgical pathology of the thyroid. Philadelphia: W.B. Saunders; 1990.
6. Riazmontazer N, Bedayat G. Psammoma bodies in fine needle aspirates from thyroids containing nontoxic hyperplastic nodular goiters. Acta Cytol. 1991;35:563–6.
7. Hunt JL, Barnes EL. Non-tumor-associated psammoma bodies in the thyroid. Am J Clin Pathol. 2003;119:90–4.
8. Hosoya T, Sakamoto A, Kasai N, Sakurai K. Nodal psammoma body in thyroid cancer as an indicator of cancer metastasis to the lymph node. Gan No Rinsho. 1983;29:1336–9.
9. Isarangkul W. Dense fibrosis. Another diagnostic criterion for papillary thyroid carcinoma. Arch Pathol Lab Med. 1993;117:645–6.
10. Qiu Y, Korteweg C, Chen Z, Li J, Luo J, Huang G, Gu J. Immunoglobulin G expression and its colocalization with complement proteins in papillary thyroid cancer. Mod Pathol. 2011.
11. Fusco A, Chiappetta G, Hui P, Garcia-Rostan G, Golden L, Kinder BK, Dillon DA, Giuliano A, Cirafici AM, Santoro M, Rosai J, Tallini G. Assessment of RET/PTC oncogene activation and clonality in thyroid nodules with incomplete morphological evidence of papillary carcinoma: a search for the early precursors of papillary cancer. Am J Pathol. 2002;160:2157–67.
12. Hunt JL, LiVolsi VA, Baloch ZW, Barnes EL, Swalsky PA, Niehouse L, Finkelstein SD. Microscopic papillary thyroid carcinoma compared with clinical carcinomas by loss of heterozygosity mutational profile. Am J Surg Pathol. 2003;27:159–66.
13. Petkov R, Gavrailov M, Mikhailov I, Todorov G, Kutev N. Differentiated thyroid cancer – a study of the pathomorphological variants in 216 patients. Khirurgiia. 1995;48:11–2.
14. Mazzaferi EYR. Papillary thyroid carcinoma: a 10-year follow-up report of the impact of therapy in 576 patients. Am J Med. 1981; 70:511–8.
15. LiVolsi VA. Papillary neoplasms of the thyroid. Pathologic and prognostic features. Am J Clin Pathol. 1992;97:426–34.
16. Akslen LA, LiVolsi VA. Prognostic significance of histologic grading compared with subclassification of papillary thyroid carcinoma. [see comments]. Cancer. 2000;88:1902–8.
17. Akslen LA, LiVolsi VA. Poorly differentiated thyroid carcinoma – it is important. Am J Surg Pathol. 2000;24:310–3.
18. Carcangiu ML, Steeper T, Zampi G, Rosai J. Anaplastic thyroid carcinoma. A study of 70 cases. Am J Clin Pathol. 1985;83: 135–58.
19. Tachikawa T, Kumazawa H, Kyomoto R, Yukawa H, Yamashita T, Nishikawa M. Clinical study on prognostic factors in thyroid carcinoma. Nippon Jibiinkoka Gakkai Kaiho [J Oto-Rhino-Laryngol Soc Jpn]. 2001;104:157–64.
20. Baloch Z, LiVolsi VA. Pathology of the thyroid gland. Philadelphia: Churchill Livingston; 2002.
21. Prasad ML, Pellegata NS, Huang Y, Nagaraja HN, Chapelle Ade L, Kloos RT. Galectin-3, fibronectin-1, CITED-1, HBME1 and cytokeratin-19 immunohistochemistry is useful for the differential diagnosis of thyroid tumors. Mod Pathol. 2005;18:48–57.
22. Casey MB, Lohse CM, Lloyd RV. Distinction between papillary thyroid hyperplasia and papillary thyroid carcinoma by immunohistochemical staining for cytokeratin 19, galectin-3, and HBME-1. Endocr Pathol. 2003;14:55–60.
23. Cheung CC, Ezzat S, Freeman JL, Rosen IB, Asa SL. Immunohistochemical diagnosis of papillary thyroid carcinoma. Mod Pathol. 2001;14:338–42.
24. Eimoto T, Naito H, Hamada S, Masuda M, Harada T, Kikuchi M. Papillary carcinoma of the thyroid. A histochemical, immunohistochemical and ultrastructural study with special reference to the follicular variant. Acta Pathol Jpn. 1987;37:1563–79.
25. van Hoeven KH, Kovatich AJ, Miettinen M. Immunocytochemical evaluation of HBME-1, CA 19-9, and CD-15 (Leu-M1) in fine-needle aspirates of thyroid nodules. Diagn Cytopathol. 1998;18: 93–7.
26. Baloch ZW, Abraham S, Roberts S, LiVolsi VA. Differential expression of cytokeratins in follicular variant of papillary carcinoma: an immunohistochemical study and its diagnostic utility. Hum Pathol. 1999;30:1166–71.
27. Kini SR. Thyroid cytopathology an atlas and text. 1st ed. Philadelphia: Lippincott Williams & Wilkins; 2008.
28. Baloch ZW, Livolsi VA. Follicular-patterned lesions of the thyroid: the bane of the pathologist. Am J Clin Pathol. 2002;117:143–50.
29. Mizukami Y, Nonomura A, Michigishi T, Ohmura K, Noguchi M, Ishizaki T. Diffuse follicular variant of papillary carcinoma of the thyroid. Histopathology. 1995;27:575–7.
30. Ivanova R, Soares P, Castro P, Sobrinho-Simoes M. Diffuse (or multinodular) follicular variant of papillary thyroid carcinoma: a clinicopathologic and immunohistochemical analysis of ten cases of an aggressive form of differentiated thyroid carcinoma. Virchows Arch. 2002;440:418–24.
31. Liu Z, Zhou G, Nakamura M, Koike E, Li Y, Ozaki T, Mori I, Taniguchi E, Kakudo K. Encapsulated follicular thyroid tumor with equivocal nuclear changes, so-called well-differentiated tumor of uncertain malignant potential: a morphological, immunohistochemical, and molecular appraisal. Cancer Sci. 2011;102:288–94.
32. Baloch Z, LiVolsi VA, Henricks WH, Sebak BA. Encapsulated follicular variant of papillary thyroid carcinoma. Am J Clin Pathol. 2002;118:603–5; discussion 605–06.
33. LiVolsi VA, Baloch ZW. Follicular neoplasms of the thyroid: view, biases, and experiences. Adv Anat Pathol. 2004;11:279–87.
34. Williams ED, Abrosimov A, Bogdanova TI, Rosai J, Sidorov Y, Thomas GA. Two proposals regarding the terminology of thyroid tumors. Guest editorial. Int J Surg Pathol. 2000;8:181–3.
35. Giordano TJ, Kuick R, Thomas DG, Misek DE, Vinco M, Sanders D, Zhu Z, Ciampi R, Roh M, Shedden K, Gauger P, Doherty G, Thompson NW, Hanash S, Koenig RJ, Nikiforov YE. Molecular classification of papillary thyroid carcinoma: distinct BRAF, RAS, and RET/PTC mutation-specific gene expression profiles discovered by DNA microarray analysis. Oncogene. 2005;24:6646–56.
36. Wreesmann VB, Ghossein RA, Hezel M, Banerjee D, Shaha AR, Tuttle RM, Shah JP, Rao PH, Singh B. Follicular variant of papillary

thyroid carcinoma: genome-wide appraisal of a controversial entity. Genes Chromosomes Cancer. 2004;40:355–64.
37. Zhu Z, Gandhi M, Nikiforova MN, Fischer AH, Nikiforov YE. Molecular profile and clinical-pathologic features of the follicular variant of papillary thyroid carcinoma. An unusually high prevalence of ras mutations. Am J Clin Pathol. 2003;120:71–7.
38. Gallagher J, Oertel YC, Oertel JE. Follicular variant of papillary carcinoma of the thyroid: fine-needle aspirates with histologic correlation. Diagn Cytopathol. 1997;16:207–13.
39. Baloch ZW, Shafique K, Flannagan M, Livolsi VA. Encapsulated classic and follicular variants of papillary thyroid carcinoma: comparative clinicopathologic study. Endocr Pract. 2010;16:952–9.
40. de los Santos ET, Keyhani-Rofagha S, Cunningham JJ, Mazzaferri L. Cystic thyroid nodules. The dilemma of malignant lesions. Arch Intern Med. 1990;150:1422–7.
41. Ruiz-Velasco R, Waisman J, Van Herle AJ. Cystic papillary carcinoma of the thyroid gland. Diagnosis by needle aspiration with transmission electron microscopy. Acta Cytol. 1978;22:38–42.
42. Ford L, Rasgon BM, Hilsinger Jr RL, Cruz RM, Axelsson K, Rumore GJ, Schmidtknecht TM, Puligandla B, Sawicki J, Pshea W. Comparison of ThinPrep versus conventional smear cytopreparatory techniques for fine-needle aspiration specimens of head and neck masses. Otolaryngol Head Neck Surg. 2002;126:554–61.
43. Busseniers AE, Oertel YC. "Cellular adenomatoid nodules" of the thyroid: review of 219 fine-needle aspirates. Diagn Cytopathol. 1993;9:581–9.
44. Oertel YC. Fine-needle aspiration and the diagnosis of thyroid cancer. Endocrinol Metab Clin North Am. 1996;25:69–91.
45. Koo JS, Kwak JY, Jung W, Hong S. Importance of foamy macrophages only in fine needle aspirates to cytologic diagnostic accuracy of cystic metastatic papillary thyroid carcinoma. Acta Cytol. 2010;54:249–54.
46. Castro-Gomez L, Cordova-Ramirez S, Duarte-Torres R, Alonso de Ruiz P, Hurtado-Lopez LM. Cytologic criteria of cystic papillary carcinoma of the thyroid. Acta Cytol. 2003;47:590–4.
47. Hay ID, Grant CS, van Heerden JA, Goellner JR, Ebersold JR, Bergstralh EJ. Papillary thyroid microcarcinoma: a study of 535 cases observed in a 50-year period. Surgery. 1992;112:1139–46; discussion 1146–37.
48. Rodriguez JM, Moreno A, Parrilla P, Sola J, Soria T, Tebar FJ, Aranda F. Papillary thyroid microcarcinoma: clinical study and prognosis. Eur J Surg. 1997;163:255–9.
49. Braga M, Graf H, Ogata A, Batista J, Hakim NC. Aggressive behavior of papillary microcarcinoma in a patient with Graves' disease initially presenting as cystic neck mass. J Endocrinol Invest. 2002;25:250–3.
50. Chan JK, Carcangiu ML, Rosai J. Papillary carcinoma of thyroid with exuberant nodular fasciitis-like stroma. Report of three cases. Am J Clin Pathol. 1991;95:309–14.
51. Carcangiu ML, Bianchi S. Diffuse sclerosing variant of papillary thyroid carcinoma. Clinicopathologic study of 15 cases. Am J Surg Pathol. 1989;13:1041–9.
52. Gomez-Morales M, Alvaro T, Munoz M, Garcia del Moral R, Aguilar D, Caballero T, Aneiros J. Diffuse sclerosing papillary carcinoma of the thyroid gland: immunohistochemical analysis of the local host immune response. Histopathology. 1991;18:427–33.
53. Berho M, Suster S. The oncocytic variant of papillary carcinoma of the thyroid: a clinicopathologic study of 15 cases. Hum Pathol. 1997;28:47–53.
54. Beckner ME, Heffess CS, Oertel JE. Oxyphilic papillary thyroid carcinomas. Am J Clin Pathol. 1995;103:280–7.
55. Apel RL, Asa SL, LiVolsi VA. Papillary Hurthle cell carcinoma with lymphocytic stroma. "Warthin-like tumor" of the thyroid. Am J Surg Pathol. 1995;19:810–4.
56. Baloch ZW, LiVolsi VA. Warthin-like papillary carcinoma of the thyroid. Arch Pathol Lab Med. 2000;124:1192–5.
57. Asanuma K, Sugenoya A, Ohashi T, Nagai N, Itoh N, Kobayashi S, Amano J. Pure clear cell papillary thyroid carcinoma with chronic thyroiditis: report of a case. Surg Today. 1998;28:464–6.
58. Carcangiu ML, Sibley RK, Rosai J. Clear cell change in primary thyroid tumors. A study of 38 cases. Am J Surg Pathol. 1985;9:705–22.
59. Ghossein R, Livolsi VA. Papillary thyroid carcinoma tall cell variant. Thyroid. 2008;18:1179–81.
60. Ghossein RA, Leboeuf R, Patel KN, Rivera M, Katabi N, Carlson DL, Tallini G, Shaha A, Singh B, Tuttle RM. Tall cell variant of papillary thyroid carcinoma without extrathyroid extension: biologic behavior and clinical implications. Thyroid. 2007;17:655–61.
61. Bronner MP, LiVolsi VA. Spindle cell squamous carcinoma of the thyroid: an unusual anaplastic tumor associated with tall cell papillary cancer. Mod Pathol. 1991;4:637–43.
62. Gopal PP, Montone KT, Baloch Z, Tuluc M, Livolsi V. The variable presentations of anaplastic spindle cell squamous carcinoma associated with tall cell variant of papillary thyroid carcinoma. Thyroid. 2011;21:493–9.
63. Solomon A, Gupta PK, LiVolsi VA, Baloch ZW. Distinguishing tall cell variant of papillary thyroid carcinoma from usual variant of papillary thyroid carcinoma in cytologic specimens. Diagn Cytopathol. 2002;27:143–8.
64. Tscholl-Ducommun J, Hedinger CE. Papillary thyroid carcinomas. Morphology and prognosis. Virchows Arch A Pathol Anat Histol. 1982;396:19–39.
65. Tennvall J, Biorklund A, Moller T, Ranstam J, Akerman M. Prognostic factors of papillary, follicular and medullary carcinomas of the thyroid gland. Retrospective multivariate analysis of 216 patients with a median follow-up of 11 years. Acta Radiol Oncol. 1985;24:17–24.
66. Pilotti S, Collini P, Manzari A, Marubini E, Rilke F. Poorly differentiated forms of papillary thyroid carcinoma: distinctive entities or morphological patterns? Semin Diagn Pathol. 1995;12:249–55.
67. Mizukami Y, Noguchi M, Michigishi T, Nonomura A, Hashimoto T, Otakes S, Nakamura S, Matsubara F. Papillary thyroid carcinoma in Kanazawa, Japan: prognostic significance of histological subtypes. Histopathology. 1992;20:243–50.
68. Ostrowski M, Merino MJ. Tall cell variant of papillary thyroid carcinoma: a reassessment and immunohistochemical study with comparison to usual type of papillary carcinoma of the thyroid. Am J Surg Pathol. 1996;20:964–74.
69. Harach HR, Williams ED. Childhood thyroid cancer in England and Wales. Br J Cancer. 1995;72:777–83.
70. Nikiforov YE, Erickson LA, Nikiforova MN, Caudill CM, Lloyd RV. Solid variant of papillary thyroid carcinoma: incidence, clinical- pathologic characteristics, molecular analysis, and biologic behavior. Am J Surg Pathol. 2001;25:1478–84.
71. Thomas GA, Bunnell H, Cook HA, Williams ED, Nerovnya A, Cherstvoy ED, Tronko ND, Bogdanova TI, Chiappetta G, Viglietto G, Pentimalli F, Salvatore G, Fusco A, Santoro M, Vecchio G. High prevalence of RET/PTC rearrangements in Ukrainian and Belarussian post-Chernobyl thyroid papillary carcinomas: a strong correlation between RET/PTC3 and the solid-follicular variant. J Clin Endocrinol Metab. 1999;84:4232–8.
72. Evans HL. Columnar-cell carcinoma of the thyroid. A report of two cases of an aggressive variant of thyroid carcinoma. Am J Clin Pathol. 1986;85:77–80.
73. Evans HL. Encapsulated columnar-cell carcinoma of the thyroid. A report of four cases suggesting a favorable outcome. Am J Surg Pathol. 1996;20:1205–11.
74. Akslen LA, Varhaug JE. Thyroid carcinoma with mixed tall-cell and columnar-cell features. Am J Clin Pathol. 1990;94:442–5.
75. Mizukami Y, Nonomura A, Michigishi T, Noguchi M, Nakamura S, Hashimoto T. Columnar cell carcinoma of the thyroid gland: a case

report and review of the literature. Hum Pathol. 1994;25: 1098–101.
76. Sobrinho-Simoes M, Nesland JM, Johannessen JV. Columnar-cell carcinoma. Another variant of poorly differentiated carcinoma of the thyroid. Am J Clin Pathol. 1988;89:264–7.
77. Jayaram G. Cytology of columnar-cell variant of papillary thyroid carcinoma. Diagn Cytopathol. 2000;22:227–9.
78. Putti TC, Bhuiya TA, Wasserman PG. Fine needle aspiration cytology of mixed tall and columnar cell papillary carcinoma of the thyroid. A case report. Acta Cytol. 1998;42:387–90.
79. Perez F, Llobet M, Garijo G, Barcelo C, Castro P, Bernado L. Fine-needle aspiration cytology of columnar-cell carcinoma of the thyroid: report of two cases with cytohistologic correlation. Diagn Cytopathol. 1998;18:352–6.
80. Vergilio J, Baloch ZW, LiVolsi VA. Spindle cell metaplasia of the thyroid arising in association with papillary carcinoma and follicular adenoma. Am J Clin Pathol. 2002;117: 199–204.
81. Bisi H, Longatto Filho A, de Camargo RY, Fernandes VS. Thyroid papillary carcinoma lipomatous type: report of two cases. Pathologica. 1993;85:761–4.
82. Schroder S, Bocker W. Lipomatous lesions of the thyroid gland: a review. Appl Pathol. 1985;3:140–9.
83. Cameselle-Teijeiro J, Chan JK. Cribriform-morular variant of papillary carcinoma: a distinctive variant representing the sporadic counterpart of familial adenomatous polyposis-associated thyroid carcinoma? Mod Pathol. 1999;12:400–11.
84. Hirokawa M, Kuma S, Miyauchi A, Qian ZR, Nakasono M, Sano T, Kakudo K. Morules in cribriform-morular variant of papillary thyroid carcinoma: immunohistochemical characteristics and distinction from squamous metaplasia. APMIS. 2004;112:275–82.
85. Lloyd RV, Erickson LA, Asioli S. Papillary thyroid carcinoma with prominent hobnail features: a new aggressive variant of moderately differentiated papillary carcinoma. A clinicopathologic, immunohistochemical, and molecular study of 8 cases. Am J Surg Pathol. 2010;34:44–52.

Part V

Postoperative Management

33 Remnant Ablation, Adjuvant Treatment and Treatment of Locoregional Metastases with ^{131}I

Douglas Van Nostrand

Introduction

The two major areas of controversy in the management of patients with differentiated thyroid cancer are when to administer an ^{131}I therapy and, if administered, what should be the amount of prescribed activity of ^{131}I that is administered. Although one of the more frequent factors that is cited for the two controversies is the lack of good prospective studies, these two controversies are complicated by many other factors such as (1) the use of the same terms with different definitions, (2) the use of the same terms with different objectives (e.g., destruction of remnant tissue, reduced recurrence, or decreased disease-specific mortality), (3) the use of a term with the same definition and objectives but different end points as the measure of success for those objectives (e.g., uptake, scan, stimulated or non-stimulated thyroglobulin blood level, recurrence, and/or structural evidence of disease), (4) the end points are measured at different follow-up times (e.g., 6, 9, 12 months), and (5) variability in the extent of initial surgery and different staging systems (risk assessment tools).

To demonstrate the variability of only one of the above factors – specifically the end point used to evaluate the success of the terms "remnant ablation" and "ablation" – 3 meta-analyses and 160 articles were reviewed. Forty-one articles were selected based on the authors reporting that they were evaluating the success of the various amounts of prescribed activity of ^{131}I for the terms, "remnant ablation" and "ablation" [1]. The end points are noted in Table 33.1. In addition, the end points described in Table 33.1 were measured at variable times after "remnant ablation" or ablation" from months to 1 year or even several years, and the level of uptake, scan findings, and thyroglobulin blood levels used to determine success were variable, and these were also all before the incorporation of ultrasound as one of the criteria for success. Although it is natural to turn to the guidelines and recommendations of the various professional organizations for guidance, a review of the various guidelines' recommendations in Table 33.2 also demonstrates the variable use of the terms [2–6]. The second controversy is the prescribed activity of ^{131}I to be administered, and this controversy has many of the same issues.

So, what is one to do? The first step is to better define the terms that we all use. The second is to distinguish prognosis from objective, albeit they are intimately related, and the third step is to stage the patient (i.e., risk assessment) as completely as reasonable. The final step is the performance and publication of prospective studies, and significant progress has been made in all of these areas.

Accordingly, the objectives of this chapter are (1) to better define terms regarding ^{131}I therapy including the objectives; (2) to discuss prognosis versus objectives; (3) to discuss various professional organizational guidelines and literature regarding whether or not to administer ^{131}I for remnant ablation, adjuvant treatment, and locoregional metastatic treatment; and (4) if ^{131}I is to be administered, to discuss what is the amount, or at least the range, of the prescribed activity of ^{131}I that has been proposed. Staging and risk assessment have already been discussed elsewhere in Chaps. 9 and 29. This chapter does not discuss the use of ^{131}I for the treatment of distant metastases of DTC, for which, the reader is referred to Chap. 56. This chapter will conclude with a discussion of fractionation of the administration of therapeutic prescribed activity of ^{131}I and the use of diuretics.

Terminology for ^{131}I Therapy for Differentiated Thyroid Cancer

It is important to define terms and to articulate the objectives of those terms. By defining terms, knowing the objectives, and assessing the patient's prognosis based on the staging

D. Van Nostrand, MD, FACP, FACNM (✉)
Nuclear Medicine Research, MedStar Research Institute and Washington Hospital Center, Georgetown University School of Medicine, Washington Hospital Center, 110 Irving Street, N.W., Suite GB 60F, Washington, DC 20010, USA
e-mail: douglasvannostrand@gmail.com

L. Wartofsky, D. Van Nostrand (eds.), *Thyroid Cancer*, DOI 10.1007/978-1-4939-3314-3_33

Table 33.1 Variable end points for studies evaluating the success of the terms "remnant ablation" and/or "ablation" [1]

Uptake and scan in 56 % (23/41)
Thyroglobulin blood level only in 2 % (1/41)
Uptake, scan, and thyroglobulin blood level in 27 % (11/41)
Recurrence in 15 % (6/41) of studies

Table 33.2 End point for remnant ablation

Organization	Recommendation
ATA [2]	"Successful remnant ablation can be defined by an undetectable stimulated serum Tg, in absence of interfering Tg antibodies, with or without confirmatory nuclear or other imaging studies." If Tg antibodies are present, then ". . . absence of visible RAI uptake on a subsequent diagnostic RAI scan."
EC [3]	"At present, the best definition of successful ablation is an undetectable serum Tg level following TSH stimulation and normal neck ultrasound"
BTA [4]	Stimulated Tg and specialized neck ultrasound should be performed in preference to a diagnostic ^{131}I whole-body scan between 9 and 12 months after remnant ablation. However, these guidelines have objectives of destroying normal thyroid tissue and prolonged survival eradication of remaining thyroid cancer cells
NCCN [5][a]	Stimulated Tg, ultrasound, and whole-body ^{131}I imaging listed for detecting recurrent or residual disease, but no specific criteria for successful remnant ablation given
SNM [6]	Not defined

[a]"The 3 general, but overlapping, functions of postoperative RAI administration include: 1) ablation of the normal thyroid remnant, which may help in surveillance for recurrent disease; 2) adjuvant therapy to try to eliminate suspected micrometastases; or 3) RAI therapy to treat know persistent disease."

system one chooses, the controversy regarding the selection of lower and higher amounts of prescribed activity of ^{131}I can be reduced. However, even if the controversy is not eliminated, then hopefully, the reason for the difference of opinions between physicians may be more appropriately identified such as a difference in opinion by the physicians of the patient's likelihood of recurrence or death and/or whether or not that perceived prognosis warrants higher or lower amounts of prescribed activity of ^{131}I, and thus increased or decreased risk of side effects. This may also help patients understand the differences of opinions among expert physicians regarding the management of their differentiated thyroid cancer.

Publications by Haugen et al. [2] and Van Nostrand [7] have proposed definitions of the above terms, and except for the interchange of the terms of *treatment* and *therapy*, the definitions and objectives are essentially identical.

Remnant ablation "...is the use of ^{131}I to destroy residual functioning thyroid tissue after thyroidectomy. Its objectives are to (1) facilitate the interpretation of subsequent serum thyroglobulin levels, (2) increase the sensitivity of detection of loco-regional disease and/or metastatic disease on any subsequent follow-up radioiodine whole-body scan, (3) maximize the therapeutic effect of any subsequent ^{131}I therapies, and (4) allow a post-therapy scan that may identify metastases that were not identified on the pre-therapy scan or when a pre-therapy scan had not been performed." Although *remnant ablation* typically refers to the first ^{131}I therapy, it may be repeated, and other terms of ^{131}I therapy may be used in combination with *remnant ablation,* which will depend on the objectives of the therapy.

Adjuvant treatment "...is the use of ^{131}I to destroy *unknown* microscopic thyroid cancer and/or *suspected but unproven* remaining thyroid cancer with the objective of potentially decreasing recurrence and/or mortality from thyroid cancer."

Treatment "... is the use of ^{131}I to destroy *known* loco-regional and/or distant metastasis with the objectives of potential cure, increased progression-free survival, increased overall survival,or palliation." The use of the adjectives *locoregional* and *distant metastatic* may be used to modify the term *treatment.* Although *locoregional* or *distant metastatic treatment* would typically be performed after *remnant ablation*, it is possible that one is performing both *remnant ablation* and *treatment* simultaneously with the first ^{131}I therapy."

Therapy "...is any generic use of ^{131}I including ^{131}I *remnant ablation*, ^{131}I *adjuvant treatment*, or ^{131}I *locoregional* or *distant metastatic treatment*." Cooper et al. [2] in the American Thyroid Association Guidelines for patients with thyroid nodules and differentiated thyroid cancer use the terms *treatment* and *therapy* in reverse relative to the definitions herein. Although a minor point, I believe that the usage of these terms as noted in this chapter is more consistent with the usage of the terms in oncology and radiation therapy. When one is referring generically to therapy with oncological drugs, I would submit that the more frequently used term is *chemotherapy* and not *chemotreatment.* Although the terms therapy and treatment are used more interchangeably in radiation therapy, I would still submit that generally, *radiotherapy* is more frequently employed than *radiotreatment*, and *radiation therapy* refers more to the overall course of multiple *radiation treatments*.

Prognosis and Objectives

In the usage of the above terms, it is important to distinguish prognosis from objectives, albeit they are intimately related. *Prognosis* as defined by Wikipedia "...is a medical term for predicting the likely outcome of one's current standing." It is of Greek origin literally meaning "foreknowing" or "foreseeing" [8]. *Objective* is a goal of "...a desired result a person or a system envisions, plans, and commits to achieve..."[9]. Although many readers might comment that the distinction between these two terms is self-evident, not infrequently when two physicians advocate different management plans for the same patient, the difference of opinion of management is due to a difference of the two physicians' opinions of either prognosis or objective. As an example, two physicians may agree on the prognosis but disagree on the objective for an ^{131}I therapy. Alternatively, the two physicians may agree on the objective for managing a patient with a specific prognosis, but they may disagree on the prognosis in a specific patient. Distinguishing prognosis from objective will help physicians clarify their management approach as well as their differences of opinion with their colleagues. Even more important is that this may also help the patient and/or patients' family and friends who may be confused by what are two completely different recommendations from two thyroid cancer experts. If physicians can help the patient understand their different perceptions of his or her prognosis and/or the physicians' different objectives, then the patient will not only better understand the discordant opinions and recommendations of the two so-called experts, but the patient may also be able to help make his/her own decision. Finally, even when physicians agree on the prognosis as well as the objectives, some patients will accept much higher risks of side effects from the ^{131}I therapy for a lower likelihood of benefits, while other patients may be willing to give up significant potential benefits to minimize the risks of side effects. Of course, this is not an issue of right or wrong; it is an issue of patient preference.

Remnant Ablation

To ablate or not to ablate with ^{131}I? With the definitions and objectives as noted above and emphasizing that remnant ablation is the destruction of normal remaining thyroid tissue, the question becomes what is the prognosis of the patient and how important is it to destroy the normal remaining thyroid tissue to potentially improve the use of serum thyroglobulin levels as a blood "tumor marker," increase the sensitivity of a radioiodine whole-body scan that might be used in the patient's future follow-up, maximize the therapeutic effect of a subsequent potential ^{131}I therapy, and/or perform a post-therapy ^{131}I scan to complete staging? Again, this does not include the objectives of decreasing local recurrence, decreasing the frequency of distant metastases, and/or increasing disease-free survival. Again, many articles have been published using various definitions, objectives, and end points. Only a few are cited here [10–31], and the guidelines of several of the professional organizations are noted in Table 33.3. As is the case for the published articles, these various professional organizational guidelines are complicated by the use of the terms ablation, remnant ablation, and adjuvant treatment with different objectives and end points.

In those patients with an excellent prognosis (very low risk), the consensus is that no ^{131}I remnant ablation is recommended. This includes any patient with a tumor size less than 1 cm, no tumor invasion, clear margins, negative lymph nodes, and no histology that is associated with a more aggressive behavior such as tall cell variant, insular, columnar, squamous cell, diffuse sclerosing, Hürthle cell, or poorly differentiated thyroid cancer. If the tumor is greater than 1 cm but less than 2 cm, the role of ^{131}I remnant ablation becomes controversial. Some physicians will again not perform ^{131}I remnant ablation, and some will offer remnant ablation or even adjuvant treatment with ^{131}I. This is a result that some physicians believe that despite the staging system that the physicians use to classify these patients as Stage 1 (e.g., by TNM), the prognosis is not as good as a patient whose primary tumor size is less than 1 cm, and thus, it is more important to ablate normal remaining thyroid tissue for the objectives listed. I anticipate that in the future, this controversy will extend to even larger tumors.

The range of prescribed activity for remnant ablation has also been very controversial with many publications of which only a few are referenced here [15, 25–28, 32–35]. The guidelines of several of the professional organizations for prescribed activity of ^{131}I for remnant ablation are noted in Table 33.4, and again, different definitions are used by the various organizations.

Importantly, two prospective, large, multi-institutional studies have been published recently that evaluated two amounts of prescribed activity of ^{131}I and compared the patient preparation with recombinant human thyroid-stimulating hormone (rhTSH) to thyroid hormone withdrawal for remnant ablation. Mallick et al. [36] in a prospective randomized non-inferiority trial involving 29 institutions in the United Kingdom evaluated 421 patients comparing low prescribed activity of 1.1 GBq (30 mCi) to high prescribed activity of 3.7 GBq (100 mCi) of ^{131}I in combination with preparation by thyroid hormone withdrawal (rhTSH) or rhTSH injections for ^{131}I remnant ablation. The major end point for the study was remnant ablation, and successful remnant ablation was defined as both a negative scan (<0.1 % uptake on the basis of the region-of-interest method drawn over the thyroid bed) and a stimulated thyroglobulin level of <2.0 ng/ml at 6–9 months. If data on one of these criteria was not available, then only the other criterion was used. Recurrence- or progression-free survival was not one of the end points for either the definition of remnant ablation or their study. For remnant ablation, they found that the low prescribed activity 1.1 GBq (30 mCi) of ^{131}I was equally effective as the high prescribed activity 3.7 GBq (100 mCi) of ^{131}I with successful ablation achieved in 85.0 % (182/214) of patients with low prescribed activity of ^{131}I compared to 88.9 % (184/207) for patients receiving high prescribed activity of ^{131}I.

Table 33.3 Guidelines of various professional organizations for ^{131}I remnant ablation, and/or adjuvant treatment

Organization	Recommendation
ATA [2]	"RAI remnant ablation is not routinely recommended after thyroidectomy for ATA lowrisk DTC patients. Consideration of specific features of the individual patient that couldmodulate recurrence risk, disease follow-up implications, and patient preferences, are relevant to RAI decision-making."
	"RAI remnant ablation is not routinely recommended after lobectomy or total thyroidectomy for patients with unifocal papillary microcarcinoma, in the absence of other adverse features."
	"RAI remnant ablation is not routinely recommended after thyroidectomy for patients with multi-focal papillary microcarcinoma, in absence of other adverse features. Consideration of specific features of the individual patient that could modulate recurrence risk, disease followup implications, and patient preferences, are relevant to RAI decision-making."
	RAI adjuvant therapy is routinely recommended after total thyroidectomy for ATA high risk differentiated thyroid cancer patients.
EC [3] They designated this section as "Postsurgical radioiodine administration (thyroid ablation)"	Very low-risk group, which are patients with complete surgery, favorable histology, unifocal microcarcinoma (≤1 cm) with no extension beyond the thyroid capsule and without lymph node or distant metastases: "No benefit of post-operative ^{131}I"
	High-risk group, which are patients with documented distant metastases, persistent disease, incomplete tumor resection, tumor extension beyond the thyroid capsule, and high risk of persistent or recurrent disease or mortality: "Postoperative ^{131}I administration reduces the recurrence rate and possibly prolongs survival; it also permits early detection of persistent disease." (Author's comment: Again, although remnant ablation may be warranted with the above, the objective is that of adjuvant treatment or treatment)
	Low-risk group, which includes all other patients: "No consensus; benefits are controversial and there are still uncertainties as to whether it should be administered to all patients or only to selected patients. Many clinicians perform ablation in this setting where completeness of thyroidectomy is uncertain." In their Table 33.1, the EC notes "probably indication" for "…less than total thyroidectomy or no lymph node dissection or age <18 years or T1 >1 cm and T2, NO MO…or unfavorable histology"
BTA [4]	Definite indication
	Tumor >4 cm or any tumor size with gross extrathyroidal extension (pT4) or distant metastases present
	No indication
	Tumor ≤1 cm unifocal or multifocal and on histology classical papillary or follicular variant or follicular minimally invasive without angioinvasion and no invasion of thyroid capsule
	Uncertain indications
	All other cases
	One or more of the following risk factors may identify patients at higher risk of recurrence who may benefit radioiodine remnant ablation
	Large tumor size, extrathyroidal extension, unfavorable histological cell type, widely invasive histology, multiple metastatic lymph nodes, large size of involved lymph nodes, high ratio of positive to negative nodes, extra capsular nodal involvement

NCCN [5][a]	"RAI ablation is not required in patients with classic PTC that have T1b/T2 (1-4 cm) cNO disease or small-volumes N1a disease (fewer than 3-5 metastatic lymph nodes with 2-5 mm of focus of cancer in node), particularly if the postoperative Tg is <1 ng/mL in the absence of interfering anti-Tg antibodies."
	"RAI ablation is recommended when the combination of individual clinical factors (such as the size of the primary tumor, histology, degree of lymphovascular invasion, lymph node metastases, postoperarive Tg, and age at diagnosis) predicts a significant risk of recurrence, distant metastases, or disease-specific mortality."
	^{131}I typically recommended: ". .. paatients at high risk of having persistent disease remaining after total thyroidectomy and includes patients with any of the following factors: 1) gross extrathyroidal extension; 2) a primary tumor greater than 4 cm; or 3) postoperative unstimulated Tg greater than 5 to 10 ng/ml."
	^{131}I recommended in selected patients: ". . . who are at greater risk for recurrence with any of the following clinical indications such as primary tumor 1 to 4 cm, high-risk histology, lymphovascular invasion, cervical lymph node metastases, macroscopc mutifocality (one focus > 1 cm), presistence of anti-Tg antibodes, or unstimulated postoperative serum Tg (<5-10 ng/ml)."
	^{131}I is not routinely recommended for " . . . .patients with all of the following factors: 1) either unifocal or multifocal classic papillary microcarcinomas (<1 cm) confined to the thyroid; 2) no detectable anti-Tg antibodies; or 3) postoperative unstimulated Tg less than 1 ng/ml."
SNM [6]	"^{131}I ablative or tumoricidal [adjuvant] treatment of DTC with radioiodine should be considered in the postsurgical management of patients with a maximum tumor diameter greater than 1.0 cm or with a maximum tumor diameter less than 1.0 cm in the presence of high-risk features such as aggressive histology (Hürthle cell, insular, diffuse sclerosing, tall cell, columnar cell, trabecular, solid, and poorly differentiated subtypes of papillary carcinoma), lymphatic or vascular invasion, lymph node or distant metastases, multifocal disease, capsular invasion or penetration, perithyroidal soft-tissue involvement or an elevated antithyroglobulin antibody level after thyroidectomy…"
	"The treatment of very low and low-risk thyroid cancers with ^{131}I is controversial as most data suggest no statistically significant improvements in disease-specific survival, although the recurrence rates may decrease." Very low risk was defined as patients without high-risk histopathology as noted above and vascular invasion. "In patients under the age of 45 y, this category includes unifocal or multicentric microcarcinoma (<1 cm), tumors smaller than 4 cm confined to the thyroid"

[a])"The 3 general, but overlapping, functions of postoperative RAI administration include: 1) ablation of the normal thyroid remnant, which may help in surveillance for recurrent disease; 2) adjuvant therapy to try to eliminate suspected micrometastases; or 3) RAI therapy to treat know persistent disease."

Table 33.4 Professional organizational guidelines for the prescribed activity for ^{131}I for remnant ablation

Organization	Recommendation
ATA [2]	*Recommendation 55*
	". . . A low administered dose activity of approximately of 30 mCi is generally favored over higher administered dose activities.
	"Higher administered activities may need to be considered for patients receiving less than a total or near-total thyroidectomy where a larger remnant is suspected or where adjuvant therapy is intended."
EC [3]	"The administered ^{131}I activity among centers ranges between 1,110 MBq (30 mCi) (low activity) and 3,700 MBq (100 mCi) or even more (high activity)"
	For the European Consensus, thyroid ablation refers to "...the postsurgical administration of ^{131}I, whose aim is to destroy any thyroid residue in the thyroid bed." The meaning of residue is not further defined but may be considered by some to be just destroying normal residual thyroid tissue or residue of suspected but unproven cancer or even known cancer
BTA [4]	They combine objectives of remnant ablation and adjuvant treatment into the term "radioiodine remnant ablation"
	pT1-2, N0 with resection with no microscopic residual disease should receive 1.1 GBq
	pT3 and/or N1 disease, the ^{131}I activity should be decided by the multidisciplinary team on an individual case basis
NCCN [5]	1.11 GBq (30 mCi) in patients at low risk. This prescribed activity". . . may be considered in patients at slightly higher risk." (Although this guideline differentiates the objectives of *remnant ablation* and *adjuvant treatment*, in this section for prescribed activity the guideline uses the term *ablation* and does not further differentiated prescribed activity for *adjuvant treatment* vs *remnant ablatio*n. For lymph node metastases with RAI uptake, one ". . . may treat with about 100-175 mC.")
SNM [6]	"Range of 1.11–3.7 GBq (30–100 mCi) is typically prescribed, depending on the radioiodine uptake measurement and amount of residual function tissue present"

Of note, although N1 disease was included in this study, this study was again only evaluating the end point of remnant ablation – not frequency of recurrence, which Mallick et al. recognized. As noted above, an additional objective of the study was to assess the outcome relative to patient preparation by either rhTSH injections or THW, and Mallick et al. demonstrated no difference in achieving successful remnant ablation with rhTSH injections to THW while significantly reducing the side effects of THW. This is discussed in more detail in Chap. 34.

The second study by Schlumberger et al. [37] was a prospective randomized trial involving 25 centers in France and evaluated 684 patients, again comparing low prescribed activity of 1.1 GBq (30 mCi) to high prescribed activity of 3.7 GBq (100 mCi) of ^{131}I as well as comparing the patient preparation of rhTSH injections to THW for ^{131}I remnant ablation. Successful remnant thyroid ablation using the definition of "normal" ultrasonography was 97 % (334/346) for 1.1 GBq (30 mCi) and 94 % (318/339) for 3.7 GBq (100 mCi) and using the definition of stimulated thyroglobulin level of <1 ng/ml was 91 % (301/330) for 1.1 GBq (30 mCi) and 93 % (299/320) for 3.7 GBq (100 mCi). The low activity of 1.1 GBq (30 mCi) was equally effective as the higher 3.7 GBq (100 mCi) of prescribed activity of ^{131}I for remnant ablation. Again, the rate of successful remnant ablation was not statistically different in patient prepared with rhTSH injections relative to THW, but hypothyroidism was eliminated with rhTSH injections relative to THW. This is discussed again in greater detail in Chap. 34. However, in summary, remnant ablation as defined herein for selected patients should be successfully achieved with as little as 1.11 GBq (30 mCi) of ^{131}I.

Adjuvant Treatment

Adjuvant treatment, as defined in more detail at the beginning of this chapter, is to destroy suspected but unproven residual differentiated thyroid cancer with the objective of reducing recurrence and/or increasing survival. The guidelines of several of the professional organizations for prescribed activity of ^{131}I for adjuvant treatment are noted in Table 33.5. Although the above studies of Mallick et al. and Schlumberger et al. are important publications in resolving the issue of the amount of prescribed activity for remnant ablation, these articles do not address prescribed activity for adjuvant treatment. Mallick et al. [36] note, "...our findings relate to [remnant] ablation success at 6 to 9 months and do not address future recurrences." Schlumberger et al. [37] note, "...whether 1.1-GBq of ^{131}I radioactivity affects long-term outcomes will be revealed only by following patients over time." The issue of residual or recurrent disease then refers to the objective of adjuvant treatment rather than remnant ablation. Certainly, with these large prospective studies of patients with low and intermediate risk of disease, the opportunity will be available to follow these patients, which has the potential to not only further evaluate low 1.1 GBq (30 mCi) prescribed activity to higher prescribed activity (i.e., 3.7 GBq (100 mCi)) of ^{131}I but also patient preparation by THW vs. rhTSH injections. However, an important caveat will be that this follow-up will only evaluate the similarities or differences of 1.1 GBq (30 mCi) vs. 3.7 GBq (100 mCi) of ^{131}I in being effective or ineffective in reducing long-term recurrence. This will not assess effectiveness or ineffectiveness of empiric prescribed activities of 5.55 GBq (150 mCi) or more or dosimetrically determined prescribed activities of

Table 33.5 Professional organizational guidelines for the prescribed activity for ^{131}I for adjuvant treatment

Organization	Recommendation
ATA [2]	*Recommendation 56*
	"When RAI is intended for initial adjuvant therapy to treat suspected microscopic residual disease, administered activities above those used for remnant ablation up to 150 mCi are generally recommended (in absence of known distant metastases)."
EC [3]	3.7 GBq (100 mCi)
BTA [4]	See Tables 33.3 and 33.4
NCCN [5]	Although this guideline differentiates the objectives of *remnant ablation* and *adjuvant treatment*, in this section for prescribed activity the guideline uses the term ablation and does not further differentiated prescribed activity for *adjuvant treatmen*t vs *remnant ablation*. For lymph node metastases with RAI uptake, one ". . . may treat with about 100-175 mC.")
SNM [6]	A category of "adjuvant treatment" of ^{131}I for suspected but not documented locoregional disease was not specifically addressed

^{131}I in reducing recurrence. For example, Castagna et al. [38] reported that their "...study provides the first evidence that in patients who are at intermediate risk, high RAI activities (e.g., 3.7 GBq (100 mCi)) at ablation (really meaning adjuvant treatment) has no major advantage over low activities (e.g., 1.11 GBq (30 mCi))." At 6–18-month follow-up, they reported rates for 3.7 GBq (100 mCi) vs. 1.11 GBq (30 mCi) of 60 % vs. 60 % for remission, 18.8 % vs. 14.3 % for biochemical (Tg) disease, and 21.2 % vs. 25.7 % for metastatic disease, respectively. At the last follow-up of their patients, they reported rates for remission of 76.5 % vs. 72.1 %, recurrent disease 2.4 % vs. 2.1 %, persistent disease 18.8 % vs. 23.6 %, and death 2.4 % and 2.1 %. This may indeed mean there is no advantage to a prescribed activity of 3.7 GBq (100 mCi) vs. 1.11 GBq (30 mCi) of ^{131}I, but this may also mean that they are *equally ineffective*. Indeed, their data could be interpreted as one needs to administer more GBq (mCi) of ^{131}I to improve their remission rate of ~75 %. A further discussion regarding delivering enough radiation absorbed dose is presented below. On the other hand, Han et al. [39] evaluated 176 patients with small (≤2 cm) lesions, microscopic extrathyroidal extension, and no cervical LN metastases and reported that the low prescribed activity (1.11 GBq (30 mCi)) was sufficient to treat these patients relative to a prescribed activity of 5.55 GBq (150 mCi). However, this was a retrospective study, over half the patients had a tumor ≤1 cm, and the definition of "sufficient to treat" needed to be clarified. If they meant "remnant ablation," then this has already been shown, and the retrospective study of Han et al. just further substantiates the larger, prospective studies of Mallick et al. and Schlumberger et al. If Han et al. use the phrase "sufficient to treat" to mean adjuvant treatment, and this author believes that this is the case from the criteria in the method section, then rather than concluding that 1.11 GBq (30 mCi) is sufficient for adjuvant treatment, they may have concluded that no adjuvant treatment is needed. In other words, neither 1.11 GBq (30 mCi) nor 5.55 GBq (150 mCi) accomplished any significant reduction in the recurrence rate because the recurrence rate was already very low. Again, my concern is that when a study demonstrates that there is no difference between outcomes of recurrence between the choices of ^{131}I therapy such as with 1.1 GBq (30 mCi) or 3. 7 GBq (100 mCi), that study may not have been designed to address potentially more more beneficial alternatives. In patients with N1a or N1b disease, perhaps higher prescribed activities of 5.55 GBq (150 mCi), 6.6 GBq (175 mCi), 7.4 (200 mCi), and/or dosimetrically determined prescribed activities of ^{131}I would be more effective and should be evaluated. Alternatively, perhaps no adjuvant treatment should be performed. Then the only decision remaining would be whether or not remnant ablation activities of ^{131}I should be administered.

In our efforts to determine the most appropriated prescribed activity for a specific patient or to study the various patient risk groups, we focus on two major appropriate criteria: side effects and outcomes. However, we still need to keep several additional fundamental tenets in mind. First, to destroy suspected residual cancer, it is important to emphasize that generally a higher prescribed activity is required to deliver a lethal radiation absorbed dose to the cancer than is required to destroying normal thyroid tissue. This may be the result of many factors such as the radioiodine in thyroid cancer cells may have lower uptake, shorter residence time, more inhomogeneous uptake, and/or less "cross-fire" effect than normal thyroid tissue. The second fundamental tenet is that to destroy the entire metastases such as in a lymph node, one needs to deliver a lethal radiation dose to the metastases. Maxon et al. [22, 40–43] evaluated the radiation absorbed dose to destroy metastatic lymph nodes with metastatic disease and demonstrated that if one could deliver at least 85 Gy (8,500 rad), one would be successful; however, if one delivered less than 30 Gy (3,000 rad), the success rate would be lower. O'Connell et al. [44] also reported that cumulative radiation absorbed doses of 100 Gy (10,000 rad) eradicated cervical node metastases. In a retrospective study of patients with known cervical metastases, Klubo-Gwiezdzinska et al. [45] demonstrated a statistical significant response to dosimetrically determined prescribed activities of ^{131}I relative to empiric prescribed activities. In the interim, the selection of the prescribed activity of ^{131}I whether empirically determined (e.g., 1.1 GBq (30 mCi), 3.7 GBq (100 mCi), or 5.55 GBq (150 mCi)) or dosimetrically determined for adjuvant treatment or even whether or not to administer ^{131}I at all to reduce recurrence in patients with various risks will remain controversial. However, although certainly lower prescribed activity is well intended to reduce the frequency and severity of side effects, one still needs to go back to the fundamental tenets of any treatment option: weighing the benefits vs. risks in the various patient risk groups. In addition, the decision based on benefits vs. risks is not always a scientific decision as one patient may accept more potential benefit with more risk and another patient may accept less potential benefit with lower risks.

Known Locoregional Metastatic Treatment

The treatment for known locoregional metastatic and specifically the role of ^{131}I treatment for known locoregional metastases of DTC involves even more controversies. The first controversy relates to what the indications are for the various treatment options for the management of known locoregional metastatic disease including additional surgery, the extent of additional surgery, how many times should additional surgery be performed, ^{131}I therapy, external radiation therapy, alcohol injections, or no intervention with careful follow-up ("active surveillance"). A discussion of all of the various options and their indications is beyond the scope of this chapter, but the recommendations of the various professional organizations for ^{131}I treatment of locoregional disease are noted in Table 33.6. The recommendations are again complicated by the use of different terms as well as the use of different definitions and/or objectives for the same term. The second controversy is if ^{131}I is selected, what is the method (empiric vs. dosimetric) for the selection of the prescribed activity of ^{131}I to be administered? The controversy of empirically determined and dosimetrically determined amounts of prescribed activity of ^{131}I has been discussed in more detail in Chap. 58 on dosimetry and Chap. 56 on the ^{131}I treatment of distant metastases. However, in this situation, it is no longer a question of how "low can we go" in prescribed activity of ^{131}I for remnant ablation, but rather as Maxon et al. [22] has pointed out, it is a question of whether or not we can administer a prescribed activity of ^{131}I that delivers the necessary radiation absorbed dose to the thyroid cancer cells in the lymph nodes (or distant metastases) to kill those cells, and this also includes the objective of not exceeding an unacceptable frequency and severity of untoward effects of the ^{131}I. The third controversy is that if an empiric amount of prescribed activity of ^{131}I is to be selected, how does one select that empiric amount, and again, what are acceptable frequency and/or severity of side effects?

For empiric amounts of prescribed activity of ^{131}I for the treatment of locoregional metastases or distant metastases, the spectrum ranges typically from 3.7 to 11.1 GBq (100–300 mCi) (see Chap. 56), but no large prospective study has been published. However, prospective studies are difficult to perform because it is difficult to control the many factors that affect the radiation absorbed dose to the locoregional disease (see Table 33.7). In addition, in choosing a higher empiric prescribed activity with the objective of trying to increase the likelihood of delivering a therapeutic radiation absorbed dose, the potential frequency and severity of untoward effects are more likely to be increased. As pointed out by Leeper [46], Kulkarni et al. [47], and Tuttle et al. [48], as many as 10–20 % of patients may exceed 200 cGy (rad) to the bone marrow with empiric prescribed activities of 3.7–7.4 MBq (100–200 mCi). Again, Maxon et al. [22, 40–43] evaluated lesional dosimetry performed with planar images, but few institutions routinely use such techniques and few publications have subsequently reported on the use of ^{131}I lesional dosimetry with planar images. Instead, whole-body dosimetry has been performed more frequently to assess the *maximum tolerable activity* (MTA), which is also called the *maximum treatment activity* (MTA), *maximum allowable activity* (MAA), or *maximum safe activity* (MSA). As recommended by Leeper et al. [49], for patients who have locoregional disease without pulmonary metastases, the MTA should be reduced when the 48 h whole-body retention exceeds 4.44 GBq (120 mCi). The MTA may also be modified based on the specific situation of the individual patient such as presence of a low absolute neutrophil count, low platelet count, the response of the absolute neutrophil (ANC) and platelet count after prior ^{131}I treatment(s), total cumulative ^{131}I activity, time from last treatment, etc. (see Chap. 56.)

Table 33.6 Professional organizational guidelines for the prescribed activity for ^{131}I for treatment of locoregional metastases

Organization	Recommendation
ATA [2]	*Recommendation 52*
	"(a) In the treatment of locoregional or metastatic disease, no recommendation can be made about the superiority of one method of RAI administration over another (empiric high dose vs. blood and/or body dosimetry vs. lesional dosimetry.) Recommendation rating: I
	(b) Empirically administered amounts of ^{131}I exceeding 200 mCi that often potentially exceed the maximum tolerable tissue dose should be avoided in patients over age 70 years. Recommendation rating: A"
EC [3]	3.7 GBq (100 mCi)
BTA [4]	"The optimal ^{131}I therapeutic activity for persistent neck disease or metastatic disease is uncertain. Most of the evidence for a benefit of ^{131}I therapy… derives from studies where empirical activities of ^{131}I were used. The role of dosimetry and its impact on clinical outcomes, compared to empirical use of ^{131}I therapy is unclear"
NCCN [5]	3.7 GBq (100 mCi) to 7.4 GBq (200 mCi)
SNM [6]	"For treatment of thyroid cancer in the cervical or mediastinal lymph nodes, activity in the range of 5.55–7.4 GBq (150–200 mCi) is typically administered. Patients with advanced local or regional disease may be treated first with surgical debulking, then with ^{131}I and, if clinically indicated, external beam radiation"

Table 33.7 Factors that may affect response of thyroid tissue to radiation absorbed dose from ^{131}I

Uptake
Residence time
Dose rate
Tissue sensitivity to radiation
Cross-fire effect (e.g., degree of heterogeneity vs. homogeneity of uptake)
Administered prescribed activity of ^{131}I

In comparing empirically determined vs. dosimetrically determined activities or comparing the various levels of empiric activities for the treatment of locoregional metastases, no prospective study has been published. However, Klubo-Gwiezdzinska et al. [45] in a retrospective study reported that patients with known locoregional disease had a statistically better outcome when the amount of ^{131}I administered was dosimetrically determined rather than empirically determined. Again, for a more in-depth discussion of dosimetrically determined and empirically determined prescribed activity of ^{131}I for therapy, the reader is referred to the discussion in Chap. 58 regarding the argument for dosimetry rather than empirically determined activities for ^{131}I treatment of either locoregional or distant metastases. Alternative simplified methods of dosimetry are now available to help determine when an empiric amount of ^{131}I may exceed 200 cGy (200 rad) to the bone marrow, when it should be reduced, or when and how much an empiric amount of ^{131}I may be increased to help maximize the administered radiation dose to the locoregional metastasis while not exceeding 200 cGy (rad) to the bone marrow, and this is discussed further in Chap. 59.

Distillation of Guidelines

In an attempt to distill as well as to consolidate the guidelines from the various professional organizations noted herein regarding the indications for remnant ablation, adjuvant treatment, and locoregional treatment as well as the two recent prospective studies, see Table 33.8. This table presents several scenarios, but it cannot cover all patient scenarios and factors.

Pediatric Prescribed Activity

The indications for ^{131}I therapy and the prescribed activities of ^{131}I for pediatric patients with differentiated thyroid cancer for remnant ablation, adjuvant treatment, and treatment of known locoregional disease and/or distant metastases are even more problematic and beyond the scope of this chapter. Please see the separate chapter entitled "Thyroid cancer in children and adolescents" (Chap. 42 and 77). Most authorities agree that the prescribed activities of ^{131}I for remnant ablation and adjuvant treatment in pediatric patients should be reduced relative to adult prescribed activities. One such method for calculating the reduced prescribed activities of ^{131}I was presented by Reynolds et al. (see Table 33.9) [75]. Although it is understandable that Mallick et al. [36] and Schlumberger et al. [37] did not evaluate the success of remnant ablation using low and high prescribed activities of ^{131}I in pediatric patients, I propose that the selection of a pediatric prescribed activity for remnant ablation may be reduced based on Reynolds' approach using an adult prescribed activity.

For locoregional metastases and distant metastases in pediatric patients, I encourage that a maximum prescribed activity be determined whenever possible with full ^{131}I dosimetry such as the Benua and Leeper approach [46, 50], the MIRD approach [51, 52] or a simplified alternative dosimetry method such as described by Van Nostrand et al. [53] or Hänscheid et al. [54]. However, this does not mean that a dosimetrically determined maximum tolerated activity should be administered, but it does permit a calculation of the prescribed activity that one should not exceed until further studies demonstrate otherwise. This is discussed further in the chapter entitled "Dosimetrically-determined prescribed activity of ^{131}I for the treatment of metastatic differentiated thyroid carcinoma" (see Chap. 58).

Fractionation

Fractionation of the administration of ^{131}I for well-differentiated thyroid cancer has been proposed to reduce the severity and frequency of the side effects of ^{131}I, allow compliance with various radiation safety regulations in different countries, and/or save on the expense of hospitalization. Dose fractionation is "…when the total dose of radiation is divided into several, smaller doses…[administered]…over a period of [time]" [55]. Fractionation is frequently used in external beam radiation therapy. Typically, cancer cells have higher rates of mitosis, and thus, there is a higher likelihood that the cancer cell relative to normal cells will be in the phase of mitosis that is most vulnerable to radiation, thereby increasing the damage to the DNA in the cancer cells relative to the normal cells. Thus, rather than administering the entire radiation absorbed dose at one time, fractionation allows time for the normal cells, which had less damage relative to the cancer cells, to repair themselves, thereby reducing the side effects in normal tissue relative to the desired damage to the cancer cells.

Although fractionation of the therapeutic administration of radiopharmaceuticals may reduce side effects to normal

Table 33.8 Distilledguidelines for first-time ^{131}I therapy for six scenarios

Selected scenarios	Spectrum of Recommendations
T1a (unifocal or multifocal) N0, NX, M0, no thyroid extension beyond capsule, and no aggressive histologic subtypes[a, b].	No ^{131}I remnant ablation[c]
T1b or T2, NX, N0, M0, no thyroid extension beyond capsule, no aggressive histologic subtypes[a, b].	Controversial including
	1. No ^{131}I remnant ablation
	2. ^{131}I remnant ablation with 1.1 GBq (30 mCi) of ^{131}I
T3, NX, N0, M0[a, b].	Controversial including
	1. ^{131}I remnant ablation with 1.1 GBq (30 mCi) of ^{131}I
	2. ^{131}I adjuvant treatment[c] with prescribed activity ranging from 1.1 GBq (30 mCi) to 5.55 GBq (150 mCi)
T4, NX, N0, M0[a, b].	1. This is not remnant ablation or adjuvant treatment
	2. ^{131}I treatment[c]. The empiric prescribed activities range as high as 5.55 GBq (150 mCi) or prescribed activity determined by whole-body dosimetry or simplified alternative whole-body dosimetry
T1b or T2, with either N1, thyroid extension beyond capsule, or aggressive histologic subtypes, and M0[a, b].	Controversial and depending on factors such as number of involved lymph nodes, size of metastases in lymph nodes, degree of extension, etc.
	1. ^{131}I remnant ablation with prescribed activity of 1.1 GBq (30 mCi) ^{131}I
	2. ^{131}I adjuvant treatment with prescribed activity ranging as high as 5.55 GBq (150 mCi)
T3 with any N, thyroid extension beyond capsule, and/or aggressive histologic subtypes[a, b].	1. ^{131}I adjuvant treatment or treatment with prescribed activity ranging as high as 5.55 GBq (150 mCi) of ^{131}I or prescribed activity determined by whole-body dosimetry or simplified alternative whole-body dosimetry

TNM staging system		
Tumor size:	TX	Primary tumor cannot be assessed
	T0	No evidence of primary tumor
	T1	Tumor less than 2 cm in greatest dimension limited to thyroid
		T1a <1 cm
		T1b ≥1 <2 cm
	T2	Tumor ≥2 cm but <4 cm in greatest dimension and limited to the thyroid
	T3	Tumor ≥4 cm in greatest dimension limited to the thyroid or tumor of any size with minimal extrathyroidal extension (e.g., to sternothyroid muscle or perithyroidal soft tissues)
	T4a	Tumor of any size extending beyond the thyroid capsule and invading local soft tissues, larynx, trachea, esophagus, or recurrent laryngeal nerve
	T4b	Tumor invading prevertebral fascia, mediastinal vessels, or encasing carotid artery in the neck

TNM staging system		
Nodes	NX	Regional nodes cannot be assessed
	N0	No metastases to regional nodes
	N1	Metastases to regional nodes are present
	N1A	To Level VI (pretracheal, paratracheal, prelaryngeal, and Delphian lymph nodes)
	N1B	In other unilateral, bilateral, or contralateral cervical or mediastinal lymph nodes
Metastases:	MX	Presence of distant metastases cannot be assessed
	M0	No distant metastases
	M1	Distant metastases are present

	Impact of age on TNM staging[d]	
	Age less than 45 years of age	Age of 45 years or older
Stage I	Any T, any N, M0	T1, N0, M0
Stage II	Any T, any N, M1	T2, N0, M0
Stage III	N/A	T3, N0, M0 or T1-T3, N1A, M0
Stage IV A	N/A	T1-T3, N1B, M1
		T4a, N0-N1, M0
Stage IV B		T4b, Nx, M0
Stage IV C		TX, NX, M1

[a]Aggressive histologic subtypes include but are not limited to tall cell, insular, columnar, diffusesclerosing, squamous cell, Hürthle cell, and poorly differentiated

[b] Any age

[c]For definitions of ^{131}I remnant ablation, adjuvant treatment, locoregional treatment, and therapy, see the text

[d] The staging for differentiated thyroid cancer is designated as stage I, II, III, or IV based upon the TNM status and the age of the patient

Table 33.9 Modification factors of prescribed activity for treatment for children

Factor	Body weight (kg)	Body surface area (m^2)
0.2	10	0.4
0.4	25	0.8
0.6	40	1.2
0.8	55	1.4
1.0	77	1.7

Source: refs. [42, 75]

Body surface area = 0.1 × (weight in kg)$^{0.67}$

tissue, help compliance with local regulations, and/or save the cost of hospitalization, fractionation of ^{131}I therapies has several major disadvantages. First, the effectiveness of a ^{131}I therapy is very dependent on uptake of ^{131}I into the thyroid cancer cell. Unfortunately, the first fractionated ^{131}I therapy may significantly reduce the uptake of ^{131}I in the cancer cell from the subsequent fractionated therapies, and thus, the radiation absorbed dose delivered to the cancer from the second or any subsequent fractionated ^{131}I therapies may be significantly reduced. A second potential disadvantage is that by fractionating the prescribed activity of ^{131}I, the *radiation dose rate* (i.e., cGy per hour [rad/h]) for each therapy is reduced. Although this decreases the biologic effects to normal tissues, it also reduces the biologic effects to the thyroid cancer, thereby increasing the time for the potential repair of the damage of the DNA in the cancer cell [56]. Third, for fractionated doses to be administered, the patients must either extend their period of thyroid hormone withdrawal and thus extend the duration of their hypothyroidism or the patient must receive additional injections of rhTSH. If low-iodine diets are recommended, these would also have to be extended.

Arad et al. [57] evaluated fractionated dose of ^{131}I for remnant ablation using two to three separate doses of 1.1 GBq (30 mCi) of ^{131}I administered weekly. Twenty patients received single doses of ^{131}I with a mean of 5.3 GBq (142.2 mCi) (range of 1.85–5.55 GBq (50–150 mCi)), and 12 patients received fractionated doses with a mean total prescribed activity of 3.1 GBq (83.6 mCi) (range of 2.2–4.1 GBq (60–111 mCi)) with individual doses ranging from 1.1 to 1.85 GBq (30–50 mCi). Remnant ablation was considered successful if the follow-up scan after 6 months demonstrated no radioiodine uptake in the thyroid bed. Remnant ablation was achieved in 80 % of the patients receiving the unfractionated doses and 75 % of the patients receiving fractionated doses. Wang et al. [58] evaluated 99 patients who received fractionated doses of ^{131}I for remnant ablation. A total of approximately 3.7 GBq (100 mCi) of ^{131}I was given in approximately equal doses every week for 3 weeks. Successful ablation, which was defined as absence of any residual thyroid uptake on follow-up scan done at least 6 months after ^{131}I remnant ablation, was achieved in 72 % (71) patients. Wu et al. [59] evaluated 35 patients who were administered 4.44 GBq (120 mCi) of ^{131}I in three fractions over 3 weeks. They performed two ^{131}I whole-body scans. The mean uptake on the first scan performed 7 days after the first administration of ^{131}I was 2.7 %, and the mean uptake on the second scan performed 7 days after the second administration was 0.26 %. The mean decrease in uptake was 81 %. Interestingly, in two patients with lung metastases, the uptake increased after the second ^{131}I therapy. Their conclusion was that they did not recommend fractionated ablative doses and further study was warranted in patients with lung metastases. Czepczyński et al. [60] compared a group of 113 patients receiving a single dose of ^{131}I of 2.2 GBq (60 mCi) to a group of 273 patients who received fractionated doses of 1.1 GBq administered at 24 h intervals. The patients were evaluated 6–8 months later with radioiodine whole-body scan and uptake, thyroglobulin, and neck ultrasound, and the results were categorized as complete remission (CR) and no complete remission (NCR). The frequencies of CR and NCR were not statistically different with 69 (61 %) and 172 (63 %) of the patients in CR in group 1 and group 2, respectively. Clerc et al. [61] administered two 7.4 GBq (20 mCi) approximately 6–18 months apart, obtaining successfully ablation after the second ^{131}I therapy in 92 % of the patients. With shorter interval between fractionated administrations of ^{131}I, this may avoid the issue of stunning and/or partial treatment resulting in reduced ^{131}I uptake of the second therapy. As a result, this may be satisfactory in countries that restrict the amount of radioiodine retained at any one time in a patient.

Despite the above, Mallick et al. and Schlumberger et al. demonstrated that 1.1 GBq (30 mCi) is adequate for remnant ablation in low- and some intermediate-risk patients, and therefore fractionated doses are not necessary for remnant ablation. Instead, the question becomes whether or not fractionated doses for adjuvant therapy or treatment for known locoregional or distant metastases are equivalent to single doses. Although Arab et al. [57] reported that none of their patients in either group had evidence of local recurrence during the follow-up period of 1–7 years (mean 3.7 years), the number of patients was low, few demographics were reported, and the follow-up period was short.

In summary, fractionation of ^{131}I therapies may help meet radiation safety requirements, reduce the costs of hospitalization, and/or even theoretically reduce side effects. However, with the recent data from Mallick et al. and Schlumberger et al. regarding the effectiveness of 1.11 GBq (30 mCi) prescribed activity for remnant ablation, fractionation is not necessary for remnant ablation. Although the benefit of fractionated higher prescribed activity of ^{131}I (i.e., >3.7 GBq (100 mCi) or even higher) for adjuvant treatment or treatment of known locoregional or distant metastases is not well studied, there are potentially significant disadvantages such as a significantly lower subsequent uptake of ^{131}I for the subsequent fractionated therapies, lower radiation dose rate delivered, longer periods of hypothyroidism, and/or increased costs of rhTSH injections. Accordingly, it is important for the patient and treating physician to understand their priorities, the motivation behind their priorities, and the subsequent advantages and disadvantages of using a fractionated protocol for ^{131}I therapies.

Diuretics

Diuretics such as furosemide (Lasix®) have been evaluated by multiple authors to facilitate the renal clearance of ^{131}I from the whole body after ^{131}I therapy, but the results are controversial [62–73]. Seabold et al. [63] recommended furosemide on the basis of its acceleration of iodide excretion. Maruca et al. [64] reported that a low-iodine diet was more important than furosemide, and Kapucu et al. [67] observed that furosemide prior to radioiodine administration increased radioiodine uptake more than a low-iodine diet. Matovic et al. [72] compared urinary radioiodine excretion after furosemide and potassium administration in 23 patients relative to 20 patients who did not receive furosemide and potassium. The former group had a significant decrease in urinary excretion of radioiodine and higher blood concentrations, and therefore, they did not recommend the use of furosemide. However, Barbaro et al. [73] evaluated 201 patients divided into two groups. Group 1 had stages I–II and was treated with 1.11 GBq (30 mCi) of ^{131}I and group 2 included patients with stages III–IV and were treated with 3.7 GBq (100 mCi). These two groups were each further subdivided into subgroups A, B, and C. All were pretreated with rhTSH injections as well as a 4-day withdrawal of thyroid hormone. Group 1A had 45 patients and group 2A had 22 patients, and none of these patients were pretreated with furosemide or treated after therapy with lithium. Group 1B had 45 patients and group 2B had 22 patients, and all of these patients received furosemide (25 mg/day orally) for 3 days prior to ^{131}I therapy. Group 1C also had 45 patients and group 2C had 22 patients, and all of these patients received furosemide (25 mg/day orally) 3 days prior to ^{131}I therapy and lithium (450 mg/day orally) during the 3 days following ^{131}I therapy. A control group of 20 patients who had very low-risk cancer were treated with 1.11 GBq (30 mCi) of ^{131}I with the same rhTSH and thyroid hormone withdrawal protocol as the other groups. In the patients from group 1, those who received furosemide and/or furosemide with lithium had a better outcome of ablation based on percent of undetectable TG values and negative whole-body scans, but these findings were not observed in group 2 patients. They concluded that pretreatment with furosemide appeared to improve the outcome of ablation by reducing the iodine pool. Further study is warranted.

Lithium

Adjunctive treatment of lithium is discussed in Chap. 61.

Redifferentiation

Redifferentiation is beyond the scope of this chapter. Suffice it to mention that a recent publication by Ho et al. [74] evaluated the potential utility of selumetinib to stimulate or increase ^{131}I uptake in patients with iodine-refractory metastatic DTC (see Chap. 68).

Summary

With better and more universal definitions of various terms, better understanding of prognosis and objectives, better staging, and two recent noteworthy prospective studies, significant progress has been made in the clarification of the management of patients and the therapeutic use of ^{131}I for remnant ablation in patients with differentiated thyroid cancer. However, much work remains to be done. Further study is needed to compare the recurrence rate and survival of various options for the management of *suspected but unknown* locoregional metastases (adjuvant treatment) as well as *known* locoregional metastases, and more studies are needed to identify and validate methods to *maximize* the radiation absorbed dose to the thyroid cancer cell per GBq (mCi) administered and to determine the best rate of cGy(rad) /unit time delivered, while minimizing the radiation absorbed dose to normal tissues.

References

1. Khorjekar G, Van Nostrand D, Kharazi P, Kulkarni K, Garcia C, Acio E, Atkins F. Division of Nuclear Medicine, Washington Hospital Center. Washington, D.C. Can the controversy regarding selecting the prescribed activity of ^{131}I for first-time therapies in patient with differentiation thyroid cancer be reduced by defining the terms? An educational exhibit. J Nucl Med. 2011;52S(abstract).
2. Haugen BR, Alexander EA, Bible KC, Doherty G, Mandel SJ, Nikiforov YE, Pacini F, Randolph GW, Sawka AM, Schlumberger M, Schuff K, Sherman SI, Sosa JA, Steward DL, Tuttle RM, Wartofsky L. 2015 American Thyroid Association Management Guidelines for Adult Patients with Thyroid Nodules and Differentiated Thyroid Cancer. Thyroid. 2016;26:1–133.
3. Pacini F, Schlumberger M, Dralle H, Elisei R, Smit JWA, Wiersinga W, The European Thyroid Cancer Taskforce. European consensus for the management of patients with differentiated thyroid carcinoma of the follicular epithelium. Eur J Endocrinol. 2006;154:787–803.
4. Perros P, Colley S, Boelaert K, Evans C, Evans RM, Gerrard GE, Gilbert JA, Harrison B, Johnson SJ, Giles TE, Moss L, Lewington V, Newbold KL, Taylor J, Thakker RV, Watkinson J, Williams GR. British Thyroid Association guidelines for the management of thyroid cancer. Clin Endocrinol. 2014;81 Suppl 1:1–122.

5. National Comprehensive Cancer Network (NCCN). Clinical practice guidelines in oncology. Thyroid carcinoma. Follicular thyroid carcinoma. V.2.2015. www.nccn.org.
6. Silberstein E, Alavi A, Halon H, et al. The SNMMI practice guideline for therapy of thyroid disease with ^{131}I 3.0. J Nucl Med. 2012;53:1633–51.
7. Van Nostrand D. The benefits and risks of ^{131}I therapy in patients with well-differentiated thyroid cancer. Thyroid. 2009;19:1381–91.
8. Wikipedia. http://en.wikipedia.org/wiki/Prognosis. Updated 4 Dec 2014 at 22:48. Accessed 21 Dec 2014.
9. Wikipedia. http://en.wikipedia.org/wiki/Objective_(goal). Updated 11 Dec 2014 at 23:58. Accessed 21 Dec 2014.
10. Mazzaferri EL, Kloos RT. Current approaches to primary therapy for papillary and follicular thyroid cancer. J Clin Endocrinol Metab. 2001;86:1447–63.
11. Wartofsky L, Sherman SI, Gopal J, et al. Therapeutic controversy: the use of radioactive iodine in patients with papillary and follicular thyroid cancer. J Clin Endocrinol Metab. 1998;83:4195–203.
12. Beierwaltes WH, Rabbani R, Dmuchowski C, et al. An analysis of ablation of thyroid remnants" with I-131 in 511 patients from 1947–1984: experience at University of Michigan. J Nucl Med. 1984;25:1287–93.
13. Comtois R, Theriault C, Del Vecchio P. Assessment of the efficacy of iodine-131 for thyroid ablation. J Nucl Med. 1993;34:1927–30.
14. DeGroot KJ, Kaplan EL, McCormick M, Straus FH. Natural history, treatment, and course of papillary thyroid carcinoma. J Clin Endocrinol Metab. 1990;71:414–24.
15. Doi SAR, Woodhouse NJY. Ablation of the thyroid remnant and 131-I dose in differentiated thyroid cancer. Clin Endocrinol. 2000;52:765–73.
16. Heufelder AE, Gorman CA. Radioiodine therapy in the treatment of differentiated thyroid cancer: guidelines and considerations. Endocrinologist. 1991;1:273–80.
17. Hodgson DC, Brierley JD, Tsang RW, Panzarella T. Prescribing 131-I iodine based on neck uptake produces effective thyroid ablation and reduced hospital stay. Radiother Oncol. 1998;47:325–30.
18. Hung G, Tu ST, Wu IS, et al. Comparison of the effectiveness between a single low dose and fractionated doses of radioiodine in ablation of post-operative thyroid remnants. Jpn J Clin Oncol. 2004;34:469–71.
19. Klain M, Ricard M, Leboulleux S, et al. Radioiodine therapy for papillary and follicular thyroid carcinoma. Eur J Nucl Med. 2002;29 Suppl 2:S479–85.
20. Kuni CC, Klingensmith WC. Failure of low doses of I-131 to ablate residual thyroid tissue following surgery for thyroid cancer. Radiology 1980; 137:773–74. Leung SF, Law MWM, Ho SKW. Efficacy of low-dose iodine-131 ablation of postoperative thyroid remnants: a study of 69 cases. Br J Radiol. 1992; 65:905–9.
21. Logue JP, Tang RW, Brierley JD, et al. Radioiodine ablation of residual tissue in thyroid cancer: relationship between administered activity, neck uptake and outcome. Br J Radiol. 1994;67:1127–31.
22. Maxon HR, Thomas SR, Hertzberg VS, et al. Relation between effective radiation dose and outcome of radioiodine therapy for thyroid cancer. NEJM. 1983;309:937–41.
23. Mazzaferri EL. Thyroid remnant 131-I ablation for papillary and follicular thyroid carcinoma. Thyroid. 1997;7:265–71.
24. Meier DA, Brill DR, Becker DV, et al. Procedure guideline for therapy of thyroid disease with I-131. J Nucl Med. 2002;43:856–61.
25. Ramacciotti C, Pretorius HT, Line B, et al. Ablation of nonmalignant thyroid remnants with low doses of radioactive iodine: concise communication. J Nucl Med. 1982;23:483–9.
26. Samaan NA, Schultz PN, Hickey RD, et al. The results of various modalities of treatment of well-differentiated thyroid carcinoma: a retrospective review of 1599 patients. J Clin Endocrinol Metab. 1992;75:714–20.
27. Sawka AM, Tepmongkol K, Brouwers M, et al. A systematic review and meta-analysis of the effectiveness of radioactive iodine remnant ablation for well-differentiated thyroid cancer. J Clin Endocrinol Metab. 2004;89:3668–76.
28. Simpson WJ, Panzarella T, Carruthers JS, et al. Papillary and follicular thyroid cancer: impact of treatment in 1578 patients. Int J Radiat Oncol Biol Phys. 1988;104:1063–75.
29. Sisson JC. Applying the radioactive eraser: I-131 to ablate normal thyroid tissue in patients from whom thyroid cancer has been resected. J Nucl Med. 1983;24:743–5.
30. Verkooijen RB, Stokkel MPM, Smit JWA, et al. Radioactive I-131 in differentiated thyroid cancer: a retrospective analysis of an uptake-related ablation strategy. Eur J Nucl Med. 2004; 31:499–506.
31. Abdel-Hamid A, Hardman J, Macias E, Roques T, Whitaker S, Vijayn R, Alvarez P, Beare S, Forsyth S, Kadalayil L, Hackshaw A. Ablation with low-dose radioiodine and thyrotropin alfa in thyroid cancer. NEJM. 2012;366:1674–85.
32. Bal CS, Padhy AK, Jana S, et al. Prospective randomized clinical trial to evaluate the optimal dose of I-131 for remnant ablation in patients with differentiated thyroid carcinoma. Cancer. 1996;77:2574–80.
33. Bal CS, Kumar A, Pant GS. Radioiodine doses of 25 to 50 mCi are equally effective for thyroid remnant ablation in patients with thyroid carcinoma. J Clin Endocrinol Metab. 2004;89:1666–73.
34. DeGroot L, Reily M. Comparison of 30- and 50-mCi of doses of iodine-131 for thyroid ablation. Ann Intern Med. 1992;96:51–3.
35. Samuel AM, Rajashekharrao B. Radioiodine therapy for well-differentiated thyroid cancer: a quantitative dosimetric evaluation for remnant thyroid ablation after surgery. J Nucl Med. 1994;35:1944–50.
36. Mallick U, Harmer C, Yap B, Wadsley J, Clarke S, Moss L, Nicol A, Clarke PM, Franell K, McCready R, Smellie J, Frankly JA, John R, Nutting CM, Newbodl K, Lemon C, Gerrard G. NEJM. 2012;366:1674-85.
37. Schlumberger M, Catargi B, Borget I, Deandreis D, Zerdoud S, Bridji B, Bardet S, Leenhardt L, Bastie D, Schvartz C, Vera P, Morel O, Benisvy D, Bournaud C, Bonichon F, Dejax C, Toubert ME, Leboulleux S, Ricard M, Benhamou E. Strategies of radioiodine ablation in patients with low-risk thyroid cancer. NEJM. 2012;366:1663–73.
38. Castagna MG, Cevenini G, Theodoropoulou A, Maino F, Memmo S, Claudia C, Belardini V, Brianzoni E, Pacini F. Post-surgical thyroid ablation with low or high radioiodine activities results in similar outcomes in intermediate risk differentiated thyroid cancer patients. Eur J Endocrinol. 2013;169:23–9.
39. Han JM, Kim WG, Kim TY, Jeon MJ, Ryu JS, Song DE, Hong SJ, Shong YK, Kim WB. Effects of low-dose and high-dose postoperative radioiodine therapy on the clinical outcome in patients with small differentiated thyroid cancer having microscopic extrathyroid extension. Thyroid. 2014;24(5):820–5.
40. Maxon HR, Smith HS. I-131 in the diagnosis and treatment of metastatic well differentiated thyroid cancer. Endocrinol Metab Clin N Am. 1990;19:685–718.
41. Thomas SR, Maxon HR, Kereiakes JG. In vivo quantitation of lesion radioactivity using external counting methods. Med Phys. 1976;3:253–5.
42. Maxon HR. Quantitative ^{131}I therapy in the treatment of differentiated thyroid cancer. Q J Nucl Med. 1999;43:313–23.
43. Maxon HR, Englaro EE, Thomas SR, et al. ^{131}I therapy for well differentiated thyroid cancer – a quantitative radiation dosimetric approach: outcome and validation in 85 patients. J Nucl Med. 1992;33:1132–6.
44. O'Connell MEA, Flower MA, Hinton PJ, Harmer CL, McCready VR. Radiation dose assessment in radioiodine therapy. Dose-response relationships in differentiated thyroid carcinoma using quantitative scanning and PET. Radiother Oncol. 1993;28:16–26.

45. Klubo-Gwiezdzinska J, Van Nostrand D, Atkins F, Burman K, Jonklaas J, Mete M, Wartofsky L. Efficacy of dosimetric versus empiric prescribed activity of ^{131}I for therapy of differentiated thyroid cancer. J Clin Endocrinol Metab. 2011;96(10):3217–25.
46. Leeper R. Controversies in the treatment of thyroid cancer: the New York Memorial Hospital approach. Thyroid Today. 1982; 5:1–4.
47. Kulkarni K, Van Nostrand D, Atkins FB, Aiken MJ, Burman K, Wartofsky L. The frequency with which empiric amounts of radioiodine "over-" or "under-" treat patients with metastatic well-differentiated thyroid cancer. Thyroid. 2006;16:1019–23.
48. Tuttle RM, Leboeuf R, Robbins RJ, et al. Empiric radioactive iodine dosing regimens frequently exceed maximum tolerated activity levels in elderly patients with thyroid cancer. J Nucl Med. 2006;47:1587–91.
49. Leeper RD, Shimaoka K. Treatment of metastatic thyroid cancer. Clin Endocrinol Metab. 1980;9:383–404.
50. Benua RS, Cicale NR, Sonenberg M, Rawson RW. The relation of radioiodine dosimetry to results and complications in the treatment of metastatic thyroid cancer. Am J Roentgenol Radium Ther Nucl Med. 1962;87:171–82.
51. Snyder WS, Ford MR, Warner GG, et al. "S" absorbed dose per unit cumulated activity for selected radionuclides and organs. In MIRD Pamphlet, no. 11. Reston: Society of Nuclear Medicine; 1975.
52. Zanzonico PB. Internal radionuclide radiation dosimetry: a review of basic concepts and recent developments. J Nucl Med. 2000;41:297–308.
53. Van Nostrand D, Atkins F, Moreau S, et al. Utility of the radioiodine whole-body retention at 48 hours for modifying empiric activity of 131-iodine for the treatment of metastatic well-differentiated thyroid carcinoma. Thyroid. 2009;10:1093–8.
54. Hanscheid H, Lassmann M, Luster M, et al. Blood dosimetry from a single measurement of the whole body radioiodine retention in patients with differentiated thyroid carcinoma. Endocrinol Relat Cancer. 2009;16:1283–9.
55. Wikipedia. http://en.wikipedia.org/wiki/Dose_fractionation. Updated 16 Sept 2013 at 08:17. Accessed 21 Dec 2014.
56. Hall EJ, Giaccia AJ. Fractionated radiation and the dose-rate effect. In: Hall EJ, Giaccia AJ, editors. Radiobiology for the radiologists, 2nd edn, Philadelphia: Wolters Kluwer; 2012. p. 67–85.
57. Arad E, Flannery K, Wilson GA, O'Mara R. Fractionated doses of radioiodine for ablation of postsurgical thyroid tissue remnants. Clin Nucl Med. 1990;10:676–7.
58. Wang SJ, Liu TJ. Use of fractionated doses of iodine-131 for ablation of thyroid remnants. Chin Med J (Taipei). 2002;65:336–40.
59. Wu HS, Hseu HH, Lin WY, Wang SJ, Kiu YC. Decreased uptake after fractionated ablative doses of iodine-131. Eur J Nucl Med Mol Imag. 2005;32:167–73.
60. Czepczynski R, Ziemnicka K, Baczyk M, Oleksa R, Ruchala M, Sowinski J. Fractionated dosage of radioiodine for the ablation of differentiated thyroid carcinoma. Thyroid. 2005;15:1261–5.
61. Clerc J, Bienvenu-Perrard M, Pichard de Malleray C, Dagousset F, Delbot T, Dreyfuss M, Groussin L, Marlow RJ, Leger FA, Chevalie A. Outpatient thyroid remnant ablation using repeated low 131-iodine activities (740 GBq/20mCi x 2) in patients with low-risk differentiated thyroid cancer. JCEM. 2012;97:871–80.
62. Fregly MJ, Gennaro JF. Effect of thiazides on metacorticoid hypertension and on thyroid activity of rats. Can J Physiol Pharm. 1973;43:521–30.
63. Seabold JE, Ben-Haim S, Pettit WA, et al. Diuretic enhanced I-131 clearance after ablation therapy for differentiated thyroid cancer. Radiology. 1993;187:839–42.
64. Maruca J, Santner S, Miller K, Santen RJ. Prolonged iodine clearance with a depletion regimen for thyroid carcinoma: concise communication. J Nucl Med. 1984;25:1089–93.
65. McCarthy JS, Fregly MJ, Nechay BR. Effect of diuretics on renal iodide excretion by rats and dogs. J Pharm Exp Ther. 1967;158: 294–304.
66. Fregly MJ. Effect of thiazides on the thyroid gland of rats. Toxicol Appl Pharm. 1965;8:558–66.
67. Kapucu LO, Azizoglu F, Ayvaz G, Karakoc A. Effects of diuretics on iodine uptake in non-toxic goiter-comparison with low-iodine diet. Eur J Nucl Med Mol Imaging. 2003;30:L1270–2.
68. Tepmongkol S. Enhancement of radioiodine uptake in hyperthyroidism with hydrochlorothiazide: a prospective randomized control study. Eur J Nucl Med Mol Imaging. 2002;29:1307–10.
69. Ding H, Kuang AR, Guan CT. Randomized controlled trial of hydrochlorothiazide in augmenting the dose of 131I absorbed by thyroid remnant. Sichuan Da Xue Xue Bao Yi Xue Ban. 2004;35:546–8.
70. Norfray JF, Quinn JL. Furosemide mediated elevations of thyroid uptake in the rat. Proc Soc Exp Biol Med. 1974;145:286–8.
71. Hamburger JI. Diuretic augmentation of 131-I uptake in inoperable thyroid cancer. N Eng J Med. 1969;280:1091–4.
72. Matovic M, Jankovic S, Jeremic M, Tasic Z, Vlajkovic M. Unexpected effect of furosemide on radioiodine excretion in patients with differentiated thyroid carcinomas treated with iodine 131. Thyroid. 2009;19:843–8.
73. Barbaro D, Gross M, Boni G, Lapi P, Pasquini C, Orsini P, Turco A, Meucci G, Marzola MC, Berti P, Miccoli P, Marinai G, Rubello D. Recombinant human TSH and ablation of post-surgical thyroid remnants in differentiated thyroid cancer: the effect of pre-treatment with furosemide and furosemide plus lithium. Eur J Nucl Med Mol Imaging. 2010;37:242–9.
74. Ho AL, Grewal RK, Leboeuf R, et al. Selumetinib-enhanced radioiodine uptake in advanced thyroid cancer. NEJM. 2013;2013(368): 623–32.
75. Reynolds JC. Comparison of I-131 absorbed radiation doses in children and adults; a tool for estimating therapeutic I-131 doses in children. In: Robbins J, editor. Treatment of thyroid cancer in children. Springfield: US Department of Commerce Technology Administration, National Technical Information Service; 1994. p. 127–35.

34 Thyroid Remnant Radioiodine Ablation with Recombinant Human Thyrotropin

Richard J. Robbins, Sheba Asghar, Kristoffer Seelbach, and Robert Michael Tuttle

Introduction

Initial treatment for most patients with differentiated thyroid cancer seeks to eliminate the entire primary tumor, to obtain sufficient material to properly stage the tumor, and to prepare the patient for a comprehensive surveillance program [1]. This often includes a total thyroidectomy and radioactive iodine (RAI) remnant ablation (RRA). The goal of RRA is to eliminate not only normal thyroid cells but also to destroy any residual microscopic thyroid carcinoma that may remain following total thyroidectomy and appropriate lymph node dissection. RAI uptake into thyroid cells is enhanced by a preparatory low-iodine diet and elevated levels of thyrotropin (TSH). For the past 40–50 years, endogenous TSH production was stimulated by several weeks of a hypothyroid state induced by thyroid hormone withdrawal (THW) prior to RAI. However, moderate to severe hypothyroid symptoms significantly reduce the quality of life for many patients and delay the clearance of radioiodine from the whole body.

Exogenous TSH (bovine TSH) was used to stimulate RAI uptake in thyroid cancer patients over 40 years ago but fell out of favor due to the development of neutralizing antibodies and allergic reactions with repeated exposures [2–6]. As reviewed in Chap. 10, the FDA approved recombinant human TSH (rhTSH; Thyrogen®, Genzyme Corporation) in 1998 for diagnostic whole-body RAI scanning and stimulated thyroglobulin measurements in the follow-up of patients with differentiated thyroid cancer [7, 8]. In 2007, the US FDA extended the indications of Thyrogen® to include preparation for RRA in patients with differentiated thyroid carcinoma without distant metastases. This chapter reviews the published data on rhTSH-stimulated RAI for remnant ablation and describes current practices for using rhTSH in clinical practice.

rhTSH as Preparation for RRA: Initial Studies

Before rhTSH became commercially available in December 1998, many patients received rhTSH-stimulated RAI treatments as part of the Genzyme Corporation's Compassionate Use Program [9–11]. Although most of these patients were receiving RAI for treatment of recurrent/persistent disease, rhTSH was used for RRA in at least 15 patients. These reports provided information on safety and RAI uptake into the thyroid remnants at the time of remnant ablation but with little information on results of the follow-up diagnostic scans.

In addition to diagnostic whole-body RAI scanning, a group of patients at the Memorial Sloan Kettering Cancer Center who received rhTSH stimulation were offered whole-body and blood dosimetry studies to determine the maximal tolerable activity (MTA) of RAI therapy that could be administered if a therapy was required. As dosimetry studies conducted in the euthyroid state (with rhTSH) were significantly different from the hypothyroid state, it was not possible to use the MTA calculations following rhTSH to predict a safe maximum dose of RAI following thyroid hormone withdrawal. Therefore, selected patients were offered the option of rhTSH-assisted RRA based on their individual dosimetry results, as an alternative to repeating the dosimetry studies in

R.J. Robbins, MD (✉)
Chairman, Department of Medicine, The Methodist Hospital, 6550 Fannin Street, Suite SM 1001, Houston, TX 77030, USA
e-mail: rjrobbins@tmhs.org

S. Asghar, MD
Division of Endocrinology, Metabolism and Lipids, Emory University School of Medicine, Atlanta, GA, USA
e-mail: sheba.asghar@emory.edu

K. Seelbach, MD
Endocrinology Division, Department of Medicine, The Methodist Hospital and Institute for Academic Medicine, Houston, TX, USA

R.M. Tuttle, MD
Department of Medicine, Memorial Sloan Kettering Cancer Center, New York, NY, USA
e-mail: tuttlem@mskcc.org

L. Wartofsky, D. Van Nostrand (eds.), *Thyroid Cancer*, DOI 10.1007/978-1-4939-3314-3_34

Table 34.1 Full whole-body and blood dosimetry in preparation for rhTSH-stimulated RRA [12]

	Monday	Tuesday	Wednesday	Thursday	Friday	Saturday
Week 1	rhTSH 0.9 mg	rhTSH 0.9 mg	^{131}Iodine 2–5 mCi	Dosimetry	Dosimetry	Dosimetry WBS
Week 2	rhTSH 0.9 mg	rhTSH 0.9 mg	Ablation			
Week 3			Post-therapy WBS			

rhTSH, 0.9 mg intramuscular; dosimetry, blood, and whole-body dosimetry measurements; ablation, amount administered range = 75–150 mCi ^{131}I; *WBS* diagnostic whole-body scan

the hypothyroid state before proceeding with RRA. Each of these initial patients received 0.9 mg of rhTSH for two consecutive days (during week 1) to allow for full dosimetry studies and two additional rhTSH injections (during week 2) to prepare for RRA (see Table 34.1). Complete absence of visible thyroid bed uptake on a follow-up diagnostic scan done 5–13 months after administering a mean activity of 110 mCi (range 30–250 mCi) was reported in all ten patients in our initial series [12]. Although RAI activity in the thyroid bed was the primary endpoint of this initial study, two patients had uptake outside of the thyroid bed (presumably cervical lymph node metastases), which was no longer visible at the time of the follow-up diagnostic whole-body scan.

In a subsequent nonrandomized retrospective analysis, we directly compared RRA following THW ($n=42$) with rhTSH simulation ($n=45$) [13]. In this larger cohort, complete resolution of visible thyroid bed uptake on the 1 year follow-up whole-body diagnostic RAI scan was seen in 84 % of those prepared with rhTSH and 81 % prepared with THW ($p>0.05$). The mean administered ^{131}I activity after rhTSH preparation was 110±65 mCi (range 30–330 mCi) compared to 129±74 mCi (range 30–300 mCi) following THW. In 2002, Pacini et al. reported the results of a nonrandomized, consecutive block design study comparing the effectiveness of 30 mCi of ^{131}I after THW, or rhTSH, as preparation for RRA [14]. The rate of successful RRA (defined by absence of uptake in the thyroid bed on the 1-year diagnostic whole-body scan) was significantly higher in the 50 patients prepared with THW (84 %), compared to euthyroid patients prepared with rhTSH (54 %, $p<0.01$). Unlike previously published studies in which the RAI was administered 24 h after the second rhTSH injection, the ablative dose of RAI in this study was given 48 h after the second injection of rhTSH.

To assess the impact of the obligate intake of stable iodine associated with the continuation of levothyroxine during rhTSH-stimulated RRA, Barbaro et al. designed a study to evaluate the effect of short-term levothyroxine withdrawal (4 days) at the time of RAI dosing for RRA [15]. In the rhTSH-stimulated RRA arm, levothyroxine therapy was initiated at the time of total thyroidectomy and discontinued 24 h prior to the first injection of rhTSH (0.9 mg for two consecutive days). The ablative dose of 30 mCi of ^{131}I was administered 24 h after the second injection of rhTSH. Levothyroxine therapy was restarted 24 h after administration of the ablative dose of RAI. At the 1-year follow-up diagnostic whole-body scan, no visible uptake in the thyroid bed was seen in 88 % (14 of 18) of patients prepared with rhTSH and 4 days THW, compared to 75 % (18 of 24) of patients prepared with traditional THW. When successful RRA ablation was defined as absence of uptake in the thyroid bed and undetectable serum thyroglobulin, similar success rates were reported (81 % with rhTSH, 75 % with THW; p = not significant). The urinary iodine values were significantly lower in the rhTSH with 4 days THW (47±4 μg/L) and a traditional THW group (39±4 μg/L) than in an additional control group undergoing diagnostic rhTSH scanning without discontinuation of levothyroxine (76±9 μg/L).

rhTSH as Preparation for RRA: Recent Studies

Overall, the studies prior to 2006 were promising but lacked scientific rigor as they were largely retrospective and had very short follow-up intervals. However, they served as the theoretical basis for larger and randomized studies that sought to prove the hypothesis that preparation by rhTSH was equal to preparation by THW. The first prospective, randomized trial examining traditional THW vs. rhTSH stimulation in low-risk differentiated thyroid cancer patients for RRA was published by Pacini et al. in 2006 [16]. This multicenter study enrolled 63 patients in nine centers in Europe, Canada, and the United States. All patients received 100 mCi (3.7 GBq) of ^{131}I for RRA. At the follow-up diagnostic rhTSH whole-body scan 1 year later, all patients in both arms had less than 0.1 % uptake in the thyroid bed. The rhTSH-stimulated serum thyroglobulin level was <2 ng/ml in 96 % of the rhTSH-prepared patients and in 86 % of the THW-prepared patients. The rhTSH-prepared patients remained euthyroid throughout the treatment protocol and had one third lower radiation dose to blood compared to the hypothyroid cohort ($p<0.001$). A longer term follow-up of these patients was published in 2009 by Elisei et al. [17]. After a median of an additional 3.7 years, there were no deaths in either group, and no recurrences in any that were deemed to be disease free at the 1 year follow-up point. The frequency of recurrence (or persistence) of disease was comparable between the two groups.

A 2012 prospective, randomized multicenter study by Schlumberger et al. [18] compared ablation success rates, 8 months after RRA, in 332 patients prepared by rhTSH, and in 318 prepared by THW. They determined that 92 % of the rhTSH patients and 93 % of the THW patients had successful remnant ablation (p = NS). Using a different definition of ablation success, the HiLo United Kingdom study group [19] published a similar multicenter prospective randomized study comparing rhTSH and THW preparation for RRA. They found successful remnant ablation in 87.1 % of those prepared by rhTSH and in 86.7 % of those who had THW. They concluded that the rhTSH preparation was not inferior to the THW preparation.

Tuttle et al. [20] reported on medium term (i.e., median 2.5 years) disease recurrence in 394 thyroid cancer survivors who underwent RRA following either rhTSH preparation or THW. Clinically evident disease recurred in 4 % of those who had RRA following rhTSH and in 7 % of those who had RRA following THW (p = NS). In this retrospective study, however, the levels of thyroglobulin were significantly lower in the rhTSH prepared group at the 2.5 year follow-up time point. Overall, they concluded that recurrence and disease persistence were comparable between the two groups.

With regard to whole-body radiation exposure in the euthyroid state with rhTSH, Frigo et al. [21] reported in 2009 that the rate of chromosomal abnormalities was significantly higher in lymphocytes from RRA patients who were prepared by THW compared to those prepared by rhTSH. In addition, Taieb also found lower whole-body radiation exposure and increased remnant half-life in RRA patients prepared with rhTSH [22]. Finally, Vallejo Casas et al. [23] and Carvalho et al. [24] also found a significantly lower whole-body radiation exposure in RRA patients following rhTSH compared to THW.

A recent study by Hugo et al. [25] addressed the utility of rhTSH preparation in intermediate to high-risk thyroid cancer survivors. They reported a retrospective study of RRA in THW patients ($n = 321$) and in euthyroid patients prepared by rhTSH ($n = 265$). Administered activity was a median of 134 mCi of ^{131}I for each group. Although they found that the ablation success rate was better in those prepared by rhTSH, the final clinical outcomes (at a median of 9 years) were not significantly different in terms of recurrence or persistence of thyroid cancer. They concluded that rhTSH-assisted RRA was a reasonable approach for higher-risk thyroid cancer survivors. Finally, a new study by the thyroid cancer group from Pisa, Italy, did a 10-year follow-up study on the patient previously reported by Pacini et al. [16]. They report no difference in long-term recurrence or persistence of disease between those prepared for RRA with rhTSH or with THW (personal communication).

Quality of Life When Hypothyroid

Several investigators have evaluated the frequency and intensity of the symptoms that differ between patients who had THW and those who remained euthyroid during RRA. Taieb et al. [26] reported on 74 patients who were randomized to prepare for RRA with either THW or with rhTSH while remaining on thyroxine. Using several different quality of life (QOL) instruments (e.g., FACIT-F and FACT-G), they found a significant decrease in QOL in the THW group compared to baseline, which resolved when thyroid hormone replacement had resumed. Lee et al. [27] also found a better preserved QOL at the time of RRA in those who were euthyroid receiving rhTSH compared to those who were undergoing THW. Dueren et al. [28] compared the clinical symptoms and the SF-12 Health Survey outcomes in thyroid cancer patients who were initially made hypothyroid in preparation for a diagnostic whole-body RAI scan and again in the same patients (6–12 months later) who were then prepared for a similar scan with rhTSH while remaining on thyroxine. They found a highly significant improvement in clinical symptoms and the ability to manage daily life when the patients remained on thyroxine, including less time off from work. The significantly reduced QOL in THW patients compared to rhTSH-prepared patients was also confirmed in a 2012 study of 438 patients from the UK National Research Network [19]. Late complications of radioiodine itself also diminish QOL. Rosario et al. [29] reported that rates of salivary and lacrimal gland dysfunction were lower in 148 thyroid cancer patients who underwent RRA with rhTSH assistance compared to published rates from previous reports in those prepared for RRA by THW. In a multicenter UK study, Malick et al. [19] found that, 3 months after receiving radioiodine for RRA, 27 % of those prepared by rhTSH and 24 % of those prepared by THW had adverse events (e.g., neck pain, nausea). They also found a significantly diminished QOL in the THW group prior to the RRA. In the recent French multicenter trial, Schlumberger et al. [18] reported that salivary gland problems were no different between the rhTSH group and the THW group; however, excessive tearing was significantly higher, 8 months after RRA, in those who were prepared by THW.

Cost of THW versus rhTSH Preparation for RRA

There are many direct and indirect costs of having thyroid carcinoma. If we try to focus solely on those costs related to RRA, we find that several reports have compared costs of preparation by THW as opposed to remaining on thyroid hormone replacement and receiving rhTSH. The drug itself costs approximately $2,400 (USD), and it is covered by all of the major American insurance carriers for thyroid cancer diagnosis and/or remnant ablation. Depending on deductibles and type of insurance policy, some of this cost is borne directly by the patient. In many countries, it is not covered by national or private insurers. Time lost from work or other activities when one is suffering from hypothyroidism is also a significant, but difficult to quantitate, metric. Finally, the lower whole-body radiation exposure is likely to result in fewer secondary malignancies in thyroid cancer survivors. Using a lifetime Markov model with a Monte Carlo simulation of 100,000 patients, Mernagh et al. [30] reported that rhTSH preparation for RRA resulted in higher-quality-adjusted life years (QALY) with an incremental cost per QALY of 958 euros (or $1,520 Canadian dollars). They concluded that rhTSH preparation represents good value for money with benefits to the patient and to society, at modest cost. Vallejo Casas et al. [23] and Borget et al. [31] found that rhTSH preparation for RRA was associated with a significantly shorter treatment room stay than THW preparation. Dueren et al. [28] found that their patients lost a median of 10 days of work when prepared by THW compared to 4 days of work when prepared by rhTSH. Wang et al. [32] used a Markov decision model to evaluate the cost-utility of using rhTSH preparation for RRA in a group of low-risk thyroid cancer survivors. They found that the rhTSH preparation yielded an incremental societal cost of $1,365 (USD) per patient. The main variables being out of pocket costs for the Thyrogen® and days of work lost. In the UK HiLo study, treatment costs (including the NHS tariff and cost of Thyrogen®) were much higher in those who were prepared by rhTSH. However, those prepared by rhTSH lost 1 day of work on average, compared to five lost work days for those who were hypothyroid [19]. On balance, it appears that the improved quality of life offsets the additional cost of rhTSH and where available and affordable, rhTSH would be the first option for RRA preparation.

How Much ^{131}I Should Be Administered in rhTSH-Assisted RRA?

Recent studies suggest that rhTSH preparation method alters the amount of radiation delivered to the remnant as well as the whole body. Most of the early studies on RRA, by tradition, administered 3.7 GBq (100 mCi) of ^{131}I. However, Pilli et al. [33] reported that administration of 1.85 GBq (50 mCi) was as successful as 3.7 GBq (100 mCi) in ablating thyroid remnants in euthyroid patients prepared with rhTSH. Chianelli et al. [34] studied RRA success following either THW or rhTSH preparation and administration of a lower activity of ^{131}I (2 GBq; 54 mCi). This group reported successful ablation in 95.2 % of the THW patients and in 90.5 % of the rhTSH patients (p = NS). Schlumberger et al. [18] performed a prospective randomized study of two different administered activities (1.1 or 3.7 GBq; 30 or 100 mCi) for RRA in rhTSH-prepared low-risk thyroid cancer patients. Six to 10 months later there was no significant difference in neck ultrasonography or serum thyroglobulin levels between the groups. Based on radioiodine imaging, 93 % of the 3.7 GBq group and 90 % of the 1.1 GBq group were judged to have complete ablation (p = NS). In a similar study, Mallick et al. [19] conducted a randomized non-inferiority trial comparing 1.1 and 3.7 GBq of ^{131}I to ablate thyroid remnants in low-risk thyroid cancer survivors following preparation by rhTSH. Ablation success rates were 84.3 % in the 1.1 GBq group and 90.2 % in the 3.7 GBq ($p=0.2$). However, adverse events were present in only 16 % of the 1.1 GBq group compared to 30 % in the 3.7 GBq group ($p=0.01$). The issue of which thyroid cancer patients benefit from RRA is an important one that is discussed in depth in Chap. 19. For those patients who chose to proceed with RRA, the published literature would support the use of 1.1 GBq (30 mCi) following total thyroidectomy in patients without obvious metastatic disease. The specific activity of ^{131}I required for patients at high risk of having microscopic residual metastases (local or distant) remains to be defined, as the endpoints of the "low" dose studies have focused on effectiveness of remnant ablation, rather than on clinical recurrence or survival.

Summary

Based upon a strong series of prospective and retrospective studies, the use of rhTSH to prepare patients for RRA has moved from an off-label use in rare selected patients to a mainstream, validated approach. Many small variations in clinical practice still exist between different medical centers – but a consensus protocol is well established (Table 34.2). Most patients without distant metastases who have all gross disease removed from the neck (regardless of AJCC stage) are candidates for rhTSH-assisted RRA while remaining on thyroxine replacement. This approach has been reproduced in many different countries with similar results. It is clear that the patient's quality of life is significantly better; the patients are exposed to much less whole-body radiation; their length of stay in the nuclear medicine unit is lower; they are able to maintain their work or family life essentially unchanged; and the incidence of late side effects of radioiodine seem to be lower than patients who get RRA while hypothyroid. Emerging evidence now suggests that lower activities of ^{131}I following rhTSH may yield high (>90 %) ablation rates, with levels of recurrence over the next 4–9 years comparable to hypothyroid RRA. One issue that is still unresolved is the dose and schedule of the rhTSH injections

Table 34.2 A modern simplified approach to rhTSH-stimulated RRA ablation in low-risk patients

RRA: 4–6 weeks following total thyroidectomy – on a stable replacement dose of thyroxine
1. Begin a low-iodine diet 7–10 days prior to therapeutic administration of ^{131}I
2. Inject 0.9 mg of rhTSH IM on Day 1 in AM
3. Inject 0.9 mg of rhTSH IM on Day 2 in AM
4. Administer diagnostic activity of ^{123}I on Day 2 in AM
5. Radionuclide whole-body scan in AM on Day 3;
6. Administer therapeutic ^{131}I activity on Day 3 – based on pathology and scan result
7. Patient to follow standard isolation policy and drink extra water for 2 days
8. Perform post-therapy whole-body scan on day 6 or 7

The diagnostic whole-body scan (steps 3 and 4) can be omitted in low-risk patient who have a total thyroidectomy and removal of all gross disease, by an experienced thyroid surgeon. *IM* intramuscular

themselves. It is possible that much less or more, rhTSH may yield very different outcomes with regard to remnant ablation, whole body clearance rates, radioiodine dwell time in (benign or malignant) thyroid cells, and eradication of microscopic thyroid cancer deposits in cervical lymph nodes. Fortunately, the morbidity and mortality of thyroid carcinoma is only a fraction of that compared to other solid tumors, which enables the construction of prospective randomized trials in these patients, as have been achieved in Europe and the United Kingdom. Recombinant human thyrotropin has been a true success story made possible by the sequencing of the alpha and beta chains of human TSH, advances in DNA biochemistry, and a close collaboration between the biotech industry and academic endocrinologists.

References

1. Haugen BR, Alexander EK, Bible KC, Doherty GM, Mandel SJ, et al. 2015 American Thyroid Association Management Guidelines for Adult Patients with Thyroid Nodules and Differentiated Thyroid Cancer: The American Thyroid Association Guidelines Task Force on Thyroid Nodules and Differentiated Thyroid Cancer Thyroid 2016;26:1–133.
2. Benua RS, Sonenberg M, Leeper RD, Rawson RW. An 18 year study of the use of beef thyrotropin to increase I131 uptake in metastatic thyroid cancer. J Nucl Med Off Publ Soc Nucl Med. 1964;5:796–801.
3. Kirkpatrick CH, Meek JC, Rich RR. Mechanism of allergy to components of commercial bovine thyrotropin. J Allergy Clin Immunol. 1973;51:296–302.
4. Melmed S, Harada A, Hershman JM, Krishnamurthy GT, Blahd WH. Neutralizing antibodies to bovine thyrotropin in immunized patients with thyroid cancer. J Clin Endocrinol Metab. 1980;51:358–63.
5. Robbins J. Pharmacology of bovine and human thyrotropin: an historical perspective. Thyroid. 1999;9:451–3.
6. Seidlin SM, Oshry E, Yalow AA. Spontaneous and experimentally induced uptake of radioactive iodine in metastases from thyroid carcinoma; a preliminary report. J Clin Endocrinol Metab. 1948;8:423–32.
7. Woodmansee WW, Haugen BR. Uses for recombinant human TSH in patients with thyroid cancer and nodular goiter. Clin Endocrinol (Oxf). 2004;61:163–73.
8. Robbins RJ, Robbins AK. Clinical review 156: recombinant human thyrotropin and thyroid cancer management. J Clin Endocrinol Metab. 2003;88:1933–8.
9. Perros P. Recombinant human thyroid-stimulating hormone (rhTSH) in the radioablation of well-differentiated thyroid cancer: preliminary therapeutic experience. J Endocrinol Invest. 1999;22:30–4.
10. Berg G, Lindstedt G, Suurkula M, Jansson S. Radioiodine ablation and therapy in differentiated thyroid cancer under stimulation with recombinant human thyroid-stimulating hormone. J Endocrinol Invest. 2002;25:44–52.
11. Luster M, Lassmann M, Haenscheid H, Michalowski U, Incerti C, Reiners C. Use of recombinant human thyrotropin before radioiodine therapy in patients with advanced differentiated thyroid carcinoma. J Clin Endocrinol Metab. 2000;85:3640–5.
12. Robbins RJ, Tuttle RM, Sonenberg M, Shaha A, Sharaf R, Robbins H, Fleisher M, Larson SM. Radioiodine ablation of thyroid remnants after preparation with recombinant human thyrotropin. Thyroid. 2001;11:865–9.
13. Robbins RJ, Larson SM, Sinha N, Shaha A, Divgi C, Pentlow KS, Ghossein R, Tuttle RM. A retrospective review of the effectiveness of recombinant human TSH as a preparation for radioiodine thyroid remnant ablation. J Nucl Med. 2002;43:1482–8.
14. Pacini F, Molinaro E, Castagna MG, Lippi F, Ceccarelli C, Agate L, Elisei R, Pinchera A. Ablation of thyroid residues with 30 mCi (131)I: a comparison in thyroid cancer patients prepared with recombinant human TSH or thyroid hormone withdrawal. J Clin Endocrinol Metab. 2002;87:4063–8.
15. Barbaro D, Boni G, Meucci G, Simi U, Lapi P, Orsini P, Pasquini C, Piazza F, Caciagli M, Mariani G. Radioiodine treatment with 30 mCi after recombinant human thyrotropin stimulation in thyroid cancer: effectiveness for postsurgical remnants ablation and possible role of iodine content in L-thyroxine in the outcome of ablation. J Clin Endocrinol Metab. 2003;88:4110–5.
16. Pacini F, Ladenson PW, Schlumberger M, Driedger A, Luster M, Kloos RT, Sherman S, Haugen B, Corone C, Molinaro E, Elisei R, Ceccarelli C, Pinchera A, Wahl RL, Leboulleux S, Ricard M, Yoo J, Busaidy NL, Delpassand E, Hanscheid H, Felbinger R, Lassmann M, Reiners C. Radioiodine ablation of thyroid remnants after preparation with recombinant human thyrotropin in differentiated thyroid carcinoma: results of an international, randomized, controlled study. J Clin Endocrinol Metab. 2006;91:926–32.
17. Elisei R, Schlumberger M, Driedger A, Reiners C, Kloos RT, Sherman SI, Haugen B, Corone C, Molinaro E, Grasso L, Leboulleux S, Rachinsky I, Luster M, Lassmann M, Busaidy NL, Wahl RL, Pacini F, Cho SY, Magner J, Pinchera A, Ladenson PW. Follow-up of low-risk differentiated thyroid cancer patients who underwent radioiodine ablation of postsurgical thyroid remnants after either recombinant human thyrotropin or thyroid hormone withdrawal. J Clin Endocrinol Metab. 2009;94:4171–9.
18. Schlumberger M, Catargi B, Borget I, Deandreis D, Zerdoud S, Bridji B, Bardet S, Leenhardt L, Bastie D, Schvartz C, Vera P, Morel O, Benisvy D, Bournaud C, Bonichon F, Dejax C, Toubert ME, Leboulleux S, Ricard M, Benhamou E, Tumeurs de la Thyroide Refractaires Network for the Essai Stimulation Ablation Equivalence Trial. Strategies of radioiodine ablation in patients with low-risk thyroid cancer. N Engl J Med. 2012;366:1663–73.
19. Mallick U, Harmer C, Yap B, Wadsley J, Clarke S, Moss L, Nicol A, Clark PM, Farnell K, McCready R, Smellie J, Franklyn JA, John R, Nutting CM, Newbold K, Lemon C, Gerrard G, Abdel-Hamid A, Hardman J, Macias E, Roques T, Whitaker S, Vijayan R, Alvarez P, Beare S, Forsyth S, Kadalayil L, Hackshaw A. Ablation with low-dose radioiodine and thyrotropin alfa in thyroid cancer. N Engl J Med. 2012;366:1674–85.

20. Tuttle RM, Brokhin M, Omry G, Martorella AJ, Larson SM, Grewal RK, Fleisher M, Robbins RJ. Recombinant human TSH-assisted radioactive iodine remnant ablation achieves short-term clinical recurrence rates similar to those of traditional thyroid hormone withdrawal. J Nucl Med. 2008;49:764–70.
21. Frigo A, Dardano A, Danese E, Davi MV, Moghetti P, Colato C, Francia G, Bernardi F, Traino C, Monzani F, Ferdeghini M. Chromosome translocation frequency after radioiodine thyroid remnant ablation: a comparison between recombinant human thyrotropin stimulation and prolonged levothyroxine withdrawal. J Clin Endocrinol Metab. 2009;94:3472–6.
22. Taieb D, Sebag F, Farman-Ara B, Portal T, Baumstarck-Barrau K, Fortanier C, Bourrelly M, Mancini J, De Micco C, Auquier P, Conte-Devolx B, Henry JF, Mundler O. Iodine biokinetics and radioiodine exposure after recombinant human thyrotropin-assisted remnant ablation in comparison with thyroid hormone withdrawal. J Clin Endocrinol Metab. 2010;95:3283–90.
23. Vallejo Casas JA, Mena Bares LM, Galvez MA, Marlowe RJ, Latre Romero JM, Martinez-Paredes M. Treatment room length-of-stay and patient throughput with radioiodine thyroid remnant ablation in differentiated thyroid cancer: comparison of thyroid-stimulating hormone stimulation methods. Nucl Med Commun. 2011;32:840–6.
24. Carvalho MR, Ferreira TC, Leite V. Evaluation of whole-body retention of iodine-131 ((131)I) after postoperative remnant ablation for differentiated thyroid carcinoma – thyroxine withdrawal versus rhTSH administration: a retrospective comparison. Oncol Lett. 2012;3:617–20.
25. Hugo J, Robenshtok E, Grewal R, Larson S, Tuttle RM. Recombinant human thyroid stimulating hormone-assisted radioactive iodine remnant ablation in thyroid cancer patients at intermediate to high risk of recurrence. Thyroid. 2012;22:1007–15.
26. Taieb D, Sebag F, Cherenko M, Baumstarck-Barrau K, Fortanier C, Farman-Ara B, De Micco C, Vaillant J, Thomas S, Conte-Devolx B, Loundou A, Auquier P, Henry JF, Mundler O. Quality of life changes and clinical outcomes in thyroid cancer patients undergoing radioiodine remnant ablation (RRA) with recombinant human TSH (rhTSH): a randomized controlled study. Clin Endocrinol (Oxf). 2009;71:115–23.
27. Lee J, Yun MJ, Nam KH, Chung WY, Soh EY, Park CS. Quality of life and effectiveness comparisons of thyroxine withdrawal, triiodothyronine withdrawal, and recombinant thyroid-stimulating hormone administration for low-dose radioiodine remnant ablation of differentiated thyroid carcinoma. Thyroid. 2010;20: 173–9.
28. Dueren C, Dietlein M, Luster M, Plenzig F, Steinke R, Grimm J, Groth P, Eichhorn W, Reiners C. The use of thyrogen in the treatment of differentiated thyroid carcinoma: an intraindividual comparison of clinical effects and implications of daily life. Exp Clin Endocrinol Diabetes. 2010;118:513–9.
29. Rosario PW, Calsolari MR. Salivary and lacrimal gland dysfunction after remnant ablation with radioiodine in patients with differentiated thyroid carcinoma prepared with recombinant human TSH. Thyroid. 2013; 23:617–619.
30. Mernagh P, Campbell S, Dietlein M, Luster M, Mazzaferri E, Weston AR. Cost-effectiveness of using recombinant human TSH prior to radioiodine ablation for thyroid cancer, compared with treating patients in a hypothyroid state: the German perspective. Eur J Endocrinol. 2006;155:405–14.
31. Borget I, Remy H, Chevalier J, Ricard M, Allyn M, Schlumberger M, De Pouvourville G. Length and cost of hospital stay of radioiodine ablation in thyroid cancer patients: comparison between preparation with thyroid hormone withdrawal and thyrogen. Eur J Nucl Med Mol Imaging. 2008;35:1457–63.
32. Wang TS, Cheung K, Mehta P, Roman SA, Walker HD, Sosa JA. To stimulate or withdraw? A cost-utility analysis of recombinant human thyrotropin versus thyroxine withdrawal for radioiodine ablation in patients with low-risk differentiated thyroid cancer in the United States. J Clin Endocrinol Metab. 2010;95: 1672–80.
33. Pilli T, Brianzoni E, Capoccetti F, Castagna MG, Fattori S, Poggiu A, Rossi G, Ferretti F, Guarino E, Burroni L, Vattimo A, Cipri C, Pacini F. A comparison of 1850 (50 mCi) and 3700 MBq (100 mCi) 131-iodine administered doses for recombinant thyrotropin-stimulated postoperative thyroid remnant ablation in differentiated thyroid cancer. J Clin Endocrinol Metab. 2007;92:3542–6.
34. Chianelli M, Todino V, Graziano FM, Panunzi C, Pace D, Guglielmi R, Signore A, Papini E. Low-activity (2.0 GBq; 54 mCi) radioiodine post-surgical remnant ablation in thyroid cancer: comparison between hormone withdrawal and use of rhTSH in low-risk patients. Eur J Endocrinol. 2009;160:431–6.

Part VI

Follow-Up and Surveillance

Follow-Up Strategy in Papillary Thyroid Cancer

35

Merica Shrestha and Henry B. Burch

Introduction

Effective surveillance for recurrent papillary thyroid cancer begins with an assessment of the risk of recurrence or death from disease. This information is used to determine an appropriate level of follow-up, which may vary from as little as an annual neck examination on replacement thyroid hormone therapy for very low-risk lesions to annual or semiannual thyrotropin (TSH)-stimulated whole-body scan (WBS) and thyroglobulin (Tg) measurement for high-risk patients. Additionally, the patients' response to initial therapy further modulates the surveillance strategy. Effective follow-up is also contingent upon a current understanding of the strengths and limitations of the tools available for thyroid cancer surveillance. This chapter focuses on the rationale used to determine the method and frequency of follow-up for patients with papillary thyroid cancer (PTC) and reviews current guidelines regarding surveillance for persistent or recurrent disease.

Defining the Risk Level

The factors used to determine a given patient's risk category and, hence, an appropriate level of surveillance are: (1) patient characteristics, including age and sex; (2) tumor features such as size, multifocality, histological grade, or subtype and the presence of extrathyroidal extension or distant metastases; (3) the extent of prior surgery and radioiodine therapy; and (4) tumor response to initial therapy. A number of scoring and staging systems have been derived from retrospective analysis of large patient cohorts studying differentiated thyroid cancer (DTC) (see Chap. 29). Although it is tempting to assign a numerical score to an individual patient and use this to design an appropriate level of surveillance, realistically, patients from all stages of disease may experience recurrence and death [1], and the onus is therefore on the clinician to provide an adequate approach to detect not only the typical but the atypical patient as well.

Defining Recurrent and Persistent Disease

The cited rates for persistent or recurrent differentiated thyroid cancer (DTC) vary considerably between centers and depend on the definitions used for these terms and the duration of follow-up. Reports originating from quaternary referral centers are biased towards patients with more aggressive disease and higher recurrence rates. Biochemical persistent or recurrent disease is defined as a stimulated or unstimulated serum thyroglobulin level of >2 ng/mL in a patient previously treated with total thyroidectomy and radioiodine remnant ablation (RRA) and in the absence of identifiable disease on cross-sectional imaging. A clinical or anatomical recurrence implies new evidence of disease on cross-sectional imaging or tissue biopsy in a patient who was previously disease-free following initial therapy. One large cohort of 1,528 patients followed for up to 40 years was

Disclaimer: The opinions expressed in this chapter reflect the personal views of the authors and not the official views of the United States Army or the Department of Defense.

M. Shrestha, MD
Endocrinology Service, Dwight David Eisenhower Army Medical Center, Ft. Gordon, GA, USA
e-mail: merica.shrestha@us.army.mil

H.B. Burch, MD, FACE (✉)
Endocrinology Division, Uniformed Services University of the Health Sciences, Walter Reed National Military Medical Center, 8901 Wisconsin Avenue, American Building, Room 5053, Bethesda, MD 20889, USA
e-mail: Henry.burch@med.navy.mil

L. Wartofsky, D. Van Nostrand (eds.), *Thyroid Cancer*, DOI 10.1007/978-1-4939-3314-3_35

found to have an overall anatomic recurrence rate of 23.5 % at a median of 16.6 years [1]. In contrast, a recent report of 1,503 patients treated with total (TT) or near-total thyroidectomy (NTT) plus RRA reported an anatomic recurrence rate of only 0.6 %, but a persistent disease rate of nearly 14 %, suggesting an improved means of detecting initially persistent disease and an overall relatively high rate of disease persistence/recurrence [2].

Level of Surveillance

A great deal of variability exists among thyroidologists in the level and frequency of follow-up in patients with PTC [3]. This evaluation should be individualized, with more rigorous and frequent monitoring in those patients deemed likely to experience a recurrence or death from disease and less intense surveillance for patients with a low risk of an adverse outcome. Twenty-year survival in a group of 585 low-risk patients has been reported as 97.8 % compared to 61.3 % in 142 high-risk patients at the same institution [4]. Increased surveillance has been emphasized in multifocal PTC, even if microscopic. These patients have been shown to have an increased risk of recurrence compared to those with unifocal disease [5, 6], particularly in those with less than a TT/NTT [7]. Interestingly, RRA does not affect recurrence rates in these patients [5, 7], but RRA does allow identification of recurrence more readily when it occurs [8]. Generally, patients with one or more poor prognostic factors (see Chap. 33) are more likely to be treated with RRA and also more likely to undergo more frequent and sustained surveillance testing. A common approach to patients with papillary thyroid cancers larger than 1.5 cm in diameter is to recommend near-total thyroidectomy, followed by radioiodine ablation with 30–150 mCi of ^{131}I [3], and then serial surveillance for recurrent disease.

Recent guidelines published by the American Thyroid Association (ATA) recommended the use of the American Joint Cancer Committee/Union Internationale Contre le Cancer (AJCC/UICC) staging system in all patients with DTC [8, 9]. In addition, the ATA proposed a new staging system that classifies patients as low, intermediate, or high risk of recurrent/persistent disease based on several disease characteristics (e.g., presence of local invasion, local/distant metastases, aggressive histology, incomplete tumor resection) [8]. These staging systems do not involve re-stratification of patients based on response to initial therapy. It makes intuitive sense that DTC in patients responding poorly to initial therapy recurs or persists at a higher rate than in those with a good response. A recent retrospective study of 588 patients with DTC with a median follow-up of 7 years validated the ATA recurrence classification system and further demonstrated that re-stratification based on initial response to therapy allowed a more accurate prediction of persistent disease at last follow-up [10].

Role for Imaging and Serum Thyroglobulin

Literature over the past decade has suggested that the WBS adds limited information to the stimulated Tg level in most patients with DTC [11, 12], particularly in low-risk patients in whom a prior WBS was negative [13], and on the other hand, cervical ultrasound (US) significantly augments stimulated Tg levels in detecting and localizing recurrent DTC. In a French study, among 256 patients with DTC of various AJCC stages undergoing withdrawal scanning 6–12 months after thyroidectomy and remnant ablation, the WBS did not detect disease outside the thyroid bed in a single case, including 46 patients with stimulated serum Tg levels greater than 1 ng/mL [11]. In a smaller study, among 108 patients 1–35 years after initial therapy, a rhTSH WBS using 3–5 mCi of ^{131}I showed no activity outside the thyroid bed, including 20 patients with stimulated serum Tg levels more than 2.0 ng/mL [12]. Conversely, a third study examined rhTSH scanning in 109 low-risk DTC patients and found WBS evidence of metastatic disease in 8 % of cases, with a stimulated serum Tg level of less than 2.0 ng/mL [13]. However, when these authors confined their analysis to those patients whose last WBS was negative, the current WBS was never informative if the stimulated Tg level was less than 2.0 ng/mL. There are important factors to consider before omitting the WBS from a given patient's surveillance regimen. First, the patient should not have anti-Tg antibodies—a caveat that may exclude up to 25 % of DTC patients [14]. Second, the Tg assay must have sufficient sensitivity to detect low levels of Tg elevation (a functional sensitivity of 1.0 ng/mL is recommended) [15]. Third, the patient should have had a negative WBS on the last WBS [13, 16]. Finally, the patient should be in a group with a low-pretest probability of metastatic disease, i.e., a low-risk group, as discussed below [15]. Recent guidelines recommend the use of WBS in the long-term follow-up of patients with a positive serum Tg or for patients in an intermediate or high-risk category [8, 16].

The use of ultrasound (US) with or without fine-needle aspiration biopsy (FNAB) and Tg-needle washout has been found to be useful in detecting recurrent thyroid cancer in both the thyroid bed and in regional lymph nodes. A retrospective study of 494 patients with DTC previously treated with TT and RRA found recurrence in 10.3 % of patients after a mean of 45 months based on FNAB or histologic results of new neck lesions. Many patients with recurrent disease had unstimulated serum Tg <2 ng/mL, as the sensitivity of serum Tg ≥ 2 ng/mL was 56.8 %, and most were without evidence of disease on WBS (sensitivity 45.1 %). US had a sensitivity of 94.1 % [17]. Patients with microscopic

PTC (<1 cm) were found in one study to have a 20-year risk of recurrence of 5.7 %, and 80 % of these occurred in the central lymph nodes [5]. In a cohort of 456 patients with microscopic PTC, serum Tg levels were found to correlate with the ultrasound-measured mass of the metastatic disease. In this study, US but not WBS was able to localize small neck lymph node metastases in some Tg-negative patients [18]. Further, the negative predictive value (NPV) of a thyroid hormone withdrawal (THW) thyroglobulin <1 ng/mL plus a negative neck ultrasound was 98.8 % at 12 months follow-up, and WBS did not add any information. The finding of US superiority over WBS in the follow-up of these low-risk patients with undetectable serum Tg has been observed in additional studies as well [19–21].

The complete assessment of specific US characteristics of lymph nodes and thyroid bed nodules in the detection of recurrence cannot be overstated. After TT, the absence of suspicious thyroid bed US features to include microcalcifications, hypoechogenicity, and increased vascularity has been shown to have a NPV of 97 % [22]. In the same study, the NPV of an absence of abnormal lymph nodes was 94 % and of the absence of rising serum thyroglobulin was 93 %. The experience of the ultrasonographer should be considered when relying on this modality for surveillance. At smaller, low-volume centers, abnormal lymph node characteristics such as microcalcifications, cystic changes, peripheral vascularity, and loss of the fatty hilum should specifically be queried. Further, patients with an undetectable stimulated Tg and negative TgAb who have minimal LN enlargement without additional features of LN metastases noted above should not be assumed to have recurrent PTC without cytologic evidence.

The application of rhTSH to thyroid cancer surveillance represents a major quality-of-life improvement for patients with thyroid cancer and has even been shown to significantly reduce number of sick leave days in comparison to traditional THW [23]. The use of rhTSH-stimulated Tg alone to manage patients with low-risk DTC was examined by Wartofsky and colleagues in a multicenter study [24]. Patients with prior NTT and remnant ablation, with a thyroid hormone suppressive therapy (THST)-Tg of less than 5.0 ng/mL, were included. At baseline, 89 % of 300 eligible patients had THST-Tg levels of less than 1.0 ng/mL. For the whole group, 53 of 300 (18 %) had Tg increments of more than 2 ng/mL after rhTSH administration. Among these patients, WBS was positive (thyroid bed or metastases) in approx 50 %. Patients with American Joint Commission on Cancer (AJCC) stage III disease were more likely to have positive stimulated Tg values than were lower stage patients. Interestingly, among 14 patients with a stimulated Tg less than 2, but in whom WBS was also obtained, 9 had positive WBS, including 5 with metastatic disease. Considered together, these data suggest that elevated rhTSH-stimulated Tg levels greater than 2 ng/mL frequently signify persistent or recurrent disease, whereas a negative Tg response does not always guarantee that the patient is disease-free [24]. A subsequent prospective study of 107 DTC patients with a median follow-up of about 3 years showed that a single rhTSH-Tg of <0.5 ng/mL had an approximately 98 % likelihood of identifying patients free of disease. The authors concluded that this set of patients could be followed with annual THST-Tg and less frequent neck US [25]. Extended follow-up of this same cohort for an average of 7–10 years found that patients whose initial surveillance stimulated Tg was < 0.5 ng/mL had a 3 % subsequent recurrence rate, compared to 11 % and 80 %, respectively, when the stimulated Tg was 0.6–2.0 ng/ml or greater than 2.0 ng/mL, respectively [26].

The value of a second rhTSH-Tg after one undetectable result during follow-up has been the subject of two recent studies [27, 28]. In the first of these studies, 67 patients who underwent TT and remnant ablation and had one negative rhTSH-Tg within 1 year of therapy were tested again at an average follow-up of 36 months. Of 67 patients, 66 (98.5 %) had a rhTSH-Tg <1 ng/mL plus negative neck US. This suggests that a second rhTSH-Tg is generally only necessary in those patients whose first rhTSH-Tg is positive and THST-Tg remains undetectable [27]. In a second larger study, among 278 patients with a negative-stimulated thyroglobulin 12 months after initial treatment for DTC, a negative predictive value of 97.8 % after the first negative-stimulated Tg rose to 99.6 % and 100 % after a second and third negative-stimulated Tg, respectively [28].

Recent literature has documented that the doubling time of Tg (Tg-DT) during follow-up can give important prognostic information. In a small cohort of 137 patients who underwent TT, cause-specific survival at 10 years was 100 % if Tg-DT was >3 years, but dropped to only 50 % if the Tg-DT was <1 year. Tg-DT was a better predictor of survival, distant metastases, and locoregional recurrence when compared to other classical prognosticators like TNM staging, age, and gender [29]. This follow-up strategy could potentially be useful in patients with history of TT but without remnant ablation, as clear guidelines do not exist for this population.

Clinical Practice Guidelines

Over the past several years, many groups have released clinical practice guidelines (CPGs) to assist the management of patients with thyroid cancer [8, 16, 30]. In 2006, the American Thyroid Association delegated an international task force of thyroid cancer experts to create a set of management guidelines for DTC, and these were revised in 2009 and again in 2015 [8]. Specific recommendations were made for follow-up. Low-risk patients who have had an undetectable suppressed Tg and negative cervical US within the first year after treatment should have serum Tg measured after withdrawal or rhTSH 12 months after ablation. If negative, they can be followed annually with neck exam and THST-Tg. These patients do not require WBS during follow-up assuming anti-Tg antibodies are negative. In intermediate to high-risk patients, on the other hand, WBS following withdrawal or rhTSH 6–12 months after remnant ablation is recommended with ^{123}I or low activity ^{131}I. Cervical US at 6–12 months is considered to be highly sensitive for recurrent disease. Suspicious lymph nodes greater than 5–8 mm should be biopsied for cytology and Tg measurement in the needle washout fluid, as this enhances sensitivity. The frequency of follow-up with ultrasound should be based on the patient's risk of recurrence. Fluorodeoxyglucose positron emission tomography scanning (18-FDG-PET) is recommended in Tg-positive, RAI scan-negative patients with an elevated Tg >10 ng/mL in order to localize recurrence. Additional uses for 18-FDG-PET can also be considered such as in initial staging and follow-up of high-risk patients with poorly differentiated, non-iodine avid thyroid cancers and as a measurement of posttreatment response following external beam irradiation, surgical resection, embolization, or systemic therapy.

The National Comprehensive Cancer Network (NCCN) CPGs, updated annually and available online [16], also provide organized, specific, and evidence-based recommendations for the management of thyroid cancer. These guidelines were developed by experts from many large cancer centers in the United States and provide separate sections for the treatment of patients with papillary, follicular, Hürthle cell, and medullary thyroid cancer. According to the NCCN guidelines, routine follow-up for a patient with papillary thyroid cancer who has had near-total thyroidectomy and remnant ablation should consist of a neck exam, THST-Tg, and anti-Tg antibody measurement at 6 and 12 months and annually thereafter if disease-free. In low-risk patients, periodic neck US is recommended only if there is suspicion for recurrence. A TSH-stimulated Tg is recommended in patients with negative THST-Tg and anti-Tg antibody. WBS should be considered in patients with T3-4 or M1 at initial staging, abnormal Tg levels, abnormal anti-Tg antibody levels, or abnormal US. If there is suspicion for recurrence based on these tests, repeat WBS every 12–24 months until negative is recommended. Additional imaging (e.g., 18-FDG-PET/CT) should be performed if a stimulated Tg is detectable and WBS is negative.

A consensus statement on the role of serum Tg as a primary monitoring method for low-risk patients with papillary thyroid cancer was published in 2003 [15]. This group of thyroid cancer experts addressed such issues as the minimal acceptable Tg assay standards, a comparison of the sensitivity of the WBS with the stimulated Tg level, and whether THST-Tg alone is sufficiently sensitive to either detect persistent disease initially or to follow patients once they are noted to have a negative-stimulated Tg test. A low-risk patient was defined as generally having AJCC stage I or II disease, no distant metastases, a prior total thyroidectomy with remnant ablation, no clinical evidence of disease, and a THST-Tg level less than 1 ng/mL. It was concluded that Tg assays used to follow thyroid cancer patients should have a functional sensitivity of 1 ng/mL and that the WBS generally added little to the information provided by a stimulated Tg level. THST-Tg was deemed too insensitive to detect persistent disease, but in low-risk patients with a prior stimulated Tg level less than 1 ng/mL, the consensus was that an *annual* stimulated Tg level was not necessary. The group was unable to determine how often, if at all, stimulated Tg testing was required in this group of patients once a single negative-stimulated Tg level is obtained [15]. Other workers [31] also have found that a WBS added very little to information provided by rhTSH-stimulated thyroglobulin levels.

Recommended Approach to Follow-Up in PTC

Because most recurrences from papillary thyroid cancer occur within the first 15 years of diagnosis [32–34], it seems prudent to continue to perform stimulated Tg testing at increasing intervals until the risk of recurrence is low enough to justify the use of THST-Tg and neck US as primary surveillance methods. Figure 35.1 reviews an algorithmic approach to the follow-up of DTC, applicable to patients who have undergone near-total thyroidectomy and remnant ablation. Withdrawal or rhTSH scanning and Tg measurement with neck ultrasound is performed at 12 months (6 months for patients in high-risk categories). The majority of patients will have stimulated Tg less than 2 ng/mL and a negative WBS for metastatic disease. Patients in higher risk categories but favorable thyroglobulin results at 1 year may be managed with serial rhTSH-stimulated Tg alone, which is performed at 3, 5, 10, and 15 years, after which surveillance consists of neck exam and THST-Tg administration. Patients deemed to be at low risk (younger patients with small primary tumors and negative initial testing) may be advanced to THST-Tg testing alone earlier in this course. According to this algorithm, patients with stimulated Tg levels greater than 2 ng/mL or who have metastatic disease on WBS are considered as Tg positive/WBS positive or Tg positive/WBS negative. Patients in the former group with cervical lymph node metastases on scan and surgical targets identified on neck ultrasound should be referred for neck dissection, followed by radioiodine therapy. Patients with distant metastases are generally treated with higher doses of radioiodine, which may be determined using dosimetry. Tg-positive/ scan-negative patients with Tg levels greater than 10–15 ng/

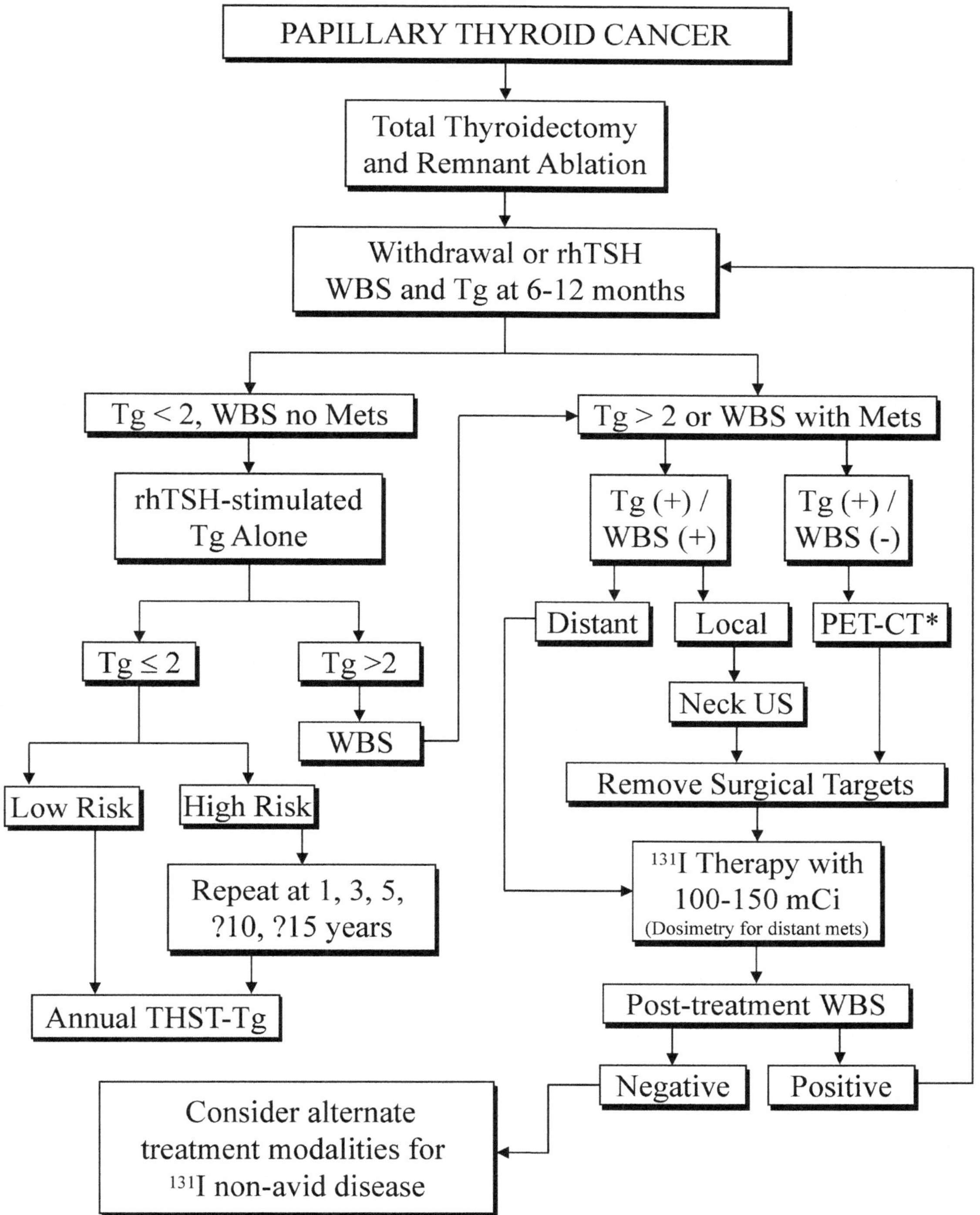

Fig. 35.1 An algorithmic approach to the follow-up of DTC after a near-total thyroidectomy and remnant ablation therapy. Patients with negative serum Tg levels and WBS at 6–12 months are followed with rhTSH-stimulated Tg levels alone, which based on risk assessment (initial and ongoing) is ultimately supplanted by annual THST-Tg monitoring. Patients with evidence of persistent disease at 12 months are distinguished on the basis of Tg and WBS status. Tg-positive/WBS-negative patients are assessed for surgical targets using fluorodeoxyglucose positron emission tomography (PET) uptake, which is the most sensitive when Tg levels are higher than 10 ng/mL. Tg-positive/WBS-positive patients require further evaluation to assess for surgical targets (WBS uptake in the neck), followed by radioiodine ablation, or they are treated with high-dose radioiodine directly if distant metastases are seen on WBS. *US* ultrasound, *CT* computed tomography

mL are candidates for fluorodeoxyglucose positron emission tomography scanning [35–38], preferably with computed tomography colocalization, with the objective of identifying and removing surgical targets [39]. By definition, these patient's tumors have less iodine avidity and are unlikely to respond to radioiodine [40]. A negative post-therapy WBS in patients with known persistent or recurrent disease should prompt consideration of other treatment modalities, such as external radiation therapy [16].

References

1. Mazzaferri EL, Kloos RT. Clinical review 128: current approaches to primary therapy for papillary and follicular thyroid cancer. J Clin Endocrinol Metab. 2001;86:1447–63.
2. Scuito R, Romano L, Rea S, et al. Natural history and clinical outcome of differentiated thyroid carcinoma: a retrospective analysis of 1503 patients treated at a single institution. Ann Oncol. 2009;20:1728–35.
3. Solomon BL, Wartofsky L, Burman KD. Current trends in the management of well differentiated papillary thyroid carcinoma. J Clin Endocrinol Metab. 1996;81:333–9.
4. Kim S, Wei JP, Braveman JM, et al. Predicting outcome and directing therapy for papillary thyroid carcinoma. Arch Surg. 2004; 139:390–4.
5. Hay ID, Hutchinson ME, Gonzalez-Losada T, et al. Papillary thyroid microcarcinoma: a study of 900 cases observed in a 60-year period. Surgery. 2008;144:980–8.
6. Lin J-D, Chao T-C, Hsueh C, et al. High recurrent rate of multicentric papillary thyroid carcinoma. Ann Surg Oncol. 2009;16: 2609–16.
7. Ross DS, Litofsky D, Ain KB, et al. Recurrence after treatment of micropapillary thyroid cancer. Thyroid. 2009;19:1043–8.
8. American Thyroid Association Guidelines Task Force on Thyroid Nodules and Differentiated Thyroid Cancer. Haugen BR, Alexander EK, Bible KC, Doherty GM, Mandel SJ, Nikiforov YE, Pacini F, Randolph GW, Sawka AM, Schlumberger M, Schuff KG, Sherman SI, Sosa JA, Steward DL, Tuttle RM, Wartofsky L. 2015 American Thyroid Association Management Guidelines for Adult Patients with Thyroid Nodules and Differentiated Thyroid Cancer. Thyroid 2016; 26:1–133.
9. Edge SB, Byrd DR, Compton CC, et al. AJCC cancer staging manual. 7th ed. New York: Springer; 2009.
10. Tuttle RM, Tala H, Shah J, et al. Estimating risk of recurrence in differentiated thyroid cancer after total thyroidectomy and radioactive iodine remnant ablation: using response to therapy variables to modify the initial risk estimates predicted by the new American Thyroid Association staging system. Thyroid. 2010;20:1341–9.
11. Cailleux AF, Baudin E, Travagli JP, et al. Is diagnostic iodine-131 scanning useful after total thyroid ablation for differentiated thyroid cancer? J Clin Endocrinol Metab. 2000;85:175–8.
12. Mazzaferri EL, Kloos RT. Is diagnostic iodine-131 scanning with recombinant human TSH useful in the follow-up of differentiated thyroid cancer after thyroid ablation? J Clin Endocrinol Metab. 2002;87:1490–8.
13. Robbins RJ, Chon JT, Fleisher M, et al. Is the serum thyroglobulin response to recombinant human thyrotropin sufficient, by itself, to monitor for residual thyroid carcinoma? J Clin Endocrinol Metab. 2002;87:3242–7.
14. Torrens JI, Burch HB. Serum thyroglobulin measurement. Utility in clinical practice. Endocrinol Metab Clin N Am. 2001;30:429–67.
15. Mazzaferri EL, Robbins RJ, Spencer CA, et al. A consensus report of the role of serum thyroglobulin as a monitoring method for low-risk patients with papillary thyroid carcinoma. J Clin Endocrinol Metab. 2003;88:1433–41.
16. Tuttle RM, Ball DW, Byrd D, et al. Thyroid carcinoma. J Natl Compr Cancer Netw. 2010;8:1228–74.
17. Frasoldati A, Pesenti M, Gallo A, et al. Diagnosis of neck recurrences in patients with differentiated thyroid carcinoma. Cancer. 2003;97:90–6.
18. Torlontano M, Attard M, Crocetti U, et al. Follow-up of low risk patients with papillary thyroid cancer: role of neck ultrasonography in detecting lymph node metastases. J Clin Endocrinol Metab. 2004;89:3402–7.
19. Schlumberger M, Berg G, Cohen O, et al. Follow-up of low-risk patients with differentiated thyroid carcinoma: a European perspective. Eur J Endocrinol. 2004;150:105–12.
20. Torlontano M, Crocetti U, Augello G, et al. Comparative evaluation of recombinant human thyrotropin-stimulated thyroglobulin levels, ^{131}I whole-body scintigraphy, and neck ultrasonography in the follow-up of patients with papillary thyroid microcarcinoma who have not undergone radioiodine therapy. J Clin Endocrinol Metab. 2006;91:60–3.
21. Durante C, Attard M, Torlontano M, et al. Identification and optimal postsurgical follow-up of patients with very low-risk papillary thyroid microcarcinomas. J Clin Endocrinol Metab. 2010;95:4882–8.
22. Rondeau G, Fish S, Hann LE, et al. Ultrasonographically detected small thyroid bed nodules identified after total thyroidectomy for differentiated thyroid cancer seldom show clinically significant structural progression. Thyroid. 2011;21:845–53.
23. Borget I, Corone C, Nocaudie M, et al. Sick leave for follow-up control in thyroid cancer patients: comparison between stimulation with Thyrogen and thyroid hormone withdrawal. Eur J Endocrinol. 2007;156:531–8.
24. Wartofsky L. Management of low-risk well-differentiated thyroid cancer based only on thyroglobulin measurement after recombinant human thyrotropin. Thyroid. 2002;12:583–90.
25. Kloos RT, Mazzaferri EL. A single recombinant human thyrotropin-stimulated serum thyroglobulin measurement predicts differentiated thyroid carcinoma metastases three to five years later. J Clin Endocrinol Metab. 2005;90:5047–57.
26. Kloos RT. Thyroid cancer recurrence in patients clinically free of disease with undetectable or very low serum thyroglobulin values. J Clin Endocrinol Metab. 2010;95:5241–8.
27. Castagna MG, Brilli L, Pilli T, et al. Limited value of repeat recombinant human thyrotropin (rhTSH)-stimulated thyroglobulin testing in differentiated thyroid carcinoma patients with previous negative rhTSH-stimulated thyroglobulin and undetectable basal serum thyroglobulin levels. J Clin Endocrinol Metab. 2008;93:76–81.
28. Klubo-Gwiezdzinska J, Burman KD, Van Nostrand D, Wartofsky L. Does an undetectable rhTSH-stimulated Tg level 12 months after initial treatment of thyroid cancer indicate remission? Clin Endocrinol (Oxf). 2011;74(1):111–7.
29. Miyauchi A, Kudo T, Miya A, et al. Prognostic impact of serum thyroglobulin doubling-time under thyrotropin suppression in patients with papillary thyroid carcinoma who underwent total thyroidectomy. Thyroid. 2011;21:707–16.
30. Kendall-Taylor P. Guidelines for the management of thyroid cancer. Clin Endocrinol. 2003;58:400–2.
31. David A, Blotta A, Rossi R, et al. Clinical value of different responses of serum thyroglobulin to recombinant human thyrotropin in the follow-up of patients with differentiated thyroid carcinoma. Thyroid. 2005;15:267–73.
32. Ain KB. Papillary thyroid carcinoma. Etiology, assessment, and therapy. Endocrinol Metab Clin N Am. 1995;24:711–60.
33. Mazzaferri EL. Long-term outcome of patients with differentiated thyroid carcinoma: effect of therapy. Endocr Pract. 2000;6:469–76.

34. Hay ID. Papillary thyroid carcinoma. Endocrinol Metab Clin N Am. 1990;19:545–76.
35. Grunwald F, Schomburg A, Bender H, et al. Fluorine-18 fluorodeoxyglucose positron emission tomography in the follow-up of differentiated thyroid cancer. Eur J Nucl Med. 1996;23:312–9.
36. Sisson JC, Ackermann RJ, Meyer MA, Wahl RL. Uptake of 18-fluoro2-deoxy-D-glucose by thyroid cancer: implications for diagnosis and therapy. J Clin Endocrinol Metab. 1993;77:1090–4.
37. Chung JK, So Y, Lee JS, et al. Value of FDG PET in papillary thyroid carcinoma with negative ^{131}I whole-body scan. J Nucl Med. 1999;40:986–92.
38. Chin BB, Patel P, Cohade C, et al. Recombinant human thyrotropin stimulation of fluoro-D-glucose positron emission tomography uptake in well-differentiated thyroid carcinoma. J Clin Endocrinol Metab. 2004;89:91–5.
39. Yeo JS, Chung JK, So Y, et al. F-18-fluorodeoxyglucose positron emission tomography as a presurgical evaluation modality for I-131 scan-negative thyroid carcinoma patients with local recurrence in cervical lymph nodes. Head Neck. 2001; 23:94–103.
40. Wang W, Larson SM, Fazzari M, et al. Prognostic value of [18F] fluorodeoxyglucose positron emission tomographic scanning in patients with thyroid cancer. J Clin Endocrinol Metab. 2000;85:1107–13.

Thyroid Hormone Therapy and Thyrotropin Suppression

36

Leonard Wartofsky

Introduction

Levothyroxine (L-T4) is arguably the most prescribed medication in the United States, with its most common therapeutic indication being for hypothyroidism due to chronic thyroiditis or Hashimoto's disease [1]. Such patients are candidates for so-called replacement dosage, with the administered dosage of L-T4 titrated to a target thyrotropin (TSH) level within the normal reference range of 0.4–3.0 mU/L. Patients with thyroid cancer who have had near-total to total thyroidectomy and have suspected residual disease are usually candidates for suppressive levothyroxine dosage, which is so-called because the aim of therapy is to give a slightly supraphysiologic dosage of thyroxine to suppress TSH [2]. The rationale for suppressive therapy is based on studies indicating that TSH stimulation enhances tumor growth, TSH serving as a growth factor or mitogen for thyroid malignancies with observations of more rapid tumor growth seen clinically after thyroxine withdrawal. The growth-promoting property of TSH is presumed to be from the presence of TSH receptors on thyroid cancer cells [3]; however, non-TSH receptor-mediated growth is certainly a property of undifferentiated thyroid cancers. In patients presenting with a thyroid nodule, the likelihood that the nodule may be malignant correlates directly to the level of serum TSH [4–10], and thyroid cancer patients with elevated TSH levels may be more likely to have more advanced disease or evidence of extrathyroidal extension [11] at time of presentation.

An early study by Mazzaferri and Jhiang [12] demonstrated that thyroid hormone therapy had a salutary effect on the survival of patients with papillary thyroid cancer. Although a clear relationship between the magnitude of TSH suppression and mortality has not been definitively shown, observational studies tend to suggest lower rates of both tumor recurrence and cancer-specific death in patients on suppressive dosage. One retrospective study concluded that improved prognosis and outcome were associated with full TSH suppression, in contrast to outcomes in patients with lesser degrees of TSH suppression [13]. Those patients with TSH levels of less than 0.5 mU/L had more prolonged disease-free intervals than those with a higher mean TSH level, making the TSH level an independent predictive factor for recurrence. However, while the degree of TSH suppression may not matter with stage I or II well-differentiated thyroid cancer, this does not appear to be the case for stage III or IV patients as Cooper et al. [14] observed better outcomes in patients with more advanced disease when they were treated with greater degrees of TSH suppression. Similar observations were made by Jonklaas et al. [15] and Hovens et al. [16] indicating that while full suppression may be required in high-risk patients, only moderate TSH suppression appears to be necessary in low-risk patients. Even for high-risk patients, there appears to be a limit on the degree of suppression required, with levels of suppression down as low as <0.03 mU/L offering no additional benefit [17].

An earlier iteration of the National Comprehensive Cancer Network (NCCN) guidelines [18] did not stipulate what degree of TSH suppression should be achieved, whereas the more recent NCCN guidelines [19] recommend suppression to less than 0.1 mU/L or to undetectable levels in a sensitive assay for high-risk patients as do the British Thyroid Association guidelines [20]. The NCCN guidelines recommend maintaining the TSH between 0.1 and 0.5 mU/L in low-risk patients without evidence of residual disease and adjusting levothyroxine dosage to allow TSH to rise into the normal reference range for those patients who are clearly free of disease [19]. The NCCN guidelines also recommend calcium (1,200 mg/day) and vitamin D supplementation (1,000 units/day) should full suppression be required on a long-term basis. A more recent study by Sugitani et al. has

L. Wartofsky, MD, MACP (✉)
Department of Medicine, MedStar Washington Hospital Center, Georgetown University School of Medicine, 110 Irving Street, N.W., Washington, DC 20010-2975, USA
e-mail: leonard.wartofsky@medstar.net

L. Wartofsky, D. Van Nostrand (eds.), *Thyroid Cancer*, DOI 10.1007/978-1-4939-3314-3_36

raised question on the need for any degree of TSH suppression in low-risk patients [21] indicating that disease-free survival was the same whether or not TSH suppression was achieved. Although this was a randomized controlled trial, the extent of postoperative disease was unclear because total thyroidectomy or radioiodine ablation was not done in all subjects and the Tg levels were not reported. Nevertheless, the latter study has provoked a great deal of renewed interest in how much TSH suppression is really required.

With levothyroxine therapy, only once daily dosing is required because of the long (6–7 days) half-life of thyroxine. Other thyroid hormone preparations are available and include desiccated thyroid extract USP, a triiodothyronine (T3) preparation, and a mixture of thyroxine (T4) and T3 (liotrix). Although once in popular use, the desiccated thyroid extract preparation is not generally recommended because of its T3 content, which is so rapidly absorbed that the resultant high-serum T3 can cause tachycardias or arrhythmias in elderly patients or those with underlying cardiac disease. Notwithstanding these concerns, one recent study employing desiccated thyroid extract did not observe any significant adverse effects, and some patients did enjoy modest weight loss although there was no overall improvement in quality of life compared to T4 therapy [22]. The T4 products are more stable with a longer and more predictable shelf life. As T4 is converted to T3, near-normal concentrations of serum T3 can be restored ultimately by administering T4 alone. Target goals for TSH suppression vary within clinical centers and among thyroid cancer experts but are generally linked to risk stratification, stage of disease, and the presence or absence of residual or recurrent tumor. If not indicated, oversuppression should be avoided because of the known deleterious effects of excessive thyroid hormone levels on both the heart [23–28] and bone mineral density [29–31]. Even in thyroid cancer patients who have evidence of residual cancer, there should be careful dosage titration and avoidance of overly judicious suppression, particularly in elderly patients with underlying cardiovascular disease, osteopenia, or osteoporosis. Moreover, there is a subpopulation of patients who, for unknown reasons, appear to be extremely sensitive to minor fluctuations (either increases or decreases) in their L-T4 levels. For all of these reasons, it is important for patients to be taking L-T4 tablets of precise levothyroxine content, potency, and bioequivalence [32, 33]. The Thyroid Foundation of America has warned patients of potential untoward effects of a change or "switch" in L-T4 preparations that are not truly bioequivalent [34], along with the American Thyroid Association, Endocrine Society, and the American Association of Clinical Endocrinologists [35]. These organizations recommend that patients remain on the same branded levothyroxine preparation and are not prescribed generic levothyroxine because pharmacists dispense different generics as refills from 1 month to the next, preparations that have not been proven bioequivalent to each other. If a change in brand is necessary, the professional organizations recommend remeasurement of TSH in 6 weeks and retitration of the levothyroxine dose to the desired level.

For individuals with no history of thyroid cancer, a normal metabolic state is associated with normalization of the TSH level with replacement levothyroxine to a TSH range of 0.5–1.5 mU/L; on average, this equates to a daily dose of L-T4 of approx 1.7 μg/kg. Patients who have had a total thyroidectomy, e.g., for thyroid malignancy, especially when surgery was followed by radioiodine ablation, will have no residual thyroid tissue, and their requirement will be closer to 2.1 μg/kg/day. Clearly, dosage adjustments should not be based solely on such approximations and are best determined by clinical criteria and TSH measurement. In high-risk thyroid cancer patients with evidence of residual disease, we would generally prescribe dosage targeted to keep TSH levels at less than 0.02 mU/L, whereas intermediate-risk patients with the possibility of residual disease might be kept between 0.05 and 0.1 mU/L. Within the first 5 years of diagnosis, thyroid cancer patients at low risk of recurrence and who have been proven free of residual disease do not need to have their TSH levels fully suppressed and may have their L-T4 dose reduced to the replacement level range of 0.2–0.6 mU/L. Finally, patients with negative recombinant human TSH-stimulated thyroglobulin levels and isotope scans, and negative ultrasonographic imaging more than 5 years since diagnosis, may have their dosage reduced to achieve normal-range TSH levels of 0.9–2.0 mU/L. In either case, careful and precise L-T4 dose titration is mandatory to achieve a specific end point for the therapy, whether it is a normal-range level of TSH or is just suppressed into the undetectable range.

Although there are no specific studies designed to assess what degree of TSH suppression may be required for individual patients with thyroid cancer, the analysis by Cooper et al. [14] of 683 patients with differentiated thyroid cancer provided useful insights into this issue. Examination of patient records of a multicenter thyroid cancer registry revealed that most patients did not have fully suppressed TSH levels at all visits, but suppression appeared to be more uniform for patients with follicular thyroid cancer. Importantly, no relationship between cancer progression and degree of TSH suppression was found for stage I or stage II papillary cancer, the staging indicating that the risk of recurrence was low; hence, the degree of TSH suppression should not matter. However, this was not the case for stage III or IV patients, whose outcomes were improved by greater degrees of TSH suppression. Similar conclusions have been reached by subsequent studies [15, 16]. The data from these latter studies serve to provide the basis for the recommendations in the revised guidelines for the management of thyroxine therapy in patients with thyroid cancer of the American Thyroid Association which are now based on risk stratification on how aggressive to be with TSH suppression [36]. A growing trend to moderating LT4 dosage in low-risk patients has derived from a number of studies such as the randomized controlled trial from Japan that concluded that there was little difference achieved in disease-free survival if postoperative TSH-suppressive therapy was given or not given in low-risk patients [21]. The most comprehensive, measured approach to levothyroxine therapy in thyroid cancer patients was outlined by Biondi and Cooper who proposed a stratified system of dosage based upon balancing cancer risk versus potential adverse effects [28].

In some circumstances, a previously stable dosage of levothyroxine may have to be increased or decreased for a variety of reasons. Of course, the most common explanation for an inappropriately high TSH is nonadherence to the prescribed regimen, but occasionally, there may be other explanations. For example, a rising TSH could signal a reduction in gastrointestinal thyroxine absorption. This could be owing to concomitant ingestion of L-T4 with food or certain other pharmacologic agents that interfere with gastrointestinal absorption (e.g., calcium, cholestyramine, colestipol, kayexalate, antacids, sucralfate, iron, and so on) or that enhance the metabolic clearance of levothyroxine (e.g., carbamazepine and phenytoin).

Most manufacturers of levothyroxine products provide a wide range of dosage strengths: 25, 50, 75, 88, 100, 112, 125, 137, 150, 175, 200, and 300 μg per tablet. Theoretically, the availability of these multiple-dosage strengths allows the clinician to precisely titrate a given patient's levothyroxine requirement to a desired metabolic and serum TSH level. Recent changes in regulations governing bioavailability and bioequivalence of the levothyroxine preparations by the US Food and Drug Administration (FDA) have led to a flurry of new L-T4 preparations, including generic or nonbranded forms of L-T4 with presumed therapeutic interchange of one preparation for another [33]. In the current era of pressures on clinicians for the most cost-effective medicine, a lower cost preparation is obviously desirable but is acceptable only if shown to be of proven equivalent potency and pharmacodynamics. Some older studies have suggested similar bioequivalence between various levothyroxine preparations, whereas other reports have found differences. Practical application of the conclusions, or definitive interpretation of the results, taken from these earlier reports is difficult because of methodologic defects in patient selection or study design that have become appreciated only in retrospect.

Apart from factors of cost and industry competition, the issue of therapeutic equivalence is obviously important in regard to the quality of patient care. The American Thyroid Association (ATA) and the American Association of Clinical Endocrinologists (AACE) have published management guidelines, indicating that the various levothyroxine products may not be therapeutically equivalent [35, 37, 38]. The literature is replete with examples of the lack of interchangeability and varying potency of the different preparations, available as either branded or generic formulations. Consequently, repetitive measurements of serum TSH and appropriate dosage retitration are recommended by the ATA and other experts when patients or their physicians may decide to switch from one preparation to another [37, 38]. The costs and inconvenience of retesting and retitration understandably may vitiate any cost savings from switching to a less expensive preparation. Hence, for an alternative product to be affirmed as cost-effective, proof of bioequivalence would be required. The ATA recommendation for retitration after switching preparations implies that the various levothyroxine preparations have not been shown to be therapeutically equivalent and interchangeable.

The Role of T3 Therapy

Interest in combined T3 and T4 therapy for hypothyroidism is based on the long-standing concern whether hypothyroid patients can be optimally replaced by treatment with T4 alone. This topic has been reviewed in editorials [39, 40], and similar questions often arise in patients with thyroid cancer. To more closely mimic thyroidal T3 secretion and normal blood levels, oral supplements of triiodothyronine would need to be given in frequent and divided dosage—a regimen that makes patient compliance problematic. Moreover, convincing arguments or data demonstrating benefit of concomitant T3 administration are lacking. A small fraction of patients continue to complain of persistent nonspecific symptoms, such as easy fatigue, and these complaints tend to be more prominent in patients with autoimmune thyroid disease (Hashimoto's thyroiditis or Graves' disease postablative therapy) than in thyroidectomized thyroid cancer patients. Depending on patient responses to symptom questionnaires, studies indicate that patients tend to feel better, at least transiently, when mildly thyrotoxic, whether by T4 therapy [41] or by T3 [42]. Perhaps thyroid cancer patients complain less because higher doses of thyroxine are administered to suppress their TSH levels.

Much interest in the concept that concomitant T3 therapy was necessary to restore euthyroidism at the tissue level was the result of the experimental rat studies by Escobar-Morreale et al. [43] who examined whether T4 therapy alone might provide insufficient intracellular levels of T3, irrespective of serum levels of either T3 or TSH. They found that no dose of T4 by itself simultaneously normalized both T4 and T3 levels in tissues, but there are no precisely comparable studies in humans. The same group [44] did perform a crossover clinical trial of combination T3/T4 versus T4 alone in humans, and although many of the patients preferred the combination, there was no objective advantage observed. A clinical study that ostensibly demonstrated a greater clinical benefit from combined T3/T4 therapy than that achieved with T4 alone was reported by Bunevicius and coworkers

[42]. Possible deficiencies in their study design and criticism of their methods and conclusions have been published [39, 40, 44]. Analysis of the data indicates that it was the thyroid cancer patients, not the Hashimoto's patients, who seemed to derive benefit from the T3 combination, suggesting that it was the overdosage that was responsible, as seen in other studies. The validity of subsequent skepticism in their results appears supported by six more recent reports of studies, all of which indicated no benefit with combined L-T4 and L-T3 therapy [45–51].

The multiple single studies have been analyzed in several meta-analyses. In one such analysis by Ma [52], of 1,243 patients, there was a suggestion that combination therapy was beneficial for the psychological and physical well-being of patients who had been treated previously with only levothyroxine. No statistically significant difference in other variables was noted. However, a second meta-analysis by Joffe [53] of nine controlled studies found no significant differences on psychiatric symptoms of combined T3/T4 therapy versus levothyroxine alone. In most cases, the study designs in these clinical trials did not provide optimally physiologic doses of T3. The argument can be readily made that those patients showing some ostensible benefit from T3 coadministration received supraphysiologic dosage of T3. One published study on combination T4/T3 therapy did examine the question of possible benefit in doses given in a more appropriate molar ratio, i.e., 14:1 [50], but again, the authors concluded that there was no benefit to T4/T3 and potential risk from subclinical hyperthyroidism. A delayed-release vehicle for the T3 could provide a real test of efficacy of combined L-T3/L-T4 therapy. Current preparations are problematic because using current T3 preparations to achieve a premorbid normal profile of thyroid function tests might require administering small doses of T3 on a TID or perhaps QID basis, certainly not an optimal regimen for thyroid cancer patients. As a result of missing the occasional second or third daily dose, patients will ingest less than that required for the desired suppression of their TSH levels, with resultant inadequately treated cancer and greater risk of recurrence. For all of these reasons, there does not appear to be a role in thyroid cancer patients for combined T3/T4 therapy. Rather, the evidence of therapeutic benefit from the administration of exogenously administered T3 vs. endogenous T3 derived from T4 has been unconvincing as was indicated by a trial by Regalbuto et al. [54].

One of the very few studies demonstrating some benefit of combination therapy came from the group of Nygaard et al. [55]. This was a randomized, double-blind controlled study in which 59 patients were treated for consecutive 12-week intervals of T4/T3 combination therapy vs. T4 monotherapy. The patients' usual L-T4 dose was substituted with either 20 or 50 mcg of L-T3 with adjustments in L-T4 dose as required to maintain TSH levels between 0.1 and 5.0 mU/L. Several symptom questionnaires were performed at baseline and after each treatment period assessing quality of life and other parameters; significant differences were seen in 7 of 11 scores suggesting superior outcomes with combination therapy. With no differences in serum TSH, 49 % of the patients preferred T3/T4 therapy compared to only 15 % who preferred T4 monotherapy ($p = < 0.002$), although blinding was not considered complete. The strengths of this study include its crossover design, the large number of subjects, and the stability maintained in TSH levels. However, given the dosage titration method employed, patients were treated with relatively more T3 daily than in most prior studies, averaging 7.5–12.5 mcg daily with ratios of T4/T3 that ranged from 2.5:1 to 8:1.

While the earlier Bunevicius study [42] has not been confirmed, a recent study by Celi et al. [56] suggests that all of the reported symptomatically beneficial clinical responses of T3 treatment [44–50] may need to be reassessed. Celi et al. did not study combination T3/T4 therapy, but rather compared a T3 only regimen to a T4-only regimen by administering either medication on a TID basis in a ratio of 1:3. Compared to treatment with L-T4, patients on T3 were found to have no differences in serum TSH, heart rate, blood pressure, exercise tolerance, flow-mediated vasodilatation, fasting glucose, insulin sensitivity, or responses to the SF-36 or health-related QOL questionnaires. On the positive side, T3-treated patients demonstrated significant weight loss without change in body fat mass, as well as reduced total cholesterol, low-density lipoprotein cholesterol and apolipoprotein B, and increased SHBG levels.

Insight into a rationale for combination T4/T3 therapy may be gained by considering the deiodinase isoforms, especially deiodinase type 2 (D2) which is present in the brain, pituitary gland, skeletal muscle, heart, brown adipose tissue, and thyroid [57]. The pituitary response to hypothyroidism is governed by intracellular T4 to T3 activation within the pituitary. Conceptually, there could be tissue hypothyroidism secondary to relatively low serum T3 in the face of "normal" serum TSH levels when those TSH levels are being maintained by intrapituitary conversion of T4 to T3. Some studies indicate that higher serum T4 levels are necessary in thyroidectomized patients in order to generate normal serum T3 concentrations [58] and thereby compensate for the absence of the 20 % fraction of circulating T3 normally derived from the thyroid.

Given the importance of deiodinases in maintaining the euthyroid state, any genetic polymorphisms in the deiodinase genes will affect serum and tissue hormone concentrations in general, and in the pituitary gland in particular. Such polymorphism in the D2 gene has been described [59–64] and to be associated with reduced T4 to T3 activation. The identification of these deiodinase polymorphisms has given some support to the concept that at least a fraction of individuals may have varying needs for thyroid hormone replacement based upon the polymorphisms present. For example, a D2 polymorphism was found in 16 % of a study population and patients with this polymorphism taking T4 had worse baseline GHQ scores that improved on combination T4/T3 therapy.

In the small percentage of patients in whom a trial of T3 might be of interest, imprecise dosing with current T3 preparations is undesirable considering the risks of underdosage of a thyroid cancer patient in whom full suppression is indicated or the risk of overdosage when not warranted, causing subclinical hyperthyroidism. Availability of a more physiologic slow-release T3 product may prove to be of interest, but at the present time, the best management for both thyroid hormone replacement and TSH suppression in thyroid cancer patients continues to be L-T4 alone [65, 66]. When faced with high-risk patients with residual tumor, full-suppressive dosage of levothyroxine is warranted. Despite the risks to the heart and bone of full thyrotropin suppression, outcome analysis suggests that suppression therapy in such patients is associated with a reduction in adverse clinical events [67].

References

1. Biondi B, Wartofsky L. Treatment with Thyroid Hormone. Endocrine Reviews, published ahead of print: doi:10/1210/er.2013-1083; 2014;35:433–512.
2. Brabant G. Thyrotropin suppressive therapy in thyroid carcinoma: what are the targets? J Clin Endocrinol Metab. 2008;93:1167–9.
3. Carayon P, Thomnas-Morvan C, Castan E, Tubiana M. Human thyroid cancer: membrane thyrotropin binding and adenylate cyclase activity. J Clin Endocrinol Metab. 1980;51:915–20.
4. Derwahl M, Broecker M, Kraiem Z. Thyrotropin may not be the dominant growth factor in benign and malignant thyroid nodules. J Clin Endocrinol Metab. 1999;84:829–34.
5. Boelaert K, Horacek J, Holder RL, Watkinson JC, Sheppard MC, Franklyn JA. Serum thyrotropin concentration as a novel predictor of malignancy in thyroid nodules investigated by fine-needle aspiration. J Clin Endocrinol Metab. 2006;91:4295–301.
6. Jin J, Machekano R, McHenry CR. The utility of preoperative serum thyroid-stimulating hormone level for predicting malignant nodular thyroid disease. Am J Surg. 2010;199:294–7.
7. Jonklaas J, Nsouli-Maktabi H, Soldin SJ. Endogenous thyrotropin and triiodothyronine concentrations in individuals with thyroid cancer. Thyroid. 2008;18:943–52.
8. Fiore E, Rago T, Provenzale MA, et al. Lower levels of TSH are associated with a lower risk of papillary thyroid cancer in patients with thyroid nodular disease: thyroid autonomy may play a predictive role. Endocr-Relat Cancer. 2009;16:1251–60.
9. Fiore E, Vitti P. Serum TSH and risk of papillary thyroid cancer in nodular thyroid disease. J Clin Endocrinol Metab. 2012;97:1134–45.
10. McLeod DS, Watters KF, Carpenter AD, Ladenson PW, Cooper DS, Ding EL. Thyrotropin and thyroid cancer diagnosis: a systematic review and dose-response meta-analysis. J Clin Endocrinol Metab. 2012;97:2682–92.
11. Haymart MR, Repplinger DJ, Leverson GE, Elson DF, Sippel RS, Jaume JC, Chen H. Higher serum thyroid stimulating hormone level in thyroid nodule patients is associated with greater risks of differentiated thyroid cancer and advanced tumor stage. J Clin Endocrinol Metab. 2008;93:809–14.
12. Mazzaferri EL, Jhiang SM. Long-term impact of initial surgical and medical therapy on papillary and follicular thyroid cancer. Am J Med. 1994;97:418–28.
13. Pujol P, Daures J-P, Nsakala N, et al. Degree of thyrotropin suppression as a prognostic determinant in differentiated thyroid cancer. J Clin Endocrinol Metab. 1996;81:4318–22.
14. Cooper DS, Specker B, Ho M, et al. Thyrotropin suppression and disease progression in patients with differentiated thyroid cancer: results from the National Thyroid Cancer Treatment Cooperative Registry. Thyroid. 1998;9:737–44.
15. Jonklaas J, Sarlis NJ, Litofsky D, et al. Outcomes of patients with differentiated thyroid carcinoma following initial therapy. Thyroid. 2006;16:1229–42.
16. Hovens GC, Stokkel MP, Kievit J, et al. Associations of serum thyrotropin concentrations with recurrence and death in differentiated thyroid cancer. J Clin Endocrinol Metab. 2007;92:2610–5.
17. Diessl S, Holzberger B, Mader U, Grelle I, Smit JW, Buck AK, Reiners C, Verburg FA. Impact of moderate vs. Stringent TSH suppression on survival in differentiated thyroid carcinoma. Clin Endocrinol. 2012;76:586–92.
18. National Comprehensive Cancer Network (NCCN). Thyroid carcinoma: clinical practice guidelines 2013. J Natl Compr Cancer Netw. 2013;3:404–57.
19. Tuttle RM, Ball DW, Byrd D, et al. National Comprehensive Cancer Network (NCCN) thyroid carcinoma: clinical practice guidelines, version 3.2011. J Natl Compr Cancer Netw. 2010; 8:1228–74.
20. British Thyroid Association. Guidelines for the management of differentiated thyroid cancer in adults. Available at: www.british-thyroidassociation.org/guidelines.htm, 2002.
21. Sugitani I, Fujimoto Y. Does postoperative thyrotropin suppressive therapy truly decrease recurrence in papillary thyroid carcinoma? A randomized controlled trial. J Clin Endocrinol Metab. 2010; 95:4576–83.
22. Hoang TD, Olsen CH, Mai VQ, Clyde PW, Shakir MK. Desiccated thyroid extract compared with levothyroxine in the treatment of hypothyroidism: a randomized double-blind, crossover study. J Clin Endocrinol Metab. 2013;98:1982–90.
23. Sawin CT, Geller A, Wolf PA, et al. Low serum thyrotropin concentrations as a risk factor for atrial fibrillation in older persons. N Engl J Med. 1994;331:1249–52.
24. Parle JV, Maisonneuve P, Sheppard MC, et al. Prediction of all-cause and cardiovascular mortality in elderly people from one low serum thyrotropin result: a 10-year cohort study. Lancet. 2001;358:861–5.
25. Fazio S, Palmieri EA, Lombardi G, Biondi B. Effects of thyroid hormone on the cardiovascular system. Recent Prog Horm Res. 2004;59:31–50.
26. Biondi B, Palmieri EA, Lombardi G, Fazio S. Effects of subclinical thyroid dysfunction on the heart. Ann Intern Med. 2002;137: 904–14.
27. Shargorodsky M, Serov S, Gavish D, et al. Long-term thyrotropin-suppressive therapy with levothyroxine impairs small and large artery elasticity and increases left ventricular mass in patients with thyroid carcinoma. Thyroid. 2006;16:381–6.
28. Biondi B, Cooper DS. Benefits of thyrotropin suppression versus the risks of adverse effects in differentiated thyroid cancer. Thyroid. 2010;20:135–46.
29. Stathatos N, Wartofsky L. Effects of thyroid hormone on bone. Clin Rev Bone Miner Metab. 2004;2:135–50.
30. Mikosch P, Obermayer-Pietsch B, Jost R, et al. Bone metabolism in patients with differentiated thyroid carcinoma receiving suppressive levothyroxine treatment. Thyroid. 2003;13:347–56.
31. Chen CH, Chen JF, Yang B, Liu RT, Tung SC, Chien WY, et al. Bone mineral density in women receiving thyroxine suppressive therapy for differentiated thyroid carcinoma. J Formos Med Assoc. 2004;103:442–7.
32. Katz M, Rosen DL, Wartofsky L. Issues in bioequivalence and therapeutic equivalence of levothyroxine products. US Pharm. 2003;9(Suppl):2–14.

33. Wartofsky L. Levothyroxine: therapeutic use and regulatory issues related to bioequivalence. Expert Opin Pharmacother. 2002;3:727–32.
34. Thyroid Foundation of America. Advice to patients from the thyroid foundation of America. Thyroid. 2004;14:487.
35. American Thyroid Association, Endocrine Society, American Association of Clinical Endocrinologists. Joint statement on the U.S. Food and Drug Administration's decision regarding bioequivalence of levothyroxine sodium. Thyroid. 2004;14:486.
36. American Thyroid Association Guidelines Task Force on Thyroid Nodules and Differentiated Thyroid Cancer, Haugen BR, Alexander EK, Bible KC, Doherty GM, Mandel SJ, Nikiforov YE, Pacini F, Randolph GW, Sawka AM, Schlumberger M, Schuff KG, Sherman SI, Sosa JA, Steward DL, Tuttle RM, Wartofsky L. 2015 American Thyroid Association management guidelines for adult patients with thyroid nodules and differentiated thyroid cancer. Thyroid. 2016;26:1–133.
37. AACE/AAES Medical/Surgical guidelines for clinical practice: management of thyroid carcinoma. Endocr Pract. 2001;7:1–19.
38. Singer PA, Cooper DA, Daniels GH, et al. Treatment guidelines for patients with thyroid nodules and well differentiated thyroid cancer. Arch Intern Med. 1996;156:2165–72.
39. Cooper DS. Combined T4 and T3 therapy—back to the drawing board. JAMA. 2003;290:3002–4.
40. Kaplan MM, Sarne DH, Schneider AB. Editorial: In search of the impossible dream? Thyroid hormone replacement therapy that treats all symptoms in all hypothyroid patients. J Clin Endocrinol Metab. 2003;88:4540–2.
41. Carr D, McLeod DT, Parry G, et al. Fine adjustment of thyroxine replacement dosage: comparison of thyrotrophin releasing hormone test using a sensitive thyrotrophin assay with measurement of free thyroid hormones and clinical assessment. Clin Endocrinol. 1988;28:325–33.
42. Bunevicius R, Kazanavicius G, Zalinkevicius R, Prange Jr AJ. Effects of thyroxine as compared with thyroxine plus triiodothyronine in patients with hypothyroidism. N Engl J Med. 1999;340:424–9.
43. Escobar-Morreale HF, Escobar del Rey FE, Obregon MJ, Morreale de Escobar G. Only the combined treatment with thyroxine and triiodothyronine ensures euthyroidism in all tissues of the thyroidectomized rat. Endocrinology. 1996;137:2490–502.
44. Escobar-Morreale HF, Botella-Carretero JI, Gomez-Bueno M, et al. Thyroid hormone replacement therapy in primary hypothyroidism: a randomized trial comparing L-thyroxine plus liothyronine with L-thyroxine alone. Ann Intern Med. 2005;142:412–24.
45. Toft AD. Thyroid hormone replacement—one hormone or two? N Engl J Med. 1999;340:469–70.
46. Clyde PW, Harari AE, Getka EJ, Shakir KMM. Combined levothyroxine plus liothyronine compared with levothyroxine alone in primary hypothyroidism. JAMA. 2003;290:2952–8.
47. Levitt A, Silverberg J. T4 plus T3 treatment for hypothyroidism: a double-blind comparison with usual T4. Los Angeles, CA: Program 74th Annual Meeting, American Thyroid Association, 2002, 112.
48. Sawka AM, Gerstein HC, Marriott MJ, et al. Does a combination regimen of thyroxine (T4) and 3,5,3′-triiodothyronine improve depressive symptoms better than T4 alone in patients with hypothyroidism? Results of a double-blind, randomized, controlled trial. J Clin Endocrinol Metab. 2003;88:4551–5.
49. Walsh JP, Shiels L, Lim EM, et al. Combined thyroxine/liothyronine treatment does not improve well-being, quality of life, or cognitive function compared to thyroxine alone: a randomized controlled trial in patients with primary hypothyroidism. J Clin Endocrinol Metab. 2003;88:4543–50.
50. Cassio A, Cacciari E, Cicognani A, et al. Treatment for congenital hypothyroidism: thyroxine alone or thyroxine plus triiodothyronine? Pediatrics. 2003;111:1055–60.
51. Siegmund W, Spieker K, Weike AI, et al. Replacement therapy with levothyroxine plus triiodothyronine (bioavailable molar ratio 14:1) is not superior to thyroxine alone to improve well-being and cognitive performance in hypothyroidism. Clin Endocrinol. 2004;60:750–7.
52. Ma C, Xie J, Huang X, Wang G, Wang Y, Wang X, Zuo S. Thyroxine alone or thyroxine plus triiodothyronine replacement therapy for hypothyroidism. Nucl Med Commun. 2009;30:586–93.
53. Joffe RT, Brimacombe M, Levitt AJ, Stagnaro-Green A. Treatment of clinical hypothyroidism with thyroxine and triiodothyronine: a literature review and metaanalysis. Psychosomatics. 2007;48:379–84.
54. Regalbuto C, Maiorana R, Alagona C, et al. Effects of either LT4 monotherapy or LT4/LT3 combined therapy in patients totally thyroidectomized for thyroid cancer. Thyroid. 2007;17:323–31.
55. Nygaard B, Jensen EW, Kvetny J, Jarlov A, Faber J. Effect of combination therapy with thyroxine (T4) and 3,5,3′-triiodothyronine versus T4 monotherapy in patients with hypothyroidism, a double-blind, randomised cross-over study. Eur J Endocrinol. 2009;161:895–902.
56. Celi FS, Zemskova M, Linderman JD, Smith S, et al. Metabolic effects of liothyronine therapy in hypothyroidism: a randomized, double-blind, crossover trial of liothyronine versus levothyroxine. J Clin Endocrinol Metab. 2011;96:3466–74.
57. Bianco AC, Salvatore D, Gereben B, Berry MJ, Larsen PR. Biochemistry, cellular and molecular biology, and physiological roles of the iodothyronine selenodeiodinases. Endocr Rev. 2002;23:38–89.
58. Jonklaas J, Davidson B, Bhagat S, Soldin SJ. Triiodothyronine levels in athyreotic individuals during levothyroxine therapy. JAMA. 2008;299:769–77.
59. Butler PW, Smith SM, Linderman JD, Brychta RJ, Alberobello AT, Dubaz OM, et al. The Thr92Ala 5′ type 2 deiodinase gene polymorphism is associated with a delayed triiodothyronine secretion in response to the thyrotropin-releasing hormone-stimulation test: a pharmacogenomic study. Thyroid. 2010;20:1407–12.
60. Panicker V, Saravanan P, Vaidya B, Evans J, Hattersley AT, Frayling TM, Dayan CM. Common variation in the DIO2 gene predicts baseline psychological well-being and response to combination thyroxine plus triiodothyronine therapy in hypothyroid patients. J Clin Endocrinol Metab. 2009;94:1623–9.
61. Appelhof BC, Peeters RP, Wiersinga WM, Visser TJ, Wekking EM, Huyser J, et al. Polymorphisms in type 2deiodinase are not associated with well-being, neurocognitive functioning, and preference for combined thyroxine/3,5,3′-triiodothyronine therapy. J Clin Endocrinol Metab. 2005;90:6296–9.
62. Heemstra KA, Hoftijzer HC, van der Deure WM, Peeters RP, Fliers E, Appelhof BC, et al. Thr92Ala polymorphism in the type 2 deiodinase is not associated with T4 dose in athyroid patients or patients with Hashimoto thyroiditis. Clin Endocrinol. 2009;71:279–83.
63. Torlontano M, Durante C, Torrente I, Crocetti U, Augello G, Ronga G, et al. Type 2 deiodinase polymorphism (threonine 92 alanine) predicts L-thyroxine dose to achieve target thyrotropin levels in thyroidectomized patients. J Clin Endocrinol Metab. 2008;93:910–3.
64. Vargens DD G, Neves RR, Bulzico DA, Ojopi EB, Meirelles RM, Pessoa CN, et al. Association of the UGT1A1-53(TA)n polymorphism with L-thyroxine doses required for thyrotropin suppression in patients with differentiated thyroid cancer. Pharmacogenet Genomics. 2011;21:341–3.
65. Biondi B, Wartofsky L. Combination treatment with T4 and T3: toward personalized replacement therapy in hypothyroidism. J Clin Endocrinol Metab. 2012;97:2256–71.
66. Wartofsky L. Combination therapy with L-triiodothyronine and L-thyroxine for hypothyroidism. Curr Opin Endocrinol Diabetes Obes. 2013;20:460–6.
67. Hay ID, Charbonneau JW, Lewis BD, et al. Successful ultrasound-guided percutaneous ethanol ablation of neck metastases in 20 patients with postoperative TNM stage I papillary thyroid carcinoma resistant to conventional therapy. (abstract). In: 74th meeting ATA. Los Angeles; 2002. p. 176.

Thyroglobulin for Differentiated Thyroid Cancer: Measurement and Interferences

37

D. Robert Dufour

Thyroglobulin and Its Measurement

Thyroglobulin

Thyroglobulin, an approximately 670 kD glycoprotein, is the major protein product of thyroid follicular cells; its rate of synthesis is increased by TSH. After synthesis, it is modified by attachment of iodine to selected tyrosine residues, which undergo rearrangement to form iodothyronines, particularly T4 and, to a lesser extent, T3. A number of other modifications of thyroglobulin also occur, including glycation and sulfation [1]. The degree of TSH stimulation affects the extent of branching of carbohydrate side chains [2]. Variable processing of thyroglobulin occurs, creating a family of proteins with differing molecular structures around a common core peptide backbone. Interestingly, there is less variability in thyroglobulin structure in thyroid cancer than in other thyroid diseases [3]. There is reduced iodine content in thyroglobulin from persons with thyroid malignancy [4], which can lead to different recognition by monoclonal antibodies [5]. In addition, the carbohydrate content of thyroglobulin differs in thyroid cancer, affecting binding of thyroglobulin to lectins, particularly the Lens culinaris lectin [6]. This structural heterogeneity creates a challenge for thyroglobulin immunoassays, and results often differ significantly when samples from an individual are measured using different thyroglobulin methods [7]. With newer immunoassays, the use of better antibodies has reduced this variation, which still exists. In one study of seven thyroglobulin assays, results were most variable at high concentrations, but were similar at concentrations near the lower limit of measurement with all assays [8].

D.R. Dufour, MD (✉)
Clinical Pathology, Veterans Affairs Medical Center, 50 Irving Street NW, Washington, DC 20422, USA
e-mail: chemdoctorbob@earthlink.net

Normally, only small amounts of intact thyroglobulin reach the circulation, in proportion to thyroid mass. It has been estimated that 1 g of thyroid tissue increases serum thyroglobulin by 1 μg/L (ng/mL) under normal TSH stimulation, and 0.5 μg/L (ng/mL) during suppression of TSH. Reference intervals for thyroglobulin, based on healthy, ambulatory individuals with normal iodide intake, typically range from 3 to 40 μg/L (ng/mL). Increased thyroglobulin is also released in response to inflammation as in thyroiditis. Other factors that increase thyroglobulin include low iodide intake and cigarette smoking. After complete thyroidectomy and remnant ablation by radioactive iodine, thyroglobulin concentration should be below the detection limit of the assay. This forms the basis for use of thyroglobulin as a marker for residual differentiated thyroid cancer.

Thyroglobulin Immunoassays

Thyroglobulin is currently measured in the laboratory by use of antibodies to thyroglobulin. There are two principal assay formats: competitive (single antibody) methods and sandwich (double antibody) methods. Generally, the laboratory does not indicate the type of assay used on its reports. It is important for the endocrinologist to be aware of the method(s) used by the laboratory, especially for thyroglobulin measurements [9]. The two types of assay formats differ in the lowest amount of thyroglobulin detectable, the likelihood of interference from anti-thyroglobulin antibodies and other potentially interfering substances (particularly heterophile antibodies and rheumatoid factor), and the direction of change in apparent concentration caused by these interferences.

Development of Thyroglobulin Antibodies

The process of developing antibodies to use in the assay involves immunization of animals with thyroglobulin. As a large, complex molecule, thyroglobulin has many epitopes

L. Wartofsky, D. Van Nostrand (eds.), *Thyroid Cancer*, DOI 10.1007/978-1-4939-3314-3_37

that can be recognized by the immune system of the injected animal. Each host genetic structure allows varying recognition of differing epitopes. Antibodies produced are harvested and processed in one of two main methods. In the simplest, serum from the animal is processed by absorbing with human samples devoid of thyroglobulin and tested for its ability to react with thyroglobulin. Strongly reacting animals can then be bled repetitively (after booster injections with thyroglobulin) as a source of antibody. This produces a mixture of antibodies produced by several clones of plasma cells (polyclonal antibody) to different epitopes on thyroglobulin. A single animal produces the same relative mixture of polyclonal antibodies that recognize varying epitopes differently. Nonidentical animals, even from the same species, produce differing mixtures of antibodies that may have varying recognition of different thyroglobulin epitopes. Combined with the varying structures of thyroglobulin molecules, this creates different binding of thyroglobulin to antibody in kits containing antibody from different animals. This will be true even of kits from the same manufacturer, since the antibody used in the kits will differ as one animal dies and is replaced by another.

Alternatively, plasma cells from the injected animal are harvested and individual cells fused with myeloma cell lines to produce hybridomas; each hybridoma produces a monoclonal antibody product. The monoclonal immunoglobulins derived from cell culture supernates of the hybridoma line are then absorbed with thyroglobulin-deficient human samples and tested for reactivity against thyroglobulin. The advantages of monoclonal antibodies include reproducible production of antibody by the immortalized cell line and recognition of only a single epitope of the molecule, minimizing differences between kits prepared by the same manufacturer. Kits from different manufacturers have different monoclonal antibodies.

Competitive (One Step) Immunoassays for Thyroglobulin

The earliest assays for measuring thyroglobulin were based on competitive immunoassay formats, illustrated in Fig. 37.1. In general, competitive immunoassays cannot detect low concentrations of thyroglobulin as well as sandwich methods. In a review of thyroglobulin assays, the functional sensitivity (defined as the level at which reproducibility between repeated measurements of the same sample was at an acceptable limit of 20 %) of competitive assays ranged from 0.7 to 2.0 μg/L (ng/mL), while the functional sensitivity of sandwich assays ranged from 0.2 to 0.6 μg/L (ng/mL) [10]. Competitive assays may produce falsely high results in the presence of anti-thyroglobulin antibodies, as discussed in more detail in Chap. 38 and illustrated in Fig. 37.2.

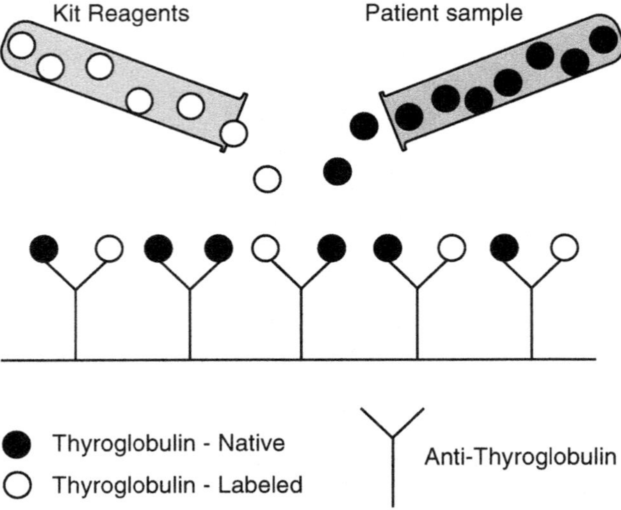

Fig. 37.1 Principle of competitive immunoassay for thyroglobulin – the principle of the assay is to use a limited amount of antibody to thyroglobulin, along with a limited amount of a labeled form of thyroglobulin; the label can be a radioactive isotope, an enzyme, or a fluorescent compound. By adding known amounts of unlabeled thyroglobulin, a calibration curve is created in which the amount of labeled thyroglobulin bound to the antibody is inversely related to the amount of unlabeled thyroglobulin in the sample tested. Unknown patient samples are then evaluated using the calibration curve to determine their concentration of thyroglobulin

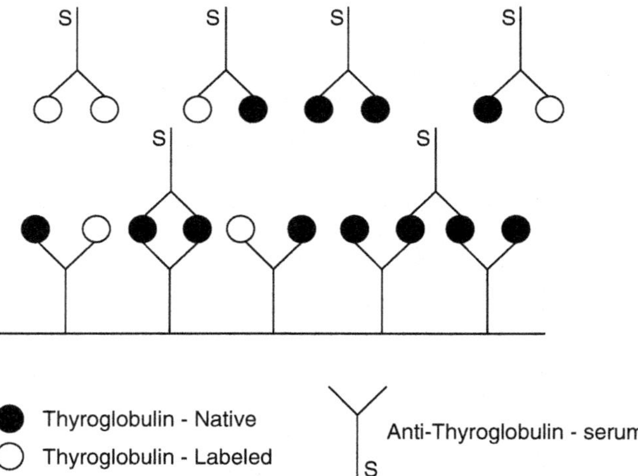

Fig. 37.2 Mechanism of interference of thyroglobulin antibodiesin competitive immunoassay for thyroglobulin – thyroglobulin antibodies likely interfere with competitive assays by one or both of two mechanisms. Thyroglobulin levels in the blood stream are actually increased because of reduced clearance when bound to antibody. Additionally, free antibody can bind labeled thyroglobulin in the reagent. Both phenomena reduce the amount of labeled thyroglobulin bound to the reagent antibody, falsely increasing reported thyroglobulin concentration

Sandwich (Two Step, Double Antibody) Immunometric Assays for Thyroglobulin

Most current thyroglobulin assays are based on sandwich or immunometric assays, as illustrated in Fig. 37.3. The two major advantages of sandwich assays are enhanced ability to detect low concentrations of thyroglobulin and ability to measure a wide range of concentrations without the need for sample dilution. Most sandwich assays also employ at least two monoclonal antibodies, allowing more reproducible measurement of thyroglobulin over time with use of the same manufacturer's method. Sandwich assays are subject to interference by the presence of heterophile antibodies and rheumatoid factor, producing falsely high results [11–14]. One study found such interference in 3 % of samples tested for thyroglobulin [15]. Although manufacturers have modified their kits to minimize heterophile antibody interference, the effectiveness of such modifications is variable, even in kits from the same manufacturer [16]. Some laboratories use tubes that absorb such heterophile antibodies. One multicenter study of sandwich assays (usually not for thyroglobulin) found that use of such binding tubes (along with the manufacturer's approaches to minimize interference) failed to prevent 49 % of clinically important interferences [16]. As illustrated in Fig. 37.4, and discussed in more detail in Chap. 38, anti-thyroglobulin antibodies in a patient sample cause falsely low results in sandwich assays.

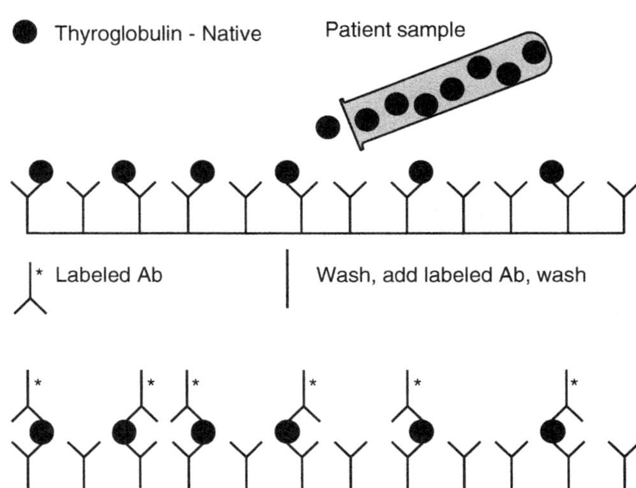

Fig. 37.3 Principle of sandwichimmunometric assays for thyroglobulin – a known, excess amount of antibody to thyroglobulin is fixed to a solid support. Known calibrators or unknown patient samples are incubated with the antibody-labeled support, which is then washed to remove any unbound thyroglobulin. A second anti-thyroglobulin antibody (often directed against a separate part of the thyroglobulin molecule), labeled with a radioactive isotope, enzyme, or fluorescent compound, is then added to the solid support. The amount of label remaining on the solid support (after a second wash) is directly related to the number of antigen-antibody complexes formed. Because the number of antigen-antibody complexes decreases when the amount of antigen exceeds the amount of antibody, sandwich assays may produce falsely low results at very high thyroglobulin concentration, a phenomenon known as the "high-dose hook effect"

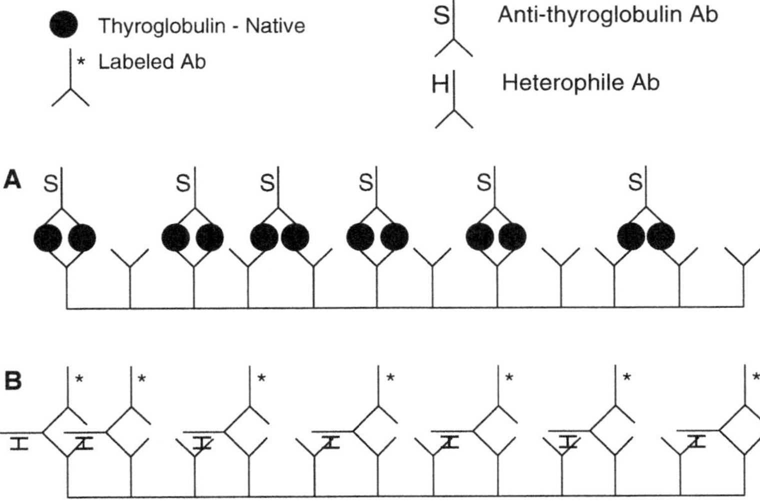

Fig. 37.4 Mechanisms of interference in sandwich immunometric assays for thyroglobulin (**a**). Thyroglobulin antibody interference – thyroglobulin antibodies likely interfere in sandwich assays by attaching to thyroglobulin linked to the bound antibody. This leads to steric inhibition of binding by the labeled antibody and falsely low thyroglobulin concentrations. – (**b**) Heterophile antibody interference – heterophile antibodies are human antibodies that react with the Fc portion of immunoglobulin molecules of other species; most commonly, anti-mouse antibodies are the cause of interference, since mouse cells are used to produce most monoclonal antibodies. (in the figure, for space reasons, the antibodies are shown as if they attach to the Fab portion of the antibody molecule). After attaching to the bound antibody, they retain one binding site to which the labeled antibody can attach, producing falsely high values. While less commonly encountered, rheumatoid factor (which attaches to the Fc portion of human and animal immunoglobulins) can produce the same pattern of interference

Other Methods for Measurement of Thyroglobulin

Two other approaches to thyroglobulin measurement have been described. One method, only available in research applications, takes advantage of the altered carbohydrate residues on thyroglobulin in patients with thyroid cancer and measures binding of thyroglobulin to Lens culinaris lectin. In a single study of this approach, 38 patients with thyroid cancer (10 of whom had metastatic disease) had total thyroglobulin and lectin-reactive thyroglobulin measured, and these were compared to healthy volunteers and patients with benign thyroid tumors. While total thyroglobulin was similar in all three thyroid tumor groups, those with metastatic thyroid cancer had significantly reduced lectin-bound thyroglobulin, but only in samples where the total thyroglobulin was >200 μg/L (ng/mL) [17]. Thus, this method seems to have limited promise for use in managing thyroid cancer.

A novel approach involves a combination of peptide detection, immune binding of thyroglobulin-derived peptides, and quantification of the peptides using mass spectrometry [18]. Theoretically, such an approach would also digest thyroglobulin antibodies and eliminate interference, allowing easier monitoring and greater reliability in the high percentage of patients with thyroid cancer who have such antibodies. However, this was not directly evaluated in the initial study. In addition, the method described had a lower detection limit of 2.6 μg/dL, higher than is desirable for post-ablation monitoring. Two additional studies of mass spectrometry have since been published and have led to introduction of tests available through two of the largest commercial reference laboratories [19, 20]. Both of these studies evaluated persons with detectable anti-thyroglobulin. The study by Kushnir [20] involved 71 patients with undetectable thyroglobulin by immunometric assay; 23 % had detectable (>0.5 ng/mL) thyroglobulin by the mass spectrometry-based assay. The study by Clarke [19] does not identify the number of samples tested, but used two approaches to evaluate for lack of antibody interference. In one, they added thyroglobulin to antibody-negative and antibody-positive sera and got similar recovery approximating 100 %. In the other, they compared results from their assay to results from immunometric assay and competitive immunoassay in samples from patients with or without anti-thyroglobulin. In antibody-negative samples, results by the three methods agreed well. In thyroglobulin antibody-positive samples, results from the mass spectrometry-based assay were always higher than those from the immunometric assay, and in about half of samples were lower than those from the competitive immunoassay (with the remainder having similar results); one sample was about 50 % higher by the mass spectrometry-based assay. The lower limit of quantitation by this assay was 0.4 ng/mL. Thus, these assays seem to have the potential to allow reliable measurement of thyroglobulin even in patients with anti-thyroglobulin; however, as emphasized in a review by Hoofnagle, it will be important to validate these assays in prospective studies of patients and to correlate results with clinical outcomes [21].

Issues and Interferences in Thyroglobulin Measurement

There are a number of other issues that limit the utility of thyroglobulin measurements for monitoring thyroid cancer. In addition to the interferences from thyroglobulin and heterophile antibodies, there are two other major issues in thyroglobulin measurement, as outlined by Spencer [22]: variation between thyroglobulin methods and detection limits of assays for identifying recurrent cancer.

Standardization Does Not Eliminate Between-Assay Differences in Thyroglobulin Level

To measure thyroglobulin by immunoassay, the amount of thyroglobulin bound to antibody in a patient sample is compared to that in samples containing known amounts of a standard preparation of thyroglobulin. The process of comparing the amount of antibody bound to samples containing the standard preparation of thyroglobulin is termed assay calibration. Because of the varying structures of thyroglobulin, it is critical that assays use the same "standard" preparation of thyroglobulin for calibration. Currently, a Certified Reference Material (CRM-457) [23], available through the Community Bureau of Reference of the Commission of the European Communities, is considered the preferred standard preparation [10]. One potential drawback to this standard is that it is derived from normal thyroid tissue and may not accurately reflect forms found in persons with thyroid malignancy [24]. In addition, although all current methods use this reference standard, results do differ between assays even when CRM-457 is measured by them [8, 25, 26]. Currently, there are many kits for performing thyroglobulin measurement commercially available in North America. As a result, it is advisable to try to always use the same thyroglobulin assay when testing the same individual. If this is not possible, the endocrinologist should attempt to have one sample analyzed on whatever new method will be used going forward as well as the previous assay; this will provide a frame of reference for comparing the new assay's results with those obtained with the old assay [7]. This requires close cooperation between the endocrinologist and the laboratory he or she routinely uses. For their part, laboratorians should always communicate to the physicians using their services when they plan to change assays for thyroglobulin (and other tumor markers) before instituting such a change to allow for this "re-baselining" procedure. While it has been suggested that laboratories save samples and run old samples at the same time as new ones to allow better detection of differences in concentration [22], this is impractical for most laboratories.

Lower Limit of Detection of Assays

The lowest amount of thyroglobulin that can be measured differs among different assays. In one study of seven currently available assays, the lower limit for detection differed between 0.02 and 0.9 μg/L (ng/mL). In this study, sensitivity for detecting residual thyroid tissue post-remnant ablation using baseline thyroglobulin was higher in the two assays with the lowest detection limit; assays with the highest detection limits had "normal" thyroglobulin on T4 suppression in about half of those with detectable thyroglobulin using the most sensitive assays. On the other hand, almost half of those who had detectable thyroglobulin using the most sensitive assays did not develop recurrent disease. The authors found that the best cutoff value for thyroglobulin with the most sensitive assays was between 0.22 and 0.27 μg/L (ng/mL) [8]. Another study compared two assays, one with a detection limit of 0.18 μg/L (ng/mL) and the other with a detection limit of 1.0 μg/L (ng/mL); the more sensitive assay detected 11 additional patients (29 %) with positive basal thyroglobulin on suppression. In addition, 20 % of patients with undetectable baseline thyroglobulin showed an increase using the more sensitive assay that was not detected by the other assay [27]. Use of a very sensitive assay, with detection limit of 0.03 μg/L (ng/mL) compared to a conventional assay with a detection limit of 0.6 μg/L (ng/mL), found increased basal thyroglobulin in 7/139 using the conventional assay, but 106/139 using the more sensitive assay. None of the additional persons found to have detectable thyroglobulin had evidence of residual thyroid tissue, even using PET scan [28]. While more studies using highly sensitive assays are clearly needed, it is not clear at this time that they will be more clinically useful.

Spencer has advocated adopting new approaches to evaluate the ability of a method to detect low levels of thyroglobulin [22]. She proposes to employ the concept of "generations," currently used to describe functional sensitivity of TSH assays. In this nomenclature, assays with detection limits (functional sensitivity) less than one log below the lower reference limit would be termed first generation, while those with a one to two log difference between lower reference limit and functional sensitivity would be termed second generation and those with two to three log difference third generation. It is not clear currently whether lower detection limits will improve ability to recognize residual thyroid cancer, or will prove too sensitive to detecting minute amounts of residual normal thyroid tissue.

Guidelines for Laboratories Performing Thyroglobulin Assays

The National Academy of Clinical Biochemistry (NACB) has published extensive guidance for laboratories performing thyroid related tests, including a number pertaining to thyroglobulin [10]. These guidelines were peer reviewed, not only by the laboratory community but by all of the international thyroid societies. The most important of these are summarized in Table 37.1. Laboratories performing thyroglobulin measurement should be aware of these recommendations, and endocrinologists should assure that their laboratories are aware of and using them.

Interferences in Thyroglobulin Immunoassays

Thyroglobulin Antibodies

As discussed in more detail in Chap. 38, thyroglobulin antibodies are commonly present in patients with differentiated thyroid cancer. As mentioned earlier, thyroglobulin antibodies can interfere with the measurement of thyroglobulin. With the typically used sandwich (immunometric assays), thyroglobulin is falsely low in persons with thyroglobulin antibodies. In individuals with detectable thyroglobulin antibodies, an undetectable thyroglobulin is thus not reassurance that there is no residual thyroid cancer. It is difficult to predict the degree of interference that will occur in a given patient. In one study [29], ten different sera containing thyroglobulin antibodies resulted in a decrease in measured thyroglobulin

Table 37.1 Selected NACB recommendations for thyroglobulin testing

There is no "normal" range for thyroglobulin for a thyroidectomized patient; it is misleading to cite the normal euthyroid reference interval for thyroidectomized patients
Serum thyroglobulin values for anti-thyroglobulin-positive specimens should not be reported if the method gives inappropriately undetectable values
Recovery tests should be eliminated (to detect thyroglobulin antibody interference); discordance between immunoassay and immunometric assay suggests interference (if values are concordant in antibody-negative specimens)
If laboratories change their thyroglobulin method, they should consult with physician users and compare results between old and new method in both thyroglobulin antibody-negative and thyroglobulin antibody-positive patients. If results are more than 10 % different between methods in antibody-negative patients, physicians should be notified to allow retesting (re-baselining) critical patients
If thyroglobulin results are reported for antibody-positive patients, an appropriate cautionary comment should be displayed on each laboratory report

From reference [6]

between 24 % and 79 % when mixed with a sample containing no thyroglobulin antibodies. In the same study, samples from ten patients lacking thyroglobulin antibodies were mixed with four different samples containing thyroglobulin antibodies. The reduction in measured thyroglobulin varied for each patient when mixed with different thyroglobulin antibodies, and the percentage reduction produced by each thyroglobulin antibody was different when mixed with different forms of thyroglobulin.

In contrast, when thyroglobulin is measured by competitive immunoassays, the pattern of interference is unpredictable [30]. Results are most commonly falsely increased or unaffected, but may be falsely decreased. It is unusual for thyroglobulin to be undetectable by competitive immunoassay when thyroglobulin antibodies are present.

This has led to suggestions that, when antibodies to thyroglobulin are present, it may be possible to evaluate the degree of interference by measuring thyroglobulin by both a competitive immunoassay and the widely used immunometric methods. Spencer has proposed that a ratio of thyroglobulin as measured by immunometric assay to that reported by competitive immunoassay of <0.75 indicates falsely low results by the immunometric method [31]. Crane recently published data on 576 patients with differentiated thyroid cancer in whom thyroglobulin was measured by both immunometric assay and competitive immunoassay and found discordant results in 12.2 %. They based "discordance" on a difference in results more than 2 sd from the average difference observed between the two methods and found that the average difference differed when using different immunometric assays. Most of the discordant results were in patients who did not have detectable thyroglobulin antibodies and in almost 10 % the immunometric assay gave higher results (1 of 4 had recurrent thyroid carcinoma); only 4 of the 49 patients with higher results by competitive immunoassay had evidence of recurrent carcinoma [32].

As discussed in more detail in Chap. 38, a consensus document was developed by members of the European Thyroid Association, and they have recommended that more data is required for evidence-based guidelines. In the interim, they suggest that no method is free of interference from anti-thyroglobulin [33].

Human Anti-Mouse Antibodies, Heterophile Antibodies, and Rheumatoid Factor

Other interferences may also affect thyroglobulin measurement in a nonspecific fashion. The most common of these is the presence of antibodies that have immunoglobulin molecules as their antigenic target. Immunoglobulins in the reagent of the thyroglobulin assay bind to these antibodies, which can affect the apparent results. With immunometric assays, results are almost always falsely positive in the presence of such antibodies, while (as is true with antibodies to thyroglobulin) effects are more variable when competitive immunoassays are used.

Many immunoassays now utilize monoclonal antibodies, which are typically produced by mouse myeloma hybridomas. Human antibodies to mouse immunoglobulins are relatively common in the population, although titers high enough to cause significant interference in immunoassays are generally found in about 0.1 % of the population [11]. To minimize this problem, manufacturers of immunometric assays often used antibodies from more than one species. However, human antibodies to immunoglobulins from a variety of species (collectively termed heterophile antibodies) are also sometimes seen. Finally, rheumatoid factor (a human immunoglobulin directed against IgG) may also react with IgG molecules from other species.

The frequency with which such anti-immunoglobulin interferences occur in thyroglobulin assays is low. Using tubes containing excess animal immunoglobulins, two studies found interference in 0.4–1.0 % of samples [34, 35]. Rheumatoid factor has rarely been reported to cause falsely high thyroglobulin [36]. In addition to the use of such commercially available heterophile-blocking tubes, there are other approaches that can suggest the presence of such interference. One is to perform serial dilution of the sample; a similar approach involves mixing a sample suspected of having interference with an equal amount of a sample free of thyroglobulin antibodies. In both cases, results will be higher than expected in the presence of anti-immunoglobulin antibodies.

Sample Stability on Storage

Limited data exist on thyroglobulin stability when samples are not analyzed rapidly by the laboratory, a situation that can exist when samples are sent to a reference laboratory. One study found that thyroglobulin increased by about 20 % when stored in a refrigerator for 48 h, but decreased by 20–30 % when stored frozen for several months [37]. While sample storage may affect results, as long as samples are handled in a similar manner each time, this should cause minimal problems with interpretation.

Thyroglobulin in Differentiated Thyroid Cancer

Current treatment for differentiated thyroid cancer (total or near-total thyroidectomy, followed by radioiodine ablation) should eradicate thyroglobulin production. Thyroglobulin is thus a highly sensitive marker for recurrent or metastatic thyroid cancer. Rarely, thyroid tumors may fail to produce thyroglobulin. In two large studies, 1–3 % of patients with recurrent thyroid cancer or residual thyroid tissue had undetectable thyroglobulin that was not due to interferences [38, 39].

There are several potential situations where thyroglobulin measurement could be of use in diagnosis and management of thyroid cancer, discussed in detail below. The diagnostic utility of thyroglobulin measurement is impaired in persons with thyroglobulin antibodies; for that reason, thyroglobulin measurements should always be accompanied by tests for thyroglobulin antibodies. As a practical matter, results of thyroglobulin measurement in the presence of thyroglobulin antibodies can be interpreted accurately (as to presence or absence of residual thyroid tumor) in some circumstances. For example, a detectable thyroglobulin by immunometric assay in a person with thyroglobulin antibodies indicates residual thyroid tumor, while undetectable stimulated thyroglobulin supports complete ablation of thyroid tumor when measured by immunoassay [10]. Because changes in titer of thyroglobulin antibodies affect the degree of interference, it is not possible to use serial thyroglobulin measurement to assess changes in tumor volume or response to therapy until such time as thyroglobulin antibodies become undetectable. As discussed in Chap. 38, falling titers indicate a favorable prognosis, while rising titers suggest recurrent thyroid malignancy.

Thyroglobulin Before Surgery

Thyroglobulin is produced by most differentiated thyroid cancers. While guidelines do not recommend thyroglobulin for preoperative diagnosis of thyroid cancer [40, 41], there may be limited benefit to preoperative thyroglobulin measurement. Thyroid cancers tend be associated with higher preoperative thyroglobulin levels than benign thyroid nodules, particularly when interpreted relative to nodule size [42–46]; however, the predictive value of preoperative thyroglobulin measurement is low. One retrospective case-control study found a relative risk of seven for development of differentiated thyroid cancer in persons with elevated thyroglobulin measured up to 23 years before diagnosis [47]. Normal thyroglobulin in a thyroglobulin antibody-negative individual preoperatively may, however, indicate that the tumor does not produce thyroglobulin and indicate the need for other approaches to follow thyroid cancer [10]. Since this is an uncommon finding, however, it is unlikely to be beneficial for routine care.

Thyroglobulin after Resection, but before Remnant Ablation

Current guidelines for use of thyroglobulin do not recommend its measurement before performing radioiodine ablation, when indicated [9, 41]. Several studies have suggested that its measurement provides additional information to thyroglobulin measurements performed after ablation. Some studies have evaluated thyroglobulin levels obtained during thyroxine suppression and have found that elevated levels (generally above 1–2 μg/L (ng/mL)) are associated with increased likelihood of metastatic disease or failure of radioiodine ablation [48, 49]. Other studies have looked at thyroglobulin levels off of thyroxine therapy at times when TSH is increased; these studies have also found high likelihood of metastatic disease and failure of ablation in those with high levels, generally above 10–15 μg/L (ng/mL) [50–52]. One study evaluated the ratio of thyroglobulin level to the percent radioiodine uptake in the thyroid bed and found that those with ratios more than 5.7 were associated with high likelihood of metastasis or radioiodine failure [53]. A meta-analysis by Webb found that 70 % of individuals had pre-ablation thyroglobulin below the detection limit and that the negative predictive value for residual or recurrent disease was 94 % [54]. These consistent findings suggest that routine measurement of thyroglobulin (either on or off thyroxine) prior to radioiodine ablation provides additional information and is worth measurement.

Thyroglobulin after Radioiodine Ablation of Thyroid Remnant

After total thyroidectomy for thyroid cancer, thyroglobulin falls with a half-life of 1–3 days [55, 56], and thyroglobulin levels typically become undetectable after about 1 month [55]. Measurements are still useful in patients who have not undergone complete thyroidectomy, but are more difficult to interpret, as thyroglobulin is typically still present [57].

Thyroglobulin During TSH Suppression

When TSH is suppressed below the lower limits of normal by thyroid hormone, thyroglobulin production indicates residual or metastatic disease with a high degree of specificity [9]. Since thyroglobulin production is stimulated by TSH, measurement in this situation is not sensitive enough to exclude residual thyroid carcinoma, however. In the initial studies of recombinant TSH, 23 % of those with thyroglobulin levels over 2 μg/L (ng/mL) after stimulation had undetectable basal levels [58]. A number of studies have shown that, in thyroglobulin antibody-negative individuals, if thyroglobulin remains very low to undetectable (typically <0.1–0.2 μg/L (ng/mL)) after the first stimulated measurement, that continuing undetectable thyroglobulin on TSH suppression indicates very low likelihood of recurrent or metastatic disease [59–65]. Current guidelines from the American Thyroid Association recommend at least one repeat TSH-stimulated thyroglobulin measurement in those with an initial negative result and very low baseline thyroglobulin on thyroxine replacement [41];

however, these guidelines were prepared before most of the studies mentioned were published. Based on more recent evidence, it seems reasonable to not require repeat of stimulated thyroglobulin measurement if initial stimulation had thyroglobulin <2 μg/L (ng/mL) and suppressed thyroglobulin remains at very low levels.

While the sensitivity of suppressed thyroglobulin for residual disease is high, the specificity of such low cutoffs is less than ideal. As noted earlier, most individuals who have thyroglobulin between 0.1–0.2 and 1.0 μg/L (ng/mL) do not have residual disease. However, using a cutoff of 1.0 μg/L (ng/mL) is not sensitive enough to identify almost all patients who do turn out to have residual disease.

TSH-Stimulated Thyroglobulin

The most sensitive method for detecting residual thyroid cancer is to measure thyroglobulin during TSH stimulation. This is particularly true for low-risk patients, in whom sensitive testing is important for detecting the relatively small number of patients who need additional treatment. Several studies have shown that about 20–25 % of persons with undetectable thyroglobulin during suppression of TSH will show a rise in thyroglobulin to ≥2.0 μg/L (ng/mL) under TSH stimulation, a level considered in most guidelines as clinically significant [9, 10, 41]. Historically, TSH stimulation was achieved by withdrawing thyroid hormone therapy to produce hypothyroidism. With the availability of recombinant TSH (rh-TSH), administration is an alternative approach. There is consensus that this is now the preferred method to evaluate patients for residual thyroid cancer if non-stimulated thyroglobulin is undetectable [9, 10, 41]. While thyroid hormone withdrawal produces greater increases in TSH and thyroglobulin than does administration of rh-TSH [66, 67], an analysis of eight comparison studies showed equivalent sensitivity of the two approaches for detecting residual cancer [10]. In the recommended protocol, 0.9 mg of rh-TSH is given on day 1 and 2, and thyroglobulin is measured on day 4. While one study suggests that this is not always the time of peak TSH or thyroglobulin and that weight-based dosing may be more accurate [67], consensus guidelines suggest the simpler protocol is adequate. A rise in thyroglobulin to >2 μg/L (ng/mL) identifies almost all individuals with persistent disease, but about two-third of those with results above this value will not turn out to have identifiable residual disease on follow-up studies [41]. Minor increases between the detection limit and 2.0 μg/L (ng/mL) are currently felt to be of no clinical significance.

References

1. van de Graaf S, Ris-Stalpers C, Pauws E, Mendive F, Targovnik H, de Vijlder J. Up to date with human thyroglobulin. J Endocrinol. 2001;170:307–21.
2. Di Jeso B, Liguoro D, Ferranti P, et al. Modulation of the carbohydrate moiety of thyroglobulin by thyrotropin and. J Biol Chem. 1992;267:1938–44.
3. Druetta L, Croizet K, Bornet H, Rousset B. Analyses of the molecular forms of serum thyroglobulin from patients with Graves' disease, subacute thyroiditis or differentiated thyroid cancer by velocity sedimentation on sucrose gradient and Western blot. Eur J Endocrinol. 1998;139:498–507.
4. Schneider A, Ikekubo K, Kuma K. Iodine content of serum thyroglobulin in normal individuals and patients. J Clin Endocrinol Metab. 1983;57:1251–6.
5. Kohno Y, Tarutani O, Sakata S, Nakajima H. Monoclonal antibodies to thyroglobulin elucidate differences in protein. J Clin Endocrinol Metab. 1985;61:343–50.
6. Shimizu K, Nakamura K, Kobatake S, et al. Discrimination of thyroglobulin from thyroid carcinoma tissue and that from benign thyroid tissues with use of competitive assay between lectin and anti-thyroglobulin antibody. Rinsho Byori. 2007;55:428–33.
7. Spencer C, Wang C. Thyroglobulin measurement. Techniques, clinical benefits, and pitfalls. Endocrinol Metab Clin North Am. 1995;24:841–63.
8. Schlumberger M, Hitzel A, Toubert M, et al. Comparison of seven serum thyroglobulin assays in the follow-up of papillary and follicular thyroid cancer patients. J Clin Endocrinol Metab. 2007;92:2487–95.
9. Mazzaferri E, Robbins R, Spencer C, et al. A consensus report of the role of serum thyroglobulin as a monitoring method for low-risk patients with papillary thyroid carcinoma. J Clin Endocrinol Metab. 2003;88:1433–41.
10. Demers L, Spencer C. Laboratory support for the diagnosis and monitoring of thyroid disease. Thyroid. 2003;13:3–126.
11. Kricka L. Human anti-animal antibody interferences in immunological assays. Clin Chem. 1999;45:942–56.
12. Levinson S, Miller J. Towards a better understanding of heterophile (and the like) antibody interference with modern immunoassays. Clin Chim Acta. 2002;325:1–15.
13. Ward G, McKinnon L, Badrick T, Hickman P. Heterophilic antibodies remain a problem for the immunoassay laboratory. Am J Clin Pathol. 1997;108:417–21.
14. Weber T, Kapyaho K, Tanner P. Endogenous interference in immunoassays in clinical chemistry. A review. Scand J Clin Lab Invest Suppl. 1990;201:77–82.
15. Preissner C, O'Kane D, Singh R, Morris J, Grebe S. Phantoms in the assay tube: heterophile antibody interferences in serum thyroglobulin assays. J Clin Endocrinol Metab. 2003;88:3069–74.
16. Marks V. False-positive immunoassay results: a multicenter survey of erroneous immunoassay results from assays of 74 analytes in 10 donors from 66 laboratories in seven countries. Clin Chem. 2002;48:2008–16.
17. Shimizu K, Nakamura K, Kobatake S, et al. The clinical utility of Lens culinaris agglutinin-reactive thyroglobulin ratio in serum for distinguishing benign from malignant conditions of the thyroid. Clin Chim Acta. 2007;379:101–4.
18. Hoofnagle A, Baker J, Wener M, Heinecke J. Quantification of thyroglobulin, a low-abundance serum protein, by immunoaffinity peptide enrichment and tandem mass spectrometry. Clin Chem. 2008;54:1796–804.
19. Clarke NJ, Zhang Y, Reitz RE. A novel mass spectrometry–based assay for the accurate measurement of thyroglobulin from patient

samples containing antithyroglobulin autoantibodies. J Invest Med. 2012;60:1157–63.
20. Kushnir MM, Rockwood AL, Roberts WL, Abraham D, Hoofnagle AN, Meikle AW. Measurement of thyroglobulin by liquid chromatography–tandem mass spectrometry in serum and plasma in the presence of antithyroglobulin autoantibodies. Clin Chem. 2013;59:982–90.
21. Hoofnagle AN, Roth MY. Improving the measurement of serum thyroglobulin with mass spectrometry. J Clin Endocrinol Metab. 2013;98:1343–52.
22. Spencer C. New insights for using serum thyroglobulin (Tg) measurement for managing patients with differentiated thyroid carcinomas. Thyroid Int. 2003;4:3–14.
23. Feldt-Rasmussen U, Profilis C, Colinet E, et al. Human thyroglobulin reference material (CRM 457). 2nd Part Physicochemical characterization and certification. Ann Biol Clin (Paris). 1996;54: 343–8.
24. Whitley R, Ain K. Thyroglobulin: a specific serum marker for the management of thyroid. Clin Lab Med. 2004;24:29–47.
25. Spencer C, Takeuchi M, Kazarosyan M. Current status and performance goals for serum thyroglobulin assays. Clin Chem. 1996;42:164–73.
26. Ferrari L, Biancolini D, Seregni E, et al. Critical aspects of immunoradiometric thyroglobulin assays. Tumori. 2003;89:537–9.
27. Fugazzola L, Mihalich A, Persani L, et al. Highly sensitive serum thyroglobulin and circulating thyroglobulin mRNA evaluations in the management of patients with differentiated thyroid cancer in apparent remission. J Clin Endocrinol Metab. 2002;87:3201–8.
28. Wunderlich G, Zophel K, Crook L, Smith S, Smith B, Franke W. A high-sensitivity enzyme-linked immunosorbent assay for serum thyroglobulin. Thyroid. 2001;11:819–24.
29. Madureira D, Prazeres S, Pedro M, Pereira T, Font A, Bugalho M. In vitro assays to test the interference of anti-thyroglobulin antibodies on thyroglobulin measurement. Endocrine. 2008;33:40–4.
30. Spencer C. Clinical utility of thyroglobulin antibody (TgAb) measurements for patients with differentiated thyroid cancers (DTC). J Clin Endocrinol Metab. 2011;96:3615–27.
31. Spencer CA, Petrovic I, Fatemi S. Current thyroglobulin antibody (TgAb) assays often fail to detect interfering TgAb that can result in the reporting of falsely low/undetectable serum Tg IMA values for patients with differentiated thyroid cancer. J Clin Endocrinol Metab. 2011;96:1283–91.
32. Crane MS, Strachan MW, Toft AD, Beckett GJ. Discordance in thyroglobulin measurements by radioimmunoassay and immunometric assay: a useful means of identifying thyroglobulin assay interference. Ann Clin Biochem. 2013;50:421–32.
33. Verburg FA, Luster M, Cupini C, et al. Implications of thyroglobulin antibody positivity in patients with differentiated thyroid cancer: a clinical position paper. Thyroid 2013 (published 19 Aug 2013 ahead of print).
34. Verburg F, Wäschle K, Reiners C, Giovanella L, Lentjes E. Heterophile antibodies rarely influence the measurement of thyroglobulin and thyroglobulin antibodies in differentiated thyroid cancer patients. Horm Metab Res. 2010;42:736–9.
35. Giovanella L, Keller F, Ceriani L, Tozzoli R. Heterophile antibodies may falsely increase or decrease thyroglobulin measurement in patients with differentiated thyroid carcinoma. Clin Chem Lab Med. 2009;47:952–4.
36. Massart C, Corcuff J, Bordenave L. False-positive results corrected by the use of heterophilic antibody-blocking reagent in thyroglobulin immunoassays. Clin Chim Acta. 2008;338:211–3.
37. Locsei Z, Toldy E, Szabolcs I, Rácz K, Kovács G. The effect of sample storage on the reliability of thyroglobulin and thyroglobulin-antibody measurements. Clin Biochem. 2009;42:225–8.
38. Westbury C, Vini L, Fisher C, Harmer C. Recurrent differentiated thyroid cancer without elevation of serum thyroglobulin. Thyroid. 2000;10:171–6.
39. Giovanella L, Suriano S, Ceriani L, Verburg F. Undetectable thyroglobulin in patients with differentiated thyroid carcinoma and residual radioiodine uptake on a postablation whole-body scan. Clin Nucl Med. 2011;36:109–12.
40. Sager P, Cooper D, Daniels G, et al. Treatment guidelines for patients with thyroid nodules and well-differentiated thyroid cancer. Arch Intern Med. 1996;256:2165–72.
41. Cooper D, Doherty G, Haugen B, et al. Revised American Thyroid Association management guidelines for patients with thyroid nodules and differentiated thyroid cancer. Thyroid. 2009;19: 1167–214.
42. Tamizu A, Okumura Y, Sato S, et al. The usefulness of serum thyroglobulin levels and Tl-201 scintigraphy in differentiating between benign and malignant thyroid follicular lesions. Ann Nucl Med. 2002;16:95–101.
43. Hocevar M, Auersperg M. Role of serum thyroglobulin in the preoperative evaluation of follicular thyroid tumours. Eur J Surg Oncol. 1998;24:553–7.
44. Sharma A, Sarda A, Chattopadhyay T, Kapur M. The role of estimation of the ratio of preoperative serum thyroglobulin to the thyroid mass in predicting the behaviour of well differentiated thyroid cancers. J Postgrad Med. 1996;42:39–42.
45. Sands N, Karls S, Rivera J, et al. Preoperative serum thyroglobulin as an adjunct to fine-needle aspiration in predicting well-differentiated thyroid cancer. J Otolaryngol Head Neck Surg. 2010;39:669–73.
46. Lee EK, Chung K-W, Min HS, et al. Preoperative serum thyroglobulin as a useful predictive marker to differentiate follicular thyroid cancer from benign nodules in indeterminate nodules. J Korean Med Sci. 2012;27:1014–8.
47. Hrafnkelsson J, Tulinius H, Kjeld M, Sigvaldason H, Jonasson J. Serum thyroglobulin as a risk factor for thyroid carcinoma. Acta Oncol. 2000;39:973–7.
48. Giovanella L, Ceriani L, Suriano S, Ghelfo A, Maffioli M. Thyroglobulin measurement before rhTSH-aided 131I ablation in detecting metastases from differentiated thyroid carcinoma. Clin Endocrinol (Oxf). 2008;69:659–63.
49. Lima N, Cavaliere H, Tomimori E, Knobel M, Medeiros-Neto G. Prognostic value of serial serum thyroglobulin determinations after total thyroidectomy for differentiated thyroid cancer. J Endocrinol Invest. 2002;25:110–5.
50. Lee H, Rha S, Jo Y, et al. Predictive value of the preablation serum thyroglobulin level after thyroidectomy is combined with postablation 131I whole body scintigraphy for successful ablation in patients with differentiated thyroid carcinoma. Am J Clin Oncol. 2007;30:63–8.
51. Lin Y, Li T, Liang J, et al. Predictive value of preablation stimulated thyroglobulin and thyroglobulin/thyroid-stimulating hormone ratio in differentiated thyroid cancer. Clin Nucl Med. 2011;36:1102–5.
52. Ronga G, Filesi M, Ventroni G, Vestri A, Signore A. Value of the first serum thyroglobulin level after total thyroidectomy for the diagnosis of metastases from differentiated thyroid carcinoma. Eur J Nucl Med. 1999;26:1448–52.
53. Grunwald F, Menzel C, Fimmers R, Zamora P, Biersack H. Prognostic value of thyroglobulin after thyroidectomy before ablative radioiodine therapy in thyroid cancer. J Nucl Med. 1996;37:1962–4.
54. Webb RC, Howard RS, Stojadinovic A, et al. The utility of serum thyroglobulin measurement at the time of remnant ablation for predicting disease-free status in patients with differentiated thyroid cancer: a meta-analysis involving 3947 patients. J Clin Endocrinol Metab. 2012;97:2754–63.

55. Hocevar M, Auersperg M, Stanovnik L. The dynamics of serum thyroglobulin elimination from the body after thyroid surgery. Eur J Surg Oncol. 1997;23:208–10.
56. Giovanella L, Ceriani L, Maffioli M. Postsurgery serum thyroglobulin disappearance kinetic in patients with differentiated thyroid carcinoma. Head Neck. 2010;32:568–71.
57. Van Wyngaarden K, McDougall I. Is serum thyroglobulin a useful marker for thyroid cancer in patients who have not had ablation of residual thyroid tissue? Thyroid. 1997;7:343–6.
58. Haugen B, Pacini F, Reiners C, et al. A comparison of recombinant human thyrotropin and thyroid hormone withdrawal for the detection of thyroid remnant or cancer. J Clin Endocrinol Metab. 1999;84:3877–85.
59. Malandrino P, Latina A, Marescalco S, et al. Risk-adapted management of differentiated thyroid cancer assessed by a sensitive measurement of basal serum thyroglobulin. J Clin Endocrinol Metab. 2011;96:1703–9.
60. Spencer C, Fatemi S, Singer P, Nicoloff J, Lopresti J. Serum basal thyroglobulin measured by a second-generation assay correlates with the recombinant human thyrotropin-stimulated thyroglobulin response in patients treated for differentiated thyroid cancer. Thyroid. 2010;20:587–95.
61. Kloos R. Thyroid cancer recurrence in patients clinically free of disease with undetectable or very low serum thyroglobulin values. J Clin Endocrinol Metab. 2010;95:5241–8.
62. Rosario P, Purisch S. Does a highly sensitive thyroglobulin (Tg) assay change the clinical management of low-risk patients with thyroid cancer with Tg on T4<1 ng/ml determined by traditional assays? Clin Endocrinol (Oxf). 2008;68:338–42.
63. Pelttari H, Laitinen K, Schalin-Jäntti C, Välimäki M. Long-term outcome of 495 TNM stage I or II patients with differentiated thyroid carcinoma followed up with neck ultrasonography and thyroglobulin measurements on T4 treatment. Clin Endocrinol (Oxf). 2008;69:323–31.
64. Castagna M, Brilli L, Pilli T, et al. Limited value of repeat recombinant human thyrotropin (rhTSH)-stimulated thyroglobulin testing in differentiated thyroid carcinoma patients with previous negative rhTSH-stimulated thyroglobulin and undetectable basal serum thyroglobulin levels. J Clin Endocrinol Metab. 2008;93:76–81.
65. Smallridge R, Meek S, Morgan M, et al. Monitoring thyroglobulin in a sensitive immunoassay has comparable sensitivity to recombinant human TSH-stimulated thyroglobulin in follow-up of thyroid cancer patients. J Clin Endocrinol Metab. 2007;92:82–7.
66. Pacini F, Molinaro E, Castagna M, et al. Recombinant human thyrotropin-stimulated serum thyroglobulin combined with. J Clin Endocrinol Metab. 2003;88:3668–73.
67. Pellegriti G, Scollo C, Regalbuto C, et al. Recombinant human thyrotropin-stimulated serum thyroglobulin combined with neck ultrasonography has the highest sensitivity in monitoring differentiated thyroid carcinoma. Clin Endocrinol (Oxf). 2003;58:556–61.

38 Thyroglobulin Antibodies and Their Measurement

D. Robert Dufour

Thyroglobulin Antibodies: Clinical Significance

Thyroglobulin antibodies are one of the more commonly encountered autoantibodies. In a study of a representative sample of the US population, they were found in 11.5 % of those over age 12 (10.4 % in those with no evidence of thyroid dysfunction). Prevalence of thyroglobulin antibodies was twice as high in women (15.2 %) as in men (7.6 %) and rose from presence in 6.3 % of teenagers to 21.6 % of those over age 80 [1]. Interestingly, in this study, the presence of thyroglobulin antibodies did not correlate with the presence of thyroid dysfunction, while thyroid peroxidase antibodies did [1].

Prevalence of Thyroglobulin Antibodies in Differentiated Thyroid Cancer

Thyroglobulin antibodies are even more commonly encountered in patients with thyroid cancer than in the general population. At the time of diagnosis, thyroglobulin antibodies are found in a greater proportion of patients with thyroid cancer than in the general population, with an average prevalence of 25 % [2]; however, some studies have found prevalence as low as 10 % [3, 4]. As in healthy individuals, thyroglobulin antibodies are more commonly found in women than in men [5]. As will be discussed in greater detail later, some of this difference is likely due to differences in the ability of different assays to detect thyroglobulin antibodies [6].

One reason for the increased frequency of thyroglobulin antibodies in patients with thyroid cancer is the increased frequency of associated thyroiditis. In two review articles, the reported frequency of thyroiditis in patients with papillary thyroid cancer varied between 0.5 % and 58 % [7, 8]. Latrofa studied six different assays for thyroglobulin antibodies and found them in 29–50 % of persons with papillary carcinoma and evidence of thyroiditis in the resected gland, but only 2–7 % of those with carcinoma and no thyroiditis [9]. The reason for such an association is not known; theories have speculated that thyroiditis increases the risk of thyroid carcinoma, that carcinoma triggers autoimmune thyroiditis, or that the high TSH that accompanies thyroiditis is carcinogenic. The frequency seems to be higher for papillary cancer than for other forms of differentiated thyroid cancer (such as follicular carcinoma or Hürthle cell carcinoma). This association also holds true for thyroglobulin antibodies, which are more frequently found in papillary carcinoma patients than in those with other forms of differentiated thyroid cancer [7, 8]. A similar association between thyroid carcinoma and Graves' disease has been found [10, 11], lending support to the theory that stimulation of thyroid cells by TSH (or thyroid-stimulating immunoglobulin) is responsible for the increased risk of papillary cancer.

Thyroglobulin Antibody Measurement

As discussed in Chap. 37, thyroglobulin antibodies are a major cause for erroneous thyroglobulin results. Current guidelines call for measurement of thyroglobulin antibodies routinely whenever thyroglobulin is ordered for monitoring of thyroid cancer, even if the antibodies were previously undetectable [12, 13]. There are a number of issues with thyroglobulin antibody measurement that are not directly addressed by the guidelines but that are important in the interpretation of results. An international consensus statement has addressed many of these issues and made recommendations [14], but Spencer has criticized a number of the recommendations [15], so there is no widespread consensus on all issues.

D.R. Dufour, MD (✉)
Clinical Pathology, Veterans Affairs Medical Center, 50 Irving Street NW, Washington, DC 20422, USA
e-mail: chemdoctorbob@earthlink.net

L. Wartofsky, D. Van Nostrand (eds.), *Thyroid Cancer*, DOI 10.1007/978-1-4939-3314-3_38

Method of Measurement of Thyroglobulin Antibodies

Currently, many assays in use employ a variation of the immunometric method discussed in Chap. 37. Instead of a capture antibody immobilized to a solid support, thyroglobulin is immobilized. After incubation with patient serum, the plate is washed, and a labeled antibody to human immunoglobulin is added. The amount of label bound to the solid support is directly proportional to the amount of thyroglobulin antibody present in the sample. However, a variety of formats are actually used to detect the interaction between thyroglobulin and the antibody in the patient's serum [6]. Older methods for thyroglobulin antibodies used less sensitive techniques, such as hemagglutination inhibition. This technique is less sensitive than more automated immunoassay formats [16], and as long ago as 2003, guidelines recommended against its use to measure thyroglobulin antibodies [17, 18]. The consensus statement recommends measurement of thyroglobulin and thyroglobulin antibodies using assays from the same manufacturer [14]. It is not clear that this recommendation is necessary or appropriate, however [15]. There are significant differences in the expression of antigenic epitopes of thyroglobulin produced in different persons [19], as well as differences in ability of assays for thyroglobulin to detect different epitopes [20].

Selection of Cutoff Points for Positive Thyroglobulin Antibodies

To gain Food and Drug Administration approval, manufacturers must perform experiments that show equivalency in diagnostic performance to a "gold standard" method. Typically, cutoff points to determine positive results are based on comparison to a standard reference material, derived from patients with autoimmune thyroiditis (World Health Organization International Reference Preparation 65/93) [21]; however, different manufacturers use different standards [22]. Thus, cutoff points are optimized to detect antibodies in patients with autoimmune thyroid disease and do not necessarily agree with each other. Use of the same international reference preparation improves correlation between methods on measurements of this material but does not eliminate differences between methods in samples in patients with thyroid cancer [23]. The epitopes in the thyroglobulin molecule that are targeted by antibodies are different in normal persons and in those with autoimmune thyroid disease, in which reactivity is limited to a distinct set of epitopes [24]; the pattern is different in persons with thyroid cancer and thyroiditis than in those with thyroid cancer alone [20]. In patients with thyroid cancer, varying patterns are seen, with some having antibody to a restricted set of epitopes, while others have more broad-scale reactivity [25, 26]. This translates to a practical issue with differences in the ability of different assays to detect thyroglobulin antibodies [6, 20, 22, 27–29]. Current recommendations are to use the lowest reliably reproducible cutoff value to classify results as positive in patients with thyroid cancer [14, 15].

Stability of Thyroglobulin Antibodies on Storage

Limited data exist on the effects of storage on thyroglobulin antibodies. A single study found that storage in a refrigerator for 2 days, or storage in a freezer for 2–3 weeks, resulted in decrease in measured thyroglobulin antibody by 15–25 % [30]. Although the number of samples evaluated in this study was small, in none of the samples did it appear that antibody became undetectable on storage. From a practical standpoint, this should not commonly lead to misdiagnosis of a sample as antibody negative. However, if samples are being evaluated serially to evaluate for declining antibody levels, it is possible that sample storage may be a variable to consider in interpreting results.

Lower Limits of Detection

The main significance of the detection limit is that it affects the ability to recognize samples that will show interference in thyroglobulin measurement. In the most detailed study to date, 785 samples from patients with thyroid cancer were analyzed for thyroglobulin antibodies, of which 556 were tested by four different thyroglobulin antibody methods [6]. In 40–60 % of the samples, results that were considered positive by the "reference" method were classified as negative by the other assays, using the manufacturer's cutoff values. When comparing thyroglobulin levels measured by immunometric assay and competitive immunoassay (with a ratio of the two results <0.75 considered to indicate significant interference), 21–44 % of samples that were "thyroglobulin antibody negative" using the manufacturer's cutoff value showed interference, including 4–10 % of samples having undetectable thyroglobulin by the immunometric assay. However, for two of the methods, considering the lowest level of thyroglobulin antibody that could be detected (which was about 1/10 of the value recommended by the manufacturer) as "positive" prevented falsely undetectable thyroglobulin results. In the two assays in which this approach did not eliminate undetectable thyroglobulin results, the lowest value that could be measured was close to or equal to the manufacturer's recommended lowest reportable value. In another study of five thyroglobulin antibody methods (only one of which was evaluated in the larger study), the lowest measurable value was markedly lower than the manufacturer's recommended cutoff for three of the five assays, while it was close to it in the other two [28]. Several other studies have shown that using these lower cutoffs improves detection of samples that show interference in thyroglobulin measurement [27, 29].

Agreement Between Different Methods

The frequency with which samples are positive for thyroglobulin antibodies differs with different methods. In one study, only 3 of 54 samples detected as having thyroglobulin antibodies were positive by all three methods evaluated [22]. Individual results vary significantly even when positive. In one study of five methods compared to a "reference" method, thyroglobulin antibody levels (expressed in the same kIU/L terms) ranged from half of the reference method to ten times the reference method results [28]. Current guidelines and review articles recommend always measuring thyroglobulin antibodies in a given patient with the same assay to be able to detect changes in antibody levels [13, 14, 18, 31, 32]. As might be deduced from the marked differences seen with different methods, the absolute value is not as important as whether it is positive or negative and as whether it is declining or increasing. Strength of reaction, either titer (using older assays) or relative signal in ELISA assays, does not predict samples that yield erroneous results for thyroglobulin measurement, however [2, 6, 33]. Some samples with high-level antibodies show no difference between immunoassays and sandwich assays, while some samples with weakly positive antibodies (even below the detection limit of some assays) show clinically important differences [6, 34]. In addition, the type of thyroglobulin assay that is used also affects the ability to detect the presence of thyroglobulin; in one study, newer thyroglobulin assays with lower detection limits showed less interference from thyroglobulin antibodies [35].

Recovery Experiments

As mentioned in Chap. 37, an alternative approach to detecting samples with interfering antibodies is to perform recovery experiments, which involve adding a known amount of thyroglobulin to a serum sample and measuring the increase of thyroglobulin compared to the expected increase predicted by the amount added. Some studies have suggested that recovery of close to 100 % of added thyroglobulin can predict levels of antibody that do not interfere with thyroglobulin measurement [36, 37]. Unfortunately, samples that show high recovery often still show significantly higher thyroglobulin with immunoassays compared to sandwich assays, indicating a clinically important interference [2, 38, 39]. Current guidelines do not recommend use of recovery studies [12, 18]. Typically, a large amount of thyroglobulin (concentrations of 50 ng/mL) has been used. More recently, use of lower amounts of thyroglobulin ("mini-recovery") has been found to more sensitively detect such interference [40], and a commercial assay using a thyroglobulin concentration of 1 ng/mL has been developed. Its sensitivity in detecting interfering samples was slightly higher than thyroglobulin antibody assay alone and was also capable of detecting interference from heterophile antibodies [41]. The use of such an assay has been evaluated in too few patients to be advocated in consensus guidelines [14].

Clinical Significance of Thyroglobulin Antibodies in Thyroid Cancer

Thyroglobulin Antibodies before Thyroidectomy

Although, as with thyroglobulin, current guidelines do not recommend measurement of thyroglobulin antibodies before surgery [12, 13], a study of over 1,600 patients found that thyroid cancers were 60 % more likely in patients with thyroid nodules who also had thyroglobulin antibodies present [42].

Thyroglobulin Antibodies After Thyroidectomy

In addition to detecting samples in which thyroglobulin measurements are likely to be unreliable, thyroglobulin antibodies have been utilized to monitor patients with thyroid cancer. Several studies have found a higher likelihood of metastatic disease in those with high levels of thyroglobulin antibodies [3, 4, 43] or in those whose levels either do not fall or increase [44, 45]. Loss of thyroglobulin antibodies is associated with a favorable prognosis and a low likelihood of recurrent or metastatic thyroid cancer [21, 44, 45]. With successful eradication of thyroid cancer, levels of thyroglobulin antibodies decrease and usually become undetectable by 1–3 years after successful treatment [46, 47]. In the best serial study, antibody became undetectable by 1–1.5 years in half of those initially positive, but in one-third of patients, antibody persisted for over 3 years [47]. Levels may transiently rise after remnant ablation in about 15 % of patients, even becoming positive in some in whom they were initially undetectable after surgery [5, 47]. The half-life for disappearance in those who ultimately become negative is about 10 weeks [47]. Patients with detectable thyroglobulin antibodies after surgery were found to be more likely to have residual disease in some studies [3, 43, 44, 48], but not in others [5, 47].

The evidence is more consistent that falling levels of thyroglobulin antibody after surgery are associated with absence of residual thyroid cancer and that these levels can be used as an alternate "tumor marker" for monitoring antibody-positive patients with thyroid cancer [5, 44, 46]. In one study with 2-year follow-up, patients with a decrease of <50 % were just as likely to have residual tumor as those whose antibody levels increased [45], and Spencer has recommended this cutoff point to identify individuals who merit closer evaluation [15]. In contrast to thyroglobulin, however, levels are not directly related to tumor mass, making them imprecise as a tumor marker [14]. Although, as mentioned earlier, differences in results using different assays make it difficult to follow patients with different assays, serial results in individual patients show parallel changes in results when tested with different assays [21]. Thus, it does not seem to matter which thyroglobulin antibody assay is used, as long as the same assay is always utilized for following the patient.

References

1. Hollowell J, Staehling N, Flanders W, et al. Serum TSH, T(4), and thyroid antibodies in the United States population (1988 to 1994): National Health and Nutrition Examination Survey (NHANES III). J Clin Endocrinol Metab. 2002;87:489–99.
2. Spencer C, Takeuchi M, Kazarosyan M, et al. Serum thyroglobulin autoantibodies: prevalence, influence on serum thyroglobulin measurement, and prognostic significance in patients with differentiated thyroid carcinoma. J Clin Endocrinol Metab. 1998;83: 1121–7.
3. Hjiyiannakis P, Mundy J, Harmer C. Thyroglobulin antibodies in differentiated thyroid cancer. Clin Oncol (R Coll Radiol). 1999; 11:240–4.
4. Rubello D, Girelli M, Casara D, Piccolo M, Perin A, Busnardo B. Usefulness of the combined antithyroglobulin antibodies and thyroglobulin assay in the follow-up of patients with differentiated thyroid cancer. J Endocrinol Invest. 1990;13:737–42.
5. Kumar A, Shah D, Shrihari U, Dandekar S, Vijayan U, Sharmak S. Significance of antithyroglobulin autoantibodies in differentiated thyroid carcinoma. Thyroid. 1994;4:199–202.
6. Spencer CA, Petrovic I, Fatemi S. Current thyroglobulin antibody (TgAb) assays often fail to detect interfering TgAb that can result in the reporting fo falsely low/undetectable serum Tg IMA values for patients with differentiated thyroid cancer. J Clin Endocrinol Metab. 2011;96:1283–91.
7. Feldt-Rasmussen U, Rasmussen A. Autoimmunity in differentiated thyroid cancer: significance and related clinical problems. Hormones. 2010;9:109–17.
8. Cunha L, Ferreira R, Marcello M, Vassallo J, Ward L. Clinical and pathological implications of concurrent autoimmune thyroid disorders and papillary thyroid cancer. J Thyroid Res. 2011;2011:387062.
9. Latrofa F, Ricci D, Montanelli L, et al. Lymphocytic thyroiditis on histology correlates with serum thyroglobulin autoantibodies in patients with papillary thyroid carcinoma: impact on detection of serum thyroglobulin. J Clin Endocrinol Metab. 2012;97:2380–7.
10. El M. Thyroid cancer and Graves' disease. J Clin Endocrinol Metab. 1999;70:826–9.
11. Belfiore A, Russo D, Vigneri R, Filetti S. Graves' disease, thyroid nodules and thyroid cancer. Clin Endocrinol (Oxf). 2001;55:711–8.
12. Pacini F, Schlumberger M, Dralle H, et al. European consensus for the management of patients with differentiated thyroid carcinoma of the follicular epithelium. Eur J Endocrinol. 2006;154:787–803.
13. Haugen BR, Alexander EK, Bible KC, Doherty GM, Mandel SJ, Nikiforov Y, Pacini F, Randolph G, Sawka A, Shepard D, Sosa J, Tuttle RM, Wartofsky L. 2015 American Thyroid Association Management Guidelines for adult patients with thyroid nodules and differentiated thyroid cancer. Available online at Thyroid 25: DOI:10.1089/thy.2015.0020; print version in Thyroid 26:1–133, 2016.
14. Verburg FA, Luster M, Cupini C, et al. Implications of thyroglobulin antibody positivity in patients with differentiated thyroid cancer: a clinical position paper. Thyroid. 2013;23:1211–25.
15. Spencer CA. Commentary on: implications of thyroglobulin antibody positivity in patients with differentiated thyroid cancer: a clinical position paper. Thyroid. 2013;23:1190–2.
16. Lindberg B, Svensson J, Ericsson U, Nilsson P, Svenonius E, Ivarsson S. Comparison of some different methods for analysis of thyroid autoantibodies: importance of thyroglobulin autoantibodies. Thyroid. 2001;11:265–9.
17. Mazzaferri E, Robbins R, Spencer C, et al. A consensus report of the role of serum thyroglobulin as a monitoring method for low-risk patients with papillary thyroid carcinoma. J Clin Endocrinol Metab. 2003;88:1433–41.
18. Demers L, Spencer C. Laboratory support for the diagnosis and monitoring of thyroid disease. Thyroid. 2003;13:3–126.
19. Latrofa F, Ricci D, Grasso L, et al. Characterization of thyroglobulin epitopes in patients with autoimmune and non-autoimmune thyroid diseases using recombinant human monoclonal thyroglobulin autoantibodies. J Clin Endocrinol Metab. 2008;93:591–6.
20. Latrofa F, Ricci D, Montanelli L, et al. Thyroglobulin autoantibodies in patients with papillary thyroid carcinoma: comparison of different assays and evaluation of causes of discrepancies. J Clin Endocrinol Metab. 2012;97:3974–82.
21. Spencer C. Clinical utility of thyroglobulin antibody (TgAb) measurements for patients with differentiated thyroid cancers (DTC). J Clin Endocrinol Metab. 2011;96:3615–27.
22. Krahn J, Dembinski T. Thyroglobulin and anti-thyroglobulin assays in thyroid cancer monitoring. Clin Biochem. 2009;42:416–9.
23. Pickett AJ, Jones M, Evans C. Causes of discordance between thyroglobulin antibody assays. Ann Clin Biochem. 2012;49:463–7.
24. Okosieme O, Parkes A, Premawardhana L, Evans C, Lazarus J. Thyroglobulin: current aspects of its role in autoimmune thyroid disease and thyroid cancer. Minerva Med. 2003;94:319–30.
25. Okosieme O, Evans C, Moss L, et al. Thyroglobulin antibodies in serum of patients with differentiated thyroid cancer: relationship between epitope specificities and thyroglobulin recovery. Clin Chem. 2005;51:729–34.
26. Rose N, Burek C. Autoantibodies to thyroglobulin in health and disease. Appl Biochem Biotechnol. 2000;83:245–51; discussion 51-4.
27. Taylor K, Parkington D, Bradbury S, Simpson H, Jefferies S, Halsall D. Concordance between thyroglobulin antibody assays. Clin Biochem. 2011;48:367–9.
28. La'ulu S, Slev P, Roberts W. Performance characteristics of 5 automated thyroglobulin autoantibody and thyroid peroxidase autoantibody assays. Clin Chim Acta. 2007;376:88–95.
29. Nygaard B, Bentzen J, Laurberg P, et al. Large discrepancy in the results of sensitive measurements of thyroglobulin antibodies in the follow-up on thyroid cancer: a diagnostic dilemma. Eur Thyroid J. 2012;1:193–7.
30. Locsei Z, Toldy E, Szabolcs I, Rácz K, Kovács G. The effect of sample storage on the reliability of thyroglobulin and thyroglobulin-antibody measurements. Clin Biochem. 2009;42:225–8.
31. Spencer C, Lopresti J. Measuring thyroglobulin and thyroglobulin autoantibody in patients with differentiated thyroid cancer. Nat Clin Pract Endocrinol Metab. 2008;4:223–33.
32. Ringel MD, Nabhan F. Approach to follow-up of the patient with differentiated thyroid cancer and positive anti-thyroglobulin antibodies. J Clin Endocrinol Metab. 2013;98:3104–10.
33. Madureira D, Prazeres S, Pedro M, Pereira T, Font A, Bugalho M. In vitro assays to test the interference of anti-thyroglobulin antibodies on thyroglobulin measurement. Endocrine. 2008;33:40–4.
34. Cubero J, Rodriguez-Espinosa J, Gelpi C, Estorch M, Corcoy R. Thyroglobulin autoantibody levels below the cut-off for positivity can interfere with thyroglobulin measurement. Thyroid. 2003;13: 659–61.
35. Giovanella L, Ceriani L. Comparison of thyroglobulin antibody interference in first- and second-generation thyroglobulin immunoassays. Clin Chem Lab Med. 2011;49:1025–7.

36. Erali M, Bigelow R, Miekle A. ELISA for thyroglobulin in serum: recovery studies to evaluate autoantibody interference and reliability of thyroglobulin value. Clin Chem. 1996;42:766–70.
37. Bourrel F, Hoff M, Regis H, Courriere P, Caron P. Immunoradiometric assay of thyroglobulin in patients with differentiated thyroid carcinomas: need for thyroglobulin recovery tests. Clin Chem Lab Med. 1998;36:725–30.
38. Massart C, Maugendre D. Importance of the detection method for thyroglobulin antibodies for the validity of thyroglobulin measurements in sera from patients with Graves disease. Clin Chem. 2002;48:102–7.
39. Mariotti S, Barbesino G, Caturegli P, et al. Assay of thyroglobulin in serum with thyroglobulin autoantibodies: an unobtainable goal? J Clin Endocrinol Metab. 1995;80:468–72.
40. Verburg F, Hartmann D, Grelle I, Giovanella L, Buck A, Reiners C. Relationship between antithyroglobulin autoantibodies and thyroglobulin recovery rates using different thyroglobulin concentrations in the recovery buffer. Horm Metab Res. 2013;45:728–35.
41. Giovanella L, Imperiali M, Verburg F, Ceriani L. Evaluation of the BRAHMS Kryptor® thyroglobulin minirecovery test in patients with differentiated thyroid carcinoma. Clin Chem Lab Med. 2012; 51:449–53.
42. Kim E, Lim D, Baek K, et al. Thyroglobulin antibody is associated with increased cancer risk in thyroid nodules. Thyroid. 2010;20:885–91.
43. Chung J, Park Y, Kim T, et al. Clinical significance of elevated level of serum antithyroglobulin antibody in patients with differentiated thyroid cancer after thyroid ablation. Clin Endocrinol (Oxf). 2002;57:215–21.
44. Kim W, Yoon J, Kim W, et al. Change of serum antithyroglobulin antibody levels is useful for prediction of clinical recurrence in thyroglobulin-negative patients with differentiated thyroid carcinoma. J Clin Endocrinol Metab. 2008;93:4683–9.
45. Tsushima Y, Miyauchi A, Ito Y, et al. Prognostic significance of changes in serum thyroglobulin antibody levels of pre-and post-total thyroidectomy in thyroglobulin antibody-positive papillary thyroid carcinoma patients. Endocr J. 2013;60:871–6.
46. Chiovato L, Latrofa F, Braverman L, et al. Disappearance of humoral thyroid autoimmunity after complete removal of thyroid antigens. Ann Intern Med. 2003;139:346–51.
47. Görges R, Maniecki M, Jentzen W, et al. Development and clinical impact of thyroglobulin antibodies in patients with differentiated thyroid carcinoma during the first 3 years after thyroidectomy. Eur J Endocrinol. 2005;153:49–55.
48. Pedrazzini L, Baroli A, Lomuscio G, Marzoli L. Prevalence, clinical significance and prognostic value of anti-thyroglobulin antibodies in the follow-up of patients with differentiated thyroid carcinoma: a retrospective study. Minerva Endocrinol. 2009;34: 195–203.

Diagnosis of Recurrent Thyroid Cancer in Patients with Anti-thyroglobulin Antibodies

39

Matthew D. Ringel and Jennifer A. Sipos

Whole-body radioiodine scanning, measurement of serum thyroglobulin, and a number of different radiographic methods are used to monitor patients with thyroid cancer for recurrence of their tumors. Over the past decade, substantial improvements in thyroglobulin immunoassays and a greater recognition of the limitations of I-131 scanning, particularly regarding its relatively low sensitivity for neck recurrences, have led to recommendations that rely primarily on accurate thyroglobulin measurements and neck ultrasound [1, 2]. However, there are some limitations of current thyroglobulin immunoassays, including inadequate sensitivity during L-T4 therapy depending on the particular assay and the presence of interfering anti-thyroglobulin antibodies in approximately 20 % of patients. Because circulating anti-thyroglobulin antibodies interfere with accurate thyroglobulin measurement, there is increased reliance on radiographic testing to monitor patients with detectable anti-thyroglobulin antibodies. In this chapter, potential alternative approaches to blood-based monitoring methods in patients with circulating anti-thyroglobulin antibodies will be discussed. The use of imaging modalities in thyroid cancer is only briefly discussed in this chapter as they are unaffected by anti-thyroglobulin antibodies. Various imaging methods are part of a general approach to monitoring patients, however, and are discussed in detail in other sections of the book.

M.D. Ringel, MD (✉)
Department of Internal Medicine, Division of Endocrinology, Diabetes and Metabolism, Wexner Medical Center, The Ohio State University, 565 McCampbell Hall, 1581 Dodd Drive, Columbus, OH 43210, USA
e-mail: matthew.ringel@osumc.edu

J.A. Sipos
Department of Endocrinology, The Ohio State University, Columbus, OH, USA
e-mail: jennifer.sipos@osumc.edu

Thyroglobulin Antibodies

Thyroglobulin is a thyroid-specific 660 KD protein that serves as a precursor and storage protein in thyroid hormone biosynthesis that is produced by normal thyroid cells and well-differentiated thyroid cancer cells. Its presence is therefore specific for thyroid cancer only in patients who are devoid of normal thyroid tissue. Patients who have a history of thyroid cancer and who are not completely athyreotic may have detectable levels that reflect the presence of remaining nonmalignant thyroid tissue. The quantitative amount of circulating thyroglobulin usually correlates with the extent of disease and the amount of residual or recurrent tissue, enhancing the clinical usefulness of the assay [3]. Similar to I-131 uptake, thyroglobulin production and release are regulated by thyrotropin (TSH). Consequently, TSH-stimulated thyroglobulin measurements are often performed in order to maximize sensitivity in recently diagnosed or high-risk patients. In this setting, the assay retains its specificity and becomes even more sensitive for disease detection. For these reasons, over the past 10–20 years, thyroglobulin monitoring has become an integral part of thyroid cancer monitoring.

Circulating anti-thyroglobulin antibodies are the major limitation of modern thyroglobulin immunoassays. Thyroglobulin is a large protein with numerous antigenic epitopes, many of which can induce antibody formation within an individual patient [4]. Major efforts have been made to circumvent the effects of these heterogenic antibodies on the thyroglobulin assays, but to date, none have proven successful for clinical practice. For this reason, it is recommended that anti-thyroglobulin antibodies are measured on the same serum sample as thyroglobulin to assess the validity of the thyroglobulin measurement. The accuracy of the anti-thyroglobulin antibody measurement is critical for clinical decision-making, a topic that is receiving increased scrutiny over the past few years and will be discussed below. Most laboratories now measure antibody presence using a sensitive

L. Wartofsky, D. Van Nostrand (eds.), *Thyroid Cancer*, DOI 10.1007/978-1-4939-3314-3_39

immunoassay and a standard antibody preparation, rather than determining antibody titers [3]. Results between different anti-thyroglobulin antibodies are not always consistent, thus if possible the same assay system should be used over time for individual patients. Some authors have advocated the use of "recovery" assays to measure the degree of interference by anti-thyroglobulin antibodies, since not all antibodies may interfere with thyroglobulin measurement to the same degree. Another approach to identify non-interfering but detectable anti-Tg antibodies is to perform both RIA and IRMA assays on the same sample to identify concordant results. However, since the majority of anti-thyroglobulin antibodies appear to interfere with measurement [5], recovery assays and performing multiple types of thyroglobulin assays on patient samples are not routinely performed by most clinical laboratories.

Anti-thyroglobulin autoantibodies themselves are a marker of autoimmune thyroid disease in patients who are hypo- or hyperthyroid, but their specificity for predicting disease is not clear as they may also be seen in euthyroid adults. Their presence was recently reported in 4–10 % of unselected women and 1–3 % of unselected men in a large US population [6, 7]. For uncertain and highly debated reasons, patients with thyroid cancer have a much greater incidence of detectable anti-thyroglobulin antibodies with most studies reporting an incidence of approximately 20 % [1, 8]. It is uncertain whether the presence of thyroid autoantibodies is a cause or an effect of thyroid cancer. In some cases, the presence of circulating anti-thyroglobulin antibodies correlates with the presence of intrathyroidal autoimmunity as evidenced by the presence of chronic lymphocytic thyroiditis or a peritumoral lymphocytic infiltration on histopathology of the thyroid gland. The correlation between anti-thyroglobulin antibodies and thyroid autoimmunity has led to speculation that patients with detectable anti-thyroglobulin antibodies may have a better prognosis due to an enhanced anti-thyroid cancer cell immune response [9, 10]; however, correlation studies have reported inconsistent results [11–13]. The lack of consensus on this relationship may be, in part, due to a lack of distinction between patients with generalized lymphocytic infiltration associated with Hashimoto's thyroiditis and those with peritumoral lymphocytic infiltration. The latter is a well-recognized immune response to the presence of tumor and may be seen in various malignancies.

An additional confounding factor in the reliability of thyroglobulin measurement is heterophile antibodies; their presence may result in a false elevation of thyroglobulin levels [14]. Heterophile antibodies are those that can bind to animal antigens used in the immunoassay. One study reported the presence of interfering heterophilic anti-thyroglobulin antibodies in up to 3 % of thyroglobulin antibody-negative thyroid cancer serum samples [14]. More recent studies, however, have found the prevalence of such heterophile antibodies to be significantly lower [15, 16]. Testing for the presence of heterophile antibodies requires the use of heterophile-blocking tubes. Current assays may be less likely to be affected by such interfering substances as most laboratories routinely use additives to reduce heterophile interference. Nonetheless, their presence should be suspected when the serum thyroglobulin is elevated in the setting of low clinical suspicion of disease and the absence of radiographic abnormalities.

Alternative Laboratory Tests for Thyroid Cancer

Thyroglobulin Antibody Levels

Because thyroglobulin antibodies represent a response to a thyroid-specific antigenic stimulus, it has been speculated that the reduction and/or disappearance of anti-thyroglobulin antibodies in peripheral blood would correlate with a reduced antigenic burden, i.e., the remission and/or cure of thyroid cancer in patients with anti-thyroglobulin antibodies. In support of this concept, several studies have correlated the reduction and disappearance of anti-thyroglobulin antibodies with reduced tumor burden [5, 8, 17, 18]. One study found that the median time to disappearance of thyroglobulin antibodies after initial treatment was 3 years and that the coexistence of autoimmune thyroid disease did not modify the pattern of disappearance of thyroid antibody compared to those with focal lymphocytic infiltration [19]. Taken together, it appears that the loss of detectable anti-thyroglobulin antibodies in an individual with differentiated thyroid cancer who has a history of circulating anti-thyroglobulin antibodies reflects an improvement in disease burden and enhances the ability to accurately measure thyroglobulin. Conversely, the appearance of thyroglobulin antibodies in a previously negative anti-thyroglobulin antibody patient suggests the possibility of persistent or recurrent disease [5]. Therefore, it is reasonable to monitor thyroglobulin and anti-thyroglobulin antibodies in these patients [20].

Importantly, recent studies have suggested that there is variability in the sensitivity of various IMA assays to detect the presence of thyroglobulin antibodies [21]. Laboratories may adopt the manufacturers' cutoff for a "detectable" anti-thyroglobulin antibody which was created to detect thyroid autoimmunity and is insensitive for detecting interference with thyroglobulin measurements. Consequently, specimens may be incorrectly classified as anti-thyroglobulin antibody negative. Importantly, even a low anti-thyroglobulin antibody level has the potential to interfere with the measurement of thyroglobulin [21]. Such false results have the potential to influence patient management. It is imperative, therefore, that the clinician has a high index of suspicion for the presence of interfering antibodies in any patient with clinically or radiographically detectable differentiated thyroid cancer but undetectable levels of thyroglobulin and anti-thyroglobulin antibodies.

Serum Levels of Other Cancer-Related Proteins

There has been interest in the development of new markers for recurrent thyroid cancer because of antibody interference, TSH dependency, lack of cancer specificity, and the loss of thyroglobulin production in some poorly differentiated cancers. A number of growth factors are crucial to thyroid cancer growth and progression, including basic fibroblast growth factor (bFGF) and vascular endothelial growth factor (VEGF). Expression of bFGF and VEGF has been described in thyroid cancer and is associated with tumor aggressiveness [22–24]. For this reason, several groups have evaluated the utility of serum levels of these two proteins in peripheral blood of patients with thyroid cancer. Serum VEGF levels appear to be elevated in patients with progressive and metastatic thyroid cancer in comparison to those free of clinically detectable disease [25–29]. In these studies, the response of serum VEGF levels to recombinant human TSH administration was reported to be either unchanged or reduced. Similar results have been reported for serum bFGF levels and also levels of matrix metalloproteinase-9 [26], intracellular adhesion molecule-1 [30–32], and oncofetal fibronectin [33].

Another approach to serum markers is to identify global changes in serum protein expression in patients with metastatic cancer, due either to tumor cells or to responses to metastatic cancer. Indeed, it has been recently reported that the patterns of protein expression among patients with benign thyroid nodules and patients with papillary thyroid cancer differ significantly. This technology even identified a pattern that distinguished different stages of the cancer [34]. Further analysis has identified additional biomarkers, improving the sensitivity and specificity (95 % and 94 %, respectively) of this promising field [35]. Additional studies are needed in larger cohorts of patients to determine if protein expression profiles can be used to predict remission or recurrence of disease.

DNA- and RNA-Based Assays

Because of antibody interference, and the potential for enhanced assay sensitivity, there has been an interest in developing DNA- and RNA-based assays for thyroid cancer monitoring using polymerase chain reaction (PCR, for DNA) or reverse transcription PCR (RT-PCR, for RNA). These types of assays do not rely on antibodies to detect protein, and thus are unaltered by anti-thyroglobulin antibodies and are more sensitive than immunoassays. The sensitivity of these assays is due to the inherent nature of PCR which logarithmically amplifies the target DNA (or cDNA if starting with RNA). More recently, the ability to accurately quantify RT-PCR reactions using probes that are specific for the gene that is being detected (real-time PCR) has generated even greater interest in these techniques. The potential for circulating DNA- and RNA-based detection for thyroid cancer has been mirrored for many other hematologic and solid malignancies for similar reasons. For DNA assays, detection of a somatically mutated gene (e.g., BRAF V600E) in peripheral blood has been thought to imply the presence of circulating thyroid cancer cells [36]. Thus, this approach would be applicable for those patients with tumors in which a mutation can be defined. Specificity may be limited by the presence of another occult cancer that might harbor the same mutation. For RNA assays, the principle has been used to detect thyroid-specific RNAs in the circulation similar to use of serum Tg protein assays. Because of the high sensitivity of RT-PCR, the principal issues in developing accurate thyroid-specific or thyroid cancer-specific RNA-based assays relate to specificity and also to the relative instability of isolated RNA.

Studies from a number of groups have been reported using several thyroid-specific markers, such as thyroglobulin, thyroid peroxidase, and TSH receptor mRNA, and also thyroid cancer-specific markers such as BRAF V600E or RET/PTC. Using qualitative methods, initial studies suggested that the presence of circulating thyroglobulin mRNA correlated with the presence of thyroid cancer and was absent in the setting of a normal thyroid [37, 38]. Follow-up studies demonstrated that thyroglobulin mRNA could be detected in most patients with thyroid tissue (benign or malignant) but rarely in patients who were athyreotic [39]. The subsequent results from multiple investigators have been highly varied, some supporting a relationship with thyroid cancer and others demonstrating no relationship [40–44]. The differences in results are likely due to enhanced assay sensitivity, alternative PCR primer design, or other methodologic differences as reviewed in detail elsewhere [45]. More recently, one group has reported utility in the preoperative diagnosis of thyroid cancer using their TSH receptor and thyroglobulin mRNA method [41, 46, 47].

In an effort to determine whether patients with greater tumor burden or extent of disease can be identified based upon their thyroid mRNA levels, several groups have attempted to quantify circulating thyroid mRNA transcripts [44, 48–53]. Overall, the results of these studies are also highly varied. In all published reports there is considerable overlap between patients with different stages of disease suggesting that none would be useful for individual patients on a routine basis. Further, all studies using the highly sensitive techniques of real-time RT-PCR have unequivocally demonstrated the presence of low levels of thyroglobulin mRNA variants in patients without evidence of thyroid tissue, leading to important questions regarding the specificity of "thyroid-specific" transcripts when detected using this highly sensitive method.

As noted above, one of the key assumptions for either DNA- or RNA-based detection of thyroid cancer is that the circulating nucleic acids are contained and protected within circulating thyroid cells. However, over the past several years, it has become apparent that not all circulating DNA and RNAs are carried in circulating tumor cells. For example, cancer cells (and other cells) secrete exosomes and microvesicles into the circulation. Exosomes are lipid bilayer structures that contain and protect mRNA, microRNA, and DNA [54]. Assays in which DNA and RNA are isolated and analyzed from circulating exosomes are being developed and studied at present in different cancers [55]. The detection of exosome-derived tumor-specific DNA or RNA species may be a potential marker of residual or recurrent thyroid cancer that could be developed for patients with anti-Tg antibodies.

Circulating Tumor Cells

Direct detection of circulating tumor cells (CTCs) has been reported for a variety of cancers and has been FDA approved for breast cancer [56]. The approach that is approved identifies cells based on expression of epithelial cell marker in a "buffy coat" preparation. This approach, or the use of more specific thyroid cell surface markers, has not yet been systematically applied to a thyroid cancer population but holds promise as an alternative to detect the potential for distant metastases or monitoring patients with metastatic disease with anti-Tg antibodies.

New Approaches to Thyroglobulin Measurement

Although thyroglobulin is a large protein, there are now alternative approaches to measuring proteins that do not rely on antibodies. These approaches, used in laboratories for years, are now being developed for clinical assay systems. One approach is mass spectroscopy which has been explored for measuring circulating thyroglobulin [57]. Although there are technical issues [58], such a detection system may represent the most promising approach for thyroglobulin measurement in patients with anti-thyroglobulin antibodies as it directly identifies proteins in a sample and does not rely on antibody-based systems prone to interference by competing antibodies.

Approach to Disease Monitoring for Patients with Anti-thyroglobulin Antibodies

Because of the difficulties in reliable serum testing for thyroid cancer monitoring in patients with anti-thyroglobulin antibodies, there is a greater reliance on radiographic testing. This includes the use of I-131 scanning, neck ultrasound, and chest CT scanning. In addition, for patients with aggressive tumors, PET scanning with [18] FDG also plays a potentially important role. The utility of these studies is not different in patients with anti-thyroglobulin antibodies and is discussed in detail in other chapters in this text. However, it is important to recognize that current proposed algorithms that rely heavily on measurement of serum thyroglobulin exclude patients with circulating anti-thyroglobulin antibodies and therefore do not apply to this population. As a result, one approach is to monitor patients with both quantitative thyroglobulin and anti-thyroglobulin antibody measurements as tumor markers and to perform neck ultrasonography and I-131 scanning yearly for the first several years after diagnosis, depending on the initial extent of the tumor. Additional radiographic studies, such as chest CT scans and PET scans, may be needed in high-risk patients. Advances in the evaluation of alternative serum markers, global analysis of peripheral blood proteins, the development of non-antibody-dependent serum Tg assays, and molecular diagnostics are promising areas of future research to aid in the management of patients with anti-thyroglobulin antibodies.

References

1. Mazzaferri EL, Robbins RJ, Spencer CA, et al. A consensus report of the role of serum thyroglobulin as a monitoring method for low-risk patients with papillary thyroid carcinoma. J Clin Endocrinol Metab. 2003;88(4):1433–41.
2. Schlumberger M, Berg G, Cohen O, et al. Follow-up of low-risk patients with differentiated thyroid carcinoma: a European perspective. Eur J Endocrinol. 2004;150(2):105–12.
3. Baloch Z, Carayon P, Conte-Devolx B, et al. Laboratory medicine practice guidelines. Laboratory support for the diagnosis and monitoring of thyroid disease. Thyroid. 2003;13(1):3–126.
4. Benvenga S, Burek CL, Talor M, Rose NR, Trimarchi F. Heterogeneity of the thyroglobulin epitopes associated with circulating thyroid hormone autoantibodies in hashimoto's thyroiditis and non-autoimmune thyroid diseases. J Endocrinol Invest. 2002;25(11):977–82.
5. Spencer CA, Takeuchi M, Kazarosyan M, et al. Serum thyroglobulin autoantibodies: prevalence, influence on serum thyroglobulin measurement, and prognostic significance in patients with differentiated thyroid carcinoma. J Clin Endocrinol Metab. 1998; 83(4):1121–7.
6. Canaris GJ, Manowitz NR, Mayor G, Ridgway EC. The Colorado thyroid disease prevalence study. Arch Intern Med. 2000;160(4): 526–34.
7. Hollowell JG, Staehling NW, Flanders WD, et al. Serum TSH, T(4), and thyroid antibodies in the United States population (1988 to 1994):

National Health and Nutrition Examination Survey (NHANES III). J Clin Endocrinol Metab. 2002;87(2):489–99.
8. Hjiyiannakis P, Mundy J, Harmer C. Thyroglobulin antibodies in differentiated thyroid cancer. Clin Oncol (R Coll Radiol). 1999; 11(4):240–4.
9. Cunha LL, Soares FA, Vassallo J, Ward LS. The role of tumor-infiltrating lymphocytes in papillary thyroid carcinomas. J Endocrinol Invest. 2011;34(9):733.
10. Romaldini J, Villagelin D, Santos R. Is diffuse and peritumoral lymphocyte infiltration in papillary thyroid cancer a marker of good prognosis? J Endocrinol Invest. 2011;34:e403–8.
11. Kebebew E, Treseler PA, Ituarte PH, Clark OH. Coexisting chronic lymphocytic thyroiditis and papillary thyroid cancer revisited. World J Surg. 2001;25(5):632–7.
12. Kumar A, Shah DH, Shrihari U, Dandekar SR, Vijayan U, Sharma SM. Significance of antithyroglobulin autoantibodies in differentiated thyroid carcinoma. Thyroid. 1994;4(2):199–202.
13. McConahey WM, Hay ID, Woolner LB, van Heerden JA, Taylor WF. Papillary thyroid cancer treated at the Mayo Clinic, 1946 through 1970: initial manifestations, pathologic findings, therapy, and outcome. Mayo Clin Proc. 1986;61(12):978–96.
14. Preissner CM, O'Kane DJ, Singh RJ, Morris JC, Grebe SK. Phantoms in the assay tube: heterophile antibody interferences in serum thyroglobulin assays. J Clin Endocrinol Metab. 2003; 88(7):3069–74.
15. Giovanella L, Keller F, Ceriani L, Tozzoli R. Heterophile antibodies may falsely increase or decrease thyroglobulin measurement in patients with differentiated thyroid carcinoma. Clin Chem Lab Med. 2009;47(8):952–4.
16. Verburg FA, Waschle K, Reiners C, Giovanella L, Lentjes EG. Heterophile antibodies rarely influence the measurement of thyroglobulin and thyroglobulin antibodies in differentiated thyroid cancer patients. Horm Metab Res. 2010;42(10):736–9.
17. Chung JK, Park YJ, Kim TY, et al. Clinical significance of elevated level of serum antithyroglobulin antibody in patients with differentiated thyroid cancer after thyroid ablation. Clin Endocrinol (Oxf). 2002;57(2):215–21.
18. Spencer CA. Challenges of serum thyroglobulin (Tg) measurement in the presence of Tg autoantibodies. J Clin Endocrinol Metab. 2004;89(8):3702–4.
19. Chiovato L, Latrofa F, Braverman LE, et al. Disappearance of humoral thyroid autoimmunity after complete removal of thyroid antigens. Ann Intern Med. 2003;139(5 Pt 1):346–51.
20. American Thyroid Association Guidelines Task Force on Thyroid Nodules and Differentiated Thyroid Cancer. Haugen BR, Alexander EK, Bible KC, Doherty GM, Mandel SJ, Nikiforov YE, Pacini F, Randolph GW, Sawka AM, Schlumberger M, Schuff KG, Sherman SI, Sosa JA, Steward DL, Tuttle RM, Wartofsky L. 2015 American Thyroid Association Management Guidelines for Adult Patients with Thyroid Nodules and Differentiated Thyroid Cancer. Thyroid 2016;26:1–133.
21. Spencer C, Petrovic I, Fatemi S. Current thyroglobulin autoantibody (TgAb) assays often fail to detect interfering TgAb that can result in the reporting of falsely low/undetectable serum Tg IMA values for patients with differentiated thyroid cancer. J Clin Endocrinol Metab. 2011;96(5):1283–91.
22. Hung CJ, Ginzinger DG, Zarnegar R, et al. Expression of vascular endothelial growth factor-C in benign and malignant thyroid tumors. J Clin Endocrinol Metab. 2003;88(8):3694–9.
23. Klein M, Vignaud JM, Hennequin V, et al. Increased expression of the vascular endothelial growth factor is a pejorative prognosis marker in papillary thyroid carcinoma. J Clin Endocrinol Metab. 2001;86(2):656–8.
24. Viglietto G, Romano A, Manzo G, et al. Upregulation of the angiogenic factors PlGF, VEGF and their receptors (Flt-1, Flk-1/KDR) by TSH in cultured thyrocytes and in the thyroid gland of thiouracil-fed rats suggest a TSH-dependent paracrine mechanism for goiter hypervascularization. Oncogene. 1997;15(22):2687–98.
25. Karaca Z, Tanriverdi F, Unluhizarci K, et al. VEGFR1 expression is related to lymph node metastasis and serum VEGF may be a marker of progression in the follow-up of patients with differentiated thyroid carcinoma. Eur J Endocrinol. 2011;164(2):277–84.
26. Lin SY, Wang YY, Sheu WH. Preoperative plasma concentrations of vascular endothelial growth factor and matrix metalloproteinase 9 are associated with stage progression in papillary thyroid cancer. Clin Endocrinol (Oxf). 2003;58(4):513–8.
27. Pasieka Z, Stepien H, Komorowski J, Kolomecki K, Kuzdak K. Evaluation of the levels of bFGF, VEGF, sICAM-1, and sVCAM-1 in serum of patients with thyroid cancer. Recent Results Cancer Res. 2003;162:189–94.
28. Sorvillo F, Mazziotti G, Carbone A, et al. Recombinant human thyrotropin reduces serum vascular endothelial growth factor levels in patients monitored for thyroid carcinoma even in the absence of thyroid tissue. J Clin Endocrinol Metab. 2003;88(10):4818–22.
29. Tuttle RM, Fleisher M, Francis GL, Robbins RJ. Serum vascular endothelial growth factor levels are elevated in metastatic differentiated thyroid cancer but not increased by short-term TSH stimulation. J Clin Endocrinol Metab. 2002;87(4):1737–42.
30. Buitrago D, Keutgen XM, Crowley M, Filicori F, Aldailami H, Hoda R, Liu YF, Hoda RS, Scognamiglio T, Jin M, Fahey TJ 3rd, Zarnegar R. Intercellular adhesion molecule-1 (ICAM-1) is upregulated in aggressive papillary thyroid carcinoma. Annals of Surgical Oncology. 2012;19(3):973–80.
31. Liang H, Zhong Y, Luo Z, et al. Assessment of biomarkers for clinical diagnosis of papillary thyroid carcinoma with distant metastasis. Int J Biol Markers. 2010;25(1):38–45.
32. Pasieka Z, Kuzdak K, Czyz W, Stepien H, Komorowski J. Soluble intracellular adhesion molecules (sICAM-1, sVCAM-1) in peripheral blood of patients with thyroid cancer. Neoplasma. 2004; 51(1):34–7.
33. Wehmeier M, Petrich T, Brand K, Lichtinghagen R, Hesse E. Oncofetal fibronectin mRNA is highly abundant in the blood of patients with papillary thyroid carcinoma and correlates with high-serum thyroid-stimulating hormone levels. Thyroid. 2010; 20(6):607–13.
34. Wang JX, Yu JK, Wang L, Liu QL, Zhang J, Zheng S. Application of serum protein fingerprint in diagnosis of papillary thyroid carcinoma. Proteomics. 2006;6(19):5344–9.
35. Fan Y, Shi L, Liu Q, et al. Discovery and identification of potential biomarkers of papillary thyroid carcinoma. Mol Cancer. 2009;8:79.
36. Cradic KW, Milosevic D, Rosenberg AM, Erickson LA, McIver B, Grebe SK. Mutant BRAF(T1799A) can be detected in the blood of papillary thyroid carcinoma patients and correlates with disease status. J Clin Endocrinol Metab. 2009;94(12):5001–9.
37. Ditkoff BA, Marvin MR, Yemul S, et al. Detection of circulating thyroid cells in peripheral blood. Surgery. 1996;120(6):959–64. discussion 964-955.
38. Tallini G, Ghossein RA, Emanuel J, et al. Detection of thyroglobulin, thyroid peroxidase, and RET/PTC1 mRNA transcripts in the peripheral blood of patients with thyroid disease. J Clin Oncol. 1998;16(3):1158–66.
39. Ringel MD, Ladenson PW, Levine MA. Molecular diagnosis of residual and recurrent thyroid cancer by amplification of thyroglobulin messenger ribonucleic acid in peripheral blood. J Clin Endocrinol Metab. 1998;83(12):4435–42.
40. Bojunga J, Kusterer K, Schumm-Draeger PM, Usadel KH. Polymerase chain reaction in the detection of tumor cells: new approaches in diagnosis and follow-up of patients with thyroid cancer. Thyroid. 2002;12(12):1097–107.
41. Chinnappa P, Taguba L, Arciaga R, et al. Detection of thyrotropin-receptor messenger ribonucleic acid (mRNA) and thyroglobulin mRNA transcripts in peripheral blood of patients with thyroid disease: sensitive and specific markers for thyroid cancer. J Clin Endocrinol Metab. 2004;89(8):3705–9.

42. Fugazzola L, Mihalich A, Persani L, et al. Highly sensitive serum thyroglobulin and circulating thyroglobulin mRNA evaluations in the management of patients with differentiated thyroid cancer in apparent remission. J Clin Endocrinol Metab. 2002;87(7):3201–8.
43. Grammatopoulos D, Elliott Y, Smith SC, et al. Measurement of thyroglobulin mRNA in peripheral blood as an adjunctive test for monitoring thyroid cancer. Mol Pathol. 2003;56(3):162–6.
44. Span PN, Sleegers MJ, van den Broek WJ, et al. Quantitative detection of peripheral thyroglobulin mRNA has limited clinical value in the follow-up of thyroid cancer patients. Ann Clin Biochem. 2003;40(Pt 1):94–9.
45. Ringel MD. Molecular detection of thyroid cancer: differentiating "signal" and "noise" in clinical assays. J Clin Endocrinol Metab. 2004;89(1):29–32.
46. Gupta M, Taguba L, Arciaga R, Siperstein A, Faiman C, Mehta A, Sethu S. Detection of circulating thyroid cancer cells by reverse transcription-PCR for thyroid-stimulating hormone receptor and thyroglobulin: the importance of primer selection. Clin Chem. 2002;48(10):1862–5.
47. Milas M, Shin J, Gupta M, et al. Circulating thyrotropin receptor mRNA as a novel marker of thyroid cancer: clinical applications learned from 1758 samples. Ann Surg. 2010;252(4):643–51.
48. Bellantone R, Lombardi CP, Bossola M, et al. Validity of thyroglobulin mRNA assay in peripheral blood of postoperative thyroid carcinoma patients in predicting tumor recurrences varies according to the histologic type: results of a prospective study. Cancer. 2001;92(9):2273–9.
49. Elisei R, Vivaldi A, Agate L, et al. Low specificity of blood thyroglobulin messenger ribonucleic acid assay prevents its use in the follow-up of differentiated thyroid cancer patients. J Clin Endocrinol Metab. 2004;89(1):33–9.
50. Eszlinger M, Neumann S, Otto L, Paschke R. Thyroglobulin mRNA quantification in the peripheral blood is not a reliable marker for the follow-up of patients with differentiated thyroid cancer. Eur J Endocrinol. 2002;147(5):575–82.
51. Ringel MD, Balducci-Silano PL, Anderson JS, et al. Quantitative reverse transcription-polymerase chain reaction of circulating thyroglobulin messenger ribonucleic acid for monitoring patients with thyroid carcinoma. J Clin Endocrinol Metab. 1999;84(11):4037–42.
52. Savagner F, Rodien P, Reynier P, Rohmer V, Bigorgne JC, Malthiery Y. Analysis of Tg transcripts by real-time RT-PCR in the blood of thyroid cancer patients. J Clin Endocrinol Metab. 2002;87(2):635–9.
53. Wingo ST, Ringel MD, Anderson JS, et al. Quantitative reverse transcription-PCR measurement of thyroglobulin mRNA in peripheral blood of healthy subjects. Clin Chem. 1999;45(6 Pt 1): 785–9.
54. Yang C, Robbins PD. The roles of tumor-derived exosomes in cancer pathogenesis. Clin Dev Immunol. 2011;2011:842849.
55. Ringel MD. Metastatic dormancy and progression in thyroid cancer: targeting cells in the metastatic frontier. Thyroid. 2011;21(5):487–92.
56. Cristofanilli M, Budd GT, Ellis MJ, et al. Circulating tumor cells, disease progression, and survival in metastatic breast cancer. N Engl J Med. 2004;351(8):781–91.
57. Hoofnagle AN, Becker JO, Wener MH, Heinecke JW. Quantification of thyroglobulin, a low-abundance serum protein, by immunoaffinity peptide enrichment and tandem mass spectrometry. Clin Chem. 2008;54(11):1796–804.
58. Dufour DR. Thyroglobulin antibodies – failing the test. J Clin Endocrinol Metab. 2011;96(5):1276–8.

Ultrasound of the Neck Lymph Nodes

40

Andrea Frasoldati, Claudio Maurizio Pacella,
Enrico Papini, and Laszlo Hegedüs

Neck Lymph Node Anatomy and Topographic Classification

Cervical lymph nodes are classified into different subgroups according to their location. The scheme proposed by the American Academy of Otolaryngology – Head and Neck Surgery to unify the terminology in neck dissection procedures identifies two main topographic districts: the lateral (right and left) and the central neck compartments, which are in turn subdivided into a number of regions, called levels [1–7] (Fig. 40.1). This scheme has gained worldwide acceptance, is endorsed by the American Joint Committee on Cancer (AJCC), and is incorporated in the pTNM classification of thyroid cancer [8, 9]. Grossly, the lateral neck compartments (levels II–V) correspond to the areas bounded anteromedially by the carotid arteries and posterolaterally by the anterior margin of the trapezius muscles. The central neck compartment (levels VI–VII) extends from the hyoid bone, superiorly, to the innominate artery on the right and to the corresponding axial plane on the left, inferiorly, with the carotid arteries and the trachea marking its lateral and medial boundaries, respectively [1–7, 10]. Level I, delimited superiorly by the mandible, posteriorly by the stylohyoid muscle and anteriorly by the anterior belly of the digastric muscle, is neither included in the lateral nor in the central compartment neck dissections routinely adopted in the surgical management of patients with thyroid cancer. In fact, metastatic spread by thyroid cancer to the submental (level Ia) and submandibular (level Ib) lymph nodes, contained in level I, is extremely rare [1, 11]. In the lateral neck compartment, level II extends from the skull base to the lower margin of the hyoid bone, with the stylohyoid muscle and the posterior margin of the sternocleidomastoid muscle marking its anterior and posterior boundaries, respectively. Level II, in turn, is subdivided by the oblique course of the spinal accessory nerve into the upper and posterior level IIb and into the lower and anterior level IIa [2–4]. Lymph nodes located in level II, also known as the upper jugular nodes, are more likely to be involved by metastases from thyroid cancers located in the upper third of the thyroid lobes and from tumors of the oral and nasal cavity, pharynx, larynx, and parotid glands [11]. Levels III and IV encompass the area located between the hyoid bone and the lower margin of the cricoid cartilage and the area between this landmark and the clavicle, respectively, while the sternohyoid and the sternocleidomastoid muscle (posterior margin) mark the anterior and posterior boundaries of both levels [1–7]. Lymph nodes in levels III and IV, also referred to as mid- and lower jugular nodes, are frequently involved by metastases from thyroid cancer [12–21], as well as from tumors of the oral cavity, pharynx, larynx, and cervical esophagus [3, 11]. Level V coincides with the posterior triangle of the neck, located between the posterior margin of the sternocleidomastoid muscle, anteriorly, and the trapezius muscle, posteriorly, with the clavicle as the inferior and the muscle convergence as the superior boundary. A plane passing across the lower margin of the cricoid subdivides level

A. Frasoldati, MD, PhD
Endocrinology Unit, Arcispedale S. Maria Nuova - IRCCS, Reggio Emilia, Italy
e-mail: frasoldati.andrea@asmn.re.it

C.M. Pacella, MD
Department of Diagnostic Imaging and Interventional Radiology, Regina Apostolorum Hospital, Rome, Albano Laziale, Italy
e-mail: claudiomauriziopacella@gmail.com; claudiomaurizio.pacella@fastwebnet.it

E. Papini, MD, FACE
Endocrinology Unit, Regina Apostolorum Hospital, Rome, Albano Laziale, Italy
e-mail: enrico.papini@fastwebnet.it

L. Hegedüs, MD, DMSc (✉)
Department of Endocrinology and Metabolism, Odense University Hospital and University of Southern Denmark,
Kloevervaenget 6, 6th floor, Odense, Funen 5000 C, Denmark
e-mail: laszlo.hegedus@rsyd.dk

L. Wartofsky, D. Van Nostrand (eds.), *Thyroid Cancer*, DOI 10.1007/978-1-4939-3314-3_40

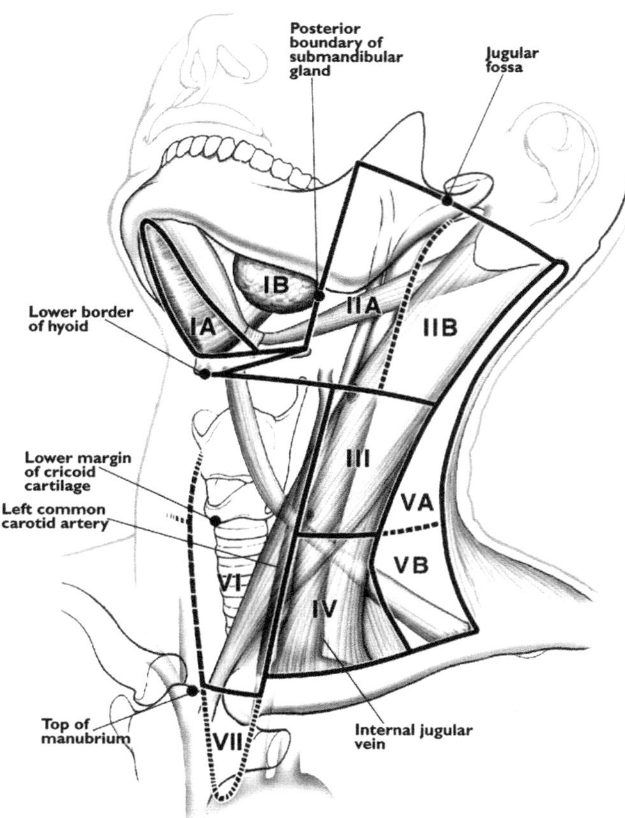

Fig. 40.1 American Academy of Otolaryngology – Head and Neck Surgery classification scheme for neck lymph node location

V into an upper (level VA) and a lower (level VB) region. Involvement of level V lymph nodes by thyroid malignancy occurs in a minority of patients, who usually present with level II–V metastases [20, 22, 23].

In the central neck compartment, level VI is defined by the carotid arteries laterally, the hyoid bone superiorly, and the suprasternal notch inferiorly. Level VI harbors the pre- and paratracheal lymph nodes, the parathyroidal nodes, and the so-called Delphian node, located on the cricothyroid membrane [1–7, 24]. The cranial portion of the anterosuperior mediastinum, immediately above the innominate artery, is also indicated as level VII. The innominate (or brachiocephalic) artery on the right and the corresponding axial plane on the left mark the lower border of the central compartment. In the clinical setting, the central compartment is often subdivided into two (left and right) or three (left, right, and median) sides, a distinction useful to direct surgical procedures as well as US examinations. However, viewed anatomically, this subdivision is somewhat arbitrary as the lymphatic drainage from the thyroid gland does not follow a strictly lateralized pathway [5].

Technique

For the purpose of US examination, lymph nodes belonging to the lateral neck compartment (levels II–V) are found in the triangular region covered anteriorly by the sternocleidomastoid muscle, while lymph nodes of the central neck compartment (levels VI–VII) are located in contiguity with the thyroid gland and the tracheal and esophageal walls.

The adoption of the bi-compartmental model as a reference point, when performing neck US, offers two major advantages. Firstly, the metastatic involvement of the lateral versus the central compartment is clinically relevant and may direct different surgical procedures [23, 25–31]. Secondly, it helps the sonographer to perform a systematic and accurate examination, minimizing the risk of overlooking any relevant findings. Usually, the inspection of the lateral compartment is more easily accomplished (perhaps with the exception of the posterior triangle) as compared to the central compartment, where the thyroid gland is a major obstacle for the complete ultrasonographic visualization of the lymph nodes located in level VI. In order to thoroughly evaluate levels VI and VII, the head of the patient needs to be fully hyperextended. Furthermore, the accuracy of the examination may be enhanced by various tactics, such as asking the patient to turn the head laterally, swallow, or perform a Valsalva maneuver [32–40].

Initially, the neck region should be examined using transverse planes from the midline to the carotid arteries (central compartment) and from the vascular axis to the posterior triangle (lateral compartment), on both sides. Transverse planes are more useful to obtain a panoramic view of the area and often allow the immediate recognition of major structural abnormalities. Along with midline to lateral shift, the probe should be directed on- and backward along a cranio-caudal direction, from level I to levels VI–VII (central compartment) and from levels II to level IV (lateral compartment). All the relevant findings will then be focused by gently changing the probe orientation in order to gain a detailed view of the object in the longitudinal plane. In case of enlarged and/or suspicious lymph nodes, size, US texture, and vascular architecture should be recorded along with a detailed topographic reference (level definition plus any relationship to a major anatomical structure, e.g., carotid artery, sternocleidomastoid muscle, thyroid capsule, etc.) [10, 32–40].

US Examination of Neck Lymph Nodes: Signs of Malignancy

US examination of neck lymph nodes is essentially based on the evaluation of their size, shape, texture, and vascular pattern. Sensitivity, specificity, and positive predictive value of most common US signs of malignancy are given in

Table 40.1. However, it should be emphasized that none of these parameters, when taken singularly, is 100 % specific and the perception of a lymph node as benign or suspicious is usually driven by the aggregate of all the characteristics [32, 33, 38, 39, 41–54]. At US examination, benign lymph nodes normally show a well-defined, oval-shaped profile. The US texture is typically homogeneous, mostly hypoechoic, with the exception of the echoic hilum structure (Fig. 40.2a). A clearly visible hilum can reliably be considered as a sign of benignity. Yet, the absence of a hilum is frequent and found in at least 40–50 % of benign lymph nodes [46]. The topographic location may also influence the relevance of the "hilum" sign. Thus, in the lateral neck compartment, the absence of a hilum is markedly more specific as a sign of malignancy, as compared to the central neck compartment [51]. In addition, a careful study by color-flow mapping may reveal the reassuring structure of a vascular hilum in most nodes which at first glance seem without a hilum [53]. It follows that the specificity of this sign is far from absolute, although in some studies the positive predictive value of the US absence of a hilum has been reported to be as high as 92 % [50].

Table 40.1 Sensitivity, specificity, and positive predictive value (PPV) of different US signs in the diagnosis of neck lymph node metastases from differentiated thyroid cancer

	Sensitivity (%)	Specificity (%)	PPV (%)
Hilum absence	31.6–100.0	29.0–90.0	54.0–92.0
Round shape	23.8–80.0	64.0–89.0	66.7–94.0
Irregular echogenicity	53.0–86.0	42.9–95.5	78.9–96.0
Cystic structure	11.0–38.0	87.0–100.0	97.0–100.0
Calcifications	3.0–49.5	91.0–100	95.0–100.0
Abnormal vascularization	47.0–86.0	57.1–99.0	76.9–97.0

Data obtained from references [42, 44, 46, 48–50]

Malignant lymph nodes are usually bigger than benign lymph nodes [46]. It is important to bear in mind that the size of benign inflammatory lymph nodes may be considerably increased as well, especially in young patients and in the lateral neck compartments. On the other hand, small (longest axis <10 mm) metastatic lymph nodes may often be detected in the central neck compartment. Therefore, the generic report of an enlarged lymph node cannot be claimed as suspicious, and no reliable cutoff value for the longest lymph node axis (i.e., the maximum diameter) can be regarded as proof of malignancy. Instead, the measurement of the shortest axis (i.e., the minimum diameter) seems clinically more relevant. Thus, a >7 mm shortest axis for level II lymph nodes and a >6 mm shortest axis for the rest of the neck have been reported to indicate malignancy with a 88.5 % accuracy [50]. In a retrospective series of 578 lymph nodes from 631 patients with thyroid cancer, nearly all (96.9 %) benign nodes and only half of the metastatic nodes showed a ≤1 cm minimum diameter [46]. In general, a ≥0.5 shortest to longest (S:L) axis ratio, also expressed as a ≤2 L:T (longitudinal to transverse diameter) ratio, typical of round-shaped lymph nodes, is a more reliable index of malignancy than the measurement of any single axis/diameter [10, 32, 41, 44, 46, 52, 55]. Again, the diagnostic accuracy of this sign may vary according to the neck district examined. In a series of 94 patients awaiting surgery for PTC, the specificity and PPV of the "round-shaped appearance" criteria were 90.2 % and 66.7 %, respectively, in level II–V lymph nodes, while these variables decreased to 11.3 % and 30.9 %, respectively, in level VI lymph nodes [51]. In fact, in patients with chronic autoimmune thyroiditis, small benign lymph nodes in the central compartment presenting with a round-shaped appearance are not infrequently observed [44, 56].

As a practical rule, any change in the usual lymph node size, profile, and/or structure detected during the course of

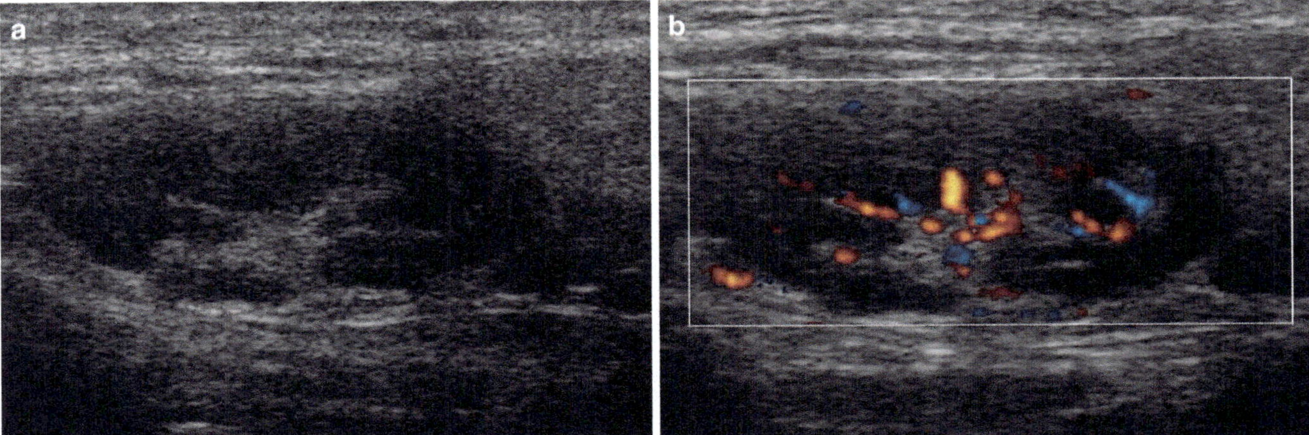

Fig. 40.2 Benign inflammatory lymph node. The shape is typically oval and elongated. The white hilum structure is quite evident in the frame of the hypoechoic and homogeneous node texture (Panel **a**). The vascular architecture (Panel **b**) resembles the branch of a tree

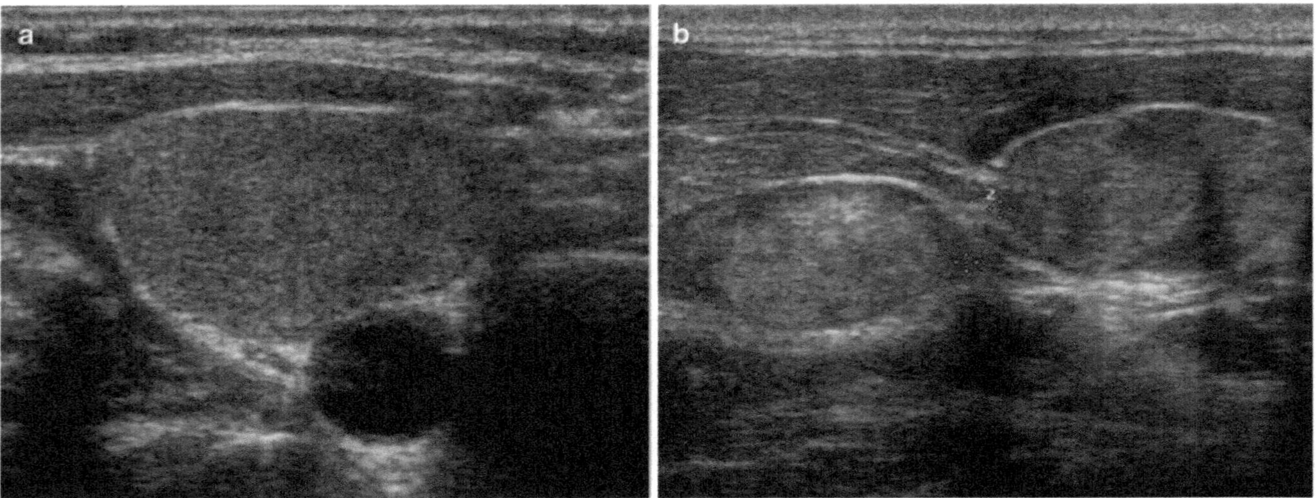

Fig. 40.3 (Panel **a**) Large metastatic lymph node in the lateral compartment, anterior to the carotid artery. US texture resembles that of the thyroid gland tissue. (Panel **b**) A couple of contiguous metastatic lymph nodes featuring a solid, inhomogeneous texture, a bumpy profile, and sharp borders

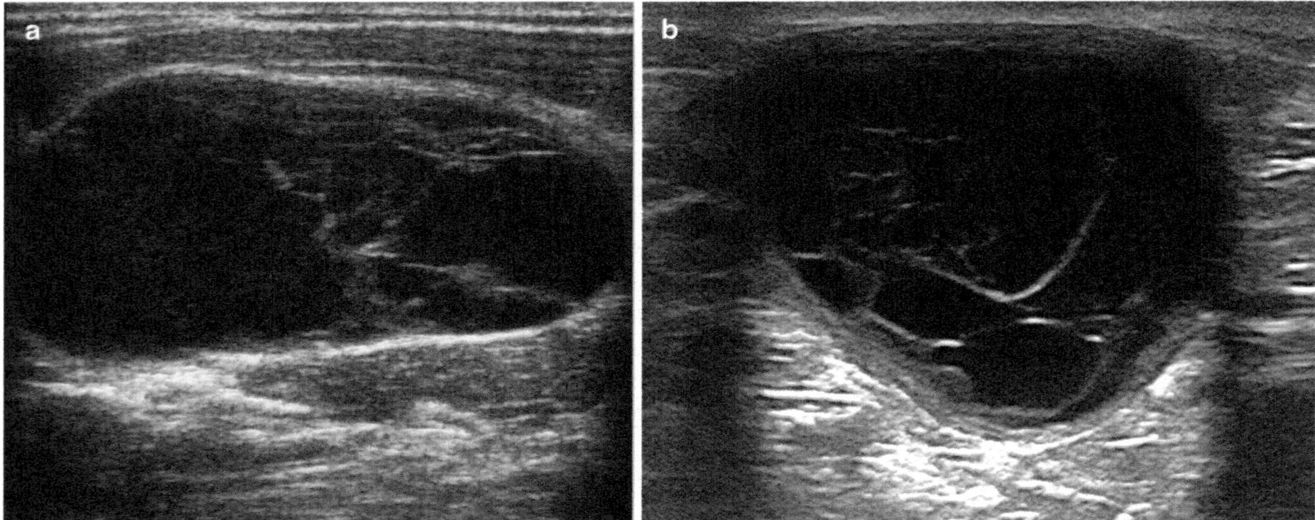

Fig. 40.4 (Panel **a**) Lymph node metastasis from papillary thyroid cancer. The node is frankly enlarged and shows a cystic content. (Panel **b**) Large branchial cleft cyst. Exemplifies that the differential diagnosis vis-à-vis a metastatic cystic lymph node may be challenging

neck US examinations warrants alertness. The attention of the US examiner may be caught by lymph nodes featuring a hyperechoic, parenchymatous-like texture, to some extent resembling the appearance of an "ectopic" thyroid nodule [45, 46, 49, 52] (Fig. 40.3). Interestingly, this sign has been more frequently observed in metastatic lymph nodes located in the lateral neck compartment [51]. A well-demarcated echogenic focus in the frame of the hypoechoic texture has also been described in lymph node metastases. The latter finding, likely to be erroneously interpreted as a thickened, irregular hilum, has been related to intranodal changes due to coagulation necrosis [49]. Microcalcifications, appearing as sparse hyperechoic speckles or isolated spots with posterior shadowing, may be detected in a minority of lymph node metastases from thyroid cancer [45, 46, 52]. As for thyroid nodules, this sign is quite specific, but its sensitivity, although variable in different studies, is generally low (Table 40.1). Lymph nodes exhibiting a mixed texture due to a fluid component, when not a frankly cystic appearance (Fig. 40.4a), should always be regarded as highly suspicious for thyroid cancer metastases, even in the absence of evident thyroid nodules. The finding of a cystic metastatic lymph node may in fact be the only US evidence of a papillary microcarcinoma [57–61]. In neck lymph nodes, cystic changes suggest metastases from thyroid cancer with 95–100 % specificity, with tuberculosis infection as the main differential diagnosis

[61–64]. Lymphomatous neck nodes may assume a pseudocystic balloon appearance, mimicking a cystic metastasis from thyroid cancer [65, 66]. Finally, metastatic lymph nodes may present with a thickened capsule, resulting in a well-defined and sharp border on US examination [49, 51], although this observation has been replicated only in a few studies and its clinical relevance remains to be fully elucidated. On the other hand, it has been suggested that the finding of ill-defined borders in a proven metastatic node may indicate extracapsular spread [48].

The evaluation of color-flow mapping may provide additional information, likely to become more relevant when the results from gray-scale US are equivocal [67]. On power Doppler US, a large percentage of normal lymph nodes will show an identifiable vascular architecture, with a predominantly hilar pattern [49, 55, 67, 68]. This usually appears as a centrally located, longitudinally oriented structure or, alternatively, as a dot-like polar vessel, with minor, symmetric radial branches originating from the hilar axis [67, 68]. Vascular mapping in benign lymph nodes may be extremely intense, occasionally quite scanty and faint, and even absent. Inflammatory lymph nodes sometimes exhibit a vascular arborization which is quite rich and diffuse but still with a preserved regular configuration [49, 67] (Fig. 40.2b). In contrast, malignant cervical nodes typically show an anarchical, multifocal vascular pattern, which is characterized by a mixed, peripheral and central, color-flow mapping. In particular, the finding of peripheral vascularity is considered a quite specific sign of malignancy [49, 51, 68] (Fig. 40.5). According to morphological studies, all these changes reflect neo-angiogenetic events in tumoral nests and neoplastic destruction of normal lymph node architecture [67–69]. The measurement of Doppler waveform parameters (e.g., resistance index = RI and pulsatility index = PI) does not offer additional clues and is of questionable relevance in a clinical context [49]. As a final remark, lymph node position is not an irrelevant factor in the assessment of potential malignancy. In fact, in patients with thyroid cancer, the majority of metastatic lymph nodes are found in the mid- to low jugular area (levels III–IV), while lymph nodes detected in levels I–II are more likely to be benign [46].

Other Neck Masses

Lymph nodes are usually easily recognized during US examination. But in the neck region, some lumps and masses may occasionally be encountered which offer differential diagnostic challenge vis-à-vis enlarged, suspicious lymph nodes [33, 55, 70–75]. Branchial cleft cysts (BCC) [66, 70, 76–78], originating from the second branchial pouch, are usually found in proximity of the mandibular angle and the submandibular salivary gland, superficially to the carotid artery and the internal jugular vein. The structure may appear as completely anechoic, due to pure fluid content, or pseudo-solid in case of cell debris, mucus, or blood clots (Fig. 40.4b). Although these lesions may be detected in asymptomatic patients, their enlargement is usually due to hemorrhagic or

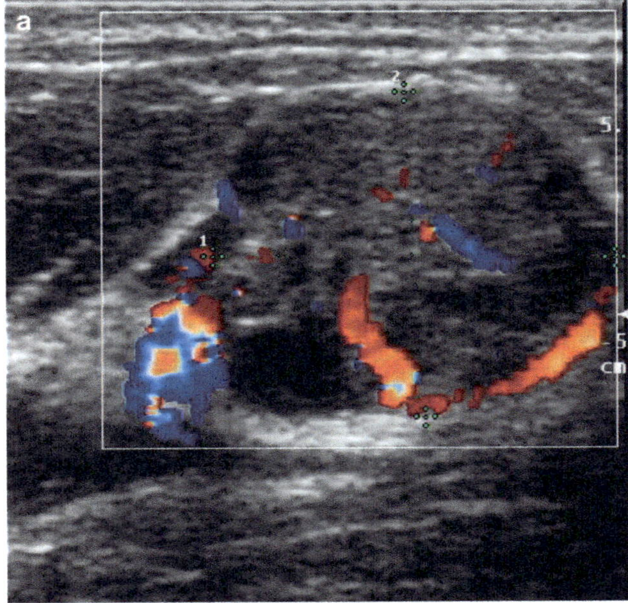

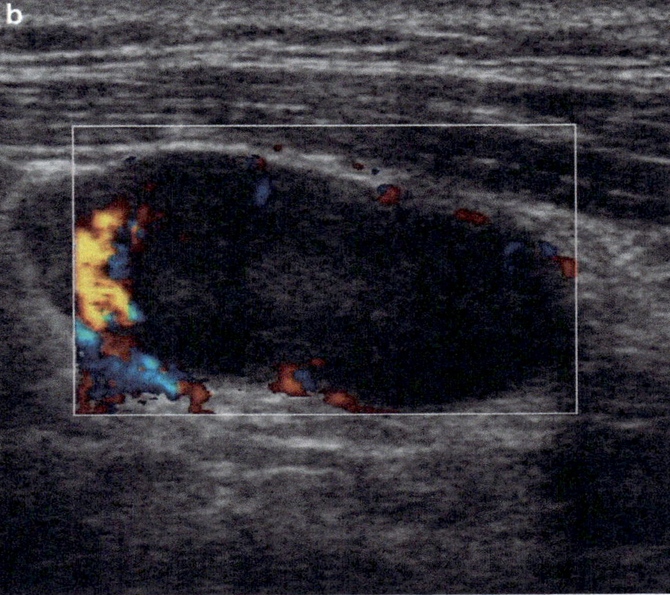

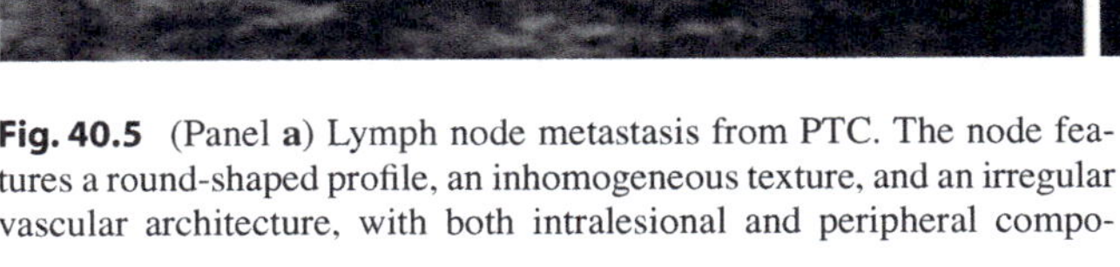

Fig. 40.5 (Panel **a**) Lymph node metastasis from PTC. The node features a round-shaped profile, an inhomogeneous texture, and an irregular vascular architecture, with both intralesional and peripheral components. (Panel **b**) Lymph node metastasis from PTC. The node is hypoechoic, without a visible hilum, and shows a clear peripheral vascular pattern

infectious complications, possibly causing discomfort, respiratory distress, or fever. BCC may also originate from the first branchial apparatus, but their location, usually within or strictly close to the parotid gland, may be more easily mistaken for salivary lesions (e.g., a Warthin tumor). Thyroglossal duct cysts (TDCs) [66, 70, 79–82] are usually located at the level of the hyoid bone (levels I–II), along or slightly lateral to the midline. Due to their position, TDCs are less likely to be misdiagnosed as abnormal lymph nodes. As for BCCs, their content may be purely fluid or show a solid component, which may require cytological sampling. TDCs are usually asymptomatic but may become infected with systemic bacteremia and manifest associated complications. Schwannomas and neurofibromas originating from the vagus nerve, the cervical sympathetic chain, or the cervical nerve roots, may present as oval hypoechoic neck lumps, sometimes endowed with a cystic component and posterior enhancement [66, 70, 74]. In patients treated with lateral neck dissection, postsurgical neuromas (Fig. 40.6), usually located along the surgical scar, may mimic metastatic lymph nodes, thus causing a false-positive US examination [83, 84]. As for schwannomas, a possible clue to the correct diagnosis comes from the detection of an elongated, rail track-like structure corresponding to the thickened nerve structure at one pole of the lesion. Moreover, FNA of these lesions may trigger an intense exacerbating pain accompanied by paresthesia, which is commonly considered diagnostic [70, 84]. Lymphangiomas and hemangiomas [70, 75], which usually appear as large, hypoechoic, and inhomogeneous masses, are a rare finding. Jugular vein thrombosis complicating a regionally aggressive thyroid tumor is another abnormal US finding which may be mistaken for a cystic metastatic neck node of the lateral compartment. Occasionally, a parathyroid adenoma may cause some challenges and mimic a metastatic lymph node in the central neck compartment.

Neck Ultrasonography in Thyroid Cancer Patients

Preoperative Neck US

US examination of the neck is fundamental in patients with newly diagnosed thyroid cancer awaiting surgery, as the surgical planning relies heavily on the information provided by US [24–27, 30, 85–87]. In fact, US is the most sensitive technique for detecting metastatic neck lymph nodes, showing an equal or superior accuracy as compared to computed tomography (CT) [36, 38, 86, 88, 89]. Based on this evidence, the systematic adoption of preoperative US followed by compartment-oriented surgery has effectively decreased recurrence rates [26, 27, 30, 31, 90]. In patients referred to surgery for thyroid cancer, US neck examination should aim at achieving a preoperative tumor staging [51, 89, 91, 92] and provide detailed information regarding both the primary tumor and neck lymph node status. In the following paragraphs, these two main components of US preoperative staging will be referred to as $_{u}T$ and $_{u}N$, respectively.

Firstly, US examination should be focused on $_{u}T$. Size and location of each thyroid nodule with a positive or suspicious cytology should be accurately reported, as this information may become relevant in the surgical planning as well as during surgery, should a frozen section be required. US signs of thyroid capsule infiltration or extracapsular tumor extension also need careful assessment together with signaling any clues suggestive of tumor multifocality and bilateral involvement. Although minimal extracapsular invasiveness, as well as microscopic multifocality, can neither reliably be ascertained nor completely ruled out by US, recent studies have reported encouraging results for US staging, with a 54.3–80.4 % and a 71.4–100.0 % PPV for extrathyroidal (pT3) and multifocal bilateral involvement, respectively [51, 52, 86, 91, 92].

The evaluation of $_{u}N$ is probably the major goal of preoperative US staging. Central and lateral neck compartments should be carefully assessed, taking into account fundamental knowledge regarding the patterns of metastatic spread in lymph node stations from thyroid cancer:

- The central neck compartment (level VI) is the most common site for thyroid cancer metastases. About 60–65 % of LNMs are found in the central compartment with pretracheal and ipsilateral paratracheal lymph nodes being most frequently involved [13, 20, 21, 93, 94]. However, the diagnostic performance of US, in this neck area, is far from optimal, and prophylactic central neck dissection often reveals LNM not apparent even to the most detailed and analytical presurgical US examination [26, 27, 51, 95, 96].
- The lateral neck compartment is affected in 15–25 % of patients with thyroid cancer. In order of prevalence, levels III, IV, and II are the most commonly involved [13, 15, 17, 19–21]. Level I metastases are quite rare. Level V metastases may be found only in a minority of patients, usually when levels II to IV are massively and/or bilaterally involved [20, 22, 23]. Although the involvement of the jugular chain is usually secondary to metastatic spread in the central compartment, skip metastases, defined as lateral lymph node metastases in the absence of central compartment involvement, may occur in a minor fraction (5–9 %) of N1 patients [20, 21, 87, 97–99]. From a clinical point of view, US examination of the lateral neck compartment is extremely relevant and any suspicious finding must be considered carefully and possibly be referred for FNA, as the presurgical evidence of LNM in the lateral compartment is a prerequisite for lateral neck dissection [25–27, 30, 85–87, 100].

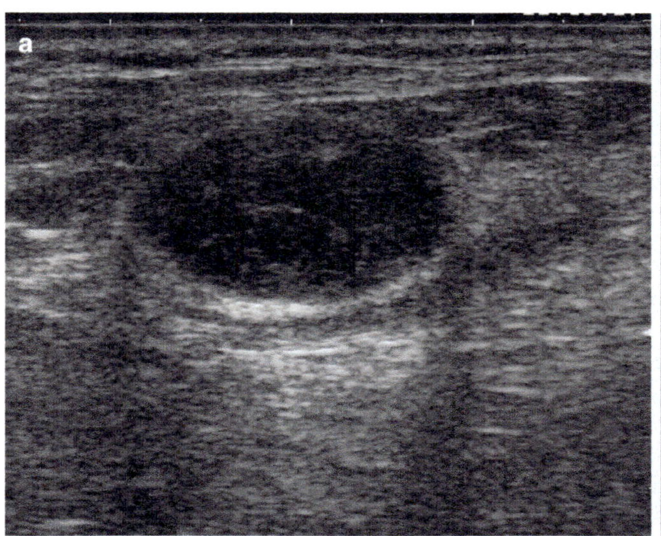

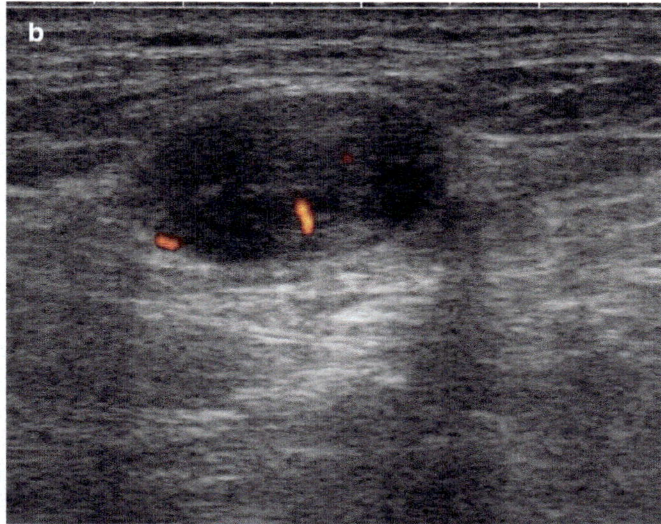

Fig. 40.6 Postsurgical neuroma in a patient previously treated by thyroidectomy and lateral neck dissection. The lesion is superficially located and appears as an oval, slightly inhomogeneous lump, with a hyperechoic posterior margin (Panel **a**). At one pole, the hypoechoic and almost avascular structure continues in an elongated tail (Panel **b**)

- Although a higher risk of lateral compartment involvement has been reported for tumors located in the upper third of thyroid lobes, the location of the primary tumor does not seem to be a critical factor in determining the pattern of lymph node metastases [93]. A higher frequency of bilateral spread has been suggested for tumors located in the isthmus, a finding not confirmed in other studies [93, 101, 102].

US signs and patterns which guide the evaluation and the interpretation of neck lymph nodes have been concisely reviewed in paragraph 2.1.3. Again, it should be emphasized that most available data concerning US appearance of LNM in thyroid cancer have been collected in series of patients with differentiated thyroid cancer. In medullary thyroid carcinoma, the US performance in the detection of LNM may to some extent be lower [25]. Nevertheless, further studies are needed to better clarify this issue. As already mentioned, the in situ thyroid gland constitutes a major limitation of the US inspection of the central neck compartment. In patients awaiting thyroidectomy, US sensitivity in detecting LNM located in the central neck compartment is remarkably lower as compared to the lateral neck compartment (about 25–50 % vs. 75–90 %, respectively) [35, 51, 53, 86, 91, 103]. In practice, this means that US, followed by FNA, usually permits a trustworthy presurgical diagnosis of LNM in the lateral compartment (Fig. 40.7), although the risk of a false-negative examination should always be taken into account, especially in case of a large, invasive primary tumor [104]. In contrast, the occurrence of LNM in the central compartment cannot be reliably excluded by a negative US study [88–92, 103]. On the other hand, US evidence of LNM in the central compartment (Fig. 40.8) usually indicates a higher risk of lateral compartment involvement, prompting for a more careful US examination of levels II–V. False-positive findings in the lateral neck compartment are usually due to enlarged inflammatory lymph nodes, but other causes of lymph node malignancy or neck masses may also be encountered [43, 49, 55, 66, 89]. Not to be forgotten, chronic autoimmune thyroiditis is a common cause of enlarged lymph nodes in the central neck compartment [44, 56].

Neck US in the Follow-Up of Thyroid Cancer: Why, When, and How?

Patients with thyroid cancer have a high frequency of neck recurrences (NRs), usually amenable to surgical treatment [105–108]. Since it has unanimously been recognized as a highly sensitive diagnostic tool for NR detection, neck US has therefore become a fundamental first-line tool in the postsurgical follow-up of patients with thyroid cancer [10, 34, 35, 55, 87, 109–117]. The importance of careful and regular neck US surveillance has further been stressed by the fact that NR from differentiated thyroid cancer may occur in the absence of detectable serum thyroglobulin (TG) or TG antibody (TGAb) levels [114, 118–120]. The term neck recurrence (NR) generally covers "any mass or lump unequivocally related to the thyroid tumor detected either in the thyroidal bed or in the lateral neck compartment, in patients under postsurgical surveillance." This definition is also adopted in the present paragraph. As a matter of fact, NR is often a sign of persistent disease rather than recurrent disease, since the majority of NRs are actually unrecognized

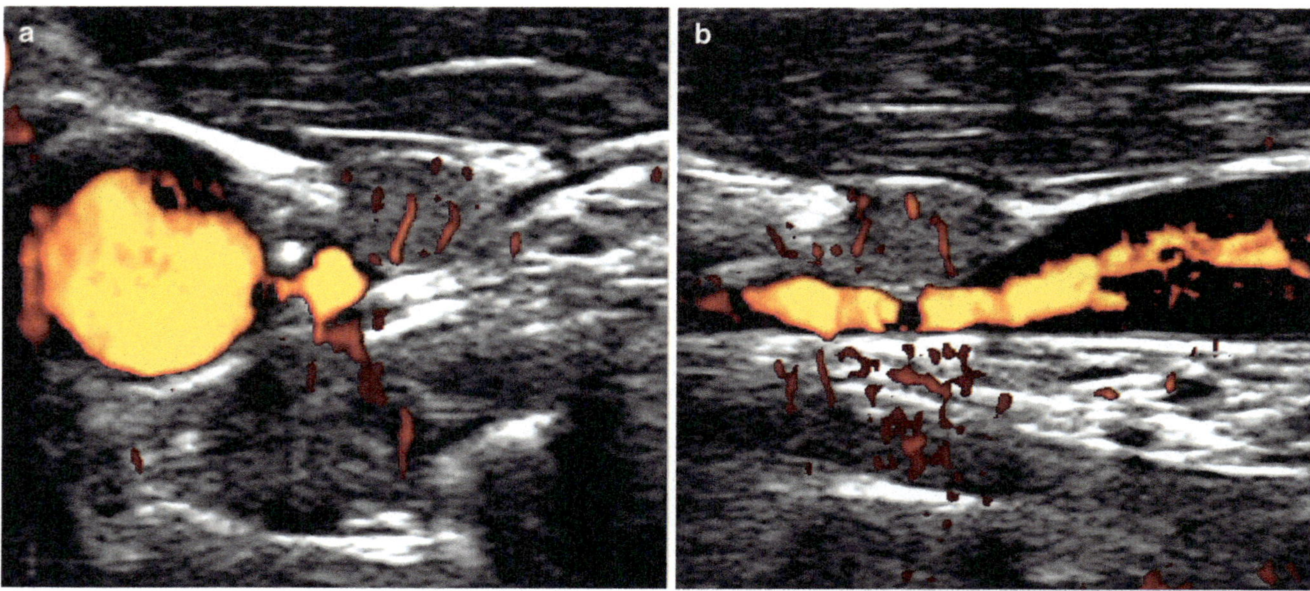

Fig. 40.7 Small (5 mm in diameter) metastatic lymph node in the left lateral neck compartment. The lesion is close to the carotid artery and anterior to the jugular vein (Panel **a**). The jugular walls are compressed with a narrowing of the vascular lumen (Panel **b**)

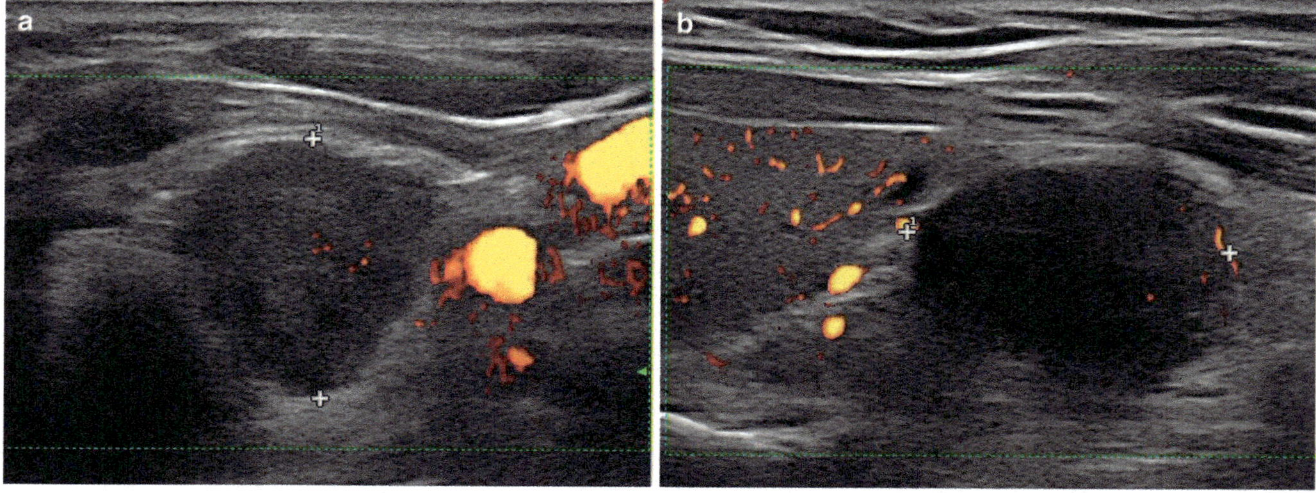

Fig. 40.8 Lymph node metastasis from MTC in the central neck compartment. The lesion is in tight contact with the tracheal wall (transverse scan, Panel **a**) and is located inferiorly to the lower pole of the left thyroid lobe (longitudinal scan, Panel **b**)

LNM at the preoperatory US staging or undetected during the course of neck surgery. While the role of neck US in the postsurgical follow-up of DTC has been addressed in many studies based on large series of patients, the evidence concerning US in the surveillance of MTC is much more limited. Accordingly, most data presented here concern DTC patients.

In patients undergoing postsurgical surveillance for DTC, the first US evaluation is commonly performed 2–3 months after initial surgery, at the time when patients who are candidates for radioiodine are going to receive ^{131}I-ablation treatment. Subsequent US controls are routinely scheduled on a 6–18-month basis, dependent on histology, pTNM staging, and the response to initial treatment testified by post-ablative whole body scintigraphy (WBS) results, serum TG levels, and previous US findings [109–112]. Indeed, all of these data are crucial for an accurate definition of the risk of recurrence in the individual patient [121–124]. Worth noting, although low-risk patients are obviously less prone to develop NR, at least 50 % of NR described in some series occur in low- and/or intermediate-risk patients [117].

The US technique in patients undergoing surveillance for thyroid cancer has previously been thoroughly reviewed [38, 55, 115–117, 125–127]. The procedure does not pose major difficulties, once the sonographer has become familiar with the anatomical changes secondary to thyroid excision, primarily the displacement of both jugular-carotid axes medially toward the trachea. Usually, while the right carotid artery comes into close contact with the tracheal wall, the left carotid artery is kept in a more lateral position by the esophagus. In the thyroidectomized patient, the trachea silhouette, the vascular axes, and the esophagus, along with muscular structures (pre-thyroidal muscles anteriorly, sternocleidomastoid and scalene muscles laterally, and longus colli muscles posteriorly), become the basic landmarks guiding the US examination [10, 55, 116, 126, 127]. For an accurate US examination, the sonographer should focus, in sequence, on the central and the lateral neck compartments, using both transverse and longitudinal scanning planes. The transverse planes are preferentially used to spot any lesion worthy of careful examination, while the longitudinal planes are useful to obtain more detailed and complete data (e.g., size, shape, color-flow mapping) of any lesion detected. The accuracy of US examination will be enhanced by a methodical approach by the sonographer, with all the neck regions inspected through a succession of contiguous transverse planes from the midline to both the right and the left vascular axes (the central compartment) and from the vascular axes to the posterior triangle (the lateral compartments). Obviously, along with gently shifting the transducer from the medial to the lateral direction, the sonographer should also continuously move the probe along the cranio-caudal axis (e.g., from the hyoid bone to the sternal notch in the central compartment and from the mandibular angle to the supraclavicular region in the lateral compartments) with a movement imitating that of painting a fence. This ensures that the whole neck is fully explored.

Neck Recurrence of Thyroid Cancer: US and Clinical Aspects

According to the data acquired from most series of patients under postsurgical surveillance for thyroid cancer, the majority of NR seems to occur in the central neck compartment [128]. NR in the central neck compartment usually develops from level VI to VII (pre- and/or paratracheal) lymph nodes, although for lesions located in the more lateral portion of the thyroidal bed close to the carotid artery, an origin from lateral compartment lymph nodes slid medially after thyroid excision has also been reported [117]. A minority of NRs do not originate from lymph nodes, but represent either "true" recurrences of the primary tumor or soft tissue metastases. Such cases, although admittedly few, have a poorer prognosis.

At US examination, central compartment NR typically appears as small (<10 mm in diameter) round-shaped, homogeneous hypoechoic lumps (Fig. 40.9a), with a faint vascularity at color-flow mapping. Inhomogeneous texture, cystic changes, and calcifications may also be seen [115–117, 125]. As recently suggested, an internally vascularized, >6 mm in diameter, hypoechoic lesion, located in the thyroidal bed, is to be considered as highly predictive of NR [127]. However, no US signs allow distinguishing, with absolute certainty, NR from a number of benign lesions (e.g., thyroid remnants, scar tissue, suture granulomata, enlarged parathyroid glands, benign lymph nodes, and esophageal diverticulas), which may be seen in the thyroidal bed [115, 117, 125, 127, 129–131]. Therefore, as a rule, FNA is required to achieve a reliable diagnosis. Of course, the significance of US findings need always to be weighed in the clinical context, taking into account the patient's history, prognosis, and the complete clinical data set. NR presenting with the above

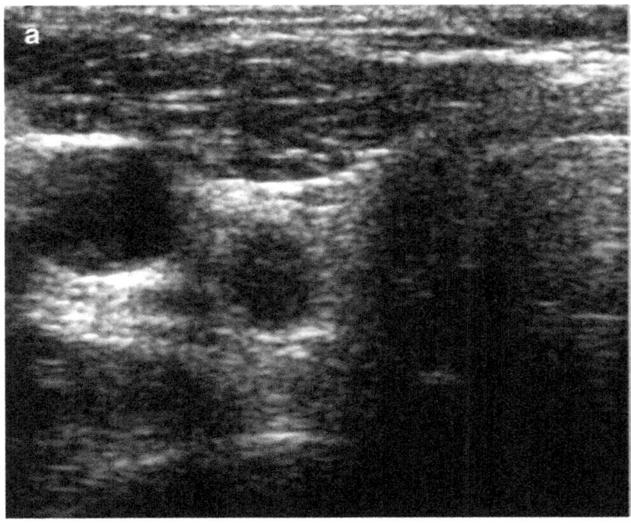

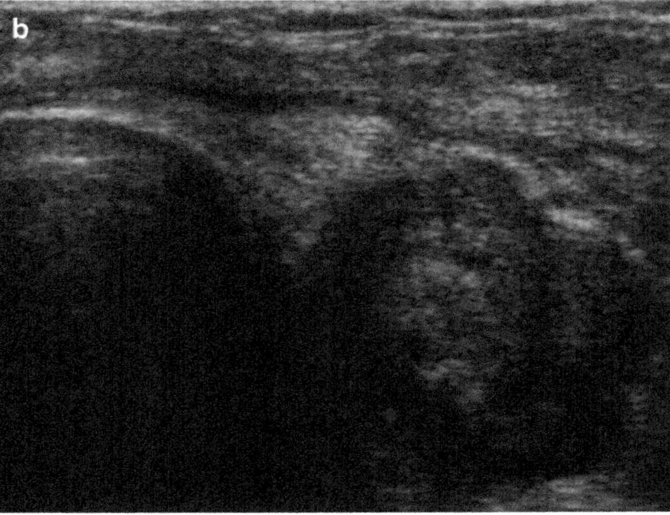

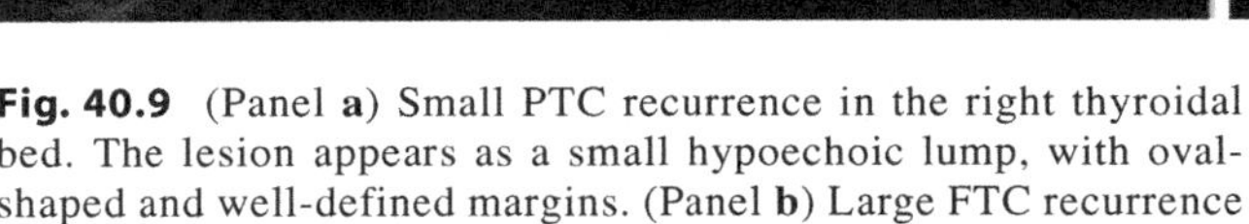

Fig. 40.9 (Panel **a**) Small PTC recurrence in the right thyroidal bed. The lesion appears as a small hypoechoic lump, with oval-shaped and well-defined margins. (Panel **b**) Large FTC recurrence in the left thyroidal bed. The lesion has an inhomogeneous texture, mostly hypoechoic, and an irregular shape with lobulated margins

depicted features should not always be perceived as clinically threatening. In general, following a diagnosis of NR, the choice between aggressive management and, alternatively, a wait and see strategy depends on a number of factors. Thus, the natural history of the disease, the perceived prognosis and comorbidity, and the hazards related to the available treatments all need to be evaluated. In most low- or intermediate-risk patients with PTC, the finding of a 4–5 mm neck node metastasis in the central compartment may not warrant immediate surgical treatment [112, 117, 127, 128]. Instead, in patients under surveillance for more dangerous histological types or variants of thyroid cancer (e.g., tall cell variant of PTC, widely invasive FTC, MTC, etc.), NR in the thyroidal bed may correspond to a rapidly growing lesion, likely to infiltrate the nearby anatomical structures (Fig. 40.9b). Based on this, finding a large, irregular-shaped lesion, possibly exhibiting a marked diffuse vascularization, in a patient undergoing surveillance for a high-risk thyroid cancer should, without undue hesitation, undergo imaging studies (e.g., CT or MR) to better clarify the true nature of the signs of local invasion and, if necessary, offer prompt treatment [117, 127, 128].

In most cases, NR located in the lateral neck compartment corresponds to level II–IV LNM, featuring suspicious US signs as those previously described. Although their identification does not usually pose major problems, in a minority of patients, NR in the lateral neck compartment may either be located in less frequently involved sites (e.g., the mandibular angle or the posterior neck triangle) or have a less typical appearance, thereby representing a major diagnostic challenge even to an experienced sonographer. US cannot distinguish, with 100 % accuracy, benign from malignant lesions in the neck lymph nodes. Also, the detection of enlarged clearly suspicious lymph nodes in a patient with a history of thyroid cancer does not automatically indicate metastases from a thyroid tumor. Other causes for malignant lymphadenopathy should always be considered and be clarified by FNA [52, 55, 132–134].

US-Guided FNA of Neck Lymph Nodes

Technique

In most institutions, FNA is routinely performed under US guidance using a 7.5–15 mHz frequency probe mounted on a digital US scanner equipped with a needle pointing device. Alternatively, the FNA procedure may be performed under US assistance, i.e., without a pointing device as a guide to the needle insertion, using either a transverse or a longitudinal approach. Both procedures are reported to be equally accurate and safe. The US-guided procedure allows a precise targeting of the lesion, with the limitation that the needle track is substantially specific and major correction is not possible once the needle has been inserted. US-assisted procedures require caution during the needle insertion, but offer the advantage of allowing major adjustments of the needle tracking to and within the lesion. A 23–26 gauge needle is usually inserted into the lymph node under visual US control. Aspiration may be facilitated by connecting the needle to a 20 ml Cameco®-mounted syringe. The FNA procedure is well tolerated by all patients and devoid of major complications. Mild subcutaneous bleeding may be observed in a minority of patients but no treatment apart from application of an ice pack is usually required. In patients with thyroid cancer metastases, seeding of malignant cells into the surrounding tissues due to the FNA maneuver has never been demonstrated. US-guided FNAB is a safe and accurate technique for identifying malignant lymph nodes [132–134]. Unfortunately, in some series up to 15–25 % of cytological smears have been reported as nondiagnostic, mainly due to scarcity of cellular material and/or blood cell contamination [52, 55, 135, 136]. The issue of a nondiagnostic cytological sample is particularly relevant in case of cervical cystic lesion [55, 136–138]. Given this problem, measurement of thyroid cancer "markers" (e.g., Tg or calcitonin) in the needle washout has proved to be a simple and effective tool for enhancing the diagnostic accuracy of FNA in patients with a history of thyroid cancer.

Tumor Marker Assays in the Needle Washout

The measurement of Tg levels in the needle washout (FNA-Tg) is a useful adjunct to cytology in the diagnosis of locoregional metastases of DTC, both in patients awaiting surgery and in those under postsurgical surveillance. FNA-Tg, originally proposed in the 1990s [139, 140], enhances the sensitivity and specificity of the procedure. It allows bypassing the limitations of cytology, due to possible scarcity of cellular material and/or blood cell contamination. In a series of 70 patients with DTC (122 lymph nodes) and 60 patients without thyroid disease (94 lymph nodes), the combination of cytology and FNA-Tg achieved a 92.0 % sensitivity versus the 84.0 % sensitivity of cytology alone [141]. Other studies report a 100 % sensitivity of cytology plus FNA-Tg in the diagnosis of cervical metastases [138–140, 142–147]. The major problem with FNA-Tg is the lack of standardized cutoff values. Different FNA-Tg thresholds, ranging from 1.0 to 36.0 ng/ml, have been proposed in various studies. All of them show good accuracy [141–156] (Table 40.2).

This issue is not yet laid to rest. For instance, the variation in the analytical performance of different Tg assays [144, 157] is still a matter of controversy. Furthermore, provided the sample is diluted in a constant volume of saline (1.0 ml

Table 40.2 FNA-Tg: cutoff values and diagnostic sensitivity and specificity reported in different studies

	Patients	Cutoff definition	Cutoff values (ng/ml)	Sensitivity (%)	Specificity (%)	LNM with inconclusive or negative cytology (%)
Frasoldati et al. [140]	70 (pre- and post-Tx)	97.5 percentile	39.3[a]	92	100	16.0
			1.1[b]			
Boi et al. [149]	73 (pre-and post-Tx)	> peak level in control samples	36[a]	100	100	14.8
			1.7[b]			
Cunha et al. [142]	67 (pre-and post-Tx)	Mean ± 2SD control group	0.9	100[c]	100	34.2
Snozek et al. [143]	88 (post-Tx)	ROC curve	1.0	100	96.2	15.9
Kim et al. [152]	168 (pre- and post-Tx)	ROC curve	10[d]	90.8	89.8	36.0
Jeon et al. [151]	161 (pre- and post-Tx)	> serum Tg levels	36[e]	94.6	90.0	19.6
Lee et al. [153]	40 (post-Tx)	ROC curve	4.1	100	100	40.0
Giovanella et al. [144]	108 (post-Tx)	ROC curve	1.1	100	100	23.0
Salmashoglu et al. [145]	225 (pre- and post-Tx)	ROC curve	28.5	100	96.0	5.0
Kim et al. [156]	68 (pre- and post-Tx)	Reference value of serum Tg	50.0	92	90.5	16.5
Jung et al. [147]	161 (pre- and post-Tx)	ROC curve	1.8	96.1	94.0	15.6
Moon et al. [146]	419 (pre- and post-Tx)	ROC curve	1.0	93.2	95.9	13.9

Pre-Tx pts patients awaiting thyroidectomy, *Post-Tx pts* thyroidectomized patients
[a]Cutoff values calculated in pre-Tx patients
[b]Cutoff values calculated in post-Tx patients
[c]Sensitivity was lower when also patients with poorly differentiated and anaplastic thyroid cancer were considered
[d]Sensitivity and specificity values reported here are calculated using 10 ng/ml as FNA-Tg cutoff values. In the study by Kim et al. [141], diagnostic performance of FNA-Tg, using different cutoff values (e.g., 1.0 ng/ml and 100 ng/ml), is also reported
[e]This FNA-Tg cutoff value was used in the study by Jeon et al. [140], when serum Tg levels were not available

in most studies), the amount of cell material collected in the needle cannot be precisely quantified. This unavoidable limitation renders FNA-Tg a semiquantitative technique. Notwithstanding, some conclusions can be drawn from the available literature and everyday experience. Firstly, the result of FNA-Tg measurements should always be balanced against serum Tg, and FNA-Tg levels can only be considered as “positive” if significantly higher than the corresponding serum Tg levels. This is to say that in a patient with high serum Tg levels (e.g., 500 ng/ml due to distant metastases), a 550 ng/ml FNA-Tg result could be due to blood contamination, not necessarily implying the presence of thyroid cells in the sampled material. Similarly, in thyroidectomized patients with low, yet detectable, serum Tg levels (e.g., 2–5 ng/ml), the finding of slightly higher FNA-Tg values (e.g., 7.5–10 ng/ml) should not at face value be viewed as a positive result. Interestingly, data obtained in two series of patients who underwent total thyroidectomy and subsequent radioiodine ablation have shown that the adoption of a 1.0–1.1 ng/ml FNA-Tg threshold may allow an accurate diagnosis in all cases with a nondiagnostic cytology [143, 144]. However, metastatic lymph nodes usually exhibit frankly elevated (e.g., 1,000–10.000 ng/ml) FNA-Tg levels. This implies that a cautious interpretation of low (e.g., 1–10 ng/ml) FNA-Tg levels is advisable, even in patients with undetectable serum Tg levels. In case of uncertain results, detection of thyroglobulin mRNA in the needle washouts has also been proposed [158, 159].

Although rarely, FNA-Tg may provide both false-negative and false-positive results. False-negative results may be due to the hook effect observed with immunometric assays at exceedingly high analyte concentrations or may occasionally be due to dedifferentiation of the neoplastic tissue [149, 150, 154]. Instead, even high titers of circulating TgAb have been shown not to cause any interference in FNA-Tg measurements [135–149]. False-positive results may also be generated by laboratory artifacts, e.g., heterophilic antibodies. However, they are more easily observed in case a thyroid remnant is targeted by FNA. Hence, it must be undescored that even clearcut (e.g., >2,000 ng/ml) FNA-Tg levels cannot be taken as indicative of NR when obtained from a lesion located in the thyroidal bed. Under such circumstances, FNA-Tg results should be carefully weighed in the context of US findings and cytological results [160].

Studies focusing on the diagnostic accuracy of calcitonin (CT) measurement in the needle washouts (FNA-CT) are quite few and only reported in small series of patients. Moreover, most of them are focused on the diagnosis of the primary tumor and do not specifically address the utility of this technique in LNM or NR from MTC [161–164].

Nevertheless, the results obtained are in line with those related to FNA-Tg. The technique is reliable, with a reported 100 % sensitivity and a 100 % specificity versus a 61.9 % sensitivity and a 80.0 % specificity of cytology alone [161]. On this basis, FNA-CT has been recommended as a useful tool in the evaluation of thyroid nodules as well as neck lymph nodes suspected of primary or metastatic MTC [112, 113, 165].

References

1. Robbins KT, Medina JE, Wolfe GT, et al. Standardizing neck dissection terminology. Official report of the Academy's Committee for head and neck surgery and oncology. Arch Otolaryngol Head Neck Surg. 1991;117:601–5.
2. Som PM, Curtin HD, Mancuso AA. Imaging-based nodal classification for evaluation of neck metastatic adenopathy. Am J Roentgenol. 2000;174:837–44.
3. Robbins KT, Clayman G, Levine PA, et al. Neck dissection classification update: revisions proposed by the American Head and Neck Society and the American Academy of Otolaryngology-Head and Neck Surgery. Arch Otolaryngol Head Neck Surg. 2002;128:751–8.
4. Robbins KT, Shaha AR, Medina JE, et al. Consensus statement on the classification and terminology of neck dissection: committee for neck dissection classification, American Head and Neck Society. Arch Otolaryngol Head Neck Surg. 2008;134:536–8.
5. Carty SE, Cooper DS, Doherty GM, et al. Consensus statement on the terminology and classification of central neck dissection for thyroid cancer. Thyroid. 2009;19:1153–8.
6. Orloff and Kuppersmith American Thyroid Associations. Central neck dissection terminology and classification for thyroid cancer consensus statement. Otolaryngol Head Neck Surg. 2010;142:4–5.
7. Ruggiero FP, Meyers AD. Neck dissection, classification. http://emedicine.medscape.com/article/849834-overview. Updated: 29 July 2008.
8. Shaha AR. TNM classification of thyroid carcinoma. World J Surg. 2007;31:879–87.
9. Edge SB, Byrd DR, Compton CC, et al., editors. AJCC cancer staging manual. 7th ed. New York: Springer; 2010. p. 87–96.
10. Randolph G, Sacks B, Baskin HJ. Ultrasound and mapping of the neck lymph nodes. In: Baskin HJ, Duick DS, Levine RA, editors. Thyroid ultrasound and ultrasound-guided FNA. 3rd ed. New York: Springer; 2013. p. 149–77.
11. Pfister DG, Ang K-K, Brizel DM, et al. Head and neck cancers. Clinical practice guidelines in oncology. J Natl Comp Cancer Netw. 2011;6:596–650.
12. Shaha AR, Shah JP, Loree TR. Patterns of nodal and distant metastasis based on histological varieties in differentiated carcinoma of the thyroid. Am J Surg. 1996;172:692–4.
13. Gimm O, Rath FW, Fralle H. Pattern of lymph node metastases in papillary thyroid carcinoma. Br J Surg. 1998;85:252–4.
14. Moley JF, Debenedetti MK. Patterns of nodal metastases in palpable medullary thyroid carcinoma: recommendations for extent of node dissection. Ann Surg. 1999;299:880–8.
15. Sivanandan R, Soo KC. Pattern of cervical lymph node metastases from papillary carcinoma of the thyroid. Br J Surg. 2001;88:1241–4.
16. Machens A, Hinze R, Thomusch O, et al. Pattern of nodal metastasis for primary and reoperative thyroid cancer. World J Surg. 2002;26:22–8.
17. Wada N, Duh QY, Sugino K, et al. Lymph node metastasis from 259 papillary thyroid microcarcinomas: frequency, pattern of occurrence and recurrence, and optimal strategy for neck dissection. Ann Surg. 2003;237:399–407.
18. Kupferman ME, Patterson M, Mandel SJ, et al. Patterns of lateral neck metastasis in papillary thyroid carcinoma. Arch Otolaryngol Head Neck Surg. 2004;130:857–60.
19. Caron NR, Tan YY, Ogilvie JB, et al. Selective modified radical neck dissection for papillary thyroid cancer – is level I, II and V dissection always necessary? World J Surg. 2006;30:833–40.
20. Roh J-L, Kim J-M, Park C. Lateral cervical lymph node metastases from papillary thyroid carcinoma: pattern of nodal metastases and optimal strategy for neck dissection. Ann Surg Oncol. 2008;15:1177–82.
21. Yüce I, Çağlı S, Ali Bayram A, et al. Regional metastatic pattern of papillary thyroid carcinoma. Eur Arch Otorhinolaryngol. 2010;267:437–41.
22. Yanir Y, Doweck I. Regional metastases in well-differentiated thyroid carcinoma: pattern of spread. Laryngoscope. 2008;118:433–6.
23. Kupferman ME, Weinstock YE, Santillan AA, et al. Predictors of level V metastasis in well-differentiated thyroid cancer. Head Neck. 2008;30:1469–74.
24. Oh EM, Chung YS, Lee YD. Clinical significance of Delphian lymph node metastasis in papillary thyroid carcinoma. World J Surg. 2013.37:2594-9.
25. Kouvaraki MA, Shapiro SE, Fornage BD, et al. Role of preoperative ultrasonography in the surgical management of patients with thyroid cancer. Surgery. 2003;134:946–54.
26. Ito Y, Tomoda C, Uruno T, et al. Preoperative ultrasonographic examination for lymph node metastasis: usefulness when designing lymph node dissection for papillary microcarcinoma of the thyroid. World J Surg. 2004;28:498–501.
27. Sugitani I, Fujimoto Y, Yamada K, et al. Prospective outcomes of selective lymph node dissection for papillary thyroid carcinoma based on preoperative ultrasonography. World J Surg. 2008;32:2494–502.
28. Hartl DM, Travagli J-P. The updated American Thyroid Association guidelines for management of thyroid nodules and differentiated thyroid cancer: the surgical perspective. Thyroid. 2009;19:1149–51.
29. Roh JL, Park JY, Kim JM, et al. Use of preoperative ultrasonography as guidance for neck dissection in patients with papillary thyroid carcinoma. J Surg Oncol. 2009;99:28–31.
30. Grant CS, Stulak JM, Thompson GB, et al. Risks and adequacy of an optimized surgical approach to the primary surgical management of papillary thyroid carcinoma treated during 1999–2006. World J Surg. 2010;34:1239–46.
31. Clark OH. Thyroid cancer and lymph node metastases. J Surg Oncol. 2011;103:615–8.
32. Haber RS. Role of ultrasonography in the diagnosis and management of thyroid cancer. Endocr Pract. 2000;6:396–400.
33. Wong KT, Ahuja AT. Ultrasound of thyroid cancer. Cancer Imaging. 2005;5:157–66.
34. Fish SA, Langer JE, Mandel SJ. Sonographic imaging of thyroid nodules and cervical lymph nodes. Endocrinol Metab Clin N Am. 2008;37:401–17.
35. Langer JE, Mandel SJ. Sonographic imaging of cervical lymph nodes in patients with thyroid cancer. Neuroimaging Clin N Am. 2008;18:479–89.
36. King AD. Imaging for staging and management of thyroid cancer. Cancer Imaging. 2008;8:57–69.
37. Sipos JA. Advances in ultrasound for the diagnosis and management of thyroid cancer. Thyroid. 2009;9:1363–72.
38. Lew JI, Solorzano CC. Use of ultrasound in the management of thyroid cancer. Oncologist. 2010;15:253–8.

39. Lee K, Kawata R, Nishikawa S, et al. Diagnostic criteria of ultrasonographic examination for lateral node metastasis of papillary thyroid carcinoma. Acta Otolaryngol. 2010;130:161–6.
40. Sheth S. Role of ultrasonography in thyroid disease. Otolaryngol Clin N Am. 2010;43:239–55.
41. Ahuja AT, Chow L, Chick W, et al. Metastatic cervical nodes in papillary carcinoma of the thyroid: ultrasound and histological correlation. Clin Radiol. 1995;50:229–31.
42. Ying M, Ahuja A. Sonography of neck lymph nodes. I. Normal lymph nodes. Clin Radiol. 2003;58:351–8.
43. Ahuja A, Ying M. Sonography of neck lymph nodes. II. Abnormal lymph nodes. Clin Radiol. 2003;58:359–66.
44. Frasoldati A, Valcavi R. Challenges in neck ultrasonography: lymphadenopathy and parathyroid glands. Endocr Pract. 2004;10:261–8.
45. Ahuja AT, Ying M. Sonographic evaluation of cervical lymph nodes. AJR Am J Roentgenol. 2005;184:1691–9.
46. Kuna SK, Bracic I, Tesic V, et al. Ultrasonographic differentiation of benign from malignant neck lymphadenopathy in thyroid cancer. J Ultrasound Med. 2006;25:1531–7.
47. Chan JM, Shin LK, Jeffrey RB. Ultrasonography of abnormal neck lymph nodes. Ultrasound Q. 2007;23:47–54.
48. Leboulleux S, Girard E, Rose M, et al. Ultrasound criteria of malignancy for cervical lymph nodes in patients followed up for differentiated thyroid cancer. J Clin Endocrinol Metab. 2007;92:3590–4.
49. Ahuja AT, Ying M, Ho SY, et al. Ultrasound of malignant cervical lymph nodes. Cancer Imaging. 2008;8:48–56.
50. Sousa do Rosario PW, de Faria S, Bicalho L, et al. Ultrasonographic differentiation between metastatic and benign lymph nodes in patients with papillary thyroid carcinoma. J Ultrasound Med. 2005;24:1385–9.
51. Park JS, Son KR, Na DG, et al. Performance of preoperative sonographic staging of papillary thyroid carcinoma based on the sixth edition of the AJCC/UICC TNM classification system. AJR Am J Roentgenol. 2009;192:66–72.
52. Sohn Y-M, Kwak JY, Kim E-K, et al. Diagnostic approach for evaluation of lymph node metastasis from thyroid cancer using ultrasound and fine-needle aspiration biopsy. AJR Am J Roentgenol. 2010;194:38–43.
53. Wu LM, Gu HY, Qu XH, et al. The accuracy of ultrasonography in the preoperative diagnosis of cervical lymph node metastasis in patients with papillary thyroid carcinoma: a meta-analysis. Eur J Radiol. 2012 Aug;81(8):1798-80
54. Ahuja A, Ying M, King A, Yuen HY. Lymph node hilus: gray scale and power Doppler sonography of cervical nodes. J Ultrasound Med. 2001;20:987–92.
55. Johnson NA, Tublin ME. Postoperative surveillance of differentiated thyroid carcinoma: rationale, techniques, and controversies. Radiology. 2008;249:429–44.
56. Paksoy N, Yazal K. Cervical lymphadenopathy associated with Hashimoto's thyroiditis: an analysis of 22 cases by fine needle aspiration cytology. Acta Cytol. 2009;53:491–6.
57. Ahuja A, Ng C, King W, Metreweli C. Solitary cystic nodal metastasis from occult papillary carcinoma of the thyroid mimicking a branchial cyst: a potential pitfall. Clin Radiol. 1998;53:61–3.
58. Verge J, Guixá J, Alejo M, et al. Cervical cystic lymph node metastasis as first manifestation of occult papillary thyroid carcinoma: report of seven cases. Head Neck. 1999;21:370–4.
59. Monchik JM, De Petris G, De Crea C. Occult papillary carcinoma of the thyroid presenting as a cervical cyst. Surgery. 2001;129:429–32.
60. Seven H, Gurkan A, Cinar U, et al. Incidence of occult thyroid carcinoma metastases in lateral cervical cysts. Am J Otolaryngol. 2004;25:11–7.
61. Wunderbaldinger P, Harisinghani M, Hahn P, et al. Cystic lymph node metastases in papillary thyroid carcinoma. AJR Am J Roentgenol. 2002;178:693–7.
62. Kessler A, Rappaport Y, Blank A, et al. Cystic appearance of cervical lymph nodes is characteristic of metastatic papillary thyroid carcinoma. J Clin Ultrasound. 2003;31:21–5.
63. Landry CS, Grubbs EG, Busaidy NL, et al. Cystic lymph nodes in the lateral neck as indicators of metastatic papillary thyroid cancer. Endocr Pract. 2011;17:240–4.
64. Choi EC, Moon WJ, Lim YC. Case report. Tuberculous cervical lymphadenitis mimicking metastatic lymph nodes from papillary thyroid carcinoma. Br J Radiol. 2009;82:208–11.
65. Ahuja AT, Ying M, Yuen HY, Metreweli C. 'Pseudocystic' appearance of non-Hodgkin's lymphomatous nodes: an infrequent finding with high-resolution transducers. Clin Radiol. 2001;56:111–5.
66. Wong KT, Lee YY, King AD, et al. Imaging of cystic or cyst-like neck masses. Clin Radiol. 2008;63:613–22.
67. Ahuja AT, Ying M. Evaluation of cervical lymph node vascularity: a comparison of colour Doppler, power Doppler and 3-D power Doppler sonography. Ultrasound Med Biol. 2004;30:1557–64.
68. Na DG, Lim HK, Byun HS, et al. Differential diagnosis of cervical lymphadenopathy: usefulness of color Doppler sonography. AJR Am J Roentgenol. 1997;168:1311–6.
69. Lyshchik A, Higashi T, Asato R, et al. Cervical lymph node metastases: diagnosis at sonoelastography—initial experience. Radiology. 2007;243:258–67.
70. Gritzmann N, Hollerweger A, Macheiner P, et al. Sonography of soft tissue masses of the neck. J Clin Ultrasound. 2002;6:356–73.
71. Schwetschenau E, Kelley DJ. The adult neck mass. Am Fam Physician. 2002;66:831–8.
72. Bhatia, et al. Imaging of palpable masses in the head and neck: a practical approach using high resolution ultrasound. Imaging. 2007;19:1–13.
73. Lee J, Fernandes R. Neck masses: evaluation and diagnostic approach. Oral Maxillofac Surg Clin N Am. 2008;20:321–37.
74. Donatini G, Iacconi P, de Bartolomeis C, et al. Neck lesions mimicking thyroid pathology. Langenbecks Arch Surg. 2009;394:435–40.
75. Sofferman RA. Ultrasound of salivary glands and the non-endocrine neck. In: Baskin HJ, Duick DS, Levine RA, editors. Thyroid ultrasound and ultrasound-guided FNA. 3rd ed. New York: Springer; 2013. p. 219–66.
76. Ahuja AT, King AD, Metreweli C. Second branchial cleft cysts: variability of sonographic appearances in adult cases. AJNR Am J Neuroradiol. 2000;21:315–9.
77. Gross E, Sichel JY. Congenital neck lesions. Surg Clin N Am. 2006;86:383–92.
78. Rosenberg TL, Brown JJ, Jefferson GD. Evaluating the adult patient with a neck mass. Med Clin N Am. 2010;94:1017–29.
79. Wadsworth DT, Siegel MJ. Thyroglossal duct cysts: variability of sonographic findings. AJR Am J Roentgenol. 1994;163:1475–7.
80. Ahuja AT, King AD, King W, et al. Thyroglossal duct cysts: sonographic appearances in adults. AJNR Am J Neuroradiol. 1999;20:579–82.
81. Ahuja AT, King AD, Metreweli C. Sonographic evaluation of thyroglossal duct cysts in children. Clin Radiol. 2000;55:770–4.
82. Kutuya N, Kurosaki Y. Sonographic assessment of thyroglossal duct cysts in children. J Ultrasound Med. 2008;27:1211–9.
83. Yabuuchi H, Kuroiwa T, Fukuya T, et al. Traumatic neuroma and recurrent lymphadenopathy after neck dissection: comparison of radiologic features. Radiology. 2004;233:523–9.
84. Kwak JY, Kim E-K, Kim MJ, et al. Sonographic features of traumatic neuromas after neck dissection. J Clin Ultrasound. 2009;37:189–93.

85. Stulak JM, Grant CS, Farley DR, et al. Value of preoperative ultrasonography in the surgical management of initial and reoperative papillary thyroid cancer. Arch Surg. 2006;141:489–94. discussion 494–496.
86. González HE, Cruz F, O'Brien A, et al. Impact of preoperative ultrasonographic staging of the neck in papillary thyroid carcinoma. Arch Otolaryngol Head Neck Surg. 2007;133:1258–62.
87. Chung YS, Kim JY, Bae JS, et al. Lateral lymph node metastasis in papillary thyroid carcinoma: results of therapeutic lymph node dissection. Thyroid. 2009;19:241–6.
88. Kim E, Park JS, Son KR, et al. Preoperative diagnosis of cervical metastatic lymph nodes in papillary thyroid carcinoma: comparison of ultrasound, computed tomography, and combined ultrasound with computed tomography. Thyroid. 2008;18:411–8.
89. Choi JS, Kim J, Kwak JY, et al. Preoperative staging of papillary thyroid carcinoma: comparison of ultrasound imaging and CT. AJR Am J Roentgenol. 2009;193:871–8.
90. Marshall CL, Lee JE, Xing Y, et al. Routine pre-operative ultrasonography for papillary thyroid cancer: effects on cervical recurrence. Surgery. 2009;146:1063–72.
91. Moon HJ, Yoon JH, Kwak JY, et al. Positive predictive value and interobserver variability of preoperative staging sonography for thyroid carcinoma. AJR Am J Roentgenol. 2011;197:W324–30.
92. Choi JS, Chung WY, Kwak JY, et al. Staging of papillary thyroid carcinoma with ultrasonography: performance in a large series. Ann Surg Oncol. 2011 Dec;18(13):3572-8
93. Mirallié E, Visset J, Sagan C, et al. Localization of cervical node metastasis of papillary thyroid carcinoma. World J Surg. 1999;23:970–3. discussion 973–4.
94. Takada H, Kikumori T, Imai T, et al. Patterns of lymph node metastases in papillary thyroid carcinoma: results from consecutive bilateral cervical lymph node dissection. World J Surg. 2011;35:1560–6.
95. Agarwal S, Chand G, Jaiswal S, et al. Pattern and risk factors of central compartment lymph node metastasis in papillary thyroid cancer: a prospective study from an endocrine surgery centre. J Thyroid Res. 2012, 2012:436243, 1–7.
96. Mulla M, Schulte K-M. Central cervical lymph node metastases in papillary thyroid cancer: a systematic review of imaging-guided and prophylactic removal of the central compartment. Clin Endocrinol. 2012;76:131–6.
97. Machens A, Holzhausen H-J, Dralle H. Skip metastases in thyroid cancer leaping the central lymph node compartment. Arch Surg. 2004;139:43–5.
98. Lim YC, Koo BS. Predictive factors of skip metastases to lateral neck compartment leaping central neck compartment in papillary thyroid carcinoma. Oral Oncol. 2012;48:262–5.
99. Lee YS, Shin S-C, Lim YS, et al. Tumor location-dependent skip lateral cervical lymph nodes metastasis in papillary thyroid cancer. Head Neck. 2014;36:887-91
100. Dralle H, Machens A. Surgical management of the lateral compartment fro metastatic thyroid cancer. Curr Opin Oncol. 2013;25:20–6.
101. Noguchi M, Kumaki T, Taniya T, et al. Bilateral cervical lymph node metastases in well differentiated thyroid cancer. Arch Surg. 1990;125:804–6.
102. Lee YS, Jeong JJ, Nam K-H, et al. Papillary carcinoma located in the thyroid isthmus. World J Surg. 2010;34:36–9.
103. Wu L-M, Gu H-Y, Qu X-H, et al. The accuracy of ultrasonoraphy in the preoperative diagnosis of cervical lymph node metastasis in patients with papillary thyroid carcinoma: a meta-analysis. Eur J Radiol. 2012;81:1798–805.
104. Mulla MG, Knoefel WT, Gilbert J, et al. Lateral cervical lymph node metastases in papillary thyroid cancer: a systematic review of imaging-guided and prophylactic removal of the lateral compartment. Clin Endocrinol. 2012;77:126–31.
105. Al-Saif O, Farrar WB, Bloomston M, et al. Long-term efficacy of lymph node reoperation for persistent papillary thyroid cancer. J Clin Endocrinol Metab. 2010;95:2187–94.
106. Baek SK, Jung KY, Kang SM, et al. Clinical risk factors associated with cervical lymph node recurrence in papillary thyroid carcinoma. Thyroid. 2010;20:147–52.
107. Schuff KG. Management of recurrent/persistent papillary thyroid carcinoma: efficacy of the surgical option. J Clin Endocrinol Metab. 2011;96:2038–9.
108. Yim JH, Kim WB, Kim EY, et al. The outcomes of first reoperation for locoregionally recurrent/persistent papillary thyroid carcinoma in patients who initially underwent total thyroidectomy and remnant ablation. J Clin Endocrinol Metab. 2011;96:2049–56.
109. Mazzaferri EL. An overview of the management of papillary and follicular thyroid carcinoma. Thyroid. 1999;9:421–7.
110. Schlumberger M, Pacini F, Wiersinga WM, et al. Follow-up and management of differentiated thyroid carcinoma: a European perspective in clinical practice. Eur J Endocrinol. 2004;151:539–48.
111. Pacini F, Castagna MG, Brilli L, et al. Thyroid cancer: ESMO clinical practice guidelines for diagnosis, treatment and follow-up. Ann Oncol. 2010;21 suppl 5:v214–9.
112. Haugen BR, Alexander EK, Bible KC, Doherty GM, Mandel SJ, Nikiforov Y, Pacini F, Randolph G, Sawka A, Shepard D, Sosa J, Tuttle RM, Wartofsky L. 2015 American Thyroid Association Management Guidelines for adult patients with thyroid nodules and differentiated thyroid cancer. Available online at Thyroid 25: DOI:10.1089/thy.2015.0020; print version in Thyroid 26:1–133, 2016.
113. Kloos RT, Eng C, Evans DB, et al. Medullary thyroid cancer: management guidelines of the American Thyroid Association. Thyroid. 2009;19:565–612.
114. Souza do Rosario PW, Fagundes TA, et al. Sonography in the diagnosis of cervical recurrence in patients with differentiated thyroid carcinoma. J Ultrasound Med. 2004;23:915–20.
115. Shin JH, Han BK, Ko EY, et al. Sonographic findings in the surgical bed after thyroidectomy: comparison of recurrent tumors and nonrecurrent lesions. J Ultrasound Med. 2007;26:1359–66.
116. Sheth S, Hamper UM. Role of sonography after total thyroidectomy for thyroid cancer. Ultrasound Q. 2008;24:147–54.
117. Frates MC. Ultrasound in recurrent thyroid disease. Otolaryngol Clin N Am. 2008;41:1107–16.
118. Antonelli A, Miccoli P, Ferdeghini M, et al. Role of neck ultrasonography in the follow-up of patients operated on for thyroid cancer. Thyroid. 1995;5:25–8.
119. Frasoldati A, Pesenti M, Gallo M, et al. Diagnosis of neck recurrences in patients with differential thyroid carcinoma. Cancer. 2003;97:90–6.
120. Torlontano M, Attard M, Crocetti U, et al. Follow-up of low risk patients with papillary thyroid cancer: role of neck ultrasonography in detecting lymph node metastases. J Clin Endocrinol Metabol. 2004;89:3402–7.
121. Tuttle RM, Leboeuf R, Shaha AR. Medical management of thyroid cancer: a risk adapted approach. J Surg Oncol. 2008;97:712–6.
122. Crocetti U, Durante C, Attard M, et al. Predictive value of recombinant human TSH stimulation and neck ultrasonography in differentiated thyroid cancer patients. Thyroid. 2008;18:1049–53.
123. Tuttle RM, Tala H, Shah J, et al. Estimating risk of recurrence in differentiated thyroid cancer after total thyroidectomy and radioactive iodine remnant ablation: using response to therapy variables to modify the initial risk estimates predicted by the new american thyroid association staging system. Thyroid. 2010;20:1341–9.
124. Verburg FA, Reiners C. Cancer: continuous re-evaluation in differentiated thyroid carcinoma. Nat Rev Endocrinol. 2011;7:127–8.
125. Ko MS, Lee JH, Shong YK, et al. Normal and abnormal sonographic findings at the thyroidectomy sites in postoperative patients with thyroid malignancy. AJR Am J Roentgenol. 2010;194:1596–609.

126. Bieker T Scanning the post-thyroidectomy neck: appearance and technique. J Diagn Med Sonography. 2010;26:215–23.
127. Kamaya A, Gross M, Akatsu H, et al. Recurrence in the thyroidectomy bed: sonographic findings. AJR Am J Roentgenol. 2011;196:66–70.
128. Udelsman R. Treatment of persistent or recurrent papillary carcinoma of the thyroid. The good, the bad and the unknown. J Clin Endocrinol Metab. 2010;95:2061–3.
129. Langer JE, Luster E, Horii SC, et al. Chronic granulomatous lesions after thyroidectomy: imaging findings. AJR Am J Roentgenol. 2005;185:1350–4.
130. Lee JH, Lee HK, Lee DH, et al. Ultrasonographic findings of a newly detected nodule on the thyroid bed in postoperative patients for thyroid carcinoma: correlation with the results of ultrasonography-guided fine-needle aspiration biopsy. Clin Imaging. 2007;31:109–13.
131. Rettenbacher T, Macheiner P, Hollerweger A, Gritzmann N, Weismann C, Todoroff B. Suture granulomas: sonography enables a correct preoperative diagnosis. Ultrasound Med Biol. 2001;27:343–50.
132. Sutton RT, Reading CC, Charboneau JW, James EM, Grant CS, Hay ID. Us-guided biopsy of neck masses in postoperative management of patients with thyroid cancer. Radiology. 1988;168:769–72.
133. Boland GW, Lee MJ, Mueller PR, Mayo-Smith W, Dawson SL, Simeone JF. Efficacy of sonographically guided biopsy of thyroid and cervical lymph nodes. Am J Roentgenol. 1993;161:1053–6.
134. Knappe M, Louw M, Gregor RT. Ultrasonography-guided fine-needle aspiration for the assessment of cervical metastases. Arch Otolaryngol Head Neck Surg. 2000;126:1091–6.
135. Baskin J. Detection of recurrent papillary thyroid carcinoma by thyroglobulin assessment in the needle washout after fine-needle aspiration of suspicious lymph nodes. Thyroid. 2004;14:959–63.
136. Baloch ZW, Barroeta JE, Walsh J, et al. Utility of thyroglobulin measurement in fine-needle specimens of lymph nodes in the diagnosis of recurrent thyroid carcinoma. Cytojournal. 2008;5:1–5.
137. Ustun M, Risberg B, Davidson B, et al. Cystic change in metastatic lymph nodes: a common diagnostic pitfall in fine-needle aspiration cytology. Diagn Cytopathol. 2002;27:387–92.
138. Cignarelli M, Ambrosi A, Marino A, et al. Diagnostic utility of thyroglobulin detection in fine-needle aspiration of cervical cystic metastatic lymph nodes from papillary thyroid cancer with negative cytology. Thyroid. 2003;13:1163–7.
139. Pacini F, Fugazzola I, Lippi F, et al. Detection of thyroglobulin in the needle aspirates of nonthyroidal neck masses: a clue to the diagnosis of metastatic differentiated thyroid cancer. J Clin Endocrinol Metabol. 1992;74:1401–4.
140. Lee MJ, Ross DS, Mueller PR, et al. Fine-needle biopsy of cervical lymph nodes in patients with thyroid cancer: a prospective comparison of cytopathologic and tissue marker analysis. Radiology. 1993;187:851–4.
141. Frasoldati A, Toschi E, Zini M, et al. Role of thyroglobulin measurement in fine-needle aspiration biopsies of cervical lymph nodes in patients with differentiated thyroid cancer. Thyroid. 1999;9:105–11.
142. Cunha N, Rodrigues F, Curado F, et al. Thyroglobulin detection in fine-needle aspirates of cervical lymph nodes: a technique for the diagnosis of metastatic differentiated thyroid cancer. Eur J Endocrinol. 2007;157:101–7.
143. Snozek CLH, Chambers EP, Reading CC, et al. Serum Thyroglobulin, high resolution ultrasound and lymph node thyroglobulin in diagnosis of differentiated thyroid carcinoma nodal metastases. J Clin Endocrinol Metab. 2007;92:4278–81.
144. Giovanella L, Ceriani L, Suriano S. Lymph node thyroglobulin measurement in diagnosis of neck metastases of differentiated thyroid carcinoma. J Thyroid Res. 2011;2011:6218–39.
145. Salmaslıoğlu A, Erbil Y, Cıtlak G, et al. Diagnostic value of thyroglobulin measurement in fine-needle aspiration biopsy for detecting metastatic lymph nodes in patients with papillary thyroid carcinoma. Langenbecks Arch Surg. 2011;396:77–81.
146. Moon JH, Kim II Y, Lim JA, et al. Thyroglobulin in washout fluid from lymph node fine-needle aspiration biopsy in papillary thyroid cancer: large scale validation of the cutoff value to determine malignancy and evaluation of discrepant results. J Clin Endocrinol Metab. 2013;98:1061–8.
147. Jung JY, Shin J-H, Han B-K, et al. Optimized cutoff value and indication for washout thyroglobulin level according to ultrasound findings in patients with well-differentiated thyroid cancer. Am J Neuroradiol. 2013;34:2349-53.
148. Uruno T, Miyauchi A, Shimizu K, et al. Usefulness of thyroglobulin measurement in fine-needle aspiration biopsy specimens for diagnosing cervical lymph node metastasis in patients with papillary thyroid cancer. World J Surg. 2005;29:483–5.
149. Boi F, Baghino G, Atzeni F, et al. The diagnostic value for differentiated thyroid carcinoma metastases of thyroglobulin (Tg) measurement in washout fluid from fine-needle aspiration biopsy of neck lymph nodes is maintained in the presence of circulating anti-Tg antibodies. J Clin Endocrinol Metabol. 2006;91:1364–9.
150. Borel A-L, Boizel R, Faure P, et al. Significance of low levels of thyroglobulin in fine needle aspirates from cervical lymph nodes of patients with a history of differentiated thyroid cancer. Eur J Endocrinol. 2008;158:691–8.
151. Jeon SJ, Kim E, Park JS, et al. Diagnostic benefit of thyroglobulin measurement in fine-needle aspiration for diagnosing metastatic cervical lymph nodes from papillary thyroid cancer: correlations with US features. Korean J Radiol. 2009;10:106–11.
152. Kim MJ, Kim EK, Kim BM, et al. Thyroglobulin measurement in fine-needle aspirate washouts: the criteria for neck node dissection for patients with thyroid cancer. Clin Endocrinol. 2009;70:145–51.
153. Lee YH, Seo HS, Suh S, et al. Cut-off value for needle washout thyroglobulin in athyrotropic patients. Laryngoscope. 2010;120:1120–4.
154. Bournaud C, Charrié A, Nozières C, et al. Thyroglobulin measurement in fine-needle aspirates of lymph nodes in patients with differentiated thyroid cancer: a simple definition of the threshold value, with emphasis on potential pitfalls of the method. Clin Chem Lab Med. 2010;48:1171–7.
155. Soon Y-M, Kim MJ, Kim E-K, et al. Diagnostic performance of thyroglobulin value in indeterminate range in fine needle aspiration washout fluid from lymph nodes of thyroid cancer. Yonsei Med J. 2012;53:126–31.
156. Kim D-W, Jeon SJ, Kim CG. Usefulness of thyroglobulin measurement in needle washouts of fine-needle aspiration biopsy for the diagnosis of cervical lymph node metastases from papillary thyroid cancer before thyroidectomy. Endocrine. 2012;42:399–403.
157. Giovanella L, Bongiovanni M, Trimboli P. Diagnostic value of thyroglobulin assay in cervical lymph node fine-needle aspirations for metastatic differentiated thyroid cancer. Curr Opin Oncol. 2013;25:6–13.
158. Arturi F, Russo D, Giuffrida D, et al. Early diagnosis by genetic analysis of differentiated thyroid cancer metastases in small lymph nodes. J Clin Endocrinol Metab. 1997;82:1638–41.
159. Lee MT, Lin SY, Yang HJ, et al. Early detection of occult thyroid cancer metastases in small cervical lymph node by genetic analysis of fine-needle aspiration specimens. J Otolaryngol. 2000;29:322–6.
160. Bishop JA, Owens CL, Shum CH, et al. Thyroid bed fine-needle aspiration. Experience at a large tertiary care center. Am J Pathol. 2010;134:335–9.
161. Boi F, Maurelli I, Pinna G, et al. Calcitonin measurement in washout fluid from fine needle aspiration of neck masses in patients with primary and metastatic medullary thyroid carcinoma. J Clin Endocrinol Metab. 2007;92:2115–8.
162. Kudo T, Miyauchi A, Ito Y, et al. Diagnosis of medullary thyroid carcinoma by calcitonin measurement in fine-needle aspiration biopsy specimens. Thyroid. 2007;17:635–8.

163. Abraham D, Gault PM, Hunt J, et al. Calcitonin estimation in neck lymph node fine-needle aspirate fluid prevents misinterpretation of cytology in patients with metastatic medullary thyroid cancer. Thyroid. 2009;19:1015–6.
164. Trimboli P, Rossi F, Baldelli R, et al. Measuring calcitonin in washout of the needle in patients undergoing fine needle aspiration with suspicious medullary thyroid cancer. Diagn Cytopathol. 2012;40:394–8.
165. Wartofsky L. Highlights of the American Thyroid Association guidelines for patients with thyroid nodules or differentiated thyroid carcinoma: the 2009 revision. Thyroid. 2009;19:1139–43.

Surveillance Radioiodine Whole Body Scans

41

Douglas Van Nostrand

Introduction

Surveillance radioiodine whole body scans have been used for many years in the follow-up of patients with differentiated thyroid cancer. However, the term "surveillance whole body scan" has been used in different ways. This chapter (1) differentiates surveillance scans from baseline scans and pre-therapy scans, (2) presents the objectives of surveillance scans, (3) presents an overview of the guidelines of various organizations for the utility of surveillance scans, and (4) presents a proposed guideline for the use of surveillance scans.

Radioiodine Surveillance Scans vs Follow-Up Baseline Scans and Pre-therapy Scans

Surveillanceradioiodine scans should be differentiated from *follow-up baseline scans* and *pre-therapy scans. A surveillance scan* is a radioiodine whole body scan performed at a routine interval, which is typically 6 months to 1–2 years after ^{131}I therapy. Its primary objective is to *screen* for functioning recurrence or metastatic differentiated thyroid cancer, thereby either helping to confirm that the patient is in clinical remission or helping to detect recurrence and/or metastasis.

A *follow-up baseline scan* is performed approximately 12–18 months after a ^{131}I therapy such as remnant ablation, adjuvant treatment, or treatment for locoregional and/or distant metastases. This scan is performed in order to establish a new baseline scan to be used for future comparison. For example, if a patient has an intermediate risk of recurrence, returns with a rising thyroglobulin blood level, and has a foci of uptake in his/her thyroid bed on his/her new radioiodine whole body scan, a comparison of that scan to a prior follow-up baseline scan may help determine whether or not that foci of uptake represents persistent thyroid tissue that was not completely ablated and had been present all the time prior to the Tg rising. As Cailleux et al. noted, a diagnostic radioiodine scan does confirm the completeness of thyroid ablation [1]. Of course, further study is warranted regarding the cost-effectiveness of a follow-up baseline scan, especially if the patient must undergo thyroid hormone withdrawal. However, if a patient is already scheduled to have obtained a rhTSH-stimulated Tg blood level, the addition of a radioiodine follow-up baseline scan adds only a modest expense relative to the rhTSH injections. If one is not already administering the rhTSH injections, then this author submits that the potential benefit of performing a new follow-up "baseline" scan relative to the additional expense of rhTSH injections is more problematic.

Apre-therapy scan is a radioiodine whole body scan performed in "anticipation" of a ^{131}I therapy in patients who are suspected of having or are already known to have recurrent local regional or distant metastases. Again, the objectives of a pre-therapy scan for anticipation of a ^{131}I therapy are to help: (1) localize sites of metastasis; (2) localize lesions for treatment options such as additional surgery, radiofrequency ablation, embolization, cryotherapy, or external radiotherapy; (3) determine whether or not ^{131}I is a therapeutic option (e.g., in those facilities that use visual uptake of radioiodine as a criteria for ^{131}I therapy); (4) identify patterns of radioiodine uptake that would alter the prescribed activity for ^{131}I therapy (e.g., diffuse lung metastases, bone metastasis, and/or brain metastasis); and/or (5) perform lesional dosimetry, whole-body dosimetry, and/or simplified dosimetry, which could alter prescribed activity for ^{131}I therapy.

D. Van Nostrand, MD, FACP, FACNM (✉)
Nuclear Medicine Research, MedStar Research Institute and Washington Hospital Center, Georgetown University School of Medicine, Washington Hospital Center, 110 Irving Street, N.W., Suite GB 60F, Washington, DC 20010, USA
e-mail: douglasvannostrand@gmail.com

L. Wartofsky, D. Van Nostrand (eds.), *Thyroid Cancer*, DOI 10.1007/978-1-4939-3314-3_41

With surveillance whole body scans described above, strong arguments have been presented that surveillance scans in selected patients are no longer cost-effective [1–11]. These arguments are further strengthened when the patient must undergo thyroid hormone withdrawal to prepare for the surveillance scan resulting in a potential prolonged period of hypothyroidism for the patient. As a result, fewer facilities perform routine surveillance scans for screening low-risk patients with no evidence of disease on physical exam and undetectable serum thyroglobulin levels on thyroid hormone suppression. As early as 2002, Mazzaferri and Kloos [3] suggested that a surveillance scan added little to no diagnostic information to rhTSH-stimulated thyroglobulin levels. In high-risk patients, de Meer et al. evaluated 112 high-risk patients, and diagnostic whole body scan offered no additional screening information to a rhTSH-stimulated thyroglobulin level [12]. Thus, as a result of these publications, surveillance scans are no longer routinely recommended in low-risk patients as noted in the American Thyroid Association (ATA) guidelines, European Consensus (EC), National Comprehensive Cancer Network (NCCN), and British Thyroid Association (BTA) guidelines in Table 41.1. In Table 41.2, this author summarizes the guidelines of the various professional organizations for surveillance scans and includes several proposals for the use of a "follow-up" baseline scan.

Table 41.1 Various professional organizational guidelines

Organization	Guideline	Rating
ATA [8]	RECOMMENDATION 66: "After the first post-treatment WBS performed following RAI remnant ablation or adjuvant therapy, low-risk and intermediate-risk patients (lower risk features) with an undetectable Tg on thyroid hormone with negative antithyroglobulin antibodies and a negativeUS (excellent response to therapy) do not require routine diagnostic WBS during follow-up."	Strong recommendation Moderate-quality evidence
	RECOMMENDATION 67: "Diagnostic WBS . . . 6-12 months after remnant ablation [or] adjuvant RAI therapy can be useful in the follow-up of patients with high or intermediate risk (higher risk feature) of persistence disease and . . . and should be done with ^{123}I or low activity ^{131}I."	Strong recommendation Low-quality evidence
EC [9]	"A diagnostic WBS will demonstrate foci of uptake outside the thyroid bed only in patients with detectable serum Tg levels following TSH stimulation. In addition, cervical node metastases are best seen by neck US. Thus, if there is no evidence of persistent disease, a diagnostic control WBS is usually not indicated."	
	"Diagnostic WBS is indicated by some authors in high-risk patients or when the post-ablation WBS was poorly informative due to high uptake in thyroid remnants or when it disclosed suspicious uptake."	
NCCN [10]	"RAI imaging . . . can be considered in patients at high risk for persistent or recurrent disease, distant metastases or disease-specific mortality; patients with previous RAI-avid metastases; or patients with abnormal Tg levels, stable or increasing anti-Tg antibodies, or abnormal ultrasound results."	
BTA [11]	"In patients selected for monitoring with RAI imaging, it is recommended every 12-24 months until no clinically significant response is seen to RAI treatment in patients with iodine-responsive tumors and detectable Tg, distant metastases, or soft tissue invasion on initial staging."	
	A diagnostic radioiodine scan (in conjunction with stimulated serum Tg measurement) should be performed in all other cases.	B = "Requires availability of well-conducted clinical studies but no randomized clinical trials on the topic of recommendation."
	"Patients with high-risk disease and with Tg antibodies (TgAb) interfering with serum Tg measurements may need additional radioiodine, ultrasound or other cross-sectional (e.g., CT or MRI) scans."	
	"No further diagnostic radioiodine scans are required for other groups of patients, unless there are indications of disease progression, such as a rising serum Tg, clinical or radiological evidence of progression."	
	"A single diagnostic WBS performed 6–8 months (but not sooner than 6 months) after ^{131}I ablation is generally indicated except in those with low-risk disease. If this is negative, further WBS is not usually required, depending on results of monitoring by measurement of serum Tg."	*Recommendation III, B*

Table 41.2 Proposed guidelines for surveillance scans and one-time "follow-up baseline scan"

If	Then
Low-risk patient who received an ^{131}I remnant ablation with normal subsequent physical exam, negative ultrasound, undetectable or low (<1.0) serum thyroglobulin (Tg) level on thyroid hormone suppression without anti-Tg antibodies, and pre-therapy/post-therapy scan showing only uptake that is most likely normal functioning thyroid tissue	"Surveillance scans" for periodic screening not recommended. If the patient is going to have a TSH-stimulated thyroglobulin level at 6–12 months after initial ^{131}I remnant ablation, consider a one-time ^{123}I or ^{131}I "baseline scan."
Low-risk patient who received an ^{131}I remnant ablation and has antithyroglobulin antibodies	If the patient is already having a TSH-stimulated thyroglobulin level obtained at 6–12 months after initial ^{131}I therapy, then consider performing a one-time follow-up rhTSH- stimulated ^{123}I or ^{131}I scan both for a one-time *surveillance scan* and to act as a new *baseline scan* to be used for any future comparison
	If the patient is not having a rhTSH-stimulated thyroglobulin level obtained at 6–12 months after initial ^{131}I therapy, then perform no follow-up *surveillance* or *baseline scan* (see text)
Intermediate - risk patient who received an ^{131}I remnant ablation or adjuvant treatment	Perform one TSH-stimulated ^{123}I or ^{131}I follow-up for a one-time *surveillance* scan and to establish a new *baseline scan* to be used for any future comparison
	Perform no further routine periodic *surveillance scans* for screening thereafter[a]
High - risk patients who received an ^{131}I therapy	Perform ^{123}I or ^{131}I follow-up scan with TSH stimulation at 6–12 months for a one-time *surveillance* scan and to establish a new *baseline scan* to be used for any future comparisons[a]
	Any subsequent routine periodic *surveillance scans* for screening should be determined on a patient-by-patient basis

[a]However, if there is evidence of recurrence such as suggested by a rising Tg and/or abnormal diagnostic ultrasound, computer tomography, etc., then a ^{123}I or ^{131}I *diagnostic pre-therapy scan* should be considered

Summary

Surveillance radioiodine whole body scans should be differentiated from follow-up baseline scans and pre-therapy scans, and the objectives of these three types of scans are significantly different. However, radioiodine surveillance scans are no longer routinely indicated in low-risk patients with an undetectable Tg on thyroid hormone with negative anti-thyrogolublin antibodies and a negative ultrasound. Surveillance scans may be considered in patients who have an intermediate or high risk of persistent or recurrent disease and/or antithyroglobulin antibodies. Further evaluation of the utility of follow-up baseline scans and screening surveillance scans in patients with high-risk disease is warranted.

References

1. Cailleux AF, Baudin E, Travagli JP, Schlumberger RM. Is diagnostic iodine-131 scanning useful after total thyroid ablation for differentiated thyroid cancer? J Clin Endocrinol Metab. 2000;85:175–8.
2. Wartofsky L. Management of low risk well differentiated thyroid cancer based only upon thyroglobulin measurement after recombinant human thyrotropin. Thyroid. 2002;12:583–92.
3. Mazzaferri EL, Kloos RT. Is diagnostic iodine-131 scanning with recombinant human TSH useful in the follow-up of differentiated thyroid cancer after thyroid ablation? J Clin Endocrinol Metab. 2002;87:1490–8.
4. Wartofsky L. Using baseline and recombinant human TSH-stimulated Tg measurements to manage thyroid cancer without diagnostic I-131 scanning. J Clin Endocrinol Metab. 2002;87:1486–9.
5. Pacini F, Capezzone M, Elisei R, et al. Diagnostic 131-iodine whole body scan may be avoided in thyroid cancer patients who have undetectable stimulated serum Tg levels after initial treatment. J Clin Endocrinol Metab. 2002;87:1499–501.
6. Fatemi S, Nicoloff J, Lo Presti J, Spencer S. TSH-stimulated serum thyroglobulin in the 1–10 ng/ml range suggests a low long-term recurrence risk for papillary thyroid cancer (PTC). Washington, DC: Program of the 73rd annual meeting of the American Thyroid Association, 2001, 290 (Abstract 194).
7. Pacini F, Molinaro E, Lippi F, et al. Prediction of disease status by recombinant human TSH-stimulated serum thyroglobulin in the post surgical follow-up of differentiated thyroid carcinoma. J Clin Endocrinol Metab. 2001;86:5686–90.
8. American Thyroid Association Guidelines Task Force on Thyroid Nodules and Differentiated Thyroid Cancer, Haugen BR, Alexander EK, Bible KC, Doherty GM, Mandel SJ, Nikiforov YE, Pacini F, Randolph GW, Sawka AM, Schlumberger M, Schuff KG, Sherman SI, Sosa JA, Steward DL, Tuttle RM, Wartofsky L. 2015 American Thyroid Association management guidelines for adult patients with thyroid nodules and differentiated thyroid cancer. Thyroid. 2016;26:1–133.
9. Pacini F, Schlumberger M, Dralle H, Elisei R, Smit JWA, Wiersinga W, the European Thyroid Cancer Taskforce. European consensus for the management of patients with differentiated thyroid carcinoma of the follicular epithelium. Eur J Endocrinol. 2006;154:787–803.
10. National Comprehensive Cancer Network (NCCN) Clinical practice guidelines in oncology. thyroid carcinoma. Follicular Thyroid Carcinoma. V.2.2015.
11. British Thyroid Association and Royal College of Physicians. Guidelines for the management of thyroid cancer. 2nd ed. Available at: http://www.british-thyroid-ssociation.org/news/Docs/Thyroid_cancer_guidelines_2007.pdf.
12. de Meer S, Vriens MR, Zelissen PM, Borel Rinkes IH, de Keizer B. The role of routine diagnostic radioiodine whole-body scintigraphy in patients with high-risk differentiated thyroid cancer. J Nucl Med. 2011;52:56–9.

Radionuclide Imaging and Treatment of Children with Thyroid Cancer

42

Steven G. Waguespack and Gary L. Francis

Radioactive iodine (RAI) was first proposed as a specific therapy for differentiated thyroid cancer (DTC) by Seidlin et al. in 1946 [1]. Since then, RAI has been incorporated into therapy protocols for both adults and children with DTC [2, 3]. Remnant ablation and adjuvant RAI treatment may improve disease-free survival in young adults (including some adolescents), but this has not been universally shown for those with small, stage 1 lesions who enjoy a good prognosis without RAI ablation [4]. Recent therapy guidelines from the American Thyroid Association support the selective rather than universal administration of RAI for young patients (<45 years of age) with small, intra-thyroidal cancers [2]. Until recently, however, studies specifically examining the benefits of RAI in children have been difficult to perform because the number of patients is small and the prognosis is favorable for almost all children, regardless of remnant ablation and/or adjuvant therapy [5–16].

The American Thyroid Association and American Association of Clinical Endocrinologists have published practice guidelines for the management of thyroid cancer in adults, but the therapy of thyroid cancer in children remains controversial [2, 17–19]. A number of questions regarding the use of RAI in children are still unresolved. Which children are most likely to benefit from RAI therapy? What is the optimal dosage of RAI for children? What are the long-term risks and complications from RAI use in young patients? What are acceptable end points for RAI therapy in children?

S.G. Waguespack, MD
Endocrine Neoplasia and Hormonal Disorders, The University of Texas MD Anderson Cancer Center, Houston, TX, USA
e-mail: swagues@mdanderson.org

G.L. Francis, MD, PhD (✉)
Division of Pediatric Endocrinology, Department of Pediatrics, Children's Hospital of Richmond Virginia Commonwealth University, 1001 E Marshall St, Richmond, VA 23298, USA
e-mail: glfrancis@vcu.edu

Introduction

Differentiated thyroid cancers (DTCs) arise from the follicular epithelium and are generally divided into papillary (PTC) and follicular (FTC) carcinomas. Although the histologic features of PTC and FTC are similar across all ages, the prognosis is much more favorable for children than for adults with similar histology and extent of disease [5–16]. Most studies are beginning to recognize important clinical differences between two subgroups of children with DTC: those <10 years of age who generally have the highest risk for regional lymph node involvement, pulmonary metastases, and persistent disease and those >10 years of age for whom the risks of regional lymph node involvement, pulmonary metastases, and persistent disease are substantially less [12, 17, 20]. In fact, some experts recommend that adolescents could be treated using protocols designed for low-risk adults (<45 years of age) [17]. At diagnosis, the majority of thyroid cancers in young children (70 %) have invaded beyond the thyroid capsule or into the regional lymph nodes, and 10–28 % of patients already have pulmonary metastases [16, 21–24, 24b, 25–28]. Despite such widespread disease, children are much less likely to die from PTC than are adults with overall mortality reported by Hay et al. [24] as 2 % and by Markovina et al. [24b] as 0 % at 20 years and 5.6 % at 30 years. Most importantly, about half of children with pulmonary metastases persist with stable disease following therapy, and other studies show a continued fall in serum thyroglobulin (Tg) after discontinuation of RAI therapy [29–31]. These favorable outcomes as well as the potential long-term sequelae of overzealous therapy with RAI during childhood are major factors that lead to the debate about RAI therapy and its use in children with DTC.

L. Wartofsky, D. Van Nostrand (eds.), *Thyroid Cancer*, DOI 10.1007/978-1-4939-3314-3_42

Which Children Are Most Likely to Benefit from RAI Therapy?

Although children are less likely to die from DTC than adults, 20–40 % have persistent/recurrent disease following initial therapy [4, 5, 7, 13, 15, 16, 21, 24, 26, 27], and in a recent report by Markovina [24b], the progression-free survival at 10, 20, and 30 years was 71 %, 62 %, and 55 %, respectively. Attempts to determine if remnant ablation or adjuvant treatment will improve these outcomes in children have been limited by small patient populations, reliance on retrospective analyses, and conflicting results [4, 5, 7, 13, 15, 16, 21, 24, 26, 27, 32, 32c]. This is exemplified by the contrast in outcome for several such studies. Jarzab et al. reported their experience with 102 children and adolescents with DTC [32]. RAI therapy decreased the relative risk of recurrence fivefold, but despite the magnitude of this improvement, it failed to achieve statistical significance ($p=0.07$). Mihailovic et al. [32c] reviewed their experience of 50 patients with juvenile differentiated thyroid carcinoma, and three factors were predictive for a significant increased risk of recurrence—younger age, tumor multifocality, and initial treatment. Patients who underwent total thyroidectomy and ^{131}I therapy had a lower probability of recurrence than those who had subtotal thyroidectomy and less intensive ^{131}I therapy. In direct contrast, Hay et al. reported on a large group of children and adolescents with DTC and found almost identical recurrence risks for those who were treated or not treated with RAI [24]. In their study, RAI remnant ablation failed to diminish the 25-year regional recurrence rate when compared to that of total thyroidectomy alone ($p=0.86$).

On the other hand, others find that selected children at high risk for recurrence do appear to benefit from RAI therapy. Chow et al. found statistically significant improvement in recurrence-free survival for high-risk children treated with RAI (71.9–86.5 %, $p=0.04$) [21]. Their patients had tumors with a diameter of more than 1 cm, extrathyroidal extension, residual neck disease, or distant metastases. It is possible that the benefit or lack of benefit from RAI in various studies could be related not only to the proportion of patients with high- and low-risk tumors but also to the extent of initial surgery [33].

Compartment focused, standardized neck dissection has been shown to reduce the risk of regional recurrence compared to selective lymph node removal, and it is possible that the extent of neck dissection might have been less in those studies showing benefit from RAI [32]. Most young children (70 % or more in many series) have disease in the regional lymph nodes, but only about 50 % of involved lymph nodes can be identified during surgery [7, 15, 34]. It is therefore difficult to identify all patients with lymph node involvement unless they undergo a neck dissection. A level VI lymph node dissection should always be performed in the presence of documented lateral or central compartment disease [18]. With no consensus regarding the potential benefits of universal RAI therapy for all children with DTC, contemplation of RAI therapy for each individual child should also include consideration of the potential risks of RAI therapy.

What Are the Long-Term Risks and Complications from RAI Use in Young Patients?

One of the major unknown factors surrounding the use of RAI therapy for children with DTC is the paucity of data concerning long-term risks. Several clinical observations and in vitro data bring doubt into the debate concerning the long-term safety of RAI therapy in children. Although RAI use in adults has rarely been associated with secondary malignancies or leukemia, the thyroid (and presumably other tissues) in children is more susceptible to radiation-induced injury, especially in those under 10 year of age [35–37]. A growing body of evidence supports the notion that RAI may be associated with an increased risk for second malignancies in thyroid cancer survivors who had received RAI.

A study by Rubino et al. followed approximately 6,000 patients with thyroid cancer from the combined Swedish, Italian, and French tumor registries. They reported a significant and dosage-dependent increase in the risk of second malignancy among these patients [38]. In their study, 344 patients were less than 20 years of age at diagnosis, and 13 patients developed second malignancies. The risk for all cancers (relative risk [RR] = 2.5), specifically breast cancers (RR=3.4), was significantly increased when compared to the general population. Overall, 61 % of the young patients received RAI, suggesting that RAI might have had a role in this rise. However, when the patients who received RAI were compared to those who did not, there was no added risk from RAI administration (RR=1.1). The number of subjects ($n=344$) may have been too small to identify an increase in the incidence of rare complications, such as second malignancy.

Hay et al. similarly reported that children with DTC who were treated with radiation [external beam radiation (XRT), RAI, and/or radium implants] developed a variety of second cancers (leukemia, stomach, bladder, colon, salivary gland, and breast) and had increased mortality compared with the general population [24]. Whether this resulted from either aggressive therapy, an underlying predisposition to cancer or from a direct effect of RAI is unknown. Another study by Brown et al. reviewed data from over 30,000 subjects and found a statistically significant increase in risk of second malignancy for patients treated with RAI (RR 1.16, $p<0.05$) and remarked that the risk was even greater for younger patients [39]. Not all data, however, have supported an increased risk for second cancers, and an analysis of 39,000 cases in the SEER database found no increase in second malignancy for patients treated with RAI [40].

In concert with these clinical observations, chromosomal analyses indicate that RAI therapy can induce specific genetic aberrations [41–43]. A highly significant increase in the number of dicentric chromosomes was observed in peripheral lymphocytes during the first week after RAI therapy. More importantly, chromosomal aberrations involving chromosomes 1, 4, and 10 were more prevalent, even after 4 years [42]. The long-term implications of these alterations are not yet known, but they do raise questions about the potential for late genetic effects from RAI therapy.

Other possible side effects from RAI include direct damage to tissues that take up RAI, such as the salivary glands. Sialadenitis, xerostomia, dental caries, stomatitis, and oral candidiasis have all been reported [44]. Other tissues in the head and neck may be affected, inducing edema, ocular dryness, and nasolacrimal duct obstruction [45, 46]. Gonadal damage has been reported in both women (temporary ovarian failure) and men (oligospermia with elevated follicular-stimulating hormone [FSH] levels) [47, 48]. The risk of ovarian failure appears to increase with age, suggesting that young patients might be less susceptible. A study by Smith et al. is particularly relevant to the use of RAI in children [49]. They evaluated 35 women who received RAI for thyroid remnant ablation during childhood or adolescence. Patients received an average RAI dosage of 5.5 GBq (150 mCi) with a range of 2.9–9.24 GBq (77.2–250 mCi) and were followed from 5.6 to 39.8 years. Three developed infertility (8.6 %). Two children with fatal birth defects were born to this cohort, and both had been conceived within 1 year of RAI therapy. From these data, the authors suggested that the risks of infertility and birth defects were similar to the general population, but they cautioned against conception during the first year after RAI therapy. Although fertility appeared to be intact in this cohort, long-term follow-up would be required to determine if late complications (e.g., premature menopause) might develop as treated children approach middle age and beyond. Elevated serum FSH levels have been reported in males after administration of as little as 1.85 GBq (50 mCi) of RAI, and only partial recovery of gonadal function was seen in a single patient after more than 2 years of follow-up [47]. These data suggest that adolescents and younger children might be at risk for gonadal damage. Consideration should be given to the possibility of sperm banking, especially in those patients who require more than a single administration of RAI.

Collectively, these data underscore the possibility of long-term complications and second malignancies potentially associated with the use of RAI in children and have led to an increase in the "selective use" of RAI for children who are most likely to benefit from RAI accompanied by "deferral" of RAI therapy for low-risk patients [18]. Low-risk patients would include those without extensive cervical lymph node involvement [18] and adolescents who are less likely to have metastases than are younger children [16, 17]. This concept is supported by the fact that disease-specific morbidity and mortality is low, even for those children who subsequently develop recurrence [24, 50]. This approach would allow detection and treatment of later recurrence with surgery or RAI as indicated [18].

Overall, however, RAI therapy is indicated for children with known or presumed iodine-avid distant metastases. However, the routine use of RAI for children with stage I DTC is debatable. RAI may lower recurrence and disease-specific mortality, but low-risk adults appear not to benefit from routine RAI therapy [2]. For children with DTC, the possible benefits must be weighed against the risks. Defining the "level of risk" for children is problematic. Compared with adults, they have increased risk for recurrence and a longer remaining period of follow-up, but they also have low risk for disease-specific morbidity and mortality and possibly life-altering complications from overzealous therapy. Current data support the notion that RAI therapy can be deferred for many children with stage I DTC. If DTC recurs when RAI has been deferred during initial management, recurrence is usually in the cervical lymph nodes and can be surgically managed without a negative impact on short-term mortality. For that reason, the universal prescription of RAI therapy is no longer recommended by many experts, but rather, selective prescription of RAI is undertaken for aggressive histologies, TNM stage T4 tumors, extensive cervical lymph node disease, and/or pulmonary or other distant metastases [18].

If RAI Therapy Were to Be Given Only to Children at High Risk, How Could This Be Reasonably Achieved?

It is essential to determine the extent of disease in children through preoperative and postoperative staging [18]. Preoperative staging generally includes a chest radiograph (CXR) to assess for macroscopic lung metastases and a comprehensive neck US to evaluate the contralateral thyroid lobe and the central and lateral lymph nodes [51]. Cross-sectional imaging of the neck is considered for bulky lymph node or fixed disease in order to facilitate surgical planning and hopefully improve outcome. Several staging systems have been used to estimate mortality risk, but the TNM (tumor-node-metastasis) classification is the most widely used [52]. The majority of young patients (<45 years of age) will be TNM stage I and only those few with distant metastases will be classified as stage II. All stage I pediatric patients have a low risk for disease-specific mortality, but the risk of recurrence is much greater (53 %) for children with cervical node involvement or direct tumor extension [53, 54]. Therefore, the absence of cervical node metastases is a powerful indicator of low recurrence risk and suggests that children without cervical node involvement could be managed by "deferral" of RAI until recurrence occurs (70 % will not recur), thereby sparing the majority of children from the potential risks of RAI.

To reduce the recurrence risk for children with PTC, operative staging requires a comprehensive and compartment-based lymph node dissection [12, 55] instead of "berry picking" alone [56]. Surgical risks are minimized when performed by a "high-volume" surgeon, underscoring the need to identify a qualified surgeon to treat pediatric DTC [33, 57, 58]. A level VI lymph node dissection should always be performed in the presence of documented lateral or central compartment disease [2, 59]. What remains more controversial is the prophylactic dissection of level VI lymph nodes in the absence of clinical disease. It is not uncommon for metastatic disease to be present in central neck lymph nodes [60–62] and so a prophylactic level VI lymph node dissection should be considered in children with PTC, who already are at increased risk for lymph node disease. Some groups suggest routinely considering a prophylactic central neck dissection, particularly for larger tumors [2, 63, 64], whereas others suggest making this decision based upon intraoperative findings [65]. In either case, level VI lymphadenectomy should only be performed by a surgeon highly experienced in the procedure.

Postoperative staging requires that patients be evaluated for persistent disease. In patients at low risk for recurrence, US of the thyroid bed and cervical lymph nodes and measurement of a suppressed serum thyroglobulin (Tg) level may be adequate. Patients at high risk for residual disease are generally taken off thyroid hormone or administered recombinant human TSH to prepare for a stimulated Tg and diagnostic RAI whole-body scan.

Special Cases

One third of PTC in adults are now incidental micro-PTC (<1 cm in diameter) [57] and are managed as low-risk lesions [66, 67]. However, because lymph node metastases do develop in micro-PTC, recurrence rates may be similar to larger lesions [68, 69] and even fatal cases of micro-PTC have been reported [70]. Very few data address the management of micro-PTC in children. Many clinicians perform an US of the contralateral lobe and cervical lymph nodes. Those without evidence of disease in those locations are generally treated with lobectomy alone and close follow-up. Those with lymph node involvement are treated as would a larger PTC.

True FTC is uncommon in children (<10 % of all cases of DTC) and is divided into those with only capsular invasion (minimally invasive FTC) and those with capsular and vascular invasion. Vascular invasion increases the risk of recurrence and metastasis. Because hematogenous spread in FTC occurs without regional lymph node disease, most patients with vascular-invasive FTC are treated with total thyroidectomy and RAI [18, 71]. The management of minimally invasive FTC is controversial [72, 73]. Many consider lobectomy sufficient. In a study of 37 patients <45 years of age with minimally invasive FTC, 10-year disease-free survival was 92 %, and none of the patients developed distant metastases [72].

What Are the Optimal Dosages of RAI for Children with DTC?

When RAI is to be administered, the TSH should be above 30 hIU/ml [2, 74–76]. In patients at high risk for disease, this is commonly induced by short-term thyroid hormone withdrawal [77]. Recombinant human TSH (rhTSH) has been used for remnant ablation in low-risk patients and may result in a lower-absorbed dosage to the blood [78]. However, data regarding rhTSH in children remain limited [79, 80]. A low-iodine diet is generally prescribed for 2 weeks prior to therapy. In children who received iodinated contrast during preoperative staging, it may take 2–3 months for the "cold" iodine to clear before being able to perform a diagnostic RAI thyroid scan and RAI ablation.

There are no standardized dosages of RAI for children. Some adjust ^{131}I dosages according to weight or body surface area (BSA) and give a fraction (e.g., child's weight in kg/70 kg) of the typical dosage used to treat adults with similarly extensive disease [75, 77]. Others base ^{131}I dosages on body weight alone with doses ranging from 37 to 55.5 MBq/kg (1.0–1.5 mCi/kg) up to 99.9 MBq/kg (2.7 mCi/kg) [81–84]. Dosimetry may be used to limit whole-body retention to <3.0 GBq (<80 mCi) at 48 h and blood/bone marrow exposure to <200 cGy (rad) and is most useful for small children and children with diffuse lung uptake [85, 86]. Although total body dosimetry calculates the absorbed dosage to bone marrow and blood, the lung is actually the dosage-limiting organ in 10 % of cases [87]. Unfortunately, dosimetry also has its limitations and disadvantages. Dosimetry requires administering a small dosage of RAI a few days before ablation and has the potential for stunning, which could reduce the efficacy of follow-up treatment dosages [88, 89]. Based on blood levels and whole-body retention, the exposure of each organ, especially the bone marrow, is calculated using simulations based on adult models. Thus, the RAI distribution in children, who have different lean body/fat mass ratios at all ages and generally distribute charged ions differently than adults, might not be accurately predicted. This difference might induce error into the calculations of organ exposure using standard dosimetry programs. Finally, dosimetry is not widely available, which limits its use in children.

Lesional dosimetry can also be used to guide selection of optimal dosages of RAI in selected cases where total accumulated RAI dosages are high or response to RAI has been minimal [25, 82, 90–92]. Tuttle et al. have shown that individual lesions in the same patient and at the same time have widely variable iodine uptake. Uptake can be so variable that while some lesions could be treated with RAI while others will not absorb sufficient RAI to have an effect, alternative treatments might be more appropriately considered [93].

Thyroid Hormone Suppression and Follow-Up

TSH suppression is prescribed for children with DTC, but the level and duration of suppression are debated [94]. Some recommend initial suppression of TSH to <0.1 μIU/ml followed by relaxation to 0.5 μIU/ml, once children enter remission [81]. Prior American Thyroid Association guidelines are also followed by many practitioners [2].

Follow-up should be lifelong. Most data in children are retrospective and previous studies used diagnostic RAI scans to define disease status. However, RAI scans are not as sensitive as ultrasound (US) and serum Tg. In adults, an undetectable TSH-stimulated Tg generally indicates remission [95–97], while Tg levels >5 ng/mL indicate residual disease [98]. Most adults with a rhTSH-stimulated Tg value of 2–10 ng/ml will have disease identified within 5 years, although in some patients, Tg may become undetectable without additional intervention [99]. ATA guidelines suggest that patients with a stimulated Tg >5–10 ng/ml can be empirically treated with ^{131}I as treatment has led to a decline in Tg in some cases [2, 100, 101]. Whether or not this improves long-term outcomes is unknown and the risks of empiric therapy in children likely outweigh potential benefits, although good data are lacking. A significant serial increase in Tg levels indicates disease that likely should be treated, assuming that the likelihood for iodine-avid disease is demonstrated [102, 103].

It is not yet clear if the abovementioned correlations of Tg levels to presence or absence of disease in adults have a similar prognostic value for children. Because survival data for children in older studies have generally been based on negative RAI scans and not serum Tg levels [104], the outcomes in children who are identified to have residual/recurrent disease based solely upon highly sensitive Tg assays are unknown. Hence, we do not know how aggressive we should be in treating disease detected solely by measurable serum Tg levels. Some treat young patients until a negative ^{131}I scan is achieved [105]. This "treat-to-negative-scan" approach is commonly used but does not take full advantage of Tg and US, which have detected disease in 23 % of children with a negative scan [106]. It should also be noted that Tg levels may decline over long periods of time in children previously treated with RAI [29]. Undetectable Tg levels may also not be a tenable goal for all children with pulmonary metastases [107–110] as many will develop stable but persistent disease after RAI therapy [9]. For these reasons, the decision to treat or not to treat a low but detectable Tg level with RAI must be individualized and should be based on prior behavior of the tumor and clinical response to previous RAI therapy. In general, empiric RAI treatment of a low but detectable Tg in the absence of other data suggesting progressive disease is discouraged.

Tg antibodies are detected in almost 25 % of patients with DTC and interfere with Tg assays [111]. For these patients, a decline in Tg antibody titers is believed to indicate a declining disease burden, but it takes a median of 3 years to clear Tg antibody levels after cure from DTC [112]. A large rise in Tg antibodies likely suggests disease progression and warrants further evaluation and possible treatment. Once children become Tg antibody negative, they are routinely followed similar to those children who were antibody negative from the outset.

Treatment of Residual/Recurrent Disease

Recurrent PTC develops in 30 % of children, most commonly in cervical lymph nodes [24]. In most cases, cervical disease can be successfully addressed with repeat surgery [113]. Up to 20 % of children with DTC have pulmonary metastases [16, 23, 24, 114–119], and these patients generally also have extensive cervical node involvement [18]. RAI is indicated for children with pulmonary metastases that are known or presumed to be iodine avid, but care must be given to select a dosage that will not result in pulmonary fibrosis. Therapy should be based on RAI uptake and tumor burden as well as patient's age and body size, complemented by dosimetry in select cases when available. A history of prior use of RAI is important because uptake may decline after each successive dosage [85]. Multiple dosages of RAI are frequently effective for pulmonary metastases but should only be given to children who are likely to benefit [81]. Durante et al. treated 37 young patients with pulmonary metastases [105]. Most (79 %) had negative RAI scans after RAI therapy and the 10-year (100 %) and 20-year (87 %) survival were excellent. Biko et al. treated 20 children and found that Tg levels continued to decline even after cessation of RAI therapy [29]. Further study is needed regarding the optimal dosing, timing, and duration of RAI therapy for children with DTC and iodine-avid pulmonary metastases. Regardless, the decision to treat should always be individualized, particularly in those patients who have already received multiple high dosages of RAI [38].

What Are Acceptable End Points for RAI Therapy in Children?

Given the potential risks of RAI therapy, and the probability that many children with pulmonary metastases will develop stable but persistent disease over many years, what should be the ultimate goal for RAI administration? Should one strive for undetectable serum Tg levels and no evidence of disease, or should one settle for stable but persistent disease? It will be obvious from the previous discussions that the answers to these questions are not yet known.

Advocates for rendering patients free from disease, as evidenced by undetectable serum Tg, base their recommendation on theoretical concerns involving RAI uptake by tumor cells, risks of dedifferentiation, and the physics of tissue destruction that correlate with RAI incorporation per gram of malignant tumor [25]. Intuitively, RAI should be more effective earlier in therapy, when the tumor burden is small and tumor cells demonstrate more avid RAI uptake and incorporation [28]. However, in a series of articles, Vassilopoulou-Sellin et al. showed that children can persist with stable disease despite therapy and that death from disease was no more frequent than death from complications of therapy [120–122], and Biko et al. [29] showed that serum Tg levels and presumably the extent of disease may decline for years after cessation of RAI therapy. It would seem prudent, therefore, to suggest that treatment of children with repeated dosages of RAI should be considered on an individual basis and that the frequency of therapy should probably be decreased from what is currently done at most centers. For patients with persistent iodine-avid pulmonary metastases, increasing caution is suggested as more than two RAI dosages are considered. Ideally, efficacy should be documented for each individual RAI therapy by a decrease in serum Tg level, a decrease in RAI uptake over the lung fields, or a decrease in tumor mass by other imaging techniques. In the absence of such evidence, or in the case of a low but detectable serum Tg level with a negative diagnostic RAI whole-body scan (WBS), continued treatment of young patients is controversial [17, 18, 30, 123].

Imaging

WBSs with RAI are unable to distinguish benign from malignant lesions during the preoperative evaluation of children with thyroid neoplasia [124–127]. However, the RAI WBS was, for decades, the "gold standard" for detecting residual thyroid cancer after thyroidectomy in adults and children [11, 16]. Recent data in adults have shown that serum Tg levels are a more sensitive indicator of disease, particularly when obtained after stimulation with synthetic recombinant human thyrotropin (rhTSH) or thyroid hormone withdrawal [97, 103, 128]. Because rhTSH is not yet approved for use in children, similar comparative studies of rhTSH-stimulated serum Tg and WBS are lacking in the pediatric age group. Despite that, we believe that serum Tg levels are a sensitive and specific marker of persistent or recurrent DTC in children. Whether the diagnostic WBS will provide additional benefit in the follow-up of children with treated DTC remains to be seen. In general, however, a diagnostic WBS continues to be useful for monitoring the anatomic location, treatment response, and extent of disease in children. The incorporation of single-photon emission computed tomography with fusion with non-contrast computed tomography (SPECT/CT) can also enhance the anatomic localization and determine the clinical significance of iodine-avid lesions, in addition to possibly guiding the decision to treat with RAI in the first place (see Chaps. 14 and 15) [129].

US has long been used in the successful preoperative evaluation of thyroid lesions in children [127]. However, neck US has also been introduced into routine follow-up of the patient with DTC [95, 130]. A study by Frasoldati et al. found that neck US was the most sensitive procedure for detecting local-regional recurrence in the neck of patients with DTC [130]. The sensitivity of US (94 %) was superior to that of either serum Tg values (57 %) or WBS (45 %). Based on the general availability, sensitivity, and noninvasive characteristics of US, neck US may prove to be of great benefit in the long-term follow-up of children with DTC [18].

Children with detectable serum Tg, but negative RAI diagnostic WBS, reflect a particularly vexing problem. Attempts have been made to identify and localize recurrent or persistent disease using computerized tomographic imaging, magnetic resonance imaging, and, more recently, ^{18}F fluorodeoxyglucose (^{18}F-FDG) positron emission tomography scanning (PET). In adults with thyroid cancer, ^{18}F-FDG-PET had a 71–93.9 % sensitivity and similar specificity [131–135]. Unfortunately, reactive lymphadenopathy can also be imaged with this technique [136, 137], which is particularly problematic in the younger population in whom reactive lymphadenopathy is common. These findings suggest the need for additional studies in children before this technique can be strongly recommended.

Summary

In summary, RAI has been widely used for the therapy of children and adolescents with DTC and continues to be recommended for those with iodine-avid distant metastases, a group most likely to benefit from RAI therapy. RAI may also reduce the recurrence risk for children and adolescents with DTC who are at high risk, including those with large tumors, extensive lymph node involvement, and incomplete resection but possibly not for those with less extensive disease.

An increasing body of evidence suggests that children appear to be at increased risk for second malignancies if treated with RAI, prompting some experts to advocate for "deferred" RAI therapy of low-risk children. In all cases, follow-up is lifelong in order to detect subsequent recurrence that could be treated with surgery (cervical node recurrence), RAI (iodine-avid distant metastases), or medically (tyrosine kinase inhibitors).

References

1. Seidlin SM, Marinelli LD, Oshry E. Radioactive iodine therapy: effect on functioning metastases of adenocarcinoma of thyroid. JAMA. 1946;132:838–47.
2. Cooper DS, Doherty GM, Haugen BR, Kloos RT, Lee SL, Mandel SJ, Mazzaferri EL, McIver B, Pacini F, Schlumberger M, et al. Revised American Thyroid Association management guidelines for patients with thyroid nodules and differentiated thyroid cancer. Thyroid. 2009;19:1167–214.
3. Singer PA, Cooper DS, Daniels GH, Ladenson PW, Greenspan FS, Levy EG, Braverman LE, Clark OH, McDougall IR, Ain KV, et al. Treatment guidelines for patients with thyroid nodules and well-differentiated thyroid cancer. American Thyroid Association. Arch Intern Med. 1996;156:2165–72.
4. DeGroot LJ, Kaplan EL, McCormick M, Straus FH. Natural history, treatment, and course of papillary thyroid carcinoma. J Clin Endocrinol Metab. 1990;71:414–24.
5. Feinmesser R, Lubin E, Segal K, Noyek A. Carcinoma of the thyroid in children – a review. J Pediatr Endocrinol Metab. 1997;10:561–8.
6. Geiger JD, Thompson NW. Thyroid tumors in children. Otolaryngol Clin N Am. 1996;29:711–9.
7. Gorlin JB, Sallan SE. Thyroid cancer in childhood. Endocrinol Metab Clin N Am. 1990;19:649–62.
8. Landau D, Vini L, A'Hern R, Harmer C. Thyroid cancer in children: the Royal Marsden Hospital experience. Eur J Cancer. 2000;36:214–20.
9. LaQuaglia M, Black T, Holcomb G, Sklar C, Azizkhan R, Haase G, Newman K. Differentiated thyroid cancer: clinical characteristics, treatment, and outcome in patients under 21 years of age who present with distant metastases. A report from the Surgical Discipline Committee of the Children's Cancer Group. J Pediatr Surg. 2000;35:955–9.
10. LaQuaglia M, Telander R. Differentiated and medullary thyroid cancer in children and adolescence. Semin Pediatr Surg. 1997;6:42–9.
11. McClellan DR, Francis GL. Thyroid cancer in children, pregnant women, and patients with Graves' disease. Endocrinol Metab Clin N Am. 1996;25:27–48.
12. Newman KD, Black T, Heller G, Azizkhan RG, Holcomb 3rd GW, Sklar C, Vlamis V, Haase GM, La Quaglia MP. Differentiated thyroid cancer: determinants of disease progression in patients <21 years of age at diagnosis: a report from the Surgical Discipline Committee of the Children's Cancer Group. Ann Surg. 1998;227:533–41.
13. Poth M. Thyroid cancer in children and adolescents. In: Wartofsky L, editor. Thyroid cancer: a comprehensive guide to clinical management. Totowa: Humana Press; 2000. p. 121–8.
14. Skinner MA. Cancer of the thyroid gland in infants and children. Semin Pediatr Surg. 2001;10:119–26.
15. Tronko MD, Bogdanova TI, Komissarenko IV, Epstein OV, Oliynyk V, Kovalenko A, Likhtarev IA, Kairo I, Peters SB, LiVolsi VA. Thyroid carcinoma in children and adolescents in Ukraine after the Chernobyl nuclear accident: statistical data and clinicomorphologic characteristics. Cancer. 1999;86:149–56.
16. Welch Dinauer CA, Tuttle RM, Robie DK, McClellan DR, Svec RL, Adair C, Francis GL. Clinical features associated with metastasis and recurrence of differentiated thyroid cancer in children, adolescents and young adults. Clin Endocrinol (Oxf). 1998;49:619–28.
17. Rivkees SA, Mazzaferri EL, Verburg FA, Reiners C, Luster M, Breuer CK, Dinauer CA, Udelsman R. The treatment of differentiated thyroid cancer in children: emphasis on surgical approach and radioactive iodine therapy. Endocr Rev. 2011; 32:798–826.
18. Waguespack SG, Francis G. Initial management and follow-up of differentiated thyroid cancer in children. J Natl Compr Cancer Netw. 2010;8:1289–300.
19. Thyroid, Carcinoma, Task, and Force. AACE/AAES medical/surgical guidelines for clinical practice: management of thyroid carcinoma. American Association of Clinical Endocrinologists. American College of Endocrinology. Endocr Pract. 2001; 7:202–20.
20. Lazar L, Lebenthal Y, Steinmetz A, Yackobovitch-Gavan M, Phillip M. Differentiated thyroid carcinoma in pediatric patients: comparison of presentation and course between pre-pubertal children and adolescents. J Pediatr. 2009;154:708–14.
21. Chow S, Law S, Mendenhall W, Au S, Yau S, Mang O, Lau W. Differentiated thyroid carcinoma in childhood and adolescence – clinical course and role of radioiodine. Pediatr Blood Cancer. 2004;42:176–83.
22. Fassina AS, Rupolo M, Pelizzo MR, Casara D. Thyroid cancer in children and adolescents. Tumori. 1994;80:257–62.
23. Harness JK, Thompson NW, McLeod MK, Pasieka JL, Fukuuchi A. Differentiated thyroid carcinoma in children and adolescents. World J Surg. 1992;16:547–53; discussion 553–544.
24. Hay ID, Gonzalez-Losada T, Reinalda MS, Honetschlager JA, Richards ML, Thompson GB. Long-term outcome in 215 children and adolescents with papillary thyroid cancer treated during 1940 through 2008. World J Surg. 2010;34:1192–202.

24b. Markovina S, Grigsby P, Schwarz JK, DeWees T, Moley JF, Siegel BJ, Perkins SM. Treatment approach, surveillance, and outcome of well-differentiated thyroid cancer in childhood and adolescence. Thyroid. 2014;24:1121–6.

25. Maxon HR. The role of radioiodine in the treatment of childhood thyroid cancer – a dosimetric approach. In: Jacob Robbins M, editor. Treatment of thyroid cancer in childhood. Bethesda: NIDDK, National Institutes of Health; 1992. p. 109–26.
26. Samuel AM, Rajashekharrao B, Shah DH. Pulmonary metastases in children and adolescents with well- differentiated thyroid cancer. J Nucl Med. 1998;39:1531–6.
27. Samuel AM, Sharma SM. Differentiated thyroid carcinomas in children and adolescents. Cancer. 1991;67:2186–90.
28. Yeh SD, La Quaglia MP. ^{131}I therapy for pediatric thyroid cancer. Semin Pediatr Surg. 1997;6:128–33.
29. Biko J, Reiners C, Kreissl MC, Verburg FA, Demidchik Y, Drozd V. Favourable course of disease after incomplete remission on (131)I therapy in children with pulmonary metastases of papillary thyroid carcinoma: 10 years follow-up. Eur J Nucl Med Mol Imaging. 2011;38:651–5.
30. La Quaglia MP, Black T, Holcomb GW, Sklar C, Azizkhan RG, Haase GM, Newman KD. Differentiated thyroid cancer: clinical characteristics, treatment, and outcome in patients under 21 years of age who present with distant metastases. A report from the Surgical Discipline Committee of the Children's Cancer Group. J Pediatr Surg. 2000;35:955–60.
31. Pawelczak M, David R, Franklin B, Kessler M, Lam L, Shah B. Outcomes of children and adolescents with well-differentiated

thyroid carcinoma and pulmonary metastases following ^{131}I treatment: a systematic review. Thyroid. 2010;20:1095–101.
32. Jarzab B, Handkiewicz Junak D, Wloch J, Kalemba B, Roskosz J, Kukulska A, Puch Z. Multivariate analysis of prognostic factors for differentiated thyroid carcinoma in children. Eur J Nucl Med. 2000;27:833–41.
32b. Enomoto K, Enomoto K, Uhino S, Shibuya H, Watanabe S, et al. Clinical features, treatment and long term outcome of papillary thyroid cancer in children and adolescents without radiation exposure. World J Surg. 2012;36:1241–6.
32c. Mikhailovic J, Nikoletic K, Srbovan D. Recurrent disease in juvenile differentiated thyroid carcinoma; prognostic factors, treatments, and outcomes. J Nucl Med. 2014;55:710–717.9.
33. Thompson GB, Hay ID. Current strategies for surgical management and adjuvant treatment of childhood papillary thyroid carcinoma. World J Surg. 2004;28:1187–98.
34. Tisell LE, Nilsson B, Molne J, Hansson G, Fjalling M, Jansson S, Wingren U. Improved survival of patients with papillary thyroid cancer after surgical microdissection. World J Surg. 1996; 20:854–9.
35. Schlumberger M, De Vathaire F. 131 iodine: medical use. Carcinogenic and genetic effects. Ann Endocrinol. 1996;57: 166–76.
36. Shore RE. Issues and epidemiological evidence regarding radiation-induced thyroid cancer. Radiat Res. 1992;131:98–111.
37. Thompson DE, Mabuchi K, Ron E, Soda M, Tokunaga M, Ochikubo S, Sugimoto S, Ikeda T, Terasaki M, Izumi S, et al. Cancer incidence in atomic bomb survivors. Part II: Solid tumors, 1958–1987 [published erratum appears in Radiat Res 1994 Jul;139(1):129]. Radiat Res. 1994;137:S17–67.
38. Rubino C, de Vathaire F, Dottorini ME, Hall P, Schvartz C, Couette JE, Dondon MG, Abbas MT, Langlois C, Schlumberger M. Second primary malignancies in thyroid cancer patients. Br J Cancer. 2003;89:1638–44.
39. Brown AP, Chen J, Hitchcock YJ, Szabo A, Shrieve DC, Tward JD. The risk of second primary malignancies up to three decades after the treatment of differentiated thyroid cancer. J Clin Endocrinol Metab. 2008;93:504–15.
40. Sandeep TC, Strachan MW, Reynolds RM, Brewster DH, Scelo G, Pukkala E, Hemminki K, Anderson A, Tracey E, Friis S, et al. Second primary cancers in thyroid cancer patients: a multinational record linkage study. J Clin Endocrinol Metab. 2006;91:1819–25.
41. Baugnet-Mahieu L, Lemaire M, Leonard E, Leonard A, Gerber G. Chromosome aberrations after treatment with radioactive iodine for thyroid cancer. Radiat Res. 1994;140:429–31.
42. Puerto S, Marcos R, Ramirez M, Galofre P, Creus A, Surrales J. Equal induction and persistence of chromosome aberrations involving chromosomes 1, 4, and 10 in thyroid cancer patients treated with radioactive iodine. Mutat Res Gene Toxicol Environ Mutagen. 2000;469:147–58.
43. Richter HE, Lohrer HD, Hieber L, Kellerer AM, Lengfelder E, Bauchinger M. Microsatellite instability and loss of heterozygosity in radiation- associated thyroid carcinomas of Belarussian children and adults. Carcinogenesis. 1999;20:2247–52.
44. Mandel SJ, Mandel L. Radioactive iodine and the salivary glands. Thyroid. 2003;13:265–71.
45. Goolden AW, Kam K, Fitzpatrick M, Munro A. Oedema of the neck after ablation of the thyroid with radioactive iodine. Br J Radiol. 1986;59:583–6.
46. Kloos R, Duvuuri V, Jhiang S, Cahill K, Foster J, Burns J. Nasolacrimal drainage system obstruction from radioactive iodine therapy for thyroid carcinoma. J Clin Endocrinol Metab. 2002;87:5817–20.
47. Handelsman DJ, Turtle JR. Testicular damage after radioactive iodine (I-131) therapy for thyroid cancer. Clin Endocrinol (Oxf). 1983;18:465–72.
48. Raymond JP, Izembart M, Marliac V, Dagousset F, Merceron R, Vulpillat M, Vallee G. Temporary ovarian failure in thyroid cancer patients after thyroid remnant ablation with radioactive iodine. J Clin Endocrinol Metab. 1989;69:186–90.
49. Smith MB, Xue H, Takahashi H, Cangir A, Andrassy RJ. Iodine 131 thyroid ablation in female children and adolescents: long-term risk of infertility and birth defects. Ann Surg Oncol. 1994;1:128–31.
50. Powers PA, Dinauer CA, Tuttle RM, Francis GL. Treatment of recurrent papillary thyroid carcinoma in children and adolescents. J Pediatr Endocrinol Metab. 2003;16:1033–40.
51. Kouvaraki MA, Shapiro SE, Fornage BD, Edeiken-Monro BS, Sherman SI, Vassilopoulou-Sellin R, Lee JE, Evans DB. Role of preoperative ultrasonography in the surgical management of patients with thyroid cancer. Surgery. 2003;134:946–54; discussion 954–945.
52. Shaha AR. TNM classification of thyroid carcinoma. World J Surg. 2007;31:879–87.
53. Borson-Chazot F, Causeret S, Lifante JC, Augros M, Berger N, Peix JL. Predictive factors for recurrence from a series of 74 children and adolescents with differentiated thyroid cancer. World J Surg. 2004;28:1088–92.
54. Wada N, Sugino K, Mimura T, Nagahama M, Kitagawa W, Shibuya H, Ohkuwa K, Nakayama H, Hirakawa S, Yukawa N, et al. Treatment strategy of papillary thyroid carcinoma in children and adolescents: clinical significance of the initial nodal manifestation. Ann Surg Oncol. 2009;16:3442–9.
55. Demidchik IE, Kontratovich VA. Repeat surgery for recurrent thyroid cancer in children. Vopr Onkol. 2009;49:366–9.
56. Musacchio MJ, Kim AW, Vijungco JD, Prinz RA. Greater local recurrence occurs with "berry picking" than neck dissection in thyroid cancer. Am Surg. 2003;69:191–6; discussion 196–197.
57. Arora N, Turbendian HK, Kato MA, Moo TA, Zarnegar R, Fahey TJ. Papillary thyroid carcinoma and microcarcinoma: is there a need to distinguish the two? Thyroid. 2009;19:473–7.
58. Sosa JA, Tuggle CT, Wang TS, Thomas DC, Boudourakis L, Rivkees S, Roman SA. Clinical and economic outcomes of thyroid and parathyroid surgery in children. J Clin Endocrinol Metab. 2008;93:3058–65.
59. The NCCN Clinical Practice Guidelines in Oncology, Thyroid Carcinoma (Version 1.2010). National Comprehensive Cancer Network; 2010.
60. Gimm O, Rath FW, Dralle H. Pattern of lymph node metastases in papillary thyroid carcinoma. Br J Surg. 1998;85:252–4.
61. Salter KD, Andersen PE, Cohen JI, Schuff KG, Lester L, Shindo ML, Sauer D, Gross ND. Central nodal metastases in papillary thyroid carcinoma based on tumor histologic type and focality. Arch Otolaryngol Head Neck Surg. 2010;136:692–6.
62. Vergez S, Sarini J, Percodani J, Serrano E, Caron P. Lymph node management in clinically node-negative patients with papillary thyroid carcinoma. Eur J Surg Oncol. 2010;36:777–82.
63. Sywak M, Cornford L, Roach P, Stalberg P, Sidhu S, Delbridge L. Routine ipsilateral level VI lymphadenectomy reduces postoperative thyroglobulin levels in papillary thyroid cancer. Surgery. 2006;140:1000–5; discussion 1005–1007.
64. Grubbs EG, Rich TA, Li G, Sturgis EM, Younes MN, Myers JN, Edeiken-Monroe B, Fornage BD, Monroe DP, Staerkel GA, et al. Recent advances in thyroid cancer. Curr Probl Surg. 2008; 45:156–250.
65. Shen WT, Ogawa L, Ruan D, Suh I, Duh QY, Clark OH. Central neck lymph node dissection for papillary thyroid cancer: the reliability of surgeon judgment in predicting which patients will benefit. Surgery. 2010;148:398–403.
66. Hay ID, Hutchinson ME, Gonzalez-Losada T, McIver B, Reinalda ME, Grant CS, Thompson GB, Sebo TJ, Goellner JR. Papillary

thyroid microcarcinoma: a study of 900 cases observed in a 60-year period. Surgery. 2008;144:980–7; discussion 987–988.
67. Noguchi S, Yamashita H, Uchino S, Watanabe S. Papillary microcarcinoma. World J Surg. 2008;32:747–53.
68. Hay ID, Grant CS, van Heerden JA, Goellner JR, Ebersold JR, Bergstralh EJ. Papillary thyroid microcarcinoma: a study of 535 cases observed in a 50-year period. Surgery. 1992;112:1139–46; discussion 1146–1137.
69. Lo CY, Chan WF, Lang BH, Lam KY, Wan KY. Papillary microcarcinoma: is there any difference between clinically overt and occult tumors? World J Surg. 2006;30:759–66.
70. Marcy PY, Thariat J, Peyrottes I, Benezery K, Benisvy D, Dassonville O, Santini J. Fulminant lethal spread of occult papillary microcarcinoma of the thyroid. Thyroid. 2010;20:445–8.
71. Taylor T, Specker B, Robbins J, Sperling M, Ho M, Ain K, Bigos ST, Brierley J, Cooper D, Haugen B, et al. Outcome after treatment of high-risk papillary and non-Hurthle-cell follicular thyroid carcinoma. Ann Intern Med. 1998;129:622–7.
72. Asari R, Koperek O, Scheuba C, Riss P, Kaserer K, Hoffmann M, Niederle B. Follicular thyroid carcinoma in an iodine-replete endemic goiter region: a prospectively collected, retrospectively analyzed clinical trial. Ann Surg. 2009;249:1023–31.
73. Zou CC, Zhao ZY, Liang L. Childhood minimally invasive follicular carcinoma: clinical features and immunohistochemistry analysis. J Paediatr Child Health. 2010;46:166–70.
74. Rachmiel M, Charron M, Gupta A, Hamilton J, Wherrett D, Forte V, Daneman D. Evidence-based review of treatment and follow up of pediatric patients with differentiated thyroid carcinoma. J Pediatr Endocrinol Metab. 2006;19:1377–93.
75. Dinauer C, Francis GL. Thyroid cancer in children. Endocrinol Metab Clin N Am. 2007;36:779–806, vii.
76. Spoudeas HA, editor. Paediatric endocrine tumours. West Sussex: Novo Nordisk Ltd; 2005.
77. Kuijt WJ, Huang SA. Children with differentiated thyroid cancer achieve adequate hyperthyrotropinemia within 14 days of levothyroxine withdrawal. J Clin Endocrinol Metab. 2005;90:6123–5.
78. Hanscheid H, Lassmann M, Luster M, Thomas SR, Pacini F, Ceccarelli C, Ladenson PW, Wahl RL, Schlumberger M, Ricard M, et al. Iodine biokinetics and dosimetry in radioiodine therapy of thyroid cancer: procedures and results of a prospective international controlled study of ablation after rhTSH or hormone withdrawal. J Nucl Med. 2006;47:648–54.
79. Lau WF, Zacharin MR, Waters K, Wheeler G, Johnston V, Hicks RJ. Management of paediatric thyroid carcinoma: recent experience with recombinant human thyroid stimulating hormone in preparation for radioiodine therapy. Intern Med J. 2006;36: 564–70.
80. Luster M, Handkiewicz-Junak D, Grossi A, Zacharin M, Taieb D, Cruz O, Hitzel A, Casas JA, Mader U, Dottorini ME. Recombinant thyrotropin use in children and adolescents with differentiated thyroid cancer: a multicenter retrospective study. J Clin Endocrinol Metab. 2009;94:3948–53.
81. Leboulleux S, Baudin E, Hartl DW, Travagli JP, Schlumberger M. Follicular cell-derived thyroid cancer in children. Horm Res. 2005;63:145–51.
82. Reynolds JC. Comparison of I-131 absorbed radiation doses in children and adults: a tool for estimating therapeutic I-131 doses in children. In: Jacob Robbins M, editor. Treatment of thyroid cancer in childhood. Bethesda: NIDDK, National Institutes of Health; 1992. p. 127–35.
83. Van Nostrand D, Atkins F. Pediatric differentiated thyroid cancer: can the prescribed activity of I-131 be increased? J Clin Endocrinol Metab. 2011;96:2401–3.
84. Verburg FA, Biko J, Diessl S, Demidchik Y, Drozd V, Rivkees SA, Reiners C, Hanscheid H. I-131 activities as high as safely administrable (AHASA) for the treatment of children and adolescents with advanced differentiated thyroid cancer. J Clin Endocrinol Metab. 2011;96:E1268–71.
85. Lassmann M, Reiners C, Luster M. Dosimetry and thyroid cancer: the individual dosage of radioiodine. Endocr Relat Cancer. 2010;17:R161–72.
86. Tuttle RM, Leboeuf R, Robbins RJ, Qualey R, Pentlow K, Larson SM, Chan CY. Empiric radioactive iodine dosing regimens frequently exceed maximum tolerated activity levels in elderly patients with thyroid cancer. J Nucl Med. 2006;47:1587–91.
87. Dorn R, Kopp J, Vogt H, Heidenreich P, Carroll R, Gulec S. Dosimetry-guided radioactive iodine treatment in patients with metastatic differentiated thyroid cancer: largest safe dose using a risk-adapted approach. J Nucl Med. 2003;44:451–6.
88. Kao CH, Yen TC. Stunning effects after a diagnostic dose of iodine-131. Nuklearmedizin. 1998;37:30–2.
89. Leger FA, Izembart M, Dagousset F, Barritault L, Baillet G, Chevalier A, Clerc J. Decreased uptake of therapeutic doses of iodine-131 after 185-MBq iodine-131 diagnostic imaging for thyroid remnants in differentiated thyroid carcinoma. Eur J Nucl Med. 1998;25:242–6.
90. Maxon HR, Thomas SR, Hertzberg VS, Kereiakes JG, Chen IW, Sperling MI, Saenger EL. Relation between effective radiation dose and outcome of radioiodine therapy for thyroid cancer. N Engl J Med. 1983;309:937–41.
91. Reynolds JC, Robbins J. The changing role of radioiodine in the management of differentiated thyroid cancer. Semin Nucl Med. 1997;27:152–64.
92. Tuttle RM, Grewal RK, Larson SM. Radioactive iodine therapy in poorly differentiated thyroid cancer. Nat Clin Pract Oncol. 2007;4:665–8.
93. Waguespack SG, Sherman SI, Williams MD, Clayman GL, Herzog CE. The successful use of sorafenib to treat pediatric papillary thyroid carcinoma. Thyroid. 2009;19:407–12.
94. Biondi B, Filetti S, Schlumberger M. Thyroid-hormone therapy and thyroid cancer: a reassessment. Nat Clin Pract Endocrinol Metab. 2005;1:32–40.
95. Pacini F, Molinaro E, Castagna MG, Agate L, Elisei R, Ceccarelli C, Lippi F, Taddei D, Grasso L. Recombinant human thyrotropin-stimulated serum thyroglobulin combined with neck ultrasonography has the highest sensitivity in monitoring differentiated thyroid carcinoma. J Clin Endocrinol Metab. 2003;88:3668–73.
96. Pacini F, Capezzone M, Elisei R, Ceccarelli C, Taddei D, Pinchera A. Diagnostic 131-iodine whole-body scan may be avoided in thyroid cancer patients who have undetectable stimulated serum Tg levels after initial treatment. J Clin Endocrinol Metab. 2002;87:1499–501.
97. Robbins RJ, Chon JT, Fleisher M, Larson SM, Tuttle RM. Is the serum thyroglobulin response to recombinant human thyrotropin sufficient, by itself, to monitor for residual thyroid carcinoma? J Clin Endocrinol Metab. 2002;87:3242–7.
98. Cailleux AF, Baudin E, Travagli JP, Ricard M, Schlumberger M. Is diagnostic iodine-131 scanning useful after total thyroid ablation for differentiated thyroid cancer? J Clin Endocrinol Metab. 2000;85:175–8.
99. Kloos RT, Mazzaferri EL. A single recombinant human thyrotropin-stimulated serum thyroglobulin measurement predicts differentiated thyroid carcinoma metastases three to five years later. J Clin Endocrinol Metab. 2005;90:5047–57.
100. Pacini F, Agate L, Elisei R, Capezzone M, Ceccarelli C, Lippi F, Molinaro E, Pinchera A. Outcome of differentiated thyroid cancer with detectable serum Tg and negative diagnostic ^{131}I whole body scan: comparison of patients treated with high (131)I activities versus untreated patients. J Clin Endocrinol Metab. 2001;86: 4092–7.
101. Pineda JD, Lee T, Ain K, Reynolds JC, Robbins J. Iodine-131 therapy for thyroid cancer patients with elevated thyroglobulin

and negative diagnostic scan. J Clin Endocrinol Metab. 1995;80:1488–92.
102. Baudin E, Do Cao C, Cailleux AF, Leboulleux S, Travagli JP, Schlumberger M. Positive predictive value of serum thyroglobulin levels, measured during the first year of follow-up after thyroid hormone withdrawal, in thyroid cancer patients. J Clin Endocrinol Metab. 2003;88:1107–11.
103. Mazzaferri EL, Robbins RJ, Spence CA, Braverman LE, Pacini F, Wartofsky L, Haugen BR, Sherman SI, Cooper DS, Braunstein GD, et al. A consensus report of the role of serum thyroglobulin as a monitoring method for low-risk patients with papillary thyroid carcinoma. J Clin Endocrinol Metab. 2003;88:1433–41.
104. Bauer AJ, Tuttle RM, Francis G. Thyroid nodules and thyroid carcinoma in children. In: Pescovitz O, Eugster E, editors. Pediatric endocrinology: mechanisms, manifestations, and management. Philadelphia: Lippincott; 2004.
105. Durante C, Haddy N, Baudin E, Leboulleux S, Hartl D, Travagli JP, Caillou B, Ricard M, Lumbroso JD, De Vathaire F, et al. Long-term outcome of 444 patients with distant metastases from papillary and follicular thyroid carcinoma: benefits and limits of radioiodine therapy. J Clin Endocrinol Metab. 2006;91:2892–9.
106. Antonelli A, Miccoli P, Fallahi P, Grosso M, Nesti C, Spinelli C, Ferrannini E. Role of neck ultrasonography in the follow-up of children operated on for thyroid papillary cancer. Thyroid. 2003;13:479–84.
107. Dottorini ME, Vignati A, Mazzucchelli L, Lomuscio G, Colombo L. Differentiated thyroid carcinoma in children and adolescents: a 37-year experience in 85 patients. J Nucl Med. 1997;38:669–75.
108. Samuel AM, Rajashekharrao B, Shah DH. Pulmonary metastases in children and adolescents with well-differentiated thyroid cancer. J Nucl Med. 1998;l39:1531–6.
109. Demidchik YE, Saenko VA, Yamashita S. Childhood thyroid cancer in Belarus, Russia, and Ukraine after Chernobyl and at present. Arq Bras Endocrinol Metabol. 2007;51:748–62.
110. Brink JS, van Heerden JA, McIver B, Salomao DR, Farley DR, Grant CS, Thompson GB, Zimmerman D, Hay ID. Papillary thyroid cancer with pulmonary metastases in children: long-term prognosis. Surgery. 2000;128:881–6; discussion 886–887.
111. Spencer CA, Takeuchi M, Kazarosyan M, Wang CC, Guttler RB, Singer PA, Fatemi S, LoPresti JS, Nicoloff J. Serum thyroglobulin autoantibodies: prevalence, influence on serum thyroglobulin measurement, and prognostic significance in patients with differentiated thyroid carcinoma. J Clin Endocrinol Metab. 1998;83:1121–7.
112. Chiovato L, Latrofa F, Braverman LE, Pacini F, Capezzone M, Masserini L, Grasso L, Pinchera A. Disappearance of humoral thyroid autoimmunity after complete removal of thyroid antigens. Ann Intern Med. 2003;139:346–51.
113. Clayman GL, Shellenberger TD, Ginsberg LE, Edeiken BS, El-Naggar AK, Sellin RV, Waguespack SG, Roberts DB, Mishra A, Sherman SI. Approach and safety of comprehensive central compartment dissection in patients with recurrent papillary thyroid carcinoma. Head Neck. 2009;31:1152–63.
114. Zimmerman D, Hay ID, Gough IR, Goellner JR, Ryan JJ, Grant CS, McConahey WM. Papillary thyroid carcinoma in children and adults: long-term follow-up of 1039 patients conservatively treated at one institution during three decades. Surgery. 1988;104:1157–66.
115. Vassilopoulou-Sellin R, Klein MJ, Smith TH, Samaan NA, Frankenthaler RA, Goepfert H, Cangir A, Haynie TP. Pulmonary metastases in children and young adults with differentiated thyroid cancer. Cancer. 1993;71:1348–52.
116. Schlumberger M, De Vathaire F, Travagli JP, Vassal G, Lemerle J, Parmentier C, Tubiana M. Differentiated thyroid carcinoma in childhood: long term follow-up of 72 patients. J Clin Endocrinol Metab. 1987;65:1088–94.
117. Bal CS, Kumar A, Chandra P, Dwivedi SN, Mukhopadhyaya S. Is chest x-ray or high-resolution computed tomography scan of the chest sufficient investigation to detect pulmonary metastasis in pediatric differentiated thyroid cancer? Thyroid. 2004;14:217–25.
118. Demidchik YE, Demidchik EP, Reiners C, Biko J, Mine M, Saenko VA, Yamashita S. Comprehensive clinical assessment of 740 cases of surgically treated thyroid cancer in children of Belarus. Ann Surg. 2006;243:525–32.
119. O'Gorman CS, Hamilton J, Rachmiel M, Gupta A, Ngan BY, Daneman D. Thyroid cancer in childhood: a retrospective review of childhood course. Thyroid. 2010;20:375–80.
120. Vassilopoulou-Sellin R. Long-term outcome of children with papillary thyroid cancer. Surgery. 2001;129:769.
121. Vassilopoulou-Sellin R, Goepfert H, Raney B, Schultz PN. Differentiated thyroid cancer in children and adolescents: clinical outcome and mortality after long-term follow-up. Head Neck. 1998;20:549–55.
122. Vassilopoulou-Sellin R, Schultz PN, Haynie TP. Clinical outcome of patients with papillary thyroid carcinoma who have recurrence after initial radioactive iodine therapy. Cancer. 1996;78:493–501.
123. La Quaglia MP, Telander RL. Differentiated and medullary thyroid cancer in childhood and adolescence. Semin Pediatr Surg. 1997;6:42–9.
124. Belfiore A, Giuffrida D, La Rosa GL, Ippolito O, Russo G, Fiumara A, Vigneri R, Filetti S. High frequency of cancer in cold thyroid nodules occurring at young age. Acta Endocrinol (Copenh). 1989;121:197–202.
125. Hopwood NJ, Kelch RP. Thyroid masses: approach to diagnosis and management in childhood and adolescence. Pediatr Rev. 1993;14:481–7.
126. Hung W. 1Nodular thyroid disease and thyroid carcinoma. Pediatr Ann. 1992;21:50–7.
127. Lugo-Vicente H, Ortiz VN. Pediatric thyroid nodules: insights in management. Bol Asoc Med P R. 1998;90:74–8.
128. Mazzaferri EL, Kloos RT. Is diagnostic iodine-131 scanning with recombinant human TSH useful in the follow-up of differentiated thyroid cancer after thyroid ablation? J Clin Endocrinol Metab. 2002;87:1490–8.
129. Blum M, Tiu S, Chu M, Goel S, Friedman K. I-131 SPECT/CT elucidates cryptic findings on planar whole-body scans and can reduce needless therapy with I-131 in post-thyroidectomy thyroid cancer patients. Thyroid. 2011;21:1235–47.
130. Frasoldati A, Pesenti M, Gallo M, Caroggio A, Salvo D, et al. Diagnosis of neck recurrences in patients with differentiated thyroid carcinoma. Cancer. 2003;97:90–6.
131. Alnafisi NS, Driedger AA, Coates G, Moote DJ, Raphael SJ. FDG PET of recurrent or metastatic 131I-negative papillary thyroid carcinoma. J Nucl Med. 2000;41:1010–5.
132. Chung JK, So Y, Lee JS, Choi CW, Lim SM, Lee DS, Hong SW, Youn YK, Lee MC, Cho BY. Value of FDG PET in papillary thyroid carcinoma with negative ^{131}I whole-body scan. J Nucl Med. 1999;40:986–92.
133. Wang W, Larson SM, Fazzari M, Tickoo SK, Kolbert K, Sgouros G, Yeung H, Macapinlac H, Rosai J, Robbins RJ. Prognostic value of [^{18}F]fluorodeoxyglucose positron emission tomographic scanning in patients with thyroid cancer. J Clin Endocrinol Metab. 2000;85:1107–13.
134. Wang W, Macapinlac H, Larson SM, Yeh SD, Akhurst T, Finn RD, Rosai J, Robbins RJ. [^{18}F]-2-fluoro-2-deoxy-D-glucose positron emission tomography localizes residual thyroid cancer in patients with negative diagnostic (131)I whole body scans and elevated serum thyroglobulin levels. J Clin Endocrinol Metab. 1999;84:2291–302.

135. Yeo JS, Chung JK, So Y, Kim S, Lee E, Lee DS, Youn YK, Hong SJ, Ahn IM, Lee MC, et al. F-18-fluorodeoxyglucose positron emission tomography as a presurgical evaluation modality for I-131 scan-negative thyroid carcinoma patients with local recurrence in cervical lymph nodes. Head Neck. 2001;23:94–103.
136. Frilling A, Gorges R, Tecklenborg K, Gassmann P, Bockhorn M, Clausen M, CE B. Value of preoperative diagnostic modalities in patients with recurrent thyroid carcinoma. Surgery. 2000;128:1067–74.
137. Frilling A, Tecklenborg K, Gorges R, Weber F, Clausen M, Broelsch E. Preoperative diagnostic value of [(18)F] fluorodeoxyglucose positron emission tomography in patients with radioiodine-negative recurrent well-differentiated thyroid carcinoma. Ann Surg. 2001;234:804–11.

Positron Emission Tomography-Computed Tomography (PET-CT and PET) in Well-Differentiated Thyroid Cancer

43

Andrei Iagaru and Iain Ross McDougall

Introduction

Positron emission tomography-computed tomography (PET-CT) is a diagnostic technique that has become very important in oncology [1]. The objective of this chapter is to present an overview of the following topics: PET physics and scanners, radiopharmaceutical for PET and indications, imaging technique, normal findings and variations, interpretation of PET-CT scans, false-positive findings, ^{18}F-FDG PET-CT and PET scanning in differentiated thyroid cancer (DTC), role in thyroglobulin (Tg)-positive and iodine-negative patients, prognostic value of ^{18}F-FDG PET scans, and the role of TSH in ^{18}F-FDG PET scanning. The chapter concludes with a brief introduction to ^{124}I PET scanning and other PET-CT radiopharmaceuticals.

PET Physics and Scaners

The basis for a PET scan is the injection of a positron-emitting radiopharmaceutical into the patient that localizes in cancers and can be imaged. A positron is a positive electron, and when emitted from the radioisotope, it travels up to a few millimeters before coming in contact with an electron that has a negative charge. These particles of equal mass and opposite charges annihilate one another. The annihilation of the masses of the positive and negative electrons produces two photons, each with an energy of 511 keV. This is derived from the equation $e = mc^2$. The photons travel in opposite directions with an angle of 180°. A positron camera usually consists of a ring of detectors designed to identify photons interacting at precisely the same time on opposite positions on the ring (180°). These are called coincident events. Millions of coincident events can be reconstructed into images of the distribution of the positron-emitting radiopharmaceutical within the patient.

However, an important problem for imaging positron-emitting radiopharmaceuticals is the correction of attenuation of those photons by the tissue. Specifically, coincident photons arising from different parts of the patient travel through different lengths of the body before reaching the ring of detectors. Thus, when a positron is emitted from a lesion in the skin on a shoulder, one photon travels through millimeters of tissue and then strikes the detector whereas the other photon has to travel through the width of the patient before interacting with the opposing detector. However, more of the photons that have to travel the longer distance through tissue will be absorbed (thus more attenuation) than those that have to travel the shorter distance—attenuation. In order to take this into account, the attenuation of the photons by the tissues of the body must be corrected. Historically, this has been obtained by repeating the scan using a source of radiation such as germanium (^{68}Ge) outside the patient, which in turn allows a measure of the different amounts of attenuation present. Over the past several years, improved technology has resulted in a PET scanner that has been combined with a CT scanner (PET-CT) [2]. The CT images are now used routinely for attenuation correction and for providing an anatomic correlation with the functional PET images. Currently, most companies manufacture predominately hybrid PET-CT scanners, and now, the first clinical PET-MR hybrid scanner has been installed. Because the positron detector is about 15 cm long, the detector must be moved to six to seven positions, called bed positions, in order to image the entire head, neck, and trunk areas. A PET scan takes approximately 30 min to complete. The extrinsic attenuation

A. Iagaru, MD (✉)
Department of Radiology, Nuclear Medicine, Stanford University Medical Center, Stanford School of Medicine,
300 Pasteur Dr, H2230 MC 5281, Stanford, CA 94305, USA
e-mail: aiagaru@stanford.edu

I.R. McDougall, MD, PhD, FRCP
Department of Radiology, Nuclear Medicine, Stanford University Hospital and Clinics, Stanford, CA USA
e-mail: RossMcDougall@Stanford.edu

L. Wartofsky, D. Van Nostrand (eds.), *Thyroid Cancer*, DOI 10.1007/978-1-4939-3314-3_43

Table 43.1 Positron-emitting radionuclides for thyroid studies

Characteristic	^{18}F	^{124}I	^{120}I	^{122}I	^{68}Ga
Half-life	110 min	4.18 days	1.35 h	3.6 min	68 min
B^{+} yield %	97	23	46	77	88
E_{B+}	635 keV	1.5 MeV	4.6 MeV	3.1 MeV	1.9 MeV
Daughter product	^{18}O	^{124}Te	^{120}Te	^{122}Te	^{68}Zn

correction by the older technique (i.e., ^{68}Ge) required a further 20–30 min, but this is reduced to about 1–2 min for combined PET-CT. Therefore, the combined PET-CT scan provides better attenuation correction, additional anatomic information, and faster throughput of patients.

Prior to the widespread sale and installation of hybrid PET-CT scanners, several companies produced scintigraphic gamma cameras. These were conventional whole-body gamma cameras with two detectors whose primary functions were to produce anterior and whole-body scintiscans or single-photon tomographic images. The two heads could also be used for detecting coincident gamma rays, and therefore, they could be used for PET imaging [3–5]. Unfortunately, these cameras had several disadvantages, the most important of which was the reduced counting ability of the two detectors versus the ring format of a dedicated PET instrument. Secondly, these cameras also had significantly reduced resolution, whereas one of the important benefits of a PET scanner is the excellent resolution. The future will be in the dedicated PET scanners combined with CT.

Radiopharmaceuticals for PET and Indications

In oncology, the PET radiopharmaceutical that is most frequently employed is ^{18}F-fluorodeoxyglucose (^{18}F-FDG). ^{18}F-FDG is taken into cells by Glut transporters where it is acted on by hexokinase. However, thereafter, it is not metabolized as rapidly as glucose and remains within the cells. Cancer cells have an increase in Glut and hexokinase. Images are obtained 1–2 h after intravenous injection of ^{18}F-FDG and demonstrate cells that have taken up and retained this radio-agent.

The main role of PET using ^{18}F-FDG is in areas of oncology distinct from thyroid cancer, and these include differentiating a benign from malignant lung nodule, in staging and evaluating the response to therapy of non-small cell lung cancer, lymphoma, head and neck cancer, esophageal and recurrent colorectal cancer, and melanoma or breast cancer [6–10]. PET-CT imaging of the brain is also important not only for cancers but in diagnosis of degenerative diseases such as Alzheimer's, multi-infarct dementia, and Parkinson's disease. PET-CT also has a role in defining whether or not ischemic myocardium is viable. In the management of patients with differentiated thyroid cancer, its main indication is the evaluation of patients who have an elevated thyroglobulin (Tg) blood level and a negative whole-body ^{131}I and/or ^{123}I diagnostic scan and/or ^{131}I post-therapy scan. ^{18}F-FDG is approved for this purpose in the United States. It is also valuable in the patient who has a positive radioiodine scan but where the thyroglobulin is disproportionally high (e.g., a small remnant with uptake <1 % seen on scintiscan associated with a Tg >1000 ng/ml). Another use, albeit a minor one, is to differentiate a benign from a malignant thyroid nodule, but the reliability and cost-effectiveness argue against this approach (see Chap. 25). ^{18}F-FDG PET-CT has a limited role in pretreatment staging of patient with newly diagnosed cancer, but it is useful for such in patients who have primary lymphoma of the thyroid or anaplastic thyroid cancer and is discussed in the relevant chapters (see Chaps. 43, 76, 87, 93, and 97).

In the case of thyroid cancer, there is a second positron emitter, ^{124}I, that has valuable properties and will have an increasing role in the management of differentiated thyroid cancer. ^{120}I and ^{122}I are also positron emitters but have not been introduced into clinical practice [11]. Table 43.1 provides the physical characteristics of these positron emitters, and ^{124}I is briefly discussed near the end of this chapter as well as in Chap. 103.

Imaging Technique

^{18}F-FDG is injected intravenously, and imaging is initiated approximately 1 h later. The patient should fast for at least 6 h before the injection, and the patient should typically be NPO after midnight. The patient should not exercise vigorously for 24 h prior to the study. In the United States, most authorities recommend measuring serum glucose prior to the injection of ^{18}F-FDG because high levels alter the distribution of the radiopharmaceutical and lower the sensitivity of the scan. In countries where the incidence of latent and prediabetic patients is low, this is not necessary. When the glucose is greater than 200 mg/dl, we advise canceling the procedure until the blood glucose is normal. ^{18}F-FDG PET imaging in diabetics requires the involvement of the patient, referring physician, and nuclear medicine technologist and physician in achieving safely an appropriate level of glucose.

After injection of ^{18}F-FDG, the patient should rest in a quiet, warm, and comfortable room for the hour between the injection of ^{18}F-FDG and imaging. The patient should not talk or chew. The reason for these precautions is that active muscles take up ^{18}F-FDG, and the uptake can cause difficulty in interpretation, which may result in false-positive findings (see below). In some patients, uptake of ^{18}F-FDG in brown fat in the neck can be misinterpreted as metastases to nodes. However, as reported by Garcia et al. [12], brown fat uptake can be essentially eliminated by keeping the patient warm several hours before the scan, and we and others have found that a single dose of propranolol 1 h before injection of ^{18}F-FDG may also help [12]. Some authorities delay scanning for 90–120 min. The extra time allows more of the background activity to be excreted through the kidneys thus making the lesions easier to detect. For thyroid cancer, this is seldom necessary, and for a steady throughput of patients, the delay of 1 h is the best compromise for accuracy and efficiency.

Normal Findings and Variations

The brain highly concentrates ^{18}F-FDG because the brain depends on a significant amount of glucose for function. ^{18}F-FDG is excreted through the kidneys and the bladder, and these areas may appear to have significant uptake. There is varying uptake in muscles and myocardium, but in a patient who has fasted and been inactive and has a normal fasting glucose, these structures should have modest uptake and allow anatomic correlation without interfering with the interpretation. ^{18}F-FDG may concentrate diffusely in the liver.

Although the thyroid is a metabolically active gland, somewhat surprisingly, the normal thyroid is typically not observed or is only faintly observed on ^{18}F-FDG scan 1 h after injection (*see also* Chap. 25). PET-CT allows the thyroid anatomy to be defined by the CT and frequently in patients being scanned for non-thyroidal cancer, the normal thyroid cannot be identified on ^{18}F-FDG PET (Fig. 43.1) When there is diffusely increased uptake in the thyroid, the patient usually has autoimmune thyroid disease, most often chronic lymphocytic thyroiditis, and less frequently Graves' hyperthyroidism (Fig. 43.2) [14–17]. In the occasional patient with autoimmune thyroid disease, the uptake of ^{18}F-FDG can be focal and misinterpreted as a malignancy in the thyroid [16].

Focal uptake of ^{18}F-FDG in the thyroid in a patient being evaluated for a non-thyroidal disease has about 10–50 % chance of being a thyroid cancer. The wide range depends on patient selection for a pathological diagnosis [18]. Cancer detected this way is usually a differentiated primary thyroid lesion, but metastasis from the non-thyroidal cancer can also occur. The latter happens most frequently in patients with melanoma and lung, renal cell, breast, or bowel cancer. In an analysis of more than 4500 ^{18}F-FDG PET scans, 2.3 % showed some abnormality in the thyroid [13]. In 87 patients, this was not pursued because of the severity of their primary cancer. However, 15 patients had a biopsy and 7 (47 %) of these were thyroid cancer. Kang et al. also reported that 2.2 % of scans showed a thyroid "incidentaloma" [14]. Some of these were diffuse and consistent with thyroiditis, but 4 of 15 (27 %) focal lesions were malignant. Several reports indicated a risk of cancer of 50 % or greater [15]. In an unpublished interinstitutional investigation, we and other colleagues identified 15 focally "hot" lesions. Nine patients were referred for operation and eight cancers were diagnosed histologically (Fig. 43.3). Ho et al. found a prevalence of thyroid uptake on ^{18}F-FDG PET-CT of 3.7 % in their retrospective review of 5877 subjects with no previous history of thyroid malignancy. Of patients who had verification by cytology or histology, 14 % (8/55) were found to have thyroid malignancies [16]. In a separate study, focal thyroidal uptake was identified in 76 of 6241 (1.2 %) [17]. Only 14 patients (18 %) had a biopsy and 4 (28.6 %) had papillary thyroid carcinoma. This begs the question of how many of the remaining 62 had cancer. Are et al. evaluated 16,300 PET scans in 8800 patients [18]. They found 263 thyroidal abnormalities (1.6 % of scans, 2.9 % of patients). Fifty-seven of the patients had fine needle aspiration (FNA), and 24 cancers were found (42 %). The incidence of thyroid cancer was 72 % in 27 patients who had thyroidectomy, and 19/20 patients had papillary cancer with the remaining patient having a lymphoma.

The term incidentaloma has been challenged for two reasons. As noted, a meaningful proportion is cancer and the lesions are functioning; hence, they prefer the term "metaboloma."

Some investigators note the degree of uptake in a metaboloma does not predict histology and underpins the importance of further investigations, in particular FNA, to exclude thyroid cancer. Others suggest that the intensity of ^{18}F-FDG uptake and the CT attenuation pattern significantly improve the accuracy of PET-CT for differentiating benign from malignant focal thyroid lesions. Benign nodules had a mean standardized uptake value (SUV) of 6.7± 5.5 whereas malignant ones had a mean value of 10.7 ± 7.8 ($P<0.05$) [19]. SUV is a quantitative measurement of the glucose uptake in regions of interest that can be selected on the image of the patient when viewed on the console of a computer. Researchers also evaluated ^{18}F-FDG PET performed for screening in healthy subjects. Chen et al. reported that thyroid metabolomas were identified in 1.2 % (60/4803) of patients, and that of those who underwent FNA and surgery, 14 % (7/50) metaboloma were found to be malignant [20].

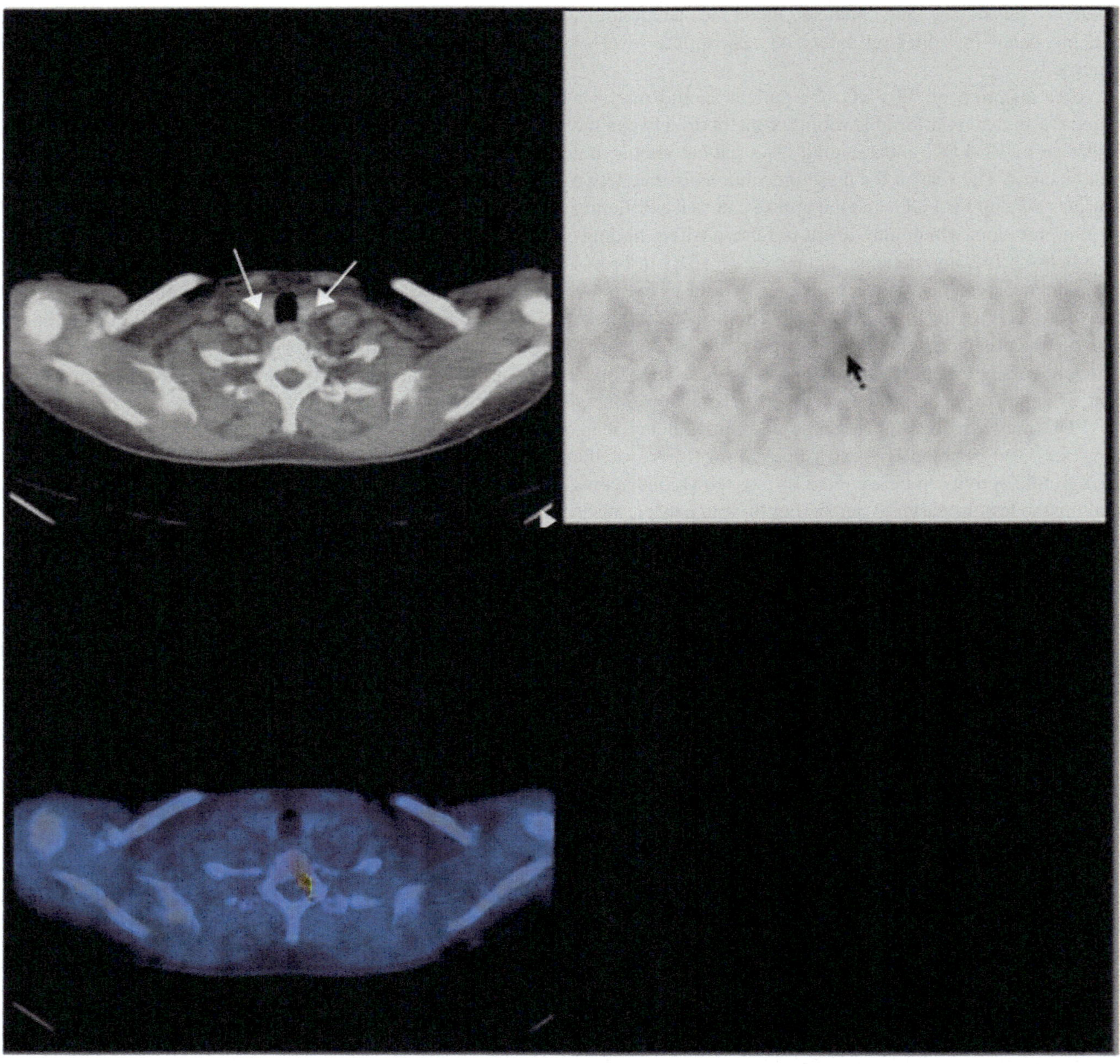

Fig. 43.1 A transaxial scan showing PET (*upper right*), CT (*upper left*), and combined PET and CT (*lower panel*). The *white arrows* show the thyroid on CT, and the *black arrow* shows a vertebra on PET scan. The thyroid has no uptake of FDG scan

Because undiagnosed thyroid cancer can appear as focally "hot" on ^{18}F-FDG scan, there was hope that ^{18}F-FDG PET would differentiate a malignant from a benign nodule. The technology is expensive and even if perfect would not replace FNA. In a study of nine patients, three cancers were PET positive but four of six benign lesions showed focal uptake [21]. Uematsu et al. using an SUV of five were able to separate four cancerous nodules from six benign ones but a patient with thyroiditis had an SUV of 6.3 [22]. In a small series of 15 patients with indeterminate cytopathology, ^{18}F-FDG PET-CT was positive in eight and negative in seven [23]. Of the eight positive cases, four were cancer, whereas three of the seven patients with negative ^{18}F-FDG PET-CT scans did subsequently have cancer confirmed. These results are equivalent to tossing a coin.

Therefore, not all focal ^{18}F-FDG PET-positive lesions in the thyroid are cancerous and an FNA, or ultrasound (US)-guided FNA, is appropriate to establish the diagnosis in most patients [24, 25]. Theoretically, ^{18}F-FDG PET might have a role in the indeterminate microfollicular lesion where the a

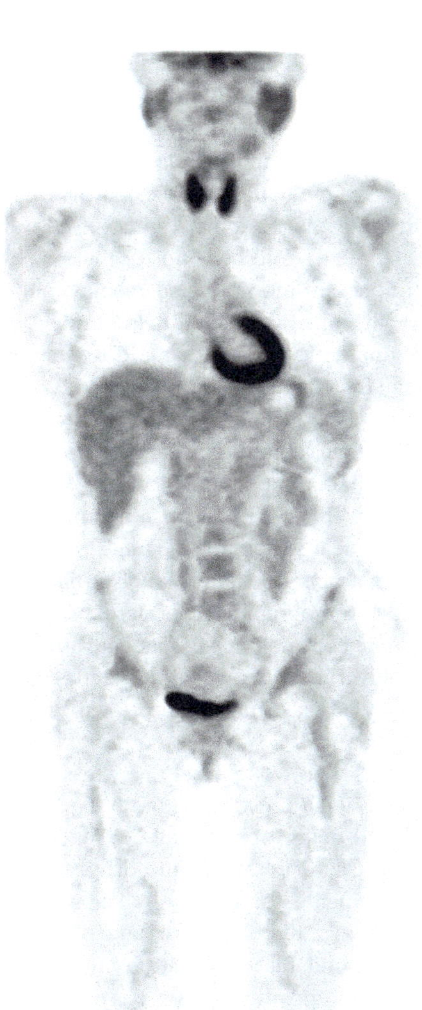

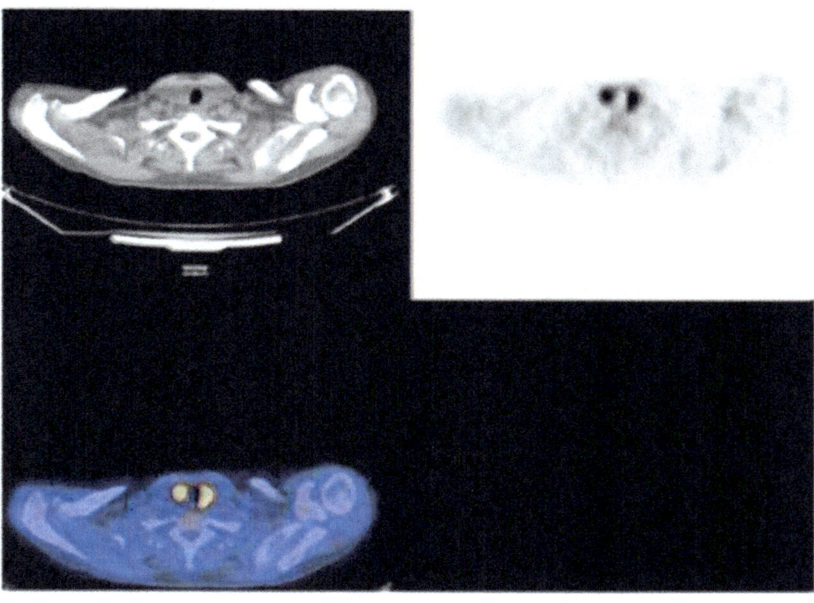

Fig. 43.2 A coronal PET scan (*left*). The image on the *right* is the transaxial images of the PET scan, CT, and combined PET-CT, as oriented in Fig. 43.1 and at the thyroid level. The thyroid has intense uptake of FDG. The patient had Hashimoto's thyroiditis

priori likelihood of cancer is greater than in nodules in general. A different group of investigators conducted ^{18}F-FDG PET-CT in 88 patients with nondiagnostic cytology [26]. Every patient had surgery and pathological confirmation and none of 41 patients (46 %) with a negative ^{18}F-FDG PET-CT had cancer. Thus, a negative ^{18}F-FDG PET could be more helpful than a positive one. In summary, the degree of focal ^{18}F-FDG uptake in a metaboloma does not predict histology and underpins the importance of further investigations—in particular FNA—to exclude thyroid cancer, and even in the indeterminate case, a focal "hot" spot on ^{18}F-FDG PET is not necessarily a cancer. However, a negative scan appears to exclude that diagnosis [27]. Again, further reading is available in Chap. 25.

Interpretation of PET-CT Scan

Regions of abnormal uptake of ^{18}F-FDG in recurrent or metastatic cancer are usually easy to identify. Combined PET-CT allows the exact anatomic site to be defined. Many authorities simply report on the findings on the scan. The optimal results are obtained by interpreting the results while sitting at a computer terminal and viewing systematically the coronal, sagittal, and transaxial projections. It is helpful to scroll through images of regions where an abnormality is identified or suspected. Some experts use a quantitative numeric result, which determines the uptake in the lesions compared to the amount of radiopharmaceutical injected. This is called the

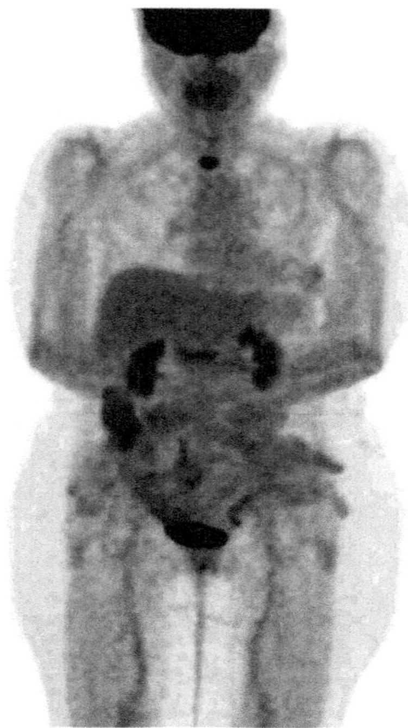

Fig. 43.3 A coronal projection showing a focal lesion in the thyroid that concentrates FDG. This was confirmed as an unsuspected papillary cancer

standardized uptake value (SUV). In general, a lesion with an SUV >2.5 is frequently accepted as being due to cancer; however, in one study discussed previously, the cutoff between malignant and benign thyroid nodule was five. In practice, the SUV is not very helpful to establish whether or not cancer is present in the thyroid, and it has also been referred to as the "silly uptake value" [28]. Locoregional and distant thyroid metastases are usually recognized visually, and the SUV is important as a baseline for comparison with subsequent scans to judge the response to treatment. SUVs may also have prognostic value as discussed below. Other investigators use the ratio of uptake in the cancer to background activity instead of the SUV. When a comparison of quantitative measurements is made between two studies, it is important to ensure they were conducted under identical conditions and that the SUV is not interpreted with an uptake ratio.

False-Positive Findings

^{18}F-FDG uptake on a PET-CT scan is not specific for thyroid cancer, and thus, ^{18}F-FDG PET-CT scans performed to evaluate for thyroid cancer may have false-positive uptake due to other malignant or active cells [29, 30]. Accordingly, it would be for a patient with thyroid cancer to also have another cancer. As discussed above, about 1–3 % of PET or PET-CT scans conducted in patients with non-thyroidal cancers show a focal thyroidal abnormality of which somewhere between 10 and 50 % are cancers. The percentage of patients with thyroid cancer who are found to have a non-thyroidal cancer diagnosed by PET-CT is not known with certainty. The distribution of any abnormal uptake should be carefully evaluated to make sure that it is consistent with the expected spread of thyroid cancer. The common sites of residual cancer would be the thyroid bed and for metastases to the regional lymph nodes in the neck and mediastinum, and distant metastases to the lungs and skeleton. Inflammatory conditions including tuberculosis and sarcoidosis show abnormal uptake, but the distribution is not likely to be confused with thyroid cancer.

There are additional specific conditions that are important in the interpretation of PET scans conducted for thyroid cancer. The first is uptake of ^{18}F-FDG in active neck muscles. Although the muscles are linear structures, the muscle uptake can result in what appears to be globular uptake similar to a lymph node. This is due to tomographic slices across muscle bellies. The finding is more common in patients who are nervous and trembling or shivering. This was first identified by Barrington et al. and they advised diazepam prior to injection of the radiopharmaceutical [31]. This requires knowledge a priori of the patients who would likely be stressed. In the United States, the physician prescribing the tranquilizer is responsible for the well-being of the patient. When the physician conducting the scan prescribes the drug, he/she must have all the requirements for conscious sedation in place. As a result, he/she is usually reluctant to take this step. Not all physicians have found that medications to reduce anxiety help reduce the false positives [38]. The poor response to anxiolytic medication most likely results from a different but more common cause of a false-positive uptake of ^{18}F-FDG in brown fat (Fig. 43.4) [32–35]. Superficially, this looks similar to the muscle uptake, but the distribution follows the shape of the neck being narrower at the level of the chin and wider at the thoracic inlet. In contrast, the muscle uptake follows the contour of the sternocleidomastoid and is therefore narrower at the manubrium. Uptake in brown fat is thought to be increased in cold temperature [33]. Our experience is that it is more common in thin women and in winter. A recent laboratory study in rats confirms that the ^{18}F-FDG uptake is increased by cold temperature, and it could be reduced by propranolol, and in one study, 90 % of the patients showed a reduction after 40 mg of propranolol orally 1 h prior to injection of ^{18}F-FDG [12, 36]. Garcia et al. demonstrated that virtually all ^{18}F-FDG uptake in brown fat can be eliminated with control of the ambient temperature around the patient prior to injection of the ^{18}F-FDG [12]. Brown fat is also localized along the vertebrae and around the diaphragm, and it can also take up on ^{18}F-FDG PET. The third abnormality that can be incorrectly diagnosed as cancer is

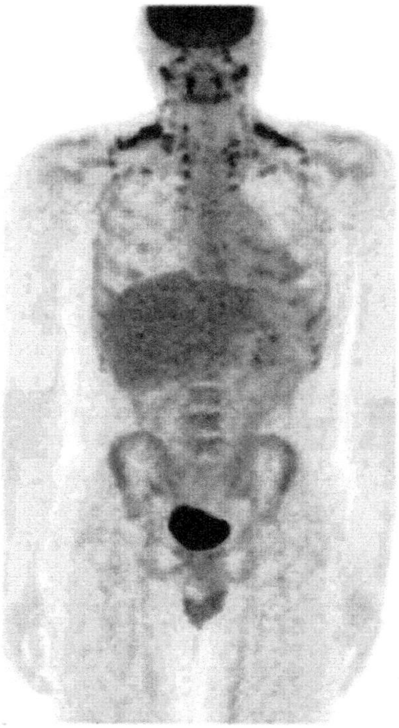

Fig. 43.4 A coronal section made 1 h after injection of 15 mCi (550 MBq) of FDG, showing symmetric uptake in the supraclavicular areas as a result of uptake in brown fat

asymmetric uptake in the functional muscles of one vocal cord when the contralateral nerve was damaged during thyroidectomy [37, 38]. A similar finding has been reported in a granulomatous foreign body reaction around a Teflon® implant to improve a paralyzed vocal cord [39]. Uptake of ^{18}F-FDG in the thymus has also been reported [40–45]. This is more common in younger patients and in those who have recently been treated with chemotherapy and perhaps after therapeutic ^{131}I. Although the bilobed shape is characteristic, this can be misinterpreted as mediastinal metastases. Combining PET-CT usually allows the differentiation of these false positives from metastatic cancer considerably easier.

^{18}F-FDG PET-CT and PET Scanning in Differentiated Thyroid Cancer: Role in Tg-Positive and Iodine-Negative Patients

The consensus for the optimal treatment for differentiated thyroid cancer is total or near total thyroidectomy and ^{131}I therapy in selected patients excluding those with small primary cancers [46]. The combination of surgery and ^{131}I therapy removes all functioning thyroid and allows for follow-up using measurement of serum Tg and in selected patients whole-body scan with ^{123}I. When the therapy has been successful, both follow-up studies are negative. When there is residual or recurrent disease, both scans are typically abnormal and allow a decision to be made about retreating with ^{131}I. However, in 15–30 % of patients with residual or recurrent disease, there is a discrepancy between the scans usually with Tg being measurable and the diagnostic radioiodine scan being negative. The reasons for this could be that there are too few cells to be identified on scan or a defect in the function or location of the sodium-iodide symporter (NIS). This is a difficult and trying problem for the patient and physician, and it has led to differences in philosophies about management (see Chap. 47). Some take the position that a therapeutic administration of ^{131}I will deliver sufficient radiation to seek out, localize in, and kill the cells producing the Tg [47, 48]. But not all physicians caring for these patients accept this approach [49–52]. An alternative approach is to employ imaging scans that are not dependent on the NIS for identifying the thyroid tissue. Imaging could include US of the neck, CT, MRI, and a range of nuclear medicine procedures (see Chap. 44). Taking the nuclear medicine scans in their historical sequence, thallium 201 (^{201}Tl) is a large atom that is taken up by the sodium potassium channel of cells. It is valuable for evaluating myocardial perfusion. Thallium is concentrated by some cancers including thyroid cancer and became popular for imaging patients with thyroid cancer [53–56]. Because of the low energy of the emitted photons and the high absorbed radiation, the small injected activity results in ^{201}Tl images that are poor in comparison to those made with radiopharmaceuticals containing technetium 99m (^{99m}Tc). As a result, ^{201}Tl is presently not used in patients with thyroid cancer. When ^{99m}Tc-labeled radiopharmaceuticals were developed for studying myocardial perfusion, they were investigated in oncology and found to be valuable in identifying sites of metastatic thyroid cancer. The images are superior to ^{201}Tl because the emitted photons have a higher energy that is suited for current gamma cameras. In addition, a larger quantity of radioactivity can be injected. The two radiopharmaceuticals are sestamibi and tetrofosmin [57]. In one report of 110 scans in 99 patients, ^{99m}Tc sestamibi and Tg agreed in 96 % [58]. However, in most of the patients, both scans were negative. There were only 16 patients with abnormal results who had a whole-body radioiodine scan. In four (25 %) of the patients, the ^{99m}Tc sestamibi scan demonstrated a lesion not seen on ^{131}I images. Similarly, ^{99m}Tc tetrofosmin has been demonstrated to identify iodine-negative cancer. Gallowitsch et al. identified 39 of 44 lesions on ^{99m}Tc tetrofosmin scans compared with 19 on whole-body ^{131}I scans [59]. Subsequent publications from these and other investigators confirm these findings [60–63]. Finally, thyroid cancer may have somatostatin receptors [64], and the somatostatin receptor imaging agent, ^{111}In pentetreotide, has also been used, but the sensitivity does not make it a powerful scan [65, 66]. This has been discussed further in Chap. 44. It is surprising to

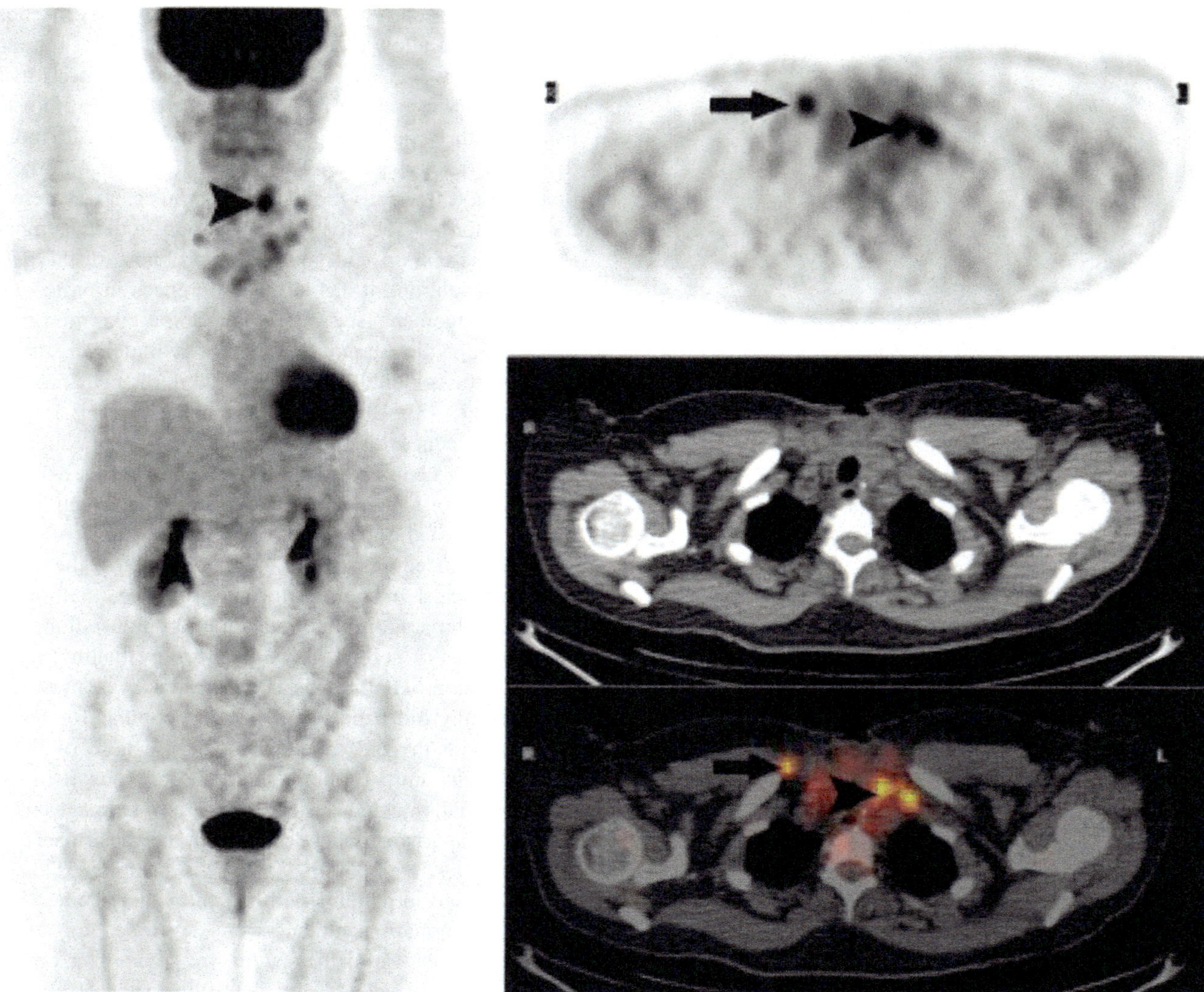

Fig. 43.5 The *left panel* shows an ^{18}F-FDG PET scan in a patient who has had thyroidectomy and ^{131}I therapy. The *arrowhead* shows a small area of ^{18}F-FDG uptake in the region of residual left lobe. Several other areas of uptake in the neck are metastases in lymph nodes. The *right panel* shows transaxial images at the level of the thyroid with a PET image at the *top*, CT image in the *middle*, and fused PET-CT image at the *bottom*. The *arrowhead* shows the same spot and the *arrow* shows one of the nodal metastasis

report that the first publication of ^{18}F-FDG PET scan for thyroid cancer dates from as early as 1987 [67]. Then, there was a delay of almost a decade after which several subsequent reports appeared. Presently, many articles have been published addressing the role and value of ^{18}F-FDG PET scan in adult patients who have measurable Tg but negative radioiodine studies [68–77]. In addition, several editorials and reviews have been published attesting to the value of ^{18}F-FDG PET [78–82]. We and other authors have found this also to be of value in children [83]. The images are superior to scans from all the other radiopharmaceuticals discussed briefly above, and the combination of PET with CT provides anatomic information that increases both sensitivity and specificity. In general, the interpretation can be reached with confidence.

It has become apparent that the less differentiated the thyroid cancer is, the more likely the ^{18}F-FDG PET scan will be positive. Very well-differentiated cancers show less or even no uptake of ^{18}F-FDG while having excellent ^{131}I uptake. This has been called a "flip/flop" phenomenon [84, 85]. Evidence for this is the comparison of ^{18}F-FDG and ^{131}I in 47 lesions [86]. Thirty-three lesions were iodine-positive but 20 (61 %) of these were ^{18}F-FDG PET negative. Conversely, there were 9 ^{18}F-FDG PET positive lesions from 14 (64 %) iodine-negative lesions. Figure 43.5 shows an abnormal ^{18}F-FDG PET-CT scan.

Table 43.2 Sensitivity of ^{18}F-FDG PET and PET-CT scans in Tg-positive, iodine-negative patients

Author reference	Number of patients	Women %	Men %	Ages	Sensitivity %	Specificity %	Altered treatment %
18F-FDG PET							
Alnafisi et al. [70]	11	73	27	19–66	100		64
Chung et al. [137]	54	78	22	24–72	94	95	
Dietlin et al. [138]	58	74	26	19–72	82		
Goshen et al. [104]	20	75	25	19–77	94		30
Grunwalt et al. [139]	222	68	32	NA	75	90	
Grunwalt et al. Tg >5 [139]					76	100	
Grunwalt et al. Iodine neg [139]					85	90	
Wang et al. [108]	37	62	38	16–83	71		51
Stokkel et al. [140]	11	55	45	26–73	100	100	
Helal et al. [141]	37	49	51	27–78	100	73	78
Schluter et al. [90]	64	61	39	21–81	65	42	11
18F-FDG PET-CT							
Mirallie et al. [92]	45	7	29	14–80	100	67	
Freudenberg et al. [142]	36	53	47	21–80	95	93	14
Ong et al. [143] [7]	17	65	45	35–73	100	100	
Kim et al. [144]	20	80	20	4–56	100	100	
Palmedo et al. [91]	40			56+16	95	90	61
Iagaru et al. [95]	76	57	43	20–81	89	89	
Rieman et al. [76]	327	209	118	53±18	92	95	43
van Dijk et al. [77]	52	36	16	44.6±16.5	69	94	13
Ozkan et al. [82]	59	44	15	48.2±22.6	82	30	

The original studies evaluated ^{18}F-FDG PET in a spectrum of patients some who had a remnant after surgery, some who had metastases that could be imaged with radioiodine, and some who had iodine-negative scans but measurable Tg. These investigations confirmed that the overall sensitivity of ^{18}F-FDG PET was low and the scan was not useful for "all-comers" [87]. However, when the Tg-positive/iodine-negative patients were analyzed separately, the sensitivity increased and the specificity remained powerful. Table 43.2 provides data from several publications including recent ones using ^{18}F-FDG PET-CT. It is apparent that the sensitivity varies from about 60 % to as high as 100 %. The high sensitivities are most likely due to the small number of patients being studied who had extensive disease. As the scan has become more widely used, patients with smaller volumes of cancer are being studied, and it is not surprising that the sensitivity has fallen. To determine specificity, it is not possible in many of these reports because all the patients studied had an elevated Tg; in other words, there were no patients who could be defined as being free of disease. In many reports, there is a relationship to the level of Tg, but there is no cutoff above which all ^{18}F-FDG PET scans are positive or below which they are all negative. In the United States, the current approved indication for PET is a Tg value of >10 ng/ml in a patient who has been treated by thyroidectomy and ^{131}I and who has a negative radioiodine scan. Although the Tg value of >10 ng/ml is arbitrary, publications do support that patients with Tg >10 ng/ml are more likely to have positive ^{18}F-FDG PET scans. Bertagna et al. in a study of 52 patients found there was a significant positive correlation between ^{18}F-FDG PET-CT-positive results and Tg levels [88]. They did not note any statistically significant correlation between ^{18}F-FDG PET-CT results and TSH levels. They found the highest accuracy was achieved when Tg was above 21 ng/ml. ^{18}F-FDG PET or ^{18}F-FDG PET-CT is not usually positive in patients with Tg levels below 2 ng/ml; however, there is usually no indication for the scan in that setting [89]. One benefit of ^{18}F-FDG PET is to identify surgically resectable sites of disease when clinical information or other imaging scans show one site of disease and ^{18}F-FDG PET shows several [90]. This prevents performing surgery only to be followed by identification of "new" recurrence.

In regard to ^{18}F-FDG PET-CT vs. ^{18}F-FDG PET alone, the former is more accurate than the latter. Palmedo et al. found that ^{18}F-FDG PET-CT has a diagnostic accuracy of 93 % and an improvement of 15 % over ^{18}F-FDG PET alone [91]. Mirallie et al. showed that ^{18}F-FDG PET-CT increased the diagnostic performance considerably over that of ^{18}F-FDG PET or CT alone with a sensitivity of 96 % for ^{18}F-FDG PET-CT, 82 % for ^{18}F-FDG PET, and 73 % for CT [92].

In a study with 50 patients with differentiated thyroid cancer, Esteva et al. found that the size of the cancer ($p<0.05$) and thyroid capsular invasion ($p<0.05$) were significantly associated with positive ^{18}F-FDG PET studies [93]. Choi et al. concluded that the absence of perithyroidal and lymphovascular invasion was an independent variable for false-negative findings on initial ^{18}F-FDG PET-CT in patients with papillary thyroid cancer [94].

Our group reviewed 98 ^{18}F-FDG PET-CTs in 76 patients and determined sensitivities per patient and per lesion of 87 % and 89 %, respectively, in patients with differentiated thyroid cancer [95]. We also reported that metastases in small cervical nodes might be missed due to the limitations of spatial resolution of PET. The most frequent sites of recurrent differentiated thyroid cancer are lymph nodes (53 %) and the thyroid bed (28 %). A study adding a higher resolution delayed dedicated neck ^{18}F-FDG PET-CT acquisition showed an increase number of abnormal foci in 29 % of the studies [96]. This increase was statistically significant. Kaneko et al. compared ^{18}F-FDG PET-CT and ^{131}I in nine patients with 33 lesions [97]. They identified all lesions by ^{18}F-FDG PET-CT but only 58 % with radioiodine. They confirm the SUV was statistically higher in lesions that did not take up iodine (6.6 ± 2.8 vs. 4.2 ± 1.8; $P=0.007$), and as expected, Tg values were significantly higher in patients with metastases to lymph nodes.

Choi et al. investigated ^{18}F-FDG PET-CTs for the initial staging of patients with papillary thyroid cancer and concluded that it did not provide additional information compared to neck sonography [98]. ^{18}F-FDG PET-CT showed lower sensitivity and higher specificity than sonography for detection of cervical node metastasis; however, no statistically significant difference was noted in their study ($p>0.99$). Even when the radioactive scans show iodine-avid disease, ^{18}F-FDG PET-CT may alter the management of some patients. Piccardo et al. showed that ^{18}F-FDG PET-CT detects more metastases in 45 % of patients with advanced differentiated thyroid cancer and a rising Tg in comparison with whole-body radioiodine and bone scans [99].

False-negative findings occur in well-differentiated cancer that retains ability to take up iodine avidly and in lesions that are too small to be resolved with modern dedicated ^{18}F-FDG PET-CT scanners that are less than about 6–8 mm. It should be emphasized that the PET and CT and combined PET-CT images should be studied since occasionally an abnormality can be identified on the CT images but not the ^{18}F-FDG PET.

Meta-analyses confirm the value of ^{18}F-FDG PET and ^{18}F-FDG PET-CT in differentiated thyroid cancer where radioiodine images are negative in particular when Tg is elevated [100–102]. In one analysis of ^{18}F-FDG PET and ^{18}F-FDG PET-CT for only papillary cancer, sensitivities calculated by two methods were 77 % and 84 % and specificities 85 % and 84 %, respectively [101]. In another, Dong et al. reviewed 549 abstracts from which they selected 195 publications, and after determining which ones met criteria of careful design, defined patient population, indications for ^{18}F-FDG PET or ^{18}F-FDG PET-CT, and confirmation of diagnosis, they were left with 25 articles, 6 of which dealt with F-FDG PET-CT [102]. Overall, the sensitivity in patients with measurable Tg and a negative ^{131}I scan was 0.885 (95 % CI: 0.828–0.929) and specificity 0.847 (95 % CI: 0.715–0.934). In the six investigations dealing with ^{18}F-FDG PET-CT, the sensitivity and specificity were 0.935 (95 % CI: 0.870–0.973) and 0.839 (95 % CI: 0.723–0.920), respectively.

Prognostic Value of ^{18}F-FDG PET Scans

A very abnormal ^{18}F-FDG PET scan with lesions showing a high SUV is a harbinger of a bad outcome [103]. In a study of 125 patients followed for 41 months, 14 patients died from thyroid cancer. The most important predictors were high SUV and a volume of cancer greater than 125 ml. In those with smaller tumor volumes, the 3-year survival was 96 %, and even patients with distant metastases who were ^{18}F-FDG PET negative all survived. This again reflects the "flip/flop" phenomenon. Well-differentiated cancer cells take up iodine and are amenable to ^{131}I therapy; less well-differentiated cancer cells do not take up iodine but do concentrate ^{18}F-FDG. In contrast, patients who are iodine negative as well as ^{18}F-FDG PET negative appear to have a good prognosis. In our experience, no patient has died and the recurrence rate is low.

As already discussed above, a positive ^{18}F-FDG PET scan can alter the management. Alnafisi et al. found that PET changed management in 7 of 11 patients, and Goshen et al. reported change in management in 6 of 20 [70, 104]. For example, when the radioiodine scan was negative, identification of a focal ^{18}F-FDG PET lesion can make surgery an option. A lesion in a vertebral body can be considered for surgical or external beam radiation. Our approach for lesions in the neck that are identified using ^{18}F-FDG PET is to obtain an US for precise anatomic localization and for US-guided FNA. The patient is operated on using intraoperative US to re-identify the site and to ensure it is excised [105]. All patients had a decrease in Tg and 64 % achieved undetectable values.

Ota et al. explored in a pilot study the use of ^{18}F-FDG PET-CT for detection of bone metastases from differentiated thyroid carcinoma. The sensitivities of ^{18}F-fluoride PET-CT and ^{99m}Tc bone scintigraphy were significantly higher than that of ^{18}F-FDG PET-CT in their report [106]. Nakajo et al. conducted a comparison of ^{18}F-FDG PET-CT vs. ^{18}F-FLT PET-CT in 20 patients with postoperative differentiated thyroid cancer, evaluating the images of lymph node and distant metastases. In a per-patient-based analysis, the sensitivity, specificity, and accuracy were 92 %, 86 %, and 90 %, respectively, for ^{18}F-FDG PET-CT and 69 %, 29 %, and 55 %, respectively, for ^{18}F-FLT PET-CT. The accuracy of ^{18}F-FDG PET-CT was significantly better than that of ^{18}F-FLT PET-CT ($P=0.023$) [107].

The Role of TSH in ^{18}F-FDG PET Scanning

The vast majority of ^{18}F-FDG studies in oncology including patients with thyroid cancer are conducted when the patient is euthyroid or, in some patients with thyroid cancer, when they are biochemically slightly hyperthyroid because of a desire to completely suppress the patient's TSH blood level. However, whether or not elevated TSH blood levels significantly improve detection of thyroid cancer on ^{18}F-FDG PET scans is controversial. Anecdotal patients who were studied twice—once when euthyroid and once with an elevated TSH—showed no difference in detection of lesions in those case reports [108, 109]. In contrast, Sisson reported increased uptake under TSH stimulus [110]. Several publications confirm this finding. This is in keeping with in vitro studies showing that TSH increases glucose uptake into thyroid cells [111]. In a study of 17 patients imaged when TSH was <0.05 μU/ml and again when the TSH was >22 μU/ml (on average 42 days later), the lesion-to-background ratio increased by an average of 63.1 % [112]. In three out of ten patients, new lesions were identified. In a similar experiment, 30 patients who had negative or equivocal ^{131}I scans and abnormal or equivocal Tg were studied before and after injection of recombinant human thyrotropin (rhTSH) [113]. When the TSH was low, a total of 45 lesions were seen in nine patients, and after administration of rhTSH, 78 lesions were seen in 19 patients. Therefore, many more lesions were diagnosed and some ^{18}F-FDG PET-negative patients became ^{18}F-FDG PET positive. These investigators did calculate an increase in SUV or lesion-to-background ratio. In a smaller study of seven patients, only one patient changed from ^{18}F-FDG PET negative to positive after injection of rhTSH [114].

In a study with 76 patients, we concluded that TSH levels at the time of ^{18}F-FDG PET-CT did not appear to impact the ability to detect disease or the ^{18}F-FDG uptake [95]. In a meta-analysis study, Ma et al. found statistically significant patient-based and lesion-based differences of ^{18}F-FDG uptake under TSH stimulation with enhanced tumor-to-background ratios compared with studies conducted when TSH was suppressed [115]. Management was altered in 9 % of patients. They also reported that the clinical significance of TSH-stimulated ^{18}F-FDG PET also depended on the knowledge of the range of possible treatments as well as cost and side effects. Of note, no end points such as survival and mortality were reported. A study comparing ^{18}F-FDG PET-CT performed before and 24 h after rhTSH administration in 63 patients indicated that rhTSH-stimulated ^{18}F-FDG PET-CT was significantly more sensitive than non-stimulated PET-CT for the detection of lesions (95 % vs. 81 %; $p=0.001$) and tended to be more sensitive for the detection of involved organs (94 % vs. 79 %; $p=0.054$). However, the number of patients in whom any lesion was detected was not different between the two groups. Management was altered in 6 % of patients [116]. In a study with 44 patients, Vera et al. also concluded that rhTSH-stimulated ^{18}F-FDG PET-CT has low sensitivity; however, the patients studied had relatively low Tg values [117]. They found no correlation between ^{18}F-FDG PET-CT and Tg levels, and positive scans were found in 20 % of patients with Tg levels lower than 10 ng/ml.

These data present a problem. Should all patients be studied with an elevated TSH? If yes, then should they be hypothyroid or euthyroid and injected with rhTSH? RhTSH has not been approved for ^{18}F-FDG PET scanning. One possible solution is to obtain a TSH-stimulated ^{18}F-FDG PET scan when the patient receives his/her rhTSH for a diagnostic radioiodine scan. The rhTSH injections could be made on Monday and Tuesday. The ^{18}F-FDG PET scan could then be obtained on Wednesday morning after a 6-h fast and then the tracer of radioiodine could be administered. Neither scan would interfere with the other. This ^{18}F-FDG PET scan could be performed when a high index of suspicion for disease still exists after a negative standard ^{18}F-FDG PET scan was performed with a low TSH.

^{124}I PET Scanning (See Also Chap. 103)

^{124}I has a half-life ($T_{1/2}$) of 4.2 days. It can be employed for PET imaging analogous to the use of ^{123}I and ^{131}I for planar and single-photon tomographic imaging [118]. PET always provides tomographic information and the images have superior resolution, and they can be used to determine volumes with accuracy. The combination of PET-CT allows images to be obtained faster, produces excellent correction for attenuation of 511 keV photons, and provides anatomic correlation (Fig. 43.6). There were theoretical concerns that the high-energy positrons and complex decay scheme with high-energy gamma photons of ^{124}I would not allow high-quality images to be obtained. Experimental studies with phantoms show that high-quality, well-resolved, images of ^{124}I are possible using a dedicated PET camera. This radioisotope of iodine is not easy to produce and is not widely used.

^{124}I has been of value in benign conditions of the thyroid, for example, in obtaining an accurate measurement of the volume of tissue to allow calculation of a specific absorbed radiation dose when treating Graves' disease [119–121]. One study showed an excellent correlation to the volume

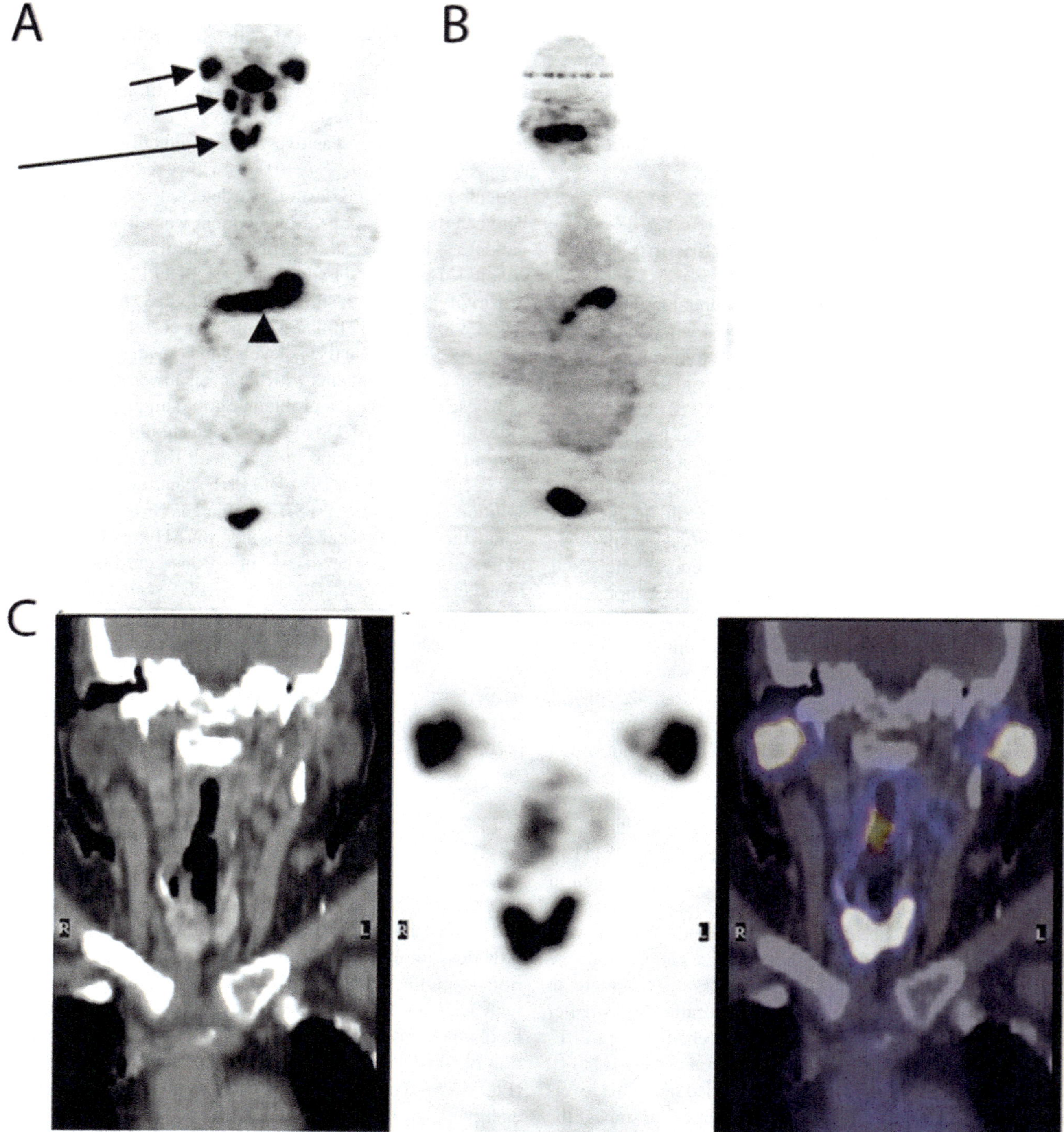

Fig. 43.6 (**a**) The *upper panel* on *left* shows anterior whole-body ^{124}I scan in patient after thyroidectomy. Significant residual thyroid is present bilaterally (*long black arrow*). There is also uptake of ^{124}I in the salivary glands (*short black arrows*) and stomach (*arrowhead*). (**b**) The *upper panel* on the *right* shows follow-up scan 1 year later with ^{131}I ablation of thyroid. (**c**) The *lower* three images represent coronal tomographic images of the lower head, neck, and thyroid area, which were obtain at the same time as (**a**) *above*. The *left*, *center*, and *right* images are CT, ^{124}I PET, and fused PET-CT, respectively

determined by US [122]. PET has the advantage of demonstrating functioning tissue as well as total volume. The role of ^{124}I in management of thyroid cancer is in development, but ^{124}I has significant potential because volumetric calculation of lesions can be obtained and the 4.2-day $T_{1/2}$ allows measurements to be made over time to measure total body clearance and $T_{1/2}$ in metastases. This allows more accurate dosimetry to be calculated, and quoting one group of investigators "is a useful procedure especially in advanced DTC, and allows the administration of safer and more effective radioiodine activities as well as earlier multimodal interventions compared to standard empirical protocols" [123]. This is expanded below and in Chap. 103.

In comparing uptake and clearance of ^{124}I and ^{131}I, Eschmann et al. [124] evaluated 3 patient and Atkins et al. [128] evaluated 25 patients, and both studies demonstrated good concordance.

Multiple studies have now been published comparing lesion detection of ^{124}I and ^{131}I, and this is discussed in more detail in Chap. 103. Freudenberg et al. [125, 126] reported twelve patients who were imaged 24 h after an average prescribed activity of 84 MBq (2.3 mCi) ^{124}I. The patients had ^{124}I PET scan, combined PET-CT, CT, and post-therapy ^{131}I scans. The detectability of lesions was 87 %, 100 %, 56 %, and 83 %, respectively.

In a study with 69 patients, Capoccetti et al. compared total body ^{124}I PET-CT and whole-body scintigraphy conducted before and after therapy with ^{131}I [127]. The two scans matched in 86.6 % of the studies. ^{124}I PET-CT detected more disease in 7 % of the patients, mostly in lymph nodes, and ^{131}I whole-body scan detected more disease in 4.9 %, mostly in disseminated ^{131}I-avid lung metastases. Another study involving 70 patients compared the ability of ^{124}I PET-CT to detect iodine-avid lung metastases and found that only 1 of 7 patients with disseminated lung metastases on the ^{131}I whole-body scan had uptake on the ^{124}I PET-CT [128]. This issue is particularly concerning if one is to use ^{124}I PET-CT for evaluation of extent of disease and prescribed activity calculation prior to ^{131}I therapy.

Comparing ^{124}I PET-CT with ^{131}I planar whole-body scan for the detection of residual and metastatic well-differentiated thyroid cancer, Van Nostrand et al. found that ^{124}I PET-CT identified 50 % more foci of radioiodine uptake suggestive of additional residual thyroid tissue and/or metastases in 32 % patients [129]. Freudenberg et al. compared ^{124}I PET-CT and ^{18}F-FDG PET-CT in the detection of recurrent differentiated thyroid carcinoma in patients with rising Tg values. They found sensitivities of 80 % and 70 % for ^{124}I PET-CT and ^{18}F-FDG PET-CT, respectively [130]. One third of the lesions demonstrated uptake with both tracers, while two thirds were positive on only one. Using both tracers, the sensitivity was 91 %.

^{124}I has also been studied for dosimetric calculations. The advantage is that high-resolution three-dimensional (3D) images can be acquired and the uptake, residence time, and volume of distribution determined. Sgouros et al. imaged 15 patients at 4, 20, 44 h and 4–6 days after prescribed activities from 74 to 148 MBq (2-4 mCi) of ^{124}I [131]. The results demonstrated that the method is feasible, and sequential PET scans can be used to obtain cumulated activity images for 3D dosimetry. Because the distribution of radioiodine within a lesion can be inhomogeneous, an accurate measurement of the radiation absorbed dose in different regions within cancer can be determined. The variability of the radiation absorbed dose is considerable and knowledge that regions of cancer are not going to receive an adequate dose would be the reason to consider additional treatment such as external radiation. It has been possible to obtain real-time three-dimensional radiobiological dosimetry using a software package, and although the researchers indicated this is unlikely to be used routinely, it certainly would be valuable in patients with extensive disease [132]. ^{124}I has been used to monitor the response to the MAPK kinase (MEK) 1 and MEK2 inhibitor selumetinib and to evaluate if the drug could reverse refractoriness to radioiodine in patients with metastatic thyroid cancer. In their study of 20 participants, Ho et al. report that selumetinib produces clinically meaningful increases in iodine uptake and retention in a subgroup of patients with thyroid cancer that is refractory to radioiodine. [133].

It should be noted that historically ^{124}I was used therapeutically [134]. This radioisotope deposits significant radiation; therefore, the diagnostic tracer could theoretically cause "stunning," a controversial topic debated elsewhere in this textbook (Chaps. 16, 17, and 18). Researchers using ^{124}I should study this possibility by comparing ^{124}I and ^{131}I post-therapy scans.

^{124}I has been used to label peptides, antibodies, and other compounds and appears to be a suitable tracer for both quantitative and imaging pharmacological investigations [135].

Other PET-CT Radiopharmaceuticals (See Chap. 44)

Somatostatin receptor scintigraphy using predominantly ^{111}In-labeled tracers has been used to evaluate differentiated thyroid cancers that have reduced or absent uptake of radioiodine. Somatostatin receptor analogues have also been labeled with positron emitters. ^{68}Ga DOTATOC is a PET tracer that has a high affinity for somatostatin receptors 2 and 5. Middendorp et al. compared ^{68}Ga DOTATOC and ^{18}F-FDG PET-CT in patients with suspected recurrent DTC [136]. The data indicates that ^{18}F-FDG PET-CT is better than

^{68}Ga DOTATOC in the detection of recurrent disease that is radioiodine negative. Specifically, it is more accurate in detecting lung and bone metastases. In radioiodine-positive cancers, both tracers are equivalent.

Summary

PET-CT scanning with ^{18}F-FDG is a very valuable scan for managing patients with well-differentiated thyroid cancer and specifically patients who have an elevated Tg and whose cancers cannot take up radioiodine. The sensitivity of the scan is high and the images identify sites of cancer that lead to a change in management in 20–60 %. Newer PET radionuclides such as ^{124}I have potential for better lesion detection and more accurate dosimetry prior to therapy with ^{131}I.

References

1. Fletcher JW, Djulbegovic B, Soares HP, Siegel BA, Lowe VJ, Lyman GH, et al. Recommendations on the use of ^{18}F-FDG PET in oncology. J Nucl Med. 2008;49:480–508.
2. Beyer T, Townsend DW, Brun T, Kinahan PE, Charron M, Roddy R, et al. A combined PET/CT scanner for clinical oncology. J Nucl Med. 2000;41:1369–79.
3. Patton J, Turkington TG. Coincidence imaging with a dual-head scintillation camera. J Nucl Med. 1999;40:432–41.
4. Chowdhury FU, Scarsbrook AF. The role of hybrid SPECT-CT in oncology: current and emerging clinical applications. Clin Radiol. 2008;63:241–51.
5. Maurer AH. Combined imaging modalities: PET/CT and SPECT/CT. Health Phys. 2008;95:571–6.
6. Huebner RH, Park KC, Shepherd JE, et al. A meta-analysis of the literature for whole-body FDG PET detection of recurrent colorectal cancer. J Nucl Med. 2000;41:1177–89.
7. Weihrauch MR, Dietlein M, Schicha H, Diehl V, Tesch H. Prognostic significance of 18F-fluorodeoxyglucose positron emission tomography in lymphoma. Leuk Lymphoma. 2003;44:15–22.
8. Schiepers C, Filmont JE, Czernin J. PET for staging of Hodgkin's disease and non-Hodgkin's lymphoma. Eur J Nucl Med Mol Imaging. 2003;30 Suppl 1:S82–8.
9. Gambhir SS. Molecular imaging of cancer with positron emission tomography. Nat Rev Cancer. 2002;2:683–93.
10. Lin M. Molecular imaging using positron emission tomography in colorectal cancer. Discov Med. 2011;11:435–47.
11. Moerlein SM, Mathis CA, Brennan KM, Budinger TF. Synthesis and in vivo evaluation of ^{122}I- and ^{131}I-labelled iodoperidol, a potential agent for the tomographic assessment of cerebral perfusion. Int J Rad Appl Instrum B. 1987;14:91–8.
12. Agrawal A, Nair N, Baghel NS. A novel approach for reduction of brown fat uptake on FDG PET. Br J Radiol. 2009;82:626–31.
13. Cohen MS, Arslan N, Dehdashti F, et al. Risk of malignancy in thyroid incidentalomas identified by fluorodeoxyglucose-positron emission tomography. Surgery. 2001;130:941–6.
14. Kang KW, Kim SK, Kang HS, et al. Prevalence and risk of cancer of focal thyroid incidentaloma identified by ^{18}F-fluorodeoxyglucose positron emission tomography for metastasis evaluation and cancer screening in healthy subjects. J Clin Endocrinol Metab. 2003;88:4100–4.
15. Ramos CD, Chisin R, Yeung HW, Larson SM, Macapinlac HA. Incidental focal thyroid uptake on FDG positron emission tomographic scans may represent a second primary tumor. Clin Nucl Med. 2001;26:193–7.
16. Ho TY, Liou MJ, Lin KJ, Yen TC. Prevalence and significance of thyroid uptake detected by ^{18}F-FDG PET. Endocrine. 2011;40:297–302.
17. Chu QD, Connor MS, Lilien DL, Johnson LW, Turnage RH, Li BD. Positron emission tomography (PET) positive thyroid incidentaloma: the risk of malignancy observed in a tertiary referral center. Am Surg. 2006;72:272–5.
18. Are C, Hsu JF, Schoder H, Shah JP, Larson SM, Shaha AR. FDG-PET detected thyroid incidentalomas: need for further investigation? Ann Surg Oncol. 2007;14:239–47.
19. Choi JY, Lee KS, Kim HJ, Shim YM, Kwon OJ, Park K, Baek CH, et al. Focal thyroid lesions incidentally identified by integrated ^{18}F-FDG PET/CT: clinical significance and improved characterization. J Nucl Med. 2006;47:609–15.
20. Chen YK, Ding HJ, Chen KT, Chen YL, Liao AC, Shen YY, et al. Prevalence and risk of cancer of focal thyroid incidentaloma identified by ^{18}F-fluorodeoxyglucose positron emission tomography for cancer screening in healthy subjects. Anticancer Res. 2005;25:1421–6.
21. Adler LP, Bloom AD. Positron emission tomography of thyroid masses. Thyroid. 1993;3:195–200.
22. Uematsu H, Sadato N, Ohtsubo T, et al. Fluorine-18-fluorodeoxyglucose PET versus thallium-201 scintigraphy evaluation of thyroid tumors. J Nucl Med. 1998;39:453–9.
23. Hales NW, Krempl GA, Medina JE. Is there a role for fluorodeoxyglucose positron emission tomography/computed tomography in cytologically indeterminate thyroid nodules? Am J Otolaryngol. 2008;29:113–8.
24. Gianoukakis AG, Karam M, Cheema A, Cooper JA. Autonomous thyroid nodules visualized by positron emission tomography with ^{18}F-fluorodeoxyglucose: a case report and review of the literature. Thyroid. 2003;13:395–9.
25. Park CH, Lee EJ, Kim JK, Joo HJ, Jang JS. Focal F-18 FDG uptake in a nontoxic autonomous thyroid nodule. Clin Nucl Med. 2002;27:136–7.
26. Giovanella L, Suriano S, Maffioli M, Ceriani L. 18FDG-positron emission tomography/computed tomography (PET/CT) scanning in thyroid nodules with nondiagnostic cytology. Clin Endocrinol (Oxf). 2011;74:644–8.
27. Wong C, Lin M, Chicco A, Benson R. The clinical significance and management of incidental focal FDG uptake in the thyroid gland on positron emission tomography/computed tomography (PET/CT) in patients with non-thyroidal malignancy. Acta Radiol. 2011;52:899–904.
28. Keyes Jr JW. SUV: standard uptake or silly useless value? J Nucl Med. 1995;36:1836–9.
29. Cook G, Maisey MN, Fogelman I. Normal variants, artefacts and interpretative pitfalls in PET with 18-fluoro-2-deoxyglucose and carbon-11 methionine. Normal variants, artefacts and interpretative pitfalls in PET with 18-fluoro-2-deoxyglucose and carbon-11 methionine. Eur J Nucl Med. 1999;26:1363–78.
30. Cook G, Wegner EA, Fogelman I. Pitfalls and artifacts in ^{18}FDG PET and PET/CT oncologic imaging. Semin Nucl Med. 2004;XXXIV:122–33.
31. Barrington S, Maisey MN. Skeletal muscle uptake of fluorine-18 FDG: effect of oral diazepam. J Nucl Med. 1996;37:1127–9.
32. Hany TF, Gharehpapagh E, Kamel EM, Buck A, Himms-Hagen J, von Schulthess GK. Brown adipose tissue: a factor to consider in symmetrical tracer uptake in the neck and upper chest region. Eur J Nucl Med Mol Imaging. 2002;29:1393–8.
33. Cohade C, Mourtzikos KA, Wahl RL. "USA-Fat": prevalence is related to ambient outdoor temperature-evaluation with 18F-FDG PET/CT. J Nucl Med. 2003;44:1267–70.

34. Cohade C, Osman M, Pannu HK, Wahl RL. Uptake in supraclavicular area fat ("USA-Fat"): description on ^{18}F-FDG PET/CT. J Nucl Med. 2003;44:170–6.
35. Yeung HW, Grewal RK, Gonen M, Schoder H, Larson SM. Patterns of ^{18}F-FDG uptake in adipose tissue and muscle: a potential source of false-positives for PET. J Nucl Med. 2003;44:1789–96.
36. Tatsumi M, Engles JM, Ishimori T, Nicely O, Cohade C, Wahl RL. Intense ^{18}F-FDG uptake in brown fat can be reduced pharmacologically. J Nucl Med. 2004;45:1189–93.
37. Igerc I, Kumnig G, Heinisch M, et al. Vocal cord muscle activity as a drawback to FDG-PET in the followup of differentiated thyroid cancer. Thyroid. 2002;12:87–9.
38. Zhu Z, Chou C, Yen TC, Cui R. Elevated F-18 FDG uptake in laryngeal muscles mimicking thyroid cancer metastases. Clin Nucl Med. 2001;26:689–91.
39. Yeretsian RA, Blodgett TM, Branstetter BF, Roberts MM, Meltzer CC. Teflon-induced granuloma: a false-positive finding with PET resolved with combined PET and CT. AJNR Am J Neuroradiol. 2003;24:1164–6.
40. Alibazoglu H, Alibazoglu B, Hollinger EF, et al. Normal thymic uptake of 2-deoxy-2[F-18]fluoro-D-glucose. Clin Nucl Med. 1999;24:597–600.
41. Kawano T, Suzuki A, Ishida A, et al. The clinical relevance of thymic fluorodeoxyglucose uptake in pediatric patients after chemotherapy. Eur J Nucl Med Mol Imaging. 2004;31:831–6.
42. Rini JN, Leonidas JC, Tomas MB, Karayalcin G, Tronco GG, Palestro CJ. FDG uptake in the anterior mediastinum. Physiologic thymic uptake or disease? Clin Positron Imaging. 1999;2:332.
43. Wittram C, Fischman AJ, Mark E, Ko J, Shepard JA. Thymic enlargement and FDG uptake in three patients: CT and FDG positron emission tomography correlated with pathology. AJR Am J Roentgenol. 2003;180:519–22.
44. Nakahara T, Fujii H, Ide M, et al. FDG uptake in the morphologically normal thymus: comparison of FDG positron emission tomography and CT. Br J Radiol. 2001;74:821–4.
45. Patel PM, Alibazoglu H, Ali A, Fordham E, LaMonica G. Normal thymic uptake of FDG on PET imaging. Clin Nucl Med. 1996;21:772–5.
46. Cooper DS, Doherty GM, Haugen BR, Kloos RT, Lee SL, Mandel SJ, et al. Revised American Thyroid Association management guidelines for patients with thyroid nodules and differentiated thyroid cancer. Thyroid. 2009;19:1167–214.
47. Pineda J, Lee T, Ain K, Reynolds JC, Robbins J. Iodine-131 therapy for thyroid cancer patients with elevated thyroglobulin and negative diagnostic scan. J Clin Endocrinol Metab. 1995;80: 1488–92.
48. Schlumberger M, Mancusi F, Baudin E, Pacini F. ^{131}I therapy for elevated thyroglobulin levels. Thyroid. 1997;7:273–6.
49. Wartofsky L. Management of scan negative thyroglobulin positive differentiated thyroid carcinoma. J Clin Endocrinol Metab. 1998;83:4195–9.
50. McDougall I. ^{131}I treatment of ^{131}I negative whole body scan, and positive thyroglobulin in differentiated thyroid carcinoma: what is being treated? Thyroid. 1997;7:669–72.
51. Fatourechi V, Hay ID, Javedan H, Wiseman GA, Mullan BP, Gorman CA. Lack of impact of radioiodine therapy in tg-positive, diagnostic whole-body scan-negative patients with follicular cell-derived thyroid cancer. J Clin Endocrinol Metab. 2002;87: 1521–6.
52. McDougall IR. Management of thyroglobulin positive/whole-body scan negative: is Tg positive/I therapy useful? J Endocrinol Invest. 2001;24:194–8.
53. Hoefnagel B, Delprat CC, Marcuse HR, Vijlder JJM. Role of thallium-201 total-body scintigraphy in follow-up of thyroid carcinoma. J Nucl Med. 1986;27:1854–7.
54. Iida Y, Hidaka A, Hatabu H, Kasagi K, Konishi J. Follow-up study of postoperative patients with thyroid cancer by thallium-201 scintigraphy and serum thyroglobulin measurement. J Nucl Med. 1991;32:2098–100.
55. Nakada K, Katoh C, Kanegae E, et al. Thallium-201 scintigraphy to predict therapeutic outcome of iodine-131 therapy of metastatic thyroid carcinoma. J Nucl Med. 1998;39:807–10.
56. Brandt-Mainz K, Muller SP, Reiners C, Bockisch A. Relationship between thyroglobulin and reliability of thallium 201 scintigraphy in differentiated thyroid cancer. Nuklearmedizin. 2000;39:20–5.
57. Yen TC, Lin HD, Lee CH, Chang SL, Yeh SH. The role of technetium-99m sestamibi whole-body scans in diagnosing metastatic Hurthle cell carcinoma of the thyroid gland after total thyroidectomy: a comparison with iodine-131 and thallium-201 whole-body scans. Eur J Nucl Med. 1994;21:980–3.
58. Almeida-Filho P, Ravizzini GC, Almeida C, Borges-Neto S. Whole-body Tc-99m sestamibi scintigraphy in the follow-up of differentiated thyroid carcinoma. Clin Nucl Med. 2000;25:443–6.
59. Gallowitsch H, Mikosch P, Kresnik E, Unterweger O, Gomez I, Lind P. Thyroglobulin and low-dose iodine-131 and technetium-99m-tetrofosmin whole-body scintigraphy in differentiated thyroid carcinoma. J Nucl Med. 1998;39:870–5.
60. Lind P, Gallowitsch HJ, Langsteger W, et al. Technetium-99m-tetrofosmin whole-body scintigraphy in the follow-up of differentiated thyroid carcinoma. J Nucl Med. 1997;38:348–52.
61. Lind P. Multi-tracer imaging of thyroid nodules: is there a role in the preoperative assessment of nodular goiter? Eur J Nucl Med. 1999;26:795–7.
62. Lind P, Gallowitsch HJ, Mikosch P, et al. Comparison of different tracers in the follow up of differentiated thyroid carcinoma. Acta Med Austriaca. 1999;26:115–7.
63. Drac-Kaniewska J, Kozlowicz-Gudzinska I, Tomaszewicz-Kubasik H, et al. 99mTc Tetrofosmin in diagnosis of distant metastases from differentiated thyroid cancer. Wiad Lek. 2001;54 Suppl 1:357–62.
64. Ahlman H, Tisell LE, Wangberg B, et al. The relevance of somatostatin receptors in thyroid neoplasia. Yale J Biol Med. 1997;70:523–33.
65. Sarlis NJ, Gourgiotis L, Guthrie LC, et al. In-111 DTPA-octreotide scintigraphy for disease detection in metastatic thyroid cancer: comparison with F-18 FDG positron emission tomography and extensive conventional radiographic imaging. Clin Nucl Med. 2003;28:208–17.
66. Baudin E, Schlumberger M, Lumbroso J, Travagli JP, Caillou B, Parmentier C. Octreotide scintigraphy in patients with differentiated thyroid carcinoma; contribution for patients with negative radioiodine scans. J Clin Endocrinol Metab. 1996;81:2541–4.
67. Joensuu H, Ahonen A. Imaging of metastases of thyroid carcinoma with fluorine-18 fluorodeoxyglucose. J Nucl Med. 1987;28:910–4.
68. Adams S, Baum RP, Hertel A, Schumm-Draeger PM, Usadel K-H, Hor G. Comparison of metabolic and receptor imaging in recurrent medullary thyroid carcinoma with histopathological findings. Eur J Nucl Med. 1998;25:1277–83.
69. Adams S, Baum R, Rink T, Schumm-Drager PM, Usadel KH, Hor G. Limited value of fluorine-18 fluorodeoxyglucose positron emission tomography for the imaging of neuroendocrine tumours. Eur J Nucl Med. 1998;25:79–83.
70. Alnafisi N, Driedger AA, Coates G, Moote DJ, Raphael SJ. FDG PET of recurrent or metastatic ^{131}I-negative papillary thyroid carcinoma. J Nucl Med. 2000;41:1010–5.
71. Altenvoerde G, Lerch H, Kuwert T, Matheja P, Schafers M, Schober O. Positron emission tomography with F-18-deoxyglucose in patients with differentiated thyroid carcinoma, elevated thyroglobulin levels, and negative iodine scans. Langenbecks Arch Surg. 1998;383:160–3.

72. Berger F, Knesewitsch P, Tausig A, et al. [18F] Fluorodeoxyglucose hybrid PET in patients with differentiated thyroid cancer: comparison with dedicated PET. Eur Ass Nucl Med Congress Paris 2000. 2000.
73. Boer A, Szakall Jr S, Klein I, et al. FDG PET imaging in hereditary thyroid cancer. Eur J Surg Oncol. 2003;29:922–8.
74. Boerner AR, Petrich T, Weckesser E, et al. Monitoring isotretinoin therapy in thyroid cancer using 18F-FDG PET. Eur J Nucl Med Mol Imaging. 2002;29:231–6.
75. Brandt-Mainz K, Muller SP, Gorges R, Saller B, Bockisch A. The value of fluorine-18 fluorodeoxyglucose PET in patients with medullary thyroid cancer. Eur J Nucl Med. 2000;27:490–6.
76. Riemann B, Uhrhan K, Dietlein M, et al. Diagnostic value and therapeutic impact of (18)F-FDG-PET/CT in differentiated thyroid cancer. Results of a German multicentre study. Nucl Med. 2013;52:1–6.
77. van Dijk D, Plukker JTM, Phan HTT, et al. 18-fluorodeoxyglucose positron emission tomography in the early diagnostic workup of differentiated thyroid cancer patients with a negative post-therapeutic iodine scan and detectable thyroglobulin. Thyroid. 2013;23:1003–9.
78. Macapinlac HA. Clinical usefulness of FDG PET in differentiated thyroid cancer. J Nucl Med. 2001;42:77–8.
79. Wong CO, Dworkin HJ. Role of FDG PET in metastatic thyroid cancer. J Nucl Med. 1999;40:993–4.
80. Khan N, Oriuchi N, Higuchi T, Zhang H, Endo K. PET in the follow-up of differentiated thyroid cancer. Br J Radiol. 2003; 76:690–5.
81. Crippa F, Alessi A, Gerali A, Bombardieri E. FDG-PET in thyroid cancer. Tumori. 2003;89:540–3.
82. Ozkan E, Aras G, Kucuk NO. Correlation of ^{18}F-FDG PET/CT findings with histopathological results in differentiated thyroid cancer patients who have increased thyroglobulin or antithyroglobulin antibody levels and negative ^{131}I whole-body scan results. Clin Nucl Med. 2013;38:326–31.
83. Armstrong S, Worsley D, Blair GK. Pediatric surgical images: PET evaluation of papillary thyroid carcinoma recurrence. J Pediatr Surg. 2002;37:1648–9.
84. Joensuu H, Klemi PJ, Eerola E. Diagnostic value of flow cytometric DNA determination combined with fine needle aspiration biopsy in thyroid tumors. Anal Quant Cytol Histol. 1987;9: 328–34.
85. Feine U, Lietzenmayer R, Hanke JP, Wohrle H, Muller-Schauenburg W. ^{18}FDG whole-body PET in differentiated thyroid carcinoma. Flipflop in uptake patterns of ^{18}FDG and ^{131}I. Nuklearmedizin. 1995;34:127–34.
86. Shiga T, Tsukamoto E, Nakada K, et al. Comparison of ^{18}F-FDG, ^{131}I-Na, and ^{201}Tl in diagnosis of recurrent or metastatic thyroid carcinoma. J Nucl Med. 2001;42:414–9.
87. Dietlein M, Moka D, Scheidhauer K, et al. Follow-up of differentiated thyroid cancer: comparison of multiple diagnostic tests. Nucl Med Commun. 2000;21:991–1000.
88. Bertagna F, Bosio G, Biasiotto G, Rodella C, Puta E, Gabanelli S, Lucchini S, et al. F-18 FDG-PET/CT evaluation of patients with differentiated thyroid cancer with negative I-131 total body scan and high thyroglobulin level. Clin Nucl Med. 2009;34: 756–61.
89. Iagaru A, Masamed R, Singer PA, Conti PS. 2-Deoxy-2-[18F] fluoro-D-glucose-positron emission tomography and positron emission tomography/computed tomography diagnosis of patients with recurrent papillary thyroid cancer. Mol Imaging Biol. 2006;8:309–14.
90. Schluter B, Bohuslavizki KH, Beyer W, Plotkin M, Buchert R, Clausen M. Impact of FDG PET on patients with differentiated thyroid cancer who present with elevated thyroglobulin and negative ^{131}I scan. J Nucl Med. 2001;42:71–6.
91. Palmedo H, Bucerius J, Joe A, Strunk H, Hortling N, Meyka S, Roedel R, et al. Integrated PET/CT in differentiated thyroid cancer: diagnostic accuracy and impact on patient management. J Nucl Med. 2006;47:616–24.
92. Mirallie E, Guiana T, Bridji B, Resche I, Rousseau C, Ansquer C, Bodet-Milin C, et al. Therapeutic impact of ^{18}FDG-PET/CT in the management of iodine-negative recurrence of differentiated thyroid carcinoma. Surgery. 2007;142:952–8; discussion 952–8.
93. Esteva D, Muros MA, Llamas-Elvira JM, Jimenez Alonso J, Villar JM, Lopez de la Torre M, Muros T. Clinical and pathological factors related to ^{18}F-FDG-PET positivity in the diagnosis of recurrence and/or metastasis in patients with differentiated thyroid cancer. Ann Surg Oncol. 2009;16:2006–13.
94. Choi JW, Yoon YH, Kim SM, Koo BS. Characteristics of primary papillary thyroid carcinoma with false-negative findings on initial ^{18}F-FDG PET/CT. Ann Surg Oncol. 2011;18:1306–11.
95. Iagaru A, Kalinyak JE, McDougall IR. F-18 FDG PET/CT in the management of thyroid cancer. Clin Nucl Med. 2007;32:690–5.
96. Davison JM, Stocker DJ, Montilla-Soler JL, Jurgens JS, Allen TW, Holley TS, Stack AL. The added benefit of a dedicated neck F-18 FDG PET-CT imaging protocol in patients with suspected recurrent differentiated thyroid carcinoma. Clin Nucl Med. 2008;33:464–8.
97. Kaneko K, Abe K, Baba S, et al. Detection of residual lymph node metastases in high-risk papillary thyroid cancer patients receiving adjuvant I-131 therapy: the usefulness of F-18 FDG PET/CT. Clin Nucl Med. 2010;35:6–11.
98. Choi WH, Chung YA, Han EJ, Sohn HS, Lee SH. Clinical value of integrated [18F]fluoro-2-deoxy-D-glucose positron emission tomography/computed tomography in the preoperative assessment of papillary thyroid carcinoma: comparison with sonography. J Ultrasound Med. 2011;30:1267–73.
99. Piccardo A, Arecco F, Morbelli S, Bianchi P, Barbera F, Finessi M, Corvisieri S, et al. Low thyroglobulin concentrations after thyroidectomy increase the prognostic value of undetectable thyroglobulin levels on levo-thyroxine suppressive treatment in low-risk differentiated thyroid cancer. J Endocrinol Invest. 2010;33:83–7.
100. Stokkel MP, Duchateau CS, Dragoiescu C. The value of FDG-PET in the follow-up of differentiated thyroid cancer: a review of the literature. Q J Nucl Med Mol Imaging. 2006;50:78–87.
101. Miller ME, Chen Q, Elashoff D, Abemayor ES, John M. Positron emission tomography and positron emission tomography-CT evaluation for recurrent papillary thyroid carcinoma: meta-analysis and literature review. Head Neck. 2011;33:562–5.
102. Dong MJ, Liu ZF, Zhao K, Ruan LX, Wang GL, Yang SY, Sun F, Luo XG. Value of ^{18}F-FDG-PET/PET-CT in differentiated thyroid carcinoma with radioiodine-negative whole-body scan: a meta-analysis. Nucl Med Commun. 2009;30:639–50.
103. Wang W, Larson SM, Fazzari M, et al. Prognostic value of [18F] fluorodeoxyglucose positron emission tomographic scanning in patients with thyroid cancer. J Clin Endocrinol Metab. 2000; 85:1107–13.
104. Goshen E, Cohen O, Rotenberg G, Oksman Y, Karasik A, Zwas ST. The clinical impact of ^{18}F-FDG gamma PET in patients with recurrent well differentiated thyroid carcinoma. Nucl Med Commun. 2003;24:959–61.
105. Karwowski J, Jeffrey RB, McDougall IR, Weigel RJ. Intraoperative ultrasonography improves identification of recurrent thyroid cancer. Surgery. 2002;132:924–8.
106. Ota N, Kato K, Iwano S, et al. Comparison of ^{18}F-fluoride PET/CT, ^{18}F-FDG PET/CT, and bone scintigraphy (planar and SPECT) in detection of bone metastases of differentiated thyroid cancer: a pilot study. Br J Radiol. 2014;87:20130444.
107. Nakajo M, Jinguji M, Tani A, et al. Diagnosis of metastases from postoperative differentiated thyroid cancer: comparison between FDG and FLT PET/CT studies. Radiology. 2013;267:891–901.

108. Wang W, Macapinlac H, Larson SM, Yeh SD, Akhurst T, Finn RD, Rosai J, Robbins RJ. [18F]-2-fluoro-2-deoxy-D-glucose positron emission tomography localizes residual thyroid cancer in patients with negative diagnostic (131)I whole body scans and elevated serum thyroglobulin levels. J Clin Endocrinol Metab. 1999;84:2291–302.
109. Grunwald F, Schomburg A, Bender H, et al. Fluorine-18 fluorodeoxyglucose positron emission tomography in the follow-up of differentiated thyroid cancer. Eur J Nucl Med. 1996;23:312–9.
110. Sisson JC, Ackermann RJ, Meyer MA, Wahl RL. Uptake of 18-fluoro-2-deoxy-D-glucose by thyroid cancer: implications for diagnosis and therapy. J Clin Endocrinol Metab. 1993; 77:1090–4.
111. Filetti S, Damante G, Foti D. Thyrotropin stimulates glucose transport in cultured rat thyroid cells. Endocrinology. 1987; 120:2576–81.
112. Moog F, Linke R, Manthey N, et al. Influence of thyroid-stimulating hormone levels on uptake of FDG in recurrent and metastatic differentiated thyroid carcinoma. J Nucl Med. 2000;41:1989–95.
113. Petrich T, Borner AR, Otto D, Hofmann M, Knapp WH. Influence of rhTSH on [(18)F]fluorodeoxyglucose uptake by differentiated thyroid carcinoma. Eur J Nucl Med Mol Imaging. 2002; 29:641–7.
114. Chin BB, Patel P, Cohade C, Ewertz M, Wahl R, Ladenson P. Recombinant human thyrotropin stimulation of fluoro-D-glucose positron emission tomography uptake in well-differentiated thyroid carcinoma. J Clin Endocrinol Metab. 2004;89:91–5.
115. Ma C, Xie J, Lou Y, Gao Y, Zuo S, Wang X. The role of TSH for 18F-FDG-PET in the diagnosis of recurrence and metastases of differentiated thyroid carcinoma with elevated thyroglobulin and negative scan: a meta-analysis. Eur J Endocrinol. 2010;163: 177–83.
116. Leboulleux S, Schroeder PR, Busaidy NL, Auperin A, Corone C, Jacene HA, et al. Assessment of the incremental value of recombinant thyrotropin stimulation before 2-[18F]-Fluoro-2-deoxy-D-glucose positron emission tomography/computed tomography imaging to localize residual differentiated thyroid cancer. J Clin Endocrinol Metab. 2009;94:1310–6.
117. Vera P, Kuhn-Lansoy C, Edet-Sanson A, Hapdey S, Modzelewski R, Hitzel A, et al. Does recombinant human thyrotropin-stimulated positron emission tomography with [18F]fluoro-2-deoxy-D-glucose improve detection of recurrence of well-differentiated thyroid carcinoma in patients with low serum thyroglobulin? Thyroid. 2010;20:15–23.
118. Lambrecht RM, Woodhouse N, Phillips R, et al. Investigational study of iodine-124 with a positron camera. Am J Physiol Imaging. 1988;3:197–200.
119. Flower M, Al-Saadi A, Harmer CL, et al. Dose response study on thyrotoxic patients undergoing positron emission tomography and radioiodine therapy. Eur J Nucl Med. 1994;21:531–6.
120. Frey P, Townsend D, Jeavons A, Donath A. In vivo imaging of the human thyroid with a positron camera using I-124. In vivo imaging of the human thyroid with a positron camera using I-124. Eur J Nucl Med. 1985;10:472–6.
121. Frey P, Townsend D, Flattet A, et al. Tomographic imaging of the human thyroid using ^{124}I. J Clin Endocrinol Metab. 1986; 63:918–27.
122. Crawford DC, Flower MA, Pratt BE, et al. Thyroid volume measurement in thyrotoxic patients: comparison between ultrasonography and iodine-124 positron emission tomography. Eur J Nucl Med. 1997;24:1470–8.
123. Freudenberg LS, Jentzen W, Stahl A, Bockisch A, Rosenbaum-Krumme SJ. Clinical applications of ^{124}I-PET/CT in patients with differentiated thyroid cancer. Eur J Nucl Med Mol Imaging. 2011;38 Suppl 1:S48–56.
124. Eschmann SM, Reischl G, Bilger K, et al. Evaluation of dosimetry of radioiodine therapy in benign and malignant thyroid disorders by means of iodine-124 and PET. Eur J Nucl Med Mol Imaging. 2002;29:760–7.
125. Freudenberg LS, Antoch G, Gorges R, et al. Combined PET/CT with iodine-124 in diagnosis of spread metastatic thyroid carcinoma: a case report. Eur Radiol. 2003;13 Suppl 4:L19–23.
126. Freudenberg LS, Antoch G, Jentzen W, et al. Value of ^{124}I-PET/CT in staging of patients with differentiated thyroid cancer. Eur Radiol. 2004;14:2092–8.
127. Capoccetti F, Criscuoli B, Rossi G, Ferretti F, Manni C, Brianzoni E. The effectiveness of ^{124}I PET/CT in patients with differentiated thyroid cancer. Q J Nucl Med Mol Imaging. 2009;53:536–45.
128. Freudenberg LS, Jentzen W, Muller SP, Bockisch A. Disseminated iodine-avid lung metastases in differentiated thyroid cancer: a challenge to ^{124}I PET. Eur J Nucl Med Mol Imaging. 2008; 35:502–8.
129. Van Nostrand D, Moreau S, Bandaru VV, Atkins F, Chennupati S, Mete M, Burman K, Wartofsky L. ^{124}I positron emission tomography versus ^{131}I planar imaging in the identification of residual thyroid tissue and/or metastasis in patients who have well-differentiated thyroid cancer. Thyroid. 2010;20:879–83.
130. Freudenberg LS, Antoch G, Frilling A, Jentzen W, Rosenbaum SJ, Kuhl H, Bockisch A, Gorges R. Combined metabolic and morphologic imaging in thyroid carcinoma patients with elevated serum thyroglobulin and negative cervical ultrasonography: role of ^{124}I-PET/CT and FDG-PET. Eur J Nucl Med Mol Imaging. 2008;35:950–7.
131. Sgouros G, Kolbert KS, Sheikh A, Pentlow KS, Mun EF, Barth A, Robbins RJ, Larson SM. Patient-specific dosimetry for ^{131}I thyroid cancer therapy using ^{124}I PET and 3-dimensional-internal dosimetry (3D-ID) software. J Nucl Med. 2004;45:1366–72.
132. Sgouros G, Hobbs RF, Atkins FB, Van Nostrand D, Ladenson PW, Wahl RL. Three-dimensional radiobiological dosimetry (3D-RD) with ^{124}I PET for ^{131}I therapy of thyroid cancer. Eur J Nucl Med Mol Imaging. 2011;38 Suppl 1:S41–7.
133. Ho A, Grewal R, Leboeuf R, et al. Selumetinib-enhanced radioiodine uptake in advanced thyroid cancer. N Engl J Med. 2013;368:623–32.
134. Dyson N, Francois PE. Some observations on the decay of iodine-124 and their implications in radioiodine therapy. Phys Med Biol. 1958;3:111.
135. Belov VV, Bonab AA, Fischman AJ, Heartlein M, Calias P, Papisov MI. Iodine-124 as a label for pharmacological PET imaging. Mol Pharm. 2011;8:736–47.
136. Middendorp M, Selkinski I, Happel C, Kranert WT, Grunwald F. Comparison of positron emission tomography with [^{18}F]FDG and [^{68}Ga]DOTATOC in recurrent differentiated thyroid cancer: preliminary data. Q J Nucl Med Mol Imaging. 2010;54:76–83.
137. Chung J-K, So Y, Lee JS, et al. Value of FDG PET in papillary thyroid carcinoma with negative ^{131}I whole-body scan. J Nucl Med. 1999;40:486–92.
138. Dietlein M, Scheidhauer K, Voth E, Theissen P, Schicha H. Fluorine-18 fluorodeoxyglucose positron emission tomography and iodine-131 whole-body scintigraphy in the follow-up of differentiated thyroid cancer. Eur J Nucl Med. 1997;24:1342–8.
139. Grunwald F, Kalicke T, Feine U, et al. Fluorine-18 fluorodeoxyglucose positron emission tomography in thyroid cancer: results of a multicentre study. Eur J Nucl Med. 1999;26:1547–52.
140. Stokkel MP, de Klerk JH, Zelissen PM, Koppeschaar HP, van Rijk PP. Fluorine-18 fluorodeoxyglucose dual-head positron emission tomography in the detection of recurrent differentiated thyroid cancer: preliminary results. Eur J Nucl Med. 1999;26:1606–9.
141. Helal BO, Merlet P, Toubert ME, Franc B, Schvartz C, Gauthier-Koelesnikov H, Prigent A, Syrota A. Clinical impact of ^{18}F-FDG PET in thyroid carcinoma patients with elevated thyroglobulin

levels and negative ^{131}I scanning results after therapy. J Nucl Med. 2001;42:1464–9.

142. Freudenberg LS, Frilling A, Kuhl H, Muller SP, Jentzen W, Bockisch A, Antoch G. Dual-modality FDG-PET/CT in follow-up of patients with recurrent iodine-negative differentiated thyroid cancer. Eur Radiol. 2007;17:3139–47.
143. Ong SC, Ng DC, Sundram FX. Initial experience in use of fluorine-18-fluorodeoxyglucose positron emission tomography/computed tomography in thyroid carcinoma patients with elevated serum thyroglobulin but negative iodine-131 whole body scans. Singapore Med J. 2005;46:297–301.
144. Kim SJ, Lee TH, Kim IJ, Kim YK. Clinical implication of F-18 FDG PET/CT for differentiated thyroid cancer in patients with negative diagnostic iodine-123 scan and elevated thyroglobulin. Eur J Radiol. 2009;70:17–24.

Alternative Thyroid Imaging

44

Anca M. Avram, Karen C. Rosenspire, Stewart C. Davidson, John E. Freitas, Ka Kit Wong, and Milton D. Gross

Introduction

Radioiodine (^{131}I and ^{123}I) remains the most frequently used radionuclide for thyroid imaging in the diagnosis and treatment of well-differentiated thyroid cancer (WDTC). However, an estimated 20–30 % of WDTCs do not accumulate radioiodine at the time of initial clinical presentation, and many WDTCs that are initially radioiodine avid will dedifferentiate and lose their ability to concentrate radioiodine. This is especially true following radioiodine therapy. In addition, medullary and anaplastic thyroid carcinomas do not accumulate radioiodine.

A.M. Avram, MD (✉)
Division of Nuclear Medicine, Department of Radiology, University of Michigan, 1500 E. Medical Center Drive, Ann Arbor, MI 48109, USA

BIG505G University Hospital, Ann Arbor, MI 48109, USA
e-mail: ancaa@umich.edu

K.C. Rosenspire, MD, PhD
Department of Radiology, Wayne State University, Detroit, MI, USA

S.C. Davidson, MBBS
Northeast Nuclear Medicine, Mooloolaba, QLD, Australia

J.E. Freitas, MD
Department of Radiology, St. Joseph Mercy Health System, Ypsilanti, MI, USA

K.K. Wong, MBBS, FRACP
Division of Nuclear Medicine, Department of Radiology, University of Michigan Health System, Ann Arbor, MI, USA

M.D. Gross, MD
Division of Nuclear Medicine, Department of Radiology, University of Michigan Medical School, Ann Arbor, MI, USA

Nuclear Medicine and Radiation Safety Service, Department of Veterans Affairs Health Systems, Washington, DC (field based) and Ann Arbor, MI, USA

Because many thyroid cancers are not radioiodine avid, other radiopharmaceuticals that have different mechanisms of accumulation have been used for thyroid cancer imaging (Table 44.1). Although many radiopharmaceuticals have been studied as potential thyroid cancer–imaging agents with variable success, this discussion is limited to ^{201}Tl chloride, ^{99m}Tc sestamibi, ^{99m}Tc tetrofosmin, and ^{111}In pentetreotide as alternative thyroid-imaging agents.

^{201}TL Chloride

^{201}Tl chloride, a potassium analogue, is accumulated in thyroid tissues by an active transport mechanism—the Na+/K+ ATPase transporter [1]. This transport mechanism is present in many normal tissues, particularly the myocardium, but the ATPase transporter has been identified in a wide variety of neoplasms, including thyroid, breast, liver, and esophageal cancer, as well as lymphoma [2]. Differential accumulation and washout of ^{201}Tl in malignant thyroid tissues, compared to adjacent benign thyroid nodules, have been used to distinguish these entities [3]. However, ^{18}F-fluoro-2-deoxyglucose positron emission tomography (FDG PET) appears better than ^{201}Tl for this indication [4]. Tumor uptake of ^{201}Tl is because of multiple factors, e.g., increased blood flow, tumor type, and Na+/K+ transporter, among others [5].

Despite the potential role for ^{201}Tl as an imaging agent for WDTC, the reported sensitivity of ^{201}Tl uptake varies significantly. Sensitivities range from 39 to 94 %, with consistently high specificities ranging from 84 to 94 %, with imaging usually performed 10–90 min after the ^{201}Tl injection [2, 5–13]. Washout of ^{201}Tl from tumor tissue does occur with time, and shorter time intervals from injection to imaging tend to achieve better sensitivity for all sites.

^{201}Tl has been used to evaluate the extent of recurrent or metastatic disease in WDTC. Because ^{201}Tl has lower uptake than ^{131}I in normal residual thyroid tissue, ^{201}Tl may help differentiate recurrent tumor from normal residual thyroid

L. Wartofsky, D. Van Nostrand (eds.), *Thyroid Cancer*, DOI 10.1007/978-1-4939-3314-3_44

Table 44.1 Alternative thyroid-imaging agents

Well-differentiated thyroid cancer	^{201}Tl chloride
	^{99m}Tc sestamibi
	^{111}In octreotide
	^{111}In-DOTA lanreotide
	^{99m}Tc EDDA/HYNIC TOC
	^{99m}Tc EDDA/HYNIC TATE
	^{99m}Tc depreotide
	^{99m}Tc tetrofosmin
	^{99m}Tc pertechnetate
	^{99m}Tc HMPAO
Medullary thyroid cancer	^{111}In octreotide
	^{99m}Tc EDDA/HYNIC TOC
	^{131}I MIBG
	^{99m}Tc (V) DMSA
	^{111}In or ^{99m}Tc CCK
	^{131}I or ^{99m}Tc CEA
	^{201}Tl chloride
Anaplastic thyroid cancer	^{67}Ga citrate
Hürthle cell cancer	^{131}I or ^{99m}Tc CEA
	^{111}In pentetreotide
	^{99m}Tc sestamibi

DOTA 1,4,7,10-tetraazacyclododecane-1,4,7,10-tetraacetic acid, *EDDA* ethylenediamine diacetic acid, *TOC* Tyr^3-octreotide, *HMPAO* hexamethylpropyleneamineoxime, *MIBG* metaiodobenzylguanidine, *DMSA* dimercaptosuccinic acid, *CCK* cholecystokinin, *CEA* carcinoembryonic antigen

tissue. It may also detect nodal metastasis, with a sensitivity of 66–68 % [7]. Although ^{131}I is superior to ^{201}Tl in the detection of lung metastasis, ^{201}Tl may detect metastases not visualized with ^{131}I, and the sensitivity of planar ^{201}Tl may be improved with single-photon emission computed tomography (SPECT) from 60 to 85 % sensitivity [9]. Nevertheless, lesions <1.5 cm in size are rarely seen with either radionuclide. The lack of ^{201}Tl uptake in posttherapy scans has been shown to be a good predictor of response to radioiodine therapy [14]. Intense ^{201}Tl uptake (>2.1 tumor-to-background ratio) in known metastases, regardless of ^{131}I uptake, predicts a failure of subsequent ^{131}I therapy. Conversely, if ^{201}Tl uptake is low with intense ^{131}I uptake, most patients (88 %) responded to ^{131}I therapy. This may be similar to the findings with FDG PET (see Chap. 43).

Imaging with ^{201}Tl has been of value when ^{131}I scans are negative in the presence of known thyroid cancer. ^{201}Tl has been shown to be useful in following patients with WDTC and elevated serum thyroglobulin levels, despite a negative ^{131}I scan [6, 10–12, 14]. Furthermore, ^{201}Tl has been used for localizing metastases from medullary thyroid cancer, which typically does not accumulate ^{131}I [2].

Both ^{201}Tl and ^{99m}Tc sestamibi can visualize thyroid tissue in patients who are taking thyroid hormone with suppressed serum thyrotropin (TSH; [15]). Whereas radioiodine imaging of thyroid tissue necessitates either thyroid hormone withdrawal or the use of recombinant TSH stimulation, imaging with ^{201}Tl can be accomplished without either requirement.

Multiple studies have compared ^{201}Tl with other agents, such as ^{99m}Tc sestamibi, ^{99m}Tc tetrofosmin, and FDG [16–18]. Although these agents all compared favorably in detecting thyroid cancer, the image quality of ^{99m}Tc radiopharmaceuticals and FDG is significantly better than ^{201}Tl.

Sestamibi

^{99m}Tc sestamibi is a cationic, lipophilic complex developed for myocardial perfusion imaging, which has been reported to accumulate in thyroid, lung, brain, breast, parathyroid, and bone tumors [19–21]. Although ^{99m}Tc sestamibi accumulates in WDTC, it is not specific for WDTC and may accumulate in Graves' disease, thyroid lymphoma, thyroid adenoma, and medullary thyroid carcinoma [22]. Uptake has been suggested as related to abundant mitochondria and is influenced by tumor blood flow and vascularization, cellular metabolism, and tissue viability. ^{99m}Tc sestamibi is a substrate for the membrane efflux pumps—permeability glycoprotein and multidrug resistance protein—which may influence cellular retention [23, 24]. Generally, the procedure involves injection of 10–15 mCi (370–555 MBq) of ^{99m}Tc sestamibi with whole-body and planar imaging at 30 min, but some authors have suggested immediate imaging to detect lesions that have rapid washout [25].

^{99m}Tc sestamibi has many advantages relative to other radionuclides and conventional imaging. Unlike radioiodine (and as already noted), ^{99m}Tc sestamibi does not require withdrawal of thyroid hormone or recombinant TSH stimulation. However, improved ^{99m}Tc sestamibi uptake in patients who are hypothyroid has been observed [26]. In comparison to both ^{201}Tl and ^{131}I, ^{99m}Tc sestamibi has a photon energy that is more suitable for γ gamma cameras, and ^{99m}Tc frequently achieves higher tumor-to-background ratios than ^{131}I, which enables SPECT imaging. ^{99m}Tc sestamibi has lower radiation exposure than ^{201}Tl or ^{131}I. Compared to conventional imaging, such as computed tomography (CT), magnetic resonance imaging (MRI), and ultrasound, ^{99m}Tc sestamibi whole-body scintigraphy may help differentiate viable tumor from fibrotic tissue.

^{99m}Tc sestamibi has also been used to assess thyroid nodules in the thyroid gland, but ^{99m}Tc sestamibi uptake is not specific for malignancy, and its utility is limited [27–30]. Foldes et al. studied 58 patients with 77 nodules and showed no relationship between ^{99m}Tc sestamibi uptake and malignancy, indicating uptake depended mainly on tissue viability [27]. Nakahara et al. found ^{99m}Tc sestamibi and ^{201}Tl to be less sensitive than aspiration cytology in differentiating malignant from benign nodules [29]. Kresnik et al. [28] and

Wei et al. [30] reported similar results, suggesting increased ^{99m}Tc sestamibi uptake is more likely to represent thyroid adenoma than malignant tumor. Casara et al. recommended ^{99m}Tc sestamibi imaging should be reserved for those patients who had: (1) a high-pretest probability of malignancy and nondiagnostic cytology, (2) doubtful cytology and high-operative risk, and (3) a large locally aggressive tumor with the need to determine preoperative chemotherapy [31]. Hürthle cell tumors are rich in mitochondria, and although authors have reported intense, persistent uptake of ^{99m}Tc sestamibi in Hürthle cell tumors (Fig. 44.1), the specificity was low [32–35].

Numerous studies have investigated the role of ^{99m}Tc sestamibi in both ^{131}I-avid and non-avid WDTC [19–22, 25, 26, 36–53]. Ng et al. compared ^{99m}Tc sestamibi and ^{131}I scintigraphy in 360 patients with WDTC and found that ^{131}I whole-body scintigraphy detected more abnormalities than ^{99m}Tc sestamibi whole-body scintigraphy. ^{131}I particularly detected more thyroid remnants, as well as bone and lung metastases [54]. In comparing ^{131}I and ^{99m}Tc sestamibi whole-body scintigraphy, Dadparvar et al. found poor sensitivity (36 %) and high specificity (89 %) for ^{99m}Tc sestamibi [19]. Low sensitivity of ^{99m}Tc sestamibi for pulmonary metastases, along with high sensitivity for lymph node metastases, has been confirmed by several studies [20, 26, 49].

Despite the superiority of ^{131}I, ^{99m}Tc sestamibi is an alternative to radioiodine for detecting non-radioiodine–avid metastases (Fig. 44.2). Nemec et al. studied 200 patients with ^{131}I negative thyroid cancer patients with ^{99m}Tc sestamibi. The sensitivity and specificity were 100 % and 99 % for bone metastases, 95 % and 95 % for lung metastases, and 81 % and 71 % for locoregional disease, respectively [50]. Seabold et al. compared ^{99m}Tc sestamibi and ^{201}Tl after a negative or an equivocal ^{131}I whole-body scan (WBS). Sensitivity, specificity, and accuracy for both were 53 %, 100 %, and 69 %, with a positive predictive value of 100 % and a negative predictive value of 51 %. Interestingly, three patients converted from negative to positive ^{99m}Tc sestamibi or ^{201}Tl scans after induction of a hypothyroid state,

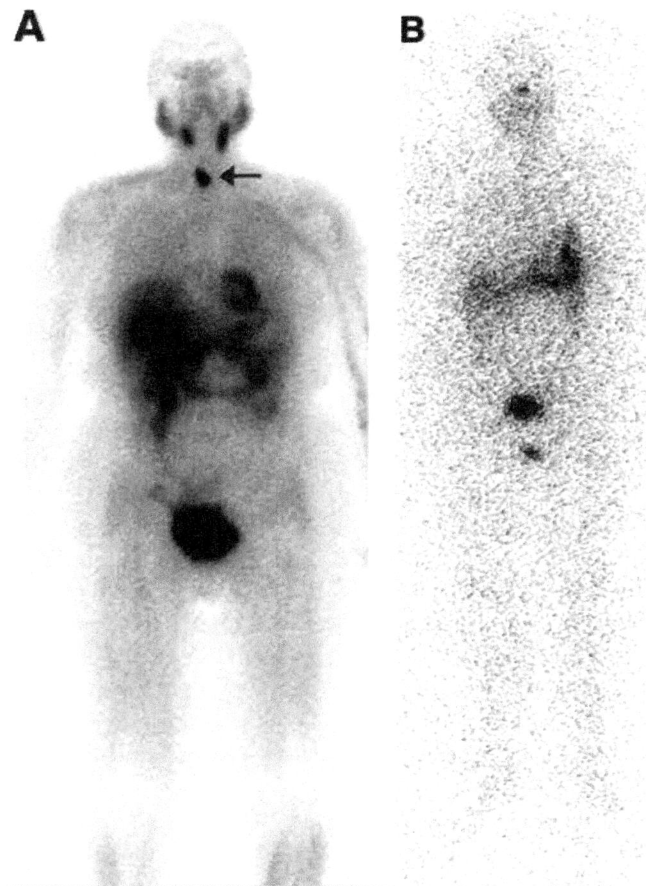

Fig. 44.1 This patient is a 69-year-old female with Hürthle cell carcinoma recurrence in the neck area. Her ^{99m}Tc sestamibi anterior whole-body scan (**a**) was performed 30 min after injection, and the patient was on thyroid hormone suppression. Intense ^{99m}Tc sestamibi uptake is present in the neck indicating the area of the recurrence (*arrow*). However, her radioiodine scan (**b**), which was performed 48 h after the administration of 2.5 mCi (92.5 MBq) ^{131}I and after thyroid hormone withdrawal, demonstrated no radioiodine accumulation. Surgical resection was subsequently performed

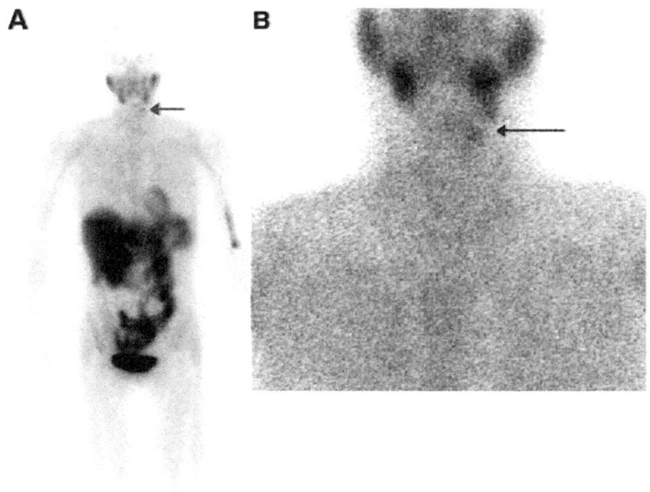

Fig. 44.2 This patient is a 53-year-old female who had papillary thyroid cancer and was ablated with radioiodine. At the time of follow-up and after thyroid hormone withdrawal, her serum thyroglobulin was elevated (26 ng/mL), and her radioiodine scan was negative (not shown). However, her whole-body ^{99m}Tc sestamibi scan (**a**) demonstrated faint uptake in the left neck area (**b**). A camera "spot" view better demonstrated this abnormal uptake in the left neck region (*arrow*), which was surgically removed using a γ gamma probe and confirmed as a 0.6-cm recurrence of thyroid cancer. The ^{99m}Tc sestamibi scan was instrumental in the localization of this recurrence

suggesting that TSH stimulation improves lesion detection in some patients [26]. Rubello et al. performed dual-phase ^{99m}Tc sestamibi scintigraphy, neck ultrasound, CT (87 patients), or MRI (35 patients) in 122 patients who had high serum thyroglobulin and negative high-dose (100 mCi [3.7 GBq]) ^{131}I scan. Positive or suspicious cases underwent fine-needle aspiration cytology. The combination of ^{99m}Tc sestamibi and ultrasound had a combined sensitivity of 98 % in detecting cervical lymph node metastases, and ^{99m}Tc sestamibi showed higher sensitivity (100 %) than CT/MRI (58 %) for detecting mediastinal lymph node metastases [55]. Comparative studies report FDG PET to be superior to ^{99m}Tc sestamibi [40, 42].

^{99m}Tc sestamibi has also been used for radioguided surgery in patients with radioiodine-negative metastases (Fig. 44.2 [56–61]). Following initial evaluation and confirmation that the radioiodine-negative metastasis accumulates ^{99m}Tc sestamibi scintigraphy, an additional 1 mCi (37 MBq) of ^{99m}Tc sestamibi is injected immediately prior to surgery. During the surgery, the metastasis is localized with the help of the intraoperative γ gamma probe. A prompt decline in neck activity after excision has been associated with normalization of elevated thyroglobulin levels [58]. A similar technique using ^{111}In has also been described in medullary thyroid carcinomas [62].

Tetrofosmin

^{99m}Tc tetrofosmin is a lipophilic phosphine used for myocardial perfusion imaging and has similar biodistribution and imaging qualities to ^{99m}Tc sestamibi. Numerous reported studies on the role of ^{99m}Tc tetrofosmin in evaluation of thyroid nodules [17, 63, 64] and imaging of WDTC suggest results similar to ^{99m}Tc sestamibi [65–81]. Comparative studies have found FDG PET is more sensitive than ^{99m}Tc tetrofosmin [65, 75, 76, 81].

Somatostatin Receptor Scintigraphy

In the past 10 year, somatostatin receptor scintigraphy (SRS) has been used for the imaging of radioiodine-negative metastatic WDTC, as well as to explore the option of somatostatin receptor–mediated therapy (see Chap. 47).

The molecular basis of SRS in WDTC is the expression of somatostatin receptors (sstr) on normal thyroid cells and thyroid carcinoma cells. Five human somatostatin receptor subtypes have been identified, and these interact with different G proteins to mediate effects via inhibition of adenylate cyclase activity. In vitro studies have demonstrated the presence of all subtypes (sstr-1–sstr-5) on Hürthle cell carcinoma tumors, but normal thyroid tissue selectively lacked sstr-2 [82]. Ain et al. reported that normal thyroid tissue has a high expression of sstr-3 and sstr-5 and a significantly weak expression of sstr-1 and sstr-2. The sstr-2 was only found in medullary and Hürthle cell carcinomas. Papillary and follicular thyroid carcinomas demonstrated a high expression of sstr-3, sstr-4, and sstr-5 [83, 84].

^{111}In pentetreotide is a somatostatin analogue that displays a high affinity for sstr-2, a lower affinity for sstr-3 and sstr-5, and notably weak affinity for sstr-1 and sstr-4 (50). Several groups have reported the use of SRS using ^{111}In pentetreotide (octreotide) to detect residual or recurrent disease in WDTC (Fig. 44.3) [85–92]. SRS has also been used for imaging Hürthle cell thyroid cancer with high sensitivity [93, 94]. For WDTC, Baudin et al. reported a sensitivity of 80 % (20 of 25) in patients, regardless of whether the radioiodine scan was positive or negative. In patients who had radioiodine-negative scans, the octreotide scans were positive in 75 % (12 of 16). In patients with radioiodine-positive scans, the octreotide scans were positive in 89 % (8 of 9; [85]). Postema et al. reported a 75 % sensitivity of SRS for the detection of metastatic WDTC [89]. These results are confirmed by Stokkel et al., who prospectively evaluated the diagnostic and prognostic value of ^{111}In pentetreotide scintigraphy in 23 patients with negative posttherapy ^{131}I scans and progressive thyroid carcinoma [92]. There were 13 papillary, eight follicular, and two Hürthle cell carcinomas; 19 of 23 patients had advanced disease as defined by T3 and T4 tumor stage and/or presence of distant metastases (M1). The uptake within tumor metastases on ^{111}In pentetreotide scans was visually quantified and scored ranging from 0 (no uptake) to 4 (intense uptake). The overall sensitivity of SRS for detection of metastases was 74 %. The sensitivity was better in patients in whom posttherapy ^{131}I WBS did not show any abnormal radioiodine uptake (82 %) than those with minimal uptake (50 %). Additionally, this study demonstrated that ^{111}In pentetreotide uptake was inversely correlated with survival. The 10-year survival rate was 33 % in patients with moderate-to-intense uptake (radioactivity scores of 2–4), compared to 100 % in patients with absent or slight uptake (radioactivity scores of 0 or 1). These results suggest that WDTC tumors with a high level of sstr expression display a more aggressive behavior.

Gorges et al. reported on 48 patients with metastatic WDTC undergoing ^{111}In pentetreotide studies [88]. The histopathology was papillary in 9, follicular in 9, insular (poorly differentiated) in 1, and Hürthle cell in 29 patients. Radioiodine scintigraphy results of diagnostic (10–27 mCi [370–999 MBq]) or posttherapeutic (80–270 mCi [2.96–9.99 GBq]) ^{131}I WBS were available for 45 patients. There were 15 patients with radioiodine-negative tumors in which SRS was performed as an alternative imaging modality to help select patients for radionuclide therapy with ^{90}Y-DOTA-D-Phe-1-Thy-3-octreotide (^{90}Y-DOTATOC). There were 30

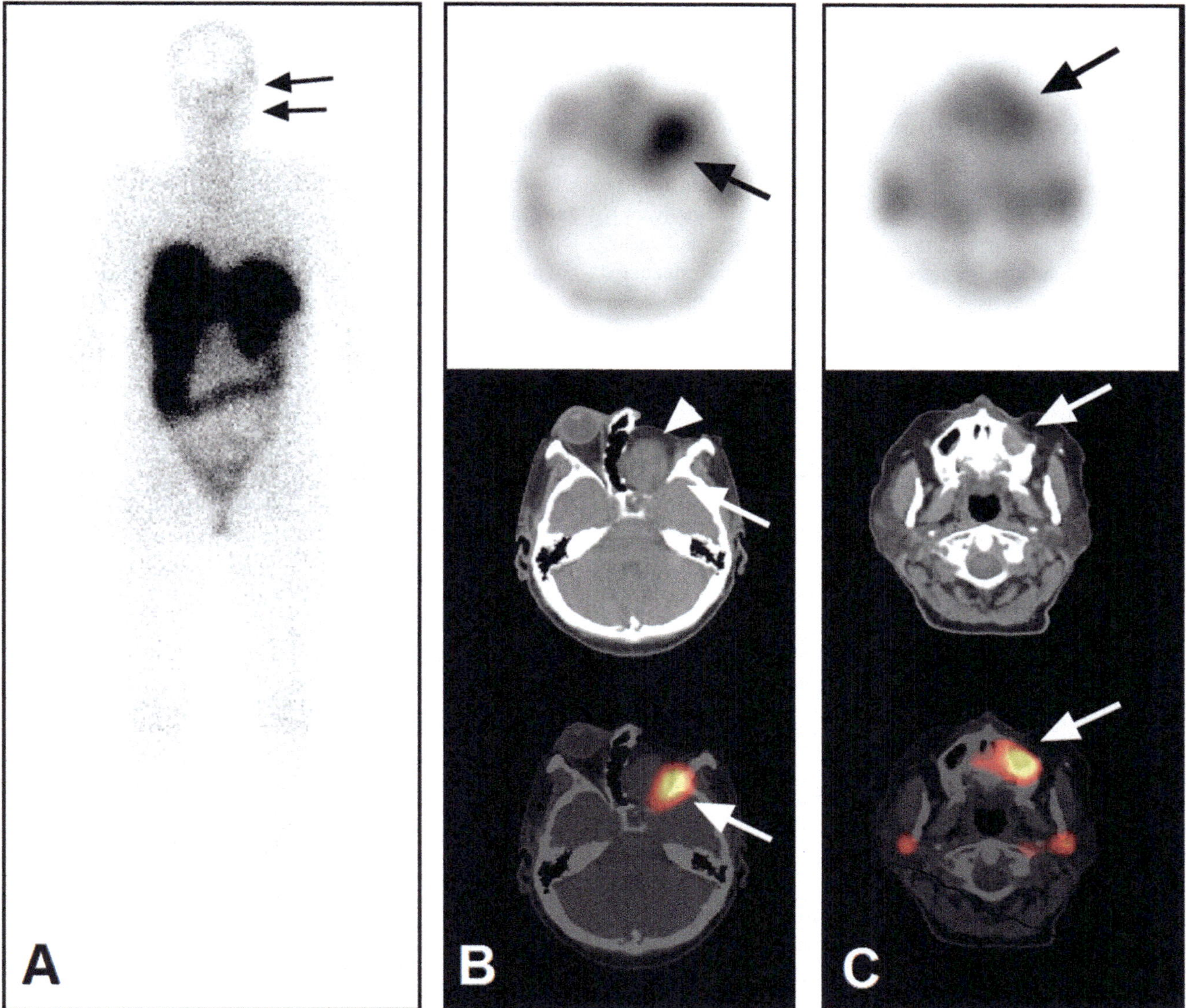

Fig. 44.3 ^{111}In pentetreotide SPECT/CT scan in a 68-year-old woman with a history of Hürthle cell carcinoma, metastatic to the left orbit, treated with orbital exenteration, anterior skull base resection, partial maxillectomy, and flap repair. Her thyroglobulin was elevated at 5.9 ng/mL. Her FDG PET scan was compatible with recurrent tumor at the skull base and left maxilla. Her radioiodine scan was negative. She was being considered for clinical trial of tyrosine kinase inhibitor and possible somatostatin treatment. Her whole-body ^{111}In pentetreotide planar scan (**a**) shows two faint foci overlying the left orbital and left maxillary regions. Axial SPECT, CT, and fusion SPECT/CT images at two axial levels demonstrate focal uptake at the (**b**) left sphenoid wing/skull base (*arrows*); note the orbital flap repair (*arrowhead*), and radiotracer uptake at the (**c**) margin of the left maxilla (*arrows*). SPECT/CT improves lesion conspicuity, precisely localizes radioactivity, and confirms tumor expression of somatostatin receptors

patients with radioiodine-positive metastases in whom the results of ^{111}In pentetreotide and ^{131}I scans were compared. The sensitivity of ^{111}In pentetreotide scintigraphy was 74 % (37 of 50 patients). For localization of metastatic disease, ^{111}In pentetreotide scintigraphy demonstrated a sensitivity of 87 % for skeletal metastases, 79 % for cervical and mediastinal lymph nodal metastases, 68 % for pulmonary or distant soft tissue metastases, and 56 % for abdominal or retroperitoneal metastases. ^{111}In pentetreotide accumulation did not correlate with tumor size. The smallest visualized tumor sites were about 8 mm in diameter.

The effect of serum thyroglobulin levels measured on thyroxine suppressive therapy on sensitivity of ^{111}In pentetreotide scintigraphy has been assessed. In patients with thyroglobulin <10 ng/mL, ^{111}In pentetreotide scintigraphy was positive in 27 % of patients, whereas in patients with thyroglobulin >10 ng/mL, SRS was positive in 85 % of patients. The maximal uptake was observed in Hürthle cell carcinomas, and

95 % of scans were positive when the thyroglobulin exceeded 10 ng/mL. The ^{111}In pentetreotide scan was positive in 45 % of papillary thyroid carcinomas and 78 % of follicular thyroid carcinomas. This study also reported the results of ^{90}Y-DOTATOC therapy (up to 9.3 GBq/250 mCi per four cycles) in three patients with negative ^{131}I WBS and progressive metastatic disease. ^{90}Y-DOTATOC displays sstr affinity profile similar to diagnostic ^{111}In pentetreotide and delivers β beta particles with a maximum range of 10 mm and mean range of 2.8 mm in targeted tumor tissues. Unfortunately, tumor progression, as demonstrated by a continuous rise in thyroglobulin levels and progressive radiological changes, could not be stopped in any patients treated with ^{90}Y-DOTATOC, and efficacy of this treatment to date has been modest [88, 95–99].

The sensitivity of ^{111}In pentetreotide scintigraphy was compared with FDG PET and conventional radiographic imaging (CRI) in 21 patients with metastatic thyroid carcinoma [90]. CRI included non-contrast CT, MRI from head to pelvis, neck ultrasonography, and bone radiographic survey. A total of 105 lesions were detected by the combined use of CRI, FDG PET, and SRS imaging in 21 patients. The lesion detection rates (sensitivity) for each method was as follows: CRI, 76.2 %; FDG PET, 67.6 %; and SRS, 49.5 %. In 9.5 % (2 of 21) of patients, SRS detected five unexpected lesions, which were not seen by either CRI or FDG PET (4.8 % of all lesions). These unexpected lesions were initially negative on ^{131}I diagnostic WBS but confirmed as functioning metastatic thyroid tissue on posttherapy radioiodine scans. Thus, FDG PET imaging was superior to SRS for the detection of metastatic radioiodine-negative WDTC, but SRS did reveal unexpected lesions and can be used in conjunction with conventional radiologic techniques for follow-up of patients with clinical and biochemical evidence of progression. Other comparative studies have confirmed FDG PET/CT to have higher sensitivity for detection of non-iodine–avid disease, compared to ^{111}In octreotide [87, 90]. Therefore, FDG PET when available is usually used in preference to alternative imaging radiotracers.

Newer somatostatin analogues utilizing DOTA or EDDA/HYNIC as the chelator rather than DTPA have shown slightly higher sensitivities than FDG PET for thyroid cancer imaging [93, 100–104]. Gabriel et al. found ^{99m}Tc-EDDA/HYNIC TOC had sensitivity of 66 % in iodine-negative WDTC similar to FDG PET [100]. Rodrigues et al. reported ^{99m}Tc depreotide with sensitivity 90 % compared to FDG PET with sensitivity 70 % [102]. In another study reporting similar findings, ^{111}In-DOTA lanreotide and ^{111}In-DOTATOC both had sensitivity of 94 % comparing favorably to FDG PET sensitivity of 83 % [103]. In 20 patients with differentiated thyroid cancer, studied with either ^{99m}Tc-EDDA/HYNIC TOC or ^{99m}Tc-EDDA/HYNIC TATE scintrigraphy, overall sensitivity was 75 % [105]. Therefore, further studies of SRS using newer somatostatin analogues are required, with a complementary role to FDG PET proposed by some authors. Recently, Ga-68 DOTA-TATE and Ga-68 DOTA-NOC PET imaging were performed in 13 patients with iodine-negative thyroglobulin-positive thyroid cancer, nine with papillary thyroid cancer, three with Hürthle cell carcinoma, and one with follicular thyroid carcinoma. Both Ga-68 DOTA-TATE and Ga-68 DOTA-NOC PET images gave comparable results with positive results in 62 % of patients, demonstrating potential utility of PET imaging with somatostatin analogues [106].

Although not a primary modality for imaging WDTC, SRS has a role in the evaluation of radioiodine-negative tumors, with a sensitivity ranging from 50 % to 85 %, and higher with newer somatostatin analogues 90–94 %, depending on the patient selection, thyroglobulin levels, and histopathology of the primary tumor [85–92]. The highest sensitivity was reported for Hürthle cell carcinomas, which are less frequently visualized with ^{131}I scintigraphy [88]. In approx 65 % of patients with radioiodine-negative metastatic WDTC, the disease is limited to the neck or mediastinum [92], and localization of metastatic deposits with alternative thyroid-imaging modalities assists in guiding surgical intervention. Confirmation of somatostatin receptor expression using SRS can also be useful to select patients more likely to benefit from radionuclide-labeled somatostatin analogue therapy [98, 99].

References

1. Kishida T. Mechanisms of thallium-201 accumulation in the thyroid gland—clinical usefulness of the dynamic study in thallium-201 chloride scintigraphy for the differential diagnosis of thyroid nodules. Kaku Igaku. 1987;24:991–1004.
2. Hoefnagel CA, Delprat CC, Marcuse HR, de Vijlder JJ. Role of thallium-201 total-body scintigraphy in follow-up of thyroid carcinoma. J Nucl Med. 1986;27:1854–7.
3. Yada H, Hozumi Y, Kanazawa K, Nagai H. Quantitative estimation and clinical significance of accumulation and washout of thallium-201 chloride in follicular thyroid neoplasm. Endocr J. 2002;49:55–60.
4. Uematsu H, Sadato N, Ohtsubo T, et al. Fluorine-18-fluorodeoxyglucose PET versus thallium-201 scintigraphy evaluation of thyroid tumors. J Nucl Med. 1998;39:453–9.
5. Ramanna L, Waxman A, Braunstein G. Thallium-201 scintigraphy in differentiated thyroid cancer: comparison with radioiodine scintigraphy and serum thyroglobulin determinations. J Nucl Med. 1991;32:441–6.
6. Brandt-Mainz K, Muller SP, Reiners C, Bockisch A. Relationship between thyroglobulin and reliability of thallium 201 scintigraphy in differentiated thyroid cancer. Nuklearmedizin. 2000;39:20–5.
7. Brendel AJ, Guyot M, Jeandot R, Lefort G, Manciet G. Thallium-201 imaging in the follow-up of differentiated thyroid carcinoma. J Nucl Med. 1988;29:1515–20.
8. Carril JM, Quirce R, Serrano J, et al. Total-body scintigraphy with thallium-201 and iodine-131 in the follow-up of differentiated thyroid cancer. J Nucl Med. 1997;38:686–92.
9. Charkes ND, Vitti RA, Brooks K. Thallium-201 SPECT increases detectability of thyroid cancer metastases. J Nucl Med. 1990;31:147–53.

10. Harder W, Lind P, Molnar M, et al. Thallium-201 uptake with negative iodine-131 scintigraphy and serum thyroglobulin in metastatic oxyphilic papillary thyroid carcinoma. J Nucl Med. 1998;39:236–8.
11. Lin JD, Kao PF, Weng HF, Lu WT, Huang MJ. Relative value of thallium-201 and iodine-131 scans in the detection of recurrence or distant metastasis of well differentiated thyroid carcinoma. Eur J Nucl Med. 1998;25:695–700.
12. Nakada K, Katoh C, Kanegae K, et al. Thallium-201 scintigraphy to predict therapeutic outcome of iodine-131 therapy of metastatic thyroid carcinoma. J Nucl Med. 1998;39:807–10.
13. Nakada K, Katoh C, Morita K, et al. Relationship among ^{201}T1 uptake, nuclear DNA content and clinical behavior in metastatic thyroid carcinoma. J Nucl Med. 1999;40:963–7.
14. Maxon HR. Detection of residual and recurrent thyroid cancer by radionuclide imaging. Thyroid. 1999;9:443–6.
15. Erdil TY, Onsel C, Kanmaz B, et al. Comparison of ^{99m}Tc-methoxyisobutyl isonitrile and 201T1 scintigraphy in visualization of suppressed thyroid tissue. J Nucl Med. 2000;41:1163–7.
16. Alper E, Akbunar T, Tamgac F. Visualization of papillary thyroid carcinoma and its metastatic lymph nodes. Images with Tc-99m pertechnetate, Tl-201, and Tc-99m sestamibi. Clin Nucl Med. 1996;21:815–6.
17. Klain M, Maurea S, Cuocolo A, et al. Technetium-99m tetrofosmin imaging in thyroid diseases: comparison with Tc-99m-pertechnetate, thallium-201 and Tc-99m-methoxyisobutylisonitrile scans. Eur J Nucl Med. 1996;23:1568–74.
18. Shiga T, Tsukamoto E, Nakada K, et al. Comparison of ^{18}F-FDG, ^{131}I-Na, and ^{201}Tl in diagnosis of recurrent or metastatic thyroid carcinoma. J Nucl Med. 2001;42:414–9.
19. Dadparvar S, Chevres A, Tulchinsky M, Krishna-Badrinath L, Khan AS, Slizofski WJ. Clinical utility of technetium-99m methoxyisobutylisonitrile imaging in differentiated thyroid carcinoma: comparison with thallium-201 and iodine-131 Na scintigraphy, and serum thyroglobulin quantitation. Eur J Nucl Med. 1995;22:1330–8.
20. Dietlein M, Scheidhauer K, Voth E, Theissen P, Schicha H. Follow-up of differentiated thyroid cancer: what is the value of FDG and sestamibi in the diagnostic algorithm? Nuklearmedizin. 1998;37:12–7.
21. Yen TC, Lin HD, Lee CH, Chang SL, Yeh SH. The role of technetium-99m sestamibi whole-body scans in diagnosing metastatic Hurthle cell carcinoma of the thyroid gland after total thyroidectomy: a comparison with iodine-131 and thallium-201 whole-body scans. Eur J Nucl Med. 1994;21:980–3.
22. Sarikaya A, Huseyinova G, Irfanoglu ME, Erkmen N, Cermik TF, Berkarda S. The relationship between 99Tc(m)-sestamibi uptake and ultrastructural cell types of thyroid tumours. Nucl Med Commun. 2001;22:39–44.
23. Van de Wiele C, Rottey S, Goethals I, et al. ^{99m}Tc sestamibi and ^{99m}Tc tetrofosmin scintigraphy for predicting resistance to chemotherapy: a critical review of clinical data. Nucl Med Commun. 2003;24:945–50.
24. Saggiorato E, Angusti T, Rosas R, et al. ^{99m}Tc-MIBI imaging in the presurgical characterization of thyroid follicular neoplasms: relationship to multidrug resistance protein expression. J Nucl Med. 2009;50:1785–93.
25. Almeida-Filho P, Ravizzini GC, Almeida C, Borges-Neto S. Whole-body Tc-99m sestamibi scintigraphy in the follow-up of differentiated thyroid carcinoma. Clin Nucl Med. 2000;25:443–6.
26. Seabold JE, Gurll N, Schurrer ME, Aktay R, Kirchner PT. Comparison of 99mTc-methoxyisobutyl isonitrile and ^{201}Tl scintigraphy for detection of residual thyroid cancer after ^{131}I ablative therapy. J Nucl Med. 1999;40:1434–40.
27. Foldes I, Levay A, Stotz G. Comparative scanning of thyroid nodules with technetium-99m pertechnetate and technetium-99m methoxyisobutylisonitrile. Eur J Nucl Med. 1993;20:330–3.
28. Kresnik E, Gallowitsch HJ, Mikosch P, Molnar M, Lind P. Tetrofosmin scintigraphy of thyroid disease. Eur J Nucl Med. 1997;24:1332.
29. Nakahara H, Noguchi S, Murakami N, et al. Technetium-99m-sestamibi scintigraphy compared with thallium-201 in evaluation of thyroid tumors. J Nucl Med. 1996;37:901–4.
30. Wei JP, Burke GJ. Characterization of the neoplastic potential of solitary solid thyroid lesions with Tc-99m-pertechnetate and Tc-99m-sestamibi scanning. Ann Surg Oncol. 1995;2:233–7.
31. Casara D, Rubello D, Saladini G. Role of scintigraphy with tumor-seeking agents in the diagnosis and preoperative staging of malignant thyroid nodules. Biomed Pharmacother. 2000;54:334–6.
32. Boi F, Lai ML, Deias C, et al. The usefulness of 99mTc-SestaMIBI scan in the diagnostic evaluation of thyroid nodules with oncocytic cytology. Eur J Endocrinol. 2003;149:493–8.
33. Vattimo A, Bertelli P, Cintorino M, Burroni L, Volterrani D, Vella A. Identification of Hurthle cell tumor by single-injection, double-phase scintigraphy with technetium-99m-sestamibi. J Nucl Med. 1995;36:778–82.
34. Vattimo A, Bertelli P, Cintorino M, et al. Hurthle cell tumor dwelling in hot thyroid nodules: preoperative detection with technetium-99m-MIBI dual-phase scintigraphy. J Nucl Med. 1998;39:822–5.
35. Chamnanrabiabkij E, Welch A, Jayapaul MK, Perros P. Detection of Hurthle cell carcinoma using sestamibi. Thyroid. 2008;18:575–6.
36. Campenni A, Violi MA, Ruggeri RM, et al. Clinical usefulness of 99mTc-MIBI scintigraphy in the postsurgical evaluation of patients with differentiated thyroid cancer. Nucl Med Commun. 2010;31:274–9.
37. Elser H, Henze M, Hermann C, Eckert W, Mende U. 99m-Tc-MIBI for recurrent and metastatic differentiated thyroid carcinoma. Nuklearmedizin. 1997;36:7–12.
38. Fridrich L, Messa C, Landoni C, et al. Whole-body scintigraphy with ^{99m}Tc-MIBI, ^{18}F-FDG and ^{131}I in patients with metastatic thyroid carcinoma. Nucl Med Commun. 1997;18:3–9.
39. Fujie S, Okumura Y, Sato S, et al. Diagnostic capabilities of I-131, TI-201, and Tc-99m-MIBI scintigraphy for metastatic differentiated thyroid carcinoma after total thyroidectomy. Acta Med Okayama. 2005;59:99–107.
40. Grunwald F, Menzel C, Bender H, et al. Comparison of ^{18}FDG-PET with ^{131}iodine and ^{99m}Tc-sestamibi scintigraphy in differentiated thyroid cancer. Thyroid. 1997;7:327–35.
41. Hsu CH, Liu FY, Yen RF, Kao CH. Tc-99m MIBI SPECT in detecting metastatic papillary thyroid carcinoma in patients with elevated human serum thyroglobulin levels but negative I-131 whole body scan. Endocr Res. 2003;29:9–15.
42. Iwata M, Kasagi K, Misaki T, et al. Comparison of whole-body ^{18}F-FDG PET, ^{99m}Tc-MIBI SPET, and post-therapeutic ^{131}I-Na scintigraphy in the detection of metastatic thyroid cancer. Eur J Nucl Med Mol Imaging. 2004;31:491–8.
43. Kaya M, Cermik TF. Tc-99m MIBI scintigraphy in tall cell variant of papillary thyroid carcinoma with negative radioiodine scan. Clin Nucl Med. 2008;33:615–8.
44. Kobayashi M, Mogami T, Uchiyama M, et al. Usefulness of 99mTc-MIBI SPECT in the metastatic lesions of thyroid cancer. Nippon Igaku Hoshasen Gakkai Zasshi. 1997;57:127–32.
45. Kresnik E, Gallowitsch HJ, Mikosch P, Lind P. MIBI and thyroid tumors. J Nucl Med. 1997;38:1501.
46. Kucuk NO, Kulak HA, Aras G. Clinical importance of technetium-99m-methoxyisobutylisonitrile (MIBI) scintigraphy in differentiated thyroid carcinoma patients with elevated thyroglobulin levels and negative I-131 scanning results. Ann Nucl Med. 2006;20:393–7.
47. Kucuk ON, Aras G, Kulak HA, Ibis E. Clinical importance of anti-thyroglobulin auto-antibodies in patients with differentiated thyroid carcinoma: comparison with ^{99m}Tc-MIBI scans. Nucl Med Commun. 2006;27:873–6.

48. Kucuk ON, Gultekin SS, Aras G, Ibis E. Radioiodine whole-body scans, thyroglobulin levels, ^{99m}Tc-MIBI scans and computed tomography: results in patients with lung metastases from differentiated thyroid cancer. Nucl Med Commun. 2006;27:261–6.
49. Miyamoto S, Kasagi K, Misaki T, Alam MS, Konishi J. Evaluation of technetium-99m-MIBI scintigraphy in metastatic differentiated thyroid carcinoma. J Nucl Med. 1997;38:352–6.
50. Nemec J, Nyvltova O, Blazek T, et al. Positive thyroid cancer scintigraphy using technetium-99m methoxyisobutylisonitrile. Eur J Nucl Med. 1996;23:69–71.
51. Ronga G, Ventroni G, Montesano T, et al. Sensitivity of [99mTc] methoxyisobutylisonitrile scan in patients with metastatic differentiated thyroid cancer. Q J Nucl Med Mol Imaging. 2007;51: 364–71.
52. Sriprapaporn J, Toopmongkol C, Satayaban B, Chantamoon N. Technetium-99m methoxyisobutylisonitrile imaging in the follow-up of differentiated thyroid carcinoma. Ann Acad Med Singapore. 2002;31:195–8.
53. Ugur O, Kostakoglu L, Caner B, et al. Comparison of ^{201}Tl, ^{99m}Tc-MIBI and ^{131}I imaging in the follow-up of patients with well-differentiated thyroid carcinoma. Nucl Med Commun. 1996;17:373–7.
54. Ng DC, Sundram FX, Sin AE. ^{99m}Tc-sestamibi and ^{131}I whole-body scintigraphy and initial serum thyroglobulin in the management of differentiated thyroid carcinoma. J Nucl Med. 2000;41:631–5.
55. Rubello D, Mazzarotto R, Casara D. The role of technetium-99m methoxyisobutylisonitrile scintigraphy in the planning of therapy and follow-up of patients with differentiated thyroid carcinoma after surgery. Eur J Nucl Med. 2000;27:431–40.
56. Meller B, Sahlmann C, Horstmann O, Gerl J, Baehre M, Meller J. Conventional gamma and high energy probe for radioguided dissection of metastases in a patient with recurrent thyroid carcinoma with ^{99m}Tc-MIBI and ^{18}F-FDG. Nuklearmedizin. 2005;44: N23–5.
57. Rubello D, Pelizzo MR, Casara D, et al. Radio-guided surgery for non-^{131}I-avid thyroid cancer. Thyroid. 2006;16:1105–11.
58. Rubello D, Piotto A, Pagetta C, Pelizzo MR, Casara D. ^{99m}Tc-MIBI radio-guided surgery for recurrent thyroid carcinoma: technical feasibility and procedure, and preliminary clinical results. Eur J Nucl Med Mol Imaging. 2002;29:1201–5.
59. Rubello D, Salvatori M, Casara D, et al. ^{99m}Tc-sestamibi radio-guided surgery of loco-regional ^{131}Iodine-negative recurrent thyroid cancer. Eur J Surg Oncol. 2007;33:902–6.
60. Rubello D, Salvatori M, Pelizzo MR, et al. Radio-guided surgery of differentiated thyroid cancer using ^{131}I or ^{99m}Tc-Sestamibi. Nucl Med Commun. 2006;27:1–4.
61. Boz A, Arici C, Gungor F, Yildiz A, Colak T, Karayalcin B. Gamma probe-guided resection and scanning with TC-99m MIBI of a local recurrence of follicular thyroid carcinoma. Clin Nucl Med. 2001;26:820–2.
62. Waddington WA, Kettle AG, Heddle RM, Coakley AJ. Intraoperative localization of recurrent medullary carcinoma of the thyroid using indium-111 pentetreotide and a nuclear surgical probe. Eur J Nucl Med. 1994;21:363–4.
63. Gallegos-Hernandez JF, Pichardo-Romero P, Esparza-Perez H, Resendiz-Colosia JA, Minauro-Munoz GG, Hernandez-Hernandez DM. Value of ^{99m}Tc tetrofosmin scan in well-differentiated thyroid cancer. Cir Cir. 2009;77:275–8, 257–79.
64. Kanmaz B, Erdil TY, Yardi OF, et al. The role of ^{99m}Tc-tetrofosmin in the evaluation of thyroid nodules. Nucl Med Commun. 2000;21:333–9.
65. Chen YK, Liu FY, Yen RF, Kao CH. Compare FDG-PET and Tc-99m tetrofosmin SPECT to detect metastatic thyroid carcinoma. Acad Radiol. 2003;10:835–9.
66. Degirmenci B, Aydin A, Comlekci A, Ozdogan O, Bekis R. Technetium-99m tetrofosmin uptake in insular thyroid carcinoma. A comparison with iodine-131. Clin Nucl Med. 2003;28: 385–8.
67. Erdem S, Baskan A, Bashekim C, Filiz E. Tc-99m tetrofosmin uptake by recurrent papillary carcinoma of the thyroid. Clin Nucl Med. 1998;23:189.
68. Gallowitsch HJ, Kresnik E, Mikosch P, Pipam W, Gomez I, Lind P. Tc-99m-tetrofosmin scintigraphy: an alternative scintigraphic method for following up differentiated thyroid carcinoma—preliminary results. Nuklearmedizin. 1996;35:230–5.
69. Gallowitsch HJ, Mikosch P, Kresnik E, Unterweger O, Gomez I, Lind P. Thyroglobulin and low-dose iodine-131 and technetium-99m-tetrofosmin whole-body scintigraphy in differentiated thyroid carcinoma. J Nucl Med. 1998;39:870–5.
70. Klain M, Cuocolo A, Salvatore M, Maurea S. Tetrofosmin thyroid scintigraphy. Eur J Nucl Med. 1998;25:816.
71. Klain M, Maurea S, Lastoria S, et al. Technetium-99m-tetrofosmin imaging of differentiated mixed thyroid cancer. J Nucl Med. 1995;36:2248–51.
72. Kosuda S, Yokoyama H, Katayama M, Yokokawa T, Kusano S, Yamamoto O. Technetium-99m tetrofosmin and technetium-99m sestamibi imaging of multiple metastases from differentiated thyroid carcinoma. Eur J Nucl Med. 1995;22:1218–20.
73. Lind P, Gallowitsch HJ. The use of non-specific tracers in the follow up of differentiated thyroid cancer: results with Tc-99m tetrofosmin whole body scintigraphy. Acta Med Austriaca. 1996;23:69–75.
74. Lind P, Gallowitsch HJ, Langsteger W, Kresnik E, Mikosch P, Gomez I. Technetium-99m-tetrofosmin whole-body scintigraphy in the follow-up of differentiated thyroid carcinoma. J Nucl Med. 1997;38:348–52.
75. Lind P, Gallowitsch HJ, Mikosch P, et al. Comparison of different tracers in the follow up of differentiated thyroid carcinoma. Acta Med Austriaca. 1999;26:115–7.
76. Lind P, Gallowitsch HJ, Unterweger O, Mikosch P, Starlinger M, Dinges HP. FDG PET in the follow-up of differentiated thyroid cancer. Comparison with Tc-99m Tetrofosmin and I-131 whole body scintigraphy. Clin Positron Imaging. 1998;1:237.
77. Nemec J, Nyvltova O, Preiningerova M, et al. Positive thyroid cancer scintigraphy using ^{99m}Tc-tetrofosmin (Myoview): a preliminary report. Nucl Med Commun. 1995;16:694–7.
78. Nishiyama Y, Yamamoto Y, Ono Y, et al. Comparison of ^{99m}Tc-tetrofosmin with ^{201}Tl and ^{131}I in the detection of differentiated thyroid cancer metastases. Nucl Med Commun. 2000;21:917–23.
79. Unal S, Menda Y, Adalet I, et al. Thallium-201, technetium-99m-tetrofosmin and iodine-131 in detecting differentiated thyroid carcinoma metastases. J Nucl Med. 1998;39:1897–902.
80. Wu HS, Liu FY, Huang WS, Liu YC, Chang CT, Kao CH. Technetium-99m tetrofosmin single photon emission computed tomography to detect metastatic papillary thyroid carcinoma in patients with elevated human serum thyroglobulin levels but negative I-131 whole body scan. Clin Radiol. 2003;58: 787–90.
81. Wu YJ, Wu HS, Yen RF, Shen YY, Kao CH. Detecting metastatic neck lymph nodes in papillary thyroid carcinoma by ^{18}F-2-deoxyglucose positron emission tomography and Tc-99m tetrofosmin single photon emission computed tomography. Anticancer Res. 2003;23:2973–6.
82. Tisell LE, Ahlman H, Wangberg B, et al. Expression of somatostatin receptors in oncocytic (Hurthle cell) neoplasia of the thyroid. Br J Cancer. 1999;79:1579–82.
83. Ain KB, Taylor KD, Tofiq S, Venkataraman G. Somatostatin receptor subtype expression in human thyroid and thyroid carcinoma cell lines. J Clin Endocrinol Metab. 1997;82:1857–62.

84. Virgolini I, Traub T, Novotny C, et al. Experience with indium-111 and yttrium-90-labeled somatostatin analogs. Curr Pharm Des. 2002;8:1781–807.
85. Baudin E, Schlumberger M, Lumbroso J, Travagli JP, Caillou B, Parmentier C. Octreotide scintigraphy in patients with differentiated thyroid carcinoma: contribution for patients with negative radioiodine scan. J Clin Endocrinol Metab. 1996;81:2541–4.
86. Christian JA, Cook GJ, Harmer C. Indium-111-labelled octreotide scintigraphy in the diagnosis and management of non-iodine avid metastatic carcinoma of the thyroid. Br J Cancer. 2003;89: 258–61.
87. Giammarile F, Houzard C, Bournaud C, Hafdi Z, Sassolas G, Borson-Chazot F. Diagnostic management of suspected metastatic thyroid carcinoma: clinical value of octreotide scintigraphy in patients with negative high-dose radioiodine scans. Eur J Endocrinol. 2004;150:277–83.
88. Gorges R, Kahaly G, Muller-Brand J, Macke H, Roser HW, Bockisch A. Radionuclide-labeled somatostatin analogues for diagnostic and therapeutic purposes in nonmedullary thyroid cancer. Thyroid. 2001;11:647–59.
89. Postema PT, De Herder WW, Reubi JC, et al. Somatostatin receptor scintigraphy in non-medullary thyroid cancer. Digestion. 1996;57 Suppl 1:36–7.
90. Sarlis NJ, Gourgiotis L, Guthrie LC, et al. In-111 DTPA-octreotide scintigraphy for disease detection in metastatic thyroid cancer: comparison with F-18 FDG positron emission tomography and extensive conventional radiographic imaging. Clin Nucl Med. 2003;28:208–17.
91. Stokkel MP, Reigman HI, Verkooijen RB, Smit JW. Indium-111-octreotide scintigraphy in differentiated thyroid carcinoma metastases that do not respond to treatment with high-dose I-131. J Cancer Res Clin Oncol. 2003;129:287–94.
92. Stokkel MP, Verkooijen RB, Smit JW. Indium-111 octreotide scintigraphy for the detection of non-functioning metastases from differentiated thyroid cancer: diagnostic and prognostic value. Eur J Nucl Med Mol Imaging. 2004;31:950–7.
93. Gambini JP, Quagliata A, Finozzi R, et al. Tc-99m- and Ga-68-labeled somatostatin analogues in the evaluation of hurthle cell thyroid cancer. Clin Nucl Med. 2011;36:803–4.
94. Kostoglou-Athanassiou I, Pappas A, Gogou L, Kaldrymides P. Scintigraphy with ^{111}In octreotide and ^{201}Tl in a Hurthle cell thyroid carcinoma without detectable radio-iodine uptake. Report of a case and review of the literature. Horm Res. 2003;60: 205–8.
95. Alhamarneh O, Murphy J, Atkin SL, England RJ. Somatostatin analogues have no role in the treatment of advanced differentiated thyroid cancer. J Laryngol Otol. 2004;118:653–4.
96. Kohlfuerst S, Igerc I, Gallowitsch HJ, et al. Is there a role for sandostatin treatment in patients with progressive thyroid cancer and iodine-negative but somatostatin-receptor-positive metastases? Thyroid. 2006;16:1113–9.
97. Margulies DJ, Blum M. Somatostatin receptor scintigraphy as a potential diagnostic and treatment modality for thyroid follicular-cell-derived cancers. Thyroid. 2010;20:671–2.
98. Teunissen JJ, Kwekkeboom DJ, Kooij PP, Bakker WH, Krenning EP. Peptide receptor radionuclide therapy for non-radioiodine-avid differentiated thyroid carcinoma. J Nucl Med. 2005;46: 107S–14.
99. Teunissen JJ, Kwekkeboom DJ, Krenning EP. Staging and treatment of differentiated thyroid carcinoma with radiolabeled somatostatin analogs. Trends Endocrinol Metab. 2006;17:19–25.
100. Gabriel M, Froehlich F, Decristoforo C, et al. 99mTc-EDDA/HYNIC-TOC and (18)F-FDG in thyroid cancer patients with negative ^{131}I whole-body scans. Eur J Nucl Med Mol Imaging. 2004;31:330–41.
101. Gambini JP, Nunez M, Vila R, Noble J, Alonso O. Tc-99m hynic octreotide SPECT-MRI in brain metastasis of thyroid papillary-insular cancer. Clin Nucl Med. 2009;34:920–1.
102. Rodrigues M, Li S, Gabriel M, Heute D, Greifeneder M, Virgolini I. ^{99m}Tc-depreotide scintigraphy versus ^{18}F-FDG-PET in the diagnosis of radioiodine-negative thyroid cancer. J Clin Endocrinol Metab. 2006;91:3997–4000.
103. Rodrigues M, Traub-Weidinger T, Leimer M, et al. Value of ^{111}In-DOTA-lanreotide and ^{111}In-DOTA-DPhe1-Tyr3-octreotide in differentiated thyroid cancer: results of in vitro binding studies and in vivo comparison with ^{18}F-FDG PET. Eur J Nucl Med Mol Imaging. 2005;32:1144–51.
104. Valsamaki P, Gotzamani-Psarrakou A, Tsiouris S, et al. Tc-99m depreotide imaging of I-131-negative recurrent metastatic papillary thyroid carcinoma. Int J Cancer. 2006;119:968–70.
105. Sager S, Kabasakal L, Halac M, et al. Comparison of ^{99m}Tc-HYNIC-TOC and HYNIC-TATE octreotide scintigraphy with FDG PET and ^{99m}Tc-MIBI in local recurrent or distant metastatic thyroid cancers. Clin Nucl Med. 2013;38:321–5.
106. Ocak M, Demirci E, Kabasakal L, Aygun A, Tutar RO, Araman A, Kanmaz B. Evaluation and comparison of Ga-68 DOTA-TATE and Ga-68 DOTA-NOC PET/CT imaging in well-differentiated thyroid cancer. Nuclear Medicine Communications. 2013;34:1084–9.

MR and CT Imaging of Thyroid Cancer

45

James Jelinek, Richard Young, Louis O. Smith III, and Kenneth D. Burman

This chapter discusses the role of magnetic resonance imaging (MRI) and computerized tomography (CT) in the evaluation of patients with thyroid cancer. Traditionally, patients with thyroid cancer have been diagnosed based on an evaluation initiated by clinical examination of a palpable thyroid nodule, and this accounts for around 60 % of ultimate diagnoses of thyroid cancer. An additional 20 % or more of patients are found to have thyroid cancer based on a clinical presentation with findings of adjacent involved cervical and/or supraclavicular lymph nodes. However, the increased utilization of both MRI and CT imaging of the head and neck has led to the "incidental" discovery of thyroid lesions that may account for as many as 20 % of patients being diagnosed with thyroid cancer. For example, there is widespread use of CT in the evaluation of the cervical spine in trauma, evaluation of the neck for any type of neck mass or hoarseness, and significantly increased utilization of CT in the evaluation of patients with lung disease and/or suspected pulmonary embolism. MRI is being increasingly utilized, in particular in the evaluation of pathology related to the cervical spine, specifically disk herniation and stenosis. MRI angiography is also being increasingly utilized for the evaluation of stroke to assess possible stenosis of the carotid and vertebral arteries. These studies will also demonstrate abnormalities of the thyroid gland and, when a suspected mass is seen, lead to instigation of a work-up of a potential thyroid tumor. With the increasing utilization of both MR and CT, it can be expected that an increased rate of discovery of thyroid cancer will occur.

J. Jelinek, MD, FACR
Director, Department of Radiology, MedStar Washington Hospital Center, Washington, DC, USA

R. Young, MD • L.O. Smith III, MD
Department of Radiology, Washington Hospital Center, Washington, DC, USA

K.D. Burman, MD (✉)
Director, Divisions of Endocrinology, Washington Hospital Center and Georgetown University Hospital, 110 Irving Street NW 2A-72, Washington, DC 20010, USA
e-mail: kenneth.d.burman@medstar.net

The incidental finding of thyroid masses is becoming increasingly common. Although less than 1 % of all cancers are present in the thyroid gland, thyroid nodules are found in at least 4–10 % of the adult population [1]. However, in our routine interpretation of neck and chest CT and MR, a higher percentage of the adult population have only small lesions or "incidentalomas" detected on CT, MRI, or ultrasound. These could be present in as much as 40 % of the adult population [1]. The question as to when incidental lesions should be evaluated further for a possible thyroid cancer is extremely controversial and difficult given the high prevalence of thyroid lesions detected by both CT and MRI (see Chaps. 17 and 23). However, when a nodule is greater than 1–1.5 cm in size, guidelines of our professional societies dictate that consultation should be sought regarding potential thyroid aspiration biopsy. Even smaller lesions may be biopsied in special circumstances, such as a history of neck radiation exposure or a family history of thyroid cancer. Clearly, clinical history and careful physical examination of the neck remain paramount. Ultrasound guidance for fine-needle aspiration is commonplace today (see Chap. 21), and MR and CT do not play a role in the guidance of biopsy for most thyroid nodules [1, 2]. Only a very rare incidentally diagnosed mass of the thyroid gland which is not reachable by traditional ultrasound methods (such as a mass which is substernal) should be biopsied by CT. Even small thyroid nodules which are immediately adjacent to the carotid artery and jugular veins do not preclude biopsy with ultrasound; in fact, such location may make FNA under ultrasound guidance even more strongly warranted. In our institution, the majority of fine-needle aspirations (FNAs) of palpable nodules are performed with no imaging guidance. However, of those FNAs performed with radiologic guidance, 99 % are performed with ultrasound with biopsy under CT, accounting for only an unusual subset of patients, in particular for deep cervical or infraclavicular post-thyroidectomy recurrences. It is controversial when

L. Wartofsky, D. Van Nostrand (eds.), *Thyroid Cancer*, DOI 10.1007/978-1-4939-3314-3_45

needle aspirations should be performed with any radiology guidance. In the past, the vast majority of aspirations were of palpable nodules, and the aspirations were performed by palpation. More recently, as techniques have evolved, a greater percentage of all aspirations are performed under ultrasound guidance. Obviously, all non-palpable nodules must be performed with imaging guidance.

The primary role of MR and CT in the evaluation of thyroid cancer is in the follow-up of recurrent thyroid cancer. In order to appreciate the value of MR and CT of the neck, a brief review of the anatomy of the neck would be helpful. The thyroid gland is present in the lowest part of the neck just above the sternal notch. The thyroid gland lies deep to the anterior neck muscles: the sternocleidomastoid muscle, omohyoid muscle, sternothyroid muscle, and sternohyoid muscle [3]. The thyroid gland sits like a saddle over the trachea with the thinnest portion of the thyroid gland (the isthmus) lying directly anterior to the trachea. The vital structures of the neck adjacent to the thyroid gland are all posterior. Moving from lateral to medial, the largest vital structure posterior and lateral is the internal jugular vein. The carotid artery, with its adjacent vagus nerve, typically resides directly medial to the jugular vein [3]. Due to normal variations of anatomy in patients, the internal carotid artery and jugular vein can reside relatively more lateral or even quite close to midline. Immediately between each lateral lobe of the thyroid gland and the trachea resides the recurrent laryngeal nerve. The esophagus is directly posterior to the trachea although occasionally may be slightly to the left and posterior to the trachea.

Other important structures include the phrenic nerve which is typically more posterior to the jugular vein. Posterior to these vital structures reside the muscles of the longus colli and scalene muscles. Importantly, the roots of the brachial plexus reside between the anterior and middle scalene muscles. Just cephalad to the thyroid gland are the important structures of the larynx, to include the cricoid cartilage, thyroid cartilage, and cartilage of the arytenoids, corniculate, and cuneiforms.

Lymph nodes have been classified by the American Joint Committee on Cancer (AJCC) [4]. Classification systems typically refer to the size and character of the lymph nodes. Nodes larger than 1 cm are considered more worrisome for harboring cancer, and benign nodes are typically oval shaped and have a discernible fatty hilum (see Chap. 21 on Ultrasound of Lymph Nodes). Unfortunately, it is becoming clear that thyroid cancer may be found in lymph nodes smaller than 1 cm which lack classic worrisome characteristics [5].

Level I lymph nodes have been described as being submental in location (Level Ia). However, and in particular in newer classifications [6], lymph nodes which are in the submandibular lymph node region (Level Ib) are also Level I nodes.

Level II lymph nodes are the upper internal jugular nodes, located above the level of the hyoid bone, along the carotid artery and jugular veins. Level IIa nodes are around the internal jugular vein, whereas Level IIb nodes are posterior to the vessels.

Level III lymph nodes are middle-level jugular nodes that are present at the level of the hyoid bone down to the level of the bottom of the cricoid cartilage but lateral to the carotid artery.

Level IV lymph nodes are lower jugular nodes and are below the level of the cricoid cartilage extending down to the level of the clavicle but remaining lateral to the carotid artery.

Level V lymph nodes are lymph nodes which are anterior to the trapezius muscle but posterior to the sternocleidomastoid muscle. Level Va nodes are above the cricoids and Level Vb nodes are below the cricoid cartilage.

Level VI (anterior or central compartment) nodes are midline anterior nodes between the manubrium sterni and the hyoid bone anteriorly [4].

Level VII lymph nodes are the superior mediastinal lymph nodes. Newer classifications do not always refer to Level VII nodes.

Computed Tomography (CT) Scanning

Computed tomography generates images using a series of x-ray beams and detectors. As in other areas of medicine, there have been huge strides in CT technology. Older CT studies were typically performed with slice thicknesses of 5–10 mm. Today, slice thicknesses are usually less than 3 mm, and, in many centers, 1–2 mm slice thicknesses are obtained and the set of images are not just presented in the axial plane. Using 1 mm or less slice thicknesses, there is the ability to perform isotropic images so that the neck can be imaged in any plane but most commonly in the axial, sagittal, and coronal planes. Images can also be easily presented as a full 3D color image which while spectacular to look at, when well reconstructed provides little additional diagnostic information. On the other hand, for large tumors, surgeons may find these helpful in preoperative planning.

CT scanners today are considerably faster than any other imaging modality, and in most cases, the total time of the imaging portion of the exam is less than 60 s. In particular, for the evaluation of the neck, almost all radiologists strongly prefer the use of CT contrast which contains high iodine content. Contrast is ideal to show the difference in contrast between the arteries and veins against their adjacent structures. With the infusion of iodinated contrast, there is a more

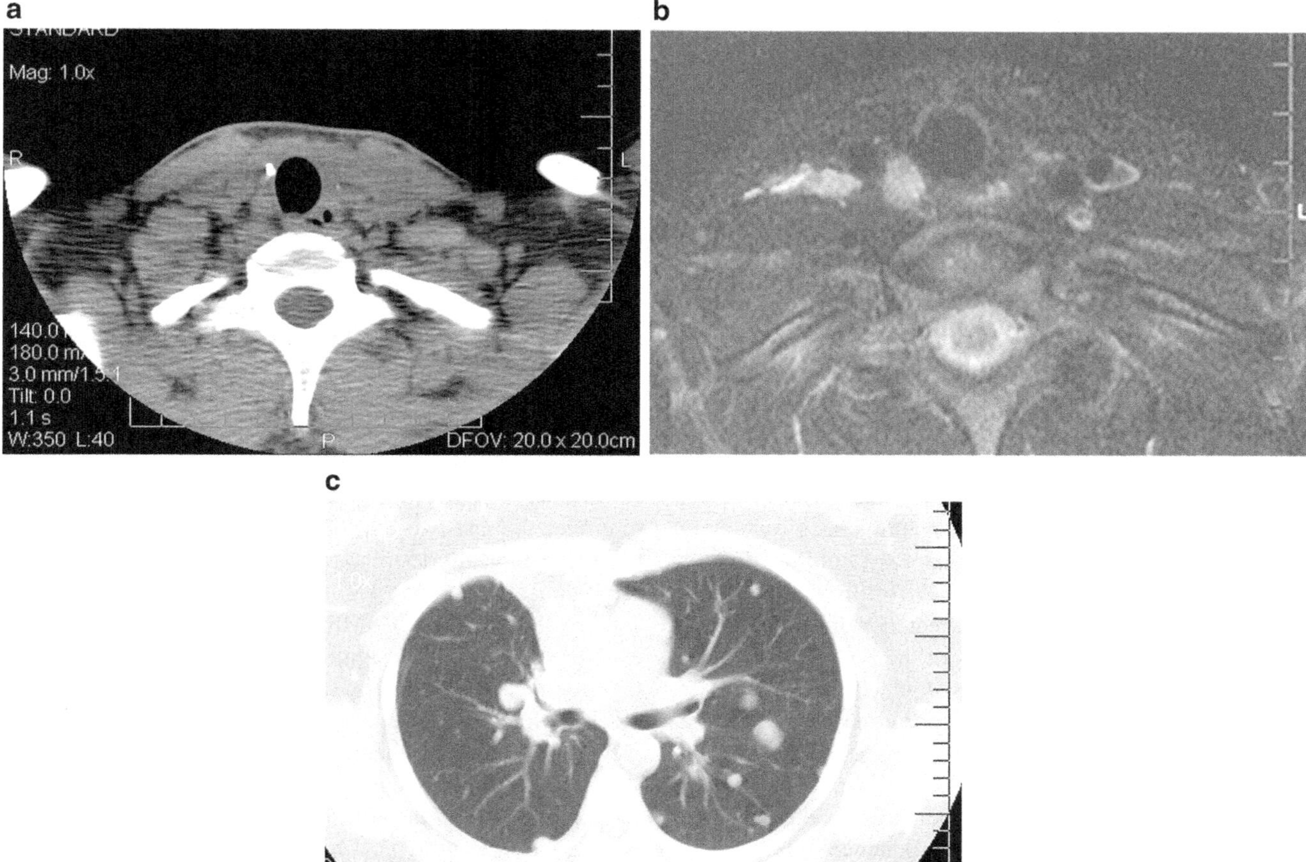

Fig. 45.1 39-year-old female with recurrent thyroid cancer. (**a**) Recurrent adenopathy is hard to assess on this non-contrast CT. (**b**) The recurrent adenopathy of the right neck is more obvious on this axial T2-weighted image. (**c**) Non-contrast CT of the lungs show multiple pulmonary nodules from metastatic disease

striking contrast of the soft tissue appearance of lymph nodes versus muscle and other adjacent tissues such as the salivary glands. Unfortunately, in patients with thyroid cancer, the ability to use iodinated contrast is restricted because of the effect of iodine excess on subsequent potential radioiodine scanning and/or therapy. Non-contrast CTs of the neck can be performed but are much more difficult to interpret and have a lower sensitivity and specificity (Fig. 45.1a). The use of contrast containing iodine may interfere with diagnostic evaluation by iodine-123 or iodine-131 as well as with the treatment of many thyroid cancers with iodine-131. For some thyroid cancers such as the anaplastic form, this may not be an issue. Nonetheless, it is prudent for all thyroid cancer patients being imaged by CT that, as a standard default, they not be given iodinated contrast unless it is explicitly stated by the physician managing their thyroid cancer that the iodinated contrast is permissible. It is unpredictable how long it may take the radio-iodinated contrast to be dissipated in a given individual, and this may be influenced by thyroid or metabolic status, renal function, etc. It is thought that iodine uptake can be blunted for from 3 to 8 weeks.

The typical advantages of CT are the widespread availability of CT scanners, the very quick scan times, the increasing ability to perform slice thicknesses of 1–3 mm, and the ability to easily generate reformatted images in any plane, including axial, sagittal, and oblique images. The major advantage of CT is the evaluation of extra thyroid invasion of adjacent structures such as the trachea, esophagus, and major blood vessels [7]. The major drawback of CT is that the CT of the soft tissue neck is markedly limited by the inability to use iodinated contrast in many thyroid cancer patients. For this reason, most centers do not use CT in the early evaluation and subsequent follow-up of patients with thyroid cancer.

Magnetic Resonance Imaging

Unlike CT scan, magnetic resonance imaging does not require the use of x-rays, and, hence, there is no ionizing radiation to the patient. Instead, MR generates electromagnetic waves and the MR images are derived from hydrogen atoms within the body. Different pulse sequences utilized are performed by applying radio-frequency pulses to the body. Typically, MR imaging has employed T1- and T2-weighted images. The two properties of T1 and T2 are difficult to explain without some details of the physics involved with radio-frequency-generated pulses and the effect on H protons, and this is beyond the scope of this book. Suffice it to say that the T1-weighted images typically show excellent anatomic boundaries between tissues. T2-weighted images are more useful in the evaluation of pathologic processes, in particular local lymph nodes and tumors. T2-weighted images typically show tumors, adenopathy, fluid, and inflammation as being "bright" [8] (Fig. 45.1b). In addition to the typical T1- and T2-weighted sequences, newer MR sequences are commonly used in other parts of the body; in particular, STIR sequences are commonly used which have suppressed fat signal intensity and "bright" appearance of water, edema, and tumor. Recent reports have suggested that STIR sequences may be quantitatively and qualitatively more sensitive and accurate in N staging of non-small cell lung cancer [9]. Whether improved turbo STIR sequences can be made applicable to the neck is an ongoing research. Other sequences such as gradient echo images are very sensitive to the detection of hemorrhage or calcification. Similar to STIR imaging, most centers do not use gradient sequences in the evaluation of the neck.

Another increasingly common MR sequence used in both stroke and oncology imaging is the use of diffusion sequences. As the name suggests, diffusion sequences show areas of restricted water diffusion and often consists of a paired set of diffusion images alongside apparent diffusion coefficient (ADC) map images. Diffusion images may be more sensitive for the detection of high-grade highly cellular tumors such as head and neck squamous cell carcinomas but show less conspicuity for lower-grade less cellular tumors [10]. With reference to thyroid tumors, diffusion images may be more helpful in the detection of anaplastic thyroid carcinoma.

Another advantage of MR is that acquisition of images can be obtained in the axial, sagittal, and coronal planes without the need for reformations.

Today, many centers, when performing oncology imaging, give MR contrast. Most MR contrast compounds represent chelates containing gadolinium which is an inert element. There are several features which make the MR contrast agent significantly better than CT contrast agents. Unlike CT contrast agents, there is no iodine and, hence, there is no contraindication for the routine imaging of patients with thyroid cancer. Other significant advantages of the MR contrast agent are the low incidence of minor and major contrast reactions. It can be anticipated with iodine-related CT contrast agents that 5 % of patients will experience minor adverse reactions such as hives, extreme warmth, or nausea. These are more uncommon with gadolinium MR contrast agents. Furthermore, the major anaphylactic reaction associated with CT contrast is almost nonexistent with MR. Nonetheless, there are very rare occasions in which MR contrast reactions do occur, but they are typically of a minor nature and include headaches and nausea. Only extremely rare case reports of severe reactions to gadolinium-based contrast agents have been reported in the worldwide literature over the last two decades. The volume of gadolinium contrast is typically 15 ml as opposed to the over 100 ml used for contrast CT.

The disadvantages to MR imaging are that the overall examination time is significantly longer than that of CT. Today's MR scanners, however, are much faster than older equipment, and examinations can frequently be completed in 30–40 min, whereas examinations performed in the 1980s and 1990s frequently took over 1 h. With today's modern equipment, the imaging techniques have also changed. While it used to be typical for imaging slice thicknesses to vary between 5 and 10 mm, on today's examination scanners, even with reduced scan time, a typical image sequence can be obtained using 3 mm slice thicknesses.

The most significant factor that would preclude a patient from having a MRI is the presence of interference from an implanted metallic device. The devices which can potentially cause problems include pacemakers, functioning implanted pumps, some implanted cochlear (ear) devices, and older aneurysm clips (most modern intracranial aneurysm clips are now made of material which is MR compatible). However, before any patient with an intracranial aneurysm clip has an MRI, it should be confirmed that the aneurysm clip is MR compatible. All patients should be first carefully screened to make sure there are no metallic substances on their body. An additional problem with MR is that there is a greater problem of claustrophobia during the procedure relative to that experienced with CT. For some patients, it may be advantageous to provide medication to decrease the anxiety of being within a closed space. Valium or other related benzodiazepines are commonly used medications to alleviate claustrophobia. Newer MR units are available in an "open" configuration. However, the "open" MR units do not have the same resolution capacity as the high field "closed" units. In particular with thyroid imaging, it is not uncommon to try to detect 2–3 mm lymph nodes. The "open" MR units will simply not be able to image to this detail. In general, the cost of CT imaging is 20–30 % less than MR. Ultrasound is significantly less expensive, but ultrasound image quality mapping and reproducibility vary greatly, depending on the skill of the ultrasonographer [11].

MR Versus CT Imaging

In the follow-up of patients with thyroid cancer, the older literature seems to indicate a preference for contrast CT over MRI [12, 13]. Most of these studies were performed in the evaluation of cervical lymph nodes in patients with primary head and neck (squamous) carcinoma [14]. No study has been performed which directly compares MR vs. CT in the evaluation of thyroid cancer; however, patients with thyroid cancer typically are not recommended to have iodinated contrast. There is little benefit of imaging by non-contrast CT over imaging by MR. Furthermore, with the newer MR equipment, higher soft tissue contrast, new pulse sequences such as turbo STIR imaging and diffusion sequences, and the use of dynamic contrast MR imaging, the literature now shows a preference for contrast MR over CT [11, 15]. For this reason, most radiologists evaluating the extent of recurrent adenopathy in the neck or chest prefer MRI both without and with contrast, and this has become the mainstay for diagnosis when advanced cross-sectional imaging is required, especially for the evaluation of recurrence in patients with thyroid cancer.

Follow-Up of Patients with Thyroid Cancer: Appropriate Use of MR and CT

Physicians following patients with thyroid cancer have at their disposal a number of different both physiologic and anatomic imaging studies [16, 17]. Typically, follow-up nuclear imaging has been performed with iodine-123 (I-123) and iodine-131 (I-131), but, in most cases, iodine-123 is preferable when available. In addition, following serum thyroglobulin levels in appropriate individuals is standard of practice. Large recurrences are easily picked up by clinical exam and ultrasound; however, it is not uncommon for patients to have abnormal I-123 uptake or increasing thyroglobulin levels and have no abnormal findings on clinical exam or ultrasound. This is typically when MRI can play a more important role in the detection of small lesions. The sensitivity and specificity of MRI will vary depending on the criteria utilized. Traditional imaging with CT and MRI has commonly used a short axis diameter dimension of 1 cm for rationalizing if an individual lymph node is either benign or malignant. However, in the evaluation of thyroid cancer, this is no longer valid. Many small local recurrent lymph nodes detected by iodine-123, rising thyroglobulin levels, or PET scanning have short axis diameters of 4–5 mm. Three-millimeter slice thicknesses are required to detect these small recurrences.

The use of positron-emission tomography (PET) using fluorodeoxyglucose (FDG) has had a significant impact on the follow-up of patients with thyroid cancer [18]. PET/CT imaging may be more sensitive and specific in the detection of early thyroid cancer [18, 19] (see Chaps. 34, 61, 71, 76, and 79] (Fig. 45.2a–c). The major drawbacks of PET/CT

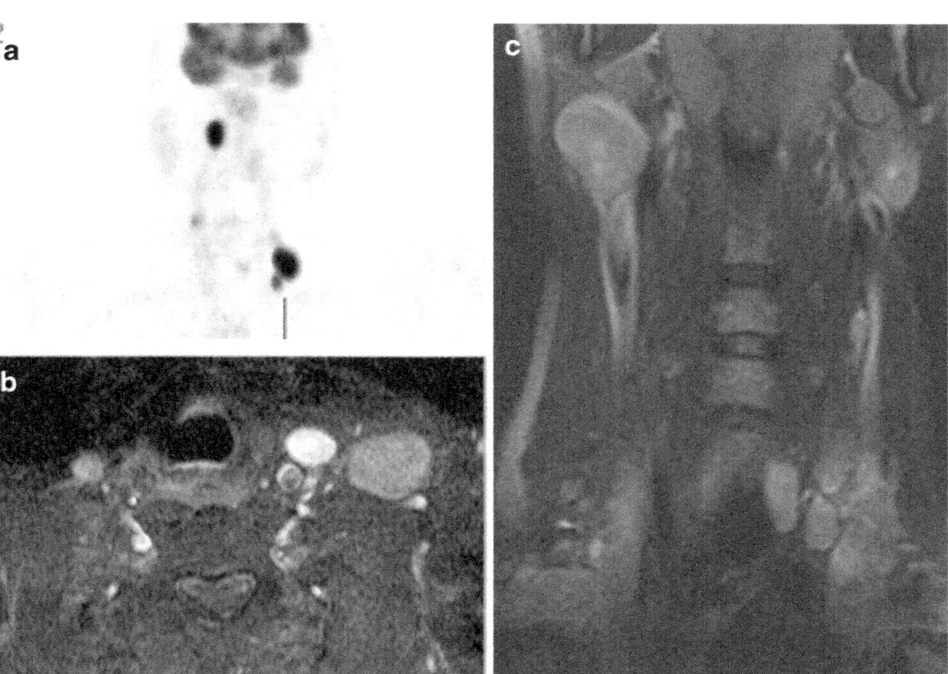

Fig. 45.2 38-year-old male with recurrent thyroid cancer. Comparison of PET and MR images. (**a**) PET image of the neck show left lower neck lymph nodes and a single large right Level II lymph node. (**b**) Axial post-contrast enhanced fat-saturated T1-weighted MR image shows recurrent left lower neck lymph nodes corresponding to the PET study. (**c**) Coronal T2-weighted MR image correlates well with the PET findings showing both left lower neck adenopathy and a single enlarged right Level II lymph node

imaging, however, are that it is not universally approved by various payers and it is significantly more expensive, is not as widely available, and third-party health coverage payors often restrict its use to only once every 6 months or less. A new exciting technology which combines the value of PET with MR is now available [14]. The combination of PET imaging with MRI using fusion software is extremely helpful to physically fuse the physiologic images of the FDG uptake with the cross-sectional images of MR in the axial, coronal, or sagittal planes. This allows a higher sensitivity and specificity. As mentioned above, the major drawback of PET-CT for patients with thyroid cancer, however, is that CT is of limited diagnostic utility in evaluating small neck nodes when no intravenous contrast can be given. But contrast-enhanced MR scan in a combined PET scanner can be extremely useful in the evaluation of lymphomas, lung cancer, and breast and colon cancer. This is not the case when using non-contrast CT in the evaluation of small lesions of the neck, in particular when there is little body fat within the neck or there are complicating factors such as postsurgical or post-radiation changes. The appropriate imaging strategies for follow-up of patients with thyroid cancer using PET with either CT or MR is evolving [17, 20].

MR and CT Findings in Patients with Thyroid Cancer

The appearance of thyroid masses or recurrent thyroid nodules can be very variable. In some cases, the thyroid cancer recurrences can be variably cystic and in other cases, in particular for papillary carcinoma, the lesions may contain focal areas of calcification [5]. In most instances, on CT or MR scan, abnormal lymph nodes rather than having a typical normal "kidney bean" shape with a narrow waist will have a more rounded, bulbous, or spherical appearance. On MRI, all lymph nodes are typically similar to muscle on T1-weighted images and bright on T2-weighted images but typically not as bright as water. A pathologically enlarged MR lymph node typically will have a more rounded appearance and be typically larger in size. A higher degree of confidence that a lymph node is malignant can be achieved if the short axis diameter is clearly greater than 1 cm. However, it can be inferred that even smaller 4–5 mm nodes may be pathologic when they appear anew together with rising serum thyroglobulin levels or positive uptake on PET scan that correlates with MR imaging by fusion software. Thus, any size lesion can potentially be a recurrent malignant lymph node although the classic usage of MR and CT has been to call a lymph node of <1 cm in size as benign.

Because lymph nodes with metastatic papillary thyroid carcinoma typically have a more rounded appearance than normal lymph nodes, the accuracy and positive predictive value of evaluating patients with recurrent papillary carcinoma are superior to that of follicular carcinoma with a positive predictive value and accuracy of 86 % and 85 %, respectively, for papillary cancer and 63 % positive predictive value and 67 % accuracy for follicular carcinoma [8]. There is, however, no specific imaging appearance on either CT or MRI which would definitively characterize lymph nodes as malignant. Abnormal uptake by iodine-123 or by PET imaging in combination with a growing size are the key predictors that a lymph node is malignant regardless of size or appearance (be it cystic or with calcification).

Typical tumor characteristics should be kept in mind in regard to imaging and follow-up of the specific types of thyroid cancers. Papillary cancers are the most common thyroid cancer accounting for approximately 70–80 % of thyroid cancers. Papillary carcinoma is multifocal in 15–30 % of cases and most commonly spreads by intraglandular spread and presents with local adenopathy. A specific feature of papillary cancer is that there may be psammoma bodies present which can give the appearance of calcification [3]. Furthermore, a mixed papillary-follicular carcinoma might also have the presence of psammomatous calcifications. The calcifications are easily picked up by CT but would not be visible on MRI. Some papillary carcinomas may also have a "cystic" appearance on both CT and MRI [5, 20]. While lymph node involvement from papillary carcinoma most commonly occurs at level IV and level VI, more distant metastatic lymph adenopathy can occur into the chest or up to the level II–III lymph nodes [20]. Because the papillary-type cancer typically takes up iodine, the radioiodine scintigrams are usually positive [16].

The second most common type of thyroid cancer, follicular carcinoma, accounts for less than 20 % of all thyroid cancers. Because follicular carcinoma is more likely to spread by the hematogenous route, regional lymph node metastases are less likely to occur. In the follow-up of follicular carcinoma, it may be more important to obtain CT scans to evaluate for lung nodules (MRI is not of significant utility in the evaluation of small pulmonary nodules). The detection of pulmonary nodules by CT does not require iodinated contrast (Fig. 45.1c). It should be emphasized that there is wide variability in the clinical manifestations of papillary and follicular thyroid cancer and individual considerations should be made for each patient. For example, papillary thyroid cancer can metastasize to the lungs with or without detectable cervical lymph node involvement.

Anaplastic carcinoma of the thyroid gland accounts for less than 10 % of thyroid cancers and is the least common, accounting for 1–4 % of thyroid cancers. Because these are much more poorly differentiated tumors, they are much more likely to attain a larger size by the time of initial diagnosis (see Chaps. 77, 78, 79, 80, and 81). In addition, because of their rapid growth, they are frequently associated with areas of hemorrhage and internal necrosis. Many cases of anaplastic carcinoma arise within a preexisting multinodular goiter or, rarely, within a more well-differentiated type of thyroid cancer.

The last common primary type of thyroid cancer is medullary carcinoma which accounts for 2–6 % of thyroid cancers (see Chaps. 67, 68, 69, 70, 71, 72, and 73). Medullary thyroid cancers may be associated with the multiple endocrine neoplasia (MEN) syndromes and are associated with elevated levels of calcitonin. The MR and CT features are not specific. Similar to that of the CT appearance of some papillary carcinoma, CT may show calcification in medullary thyroid carcinoma but it is typically denser than that seen with papillary cancer. Peripheral metastatic lesions to the lung and liver may also show calcification. When medullary thyroid cancer is familial, it may also be associated with hyperparathyroidism and pheochromocytoma.

MR and CT Imaging in the Preoperative Staging of Thyroid Cancer

Typically preoperative imaging of newly diagnosed thyroid cancer is limited for patients with isolated thyroid nodules or small cervical neck lymph nodes. Many institutions only sparingly use any preoperative imaging other than ultrasound and reserve staging with postoperative radioiodine (I^{131}) and then subsequently employ other advanced imaging modalities. While MR and CT are not routinely used in the preoperative staging of a small thyroid nodule, some large thyroid cancers may require more careful preoperative planning. In particular, large tumors which have invaded the thyroid cartilage, esophagus, or adjacent local structures need a more careful preoperative plan to determine what type of resection may be required or whether the tumor is, in fact, inoperable. MR is the ideal study for assessing the extent of tumor invasion into critical structures. MR has been assessed for its accuracy in the identification of invasion of the tracheal cartilage, involvement of the recurrent laryngeal nerve, and involvement of the esophagus. MR is typically 80–95 % sensitive for the detection of invasion of these critical structures and with a similar to slightly higher specificity [20–22]. As opposed to therapeutic approaches to other types of carcinoma, papillary cancer in particular remains the most radiosensitive. The intent of most surgical resections is to obtain a clear margin. However, a significant debulking of a thyroid papillary tumor will allow a potentially greater response to radioactive iodine. The criticality of negative surgical margins is not as stringent for the radioactive iodine-sensitive thyroid carcinomas.

Postoperative and Post-radiation Imaging of Thyroid Cancer

The most common algorithm for newly diagnosed thyroid cancer patient post thyroidectomy starts with whole-body radioiodine I^{131} or I^{123} scanning for the detection of local and metastatic disease [17]. For patients with nonpapillary/nonfollicular thyroid cancer, whole-body PET/CT is often employed in an increasing number of protocols and PET/CT is replacing I^{131} scanning [23]. Depending on the results of a metastatic survey with I^{131}, various different imaging modalities may be used. For pulmonary metastases, chest CT is the option of choice. For metastatic disease to the upper neck, brain, and bones, MRI is the most sensitive test. The postoperative imaging of residual or recurrent neck thyroid cancer is best achieved with MRI. CT, in most cases, is again limited by the inability to use iodinated contrast. With the follow-up findings of scarring, thickening, and loss of fascial planes, CT becomes even more difficult to assess for recurrent tumor [24]. The abnormal changes on MRI become easier to interpret after a latency period of 4–6 weeks in which postoperative edema subsides. For those patients receiving whole-neck external beam radiation, there will be a latency period of 4–6 months in which residual edema and swelling may be present. Because the normal anatomic planes which are usually outlined by fat between the fascia delineate the structures, loss of these normal fascial planes makes interpretation of recurrence significantly more difficult [24]. However, the further from the patient's initial surgery and the further from postoperative radiation, any new findings in the surgical bed or in the upper neck or mediastinum are more likely to represent recurrence. This is particularly true when correlated with positive findings seen on PET or radioactive iodine scanning. In many cases, initial early studies can serve as a valuable baseline for comparison on follow-up study, thereby allowing newly developing interval processes to be detected earlier and with greater specificity.

Multidisciplinary Approach to the Evaluation of Recurrent Thyroid Cancer

Perhaps in no other area of oncology imaging are there so many diverse disciplines and tools available to detect recurrent thyroid cancer. A very close working relationship

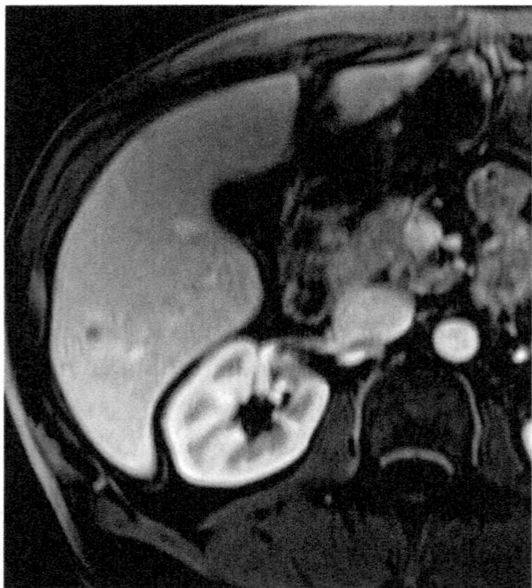

Fig. 45.3 50-year-old male with metastatic thyroid cancer to the liver. Dynamic contrast-enhanced T1 image of the liver shows a right lobe liver metastasis

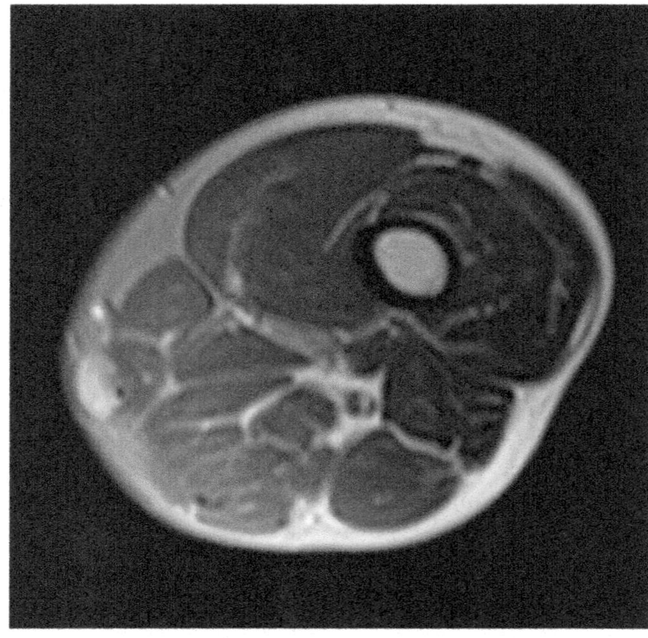

Fig. 45.4 52-year-old male with multiple sites of metastatic disease. Axial T2-weighted image through the left mid thigh shows a metastatic lesion of the left gracilis muscle

between radiologists, nuclear medicine physicians, pathologists, surgeons, and endocrinologists is optimal. Correlating PET scan findings with abnormalities detected on MR (or, less likely, CT) in combination with changing thyroglobulin levels can become challenging, particularly if each individual physician works within a vacuum. A combined multidisciplinary approach enables a much more sensitive and meaningful detection of recurrent tumors. Traditional criteria using MR or CT for thyroid cancer detection would assess for lymph nodes with a short axial diameter of 1 cm. However, when combining endocrine findings of a rising thyroglobulin level and associated positive findings on either PET/CT or I-123 or I-131, small (4 mm) lymph nodes can be identified as reflecting recurrence and, in some cases, with an experienced ultrasonographer, then undergo FNA biopsy. In other cases, positive findings by MR or PET may have other anatomic or physiologic causes not related to recurrence of thyroid cancer. Each single modality by itself can be very nonspecific or insensitive. Sorting through these different possibilities is greatly facilitated by a multidisciplinary approach.

Uncommon Sites of Metastatic Thyroid Cancer

The typical sites of metastatic thyroid cancer include neck nodes, superior mediastinal nodes, pulmonary metastases, and bone. However, virtually any organ or location has been reported with the more frequently cited uncommon locations being the brain, liver, skin, muscle, and breast [25–27]. Small lesions of the liver, skin, muscle, bone, and breast are usually best detected with MR over CT (Figs. 45.3 and 45.4). A larger lytic bone lesion may be equally well seen by either MR or CT (Fig. 45.5a,b). A small bone lesion would be better seen by MRI, whereas a larger lytic lesion may be equally well seen by either MR or CT (Fig. 45.5). While 31 % of patients with differentiated thyroid cancer *with* evidence of distant metastatic disease may have up to a 10-year survival, that is less true depending on the site of metastases [26]. Patients with CNS metastases will have a significantly shorter prognosis even with differentiated thyroid carcinoma [28, 29] (Fig. 45.6a,b).

CT Guidance for Ablation of Peripheral Metastatic Thyroid Cancer

The newest weapon in the oncologist's armamentarium against cancer is local ablative therapy (see Chap. 54). Radio-frequency ablation and cryotherapy can be used to ablate both neck recurrence and distal metastasis [30, 31]. Using CT guidance (as used for CT-guided biopsies), a large needle, such as a 14 G needle, can be placed into the center of tumor recurrence. Either a "hot" tip radio-frequency wire or a cryotherapy probe can then be guided through the needle and then the lesion either "heated" or "frozen." The ablative therapy can be either palliative or helpful in "debulking" tumor to make radioactive iodine more effective (Fig. 45.7).

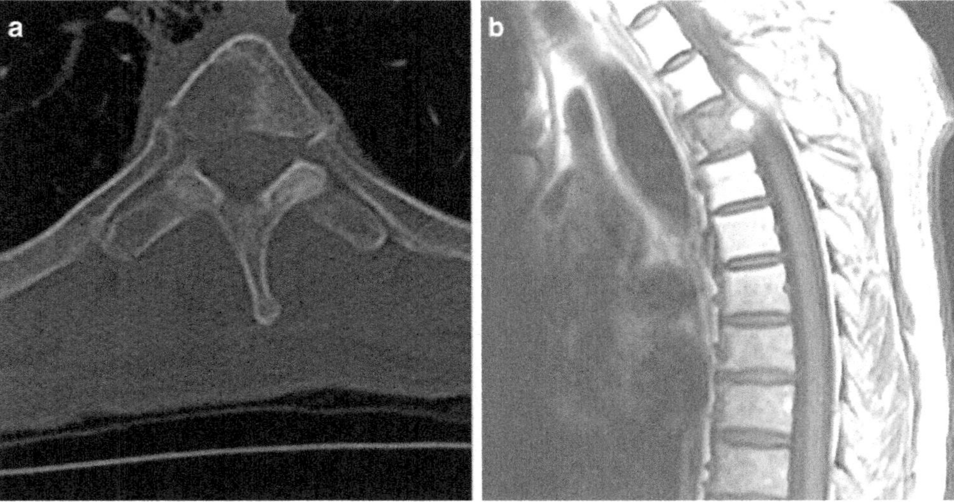

Fig. 45.5 50-year-old male with spine metastases. T3 metastasis is best seen on the MR image as compared to CT. (**a**) Axial CT shows a metastasis of the T3 vertebral body. (**b**) Sagittal T1 MR shows a metastasis of the T3 vertebral body

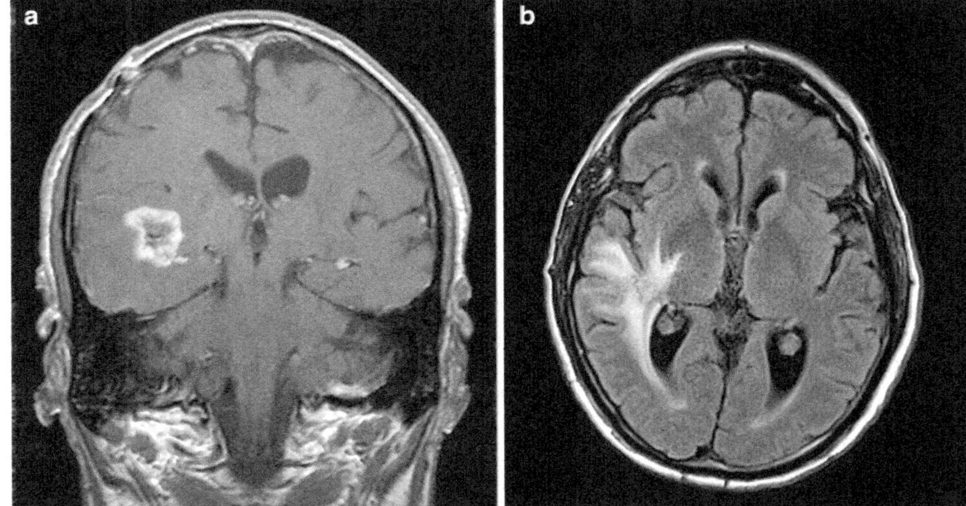

Fig. 45.6 67-year-old male with brain metastasis of the right temporal lobe. The lesions shows ring enhancement (common) and moderate vasogenic edema. (**a**) Coronal T1 post-contrast MR of the brain and (**b**) axial FLAIR image of the brain show moderate vasogenic edema surrounding a metastasis of the right temporal lobe

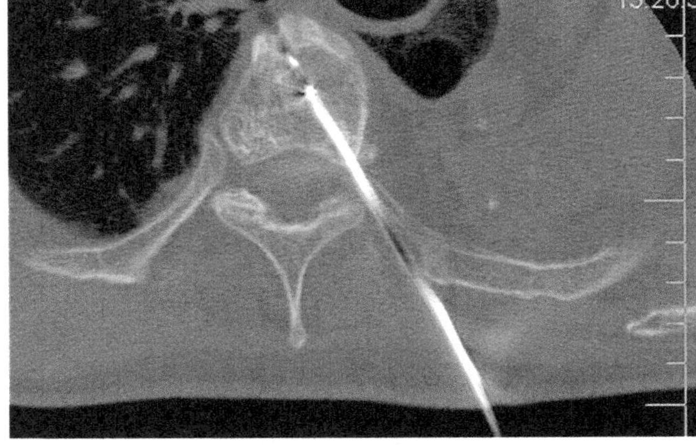

Fig. 45.7 75-year-old male with metastatic disease to thoracic spine. Axial CT image shows a biopsy needle with RF prongs deployed into the thoracic vertebral body metastasis for treatment

References

1. Weiss RE, Lado-Abeal J. Thyroid nodules: diagnosis and therapy. Curr Opin Oncol. 2002;14:46–52.
2. Blum M. Nonisotopic imaging of the neck in patients with thyroid nodules or cancer. In: Wartofsky L, editor. Thyroid cancer; a comprehensive guide to clinical management. Totowa, NJ: Humana Press; 2000. p. 9–34.
3. Smoker WRK, Harnsberger HR, Reede DL, Holliday RA, Som PM, Bergeron RT. The neck. In: Som PM, Bergeron RT, editors. Head and neck imaging. 2nd ed. St. Louis: Mosby Yearbook; 1991. p. 497–592.
4. Becker M. Other infrahyoid neck lesions. In: Mafer MF, Valvassori GE, Becker M, editors. Imaging of the head and neck. 2nd ed. Stuttgart: Thieme; 2005. p. 780–845.
5. Som PM, Brandwein M, Lidov M, et al. The varied presentations of papillary thyroid cervical nodal disease: CT and MR findings. AJNR. 1994;15:1123–8.
6. Som PM, Curtin HD, Mancuso AA. Imaging-based nodal classification for evaluation of neck metastatic adenopathy. AJR. 2000;174:837–44.
7. Seo YL, Yoon DY, Lim KJ, et al. Locally advanced thyroid cancer: can CT help in prediction of extrathyroidal invasion to adjacent structures? AJR. 2010;195:240–4.
8. Gross ND, Weissman JL, Talbot JM, Anderson PE, Wax NK, Johen JI. MRI detection of cervical metastases from differentiated thyroid carcinoma. Laryngoscope. 2001;111:1905–9.
9. Ohno Y, Koyama H, Yoshikawa T, et al. N stage disease in patients with non-small cell lung cancer: efficacy of quantitative and qualitative assessment with STIR turbo spin echo imaging, diffusion-weighted MR imaging and fluorodeoxyglucose PET/CT. Radiology. 2011;26:605–15.
10. Kim S, Loevner L, Quon H, et al. Diffusion-weighted magnetic resonance imaging for predicting and detecting early response to chemoradiation therapy of squamous cell carcinomas of the head and neck. Clin Cancer Res. 2009;15:986–94.
11. Schroder RJ, Rost B, Hidajat N, Rademaker J, Felix R, Maurer J. Value of contrast-enhanced ultrasound vs. CT and MR in palpable enlarged lymph node of the head and neck. Rofo. 2002;174:1099–106.
12. Curtin HD, Ishwaran H, Mancuso AA, et al. Comparison of CT and MR imaging in staging of neck metastases. Radiology. 1998;207:123–30.
13. Yousem DM, Som PM, Hackney DB, et al. Central necrosis and extracapsular neoplastic spread in cervical lymph nodes: MR imaging versus CT. Radiology. 1992;182:753–9.
14. Von den Brekel MWM. Lymph node metastasis: CT and MRI. Eur J Radiol. 2000;22:230–8.
15. King AD, Tse GM, Yuen EH, et al. Comparison of CT and MR imaging for the detection of extranodal neoplastic spread in metastatic neck nodes. Eur J Radiol. 2004;52:264–70.
16. James C, Starks M, MacGilloroy DC, White J. The use of imaging studies in the diagnosis and management of thyroid cancer and hyperparathyroidism. Surg Oncol Clin N Am. 1999;8:145–69.
17. Johnson NA, Tublin ME. Postoperative surveillance of differentiated thyroid carcinoma: rationale, techniques, and controversies. Radiology. 2008;249:429–44.
18. Benchaou M, Lehmann W, Slosmann DO, et al. The role of FDG-PET in the preoperative assessment of N-staging in head and neck cancer. Acta Otolaryngol. 1996;116:332–5.
19. Popperl G, Lang S, Dogdelen O. Correlation of FDG-PET and MRI/CT with histopathology in primary diagnosis, lymph node staging and diagnosis of recurrency of head and neck cancer. Rofo Fortschr. 2002;174:714–20.
20. Takashima S, Matsushita T, Takayama F, Kadoya M, Fujimori M, Kobayashi S. Prognostic significance of magnetic resonance findings in advanced papillary thyroid cancer. Thyroid. 2001;11:1153–9.
21. Takashima S, Takayama F, Wang JC, Kobayashi S, Kodoya M. Using MR imaging to predict invasion of the recurrent laryngeal nerve by thyroid cancer. AJR Am J Roentgenol. 2003;180:837–42.
22. Wang JC, Takashima S, Takayama F, Kawakami S, Saito A, Matsushita T, Matsuba H, Kobayashi S. Tracheal invasion by thyroid carcinoma: prediction using MR imaging. Am J Roentgenol. 2001;177:926–36.
23. Saab G, Driedger AA, Pavlosky W, et al. Thyroid-stimulating hormone simulated fused positron emission tomography/computed tomography in the evaluation of recurrence in I^{131}-negative papillary thyroid carcinoma. Thyroid. 2006;16:267–72.
24. Becker M, Schroth G, Zbaren P, et al. Long-term changes induced by high-dose irradiation of the head and neck region: image findings. Radiographics. 1997;17:5–26.
25. Song HJ, Xue YL, Xu YH, Qiu ZL, Luo QY. Rare metastases of differentiated thyroid carcinoma. Endocr Relat Cancer. 2011;18:R165–74.
26. Haq M, Harmer C. Differentiated thyroid carcinoma with distant metastases at presentation: prognostic factors and outcome. Clin Endocrinol. 2005;63:87–93.
27. Shammas A, Degirmenci B, Mountz JM, et al. ^{18}F-FDG PET/CT in patients with suspected or metastatic well-differentiated thyroid cancer. J Nucl Med. 2007;48:221–6.
28. Chiu AC, Delpassand ES, Sherman SI. Prognosis and treatment of brain metastasis in thyroid carcinoma. J Clin Endocrinol Metab. 1997;82:3637–42.
29. Xu YH, Song HJ, Qiu ZL, Luo QY. Brain metastases with exceptional features from papillary thyroid carcinoma; report of three cases. Hell J Nucl Med. 2011;14:56–9; nucmed.web.auth.gr/magazine/eng/jan11/10.pdf.
30. Dupuy DE, Monchick JM, Decrea C, Pisharodi L. Radio-frequency ablation of regional recurrence from well-differentiated thyroid malignancy. Surgery. 2001;130:971–7.
31. Lee JM, Jin GY, Goldberg SN, Lee YC, Chung GH, Han YM, Lee SY, Kim CS. Percutaneous radio-frequency ablation for inoperable non-small cell lung cancer and metastases: preliminary report. Radiology. 2004;230:125–34.

Thyroglobulin in Lymph Node Aspirate

46

D. Robert Dufour

Lymph Node Involvement in Thyroid Cancer

In patients with differentiated thyroid cancer, the most common site of extrathyroidal involvement is in cervical lymph nodes. As discussed in Chap. 49, nodal involvement results in changes in management, often requiring surgery for resection of involved lymph nodes to prevent locoregional recurrences.

Diagnosis of Nodal Involvement

Current guidelines for management of patients with differentiated thyroid cancer recommend the use of neck ultrasound, with fine-needle aspiration cytology of lymph nodes larger than 5–8 mm if detection of nodal involvement would change management [1, 2]. Cytologic examination of lymph nodes has fewer limitations diagnostically than does examination of thyroid nodule aspirates but (due to sampling errors) still has false-negative results. Sensitivity for recognition of nodal involvement by thyroid cancer is typically in the range of 75–85 % [3], although sensitivity is significantly lower in those with cystic lymph node involvement.

Thyroglobulin in Lymph Node Aspirates

Pacini was the first to suggest measurement of thyroglobulin in lymph node aspirates [4]. In 35 patients (23 patients with known thyroid cancer postsurgery and remnant ablation and 12 patients with lymphadenopathy of unknown cause), they found thyroglobulin detectable in the aspirate in all patients who had proven nodal metastases but also detectable in 7/21 patients who did not have nodal metastases. Levels were markedly higher in those with metastases (mean 37,000 ng/aspirate) than in those who had measurable thyroglobulin but no metastases (12.1 ng/aspirate). They found no stainable thyroglobulin by immunohistochemistry in the lymph nodes from those with measurable thyroglobulin but no metastases and found that peripheral vein thyroglobulin concentrations were similar or higher than lymph node aspirate thyroglobulin concentration in these patients. In contrast, in all but two of the patients with metastatic carcinoma in the lymph nodes, thyroglobulin levels were markedly higher in lymph node aspirate fluid than in peripheral blood (including three patients with undetectable serum thyroglobulin).

The first large study was published by Frasoldati in 1999 [5]. They evaluated lymph nodes in 130 patients, including patients with thyroid carcinoma both before and after surgery. They found that lymph node thyroglobulin concentration was higher in nodes without metastases in thyroid cancer patients who had not had surgery (mean 4.9 ng/mL) than in those who had undergone thyroidectomy (mean 0.5 ng/mL). A likely explanation for the presence of thyroglobulin at higher levels in lymph nodes of patients who have a thyroid gland is the presence of thyroglobulin in macrophages in lymph nodes draining thyroid cancers (but not in normal lymph nodes) [6]. This suggests that small amounts of thyroglobulin are released by carcinoma cells both into the peripheral blood and into lymphatic fluid. Two other studies found that a markedly higher cutoff value is needed to distinguish lymph node involvement in patients whose lymph nodes are biopsied before surgery [7, 8], although one study reported a similar cutoff value [9]; most studies have not evaluated the use of different cutoff values or only evaluated postoperative patients. Most studies did not evaluate whether remnant ablation following total thyroidectomy affected cutoff values, although in one small study, there was no difference in performance of cutoff values [10], and no studies evaluated the need for different cutoff values after partial thyroidectomy.

D.R. Dufour, MD (✉)
Clinical Pathology, Veterans Affairs Medical Center, 50 Irving Street NW, Washington, DC 20422, USA
e-mail: chemdoctorbob@earthlink.net

L. Wartofsky, D. Van Nostrand (eds.), *Thyroid Cancer*, DOI 10.1007/978-1-4939-3314-3_46

A number of other studies of measurement of thyroglobulin have been published, most in the past 5 years. These studies are summarized in Table 46.1. Current guidelines on management of thyroid cancer recommend measuring thyroglobulin in lymph node aspirate as an adjunct to cytology in recognition of nodal involvement [1, 2].

Technique for Measurement

After aspiration biopsy of lymph nodes, there is some residual fluid in the needle. A small amount of fluid is aspirated into the needle, and the fluid is then collected into a tube for transport to the laboratory. While most studies did not evaluate the effects of tube type, Giovanella [11] found that plain

Table 46.1 Diagnostic performance of lymph node thyroglobulin measurement

Author	Number patients	Sensitivity (%)	Specificity (%)	Tg cutoff (ng/mL)
Pacini [4]	35	100	67	43.4[a]
Lee [22]		91	91	3.5 (per aspirate)
Frasoldati [5]	130	84	100	78.6 (pre-op)[b]
				2.2 (post-op)
Cignarelli [23]	79	100		
Urono [24]	111	81	–	Not given
Mikosinski [25]	105	100	98	Not given
Cunha [16]	67	100	–	1.8[b]
Boi [7]	73	100[c]	100	36 (pre-op)
				1.7 (post-op)
Sigstad [17]	145	100[e]	100 (post-op)	>serum thyroglobulin
			86 (pre-op)	
Snozek [26]	73[d]	100	96	1.0
Borel [13]	73	100	100	2.0[a, b]
Jeon [27]	47	95	90	36 (pre-op)
				>serum thyroglobulin (post-op)
Kim [28]	168	95[f]	82[f]	10
Bournaud [29]	114	94	98	0.9
Lee [30]	40	100	100	8.2[b]
Zanella [31]	43	100	100	20[b]
Giovanella [32]	108	100	100	2.2[b]
Salmaslıoğlu [12]	225	99	96	6.0[g]
Kim [8]	91	80	100	50.0[b,h]
Sohn [33]	92[i]	69	83	10.0[b]
Moon [34]	528	93	96	2.0[b]
Suh [10]	47	100	69	2.0[b]
		100	84	20.0[b]
		100	69	FNA Tg >serum Tg
Li [35]	208	97	81	<0.2
		76	98	19.2[b]
Jung [9]	177	96.1	94	3.6[b,j]
		88.3	96	20.0[b,j]
Baldini [36]	32	92	83	2.0[b]

[a]Results adjusted to ng/mL (expressed as per aspirate in original article)
[b]Results adjusted based on use of 1 mL washout fluid compared to 0.5 mL in other studies
[c]Three patients with poorly differentiated or anaplastic carcinomas had undetectable lymph node thyroglobulin
[d]Number of lymph nodes; number of patients not given
[e]Results falsely negative in two samples collected into lithium heparin tubes
[f]Performance better in post-op than pre-op patients but actual statistics not provided
[g]Results adjusted based on use of 3 mL washout fluid compared to 0.5 mL in other studies
[h]Study included only patients who had not undergone thyroidectomy
[i]Study included only patients with lymph node thyroglobulin between 0.2 and 100 ng/mL; it excluded 554 patients with thyroglobulin in aspirate fluid >100 ng/mL or <0.2 ng/mL; sensitivity and specificity were 100 % in those patients
[j]Study included both preoperative (46 %) and postoperative (54 %) patients; data not reported separately, but results section indicates optimal cutoff was "similar"

tubes had significantly higher thyroglobulin levels than did serum separator (gel) tubes or lithium heparin tubes, and two patients had false-negative thyroglobulin in samples collected in lithium heparin tubes. For that reason, they advocate use of plain tubes for transport.

In two studies, thyroglobulin-free serum (reagent diluent) was used as the fluid [4, 7], but most subsequent studies have used saline. The amount of fluid used initially was 0.5 mL, but more recently, most published studies have used 1.0 mL, and in one study, 3.0 mL was used [12]. Flushing the fluid through the needle three times washes out >97 % of thyroglobulin present [13]. No direct comparison of results with different fluids has been performed, so it is impossible to state that one is preferable to another. A general issue with immunoassays is the possibility of "matrix effects," where the antigen-antibody interaction is altered by changing the makeup of the samples analyzed. Since results of published studies have shown very high sensitivity and specificity even when saline is used as a diluent, it does not appear that this is an important consideration, but it is possible that some samples that were erroneously negative or positive were actually due to such matrix effects. Future studies should involve laboratorians who are familiar with this issue to determine the optimum diluent for measurement.

All studies appear to have used immunometric (sandwich) assays for measurement of thyroglobulin, although the method used is not specified in all studies. One consideration with the use of immunometric assays is that results may be falsely low in samples with markedly elevated levels, termed the "high-dose hook effect." This phenomenon was reviewed by St. Jean as it effects various hormone measurements; they found evidence of high-dose hook effect in 6 % of patients with macroprolactinomas [14]. Although the possibility of "high-dose hook effect" causing erroneous lymph node thyroglobulin was discussed by Giovanella [11], no studies have been done to evaluate whether this might affect measured results. This could be evaluated by analyzing serial dilutions of serum; if the "'high-dose hook effect" is present, apparent results will rise in the diluted samples. Giovanella has recommended repeat measurement of low or undetectable thyroglobulin results following sample dilution [15], although most published studies have not followed this approach.

Since manufacturers do not typically provide reference intervals or procedures for measurement of thyroglobulin in lymph node aspirates, laboratories that perform this assay must perform some validation of the procedure. The Food and Drug Administration (FDA) has proposed increasing regulation of testing on nonstandard samples, and it is unclear at present what the effects of such regulation would be on the measurement of thyroglobulin in lymph node aspirates.

Effect of Thyroglobulin or Heterophile Antibodies

Since most studies have used immunometric assays, the potential exists for falsely low thyroglobulin results in patients who have thyroglobulin antibodies in serum. There have been no studies that have directly compared results of thyroglobulin measurement with immunometric and competitive assays in lymph node aspirates. Boi [7] did not find any falsely negative lymph node thyroglobulin results in patients with thyroglobulin antibodies, although serum thyroglobulin was undetectable in half, and about one-quarter of those with serum thyroglobulin antibodies had detectable antibody levels in lymph node aspirates. Two other studies did not find falsely absent thyroglobulin in patients with thyroglobulin antibodies in serum [16, 17], although two others did [18, 19]. In a single study involving one patient with misleading serum thyroglobulin due to heterophile antibodies, lymph node thyroglobulin was markedly increased with two different immunometric assays, suggesting that false-negative aspirate thyroglobulin would be unlikely [20].

Use of Recombinant TSH When Aspirate Thyroglobulin Is Negative and Thyroglobulin Antibodies Are Strongly Positive

Cappelli [18] described two patients with very strongly positive serum thyroglobulin antibodies who had negative lymph node thyroglobulin, but which became positive (at 7.1 and 9.2 ng/mL) after administration of recombinant TSH. They hypothesized that the increase in thyroglobulin production in the metastases saturated the antibody binding sites, allowing thyroglobulin to become detectable. In an accompanying letter, Giovanella [21] noted that cytology had not been documented on the initial or follow-up aspirates and that sampling could have explained the negative results. Thus, the possible role of recombinant TSH in patients with suspected negative LN aspirate cannot be determined.

References

1. Haugen BR, Alexander EK, Bible KC, Doherty GM, Mandel SJ, Nikiforov Y, Pacini F, Randolph G, Sawka A, Shepard D, Sosa J, Tuttle RM, Wartofsky L. 2015 American Thyroid Association Management Guidelines for adult patients with thyroid nodules and differentiated thyroid cancer. Available online at Thyroid 25: DOI:10.1089/thy.2015.0020; print version in Thyroid 26:1–133, 2016.
2. Pacini F, Schlumberger M, Dralle H, et al. European consensus for the management of patients with differentiated thyroid carcinoma of the follicular epithelium. Eur J Endocrinol. 2006;154(6):787–803.
3. Costante G, Filetti S. Diagnosis: thyroglobulin in fine-needle aspirates-a clue to metastasis? Nat Rev Endocrinol. 2009;5(5):249–50.
4. Pacini F, Fugazzola L, Lippi F, et al. Detection of thyroglobulin in fine needle aspirates of nonthyroidal neck masses: a clue to the diagnosis of metastatic differentiated thyroid cancer. J Clin Endocrinol Metab. 1992;74(6):1401–4.

5. Frasoldati A, Toschi E, Zini M, et al. Role of thyroglobulin measurement in fine-needle aspiration biopsies of cervical lymph nodes in patients with differentiated thyroid cancer. Thyroid. 1999;9(2): 105–11.
6. Venkatraman L, Maxwell P, McCluggage W. Thyroglobulin immunoreactivity in lymph node histiocytes: a potential diagnostic pitfall. J Clin Pathol. 2001;54(4):314–6.
7. Boi F, Baghino G, Atzeni F, Lai M, Faa G, Mariotti S. The diagnostic value for differentiated thyroid carcinoma metastases of thyroglobulin (Tg) measurement in washout fluid from fine-needle aspiration biopsy of neck lymph nodes is maintained in the presence of circulating anti-Tg antibodies. J Clin Endocrinol Metab. 2006;91(4):1364–9.
8. Kim D, Jeon S, Kim C. Usefulness of thyroglobulin measurement in needle washouts of fine-needle aspiration biopsy for the diagnosis of cervical lymph node metastases from papillary thyroid cancer before thyroidectomy. Endocrine. 2012;42(2):399–403.
9. Jung JY, Shin JH, Han B-K, Ko EY. Optimized cutoff value and indication for washout thyroglobulin level according to ultrasound findings in patients with well-differentiated thyroid cancer. Am J Neuroradiol. 2013. doi:10.3174/ajnr.A3687.
10. Suh YJ, Son EJ, Moon HJ, Kim E-K, Han KH, Kwak JY. Utility of thyroglobulin measurements in fine-needle aspirates of space occupying lesions in the thyroid bed after thyroid cancer operations. Thyroid. 2013;23(3):280–8.
11. Giovanella L, Ceriani L, Suriano S, Crippa S. Thyroglobulin measurement on fine-needle washout fluids: influence of sample collection methods. Diagn Cytopathol. 2009;37(1):42–4.
12. Salmaslıoğlu A, Erbil Y, Çıtlak G, et al. Diagnostic value of thyroglobulin measurement in fine-needle aspiration biopsy for detecting metastatic lymph nodes in patients with papillary thyroid carcinoma. Langenbecks Arch Surg. 2011;396(1):77–81.
13. Borel A, Boizel R, Faure P, et al. Significance of low levels of thyroglobulin in fine needle aspirates from cervical lymph nodes of patients with a history of differentiated thyroid cancer. Eur J Endocrinol. 2008;158:691–8.
14. St-Jean E, Blain F, Comtois R. High prolactin levels may be missed by immunoradiometric assay in patients with macroprolactinomas. Clin Endocrinol (Oxf). 1996;44(3):305–9.
15. Giovanella L, Bongiovanni M, Trimboli P. Diagnostic value of thyroglobulin assay in cervical lymph node fine-needle aspirations for metastatic differentiated thyroid cancer. Curr Opin Oncol. 2013;25(1):6–13.
16. Cunha N, Rodrigues F, Curado F, et al. Thyroglobulin detection in fine-needle aspirates of cervical lymph nodes: a technique for the diagnosis of metastatic differentiated thyroid cancer. Eur J Endocrinol. 2007;157(1):101–7.
17. Sigstad E, Heilo A, Paus E, et al. The usefulness of detecting thyroglobulin in fine-needle aspirates from patients with neck lesions using a sensitive thyroglobulin assay. Diagn Cytopathol. 2007;35(12):761–7.
18. Cappelli C, Pirola I, De Martino E, et al. Thyroglobulin measurement in fine-needle aspiration biopsy of metastatic lymph nodes after rhTSH stimulation. Head Neck. 2013;35(1):E21–3.
19. Jeon MJ, Park JW, Han JM, et al. Serum antithyroglobulin antibodies interfere with thyroglobulin detection in fine-needle aspirates of metastatic neck nodes in papillary thyroid carcinoma. J Clin Endocrinol Metab. 2013;98(1):153–60.
20. Giovanella L, Ghelfo A. Undetectable serum thyroglobulin due to negative interference of heterophile antibodies in relapsing thyroid carcinoma. Clin Chem. 2007;53(10):1871–2.
21. Giovanella L. Lymph nodes thyroglobulin measurement after rhTSH stimulation. Head Neck. 2013;35(1):146.
22. Lee M, Ross D, Mueller P, Daniels G, Dawson S, Simeone J. Fine-needle biopsy of cervical lymph nodes in patients with thyroid cancer: a prospective comparison of cytopathologic and tissue marker analysis. Radiology. 1993;187(3):851–4.
23. Cignarelli M, Ambrosi A, Marino A, et al. Diagnostic utility of thyroglobulin detection in fine-needle aspiration of cervical cystic metastatic lymph nodes from papillary thyroid cancer with negative cytology. Thyroid. 2003;13(12):1163–7.
24. Uruno T, Miyauchi A, Shimizu K, et al. Usefulness of thyroglobulin measurement in fine-needle aspiration biopsy specimens for diagnosing cervical lymph node metastasis in patients with papillary thyroid cancer. World J Surg. 2005;29(4):483–5.
25. Mikosiński S, Pomorski L, Oszukowska L, et al. The diagnostic value of thyroglobulin concentration in fine-needle aspiration of the cervical lymph nodes in patients with differentiated thyroid cancer. Endokrynol Pol. 2006;57(4):392–5.
26. Snozek C, Chambers E, Reading C, et al. Serum thyroglobulin, high-resolution ultrasound, and lymph node thyroglobulin in diagnosis of differentiated thyroid carcinoma nodal metastases. J Clin Endocrinol Metab. 2007;92(11):4278–81.
27. Jeon S, Kim E, Park J, et al. Diagnostic benefit of thyroglobulin measurement in fine-needle aspiration for diagnosing metastatic cervical lymph nodes from papillary thyroid cancer: correlations with US features. Korean J Radiol. 2009;10(2):106–11.
28. Kim M, Kim E, Kim B, et al. Thyroglobulin measurement in fine-needle aspirate washouts: the criteria for neck node dissection for patients with thyroid cancer. Clin Endocrinol (Oxf). 2009;70(1):145–51.
29. Bournaud C, Charrié A, Nozières C, et al. Thyroglobulin measurement in fine-needle aspirates of lymph nodes in patients with differentiated thyroid cancer: a simple definition of the threshold value, with emphasis on potential pitfalls of the method. Clin Chem Lab Med. 2010;48(8):1171–7.
30. Lee Y, Seo H, Suh S, et al. Cut-off value for needle washout thyroglobulin in athyrotropic patients. Laryngoscope. 2010;120(6): 1120–74.
31. Zanella A, Meyer E, Balzan L, et al. Thyroglobulin measurements in washout of fine needle aspirates in cervical lymph nodes for detection of papillary thyroid cancer metastases. Arq Bras Endocrinol Metabol. 2010;54(6):550–4.
32. Giovanella L, Ceriani L, Suriano S. Lymph node thyroglobulin measurement in diagnosis of neck metastases of differentiated thyroid carcinoma. J Thyroid Res. 2011. doi:10.4061/2011/621839.
33. Sohn Y, Kim M, Kim E, Kwak J. Diagnostic performance of thyroglobulin value in indeterminate range in fine needle aspiration washout fluid from lymph nodes of thyroid cancer. Yonsei Med J. 2012;53(1):126–31.
34. Moon JH, Kim YI, Lim JA, et al. Thyroglobulin in washout fluid from lymph node fine-needle aspiration biopsy in papillary thyroid cancer: large-scale validation of the cutoff value to determine malignancy and evaluation of discrepant results. J Clin Endocrinol Metab. 2013;98(3):1061–8.
35. Li QK, Nugent SL, Straseski J, et al. Thyroglobulin measurements in fine-needle aspiration cytology of lymph nodes for the detection of metastatic papillary thyroid carcinoma. Cancer Cytopathol. 2013;121(8):440–8.
36. Baldini E, Sorrenti S, Di Gioia C, et al. Cervical lymph node metastases from thyroid cancer: does thyroglobulin and calcitonin measurement in fine needle aspirates improve the diagnostic value of cytology? BMC Clin Pathol. 2013;13(1):7.

Management of the Patients with Negative Radioiodine Scan and Elevated Serum Thyroglobulin

47

Leonard Wartofsky

In the past two decades, significant improvements in the assays for serum thyroglobulin (Tg) have revolutionized the standard follow-up and surveillance for recurrence in patients with thyroid carcinoma [1–6]. Not infrequently, we are faced with the management dilemma presented by patients with differentiated thyroid cancer (DTC) in whom measurable or high serum Tg levels suggest residual or metastatic disease, but their radioiodine diagnostic survey scans are negative [7].

Some workers have advocated empiric high-dose radioiodine therapy in these patients, based on the Tg levels indicating disease, even when the negative scan suggests there will be little to no uptake. However, this approach has been somewhat controversial [8–14]. The National Comprehensive Cancer Network guidelines [15] are far from definitive on this issue but point out that no studies have yet demonstrated significantly reduced morbidity and mortality from radioiodine therapy given strictly for elevated serum Tg levels. The British Thyroid Association guidelines [16] are completely silent on the dilemma. Pacini and Schlumberger [17] were the first investigators to advocate this empiric high-dose 131I therapy for patients who are "scan-negative, Tg-positive," whereas Sherman and Gopal [18] advised caution in the absence of data confirming efficacy and an acceptable risk/benefit ratio. It is not likely that Pacini and Schlumberger would have the same opinion today, as members of the American Thyroid Association Cancer Guidelines Committee that recommends that radioiodine not be given for radioiodine refractory tumors, i.e., in the absence of radioiodine uptake [19].

When initially faced with this perplexing pairing of diagnostic data—positive Tg and negative scan—it is essential to first attempt to uncover a cause for a possibly false-negative scan or a false-positive elevation of serum Tg before even considering empiric radioiodine therapy. For example, a falsely positive serum Tg level could occur because of interfering anti-Tg antibodies [20–23]. Explanations for a false-negative radioiodine scan include inadequate thyrotropin (TSH) elevation, stable iodine contamination (e.g., history of recent iodine contrast radiography), dispersed microscopic metastases too small to visualize, or dedifferentiation of the tumor such that it can still produce Tg but has lost its iodide-trapping ability. It has even been speculated that there could be radioiodine-resistant remnants of normal thyroid tissue or Tg secretion from thymus gland that might account for the measurable Tg [24]. On the other hand, the failure to visualize foci of uptake on a radionuclide scan could be due to iodine excess. To rule out iodine contamination, serum or urinary iodide can be measured, and if found to be moderately elevated, a repeat total-body scan (TBS) 4–6 weeks after an iodide depletion regimen can be considered [25]. It is also possible, as has been seen in some series of patients, that patients with residual tumor may have both undetectable serum Tg and a negative scan, presumably representing dedifferentiation of these tumors [26].

In managing the patient who presents with a negative scan and measurable Tg, patient-specific clinical aspects should be taken into account before definitive action is taken to prescribe empiric radioiodine therapy. Important matters to consider include risk factors, evidence of prior metastatic or aggressive disease, and the options for employing other imaging tools, such as magnetic resonance imaging (MRI) or ultrasound to visualize potential occult disease. How the clinical context can alter the approach is illustrated by two hypothetical cases. First, in a 60-year-old man with a history of a stage III 4-cm papillary or a 2-cm invasive follicular carcinoma, the author would consider application of the earlier Pacini-Schlumberger approach of empiric treatment with high-dose radioiodine. Alternatively, in a 25-year-old woman with a history of a 2-cm stage I papillary cancer with negative nodes and only marginally measurable or slightly elevated Tg (e.g., <4 ng/mL), the author might favor a more conservative approach, at least for a period of time with continued monitoring of the patient. One

L. Wartofsky, MD, MACP (✉)
Department of Medicine, MedStar Washington Hospital Center, Georgetown University School of Medicine, 110 Irving Street, N.W., Washington, DC 20010-2975, USA
e-mail: leonard.wartofsky@medstar.net

L. Wartofsky, D. Van Nostrand (eds.), *Thyroid Cancer*, DOI 10.1007/978-1-4939-3314-3_47

argument for simply continuing to monitor is that serum Tg levels are known to fall spontaneously with time over the course of 1–5 years post-ablation [27, 28, 28a].

Whether serum Tg levels are stable or rising is very useful in the decision-making process regarding radioiodine therapy. Of course, the patient must be brought into the decision-making process and informed fully of the extent of collective knowledge, experience, and biases pertaining to that patient's specific situation. We would like to avoid treatment with aggressive high-dose radioiodine for uncertain indications and treatment that might result in harmful sequelae, such as neutropenia, xerostomia, and/or azoospermia.

As pointed out by Sherman and Gopal [18], the risks of aggressive radioiodine therapy may not be warranted given the ill-defined goals, unless there is evidence of progressive disease. Pacini et al. [17] and Schlumberger et al. [29] are not the only investigators to describe a salutary result from empiric treatment of the Tg-positive/scan-negative patient. Pineda et al. [30] reported their results in 17 Tg-positive/scan-negative patients who all had prior total thyroidectomy and radioiodine ablation. After empiric treatment with 150–300 mCi of 131I, 16 of 17 had visualization of metastases on their post-treatment scan. Tg levels decreased in 81 % of patients after their first treatment dose and decreased in 90 % and 100 % of those who received second and third doses, respectively. Although these results sound impressive [30, 31], examination of the individual patient's Tg level response is less so. Mean Tg decreased from 74–62 to 32 over 1–2 years of follow-up, and only 6 of 29 positive scans became negative.

A definite tilt toward empiric radioiodine therapy in 16 scan-negative/Tg-positive patients was evident in the report by de Keizer et al. [32] who described a decreased Tg level in 88 % of patients. The period of follow-up was too short to indicate any improvement in survival or disease-free interval; however, the authors proposed treatment of such patients with at least one dose when scans were negative. As with the Pineda and Robbins studies [30, 31], serum Tg did decline in the majority of patients but not dramatically so.

The cogent issues raised by Sherman and Gopal, and previously by McDougall [33] and Mazzaferri [34], reflect the fact that many patients treated by Schlumberger et al. and Pineda and Robbins had minimal, if any, disease that would affect their life expectancy. The empiric therapy would expose them to unwarranted doses of radiation exposure, unwarranted at least until sufficient data is obtained from well-controlled studies that confirm efficacy of therapy. Based on their own experience in 24 patients [35] and their analysis of the literature [36], Fatourechi and Hay suggested two general patient categories. The first group has a higher risk of demonstrating uptake on the scan after high-dose therapy, representing younger patients with diffuse micrometastases and negative whole-body scan and conventional imaging but moderately elevated Tg levels. Patients in the second group are likely to be older, higher risk patients with known metastases that release Tg and do not take up radioiodine but are identified by other imaging. In their experience, this latter group will not demonstrate uptake on a posttreatment scan and therefore does not warrant therapy.

Arguably, the most useful experience reported to date is that of Pacini et al. [28] who compared the outcomes in 42 scan-negative/Tg-positive patients (group 1) treated with radioiodine to 28 patients (group 2) followed without treatment, where the average follow-up was 6.7 and 11.9 years, respectively. The first posttherapy scan was positive in 30 of 42 treated patients, negative in 12, and only the patients with positive scans were given additional 131I therapy. Complete remission was seen in 10 of 30 (normalized Tg levels), partial remission (still detectable Tg) in 9 of 30, and evidence of persistent disease in 11 of 30 (measurable Tg and scans became positive). Among these 30 patients with positive posttherapy scans, when radioiodine uptake was seen in the lungs (metastatic disease) on the posttherapy scan, it resolved in 8 of 9 (89 %) cases but in only 11 of 18 cases with cervical lymph node involvement. In the remaining 12 of the 42 group 1 patients who did not have positive scans after treatment doses, 2 entered remission, 7 had persistent Tg elevations, 2 had mediastinal lymph node involvement, and only 1 died of disease during the follow-up period. The changes in Tg were not directly compared to the changes in the no-treatment group. Significantly, of these 28 patients (group 2) who were followed with no treatment, 19 of 28 (68 %) became Tg-negative, another 6 of 28 (21.4 %) were unchanged, and only 3 (11 %) had an increase in Tg levels. Pacini et al. concluded that there may be a role for empiric 131I therapy in patients with pulmonary metastases but that their data supporting empiric therapy in patients with cervical lymph nodes was far from compelling. In view of the remarkable stability in those who were not treated, they did not advocate further radioiodine therapy in those patients whose first posttherapy scan remains negative—an approach that seems to be quite balanced.

Serum Tg levels drawn soon after ablation have prognostic value in regard to future recurrence [37]. It was possible to compare the change in Tg levels in 28 treated vs 32 nonradioiodine-treated patients in the study by Koh et al. [38]. Significantly greater reductions in Tg were seen with 131-I therapy, with four patients actually becoming undetectable. Posttherapy scans became positive in 12 of 28 (43 %) of the scan-negative/Tg-positive patients. Like deKeizer et al. [32], the authors encouraged consideration of empiric radioiodine therapy, both for palliation and potential localization of lesions on the posttreatment scan.

In their review of the literature, Ma et al. [39] concluded that the decision to treat should be individualized on the basis of the extent of disease as indicated by serum Tg levels. Thus, individuals with Tg levels >10 ng/mL or patients stratified at high risk for recurrence should be treated with radioiodine with the expectation that approximately two thirds will show both a fall in Tg and a positive posttreatment scan.

It may seem easy to recommend empiric therapy based on these data indicating declines in serum Tg after treatment, but it should be noted that improvement in survival is yet to be shown. In addition to the potential untoward complications of high-dose radioiodine therapy mentioned above (and enumerated in Chap. 50), another important aspect of empiric therapy is the cost to the patient regarding either the morbidity of hypothyroidism or the dollar cost of rhTSH and the negative impact on productivity when hypothyroid, as well as the cost in health care related to hospitalization and the associated expensive technological procedures.

In the author's approach to the scan-negative/Tg-positive patient, it is important to turn at an early stage in evaluation to alternative imaging procedures. Although radioiodine therapy may not be feasible because of the lack of visible uptake on diagnostic scanning, alternative therapeutic approaches to metastatic deposits of thyroid cancer may be available. These might include surgical excision, localized ablation by ethanol instillation or radiofrequency ablation (see Chap. 54), or localized external-radiation therapy ([40, 41]; see Chap. 51), but the location of the metastases should first be identified and assessed before one of these approaches is taken. Imaging with computed tomography (CT), MRI, and ultrasound have been employed for this purpose, and alternative scanning agents may have a role in identifying lesions that are not visualized with traditional 131I whole-body scan (see Chap. 35).

Alternative Scanning Agents

Two early scanning agents used as alternatives to radioiodine were 201Tl [42] and 99mTc sestamibi [43]. In one study of patients with bone metastases documented with positive 131I scans, 201Tl was compared to the bone agent, 99mTc hydroxymethylene diphosphonate (99mTc-HMDP; [42]). The two agents had a combined sensitivity of 93.5 %. In a group of 14 patients with negative 131I scans and other evidence of thyroid malignancy, 201Tl was positive in 10 of 14, and 99mTcHMDP was positive in all 14. Carril et al. [44] found that 201Tl showed a sensitivity and specificity higher than that associated with 131I for recurrent or persistent disease. Lesions were detected in 31 of 116 patients by 201Tl but not by 131I TBS. In patients who have been ablated and show no further 131I uptake, the authors proposed continuing management with no additional 131I scans. Because 201Tl scanning does not require levothyroxine withdrawal, follow-up would be guided only by 201Tl scanning and monitoring serum Tg. Dadparvar et al. [45] compared 201Tl and scanning with 99mTc-methoxyisobutyl isonitrile (99mTc-MIBI). They found that a 131I TBS alone was satisfactory as a preablation diagnostic study, but the addition of either alternative agent increased the diagnostic yield postablation, particularly when the 131I TBS was negative. However, these results have not been universal because Lorberboym et al. [46] found 131I TBS to be more sensitive and specific than 201Tl, with the latter giving several false-positive scans. Ugur et al. [47] noted a 70 % overall concordance between 201Tl, 99mTc-MIBI, and 131I TBS but observed false-negatives with both alternative agents, concluding that they should not be used in lieu of 131I TBS. In one reported case, 201Tl scanning was positive and useful in a patient with metastatic disease with both negative 131I TBS and negative serum Tg levels [48].

Employing 99m-Tc-depreotide, Rodriques et al. [49] were able to visualize lesions in 9/10 radioiodine scan-negative patients with suspected residual disease. In studies with the agent, 99mTc sestamibi, Elser et al. [50] noted a 94 % sensitivity for the detection of positive lymph nodes and local recurrence; they detected 32 of 40 metastases with sestamibi vs only 18 of 40 with an 131I TBS. Another cationic scanning agent, 99mTc tetrafosmin, which has been used previously for myocardial perfusion imaging, was assessed for the detection of thyroid cancer [51–53]. For 12 patients with elevated serum Tg (4 with negative 131I TBS), tetrafosmin was slightly superior to 201Tl and 99mTc-MIBI. This same group of workers [53] reported that tetrafosmin successfully identified all of 21 lesions that were positive by 131I TBS, as well as an additional 17 of 23 lesions that were negative by 131I TBS. The agent had 86 % sensitivity for distant metastases and was positive in four patients with 131I-negative proven pulmonary metastases. The findings correlated with other imaging modalities for tumor identification, e.g., CT or ultrasound.

It is also significant that these alternative agents are logistically both more convenient and expedient than scanning with 131I. Along with the ability to scan patients while euthyroid and still on TSH-suppressive levothyroxine therapy, the time required for evaluation is much reduced. Instead of scanning 48–72 h after a dose of 131I, the 99mTc tetrafosmin planar scan is performed 20 min after injection of the isotope, with additional images taken by single-photon emission computed tomography of any suspicious lesions. 99mTc tetrafosmin scans were negative in all 68 patients studied by Lind et al. [53], who were free of disease on the basis of 131I TBS and serum Tg.

Fluorodeoxyglucose-Positron Emission Tomography (Chaps. 34 and 61)

Some insight into the minimal value of the above-described imaging agents is apparent from the fact that they have not been widely adopted for this group of patients over the past several years. Rather, another agent, 18-fluorine fluorodeoxyglucose (FDG), has shown the most promise and has been employed with positron emission tomography (PET) for detection of thyroid cancer with uptake of the agent related to glucose utilization by tumor tissue [54–57]. Indeed, FDG-PET scanning is rapidly becoming a part of the routine armamentarium of diagnostic imaging procedures for thyroid cancer, especially metastatic disease [58, 59], and may be the optimal imaging modality for medullary thyroid cancer [60]. Notwithstanding that several workers have recommended its routine use [61], its more widespread adoption has been limited by its relatively high cost and the reluctance of insurers to provide coverage for all but selected patient populations. One of the populations in which PET scanning has been found useful is the scan-negative/Tg-positive patients. Numerous publications testify to its utility in both individual patient case reports and small patient series [62–68].

The greatest uptake sensitivity for FDG-PET scanning has been noted with the fastest growing undifferentiated tumors. Grunwald et al. [69] compared FDG-PET to 99mTc sestamibi and 131I TBS. Of 29 studies, 11 of 29 had disease detected only with FDG-PET, 8 of 29 were detected only with 131I TBS, and 10 of 29 were detected by both. Five sites were found by FDG-PET and not by 99mTc sestamibi. FDG-PET may be useful in patients in whom 131I TBS is not feasible owing to a history of iodine exposure; similarly, its use would not preclude CT scanning (with contrast if desired) as an additional means to image tumors.

A larger study by Schluter et al. [70] described 118 PET scans in 64 scan-negative/Tg-positive patients. Of 64 patients, 44 had positive PET studies, 34 of whom were proven to be true positives, leading to an altered therapeutic approach in 19 of 34 (surgery and/or external irradiation), whereas 20 patients had negative scans. Their results indicated a positive predictive value (PPV) for PET of 83 % but a negative predictive value (NPV) of only 25 %. In seven patients, there was so much metastatic disease identified that a palliative, rather than curative, approach was taken. Yet, for the most part, they found PET to be a valuable adjunct to identify patients who could benefit from further therapy. Wang and coworkers [71] reported good results with PET scanning in 37 patients with negative 131I scans. PET identified occult lesions in 71 %, with a 92 % PPV in patients with high serum Tg and a 93 % NPV in patients with lower Tg levels. Chung et al. [72] reported excellent utility of FDG-PET scanning in 54 patients with negative 131I scans after thyroxine withdrawal, and they demonstrated a 94 % PPV and a 93 % NPV. FDG-PET may be particularly useful when both the iodine scan and serum Tg are false-negatives, and this often applies when the low-serum Tg is a result of interfering anti-thyroglobulin antibodies. Chung et al. noted that this often implied regional lymph node involvement. Although Wang et al. [71] found that FDG-PET was not that useful in detecting small degrees of residual papillary tumor in the neck, Chung et al. showed PET to be positive more often with neck disease and conventional scanning than in detecting pulmonary metastases, and Ozkan et al. found that the best success with PET imaging occurred in the patients with the highest Tg antibody levels [73]. Comparably encouraging results have been reported by Helal et al. [74] in a series of 37 scan-negative/Tg-positive patients with DTC. In a group of ten patients with known metastases via conventional imaging, PET confirmed tumor at 17 of 18 sites and identified tumors at 11 additional sites. PET was positive in 19 of 27 patients in a second group with negative imaging by other methods. These findings led to a change in treatment management in 29 of 37 patients, with 23 receiving further surgery and 14 of 23 achieving disease-free status. These authors proposed PET as the "first-line investigation" in scan-negative/Tg-positive patients. A more pessimistic view was expounded by van Tol and colleagues in a letter to the editor [75] in which they described an extraordinary high rate of false-positives (64 %) with PET and that the findings led to a significant change in management in only 1 of 11 (9 %) patients. A drawback is the lack of widespread availability of PET scanners because of their high cost, and, most importantly, these scans are currently not reimbursed by most insurers in the United States except for specific indications. (This situation has been improving steadily over the past few years.)

Fridrich et al. [76] compared FDG-PET to 99mTc-MIBI and 131I TBS and found both to be more sensitive than 131I TBS, with a slight edge in favor of 99mTc-MIBI. In addition to the benefit of good uptake, independent of the patients' serum TSH level, FDG-PET or MIBI did not have the propensity for high background in the neck, mediastinum, and chest as with 131I and could be used more effectively to detect small metastases in these areas. In contrast, the liver and brain demonstrate high FDG uptake, and the ability to detect metastases in these areas is limited with this agent. Indeed, Feine et al. [77] were able to localize and identify positive neck metastases with FDG-PET in six patients with elevated serum Tg levels. Dietlein et al. proposed a more conservative perspective regarding the utility of FDG-PET scanning [78]. They observed positive FDG-PET images in 7 of 21 patients with positive lymph node metastases but negative 131I TBS; sensitivity was 82 % in patients with high serum Tg but negative TBS. They concluded that FDG-PET should not be used in lieu of 131I-TBS but would serve as a useful adjunct or complement to evaluation, particularly when the 131I TBS was negative in conflict with a rising or elevated level of serum Tg. Altenvoerde et al. [79] performed PET studies in 12 of 32 patients with scan-negative/Tg-positive findings, and the PET scans were positive in 6 of 12. Interestingly, the mean Tg level in the six positive patients was 147 ± 90, whereas the PET-negative patients had a mean Tg of only 9 ± 7.6, suggesting that PET is most useful in those patients with more aggressive and/or larger metastases.

Similar conclusions were reached by Grunwald et al. [80] and Wang et al. [81]. In this regard, PET-positive patients with larger volume disease have a worse prognosis [71, 82]. The association of PET positivity with dedifferentiation was commented upon by Caobelli et al. in a communication [83] that discussed a report by Vural et al. [84] linking prognosis to PET findings. The latter workers described their experience with 105 scan-negative/Tg-positive patients and noted that the best prognosis was associated with Tg levels that were suppressible by levothyroxine in PET-negative patients whereas PET positivity correlated with recurrence and extrathyroidal spread. A correlation of better prognosis with negative FDG-PET was also noted by Pachon-Garrudo et al. [85].

Clearly, PET scanning may miss some types of metastases. In the report of Hung et al. [86], 20 scan-negative/Tg-positive patients underwent FDG-PET scanning with lesions detected in 17 of 20, but PET scans were negative in 2 patients proven to have miliary distribution of pulmonary micrometastases. The authors suggest imaging with chest CT scans in such cases. Most valuable has been the newest technology that combines PET scanning with CT or MRI by either fusion software or preferably within one dedicated PET/CT scanner [58, 59]. An overlay of high SUV on a CT or MR image provides much greater specificity that the imaged finding is cancer. As with many diagnostic modalities, negative findings would not preclude disease, but positive findings on PET/CT would dictate CT-guided or ultrasound-guided FNA cytology and then surgery if tumor is confirmed. As mentioned, the utility of FDG-PET scanning in this group of patients tends to correlate with the magnitude of the serum Tg level. For example, Na et al. [64] noted a sensitivity of PET of 28.6 % with Tg levels between 2 and 5, 57.1 % with levels between 5 and 10 and 86 % when Tg was equal to or greater than 20 ng/mL.

TSH Stimulation of FDG-PET

Whether FDG uptake and imaging might be enhanced by either endogenous TSH after levothyroxine withdrawal or by recombinant human TSH (rhTSH) remains somewhat controversial. It appears that the effect of TSH stimulation was best seen in patients with the highest levels of Tg suggesting greater tumor mass, and it has been proposed that FDG-PET may be most useful above a threshold Tg level of 10 ng/mL [87]. Some workers relate the basis for TSH stimulation to in vitro thyroid cell culture studies in which TSH will increase uptake of both FDG [88] and 201Tl [89]; however, that does not prove that thyroid cancer cells will respond in the same way in vivo. TSH could probably improve imaging because TSH stimulates glucose transport into the cells and cellular metabolism.

The best proof of this concept is derived from several clinical studies. For example, Chin et al. [90] evaluated seven patients who were scan-negative/Tg-positive and compared PET scans of those patients on thyroxine suppression to PET scans after rhTSH. The scans after rhTSH disclosed more lesions, and the average tumor-to-background (T:B) ratio values were higher. Similar results were seen by Petrich et al. [91] in 30 patients with largely negative radioiodine scans. rhTSH stimulation provided higher T:B ratios and uncovered more lesions in more patients. Comparing PET scans after thyroxine withdrawal (not rhTSH) to PET scans of patients on suppressive therapy, both Moog et al. [92] and van Tol et al. [93] concluded that TSH stimulation detected more lesions. Rational patient selection is needed, and clinicians and payors have to determine whether the additional cost burden of rhTSH to an already expensive PET scan will constitute a favorable cost–benefit ratio. After an analysis of seven prospective controlled clinical trials that included a total of 168 patients, Ma et al. [94] concluded that TSH stimulation was beneficial in demonstrating more PET-positive lesions but that the findings were associated with altered clinical management in less than 10 % of the patients. Notwithstanding the results of these studies indicating improved imaging with TSH stimulation, Bertagna et al. [66] found no difference in the utility of FDG-PET in patients on levothyroxine vs those with an elevated TSH level. Unrelated to PET scanning but relevant to rhTSH, there is a case report of a scan-negative/Tg-positive patient in whom radioiodine trapping was restored after a period of levothyroxine withdrawal and rhTSH stimulation [95]. Occasionally, radioiodine trapping may also be restored after chemotherapy [96], and the matter of redifferentiation is discussed in Chap. 86.

Somatostatin Imaging

Because some thyroid cancers—especially medullary thyroid cancer [97]—contain somatostatin receptors, somatostatin receptor scintigraphy (SRS) with octreotide or octreotide derivatives has been studied and reported [98, 99]. These agents have also been employed for therapy [100, 101]. Of 25 patients with DTC and elevated serum Tg levels studied by Baudin [98], 16 of 25 had negative 131I TBS, and SRS was positive in 12 of these patients as well as in 8 of 9 patients with positive 131I TBS. Stokkel et al. [102] studied ten Tg-positive/131I scan-negative patients with octreotide scanning and described multiple metastases in nine of ten. Based on octreotide uptake, the authors speculate that 111-In-labeled octreotide or its analogues might be useful for therapy of such patients as it has been shown to be for medullary thyroid carcinoma [97]. Sarlis et al. [103] compared octreotide scanning to PET and conventional imaging in 21 patients with aggressive disease, finding that octreotide had only moderate sensitivity yet detected disease in 5 patients who were negative by PET and other imaging. In preliminary studies, Sager et al. [104] examined a group of radioiodine scan-negative patients employing technetium-labeled octreotide analogues 99mTc-HYNIC-TOC and HYNIC-TATE and proposed that these agents could be used routinely in patients who are somatostatin receptor positive. In a comparison to FDG-PET scanning, Middendorp et al. [105] employed [(68)Ga]DOTATOC and found comparable diagnostic utility although FDG-PET did exhibit a slightly higher rate of lesion detection. Confirmatory studies are required, but SRS with labeled octreotide or one of these newer derivatives may represent another useful alternative to 131-I TBS or FDG-PET, with the advantage of lacking the need to withdraw TSH-suppressive levothyroxine therapy.

Surgery

As mentioned above, ultrasonography of the neck is extremely useful to identify occult metastases of papillary thyroid cancer [106, 107] and deserves to be an almost routine imaging tool for this purpose (see Chaps. 21 and 37), particularly if used in conjunction with rhTSH-stimulated thyroglobulin levels [108]. Another approach has been to proceed with cervical exploration and node dissection in the case of papillary carcinoma, even when all additional imaging studies are unrevealing. In one such series of 21 patients, Alzahrani et al. [109] performed neck dissections after confirming the presence of tumor by ultrasound-guided fine-needle aspiration cytology. Postoperatively, serum Tg fell from a mean of 185±79 to 127±59, with 4 patients who achieved remission, 13 who had persistent disease, and 4 who showed progression. They concluded that the additional surgery offered benefit in a minority of patients and that most remained stable during follow-up. In addition, the intraoperative use of ultrasound can readily improve the detection of residual or recurrent thyroid cancer [110], and there has been greater success with positive node dissections since its use by surgeons at our institution. In some hands the combined use of (18)F-FDG PET/CT imaging and gamma probe radio-guided surgery has proved successful for the localization and confirmation of metastatic lesions in the radioiodine scan-negative patient [111].

The opposite Scenario: Undetectable TG and Positive 131-I Scan

In recent years, the opposite even more puzzling scenario has been noted, that of finding patients with positive uptake seen on follow-up radionuclide scans indicating the likelihood of residual disease but having undetectable levels of serum Tg [112–114]. While this situation is relatively infrequent in our experience, it has been reported more frequently by others, with undetectable Tg levels observed in 20 % of patients who were thought to have residual benign thyroid remnants and in 8 % who were identified as having residual thyroid carcinoma [112]. Significant metastatic disease has been found in some of these patients, typically to regional lymph nodes, leading some investigators to advocate for more routine performance of survey radioiodine scans [114], perhaps as part of periodic rhTSH stimulation testing with both Tg levels and scan post-stimulation [112]. On the other hand, in a retrospective review of 389 patients of whom 44 (11.3 %) had positive scans and undetectable Tg levels, Lim et al. [115] found that long-term clinical outcomes did not differ in these patients and suggested that repetitive radioiodine scans were not necessary and that conservative monitoring would suffice for long-term follow-up.

We believe that the explanation for this clinical situation in most cases is related to false-negative results for serum Tg. In recent years, we have begun to understand better the reasons for differences in results between various ICMA or RIA methodologies for both serum Tg and anti-Tg antibodies, on the basis of differences in assay reagents or assay "hook effects," and the presence of different idiotypic antithyroglobulin antibodies in the patient's serum [116]. Both interfering anti-Tg antibodies and heterophile antibodies have been incriminated [113, 117]. Our suggestion to clinicians facing this dilemma is to obtain Tg and Tg antibody measurements in several different laboratories, by both ICMA and RIA methodology. Doing so is likely to discover the presence of antibodies detected in one system that were not detected in the original assay, thereby accounting for the discordant results.

Conclusions

In conclusion, how should the scan-negative/Tg-positive patient be managed with no underlying reason to suspect either false-negative scan or false-positive serum Tg level? Schlumberger [118, 119] has advocated empiric administration of 100 mCi 131I to any patient with a Tg level more than 10 ng/mL while off levothyroxine and would only repeat the 131I whole-body scan every 2–5 years when the Tg level is in the range of 1–10 ng/mL. As mentioned above, no studies show improved survival with this approach. On the contrary, the follow-up study of van Tol et al. [120] indicates little support for empiric therapy based on an average follow-up period of 4.2 years. Of 56 patients given a "blind" dose of 150 mCi of 131I, uptake was revealed on the posttreatment scan in 28 of 56 (50 %) of the patients with no difference in serum Tg levels. They concluded that therapy had no salutary effect on survival or reduction of tumor burden. There may be many factors that could differentiate those patients who seem to respond to empiric therapy from those who do not. One factor could be the size of the lesions as micrometastases may be more readily ablated than macrometastases [121]. At this point in our knowledge, I am attracted to the concept of individualization of empiric therapy as proposed by Ma et al. [39] based upon the height of the Tg levels and whether or not they are seen to be increasing during follow-up. Indeed, although controversial as discussed above and elsewhere [14], empiric radioiodine therapy can be attempted at least one more time in selected patients with Tg levels >10 ng/mL or rising. Posttherapy Tg levels and the posttherapy scan should be examined to assess potential benefit. In an attempt to maximize the efficacy of the radioiodine, I employ a low-iodine diet for 3 weeks prior to therapy supplemented by low-dose diuretic (20 mg/day furoseamide) and confirm the patient's adherence to the diet by measurement of urinary iodine 1 week prior to the planned therapy. We proceed with therapy if the urinary iodide is less than 50 μg/L, and most patients can achieve levels of less than 20 μg/L. In addition, radioiodine retention and presumed therapeutic benefit can be augmented by lithium carbonate therapy as discussed in Chap. 49. The growing number of reports [32, 37–39, 121, 122] indicating benefit of empiric therapy appears to justify this approach.

If radioiodine therapy is not to be given in the face of clearly measurable Tg levels, alternative imaging procedures should be encouraged. For papillary thyroid carcinoma with a propensity to regional recurrence, that could include ultrasound, CT, MRI, 99mTc-MIBI, or FDG-PET, with fine-needle aspiration cytology when feasible to confirm the diagnosis. For follicular thyroid cancer with its propensity for distant metastases (especially to bone and lung), imaging with PET/CT, 99mTc tetrafosmin, 99mTc-HMDP, or 201Tl could be attempted. Identification of isolated distant lesions by these methods would allow earlier intervention by surgical excision, a local ablative technique, or external radiotherapy instead of delaying further treatment until a subsequent 131-I TBS might become positive or serum Tg levels might increase further because of further tumor growth. In patients with higher risk disease following early total thyroidectomy and high-dose radioiodine ablation, this approach should permit effective management until more target-specific tumoricidal therapies become available.

References

1. Spencer CA. New insights for using serum thyroglobulin (Tg) measurement for managing patients with differentiated thyroid carcinomas. Thyroid Int. 2003;4:1–14.
2. Spencer CA, Fatemi S, Singer P, Nicoloff J, LoPresti J. Serum basal thyroglobulin measured by a second-generation assay correlates with the recombinant human thyrotropin-stimulated thyroglobulin response in patients treated for differentiated thyroid cancer. Thyroid. 2010;20:587–95.
3. Schlumberger M, Hitzel A, Toubert ME, et al. Comparison of seven serum thyroglobulin assays in the follow-up of papillary and follicular thyroid cancer patients. J Clin Endocrinol Metab. 2007;92:2487–95.
4. Nascimento C, Borget I, Troalen F, Al Ghuzlan A, Deandreis D, Hartl D, et al. Ultrasensitive serum thyroglobulin measurement is useful for the follow-up of patients treated with total thyroidectomy without radioactive iodine ablation. Eur J Endocrinol. 2013;169(5):689–93. doi:10.1530/EJE-13-0386.
5. Giovanella L, Teglia G, Sadeghi R, Trimboli P, Ceriani L, Verburg FA. Unstimulated high-sensitive thyroglobulin in follow-up of differentiated thyroid cancer patients: a meta-analysis. J Clin Endocrinol Metab. 2014;99:440–7.
6. Lee JI, Chung YJ, Cho BY, Chong S, Seok JW, Park SJ. Postoperative-stimulated serum thyroglobulin measured at the time of 131I ablation is useful for the prediction of disease status in patients with differentiated thyroid carcinoma. Surgery. 2013;153(6):828–35.
7. Wartofsky L. Management of scan negative thyroglobulin positive differentiated thyroid carcinoma. J Clin Endocrinol Metab. 1998;83:4195–9.
8. Giovanella L, Treglia G, Ceriani L, Verburg F. Detectable thyroglobulin with negative imaging in differentiated thyroid cancer patients: what to do with negative anatomical imaging and radioiodine scan? Nucl Med. 2014;53:1–10.
9. Clark OH, Hoelting T. Management of patients with differentiated thyroid cancer who have positive serum thyroglobulin levels and negative radioiodine scans. Thyroid. 1994;4:501–5.
10. McDougall IR. Management of thyroglobulin positive/whole-body scan negative: is 131-I therapy useful? J Endocrinol Invest. 2001;24:194–8.
11. Levy EG, Fatourechi V, Robbins R, Ringel MD. Thyroglobulin-positive, radioiodine-negative thyroid cancer. Thyroid. 2001;11: 599–602.
12. Gemsenjager E. Thyroglobulin-positive, radioiodine-negative thyroid cancer (letter to editor). Thyroid. 2003;13:833–4.
13. Hurley JR. Management of thyroid cancer: radioiodine ablation, "stunning", and treatment of thyroglobulin-positive, (131)I scan-negative patients. Endocr Pract. 2000;6:401–6.
14. Mazzaferri EL. Empirically treating high serum thyroglobulin levels. J Nucl Med. 2005;46:1079–88.
15. Tuttle RM, Ball DW, Byrd D, Dilawari RA, Doherty GM, Duh QY, et al. Thyroid carcinoma. National Comprehensive Cancer Network. 2012. Version 3.2012. Available from: http://www.nccn.org/professionals/physician_gls/pdf/thyroid.pdf. Accessed 24 Aug 2012.
16. British Thyroid Association, Royal College of Physicians. Guidelines for the management of thyroid cancer. In: Perros P, editor. Report of the thyroid cancer guidelines update group. 2nd ed. London: Royal College of Physicians; 2007.
17. Pacini F, Lippi F, Formica N, et al. Therapeutic doses of iodine-131 reveal undiagnosed metastases in thyroid cancer patients with detectable serum thyroglobulin levels. J Nucl Med. 1987;28: 1888–91.
18. Wartofsky L, Sherman SI, Gopal J, et al. The use of radioactive iodine in patients with papillary and follicular thyroid cancer. J Clin Endocrinol Metab. 1998;83:4195–203.
19. Haugen BR, Alexander EK, Bible KC, Doherty GM, Mandel SJ, Nikiforov Y, et al. 2015 American Thyroid Association Guidelines for patients with thyroid nodules and differentiated thyroid cancer. Available online at Thyroid 25: DOI:10.1089/thy.2015.0020; print version in Thyroid 26:1–133, 2016.
20. Spencer CA. Clinical utility of thyroglobulin antibody (TgAb) measurements for patients with differentiated thyroid cancers (DTC). J Clin Endocrinol Metab. 2011;96:3615–27.
21. Spencer CA, Petrovic I, Fatemi S. Current thyroglobulin autoantibody (TgAb) assays often fail to detect interfering TgAb that ca

result in the reporting of falsely low/undetectable serum Tg IMA values for patients with differentiated thyroid cancer. J Clin Endocrinol Metab. 2011;96:1283–91.
22. Verburg FA, Luster M, Cupini C, et al. Implications of thyroglobulin antibody positivity in patients with differentiated thyroid cancer: a clinical position paper. Thyroid. 2013;23:1211–25.
23. Spencer CA. Commentary on: implications of thyroglobulin antibody positivity in patients with differentiated thyroid cancer: a clinical position paper. Thyroid. 2013;23:1190–2.
24. Zanotti-Fregonara P, Keller I, Calzada-Nocaudie M, Al-Nahhas A, Devaux JY, Grassetto G, et al. Increased serum thyroglobulin levels and negative imaging in thyroid cancer patients: are there sources of benign secretion? A speculative short review. Nucl Med Commun. 2010;31(12):1054–8.
25. Maxon HR, Thomas SR, Boehringer A, et al. Low iodine diet in I-131 ablation of thyroid remnants. Clin Nucl Med. 1983;8:123–6.
26. Klutmann S, Jenicke L, Geiss-Tonshoff M, et al. Prevalence of iodine-and thyroglobulin-negative findings in differentiated thyroid cancer. A retrospective analysis of patients treated from 1951 to 1998 in university hospital. Nuklearmedizin. 2001;40:143–7.
27. Padovani RP, Robenshtok E, Brokhin M, Tuttle RM. Even without additional therapy, serum thyroglobulin concentrations often decline for years after total thyroidectomy and radioactive remnant ablation in patients with differentiated thyroid cancer. Thyroid. 2012;22:778–83.
28. Pacini F, Agate L, Elisei R, et al. Outcome of differentiated thyroid cancer with detectable serum Tg and negative diagnostic (131)I whole body scan: comparison of patients treated with high (131)I activities versus untreated patients. J Clin Endocrinol Metab. 2001;86:4092–7.
28a. Frank RW, Middleton L, Stack Jr BC, Spencer HJ, Riggs AT, Bodenner DL. Conservative management of thyroglobulin positive, nonlocalizable thyroid carcinoma. Head Neck. 2014;36:155–7.
29. Schlumberger M, Mancusi F, Baudin E, Pacini F. 131-I therapy for elevated thyroglobulin levels. Thyroid. 1997;7:273–6.
30. Pineda JD, Lee T, Ain K, et al. Iodine-131 therapy for thyroid cancer patients with elevated thyroglobulin and negative diagnostic scan. J Clin Endocrinol Metab. 1995;80:1488–92.
31. Robbins J. Management of thyroglobulin-positive, body scan-negative thyroid cancer patients: evidence for the utility of I-131 therapy. J Endocrinol Investig. 1999;22:808–10.
32. De Keizer B, Koppeschaar HP, Zelissen PM, et al. Efficacy of high therapeutic doses of iodine-131 in patients with differentiated thyroid cancer and detectable serum thyroglobulin. Eur J Nucl Med. 2001;28:198–202.
33. McDougall IR. 131-I treatment of 131-I negative whole body scan, and positive thyroglobulin in differentiated thyroid carcinoma: what is being treated? Thyroid. 1997;7:669–72.
34. Mazzaferri EL. Editorial: treating high thyroglobulin with radioiodine: a magic bullet or a shot in the dark? J Clin Endocrinol Metab. 1995;80:1485–7.
35. Fatourechi V, Hay ID, Javedan H, et al. Lack of impact of radioiodine therapy in Tg-positive, diagnostic whole-body scan-negative patients with follicular cell-derived thyroid cancer. J Clin Endocrinol Metab. 2002;87:1521–6.
36. Fatourechi V, Hay ID. Treating the patient with differentiated thyroid cancer with thyroglobulin-positive iodine-131 diagnostic scan-negative metastases: including comments on the role of serum thyroglobulin monitoring in tumor surveillance. Semin Nucl Med. 2000;30:107–14.
37. Webb RC, Howard RS, Stojadinovic A, Gaitonde DY, Wallace MK, Ahmed J, Burch HB. The utility of serum thyroglobulin measurement at the time of remnant ablation for predicting disease-free status in patients with differentiated thyroid cancer: a meta-analysis involving 3947 patients. J Clin Endocrinol Metab. 2012;97:2754–63.
38. Koh JM, Kim ES, Ryu JS, et al. Effects of therapeutic doses of 131-I in thyroid papillary carcinoma patients with elevated thyroglobulin level and negative 131-I whole-body scan: comparative study. Clin Endocrinol. 2003;58:421–7.
39. Ma C, Xie J, Kuang A. Is empiric 131-I therapy justified for patients with positive thyroglobulin and negative 131-K whole-body scanning results? J Nucl Med. 2005;46:1164–70.
40. Ford D, Giridharan S, McConkey C, et al. External beam radiotherapy in the management of differentiated thyroid cancer. Clin Oncol. 2003;15:337–41.
41. Brierley JD, Tsang RW. External-beam radiation therapy in the treatment of differentiated thyroid cancer. Semin Surg Oncol. 1999;16:42–9.
42. Alam MS, Takeuchi R, Kasagi K, et al. Value of combined technetium-99m hydroxy methylene diphosphonate and Thallium-201 imaging in detecting bone metastases from thyroid carcinoma. Thyroid. 1997;7:705–12.
43. Almeida-Filho P, Ravizzini GC, Almeida C, et al. Whole-body Tc-99m sestamibi scintigraphy in the follow-up of differentiated thyroid carcinoma. Clin Nucl Med. 2000;25:443–6.
44. Carril JM, Quirce R, Serrano J, et al. Total body scintigraphy with thallium-201 and iodine-131 in the follow-up of differentiated thyroid cancer. J Nucl Med. 1997;38:686–92.
45. Dadparvar S, Chevres A, Tulchinsky M, et al. Clinical utility of technetium-99m methoxisobutylisonitrile imaging in differentiated thyroid carcinoma: comparison with thallium-201 and iodine-131 scintigraphy and serum thyroglobulin quantitation. Eur J Nucl Med. 1995;22:1330–8.
46. Lorberboym M, Murthy S, Mechanick JI, et al. Thallium-201 and iodine-131 scintigraphy in differentiated thyroid carcinoma. J Nucl Med. 1996;37:1487–91.
47. Ugur O, Kostakoglu L, Caner B, et al. Comparison of 201-Tl, 99mTcMIBI and 131-I imaging in the follow-up of patients with well differentiated thyroid carcinoma. Nucl Med Commun. 1996;17:373–7.
48. Harder W, Lind P, Molnar M, et al. Thallium-201 uptake with negative iodine-131 scintigraphy and serum thyroglobulin in metastatic oxyphilic papillary thyroid carcinoma. J Nucl Med. 1998;39:236–8.
49. Rodrigues M, Li S, Gabriel M, Heute D, Greifendeder M, Virgolini I. 99m-Tc-depreotide scintigraphy versus 18F-FDG-PET in the diagnosis of radioiodine-negative thyroid cancer. J Clin Endocrinol Metab. 2006;91:3997–4000.
50. Elser H, Henze M, Hermann C, et al. 99m-Tc-MIBI for recurrent and metastatic differentiated thyroid carcinoma. Nuklearmedizin. 1997;36:7–12.
51. Lind P, Gallowitsch HJ. The use of non-specific tracers in the follow up of differentiated thyroid cancer: results with Tc-99m tetrofosmin whole body scintigraphy. Acta Med Aust. 1996;23:69–75.
52. Gallowitsch HJ, Kresnik E, Mikosch P, et al. Tc-99m-tetrafosmin scintigraphy: an alternative scintigraphic method for following up differentiated thyroid carcinoma—preliminary results. Nuklearmedizin. 1996;35:230–5.
53. Lind P, Gallowitsch HJ, Langsteger W, et al. Technetium-99m-tetrafosmin whole-body scintigraphy in the follow-up of differentiated thyroid carcinoma. J Nucl Med. 1997;38:348–52.
54. van Dijk D, Plukker JTM, Phan HTT, et al. 18-fluorodeoxyglucose positron emission tomography in the early diagnostic workup of differentiated thyroid cancer patients with a negative post-therapeutic iodine scan and detectable thyroglobulin. Thyroid. 2013;23(8):1003–9.
55. Iagaru A, Kalinyak JE, McDougall IR. F-18 FDG PET/CT in the management of thyroid cancer. Clin Nucl Med. 2007;32(9):690–5.
56. Choi WH, Chung YA, Han EJ, Sohn HS, Lee SH. Clinical value of integrated [18F]fluoro-2-deoxy-D-glucose positron emission tomography/computed tomography in the preoperative assess-

ment of papillary thyroid carcinoma: comparison with sonography. J Ultrasound Med. 2011;30(9):1267–73.
57. Schoder H, Yeung HWD. Positron emission imaging of head and neck cancer, including thyroid carcinoma. Semin Nucl Med. 2004;34:180–97.
58. Ota N, Kato K, Iwano S, et al. Comparison of 18F-fluoride PET/CT, 18F-FDG PET/CT, and bone scintigraphy (planar and SPECT) in detection of bone metastases of differentiated thyroid cancer: a pilot study. Brit J Radiol. 2014;87(1034):20130444.
59. Nakajo M, Jinguji M, Tani A, et al. Diagnosis of metastases from postoperative differentiated thyroid cancer: comparison between FDG and FLT PET/CT studies. Radiology. 2013;267(3):891–901.
60. deGroot JW, Links TP, Jager PL, et al. Impact of 18F-fluoro-2-D-glucose positron emission tomograph (FDG-PET) in patients with biochemical evidence of recurrent or residual medullary thyroid cancer. Ann Surg Oncol. 2004;11:786–94.
61. Bannas P, Derlin T, Groth M, Apostolova I, Adam G, Mester J, Klutmann S. Can (18)F-FDG-PET/CT be generally recommended in patients with differentiated thyroid carcinoma and elevated thyroglobulin levels but negative I-131 whole body scan? Ann Nucl Med. 2012;26(1):77–85.
62. Bertagna F, Biasiotto G, Orlando E, Bosio G, Giubbini R. Role of 18F-fluorodeoxyglucose positron emission tomography/computed tomography in patients affected by differentiated thyroid carcinoma, high thyroglobulin level, and negative 131I scan: review of the literature. Jpn J Radiol. 2010;28(9):629–36.
63. Muros MA, Llamas-Elvira JM, Ramirez-Navarro A, et al. Utility of fluorine-18-fluorodeoxyglucose positron emission tomography in differentiated thyroid carcinoma with negative radioiodine scans and elevated serum thyroglobulin levels. Am J Surg. 2000;179:457–61.
64. Na SJ, Yoo IR, O JH, Lin C, Lin Q, Kim SH, Chung SK. Diagnostic accuracy of (18)F-fluorodeoxyglucose positron emission tomography/computed tomography in differentiated thyroid cancer patients with elevated thyroglobulin and negative (131)I whole body scan: evaluation by thyroglobulin level. Ann Nucl Med. 2012;26(1):26–34.
65. Creach KM, Nussenbaum B, Siegel BA, Grigsby PW. Thyroid carcinoma uptake of 18F-fluorodeoxyglucose in patients with elevated serum thyroglobulin and negative 131I scintigraphy. Am J Otolaryngol. 2013;34(1):51–6.
66. Bertagna F, Bosio G, Biasiotto G, Rodella C, Puta E, Gabanelli S, et al. F-18 FDG-PET/CT evaluation of patients with differentiated thyroid cancer with negative I-131 total body scan and high thyroglobulin level. Clin Nucl Med. 2009;34(11):756–61.
67. Dong MJ, Liu ZF, Zhao K, Ruan LX, Wang GL, Yang SY, Sun F, Luo XG. Value of 18F-FDG-PET/PET-CT in differentiated thyroid carcinoma with radioiodine-negative whole-body scan: a meta-analysis. Nucl Med Commun. 2009;30(8):639–50.
68. Kim SJ, Lee TH, Kim IJ, Kim YK. Clinical implication of F-18 FDG PET/CT for differentiated thyroid cancer in patients with negative diagnostic iodine-123 scan and elevated thyroglobulin. Eur J Radiol. 2009;70(1):17–24.
69. Grunwald F, Menzel C, Bender H, et al. Comparison of 18FDG-PET with 131-Iodine and 99m-Tc-sestamibi scintigraphy in differentiated thyroid cancer. Thyroid. 1997;7:327–35.
70. Schluter B, Bohuslavizki KH, Beyer W, et al. Impact of FDG PET on patients with differentiated thyroid cancer who present with elevated thyroglobulin and negative 131I scan. J Nucl Med. 2001;42:71–6.
71. Wang W, Macapinlac H, Larson SM, et al. [18F]-2-fluoro-2-deoxy-Dglucose positron emission tomography localizes residual thyroid cancer in patients with negative diagnostic (131)I whole body scans and elevated serum thyroglobulin levels. J Clin Endocrinol Metab. 1999;84:2291–302.
72. Chung JK, So Y, Lee JS, et al. Value of FDG-PET in papillary thyroid carcinoma with negative 131-I whole body scan. J Nucl Med. 1999;40:986–92.
73. Ozkan E, Aras G, Kucuk NO. Correlation of 18F-FDG PET/CT findings with histopathological results in differentiated thyroid cancer patients who have increased thyroglobulin or antithyroglobulin antibody levels and negative 131I whole-body scan results. Clin Nucl Med. 2013;38(5):326–31.
74. Helal BO, Merlet P, Toubert ME, et al. Clinical impact of (18) F-FDG PET in thyroid carcinoma patients with elevated thyroglobulin levels and negative (131)I scanning results after therapy. J Nucl Med. 2001;42:1464–9.
75. van Tol KM, Jager PL, Dullaart RP, Links TP. Follow-up in patients with differentiated thyroid carcinoma with positive 18F-fluoro-2-deoxy-Dglucose-positron emission tomography results, elevated thyroglobulin levels, and negative high-dose 131I posttreatment whole body scans. J Clin Endocrinol Metab. 2000;85:2082–3.
76. Fridrich L, Messa C, Landoni C, et al. Whole-body scintigraphy with 99m-TC-MIBI, 18F-FDG and 131-I in patients with metastatic thyroid carcinoma. Nucl Med Commun. 1997;18:3–9.
77. Feine U, Lietzenmayer R, Hanke JP, et al. Fluorine-18-FDG and iodine-131 uptake in thyroid cancer. J Nucl Med. 1996;37:1468–72.
78. Dietlein M, Scheidhauer K, Voth E, et al. Fluorine-18 fluorodeoxyglucose positron emission tomography and iodine-131 whole-body scintigraphy in the follow-up of differentiated thyroid cancer. Eur J Nucl Med. 1997;24:1342–8.
79. Altenvoerde G, Lerch H, Kuwert T, et al. Positron emission tomography with F-18-deoxyglucose in patients with differentiated thyroid carcinoma, elevated thyroglobulin levels, and negative iodine scans. Langenbeck's Arch Surg. 1998;383:160–3.
80. Grunwald F, Kalicke T, Feine U, et al. (18)F-FDG PET scanning in patients with thyroid cancer: results of a multicentre study. Eur J Nucl Med. 1999;26:1547–52.
81. Wang W, Larson SM, Fazzari M, et al. Prognostic value of (18) F-FDG PET scanning in patients with thyroid cancer. J Clin Endocrinol Metab. 2000;85:1107–13.
82. Marcus CS. Prognostic significance of FDG PET/CT on the follow-up of patients of differentiated thyroid carcinoma with negative I131 whole- body scan and elevated thyroglobulin levels. Clin Nucl Med. 2013;38(3):195.
83. Caobelli F, Pizzocaro C, Guerra UP. Prognostic significance of FDG PET/CT on the follow-up of patients of differentiated thyroid carcinoma with negative I131 whole-body scan and elevated thyroglobulin levels. Clin Nucl Med. 2013;38(3):196.
84. Vural GU, Akkas BE, Ercakmak N, Basu S, Alavi A. Prognostic significance of FDG PET/CT on the follow-up of patients of differentiated thyroid carcinoma with negative 131I whole-body scan and elevated thyroglobulin levels: correlation with clinical and histopathologic characteristics and long-term follow-up data. Clin Nucl Med. 2012;37(10):953–9.
85. Pachon-Garrudo VM, Cuenca-Cuenca JI, Ruiz-Franco-Baux J, Borrego-Dorado I, Tirado-Hospital JL, Navarro-Gonzalez E, Vazquez-Albertino R. Value of the negative PET-FDG in the middle term follow-up of differentiated thyroid cancer in patients with negative 131 I-Na scan and elevated thyroglobulin serum levels. Rev Esp Med Nucl Imag Mol. 2012;31(6):315–21.
86. Hung MC, Wu HS, Kao C, et al. F18-fluorodeoxyglucose positron emission tomography in detecting metastatic papillary thyroid carcinoma with elevated human serum thyroglobulin levels but negative I-131 whole body scan. Endocr Res. 2003;29: 169–75.
87. Vera P, Kuhn-Lansoy C, Sanson AE, Hapdey S, Modzelewski R, Hitzel A, et al. Does recombinant human thyrotropin-stimulated positron emission tomography with [18F]fluoro-2-deoxy-D-glucose improve detection of recurrence of well-differentiated thyroid carcino a in patients with low serum thyroglobulin? Thyroid. 2010;20:15–23.

88. Deichen JT, Schmidt C, Prante O, et al. Influence of TSH on uptake of [18F]fluorodeoxyglucose in human thyroid cells in vitro. Eur J Nucl Med Mol Imaging. 2004;31:507–12.
89. Mruck S, Pfahlberg A, Papadopoulos T, et al. Uptake of 201TI into primary cell cultures from human thyroid tissue is multiplied by TSH. J Nucl Med. 2002;43:145–52.
90. Chin BB, Patel P, Chhade C, et al. Recombinant human thyrotropin stimulation of fluoro-d-glucose positron emission tomography uptake in well-differentiated thyroid carcinoma. J Clin Endocrinol Metab. 2004;89:91–5.
91. Petrich T, Borner AR, Otto D, et al. Influence of rhTSH on [18-F] fluorodeoxyglucose uptake by differentiated thyroid carcinoma. Eur J Nucl Med Mol Imag. 2002;29:641–7.
92. Moog F, Linke R, Manthey N, et al. Influence of thyroid-stimulating hormone levels on uptake of FDG in recurrent and metastatic differentiated thyroid carcinoma. J Nucl Med. 2000;41:1989–95.
93. van Tol KM, Jager PL, Piers DA, et al. Better yield of 18-fluorodeoxyglucose-positron emission tomography in patients with metastatic differentiated thyroid carcinoma during thyrotropin stimulation. Thyroid. 2002;12:381–7.
94. Ma C, Xie J, Lou Y, Gao Y, Zuo S, Wang X. The role of TSH for 18F-FDG-PET in the diagnosis of recurrence and metastases of differentiated thyroid carcinoma with elevated thyroglobulin and negative scan: a meta-analysis. Eur J Endocrinol. 2010;163(2):177–83.
95. Kasner DL, Spieth ME, Starkman ME, Zdor-North D. Iodine-131negative whole body scan reverses to positive after a combination thyrogen stimulation and withdrawal. Clin Nucl Med. 2002;27:772–80.
96. Morris JC, Kim CK, Padilla MLK, et al. Conversion of non-iodine concentrating differentiated thyroid carcinoma metastases into iodine-concentrating foci after anticancer chemotherapy. Thyroid. 1997;7:63–6.
97. Lodish M, Dagalakis U, Chen CC, Sinaii N, Whitcomb P, Aikin A, et al. 111-In-octreotide scintigraphy for identification of metastatic medullary thyroid carcinoma in children and adolescents. J Clin Endocrinol Metab. 2012;97:E207–12.
98. Baudin E, Schlumberger M, Lumbroso J, et al. Octreotide scintigraphy in patients with differentiated thyroid carcinoma: contribution for patients with negative radioiodine scan. J Clin Endocrinol Metab. 1996;81:2541–4.
99. Haslinghuis LM, Krenning EP, De Herder WW, et al. Somatostatin receptor scintigraphy in the follow-up of patients with differentiated thyroid cancer. J Endocrinol Invest. 2001;24:415–22.
100. Margulies DJ, Blum M. Somatostatin receptor scintigraphy as a potential diagnostic and treatment modality for thyroid follicular-cell derived cancers. Thyroid. 2010;20:671–2.
101. Teunissen JJ, Kwekkeboom DJ, Kooij PP, Bakker W, Krenning EP. Peptide receptor radionuclide therapy for non-radioiodine-avid differentiated thyroid cancer. J Nucl Med. 2005;46 Suppl 1:107S–14.
102. Stokkel MP, Reigman HI, Verkooijen RB, Smit JW. Indium-11Octreotide scintigraphy in differentiated thyroid carcinoma metastases that do not respond to treatment with high-dose I-131. J Cancer Res Clin Oncol. 2003;129:287–94.
103. Sarlis NJ, Gourgiotis L, Guthrie LC, et al. In-111 DTPA-octreotide scintigraphy for disease detection in metastatic thyroid cancer: comparison with F-18 FDG PET and extensive conventional radiographic imaging. Clin Nucl Med. 2003;28:208–17.
104. Sager S, Kabasakal L, Halac M, Maecke H, Uslu L, Onsel C, Kanmaz B. Comparison of 99mTc-HYNIC-TATE octreotide scintigraphy with FSG PET and 99mTc-MIBI in local recurrent or distant metastatic thyroid cancers. Clin Nucl Med. 2013;38:321–5.
105. Middendorp M, Selkinski I, Happel C, Kranert WT, Grunwald F. Comparison of positron emission tomography with [(18)F]FDG and [968] Ga] DOTATOC in recurrent differentiated thyroid cancer: preliminary data. Q J Nucl Med Mol Imag. 2010;54:76–83.
106. Durante C, Filetti S. Management of papillary thyroid cancer patients in absence of postoperative radioiodine remnant ablation: tailoring follow-up by neck sonography. J Clin Endocrinol Metab. 2011;96:3059–61.
107. Ito Y, Amino N, Miyauchi A. Thyroid ultrasonography. World J Surg. 2010;34:1171–80.
108. Pacini F, Molinaro E, Castagna MG, et al. Recombinant human thyrotropin-stimulated serum thyroglobulin combined with neck ultrasonography has the highest sensitivity in monitoring differentiated thyroid carcinoma. J Clin Endocrinol Metab. 2003;88: 3668–73.
109. Alzahrani AS, Raef H, Sultan A, et al. Impact of cervical lymph node dissection on serum TG and the course of disease in TG-positive, radioactive iodine whole body scan-negative recurrent/persistent papillary thyroid cancer. J Endocrinol Invest. 2002;25:526–31.
110. Karwowski JK, Jeffrey B, McDougall IR, Weigel RJ. Intraoperative ultrasonography improves identification of recurrent thyroid cancer. Surgery. 2002;132:924–9.
111. Agrawal A, Hall NC, Ringel MD, Povoski SP, Martin Jr EW. Combined use of perioperative TSH-stimulated (18)F-FDG PET/CT imaging and gamma probe radio-guided surgery to localize and verify resection of iodine scan-negative recurrent thyroid carcinoma. Laryngoscope. 2008;118(12):2190–4.
112. Cherk MH, Francis P, Topliss DJ, Bailey M, Kalff V. Incidence and implications of negative serum thyroglobulin but positive I-131 whole-body scans in patients with well-differentiated thyroid cancer prepared with rhTSH or thyroid hormone withdrawal. Clin Endocrinol. 2012;76(5):734–40.
113. Giovanella L, Suriano S, Ceriani L, Verburg FA. Undetectable thyroglobulin in patients with differentiated thyroid carcinoma and residual radioiodine uptake on a postablation whole-body scan. Clin Nucl Med. 2011;36(2):109–12.
114. Park EK, Chung JK, Lim IH, do Park J, Lee DS, Lee MC, Cho BY. Recurrent/metastatic thyroid carcinomas false negative for serum thyroglobulin but positive by posttherapy I-131 whole body scans. Europ J Nucl Med Molec Imag. 2009;36(2):172–9.
115. Lim D-J, O JH, Kim M-H, Kim J-H, Kwon H-S, Kim S-H, et al. Clinical significance of observation without repeated radioiodine therapy in differentiated thyroid carcinoma patients with positive surveillance whole-body scans and negative thyroglobulin. Korean J Intern Med. 2010;25:408–14.
116. Nygaard B, Bentzen J, Laurberg P, Pedersen SM, Bastholt L, Handberg A, et al. Large discrepancy in the results of sensitive measurements of thyroglobulin antibodies in the follow-up on thyroid cancer: a diagnostic dilemma. Eur Thyroid J. 2012;1:193–7.
117. Giovanella L. False-negative thyroglobulin measurement in recurrent/metastatic thyroid carcinomas. Eur J Nucl Med Mol Imag. 2009;36(2):326–7. author reply 328 [Letter].
118. Schlumberger MJ. Papillary and follicular thyroid carcinoma. N Engl J Med. 1998;338:297–306.
119. Schlumberger M, Hay ID. Use of radioactive iodine in patients with papillary and follicular thyroid cancer. J Clin Endocrinol Metab. 1998;83:4195–203.
120. van Tol KM, Jager PL, deVries EG, et al. Outcome in patients with differentiated thyroid cancer with negative diagnostic whole-body scanning and detectable stimulated thyroglobulin. Eur J Endocrinol. 2003;148:589–96.
121. Kabasakal L, Selcuk NA, Shafipour H, et al. Treatment of iodine-negative thyroglobulin-positive thyroid cancer; differences in outcome in patients with macrometastases and patients with micrometastases. Eur J Nucl Med Mol Imag. 2004;31:1500–4.
122. Kamel N, Corapcioglu D, Sahin M, et al. I-131 therapy for thyroglobulin positive patients without anatomical evidence of persistent disease. J Endocrinol Invest. 2004;27:949–53.

Prognosis in Papillary Thyroid Cancer

48

Henry B. Burch

Determinants of Survival in Papillary Thyroid Cancer

What features distinguish the rare patient with rapidly progressive and ultimately fatal papillary thyroid cancer from the more typical patient with an essentially normal survival? Prognostication in papillary thyroid cancer has been facilitated by the recognition of clinical and pathological features that correlate with the risk of recurrence and death from disease (Table 48.1). Numerous retrospective analyses have identified patient age older than 40–50 years, tumor size larger than 4 cm, advanced tumor grade, male sex, local tumor invasion beyond the thyroid capsule, and distant metastatic disease as having a negative impact on survival [1–5].

The Mayo Clinic provided a detailed accounting of 1500 consecutive cases of papillary thyroid cancer receiving care over 40 years [2]. The 20-year cancer-specific mortality in this cohort was 0.8 % for patients less than 50 years of age, 7 % for patients 50–59 years of age, 20 % for patients 60–69 years of age, and 47 % for patients aged 70 or higher. Likewise, mortality from thyroid cancer increased with the size of the tumor, with a 20-year mortality of 0.8 % for patients with tumors less than 2.0 cm in diameter, 6 % for tumors 2.0–3.9 cm, 16 % for tumors 4.0–6.9 cm, and 50 % for tumors greater than 7 cm. Patients with tumors extending through the thyroid capsule had a 20-year mortality of 28 %, compared to only 1.9 % of patients with tumor confined to the thyroid. The worst outcome occurred in patients with distant metastases at presentation, for whom the 10-year cancer mortality was 69 %, compared to 3 % in those patients with tumors confined to the neck. Overall mortality from thyroid cancer was 9 % for men and 4 % for women.

Mazzaferri has reported long-term follow-up on a large cohort of differentiated thyroid cancer patients, with longest follow-up now at 40 years [1, 3]. Although the cohort analysis includes patients with follicular thyroid cancer (21 % of patients in 1994), a great deal of useful information has been gleaned from this series and recently updated [1]. For the patients with papillary thyroid cancer, the overall recurrence rate at 30 years was 31 %, and the disease-specific death rate was 6 % [3]. Age at diagnosis was an important determinant of disease-specific mortality, with a 1.8 % death rate for patients less than 40 years old, 12 % for patients greater than 40 years old, and 21 % for patients greater than 50 years old at diagnosis [3]. Tumor size was an also predictive of recurrence and death, with size less than 1.5 cm yielding a recurrence rate of 11 % and tumor-specific death rate of 0.4 %, compared to 33 % and 7 %, respectively, for patients with tumors greater than 1.5 cm at diagnosis.

A series of 810 patients with papillary thyroid cancer seen at Memorial Sloan-Kettering Cancer Center from 1930 to 1985 has been examined for prognostic factors and reported in 1996, after a median follow-up duration of 20 years [5]. Patients less than 45 years old had a 4 % disease-specific death rate at 20 years, compared to 27 % in those aged greater than or equal to 45 years old. Local extension of tumor into the surrounding neck structures was associated with a 61 % cancer death rate at 20 years, compared to only 5 % in patients with no local extension, and patients with distant metastases had a 54 % cancer death rate at 20 years. Other significant predictors of mortality by multivariate analysis were tumor size greater than 4 cm and male gender, but not multifocality or positive lymph nodes. A unique feature of this paper involved the description of an intermediate-risk group, defined as either an age less than 45 but tumor greater than 4 cm or age greater than 45 but tumor less than 4 cm and without local invasion or distant metastases. These two groups of patients together comprised 39 % of all patients and appeared to have an intermediate risk of death

Disclaimer: The opinions expressed in this paper reflect the personal views of the authors and not the official views of the US Army or the Department of Defense.

H.B. Burch, MD FACE (✉)
Endocrinology Division, Uniformed Services University of the Health Sciences, Walter Reed National Military Medical Center, 8901 Wisconsin Avenue American Building, Room 5053, Bethesda, MD 20889, USA
e-mail: Henry.burch@med.navy.mil

L. Wartofsky, D. Van Nostrand (eds.), *Thyroid Cancer*, DOI 10.1007/978-1-4939-3314-3_48

Table 48.1 Consistently poor prognostic factors for papillary thyroid cancer

Patient age >40 at diagnosis
Large tumors (>4. 0 cm)
Male sex
Advanced tumor grade
Tumors with local extension
Distant metastases

(8 % at 20 years compared to 1 % for the lowest risk patients and 57 % for high risk patients) that was independent of patient age.

Lastly, a series of 269 patients with papillary thyroid cancer followed an average of 12 years after diagnosis at the University of Chicago found an overall recurrence rate of 25 % and a cancer death rate of 8.2 % [4]. Considering death from thyroid cancer, age greater than 45 years was associated with a 32-fold increased risk, a tumor larger than 3.0 cm with a 5.8-fold increased risk, extrathyroidal extension with a 7.7-fold increased risk, and distant metastases with a 47-fold increased risk of death from disease.

Although this discussion has focused on cause-specific *mortality* from thyroid cancer, many of the same prognostic indicators cited in this section are also predictive of local recurrences and distant metastases [2, 6]. Kaplan-Meier disease-specific and disease-free survival curves for differentiated thyroid cancer are shown in Fig. 48.1, indicating a low mortality, but relatively high recurrence rate in patients with this disease [7].

Determinants of Recurrence in Papillary Thyroid Cancer

In 2009, the ATA proposed a staging system for persistent or recurrent disease that classifies patients into low-, intermediate-, or high-risk categories [8]. In this system, low-risk patients are those with no known residual tumor, no local extension or metastatic disease, and no aggressive histology. Intermediate-risk patients have a history of microscopic local invasion, prior regional metastatic disease to lymph nodes, or have aggressive histology, such as the tall-cell variant. High-risk patients have persistent unresectable tumor, gross local invasion, or distant metastases. A retrospective study of 588 patients with DTC with a median follow-up of 7 years validated the ATA recurrence classification system and further demonstrated that re-stratification based on initial response to therapy allowed a more accurate prediction of persistent structural disease during subsequent follow-up [9]. As shown in Fig. 48.2, 13 % of patients deemed low risk by ATA criteria had structural evidence of disease at subsequent follow-up if their initial response to therapy was incomplete, defined as an unstimulated serum Tg level ≥1.0 ng/mL, stimulated Tg ≥10.0 ng/mL, or if there was structural evidence of disease on cross-sectional imaging during the first 2 years of follow-up. Conversely, only 14 % of patients classified by the ATA system as being at high risk of recurrence had structural disease at subsequent follow-up if their initial response to therapy was excellent, defined as a stimulated Tg <1.0 ng/mL and no structural evidence of disease in the first 2 years of follow-up, but this rate increased to 79 % in patients with an incomplete response. Although it is intuitive that patients with structural disease in the first 2 years will be more likely to have structural disease during subsequent follow-up, this study formalizes the practice of ongoing risk assessment based on response to initial therapy.

Effect of Treatment on Outcome

The extent of initial therapy for papillary thyroid cancer has value for predicting tumor recurrence and cancer-related death. In a study including 1077 patients with papillary thyroid cancer and 278 with follicular thyroid cancer, patients with tumors greater than 1.5 cm and no distant metastases had a 30-year recurrence rate of 26 % and a cancer-related mortality rate of 6 % when treated with total or near-total thyroidectomy, compared to rates of 40 % and 9 %, respectively, for patients treated with less complete surgery [3]. These same authors found that despite having more advanced disease, patients receiving postoperative radioiodine ablation for tumors greater than 1. 5 cm and no distant metastases (stages 2 and 3) had significantly lower rates of tumor recurrence (16 % versus 38 %, $P<0.001$) and cause-specific mortality (3 % versus 9 %, $P=0.03$) than patients not receiving radioiodine ablation [3]. Another study including 269 patients with papillary thyroid cancer followed for an average of 12 years found that patients with tumors greater than 1 cm in diameter had a lower incidence of recurrence and death when a total or near-total thyroidectomy was performed [4]. Likewise, this study determined that postoperative radioiodine ablation resulted in lower rates of recurrence and death from thyroid cancer, although this was of marginal statistical significance and limited to patients with tumors larger than 1 cm and confined to the thyroid or metastatic only to cervical lymph nodes [4]. Not all studies have supported the use of prophylactic radioiodine ablation following surgery for papillary thyroid. In the Mayo Clinic review of 1500 papillary thyroid cancer patients, no difference in recurrence or cause-specific mortality was found between 946 patients treated with surgery alone and 220 patients treated with surgery plus radioiodine ablation [2]. This disparity likely reflects the limitations imposed by the application of retrospective data to judge treatment efficacy for thyroid cancer. Patients treated more aggressively are likely

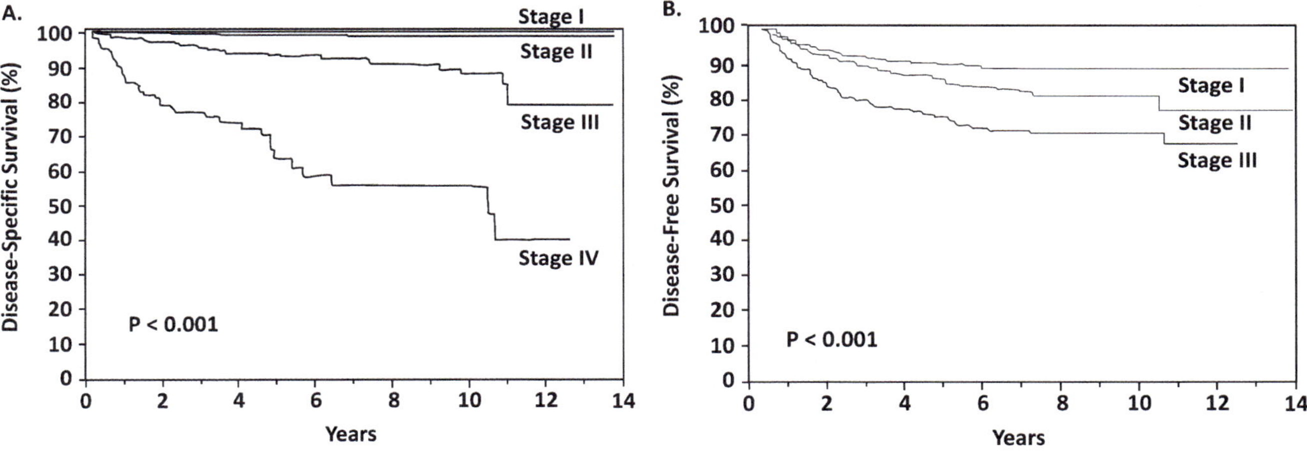

Fig. 48.1 Product-limit estimated disease-specific (**a**) and disease-free (**b**) survival in patients with differentiated thyroid cancer according to National Thyroid Cancer Treatment Cooperative Study Group Registry staging system (Adapted from Jonklass et al. [17])

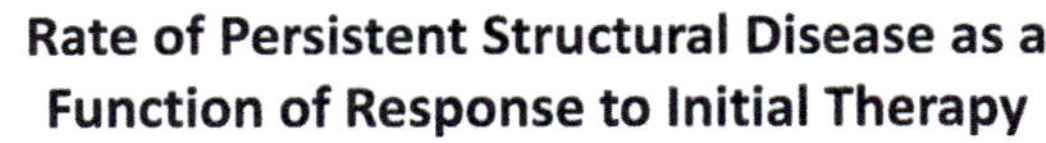

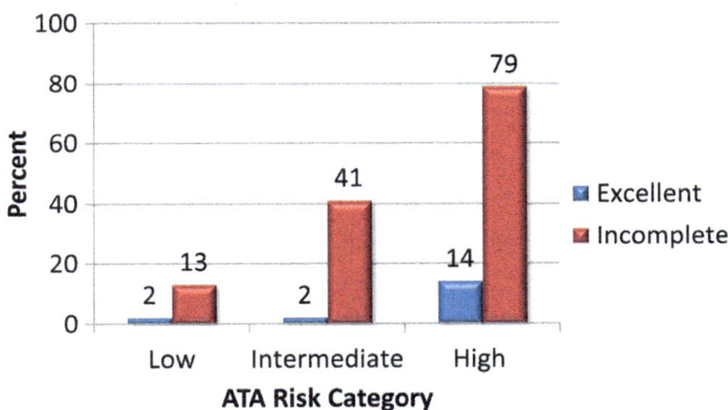

Fig. 48.2 The effect of response to initial therapy on the rate of persistent structural disease in DTC. While it is not unexpected that patients with an inadequate response to therapy will have a higher rate of persistent disease, the analysis by Tuttle et al. [9] gives a quantitative assessment of the magnitude of this effect. Hence, low-risk patients with an unexpectedly poor response to initial therapy have as high a rate of persistent structural disease (13 %) as those high-risk patients who responded to initial therapy (14 %) (Adapted from Tuttle RM et al. [9])

to have been at a higher risk for recurrence and death from disease. This confounding effect would tend to underestimate the benefit of therapy. Conversely, the inclusion of patients receiving radioiodine therapy for known residual disease in an analysis of remnant ablation would tend to overestimate the benefit of the latter practice.

Effect of Tumor Subtype

Although papillary thyroid cancer as a whole has an excellent prognosis, it is evident that certain rare subtypes of this disease have a distinctly poor prognosis. These include the tall cell variant, the columnar variant, and insular pattern thyroid carcinomas as have recently extensively reviewed [10, 11]. The follicular variant of papillary thyroid is a subtype having a microfollicular histological pattern but nuclear features and biological behavior similar to typical papillary thyroid cancer [12]. Papillary microcarcinoma is generally believed to be a more indolent form of thyroid cancer. Two recent series have shown that multifocality and positive lymph nodes in the neck are associated with a higher risk of recurrent disease [13, 14]. A study of more than 18,000 patients with papillary microcarcinoma in the SEER cancer database showed that mortality from this disease, though rare, could be predicted on the basis of clinical features. In this analysis, age greater than 45 years, male sex, minority race, node metastases, extrathyroidal invasion, and distant metastases were each found to be risk factors for increased mortality. Among 49 thyroid cancer-related deaths, 92 % of patients had at least two of these risk factors, and 51 % had three or more risk factors compared to 5.7 % in the rest of the cohort [15]. Another recent study including 445 patients with papillary microcarcinoma found that the presence of capsular invasion, extrathyroidal extension, and positive cervical lymph nodes at the time of diagnosis were each independent risk factors for future local and distant recurrence [16].

References

1. Mazzaferri EL, Kloos RT. Clinical review 128: current approaches to primary therapy for papillary and follicular thyroid cancer. J Clin Endocrinol Metab. 2001;86(4):1447–63.
2. Hay ID. Papillary thyroid carcinoma. Endocrinol Metab Clin North Am. 1990;19(3):545–76.
3. Mazzaferri EL, Jhiang SM. Long-term impact of initial surgical and medical therapy on papillary and follicular thyroid cancer. Am J Med. 1994;97(5):418–28.
4. DeGroot LJ, Kaplan EL, McCormick M, Straus FH. Natural history, treatment, and course of papillary thyroid carcinoma. J Clin Endocrinol Metab. 1990;71(2):414–24.
5. Shaha AR, Shah JP, Loree TR. Risk group stratification and prognostic factors in papillary carcinoma of thyroid. Ann Surg Oncol. 1996;3(6):534–8.
6. Ain KB. Papillary thyroid carcinoma. Etiology, assessment, and therapy. Endocrinol Metab Clin North Am. 1995;24(4):711–60.
7. Jonklaas J, Sarlis NJ, Litofsky D, et al. Outcomes of patients with differentiated thyroid carcinoma following initial therapy. Thyroid. 2006;16(12):1229–42.
8. American Thyroid Association Guidelines Task Force on Thyroid Nodules and Differentiated Thyroid Cancer. Haugen BR, Alexander EK, Bible KC, Doherty GM, Mandel SJ, Nikiforov YE, Pacini F, Randolph GW, Sawka AM, Schlumberger M, Schuff KG, Sherman SI, Sosa JA, Steward DL, Tuttle RM, Wartofsky L. 2015 American Thyroid Association Management Guidelines for Adult Patients with Thyroid Nodules and Differentiated Thyroid Cancer. Thyroid. 2016;26:1–133.
9. Tuttle RM, Tala H, Shah J, et al. Estimating risk of recurrence in differentiated thyroid cancer after total thyroidectomy and radioactive iodine remnant ablation: using response to therapy variables to modify the initial risk estimates predicted by the new American Thyroid Association staging system. Thyroid. 2010;20:1341–9.
10. Prendiville S, Burman KD, Ringel MD, et al. Tall cell variant: an aggressive form of papillary thyroid carcinoma. Otolaryngol Head Neck Surg. 2000;122(3):352–7.
11. Burman KD, Ringel MD, Wartofsky L. Unusual types of thyroid neoplasms. Endocrinol Metab Clin North Am. 1996;25(1):49–68.
12. Zidan J, Karen D, Stein M, Rosenblatt E, Basher W, Kuten A. Pure versus follicular variant of papillary thyroid carcinoma: clinical features, prognostic factors, treatment, and survival. Cancer. 2003;97(5):1181–5.
13. Hay ID, Hutchinson ME, Gonzalez-Losada T, et al. Papillary thyroid microcarcinoma: a study of 900 cases observed in a 60-year period. Surgery. 2008;144(6):980–7; discussion 987–8.
14. Ross DS, Litofsky D, Ain KB, et al. Recurrence after treatment of micropapillary thyroid cancer. Thyroid. 2009;19(10):1043–8.
15. Yu XM, Wan Y, Sippel RS, Chen H. Should all papillary thyroid microcarcinomas be aggressively treated?: an analysis of 18,445 cases. Ann Surg. 2011;254(4):653–60.
16. Mercante G, Frasoldati A, Pedroni C, Formisano D, et al. Prognostic factors affecting neck lymph node recurrence and distant metastasis in papillary microcarcinoma of the thyroid: results of a study in 445 patients. Thyroid. 2009;19(7):707–16.
17. Jonklaas J, Sarlis NJ, Litofsky D, et al. Outcomes of patients with differentiated thyroid carcinoma following initial therapy. Thyroid. 2006;16(12):1229–42.

49 Surgical Management of Lymph Node Metastases

Gerard M. Doherty

Lymph node metastases are common with some types of thyroid cancer, and less common with others. Papillary thyroid cancer quite commonly includes spread to the lymph nodes at presentation, which can be managed by operative resection, radioiodine therapy, or a combination of both. Papillary adenocarcinoma accounts for 85 % of cancers of the thyroid gland and spreads via intraglandular lymphatics and then to the subcapsular and pericapsular lymph nodes. Follicular adenocarcinoma accounts for approximately 10 % of malignant thyroid tumors and only occasionally (~5 %) metastasize to the regional lymph nodes. Hürthle cell carcinoma behaves as a clinical variant of follicular carcinoma and is more likely to involve lymph nodes than follicular carcinoma. The prognosis is not as good for either follicular or Hürthle cell cancers as with the papillary subtype [1]. Anaplastic thyroid cancer can include nodal metastases, though the lymph node spread is rarely the most significant clinical problem [2].

The treatment of differentiated thyroid carcinoma (which does not include anaplastic carcinoma or medullary thyroid cancer) is operative removal including affected lymph nodes. The management strategy for potential nodal disease depends first upon the identification of the disease when present. All patients with a preoperative diagnosis of differentiated thyroid carcinoma should have a cervical ultrasound examination in order to search for preoperative evidence of central or lateral lymph node metastasis [3]. Suspicious lymph nodes can be confirmed as thyroid cancer by ultrasound-guided aspiration for cytologic analysis and thyroglobulin measurement. The preoperative documentation of nodal disease allows the patient and the surgeon to plan appropriate intervention. If the staging ultrasound does not show node metastases, then there should be an active evaluation of the central (level 6) lymph nodes during operation for evidence of metastasis.

Patients who have affected lymph nodes should have clearance of any involved lymph node compartment known to contain metastatic disease [1]. More limited lymphadenectomy removing only the grossly involved nodes has an unacceptable rate of in-compartment recurrence. Patients known to have lateral (levels 2–5) node metastasis should have a central (level 6) dissection as a part of the procedure. The role of central neck node dissection in the absence of proven metastasis is controversial however. Some data have suggested that prophylactic dissection can improve disease-specific survival [4] local recurrence [5, 6], and posttreatment thyroglobulin levels [5, 7]. It may be that the best current uses of staging lymphadenectomy are to determine the use of adjuvant RAI [8–11] and to estimate the risk of recurrence [10, 12, 13]. If there is a difference in long-term outcome due to prophylactic dissection, then the difference is small, while the additional dissection increases the temporary hypocalcemia [11, 14–17].

The use of staging information for the planning of adjuvant therapy depends upon whether this information will affect the team-based decision-making for the individual patient [18, 19]. For these reasons, groups may elect to include prophylactic dissection in the presence of prognostic features associated with an increased risk of metastasis and recurrence (such as older or very young age, larger tumor size, multifocal disease, extrathyroidal extension) to contribute to decision-making and disease control [5, 7, 19]. In other situations, treatment teams may apply prophylactic level 6 dissection to patients with better prognostic features if the patient is to have a bilateral thyroidectomy and if the nodal staging information will be used to determine adjuvant therapy or follow-up planning [8–10]. Finally, for some groups it appears reasonable to use a selective approach that applies level 6 lymph node dissection at the time of initial operation only to patients with clinically evident disease based on preoperative physical exam, preoperative radiographic evaluation, or intraoperative demonstration of detectable disease [20–22].

G.M. Doherty, MD, FACS (✉)
Department of Surgery, Boston Medical Center, Boston University, 88 East Newton Street Collamore Building Suite 500, Boston, MA 02118, USA
e-mail: dohertyg@bu.edu

L. Wartofsky, D. Van Nostrand (eds.), *Thyroid Cancer*, DOI 10.1007/978-1-4939-3314-3_49

References

1. Cooper DS, et al. Revised American Thyroid Association management guidelines for patients with thyroid nodules and differentiated thyroid cancer. Thyroid. 2009;19(11):1167–214.
2. Smallridge RC, et al. American Thyroid Association guidelines for management of patients with anaplastic thyroid cancer. Thyroid. 2012;22(11):1104–39.
3. Kouvaraki MA, et al. Role of preoperative ultrasonography in the surgical management of patients with thyroid cancer. Surgery. 2003;134(6):946–54; discussion 954–5.
4. Barczynski M, et al. Prophylactic central neck dissection for papillary thyroid cancer. Br J Surg. 2013;100(3):410–8.
5. Popadich A, et al. A multicenter cohort study of total thyroidectomy and routine central lymph node dissection for cN0 papillary thyroid cancer. Surgery. 2011;150(6):1048–57.
6. Hartl DM, et al. Influence of prophylactic neck dissection on rate of retreatment for papillary thyroid carcinoma. World J Surg. 2013; 37(8):1951–8.
7. Sywak M, et al. Routine ipsilateral level VI lymphadenectomy reduces postoperative thyroglobulin levels in papillary thyroid cancer. Surgery. 2006;140(6):1000–5; discussion 1005–7.
8. Bonnet S, et al. Prophylactic lymph node dissection for papillary thyroid cancer less than 2 cm: implications for radioiodine treatment. J Clin Endocrinol Metab. 2009;94(4):1162–7.
9. Hartl DM, et al. Optimization of staging of the neck with prophylactic central and lateral neck dissection for papillary thyroid carcinoma. Ann Surg. 2012;255(4):777–83.
10. Laird AM, et al. Evaluation of postoperative radioactive iodine scans in patients who underwent prophylactic central lymph node dissection. World J Surg. 2012;36(6):1268–73.
11. Wang TS, et al. Effect of prophylactic central compartment neck dissection on serum thyroglobulin and recommendations for adjuvant radioactive iodine in patients with differentiated thyroid cancer. Ann Surg Oncol. 2012;19(13):4217–22.
12. Costa S, et al. Role of prophylactic central neck dissection in cN0 papillary thyroid cancer. Acta Otorhinolaryngol Ital. 2009; 29(2):61–9.
13. Ryu IS, et al. Lymph node ratio of the central compartment is a significant predictor for locoregional recurrence after prophylactic central neck dissection in patients with thyroid papillary carcinoma. Ann Surg Oncol. 2014;21(1):277–83.
14. Chisholm EJ, Kulinskaya E, Tolley NS. Systematic review and meta-analysis of the adverse effects of thyroidectomy combined with central neck dissection as compared with thyroidectomy alone. Laryngoscope. 2009;119(6):1135–9.
15. Hughes DT, et al. Influence of prophylactic central lymph node dissection on postoperative thyroglobulin levels and radioiodine treatment in papillary thyroid cancer. Surgery. 2010;148(6):1100–6; discussion 1006–7.
16. Lang BH, et al. Impact of routine unilateral central neck dissection on preablative and postablative stimulated thyroglobulin levels after total thyroidectomy in papillary thyroid carcinoma. Ann Surg Oncol. 2012;19(1):60–7.
17. Raffaelli M, et al. Prospective evaluation of total thyroidectomy versus ipsilateral versus bilateral central neck dissection in patients with clinically node-negative papillary thyroid carcinoma. Surgery. 2012;152(6):957–64.
18. Zetoune T, et al. Prophylactic central neck dissection and local recurrence in papillary thyroid cancer: a meta-analysis. Ann Surg Oncol. 2010;17(12):3287–93.
19. Sancho JJ, et al. Prophylactic central neck disection in papillary thyroid cancer: a consensus report of the European Society of Endocrine Surgeons (ESES). Langenbecks Arch Surg. 2014; 399(2):155–63.
20. Randolph GW, et al. The prognostic significance of nodal metastases from papillary thyroid carcinoma can be stratified based on the size and number of metastatic lymph nodes, as well as the presence of extranodal extension. Thyroid. 2012;22(11): 1144–52.
21. Moreno MA, et al. In papillary thyroid cancer, preoperative central neck ultrasound detects only macroscopic surgical disease, but negative findings predict excellent long-term regional control and survival. Thyroid. 2012;22(4):347–55.
22. Gyorki DE, et al. Prophylactic central neck dissection in differentiated thyroid cancer: an assessment of the evidence. Ann Surg Oncol. 2013;20(7):2285–9.

Utility of Second Surgery for Lymph Node Metastases

50

Nancy Marie Carroll

Introduction

Although most patients with differentiated thyroid cancer enjoy long survival, locoregional recurrence is common. Long-term locoregional recurrence after initial treatment of papillary thyroid cancer has been reported in up to 30 % of patients, while nodal recurrence is less common with follicular thyroid cancer [1]. Locoregional recurrence may be associated with morbidity as well as increased long-term mortality [2]. In light of the high incidence of recurrence, how to best manage nodal recurrence is an important issue in the treatment of thyroid cancer patients. This chapter addresses surgery for treatment of nodal recurrence. In general, surgery is suitable treatment when the benefit of surgery outweighs the risk of surgery. The risk of operation for nodal recurrence is low in expert hands, and our focus will be on the potential benefit of surgery as performed at major medical centers. The ideal outcome of surgery is cure. There may be a role for surgery in the palliation of nodal disease, but there is limited literature extant regarding outcomes in terms of palliation. Consequently, the following discussion addresses surgical intervention with intent to cure.

The literature on outcomes of operation for nodal recurrence is challenging to interpret. There are few published studies with large sample size and long follow-up, and the studies are difficult to compare to each other. Challenges in comparing studies largely fall into three categories: differences in patient characteristics, differences in surgical technique, and differences in the method of detection of recurrent disease. These three categories will be discussed in more detail.

N.M. Carroll, MD (✉)
Department of Surgery, MedStar Washington Hospital Center, 106 Irving Street NW, Physicians Office Building Suite 2100, North Tower, Washington, DC 20010, USA
e-mail: nancy.m.carroll@medstar.net

Disparate patient populations have been examined in various studies of series of patients who underwent operation for nodal recurrence. Differences in patient characteristics include differences in histopathology, stage at presentation, initial surgical procedure, whether or not patients received radioactive iodine, and disease-free survival prior to surgery for recurrent disease. There are studies of recurrent papillary carcinoma and studies that consider papillary and follicular recurrence together. Lumping follicular and papillary cancer together makes it impossible to appreciate differences in surgical outcomes between the two tumors which may be substantial given their generally dissimilar biologic behavior. There are no large studies of only recurrent follicular nodal disease likely due to its infrequency. In addition, some papers lump thyroid bed recurrence (from extrathyroidal extension of tumor) and nodal recurrence together. There is evidence that the prognosis of purely nodal disease is better than that of thyroid bed recurrence, and so it may be misleading to not distinguish between the two when assessing outcomes of reoperative surgery [3, 4]. There is also evidence that extranodal extension is associated with aggressive disease biology [5]. While many papers on surgical treatment of nodal recurrence note the number of nodes resected and the number harboring tumor, most do not comment on extranodal extension. As a result, the efficacy or impact on outcomes of resection of recurrent nodal disease is unknown.

Different surgical techniques have been utilized in studies of operative treatment of nodal recurrence. These have ranged from targeted surgery in which only the involved node is resected to significantly more extensive surgery in which lymph nodes in the cervical compartment with the recurrence and adjacent compartments are resected. Variability in reported results is the consequence of different surgeons having distinct approaches which they believe are minimizing morbidity while maximizing oncologic benefit. But such approaches are being performed in the absence of long-term outcome data establishing the best approach. Clearance of entire nodal compartments is generally favored

L. Wartofsky, D. Van Nostrand (eds.), *Thyroid Cancer*, DOI 10.1007/978-1-4939-3314-3_50

to minimize the chance of needing to operate again in a previously violated field. In addition, surgery has been performed with and without instruments such as intraoperative ultrasound or gamma probe isotope detectors to assist with intraoperative localization of tumor that may also impact the efficacy of surgery.

Further, published reports on the efficacy of surgery for nodal recurrence vary in how the recurrence was detected. This is an issue both in terms of when in the disease course patients were operated on for recurrent disease and how patients were classified after the surgery. Early studies used relatively crude parameters such as physical examination to detect recurrence, while more recent studies have applied more sensitive methods, such as assessment of suppressed and thyrotropin-stimulated thyroglobulin (Tg) levels and high-resolution ultrasound. It is likely that many patients in earlier studies were treated for nodal recurrence later in their disease course than were patients in more recent studies. While there are some limited data that show that a delay in the primary treatment of thyroid cancer has a negative impact on outcome [1], little is known about how delay in the treatment of recurrent nodal disease may affect outcome. In addition, the reported success rates of surgery for nodal recurrence are impacted by how thoroughly evaluated the patients were for residual or recurrent disease after the surgery. It is likely that many patients described as "free of disease" in older published series using insensitive markers would be labeled as "alive with disease" using today's diagnostic tools. The literature must be interpreted with an appreciation of how methods used to assess patients after surgery for recurrent disease may affect reported outcome.

Despite these challenges, much can be learned from the recent literature on the surgical treatment of nodal recurrence. The literature will be reviewed in chronologic order to emphasize evolution and hopefully refinements, in our surgical approaches to nodal recurrence.

Reoperative Lymph Node Surgery in the 1990s

In 1994, Coburn et al. reported a retrospective study of the survival of 74 patients with recurrent differentiated thyroid cancer diagnosed by I^{131} scan or clinical examination and chest radiograph [6]. The outcomes of patients with recurrence detected exclusively by I^{131} scan were compared to patients with clinically detected recurrence. Patients with solely scintigraphically detected disease fared better than those with clinical recurrence. Among the clinically detected cases, treatment with surgery alone was compared to surgery plus I^{131} treatment. Among clinically detected recurrences, 12 of 21 patients (57 %) treated with surgery alone had no evidence of disease at last follow-up, while the other 9 died of disease. Three of 15 patients (20 %) treated with I^{131} and surgery were without evidence of disease at last follow-up, 7 were dead of disease, and 5 were alive with disease. No data were provided regarding the characteristics of the surgery alone group versus the surgery plus radioiodine group. The worse outcome in the surgery plus radioiodine group may have been due to selection bias. Tg levels were not reported in the study.

In 1998, Travagli et al. reported using preoperative radioiodine to improve the completeness of surgical excision of persistent or recurrent differentiated thyroid carcinoma [7]. All the patients in the study had previously undergone thyroid surgery and had received radioiodine after the initial surgery. Sixty-one percent had undergone lymph node dissection. The mean time that had elapsed between initial treatment and inclusion in the study was 5 years. Fifty-four sequential patients with functioning lymph node metastases received 100 mCi ^{131}I on day zero and then underwent total-body scintigraphy on day 4. Subsequently, surgery was performed using an intraoperative gamma probe to detect radioiodine-avid lesions. Surgery consisted of complete dissection of previously undissected areas and excision of neoplastic foci only in previously dissected areas. A postoperative scan was performed on day 7. The use of the intraoperative probe was considered decisive in 20 patients as neoplastic foci were found inside sclerotic foci due to previous surgery, at unusual sites, or both. In 26 patients the probe facilitated detection of neoplastic foci. Lymph node metastases undetected by preoperative radioiodine scan or the probe were found in excised tissue in 14 patients on histologic examination supporting the performance of en bloc dissection in spite of the use of the probe. The patients were followed for a mean of 2.3 years after the probe-guided surgery. An annual clinical neck examination was normal in all patients. Tg levels were measured in 47 patients on TSH suppression three or more months after surgery. Tg levels were undetectable in 41 patients and ranged from 2 to 10 ng/ml in the other 6. Postoperative stimulated Tg levels were measured in 33 patients. They were undetectable in 25 patients, ranged from 1 to 10 ng/ml in 4 patients, and ranged from 11 to 55 ng/ml in 4 patients. Isotopic scanning techniques have been criticized for exposing patients to additional radiation dose solely for localization (as opposed to therapy) and are not widely adopted.

Reoperative Lymph Node Surgery in the 2000s

In 2002, Karwowski et al. reported the utility of intraoperative ultrasound in identifying and subsequently treating 13 patients with recurrent thyroid cancer [8]. Nodal and local (thyroid bed) recurrences were included in the study.

Recurrence was not palpable preoperatively in 12 patients. Eleven patients had complete resections and two patients were not completely resected due to local invasion. Ultrasound was required for identification of tumor in seven patients including all patients with a history of external beam radiotherapy and in patients with tumors 20 mm or less in maximal diameter. Of 11 patients with detectable Tg on suppression preoperatively, the level declined in 10 patients and became undetectable in 7 postoperatively. Intraoperative ultrasound has been more widely adopted than the gamma probe.

In the same year Alzahrani et al. reported an assessment of the impact of node dissection on the course of disease in papillary thyroid cancer patients with an elevated Tg but a negative radioiodine scan [9]. Twenty-one patients developed an elevated (greater than 10 ng/ml) Tg after initial surgery and radioactive iodine ablative therapy. All patients had a negative radioiodine scan, but the presence of recurrent/persistent disease was confirmed by ultrasound-guided FNA. The second surgery consisted of unilateral (13) or bilateral (8) modified neck dissection. The mean stimulated Tg prior to neck re-exploration was 184.8 ng/ml and declined after surgery to 127.5 ng/ml. Only four patients (19 %) achieved remission (simulated Tg less than 10 ng/ml with negative whole-body scan); the others received radioiodine treatment, external beam radiotherapy, or additional surgery (five patients). Thirteen patients continued to have persistent disease, while four demonstrated progressive disease. The mean follow-up after the second surgery was 20.7 months. Of note, poorly differentiated carcinoma was seen in none of the node dissection specimens on pathologic exam.

In 2003 Gemsenjager et al. reported a retrospective analysis of 156 patients with papillary thyroid cancer treated for cure by one surgeon [10]. Eight of the patients suffered nodal recurrence. Treatment of nodal recurrence was surgery and radioiodine, with external beam radiation administered to one patient. Two of the eight patients with nodal recurrence died, one from locoregional disease and the other with pulmonary metastases. One patient was living with regional disease at last follow-up. Details on how recurrence was detected were not provided.

In 2004 Bin Yousef et al. reported the utility of preoperative ultrasonographic mapping in treating patients with recurrent papillary thyroid cancer [11]. All patients had undergone total thyroidectomy and had received radioactive iodine. Forty-four percent of the patients had lymph node dissections at the time of initial surgery. Subsequently, the patients developed recurrent disease and presented for additional surgery. Nineteen patients who underwent regional neck dissection before the introduction of preoperative ultrasonographic mapping at the institution were compared to 26 patients who had limited lymph node resection guided by ultrasonographic mapping the morning of surgery. In the preoperative mapping group, exploration was limited to the areas with abnormal ultrasound findings, as opposed to exploring the whole affected compartment. The resected lesions were positive for papillary thyroid cancer in 89.5 % of the patients treated without preoperative mapping and 96.2 % of the patients who underwent preoperative mapping. Postoperatively, neck ultrasound became negative in 50 % of the patients without preoperative mapping and in 83.3 % of the patients who underwent preoperative mapping. Tg became undetectable in 37.5 % of the unmapped group and in 52.3 % of the mapped group. Whole-body iodine scans became negative in 16.7 % of the unmapped group and in 75 % of the mapped group. At a mean follow-up of 23.8 months, 31.6 % of the unmapped group was in remission (no clinical evidence of disease, negative whole-body scan, undetectable unstimulated Tg or stimulated Tg ≤ (less than or equal to) 5 ng/dL). At a mean follow-up of 9.8 months, 62.5 % of the mapped group was in remission. Though the follow-up is short, it appeared that the use of ultrasound for preoperative mapping contributed to improved results.

In 2005 Kloos and Mazzaferri reported a group of 107 differentiated thyroid carcinoma patients [12] who were studied to determine the accuracy of a single rhTSH-stimulated Tg level in predicting differentiated thyroid carcinoma metastases over time (3–5 years), but the data is also informative regarding the outcome of patients who underwent surgery for nodal recurrence. The patients were free of disease on the basis of clinical exam, imaging studies, and one or more undetectable or low (below 1 ng/ml) Tg measurements on suppression after initial therapy (total or near total thyroidectomy with (28 %) or without (72 %) lymph node dissection and then radioiodine therapy). The median time from initial surgery to the first round of recombinant thyrotropin-stimulated Tg measurement was 3.3 years. Patients were stratified according to their initial recombinant human thyrotropin-stimulated Tg. Group 1 had Tg less than 0.5 ng/ml, group 2 had Tg 0.6–2.0 ng/ml, and group 3 had Tg greater than 2 ng/ml. Subsequent evaluations included Tg levels drawn during thyroid hormone suppression, after recombinant human thyrotropin administration, and/or after thyroid hormone withdrawal. Patients were categorized as being free of disease if neck ultrasound was negative and they had either (1) one or more stimulated Tg levels less than 0.5 ng/ml or (2) at least two subsequent Tg levels on thyroid hormone less than 0.5 ng/ml six or more months apart. Imaging studies were performed as indicated, usually when the Tg was elevated and neck ultrasound was negative. Six patients were lost to follow-up early in the study. One of 63 patients in group 1 developed lateral adenopathy, underwent neck dissection, and was without evidence of disease at last follow-up. The rest of the group 1 patients had no evidence of disease at the end of the study. In group 2 (18 patients), 5 patients demonstrated a rise in stimulated Tg during the study. In four of these patients, no tumor was found. One patient had a positive neck ultrasound and underwent excision of malignant central nodes. At last follow-up the patient was without radiographic evidence of disease but had an elevated Tg. In group 3 (20 patients), 9 patients had persistent tumor identified at the start of the study. Four of these patients underwent surgery for cervical nodal disease. Two of these patients also received radioiodine. All four patients were without evidence of disease at the end of the study. Tumor was found in seven more group 3 patients during the study. Four of these patients underwent resection of central nodes. One patient received radioiodine in addition to surgery. Three of the four patients were without radiologic evidence of disease at the end of the study, and one patient's status was unknown. Two of the three patients without radiologic evidence of disease had detectable stimulated Tg (2.2 and 1.5 ng/ml) by the end of the follow-up period. Overall this study demonstrates the potential for good short-term results for surgery in the treatment of nodal recurrence in selected patients.

In 2007 Roh et al. investigated the utility of central neck dissection in 22 patients who underwent reoperation for lateral nodal recurrence of papillary thyroid cancer [13]. None of the patients had undergone central neck dissection at their initial surgery, while 27 % of the patients had a lateral neck dissection at initial surgery. Sixteen of the patients had received radioiodine therapy. Preoperative ultrasound examinations suggested central neck recurrence in eight patients. Four patients had recurrent tumors in the thyroid bed and two patients had evidence of lung metastases. Patients underwent comprehensive dissection of the ipsilateral (10) or bilateral (12) central neck in addition to their lateral neck dissection. Central neck nodes were involved in 86 % of patients: 82 % ipsilateral paratracheal, 32 % pretracheal, and 27 % superior mediastinal, and two patients had contralateral central nodal involvement. Lateral recurrence without central nodal involvement (skip metastasis) was observed in 14 % of patients. All patients received postoperative radioiodine therapy. The mean duration of follow-up was 32 months. Twenty of 22 patients were without evidence of disease (not precisely defined) and 2 patients were alive with lung metastases. Mean Tg measured 3.7 ng/mL at 6 months after reoperation and radioiodine therapy, down from a mean of 37 ng/mL preoperatively. There were two cases of permanent hypocalcemia postoperatively. The authors conclude that ipsilateral central and lateral neck dissection are necessary for the treatment of lateral cervical recurrence.

In 2008 Schuff et al. reported a retrospective review of central or lateral lymph node dissections performed for persistent or recurrent papillary thyroid cancer between 2004 and 2006 [14]. All patients had previously undergone total or near total thyroidectomy with or without node dissection, and the majority had received radioiodine ablation. Neck dissections were generally planned to include all compartments with evidence of disease and the compartments immediately adjacent if they had not been dissected previously. For example, if the right central compartment was involved, the right lateral and left central compartments were also dissected. This approach is more extensive than the approach described in most reports of node dissection for recurrent papillary thyroid cancer. Thirty-nine patients had Tg data available to assess response. Sixteen (41 %) resections resulted in "undetectable" postoperative stimulated Tg levels of 2 ng/dL or less. An additional 12 resections resulted in significant (greater than or equal to 50 %) reductions in suppressed or stimulated Tg. The mean number of nodes resected was 31 and the mean number of nodes involved was 6. A high rate of central compartment disease was reported (80 %), and it was unusual to have isolated lateral nodal recurrence without associated central compartment disease (11 %). These findings are similar to those of Roh et al. [13]. No clinical, pathologic, or surgical factors were predictive of benefit from surgery by binomial and multinomial logistic regression analysis. Seven percent of patients suffered permanent hypocalcemia postoperatively. The authors postulate that the high incidence of central compartment disease may explain why so many patients undergoing lateral node dissection alone in other series are not free of disease postoperatively. They advocate at least routine ipsilateral central neck dissection in patients undergoing surgery for lateral nodal disease similar to the technique employed by Roh et al. [13].

In 2009 Clayman et al. reported a retrospective analysis of consecutive patients treated by a single surgeon for recurrent papillary thyroid carcinoma in the central compartment over an 18-month period [15]. All the patients had undergone at least a prior thyroidectomy with curative intent from 6 months to 30 years prior to their recurrence. Forty-one percent of the patients had more than one prior surgery. Ninety-two percent of the patients had received one or more doses of radioiodine. Indications for surgery required progressive disease among those patients under 45 years of age (52 % of the patients) with at least one lesion exceeding 1 cm in greatest dimension. Patients who had received external beam radiation and those with only soft tissue or visceral involvement of the central compartment were excluded. Sixty-three patients underwent comprehensive dissection of levels VI and VII. Ninety-seven percent of the patients had a lateral or bilateral neck dissection in addition to the central compartment dissection. The resections were oncologically complete in all but two patients. The median number of nodes resected was 16 (range 3–52) with 7 (1–20) pathologic nodes. Soft tissue metastases or extracapsular spread from lymph nodes was present in 65 % of patients. Although postoperative Tg levels were reported as non-detectable in 71 % of informative cases, the specifics of the postoperative Tg assessments were not provided as the paper focused on surgical technique and complications.

Results of Reoperative Lymph Node Surgery Reported in the 2010s

In 2010, Al-Saif et al. reported the results of a retrospective study of the outcome of surgical resection of metastatic papillary thyroid cancer in cervical lymph nodes after the failure of initial surgery and I^{131} therapy (with or without nodal dissection) [16]. Seventy Tg antibody-negative patients underwent neck reoperation from 1999 to 2005. The median time from initial thyroidectomy to reoperation for recurrent disease was 3 years. The majority of the patients had nodal metastases and capsular invasion by tumor at the initial thyroid surgery. Biochemical complete remission was defined as undetectable TSH-stimulated Tg. Two different Tg assays were used in the study, one with a functional sensitivity of 0.5 ng/ml and the other with a functional sensitivity of 0.9 ng/ml. Biochemical complete remission was achieved initially in 12 patients (17 %). The median number of lymph nodes removed after the first reoperation was 11 (range 1–61) with median positive histology in 2 (range 0–11). Of the 58 patients with detectable post-reoperation Tg, 28 had a second reoperation, and a biochemical complete response was achieved in five (18 %). The median number of lymph nodes removed at the second reoperation was seven (range 0–55) with median positive histology in two (range 0–12). Seven patients had a third reoperation and none achieved a biochemical complete response. The total number of nodes removed, as well as the number of positive nodes, was similar between those patients who achieved a biochemical complete response and those with persistent disease. No patient who achieved a biochemical complete response had a subsequent recurrence during the follow-up period (mean 60 months). No patient developed distant metastatic disease or died of disease during the study. Two patients who initially had detectable stimulated Tg values after their first reoperation achieved a biochemical complete response during long-term follow-up without further treatment.

Of note, preoperative FNA demonstrating malignant adenopathy was not required in this study. FNA of suspicious nodes was commonly performed early in the series, but as time went on FNA was performed selectively. Fifty-three percent of the lymphadenectomies were performed based on suspicious ultrasound without cytologic confirmation. Metastatic papillary thyroid cancer was detected in 93 % of the lymphadenectomies performed using this selective FNA approach. Also of interest were the details provided on ten patients who underwent reoperation with negative histology at reoperation. None of these patients went on to achieve a biochemical complete response. Most of these patients had small (less than 11 mm in greatest diameter) target lesions. This likely reflects the difficulty of finding small malignant nodes at reoperation. The median number of nodes harvested in these patients was four (range 0–22).

Al-Saif [16] also reported outcomes in terms of postoperative stimulated Tg less than 1 ng/ml and less than 2 ng/ml. The 1 ng/ml data facilitates comparison with the series reported by Yim [17]. Twenty-three percent of patients achieved a stimulated Tg less than 1 ng/ml after the first reoperation, and 18 % of patients achieved a stimulated Tg less than 1 ng/ml after a second reoperation.

In 2011, Yim et al. reported the outcomes of 83 patients who underwent initial total thyroidectomy and nodal dissection along with radioactive iodine remnant ablation and who subsequently received reoperation for locally recurrent/persistent papillary thyroid cancer [17]. The patients underwent initial surgery between 1996 and 2004 and subsequently developed recurrent disease. Central neck dissection had been performed in 75 % of the patients as part of the initial surgery, and modified radical neck dissection had been performed as part of the initial surgery in 24 % of patients. Patients with anti-Tg antibody titers greater than 100 U/ml were excluded from the study. Clinical relapse-free survival until the first recurrence was a median of 2.3 years. TSH-stimulated Tg levels after thyroid hormone withdrawal were assessed before and after reoperation. Biochemical remission was defined as a stimulated Tg less than 1 ng/ml. Biochemical remission was achieved in 51 % of patients who underwent first reoperation. There were no significant differences between the biochemical remission group and those who did not achieve remission in terms of age, extent of reoperation, and the administration of I-131 after reoperation. A median of 4 (1–31) malignant nodes was resected in the group that did not achieve biochemical remission, and a median of 3 (1–9) malignant nodes was resected in the group that achieved biochemical remission. The stimulated Tg levels prior to reoperation were significantly lower in the biochemical remission group than in those who did not achieve remission (5.6 ng/ml versus 31.1 ng/ml). Patients with high stimulated Tg before reoperation had little chance of cure with reoperation. Only two of ten patients with pre-reoperation stimulated Tg greater than 100 ng/ml achieved biochemical remission after reoperation. It is unknown whether this high failure rate was secondary to incomplete clearance of cervical disease or the presence of occult metastatic disease.

Yim et al. also evaluated the patients in terms of clinical evidence of disease (physical exam or imaging study) exclusive of their Tg level. Seventy of the 83 patients had no clinical evidence of disease after reoperation, while 13 patients had persistent or recurrent disease after reoperation. Pre-reoperation stimulated Tg and post-reoperation stimulated Tg levels were significantly higher in the group with clinical evidence of disease than in the group that had no clinical evidence of disease (15.0 versus 31.7 and 0.32 versus 19.5, respectively). There were no significant differences between the groups in terms of age, gender, the number of removed nodes, the number of malignant nodes, and the extent of reoperation.

Of the 13 patients with a second clinical recurrence, 8 had only locoregional disease. Five of these patients underwent additional surgery, two received local ablative therapies, and one refused additional treatment. The seven treated patients had no clinical evidence of disease at the end of follow-up. Three of the 13 patients with a second clinical recurrence had undetectable stimulated Tg after the first reoperation and also at the time of their second clinical relapse. Patients with stimulated Tg levels >5 ng/ml after the first reoperation had a greater chance of a second clinical recurrence during the follow-up period (median 5.4 years). The estimated 5-year clinical recurrence-free survival rate was 94 ± 3 % in the Tg <5 ng/ml group versus 74 ± 9 % in the Tg >5 ng/ml group.

Conclusion

The percentage of patients rendered disease-free by surgery for nodal recurrence of differentiated thyroid cancer varies substantially from study to study as do the criteria that define freedom from disease. Overall surgery appears to be a reasonable option for managing nodal recurrence in the short term. Long-term studies are needed to assess the impact of surgery on survival. The optimal extent of surgery has not been determined. Because many patients are left with persistent disease even after extensive surgery, a candid preoperative dialogue with the patient is essential to achieve realistic expectations of surgery.

References

1. Mazzaferri EL, Jhiang SM. Long-term impact of initial surgical and medical therapy on papillary and follicular thyroid cancer. Am J Med. 1994;97(5):418–28.
2. Kloos RT. Papillary thyroid cancer: medical management and follow-up. Curr Treat Options Oncol. 2005;6(4):323–38.
3. Waseem Z, Palme CE, Walfish P, Freeman JL. Prognostic implications of site of recurrence in patients with recurrent well-differentiated thyroid cancer. J Otolaryngol. 2004;33(6): 339–44.
4. Yamashita H. In: Clark OH, Noguchi S, editors. Thyroid cancer: diagnosis and treatment. St Louis: Quality Medical Publishing; 2000. p. 309–26.
5. Vassilopoulou-Selllin R, Schultz PN, Haynie TP. Clinical outcome of patients with papillary thyroid carcinoma who have recurrence after initial radioactive iodine therapy. Cancer. 1996;78(3):493–501.
6. Coburn M, Teates D, Wanebo H. Recurrent thyroid cancer: role of surgery versus radioactive iodine. Ann Surg. 1994;219(6):587–95.
7. Travagli JP, Cailleux AF, Ricard M, Baudin E, Caillou B, Parmebtier, Schlumberger M. Combination of radioiodine (^{131}I) and probe-guided surgery for persistent or recurrent thyroid carcinoma. JCEM. 1998;83(8):2675–80.
8. Karwowski JK, Jeffrey RB, McDougall IR, Weigel RJ. Intraoperative ultrasonography improves identification of recurrent thyroid cancer. Surgery. 2002;132(6):924–9.
9. Alzahrani AS, Raef H, Sultan A, Al Sobhi S, Ingemansson S, Ahmed M, Al Mahfouz A. Impact of cervical lymph node dissection on serum Tg and the course of disease in Tg-positive, radioactive iodine whole body scan-negative recurrent/persistent papillary thyroid cancer. J Endocrinol Invest. 2002;25:526–31.
10. Gemsenjager E, Perren A, Seifert B, Schuler G, Schweizer I, Heitz PU. Lymph node surgery in papillary thyroid carcinoma. J Am Coll Surg. 2003;197(2):182–90.
11. Bin Yousef HM, Alzahrani AS, Al-Sobhi SS, Al Suhaibani HS, Chaudhari MA, Raef HM. Preoperative neck ultrasonographic mapping for persistent/recurrent papillary thyroid cancer. World J Surg. 2004;28(11):1110–4.
12. Kloos RT, Mazzaferri EL. A single recombinant human thyrotropin-stimulated serum thyroglobulin measurement predicts differentiated thyroid carcinoma metastases three to five years later. JCEM. 2005;90(9):5047–57.
13. Roh J, Park J, Rha KS, Park CI. Is central neck dissection necessary for the treatment of lateral cervical nodal recurrence of papillary thyroid carcinoma? Head Neck. 2007;29(10):901–6.
14. Schuff KG, Weber SM, Givi B, Samuels MH, Andersen PE, Cohen JI. Efficacy of nodal dissection for treatment of persistent/recurrent papillary thyroid cancer. Laryngoscope. 2008;118:768–75.
15. Clayman GL, Shellenberger TD, Ginsberge LE, Edeiken BS, El-Naggar AK, Sellin RV, Waguespack SG, Roberts DB, Mishra A, Sherman SI. Approach and safety of comprehensive central compartment dissection in patients with recurrent papillary thyroid carcinoma. Head Neck. 2009;31(9):1152–63.
16. Al-Saif O, Farrar WB, Bloomston M, Porter K, Ringel MD, Kloos RT. Long-term efficacy of lymph node reoperation for persistent papillary thyroid cancer. JCEM. 2010;95(5):2187–94.
17. Yim JH, Kim WB, Kim EY, Kim WG, Kim TY, Ryu J, Gong G, Hiong SJ, Shong YK. The outcomes of first reoperation for locoregionally recurrent/persistent papillary thyroid carcinoma in patients who initially underwent total thyroidectomy and remnant ablation. JCEM. 2011;96(7):2049–56.

Papillary Cancer: Special Aspects in Children

51

Andrew J. Bauer and Sogol Mostoufi-Moab

Epidemiology and General Considerations

Currently, approximately 1.8 % of thyroid cancers are diagnosed in children and adolescents, but the incidence appears to be increasing [1]. Differentiated thyroid carcinoma (papillary and follicular thyroid cancer) is now the eighth most common malignancy in adolescents and the second most common cancer in Caucasian females 15–19 years of age [2]. The most common form of thyroid malignancy in children, as in adults, is papillary thyroid cancer (PTC), accounting for approximately 70–80 % of newly diagnosed pediatric thyroid cancers [1, 3–6]. In contrast to adults, pediatric patients with PTC typically have a greater incidence of cervical lymph node (35–70 %) [7–11] and pulmonary metastasis (15–20 %) [12–15] found at the time of diagnosis and a higher incidence of recurrent or persistent disease after initial treatment [3–5, 12, 16–21]. However, despite these more invasive characteristics, 10-year survival is greater than 98 % and disease-specific mortality is extremely uncommon [10, 11, 16, 22].

Our current approach to evaluation and treatment of PTC in children and adolescents has been extrapolated from the treatment of PTC in adults [23–25]. While the histology of the cancer is the same, the clinical behavior of PTC in children is very different and the potential short- and long-term risks of complications from treatment are expressed over a greater period of time. As the pediatric community continues to search for the safest and most effective treatment options for children, one must be cognizant that our current knowledge and approach to care is based on retrospective chart reviews. These reviews often cover decades of time with great variations in age of patient, degree of iodine sufficiency, and details of surgical as well as medical evaluation and management. While the last decade has witnessed a marked increase in the number of reports on pediatric thyroid cancer, information on 30–40-year posttreatment follow-up remains quite limited [10, 11, 17, 18, 21]. These disparities and unknowns continue to create controversy in treatment as we strive to balance and individualize the use of aggressive surgical and medical treatment for a cancer that on presentation appears aggressive, with an increased frequency of regional and pulmonary metastasis, but, in contrast to adults, appears to have a more indolent, long-term natural history and lower incidence of disease-specific mortality. In 2105, in an effort to improve the evaluation and management of thyroid nodules and differentiated thyroid cancer in children and adolescents, the American Thyroid Association published pediatric specific guidelines [26].

Presentation and Evaluation

PTC in children and adolescents most commonly presents in one of three ways: an asymptomatic, solitary thyroid nodule noted during routine physical exam [9, 10, 27–30], an incidentally discovered thyroid lesion revealed during non-thyroid anatomic imaging of the head and neck [31], or incidentally discovered thyroid lesion during evaluation for persistent cervical lymphadenopathy. Palpable cervical lymphadenopathy in children and adolescents is quite common, typically benign, and most commonly associated with an infectious etiology. However, in patients with a thyroid

A.J. Bauer, MD (✉)
Division of Endocrinology and Diabetes, Department of Pediatrics, The Children's Hospital of Philadelphia, The Perelman School of Medicine, The University of Pennsylvania,
34th Street and Civic Center Boulevard, Suite 11 NW30, Philadelphia, PA 19014, USA
e-mail: bauera@chop.edu

S. Mostoufi-Moab, MD, MSCE
Divisions of Oncology and Endocrinology, Department of Pediatrics, The Children's Hospital of Philadelphia, Philadelphia, PA, USA
e-mail: moab@email.chop.edu

L. Wartofsky, D. Van Nostrand (eds.), *Thyroid Cancer*, DOI 10.1007/978-1-4939-3314-3_51

nodule(s), the presence of palpable cervical lymph nodes is significantly associated with an increased risk of PTC [32].

Irrespective of the method of discovery, a thyroid ultrasound (US) should be the initial step in evaluation. Nuclear imaging studies are rarely helpful in determining the risk of malignancy and should only be considered in the evaluation if the baseline TSH is suppressed [32–36]. Complete US interrogation and description of the thyroid aids in selecting which nodule(s) should undergo fine needle aspiration biopsy (FNA; see Chap. 27, Table 27.3 for a list of benign and malignant US features). US interrogation of the lateral neck should be included to investigate for evidence of regional metastasis [32–35]. Lymph nodes that have a rounded shape, loss of the central hilum, the presence of peripheral vascularity, cystic areas, and/or microcalcifications increase the likelihood of diagnosing a thyroid malignancy [32, 37, 38].

The sensitivity, specificity, and accuracy of FNA in diagnosing thyroid cancer are similar for both pediatric and adult patients, reported to be as high as 95 %, 86.3 %, and 90.4 %, respectively [33, 39]. The use of US-guided FNA [40], bedside confirmation of sample adequacy, and preparation and evaluation of the FNA by pathologists with expertise in thyroid disease increases the accuracy of diagnosis. Without exception, all children, and the majority of adolescent patients, should be offered, and consented for, conscious sedation.

In adults, incorporation of the Bethesda System for Reporting Thyroid Cytopathology (TBSRTC) classification scheme into clinical practice has led to improved risk assessment and diagnostic accuracy [23, 41, 42]. Within the new system, the previous category of "indeterminate" cytology has been further delineated into "follicular lesion or atypia of undetermined significance," "follicular neoplasm," and "suspicious for malignancy." Within these categories, the risk of malignancy is 5–15 %, 15–30 %, and 60–75 %, respectively [43, 44]. In adults, the combined use of cytologic and genetic tests has afforded further information into stratification of risk [45]. Preliminary reports of oncogene analysis for pediatric patients with nodules displaying indeterminate cytology also show improved preoperative prediction for malignancy [46, 47]. Additional studies and consensus are needed to validate the results and determine how to incorporate molecular testing into clinical practice in an effort to optimize surgical management.

Preoperative Staging

In patients with a high suspicion for, or biopsy-proven, PTC, cross-sectional anatomic imaging of the neck and upper mediastinum with MRI may be considered prior to surgical intervention. Due to the increased risk of complications and the commonality of reactive lymph nodes within the pediatric population, FNA of suspicious appearing LN in the lateral neck should be considered prior to a decision to perform a unilateral or bilateral lateral neck dissection. For LN with equivocal cytopathology, the addition of a thyroglobulin (Tg) level obtained from the washout fluid of the FNA needle aids in the diagnosis of PTC [48, 49].

Prior to thyroidectomy, cross-sectional imaging has higher sensitivity at detecting regional metastasis within the central neck (level VI) [50, 51], the retro- and parapharyngeal areas, and the superior mediastinum, areas not well visualized via routine US. Computerized tomography (CT) may also be considered, but disadvantages include increased exposure to diagnostic radiation and the required use of iodine-containing contrast for more defined separation of tissue density [52]. Because younger patients often require conscious sedation to obtain quality MRI images, the potential benefit of adding preoperative anatomic imaging must be weighed against the risks of sedation. Further studies are required to determine if complete preoperative staging will lead to improved surgical planning and improved outcome. There are no data to support the use of FDG-PET/CT in the evaluation or staging of PTC in children and adolescents.

Micronodular metastases to the lung are found in 6–20 % of children, nearly exclusively associated with the presence of diffuse cervical lymph node metastasis [7, 8, 12, 13, 15, 16, 19]. Chest radiographs are relatively insensitive in detecting lung metastases and are often normal even in the presence of diffuse pulmonary metastatic disease [14, 30, 53]. Whole-body scanning, whether postsurgical, post-ablation, or posttherapy, is more sensitive, but this is positively correlated to the amount of ^{123}I or ^{131}I administered and negatively correlated with the amount of thyroid tissue present in the thyroid bed or cervical region [14]. Thus, one of the arguments supporting aggressive initial surgery is based on improved sensitivity for early detection of pulmonary disease, which will afford an opportunity for more deliberate, nonempiric dosing of ^{131}I.

Risk Factors and Pathophysiology

The majority of pediatric-aged patients diagnosed with PTC will not have an identifiable risk factor or etiology found by history, physical exam, or laboratory investigation. The exception is in patients with a family history of PTC [54–58] or a tumor syndrome, including PTEN Hamartoma syndrome [59], DICER1 syndrome [60], Carney complex [61] and familial adenomatous polyposis [62, 63]. The most frequently identified and established risk factor for the development of PTC is a history of radiation exposure, typically secondary to therapeutic radiation used in the treatment of a previous non-thyroid head and neck malignancy or in a conditioning regimen as preparation for bone-marrow transplantation [64–68]. The younger the age of the patient at the time of exposure and the lower the activity of radiation (maximum risk is ≤20 Gy), the shorter the latency and the higher the risk of radiation-induced thyroid malignancy [64, 69, 70]. Exposure to internalized ionizing radiation is also associated with an increased risk of developing PTC with increased risk associated with the presence of iodine insufficiency or deficiency [71–73]. The small doses of radioiodine typically used in diagnostic studies or in the treatment of Graves' disease have not been shown to increase the risk of PTC [74].

Advances in molecular and genetic testing of patients with PTC have improved our understanding of the pathogenesis, but there has been a paucity of research in children and adolescents on how to implement these data for diagnostic or therapeutic advantage. Approximately 5 % of patients have a positive family history for PTC [75] with activation of the RAS-RAF-MEK-ERK (mitogen-activated protein kinase) pathway playing a critical role in all identified genetic mutations to date [76]. There are conflicting data and opinion on whether a family history of PTC (familial non-medullary thyroid cancer) portends a more aggressive course of disease and a worse prognosis [58, 77–80]. A similar discussion has ensued for disease behavior between pre- and postpubertal children [81, 82] as well as for patients with radiation-induced compared to sporadic PTC [83]. In practice, there does not appear to be an absolute or predictable pattern to which a subgroup of patients is at greatest risk for developing regional metastasis to the lateral neck (most commonly to levels II, III, and IV), distant metastasis to the lungs, and persistent or recurrent disease. However, while limited, the most compelling data suggest that patients less than 10 years of age appear to have an increased risk of disease-specific mortality [10, 84, 85].

With this in mind, the approach to evaluation and treatment should be based on clinical presentation rather than on any one potential risk factor. The reflex should not be to send all pediatric aged patients with a thyroid nodule for surgical resection, but to use the history, physical exam, and US and FNA data to stratify an appropriate treatment plan. Published data suggest a 1.5–2.0-fold lower rate of malignancy in operated thyroid nodules between children and adults (26 % vs. 43 %, respectively) [86–88], highlighting a need to improve selection of which pediatric patients are referred for surgery. The unrealized challenge is to reduce the potential complications of treatment without a resultant decrement in prognoses. Ultimately, this may only be accomplished through referral of patients to tertiary pediatric centers with multidisciplinary experience in thyroid cancer evaluation and treatment.

For more complete discussion on the etiology and cancer risk of thyroid nodules in children and the molecular aspects of thyroid cancer in children, please refer to Chaps. 4 and 27.

Approach to Treatment

Surgical Approach

The initial therapy of thyroid cancer in children, as in adults, involves surgical resection. Because surgical complication rates are higher in children, surgery should be performed by a skilled high-volume surgeon in an environment staffed to safely monitor and care for potential surgical complications [89–91].

For the majority of patients, total thyroidectomy (TT) is the best approach. This recommendation is based on multiple studies demonstrating an increased incidence of bilateral and multifocal disease, 30 % and 65 %, respectively, as well as a higher risk of recurrence and subsequent second procedures when less than TT is performed [3, 6, 12, 16, 17, 20, 21, 92–94]. In long-term analysis, bilateral resection compared to unilateral resection has also been shown to decrease the risk of local recurrence from 35 to 6 % over 40 years of follow-up [21]. In addition, most children with PTC have regional [7–11] as well as a greater risk for distant metastasis [12–15]. Thus, TT affords potential for improved efficacy with radioiodine (RAI) therapy [1, 17], when appropriate, and improved sensitivity and specificity for using thyroglobulin (Tg) as a marker for persistent and/or recurrent disease [95, 96].

The increased incidence of regional metastasis suggests that prophylactic central neck (level VI) dissection (CND) may be more beneficial in decreasing the chances of persistent or recurrent disease in children than in adults. Several retrospective studies in children and adolescents have reported that performing less than a TT with CND is associated with an increased relative risk of relapse, decreased disease-free survival, and increased disease progression [1, 17, 21, 92–94, 97, 98]. However, there are no prospective, randomized control trials to ascertain if prophylactic CND for all pediatric patients with PTC would result in decreased recurrent disease, improved disease-free survival, or improved quality of life (decreased second surgery and less-intense lifetime surveillance).

In the absence of a prospective study, it seems reasonable to consider that children and adolescents with multifocal disease, bilateral disease, extrathyroidal extension, and/or locoregional metastasis should undergo a TT and a therapeutic CND. For all other children, until additional data are available, one must weigh the increased risk of surgical complications associated with prophylactic CND with the potential benefit of decreasing persistent and/or recurrent disease. In the pediatric population, considerations that suggest benefit for prophylactic CND include a higher incidence of regional metastasis, a reported reoperation rate as high as 77 % [82], and a potential decrease in total radioiodine dose to achieve remission. The majority of the risks can be reduced by ensuring surgery is performed by a skilled high-volume surgeon.

Lateral neck dissection should only be performed if there is clear evidence of lateral LN metastasis. Confirmation by FNA should be considered for equivocal disease. Size of the tumor should not be used as the sole criterion for deciding on the extent of surgical resection. Although larger primary tumors are more likely to be associated with metastases, tumor size in pediatric patients is relative to the developmental size of the thyroid [99] and smaller tumors may also be associated with the presence of regional metastases [7, 19, 20]. For all LN dissections, a comprehensive and compartment-focused approach should be employed as a higher risk of recurrence is associated with "berry picking" [100].

Lobectomy and isthmusectomy may be considered in low-risk patients, defined by age >10 years, negative history of familial non-medullary thyroid cancer or radiation exposure, and with a small (<1 cm) unifocal PTC without evidence of regional metastasis as determined by physical exam and comprehensive anatomic imaging of the neck (US and/or MRI or CT) [24, 101, 102]. A frequent clinical scenario where this may be encountered is the finding of an incidental, <0.5–1.0 cm focus of PTC after lobectomy is performed for a benign thyroid disease such as an autonomous nodule. If completion thyroidectomy is not performed, one most weigh the benefit of decreased surgical complications and avoiding long-term thyroid hormone replacement, with the potential increased risk of recurrent disease and the need for lifelong surveillance of the remaining thyroid tissue.

Risks of Surgical Complications

The risk of surgical complications correlates with the age of the patient, the extent of disease and surgical resection, and the experience of the surgeon.

In a cross-sectional analysis of over 600 pediatric patients undergoing thyroid surgery, there were fewer general and endocrine-specific complications when procedures were performed by high-volume surgeons (>30 thyroid surgeries per year) compared to pediatric surgeons, 8.7 % vs. 13.4 % and 5.6 % vs. 11 %, respectively [91]. In addition, the length of hospital stay and cost were significantly lower for procedures performed by high-volume surgeons [89, 91]. Unfortunately, the majority of pediatric patients continue to have thyroid surgery in non-tertiary care settings and in hospitals where less than 23 endocrine head and neck surgeries are performed per year [103].

The most common complications after thyroidectomy are endocrine related and include transient or permanent hypoparathyroidism. With more extensive or repeat surgery, up to 46 % of patients may experience transient hypoparathyroidism [8, 22, 81, 104–109]. Permanent hypoparathyroidism occurs less frequently, with an incidence of 0–15 % [7, 17, 89, 98, 110]. If there is concern over loss of viability of the parathyroid glands during the procedure, autotransplantation of the parathyroid gland(s) will decrease the risk of permanent hypoparathyroidism [111, 112]. There are several approaches that can predict which patients are at an increased risk of hypocalcemia [82]. These include serial perioperative measurements of serum calcium [113] and intact parathyroid hormone (PTH) level. The clinical utility of postoperative PTH is fairly well established, with a level of <10–15 pg/mL correlating with an increased risk of developing clinically significant hypocalcemia [114, 115]. An elevated postoperative serum phosphorous may also be predictive [116]. An alternative to using perioperative PTH and/or phosphorous to determine which patients require calcium and/or vitamin D replacement is to place all patients that have undergone TT with or without CND on empiric calcium and/or vitamin D replacement therapy and subsequently wean off of supplemental therapy based on serial calcium measurements during the postoperative period.

Surgery-specific, non-endocrine-related complications include recurrent laryngeal nerve damage and Horner syndrome, occurring with an average rate of 1–6 % [7, 17, 89, 98, 110]. The use of intraoperative recurrent laryngeal nerve monitoring may be considered as an adjunct monitoring device and should be considered for younger patients (<10 years of age), in patients undergoing CND, and in patients undergoing repeat surgical procedures. However, the use of RLN monitoring does not obviate the need for referral to a high-volume surgeon and has not been shown to lower the incidence of RLN damage [117].

Postsurgical Staging

There are multiple staging and scoring systems to estimate the risk of death for patients with PTC [118–121]. Perhaps the most well known and utilized is the tumor, node, and metastasis (TNM), a staging system adopted by the American Joint Committee on Cancer (AJCC) and the International Union Against Cancer (UICC). The TNM system is used to divide patients into prognostic groups to help stratify treatment [23]. Age is included as part of the staging system but, unfortunately, is limited to two distinct groups: patients less than and greater than 45 years of age. Thus, by definition, all pediatric patients are limited to either stage I (any T, any N, no distant metastasis) or stage II (any T, any N, and distant metastasis) disease. Within the pediatric population, the system accurately describes a low risk of mortality but does not adequately stratify risk of recurrence or allow for stratification of treatment as patients with an incidental finding of PTC (0 % risk of recurrence) and patients with extrathyroidal extension and cervical lymph node metastasis (30–50 % risk of persistent or recurrence) would both be classified as stage I disease [21, 102].

Despite these limitations, the TNM system is widely used by pathologists to describe the extent of disease within a surgical specimen and, when combined with other clinical features, serves as an additional source of data to predict prognosis. In pediatric patients, the presence of cervical lymph node metastasis, multifocal disease, and the diffuse sclerosing variant of PTC all carry an increased risk of pulmonary metastasis, portending an increased risk of persistent and recurrent disease [102, 122].

^{131}I Therapy

The use of ^{131}I (RAI) remnant ablation may be considered for patients that have received TT or completion thyroidectomy. The goal of ablation is twofold: (1) the destruction of any residual sources of Tg secretion allowing for the use of Tg as a sensitive and specific marker of PTC persistence or recurrence and (2) improved sensitivity of post-ablation whole-body scan (WBS) to detect lung metastasis [90, 123].

Long-established recommendations are to administer an ablative dose of ^{131}I to patients with PTC 4–6 weeks after surgery. Thyroid hormone (TH) replacement is usually withheld during this time, with 2–3 weeks of withdrawal typically adequate to raise serum TSH levels to above 30 μIU/mL [124]. A higher prevalence of functional metastases with increased sodium-iodine symporter (NIS) expression [125, 126] and age-dependent differences in metabolism are likely explanations for the decreased length of time required for TH withdrawal (THw). Two weeks before receiving RAI (most commonly ^{123}I), patients are placed on a low-iodine diet in an effort to improve the sensitivity of WBS to detect residual disease [24].

In adults, recombinant human TSH (rhTSH) appears to be as efficacious as THw in achieving ^{131}I remnant ablation with the advantage of avoiding symptoms of THw and, potentially, decreasing exposure of non-thyroid tissue to the negative effects of RAI. The use of rhTSH preparation has not been associated with a need for increased dosing of RAI [127, 128] or an increased risk of higher short-term recurrence rates [129, 130]. These potential benefits are equally attractive in caring for pediatric patients, and several small studies have shown equivalent ability to raise TSH [131, 132] and effectively achieve remnant ablation [133]. However, without prospective data in children exploring recurrence rates between rhTSH and THw, rhTSH preparation should be limited to patients with low risk of metastasis (no evidence of regional metastasis on preoperative imaging) or the more unusual patient that cannot tolerate TSH withdrawal or is incapable of mounting an elevated TSH secondary to the presence of functional metastasis or hypothalamic-pituitary dysfunction (survivor of a CNS malignancy, trauma, or congenital defect).

There is no consensus on a standardized dose of RAI for remnant ablation in children. In adults, smaller activities of RAI (50 mCi vs. 100 mCi) for low-risk patients appear to be as effective for thyroid remnant ablation, even in the presence of lymph node metastasis [128]. In children, RAI activity is frequently dosed empirically, given as a fraction (child's weight in kg divided by 70 kg) of a typical adult dose or based on weight (1.0–1.5 mCi/kg) or body surface area [24, 25, 90, 134]. The dose is then adjusted based on the stimulated Tg level and the diagnostic WBS uptake and images (i.e., thyroid bed uptake only vs. evidence of regional or distant metastasis). Lower doses of RAI may suffice for patients with a low risk of persistent disease (30–50 mCi), and larger doses, usually 50–125 mCi, may serve as an initial treatment for metastatic disease [12, 90, 93]. RAI should not be used in an attempt to treat bulky, persistent disease. If this is found during the post-initial surgery, pre-RAI evaluation, repeat surgery should be pursued prior to the administration of RAI. For younger patients and patients with known pulmonary metastasis, dosimetry may be preferable, either lesional based, calculated to maximize the likelihood of tumor control, or based on the maximum activity that can be administered to limit damage to normal tissue (bone marrow and lung) [24, 25, 135]. A post-treatment WBS is obtained 5–8 days later and serves as a more sensitive indicator of metastatic disease. The addition of single-photon emission CT (SPECT) increases the specificity of localizing persistent disease [136, 137].

Multiple studies have shown a twofold or greater incidence in recurrence of locoregional or distant metastasis when patients have not received RAI remnant ablation [8, 12, 17, 30, 92, 123]. In a study of 109 children, ages 6–17 years, 74 % received total thyroidectomy with lymph node dissection, 55 % received ^{131}I ablation (60–80 mCi), and 78 % received ^{131}I (cumulative dose of 60–580 mCi). Patients that received RAI had a fivefold lower relative risk factor for relapse [17]. In addition, after 5 years of observation, 97 % of children treated with ^{131}I were disease-free, while 40 and 60 % of children without ^{131}I relapsed after 5 and 10 years, respectively [17]. Of note, all younger children ($n = 14$) in the 6–10-year age group relapsed within 5 years, supporting the observation that younger age may portend a decreased chance of disease-free survival [17]. On multivariate analysis, the use of RAI remnant ablation has been shown to have similar impact as the extent of surgery on decreasing the risk of thyroid bed and locoregional recurrence [12, 93].

Recent concerns over the risk of RAI-induced non-thyroid second primary malignancy (SPM) have led to renewed discussion over which patients may or may not benefit from its use. This concern has been highlighted in a recent report showing increased overall mortality for pediatric patients treated with radiation (external beam, radium implants, or RAI) while at the same time revealing no difference in recurrence-free survival over nearly four decades of follow-up between patients that did or did not receive RAI ablation [21]. These data add to previous reports suggesting an increased risk of SPM related to age at the time of exposure and increased cumulative dose of RAI [138–141].

Thus, similar to the trend in adult patients with PTC, we're left to question whether RAI ablation is warranted for all pediatric patients with PTC. There is no question that radiation has teratogenic effects, and the location of the SPMs is consistent with either direct exposure to the ingested dose (stomach, colon, bone marrow, bladder) or absorption in nonthyroid tissues (salivary glands, lung, breast) [138–142]. However, while the recent report by Hay et al. raises great concern [21], there are several other investigators that have reported either no increased risk related to RAI [143] or that if the association is real, it is likely small [140] and related to genetic predisposition, not related to RAI treatment [144].

In the absence of prospective data to determine the absolute risk of SPM in children, and in light of the relatively slow growth of disease and the low risk of disease-specific mortality, it is prudent to look for subgroups of children where RAI remnant ablation may not be warranted. RAI remnant ablation is clearly indicated for patients with evidence of LN and/or distant metastasis as well as histology showing multifocal disease and/or lymphovascular invasion. The challenge in the pediatric population is to accurately define "low risk" and to determine which subgroup of patients may not experience an increase in disease morbidity if RAI remnant ablation is withheld. In adults, there is general consensus that for patients with unifocal PTC, 1 cm or less in size, and no evidence of metastasis, the risk of recurrence is low (2 %) and RAI remnant ablation is not warranted [23, 145]. This "low-risk" category includes patients with incidentally found PTC discovered unexpectedly after surgical resection for benign disease. Although prospective studies have not been performed, a similar approach is likely applicable for adolescent patients. In prepubertal patients with unifocal disease and no evidence of metastasis at initial evaluation, one could also consider withholding RAI; however, tumor size must be interpreted in the context of the developmental size of the thyroid. Without definitive data, parents/caregivers should be provided full disclosure of the potential risks and benefits and their opinion considered in the final decision. An alternative option that merits further investigation is the use of rhTSH preparation and/or using lower activities of RAI, i.e., 30 mCi for adolescent and 0.5 mCi/kg for prepubertal patients, to balance the potential risks and benefits of RAI remnant ablation. While we strive to find a balance between the risks of disease and risks of therapy, the recently published ATA guidelines define pediatric-specific categories for the risk of persistent disease that provide guidance to stratify the use of postoperative RAI [26].

In patients that receive RAI, additional side effects must be kept in mind. Acute side effects include nausea, neck pain over the first 1–2 days post-ingestion, and impaired salivary gland function [90, 123]. Strategies exist to help treat or prevent RAI-related side effects [146, 147]; however, even single doses of RAI may lead to permanent salivary gland dysfunction with lifelong xerostomia, an increased incidence of dental caries, and a potential increased risk for salivary gland malignancy [142, 147]. The use of sour candy or lemon juice, with vigorous hydration over the 48 h after RAI ingestion, may protect salivary gland function. While concerns have been voiced that increasing salivary gland activity with lemon juice may further increase the risk of damage [148], this has been disputed by other more recent studies [148, 149]. The use of rhTSH has not been shown to decrease salivary gland toxicity when compared to THw [149]. While none of these prophylactic measures, or other forms of sialogogues, have been formally studied in the pediatric population, we urge our patients to follow these recommendations and encourage the use of dental sealants as a prophylactic measure to help prevent caries.

Gonadal toxicity is another potential long-term toxic effect of ^{131}I and should be discussed prior to therapy. In postpubertal males, transient rise in FSH is common and may persist for up to 18 months after RAI exposure [150, 151]. Increasing cumulative doses of RAI may lead to decreased spermatogenesis with preserved testosterone production [151–153]. Current guidelines recommend that males avoid attempts at conception for at least 4 months. Postpubertal testes appear to be more vulnerable than prepubertal testes to the toxic effects of ionizing radiation [154], so counseling for sperm banking should be offered for postpubertal male patients receiving cumulative doses in access of 400 mCi [155].

Transient amenorrhea and menstrual irregularities have been reported in up to 17 % of females under the age of 40 years, 65 % of whom were treated with a single ablative dose of 81 mCi [156]. While there does not appear to be an increase in infertility or birth defects in subsequent pregnancies after RAI [157], an increase in miscarriage rate within the year after large dose of ^{131}I has led to the recommendation for avoiding conception during the year after ^{131}I therapy [158].

Acute suppression of bone marrow may occur, but hematologic parameters are usually normalized within 60 days after RAI exposure. Untoward long-term consequences of acute, transient bone marrow suppression are extremely rare; however, there are reported incidences of leukemia after multiple high doses of ^{131}I were given over a short period of time [159]. Therefore, it is important to allow for recovery of bone marrow before retreatment with current recommendations, suggesting a minimum time of at least 6 months between RAI dosing [160].

Lastly, for pediatric patients with lung metastases, there is significant risk for either tumor- and/or RAI-induced pulmonary fibrosis with an increased risk associated with retained ^{131}I activity above 80 mCi [90, 134]. For patients with significant uptake on diagnostic WBS, dosimetry or reduced dosing should be considered. In addition, serial pulmonary function testing should be completed in order to follow pulmonary status.

Thyroid Hormone Suppression

All children with PTC will ultimately require thyroid hormone suppressive therapy irrespective of the extent of surgical resection or administration of ^{131}I ablation. Physiologic replacement dosing in children and adolescents is 1–3 μg/kg/day or 75–100 μg/m^2/day, and a dose of 2.1–4.5 μg/kg/day is usually sufficient to suppress the TSH to a goal of <0.1 μIU/mL [24, 134, 161]. One must remember that until cure has been proven, the goal is to suppress the TSH to a level below assay detection and the individual patient may require a dose greater than the dose determined by standard calculation.

While all patients will require lifelong thyroid hormone therapy, release from near-total suppression to physiologic replacement doses is considered once the patient is in remission. The time at which to decrease the dose is debatable and must be individualized with the goal of this phase of replacement therapy to keep the TSH just above the assay detection limit, typically at 0.1–0.5 μUI/mL [24, 134, 161]. This is particularly important in children as the hyperthyroidism resulting from the relatively high levels of free T_4 required for TSH suppression may result in potential negative long-term effects on bone mineral density [162, 163] and behavioral symptoms similar to attention deficit disorder [161]. The potential negative effect on bone mineral density is of particular concern during childhood and adolescence, a critical time of peak bone mass acquisition. Future research studies are needed to assess the long-term effects of suppressive thyroid hormone therapy on peak bone mass acquisition and to determine if clinically detrimental bone loss occurs.

Surveillance

Follow-up for persistent or recurrent disease, as well as the potential late effects from therapy, follows a similar approach to adult patients with PTC [23]. This includes serial measurements of Tg every 3–6 months and radiologic imaging every 6–12 months after initial therapy. Exceptions to this approach are based on the more indolent nature of the disease associated with lower disease-specific mortality and a higher incidence of recurrence [13]. Remission, defined as an undetectable Tg, with negative Tg antibodies, and negative imaging (US and/or WBS) may be achieved within 1–2 years for a subgroup of patients; however, for other patients, most commonly patients with pulmonary disease, stable persistent disease may develop that is unresponsive to repeat RAI dosing [164, 165]. Because of these realities, being "cured from PTC" is not a concept that is frequently conveyed to pediatric patients and their families. The psychosocial impact of having a chronic malignancy, requiring lifelong surveillance, is one of several areas that require further attention and investigation.

Surveillance and Follow-Up Therapy

Similar to adults, patients are reevaluated for residual disease every 3–6 months after initial RAI ablation. In the past, the conventional approach required patients to undergo thyroid hormone withdrawal, or rhTSH stimulation, along with being placed on a low-iodine diet in order to obtain a stimulated Tg and a diagnostic WBS on an annual basis. Over the last 5–10 years, there has been increased reliance on using US, with the selective addition of anatomic, cross-sectional imaging using CT or MRI, to identify patients with cervical disease rather than relying on the less-sensitive, and more cumbersome, diagnostic WBS [166, 167]. The addition of neck MRI is particularly useful in evaluating patients for potential retro- or parapharyngeal LN metastasis where US detection is less sensitive [168]. MRI appears to have equal sensitivity in detecting cervical recurrences when compared to WBS; however, the use of MRI can be associated with an increased risk of false-positive findings [169].

For patients with known, or concern for, pulmonary metastasis, WBS continues to play a central role in screening for disease. WBS has a higher sensitivity and specificity, compared to CXR or chest CT, for detecting pulmonary disease [14]. As children have a lower incidence of dedifferentiated disease, the use of WBS is associated with a lower false-negative rate when compared to adults with similar disease (7 % vs. 15–20 %, respectively) [14].

The more frequent use of US and anatomic imaging has occurred in conjunction with the development, increased availability, and increased reliance on second-generation Tg assays. The newer Tg assays have a reported functional sensitivity as low as 0.05 ng/mL (μg/L) [170]. Using these newer assays, a non-TS-stimulated (basal) Tg below 0.1 ng/mL correlates with a low likelihood of having a rhTSH-stimulated Tg above 2.0 ng/mL, the "cut-off" point associated with an increased likelihood of finding residual disease [170]. In addition, with the high, between-run precision of these newer assays, following the trend of basal-Tg levels allows for a sensitive method to monitor changes in disease burden [170, 171]. Due to marked variation in assay sensitivity and reproducibility, every attempt should be made to use the same Tg assay for a particular patient. On the same sample, assays by different laboratories can result in a three- to tenfold variation in measured Tg [170, 172]. While following basal Tg appears to be a practical approach for children, one must be aware that there are no data defining a cutoff point for basal Tg, or a predicted fold-change rate for basal or stimulated Tg, that has been validated to predict clinically significant or progressive disease in the pediatric population.

With these issues in mind, and pending further data and consensus, it is reasonable to follow a similar approach to surveillance and treatment in children as for adults [23, 24]. Patients with an undetectable basal Tg should be monitored with a basal Tg every 3–6 months for the first 2 years with subsequent decreased frequency once remission has been established. For patients with a detectable Tg at 6 months post initial therapy and no known history of pulmonary metastasis based on post-ablation WBS, repeat US imaging of the neck should be obtained with particular focus on levels II, III, IV, and VI, areas associated with the highest rate of metastasis [173]. If the US is negative, additional imaging with MRI should be considered to evaluate for abnormal LN that may have not been found on routine US to include the retro- and parapharyngeal space. The finding of pathologic lymph node(s) on imaging obviates the need for subsequent stimulated Tg and WBS imaging. In the presence of bulky cervical disease, FNA should be considered to confirm PTC, subsequently followed by compartment focused surgical resection. Unfortunately, repeat surgical procedures for recurrence are common across all pediatric ages [82]. Referral to an experienced surgeon is imperative in an effort to ensure complete dissection and to lower the risk of potential complications. If, despite this intervention, the postoperative Tg remains elevated, a stimulated Tg and WBS should be considered to evaluate for distant metastasis, particularly in the lungs. In patients with RAI-avid disease not amenable to additional surgery, repeat RAI therapy may be considered [174].

In patients with a detectable basal Tg and no evidence of persistent or recurrent cervical disease by US and/or anatomic imaging, further evaluation and follow-up are dictated by the history of pulmonary metastasis. In patients with no known history of pulmonary metastasis (negative posttreatment WBS), a stimulated Tg (THw or rhTSH) and WBS should be obtained, with repeat RAI considered based on the findings. In patients with a known history of pulmonary disease and no evidence of cervical disease, one should consider following the basal Tg trend in an effort to establish whether the patient has stable or progressive disease. Serial pulmonary function testing should also be followed, obtained every 6–12 months depending on disease status and anticipated therapy. In contrast to adults, up to 50 % of pediatric patients may develop stable, but persistent, pulmonary disease unresponsive to repeat doses of RAI [14, 16, 164, 165, 175, 176]. Fortunately, even in this setting, the disease-specific mortality remains low, <3 % [165]. The diagnosis of unresponsive disease is typically established after 2–3 doses of RAI fail to result in decreased disease burden, defined by a declining basal and/or stimulated Tg as well as WBS and/or CT imaging. For this subgroup of pediatric patients, repeat dosing of RAI will not induce remission and may lead to an increased risk of SPM as well as an increased risk of pulmonary fibrosis. Interestingly, although without a clear explanation, there is evidence to suggest that Tg levels may continue to decline years after the last dose of RAI therapy [164]. Lastly, on rare occasion, pediatric patients with pulmonary disease may develop Tg(+), WBS(−) (non-RAI avid) disease (unpublished observations). Although there are no studies in children to define the prognostic significance of dedifferentiated, FDG-PET(+), WBS(−) disease, this may be the only setting where FDG-PET may aid in evaluation and care.

A thyroglobulin antibody titer (TgAb) should be performed with every Tg level. Approximately 20 % of patients with PTC will have detectable Tg-antibody titers [96, 177]. The presence of TgAbs interferes with all renditions of the Tg immunometric (IMA) assay, typically leading to false lowering of Tg titers [178]. In TgAb+ patients, the TgAb levels may be followed serially as a surrogate of Tg levels to determine the course of disease [96]. Similar to the measurement of Tg, consistent use of the same TgAb assay is important. Alternatively, if available, Tg measurement by radioimmunoassay (RIA) may be used, as this method appears to be more resistant to interference by TgAb [172]. TgAb titers can be detected for a median of 3 years after complete ablation of thyroid tissue [179].

Conclusion

The availability of a several different prognostic scoring systems for adult patients with PTC, such as age, distant metastases, extent, and size (AMES); age, grade, extent, and size (AGES); metastasis, age, completeness of resection, invasion, and size (MACIS); and the TNM stating system, affords adult clinicians with an ability to more accurately stratify which patients may benefit from aggressive therapy [121]. In addition, the identification of BRAF as a specific marker of malignancy, as well as a maker of invasiveness, serves as an additional prognostic tool to help guide therapy [180].

In pediatric patients with PTC, the search for reliable prognostic factors useful for individualizing treatment has included the evaluation of gender, age at presentation, size of the tumor, and presence of local and/or regional disease. Unfortunately, no one or combination of these factors has been shown to be reliable [17, 18, 20]. The cutoff age of less than 40–45 years for defining low and high risk in the adult staging systems makes these systems uninformative for use in pediatric patients.

There are multiple studies demonstrating that children under the age of 10 years of age have more invasive disease at diagnosis, when compared to older children [17, 18, 20, 81], with one study reporting a 100 % recurrence rate within the initial 5 years of therapy for patients 6–10 years of age [17]. In this report, male sex, previously associated with worse prognosis [20], was not associated with a worse outcome [17]. Several other studies have not supported the observation that age (prepubertal vs. pubertal) or gender carries any prognostic significance [17, 82, 93].

Tumor size at presentation may also be associated with more advanced disease (distant metastasis) and with a lower likelihood of response to initial therapy [19]. However, other studies have not shown size to be of prognostic significance for achieving remission [5]. Thus, based on these and other data, tumor size should likewise not be used as the sole guide to decide on the extent of surgery or medical management in children.

While pediatric patients may present with widely invasive disease, with rare exception, PTC in children is associated with low disease-specific mortality. In the absence of validated markers or a validated prognostic system, the evaluation and treatment of pediatric patients with PTC should be directed at reducing the risk of recurrent disease. The cornerstone of treatment is complete surgical resection. For the majority of patients, this will include total thyroidectomy as the initial surgical approach with therapeutic CND for patients with known locoregional or distant metastasis. Referral to a high-volume surgeon can minimize the potential risks associated with TT and CND. RAI therapy should be used for all patients at increased risk of persistent or recurrent disease and withheld, or significantly reduced, for patients with a low risk of persistent, postoperative disease [26]. As an example, RAI is not indicated for patients with a small, incidentally discovered PTC and is likely of little to no benefit in patients with a postresection Tg <1–2 ng/mL and limited thyroid bed uptake on WBS. Reevaluation for persistent disease should occur at 6–12 months, with further therapy directed based on the identification of clinically significant disease, defined by an increasing trend in Tg levels (basal or rhTSH stimulated) and radiographic evidence of disease. This approach, termed delayed risk stratification (DRS) [181, 182], affords an opportunity to more accurately stratify individual risk and more thoughtfully manage future evaluation and therapy [181].

Despite the excellent long-term prognosis for children and adolescents with PTC, all patients must be followed closely for an extended period of time, perhaps for life. Recurrences may occur years after the initial diagnosis, even with appropriate treatment and apparent disease-free status. Increased efforts and collaboration are needed in order to identify potential molecular markers that may be used to predict invasive potential and to more fully explore and validate our current, and future, approach to the evaluation and care of pediatric patients with PTC.

References

1. Hogan AR, et al. Pediatric thyroid carcinoma: incidence and outcomes in 1753 patients. J Surg Res. 2009;156(1):167–72.
2. Wu X, et al. Cancer incidence patterns among adolescents and young adults in the United States. Cancer Causes Control. 2005;16(3):309–20.
3. Giuffrida D, et al. Differentiated thyroid cancer in children and adolescents. J Endocrinol Invest. 2002;25(1):18–24.
4. Kumar A, Bal CS. Differentiated thyroid cancer. Indian J Pediatr. 2003;70(9):707–13.
5. Lee YM, et al. Well-differentiated thyroid carcinoma in Hong Kong Chinese patients under 21 years of age: a 35-year experience. J Am Coll Surg. 2002;194(6):711–6.
6. Bargren AE, et al. Outcomes of surgically managed pediatric thyroid cancer. J Surg Res. 2009;156(1):70–3.
7. Demidchik YE, et al. Comprehensive clinical assessment of 740 cases of surgically treated thyroid cancer in children of Belarus. Ann Surg. 2006;243(4):525–32.
8. Frankenthaler RA, et al. Lymph node metastasis from papillary-follicular thyroid carcinoma in young patients. Am J Surg. 1990;160(4):341–3.
9. Harness JK, et al. Differentiated thyroid carcinoma in children and adolescents. World J Surg. 1992;16(4):547–53; discussion 553–4.
10. Schlumberger M, et al. Differentiated thyroid carcinoma in childhood: long term follow-up of 72 patients. J Clin Endocrinol Metab. 1987;65(6):1088–94.
11. Zimmerman D, et al. Papillary thyroid carcinoma in children and adults: long-term follow-up of 1039 patients conservatively treated at one institution during three decades. Surgery. 1988;104(6):1157–66.
12. Chow SM, et al. Differentiated thyroid carcinoma in childhood and adolescence-clinical course and role of radioiodine. Pediatr Blood Cancer. 2004;42(2):176–83.
13. Jarzab B, Handkiewicz-Junak D. Differentiated thyroid cancer in children and adults: same or distinct disease? Hormones (Athens). 2007;6(3):200–9.
14. Bal CS, et al. Is chest x-ray or high-resolution computed tomography scan of the chest sufficient investigation to detect pulmonary metastasis in pediatric differentiated thyroid cancer? Thyroid. 2004;14(3):217–25.
15. Vassilopoulou-Sellin R, et al. Pulmonary metastases in children and young adults with differentiated thyroid cancer. Cancer. 1993;71(4):1348–52.
16. Brink JS, et al. Papillary thyroid cancer with pulmonary metastases in children: long-term prognosis. Surgery. 2000;128(6):881–6; discussion 886–7.
17. Jarzab B, et al. Multivariate analysis of prognostic factors for differentiated thyroid carcinoma in children. Eur J Nucl Med. 2000;27(7):833–41.
18. Landau D, et al. Thyroid cancer in children: the Royal Marsden Hospital experience. Eur J Cancer. 2000;36(2):214–20.
19. Powers PA, et al. Tumor size and extent of disease at diagnosis predict the response to initial therapy for papillary thyroid carcinoma in children and adolescents. J Pediatr Endocrinol Metab. 2003;16(5):693–702.
20. Welch Dinauer CA, et al. Clinical features associated with metastasis and recurrence of differentiated thyroid cancer in children, adolescents and young adults. Clin Endocrinol (Oxf). 1998;49(5):619–28.
21. Hay ID, et al. Long-term outcome in 215 children and adolescents with papillary thyroid cancer treated during 1940 through 2008. World J Surg. 2010;34(6):1192–202.
22. Vassilopoulou-Sellin R, et al. Differentiated thyroid cancer in children and adolescents: clinical outcome and mortality after long-term follow-up. Head Neck. 1998;20(6):549–55.

23. Cooper DS, et al. Revised American Thyroid Association management guidelines for patients with thyroid nodules and differentiated thyroid cancer. Thyroid. 2009;19(11):1167–214.
24. Waguespack SG, Francis G. Initial management and follow-up of differentiated thyroid cancer in children. J Natl Compr Cancer Netw. 2010;8(11):1289–300.
25. Rivkees SA, et al. The treatment of differentiated thyroid cancer in children: emphasis on surgical approach and radioactive iodine therapy. Endocr Rev. 2011;32:798–826.
26. Francis GL, Waguespack SG, Bauer AJ, et al. Management guidelines for children with thyroid nodules and differentiated thyroid cancer: American Thyroid Association Guidelines Task Force. Thyroid. 2015;25(7):716–59.
27. Ceccarelli C, et al. Thyroid cancer in children and adolescents. Surgery. 1988;104(6):1143–8.
28. Jocham A, et al. Thyroid carcinoma in childhood: management and follow up of 11 cases. Eur J Pediatr. 1994;153(1):17–22.
29. Samuel AM, Sharma SM. Differentiated thyroid carcinomas in children and adolescents. Cancer. 1991;67(8):2186–90.
30. Viswanathan K, Gierlowski TC, Schneider AB. Childhood thyroid cancer. Characteristics and long-term outcome in children irradiated for benign conditions of the head and neck. Arch Pediatr Adolesc Med. 1994;148(3):260–5.
31. Avula S, et al. Incidental thyroid abnormalities identified on neck US for non-thyroid disorders. Pediatr Radiol. 2010;40(11):1774–80.
32. Corrias A, et al. Diagnostic features of thyroid nodules in pediatrics. Arch Pediatr Adolesc Med. 2010;164(8):714–9.
33. Corrias A, et al. Accuracy of fine needle aspiration biopsy of thyroid nodules in detecting malignancy in childhood: comparison with conventional clinical, laboratory, and imaging approaches. J Clin Endocrinol Metab. 2001;86(10):4644–8.
34. Croom 3rd RD, et al. Autonomously functioning thyroid nodules in childhood and adolescence. Surgery. 1987;102(6):1101–8.
35. Hopwood NJ, et al. Functioning thyroid masses in childhood and adolescence. Clinical, surgical, and pathologic correlations. J Pediatr. 1976;89(5):710–8.
36. Smith M, et al. Carcinoma of the thyroid in patients with autonomous nodules. Am Surg. 1988;54(7):448–9.
37. Frates MC, et al. Management of thyroid nodules detected at US: society of radiologists in ultrasound consensus conference statement. Ultrasound Q. 2006;22(4):231–8; discussion 239–40.
38. Fish SA, Langer JE, Mandel SJ. Sonographic imaging of thyroid nodules and cervical lymph nodes. Endocrinol Metab Clin N Am. 2008;37(2):401–17, ix.
39. Arda IS, et al. Fine needle aspiration biopsy of thyroid nodules. Arch Dis Child. 2001;85(4):313–7.
40. Izquierdo R, et al. Ultrasound-guided fine-needle aspiration in the management of thyroid nodules in children and adolescents. Thyroid. 2009;19:703–5.
41. Cibas E. Bethesda and beyond. Cancer Cytopathol. 2010;118(4):184–5.
42. Cibas ES, Ali SZ. The Bethesda system for reporting thyroid cytopathology. Thyroid. 2009;19(11):1159–65.
43. Baloch ZW, et al. Diagnostic terminology and morphologic criteria for cytologic diagnosis of thyroid lesions: a synopsis of the National Cancer Institute Thyroid Fine-Needle Aspiration State of the Science Conference. Diagn Cytopathol. 2008;36(6):425–37.
44. Cibas ES, Ali SZ. The Bethesda system for reporting thyroid cytopathology. Am J Clin Pathol. 2009;132(5):658–65.
45. Bauer AJ, Francis GL. Update on the molecular signature of differentiated thyroid cancer: clinical implications and potential opportunities. Expert Rev Endocrinol Metab. 2011;6(6):819–34.
46. Ballester LY, Sarabia SF, Sayeed H, et al. Integrating molecular testing in the diagnosis and management of children with thyroid lesions. Pediatr Dev Pathol. 2016;19(2):94–100.
47. Prasad ML, Vyas M, Horne MJ, et al. NTRK fusion oncogenes in pediatric papillary thyroid carcinoma in northeast United States. Cancer. 2016;122(7):1097–107.
48. Pacini F, et al. Detection of thyroglobulin in fine needle aspirates of nonthyroidal neck masses: a clue to the diagnosis of metastatic differentiated thyroid cancer. J Clin Endocrinol Metab. 1992;74(6):1401–4.
49. Baloch ZW, et al. Utility of thyroglobulin measurement in fine-needle aspiration biopsy specimens of lymph nodes in the diagnosis of recurrent thyroid carcinoma. Cytojournal. 2008;5:1.
50. Hwang HS, Orloff LA. Efficacy of preoperative neck ultrasound in the detection of cervical lymph node metastasis from thyroid cancer. Laryngoscope. 2011;121(3):487–91.
51. Park JS, et al. Performance of preoperative sonographic staging of papillary thyroid carcinoma based on the sixth edition of the AJCC/UICC TNM classification system. AJR Am J Roentgenol. 2009;192(1):66–72.
52. Miyakoshi A, Dalley RW, Anzai Y. Magnetic resonance imaging of thyroid cancer. Top Magn Reson Imaging. 2007;18(4):293–302.
53. Fassina AS, et al. Thyroid cancer in children and adolescents. Tumori. 1994;80(4):257–62.
54. Hemminki K, Eng C, Chen B. Familial risks for nonmedullary thyroid cancer. J Clin Endocrinol Metab. 2005;90(10):5747–53.
55. Nose V. Familial follicular cell tumors: classification and morphological characteristics. Endocr Pathol. 2010;21(4):219–26.
56. Prazeres H, et al. The familial counterparts of follicular cell – derived thyroid tumors. Int J Surg Pathol. 2010;18(4):233–42.
57. Sturgeon C, Clark OH. Familial nonmedullary thyroid cancer. Thyroid. 2005;15(6):588–93.
58. Zivaljevic V, et al. The incidence of familial nonmedullary thyroid cancer in a large case series. Acta Chir Belg. 2008;108(3):328–32.
59. Tan MH, Mester JL, Rybicki NJ, et al. Lifetime cancer risks in individuals with germline PTEN mutations. Clin Cancer Res. 2012;18(2):400–7.
60. Rutter MM, Jha P, Schultz KA, et al. DICER1 mutaitons and differentiated thyroid carcinoma: evidence of a direct association. J Clin Endocrinol Metab. 2016;101(1):1–5.
61. Sandrini F, et al. Regulatory subunit type I-alpha of protein kinase A (PRKAR1A): a tumor-suppressor gene for sporadic thyroid cancer. Gene Chromosome Cancer. 2002;35(2):182–92.
62. Brasseur B, et al. Multiple neoplasia in a 15-year-old girl with familial adenomatous polyposis. J Pediatr Hematol Oncol. 2009; 31(7):530–2.
63. Cameselle-Teijeiro J, et al. Cribriform-morular variant of papillary thyroid carcinoma: molecular characterization of a case with neuroendocrine differentiation and aggressive behavior. Am J Clin Pathol. 2009;131(1):134–42.
64. Bhatti P, et al. Risk of second primary thyroid cancer after radiotherapy for a childhood cancer in a large cohort study: an update from the childhood cancer survivor study. Radiat Res. 2010;174(6):741–52.
65. Cohen A, et al. Risk for secondary thyroid carcinoma after hematopoietic stem-cell transplantation: an EBMT Late Effects Working Party Study. J Clin Oncol. 2007;25(17):2449–54.
66. Laughton SJ, et al. Endocrine outcomes for children with embryonal brain tumors after risk-adapted craniospinal and conformal primary-site irradiation and high-dose chemotherapy with stem-cell rescue on the SJMB-96 trial. J Clin Oncol. 2008;26(7):1112–8.
67. Sigurdson AJ, et al. Primary thyroid cancer after a first tumour in childhood (the Childhood Cancer Survivor Study): a nested case-control study. Lancet. 2005;365(9476):2014–23.
68. Sklar C, et al. Abnormalities of the thyroid in survivors of Hodgkin's disease: data from the Childhood Cancer Survivor Study. J Clin Endocrinol Metab. 2000;85(9):3227–32.
69. Ron E, et al. Thyroid cancer after exposure to external radiation: a pooled analysis of seven studies. Radiat Res. 1995;141(3):259–77.

70. Ronckers CM, et al. Thyroid cancer in childhood cancer survivors: a detailed evaluation of radiation dose response and its modifiers. Radiat Res. 2006;166(4):618–28.
71. Cardis E, et al. Risk of thyroid cancer after exposure to 131I in childhood. J Natl Cancer Inst. 2005;97(10):724–32.
72. Nesterenko AV, Nesterenko VB. 14. Protective measures for activities in Chernobyl's radioactively contaminated territories. Ann N Y Acad Sci. 2009;1181:311–7.
73. Nesterenko AV, Nesterenko VB, Yablokov AV. Introduction: the difficult truth about Chernobyl. Ann N Y Acad Sci. 2009;1181:1–3.
74. Read Jr CH, Tansey MJ, Menda Y. A 36-year retrospective analysis of the efficacy and safety of radioactive iodine in treating young Graves' patients. J Clin Endocrinol Metab. 2004;89(9):4229–33.
75. Kebebew E. Hereditary non-medullary thyroid cancer. World J Surg. 2008;32(5):678–82.
76. Yamashita S, Saenko V. Mechanisms of disease: molecular genetics of childhood thyroid cancers. Nat Clin Pract Endocrinol Metab. 2007;3(5):422–9.
77. Alsanea O, et al. Is familial non-medullary thyroid carcinoma more aggressive than sporadic thyroid cancer? A multicenter series. Surgery. 2000;128(6):1043–51.
78. Capezzone M, et al. Familial non-medullary thyroid carcinoma displays the features of clinical anticipation suggestive of a distinct biological entity. Endocr Relat Cancer. 2008;15(4):1075–81.
79. Musholt TJ, et al. Familial papillary thyroid carcinoma: genetics, criteria for diagnosis, clinical features, and surgical treatment. World J Surg. 2000;24(11):1409–17.
80. Takami H, Ozaki O, Ito K. Familial nonmedullary thyroid cancer: an emerging entity that warrants aggressive treatment. Arch Surg. 1996;131(6):676.
81. Lazar L, et al. Differentiated thyroid carcinoma in pediatric patients: comparison of presentation and course between prepubertal children and adolescents. J Pediatr. 2009;154(5):708–14.
82. Machens A, et al. Papillary thyroid cancer in children and adolescents does not differ in growth pattern and metastatic behavior. J Pediatr. 2010;157(4):648–52.
83. Naing S, Collins BJ, Schneider AB. Clinical behavior of radiation-induced thyroid cancer: factors related to recurrence. Thyroid. 2009;19(5):479–85.
84. Bal CS, Padhy AK, Kumar A. Clinical features of differentiated thyroid carcinoma in children and adolescents from a sub-Himalayan iodine-deficient endemic zone. Nucl Med Commun. 2001;22(8):881–7.
85. Harach HR, Williams ED. Childhood thyroid cancer in England and Wales. Br J Cancer. 1995;72(3):777–83.
86. Niedziela M. Pathogenesis, diagnosis and management of thyroid nodules in children. Endocr Relat Cancer. 2006;13(2):427–53.
87. Oertel YC, et al. Value of repeated fine needle aspirations of the thyroid: an analysis of over ten thousand FNAs. Thyroid. 2007;17(11):1061–6.
88. Yang J, et al. Fine-needle aspiration of thyroid nodules: a study of 4703 patients with histologic and clinical correlations. Cancer. 2007;111(5):306–15.
89. Sosa JA, et al. Clinical and economic outcomes of thyroid and parathyroid surgery in children. J Clin Endocrinol Metab. 2008;93(8):3058–65.
90. Thompson GB, Hay ID. Current strategies for surgical management and adjuvant treatment of childhood papillary thyroid carcinoma. World J Surg. 2004;28(12):1187–98.
91. Tuggle CT, et al. Pediatric endocrine surgery: who is operating on our children? Surgery. 2008;144(6):869–77; discussion 877.
92. Grigsby PW, et al. Childhood and adolescent thyroid carcinoma. Cancer. 2002;95(4):724–9.
93. Handkiewicz-Junak D, et al. Total thyroidectomy and adjuvant radioiodine treatment independently decrease locoregional recurrence risk in childhood and adolescent differentiated thyroid cancer. J Nucl Med. 2007;48(6):879–88.
94. Popovtzer A, et al. Thyroid cancer in children: management and outcome experience of a referral center. Otolaryngol Head Neck Surg. 2006;135(4):581–4.
95. Pacini F, et al. Diagnostic 131-iodine whole-body scan may be avoided in thyroid cancer patients who have undetectable stimulated serum Tg levels after initial treatment. J Clin Endocrinol Metab. 2002;87(4):1499–501.
96. Spencer CA. Clinical Utility of Thyroglobulin Antibody (TgAb) measurements for patients with Differentiated Thyroid Cancers (DTC). J Clin Endocrinol Metab. 2011;96:3615–27.
97. Feinmesser R, et al. Carcinoma of the thyroid in children – a review. J Pediatr Endocrinol Metab. 1997;10(6):561–8.
98. Newman KD, et al. Differentiated thyroid cancer: determinants of disease progression in patients <21 years of age at diagnosis: a report from the Surgical Discipline Committee of the Children's Cancer Group. Ann Surg. 1998;227(4):533–41.
99. Zimmermann MB, et al. New reference values for thyroid volume by ultrasound in iodine-sufficient schoolchildren: a World Health Organization/Nutrition for Health and Development Iodine Deficiency Study Group Report. Am J Clin Nutr. 2004;79(2):231–7.
100. Musacchio MJ, et al. Greater local recurrence occurs with "berry picking" than neck dissection in thyroid cancer. Am Surg. 2003;69(3):191–6; discussion 196–7.
101. Spoudeas HA, editor. Paediatric endocrine tumours. A multi-disciplinary consensus statement of best practice from a working group convened under the auspices of the British Society of Paediatric Endocrinology & Diabetes and the United Kingdom Children's Cancer Study Group. West Sussex: Novo Nordisk Ltd; 2005.
102. Borson-Chazot F, et al. Predictive factors for recurrence from a series of 74 children and adolescents with differentiated thyroid cancer. World J Surg. 2004;28(11):1088–92.
103. Raval MV, et al. Utilization of total thyroidectomy for differentiated thyroid cancer in children. Ann Surg Oncol. 2010;17(10):2545–53.
104. Farahati J, et al. Characteristics of differentiated thyroid carcinoma in children and adolescents with respect to age, gender, and histology. Cancer. 1997;80(11):2156–62.
105. Massimino M, et al. Primary thyroid carcinoma in children: a retrospective study of 20 patients. Med Pediatr Oncol. 1995;24(1):13–7.
106. Patwardhan N, Cataldo T, Braverman LE. Surgical management of the patient with papillary cancer. Surg Clin N Am. 1995;75(3):449–64.
107. Shindo ML. Considerations in surgery of the thyroid gland. Otolaryngol Clin N Am. 1996;29(4):629–35.
108. Stael AP, et al. Total thyroidectomy in the treatment of thyroid carcinoma in childhood. Br J Surg. 1995;82(8):1083–5.
109. Raval MV, et al. Total thyroidectomy for benign disease in the pediatric patient – feasible and safe. J Pediatr Surg. 2009;44(8):1529–33.
110. Savio R, et al. The role of a more extensive surgical approach in the initial multimodality management of papillary thyroid cancer in children. J Pediatr Surg. 2005;40(11):1696–700.
111. Barczynski M, et al. Applicability of intraoperative parathyroid hormone assay during total thyroidectomy as a guide for the surgeon to selective parathyroid tissue autotransplantation. World J Surg. 2008;32(5):822–8.
112. Skinner MA, et al. Heterotopic autotransplantation of parathyroid tissue in children undergoing total thyroidectomy. J Pediatr Surg. 1997;32(3):510–3.
113. Walsh SR, Kumar B, Coveney EC. Serum calcium slope predicts hypocalcaemia following thyroid surgery. Int J Surg. 2007;5(1):41–4.
114. Grodski S, et al. Postoperative PTH measurement facilitates day 1 discharge after total thyroidectomy. Clin Endocrinol (Oxf). 2009;70(2):322–5.

115. Grodski S, Serpell J. Evidence for the role of perioperative PTH measurement after total thyroidectomy as a predictor of hypocalcemia. World J Surg. 2008;32(7):1367–73.
116. Sam AH, et al. Serum phosphate predicts temporary hypocalcaemia following thyroidectomy. Clin Endocrinol (Oxf). 2011;74(3): 388–93.
117. Angelos P. Recurrent laryngeal nerve monitoring: state of the art, ethical and legal issues. Surg Clin N Am. 2009;89(5):1157–69.
118. Grubbs EG, et al. Recent advances in thyroid cancer. Curr Probl Surg. 2008;45(3):156–250.
119. Lang BH, et al. Staging systems for papillary thyroid carcinoma: a study of 2 tertiary referral centers. Ann Surg. 2007;246(1):114–21.
120. Powers PA, et al. The MACIS score predicts the clinical course of papillary thyroid carcinoma in children and adolescents. J Pediatr Endocrinol Metab. 2004;17(3):339–43.
121. Shaha AR. TNM classification of thyroid carcinoma. World J Surg. 2007;31(5):879–87.
122. Koo JS, Hong S, Park CS. Diffuse sclerosing variant is a major subtype of papillary thyroid carcinoma in the young. Thyroid. 2009;19(11):1225–31.
123. Jarzab B, Handkiewicz-Junak D, Wloch J. Juvenile differentiated thyroid carcinoma and the role of radioiodine in its treatment: a qualitative review. Endocr Relat Cancer. 2005;12(4):773–803.
124. Kuijt WJ, Huang SA. Children with differentiated thyroid cancer achieve adequate hyperthyrotropinemia within 14 days of levothyroxine withdrawal. J Clin Endocrinol Metab. 2005;90(11):6123–5.
125. Faggiano A, et al. Age-dependent variation of follicular size and expression of iodine transporters in human thyroid tissue. J Nucl Med. 2004;45(2):232–7.
126. Patel A, et al. Differentiated thyroid carcinoma that express sodium-iodide symporter have a lower risk of recurrence for children and adolescents. Pediatr Res. 2002;52(5):737–44.
127. Pacini F, et al. Radioiodine ablation of thyroid remnants after preparation with recombinant human thyrotropin in differentiated thyroid carcinoma: results of an international, randomized, controlled study. J Clin Endocrinol Metab. 2006;91(3):926–32.
128. Pilli T, et al. A comparison of 1850 (50 mCi) and 3700 MBq (100 mCi) 131-iodine administered doses for recombinant thyrotropin-stimulated postoperative thyroid remnant ablation in differentiated thyroid cancer. J Clin Endocrinol Metab. 2007;92(9):3542–6.
129. Tuttle RM, et al. Recombinant human TSH-assisted radioactive iodine remnant ablation achieves short-term clinical recurrence rates similar to those of traditional thyroid hormone withdrawal. J Nucl Med. 2008;49(5):764–70.
130. Elisei R, et al. Follow-up of low-risk differentiated thyroid cancer patients who underwent radioiodine ablation of postsurgical thyroid remnants after either recombinant human thyrotropin or thyroid hormone withdrawal. J Clin Endocrinol Metab. 2009;94(11):4171–9.
131. Iorcansky S, et al. Serum thyrotropin (TSH) levels after recombinant human TSH injections in children and teenagers with papillary thyroid cancer. J Clin Endocrinol Metab. 2005;90(12):6553–5.
132. Luster M, et al. Recombinant thyrotropin use in children and adolescents with differentiated thyroid cancer: a multicenter retrospective study. J Clin Endocrinol Metab. 2009;94(10):3948–53.
133. Lau WF, et al. Management of paediatric thyroid carcinoma: recent experience with recombinant human thyroid stimulating hormone in preparation for radioiodine therapy. Intern Med J. 2006;36(9):564–70.
134. Rachmiel M, et al. Evidence-based review of treatment and follow up of pediatric patients with differentiated thyroid carcinoma. J Pediatr Endocrinol Metab. 2006;19(12):1377–93.
135. Van Nostrand D, Atkins F. Pediatric differentiated thyroid cancer: can the prescribed activity of I-131 be increased? J Clin Endocrinol Metab. 2011;96(8):2401–3.
136. Gelfand MJ, Lemen LC. PET/CT and SPECT/CT dosimetry in children: the challenge to the pediatric imager. Semin Nucl Med. 2007;37(5):391–8.
137. Wong KK, et al. Hybrid SPECT-CT and PET-CT imaging of differentiated thyroid carcinoma. Br J Radiol. 2009;82(982):860–76.
138. Rubino C, et al. Second primary malignancies in thyroid cancer patients. Br J Cancer. 2003;89(9):1638–44.
139. Sandeep TC, et al. Second primary cancers in thyroid cancer patients: a multinational record linkage study. J Clin Endocrinol Metab. 2006;91(5):1819–25.
140. Sawka AM, et al. Second primary malignancy risk after radioactive iodine treatment for thyroid cancer: a systematic review and meta-analysis. Thyroid. 2009;19(5):451–7.
141. Brown AP, et al. The risk of second primary malignancies up to three decades after the treatment of differentiated thyroid cancer. J Clin Endocrinol Metab. 2008;93(2):504–15.
142. Klubo-Gwiezdzinska J, et al. Salivary gland malignancy and radioiodine therapy for thyroid cancer. Thyroid. 2010;20(6): 647–51.
143. Bhattacharyya N, Chien W. Risk of second primary malignancy after radioactive iodine treatment for differentiated thyroid carcinoma. Ann Otol Rhinol Laryngol. 2006;115(8):607–10.
144. Verkooijen RB, et al. The incidence of second primary tumors in thyroid cancer patients is increased, but not related to treatment of thyroid cancer. Eur J Endocrinol. 2006;155(6):801–6.
145. Pacini F, et al. Post-surgical use of radioiodine (131I) in patients with papillary and follicular thyroid cancer and the issue of remnant ablation: a consensus report. Eur J Endocrinol. 2005;153(5): 651–9.
146. Kloos RT. Protecting thyroid cancer patients from untoward effects of radioactive iodine treatment. Thyroid. 2009;19(9):925–8.
147. Lee SL. Complications of radioactive iodine treatment of thyroid carcinoma. J Natl Compr Cancer Netw. 2010;8(11):1277–86; quiz 1287.
148. Nakada K, et al. Does lemon candy decrease salivary gland damage after radioiodine therapy for thyroid cancer? J Nucl Med. 2005;46(2):261–6.
149. Grewal RK, et al. Salivary gland side effects commonly develop several weeks after initial radioactive iodine ablation. J Nucl Med. 2009;50(10):1605–10.
150. Rosario PW, et al. Testicular function after radioiodine therapy in patients with thyroid cancer. Thyroid. 2006;16(7):667–70.
151. Sawka AM, et al. A systematic review of the gonadal effects of therapeutic radioactive iodine in male thyroid cancer survivors. Clin Endocrinol (Oxf). 2008;68(4):610–7.
152. Edmonds CJ, Smith T. The long-term hazards of the treatment of thyroid cancer with radioiodine. Br J Radiol. 1986;59(697): 45–51.
153. Hyer S, et al. Testicular dose and fertility in men following I(131) therapy for thyroid cancer. Clin Endocrinol (Oxf). 2002;56(6): 755–8.
154. Wallace WH. Oncofertility and preservation of reproductive capacity in children and young adults. Cancer. 2011;117(10 Suppl):2301–10.
155. Pacini F, et al. Testicular function in patients with differentiated thyroid carcinoma treated with radioiodine. J Nucl Med. 1994;35(9):1418–22.
156. Vini L, et al. Prognosis for fertility and ovarian function after treatment with radioiodine for thyroid cancer. Postgrad Med J. 2002;78(916):92–3.
157. Sawka AM, et al. A systematic review examining the effects of therapeutic radioactive iodine on ovarian function and future pregnancy in female thyroid cancer survivors. Clin Endocrinol (Oxf). 2008;69(3):479–90.
158. Casara D, et al. Pregnancy after high therapeutic doses of iodine-131 in differentiated thyroid cancer: potential risks and recommendations. Eur J Nucl Med. 1993;20(3):192–4.
159. Van Nostrand D, Neutze J, Atkins F. Side effects of "rational dose" iodine-131 therapy for metastatic well-differentiated thyroid carcinoma. J Nucl Med. 1986;27(10):1519–27.

160. Maxon 3rd HR, Smith HS. Radioiodine-131 in the diagnosis and treatment of metastatic well differentiated thyroid cancer. Endocrinol Metab Clin N Am. 1990;19(3):685–718.
161. Hung W, Sarlis NJ. Current controversies in the management of pediatric patients with well-differentiated nonmedullary thyroid cancer: a review. Thyroid. 2002;12(8):683–702.
162. Radetti G, et al. Bone mineral density in children and adolescent females treated with high doses of L-thyroxine. Horm Res. 1993;39(3–4):127–31.
163. Solomon BL, Wartofsky L, Burman KD. Prevalence of fractures in postmenopausal women with thyroid disease. Thyroid. 1993;3(1):17–23.
164. Biko J, et al. Favourable course of disease after incomplete remission on (131)I therapy in children with pulmonary metastases of papillary thyroid carcinoma: 10 years follow-up. Eur J Nucl Med Mol Imaging. 2010;38(4):651–5.
165. Pawelczak M, et al. Outcomes of children and adolescents with well-differentiated thyroid carcinoma and pulmonary metastases following (1)(3)(1)I treatment: a systematic review. Thyroid. 2010;20(10):1095–101.
166. Antonelli A, et al. Role of neck ultrasonography in the follow-up of children operated on for thyroid papillary cancer. Thyroid. 2003;13(5):479–84.
167. Frasoldati A, et al. Diagnosis of neck recurrences in patients with differentiated thyroid carcinoma. Cancer. 2003;97(1):90–6.
168. Kaplan SL, et al. The role of MR imaging in detecting nodal disease in thyroidectomy patients with rising thyroglobulin levels. AJNR Am J Neuroradiol. 2009;30(3):608–12.
169. Mihailovic J, et al. MRI versus (1)(3)(1)I whole-body scintigraphy for the detection of lymph node recurrences in differentiated thyroid carcinoma. AJR Am J Roentgenol. 2010;195(5):1197–203.
170. Spencer C, et al. Serum Basal thyroglobulin measured by a second-generation assay correlates with the recombinant human thyrotropin-stimulated thyroglobulin response in patients treated for differentiated thyroid cancer. Thyroid. 2010;20(6):587–95.
171. Malandrino P, et al. Risk-adapted management of differentiated thyroid cancer assessed by a sensitive measurement of basal serum thyroglobulin. J Clin Endocrinol Metab. 2011;96(6):1703–9.
172. Spencer CA, Lopresti JS. Measuring thyroglobulin and thyroglobulin autoantibody in patients with differentiated thyroid cancer. Nat Clin Pract Endocrinol Metab. 2008;4(4):223–33.
173. Carty SE, et al. Consensus statement on the terminology and classification of central neck dissection for thyroid cancer. Thyroid. 2009;19(11):1153–8.
174. Leboulleux S, et al. Follicular cell-derived thyroid cancer in children. Horm Res. 2005;63(3):145–51.
175. Dottorini ME. Differentiated thyroid carcinoma in childhood. Rays. 2000;25(2):245–55.
176. Samuel AM, Rajashekharrao B, Shah DH. Pulmonary metastases in children and adolescents with well-differentiated thyroid cancer. J Nucl Med. 1998;39(9):1531–6.
177. Corrias A, et al. Thyroid nodules and cancer in children and adolescents affected by autoimmune thyroiditis. Arch Pediatr Adolesc Med. 2008;162(6):526–31.
178. Spencer C, Petrovic I, Fatemi S. Current thyroglobulin autoantibody (TgAb) assays often fail to detect interfering TgAb that can result in the reporting of falsely low/undetectable serum Tg IMA values for patients with differentiated thyroid cancer. J Clin Endocrinol Metab. 2011;96(5):1283–91.
179. Chiovato L, et al. Disappearance of humoral thyroid autoimmunity after complete removal of thyroid antigens. Ann Intern Med. 2003;139(5 Pt 1):346–51.
180. Xing M, et al. BRAF mutation predicts a poorer clinical prognosis for papillary thyroid cancer. J Clin Endocrinol Metab. 2005;90(12):6373–9.
181. Castagna MG, et al. Delayed risk stratification, to include the response to initial treatment (surgery and radioiodine ablation), has better outcome predictivity in differentiated thyroid cancer patients. Eur J Endocrinol. 2011;165(3):441–6.
182. Tuttle RM, et al. Estimating risk of recurrence in differentiated thyroid cancer after total thyroidectomy and radioactive iodine remnant ablation: using response to therapy variables to modify the initial risk estimates predicted by the new American Thyroid Association staging system. Thyroid. 2010;20(12):1341–9.

Special Presentations of Thyroid Cancer in Thyrotoxicosis, Renal Failure, and Struma Ovarii

52

Kenneth D. Burman

Introduction

Differentiated thyroid cancer most commonly exists in euthyroid individuals, who present with a thyroid mass or who have a structural thyroidal abnormality detected on a radiologic study. In contrast to this typical presentation, there are several groups of patients who have thyroid cancer associated with other clinical circumstances and therefore may require special attention. This chapter discusses these special situations and includes patients with thyroid cancer and (1) concomitant thyrotoxicosis, (2) renal failure on dialysis, and (3) tumor origin in an ectopic site. (Patients with thyroglossal duct thyroid cancer are discussed in Chap. 53.) The general principles underlying the diagnosis and treatment of thyroid cancer in these subgroups are comparable to cancer presenting in the more typical cases, but these special circumstances require additional considerations.

Concomitant Thyrotoxicosis

The association between thyroid cancer and hyperthyroidism can occur in several different forms. Thyroid cancer, for instance, can occur in a patient with known or suspected Graves' disease. Often, this occurs when a thyroid nodule or "hypofunctioning area" is detected by sonogram, isotope scan, and/or palpation. Occasionally, a cervical lymph node is detected in combination with the thyroid nodule or as a separate and distinct finding. This topic has been reviewed by Stocker and Burch [1]. Thyroid cancer has been estimated to occur in between 1 and 9 % of Graves' disease patients. Of course, this detection rate depends on how assiduous the search is for nodules and thyroid cancer. Although controversial, it has been speculated that thyroid cancer is more aggressive when it occurs in conjunction with Graves' disease, possibly from the presence of thyrotropin (TSH) receptor-stimulating antibodies that may directly stimulate growth and differentiation of the malignant thyroid cells [1–3]. Although it is a relatively rare occurrence, it is prudent to perform both a careful thyroid and neck examination and a thyroid sonogram in patients with Graves' disease.

Recent American Thyroid Association Guidelines have recommendations regarding when to perform a thyroid fine-needle aspiration (FNA) [4]. Patients who have a history associated with high risk for thyroid cancer (e.g., history of thyroid cancer in one or more first-degree relatives; history of external beam radiation as a child; exposure to ionizing radiation in childhood or adolescence; prior hemithyroidectomy with identification of thyroid cancer, focal 18FDG avidity on PET scanning; MEN2 or familial medullary thyroid cancer, serum calcitonin >100 pg/ml) should have nodules larger than 5 mm aspirated if the nodule has suspicious sonographic features. Solid, hypoechoic nodules larger than 1 cm should also be aspirated as should iso-echoic nodules 1–1.5 cm or larger. Mixed solid-cystic nodules should be aspirated if larger than 1.5–2.0 cm, if there are suspicious sonographic features, and if larger than 2 cm without suspicious sonographic features (e.g., microcalcifications, hypoechoic, increased nodular vascularity, infiltrative margins, taller than wide on transverse view). Coexistent hyperthyroidism (as opposed to euthyroidism) does not alter the approach as recommended.

The Bethesda Classification System has become the standard method of reporting thyroid FNA's as either benign, atypia of undetermined significance, neoplasm, suspicious for malignancy, malignant, or nondiagnostic with an estimated relative likelihood of harboring cancer of <1 %, 5–10 %, 20–30 %, 50–75 %, and 100 %, respectively, with the chance of malignancy in a nondiagnostic aspirate being variable [5].

K.D. Burman, MD (✉)
Director, Divisions of Endocrinology, Washington Hospital Center and Georgetown University Hospital, 110 Irving Street NW 2A-72, Washington, DC 20010, USA
e-mail: kenneth.d.burman@medstar.net

L. Wartofsky, D. Van Nostrand (eds.), *Thyroid Cancer*, DOI 10.1007/978-1-4939-3314-3_52

If the lesion has suspicious or malignant cytology, then a thyroidectomy becomes the preferred therapy for both the suspicious nodule and the thyrotoxicosis. Molecular diagnostic techniques are becoming increasingly useful in helping to determine which suspicious or indeterminate nodules are likely to be malignant [6, 7]. Of course, the patient's hyperthyroidism should be controlled prior to surgery, usually with the use of an antithyroid agent (preferably methimazole) and β-blockers. The patient should be rendered clinically and biochemically euthyroid as rapidly as possible so as to not delay definitive therapy.

After restoring euthyroidism, it is also optimal to deplete thyroidal stores of thyroid hormone by continuing the thiourea treatment for several weeks prior to surgery. Some clinicians will utilize preoperative treatment with iodine (SSKI or Lugol's) for about 7–10 day before surgery to help reduce thyroid function quickly, possibly reduce gland vascularity, and hopefully decrease the risk of acute thyroid hormonal release at surgery. Particularly when administered for longer than several weeks, iodine preparations can actually enhance thyroid hormone release (escape from the Wolff-Chaikoff effect); thus, care must be taken when employing these agents. Radiocontrast agents, e.g., ipodate, had been utilized effectively in the preoperative treatment of thyrotoxic patients, but this agent is not presently available in the USA. Following thyroidectomy, the treatment and monitoring plans for a patient with concomitant Graves' hyperthyroidism and differentiated thyroid cancer are basically the same as if thyrotoxicosis had not been present.

Metastatic Thyroid Cancer and Thyrotoxicosis

A separate and also unusual presentation is the occurrence of thyrotoxicosis in the setting of widespread metastatic thyroid cancer, typically of the follicular type. The occurrence of this rare syndrome is related to the volume of functioning differentiated thyroid cancer cells in the patient. It occurs when there is extensive thyroidal tissue in metastatic foci that can trap iodine, synthesize iodothyronines, and then secrete sufficient thyroxine (T4) and triiodothyronine (T3) to render the patient biochemically (and usually clinically) hyperthyroid, despite a previous thyroidectomy and likely radioactive iodine ablative therapy. Generally, it is easily recognized that these patients have widespread metastases, but the appearance of hyperthyroidism may initially be thought to be associated with excessive exogenous L-thyroxine administration. When the patient remains hyperthyroid, even when the dosage of levothyroxine is reduced, the mechanism for the hyperthyroidism should become clear. Occasionally, this condition is recognized when a patient is prepared for a withdrawal ^{131}I scan. The clue is that the serum TSH fails to sufficiently rise after the withdrawal of levothyroxine therapy to perform radioisotopic scanning or therapy. This occurs because the pituitary thyrotropic cells are suppressed by the high circulating levels of thyroid hormone from the metastases. This circumstance can be differentiated from a patient who has not discontinued exogenous L-T4 as scheduled because of elevated serum thyroglobulin and the presence of metastatic lesions when a radioiodine scan is ultimately performed. Isotopic scanning and radioiodine therapy when TSH fails to rise can be achieved with the use of recombinant human TSH (Thyrogen®). The treatment of these patients is directed at the malignant lesions using ^{131}I therapy (or other direct modalities, such as surgery or external radiation as appropriate). However, attention may also have to be directed at treating the hyperthyroidism with antithyroid agents, e.g., methimazole and β-blockers.

Although this syndrome is usually due to widespread metastatic disease, it rarely may be related to minimal residual disease that is stimulated by thyroid-stimulating immunoglobulins (TSH-R-AB) in a patient with underlying Graves' disease [3, 8]. Metastatic thyroid cancer causing hyperthyroidism is seen most frequently with follicular cancer, but it has also been described with other types, including papillary and anaplastic cancer [9, 10].

Renal Failure

The presence of thyroid cancer in a patient with end-stage renal disease (ESRD) requiring hemodialysis needs special consideration because of the issue of radioactive iodine therapy and its failure to be normally excreted by functioning kidneys [11–13]. This circumstance should be managed by a multidisciplinary approach, involving endocrinologists, nuclear medicine specialists, radiation safety officers, and nurses. This discussion focuses on the use of radioactive iodine in the renal failure patient, but general medical and surgical principles should be used for the initial evaluation, diagnosis, and management of the thyroid neoplasm.

There are specific considerations regarding ^{131}I therapy because iodine clearance occurs primarily via the kidneys. Consequently, the clearance of radioiodine in an end-stage renal disease (ESRD) patient given ^{131}I therapy is managed with the use of hemodialysis. In general, our approach is to perform hemodialysis immediately prior to ^{131}I treatment and then dialyze the patient again about 24 h after the ^{131}I dose. Several review articles are available that have addressed this topic [11–13]. In general, we believe that it is preferable, if possible, to perform dosimetric therapy, a process that provides a quantitative estimate of the isotope retention and exposure in the individual patient. If this technique is not available, it seems appropriate to administer approximately 30–40 % of the usual empiric ^{131}I dose that would have been given to the patient had they not had ESRD. Based on the literature and our experience, hemodialysis can be safely performed after radioiodine therapy using the standard precautions but with some caveats. Because there is significant radioiodine removal by dialysis initially, special precautions should include using adequate distance and shielding between the dialysis technician and patient. The dialysate should be disposed of into the sewer system, preferably via a closed system. Following the first three or four dialysis procedures post-radioiodine ablation, a large fraction of the radioiodine should have been cleared from the blood, and the patient can then continue on dialysis in the usual manner. All medical health personnel involved in the patient's care should be advised of the radiation safety issues and should wear a radiation badge for exposure to be monitored and documented [14].

Ectopic Sites of Thyroid Cancer

Thyroid tissue can arise in ectopic locations, presumably from variant embryologic migration. Ectopic thyroid tissue resides most commonly in the lingual, sublingual, thyroglossal, laryngotracheal, or lateral cervical areas, although ectopic thyroid tissue has been reported in a wide variety of sites, such as mediastinum, heart, pancreas, gallbladder, and skin [15].

Such ectopic thyroid tissue is thought to have the same risk of developing thyroid cancer as thyroid tissue in its eutopic location. However, the identification of this ectopic tissue and the ability to diagnose thyroid cancer may often be difficult. Possibly the two most commonly discussed locations for ectopic thyroid tissue are in the neck and in the ovary (i.e., struma ovarii) [15]. Most ectopic thyroid tissue in the ovary is benign, but there are numerous case reports of thyroid cancer that originates in the ovaries [16]. When metastases occur from a primary ovarian thyroid carcinoma, they typically manifest as peritoneal studding; however, distant metastases to the lung and other sites (e.g., bone, brain, and liver) may also occur. Whether the struma ovarii is benign or malignant, it can produce sufficient thyroid hormone to cause biochemical or clinical thyrotoxicosis. Radioactive iodine scans may show uptake in the ovary, as well as in the normal thyroid location in the neck. However, with struma ovarii-related thyrotoxicosis, the high thyroid hormone levels will suppress TSH and there will be little if any uptake of isotope in the normal thyroid gland.

Malignant struma ovarii is typically diagnosed incidentally in the evaluation of an ovarian mass [16–29]. Occasionally, the first presentation is of the metastases, perhaps in the peritoneal or pulmonary area. Given the rarity of the condition, there are no evidence-based studies to direct what may be optimal evaluation and treatment. The general approach is to remove the ectopic cancer tissue by an oophorectomy with related surgery for local disease, such as taking multiple peritoneal and omental biopsies with common iliac and paracaval node sampling as appropriate [30]. Tumor staging with radiologic studies of the neck, chest, abdomen, pelvis, and possibly brain and bone is needed, with special attention to the thyroid gland. A thyroid sonogram may discover a thyroid nodule that requires FNA.

It is possible, albeit rare, that eutopic thyroid cancer will metastasize to the ovary [23] and there is a histologic variant of ovarian cancer that is papillary in nature [31–33] making identification of the site of origin of the primary tumor problematic. Papillary thyroid cancer will stain histochemically for thyroglobulin [29]. Ascites may occur and thyroid cancer can also elevate the ovarian tumor marker, CA 125 [21]. Primary thyroid cancer that originates within the ovary is usually papillary in nature, with a few cases of follicular and anaplastic cancer reported [20, 22, 27, 29].

In addition to appropriate surgery and staging in conjunction with radiologic assessment, ^{131}I scans, ^{131}I treatment, and monitoring via ultrasound, computed tomography, or magnetic resonance imaging and serum thyroglobulin determinations are useful in the management of patients with primary ovarian thyroid cancer [26]. Most authorities also recommend that a near-total thyroidectomy be performed when ovarian thyroid cancer is detected, which allows more accurate utilization of radioiodine treatment and monitoring. Because the ability of ectopic thyroid tissue to trap iodine may be relatively limited, recombinant TSH has been used to enhance radioiodine uptake and treatment [26].

Thyroid tissue and cancer can also occur at ectopic sites closer to the thyroid bed [15, 34]. Such tissue, either benign or harboring cancer, has been identified in the tongue [35] within the tracheal lumen [34] or in the thyroglossal duct ([36]; see Chap. 53). Thyroid cancer that arises in ectopic locations represents an unusual clinical circumstance. We believe that the same general principles guiding our approach to eutopic thyroid cancer apply to ectopic thyroid cancer, but individual variation based on the specific tumor site and other aspects of a given patient is warranted.

In conclusion, thyroid cancer linked to special circumstances, such as in conjunction with hyperthyroidism, end-stage renal failure, or in anatomically ectopic locations, should be treated similarly to eutopic thyroid cancer in euthyroid, otherwise "normal" subjects. These specific conditions are unusual but should be considered when assessing thyroid cancer patients.

References

1. Stocker DJ, Burch HB. Thyroid cancer yield in patients with Graves' disease. Minerva Endocrinol. 2003;28(3):205–12.
2. Filetti S, et al. The role of thyroid-stimulating antibodies of Graves' disease in differentiated thyroid cancer. N Engl J Med. 1988; 318(12):753–9.

3. Basaria S, Salvatori R. Thyrotoxicosis due to metastatic papillary thyroid cancer in a patient with Graves' disease. J Endocrinol Invest. 2002;25(7):639–42.
4. American Thyroid Association Guidelines Task Force on Thyroid Nodules and Differentiated Thyroid Cancer. Haugen BR, Alexander EK, Bible KC, Doherty GM, Mandel SJ, Nikiforov YE, Pacini F, Randolph GW, Sawka AM, Schlumberger M, Schuff KG, Sherman SI, Sosa JA, Steward DL, Tuttle RM, Wartofsky L. 2015 American Thyroid Association Management Guidelines for Adult Patients with Thyroid Nodules and Differentiated Thyroid Cancer. Thyroid 2016;26:1–133.
5. Baloch ZW, et al. Diagnostic terminology and morphologic criteria for cytologic diagnosis of thyroid lesions: a synopsis of the National Cancer Institute thyroid fine-needle aspiration state of the science conference. Diagn Cytopathol. 2008;36(6):425–37.
6. Nikiforov YE. Molecular diagnostics of thyroid tumors. Arch Pathol Lab Med. 2011;135(5):569–77.
7. Li H, et al. Cost-effectiveness of a novel molecular test for cytologically indeterminate thyroid nodules. J Clin Endocrinol Metab. 2011;96(11):E1719–26.
8. Guglielmi R, et al. Severe thyrotoxicosis due to hyperfunctioning liver metastasis from follicular carcinoma: treatment with (131) I and interstitial laser ablation. Thyroid. 1999;9(2):173–7.
9. Alagol F, et al. Anaplastic thyroid cancer with transient thyrotoxicosis: case report and literature review. Thyroid. 1999;9(10):1029–32.
10. Salvatori M, et al. Severe thyrotoxicosis due to functioning pulmonary metastases of well-differentiated thyroid cancer. J Nucl Med. 1998;39(7):1202–7.
11. Holst J, et al. Dosimetric analysis of radioiodine therapy for thyroid cancer and hyperthyroidism in patients with end stage renal disease on hemodialysis. Submitted for publication.
12. Jimenez RG, et al. Iodine-131 treatment of thyroid papillary carcinoma in patients undergoing dialysis for chronic renal failure: a dosimetric method. Thyroid. 2001;11(11):1031–4.
13. Mello A, et al. Management of papillary thyroid carcinoma with radioiodine in a patient with end stage renal disease on hemodialysis. Clin Nucl Med. 1992;19:776–81.
14. Murcutt G, et al. Hemodialysis of chronic kidney failure patients requiring ablative radioiodine therapy. Kidney Int. 2008;73(11): 1316–9.
15. Klubo-Gwiezdzinska J, et al. Clinical review: ectopic cervical thyroid carcinoma–review of the literature with illustrative case series. J Clin Endocrinol Metab. 2011;96(9):2684–91.
16. Takeuchi K, Murata K, Fujita I. "Malignant struma ovarii" with peritoneal metastasis: report of two cases. Eur J Gynaecol Oncol. 2000;21(3):260–1.
17. Chan SW, Farrell KE. Metastatic thyroid carcinoma in the presence of struma ovarii. Med J Aust. 2001;175(7):373–4.
18. Checrallah A, et al. Malignant struma ovarii: an unusual presentation. Thyroid. 2001;11(9):889–92.
19. Dardik RB, et al. Malignant struma ovarii: two case reports and a review of the literature. Gynecol Oncol. 1999;73(3):447–51.
20. Griffiths AN, Jain B, Vine SJ. Papillary thyroid carcinoma of struma ovarii. J Obstet Gynaecol. 2004;24(1):92–3.
21. Huh JJ, Montz FJ, Bristow RE. Struma ovarii associated with pseudo-Meigs' syndrome and elevated serum CA 125. Gynecol Oncol. 2002;86(2):231–4.
22. Hemli JM, et al. Papillary carcinoma of the thyroid arising in struma ovari – report of a case and review of management guidelines. Gynecol Endocrinol. 2001;15(3):243–7.
23. Logani S, et al. Cystic ovarian metastasis from papillary thyroid carcinoma: a case report. Thyroid. 2001;11(11):1073–5.
24. Nahn PA, Robinson E, Strassman M. Conservative therapy for malignant struma ovarii. A case report. J Reprod Med. 2002; 47(11):943–5.
25. Ribeiro-Silva A, Bezerra AM, Serafini LN. Malignant struma ovarii: an autopsy report of a clinically unsuspected tumor. Gynecol Oncol. 2002;87(2):213–5.
26. Rotman-Pikielny P, et al. Recombinant human thyrotropin for the diagnosis and treatment of a highly functional metastatic struma ovarii. J Clin Endocrinol Metab. 2000;85(1):237–44.
27. Soto Moreno A, et al. Thyroid carcinoma on an ovarian teratoma: a case report and review of the literature. Gynecol Endocrinol. 2002;16(3):207–11.
28. Utsunomiya D, et al. Struma ovarii coexisting with mucinous cystadenoma detected by radioactive iodine. Clin Nucl Med. 2003; 28(9):725–7.
29. Volpi E, et al. Malignant struma ovarii: a case report of laparoscopic management. Gynecol Oncol. 2003;90(1):191–4.
30. Marti JL, et al. Optimal surgical management of well-differentiated thyroid cancer arising in struma ovarii: a series of 4 patients and a review of 53 reported cases. Thyroid. 2012;22(4):400–6.
31. Santin AD, et al. Discrimination between uterine serous papillary carcinomas and ovarian serous papillary tumours by gene expression profiling. Br J Cancer. 2004;90(9):1814–24.
32. Soliman PT, et al. Synchronous primary cancers of the endometrium and ovary: a single institution review of 84 cases. Gynecol Oncol. 2004;94(2):456–62.
33. Ryu DR, et al. Minimal change disease in a patient with ovarian papillary serous carcinoma. Gynecol Oncol. 2004;93(2): 554–6.
34. Byrd MC, Thompson LD, Wieneke JA. Intratracheal ectopic thyroid tissue: a case report and literature review. Ear Nose Throat J. 2003;82(7):514–8.
35. Kao SY, et al. Primary ectopic thyroid papillary carcinoma in the floor of the mouth and tongue: a case report. Br J Oral Maxillofac Surg. 2002;40(3):213–5.
36. LiVolsi VA, Perzin KH, Savetsky L. Carcinoma arising in median ectopic thyroid (including thyroglossal duct tissue). Cancer. 1974; 34(4):1303–15.

Thyroglossal Duct Carcinoma

53

Leonard Wartofsky and Nikolaos Stathatos

Papillary thyroid cancer is the most common endocrine malignancy. In the vast majority of cases, it presents initially as a nodule within the thyroid gland, with or without metastatic disease (local or distal). Rarely, extrathyroidal or ectopic origin of this malignancy has been documented, typically in embryologic rests of thyroid cells. One common site is the thyroglossal duct. Although a cystic nodule within a remnant of this duct is the most typical neck mass detected during childhood, such nodules are almost always histologically benign [1].

During embryologic development, the thyroid gland descends in a caudal direction from the foramen cecum, initially forming the thyroglossal duct. In most individuals, this structure disappears completely by week 10 of gestation. In some cases, however, it fails to completely atrophy and persists, often forming a cyst of varying size and histology. These cystic remnants most often contain a lining of follicular thyroid tissue (60 % of cases; [2]). Other epithelial types have been described, such as squamous, cuboidal, columnar [3, 4], intestinal, and gastric [5]. As much as 7 % of the healthy population may have some remnant of the thyroglossal duct at postmortem [6].

Thyroglossal duct remnants are the most common neck masses diagnosed during childhood and account for about 70 % of all neck masses in children [7]. Most remain asymptomatic into adulthood, but in a few rare cases, these remnants have been the site of malignant tumors. Brentano [8] may have reported the first case of carcinoma derived in a thyroglossal duct cyst in 1911; since then, there have been about 300–350 published cases. The reported prevalence of cancer is approx 1 % of all diagnosed thyroglossal duct remnants [9, 10], although carcinoma was present in 9/139 (6.5 %) of patients in one large series [11]. Thyroid cancer may present at any age and has been reported to affect patients between 6 and 81 years of age. The most frequent presentation occurs in the fourth decade of life, with a female predominance (2:1 ratio [12]).

The origin of these cancers has brought much debate: do they arise de novo or represent metastatic disease from a primary lesion inside the thyroid gland itself? Criteria have been proposed to help with this distinction [13] and include the presence of a thyroglossal duct remnant lined with epithelial cells and the documentation of a normal thyroid gland [14, 15]. The majority of these tumors are papillary thyroid carcinomas (80 %), followed by squamous cell carcinomas (6 %) and mixed follicular tumors (4 %; 12). Even Hürthle cell and anaplastic carcinoma [16] have been reported, but our review of the literature failed to find any cases of medullary thyroid cancer in a thyroglossal duct remnant. This latter finding is probably because of the different embryologic origin of the C cells from which medullary thyroid tumors originate.

For the evaluation of these lesions, a physical exam can provide important clues. A neck mass that moves with swallowing and tongue movement is characteristic. The possibility of metastatic papillary carcinoma to a Delphian lymph node in the same midline location must be considered. Some authors advocate obtaining a thyroid nuclear scan [12] to detect ectopic thyroid tissue and to determine if there is actually a fully functioning thyroid gland prior to removing the cyst. Although this may provide such evidence, results may be difficult to interpret because of the adjacent presence of a normal thyroid gland. It may not be possible to distinguish a small ectopic focus from the thyroid gland itself. Other imaging techniques can be used to make this diagnosis, including ultrasound and magnetic resonance image (MRI).

L. Wartofsky, MD, MACP (✉)
Department of Medicine, MedStar Washington Hospital Center, Georgetown University School of Medicine, 110 Irving Street, N.W., Washington, DC 20010-2975, USA
e-mail: leonard.wartofsky@medstar.net

N. Stathatos, MD
Department of Medicine, Massachusetts General Hospital, Boston, MA, USA
e-mail: nstathatos@partners.org

L. Wartofsky, D. Van Nostrand (eds.), *Thyroid Cancer*, DOI 10.1007/978-1-4939-3314-3_53

These methods are not able to give clues to the histologic composition of the masses, but they can be helpful preoperatively for anatomic localization and evaluation of possible metastatic disease. Characteristics of malignant lesions on computerized tomography (CT) have been reported by Branstetter et al. [17] and include calcification, irregular margins, a thickened cyst wall, and dense or enhancing nodules on the cyst wall.

A more widely accepted method of testing for the presence of thyroid tissue is fine-needle aspiration (FNA) cytology of the mass [18]. Although significantly less than 100 % sensitive, it is one of the most reliable preoperative diagnostic tools, not only for detecting thyroid tissue but also for diagnosing malignancy, if present. In our view, a tissue diagnosis prior to the definitive surgical procedure should be considered mandatory. If the initial FNA is nondiagnostic, a repeated attempt with ultrasound guidance should be done with multiple aspirates. If still nondiagnostic, frozen-section analysis of the excised duct at surgery before closure has been recommended, along with careful intraoperative digital examination of the thyroid gland [19].

The most frequently used surgical therapeutic approach for these tumors is the Sistrunk procedure [20–26], which involves dissection of the thyroglossal cyst. Prior to FNA, carcinoma of the thyroglossal duct would be typically identified during the pathologic analysis of a thyroglossal duct cyst removed during a Sistrunk operation. Lymph node dissection is then performed, as needed, with lymph node metastases reported in 7–12 % of thyroglossal duct carcinomas [9, 27]. The operation involves the hyoid bone because of the embryologic development of the hyoid from the second branchial arch through which the thyroglossal duct passes. Invasion into the hyoid bone has been described in as many as 30 % of malignant cases—an estimate that some authors believe necessitates the Sistrunk procedure [28, 29]. In this procedure, the tract is dissected down to the hyoid bone, and the middle or median portion of the hyoid bone is also removed. In general, surgical approaches will vary but most workers emphasize the importance of careful surgical planning [21, 24].

A review of thyroglossal duct carcinoma cases in children [30] provides similar data to that summarized above for adults. Of 21 cases, 12 were present in girls at a mean age of 13 years old. All cases were the papillary type, except for three that were mixed papillary and follicular. The tumor was confined to the thyroglossal duct in all the patients with the thyroid gland found negative for carcinoma, but there was invasion of the duct capsule in 10 of 21 (45 %) and local invasion in 5 of 21 (23 %), one of whom had pulmonary metastases. All patients generally had surgery for a nontender, painless, asymptomatic mass with carcinoma diagnosed by pathology; no patients had FNA cytology. One patient died 8 h postoperatively, and all the others had a relatively uneventful follow-up period. The same positive and negative arguments for thyroidectomy appear to apply in children as in adults, and these authors favored management by near-total thyroidectomy, radioiodine ablation, and levothyroxine suppressive therapy.

The controversy regarding whether adult patients should have a total thyroidectomy if thyroid cancer is identified in a thyroglossal duct remnant is ongoing. Differing approaches often relate to whether one believes that these tumors arise de novo or represent metastases from a primary tumor within the thyroid gland. Support for the concept that the tumors originate in the thyroid gland is provided by findings of unsuspected thyroid cancer in up to a third of cases [21, 22, 31–33], and an incidental malignant focus in the opposite lobe of the gland is not an uncommon finding. On the other hand, one may argue that this frequency of unsuspected malignancy is approximately the same as is found on autopsy [34]. Indeed, the addition of a total thyroidectomy to a Sistrunk procedure in those patients lacking a suspicious lesion on the basis of imaging studies did not significantly improve outcome [27]. Nevertheless, it is recommended that patients with intrathyroidal cancer have a total thyroidectomy which is considered by some as the standard of care today. Although these data could suggest that the same management should apply for a tumor originating in a thyroglossal duct remnant, there has not been a sufficient number of these cases to draw a more definite conclusion. There remain cogent arguments against routine-associated thyroidectomy for papillary cancer [1], given the excellent prognosis for the overwhelming majority of small stage I lesions, particularly in young patients. However, the case for thyroidectomy is more compelling when the tumor is follicular, considering the propensity for angioinvasion and a more aggressive course of the latter cancer. Depending on the histology and extent of the primary tumor and the need for further therapy with radioactive iodine, a total thyroidectomy may be a necessary step to ensure a cure. As recommended by the American Thyroid Association guidelines [35], thyroid sonography is indicated, and the identification of nodular disease provides a strong indication for concomitant thyroidectomy. Incidence may be as high as 33 % for associated carcinoma within the thyroid gland [28, 34]. On the contrary, because many of these carcinomas have been detected in the duct without any evidence of tumor within the thyroid gland, thyroidectomy might be avoided if the thyroid has no demonstrable nodules by ultrasound, and the primary tumor is small without proof of metastasis to cervical nodes. Proponents of concomitant thyroidectomy [36] point out that there may be a high incidence of local spread of these tumors not detected at a Sistrunk procedure. The full procedure with thyroidectomy allows appropriate staging and subsequent monitoring by isotopic scans and serum thyroglobulin measurements. Moreover, a patient was reported to develop lung metastases and die following treatment with only cyst removal and without thyroidectomy [18]. On rare occasion, persistent measurable thyroglobulin may be due to coincidental presence of a thyroglossal duct remnant which can usually be readily identified by isotopic scanning [14].

The potential presence of lymph node metastases reflects another rationale for total thyroidectomy as well as lymph node dissection [15]. In one series, 12/16 (75 %) of patients presented with lymph nodes metastases identified on neck dissection [33]. The management approach suggested by Patel [27] was based on stratifying patients into either low- or high-risk categories. Low-risk patients, such as those <45 years old, with tumor <4 cms without local or distant extension may be treated solely by a Sistrunk procedure. Whereas high-risk patients, defined as >45 years of age, with tumors >4 cms, and evidence of soft tissue extension would undergo total thyroidectomy in addition to the Sistrunk procedure, with node dissection as warranted by evidence of lymph node metastases on ultrasound or at surgery, followed by radioiodine ablation. This approach was modified subsequently by Plaza et al. [37] who recommended a sole Sistrunk procedure only in patients <45 years with tumors of <1.5 cms confined to the cyst with an otherwise normal thyroid and neck on ultrasound. But in their approach, a thyroidectomy and lymph node dissection followed by radioiodine ablation would be done if there were involved lymph nodes identified.

If the tumor histology is that of squamous cell carcinoma, a more extensive surgical excision is usually required. These tumors generally have a much worse prognosis, whereas papillary thyroid carcinomas have the same excellent prognosis as those originating from the thyroid gland, depending (as always) on the stage of the disease at diagnosis. Notably, few deaths from papillary thyroid carcinoma have been reported with none noted in one series after a 10-year follow-up period [27]. This contrasts with squamous cell carcinoma, however, for which adjunctive postoperative external radiation therapy may also be warranted because of the very poor prognosis. Boswell et al. [10] reported that 3/9 patients with this tumor died within 15 months of diagnosis. As summarized by Mazzaferri [38], we may not be in a position to always make a fully rational judgment based on the data available on these tumors. However, the presence of either those characteristics associated with a more aggressive cancer course or those features associated with a good outcome will make the decision easier in many cases. As with most patients, because of the many potential complex issues surrounding each patient's presentation, an individualized approach is best.

References

1. Klubo-Gwiezdzinska J, Manes RP, Chia SH, Burman KD, Stathatos NA, Deeb ZE, Wartofsky L. Clinical review: ectopic cervical thyroid carcinoma–review of the literature with illustrative case series. J Clin Endocrinol Metab. 2011;96(9):2684–91.
2. LiVolsi V, Perzen K, Savetsky L. Carcinoma arising in median ectopic thyroid. Cancer. 1974;34:1303–13.
3. Akbari Y, Richter P, Papadakis L. Thyroid carcinoma arising in thyroglossal duct remnants. Arch Surg. 1967;94:235–9.
4. Magsalin R, Diener C, Jawadi H. Thyroglossal cyst carcinoma. J Kans Med Soc. 1982;83:426–7.
5. Chandrasoma P, Janssen M. A thyroglossal cyst lined by gastric epithelium. JAMA. 1982;247:1406.
6. Hilger AW, Thompson SD, Smallman LA. Papillary carcinoma arising in a thyroglossal cyst: a case report and literature review. J Laryngol Otol. 1995;109:1124–7.
7. Gardner D. Unusual appearance of a thyroglossal duct cyst carcinoma. J Otolaryngol. 1989;18:258–9.
8. Brentano H. Struma aberrata lingual mit drusen metastasen. Deut Med Wschr. 1911;37:665.
9. Weiss SD, Orlich CC. Primary papillary carcinoma of a thyroglossal duct cyst: report of a case and literature review. Br J Surg. 1991;78:87–9.
10. Boswell W, Zoller M, Williams J. Thyroglossal duct carcinoma. Am Surg. 1994;60:650–5.
11. Forest VI, Murali R, Clark JR. Thyroglossal duct cyst carcinoma: case series. J Otolaryngol Head Neck Surg. 2011;40:151–6.
12. Renard T, Choucair R, Stevenson W, et al. Carcinoma of the thyroglossal duct. Surg Gynecol Obstet. 1990;171:305–8.
13. Komorowski R, Joseph T. Thyroglossal duct carcinoma. Hum Pathol. 1975;6:717–29.
14. Li D, Meng Z, Zhang G, Yu T, Tan J, Dong F. Visualization of thyroglossal duct cyst in differentiated thyroid cancer patient. Clin Nucl Med. 2010;35(7):499–504.
15. Kwon JK, Lee SM, Lee HM, Lee JC. Papillary thyroid carcinoma arising from a primary thyroglossal duct cyst with cervical node metastases. Thyroid. 2012;22(3):330–1.
16. Woods RH, Saunders Jr JR, Pearlman S, et al. Anaplastic carcinoma arising in a thyroglossal duct tract. Otolaryngol Head Neck Surg. 1993;109:945–9.
17. Branstetter BF, Weissman JL, Kennedy TL, Whitaker M. The CT appearance of thyroglossal duct carcinoma. AJNR. 2000;21: 1547–50.
18. Bardales RH, Suhrland MJ, Korourian S, et al. Cytologic findings in thyroglossal duct carcinoma. Am J Clin Pathol. 1996;106:615–9.
19. Luna-Ortiz K, Hurtado-Lopez LM, Valderrama-Landaeta JL, Ruiz-Vega A. Thyroglossal duct cyst with papillary carcinoma: what must be done? Thyroid. 2004;14:363–6.
20. Sistrunk W. The surgical treatment of cysts of the thyroglossal tract. Ann Surg. 1920;71:121–2.
21. Pelligriti G, Lumera G, Malandrino P, Latina A, Masucci R, Scollo C, et al. Thyroid cancer in thyroglossal duct cysts requires a specific approach due to its unpredictable extension. J Clin Endocrinol Metab. 2013;98:458–65.
22. Park M-H, Yoon JH, Jegal YJ, Lee JS. Papillary thyroglossal duct cyst carcinoma with synchronous occult papillary thyroid microcarcinoma. Yonsei Med J. 2010;51:609–11.
23. Tachibana T, Orita Y, Fujisawa M, Ogawara Y. Papillary thyroid carcinoma arising from a median ectopic thyroid with no thyroglossal duct remnant. Acta Med Okayama. 2013;67:61–4.
24. Byeon HK, Ban MJ, Lee JM, Ha JG, Kim ES, Koh YW, Choi EC. Robot-assisted Sistrunk's operation, total thyroidectomy, and neck

dissection via a transaxillary and retroauricular (TARA) approach in papillary carcinoma arising in thyroglossal duct cyst and thyroid gland. Ann Surg Oncol. 2012;19(13):4259–61.
25. Dzodic R, Markovic I, Stanojevic B, Saenko V, Buta M, Djurisic I, et al. Surgical management of primary thyroid carcinoma arising in thyroglossal duct cyst: an experience of a single institution in Serbia. Endocr J. 2012;59(6):517–22.
26. Choi YM, Kim TY, Song DE, Hong SJ, Jang EK, Jeon MJ, et al. Papillary thyroid carcinoma arising from a thyroglossal duct cyst: a single institution experience. Endocr J. 2013;60(5):665–70.
27. Patel SG, Escrig M, Shaha AR, et al. Management of well-differentiated thyroid carcinoma presenting within thyroglossal duct cyst. J Surg Oncol. 2002;79:134–9.
28. Stephenson B, Wheeler M. Carcinoma of the thyroglossal duct. Aust N Z J Surg. 1994;64:212.
29. Dan D, Rambally R, Naraynsingh V, Maharaj R, Hariharan S. A case of malignancy in a thyroglossal duct cyst–recommendations for management. J Natl Med Assoc. 2012;104(3–4):211–4.
30. Peretz A, Leiberman E, Kapelushnik J, Hershkovitz E. Thyroglossal duct carcinoma in children: case presentation and review of the literature. Thyroid. 2004;14:777–85.
31. Heshmati HM, Fatourechi V, van Heerden JA, Hay ID, Goellner JR. Thyroglossal duct carcinoma: report of 12 cases. Mayo Clin Proc. 1997;72:315–9.
32. Cherian MP, Nair B, Thomas S, Somanathan T, Sebastian P. Synchronous papillary carcinoma in thyroglossal duct cyst and thyroid gland: case report and review of literature. Head Neck. 2009;31(10):1387–91.
33. Hartl DM, Al Ghuslan A, Chami L, Leboulleux S, Schlumberger M, Travagli JP. High rate of multifocality and occult lymph node metastases in papillary thyroid carcinoma arising in thyroglossal duct cysts. Ann Surg Oncol. 2009;16:2595–601.
34. Martinez-Tello FJ, Martinez-Cabruja R, Fernandez-Martin J, Lasso-Oria C, Ballestin-Carcavilla C. Occult carcinoma of the thyroid. A systematic autopsy study from Spain of two series performed with two different methods. Cancer. 1993;71: 4022–9.
35. Haugen BR, Alexander EK, Bible KC, Doherty GM, Mandel SJ, Nikiforov Y, et al. American thyroid association management guidelines for patients with thyroid nodules and differentiated thyroid cancer. Thyroid. 2014;24: 2014 (in press).
36. Miccoli P, Minuto MN, Galleri D, et al. Extent of surgery in thyroglossal duct carcinoma: reflections on a series of eighteen cases. Thyroid. 2004;14:121–3.
37. Plaza CPR, Lopez MED, Carrasco CEG, Meseguer LM, Perucho AD. Management of well-differentiated thyroglossal remnant thyroid carcinoma: time to close the debate? Report five new cases and proposal of a definite algorithm for treatment. Ann Surg Oncol. 2006;13:745–52.
38. Mazzaferri EL. Editorial: thyroid cancer in thyroglossal duct remnants: a diagnostic and therapeutic dilemma. Thyroid. 2004;14: 335–6.

Thyroid Cancer in Pregnancy

54

Shannon D. Sullivan

Introduction

Differentiated thyroid cancer (DTC) is most commonly diagnosed in euthyroid adults who present with a thyroid mass or structural abnormality in the thyroid gland, such as one or more nodules, which are typically confirmed by radiologic imaging. In addition to the typical presentation, there are several unique clinical circumstances under which thyroid cancer is diagnosed. One that requires special consideration and attention is a diagnosis of thyroid cancer during pregnancy. Thyroid cancer is the second most commonly diagnosed malignancy during pregnancy behind only breast cancer, with approximately 14 cases per 100,000 pregnancies [1]. The general principles of diagnosing and treating thyroid cancer in pregnant women are the same as those used in the more typical presentations; however, additional treatment restrictions and consideration of the timing of treatments are required when both a woman and her developing child will be affected. As stated by Oduncu and colleagues in their review of maternal-fetal issues related to a diagnosis of malignancy during pregnancy, "there is always a conflict between maternal optimal therapy and fetal well-being" [2]. In this chapter, special considerations that must be made when diagnosing and treating thyroid cancer during or around the time of pregnancy are discussed.

S.D. Sullivan, MD, PhD (✉)
Department of Endocrinology & Metabolism,
MedStar Washington Hospital Center,
110 Irving St., NW, Suite 2A-72, Washington, DC 20010, USA
e-mail: shannon.d.sullivan@medstar.net

Physiologic Changes in Thyroidal Economy During Pregnancy

Physiologic alterations in maternal thyroid hormone levels and thyroidal economy occur during pregnancy. The thyroid gland of the developing fetus starts producing small amounts of thyroid hormone at approximately 10 weeks of gestation, with progressively more hormone produced until fetal production plateaus at around 35 weeks [3]. Thus, particularly in the first trimester of pregnancy, the fetus is entirely dependent on thyroid hormone transferred from the mother, without which neurologic and cognitive development are severely impacted, as has been shown in the infants of hypothyroid mothers living in iodine-deficient regions [4, 5]. During pregnancy, physiologic adjustments in the maternal hypothalamic-pituitary-thyroid axis occur to ensure that fetal demands for thyroid hormone are met. Importantly, high levels of β-hCG produced by the placenta stimulate production of thyroid hormone by cross-reacting with TSH receptors in the maternal thyroid gland [6]. This leads to suppression of maternal TSH secretion from the anterior pituitary via normal negative feedback mechanisms and increased production of thyroid hormones secondary to hCG stimulation, resulting in elevated levels of free T4 and free T3. Thus, throughout pregnancy, normative ranges for TSH are lower than the normal reference range for nonpregnant women [7]. In addition, maternal thyroid hormone requirements increase substantially (25–50 %) during gestation due to multiple factors, including transfer of thyroid hormone to the fetus, increased maternal thyroxine-binding globulin (TBG) production that is stimulated by high estrogen levels, increased maternal clearance of thyroid hormone by placental deiodinase activity, and increased maternal renal clearance of thyroid hormone [3, 8, 9]. In athyreotic newborns, cord blood total thyroxine concentration is about half of the level seen in newborns with normal thyroid function, indicating that a significant amount of maternal thyroid hormone

L. Wartofsky, D. Van Nostrand (eds.), *Thyroid Cancer*, DOI 10.1007/978-1-4939-3314-3_54

passes via the placenta to provide thyroid hormone to the fetus [10]. In euthyroid pregnant women, the maternal thyroid gland is able to compensate for this increased demand. Thyroid hormone secretion returns to normal when the marked elevations in β-hCG seen in early pregnancy begin to decline. In hypothyroid women, the dose of exogenous levothyroxine replacement must be adjusted to account for the increased demand for thyroid hormone during pregnancy.

Precise regulation of thyroid hormone levels during pregnancy is crucial for achieving an optimal outcome for both mother and child. The mainstay of treatment for DTC is total thyroidectomy followed by radioiodine ablation of residual disease, which renders the patient hypothyroid and dependent on exogenous levothyroxine replacement. For this reason, maintaining a precise thyroid hormone economy is of paramount importance among women with DTC who are pregnant or planning pregnancy in order to achieve optimal outcomes with respect to both the DTC and the pregnancy. Indeed, maternal hypothyroidism is one of the most concerning complications of pregnancy, as this condition increases the risk for spontaneous miscarriage, preterm delivery, gestational hypertension, preeclampsia, placental abruption, postpartum hemorrhage, and neurologic and cognitive impairment to the offspring [11–15]. On the other hand, excess maternal thyroid hormone during pregnancy is also detrimental and can lead to abnormal fetal growth, maternal hypertension or preeclampsia, preterm delivery, and miscarriage [16, 17].

Is Risk of Thyroid Cancer Increased During Pregnancy?

There is a clear gender disparity in the prevalence of differentiated thyroid cancer, with women affected ~3 times more frequently than men, suggesting sex hormone differences may play a role [18]. In support of this hypothesis, incidence of DTC in women peaks during the reproductive years, whereas in men, incidence progressively increases with age [19]. It is hypothesized that increased DTC incidence in women of reproductive age may be due, at least in part, to high β-hCG levels during pregnancy, as β-hCG binds to and stimulates TSH receptors, resulting in growth of thyroid tissue [20]. Moreover, estradiol stimulates expression of the thyroglobulin gene in differentiated thyroid tumor cells in vitro [21], and thyroid cancer cells bind estrogen, suggesting they express estrogen receptors and are thus susceptible to stimulation by estradiol [22].

Interactions between estradiol, β-hCG, and the thyroid gland have led multiple investigators to evaluate the relationship between female reproductive history, including pregnancy history, and risk of thyroid cancer. Conflicting evidence exists regarding the risk of thyroid cancer during and following pregnancy, with some studies showing an increased risk [23, 24] and others demonstrating no change in risk [25, 26]. A population-based case-control study by Rossing and colleagues [23] compared the presentation of papillary thyroid cancer (PTC) in adult parous women to controls and found that both pregnancy and lactation may transiently increase the risk of PTC. A more recent study found that for women <45 years old, risk of thyroid cancer was increased in the first 5 years following pregnancy, again suggesting pregnancy may play a causal role [24]. Also in that study, among women >45 years old, use of estrogen replacement therapy was associated with a trend toward an increased risk of PTC, although this relationship was not statistically significant (RR 1.69, 95 % CI 0.95–2.98). On the other hand, a population-based retrospective study of reproductive and hormonal risk factors for thyroid cancer in women found no consistent link between reproductive history and thyroid cancer [25]. In the study by Mack et al., risk of thyroid cancer was not altered by use of exogenous estrogens, including oral contraceptive pills. Further, they found that increasing parity increased thyroid cancer risk only in women who suppressed lactation postpartum, while thyroid cancer risk was decreased among women who had ever breastfed, with longer duration of lactation associated with lower risk. Sakoda and colleagues [26] found no overall change in risk of thyroid cancer with a history of pregnancy, including history of pregnancy that resulted in miscarriage or elective abortion, compared to nulligravid women. They also found no association of thyroid cancer with prior use of oral contraceptives or hormone replacement therapy. On the other hand, they did find a ~2-fold increased risk among women <45 years old who reported a pregnancy within the previous 5 years [26], similar to their more recent data discussed above [24]. Indeed, when taken together, these data are conflicting regarding a role for sex hormones or pregnancy on the incidence of DTC, although sufficient evidence exists to warrant further investigations to help clarify the relationship between estrogen and β-hCG (and thus reproductive history, including pregnancy) and thyroid cancer risk.

Evaluation of Thyroid Nodules During Pregnancy

Thyroid cancer is most often detected within a thyroid nodule, and there is evidence to suggest that pregnancy is a stimulus for thyroid nodule formation, as well as for growth of preexisting nodules. Stimulation of the thyroid by elevated levels of β-hCG and estrogen, as well as negative iodine balance during pregnancy (even in iodine-sufficient areas), contributes to growth of thyroid tissue during pregnancy. In a study among women aged 36–50, 9 % of nulligravid compared to 25 % of parous women had ultrasound evidence of thyroid nodules [27]. During pregnancy, thyroid volume increases, and the volume of preexisting thyroid nodules may also increase, with a return to prepregnancy volume by 3 months postpartum [28]. Interestingly, the prevalence of thyroid nodules has been shown to increase with increasing parity in women, although this has most notably been shown in areas of iodine insufficiency [27, 28]. Accentuated iodine deficiency with subsequent pregnancies has been proposed to be a mechanism, although it is possible that increasing maternal age with increasing parity may in fact play a larger role [29]. Two studies have shown that among women with one thyroid nodule detected during the first trimester of pregnancy, up to 20 % will develop a second nodule during that pregnancy [27, 28], although it is possible that this may have been the course of thyroid nodule development irrespective of the pregnant state. Nonetheless, regardless of the specific etiology, many women will be newly diagnosed with thyroid nodules during pregnancy and therefore will need to undergo evaluation to rule out thyroid malignancy if suspicious sonographic features are present.

Any thyroid nodule detected during pregnancy should undergo similar initial evaluation as a nodule detected outside of pregnancy. Specifically, the patient should be asked about family and personal history of thyroid cancer and related syndromes [multiple endocrine neoplasia type 2 (MEN2), familial polyposis coli, etc.], history of head and neck irradiation, and clinical signs and symptoms, such as dysphagia, dysphonia, or compressive symptoms of the neck. Additionally, a complete physical examination of the neck should be performed, including evaluation of cervical lymph nodes. The best imaging modality for detecting or confirming thyroid nodules and lymph nodes and evaluating their features is ultrasound. As in nonpregnant individuals, pregnant women with thyroid nodules with sonographic features that are suspicious for malignancy and/or >1 cm should undergo fine needle aspiration (FNA) with cytological analysis. FNA of suspicious thyroid nodules can be done at any time during pregnancy, as this procedure poses no risk to the mother or fetus. That being said, FNA can also be delayed until after delivery for nodules without concerning features or for concerning nodules that are discovered late in pregnancy, as any indicated treatment will be postponed until after delivery. In addition, any pregnant (or nonpregnant) woman with a thyroid nodule should have thyroid function tested (serum TSH and free T4). An unstimulated calcitonin level should *only* be measured in women with a family history of medullary thyroid cancer (MTC) or MEN2. Use of pentagastrin for a stimulated calcitonin level is contraindicated in pregnancy [30]. Of course, radioiodine scans for evaluation of hyperfunctioning thyroid nodules and thyroid ablative treatment with radioactive iodine are contraindicated during pregnancy [30, 31].

Treatment of Thyroid Cancer in Pregnancy

According to guidelines published by the American Thyroid Association (ATA) [30] and the Endocrine Society [8], the most widely respected and utilized bodies guiding diagnosis and treatment of thyroid disease in the United States, in most cases it is appropriate to delay treatment of differentiated thyroid cancer until the postpartum period in women who are diagnosed during pregnancy. This recommendation is based on a lack of evidence of worse outcomes when treatment is delayed several months, particularly for papillary and follicular variants of thyroid cancer [30]. That being said, it is nonetheless necessary to manage each case of thyroid cancer individually based on tumor characteristics present in a given patient and patient preference. When DTC is diagnosed early in pregnancy by FNA, repeat neck examinations and neck ultrasound examinations should be performed each trimester to monitor for any growth of the lesion/s (nodule/s) and to rule out rapid growth. If the lesion(s) remains stable, surgery may be delayed until after delivery; however, if significant nodule growth is seen (defined as ≥50 % in volume or ≥20 % in diameter, in two dimensions) or LN metastases are detected, surgery is recommended in the second trimester. If DTC is not diagnosed until the second or third trimester, surgery can also be delayed until after delivery. The exception is when initial diagnosis by cytology and ultrasound indicates advanced disease, such as bulky cervical adenopathy, in which case surgery should be performed as soon as possible and ideally in the second trimester. In all cases of DTC diagnosed during pregnancy, whether or not thyroidectomy is performed during gestation, the ATA recommends starting suppressive dose of levothyroxine (LT4), with goal TSH between 0.1 and 0.5 mIU/L. Neither surgery during the second trimester nor suppressive doses of LT4 are recommended for pregnant women found to have nodules that are *suspicious* for DTC by cytology, given that ~70 % of these nodules are later proven to be benign [30].

In cases of thyroid cancer diagnosed during pregnancy in which surgical resection is indicated or desired as soon as possible, such as in aggressive forms of thyroid cancer, thyroidectomy can be performed in the second trimester. This is the earliest time point in gestation at which organogenesis is complete. However, thyroid surgery done during pregnancy is associated with higher risk of surgical complications, longer length of hospital stay, and, consequently, significantly increased overall cost compared to the same surgery performed in nonpregnant patients. An analysis of the Healthcare Cost and Utilization Project-National Inpatient Sample compared outcomes of thyroid or parathyroid surgery in 201 pregnant women with >31,000 age-matched, nonpregnant controls and found that pregnant women were twice as likely to have surgical complications, both maternal and fetal, including miscarriage [32]. The elevated risks of thyroidectomy performed during pregnancy can be explained, at least in part, by the following factors: (1) the normal increase in thyroid gland volume that occurs with pregnancy makes surgical resection more difficult, (2) the significant pregnancy-induced changes in maternal physiology complicate anesthesia, (3) there is the possibility of fetal demise, and (4) the women undergoing any surgical procedure during pregnancy represent a higher risk group by definition [32]. Anesthesia at any time during pregnancy is complicated by multiple factors, including increased maternal blood volume and cardiac output, and can result in maternal hypotension and fetal hypoperfusion. When thyroidectomy is performed in the first trimester, the spontaneous abortion rate is higher than if surgery is performed in the second or third trimester; thus first-trimester surgery should be avoided whenever possible (reviewed in [33]).

Endocrine complications specific to thyroidectomy that pose significant risks to the fetus include postoperative maternal hypoparathyroidism and maternal hypothyroidism. Hypoparathyroidism following total thyroidectomy is not uncommon, and because fetal calcium homeostasis is dependent on maternal calcium levels, maternal hypocalcemia will stimulate fetal parathyroid tissue, resulting in bone demineralization [34]. Conversely, ingestion of large doses of supplemental calcium, especially with concurrent vitamin D administration, by a pregnant woman with hypoparathyroidism may suppress fetal parathyroid function and result in fetal hypocalcemia [35]. To avoid complications of abnormal maternal calcium homeostasis following total thyroidectomy, parathyroid function should be closely monitored intra- and postoperatively.

After total thyroidectomy for DTC, replacement levothyroxine is necessary and is especially important during pregnancy, not only for suppression of residual or recurrent thyroid cancer but also for normal fetal development and optimal pregnancy outcomes. Complications associated with maternal hypothyroidism in pregnancy include spontaneous miscarriage, preterm delivery, pregnancy-induced hypertension, placental abruption, postpartum hemorrhage, and fetal neurologic and/or cognitive impairment [11–15]. Goal maternal TSH is $\leq$2.5 mIU/L during the first trimester and $\leq$3.0 mIU/L during the second and third trimesters to avoid maternal and fetal complications. It is recommended that TSH levels be followed at least every 4 weeks so that adjustments in levothyroxine dosages can be made to meet the increased requirements during pregnancy and/or optimize therapy [8, 30].

Radioactive iodine (I-131) is absolutely contraindicated during pregnancy due to the risks of exposure to radioactivity on the developing fetus [30, 36]. Therefore, in women diagnosed with DTC during pregnancy, if radioactive iodine (RAI) treatment is indicated, it should be postponed until as soon as possible in the postpartum period, also keeping in mind restrictions with respect to lactation. Breastfeeding should not be initiated or continued for at least 6 months following RAI ablation; thus many women will postpone RAI treatment until they have had an opportunity to breastfeed their infant for 3–6 months. When the plan is to proceed with RAI ablation in the early postpartum period, the patient's obstetrician should be aware of this and should be advised to avoid topical iodine solutions as antiseptic agents during delivery, as these may reduce the effectiveness of the radioiodine treatment.

Does Pregnancy Alter the Course of Differentiated Thyroid Cancer?

Several groups have investigated whether pregnancy that occurs after a woman's diagnosis and treatment of DTC poses a risk for disease progression or recurrence due to hormonal factors stimulatory to thyroid and nodular growth. Hirsch et al. [37] retrospectively reviewed charts of women diagnosed with PTC followed by at least one pregnancy and found that among women without structural or biochemical evidence of disease at conception, pregnancy did not increase the risk for recurrence within a median of 4 years of postpartum follow-up. Six of 13 women (46 %) with evidence of residual disease at conception did show progression during pregnancy. However, this study could not confirm causality, and these women, who had higher risk disease, may have shown similar progression had they not become pregnant. This study confirms findings from another recent study that monitored serum Tg levels and neck ultrasound findings before pregnancy and after delivery in 36 women who had received past treatment for DTC [38]. In that study, no disease progression was seen among women without evidence of residual disease, but two of four women with known residual or metastatic lesions prior to pregnancy did have evidence of progression in the early postpartum period, suggesting pregnancy may stimulate thyroid cancer tissue growth in the presence of persistent disease. Again, however, causality could not be proven, and advancing thyroid cancer burden may have occurred in these patients in the absence of a recent pregnancy. Finally, Rosario and colleagues also showed lack of disease recurrence in the early postpartum period among women without evidence of residual DTC at the time of conception [39]. Together, these studies indicate that, at least in the short term and for low-risk patients, pregnancy does not present a clinically significant stimulus to thyroid cancer recurrence or growth.

In women who have been diagnosed with DTC prior to pregnancy and who are already on post-thyroidectomy suppressive doses of LT4, TSH suppression should be maintained at the same level as it was prior to pregnancy in order to minimize disease progression. Maintenance of TSH suppression requires frequent monitoring of thyroid function tests (at least every 4 weeks) so that adjustments to the LT4 dose can be made if necessary. Most hypothyroid women will require increased doses of LT4 during pregnancy due to increased maternal and fetal demands, with dose increases potentially necessary during each trimester. Goal TSH for non-thyroid cancer patients during pregnancy is ≤2.5 mIU/L during the first trimester and ≤3.0 mIU/L during the second and third trimesters. In women with thyroid cancer on suppressive doses of LT4, goal TSH during pregnancy does not change from that recommended for the nonpregnant state. In that regard, there are no clinically significant negative consequences to maternal subclinical hyperthyroidism during pregnancy; thus maintaining prepregnancy TSH suppression is acceptable [30]. Because women with histories of DTC are already on suppressive doses of LT4, they will typically require smaller LT4 dose increases compared to women who are hypothyroid for other reasons, such as Hashimoto's thyroiditis [40]. Furthermore, women who are hypothyroid and dependent on LT4 replacement for any reason should take a daily prenatal multivitamin containing iodine due to increased iodine requirements during pregnancy. Total daily iodine intake is recommended to be 250–300 mcg daily in pregnancy and in lactation if breastfeeding [30, 41]. Some (but not all) prenatal multivitamins contain 150 mcg of potassium iodide, which should supplement dietary iodine intake to meet the increased daily requirements in pregnancy.

Some debate exists regarding the utility of following serum thyroglobulin (Tg) levels during pregnancy due to normal pregnancy-induced changes in Tg production. In euthyroid women, Tg levels are higher during pregnancy compared to the nonpregnant state [38], and there is data to suggest that high estrogen states such as pregnancy may increase expression of the thyroglobulin gene [42]. Soldin and colleagues [43] investigated changes in Tg levels across trimesters during pregnancy in euthyroid women and found significant differences between the first and third trimesters, suggesting trimester-specific normal ranges should be used. Levels of TSH, T4, T3, and urine iodine seem to affect serum Tg during pregnancy; thus Mazzaferri suggests that following Tg levels during pregnancy in women with thyroid cancer has little utility and cannot be used to guide clinical decision-making. Rather, serial neck ultrasound examinations and close monitoring of serum TSH during pregnancy appear to be a better follow-up strategy [33].

Outcome of Thyroid Cancer Diagnosed During Pregnancy

Thyroid cancer diagnosed during pregnancy typically means that some or all treatments will be delayed until after delivery, thus raising concern that a diagnosis of thyroid cancer during pregnancy results in greater morbidity and mortality. Mazzaferri and colleagues [44] asked this question in a study comparing long-term outcomes related to differentiated thyroid cancer between women who were diagnosed during pregnancy and age-matched women who were diagnosed outside of pregnancy. Among women diagnosed during pregnancy, thyroidectomy was performed during the second trimester in 20 % and during the postpartum period in 77 %. Comparable numbers of patients diagnosed during and outside of pregnancy received I-131 postoperatively (30 % vs. 25 %, pregnant vs. nonpregnant). Of interest, outcomes over 20 years of follow-up, including cancer recurrences, distant metastases, and cancer deaths, were similar (1) between women diagnosed during pregnancy and those diagnosed outside of pregnancy and (2) among women diagnosed during pregnancy, between those who underwent thyroidectomy in the second trimester and those who delayed thyroidectomy until the postpartum period. These data are in concert with those of Herzon and colleagues, who showed that survival rates were similar between women aged 18–46 diagnosed with DTC during pregnancy and age-matched women diagnosed outside of pregnancy [45]. A third study by Yasmeen et al. [46], a retrospective population-based cohort study using data from the California Cancer Registry and a linked statewide registry of neonatal and maternal hospital discharges, compared thyroid cancer prognosis and maternal and fetal outcomes among three groups of women: (1) women diagnosed with DTC during pregnancy or in the first postpartum year; (2) age-matched, nonpregnant women diagnosed with DTC; and (3) pregnant women without thyroid cancer. These investigators failed to find any significant differences in thyroid cancer prognosis or in any maternal or fetal outcome measures between these groups. Further, among women with DTC diagnosed around the time of pregnancy, neither the timing of diagnosis (i.e., prepartum vs. antepartum vs. postpartum) nor the timing of initial thyroidectomy (i.e., during pregnancy or in the postpartum period) affected maternal or fetal outcomes. On the other hand, Vannucchi et al. [47] found that DTC diagnosed during pregnancy or in the first postpartum year was associated with significantly higher expression of ERα within pathological thyroid specimens compared to ERα expression within thyroid tissue that was surgically removed >1 year after delivery or before pregnancy. Furthermore, these investigators found that a diagnosis of DTC during pregnancy or in the first year postpartum was a significant predictor of persistent disease [47]. Taken together with the other studies, however, the data overwhelmingly suggest that a diagnosis of thyroid cancer during or around the time of pregnancy does not have a significant impact on disease prognosis or pregnancy outcome. Thus, for most women, delaying definitive treatment of DTC until after pregnancy is an acceptable option that is not likely to lead to worsened maternal outcomes. Nevertheless, in high-risk cases of DTC such as tall cell variant or DTC involving regional lymph nodes or distant metastases, strong consideration should be made for performing thyroidectomy during pregnancy (in the second trimester if possible) to improve long-term maternal outcomes.

Fertility, Pregnancy, and Breastfeeding After I-131 Treatment of Differentiated Thyroid Cancer

Although rigorous controlled studies have not been done, several investigators have evaluated gonadal function and pregnancy outcomes after I-131 treatment in men and women with differentiated thyroid cancer. It is estimated that the radiation dose delivered to the gonads is approximately 0.14 cGy for every 1 mCi of I-131 [48]. For example, for a patient receiving 100 mCi of I-131, the gonads receive approximately 14 cGy (or 14 rads) of radioactivity, which is the radiation equivalent of approximately 14 abdominal CT scans. Radiation exposure increases when functioning metastases are located in proximity to the gonads. Likely due to gonadal insult from the increased radiation exposure, several investigators have found that I-131 treatment causes transient gonadal dysfunction in both men and women, characterized by increased serum FSH levels in both sexes, and transient menstrual cycle abnormalities in women (without permanent ovarian failure). These effects may last for up to 1 year following RAI treatment, suggesting the RAI itself causes transient gonadal dysfunction. However, in these cases, it is difficult to distinguish gonadal dysfunction that is due to radioactive iodine exposure vs. that which is due to a delay in attaining euthyroidism following total thyroidectomy, particularly when RAI ablation occurs very soon after total thyroidectomy. In that regard, both hypo- and hyperthyroidism are well-established causes of reproductive dysfunction in women and men [49]. Moreover, whether or not RAI causes transient gonadal dysfunction, I-131 has *not* been associated with decreased fertility in either sex or with worsened pregnancy outcomes, including fetal congenital abnormalities, low birth weight, preterm delivery, miscarriage, or early childhood morbidity ([50] and references within) (Table 54.1).

In a study of >2600 pregnancies among women with DTC, a 20 % miscarriage rate was observed among women who had undergone thyroidectomy alone compared to a 19 % miscarriage rate among women whose pregnancies occurred after thyroidectomy plus I-131 treatment. In that study, even women who had received either (1) large doses of I-131 or (2) I-131 during the 12 months prior to the index pregnancy had similar miscarriage rates, suggesting that I-131 treatment in the year *prior* to pregnancy poses minimal risk, at least for miscarriage. Additionally, this study showed no change in the incidence of stillbirth, preterm delivery, low birth weight, congenital malformation, death by 1 year of age, childhood thyroid disorders, or childhood cancers between women whose pregnancies occurred before or after I-131 [51]. Bal et al. [52] evaluated female fertility and pregnancy outcomes in 40 women who conceived from 7 to 120 months following RAI ablation of DTC. Similarly, they found that RAI therapy had no effect on fertility, pregnancy complications including miscarriage, or health of the offspring, even in mothers who had been treated with large and/or repeat doses of I-131 or in mothers who conceived prior to 12 months following RAI treatment [52]. Likewise, no differences in pregnancy

Table 54.1 Studies investigating pregnancy outcome after maternal I-131 ablation therapy

Study authors	Radioactivity	# Pregnancies	Miscarriage rate	Preterm births	Low birth weight	Congenital abnormalities	Infant deaths
Garsi et al. (2008) [51]	100–238 mCi	2673	10 % before I-131, 20 % after thyroidectomy, 19 % after I-131	No differences	No differences	No differences	No differences
Do Rosario et al. (2006) [69]	101–149 mCi	78	5.1 %	4	5.4	1.3	0
Balenovic et al. (2006) [70]	100 mCi or >100 mCi	49	10%	No differences	No differences	0	0
Brandao et al. (2007) [71]	30–550 mCi	66	6.3 % patients, 11.6 % controls	3	No differences	1.5	0
Fard-Esfahani et al. (2009) [72]	>100 mCi	126 post-I-131, 101 pre-I-131	26.2 % post-I-131, 16.8 % pre-I-131	No differences	0	2.4	No differences
Vini et al. (2002) [73]	81–1595 mCi	441	3.2%	0.9	No data	0	0
Chow et al. (2004) [74]	96.6 mCi	263	No differences	Significant increase ($P=0.03$)	No differences	0	0

Adapted from Sioka et al. [50]

outcomes have been demonstrated in pregnancies that occurred before or after the *fathers* were treated with I-131 therapy for DTC [53].

Although recent studies do not demonstrate adverse effects among women whose pregnancies occurred after radioiodine therapy, it is recommended that women delay pregnancy for 6 months to 1 year following I-131 [8, 30, 54] due to (1) transient effects of RAI on gonadal function and (2) older data showing increased risk of miscarriage in the year following radioiodine, which may have been due to lack of optimization of maternal thyroid hormone levels after radioablative treatment [55], and (3) to avoid significant delays if repeat RAI treatment will be indicated [54]. Studies to date that have reported on pregnancy outcomes after I-131 therapy are summarized in Table 54.1 (adapted from [50]).

As stated previously, radioactive iodine is contraindicated during pregnancy. Effects on the fetus of I-131 that is given inadvertently during pregnancy vary with the time of gestation in which the dose was administered. Exposure during organogenesis (starting at week 2 of gestation) and in particular during thyroidogenesis (starting at week 10 of gestation) can lead to major malformations and fetal thyroid ablation resulting in fetal hypothyroidism, respectively. Radioiodine exposure in utero may also result in growth retardation, cognitive decline, and perhaps increased incidence of adulthood malignancies, particularly thyroid cancer. Exposure very early in pregnancy, prior to embryo implantation, may result in embryonic death but is unlikely to cause birth defects, thyroid ablation, or neurocognitive deficits because developmental processes have not yet begun [30, 36]. In a case report published by Berg et al. [56], a woman with Graves' hyperthyroidism was treated with 13.5 mCi (500 MBq) of I-131 in the 20th week of pregnancy after a urinary β-hCG test was falsely negative. Uptake in the fetal thyroid gland was 2 % and the calculated absorbed dose was considered an ablative dose (600 Gy); thus she was treated with suppressive doses of LT4 during the remainder of her pregnancy to supply the fetus with adequate thyroid hormone. She delivered a healthy male at full term; however, cord blood TSH was markedly elevated despite maternal LT4 therapy. At the age of 8, neuropsychological testing showed an "uneven profile," low attention span, and subnormal figurative memory [56]. Another case report of inadvertent administration of RAI during pregnancy showed that after ablative treatment with 100 mCi of RAI at week 2 and again at week 22 of pregnancy in a 28-year-old woman with PTC, the fetus suffered from necrotic destruction of the thyroid gland but no chromosomal abnormalities, as determined on autopsy after the pregnancy was terminated [57]. A large, retrospective survey by Stoffer and Hamburger [58] analyzed fetal outcomes in 182 pregnancies in which RAI was given in the first or second trimester to treat hyperthyroidism. Six of the children (3.3 %) had documented hypothyroidism and/or cognitive deficiencies, and another six (3.3 %) suffered from other devastating complications, including two miscarriages and two stillbirths.

Together, these cases highlight the potentially devastating risks of inadvertent RAI administration during pregnancy and underscore the importance of measuring *serum* β-hCG prior to radioiodine therapy in all women of childbearing age, as urine pregnancy tests are less sensitive and can be falsely negative, especially in the first trimester of pregnancy. In addition, because even serum pregnancy tests may be falsely negative in the first week of pregnancy, obtaining a complete sexual and menstrual history from women prior to RAI treatment is advisable, albeit often unreliable. In the case that inadvertent fetal exposure to RAI has occurred, an attempt should be made by a nuclear medicine physicist to determine the radioiodine dose delivered to the fetus, so that this information, along with the timing of the exposure during gestation, can be used to help guide the parents and providers in the difficult decision regarding potential therapeutic abortion [54]. If the pregnancy is continued, intra-amniotic thyroxine therapy has been used to successfully treat fetal hypothyroidism in select cases, although the risk of miscarriage with this mode of thyroxine delivery must be strongly considered before deciding to initiate such treatment [59].

Little data exist regarding the transfer of radioiodine to human breast milk; however, one would expect that transfer is significant, just as natural maternal iodine is normally transferred to breast milk to fuel the infant thyroid gland. To avoid transferring radioiodine to an infant when the thyroid gland is small and highly radiosensitive, it is recommended that women avoid breastfeeding for 6 months to 1 year following I-131 treatment [30]. It is not surprising then that reports of breast uptake of I-131 have been associated with elevated prolactin levels; thus uptake is minimal to none in non-lactating breast tissue but increases when prolactin levels are high. Further, normalization of prolactin levels results in decreased breast uptake, suggesting that prolactin is a stimulus for breast accumulation of iodine [60]. The mechanism for this is increased breast sodium-iodide symporter activity [61]. To protect the developing neonatal thyroid gland, lactating women should not be treated with radioiodine unless they plan to discontinue breastfeeding. It has been suggested that, just as large doses of stable (cold) iodine block thyroidal iodine uptake, such treatment given several days after the administration of radioiodine to the mother will also block uptake of radioiodine into breast tissue and thus block transfer into breast milk [62]. However, whether treatment of the mother with cold iodine actually decreases concentration of radioiodine within a nursing infant's very radiosensitive thyroid gland has not been investigated.

Several groups have investigated radioiodine uptake into breast tissue in lactating and non-lactating women and subsequent risk of breast cancer. Epidemiological trials have failed to demonstrate an increase in breast cancer risk after treatment with I-131 for hyperthyroidism [63–65]. On the other hand, the ATA Taskforce on Radiation Safety recommends that lactating women delay I-131 treatment for a minimum of 6 weeks, and ideally for 3 months, following cessation of breastfeeding to minimize breast RAI uptake and to reduce any theoretical increase in breast cancer risk [54].

Interestingly, Hammami et al. showed that breast uptake is common in women after both diagnostic I-123 and I-131 post-ablation whole-body scans, irrespective of lactation status [66]. Of note, those women were all exposed to RAI in the hypothyroid state, which promotes hyperprolactinemia, and more than half had either mildly elevated serum prolactin levels or expressible galactorrhea. Brzozowska and colleagues demonstrated variable breast uptake of I-123 in eight postpartum women with thyroid cancer undergoing diagnostic scans and found that uptake was significantly reduced in women treated with dopamine agonists to inhibit lactation compared to untreated women. In that study, breast RAI activity was negligible as soon as 3 weeks after initiating dopaminergic agonist therapy [67].

Minimizing breast uptake of RAI is important because uptake by breast tissue may (1) in theory increase future risk of breast cancer [54] and (2) mimic lung metastases, thereby confusing the management of thyroid cancer [67, 68]. Use of dopamine agonists in recently lactating women, or in women with hyperprolactinemia for other reasons (such as a prolactin-secreting pituitary adenoma), may be warranted to minimize breast uptake, although this is an off-label use of this medication class [54, 67]. Brzozowska also suggests performing pre-ablation I-123 diagnostic scans in women to determine breast uptake and delaying RAI ablation with I-131 if necessary until there is negligible breast I-123 uptake [67]. The ATA supports this view, particularly in women who are postpartum or have recently breastfed and for whom I-131 treatment is urgent [54]. Finally, because prolactin stimulates breast uptake of iodine, and hypothyroidism is a well-established cause of hyperprolactinemia, preparation for I-131 treatment with recombinant TSH (rTSH, Thyrogen®) may be preferable to preparation by thyroid hormone withdrawal in women. Although this has not been rigorously tested to date, women who are treated with rTSH and thus remain euthyroid prior to RAI should in theory have less breast uptake compared to women who are rendered hypothyroid for several weeks prior to the radiation exposure. This may be especially applicable to women in whom prolactin levels are still mildly elevated from recent lactation because prolactin may be further elevated by hypothyroidism. To date, unfortunately, no studies have compared breast uptake of radioiodine in women after preparation by withdrawal of exogenous LT4 to breast uptake after preparation with rTSH; thus we can only speculate that RAI treatment after preparation with rTSH is the preferable method in the female DTC population.

Conclusions

DTC that is diagnosed during or near the time of pregnancy poses many challenges to the medical team caring for these patients. These complex cases should be followed closely during pregnancy and breastfeeding by a team of physicians that includes the patient's obstetrician, an endocrinologist, an endocrine surgeon, nuclear medicine specialists, and the baby's pediatrician. The standard treatment of DTC – total thyroidectomy followed by radioactive iodine ablation of residual disease – poses significant risks to a pregnancy; thus in general, definitive treatment should be delayed until the postpartum period. The majority of evidence suggests that long-term maternal outcomes are not adversely affected by this delay in treatment. However, due to the theoretical potential that a delay in treatment may worsen maternal survival, very close clinical follow-up during and after pregnancy is paramount to making the optimal clinical decisions in these unique cases.

References

1. Smith LH, Danielsen B, Allen ME, et al. Cancer associated with obstetric delivery: results of linkage with the California cancer registry. Am J Obstet Gynecol. 2003;189:1128–35.
2. Oduncu FS, Kimmig R, Hepp H, Emmerich B. Caner in pregnancy: maternal-fetal conflict. J Cancer Res Clin Oncol. 2003;129:133–46.
3. Burrow GN, Fisher DA, Larsen PR. Maternal and fetal thyroid function. NEJM. 1994;331:1072–8.
4. De Escobar GM, Obregon MJ, del Rey FE. Iodine deficiency and brain development in the first half of pregnancy. Public Health Nutr. 2007;10:1554–70.
5. Delange F. Disorders induced by iodine deficiency. Thyroid. 1994;4:107–28.
6. Yoshimura M, Hershman JM. Thyrotropic action of human chorionic gonadotropin. Thyroid. 1995;5:425–34.
7. Dashe JS, Casey BM, Wells CE, et al. Thyroid-stimulating hormone in singleton and twin pregnancy: importance of gestational age-specific reference ranges. Obstet Gynecol. 2005;106:753–7.
8. Abalovich M, Amino N, Barbour LA, et al. Management of thyroid dysfunction during pregnancy and postpartum: an Endocrine Society clinical practice guideline. J Clin Endocrinol Metab. 2007;92:S1–47.
9. Alexander EK, Marqusee E, Lawrence J, et al. Timing and magnitude of increases in levothyroxine requirements during pregnancy in women with hypothyroidism. NEJM. 2004;351:241–9.
10. Vulsma T, Gons MH, de Vijlder JJM. Maternal-fetal transfer of thyroxine in congenital hypothyroidism due to a total organifications defect or thyroid agenesis. N Engl J Med. 1989;321:13–6.
11. Krassas GE, Poppe K, Glinoer D. Thyroid function and human reproductive health. Endocr Rev. 2010;31:1–54.
12. Abalovich M, Gutierrez S, Alcaraz G, et al. Overt and subclinical hypothyroidism complicating pregnancy. Thyroid. 2002;12:63–8.
13. Davis LE, Leveno KJ, Cunningham FG. Hypothyroidism complicating pregnancy. Obstet Gynecol. 1988;72:108–12.
14. Leung AS, Miller LK, Koonings PP, et al. Perinatal outcome in hypothyroid pregnancies. Obstet Gynecol. 1993;81:349–53.
15. Pop VJ, Kujipens JL, van Baar AL, et al. Low maternal free thyroxine concentrations during early pregnancy are associated with impaired psychomotor development in infancy. Clin Endocrinol (Oxf). 1999;50:149–55.

16. Glinoer D. The regulation of thyroid function in pregnancy: pathways of endocrine adaptation from physiology to pathology. Endocr Rev. 1997;18:404–33.
17. Anselmo J, Cao D, Karrison T, et al. Fetal loss associated with excess thyroid hormone exposure. JAMA. 2004;292:691–5.
18. Rahbari R, Zhang L, Kebebew E. Thyroid cancer gender disparity. Future Oncol. 2010;6:1771–9.
19. Aschebrook-Kilfoy B, Ward MH, Sabra MM, et al. Thyroid cancer incidence patterns in the United States by histologic type, 1992–2006. Thyroid. 2011;21:125–34.
20. Yoshimura M, Nishikawa M, Yoshikawa N, et al. Mechanism of thyroid stimulation by human chorionic gonadotropin in sera of normal pregnant women. Acta Endocrinol (Copenh). 1991;124:173–8.
21. del Songo L, degli Uberti E, Hanau S, et al. In vitro effects of estrogen on tgb and c-myc gene expression in normal and neoplastic human thyroids. Mol Cell Endocrinol. 1989;63:67–74.
22. Imai Y, Yamakawa M, Matsuda M, et al. Endogenous sex hormone and estrogen binding activity in thyroid cancer. Histol Histopathol. 1989;4:39–45.
23. Rossing MA, Voigt LF, Wicklund KG, Daling JR. Reproductive factors and risk of papillary thyroid cancer in women. Am J Epidemiol. 2000;151(8):765–72.
24. Horn-Ross PL, Chang ET, Clarke CA, et al. Nativity and papillary thyroid cancer incidence rates among Hispanic women in California. Cancer Epidemiol Biomarkers Prev. 2011;20:1751–9.
25. Mack WJ, Preston-Martin S, Bernstein L, et al. Reproductive and hormonal risk factors for thyroid cancer in Los Angeles County females. Cancer Epidemiol Biomarkers Prev. 1999;8:991–7.
26. Sakoda L, Horn-Ross PL. Reproductive and menstrual history and papillary thyroid cancer risk: the San Francisco Bay Area thyroid cancer study. Cancer Epidemiol Biomarkers Prev. 2002;11:51–7.
27. Struve CW, Haupt S, Ohlen S. Influence of frequency of previous pregnancies on the prevalence of thyroid nodules in women without clinical evidence of thyroid disease. Thyroid. 1993;3:7–9.
28. Kung AW, Chau MT, Lao TT, et al. The effect of pregnancy on thyroid nodule formation. J Clin Endocrinol Metab. 2002;87:1010–4.
29. Glinoer D, Soto MF, Bourdoux P, et al. Pregnancy in patients with mild thyroid abnormalities: maternal and neonatal repercussions. J Clin Endocrinol Metab. 1991;73:421–7.
30. Stagnaro-Green A, Abalovich M, Alexander E, et al. Guidelines of the American Thyroid Association for the diagnosis and management of thyroid disease during pregnancy and postpartum. Thyroid. 2011;21:1–45.
31. Pauwels EK, Thomson WH, Blokland JAK, et al. Aspects of fetal thyroid dose following iodine-131 administration during early stages of pregnancy in patients suffering from benign thyroid disorders. Eur J Nucl Med. 1999;26:1453–7.
32. Kuy S, Roman SA, Desai R, et al. Outcomes following thyroid and parathyroid surgery in pregnant women. Arch Surg. 2009;144:399–406.
33. Mazzaferri EL. Approach to the pregnant patient with thyroid cancer. J Clin Endocrinol Metab. 2011;96:265–72.
34. Thomas AK, McVie R, Levine SN. Disorders of maternal calcium metabolism implicated by abnormal calcium metabolism in the neonate. Am J Perinatol. 1999;16:515–20.
35. Robertson Jr WC. Calcium carbonate consumption during pregnancy: an unusual cause of neonatal hypocalcemia. J Child Neurol. 2002;17:853–5.
36. Hyer SL, Pratt B, Newbold K, et al. Outcome of pregnancy after exposure to radioiodine in utero. Endocr Pract. 2011;17:1–10.
37. Hirsch D, Levy S, Tsvetov G, et al. Impact of pregnancy on outcome and prognosis of survivors of papillary thyroid cancer. Thyroid. 2010;20:1179–85.
38. Leboueuf R, Emerick LE, Martorella AJ, et al. Impact of pregnancy on serum thyroglobulin and detection of recurrent disease shortly after delivery in thyroid cancer survivors. Thyroid. 2007;17:543–7.
39. Rosario RW, Barrosa AL, Purisch S. The effect of subsequent pregnancy on patients with thyroid carcinoma apparently free of the disease. Thyroid. 2007;20:1175–6.
40. Loh JA, Wartofsky L, Jonklaas J, Burman KD. The magnitude of increased levothyroxine requirements in hypothyroid pregnant women depends upon the etiology of the hypothyroidism. Thyroid. 2009;19:269–75.
41. Delange F. Iodine requirements during pregnancy, lactation and the neonatal period and indicators of optimal iodine nutrition. Public Health Nutr. 2007;10:1571–80.
42. Akslen LA, Nilssen S, Kvale G. Reproductive factors and risk of thyroid cancer. A prospective study of 63,090 women from Norway. Br J Cancer. 1992;65:772–4.
43. Soldin OP, Tractenberg RE, Hollowell JG, et al. Trimester-specific changes in maternal thyroid hormone, thyrotropin, and thyroglobulin concentrations during gestation: trends and associations across trimesters in iodine sufficiency. Thyroid. 2004;14:1084–90.
44. Moosa M, Mazzaferri EL. Outcome of differentiated thyroid cancer diagnosed in pregnant women. J Clin Endocrinol Metab. 1997;82:2862–6.
45. Herzon FS, Morris DM, Segal MN, et al. Coexistent thyroid cancer and pregnancy. Arch Otolaryngol Head Neck Surg. 1994;120:1191–3.
46. Yasmeen S, Cress R, Romano PS, et al. Thyroid cancer in pregnancy. Int J Gynecol Obstet. 2005;91:15–20.
47. Vannucchi G, Perrino M, Rossi S, et al. Clinical and molecular features of differentiated thyroid cancer diagnosed during pregnancy. Eur J Endocrinol. 2010;162:145–51.
48. MIRD. MIRD primer for absorbed dose calculations. Reston: Society of Nuclear Medicine; 1988.
49. Krassas GE, Poppe K, Glinoer D. Thyroid function and human reproductive health. Endocr Rev. 2010;31:702–55.
50. Sioka C, Fotopoulos A. Effects of I-131 therapy on gonads and pregnancy outcome in patients with thyroid cancer. Fertil Steril. 2011;95:1552–8.
51. Garsi JP, Schlumberger M, Rubino C, et al. Therapeutic administration of I-131 for differentiated thyroid cancer: radiation dose to ovaries and outcome of pregnancies. J Nucl Med. 2008;49:845–52.
52. Bal C, Kumar A, Tripathi M, et al. High-dose radioiodine treatment for differentiated thyroid carcinoma is not associated with change in female fertility or any genetic risk to the offspring. Int J Radiat Oncol Biol Phys. 2005;63:449–55.
53. Garsi JP, Schlumberger M, Ricard M, et al. Health outcomes of children fathered by patients treated with radioiodine for thyroid cancer. Clin Endocrinol (Oxf). 2009;71:880–3.
54. Sisson JC, Freitas J, McDougall IR, et al. Radiation safety in the treatment of patients with thyroid disease by radioiodine ^{131}I: practice recommendations of the American Thyroid Association. Thyroid. 2011;21:335–46.
55. Schlumberger M, De Vathaire F, Ceccarelli C, et al. Exposure to radioactive iodine-131 for scintigraphy or therapy does not preclude pregnancy in thyroid cancer patients. J Nucl Med. 1996;37:606–12.
56. Berg GE, Nystrom EH, Jacobsson L, et al. Radioiodine treatment of hyperthyroidism in a pregnant woman. J Nucl Med. 1998;39:357–61.
57. Arndt D, Mehnert WH, Franke WG, et al. Radioiodine therapy during an unknown remained pregnancy and radiation exposure of the fetus. A case report. Strahlenther Onkol. 1994;170:408–14.
58. Stoffer SS, Hamburger JI. Inadvertent I-131 therapy for hyperthyroidism in the first trimester of pregnancy. J Nucl Med. 1975;17:146–9.
59. Abuhamad AZ, Fisher DA, Warsot SL, et al. Antenatal diagnosis and treatment of fetal goitrous hypothyroidism: case report and

review of the literature. Ultrasound Obstet Gynecol. 1995;6: 368–71.
60. Ronga G, Bruno R, Puxeddu E, et al. Radioiodine uptake in nonlactating mammary glands: evidence for a causative role of hyperprolactinemia. Thyroid. 2007;17:363–6.
61. Azizi F, Smith P. Breastfeeding and maternal and infant iodine nutrition. Clin Endocrinol (Oxf). 2009;70:803–9.
62. Simon SL, Luckyanov N, Bouville A, et al. Transfer of I131 into human breast milk and transfer coefficients for radiological dose assessments. Health Phys. 2002;82:796–806.
63. Hall P, Berg G, Bjelkengren G, et al. Cancer mortality after iodine-131 for hyperthyroidism. Int J Cancer. 1992;50:886–90.
64. Franklyn JA, Maisonneuve P, Sheppard M, et al. Cancer incidence and mortality after radioiodine treatment for hyperthyroidism: a population-based cohort study. Lancet. 1999;353:2111–5.
65. Goldman MB, Maloof F, Monson RR, et al. Radioactive iodine therapy and breast cancer. A follow-up study of hyperthyroid women. Am J Epidemiol. 1988;127:969–80.
66. Hammami MM, Bakheet S. Radioiodine breast uptake in non-breastfeeding women: clinical and scintigraphic characteristics. J Nucl Med. 1996;37:26–31.
67. Brzozowska M, Roach PJ. Timing and potential role of diagnostic I-123 scintigraphy in assessing radioiodine breast uptake before ablation in postpartum women with thyroid cancer. A case series. Clin Nucl Med. 2006;31:683–7.
68. Bakheet S, Powe J, Hammami M. Unilateral radioiodine breast uptake. Clin Nucl Med. 1998;23:170–1.
69. Do Rosario PW, Barroso AL, Rezende LL, et al. Malformations in the offspring of women with thyroid cancer treated with radioiodine for the ablation of thyroid remnants. Arq Bras Endocrinol Metabol. 2006;50:930–3.
70. Balenovic A, Vlasic M, Sonicki Z, et al. Pregnancy outcome after treatment with radioiodine for differentiated thyroid carcinoma. Coll Antropol. 2006;30:743–8.
71. Brandao CD, Miranda AE, Correa ND, et al. Radioiodine therapy and subsequent pregnancy. Arq Bras Endocrinol Metabol. 2007;51:534–40.
72. Fard-Esfahani A, Hadifar M, Fallahi B, et al. Radioiodine treatment complications to the mother and child in patients with differentiated thyroid carcinoma. Hell J Nucl Med. 2009;12:37–40.
73. Vini L, Hyer S, Al-Saadi A. Prognosis for fertility and ovarian function after treatment with radioiodine for thyroid cancer. Postgrad Med J. 2002;78:92–3.
74. Chow SM, Yau S, Lee SH, et al. Pregnancy outcome after diagnosis of differentiated thyroid carcinoma: no deleterious effect after radioactive iodine treatment. Int J Radiat Oncol Biol Phys. 2004;59:992–1000.

Part VII

Treatment

Radiation and Radioactivity

55

Richard J. Vetter and John Glenn

Introduction

^{131}I therapy may result in the patient becoming a hazard to other people. When a patient treated with ^{131}I is hospitalized, caregivers must take special precautions to protect themselves against the radiation from the ^{131}I in the patient. When patients are released immediately or shortly after treatment, they must take precautions to protect members of the public. Special governmental regulations affect the management of patients who are treated with ^{131}I, and the physician administering the ^{131}I must comply with these regulations. The treating physician must communicate to the patient the risk of radiation from the ^{131}I treatment and any special precautions the patient should take to protect others. The patient should relay the information to the patient's family, friends, and caretakers. Communication of precautions is challenging, and patients may forget what they have been told [1]. A balance must be achieved in convincing the patient to agree with these specific instructions and, at the same time, dispel unnecessary fear. For this balance, the physician may need to adopt different strategies with different patients, requiring a good working knowledge of radiation and radioactivity, ionizing and nonionizing radiation, and units of radioactivity and radiation dosage. The physician must also know the regulations for hospitalization, conditions for earlier release, radiation safety precautions during hospital stay and upon release, and the myths and fears about radioactivity. This chapter presents an overview of these topics.

R.J. Vetter, PhD, CHP (✉)
Biophysics, Mayo Medical School, Mayo Clinic and Medical School, 200, 1st Street SW Medical Sciences B-28, Rochester, MN 55902, USA
e-mail: rvetter@mayo.edu

J. Glenn, PhD
Radiation Safety, Georgetown University Hospital, Washington, DC, USA

Radiation and Radioactivity

The physician and patient should have a clear understanding of the difference between radiation and radioactivity. Both are closely related concepts, but the distinction is important to determine methods to protect patients and anyone with whom they may come in close contact.

Radiation

Radiation is the process in which energetic particles or bundles of energy travel through matter or space. There are two general types of radiation: ionizing and nonionizing. Light from a flashlight and microwaves that cook food are both nonionizing radiation The heat (infrared radiation) that warms our faces in front of the fireplace is another form of nonionizing radiation. The atomic particles released by the sun as solar wind, the particles released by radon in our homes, and the x-rays from a computed tomography (CT) machine are ionizing radiation (capable of "stripping" electrons from atoms to create chemical ions). The x-rays or γ rays, positrons, and the α or β particles released from radioactive materials are ionizing radiation. Patients who are treated with ^{131}I (a radioisotope of iodine) emit ionizing radiation, principally in the form of γ rays. People who come into close proximity to a patient treated with ^{131}I are exposed to radiation (γ rays) but are not contaminated with radioactive materials.

Radioactivity

Radioactivity is the spontaneous disintegration (decay) of the nucleus of an atom. Radioactive atoms are different from other atoms because they can release energy in the form of radiation as discussed above. The ^{131}I used to treat thyroid

L. Wartofsky, D. Van Nostrand (eds.), *Thyroid Cancer*, DOI 10.1007/978-1-4939-3314-3_55

disease contains radioactive atoms of ^{131}I. People near such a patient are exposed to radiation, while those who come in direct contact with the patient can get radioactive ^{131}I in or on themselves. Unwanted radioactive materials on a person or thing are called contamination.

Types of Radiation from Radioactive Materials

The most important types of radiation emitted by radioactive atoms are α, β, positron, and γ rays.

Alpha (α) *radiation* is the nucleus of a helium atom (two protons and two neutrons) traveling rapidly through matter. The α particle is massive (heavy) and energetic with a double positive charge. Because it is heavy, the speed at which it travels through space is relatively slow. That plus its double positive charge causes it to lose energy very rapidly. This property means that it gives high radiation-absorbed doses when ingested, injected, or otherwise inserted into tissue. However, because an α particle deposits its energy quickly over a very short path length, it almost never penetrates the skin. Thus, patients receiving radioactive material emitting only α radiation will receive high internal doses but are not a hazard to people in their vicinity.

Beta (β) *radiation* is an electron that originates in the nucleus and travels through matter at a velocity that approaches the speed of light. The β particle has a small mass, which is about 2000 times less than the smallest atom, and has a negative electric charge. The β particle loses energy less rapidly than an α particle and can penetrate tissue for a short distance of 1 or 2 cm. Thus, patients receiving radioactive material emitting only β radiation will receive moderately high internal radiation-absorbed doses. However, as a source of radiation, they are not normally a hazard to people in their vicinity because most of the energy from β radiation is deposited inside the body.

Positron is another form of radiation that nuclear medicine has recently harnessed for diagnostic purposes. The positron originates in the nucleus of certain radioactive atoms and has the same mass as a β particle or electron, but its charge is positive rather than negative like the electron. The positron is classified as the antimatter, a twin of the electron. An amazing property of antimatter/matter twins is that when they collide, they annihilate each other. All the mass is converted into pure energy, according to Einstein's famous equation ($E = mc^2$). This energy always shows up as two γ rays of identical energy, traveling in exactly opposite directions. This property allows precise spatial imaging. The imaging process is referred to as *positron emission tomography* (PET).

Gamma (γ) *radiation* is electromagnetic energy that travels through space in packets of energy called photons. γ radiation has no resting mass but a relativistic mass given by the equation, $E = mc^2$. Because γ rays are high energy and travel through matter at the speed of light, they can travel many meters before depositing their energy. γ rays give up energy (ionize matter) only when coming into close proximity with atomic electrons. Thus, individual γ rays release energy less rapidly than α or β particles and may pass through the human body depositing a low radiation dose. Patients who receive radioactive material that emits only γ radiation will receive moderately low doses, but people in their vicinity may also receive a radiation-absorbed dose from the γ radiation that passes through the tissues of the patient.

^{131}I emits both β and γ radiation. The β radiation is the major source of radiation to any remaining normal thyroid tissue and functioning metastatic thyroid cancer cells. A significant portion of the γ radiation "escapes" the patient. Although this energy can be harnessed to obtain images, γ rays can result in a radiation-absorbed dose to family and friends. Because of the γ radiation emitted from the patient, ^{131}I therapy must be monitored and controlled to minimize its effect on family, friends, caretakers, and other members of the public.

Radiation-Absorbed Dose

When ionizing radiation interacts with matter, it alters the number of electrons within the atoms of the matter. Those affected atoms are called *ions* because they have either lost or gained one or more electrons, which alters the charge of the atom. The number of ions created within matter, including the human tissue, depends on the amount of energy deposited by the ionizing radiation. This deposited energy is the *radiation-absorbed dose*. Formation of a large number of ions results in a high radiation-absorbed dose.

Ions created inside the cell can interact with other molecules and cause the cell's chemical properties to change forming free radicals with changed oxidation states. These free radicals may cause damage to the DNA molecules that control the cell's ability to replace or regulate itself. For example, DNA may undergo breaks, and the repair process may lead to errors in the nucleotide sequences or faulty repair of the broken helical strands. While nearly all damage to DNA is repaired properly, occasional errors in repair may result in cell death or propagation of the error (mutation) to the daughter cells after division.

Deterministic and Stochastic Effects

The biological effects of ionizing radiation are categorized as *deterministic* or *stochastic*. A *deterministic* effect is damage that occurs above a threshold dose, and the severity of the effect increases with dose. An example is the death of residual thyroid cells including cancer cells, which is the objective of ^{131}I therapy. The suppression of bone marrow stem cells in the ^{131}I patient is also a deterministic effect. The more ^{131}I that is deposited in the bone marrow, the higher the radiation-absorbed dose and the higher the toxicity to bone marrow. While a large radiation-absorbed dose is virtually guaranteed to cause toxicity, it may or may not cause a *stochastic* effect. A *stochastic* effect is a probability of occurrence. This probability increases with dose, but the severity of the effect does not increase with the dose, and the effect is assumed to have no threshold. Cancer induction is a stochastic effect—a DNA mutation that results in cancer is dependent on the probability of the effect occurring, rather than the severity of the effect. The higher the radiation-absorbed dose to a tissue, the higher the probability that some (but not all) cells in the tissue will become cancerous. Additional details on the patient risk from medical procedures are published by The International Commission on Radiological Protection [2].

Units of Radioactivity and Radiation Dose

Science needs to define precisely the units of measurement. A problem in the United States is our reluctance to adopt international systems, including the metric system. Thus, the physician will encounter two different systems for measuring radioactivity and radiation-absorbed dose.

International System

In the international system, named units are based on the three fundamental metric units: the meter, kilogram, and second. Radioactivity is the measure of the number of atomic nuclei disintegrating per unit of time. The fundamental unit has been named the *Becquerel* (Bq) and is defined as:

$$1 \text{ Bq} = \frac{1 \text{ disintegration}}{\text{sec}}$$

Radiation-absorbed dose is defined as the energy deposited in matter, including tissue and per unit mass, and is measured in a unit named the *gray* (Gy). One *gray* is the absorption of 1 J of energy per kilogram of matter:

$$1 \text{ Gy} = 1 \text{ J/kg} = 1 \text{m}^2 / \text{s}^2$$

Biological damage is dependent on the number of ions formed per unit path length. To account for these differences among the different types of radiation, e.g., α, β and γ, the radiation-absorbed dose is multiplied by a factor that reflects the probability of a biological effect. This radiation quantity is called the equivalent dose, and the unit for equivalent dose is called the Sievert (Sv). For the radioisotopes of iodine, e.g., ^{131}I, the adjustment factor is 1; therefore, 1 Gy = 1 Sv. For radionuclides such as ^{131}I, which are not distributed uniformly throughout the body, the equivalent dose is further adjusted for distribution of equivalent dose among the organs and the probability of stochastic effects in those organs. This produces a radiation dose for the whole body called the effective dose. The unit for effective dose is also the Sievert (Sv).

Special Units System

Regulations in the United States require use of the special units system. Radioactivity is still the measure of the number of atomic nuclei disintegrating per unit of time, but the special unit is the *Curie* (Ci) and equals the number of disintegrations in 1 g of ^{226}Ra in 1 s (s). A Curie equals 37 billion disintegrations per second.

$$1 \text{ Ci} = 37 \text{ billion Bq}$$

$$1 \text{ mCi} = 37 \text{ million Bq}$$

$$1 \text{disintegration} / \text{min} = 1 \text{disintegration} / (60 \text{s}) = 0.0167 \text{ Bq}$$

The “special units” is a hybrid system widely used in the United States but used nowhere else in the world. It is required by NRC and Agreement States for all regulatory purposes. Radiation-absorbed dose is still absorbed energy per unit mass but in cgs units. The unit of energy is a much smaller metric unit, *erg*, and the unit of mass is *gram*, rather than the kilogram. The unit of radiation-absorbed dose is the *rad*. 1 rad = 100 erg/g =100 cm^2/s^2 = 0.01 Gy

or

$$1 \text{ Gy} = 100 \text{ rad}$$

The special unit for equivalent dose and effective dose is the rem.

In this discussion, the international units will be used with the special units in parentheses.

US Regulatory Framework

The establishment of radiation standards in the United States is a federal function. The Environmental Protection Agency (EPA) is the lead agency, but several agencies participate in the standards-setting process. The Atomic Energy Act of 1954 gives the Nuclear Regulatory Commission (NRC) the statutory responsibility for all radioactive material produced by the nuclear fuel cycle, i.e., all radioactive material produced in a nuclear reactor as well as thorium and uranium processed from ore and radioactive materials enriched in fissionable materials by physical processes. In 2005, Congress created the federal Energy Policy Actgiving NRC the authority to regulate radioactive materials produced in particle accelerators. Typically, ^{123}I is produced in a particle accelerator called a cyclotron and ^{131}I is produced in a reactor, but the use of both is regulated by the NRC. The Atomic Energy Act also allows the NRC to delegate regulatory authority to states that establish a compatible regulatory program by written agreement (i.e., Agreement States). Possession and use of ^{131}I requires hospitals or clinics to obtain a license from the appropriate Agreement State or the NRC. To determine if your state is an Agreement State, the following Internet address displays a map showing NRC and Agreement States: http://nrc-stp.ornl.gov/rulemaking.html.

Before the mid-1990s, the Atomic Energy Commission, and later the NRC, had required that all patients receiving more than 1.11 billion Bq (1.11 GBq or 30 mCi) of radioactive material for therapy remain in the hospital until the radioactivity dropped below 1.11 GBq (30 mCi). Patients could also leave if the radiation-absorbed dose measured at 1 m from their bodies dropped below 0.00005 Gy/h (50 μGy/h or 5 mrad/h). These criteria were intended to make sure family and friends would not be exposed to more than 0.005 Gy (0.5 rad) from any patient receiving ^{131}I. The criteria were derived from some cautious assumptions:

- None of the radioactive material would be eliminated except by natural decay. (This assumption is contrary to real experience in cancer patients where 80–90 % of the ^{131}I may be excreted in the first 24 h.)
- The patient's body would not absorb any radiation emitted. (In practice, the patient's tissues reduce external-radiation doses from ^{131}I by a measurable amount.)
- The most exposed individual family member or friend would spend no more than 25 % of their time within 3 ft of the patient until all the radioactive material was gone from natural decay. (This is not a cautious assumption unless the patient has been advised to sleep in a separated bed for a few days.)

Based largely on comments from physicians who treat patients with radioactive materials, the NRC changed its patient-release criteria in 1997 [6]. The Agreement States had 3 years to adopt "compatible" regulations. Thus, the description of the NRC's requirements presented here may vary slightly (but not significantly) from state to state.

Instead of basing release of the patient exclusively on a specified level of radioactivity or radiation-absorbed dose rate at 1 m from the patient, the physician is required to demonstrate that no other individual, including family and friends, is likely to receive an effective dose in excess of 0.005 Sv (0.5 rem) from the patient if the patient is released from the hospital. The physician has three options on which to base the release of the patient:

1. Base release of the patient on the administered dosage (prescribed activity). The release limits for a number of radionuclides are provided by NRC in Regulatory Guide 8.39 [7]. For ^{131}I, the release limit is 0.24 GBq (33 mCi). Using the same cautious assumptions used previously, the NRC has determined that release of patients who have been administered the activity listed in Regulatory Guide 8.39 will not result in any other individual receiving a radiation-absorbed dose in excess of 0.005 Sv (0.5 rem).
2. Base release of the patient on the measured dose rate at 1 m from the surface of the patient. Acceptable dose rates for release of the patient are provided in Regulatory Guide 8.39 [7]. For ^{131}I, the acceptable dose rate for release of the patient is 0.07 mSv/h (7 mrem/h). Using the same cautious assumptions used previously, the NRC has determined that release of patients whose surface dose readings do exceed those listed in Regulatory Guide 8.39 will not result in any other individual receiving a radiation-absorbed dose in excess of 0.005 Sv (0.5 rem).
3. Base release of the patient on patient-specific-dose calculations. Using this method, the physician must calculate the maximum likely effective dose to an individual exposed to the patient on a case-by-case basis. If the estimated maximum likely effective dose to an individual does not exceed 5 mSv (0.5 rem), the patient may be released. Using this method, the physician may be able to release patients whose activity or surface dose rate at the time of release exceeds the limits in options 1 or 2. To accomplish this, the dose calculation must take into account the effective half-life of the radioactive material, an occupancy factor described in Regulatory Guide 8.39 [7], and other factors that may be relevant to the particular case. Regulatory Guide 8.39 [7] contains procedures for performing patient-specific-dose calculations.

Patient Instructions

If the total effective dose equivalent to another individual could exceed 0.001 Sv (0.1 rem), the patient must be provided instructions, including written instructions, on actions recommended to maintain doses to other individuals as low as is reasonably achievable. For physicians who do not use patient-specific calculations, Regulatory Guide 8.39 (http://pbadupws.nrc.gov/docs/ML0037/ML003739575.pdf) [7] provides a table to determine the activity or dose rate above which instructions must be given to patients. For ^{131}I, the limits are 0.24 GBq (7 mCi) or 0.02 mSv/h (2 mrem/h). The instructions should be specific to the type of treatment given, such as ^{131}I for hyperthyroidism or thyroid carcinoma. The instructions may include information for individual situations, but they should not interfere with or contradict the best medical judgment of physicians. It is advisable to include the name of a knowledgeable person to contact and that person's telephone number in case the patient has any questions or needs to verify their treatment such as for a law enforcement agent who was monitoring vehicles or individuals for high radiation exposures. If the dose to a breast-feeding infant or child could exceed 1 millisievert (100 mrem), instructions must include guidance on interruption of breast-feeding and information on the consequences of failure to follow instructions. Regulatory Guide 8.39 contains examples of instructions than can be given to patients including:

- Maintaining distance from other persons, including separate sleeping arrangements.
- Minimizing time in public places, e.g. public transportation, grocery stores, shopping center, theaters, restaurants, and sporting events.
- Precautions to reduce the spread of radioactive contamination.
- The length of time each of the precautions should be in effect.

Sample written instructions are given in Example 1 (Appendix C).

Internet Resources

The Internet offers the opportunity to access current regulations and guidance of the NRC and many Agreement States. The NRC provides a Medical Uses Licensee Toolkit with many links to help review licensing, procedures, and inspection at: www.nrc.gov/materials/miau/med-use-toolkit.html. Extensive guidance for the release of patients on ^{131}I therapy is provided in Appendix U, "Model Procedure for Release of Patients or Human Research Subjects Administered Radioactive Materials" in the NRC's *Consolidated Guidance About Materials Licenses Program—Specific Guidance About Medical Use Licenses, vol. 9*. Numerous appendices, including Appendix U can be found at: http://pbadupws.nrc.gov/docs/ML0231/ML023120214.pdf. The Conference of Radiation Control Program Directors, Inc. has posted free information on patient release at: www.crcpd.org.

Protection of People Other than Patients

Immediately after ^{131}I cancer treatment, anyone in contact with or near the patient is at risk of receiving a radiation dose from the radioactive iodine within the patient. This can occur directly from the radiation emitted from the patient's body or by ingesting or inhaling radioactive iodine that the patient sheds through breath or body fluids. The current scientific consensus about the risks from exposure to radiation has been published by the National Academy of Sciences [3].

To maintain the cancer risk to friends and family members as low as reasonably achievable—a concept radiation health experts refer to as ALARA—some patients may require hospitalization, and all patients must receive specific radiation safety instructions whether released after hospitalization or immediately after treatment. Both of these circumstances are discussed below; however, the instructions are based on radiation protection standards set by the NRC [4] or similar regulations adopted by many state agencies [5]. These instructions are intended to establish a level of risk comparable to activities normally considered "safe," like office work. Thus, the most exposed individual in contact with the patient has an estimated risk of less than 0.04 % of developing a fatal cancer from radiation in the next 10–60 years. Simply, fewer than 4 of every 100,000 people in close contact with the patient may develop a fatal cancer later in life because of radiation from the patient compared to a natural cancer mortality rate of approximately 24 % [9].

Hospitalization

Hospitalization was required for all isotope administrations above 1.11 GBq (30 mCi) before the NRC changed its regulations. Today hospitalization may not be necessary. The physician is responsible for the assessment as to when a patient requires initial hospitalization and when the patient can be released. Training of hospital staff is required for success and is necessary by regulation. A sample handout for alerting patients to hospital restrictions is included as Example 2 (Appendix C).

As time passes after the ^{131}I is administered, the risk of exposing another person to radiation decreases. Table 55.1 shows how the dose rate drops off with time for measurements made at 1 m from the patient's body. This table is calculated from the ^{131}I retention assumptions for a cancer patient in the NRC Regulatory Guide 8.39 [7].

Generally, the physician does not have to hospitalize the patient if the *measured* dose rate is less than 0.07 mSv/h (7 mrem/h). However, the physician is required to provide written instructions for:

- Guidance on the interruption or discontinuation of breast-feeding as appropriate
- Guidance on practices to reduce the radiation dose to others
- Information on the consequences of failure to follow the guidance

Table 55.1 Predicted dose rate at 1 m from the patient

Time	3.7 GBq (100 mCi)	5.55 GBq(150 mCi)	7.4 GBq (200 mCi)
	μGy/h (mrad/h)	μGy/h (mrad/h)	μGy/h (mrad/h)
0 day	500 (50)	750 (75)	1000 (100)
0.25 days	300 (30)	450 (45)	600 (60)
0.5 days	180 (18)	270 (27)	360 (36)
0.75 days	110 (11)	165 (16.5)	220 (22)
1 day	70 (7)	105 (10.5)	140 (14)
2 days	25 (2.5)	38 (3.8)	50 (5 h)
3 days	16 (1.6)	24 (2.4)	32 (3.2)
4 days	15 (1.5)	18 (1.8)	30 (3.0)
5 days	13 (1.3)	19.5 (1.95)	26 (2.6)
6 days	12 (1.2)	18 (1.8)	24 (2.4)
7 days	11 (1.1)	17 (1.7)	22 (2.2)
14 days	6 (0.6)	9 (0.9)	12 (1.2)
21 day	3 (0.3)	4.5 (0.45)	6 (0.6)

Adapted from NRC Regulatory Guide 8.39 [7]

Table 55.2 Radioactive iodine excreted by various pathways during days following dosage

Day	Perspiration[a]	Saliva[b]	Breath[b]	Urine[b]
1	925,000 Bq	1,702,000 Bq	1,665,000 Bq	2,960,000,000 Bq
	(25 μCi)	(46 μCi)	(45 μCi)	(80,000 μCi)
2	481,000 Bq	296,000 Bq	407,000 Bq	318,200,000 Bq
	(13 μCi)	(8 μCi)	(11 μCi)	(8600 μCi)
3	74,000 Bq	33,300 Bq	48,100 Bq	37,000,000 Bq
	(2 μCi)	(0.9 μCi)	(1.3 μCi)	(1000 μCi)
4	7400 Bq	3700 Bq	(7400 Bq)	3,700,000 Bq
	(0.2 μCi)	(0.11 μCi)	(0.2 μCi)	(100 μCi)
5	740 Bq	370 Bq	740 Bq	481,000 Bq
	(0.02 μCi)	(0.01 μCi)	(0.02 μCi)	(13 μCi)
6	74 Bq	37 Bq	74 Bq	74,000 Bq
	(0.002 μCi)	(0.001 μCi)	(0.002 μCi)	(2 μCi)
7	Minimal	Minimal	Minimal	7400 Bq
	Minimal	Minimal	Minimal	(0.2 μCi)
The excreted activity is Becquerel (mCi) per 3.7 GBq (100 mCi) administered				

Based on data from Ibis et al. [8]
[a]Activity on whole body
[b]Per cubic centimeter

For the release of a patient at higher measured dose rates, the physician must ask the patient questions to document that he or she is a suitable candidate for release. The physician must also ascertain that the patient does not plan any extended travel time in public transportation. A sample questionnaire is shown in Example 3 (Appendix C), which is discussed further below.

Even if the patient can maintain isolation, concern may still persist regarding the patient's potential to contaminate the living space during the first 24–36 h. However, after 2 days, the patient usually will not emit any radioactive contamination that is seriously consequential (see Table 55.2). During the first 24 h, urine, saliva, breath, and blood contain concentrations of radioactive iodine that could harm another person's thyroid. Again, the physician must seriously evaluate both the probability and consequences of an accident that could result in another person's uptake of radioactive iodine. Keeping the patient for an 18-h hospital stay or longer significantly reduces the risks associated with any accidental exposure to bodily fluids.

Radiation Safety Precautions

The medical staff, support staff, other patients, visitors, and the next patient to occupy the room must be protected from unnecessary exposure to radiation and radioactive material. The methods of achieving protection are: (1) isolation of the patient, (2) containment of radioactive material to the assigned room, (3) measurement and release of anything leaving the room, and (4) good hygiene by anyone entering and leaving the room.

Isolation

The patient is isolated from all but a few hospital staff. Hospital staff members are instructed to have as little contact as possible, consistent with the standard of care. Isolation is not required because of immediate danger to people coming in close contact with the patient, but it is to ensure the ALARA principle. In an emergency, the medical staff should provide all the necessary medical attention that the patient needs regardless of the radiation exposure to themselves. The maximum radiation-absorbed dose likely during a 1-h emergency is about equal to the radiation-absorbed dose from background radiation in 1 year: 3 mSv (300 mrem). If radiation doses to medical staff are likely to exceed 0.005 Gy (0.5 rad), personal dosimetry must be provided. Proximity to the patient, even right after treatment, should not expose a staff member to more radiation than a member of the public receives in 1 year from natural background radiation. However, that kind of radiation exposure from 20 to 40 patients in 1 year would result in relatively high radiation exposure and a small but unnecessary risk of cancer later in life.

Visitors are not permitted unless the physician managing the ^{131}I administration believes certain family members or close friends are needed to provide unique care or support. If visitors are allowed, they may need to be monitored for radiation-absorbed dose and precautions must be taken to keep doses below 5 mSv (500 mrem).

Containment

Everything that enters the room should be left in the room unless cleared by radiation safety personnel. The hospital population is not exposed to radioactive material as long as it stays in the room. Personal belongings should be limited to clothes, disposable materials, or items that can be cleaned easily. Personal possessions that cannot be cleaned and are contaminated with ^{131}I above a limit set by hospital radiation safety should be disposed of by the hospital or kept until the radioactivity decays.

Measurement and Release

Before leaving the hospital, the patient should be monitored to determine the absorbed dose rate from the patient, and all patient belongings should be monitored for radioactive contamination before leaving. After the patient has been discharged, the room contents should be monitored. There are three possibilities for contaminated belongings and room contents: (1) release, if not contaminated above the release limit, (2) held for later release after radioactive decay, and (3) disposal as radioactive waste. Preparing the room before the patient is admitted enables more rapid cleanup of the room and quicker release. Floors, door handles, telephones, and other items likely to be touched should be covered with paper or plastic to help prevent radioactive contamination.

Hygiene

Everyone who enters the patient's room should wear gloves and shoe covers and should remove their gloves and shoe covers as they leave the room. Washing their hands promptly provides additional benefit against contamination.

Conditions for Earlier Release

A patient's agreement to limit close contact within arm's length with family and friends to 3 h a day for the first few days is often enough for a licensee to justify earlier release. Under certain circumstances, an NRC licensee may immediately release a patient who has been given several GBq of ^{131}I based on that patient's ability to be isolated from other people. Many hospitals release all but a few patients within a few hours after administration of ^{131}I.

Considerations for release earlier than 18 h should include:

- Almost total isolation at home for the first day.
- Separate eating, bathing, and toilet facilities for the first few days.
- No use of public facilities or transportation for the first few days.
- No trips longer than a few hours in a private automobile and while sitting as far as possible from other passengers.
- No trips longer than 1 h sitting in contact with another passenger during the first day after administration.
- The ability of the patient to provide self-care without assistance.
- No medical need to observe the patient for the first day.

A worksheet for documenting patient release above the default values, based on the questionnaire (Example 3; Appendix C), is included as Example 4 (Appendix C). Note that the sample includes the derivation of a release criterion based only on the occupancy factor (E). Based on this derivation, the maximum acceptable dose rate at release is:

$$\frac{dD}{dt} = 1.79 / \mathrm{E\ mrem/h}$$

Other Considerations

There is a potential risk of injury to another individual's thyroid if more than 1.1 MBq (0.030 mCi) is ingested or inhaled as a result of exposure to ^{131}I from the thyroid cancer patient. Washing hands and staying at least 1 m away from other people will prevent an unhealthy dose of radiation. Certain intimate contacts could transfer more than 1.1 million Bq (0.030 mCi) in the very early days after administering radioactive iodine. Breast milk and pregnancy are particularly concerning. Women of childbearing age must avoid pregnancy during their treatment, and mothers must not nurse infants.

The amount of radioactivity shed through breath, saliva, urine, and perspiration drops rapidly with time after administration. Intimate contact should be avoided only for days, rather than weeks. As noted, Table 55.2 shows estimates of the amount of radioactivity the patient will release through perspiration, saliva, breath, and urine during each day following dosage. Other than radioactivity excreted in urine, by day 4, the levels are much smaller than 1.1 MBq (0.030 mCi) and, by day 7, are extremely small. Table 55.2 was calculated using an average of measurements made at 24 and 48 h by the Medical College of Wisconsin [8] with the assumption that the measured levels after 48 h would drop as predicted using the NRC Regulatory Guide 8.39 retention model. These measurements indicated that the levels (except for urine) are greatest at 24 h.

Evolving Recommendations

Although not connected with NRC requirements, International Atomic Energy Agency (IAEA) Safety Reports Series No. 63 *Release of Patients after Radionuclide Therapy* (http://www-pub.iaea.org/MTCD/publications/PDF/pub1417_web.pdf) provides an international perspective of release of patient following treatment with therapeutic radionuclides [10]. Clinicians in the United States are examining the criteria used to determine when a patient should be hospitalized [11]. The NRC continues to be concerned about population exposure from all regulated sources of radiation including patients who have been released following treatment with ^{131}I. Professional organizations have made recommendations based on research conducted by a number of investigators. The American Thyroid Association Task Force on Radioiodine Safety published recommendations to guide physicians and patients in safe practices after treatment with radioactive iodine [12]. Their recommendations are compatible with those of the National Council on Radiation Protection and Measurements and the International Commission on Radiological Protection and the regulations of the NRC, and they take into consideration literature generated by physicians and researchers. Tables 55.3 and 55.4 below are based on their recommendations and provide examples that may be used as guidance for release of patients.

Table 55.3 Examples of restrictions after radioiodine treatment for hyperthyroidism

	MBq (mCi) administered			
	370	555	740	1110
	(10)	(15)	(20)	(30)
Daytime restrictions (number of days)				
Maximize your distance (6 ft or more) from children and pregnant women	1	1	2	5
Avoid extended time in public places	1	1	1	3
You may return to work	1	1	2	5
Nighttime restrictions (number of days)				
Sleep in a separate (6-ft separation) bed from adults	3	6	8	11
Sleep in a separate bed from pregnant partners, infant, or child	15	18	20	23
Travel time (hours) without exceeding regulatory dose limit				
• Day 0 (beginning with treatment)	5.9	3.9	2.9	2.0
• Day 1	9.2	6.1	4.6	3.1
• Day 2	13.0	8.7	6.5	4.3
• Day 3	–	10.6	8.0	5.3

Adapted from Sisson et al. [12]
Assumes 50 % uptake by thyroid, with effective T1/2 of about 5 days. Modify examples to meet local and specific patient needs. These examples are based on dose rate of 17 uSv/h (0.17 mrem/h) per 37 MBq (1 mCi) at 1 m, 5 m
Sv (500 mrem) per year for family member and caregiver, 1 mSv (100 mrem) for pregnant women, children, and the public, and Occupancy Factors for adults of 0.25 except for sleeping 0.33. Resumption of sleeping with a partner assumes a distance of 0.3 m

Table 55.4 Examples of restrictions after radioiodine treatment for thyroid carcinoma ablation

	MBq (mCi) administered			
	18501850550	3700	5550	7400
	(50)	(100)	(150)	(200)
Nighttime restrictions (days)				
Sleep in a separate (6-ft separation) bed from adults	1	1	2	4
Sleep in a separate bed from pregnant partners, infant, or child	6	13	18	21
Daytime restrictions				
You may return to work after days shown	1	1	1	1
Maximize your distance (6 ft) from children and pregnant women	1	1	1	1
Avoid extended time in public places	1	1	1	1
Travel time (hours) without exceeding regulatory dose limit				
• Day (24-h cycles) 0 (beginning with treatment)	1.2	0.6	0.4	0.3
• Day (24-h cycles) 1	3.0	1.5	1.0	0.8
• Day (24-h cycles) 2	7.2	3.8	2.5	1.9
• Day (24-h cycles) 3	15.0	7.5	5.0	3.8
• Day (24-h cycles) 4	–	15.0	10.0	7.5

Adapted from Sisson et al. [12]
Assumes biexponential decay with early effective T1/2 of about 0.76 days and 2 % uptake in remnant with effective T1/2 of about 7.3 days. Modify examples to meet local and specific patient needs. These examples are based on dose rate of 17 uSv/h (0.17 mrem/h) per 37 MBq (1 mCi) at 1 m,5 mSv (500 mrem) per year for family member and caregiver, 1 mSv (100 mrem) for pregnant women, children, and the public, and Occupancy Factors for adults of 0.25 except for sleeping 0.33. Resumption of sleeping with a partner assumes a distance of 0.3 m.

Table 55.5 Radiation dosefrom natural and man-made sources

Source of exposure	Percentage (%)
Natural sources	50
Radon gas	36.5
Natural radioactivity in your body	4.5
Natural radioactivity in the earth	3.5
Radiation from outer space	5.5
Artificial sources	50
Medical (mostly from CT)	48
Consumer products	2
Coast-to-coast airplane roundtrip	0.2
Nuclear power	–0.002

Adapted from NCRP [9]

Myths and Fears About Radioactivity

1. *Radiation exposure will make a person radioactive.* This statement is false. A patient who has received ^{131}I is radioactive and is a source of radiation exposure only as long as radioactive iodine remains in the body. More than 99 % of the radioactive iodine administered to a thyroid cancer patient is eliminated in the first few days.
2. *Radiation exposure is unusual and is very dangerous.* In fact, most radiation exposure comes from nature, whereas the minority is man-made (see Table 55.5). A large radiation dose can cause injury or death. Large doses during pregnancy can cause developmental deficiencies. Small doses may increase the risk for cancer.
3. *If I avoid man-made sources of radiation, I will not get any extra radiation dose.* Compare living within 50 miles of a nuclear power plant (1 uSv/year) to natural radioactivity in your body (140 uSv/year).

Conclusion

This chapter has discussed the differentiation of radiation and radioactivity, ionizing and nonionizing radiation, units of radioactivity and radiation-absorbed dose, hospitalization regulations, conditions for earlier release, radiation safety precautions during the hospital stay and upon release, and myths and fears about radioactivity. Protection of the public to prevent unnecessary exposure from patients taking ^{131}I therapy requires knowledge, planning, procedures, and education. Advance communication with the patient about radiation, radioactivity, risks, regulations, hospitalization, and appropriate precautions at home will help ensure good compliance, resulting in reduced radiation exposure to family, friends, caretakers, and the general public.

References

1. Ong LM, de Haes JC, Hoos AM, Lammes FB. Doctor-patient communication: a review of the literature. Soc Sci Med. 1995;40:903–18.
2. Radiation and your patient: a guide for medical practitioners. Ann ICRP. 2001;2001:1–52.
3. National Research Council of the National Academies. Health effects from exposure to low levels of ionizing radiation: BEIR VII phase 2. Washington, DC: The National Academies Press; 2006.
4. Part 35, Medical use of byproduct material. Title 10, code of federal regulations, section 35.75.
5. Part G, Use of radionuclides in the healing arts. Suggested state regulations for control of radiation, vol. I, ionizing radiation. Conference of Radiation Control Program Directors. Inc.
6. Federal Register, 62 FR 4120, 29 Jan 1997.
7. Release of patients administered radioactive materials. Division 8, Occupational Health, Regulatory Guide 8.39, U.S. Nuclear Regulatory Commission, 1997. http://pbadupws.nrc.gov/docs/ML0037/ML003739575.pdf. Accessed 1 Jul 2014.
8. Ibis E, Wilson CR, Collier BD, et al. Iodine-131 contamination from thyroid cancer patients. Nucl Med. 1992;33:2110–5.
9. National Council on Radiation Protection and Measurements. Ionizing radiation exposure of the population of the United States. NCRP Report No. 160; Bethesda: NCRP. 2009.
10. International Atomic Energy Agency. Release of patients after radionuclide therapy. IAEA safety reports series No. 63. Vienna: IAEA; 2009 http://www-pub.iaea.org/MTCD/publications/PDF/pub1417_web.pdf. Accessed 1 Jul 2014.
11. Harolds JA. New scrutiny of outpatient therapy with I-131. Clin Nucl Med. 2011;36:206–8.
12. Sisson J, et al. Radiation safety in the treatment of patients with thyroid diseases by radioiodine ^{131}I: practice recommendations of the American Thyroid Association. Thyroid. 2011;121:335–46.

^{131}I Treatment of Distant Metastases

56

Douglas Van Nostrand

Introduction

^{131}I has been used for many years for the therapy of patients who have distant metastases derived from differentiated thyroid cancer [1]. This chapter presents an overview of the literature regarding the efficacy of ^{131}I therapy in the treatment of distant metastases and discusses the approaches to select the prescribed activity (dosage) of ^{131}I for these therapies.

Efficacy of ^{131}I Treatments for Distant Metastases

The major difficulty in assessing the efficacy of ^{131}I treatments of distant metastases is that no prospective study has been performed, and the likelihood of such is remote. However, multiple retrospective studies are available [2–49]. Selected publications for ^{131}I treatment for lung metastases are listed in Table 56.1, pulmonary and bone metastases in Table 56.2, bone metastases in Table 56.3, brain metastases in Table 56.4, and distant metastases not separated by site in Table 56.5. The numerous limitations associated with retrospective studies are listed in Table 56.6. Management of metastases to the bone is also discussed further in Chap.65.

Pulmonary Metastases

As applicable to many areas of thyroid cancer management, controversy exists regarding whether ^{131}I therapy increases survival, reduces recurrence, and/or palliates metastasis in patients with pulmonary metastases. For example, data from Ruegemer [10], Dinneen [18], and Sisson [23] show little or no evidence to suggest a therapeutic effect of ^{131}I, whereas data from Casara, [15], Schlumberger [9, 20], Samaan [7], Pacini [16], Ronga [41], and others support a therapeutic effect from ^{131}I in pulmonary metastases. Again, a summary of these publications is noted in Table 56.1, and the guidelines of various organizations and societies for the use of ^{131}I in the treatment of pulmonary metastases are noted in Table 56.7 [79–86]. Selected publications are discussed in more detail below.

Ruegemer et al. [10] from the Mayo Clinic reported that, "by univariate analysis, patient age, tumor extent ($p=0.0002$), pattern of lung involvement ($p=0.0001$), radioiodine uptake of the metastases, and ^{131}I treatment were significant prognostic factors." Naturally, potential benefit from ^{131}I therapy must depend on the presence of radioiodine uptake; in their series, mortality was lower in 19 patients with radioiodine uptake than in the 33 patients with no evidence of radioiodine uptake on scan ($p=0.016$). In addition, a higher proportion of micronodular lung involvement was present in the 19 patients (58 %) versus the 33 patients who had no radioiodine uptake (12 %; $p=0.0005$). However, Ruegemer stated, "By multivariate analysis, only age at the time of first diagnosis of distant metastases and involvement of multiple organ sites were independently associated with cancer mortality." The Cox regression model suggested that after adjustment for age and extent of metastatic involvement, ^{131}I administration did not have a significant influence on survival.

Another Mayo Clinic series, reported by Dinneen et al. [18], described 100 patients with pulmonary metastases, as well as other various distant metastases. The favorable prognostic factors by univariate analysis included the use of ^{131}I therapy ($p<0.001$), age at time of diagnosis of distant metastases, completeness of resection of the primary tumor, histological grade 1, diploid nuclear DNA, and lung as the first site of metastases. However, again, ^{131}I treatment was not identified as a favorable prognostic factor by multivariate analysis. The other favorable prognostic factors by multivariate analysis were age, site of distant metastasis, and degree

D. Van Nostrand, MD, FACP, FACNM (✉)
Nuclear Medicine Research, MedStar Research Institute and Washington Hospital Center, Georgetown University School of Medicine, Washington Hospital Center, 110 Irving Street, N.W., Suite GB 60F, Washington, DC 20010, USA
e-mail: douglasvannostrand@gmail.com

L. Wartofsky, D. Van Nostrand (eds.), *Thyroid Cancer*, DOI 10.1007/978-1-4939-3314-3_56

Table 56.1 Pulmonary metastases only

Author	Specifics	No. of patients	1-year survival	5-year survival	10-year survival	15-year survival	Remission	Comments
Brown [5]		20		63 %	54 %		65 %	
Casara [15]	Normal chest X-ray, positive ^{131}I scan	42	100 %	100 %	96 %		Complete remission 78 %	
	Abnormal chest X-ray, positive ^{131}I scan	54	~92 %	~0.55	36 %		Complete remission 3.7 %	
	Abnormal chest X-ray, negative ^{131}I scan	38	~75 %	~18 %	11 %		None	
Massin [6]	Overall	58	68 %	44 %				
	Radioiodine-treated group	24		74 %				
	Micronodular	11					9/11 considered cured	
	Macronodular	13					3/13 considered cured	
	Untreated	29	50 %	10 %				Macronodular disease, low or no ^{131}I uptake
Schlumberger [20]	Lung only	214			61 %		50 %	
Nemec [3]	All pulmonary metastases	78		29 %	12 %	36 %		Survival following diagnosis of thyroid cancer
	Fine pattern	25		76 %	59 %	39 %		4 patients had bone metastases
	Coarse pattern	33		41 %	14 %	4 %		19 patients had bone metastases
	^{131}I uptake	66		92 %	70%	35 %		
	No ^{131}I uptake	12		32 %	6 %	3 %		
Hindié [38]	Positive ^{131}I uptake	20		90 %	84 %			Average follow-up for the 17 survivors was 12.7 years
	Negative chest X-ray, positive ^{131}I scan	11			90 %		73 %	
	Abnormal chest X-ray, positive ^{131}I scan	9			78 %		22 %	
	Negative ^{131}I scan	12		33 %	0 %			
Sampson [44]		22	77 % (3-year survival)					
Sisson [23]	Micronodular ^{131}I avid	12						A complete remission occurred in only 2 of 12 patients
Llgan [42]		42	86 % (36/42) 3-year survival	76 % (32/42)				CT detects lung met in 10 out of 14 patients with normal chest X-ray Stage of disease, existence of other distant mets and CT characteristics were significant prognostic variables Lung metastases can be cured with ^{131}I therapy
Cho [50]		152			85 %	20-year survival was 71 %		

of extrathyroidal invasion of the primary tumor. In contrast to the observations of Schlumberger et al. [20] discussed below, Dinneen et al. noted no difference in survival for the time periods of 1940–1954, 1955–1969, and 1970–1989. He concluded that this indirect evidence suggested that recent advances in the diagnosis and management of distant metastasis, such as ^{131}I treatment, had no effect on survival.

Maheshwari et al. [4] from the University of Texas MD Anderson Hospital and Tumor Institute reviewed 53 patients with pulmonary metastases and 31 patients with metastases to the bone. Although specific data on these patients were not presented, Maheshwari stated, "Repeated therapy with ^{131}I did not appear to improve the patients' survival rate."

In an analysis of 12 patients, Sisson et al. [23] reported that it was uncommon to achieve complete remission of distant metastases with ^{131}I. Their administered activity ranged from 2.2 to 13 GBq (60–350 mCi) with total accumulative prescribed activity ranging from 5.2 to 29.6 GBq (140 to 800 mCi). In a subsequent report, Sisson et al. [29] questioned whether ^{131}I could deliver enough of a radiation absorbed dose to small pulmonary metastases less than 1 mm in diameter to be effective. Their concern was based on the fact that as a tumor becomes smaller and smaller, the β and γ energy deposited within the actual tumor decreases; thus, for a sphere of 0.5-mm diameter, less than 40 % of ^{131}I energy is deposited within that sphere [29]. In addition, even if a 1-mm focus of pulmonary metastasis could receive enough radiation absorbed dose to be treated successfully, that focus may have small 100–500 μ papillary projections that may not receive sufficient radiation absorbed dose.

In a multivariate analysis of 134 patients who had pulmonary metastases, Casara et al. [15] from the University of Padua and the Institute of Semeiotica Medica in Italy showed that only radioiodine uptake ($p<0.0001$), chest X-ray ($p=0.0014$), and multiple distant metastases ($p=0.01$) were significant independent variables. Univariate analysis identified radioiodine uptake ($p<000.1$), patient age ($p<0.0001$), histology ($p=0.04$), chest X-ray, and the presence of multiple distant metastases ($p<0.0001$) as prognostic factors. Casara concluded that early scintigraphic diagnosis and ^{131}I therapy of lung metastases appeared to be the most important factors associated with a significant improvement in survival rate and a prolonged disease-free time interval. Regarding the different results of Casara and Ruemeger, Casara raised the possibility that the lack of ^{131}I influence in the Mayo Clinic data may have been partly a result of the performance of only partial thyroidectomies. Casara et al. [15] further commented that: "When the pulmonary metastases were <5 mm in diameter with a negative chest X-ray, complete disease remission following ^{131}I therapy almost always occurred. When metastases were >5 mm in diameter (positive chest X-ray), the survival rate is still considered fairly good, but the probability of obtaining complete disease remission was very low despite ^{131}I uptake. Moreover, when the macronodular metastases lose the capability of radioiodine uptake, a fatal outcome was almost always observed."

In 1996, Schlumberger et al. [20] from Institut Gustave-Roussy in Villejuif, France, reported the therapeutic benefit of ^{131}I in 394 patients with distant metastases. Positive prognostic factors for survival by multivariate analysis were (1) radioiodine uptake, (2) a younger age, (3) the time of metastases detection, (4) histological type, and (5) small extent of disease. Schlumberger concluded that ^{131}I treatment was one of the factors that increased survival. Schlumberger also noted that patients who had their distant metastases discovered after 1976 had a 140 % increase in survival, relative to those patients who had their distant metastases discovered before 1960. For patients who had their distant metastases discovered between 1960 and 1977, the increase in survival was 30 %. He proposed that these improvements could relate to the introduction of ^{131}I in 1960 and serum thyroglobulin measurements in 1977. As Ruegemer noted, the discordance between the results of Ruegemer and Schlumberger may relate to a difference in patient population. Only one of Ruegemer's patients had a positive radioiodine scan and negative chest X-ray, whereas 18 % (51 of 281) of patients evaluated by Schlumberger had a positive radioiodine scan and negative chest and bone X-ray.

Samaan et al. [7] reviewed 101 patients with pulmonary metastases, who were also studied at the University of Texas MD Anderson Hospital and Tumor Institute. Samaan concluded that patients treated with ^{131}I had a longer survival than those not treated ($p<0.002$) and uptake of radioactive iodine by lung metastasis was a favorable prognostic factor, especially in patients with negative chest X-rays. However, he also observed the link between age and radioactive iodine uptake.

Hindié et al. [38] from Hôpital Saint-Antoine stated that ^{131}I had a beneficial impact on functioning pulmonary metastases. However, he questioned that the "beneficial impact" of ^{131}I in patients who had negative chest X-rays and positive radioiodine scans, compared to patients with positive chest X-rays and negative radioiodine scans, may not be the result of the ^{131}I. Rather, this impact may represent two distinct entities, or two stages, of the same disease but with different prognoses, regardless of the ^{131}I treatment.

Relating to the different results that Hindié observed in comparison to Ruegemer's findings at Mayo Clinic, Hindié suggested this might be partly explained by different stages of metastatic disease at the time of diagnosis, as well as the intensity of ^{131}I therapy. The group of 85 patients in Ruegemer's series (Mayo Clinic) did not receive ^{131}I ablation after thyroid surgery, and distant metastases were detected by chest or bone X-ray in 99 % (84 of 85) of patients. Furthermore, only 37 % of patients who subsequently received ^{131}I therapy in the Mayo Clinic series had ^{131}I uptake.

Table 56.2 Pulmonary metastases, bone metastases, and/or other distant sites

Author	Specifics	No. of patients	1-year survival	5-year survival	10-year survival		Remission	Comments
Brown [5]		11					9 %	Improvement in only 1 patient.
Schlumberger [20]		72			13 %		7 %	
Petrich [33]	Radioiodine +	41						Mean survival of 7.3 years
Dorn [37]		6						Follow-up was an average of 3.7 years (range of 1.2–7.2 years) 85 %. Survival to date, with 1 death attributable to thyroid cancer
Lee [49]	All patients diagnosed initially and after initial treatment	91	83.8[a]	72.1[a]				1. Pts with distant metastases diagnosed initially had improved DSS[b] than those diagnosed after initial treatment
								2. Complete local control was a predictor of improved OS[a] and DSS[b]
								3. Radioiodine avidity improved OS[a] and DSS[b] in pts diagnosed with distant metastases after initial treatment and only DSS[b] in pts initially diagnosed with distant metastases
			68.5[b]	26.8[b]				
Mihailovic [48]		77		58 %	48 %	40 %	40 %	Age had greater influence on survival than iodine avidity ($p<0.001$)
	Iodine avid			66.7 %	55 %	45 %	45 %	
	Non-iodine avid			18 %	18 %			
Stefanovic [51]				63 %[b]	50 %[b]			
Shoup [52]		252 (103 lung only; 80 bone only)			26 % DSS with median survival of 4.1-year DSS			34 % DSS[b] and initial 23 % DSS[b] and initial (NS)
	<45 years old				58 % DSS			
	>45 years old				13 % DSS			

(continued)

Table 56.2 (continued)

Author	Specifics	No. of patients	1-year survival	5-year survival	10-year survival	15-year survival	20-year survival	Remission	Comments
Mizukami [53]		34			70 % with ^{131}I positive mets and 40 % with ^{131}I negative mets				
Sugitani [46]		86		65 %[b]	45 %[b]				Multiple sites
									Multiple interventions other than just ^{131}I
Lin [54]		137 (24 lung, 13 bone, 13 mediastinal nodes, 18 others)		~80 %	~55 %	~15 %			Mean follow-up 5.9 years
Lee [49]		91 (62 diffuse lung; 15 bone only)		With mets at initial treatment:	With mets at initial treatment:				Complete local control was significant predictor
				84 % (OS)	72 % (OS)				
				69 % (DSS)	27 % (DSS)				In pts who developed mets after treatment, iodine avidity was positively associated with OS[a] and DSS[b]
				With mets after treatment:	With mets after treatment:				
				71 % (OS)	60 % (OS)				
				37 % (DSS)	20 % (DSS)				
Durante [43]		233 lung only			42 %	33 %	29 %		
		115 bone only, and 82 both lung and bone							

[a]Overall survival (OS)
[b]Disease-specific survival (DSS)

In Hindié's series, 63 % of patients had radioiodine uptake. Again, these discordances may be due to either a difference in the stage of disease at diagnosis or intensity of therapy.

Ronga et al. [41] from Sapienza University of Rome, Italy, evaluated 96 patients with pulmonary metastases from 1958 to 2000, concluding that the most important factors increasing survival rates were a young age at diagnosis and radioiodine uptake by metastases. The multivariate analysis demonstrated that the risk of death was 5.4 times higher in patients over age 45 years and was reduced by ^{131}I treatment to nearly 1/6. Although Ronga's data indicated that improved survival also appeared associated with a miliary versus a nodular pattern, Ronga thought this link was related to radioiodine uptake and possibly a more favorable prognosis for patients with a miliary pattern.

Nemec et al. [3] from the Research Institute of Endocrinology in Prague reviewed 78 patients with pulmonary metastases. Nemec implied survival was improved in patients who were younger and had a pattern of radioiodine uptake in the lung that was considered "fine" (<10 mm). The survival rate was worse with greater abnormalities on chest X-ray and bone metastases. He stated that the most important factor for survival was radioiodine uptake; however, he did not correct his data to include the impact of age.

Massin et al. [6] from Groupe Hospitalier Pitié-Salpétriére evaluated 58 cases of pulmonary metastases, of which 24 were treated with ^{131}I and 29 were untreated. The survival for the ^{131}I -treated group at 5 and 8 years was 74 % and 42 %, respectively, whereas the untreated survival at the same

Table 56.3 Bone metastases only

Author	Specifics	No. of patients	1-year survival[a]	3-year survival[a]	5-year survival[a]	10-year survival[a]	20-year survival[a]	Remission	Comments
Brown [5]		21			7 %	0 %		0 %	11 patients also had lung metastases
Schlumberger [20]		108				21 %		10 %	
Marocci [12]		30	98 %		65 %	18 %		10 %	3 patients with complete remission had both surgery and radioiodine treatment
Petrich [33]	Radioiodine +	60							Mean survival of 8.9 years (survival longer in those with uptake. $P<0.0005$)
	Radioiodine –	6							Mean survival of 1.2 years
Proye [14]		28	53 %					36 % responded	Combination of treatments
								7 % (2) cured	7 patients alive with follow-up of 8 months to 8 years
	Radioiodine + Radiographically –	12						2/12 cured	
Bernier [35]		109	41 %		15 %		7 %		Median survival of 3.9 years
Pittas [31]		146			25 %	13 %			1 % patients had anaplastic carcinoma, 6 had medullary carcinoma, and 3 had lymphoma
Fanchiang [30]		39			65 %				16 patients had other organ involvement. 25 patients had surgical treatment, and 18 patients received external radiotherapy
Woods [13]		37			47 %	34 %			Only 1 patient received just radioiodine intra-arterially
Zettinig [36]		41			59 %	39 %			

Dorn [37]		9						Follow-up was an average of 6.7 years (range of 1.3–10.9) 88 % survival to date, with 2 deaths not attributed to thyroid cancer	Patients may have had other non-lung metastases
Tickoo [32]		79			29 %	13 %			Patients included poorly differentiated or undifferentiated thyroid cancer (68 %) as well as anaplastic and medullary thyroid cancer (30 %)
Khorjekar [55]		30	96 %	90 %	75 %			Follow-up was an average of 4.07 years (range of 0.8–9.5)	No anaplastic or medullary thyroid cancer was included
Qui [56]		196			87 %	58 %			Only solitary bone met and ^{131}I therapy were independent factors
Sampson et al. [44]		19		56 %					Those with iodine-avid bone metastases did better than those with non-iodine-avid bone metastases

(continued)

Table 56.3 (continued)

Author	Specifics	No. of patients	1-year survival[a]	3-year survival[a]	5-year survival[a]	10-year survival[a]	20-year survival[a]	Remission	Comments
Wu [47]		44			79 %[a] (64 % for papillary and 82 % for follicular)	53 %			Pts with anaplastic (3) and medullary (3) carcinoma were included
									Surgical tx performed in 17 pts, and 5-year survival for pts with surgical was 80.2 % vs 70.6 % without surgery but not statistically significant
									Hypercalcemia associated with reduced prognosis
Hindié [57]		16		0 % (3/3 with nonfunctioning mets) 88 % (7/8 with functioning mets)	80 % (4/5 with functioning mets)				

[a]Time is from diagnosis of initial bone metastasis to death

Table 56.4 Brain metastases (BM) of differentiated thyroid cancer (DTC)

Author	No. of patients (DTC)	Histology	Survival after diagnosis of brain metastasis (BM)	Comments
Chiu [26]	Total: 32 (1.2 %) DTC	Pap: 28 Follic: 1 Hürthle cell: 3	12.4 months	Pts with BM secondary to DTC tended to have characteristics at initial presentation of older age, larger primary tumor, frequent extrathyroidal invasion, and loco- and distant mets. Single BM lesion predicted longer survival than multiple BM. Resection of at least 1 BM foci was the only modality that appeared to significantly affect survival
Chen [58]	20 total 18 DTC (9 BM, 9 skull)	Pap: 4 Follic: 4 Hürthle cell: 1	18 ± 29.2 months (8.7 ± 12.7 months for those w/o tx) (29.2 ± 40.5 months for those w/tx)	Pts with BM tend to be older, female, and present with neurological symptoms (e.g., headache, seizure, focal motor weakness, sensory deficits, and ataxia). Single lesions did much better than multiple lesions. Surgical resection greatly increased survival. No other modality could do the same. Whole-brain XRT improved survival but not statistically significant
Bernad [59]	23	Of histology reported, 9 pap, 2 Hürthle cell	Overall survival 20.8 months With SRS 37.4 months Without SRS 12.3 months	Highly recommend use of SRS
de Figueiredo [60]	21	Pap: 12 Follic: 5 Poorly diff: 4	Overall median survival 7.1 months With surgery or SRS 11.9 months Without surgery or SRS 3.6 months	Aggressive treatment with neurosurgery and/or RT
Bedikian [61]	33 (not all DTC but melanoma, breast, and lung cancers)		Median survival with glycerol + WBRT: 5.5 months	Glycerol is very effective in treating edema secondary to radiation therapy to the brain. It can be administered safely with radiotherapy and chemotherapy without compromising the immune system. It helped improve pts neurologically following brain irradiation
Samuel [62]	15	Pap: 3 Follic: 9 Folic + pap: 2 Hürthle cell: 1		Only one patient had total removal of the brain met and survived 8 years after surgery Only 2 patients showed radioiodine uptake in brain met, and 2 showed improvement

(continued)

Table 56.4 (continued)

Author	No. of patients (DTC)	Histology	Survival after diagnosis of brain metastasis (BM)	Comments
McWilliams [40]	13	Pap: 10 Follic: 2 Hürthle cell: 1	Overall average survival: 17.4 months after dx Pap (8.2 months) Follic (23.6 months) Hürthle cell (20.8 months)	Those pts with single lesions did much better than those multiple lesions. Recommended surgery for at least 1 lesion. Recommended stereotactic radiotherapy for isolated lesions in pts with high risk for open craniotomy. Recommended whole beam RT as adjuvant therapy following resection. If ^{131}I uptake, then ^{131}I potentially good option, but cautioned against ^{131}I due to complications. Does not recommend chemotherapy because no objective responses had yet to be reported
Venkatesh [63]	11	Pap: 8 Follic: 1 Hürthle cell: 2	Mean survival after development of brain metastases in the eight patients who died was 11.75 months	The longest surviving patient was alive at 75 mo and had single brain metastasis removed by surgery and treated with ^{131}I
Misaki [64]	9	Pap: 7 Follic: 2	Overall mean survival: 9.4 months 2 pts still alive (42 months and 3 months) at time of publication. Both treated with radiosurgery	WBRT response seems moderate at best. Surgical resection was not as effective as reported in other articles. Radiosurgery seems to be the best modality due to its noninvasive nature
Kim [65]	7	Pap: 7	33 months, 6 pts still living at time of publication	Recommends SRS as an effective minimally invasive strategy for BM. Smaller lesions are better because one is able to achieve higher doses. WBRT may have limited role in management but no conclusions
Ikekubo [66]	7	Pap: 7	30 months	Five tx with ^{131}I, 2 tx with SRS
Salvati [67]	6	Pap: 3 Follic: 3	Overall median survival 26 months (mean: 24 months)	Surgery best option for patients with solitary BMs. Consider WBRT postoperatively to prevent recurrence
Hjiyiannakis [68]	6	Pap: 6		Survival after diagnosis of brain met was 1–19 months. 4 had ^{131}I, 4 EBRT, and/or 1 excision
Miranda [69]	1	Follic		Aggressive surgical resection and radiotherapy should be considered in treating BM secondary to DTC
Diyora [70]	1	Pap		Pts with BM tended to be older age with larger primary and extrathyroidal invasion. Recommended treatment modalities be tailored to each patient
Izci [71]	1	Follic		
Anoop [72]	1	Follic	At 3-month follow-up, lesion size was reduced	

(continued)

Table 56.4 (continued)

Author	No. of patients (DTC)	Histology	Survival after diagnosis of brain metastasis (BM)	Comments
Datz [73]	1	Pap-follic		Seizures resulting from the radiation-induced cerebral edema are likely. Corticosteroids have been used to reduce this type of edema, though the mechanism is not fully understood. Because adrenocorticosteroids have been suggested to decrease ^{131}I uptake, Datz recommends glycerol as a better choice if giving ^{131}I
Holmquest [74]	1	Pap-follic		As opposed to treatment with ^{131}I and associated complications, consider craniotomy of mass first
Miranda [69]	1	Pap	Patient is still living at 10 years at time of publication	The combination of treatment modalities (i.e., surgery, ^{131}I, WBRT, SRS) appeared to work well in this patient
Aguiar [75]	1	Pap		Surgery combined with WBRT seems to be an effective means of treating BMs secondary to WDTC
Gkountouvas [76]	1	Pap-follic		Suggest that for elderly patients presenting with aggressive types of DTC and elevated Tg levels, use MRI or CT to check for any BMs
Pacak [77]	1	Pap		
Goolden [78]	1	Pap		

WBRT whole brain radiotherapy, *DTC* differentiated thyroid cancer, *BM* brain metastasis, *Pap* papillary, *Follic* follicular, *SRS* stereotactic radiosurgery

follow-up was 50 % and 10 %, respectively. Massin proposed that radioiodine uptake, age, and tumor invasion were favorable prognostic factors. He further suggested that the favorable prognostic aspect of the radioiodine uptake had a direct relationship to therapy with ^{131}I. However, this was not a multivariate analysis, and he stated radioiodine uptake was more likely in patients 30 years of age or younger and less likely in patients more than 80 years old.

Brown et al. [5] examined 42 patients with distant metastases at the Royal Marsden Hospital Thyroid Unit. In patients with only lung metastases, 54 % were alive and free of disease 10 years after ^{131}I treatment. The average total prescribed activity of ^{131}I administered in the entire series was 680 mCi (25.2 GBq), and seven patients received more than 1000 mCi (37 GBq). There were 13 patients (65 %) who had only pulmonary metastases that showed complete remission, which were all achieved with a total cumulative amount of ^{131}I of 800 mCi (29.6 GBq) or less. In 11 patients with lung (and bone metastases), complete resolution of the lung "deposits" was seen in 1 patient, with definite improvement in the chest X-ray in 3 patients.

Menzel et al. [21] from the University of Bonn treated 26 patients with a variety of distant metastases with an empiric activity of 300 mCi (1.11 GBq) at approx 3-month intervals. Menzel reported complete or partial remission in 35 %, stable disease in 23 %, and progressive disease in 42 %. The mean overall follow-up after the onset of metastatic spread was 52 months (range 9–157 months). He concluded that high prescribed activity with repetitive treatments of 300 mCi (11.1 GBq) and cumulative activities of up to 2000 mCi (74 GBq) of ^{131}I was beneficial in the treatment of advanced differentiated thyroid carcinoma.

Pacini et al. [16] from the Institute of Endocrinology of the University of Pisa reported on 118 patients with metastatic disease—the majority of whom had lung metastases. Specifically, 86 patients had only lung metastases, 16 had only bone metastases, 13 had lung and bone metastases, and 3 had other metastases. Although the results were not separated and analyzed by site of distant metastases, the overall "cure" rate for distant metastases was 36 % (43 of 118). They observed that the efficacy of ^{131}I therapy depended predominately on the size, location, and number of distant metastatic lesions. The best chance for a favorable response was in patients with radioiodine-positive, radiograph-negative, micronodular diffuse lung metastases. The effects of ^{131}I appeared even more favorable in children. Furthermore, they commented that early recognition and treatment of pulmonary metastases might improve the effectiveness of ^{131}I therapy.

Table 56.5 Distant metastases not separated by location

Author		No. of patients	1-year survival	5-year survival	10-year survival	15-year survival	Remission	Comments
Petrich [33]	<45 years old	8					63 % total or partial remission	
	>45 years old	99					50 % total or partial remission	
Schlumberger [20]	Complete response	124		96 %	93 %	89 %		
	No complete response	270		37 %	14 %	8 %		
	<40 years old with neg X-rays	56			96 %			
	>40 years old with macronodular lung or multiple bone metastases	156			7 %			
Pacini [16]		118					36 % cured	76 % survival at end of follow-up, with a mean survival of 5.8 years (86 lung only, 13 lung and bone, 16 bone only, and 3 other sites)
Høi [11]		91	58 %	20 %	Approx 6 % (9 years)		8 %	
Ruegemer [10]		85	76 %	42 %	33 %			
Dineen [18]		100	40 %	27 %	24 %			
Menzel [21]		26					35 % complete or partial remission	Mean follow-up of 52 months

Table 56.6 Variables limiting retrospective studies on the efficacy of ^{131}I in distant metastases

Method and depth of review
Small patient populations
Histopathology
Extent of initial surgery
Use of ^{131}I remnant ablation or adjuvant treatment
Amount of ^{131}I used for remnant ablation or adjuvant treatment
Extent of metastases
Sites of metastases
Use of ^{131}I for treatment of metastasis(es)
Amount of ^{131}I used for treatment of metastasis(es)
Length and frequency of follow-up
Definition of clinical remission

Table 56.7 Organizational guidelines for pulmonary metastases

Organization	Recommendation
ATA [79]	Recommendation 77
	"Pulmonary micrometastases should be treated with RAI therapy, and repeated every 6–12 months as long as disease continues to concentrate RAI and respond clinically, because the highest rates of complete remission are reported in these subgroups" (Strong recommendation, Moderate-quality evidence)
	Recommendation 77
	"The selection of RAI activity to administer for pulmonary micrometastases can be empiric (100–200 mCi) or estimated by dosimetry to limit whole-body retention to 80 mCi at 48 h and 200 cGy to the red bone marrow." (Strong recommendation, Moderate-quality evidence)
	Recommendation 78
	"Radioiodine-avid macronodular metastases may be treated with RAI and treatment may be repeated when objective benefit is demonstrated (decrease in the size of the lesions, decreasing Tg), but complete remission is not common and survival remains poor. The selection of RAI activity to administer can be made empirically (100–200 mCi) or by lesional dosimetry or wholebody dosimery if available in order to limit whole-body retention to 80 mCi at 48 h and 200 cGy to the red bone marrow." (Weak Recommendation, Low-quality evidence)
BTA [80]	"The size of pulmonary metastases influences the efficacy of ^{131}I therapy. Micronodular or miliary metastases are more likely to respond favourably to ^{131}I therapy than patients with pulmonary macronodular metastases, who rarely achieve a complete response"
	(i) For pulmonary metastases, repeat treatments at 6–12-month intervals are recommended provided there are continued ^{131}I uptake and evidence of ongoing benefit based on symptomatic improvement, radiological response, and reduced serum Tg concentration
CSE/CSS/CACA/CSNM [81]	Recommendation 2–19
	Post-thyroidectomy RAI treatment for metastases should be considered in selected patients. Recommendation rating: B
	"RAI therapy is indicated for inoperable metastases of functional thyroid carcinoma"
	"Microscopic or small macroscopic lung metastases may benefit more from the RAI therapy"
	Recommendation 2–20
	The first dose of ^{131}I for treating metastases should be administered at least 3 months after the RAI ablation. Repeated treatment by ^{131}I, if necessary, should be administered every 4–8 months. Recommendation rating: C
	Recommendation 2–21
	The recommended empiric RAI activity to administer for metastases is 100–200 mCi. Recommendation rating: C
	Recommendation 2–22
	There is no maximum limit to the individual or cumulative ^{131}I dose that can be given to patients with persistent disease. However, with higher individual and cumulative doses, there are increased risks of side effects. Recommendation rating: C
	Recommendation 2–47
	The preferred treatment for metastatic disease (in order) is surgical excision, RAI therapy for ^{131}I-avid disease, external beam radiation, watchful waiting with TSH suppression therapy, and experimental trials. Recommendation rating: B

(continued)

Table 56.7 (continued)

Organization	Recommendation
EANM [82]	"When radioiodine uptake is scintigraphically proven before therapy or after empiric RAIT, radioiodine treatment of non-resectable or incompletely resectable tumour, e.g. local recurrences, lymph node metastases or disseminated iodine avid lung metastases or other distant lesions, has shown in various investigations to be effective in eradicating disease, slowing disease progression or providing symptomatic relief. Indeed, outcome has been shown to be superior in patients with radioiodine-avid metastases compared to those with radioiodine-negative extra-thyroidal lesions"
	"The results of RAIT are superior for microscopic or small macroscopic tumours than for larger lesions. Therefore, the feasibility of partial or complete resection of macroscopic lesions should always be checked as a first treatment option"
	Definite indications of RAI treatment: "… Iodine-avid pulmonary micrometastases, especially before they become visible on CT…" "… Non-resectable or partially resectable iodine-avid pulmonary macrometastases…."
	Optional indications of RAI treatment: "Recurrent iodine-avid… distant metastases, as an adjuvant to surgery"
	Non-indications of RAI treatment: "… Iodine non-avid lung macrometastases…."
	"In late adolescents and adults, inoperable iodine-avid distant metastases are typically treated with multiple administrations, each 3.7–7.4 GBq or more, given every 4–8 months during the first 2 years following diagnosis of metastatic disease and at longer intervals thereafter"
	"As an alternative to the administration of fixed RAIT activities in adult or paediatric patients, pre-therapeutic dosimetry may be used to calculate an individualised activity projected to deliver a desired amount of radioactivity to tumour or extra-thyroidal compartments, or both. The generally accepted absorbed dose thresholds providing high efficacy are ≥300 Gy to remnants or ≥80 Gy to tumour deposits. The generally accepted surrogate dose threshold to avoid serious myelotoxicity is a blood absorbed dose ≤2 Gy"
EC [83]	"In the case of ^{131}I uptake, treatment consists of ^{131}I administration following prolonged withdrawal. An activity ranging between 3.7 and 7.4 GBq (or higher) is administered every 4–8 months during the first 2 years and thereafter at longer intervals"
	"A WBS performed 2–5 days after administration of ^{131}I provides assessment of response to treatment, together with serum Tg monitoring, thus guiding further treatment. Diagnostic ^{131}I WBS is not required prior to treatment, because it will not modify the indication for treatment and may induce stunning (reduction of uptake of the subsequent therapeutic activity)"
	"There is no maximum limit for the cumulative ^{131}I activity that can be given to patients with persistent disease. However, most remissions are obtained with cumulative activity equal to or lower than 22 GBq (600 mCi); above this cumulative activity the indication for further treatments should be taken on an individual basis. Lithium may be a useful adjuvant for ^{131}I treatment of metastatic well-differentiated thyroid carcinomas, increasing both the accumulation and retention of radioiodine in lesions"
ESMO [84]	Distant metastases are more successfully cured if they take up radioiodine and are of small size and located in the lungs (not visible at X-rays). Lung macronodules may benefit from radioiodine therapy but the definitive cure rate is very low)
	Chemotherapy is no longer indicated because of lack of effective results (IV, D) and should be replaced by enrollment of the patients in experimental trials with targeted therapy. Reinducing differentiation in DTC with insufficient uptake of ^{131}I has been attempted with drugs such retinoids and thiazolidinediones but till now with poor results

(continued)

Table 56.7 (continued)

Organization	Recommendation
NCCN [85]	For papillary, follicular, and Hürthle cell:
	Clinically significant structural disease should be surgically resected if possible before ^{131}I treatment.
	If radioiodine uptake, ^{131}I treatment with empiric doses of 100-200 mCi or dose adjusted by dosimetry
SNMMI [86]	"Post-thyroidectomy ^{131}I therapy is indicated for metastases of functioning thyroid carcinoma to lymph nodes, lung, bone, and, less often, brain, liver, skin, and other sites"
	"For treatment of distant metastases, an activity of 7.4 GBq (200 mCi) or more is often given. The radiation dose to the bone marrow is typically the limiting factor. It is recommended that the estimated radiation dose to the bone marrow be less than 2 Sv (200 rem). Blood and whole-body dosimetry may be indicated when a high activity of ^{131}I is planned to treat metastatic disease. Dosimetry will determine the maximum safe activity of ^{131}I and is recommended for all such patients over 50–55 years old, especially in the presence of a reduced glomerular filtration rate and when lung metastases may concentrate a large amount of ^{131}I. To reduce the risk of significant myelosuppression, retention of ^{131}I in the body at 48 h should be less than 4.44 GBq (120 mCi), or less than 2.96 GBq (80 mCi) if diffuse lung metastases are present, to reduce the risk of radiation pneumonitis as well. An adaptation of the 2.96-GBq (80-mCi) method has been published to correct for differences in patient size—for example, children versus adults"

The Chinese translation of the CSE/CSS/CACA/CSNM was performed by H. Guan and W. Teng. Dept of Endocrinology & Metabolism and Inst of Endocrinology. The First Hosp of China Med Univ, Shenyang, Liaoning Province 110001, P.R.China

ATA American Thyroid Association, *BTA* British Thyroid Association, *CSE/CSS/CACA/CSNM* Chinese Society of Endocrinology (CSE)/Chinese Society of Surgery (CSS)/Chinese Anti-Cancer Association (CACA)/Chinese Society of Nuclear Medicine (CSNM), *EANM* European Association of Nuclear Medicine, *EC* European Consensus, *ESMO* European Society of Medical Oncology, *NCCN* National Comprehensive Cancer Network, *SNMMI* Society of Nuclear Medicine and Molecular Imaging

Vassilopoulou-Sellin et al. [19] from the University of Texas MD Anderson Cancer Center reviewed 18 patients who developed distant metastases, of whom 16 had pulmonary metastases with and without other sites of metastases. Although few data are available, the one patient free of disease after 9 years of follow-up was a 6-year-old female child with radioiodine-positive, radiograph-negative lung metastases.

Høie et al. [11] from the Norwegian Radium Hospital in Norway reported on 91 patients with distant metastases, and the overall survival data after 1 year was 50 %. Of the 91 patients, 73 had intrathoracic metastases, and two types of radioiodine accumulation patterns were described. One pattern was of miliary or multiple parenchymal lesions, with either granular or nodular X-ray changes, and was observed in 48 patients. A second pattern of pulmonary infiltrations was observed in 25 patients and was associated with hilar or mediastinal enlargement and pleural effusions. However, they did not separate the survival data for patients who had only lung metastases, lung and other metastases, or non-lung metastases. Additionally, the authors did not distinguish between the results of the patients treated and not treated with ^{131}I. Postoperative ^{131}I ablation was not routine.

Leeper [2] from Memorial Sloan Kettering Cancer Center reported that 11 of 18 older patients with distant metastases from follicular carcinoma were treated with ^{131}I and six patients demonstrated tumor regression. He concluded that the survival time of patients was enhanced significantly by ^{131}I therapy. Also from Memorial Sloan Kettering Cancer Center, Robbins et al. [39] reported that after one high-dose treatment of ^{131}I, complete resolution of radioiodine uptake was achieved in 33 % of patients with pulmonary metastases.

Sampson et al. [44] evaluated 40 pts, of which 18 (45 %) patients had only lung metastasis, and the 3-year survival for only lung metastases was 77 %.

Cho et al. [50] evaluated the long-term prognosis of lung metastases and the prognostic factors for 152 patients in Korea. The 10- and 20-year survival rates were 85 % and 71 %, respectively. With a median follow-up of 11 years (range 2–41 years), *no* evidence of disease was reported in 22 %, stable disease 28 %, progressive disease 36 %, and death 14 %. A poor prognosis was associated with older age at diagnosis (≥45), primary tumor size ≥2 cm, follicular thyroid cancer, metastasis diagnosed after initial evaluation or ^{131}I remnant ablation, multiple metastases other than lung, ^{131}I non-avidity, and presence of macronodules (≥1 cm). However, the only independent predictive factor for a poor prognosis was ^{131}I non-avidity.

Kim et al. [87] evaluated the radiological characteristics in 105 patients with pulmonary metastases. Eighty-nine patients (84.9 %) demonstrated radioiodine uptake in pulmonary metastases on the post-^{131}I therapy scan, and the remaining 16 (15.2 %) patients had no radioiodine uptake. Of the patients with radioiodine uptake, 90 % and 87 % of the metastatic lesions were also visualized on the CT and ^{18}F FDG PET, respectively. On the 105 patients, 7 (6.7 %) patients had metastases that were radioiodine positive but not visualized on either CT or ^{18}F FDG PET scans. Complete remission was achieved in 5.7 % of patients, and these patients had either a negative chest CT or micronodular lesions on CT, while 6.7 % of patient had metastatic lesions not visualized on chest CT of 18F FDG PET-CT but visualized only on the post-^{131}I therapy scan.

Although the debate continues regarding the prognostic significance of the many various factors such as age, ability for complete local control (e.g., curative surgery), primary tumor size, and the effect on survival, recurrence, and palliation of patients treated with ^{131}I for lung metastases [34, 49, 88, 89], this author believes that the data support the use of ^{131}I in selected patients. This is further discussed later in the summary section of this chapter.

Bone Metastases

Many studies advocate ^{131}I as valuable in the management of bone metastases [16, 20, 22, 31, 33, 35, 37] while many others do not (see also Chap. 65) [10–13, 16, 18, 30, 36]. A summary of these publications is noted in Table 56.3. The guidelines of various organizations and societies for bone metastases are noted in Table 56.8. Again, selected publications are reviewed below.

Bernier et al. [35] evaluated 109 patients with bone metastases at the Groupe Hospitalier Pitié-Salpétriére. The survival rates after 5 and 10 years were 41 % and 15 %, respectively. Factors associated with an improved survival by univariate analysis were (1) ^{131}I therapy, (2) younger age at discovery of bone metastases, (3) bone metastases as the revealing symptom for well-differentiated thyroid cancer, and (4) surgery for bone metastasis. Prognostic features associated with an improved survival by multivariate analysis included (1) the cumulative dose of ^{131}I therapy, (2) absence of metastases in other organs, and (3) complete surgical removal of bone metastases in patients younger than 45 years old.

Pittas et al. [31] at Memorial Sloan Kettering Cancer Center analyzed 146 patients with bone metastases from thyroid carcinoma. These results did include 13 (1 %) patients with anaplastic thyroid carcinoma, six with medullary carcinoma, and three with lymphoma. The significant prognostic factors by univariate analysis of their data were (1) radioiodine uptake, (2) treatment with ^{131}I ($p = 0.001$), (3) time from initial bone metastasis, and (4) absence of non-osseous metastases. Neither surgery nor external radiotherapy was a significant factor. The major prognostic factors for improved survival by multivariate analysis were radioiodine uptake and absence of non-osseous metastases, and these were independent variables. However, after adjusting for all variables, ^{131}I treatment was not identified to affect survival. Pittas et al. concluded that the "overall survival is best in those whose lesions concentrate radioactive iodine and those who have no non-osseous metastases."

Petrich et al. [33] from Hannover University Medical School in Germany evaluated 107 patients with bone metastases. There were 60 patients who had bone metastases with radioiodine uptake, and the mean survival time was 8.9 years. In patients with both bone metastases and lung metastases without radioiodine uptake, the mean survival was 1.2 years. As other authors have noted, the data of Petrich et al. suggested that age was important, and 4 of 8 patients who were 45 years old or younger achieved complete remission, whereas only 21 of 99 patients older than 45 years achieved complete remission. Complete remission was also twice as likely to be achieved in patients with three or less sites of bone metastases, compared to those patients with more than three sites of bone metastases. Notably, no statistical difference was found in the mean survival in patients with radioiodine uptake in only bone metastases versus patients who had both bone and lung metastases (7.3 years).

In the data reported by Dorn et al. [37] from Augsburg Clinic in Germany, 15 patients who had bone metastases were selected to be treated with dosimetrically determined amounts of ^{131}I. At the time of publication, 87 % (13 of 15) of the patients had survived, with an average follow-up of 5.1 years, mean follow-up of 5.0 years, and range of 0.6–10.9 years. The two deaths at 3.2 and 10.9 years were attributed to thyroid cancer. The largest single amount of ^{131}I administered was 38.5 GBq (1040 mCi).

In 28 patients with bone metastases evaluated at the Surgical Professorial Unit at Lille University in France, Proye et al. [14] described a 1-year survival rate of 53 %; 43 % of patients with bone metastases had positive radioiodine scans. Two patients were reported to have been "cured," and six patients had a partial remission. Both patients with "normal" X-rays and the diagnosis of bone metastasis on radioiodine scans alone had a response. Bone metastases with an X-ray abnormality never disappeared with ^{131}I therapy alone. Of patients with positive radioiodine scans with or without an X-ray abnormality, the response rate was 50 % (6 of 12). Regardless of whether there was radioiodine uptake, the response rate was 36 % (8 of 22). Most patients received a combination of treatments, including ^{131}I, surgery, and external radiotherapy. Patients who had bone metastases at the time of their initial diagnosis of well-differentiated thyroid carcinoma had a worse prognosis than those patients who subsequently developed bone metastases. These data of Proye et al. suggests that overall bone metastases respond poorly to radioiodine, and bone metastases that do respond to ^{131}I were radioiodine positive and radiographically negative. Finally, they stated that surgical excision should be considered for isolated radiographically positive bone metastasis.

Zettinig et al. [36] from the University of Vienna analyzed 41 consecutive patients with bone metastases. By univariate analysis, total thyroidectomy, lymph node surgery, ^{131}I therapy, and the absence of extra-skeletal distant metastases were significant predictors of survival. However, no major prognostic factors were identified by multivariate analysis. In patients with only bone metastasis, univariate analysis determined that surgical expiration of the bone metastases was a prognostic factor for improved survival.

Marcocci et al. [12] from the Institute of Endocrinology at the University of Pisa, Italy, reported on 30 patients with bone metastases. Of these patients, 25 were administered ^{131}I with cumulative doses of 50–1810 mCi (1.85–6.7 GBq). Eleven bone metastases were radioiodine positive and radiograph negative; in six of these patients, the radioiodine uptake resolved. None of the 27 bone metastases that were radioiodine positive and radiograph positive showed a complete response. Marcocci et al. stated that apparently only surgical treatment can lead to a cure for bone metastases and is the preferred treatment for resectable bone metastases. Although Marcocci et al. suggested this was especially true for a single-bone lesion, Pittas et al. [31] indicated that other subclinical bone metastases are likely and metastatic bone disease is virtually always a multicentric process.

Fanchiang et al. [30] from Chang Gung Memorial Hospital in Taipei reported on 39 patients, of whom 32 patients had bone metastases at the time of diagnosis. Using the Kaplan-Meier method of analysis, the 5-year survival rate was estimated to be 64.9 %. A total of 31 patients had multiple bone metastases, and the radiographs were abnormal in 33 of the 39 patients. There were 25 patients who received surgical intervention, and 18 received external radiotherapy. Although 28 patients had radioiodine uptake on scan, the number of patients treated with ^{131}I was not indicated in the article, and no data were presented regarding the overall utility of ^{131}I treatment. Fanchiang et al. concluded that surgery was the recommended treatment for surgically resectable and radiographically positive bone metastases because ^{131}I could not eradicate the metastases completely.

As noted above, Pacini et al. [16] reported on 118 patients with metastatic disease, of whom 16 patients had bone metastases. However, the data of these patients was not separated from that of the patients with other sites of metastases. The authors did comment that some complete remissions were obtained in single radioiodine-positive, radiograph-negative bone metastases, but the overall response rate was poor. He proposed that, "Surgical removal of accessible bone metastases should be considered whenever possible" [16].

Woods et al. [13] from the University of Texas MD Anderson Cancer Center could not assess the effect of radioactive iodine, as only one patient received ^{131}I alone, and this was given as an intra-arterial injection into the axillary artery.

Tickoo et al. [32] evaluated 79 patients, of which 68 % had poorly differentiated or undifferentiated features in their primary and/or metastatic tumors and 10, 9, and 5 were anaplastic, Hürthle cell, and medullary carcinomas, respectively. Interestingly the metastatic tumors were better differentiated than the primary cancers in one third of the patients, and only one case showed a less differentiated metastasis. The overall 5- and 10-year survival probabilities after the bone metastases appeared were 29 % and 13 %, respectively. Tumor type and differentiation seemed to affect survival after appearance of bone metastases, and this was primarily due to the much worse prognosis in the case of anaplastic and medullary carcinoma. No difference in survival among patients up to 45 years or older than 45 years at the time of metastases was demonstrated ($p=0.31$).

Khorjekar et al. [55] reported data on 30 patients with bone metastases, but these patients not only received ^{131}I treatment but multiple other treatment modalities including external radiotherapy, surgical excision, stereotactic radiotherapy, radiofrequency ablation, cryotherapy, arterial embolization, bisphosphonates, and chemotherapy. The mean, range, and standard deviation for years of follow-up were 4.07, 0.8–9.50, and 2.6, respectively. The survival rates at 1, 2, 3, and 5 years were 30/30 (100 %), 23/24 (96 %), and 19/21 (90 %), and 9/12 (75 %), respectively. Thirty-one additional treatment modalities were received in these 30 patients. Fifteen and 5 of these 30 patients received dosimetrically determined and empiric prescribed activity of ^{131}I, respectively. Eight, three, and one patient received Zometa® infusion, Fosamax®, and Actonel®, respectively. Excellent initial survival rate was achieved with multimodality treatments.

Qiu et al. [56] evaluated 106 patients with bone metastases. Of 61 patients with painful bone metastases, 39 (64 %) patients obtained significant relief of bone pain and 37 (34.9 %) patients had a significant decrease in serum Tg. In the majority of patients (76 %), no changes in anatomic imaging of the bone metastases after ^{131}I therapy were reported. The 5- and 10-year survival rates were 86.5 and 57.9 %, respectively. Multivariate analysis showed that solitary bone metastases, only bone metastases, and ^{131}I therapy with bone surgery prior ^{131}I were independent factors associated with a better prognosis ($p=0.024$, 0.009, and 0.031, respectively).

Hindié et al. [57] reported on 16 patients, of which all 3 patients with non-^{131}I functioning bone metastases were deceased (5, 19, and 34 months). Of the 13 patients with ^{131}I functioning bone metastases, 2 (15 %) were deceased with 88 % (7/8) alive at 3 years and 80 % (4/5) at 5 years. They

Table 56.8 Organizational guidelines for bone metastases

Organization	Recommendation
ATA [79]	Recommendation 79
	"Complete surgical resection of isolated symptomatic metastases has been associated with improved survival and should be considered, especially in patients <45 years old with slowly progressive disease"
	Recommendation 79
	"RAI therapy of iodine-avid bone metastases has been associated with improved survival and should be employed, although RAI is rarely curative. (Strong recommendation, Moderate-quality evidence) The RAI activity administered can be given empirically (100–200 mCi) or determined by dosimetry." (Weak recommendation, Low-quality evidence)
	"A dosimetrically determined administered dose of RAI may be beneficial for patients with bone metastases, although this is not proven in controlled studies"
	"Patients undergoing RAI therapy for bone metastases should also be considered for directed therapy of bone metastases that are visible on anatomical imaging. This may include surgery, external beam radiation, and other focal treatment modalities. These patients should also be considered for systemic therapy with bone-directed agents."
BTA [80]	"For symptomatic solitary bone metastases consideration should be given in the first instance to complete surgical resection or high dose radiotherpay, which may be delivered using intensity modulated stereotactic radiotherapy technique or thermal ablation depending on the site of disease. ^{131}I therapy for iodine avid disease can be helpful in improving symptoms, stabilising disease and potentially improving survival but rarely achieves a complete response"
	"Extensive bone metastases are generally not curable by ^{131}I therapy alone. For solitary or a limited number of bone metastases that are not cured by ^{131}I therapy, external beam radiation therapy (EBRT) with / without resection and/or embolisation/thermal ablation or cement injection may be beneficial in selected cases. EBRT also has an important role in the management of spinal cord compression due to vertebral metastases in addition to surgery"
	"Solitary or limited bone metastases unresponsive to ^{131}I should be considered for further treatment with one or more of the following modalities: EBRT, surgical resection, embolisation, thermal ablation, cement injection"
	"Bisphosphonates or denosumab should be considered in patients with bone metastases"
CSE/CSS/CACA/CSNM [81]	Recommendation 2–19
	Treatment for metastases by RAI should be considered in selected patients. Recommendation rating: B
	"Bone metastases with bone damage rarely respond to RAI therapy, even though the lesions are iodine-avid"
	"XRT should be considered in the management of painful bone metastases or of metastases in critical locations, or of metastases that are not amenable to surgery or RAI treatment"
EANM [82]	Optional indications of RAI treatment: "Recurrent iodine-avid . . . distant metastases, as an adjuvant to surgery . . . ." "Non-resectable or partially resectable iodine-avid bone metastases, especially when symptomatic or threatening vital structures . . . ."
	Non-indications of RAI treatment: "Iodine non-avid bone metastases"
	". . . XRT should be considered in the management of painful bone metastases or of metastases in critical locations likely to result in fractures or neurological or compressive symptoms, if these lesions are not amenable to surgery. Use of RAIT in combination with XRT may increase the response, especially in painful bone lesions"

(continued)

Table 56.8 (continued)

Organization	Recommendation
EC [83]	"Bone metastases should be treated by a combination of surgery whenever possible, ^{131}I treatment if uptake is present in the metastases, and external beam radiotherapy either as resolutive treatment or as pain control. Other local treatment procedures such as the use of bisphosphonates, embolization or cement injection may be useful"
ESMO [84]	"Bone metastases have the worst prognosis even when aggressively treated by the combination of radioiodine therapy and external beam radiotherapy"
	"Chemotherapy is no longer indicated because of lack of effective results and should be replaced by enrollment of the patients in experimental trials with targeted therapy. Reinducing differentiation in DTC with insufficient uptake of ^{131}I has been attempted with drugs such retinoids and thiazolidinediones but till now with poor results"
NCCN [85]	For papillary, follicular, and Hürthle cell:
	Clinically significant structural disease should be surgically resected if possible before ^{131}I treatment
	If radioiodine uptake, ^{131}I treatment with empiric doses of 100–200 mCi or dose adjusted by dosimetry
SNMMI [86]	"Post-thyroidectomy ^{131}I therapy is indicated for metastases of functioning thyroid carcinoma to lymph nodes, lung, bone, and, less often, brain, liver, skin, and other sites"
	"Skeletal metastases that are painful or are a threat to life or function may, in addition to being treated with ^{131}I, be treated with bone-seeking beta-emitting radiopharmaceuticals (e.g., ^{89Sr} or ^{153}Sm-lexidronam) if the bone scan is positive at the painful site, although these carry a greater risk of myelosuppression than ^{131}I, external radiotherapy, or surgery"

The Chinese translation of the CSE/CSS/CACA CSNM was performed by H. *Guan H and W. Teng. Dept Endocrinology & Metabolism and Inst of Endocrinology. The First Hosp of China Med Univ, Shenyang, Liaoning Province 110001, P.R.China*
ATA American Thyroid Association, *BTA* British Thyroid Association, *CSE/CSS/CACA/CSNM* Chinese Society of Endocrinology (CSE) / Chinese Society of Surgery (CSS) / Chinese Anti-Cancer Association (CACA)/Chinese Society of Nuclear Medicine (CSNM), *EANM* European Association of Nuclear Medicine, *EC* European Consensus, *ESMO* European Society of Medical Oncology, *NCCN* National Comprehensive Cancer Network, *SNMMI* Society of Nuclear Medicine and Molecular Imaging

suggested that a substantial percentage of bone metastases can be detected early, when the Tg level may only be moderately elevated and when other radiological studies are negative, which may increase the potential for a cure.

Sampson et al. [44] evaluated 40 patients, of whom 16 (39 %) had only bone metastases and the 3-year survival was 56 %. Those patients whose bone metastases were iodine-avid did better than those with non-iodine-avid bone metastases.

Lang et al. [90] evaluated prognostic factors of 51 patients with distant metastases of whom 19 patients had bone metastases. Bone metastases and non-radioiodine uptake were independent prognostic factors. Ito et al. [91] reported in 33 patients that extrathyroidal extension, tumor size greater than 4 cm, and metastases to the lymph nodes were independent predictive factors for bone recurrence. A significant survival advantage was observed by Orita et al. [92] for 52 patients with bone metastases who had ^{131}I therapy. Greater doses of ^{131}I and operative resection of the bone metastases also appeared to be associated a better prognosis.

Complications secondary to bone metastases include spinal cord compressions and pathological fractures. Farooki et al. [93] reported that in 245 patients with bone metastases, 78 % (192) of the patients had a skeletal-related event. Ninety-seven patients had a skeletal-related event at the time of presentation, and in the remaining 114 patients, the time from identification of the bone metastases to a skeletal-related event was a median of 5 months. However, Robenshtok et al. [94] reported that in 5 % (14/288) of the patients who had bone metastases that were radioiodine positive but had no structural correlate on CT or MRI, there were no skeletal-related events and no evidence of structural bone metastases with all patients alive during the 5-year follow-up period. Their conclusion was that radioiodine-positive bone metastases with no structural correlate had no major prognostic significance. However, whether or not these metastases will become a problem for these patients sometime after 5 years and whether or not they should be aggressively managed are to be determined. However, this author agrees with Zanotti-Fregonara et al. [95] that bone metastases should be diagnosed as early as possible and individually and aggressively treated.

Interestingly, Zhao et al. [96] has reported a case of multifocal bone metastases secondary to papillary thyroid carcinoma with very low persistent thyroglobulin levels with negative anti-thyroglobulin antibodies during thyroid hormone withdrawal.

In summary, the role of ^{131}I treatment in bone metastases continues to remain controversial. However, as more studies are reported, we are becoming more adept in identifying which patients with bone metastases will or will not benefit from ^{131}I treatment. A patient who may benefit from ^{131}I is one whose bone metastasis is (1) radioiodine positive, (2) radiographically negative, (3) not associated with other organ involvement, and (4) not potentially curable from surgery or other site-specific treatment modalities such as CyberKnife radiotherapy, radiofrequency ablation, cryotherapy, or embolization. Further studies are needed to determine if ^{131}I is more effective in bone metastases with dosimetry-determined amounts of ^{131}I rather than empiric amounts. As noted elsewhere, the amounts of ^{131}I that may be given based on dosimetry are typically higher than most empiric prescribed activities. With higher quantities of prescribed activity, ^{131}I may be significantly more effective because of higher radiation absorbed doses, higher radiation absorbed dose rates, and less fractionation of treatments. Finally, combination treatments, e.g., surgery and ^{131}I with dosimetrically determined prescribed activity followed immediately by external radiotherapy, deserve further studies.

Mediastinal Metastases

Mediastinal metastases are less frequent than either lung or bone metastases from DTC [18], and no specific data exist pertaining to the effects of ^{131}I or its success on mediastinal metastases.

Of note, Massin et al. [6] suggested that mediastinal metastases are secondary from pulmonary metastases, rather than representing spread from cervical node metastases. This theory was based on their observations that (1) there was no statistical correlation between cervical and mediastinal lymph node metastases, (2) the main histological patterns were different at both sites (follicular was the most frequent histology in the mediastinal nodes, whereas papillary histology predominated in the cervical nodes), and (3) isolated mediastinal nodes were rare. Høie et al. [11] also implied that the source of mediastinal metastases was pulmonary metastases.

Irrespective of the pattern of metastatic spread, further study is needed regarding the utility of ^{131}I therapy on mediastinal metastases.

Brain Metastases

No prospective or large retrospective study has been reported on the management of brain metastases secondary to differentiated thyroid cancer. To date, over 150 cases have been reported and previously reviewed by Jordan et al. [97] and the data are summarized in Table 56.4.

The prognosis of brain metastases appears to depend on many factors with a reduced prognosis associated with such factors as an older age, a higher number of brain metastases, more extensive loco- and distant metastases elsewhere, and the presence of other significant patient health problems. For the management of brain metastases, the recommendations of various organizations are noted in Table 56.9, and the treatment options include surgical resection, stereotactic radiosurgery, whole brain radiotherapy, ^{131}I therapy, and chemotherapy. Although the management plan should be individualized, surgical resection should be considered first, especially in patients who have one or two potentially resectable lesions with minimal other health problems. Chiu et al. [26] from the University of Texas MD Anderson Cancer Center analyzed 32 patients with brain metastases from differentiated thyroid carcinoma. No evidence of survival benefit was found from ^{131}I therapy. However, resection of one or more foci of brain metastases significantly improved survival. Surgical excision improved the median disease-specific survival from the time of diagnosis of brain metastases from 3.4 to 16.7 months ($p<0.05$). McWilliams et al. [40] of the Mayo Clinic reported on 16 patients with brain metastases. Surgical excision appeared to improve the average survival after diagnosis of brain metastases from 2.7 to 20.8 months. Four received ^{131}I treatment. Of these, one patient had uptake on the radioiodine scan, and two patients had no uptake. No scan results were available for the fourth patient. None of the patients had an objective response to ^{131}I treatment.

de Figueiredo et al. [60] reported that in 21 patients with brain metastases, the median overall survival was 7.1 months. The patients had a mean number of brain metastases of 2.8 (range 1–10), and mean size of the metastases was 22.5 mm (range 3–44 mm). The overall survival was 42 and 36 % at 1 and 2 years, respectively. The overall survival after surgery or stereotactic radiosurgery was 11.9 months versus 3.6 months without either. Performance status was important with an overall survival of 27 months with performance status of <2 versus 3 months when performance status was >2. The performance status was based on the World Health Organization criteria.

For those patients who may not be good candidates for craniotomy, stereotactic radiosurgery (e.g., Gamma Knife®) would be a good alternative. Whole-brain radiotherapy may be a potential option for those with multiple brain metastases. For ^{131}I therapy, this author believes that this should be considered only when surgical resection and stereotactic radiosurgery (e.g., Gamma Knife®) are not good options and when the brain metastases have good ^{131}I uptake. "Blind" ^{131}I treatments (treating with ^{131}I when there is no radioiodine uptake on scan) are not recommended. A "blind" ^{131} treatment has the added risk of cerebral edema from the prepara-

Table 56.9 Organizational guidelines for brain metastases

Organization	Recommendation
ATA [79]	Recommendation 94 "While surgical resection and stereotactic external beam radiotherapy are the mainstays of therapy for CNS metastases, RAI can be considered if CNS metastases concentrat RAI. If RAI is being considered, stereotactic external beam radiotherapy and concomitant glucocorticoid therapy are recommeneded prior to RAI therapy to minimize the effects of a potential TSH-induced increase in tumor size and RAI-induced inflammatory response (Weak recommendation, Low-quality evidence.)"
BTA [80]	"External beam radiotherapy has an important palliative role in the management of cerebral metastases along with surgery if appropriate"
CSE/CSS/CACA/CSNM [81]	"In general, brain metastases are not indications of RAI treatment"
EANM [82]	No specific comment regarding brain metastases
EC [83]	"Whenever possible they should be resected; if not resectable and non-iodine-avid, external beam radiation may provide palliation. Usually they carry a poor prognosis"
ESMO [84]	"Surgical resection and external beam radiotherapy present the only therapeutic options. Chemotherapy is no longer indicated because of lack of effective results and should be replaced by enrollment of the patients in experimental trials with targeted therapy. Reinducing differentiation in DTC with insufficient uptake of ^{131}I has been attempted with drugs such retinoids and thiazolidinediones but till now with poor results"
NCCN [85]	"For solitary CNS lesions, either neurosurgical resection or stereotactic radiosurgery is preferred. For multiple CNS lesions, surgical resection and/or EBRT can be considered."
SNM [86]	"Patients with…distant metastases, especially those with involvement of the aerodigestive tract, brain, or spinal cord, may be treated with both ^{131}I and external-beam radiation postoperatively. Corticosteroids to prevent swelling may be required if central nervous system metastases are to be irradiated. The use of external beam radiation beforehand, or alternating with ^{131}I treatment, has not been documented to be associated with a subsequent reduction in tumor uptake of radioactive iodine. Therefore, external-beam radiation, if clinically and emergently indicated, need not be delayed"

The Chinese translation of the CSE/CSS/CACA CSNM was performed by H. *Guan H and W. Teng. Dept Endocrinology & Metabolism and Inst of Endocrinology. The First Hosp of China Med Univ, Shenyang, Liaoning Province 110001, P.R.China*
ATA American Thyroid Association, *BTA* British Thyroid Association, *CSE/CSS/CACA/CSNM* Chinese Society of Endocrinology (CSE) / Chinese Society of Surgery (CSS)/Chinese Anti-Cancer Association (CACA)/Chinese Society of Nuclear Medicine (CSNM), *EANM* European Association of Nuclear Medicine, *EC* European Consensus, *ESMO* European Society of Medical Oncology, *NCCN* National Comprehensive Cancer Network, *SNMMI* Society of Nuclear Medicine and Molecular Imaging

tion with either recombinant human thyroid-stimulating hormone (rhTSH) or thyroid hormone withdrawal (THW). However, if ^{131}I treatment is planned, this author recommends several further considerations. The maximum prescribed activity of ^{131}I should be determined with either dosimetry or simplified dosimetric methods such as percent 48 h whole-body retention [98, 99]. Although no data is available regarding whether rhTSH or THW is better for patients who are undergoing treatment with ^{131}I for brain metastases, this author proposes that rhTSH injections should be considered first. Although controversy exists regarding whether or not one maximizes the radiation absorbed dose to distant metastases by preparing the patient with rhTSH versus THW, the shorter exposure of the brain metastases to elevated TSH stimulation from rhTSH injections of several days rather than several weeks from thyroid hormone withdrawal would appear to be the safer approach to minimize the growth of the tumor and the possibility of cerebral edema. Nevertheless and in order to minimize cerebral edema, steroids, glycerol, and/or mannitol prior to either rhTSH injections or THW has been recommended (see Table 56.4), and treatment should be continued for a significant period of time after administration of the therapeutic prescribed activity of ^{131}I.

Although little data is available regarding chemotherapy, chemotherapy presently appears to have little, if any, effect.

Other Sites of Distant Metastases

Differentiated thyroid cancer may occasionally metastasize to other distant sites, and these have been reviewed in Chap. 66. However, little information is available regarding the management of these rare sites. Again, development of an individual treatment plan is warranted with consideration of surgical resection, stereotactic radiosurgery, radiofrequency ablation, cryotherapy, embolization, chemo-embolization, ^{131}I therapy, and/or chemotherapy.

In regard to liver metatases and ^{131}I treatment, very little data have been published. Brown et al. [5] reported a single patient whose only site of metastatic disease was in the liver. After ^{131}I therapy, the patient's condition was stable for 12 years, but then the patient developed gross hepatomegaly and died within several weeks.

Distant Metastases That Are Thyroglobulin Positive and Scan Negative (Tg+/Scan−) "Blind" ^{131}I Therapies

The management of patients with differentiated thyroid cancer who have metastases indicated by positive thyroglobulin levels but negative radioiodine scans has been discussed in more detail in Chap. 47, and this is problematic in many areas including whether or not to perform a "blind" ^{131}I therapy. "Blind" ^{131}I therapies are the therapeutic administration of ^{131}I when the source of the elevated thyroglobulin level cannot be identified. In the discussion of the indication, utility, and prescribed activity of a "blind" ^{131}I therapy for Tg+ and scan− distant metastases, these therapies must be considered in the context of the patients, the steps for evaluation of Tg+/scan− patients, and alternative therapeutic options. With a better understanding of these three factors, one may have a better understanding regarding the potential use of a "blind" ^{131}I therapy when in fact the data for and against the benefit of such is limited (again, see Chap. 47 [100]. The options for the amount of prescribed activity for a "blind" ^{131}I therapy are discussed later in this chapter.

First and foremost, patients who are Tg+/scan− should not be viewed as a single group. Rather, they should be seen as a wide spectrum of multiple clinical scenarios and prognoses. At the two ends of the spectrum, one patient may have a positive Tg and negative radioiodine scan, but the patient may be staged as having a very low risk with an excellent prognosis and have a low suppressed Tg (e.g., 2 ng/ml) that is stable. At the other end of the spectrum, the patient may have (1) a significantly elevated Tg, (2) rapid doubling time of the Tg, (3) known diffuse lung metastases, and (4) progression of those lung metastases on CT. In this situation, the managing physician may be considering a tyrosine kinase inhibitor (TKI). However, before initiating the TKI, one may wish to consider a "blind" ^{131}I therapy. In such a patient with progression and a poor prognosis with a short expected survival, this author submits that consideration of "blind" ^{131}I therapy may be reasonable to consider before one considers the patient to be radioiodine-refractory and administers a TKI. At the time of the publication of this textbook, two TKIs have been approved. A "blind" ^{131}I therapy may be reasonable. Again, the scenario of Tg+/scan− patient represents a wide spectrum of situations, and the patient's specific clinical situation is very important regarding whether or not one should consider a "blind" ^{131}I therapy.

Second, a "blind" ^{131}I therapy should only be considered after an appropriate evaluation of a patient who is Tg+/scan− as discussed in Chap. 47. As proposed in Fig. 56.1 and Fig. 56.2, several steps should be completed before consideration of a "blind" ^{131}I therapy. In brief, step 1 is excluding false + Tg levels such as secondary to Tg antibodies and false-negative radioiodine scans such as secondary to recent large iodine load, inadequate elevation of the TSH with thyroid hormone withdrawal, error of radiopharmaceutical administration, and/or dedifferentiation of tumor. The second step is risk stratifying the patient such as the two patients described above. The third step is a wide spectrum of potential imaging options including: ultrasound; CT of the chest, abdomen, and pelvis; ^{18}F FDG PET-CT; brain MR; ^{99m}Tc MDP; ^{18}F NaF PET-CT; ^{201}thallium; ^{99m}Tc sestamibi or tetrofosmin; and ^{111}In octreotide. Then depending on whether or not the likely source of the elevated thyroglobulin level is identified, further local therapy customized such as the location and character of the metastases should be considered. These local therapies could include but are not limited to surgical resection, external beam radiotherapy, stereotactic radiosurgery, radiofrequency ablation, cryotherapy, embolization, and/or alcohol injections. However, if the imaging studies performed identify the source of the thyroglobulin but the metastases cannot be locally managed, then again

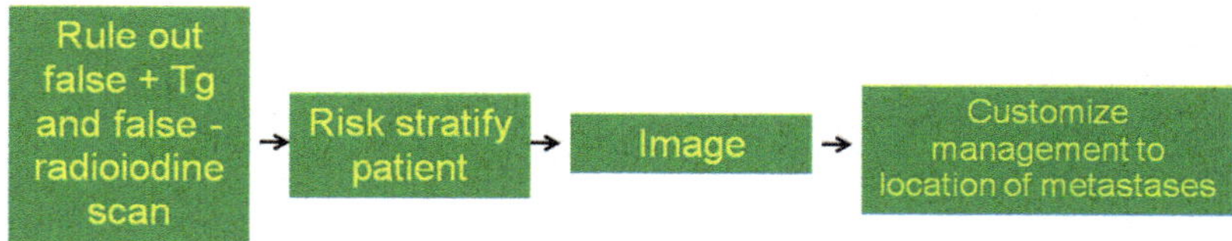

Fig. 56.1 This algorithm demonstrates a proposed four-step approach to the management of patients whose thyroglobulin level is positive but radioiodine scan is negative (Reproduced with permission of Keystone Press, Inc.)

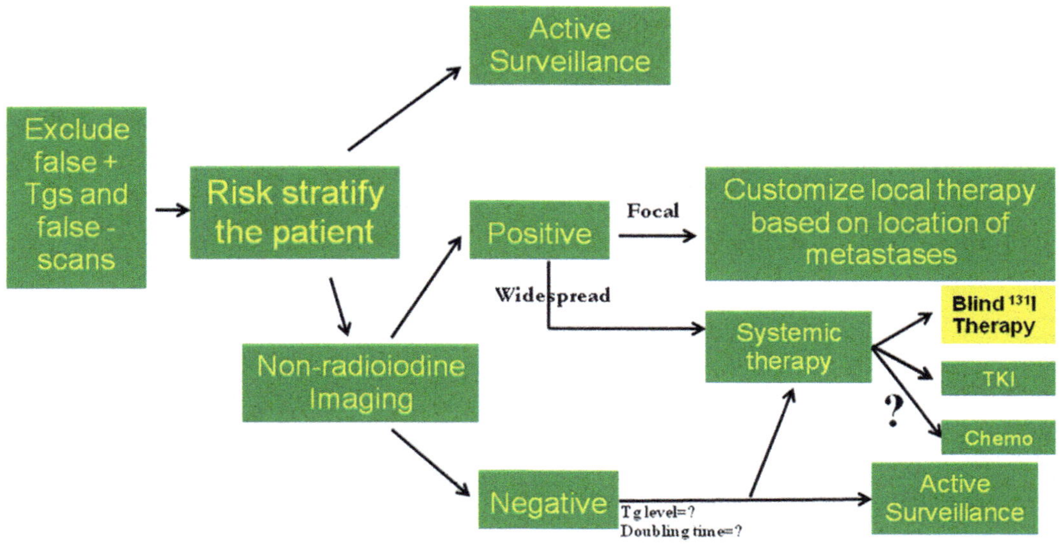

Fig. 56.2 This algorithm demonstrates not only a proposed algorithm for the approach to patients who are Tg+/scan− but also a possible role for a "blind" ^{131}I therapy. This steps again include excluding false-positive Tg levels and false-negative radioiodine scans to the best of one's ability. The patient has been risk stratified. Imaging has demonstrated that the metastases cannot be managed or easily managed by local therapy and there is significant progression of disease with a very poor prognosis. In this case, a TKI and/or "blind" ^{131}I therapy may be considered (Reproduced with permission of Keystone Press, Inc.)

depending on the patient's clinical situation, one may consider active surveillance, a TKI, or a "blind" ^{131}I therapy.

Selection of Prescribed Activity for ^{131}I Treatment of Distant Metastases

The selection of prescribed activity for ^{131}I for the treatment of distant metastases is problematic and very controversial. The selection of a prescribed ^{131}I activity for treatment of distant metastases of differentiated thyroid cancer has been based on either empiric recommendations or dosimetric calculations (see Fig. 56.3). Multiple authors have adopted various empiric prescribed activities for ^{131}I therapy of recurrent and metastatic disease with a range from 3.7 to 11.1 GBq (100–300 mCi) and using different schedules (see Fig. 56.4) [2, 5, 20, 21, 23, 33, 38]. Likewise, multiple authors have determined their prescribed activity for these treatments based on dosimetric calculations of either the lesion(s), blood (bone marrow), or both [8, 37, 101–104]. A detailed discussion of dosimetry, along with the advantages and disadvantages of empiric and dosimetrically determined prescribed activity, is presented in Chaps. 58 and 59. Although recommendations for the method of determination of prescribed activity and recommendations for specific prescribed activity are presented in guidelines from various organizations and societies (see Tables 56.7, 56.8, and 56.9), these are very general because to date only one retrospective study has been reported comparing empirically selected prescribed activity to dosimetrically determined prescribed activity [105], and no prospective study comparing any of the empiric approaches has been published.

Again, various empiric approaches are summarized in Fig. 56.4. Beierwaltes [106] proposed treatment with empiric prescribed activities of 5.55–6.48 GBq (150–175 mCi) for cervical lymph nodes metastases, 6.48–7.4 GBq (175–200 mCi) for pulmonary metastases, and 7.4 GBq (200 mCi) for bone metastases. Schlumberger et al. [20] typically treated patients with 3.7 GBq (100 mCi) every 3–6 months until the post-therapy scan was negative, with a maximum limit of ~600 mCi. If metastasis was identified on a post-therapy scan, Petrich et al. [33] would then immediately retreat with 7.4 GBq (200 mCi), and their next follow-up treatment was typically at 4–6 months with mean activity of 11.1 GBq (300 mCi). Brown et al. [5] treated patients with 5.55 GBq (150 mCi) every 3–4 months until the scan was negative or there was evidence of progression. They also had no formal limit for maximum cumulative prescribed activity. After the diagnosis of metastatic disease, Menzel et al. [21] used 11.1 GBq (300 mCi) at 3-month intervals. The maximum total activity administered in 1 year was 44.4 GBq (1200 mCi), which was given to 7 patients, and the range of total cumulative activity was 14.80–99.90 GBq (400 mCi to 2.7 Ci) in 26 patients treated for advanced thyroid cancer. Hindié et al. [38] treated patients with 3.7 GBq (100 mCi) of ^{131}I every 6 months until no uptake was present. If pulmonary uptake was still visible on the post-^{131}I therapy scan after a cumulative activity of 18.5 GBq (500 mCi), then the frequency of ^{131}I therapy was

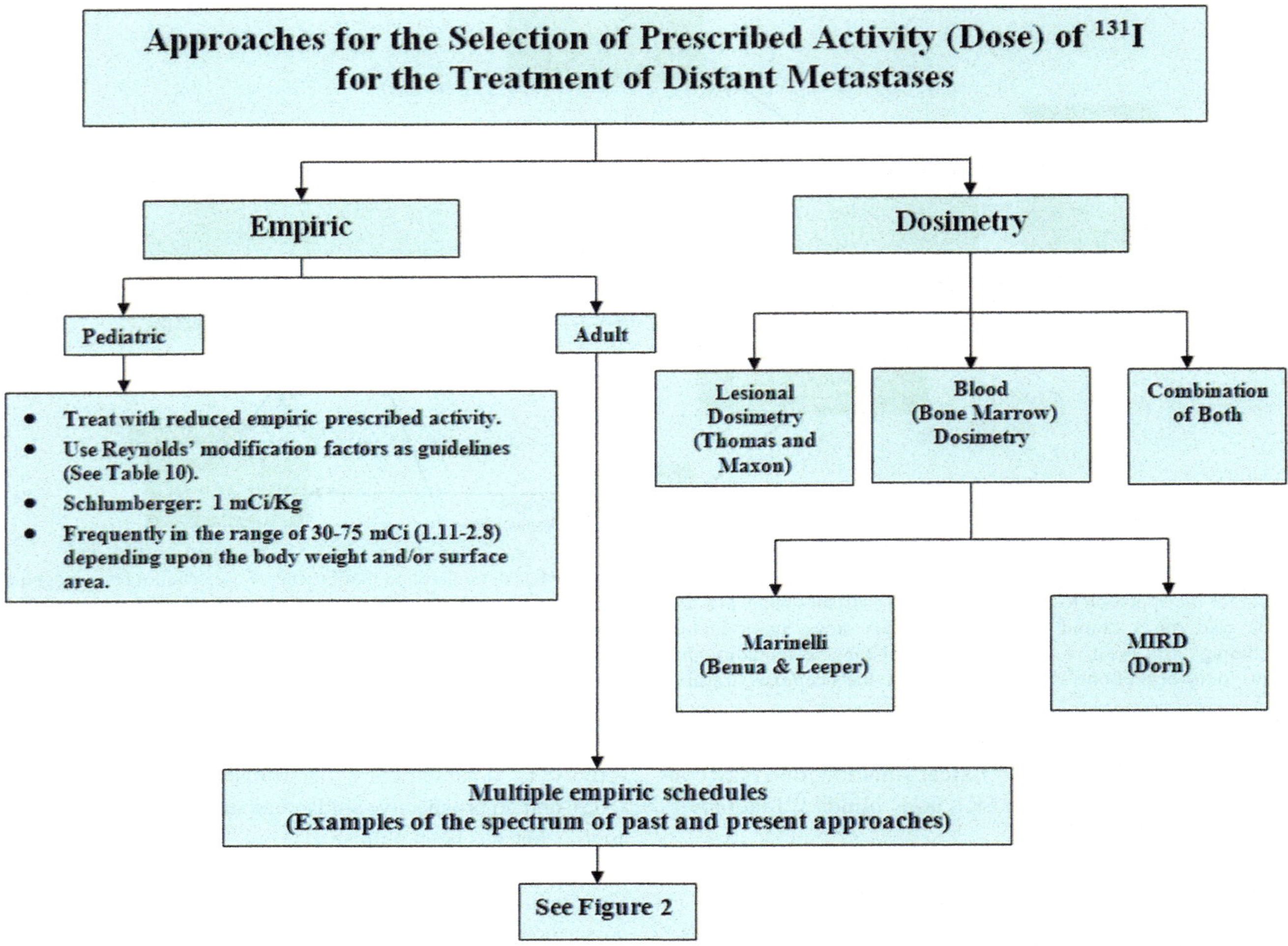

Fig. 56.3 Approaches for the selection of prescribed activity (dosage) for the treatment of distant metastases

reduced to once a year and then to once every 2 years. For patients with positive findings on chest X-ray, Hindié administered 3.7–5.55 GBq (100–150 mCi) of ^{131}I every 6 months and altered the prescribed activity and frequency according to the course of the disease. This dosage ranged from 3.7 GBq (100 mCi) once a year to 5.55 GBq (150 mCi) every 6 months. Of note and at the time of the publication of this book, these facilities may have changed their protocols.

Those facilities who determine their prescribed activity for ^{131}I treatment for metastases typically perform whole-body (e.g., blood) dosimetry for determination of maximum tolerated activity using either the Marinelli (i.e., Benua-Leeper Memorial Sloan Kettering Cancer Center approach) with 200 cGy (rad) maximum radiation absorbed dose to the blood (e.g., surrogate for the bone marrow) or the MIRD approach with 300 cGy (rad) maximum radiation absorbed dose to the blood. Once the maximum tolerated activity (MTA) is calculated, the MTA may be altered either because of prior recommended restrictions or multiple other factors (see Table 56.11). Simplified alternative approaches to full dosimetry for the determination of prescribed activity for ^{131}I treatment for metastases are also available and are discussed in further detail in Chap. 59 entitled "Simplified Methods of Dosimetry".

Strengths and Limitations of the Empiric and Dosimetric Approaches

The strengths and limitations of the empiric and dosimetric approaches have already been discussed in Chap. 58. However to summarize part of that discussion here, a major argument against the use of dosimetric approaches is that until there are prospective studies demonstrating that dosimetric approaches have superior outcomes than empiric approaches, one should use one of the various empiric approaches. Although this author agrees with the empiric selection of the prescribed activity of ^{131}I for remnant ablation and adjuvant

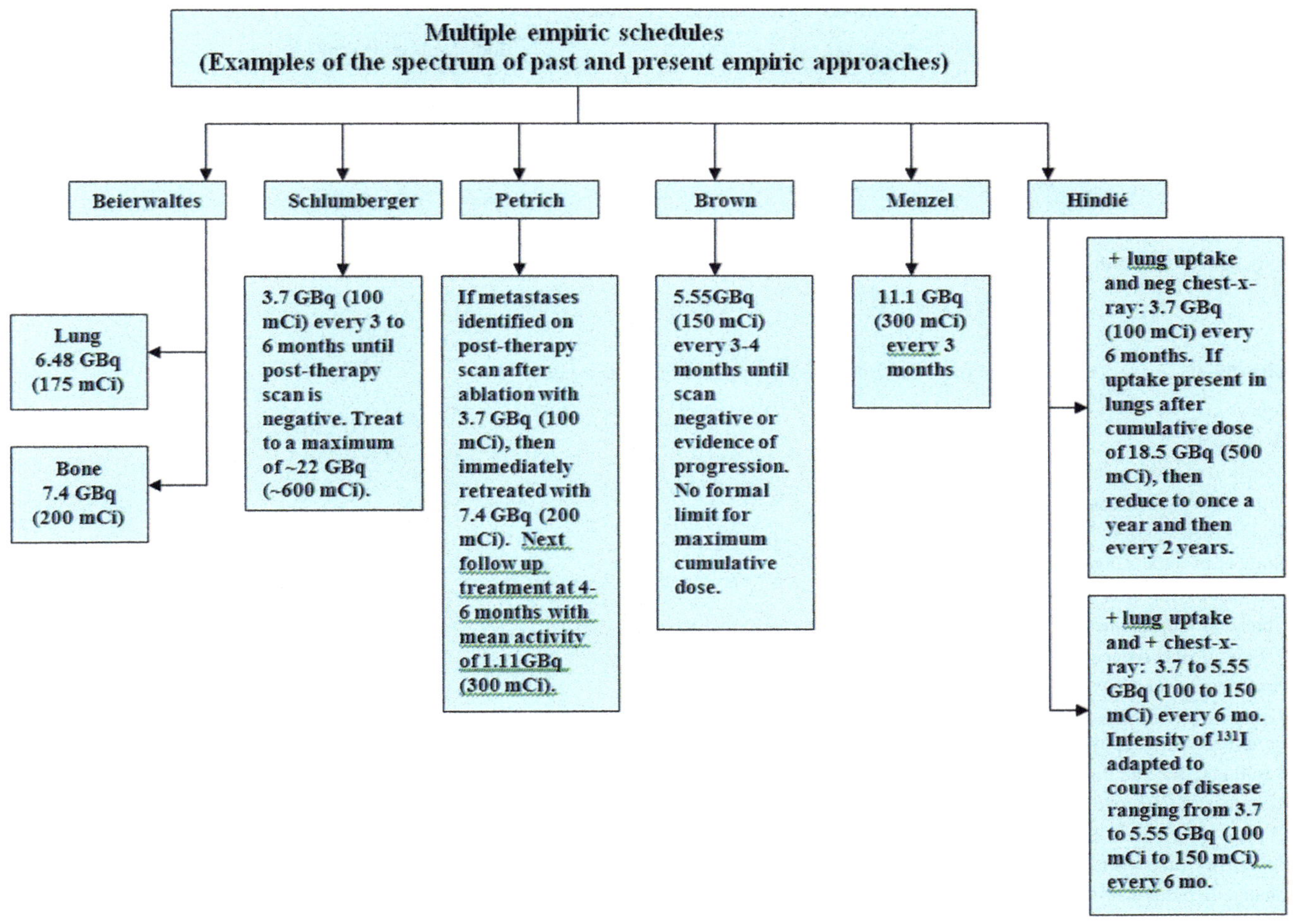

Fig. 56.4 Multiple empiric schedules (examples of the spectrum of past and present approaches)

treatment (see Chap. 33 entitled "Remnant Ablation, Adjuvant Treatment, and Treatment of Locoregional Metastases with ¹³¹I.", he does not agree with this position when selecting the prescribed activity of ¹³¹I for the treatment of *distant* metastases. Rather, this author submits that until further data are published demonstrating that the outcomes of treatment with the empiric methods are equal or superior to the dosimetric methods, one should use one of the dosimetric methods. Dosimetric methods are based on—or at least are an attempt to be based on—one or both of the two fundamental principles of radiation therapy planning. Namely, these principles are ". . . determining and delivering radiation absorbed dose to the tumor for control of the tumor as well as determining and minimizing the radiation absorbed dose to the normal tissues." None of the various empiric approaches are based on either one of these fundamental principles of radiation therapy planning. Instead, empiric fixed prescribed activities are typically based on a proposal of one or another individual at one or another facility, and ironically no prospective studies are available comparing the many different approaches of empiric prescribed activities of ¹³¹I for the treatment of distant metastatic DTC. Further, if one does accept the argument that until additional data are available to demonstrate that dosimetrically determined prescribed activity yields outcomes superior to empirically prescribed activity, then how does one select one of the empiric approaches for prescribed activity (e.g., 3.7 GBq [100 mCi], 5.55 GBq [150 mCi], 7.4 GBq [200 mCi], or even 11.1 GBq [300 mCi]) and one of the many different schedules when there is no data to demonstrate which of those prescribed activities and schedules result in superior outcomes? This seems contradictory from either deductive or inductive reasoning in that until there are data to show that dosimetric approaches have better outcomes than empiric prescribed activities and schedules, one is then free to choose any empiric method one wants to choose. Accordingly and until outcome data are published demonstrating that one empiric method has outcomes equivalent to or better than dosimetric

Table 56.10 Modification factors of prescribed activity for treatment for children

Factor	Body weight (kg)	Body surface area (m^2)
0.2	10	0.4
0.4	25	0.8
0.6	40	1.2
0.8	55	1.4
1.0	77	1.7

Source: Refs. [108, 109]
Body surface area = 0.1 × (weight in kg) 0.67

Table 56.11 Factors that individualize treatments of patients with distant metastases

Age
Histology
Location of metastases (e.g., the lung, bone, or brain)
Number of metastases
Size of metastasis(s)
Number of organs involved
Signs and symptoms secondary to metastases
Uptake of radioiodine
Radiological evidence of disease
Potential for surgical excision
Response of metastases to any previous radioiodine treatment (e.g., indicated by physical exam, radioiodine scan, chest X-ray, ultrasound, computed tomography, magnetic resonance, and serum thyroglobulin levels)
Baseline CBC[a] and differential prior to treatment with special attention to granulocytes, lymphocytes, and platelets
Response of CBC and absolute neutrophil count during the 3–6-week period after previous treatment
Change in baseline CBC and differential 6 to 12 months after previous treatment
Pulmonary function test pretreatment
Change in pulmonary function tests after treatment
Bone marrow biopsy for assessment, not for metastases but for percent cellularity and adipose tissue in the bone marrow
Concomitant disease(s)
Facilities available
Patient desire(s)

[a]*CBC* complete blood count

methods, the logical choice for this author is to select the method that is at least rationally based on one of the fundamentals of radiation therapy planning and not on one or another's individual empiric preference. In addition, dosimetry may identify those patients who may receive a larger amount of prescribed activity of ^{131}I than an empirically selected prescribed activity or dosimetry may identify those patients who may exceed 200 cGy (rad) to the bone marrow for a given empiric amount of ^{131}I for which that empiric prescribed activity should be reduced. If one's own facility is not able or willing to perform full dosimetry and if there is no facility nearby that performs full dosimetry, then one of the alternative simplified dosimetric approaches is strongly recommended [98, 99]. As discussed above, these alternative approaches can be performed in almost any nuclear medicine facility and will again identify those patients who may exceed 200 cGy (rad) to the bone marrow for a planned empiric amount of ^{131}I (see Chap. 59).

In regard to the selection of the prescribed activity for "blind" ^{131}I therapies, the above discussion regarding empiric, full dosimetry and simplified dosimetry applies. However, an additional option is proposed herein. Instead of administering either the empirically determined or dosimetrically determined prescribed activity of ^{131}I, administer 20–40 mCi (0.74 or 1.47 GBq) of ^{131}I and then image 24–36 h later. If these images, for which one has called it a "peak-a-boo" scan, demonstrate uptake in metastases, then administer the balance of the empirically or dosimetrically determined ^{131}I therapeutic prescribed activity that day. This potentially allows not only minimization of the number of patients who may be administered large empirically or dosimetrically determined doses unnecessarily, but it also potentially avoids the effects of stunning or partial therapy of the metastases by the initial 20–40 mCi (0.74 or 1.47 GBq) administration of ^{131}I. McDougal et al. have previously discussed the potential time to stunning/therapy from earlier doses of ^{131}I in Chap. 17. Unfortunately, no study to date is available evaluating the utility of our facility's additional approach, and at the time of the publication of this textbook, four patients have received this "test dose." All four were negative, and none of those patient received the balance of the empirically or dosimetrically determined therapeutic prescribed activity of ^{131}I. All four did have a subsequent scan performed 7 days after the "test dose," and one scan demonstrated uptake in metastatic disease. Development of a prospective study is under way.

Finally, in regard to the prescribed activity of ^{131}I for a metastasis of differentiated thyroid cancer, additional research is needed to maximize the uptake of ^{131}I (e.g., selumetinib), increase the *rate* of radiation absorbed dose delivered while minimizing non-thyroidal side effects, and increase the retention time of ^{131}I in the metastases (e.g., lithium and iodine).

Time of Administration of ^{131}I Therapy in Patients with Metastases

Very little data have been published regarding the timing of the administration of ^{131}I therapy in patients with metastases. Higashi et al. [107] evaluated the significance of the time from the patient's completion total thyroidectomy to ^{131}I therapy in 198 patients who had extrathyroidal extension and/or distant metastases. The risk of death in those patients who were administered their ^{131}I therapy more than 180 days after their completion thyroidectomy was 4.22 times higher than those patients who were administered their ^{131}I within 180 days. A confounding factor is that 59 of the above patients had had a prior hemithyroidectomy or sub-total thyroidectomy prior to their completion thyroidectomy. However, delay in ^{131}I therapy may be an important factor regarding prognosis in patients with distant metastatic disease.

Summary

In summary, no prospective study is available evaluating the effectiveness of ^{131}I treatment for distant metastases such as increasing survival, reducing recurrences, and/or improving palliation. The retrospective studies also do not adequately evaluate these issues. Thus, the debate continues. Similarly, when ^{131}I is used for treatment, decisions will be made with incomplete information about what is the appropriate amount of ^{131}I to administer and the method to determine that amount. However, based on the data and guidelines noted earlier in this chapter and in other chapters such as Chaps. 33, 47, 58, and 59, this author submits the following conclusions and opinions, and from these conclusions and opinions, guidelines are illustrated in Fig. 56.3.

General Comments

- The treatment of patients with distant metastases should be individualized.
- The prognosis of patients with distant metastases may be reduced by many interrelated factors. Such factors are increasing age of patient, increasing size of metastasis(es), histology, increasing number of metastases, location of metastases (e.g., the lung, bone, or brain), increasing number of organs involved, pattern of metastases (e.g., pulmonary macronodular versus micronodular, focal versus diffuse pulmonary metastases), radiological evidence of metastasis, and absence of radioiodine uptake, to list only a few.
- ^{131}I treatment can be curative in selected patients who have distant metastases.
- ^{131}I therapy can be palliative in selected patients with distant metastases.
- However, a majority of patients who have distant metastases are not cured with ^{131}I therapy, and many patients may only receive little to no palliation from ^{131}I.
- The criteria for the selection of patients for ^{131}I treatment are important.

Pulmonary Metastases

- Patients with diffuse pulmonary metastases that are not visualized on chest X-ray and computed tomography (CT) ("X-ray negative") but are seen on radioiodine scan ("radioiodine positive") are good candidates for ^{131}I treatments. The potential benefit from ^{131}I appears to decrease when the pulmonary metastases are visualized with chest X-ray/CT or ^{18}F fluorodeoxyglucose positron emission tomography, are more focal and larger, and/or do not take up radioiodine.
- Early diagnosis and treatment of selected pulmonary metastases are important to maximize the efficacy of ^{131}I therapy, to increase the probability of achieving a complete remission, and/or to increase survival. Notably, this may also be a result, at least in part, of the metastases being more radiosensitive at this stage.
- Children who have diffuse pulmonary metastases that are X-ray negative and radioiodine positive may have an excellent prognosis without any treatment, and this prognosis typically is many years. However, their life expectancy still may be reduced, and these patients are still

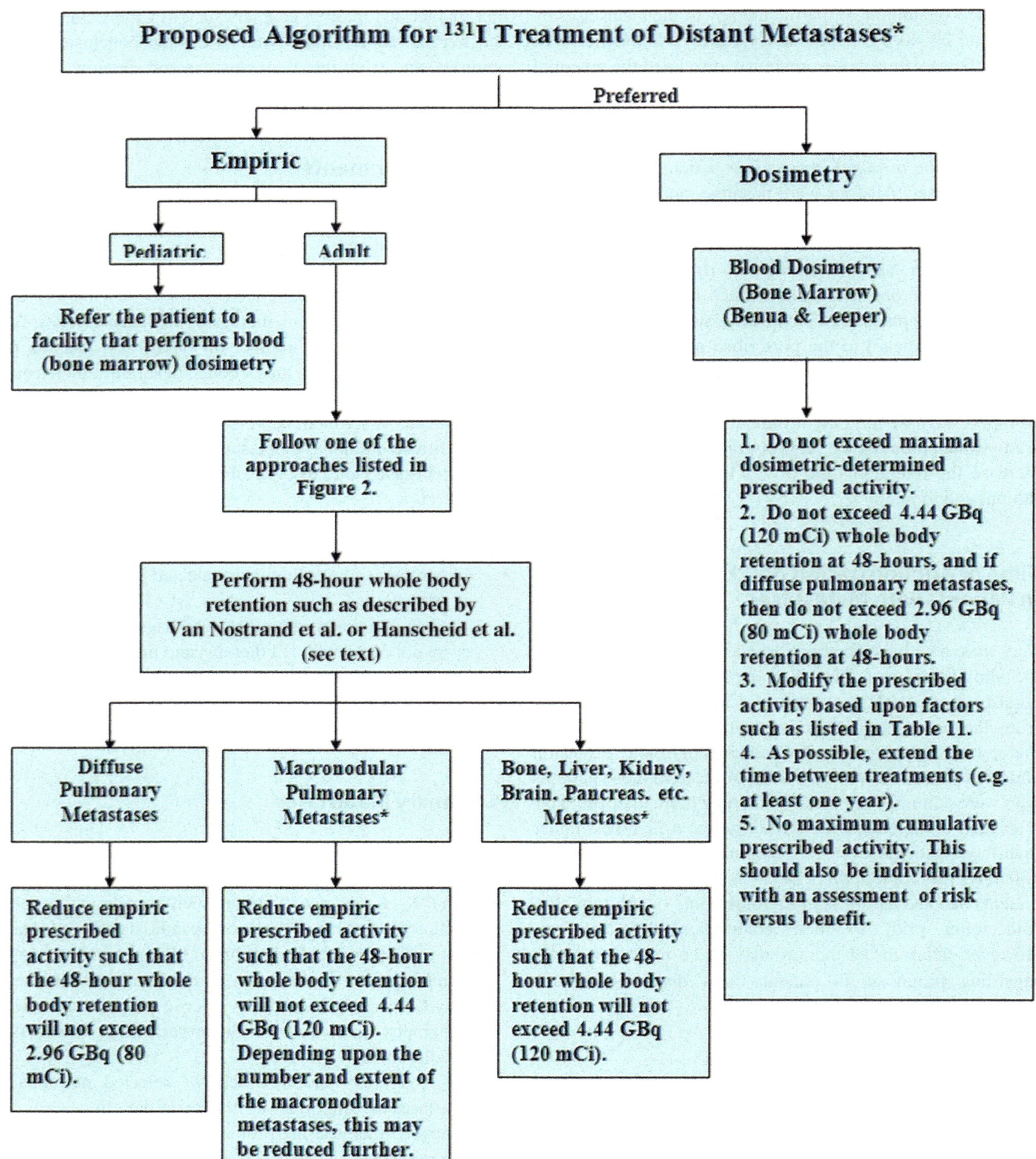

Fig. 56.5 Proposed algorithm for radioiodine treatment of distant metastases

good candidates for treatment with ^{131}I. However, considering these children's excellent prognosis, it is particularly important that every effort be made to select the appropriate amount of ^{131}I to maximize the chance for cure or to increase survival while minimizing significant side effects such as bone marrow suppression, radiation pneumonitis, and pulmonary fibrosis (Table 56.10). In addition, aggressive efforts should be made at the time of first and all subsequent ^{131}I therapies to reduce the radiation absorbed dose to other organs such as the salivary glands, gastrointestinal system, urinary bladder, etc.

- Patients who have a single pulmonary metastasis with no other evidence of distant metastases should be considered for pulmonary metastasectomy [110].
- ^{131}I alone does not significantly increase survival or achieve significant palliation for patients who have pulmonary metastases that are macronodular in size (>1 cm) on X-ray and are radioiodine negative.

Bone Metastases

- A single-bone metastasis that is X-ray negative and radioiodine positive may respond well to ^{131}I [28]. However, alternative therapies (e.g., complete surgical excision, stereotactic radiosurgery, radiofrequency ablation, cryotherapy, and arterial embolization) should be considered first (see Chap. 65). ^{131}I may be used as adjunctive therapy to the above treatment options, or if the above treatments are not options, then ^{131}I may be used as an alternative treatment.
- For patients with multiple, extensive, radioiodine-negative bone metastases, ^{131}I treatments do not significantly increase survival or achieve significant palliation.

Brain Metastases

- For patients who have brain metastases, surgical excision of the brain metastases or external radiotherapy (e.g., stereotactic radiosurgery) should be considered first. If the brain metastasis is radioiodine positive, then ^{131}I may be used as adjunctive or palliative treatment, but the probability of any significant effect is low.

"Blind Treatments" for Patients Who Have Positive Tg Levels and Negative Radioiodine Scans

1. The management of patients who have positive Tg levels and negative radioiodine is controversial. The first step is recognizing that patients with positive Tg levels and negative radioiodine scan do not represent a single entity. Rather, they represent a very wide spectrum of patients. "Blind ^{131}I treatments" are not indicated in patient such as those who have very low risk disease with low and stable Tg levels. However, "blind" ^{131}I therapies may be considered in selected patients prior to initiation of tyrosine kinase inhibitors. An example is a patient who has significantly elevated Tg levels, rapidly rising Tg levels, negative radioiodine scans, false-positive Tg levels have been excluded, false-negative radioiodine scans have been excluded, and alternative imaging studies demonstrated the source of the elevated Tg level (e.g., diffuse pulmonary metastases on CT scan) that could not be managed with site-specific therapy. As with the decision of initiating a tyrosine kinase inhibitor, the patient must clearly understand the likelihood of potential benefits and the risks of complications for a "blind" ^{131}I treatment and a tyrosine kinase inhibitor.
2. Patients with distant metastases who have a negative post-therapy scan should not be considered for any further ^{131}I treatments unless redifferentiation—reestablishment of radioiodine uptake—is achieved.

Selection of Prescribed Activity of ^{131}I for Treatment of Distant Metastases

- The method to select the amount of ^{131}I depends on the medical practice and capabilities of the specific facility and country.
- The first treatment ("first strike") of distant metastases has the highest chance of being curative [37].
- The radiation absorbed dose delivered to the tumor must exceed a minimum level to have a notable effect [103].
- The difference between a significant effect and a minimal effect from ^{131}I treatment may be a small difference in regard to the amount of radiation absorbed dose delivered and, thus, a small difference in the amount of becquerels (millicuries) administered [103].
- Higher dose *rates* (Gy/h and rad/h) are more effective [27, 111].
- For radioiodine-positive distant metastases, ^{131}I administered in a single treatment is more likely to have a greater effect on the tumor than when the same amount of ^{131}I is administered in fractionated treatments over months to several years. The lower response rate from fractionated treatments is a result of (1) low radiation absorbed dose *rates* and (2) reduced radiation absorbed doses delivered by the second and subsequent treatments because of decreased radioiodine uptake resulting from the preceding treatments).
- As the radiation absorbed doses and dose rates are increased, the frequency and severity of side effects are also increased (see Chap. 62).

- As medical treatment plans are individualized for each patient, the amount of ^{131}I to treat distant metastases should also be individualized. The purpose of this individualization is to maximize the potential radiation absorbed dose and dose rate to the tumor without exceeding the maximal tolerated radiation absorbed dose to organs such as the bone marrow, lungs, or salivary glands.
- Dosimetrically determined amounts of ^{131}I, as determined by either the Benua-Leeper or the MIRD methods (see Chaps. 58 and 59 on dosimetry), potentially allow more patients to receive higher radiation absorbed doses and higher dose rates to the metastases than empiric amounts of ^{131}I while minimizing severe side effects to the bone marrow.
- Dosimetrically determined amounts of ^{131}I can identify as many as 11–19 % of patients who would have received more than 200 cGy (rad) to the bone marrow if treated with an empiric prescribed activity of 5.5–7.4 GBq (150–200 mCi) of ^{131}I [112–115]. This percentage is even higher if the planned empiric prescribed activity is higher.
- Patients who (1) have distant metastases, (2) are going to be treated with ^{131}I, and (3) may receive multiple subsequent ^{131}I treatments should be managed *early* and *aggressively* in order to reduce the radiation absorbed dose to nontarget organs, such as the salivary glands, gastrointestinal tract, and urinary bladder (see Chap. 62).
- If dosimetry cannot be performed, then the measurement of a percent 48 h whole-body retention as suggested by Van Nostrand et al. [98] or Hanscheid et al. [99] may help identify patients who may be eligible for higher empiric amounts of ^{131}I or should have their empiric prescribed activity reduced.

Proposed Algorithms for the Selection of the Prescribed Activity of ^{131}I

Based on the above conclusions and opinions, this author proposes an algorithm for the selection of the amount of ^{131}I to be administered to patients with distant metastases (Fig. 56.5). However, there are two caveats. The algorithm in Fig. 56.5 is not for the selection of patients for ^{131}I therapy but for the selection of the prescribed activity of ^{131}I to be administered. In addition, this algorithm is not absolute. Rather, the algorithm is one physician's guidelines. The decision whether or not to treat and the amount of ^{131}I to administer must be individualized according to many factors, of which a few are listed in Table 56.11. Thus, the "practice" of medicine continues.

Acknowledgment I would like to thank our library staff for their excellent support in obtaining these references.

References

1. Seidlin SM, Marinelli LD, Oshry E. Radioactive iodine therapy: effect on functioning metastases of adenocarcinoma of the thyroid. JAMA. 1946;132:838–47.
2. Leeper RD. The effect of I-131 therapy on survival of patients with metastatic papillary or follicular thyroid carcinoma. J Clin Endocrinol Metab. 1973;36:1143–52.
3. Nemec J, Zamrazil V, Pohunkova D, Rohling S. Radioiodide treatment of pulmonary metastases of differentiated thyroid cancer: results and prognostic factors. Nucl Med. 1979;18:86–90.
4. Maheshwari YK, Stratton Hill C, Haynie TP, et al. Iodine-131 therapy in differentiated thyroid carcinoma: M.D. Anderson Hospital experience. Cancer. 1981;47:664–71.
5. Brown AP, Greening WP, McCready VR, et al. Radioiodine treatment of Metastatic thyroid carcinoma: the Royal Marsden hospital experience. Br J Radiol. 1984;57:323–7.
6. Massin JP, Savoie JC, Garnier H, et al. Pulmonary metastases in differentiated thyroid carcinoma: study of 58 cases with implications for the primary tumor treatment. Cancer. 1984; 53:982–92.
7. Samaan NA, Schultz PN, Haynie TP, Ordonez NG. Pulmonary metastasis of differentiated thyroid carcinoma: treatment results in 101 patients. J Clin Endocrinol Metab. 1985;65:376–80.
8. Leeper RD. Thyroid cancer. Med Clin North Am. 1985;69:1079–96.
9. Schlumberger M, Arcangioli O, Piekarski JD, et al. Detection of and treatment of lung metastases of differentiated thyroid carcinoma in patients with normal chest x-rays. J Nucl Med. 1988;29:1790–4.
10. Ruegemer JJ, Hay ID, Bergstralh EJ, et al. Distant metastases in differentiated thyroid carcinoma: a multivariate analysis of prognostic variables. J Clin Endocrinol Metab. 1988;67:501–8.
11. Høie J, Stenwig AE, Kullman G, Lindegaard M. Distant metastases in papillary thyroid cancer: a review of 91 patients. Cancer. 1988;61:1–6.
12. Marcocci C, Pacini F, Elisi R, et al. Clinical and biological behavior of bone metastases from differentiated thyroid carcinoma. Surgery. 1989;106:960–6.
13. Woods WJ, Singletary SE, Hickey RC. Current results of treatment for distant metastatic well-differentiated thyroid carcinoma. Arch Surg. 1989;124:1374–7.
14. Proye CAG, Dromer DHR, Carnaille BM, et al. Is it still worthwhile to treat bone metastases from differentiated thyroid carcinoma with radioactive iodine? World J Surg. 1992;16:640–6.
15. Casara D, Rubello D, Saladini G, et al. Different features of pulmonary metastases in differentiated thyroid cancer: natural history and multivariate statistical analysis of prognostic variables. J Nucl Med. 1993;34:1626–31.
16. Pacini F, Cetani F, Miccoli P, et al. Outcome of 309 patients with metastatic thyroid carcinoma treated with radioiodine. World J Surg. 1994;18:600–4.
17. Samuel AM, Rajashekharrao B. Radioiodine therapy for well-differentiated thyroid cancer: a quantitative dosimetric evaluation for remnant thyroid ablation after surgery. J Nucl Med. 1994;35:1944–50.
18. Dinneen SF, Valimaki MJ, Bergstralh EJ, et al. Distant metastases in papillary thyroid carcinoma: 100 cases observed at one institution during 5 decades. J Clin Endocrinol Metab. 1995;80:2041–5.
19. Vassilopoulou-Sellin R, Libshitz HI, Haynie TP. Papillary thyroid cancer with pulmonary metastases beginning in childhood. Clinical course over three decades. Med Pediatr Oncol. 1995;24:119–22.

20. Schlumberger M, Challeton C, De Vathaire F, et al. Radioactive iodine treatment and external radiotherapy for lung and bone metastases from thyroid carcinoma. J Nucl Med. 1996;37:598–605.
21. Menzel C, Grunwald F, Schomburg A, et al. “High-dose” radioiodine therapy in advanced differentiated thyroid carcinoma. J Nucl Med. 1996;37:1496–503.
22. Vassilopoulou-Sellin R, Schultz P, Haynie TP. Clinical outcome of patients with papillary thyroid carcinoma who have recurrence after initial radioactive iodine therapy. Cancer. 1996;78:494–501.
23. Sisson JC, Giordano TJ, Jamadar DA, et al. ^{131}I treatment of micronodular pulmonary metastases from papillary thyroid cancer. Cancer. 1996;78:2184–92.
24. McCormack KR. Bone metastases from thyroid carcinoma. Cancer. 1966;19:181–4.
25. Shaha AR, Shah JP, Loree TR. Patterns of nodal and distant metastasis based on histologic varieties in differentiated thyroid carcinoma of the thyroid. Am J Surg. 1996;172:692–4.
26. Chiu AC, Delpassand ES, Sherman SI. Prognosis and treatment of brain metastases in thyroid carcinoma. J Clin Endocrinol Metab. 1997;82:3637–42.
27. Samuel AM, Rajashekharrao B, Shah DH. Pulmonary metastases in children and adolescents with well-differentiated thyroid cancer. J Nucl Med. 1998;30:1531–6.
28. Schlumberger J, Tubiana M, De Vathaire F, et al. Long term results of treatment of 283 patients with lung and bone metastases from differentiated thyroid carcinoma. J Clin Endocrinol Metab. 1998;63:960–7.
29. Sisson JC, Jamadar DDA, Kazerooni EA, et al. Treatment of micro-nodular lung metastases of papillary thyroid cancer: are the tumors too small for effective irradiation from radioiodine? Thyroid. 1998;8:215–21.
30. Fanchiang JK, Lin JD, Huang MJ, Shih NW. Papillary and follicular thyroid carcinomas with bone metastases: a series of 39 cases during a period of 18 years. Chang Gung Med J. 1998;21:377–82.
31. Pittas AG, Adler M, Fazzari M, et al. Bone metastases from thyroid carcinoma; clinical characteristics and prognostic variables in one hundred forty six patients. Thyroid. 2000;10:261–8.
32. Tickoo SK, Pittas AG, Adler M, Fazzari M, Larson SM, Robbins RJ, Rosai J. Bone metastases from thyroid carcinoma: a histopathologic study with clinical correlates. Arch Pathol Lab Med. 2000;124:1440–7.
33. Petrich T, Widjaja A, Musholt TJ, et al. Outcome after radioiodine therapy in 107 patients with differentiated thyroid carcinoma and initial bone metastases: side effects and influence of age. Eur J Nucl Med. 2001;28:203–8.
34. Akkas BE, Demirel BB, Vural GU. Prognostic factors affecting disease-specific survival in patients with recurrent and/or metastatic differentiated thyroid carcinoma detected by positron emission tomography/computer tomography. Thyroid. 2014;24:287–95.
35. Bernier MO, Leenhardt L, Hoang C, et al. Survival and therapeutic modalities in patients with bone metastases of differentiated thyroid carcinomas. J Clin Endocrinol Metab. 2001;86:1568–73.
36. Zettinig G, Fueger B, Passier C, et al. Long-term follow-up of patients with bone metastases from differentiated thyroid carcinoma—surgery or conventional therapy? Clin Endocrinol. 2002;56:377–82.
37. Dorn R, Kopp J, Vogt H, et al. Dosimetry-guided radioactive iodine treatment in patients with metastatic differentiated thyroid cancer: largest safe dose using a risk—adapted approach. J Nucl Med. 2003;44:451–6.
38. Hindié E, Melliere D, Lange F, et al. Functioning pulmonary metastases of thyroid cancer: does radioiodine influence the prognosis? Eur J Nucl Med. 2003;30:974–81.
39. Robbins RJ, Larson SM, Pentlow KS, Tuttle RM. Treatment of thyroid cancer metastases with I-131 following thyroid hormone withdrawal or recombinant human TSH. Thyroid. 2003;13:702.
40. McWilliams RR, Giannini C, Hay ID, et al. Management of brain metastases from thyroid carcinoma: a study of 16 pathologically confirmed cases over 25 years. Cancer. 2003;98:356–62.
41. Ronga G, Filesi M, Montesano T, et al. Lung metastases from differentiated thyroid carcinoma. A 40 years' experience. Q J Nucl Med Mol Imaging. 2004;48:12–9.
42. Llgan S, Karacalioglu O, Pabuscu Y, et al. Iodine-131 treatment and high resolution CT: results in patients with lung metastases form differentiated thyroid carcinoma. Eur J Nucl Med Mol Imaging. 2004;31:825–30.
43. Durante C, Haddy N, Baudin S, et al. Long-term outcome of 44 patients with distant metastases from papillary and follicular thyroid carcinoma: benefits and limits of radioiodine therapy. J Clin Endocrinol Metab. 2006;91:2892–9.
44. Sampson E, Brierley JD, Le L, et al. Clinical management and outcome of papillary and follicular (differentiated) thyroid cancer presenting with distant metastasis at diagnosis. Cancer. 2007;110:1451–6.
45. Toubert ME, Hindié E, Rampin L, et al. Distant metastases of differentiated thyroid cancer: diagnosis, treatment and outcome. Nucl Med Rev. 2007;10:106–9.
46. Sugitani I, Fujimoto Y, Yamamoto N. Papillary thyroid carcinomas with distant metastases: survival predictors and the importance of local control. Surgery. 2007;143:35–42.
47. Wu K, Hou S-M, Huang TS, et al. Thyroid carcinoma with bone metastases: a prognostic factor study. Clin Med Oncol. 2008;2:120–34.
48. Mihailovic JM, Stefanovic LJ, Malesevic M, et al. The importance of age over radioiodine avidity as a prognostic factor in differentiated thyroid carcinoma with distant metastases. Thyroid. 2009;19:227–32.
49. Lee J, Soh EY. Differentiated thyroid carcinoma presenting with distant metastasis at initial diagnosis: clinical outcomes and prognostic factors. Ann Surg. 2010;251:114–9.
50. Cho SW, Choi HS, Yeom GJ, Lim JA, Moon JH, Park DJ, Chung JK, Cho BY, Yi KH, Park YJ. Long-term prognosis of differentiated thyroid cancer with lung metastasis in Korea and its prognostic factors. Thyroid. 2014;24:277–86.
51. Stefanović L, Gudurić B, Silapić N, et al. Protocol of the diagnostic therapy and follow-up of differentiated thyroid cancer. Med Pregl. 1993;46 Suppl 1:90–1.
52. Shoop M, Stojadinovic A, Nissan A, et al. Prognostic indicators of outcomes in patients with distant metastases from differentiated thyroid carcinoma. J Am Coll Surg. 2003;197:191–7.
53. Mizukami Y, Michigishi T, Nonomura A, et al. Distant metastases in differentiated thyroid carcinomas: a clinical and pathologic study. Hum Pathol. 1990;21:283–90.
54. Lin JD, Chao TC, Chou SC, et al. Papillary thyroid carcinoma with lung metastases. Thyroid. 2004;14:1091–6.
55. Khorjekar G, Van Nostrand D, Moreau S, Atkins F, Mete M, Burman K, Wartofsky L. Survival rate in patients diagnosed with well-differentiated thyroid cancer with bone metastases. J Nucl Med. 2010;51S:1080, (abstract).
56. Qiu ZL, Song HJ, Xu YH, et al. Efficacy and survival analysis of ^{131}I therapy for bone metastases from differentiated thyroid cancer. J Clin Endocrinol Metab. 2011;96:3078–86.
57. Hindié E, Zanotti-Fregonara P, Keller I, et al. Bone metastases of differentiated thyroid cancer: impact of early ^{131}I-based detection on outcome. Endocr-Relat Cancer. 2007;14:799–807.
58. Chen HW, Su DH, Chen HW, Chang TC. Thyroid carcinomas with brain or skull metastases. Endocrinologist. 2005;15:303–8.
59. Bernad DM, Sperduto PW, Souhami L, Jensen AW, Roberge D. Stereotactic radiosurgery in the management of brain metasta-

ses from primary thyroid cancers. J Neuro Oncol. 2010;98:249–52.
60. de Figueiredo BH, Godbert Y, Soubeyan I, Carrat X, Lagarde P, Cazeau AL, Italiano A, Sargos P, Kantor G, Loiseau H, Bonichon F. Brain metastases from thyroid carcinoma: a retrospective study of 21 patients. Thyroid. 2014;24:270–6.
61. Bedikian AY, Valdivieso M, Heilbrun LK, et al. Glycerol: a successful alternative to dexamethasone for patients receiving brain irradiation for metastatic disease. Cancer Treat Rep. 1978;62: 1081–3.
62. Samuel AM, Shah DH. Brain metastases in well-differentiated carcinoma of the thyroid. Tumori. 1997;83:608–10.
63. Venkatesh S, Leavens ME, Samaan NA. Brain metastases in patients with well-differentiated thyroid carcinoma: study of 11 cases. Eur J Surg Oncol. 1990;16:448–50.
64. Misaki T, Iwata M, Kasagi K, Konishi J. Brain metastasis from differentiated thyroid cancer in patients treated with radioiodine for bone and lung lesions. Ann Nucl Med. 2000;14:111–4.
65. Kim IY, Kondziolka D, Niranjan A, Flickinger JC, Lunsford LD. Gamma knife radiosurgery for metastatic brain tumors from thyroid cancer. J Neuro Oncol. 2009;93:355–9.
66. Ikekubo K, Hino M, Ita H, Hirao K, Ueshima M, Tanaka T, Kobayshi H, Ishihara T, Kurahachi H. Seven cases of brain metastasis from papillary thyroid carcinoma. Kaku Igaku. 2000;37:349–57.
67. Salvati M, Frati A, Rocchi G, et al. Single brain metastasis from thyroid cancer: report of twelve cases and review of the literature. J Neuro Oncol. 2001;51:33–40.
68. Hjiyiannakis P, Jefferies S, Harmer CL. Brain metastases in patients with differentiated thyroid carcinoma. Clin Oncol. 1996;8:327–30.
69. Miranda ER, Padrao EL, Silva BC, Marco L, Sarquis MS. Papillary thyroid carcinoma with brain metastases: an unusual 10-year-survival case. Thyroid. 2010;20:657–61.
70. Diyora B, Nayak N, Kamble H, Sharma A. Brain metastasis from papillary carcinoma of thyroid gland. J Neurosci Rural Pract. 2010;1:55–7.
71. Izci Y, Gonul E, Gurkanlar D, Bolu E. Brain metastasis from follicular thyroid carcinoma: case report and literature review. Turk Neurosurg. 2005;15:132–5.
72. Anoop TM, Puthukuli NM, Divya KP, Nikhil S, Jabbar PK. Thyroid follicular carcinoma presenting as intraorbital, intracranial, and subcutaneous metastasis. Am J Surg. 2010;199:e72–4.
73. Datz F. Cerebral edema following iodine-131 therapy for thyroid carcinoma metastatic to the brain. J Nucl Med. 1986;27:637–40.
74. Holmquest DL, Lakes P. Sudden hemorrhage in metastatic thyroid carcinoma of the brain during treatment with iodine-131. J Nucl Med. 1976;17:307–9.
75. Aguiar PH, Agner C, Tavares FR, Yamaguchi N. Unusual brain metastases from papillary thyroid carcinoma: case report. Neurosurgery. 2001;49:1008–13.
76. Gkountouvas A, Nikas M, Aggelopoulou A, et al. Brain metastases due to papillary thyroid carcinoma. Endocrinologist. 2010;20:100–1.
77. Pacak K, Sweeney DC, Wartofsky L, et al. Solitary cerebellar metastasis from papillary thyroid carcinoma: a case report. Thyroid. 1998;8:327–35.
78. Goolden AWG, Mclaughlin JE, Valentine AR, et al. Solitary cerebral metastasis from a papillary carcinoma of the thyroid. Postgrad Med J. 1990;66:127–9.
79. Haugen, BR, Alexander EA, Bible KC, Doherty G, Mandel SJ, Nikiforov YE, Pacini F, Randolph GW, Sawka AM, Schlumberger M, Schuff K, Sherman SI, Sosa JA, Steward DL, Tuttle RM, Wartofsky L. 2015 American Thyroid Association Management Guidelines for Adult Patients with Thyroid Nodules and Differentiated Thyroid Cancer. Thyroid. 2016;26:1–133.
80. Perros P, Colley S, Boelaert K, Evans C, Evans RM, Gerrard GE, Gilbert JA, Harrison B, Johnson SJ, Giles TE, Moss L, Lewington V, Newbold KL, Taylor J, Thakker RV, Watkinson J, Williams GR. British Thyroid Association guidelines for the management of thyroid cancer. Clin Endocrinol. 2014;81 Suppl 1:1–122.
81. Chinese Society of Endocrinology, Chinese Society of General Surgery Endocrinology Group, China Anti-Cancer Association Head and Neck Tumor Professional Committee, Chinese Society of Nuclear Medicine. The Chinese guideline for management of thyroid nodules and differentiated thyroid cancer. Chin J Endocrinol Metab. 2012;28:779–97.
82. Luster M, Clarke E, Dietlein M, et al. Guidelines for radioiodine therapy of differentiated thyroid cancer. Eur J Nucl Med Mol Imaging. 2008;35:1941–59.
83. Pacini F, Schlumberger M, Dralle H, Elisei R, Smit JWA, Wiersinga W, European Thyroid Cancer Taskforce. European consensus for the management of patients with differentiated thyroid carcinoma of the follicular epithelium. Eur J Endocrinol. 2006;154:787–803.
84. Pacini F, Castagna MG, Brilli L, et al. Thyroid cancer: ESMO clinical practice guidelines for diagnosis, treatment and follow-up. Ann Oncol. 2010;21(S5):v214–9.
85. National Comprehensive Cancer Network (NCCN). Clinical practice guidelines in oncology. Thyroid carcinoma. Follicular thyroid carcinoma. V.2.2015. www.nccn.org.
86. Silberstein EB, Alavi A, Balon HR, Clarke SEM, Divgi C, Gelfand MJ, Goldsmith SJ, Jadvar H, Marcus CS, Martin WH, Parker JA, Royal HD, Sarkar SD, Stabin M, Waxman AD. The SNMMI practice guideline for therapy of thyroid disease with ^{131}I. J Nucl Med. 2012;53:1633–51.
87. Kim DH, Jung JH, Son SY, Kim CY, Hong CM, Jeong SY, Lee SW, Lee J, Ahn BC. Difference of clinical and radiological characteristics according to radioiodine avidity in pulmonary metastases of differentiated thyroid cancer. Nucl Med Mol Imaging. 2014;48:55–62.
88. Sugino K, Ito K, Nagahama M, Kitagawa W, Shibuya H, Ohkuwa K, Yano Y, Uruno T, Akaishi J, Kameyama K, Ito K. Prognosis and prognostic factors for distant metastases and tumor mortality in follicular thyroid carcinoma. Thyroid. 2011;21:751–7.
89. Huang IC, Chou FF, Liu RT, Tung SC, Chen JF, Kuo MC, Hsieh CJ, Wang PW. Long-term outcomes of distant metastasis from differentiated thyroid carcinoma. Clin Endocrinol. 2012;76:439–47.
90. Lang BHH, Wong KP, Cheung CY, Wan KY, Lo CY. Evaluating the prognostic factors associated with cancer-specific survival of differentiated thyroid carcinoma presenting with distant metastasis. Ann Surg Oncol. 2013;2:1329–35.
91. Ito Y, Kudo T, Kobayashi K, Miya A, Ichihara K, Miyauchi A. Prognostic factors for recurrence of papillary thyroid carcinoma in the lymph nodes, lung, and bone: analysis of 5,768 patients with average 10-year follow-up. World J Surg. 2012;36:1274–8.
92. Orita Y, Sugitani L, Matsuura M, Ushiima M, Tsukahara K, Fujimoto Y, Kawabata K. Prognostic factors and the therapeutic strategy for patients with bone metastasis from differentiated thyroid carcinoma. Surgery. 2010;147:424–31.
93. Farooki A, Leung V, Tala H, Tuttle RM. Skeletal-related events due to bone metastases from differentiated thyroid cancer. J Clin Endocrinol Metab. 2012;97:2433–9.
94. Robenshtok E, Farooki A, Grewal RK, Tuttle RM. Natural history of small radioiodine-avid bone metastases that have no structural correlate on imaging studies. Endocrine. 2013;12:1–7.
95. Zanotti-Fregonara P, Rubello D, Hindié E. Bone metastases of differentiated thyroid cancer: the importance of early diagnosis and ^{131}I therapy of prognosis. J Nucl Med. 2008;49:1902–3.
96. Zhao CL, Qiu ZL, Chen LB, Yuan ZB, Judo QY. Sustained and diffuse ^{131}I avid bone metastases with low thyroglobulin levels in a patient with papillary thyroid carcinoma. Clin Nucl Med. 2013;38:375–7.

97. Jordan H, Hall JP, Van Nostrand D, Schneider M, Burman K. Brain metastases secondary to differentiated thyroid cancer: an educational exhibit. J Nucl Med. 2012;53:1052. (abstract).
98. Van Nostrand D, Atkins F, Moreau S, Aiken M, Kulkarni K, Wu JS, Burman K, Wartofsky L. Utility of the radioiodine whole body retention at 48 hours for modifying empiric activity of 131-iodine for the treatment of metastatic well-differentiated thyroid carcinoma. Thyroid. 2009;19:1093–8.
99. Hänscheid H, Lassman M, Luster M, et al. Blood dosimetry from a single measurement of the whole body radioiodine retention in patients with differentiated thyroid carcinoma. Endocr-Relat Cancer. 2009;16:1283–9.
100. Ma C, Xie J, Kuang A. Is empiric ^{131}I therapy justified for patients with positive thyroglobulin and negative ^{131}I whole-body scanning results? Nucl Med. 2005;46:1164–70.
101. Thomas SR, Maxon HR, Kereiakes JG. In vivo quantitation of lesion radioactivity using external counting methods. Med Phys. 1976;3:253–5.
102. Thomas SR, Maxon HR, Kereiakes JG, Saenger EL. Quantitative external counting techniques enabling improved diagnostic and therapeutic decisions in patients with well-differentiated thyroid cancer. Radiology. 1977;122:731–7.
103. Maxon HR, Thomas SR, Hertzbert VS, et al. Relation between effective radiation dose and outcome of radioiodine therapy for thyroid cancer. N Engl J Med. 1983;309:937–41.
104. Benua RS, Cicale NR, Sonenberg M, Rawson RW. The relation of radioiodine dosimetry to results and complications in the treatment of metastatic thyroid cancer. Am J Roentgenol Radium Ther Nucl Med. 1962;87:171–82.
105. Klubo-Gwiezdzinska J, Van Nostrand D, Atkins F, Burman K, Jonklaas J, Mete M, Wartofsky L. Efficacy of dosimetric versus empiric prescribed activity of ^{131}I for therapy of differentiated thyroid cancer. Thyroid. 2011;96:3217–25.
106. Beierwaltes WH. The treatment of thyroid carcinoma with radioactive iodine. Semin Nucl Med. 1978;8:79–94.
107. Higashi T, Nishii R, Yamada S, Nakamoto Y, Ishizu K, Kawase S, Togashi K, Itasaka S, Hiraoka M, Misaki T, Konishi J. Delayed initial radioactive iodine therapy resulted in poor survival in patients with metastatic differentiated thyroid carcinoma: a retrospective statistical analysis of 198 cases. J Nucl Med. 2011;52:683–9.
108. Reynolds JC. Comparison of I-131 absorbed radiation doses in children and adults; a tool for estimating therapeutic I-131 doses in children. In: Robbins J, editor. Treatment of thyroid cancer in children. Springfield: US Department of Commerce Technology Administration, National Technical Information Service; 1994. p. 127–35.
109. Maxon HR. Quantitative radioiodine therapy in the treatment of differentiated thyroid cancer. Q J Nucl Med. 1999;43:313–23.
110. Khan JH, McElhinney DB, Rahman SB, et al. Pulmonary metastases of endocrine origin: the role of surgery. Chest. 1998;114: 526–34.
111. Kassis AI, Adelstein SJ. Radiobiologic principles of radionuclide therapy. J Nucl Med. 2005;46:4S–12.
112. Leeper R. Controversies in the treatment of thyroid cancer: the New York Memorial Hospital approach. Thyroid Today. 1982;5:1–4.
113. Tuttle RM, Leboeuf R, Robbins RJ, et al. Empiric radioactive iodine dosing regimens frequently exceed maximum tolerated activity levels in elderly patients with thyroid cancer. J Nucl Med. 2006;47:1587–91.
114. Kulkarni K, Van Nostrand D, Atkins F, Aiken M, Burman K, Wartofsky L. The relative frequency in which empiric dosages of radioiodine would potentially overtreat or undertreat patients who have metastatic well-differentiated thyroid cancer. Thyroid. 2006;16:1019–23.
115. Esposito G, Van Nostrand D, Atkins F, Burman K, Wartofsky L, Kulkarni K. Frequency of "over" and "under" treatment with empiric dosage of I-131 in patients with and without lung metastasis secondary to well-differentiated thyroid. Cancer J Nucl Med. 2006;47(1):238P.

Treatment of Metastatic Thyroid Cancer with Radioiodine Following Preparation by Recombinant Human Thyrotropin

57

Richard J. Robbins, Leah Folb, and R. Michael Tuttle

Introduction

Complete eradication of metastatic thyroid carcinoma is difficult to achieve. This challenge is attributed to (1) the reduction in iodine uptake by thyroid cancer cells, (2) the relatively slow and unpredictable rate of progression, and (3) the generally high quality of life (QOL), even in patients with widely metastatic disease. Furthermore, relatively few studies have identified reliable predictors of the progression rate, the pattern of metastatic spread, or the sensitivity to ^{131}I therapy. Patients and their physicians often continue to administer large amounts of ^{131}I to lesions that appear iodine-avid, even in the absence of previous tumor responses. A common rationalization for this approach is that tumor progression would have been worse if another dose of ^{131}I had not been administered.

To compound this dilemma, considerable evidence suggests that thyrotropin (TSH) is a progression factor for metastatic thyroid carcinoma. Therefore, the standard management approach employs constant suppression of this pituitary hormone. Unfortunately, TSH is also the only known activator of the sodium-iodide symporter (NIS), which must be stimulated to deliver the optimal amount of ^{131}I. For many years, it has been the standard of care to withdraw patients from thyroid hormone in order to elevate endogenous TSH production, allowing TSH stimulation and possible cancer cell proliferation for 6–8 weeks. In vitro and in vivo studies provide evidence for thyroid cancer growth under TSH stimulation, and clinical examples of tumor expansion and progression have been documented in this setting [1–3].

Numerous clinicians have tried to attenuate the clinical symptoms of hypothyroidism by reducing the time of thyroid hormone withdrawal (THW) or by using triiodothyronine (T3) for a few weeks to minimize the hypothyroid state. These strategies all rely on the assumption that maximum radioiodine uptake, by neoplastic thyroid cells, occurs when the serum TSH has risen above the 25–30-mU/mL range. There is remarkably little evidence that indicates this assumption is true, despite its widespread acceptance within the community of thyroid specialists.

The advent of clinical-grade recombinant human TSH (rhTSH) provided an opportunity to examine the possibility that short-term elevations in serum TSH (i.e., 3–4 days) might enable a comparable activation of the NIS [4] in thyroid cancer tissue, without the need for prolonged TSH stimulation, which might result in disease progression. rhTSH-assisted treatment is usually given with patients taking full therapeutic doses of thyroxine (T4) following a low-iodine diet. A reduced whole-body radiation load is an additional theoretical advantage of the rhTSH approach, considering the known reduced renal iodine clearance that exists in hypothyroidism [5]. Finally, in our personal experience with thousands of thyroid cancer survivors, there is a reluctance to repeatedly withdraw from T4, because of its negative effect on their QOL [6–8]. Many patients simply choose to forgo the possible benefit of radioiodine therapy simply because they want to avoid hypothyroidism.

Immediately after the preliminary results from the phase II testing of rhTSH were announced, clinicians began requesting access to rhTSH for "unusual" patients who could not produce TSH endogenously or who were too unstable to undergo THW. Through a compassionate need program supported by the Genzyme Corporation and sanctioned by federal agencies, rhTSH (Thyrogen®) was made available to physicians on a case-by-case basis in April 1995.

R.J. Robbins, MD (✉)
Chairman, Department of Medicine, The Methodist Hospital, 6550 Fannin Street Suite SM 1001, Houston, TX 77030, USA
e-mail: rjrobbins@tmhs.org

L. Folb, MD
Endocrinology, Medical Clinic of Houston, L.L.P., 1701 Sunset Blvd., Houston, TX 77005, USA

R.M. Tuttle, MD
Department of Medicine, Memorial Sloan Kettering Cancer Center, 1275 York Ave, New York, NY 10021, USA
e-mail: tuttlem@mskcc.org

L. Wartofsky, D. Van Nostrand (eds.), *Thyroid Cancer*, DOI 10.1007/978-1-4939-3314-3_57

Case Reports (Table 57.1)

The first evidence that rhTSH could be used to stimulate ^{131}I uptake in metastatic lesions was presented at the annual meeting of the American Thyroid Association in November 1996 [9]. All four patients in this preliminary report remained on TSH suppressive doses of T4 throughout testing and therapy. Uptake of ^{131}I into metastatic lesions was demonstrated on post-therapy scans in all four patients. The initial published report on rhTSH-assisted ^{131}I therapy of metastatic thyroid carcinoma was by Rudavsky and Freedman [10]. These physicians also showed that rhTSH could substitute for endogenously produced TSH and stimulate the uptake of ^{131}I into lung and bone metastases in one patient. Their patient received 515 mCi of ^{131}I 24 h after the second of two daily 0.9-mg injections of rhTSH. Within 2 weeks, the patient had a substantial reduction in bone pain related to his metastases. His serum thyroglobulin (Tg) level fell from 7,800 ng/mL to 1,924 ng/mL over a 4-months interval. Subsequent to this report, many clinicians and investigators began to apply this approach to selected patients. Chiu et al. [1] administered 200 mCi of ^{131}I following two 0.9-mg doses of rhTSH to treat brain metastases in a patient with a tall-cell variant of papillary thyroid carcinoma and demonstrated uptake of the isotope into the lesions.

Adler et al. [2] reported that rhTSH could stimulate uptake of a therapeutic dose of ^{131}I into the brain, spine, and lung metastases. One patient had central TSH deficiency. Improvement in the lung metastases was observed in one patient. Colleran and Burge [11] reported on the use of rhTSH for a patient whose TSH level did not elevate following 7 weeks of THW, despite being clinically hypothyroid. Magnetic resonance imaging (MRI) of the pituitary revealed an empty sella. rhTSH was then used to stimulate ^{131}I uptake. Rotman-Pikielny et al. [12] used rhTSH to assist ^{131}I therapy in a patient with functioning hepatic metastases, which prevented an elevation of TSH after THW. A partial reduction in liver metastases was found 6 months after therapy.

Perros [3] reported on a patient with unstable angina who sustained a myocardial infarction following THW in preparation for radioiodine therapy for follicular thyroid carcinoma. rhTSH was then used to prepare the patient for ^{131}I administration, without any adverse cardiovascular events, on two different occasions. Risse et al. and Masiukiewicz et al. [13, 14] both reported on the use of rhTSH to assist in ^{131}I therapy of patients with hypopituitarism from thyroid cancer involvement of the pituitary gland. Vargas et al. [15] also reviewed a patient with thyroid cancer involving the pituitary region. Unfortunately, in this case, rapid expansion of the lesion following rhTSH was associated with the onset of hemiplegia. After 4 days, the patient received 304 mCi of ^{131}I. A follow-up MRI scan 2 years later documented a reduction in the size of the pituitary mass.

Mazzaferri and Kloos [16] described a patient with papillary thyroid cancer and end-stage renal failure who could not tolerate hypothyroidism. Following two doses of rhTSH, the patient was treated with ^{131}I, and the post-therapy scan revealed uptake in lung metastases that was not seen on chest X-ray. Robbins et al. [17] reported a patient with follicular thyroid cancer who developed rapid expansion of a previously undiagnosed brain metastasis associated with hemiplegia after two rhTSH injections. The patient demonstrated good uptake of ^{131}I in lung, bone, and central nervous system lesions. This patient was treated on two subsequent occasions with the assistance of rhTSH and glucocorticoids and had no neurologic complications. Aslam and Daly [18] reported on a 62-year-old man treated with radioactive iodine for widely metastatic papillary thyroid cancer that was

Table 57.1 Individual case reports of rhTSH as preparation for radioiodine therapy

Author	Metastatic sites	131i(mCi)	Side effects	Outcome
Rudavsky	Lung, bone	515	Vomiting	PR
Chiu	Brain	200	NA	NA
Adler	Brain, lung, bone	434–506	Bone pain	PR
Colleran	Neck	150	NA	NA
Perros	Neck	135, 141	None	PR
Risse	Pituitary	0	None	Not treated
Masiukiewicz	Pituitary	200	NA	NA
Vargas	Brain	304	Hemiplegia	PR
Mazzaferri	Lung	100–140	NA	PR
Robbins	Brain	154	Papilledema	PR
Rotman	Liver	65	Nausea	PR
Aslam	C-spine, neck, mediastinum	209	NA	NA
Serafini	Orbit	207	NA	NA
Goffman	Lung, neck	157	Vomiting, dyspnea	PR

PR partial response, *NA* not available

enabled by rhTSH. Serafini et al. [19] reported on a woman with papillary thyroid cancer who was unable to tolerate hypothyroidism because of severe generalized malaise. On multiple occasions, she refused to be withdrawn from thyroid hormone, and rhTSH was used to prepare her for a therapeutic dose of ^{131}I. The post-therapy scan revealed radioiodine uptake in the thyroid bed region and disclosed a new metastatic lesion in her left orbit. Finally, Goffman et al. [20] analyzed a patient with diffuse lung metastases who was considered too ill to undergo THW as preparation for ^{131}I treatment. After two rhTSH injections, she developed moderate swelling of her neck lesions and dyspnea. She then received 157 mCi of ^{131}I; 2 days later, she developed severe respiratory failure, necessitating oxygen, steroids, and antibiotics. She gradually improved, and her serum Tg level declined. The sudden deterioration in pulmonary function was thought to be most likely the result of lesional edema, partly owing to the direct effect of rhTSH. Although these reports describe a diverse set of patients and circumstances, they have established that following rhTSH:

1. Serum TSH is reliably elevated considerably higher than 30 mIU/L.
2. Uptake of radioiodine is routinely demonstrated on post-therapy scans.
3. Although rhTSH is generally well-tolerated, large metastatic lesions can rapidly swell, causing neurological, respiratory, or painful events.
4. The vast majority of patients experience no symptoms of hypothyroidism.
5. Evidence of partial response to radioiodine or stabilization of disease is often realized.

However, individual case reports do not provide the full perspective of the possible risks and benefits of this approach that become evident in larger standardized trials.

Larger Series: Initial Results (Table 57.2)

From Wurzburg, Germany, Luster et al. [21] reported their observations in ten patients with advanced metastatic thyroid carcinoma who were treated with ^{131}I after rhTSH preparation, according to a standard protocol. Patients were offered this option because of the inability to produce sufficient TSH or because of a medical contraindication to hypothyroidism. Each patient received two daily 0.9-mg rhTSH injections, and the therapeutic administration of ^{131}I was given on the third day. T4 therapy was continued throughout the procedure. Those with brain or spinal cord metastases received high-dose steroids to prevent lesion edema. At follow-up (a mean of 4.3 months), three patients had died of progressive disease. Six of the eight surviving patients had evidence of partial responses, as indicated by reductions (at least 30 % lower than baseline) in serum Tg, and the other two were stable. No major adverse events occurred; however, headache ($n=2$), bone pain ($n=1$), fever ($n=1$), and rash ($n=1$) were reported. The authors concluded that this approach was a reasonable alternative to THW in selected patients.

Mariani et al. [22] administered ^{131}I to eight thyroid cancer survivors after preparation with rhTSH, which was administered as two 0.9-mg injections per day, and the ^{131}I was administered on day 3. Post-therapy scans showed considerable radioiodine uptake in residual disease in seven of the eight patients, but no long-term follow-up data was available to analyze its efficacy. Lippi et al. from Pisa, Italy, [23] used rhTSH-assisted ^{131}I therapy for 12 patients who had differentiated thyroid carcinoma and residual metastatic disease. They used two 0.9-mg injections of rhTSH for a 4-mCi diagnostic whole-body scan (WBS), then two more injections of rhTSH within 1 week to prepare for ^{131}I therapy, which was given 24 h following the last rhTSH injection. Based on published data suggesting that blood clearance rates of iodine were 50 % slower in hypothyroid patients, they doubled their usual activity administered to compensate. Serum TSH levels rose to over 100 mIU/L in all patients. The post-therapy WBS showed radioiodine uptake into metastatic lesions in all as well. Despite relatively advanced disease and previous high doses of ^{131}I, four of ten evaluable patients had a reduction in their serum Tg. Although this approach was well-tolerated, two patients had swelling and pain in bone lesions, similar to their past experience when withdrawn from T4. As in other reports, nausea and fever in low levels were also present. The authors concluded that rhTSH-assisted treatment of metastatic thyroid carcinoma was a safe method to administer ^{131}I, preventing the debilitating effects of hypothyroidism. Berg et al. [24] also investigated the safety and efficacy of rhTSH-treated ^{131}I in 11 frail thyroid cancer patients. Patients remained on T4 and were placed on a low-iodine diet for the 2 weeks prior to therapy. After two daily 0.9-mg injections of rhTSH, the patients each received approximately 108 mCi of ^{131}I. Of the 11 patients, 8 were being treated for metastatic disease. Five of the eight patients showed partial response to the therapy, two showed no response, and one is under surveillance. The rhTSH was well tolerated, with the exception of two patients who developed lesional swelling, one with nausea and the other with bone pain. No serious adverse events occurred. The authors concluded that rhTSH-assisted ^{131}I was safe and feasible in frail elderly patients and that it offered a means to reasonable palliative therapy for those with widely metastatic disease.

De Keizer et al. [25] applied this same strategy in 16 patients who underwent 19 rhTSH-administered ^{131}I treatments for metastatic disease. All patients had total thyroidectomy with radioiodine remnant ablation and were

Table 57.2 Reports of larger series of patients who received rhTSH-assisted therapy

Author	rhTSH schedule	131I administered	Side effects	Outcomes
Luster	0.9 mg IM 48 and 24 h prior	27–200 mCi	Headache, bone pain	PR: 5
				POD: 5
Mariani	0.9 mg IM 48 and 24 h prior	NA	Mild nausea, malaise	NA
Lippi	0.9 mg IM four doses prior	100 MBq/kg	Bone pain, nausea, fever	PR: 4
				Stable: 2
				POD: 4
Berg	0.9 mg IM 48 and 24 h prior	108 mCi	Nausea, bone pain	PR: 5
				NR: 2
De Keizer	0.9 mg IM 48 and 24 h prior	200 mCi	None	PR: 3
				Stable: 2
				POD: 6
Jarzab	0.9 mg IM 48 and 24 h prior	100–200 mCi	Bone pain, lesion edema,	CR: 1
			Paresthesiae, rash	PR: 12
				Stable: 19
				POD: 15

CR complete response, *PR* partial response; *stable* stable disease, *POD* progression of disease, *NR* no response, *IM* intramuscular

being treated for residual cancer. Patients were on a low-iodine diet and received two daily 0.9-mg injections of rhTSH, then ^{131}I on day 3. The radiation to individual lesions was estimated by post-therapy scanning techniques. Tumor response was solely based on changes in serum Tg. In 11 evaluable treatments, a partial Tg response occurred in 27 %, stable disease in 18 %, and progression of disease was seen in 55 %. None of those whose disease progressed received a lesion dose of more than 30 Gy. The treatments were well tolerated, with only one patient showing spinal cord compression that responded to corticosteroid administration. The authors thought that this approach was reasonable for those with advanced disease who were not good candidates for THW.

The largest report yet on this strategy is from Jarzab et al. [26]. They used rhTSH-assisted ^{131}I therapy in 54 patients who, with a few exceptions, had a total thyroidectomy and radioiodine remnant ablation. Only 31 of the patients had radioiodine-avid metastases. Those with nonfunctional metastases were given retinoic acid prior to the rhTSH to determine if they could reinduce radioiodine avidity. All patients received twice-daily 0.9-mg rhTSH injections, followed by ^{131}I on day 3 (median, 100 mCi; range, 100–250 mCi). They were not placed on low-iodine diets. The patients who qualified for this trial had a large amount of residual cancer that was considered at risk for growth during a prolonged THW preparation. A total of 18 patients were considered to have insufficient endogenous TSH production. In 49 patients, the serum TSH at the time of treatment was significantly higher after rhTSH than in previous THW treatments (mean, 190 mIU/L vs 70 mIU/L). Bone pain occurred in 25 % of those with known bone metastases. Tumor edema in the neck was seen in three patients, tachycardia in five, and a rash occurred in two. Of 47 evaluable patients at 6-month follow-up, these investigators found 1 who had a complete response to ^{131}I treatment, 12 (26 %) had partial responses, 19 (40 %) had stable disease, 15 (32 %) had progression of disease, and 5 patients died. Of the subset ($n=20$) with non-radioiodine-avid disease following retinoids, 2 had partial responses, 11 had stable disease, and 7 had progression. In 34 patients, there was a 46 % reduction in the median serum Tg; however, this did not have statistical significance. There were 44 patients who had a previous THW-assisted ^{131}I therapy, allowing outcomes to be compared between the two methods of preparation, where patients served as their own controls. The early outcomes were found to be identical in 52 %, better after rhTSH in 32 %, and inferior following rhTSH in 16 %, compared to preparation by THW. The authors concluded that rhTSH-administered ^{131}I therapy of metastatic thyroid cancer was safe and as equally effective as THW.

Robbins et al. [27] published a retrospective experience of rhTSH-assisted RAI therapy in patients with metastatic thyroid cancer from the USA and Canada. All 115 of these patients were judged unable to produce TSH or were too medically unstable to be withdrawn from thyroid hormone. Formal evaluations were done every 3 months up to 1 year. At the 1-year time point, 73 % of the patients had decreased or undetectable serum Tg levels; overall cancer-related symptoms were judged to be improved in 24 % and stable in another 54 %. Only 2 of the 115 patients were felt to have suffered a serious adverse event related to rhTSH. Overall, many of these patients, who had no other means of receiving radioiodine therapy, benefited by the ability to use rhTSH as a preparation for radioiodine.

In aggregate, these larger series provide a clear sense that rhTSH preparation can stimulate radioiodine uptake in metastatic lesions, that the approach is generally safe, that many patients actually benefit from additional radioiodine treatment, and that steroid pretreatment should be considered in any lesions of the bone, pleura, or the central nervous system, to prevent sudden swelling. These reports also show that partial responses and/or disease stabilization is the most common short-term outcome.

Larger Series: Intermediate-Term Outcomes

Tala et al. [28] published a retrospective study on overall survival in a cohort of 175 thyroid cancer patients who were treated with high-dose radioiodine for lung and/or bone metastases. Radioiodine was administered following THW only in 35 patients; 82 patients had their initial radioiodine treatment following THW and all subsequent treatments following rhTSH preparation, while 58 of the patients received all of their radioiodine treatments following rhTSH preparation. rhTSH-prepared patients received an average of four injections of 0.9 mg rhTSH in the 2 weeks prior to a therapeutic dose of radioiodine. These patients also received the largest safe dose of ^{131}I based on formal dosimetry. After a median of 5.5 years of follow-up, there were no significant differences in overall survival among the three groups. Overall 5-survival was in the 75–80 % range. Most recently, Klubo-Gwiezdzinska et al. [29] reported a retrospective study on 56 thyroid cancer survivors who had distant metastases. Forty one patients received dosimetry-based amounts of radioiodine following THW and 15 following rhTSH preparation. Clinical features were comparable between the groups. After a mean of 72 months of follow-up, they found no differences between the two groups in rates of complete response, stable disease, or progression-free survival. Rates of adverse effects of the radioiodine were also similar between the two groups. They concluded that similar benefits occurred regardless of the method of preparation for radioiodine treatment.

Summary

The international use of rhTSH to prepare thyroid cancer patients for high-dose ^{131}I therapy of metastatic disease is growing. Given the small number of patients who die each year of thyroid cancer, it is unlikely that any federal agencies will support research analyzing the rhTSH preparation vs. THW preparation. Second, it is unlikely that any single center has sufficient patients to answer the many questions that have been raised. Therefore, it is time for leaders in the field to develop a set of guidelines regarding the appropriate use of this approach and design multicentered trials to quantify the safety and efficacy of rhTSH preparation in comparison to the traditional method of thyroid hormone withdrawal.

Issues that need to be carefully addressed include:

1. What are the optimum rhTSH doses and schedules for rhTSH-assisted ^{131}I therapy? Some studies utilize four 0.9-mg injections just prior to therapy, whereas others use only two.
2. Should strict low-iodine diets be routinely employed and should patients continue taking T4 immediately preceding the administration of ^{131}I?
3. Uniform criteria should be established to define complete and partial responses, stability, and progression of disease. A consensus on this point among the leaders in the field would be valuable, as research on this approach moves forward.
4. It is clear that radioiodine clearance from blood and bodily tissues is not the same in the hypothyroid state when compared to the slightly hyperthyroid state. The differences between blood and lesional clearance should be more carefully defined so that investigators can agree whether to adjust the therapeutic administered activity of ^{131}I. The use of ^{124}I dosimetry with PET/CT scanning may enable the determination of the exact amount of radiation that can be delivered to a specific lesion.
5. Additional studies examining longer monitoring periods (5–10 years) will be necessary before concluding that rhTSH preparation is comparable to thyroid hormone withdrawal as an adjunct to radioiodine therapy in patients with distant metastases.
6. The incidence of adverse effects should be prospectively studied in a randomized controlled trial of rhTSH preparation vs. T4 withdrawal. The evidence that repeated episodes of prolonged serum TSH elevations may foster tumor progression is only referred to anecdotally in the literature.

References

1. Chiu AC, Delpassand ES, Sherman SI. Prognosis and treatment of brain metastases in thyroid carcinoma. J Clin Endocrinol Metab. 1997;82:3637–42.
2. Adler M, Macapinlac HA, Robbins RJ. Radioiodine treatment of thyroid cancer with the aid of recombinant human thyrotropin. Endocr Pract. 1998;4:282–6.
3. Perros P. Recombinant human thyroid-stimulating hormone (rhTSH) in the radioablation of well-differentiated thyroid cancer: preliminary therapeutic experience. J Endocrinol Invest. 1999;22:30–4.
4. Dai G, Levy O, Carrasco N. Cloning and characterization of the thyroid iodide transporter. Nature. 1996;379:458–60.
5. Villabona C, Sahun M, Roca M, et al. Blood volumes and renal function in overt and subclinical primary hypothyroidism. Am J Med Sci. 1999;318:277–80.

6. Cohen O, Dabhi S, Karasik A, Zila ZS. Compliance with followup and the informative value of diagnostic whole-body scan in patients with differentiated thyroid carcinoma given recombinant human TSH. Eur J Endocrinol. 2004;150:285–90.
7. Reiners C, Lassmann M, Luster M. Recombinant human thyrotropin: safety and quality of life evaluation. J Endocrinol Invest. 2012;35(6 Suppl):30–5.
8. Klubo-Gwiezdzinska J, Burman KD, Van Nostrand D, et al. Potential use of recombinant human thyrotropin in the treatment of distant metastases in patients with differentiated thyroid cancer. Endocr Pract. 2012;27:1–26.
9. Robbins R, Macapinlac H, Yeung H, Larson S. 131-Iodine therapy of metastatic thyroid cancer with the aid of human recombinant TSH. Thyroid. 1996;6:S1–6.
10. Rudavsky AZ, Freeman LM. Treatment of scan-negative, thyroglobulin positive metastatic thyroid cancer using radioiodine 131I and recombinant human thyroid stimulating hormone. J Clin Endocrinol Metab. 1997;82:11–4.
11. Colleran KM, Burge MR. Isolated thyrotropin deficiency secondary to primary empty sella in a patient with differentiated thyroid carcinoma: an indication for recombinant thyrotropin. Thyroid. 1999;9:1249–52.
12. Rotman-Pikielny P, Reynolds JC, Barker WC, et al. Recombinant human thyrotropin for the diagnosis and treatment of a highly functional metastatic struma ovarii. J Clin Endocrinol Metab. 2000;85:237–44.
13. Risse JH, Grunwald F, Bender H, et al. Recombinant human thyrotropin in thyroid cancer and hypopituitarism due to sella metastasis. Thyroid. 1999;9:1253–6.
14. Masiukiewicz US, Nakchbandi IA, Stewart AF, Inzucchi SE. Papillary thyroid carcinoma metastatic to the pituitary gland. Thyroid. 1999;9:1023–7.
15. Vargas GE, Uy H, Bazan C, et al. Hemiplegia after thyrotropin alfa in a hypothyroid patient with thyroid carcinoma metastatic to the brain. J Clin Endocrinol Metab. 1999;84:3867–71.
16. Mazzaferri EL, Kloos RT. Using recombinant human TSH in the management of well-differentiated thyroid cancer: current strategies and future directions. Thyroid. 2000;10:767–78.
17. Robbins RJ, Voelker E, Wang W, et al. Compassionate use of recombinant human thyrotropin to facilitate radioiodine therapy: case report and review of literature. Endocr Pract. 2000;6:460–4.
18. Aslam SN, Daly RG. Use of recombinant human thyrotropin in a complicated case of metastatic papillary thyroid carcinoma. Endocr Pract. 2001;7:99–101.
19. Serafini AN, Clauss RP, Levis-Dusseau S. Protocol for the combined diagnostic and therapeutic use of recombinant human thyroid stimulating hormone. Clin Nucl Med. 2003;28:14–7.
20. Goffman T, Ioffe V, Tuttle M, et al. Near-lethal respiratory failure after recombinant human thyroid-stimulating hormone use in a patient with metastatic thyroid carcinoma. Thyroid. 2003; 13:827–30.
21. Luster M, Lassmann M, Haenscheid H, et al. Use of recombinant human thyrotropin before radioiodine therapy in patients with advanced differentiated thyroid carcinoma. J Clin Endocrinol Metab. 2000;85:3640–5.
22. Mariani G, Ferdeghini M, Augeri C, et al. Clinical experience with recombinant human thyrotrophin (rhTSH) in the management of patients with differentiated thyroid cancer. Cancer Biother Radiopharm. 2000;15:211–7.
23. Lippi F, Capezzone M, Angelini F, et al. Radioiodine treatment of metastatic differentiated thyroid cancer in patients on L-thyroxine, using recombinant human TSH. Eur J Endocrinol. 2001;144:5–11.
24. Berg G, Lindstedt G, Suurkula M, Jansson S. Radioiodine ablation and therapy in differentiated thyroid cancer under stimulation with recombinant human thyroid-stimulating hormone. J Endocrinol Invest. 2002;25:44–52.
25. de Keizer B, Brans B, Hoekstra A, et al. Tumour dosimetry and response in patients with metastatic differentiated thyroid cancer using recombinant human thyrotropin before radioiodine therapy. Eur J Nucl Med Mol Imaging. 2003;30:367–73.
26. Jarzab B, Handkiewicz-Junak D, Roskosz J, et al. Recombinant human TSH-aided radioiodine treatment of advanced differentiated thyroid carcinoma: a single-centre study of 54 patients. Eur J Nucl Med Mol Imaging. 2003;30:1077–86.
27. Robbins RJ, Driedger A, Magner J, et al. Recombinant human thyrotropin-assisted radioiodine therapy for patients with metastatic thyroid cancer who could not elevate endogenous thyrotropin or be withdrawn from thyroxine. Thyroid. 2006;16:1121–30.
28. Tala H, Robbins R, Fagin JA, et al. Five-year survival is similar in thyroid cancer patients with distant metastases prepared for radioactive iodine therapy with either thyroid hormone withdrawal or recombinant human TSH. J Clin Endocrinol Metab. 2011;96:2105–11.
29. Klubo-Gwiezdzinska J, Burman KD, Van Nostrand D, et al. Radioiodine treatment of metastatic thyroid cancer: relative efficacy and side effect profile of preparation by thyroid hormone withdrawal versus recombinant human thyrotropin. Thyroid. 2012;22:310–7.

Dosimetrically Determined Prescribed Activity of ^{131}I for the Treatment of Metastatic Differentiated Thyroid Carcinoma

58

Frank B. Atkins, Douglas Van Nostrand, and Leonard Wartofsky

Introduction

Although a favorable prognosis is typically associated with differentiated thyroid carcinoma, this is not necessarily the case for metastatic differentiated thyroid carcinoma (DTC) [1]. Consequently, modifications to the therapeutic approach, particularly with ^{131}I, may be required to achieve better outcomes in patients with metastatic DTC. ^{131}I was first shown to localize in metastatic DTC over half a century ago [2] and has been used extensively since then in the management of these patients [1, 3–5].

However, there is no consensus among clinicians managing these patients regarding what constitutes an appropriate ^{131}I prescribed activity[1] for the treatment of metastatic DTC. Several approaches to select a therapeutic prescribed activity of ^{131}I have been advocated. These can be broadly classified into two groups: (1) "empiric fixed prescribed activity" and (2) "dosimetrically determined prescribed activity." Given the heterogeneity of thyroid cancer patients, the same empiric fixed prescribed activity may not be appropriate for all patients. This chapter reviews the rationale and technique for "dosimetrically determined" prescribed activity of ^{131}I for the treatment of metastatic DTC and discusses (1) the alternatives for selection of a prescribed activity, (2) the two most common approaches for dosimetrically determining ^{131}I prescribed activity, (3) several modifications of these approaches that have been implemented over time, and (4) an overview of the literature regarding the results. The chapter then concludes with general recommendations for patient management regarding the use of dosimetry. This review does not address the use of dosimetrically determined prescribed activity of ^{131}I for the remnant ablation or adjuvant treatment. For definitions and objectives of remnant ablation, adjuvant treatment, and treatment of distant metastases, see Chaps. 33 and 34.

Empiric Fixed Prescribed Activity

Many excellent reviews of empiric fixed prescribed activity have been previously published [1, 4, 6–10]. One of the most frequently used and early guidelines for empiric fixed prescribed activities was proposed by Beierwaltes [3] and is summarized in Table 58.1. With this approach, the fixed prescribed activities are typically in the range of 5.55–7.4 GBq (150–200 mCi). However, both smaller and larger prescribed activities have also been proposed and used in practice [11, 12]. Some investigators have used repeated moderate levels of prescribed activities over short time intervals. For example, Schlumberger et al. used an initial prescribed activity of 3.7 GBq (100 mCi) of ^{131}I to treat metastasis of the lung and bone, which might be repeated every 3–6 months. The cumu-

[1]Many authors have used the word "dose" to refer either to the amount of a radiopharmaceutical to be administered for a diagnostic scan, ablation, or treatment in units of Bq (mCi) or to the amount of radiation exposure to an organ or patient in units of cGy (rad). Because this may result in confusion, the authors have used the words "prescribed activity" and "dosage" to refer to the amount of a radiopharmaceutical for diagnostic scan, remnant ablation, adjuvant treatment, and treatment of known metastases while reserving the term "dose" for the radiation exposure.

F.B. Atkins, PhD (✉)
Division, Nuclear Medicine, MedStar Washington Hospital Center, Georgetown University School of Medicine, 110 Irving Street, NW, Room GB01, Washington, DC 20010, USA
e-mail: Francis.B.Atkins@Medstar.net

D. Van Nostrand, MD, FACP, FACNM
Nuclear Medicine Research, MedStar Research Institute and Washington Hospital Center, Georgetown University School of Medicine, Washington Hospital Center, 110 Irving Street, N.W., Suite GB 60F, Washington, DC 20010, USA
e-mail: douglasvannostrand@gmail.com

L. Wartofsky, MD, MACP
Department of Medicine, MedStar Washington Hospital Center, Georgetown University School of Medicine, 110 Irving Street, N.W., Washington, DC 20010-2975, USA
e-mail: leonard.wartofsky@medstar.net

L. Wartofsky, D. Van Nostrand (eds.), *Thyroid Cancer*, DOI 10.1007/978-1-4939-3314-3_58

Table 58.1 Empiric fixed prescribed activity

Regional nodes that cannot be removed by surgery	5.6–6.5 GBq (150–175 mCi)
Pulmonary metastasis	6.5–7.4 GBq (175–200 mCi)
Bone metastasis	7.4 GBq (200 mCi)

Source: Ref. [3]

lative ^{131}I prescribed activity in this group of patients ranged from 2 to 55.5 GBq (54–1,500 mCi), with a mean of 12.5 GBq (339 mCi [±281 mCi]) [11]. Menzel adopted a more aggressive approach, employing an empiric fixed prescribed activity of 11.1 GBq (300 mCi), with intervals as short as 3 months [12]. Further discussion of the spectrum of empiric prescribed activity is discussed in Chap. 56.

"Dosimetrically Determined" Prescribed Activity

Although the simplicity of a set of empiric fixed prescribed activities is appealing and convenient, the wide spectrum of proposed protocols of empiric fixed prescribed activity with no data to show which protocol is better and the persistence of disease in a significant proportion of patients have led to attempts to improve the empiric approach to ^{131}I therapy. The ideal prescribed activity of ^{131}I to treat metastatic DTC is based on the minimum amount of ^{131}I needed to successfully treat the patient's metastases without resulting in unacceptable side effects or risks. Efforts to meet this goal have led to two major approaches, each of which addresses a different aspect of this problem. Benua et al. developed an approach based on determining the maximum activity of ^{131}I that could be administered without causing significant bone marrow suppression [13]. Thomas and Maxon developed a method to evaluate the amount of ^{131}I needed to adequately treat metastatic lymph nodes [14]. This section discusses the two basic approaches of dosimetrically determined prescribed activity and begins with a brief review of the principles involved to better understand the rationale for and the potential greater efficacy of the dosimetric approaches.

Background

Dosimetry

The term *dosimetry* has been used in a variety of contexts. It has been most commonly employed in the area of radiation oncology to describe the methodology and analysis used to calculate a treatment plan designed to deliver a prescribed radiation dose to the patient's tumor using external radiation. Within radiation safety programs and services, it has been used to describe the *monitoring* of the exposure of individuals from internal and external radiation hazards within a working environment. Finally, regarding thyroid cancer therapy with radionuclides, this terminology has been used in two contexts: (1) the calculation of a maximum tolerated activity (MTA) of ^{131}I that can be administered to a given patient, which would not exceed some empirically determined radiation dose to the blood or blood-forming components, and (2) the calculation of the radiation dose that would deliver (or has been delivered) to individually identifiable and quantifiable foci of remnant thyroid tissue or metastatic lesions. The latter conforms more closely with the traditional usage of this term within the radiation oncology community because it applies to the calculation of the dose specifically for the cancer being treated. However, just as in the case of external radiation therapy, it is the radiation dose delivered to the patient's normal tissues that frequently limits the maximum tumor dose. With ^{131}I therapy, the most radiosensitive organ of greatest concern is the patient's bone marrow.

Internal Radiation Dosimetry

When ionizing radiation is absorbed in living tissues, it can cause cellular damage because of the energy that is deposited. Different cell types will respond differently to the same amount of absorbed radiation. Nevertheless, one of the most important parameters used in the assessment of the radiation effects on any particular organ is the amount of energy deposited by the radionuclide in that organ. This calculation has come to be referred to as *internal radiation dosimetry*. When radionuclides were first used for medical purposes, at best, this type of information was fragmented. Consequently, conservative estimates were used to estimate the order of magnitude of the radiation absorbed dose to the body and other critical organs that resulted from the administration of a radionuclide. This radiation absorbed dose (to be distinguished from prescribed activity previously noted) is expressed in units of centigray (rad), which is a measure of the total amount of energy deposited per gram of tissue by all the radiation types emitted by the radionuclide. To perform this calculation, we need to know detailed information about (1) the types of radiation emitted in each disintegration (i.e., charged particles or photons), their relative abundance, and their energy; (2) how many disintegrations occur in each organ; and (3) what fraction of the energy of each radiation type that is released in any given organ is absorbed in another organ (including itself). The nuclear decay data required for the first issue can be found in the physics literature [15] based on experimental measurements performed in the laboratory. The second issue requires detailed knowledge about the uptake and clearance of the radionuclide in various organs within the patient. The third issue requires knowledge not only of the absorption and penetration characteristics of the various radiations emitted but also the size, shape, volume, and geometrical arrangements of the various organs within the patient. Ideally, direct measurements of the absorbed dose at relevant locations within each patient would be best, but this is nearly impossible. Thus, we are instead restricted to theoretical estimates according to models and measurements performed using standardized humanoid phantoms.

Classical Dosimetry

The so-called classical dosimetry method was first published in 1948 by Marinelli et al. [16]. This was refined in 1956 by Loevinger et al. [17] and soon became the standard method [18] for calculating the radiation absorbed dose from internal sources. Because charged particles (i.e., β radiation) typically only travel a few millimeters in tissue, it is generally assumed that all the energy carried by this type of radiation is locally absorbed in the organ in which the radioactive decay occurs. In the case of ^{131}I, the maximum range of β particles in tissue [19] is 2.4 mm with most traveling substantially less than this distance. The model developed by Loevinger addressed the more penetrating radiation: the γ emissions. Therefore, the radiation absorbed dose from the two components (penetrating and nonpenetrating) can be expressed as

$$D_{\beta} = 73.8C < E_{\beta} > T_{e}$$

$$D_{\gamma} = 0.0346C\,\Gamma\,gT_{e}$$

where C is the initial concentration of the radionuclide in the organ (μCi/g), $<E_{\beta}>$ is the mean energy of the β radiation, Γ is the exposure rate constant specific to ^{131}I, T_e is the effective half-life in days, and g is a geometric factor to account for variations in the organ's size, shape, and volume. The constants that appear in these equations are conversion factors, such that the dose is expressed in units of centigray (rad).

Medical Internal Radiation Dose Schema

The medical internal radiation dose (MIRD) methodology was developed by a committee within the Society of Nuclear Medicine and Molecular Imaging to provide a more sophisticated approach for calculating the radiation dose to various organs from radionuclides that are internally deposited and accumulate in other organs. The initial models were released in the mid-1970s [20] and continue to be expanded and refined with the publication of new pamphlets. A review of the basic concepts and recent developments in internal radionuclide radiation dosimetry has been published [21]. This formulation simplified the calculation of radiation absorbed dose to varying organs within the patient by separating biological parameters that describe the uptake and clearance, along with physical decay from the details of energy absorption of the radiation released in each decay. All the absorption characteristics have been lumped into a single quantity: the "S" factor. These "S" factors incorporate (1) the details of the types and energies of the radiations emitted (e.g., how many, how much energy, what type); (2) the size and shape of the organ in which the radionuclide is distributed; (3) the size, shape, and geometrical relationship of any other organ within the patient; and (4) the fraction of energy from each possible emission that would be absorbed in any given organ coming from radiation that originated in any organ. Consequently, this single factor depends on the radionuclide, the organ containing the radionuclide (source), and the organ for which the dose is calculated (target). We can then express the dose to the target organ, D_t, as follows:

$D_t = \sum \tilde{A}_s S(t \leftarrow s)$ where $\tilde{A}_s$ represents the total number of decays that occur for the radionuclide in a given source organ, s. Finally, we sum the dose contributions from all the possible source organs to the target organ, indicated by $\sum$ in this equation, which can include the target organ as one of the source organs.

Dosimetry Approaches

Based on the principles outlined above, Benua et al. [13] developed an approach that set an empirically determined upper limit for the radiation absorbed dose to the patient's blood, whereas Thomas and Maxon [14] calculated the radiation absorbed dose that could be delivered to the lesion. Previous reviews are available [22–24]

Limited Bone Marrow (Benua Approach)

Keldsen et al. noted [25] that even with a relatively conservative empiric fixed prescribed activity of ^{131}I, bone marrow depression still occurs in about one quarter of all patients treated for metastatic thyroid cancer. Unfortunately, the empiric methods do not provide any information to help predict in which patients this would occur. However, the method reported by Benua et al. [13, 26] allows an estimate to be calculated for the radiation absorbed dose that will be delivered to the hematopoietic system from each GBq (or mCi) of ^{131}I administered to a given patient. This is possible because it utilizes information obtained from data collected over the course of 4 days or more following the administration of a tracer prescribed activity of ^{131}I to the patient. Considering the time period when this methodology was first developed, the dosimetry calculations were based on the classical formulations, rather than on MIRD. Furthermore, it should be emphasized that these calculations yield the radiation absorbed dose to the whole blood compartment, not directly to the bone marrow. In their study, a total of 122 administrations in 59 patients were reviewed. However, adequate data were only available to calculate a dose in 85 of these treatments. For this group, the whole blood dose ranged from 45 to 740 cGy (rad) with a mean of 267 cGy (rad), whereas the largest single prescribed activity of ^{131}I was 22.2 GBq (600 mCi). As might be expected, several serious complications and side effects occurred in this group. However, within a patient subgroup (i.e., those that received 200 cGy (rad) or less to the blood), the side effects were not as serious. Based on these observations, a protocol was implemented by Benua and Leeper at the Memorial Sloan Kettering Cancer Center (MSKCC), in which a prescribed activity for ^{131}I treatment was selected that would restrict delivery to no more than 200 cGy (rad) to the blood [27].

Description of the Benua Protocol

Regardless of the dosimetric methodology employed, a common feature is the incorporation of the ^{131}I pharmacokinetics in a given patient into the calculations. Consequently, a tracer prescribed activity of ^{131}I is first administered to the patient, and then the uptake and clearance of this radioiodine is followed for a specified time period. The form of ^{131}I (e.g., liquid or capsule) used for the dosimetry should be the same as that used for the subsequent treatment. In the classical approach, the blood is considered the critical organ, which is irradiated either from the beta particles emitted from the activity circulating in the blood itself or from the gamma emissions originating from activity dispersed throughout the remainder of the body. Therefore, only two compartments need to be monitored for radioactivity: the blood and whole body. The activity in the blood was determined from periodic 5 ml heparinized blood samples, While the activity in the whole body (i.e., the activity remaining in the patient) was monitored redundantly using two independent techniques: 24 h urine collections and whole-body counting using a single uncollimated radiation probe in a fixed geometry with respect to the patient. In this case, the patient-to-detector distance needs to be sufficiently large as to allow the activity from the entire patient while standing to be detected, with nearly the same sensitivity from head to foot. Typically, this requires distances greater than about 3 m. A 12.7 cm diameter NaI(Tl) detector was used originally, but smaller diameter probes could be used with a corresponding increase in the acquisition time to offset the reduction in sensitivity. Benua employed an energy window of ±50 keV centered on the 364-keV γ emission. Although their original investigation followed patients for at least 6 days after the tracer prescribed activity, their protocol has been modified to typically end after 4 days. Thus, a study beginning on Monday would be completed by Friday.

Data Collection

The data collected included the following:

- Blood samples (5 ml, heparinized) at 2, 4, 24, 48, 72, and 96 h
- Whole-body counts at 0, 2, 4, 24, 48, 72, and 96 h
- Total urine collection at 24, 48, 72, and 96 h
- Activity administered to patient as tracer prescribed activity (approximately 37 MBq [1 mCi])

In addition, a standard was prepared at the onset of the procedure of 37 MBq (1 mCi) of ^{131}I to normalize the whole-body counts. This was counted at a distance comparable to that of the patient in a reproducible geometry and was used throughout the 4-day monitoring period. During the initial 4 h period following the ^{131}I administration, the patient is not allowed to urinate or defecate. Under these circumstances, essentially 100 % of the prescribed activity will be contained within the patient at any time during the initial 4 h. The maximum value at 0, 2, or 4 h is then defined to represent the 100 % value, and subsequent daily measurements are normalized to this value using this formula:

$$\text{Retention}(t) = \times \frac{\text{Patientcounts}\,(t)}{\text{Standardcounts}\,(t)} \times \frac{\text{Standardcounts@MaxTime}}{\text{Patientcounts@MaxTime}} \times 100\%$$

When used in this way, the standard will correct for variations in detector sensitivity from measurement to measurement, as well as for physical decay. Absolute calibrations are not necessary, as the patient is used as his or her reference. The blood and urine samples are counted using scintillation well-detector systems. Because the activity must be established in these samples, it is necessary to make up a calibration standard that can be counted at the same time as the blood samples. This involves the addition of a carefully assayed quantity of ^{131}I (approximately 3.7–7.4 MBq [100–200 μCi]) to a total volume of 500–1,000 ml. Such a small concentration is necessary to avoid saturating the detector. An alternative might be to use a ^{133}Ba rod source that has been cross calibrated against the ^{131}I standard. With its relatively long half-life (10.5 years) and similar γ emissions, ^{133}Ba could serve as a suitable replacement for the prepared ^{131}I standard, which simplifies the protocol. At the conclusion of the data acquisition, 2 ml aliquots of whole blood, diluted or undiluted urine, and the in vitro standard are counted. Using this information, it is possible to calculate the percent of administered dose per liter of whole blood at each timed sample. A zero time point is calculated by dividing the total prescribed activity by the patient's total blood volume. However, a patient-specific blood volume is not determined but is assumed to equal 20 % of the body weight. As indicated in the section on internal radiation dosimetry, one of the factors needed in the dose calculation is the total number of disintegrations that occur in the organ over time. This is reflected in the effective half-life T_e that appears in the first two equations. This formulation assumes that the radionuclide clearance from the organ of interest follows a single exponential curve that can be characterized by the effective half-life. Alternatively, knowing the organ activity as a function of time, and because activity is a measure of disintegrations per second, then the integral (i.e., the area under this curve) is actually a measure of the total number of disintegrations. Therefore, based on this *classical* dosimetry approach, the formula to calculate the radiation absorbed dose to the whole blood follows. The calculation of the area under these two curves is based on a mathematical fit to the data points using a multiple exponential function. Because the data collection is terminated after 4 days, these curves must then be extrapolated to infinity. A conservative estimate is employed by assuming that the clearance following the final measured data point is based simply on the physical decay. Ignoring any biological clearance beyond the last time point results in an overestimate of the area of these tails and, hence, an overestimate in the radiation absorbed dose as well. The radiation absorbed dose to the blood from the beta and gamma components expressed in cGy (rad) per MBq ^{131}I administered is then given as

$$\gamma(\text{cGy / MBq}) = 0.0000141\text{g} \times [\frac{1}{Weight(kg)}] \times [area\ under\ body\ curve]$$

$$\beta(\text{cGy / MBq}) = 0.00259 \times [area\ under\ blood\ curve]$$

Examples of two patient studies are shown in Fig. 58.1; Fig. 58.1a demonstrates rapid clearance, and Fig. 58.1b shows relatively slow clearance. The *maximum treatment prescribed activity or the maximum tolerated activity* (*MTA*) is then calculated as the activity of ^{131}I that would deliver a combined β and γ dose to the blood component of 200 cGy (200 rad) and is given by

$$\text{Treatment prescribed activity(MBq)} = 200\ \text{cGy} / (\beta[\text{cGy / MBq}] + \gamma[\text{cGy / MBq}])$$

Adjustments to the Original Protocol

To improve reliability and simplify the original dosimetry protocol, several groups have introduced a number of modifications and enhancements; the more significant ones are outlined below, and additional simplified alternatives to full dosimetry are discussed in Chap. 59.

Elimination of the Urine Collection

As previously mentioned, the urine data was used as a redundant method to determine the whole-body activity as a function of time and served as a check of the probe data. The whole-body retention was inferred from the difference between the administered activity and accumulated urine activity. Consequently, there is an inherent problem with this method: any error that may have occurred at one time point is propagated throughout *all* of the following data points as well. Particularly, some potential problems are associated with this measurement, including:

- Incomplete urine collection.
- Loss of iodine through alternative pathways, principally fecal, but also sweat, saliva, respiration, and so on.
- The high concentration of activity in the first 2 days can frequently saturate a well-counter detector, such that an additional 10:1 dilution might be required to avoid dead time counting errors.
- Errors in measuring the volume for each 24 h collection.
- Pipetting errors.

The net effect is that cumulative errors as high as factors of 2–5 in specific cases [28] can occur. Removing the urine collection step, which is a significant burden for many

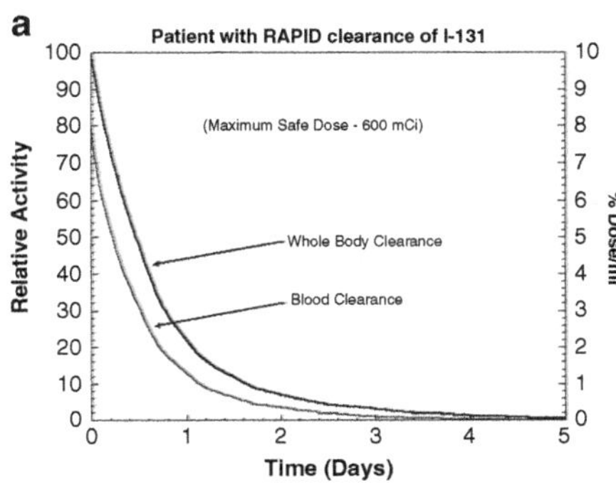

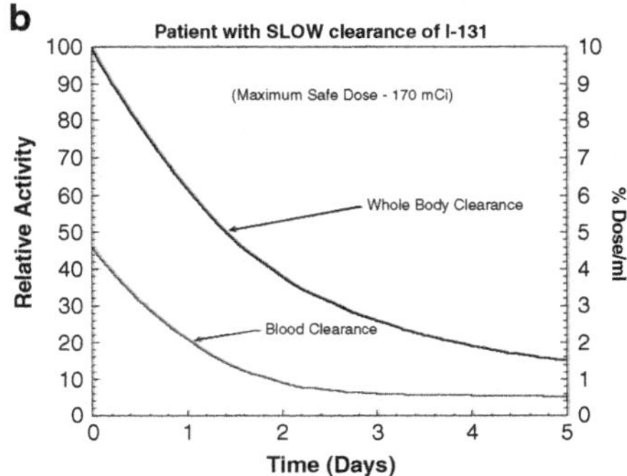

Fig. 58.1 Whole-body and blood clearance curves of ^{131}I for two dosimetry patients. In both cases, the final measured data point was determined at 4 days post-dosing. The classical dosimetry model then uses a conservative assumption of only physical decay, which can be seen as the abrupt change in the slope of the curves at this time point. The patient in **a** has rapid clearance, and little additional area under the extrapolated segment is present, which results in a calculated maximum treatment activity (MTA) of 22.6 GBq (610 mCi) to deliver 200 cGy (rad) to the blood. In contrast, in a patient with slower clearance, such as in **b**, there is a greater area under these curves, which leads to a lower calculated value for the MTA of 10.8 GBq (293 mCi)

patients, substantially reduces the complexity of this protocol by removing all the problems associated with the transport, storage, and handling of large volumes of radioactive body fluids. Furthermore, deleting the urine assay from the protocol also eliminates the possible risk to personnel due to accidental spills and radiation exposure from handling the radioactive urine. Most importantly, this simplification can be accomplished without compromising the objective.

Geometric Mean for Whole-Body Counting

A method of organ and body activity quantitation that has been widely adopted in nuclear medicine incorporates a geometric mean approach. Because the γ rays from ^{131}I are absorbed by varying amounts depending on the depth of the source in the patient, neither an anterior nor a posterior orientation alone is appropriate. This is especially the case as the radionuclide redistributes over time after the absorption from the stomach. Moreover, the geometric mean ($\sqrt{\text{ant} \times \text{post}}$) has been shown to be less sensitive to these variations [29].

Timing and Number of Data Points

Whole-body counting immediately following the ^{131}I tracer administration is generally neither practical nor useful. This is more relevant today when capsules are used instead of liquids for the isotope administration. The activity at this point in time is essentially confined to the stomach in a geometry that does not match the more diffuse body distribution at later times. In addition, a delayed sample at 4 h is inconvenient and may be difficult for the patient to avoid urinating before this measurement can be performed, which would invalidate this sample for normalization purposes. By this time (4 h), there can also be significant accumulation of activity in the bladder that can also bias this measurement. Therefore, a single data point at approximately 2 h after administration of the ^{131}I is usually sufficient for the normalization operation. Although it might seem that there is an insufficient number of time points, it has been shown [30] that a sampling scheme, such as the one outlined above, provides basically the same accuracy as more extensive sampling, at least in the case of radioimmunotherapy. The last data point is also collected at approximately 96 h post-administration of the tracer activity, provided that the whole-body retention at this time is approximately 4 % or less. If not, then an additional measurement may be performed on the following Monday (i.e., day 7).

Whole-Body Counting Using the γ Camera

As an alternative to using an external probe to measure whole-body retention, a dual detector γ camera system can be used. In this case, the patient is scanned in the whole-body mode in a reproducible geometry while lying supine on the imaging table. This method has been generally accepted for patient-specific whole-body dosimetry of ^{131}I-radiolabeled antibodies [31]. Furthermore, it has been shown to yield results comparable to those obtained using an external probe [32]. This technique has the following features:

- Simultaneous anterior and posterior images using a high-energy collimator.
- Table height, detector radii, scan length, scan speed, and energy window are standardized and reproduced for each data point.
- Scan speed can be relatively rapid (typically 30 cm/min) to complete the data acquisition in approximately 8 min and is comparable to the time required using an external probe.
- Additional scans are performed each day for background and a counting standard (vial containing about 37 MBq [1 mCi] of ^{131}I).
- Total counts in the image or fixed regions of interest encompassing the entire body are used for the calculation of whole-body retention.

Although these images are not used for diagnostic purposes, this approach has the added advantage that if for some reason there is delayed absorption of the tracer in the stomach, then the measurement could be repeated after 4 h. There are other advantages when using this technique over the probe in the dosimetry protocol. This method is easier for patients who are unable to stand for the 5–10 min, which is needed when using a probe. More importantly, it utilizes space and equipment normally found in most nuclear medicine laboratories. In most centers, a radiation probe that can be dedicated to this purpose is not available; hence, a standard thyroid uptake probe is used. These detectors typically have only a 1 in. diameter, and their geometric efficiency is therefore only 1/25 of that of the 5 in. detector used by Benua and Leeper. It is also frequently difficult to locate space where there is an unobstructed area that the probe and patient can be positioned with the required minimum separation of about 3 m. A revised classical blood dosimetry protocol, incorporating the changes discussed above, is summarized in Table 58.2.

Other Modifications

Other modifications and refinements to this dosimetry protocol have also been proposed. Furhang et al. [33] suggested an analytical curve-fitting technique to generate a more realistic extrapolation of the clearance curve beyond the final data point. Another attempt at simplifying this dosimetry protocol [34] suggested the elimination of blood samples. Their investigation examined the accuracy with which the total dose to the blood could be predicted using only the

Table 58.2 Modified classical dosimetry protocol

Whole-body counting (conjugate counting)	2, 24, 48, 72, and 96 h
	Count standard and background
	Normalize data points to 100 % using 2 h value
	Calculate γ component of dose (Gy/MBq) using classical approach
Blood sample (5 ml heparinized)	2, 24, 48, 72, and 96 h
	At conclusion of data collection, make ^{131}I counting standard with concentration of 3.7–7.4 KBq/ml (0.1–0.2 μCi/ml)
	Pipet 1 ml of whole blood from each collection and from standard
	Count duplicate samples in well counter in same run
	Convert blood data into units of % ingested dose/l
	Calculate β component of dose (Gy/MBq) using classical approach

whole-body data. Although there is a strong correlation between these two components, this method assumes that the β and γ doses are in a fixed ratio to each other. Unfortunately, there is a wide range in this value among patients, as shown in the data of Thomas et al. [34], as well as in the study by Robeson et al. [35]. Another area involves the transition from the *classical* model to the MIRD schema. For example, all the β energy released in the blood is assumed to be absorbed in the blood. Because these particles can travel several millimeters, this is likely an overestimation. More sophisticated models that account for the vascular space and geometrical configurations have suggested a value of 0.82 for the absorbed fraction [36]. The recent successes in the use of ^{131}I radioimmunotherapy for B-cell lymphoma have focused considerable attention on patient-specific dosimetry where again the radiation dose to the bone marrow is the limiting factor [37].

Hermanska et al. [38] has suggested using a biphasic model which might approximate complex multicompartmental models better than a monoexponential model. Such a biphasic model incorporates the uptake phase as well as better predicts the slower, long-term clearance phase. However, Hermanska's biphasic model requires more data points than a monoexponential model. Furthermore, the evaluation of the biphasic model was performed in patients who were receiving their first ^{131}I therapy. These patients tend to have more complicated iodine kinetics due to varying amounts of residual normal thyroid tissue compared to post-ablation patients.

Finally, Sisson and Carey [39] has suggested additional empiric modifications of dosimetrically determined prescribed activity in patients who have functioning metastasis with measurable serum thyroxine. For these patients, they have recommended reduction in their therapeutic ^{131}I prescribed activity based on hormone levels. Although further discussion of this is beyond the scope of this chapter, more extensive discussion of other simplified methods of dosimetry is discussed in Chap. 59.

Other Radioiodines for Dosimetry

Although all the discussions in this chapter involve the use of ^{131}I for conducting dosimetry, it is feasible that other radioisotopes of iodine (e.g., ^{123}I and ^{124}I) could also be used for this purpose. The primary reasons that ^{131}I has been used are that (1) it is readily available and relatively inexpensive, (2) it has a physical half-life suited for the required 4–8-day monitoring period, and (3) the γ emission, although somewhat high in energy, is appropriate for imaging with conventional scintillation cameras. Unfortunately, for the radionuclide ^{123}I, the first two requirements are unfavorable. However, a potentially significant advantage of ^{123}I over ^{131}I is that on a per millicurie basis, the radiation dose delivered to a thyroid remnant or metastatic lesion is about 100-fold less. Consequently, potential "stunning" because of the dosimetry procedure prior to treatment would be less concerning. However, the relatively short 13 h half-life of this radionuclide makes it more difficult for a prolonged biokinetic studies. However, it might be feasible to use ^{123}I in a patient for whom it is known that 4 days would be an adequate observation period if the prescribed activity could be increased to about 740 MBq (20 mCi). Of course, with current pricing for ^{123}I, this would be very expensive, even though the radiation dose would still be a fraction of that from a typical amount of activity of 74 MBq (2 mCi) ^{131}I, along with the added benefit of significantly improved image quality on the 24 and 48 h metastatic surveys.

The other potential candidate, ^{124}I, is a positron emitter and could quite possibly become the preferred radioisotope of iodine not only for dosimetry but for part or all of thyroid cancer imaging (see Chap. 103). Unfortunately, it is not approved in the United States by the Food and Drug Administration, and it also has a complicated decay scheme. However, in a study by Eschmann et al. [40], they concluded that ^{124}I, despite its complicated decay scheme, is suitable for the dosimetry of ^{131}I therapy in both benign and malignant thyroid diseases.

Lesion-Based Dosimetry (Maxon Approach)

Calculating a treatment plan based on delivering a prescribed radiation absorbed dose to the tumor is the fundamental tenet of radiotherapy, whereas the classical dosimetry approach of Benua was based on giving the maximum prescribed activity of ^{131}I that was considered safe and therefore more in line with thermotherapeutic strategies. The implicit assumption in the lesion-based dosimetry is that a treatment prescribed activity derived in this manner would achieve the maximum therapeutic effect to any metastatic disease while minimizing the risk to the patient. Numerous investigations have been performed to determine the radiation absorbed dose that would be delivered to residual thyroid and metastatic tissue, with the objective to correlate the radiation absorbed dose with the therapeutic effect. In order to perform these calculations, it is necessary to measure the uptake and clearance of ^{131}I from identifiable thyroid remnants and/or metastatic lesions. This calculation of lesion dose [41] is generally based on a classical model, which for ^{131}I is given by

Dose(cGy) = $0.63C_0T_{1/2\ \mathrm{lesion}}$ where C_0 is the initial concentration (μCi/g) of ^{131}I in the lesion and $T_{1/2\ \mathrm{lesion}}$ is the effective half-life of the lesion activity in hours. In order to determine the concentration of ^{131}I, how much activity (in absolute units) is contained in the lesion must be known. One way to ascertain this is based on an analysis of selected regions of interest on conjugate view γ camera images. These images are obtained at several time points, measured from the time of administration of the tracer prescribed activity. Typically, these images would be acquired at 24, 48, and 72 h, but later time samples might be necessary if the uptake and clearance are delayed. In addition, transmission images to correct for attenuation in the lesion area, as well as images of a standard for calibration purposes, are necessary. A curve-fitting procedure is then used to establish the assumed single-exponential half-life value and to extrapolate the curve-to-zero time to determine the lesion's initial activity. Another parameter needed to calculate the activity concentration is the lesion mass or volume. Several approaches have been suggested for this determination. For example, Maxon et al. [54] used the nonmagnified anterior images from a rectilinear scanner to determine the lesion dimensions and assumed a spherical or elliptical shape; Koral et al. [42] used both anterior and lateral pinhole camera images with corrections for magnification and an ellipsoidal shape. However, determining the lesion dimensions on a γ camera image has inherent problems. If the projected dimensions of the lesion are small compared to the spatial resolution of the imaging system, then partial volume errors are introduced. In addition, only 2D distances (e.g., the major and minor axes) are measured, and the volume is calculated from a presumed three-dimensional (3D) shape. To overcome some of these limitations, others [43] have used alternative, higher spatial resolution images, such as computed tomography or ultrasound, to determine the mass.

Many investigators have reported the effective half-life of ^{131}I in thyroid metastatic lesions as within a range of about 1–5 days. Thus, a limited number of temporal samples may not accurately predict this curve. Furthermore, in a small sampling of patients studied posttherapy [42], the uptake in the lesion did not achieve its maximum value until 1–3 days post-administration. An assumption of instantaneous uptake therefore results in an overestimate of the radiation absorbed dose. Furthermore, if the dimensions are smaller than about 5 mm (assuming that this could be accurately determined), then the range of the β particles can no longer be neglected in the dose calculation. For example, if ^{131}I is uniformly distributed at the same concentration in small spherical tissues of 0.1 or 1.0 mm in diameter, they would receive a relative radiation absorbed dose of 8.6 % and 56 % [44], respectively, compared to a 5 mm diameter lesion. Consequently, if the concentration of ^{131}I is a constant, then the absorbed dose rate initially increases as the radius of a spherical lesion increases. This curve begins to flatten off at a radius of about 7 mm and is essentially constant for lesions with radii more than 10 mm. Over the range of radii from 1 to 10 mm, there is approximately a threefold increase [45] in the dose rate. In fact, dose rate is a factor that has been generally ignored in ^{131}I therapy. It is well known in external radiation treatment that the dose rate and the total dose have an impact on cell survival. As the dose rate is reduced, more and more of the sublethal cell damage may be repaired during the course of the exposure. Below about 0.6 Gy/h (60 rad/h), there is only a little dose rate effect [46], with the residual cell killing effect from nonrepairable injury associated with the total cumulative radiation absorbed dose. However, these are realistic dose rates for ^{131}I therapy. For example, Schlesinger et al. [47] calculated that for an ^{131}I prescribed activity for treatment of 5.5 GBq (150 mCi) and a lesion uptake of 0.3 % per gram, the initial dose rate would be 1.83 Gy/h. Assuming an effective half-life of 3 days, their data showed that it would take about 5 days to reduce the dose rate to this critical value.

MIRD Dosimetry

Dosimetric approaches have improved significantly over the past 40 years and continue to evolve into more sophisticated methodologies to characterize the transport and absorption of radiation in complex biological systems. Patient-specific models employing Monte Carlo simulations have even been proposed. Indeed, it is generally believed that the MIRD methodology is a more accurate approach to dosimetry than the classical models employed in the Benua and Leeper approach. Using the MIRD methodology, it is possible to estimate the radiation absorbed dose that would be delivered not only to critical organs, such as the bone marrow and lung, but also to the lesion(s) to be treated. However, the latter is considerably more complicated and often not technically feasible if the lesion cannot be visualized with the small prescribed activity of ^{131}I used for the tracer study. Nevertheless, dosimetry-guided ^{131}I therapy for metastatic thyroid cancer has also been reported based on the MIRD methodology by Dorn et al. [48]. This group used the red marrow as the critical target organ, rather than the whole blood, which has been used as a surrogate for the bone marrow in the Benua and Leeper approach. Furthermore, for safety purposes, 3 Gy (300 rad) to the bone marrow or

30 Gy (3,000 rad) to the lungs was selected as their upper limit. Out of all their treatments with a curative intent (n=41), only 19 treatments resulted in the bone marrow receiving 3 Gy (300 rad). Based on this approach and the higher safety limit chosen, a single treatment prescribed activity of ^{131}I as high as 38.5 GBq (1,040 mCi) could be given. Although these workers claimed that such a dose limit (i.e., 3 Gy [300 rad]) to the bone marrow is safe and does not result in permanent marrow suppression, the evidence is still somewhat limited to support this conclusion. Note also that the Benua and Leeper model uses 2 Gy (200 rad) to the whole blood, not the bone marrow, as the limit. The actual radiation absorbed dose to the bone marrow is less than that delivered to the whole blood and, at most, is probably about 60–70 % of this value.

OLINDA®, 3D-ID®, and 3D-RD®

More recently, additional reports have been published in attempts to improve dosimetric calculations, and these include OLINDA®, 3D-ID®, and 3D-RD®. A detailed discussion of 3D-ID® and 3D-RD® is available in Chap. 103.

Results

Patient outcomes of ^{131}I treatment for metastatic thyroid carcinoma have been previously reported for (1) empiric fixed prescribed activity [1, 5, 49–52], (2) the Maxon dosimetric approach [14, 53, and 60], and (3) the Benua dosimetric approach [13, 24, 61]. Outcomes of ^{131}I treatments are more extensively discussed in Chaps. 33, 34, 56, 57, 60 and 75. The following is a brief overview of outcomes related to empiric fixed prescribed activity, the Maxon dosimetric approach, and the Benua dosimetric approach.

Maxon and Smith reviewed the literature regarding the effects of ^{131}I on functioning metastatic disease where the ^{131}I prescribed activities used were predominantly empiric fixed activity similar to those in Table 58.1 [5]. Complete resolution was typically defined as no evidence of disease by scan, X-ray, and clinical examination. Thyroglobulin levels were not initially available. For metastasis to the lymph nodes, complete resolution of disease was seen in 68.2 % (58 of 85), "improvement but still evident" disease in 18.8 %, and no apparent effect in 12.5 %. For metastasis to the lung, complete resolution of disease was seen in 45.9 % (134 of 292), "improvement but still evident" disease in 27.7 %, and no apparent effect in 24.5 %. For metastasis to the bone, complete resolution of disease was seen in 6.8 % (16 of 233), "improvement but still evident" disease in 35.6 %, and no apparent effect in 54.2 %. Also examining results after empiric prescribed activity, Schlumberger reported survival rates measured from the time of metastases discovery of 53 % at 5 years, 38 % at 10 year, and 30 % at 15 years. Remission was achieved in only 79 (28 %) of 283 patients once metastases were discovered [11]. Subsequently, Schlumberger indicated (1) a remission rate of 50 % with a 10-year survival rate of 61 % for lung metastasis; (2) a remission rate of 10 % with a 10-year survival rate of 21 % for bone metastasis, and (3) a remission rate of 7 % with a 10-year survival rate of 13 % for lung and bone metastasis [62]. Also using empiric fixed prescribed activity, Menzel reported clinical remission in 14 patients, partial remission in three, stable disease in 16, and progressive disease in 37 [12]. Dinneen found overall survival rates (for all causes) for distant metastasis to be 37 % at 5 years, 24 % at 10 year, and 20% at 15 years [63].

Based on the Benua dosimetry approach to selecting prescribed activity, Leeper described the status of 70 patients treated at MSKCC for metastatic differentiated thyroid cancer from 1974 to 1981 ([61]; see Table 58.3) and from 1974 to 1984 ([26]; see Table 58.4). This occurred after Benua had implemented several restrictions (see footnotes and Tables 58.3 and 58.4). Benua and Leeper administered an average single therapeutic prescribed activity of ^{131}I of 11.4 GBq (308

Table 58.3 Memorial Sloan Kettering Cancer Center 1974–1981 experience

		Number of ^{131}I treatments						
Status	Number of patients	1	2	3	4	5	6	Average total dose GBq (mCi ^{131}I)
Cured	21	13	6	1	0	0	1	14.7 GBq (463)
Died of disease	17	9	3	3	0	1	1	23.3 GBq (630)
Died of other causes	4	2	2	0	0	0	0	21.0 GBq (568)
Under treatment	19	10	6	1	2	0	0	19.0 GBq (514)
Living with disease; no further treatment	6	5	1	0	0	0	0	17.2 GBq (466)
Lost to follow-up	3	2	1	0	0	0	0	14.0 GBq (379)
Total	70	41	19	5	2	1	2	19.2 GBq (520)

Source: Ref. [61]

After implementation of restriction of maximum (a) 200 cGy (200 rad) total blood radiation, (b) 4.44 GBq (120) mCi of ^{131}I whole-body retention at 48 h, and (c) 2.96 GBq (80 mCi) of ^{131}I whole-body retention at 48 h if pulmonary metastases are present

Table 58.4 Memorial Sloan Kettering Cancer Center 1974–1984 experience

Status	Number of patients
Cured	45
Died of all causes	28
Under treatment	29
Living with disease	9
Status unknown	5
Total	116

Source: Ref. [26]
After implementation of restriction of maximum (a) 200 cGy (200 rad) total blood radiation, (b) 4.44 GBq (120 mCi) of ^{131}I whole-body retention at 48 h, and (c) 2.96 GBq (80 mCi) of ^{131}I whole-body retention at 24 h if pulmonary metastases are present

mCi) with a range of 2.6–24.2 GBq (70–654 mCi). The total cumulative prescribed activity of ^{131}I exceeded 37 GBq (1 Ci) in six patients with the largest being 77.7 GBq (2.1 Ci). In Leeper's group of patients, 19 % were treated with a prescribed activity less than 7.4 GBq (200 mCi). In most cases, each treatment delivered a calculated radiation dose of 200 cGy (200 rad) to the blood. A "cure" was defined as negative roentgenograms, clinical examination, and radioiodine scan. Thyroglobulin assays, albeit relatively insensitive by today's standards, were only used near the end of the above time period. If necessary, treatments were repeated at annual intervals. In 1984, Leeper reported that 58 % of the patients receiving one treatment were "cured." Patients younger than age 40 had a higher "cure" rate (30 of 33, 90 %) than those over age 40 (10 of 23, 43 %).

Using his quantitative, lesional dosimetry approach, Maxon et al. [53] treated 26 patients who collectively had over 67 metastatic lesions. There were 63 lesions in the neck, one in the lung, two in the mediastinum, and one in the bone. One patient had numerous abnormalities in the neck, chest, and abdomen, which were not detailed in the report. Of the 67 lesions in the other 25 patients, 59 responded to ^{131}I. None of the numerous lesions in the 26th patient responded. Based on the location of the abnormalities, the response was 58 of 63 (92 %) in the neck, one of two in the mediastinum, zero of one in the lung, and zero of one in the bone. Maxon reported that the response rate significantly increased in those lesions that received over 8,000 cGy (rad), as determined by his dosimetric approach. Little chance of a response was seen if the radiation dose to the lesion was less than 3,500 cGy (rad). In a subsequent article, Maxon et al. [54] reported successful treatment in 81 % (63 of 78) of lymph node metastases and in 74 % (17 of 23) of overall patients. Notably, some of these patients had residual thyroid tissue in the thyroid bed. The results were achieved after a single ^{131}I administration calculated to deliver a radiation dose to the lesion of at least 8,500 cGy (rad). The mean prescribed activity of ^{131}I in this group was 5.8 ± 1.9 GBq (156.7 ± 51.7 mCi), with a range of 1.8–9.1 GBq (48.6–246.3 mCi). When no residual thyroid tissue was present in the thyroid bed and no distant metastasis was noted, Maxon's treatment success increased to 90 % (26 of 29) of lymph node metastases and 86 % (6 of 7) of patients. This success was seen after a single administration of ^{131}I delivered a radiation exposure of at least 14,000 cGy (rad). The definition of "success" in this case was the absence of evident lymph node metastasis on physical examination and on a 37 MBq (2 mCi) radioiodine scan.

Despite the published outcomes for empiric fixed prescribed activity or prescribed activity determined by either the Maxon or Benua approach, a comparison of those results is difficult. The difficulties lie in the differences in the (1) definition of successful treatment, (2) changing definitions of successful treatment, (3) variability in additional treatment modalities, (4) duration of follow-up, and (5) variability in data collection. In addition, no prospective study comparing the outcomes of empiric prescribed activities to dosimetrically determined prescribed activities has been published. Obtaining adequate statistical samples with reliable follow-up over long time periods is very difficult. To date, only one publication by Klubo et al. [55] has compared dosimetrically determined prescribed activities to empiric fixed prescribed activities, and this report demonstrated a higher efficacy of dosimetrically determined prescribed activity with a similar safety profile compared to the empirical prescribed activity in high-risk patients. However, regardless of the above limitations, we believe that reasonable inferences may be drawn from the data to allow the development of guidelines for the use of dosimetry (see section "Recommendations"). A more extensive discussion of selection of ^{131}I prescribed activity for the treatment of metastatic disease is noted in Chap. 56.

At the time of this publication, the outcomes regarding dosimetry for lesions, whole body, blood, and other organs using ^{124}I are only in the development stage (see Chap. 103).

Strengths and Limitations of the Various Approaches

Empiric Fixed Prescribed Activity

The strengths of using the empiric fixed prescribed activity, such as those of Beierwaltes, are (1) convenience, (2) a long history of use, and (3) a reasonably acceptable rate and severity of complications. A theoretical strength of the higher empiric fixed prescribed activity approach (e.g., protocols using 7.4 GBq (300 mCi) of ^{131}I at 3–6 months' intervals) is improved outcome, but a limitation is the lack of significant data confirming outcomes, as well as the rate and severity of complications. In addition, empiric fixed prescribed activity permits the option of treating recurrent disease as detected by ^{123}I scans, thyroglobulin blood levels, and/or other imaging modalities without using ^{131}I diagnostically. Avoiding the use of diagnostic ^{131}I eliminates potential reduction of therapeutic ^{131}I uptake because of real or theoretical "stunning" from the diagnostic prescribed activity.

However, empiric fixed prescribed activity has its disadvantages. One major limitation of empiric fixed prescribed activity is the failure to incorporate the individual status of the patient. The ideal ^{131}I prescribed activity to treat metastatic thyroid carcinoma is the lowest possible amount of ^{131}I that still delivers a lethal dose of radiation to the *entire* metastasis while minimizing side effects. Empiric fixed prescribed activities, by their very nature, do not permit the determination of either the minimal ^{131}I that will deliver a lethal radiation absorbed dose or the reasonably safe maximum tolerated activity. In regard to the latter, Leeper [56], Tuttle et al. [57], Kulkarni et al. [58], and Esposito et al. [59] demonstrated that empiric prescribed activity of 11.1 GBq (300 mCi), 7.4 GBq (200 mCi), and even 3.7 GBq (100 mCi) may exceed 200 cGy (rad) to the blood, which may result in increased frequency and severity of complications such as bone marrow suppression and pulmonary inflammation and fibrosis. An additional limitation is that multiple empiric fixed prescribed activities (fractionated radiotherapy) may not be equivalent to the same total ^{131}I prescribed activity calculated by dosimetry administered at one time. As already discussed, dose rate (cGy/h) is also important; thus, multiple smaller prescribed activities may have less therapeutic benefit than the same total prescribed activity administered at one time. Moreover, the first empiric treatment may reduce the effects of the second empiric treatment by reducing the uptake of the ^{131}I by the metastases—one of the arguments used for not even administering diagnostic prescribed activities of ^{131}I because of stunning.

The Benua Approach

The strengths of the Benua approach are the (1) patient-specific determination of the maximal tolerated activity (MTA) of ^{131}I, (2) identification of as many as one in five patients whose MTA is less than the empiric fixed prescribed activity, (3) potential to give higher radiation absorbed doses to metastasis at one time rather than multiple treatments with lower empiric prescribed activities which have lower total effective radiation absorbed doses, (4) experience of a long history of use by Benua, Leeper, and Larson at MSKCC, (5) empiric modifications of the original protocol based on observed initial complications, and (6) reasonable complications rates relative to the disease severity after the implementation of those additional modifications.

However, the Benua approach also has several limitations. First, the approach results in increased cost and patient inconvenience. However, we believe this is reasonable and not unlike treatment programs for metastatic disease secondary to other cancers. Second, the approach does not estimate the radiation absorbed dose to the metastasis, and the MTA may be administered without any potential therapeutic effect. Third, the program requires a committed medical staff. Like any treatment program for metastatic disease, the institution must see a reasonable number of patients to establish efficiency and assure quality. Fourth, present dosimetric approaches use ^{131}I diagnostically, which may subsequently reduce uptake of the therapeutic prescribed activity and therefore reduce the radiation absorbed dose delivered to the metastasis (stunning) (see Chaps. 16, 17, and 18). But using a smaller diagnostic prescribed activity, we do not believe this is a problem.

The Maxon Approach

The strength of the Maxon approach, as originally discussed by Maxon, is "[a] more selective exposure to individual patients based upon their individual needs without an increase in radiation exposure to the total patient population and lower overall costs." This could improve the outcome in some patients and avoid complications in those patients who receive no significant benefit from the ^{131}I therapy. However, Maxon's proposed lower overall costs are less because of two factors. First, new Nuclear Regulatory Commission guidelines allow earlier release from hospitals as well as outpatient treatments that reduce costs. Second, more expensive imaging methods may be required to determine the volumes of metastases.

Some technical limitations of the Maxon approach are noted in Table 58.5. Other limitations include the following: (1) increased cost and inconvenience, albeit we again believe that these are also modest and reasonable; (2) no prospective data regarding its use in distant metastasis; and (3) potentially difficult implementation of the approach in distant metastasis.

Another potential disadvantage of the Maxon approach is whether nonvisualization of a lymph node or any distant metastasis on a 74 MBq (2 mCi) ^{131}I scan implies that the metastasis is not treatable with ^{131}I. Again, Maxon indicated that delivery of 8,000 cGy (rad) to the lymph node metastasis was associated with an excellent chance

Table 58.5 Potential problems and limitations of lesion-based dosimetry

A single-exponential model may not accurately reflect the kinetics of the radioiodine in the lesion
Assumption of instantaneous uptake and maximum at time zero
Estimation of the lesion mass
Assumption of uniform distribution of ^{131}I in the lesion
Statistical errors in the measurements
Therapeutic response relative to dose rate
Reduced radiation absorbed dose for a given prescribed activity for lesions <5 mm in diameter

of successful treatment, and doses of less than 3,500 cGy (rad) reduced the chance of effective treatment. However, does this suggest that the necessary cGy (rad) cannot be delivered to a functioning metastasis that is not visualized on a 64 MBq (2 mCi) ^{131}I scan? Arnstein et al. [64] has suggested that significant radiation absorbed dose can still be delivered to lesions even when they are not visualized on scans performed using prescribed activities of ^{131}I of 74 Bq (2 mCi) and even as high as 1.11 GBq (30 mCi). This is one of the arguments for a "blind" ^{131}I therapy when serum thyroglobulin is elevated and the pretherapy radioiodine scan is negative. Clearly, further study is warranted, and ^{124}I may be very useful in these areas of investigation.

General Limitations of All Approaches

A major downfall of all the approaches is the less than optimal definition of "success." This includes not only the criteria for complete remission and partial remission but also the length of follow-up. For example, the criteria for "success" could be merely a normal physical exam and negative radioiodine whole-body survey within less than 3 years of follow-up. These criteria may have been reasonable at the time of the original studies, but it is arguable whether these criteria and the short length of follow-up provide much information about patient outcomes, e.g., the rate of complete remission, partial remission, and length of remission. For example, diagnostic modalities other than physical exam, such as ultrasound of the neck and CT of the chest, were available and have been used since the 1970s. Additional modalities to detect residual disease have become available and were used in the 1980s and 1990s (e.g., serum thyroglobulin assays and magnetic resonance imaging [MRI]). By today's standards, the results of radioiodine whole-body surveys are poor criteria by which to judge success. For example, we now know that the lack of uptake on a 7.4 MBq (2 mCi) radioiodine scan is not necessarily evidence of successful treatment. The size and/or uptake of the metastasis may be too little to be visualized on the radioiodine scan, and/or the metastasis may have dedifferentiated and lost its functional ability to take up iodine. To simply rely on physical exam and a negative radioiodine scan is inadequate as a definition of success. In addition, the described follow-up periods of only several years to assess altered outcomes in a disease that may take significantly longer time periods to recur or progress are problematic. Accordingly, less than optimal definitions of success and short follow-up periods may have overestimated "success" as defined by earlier reports. In addition, the variability of the definitions makes meaningful comparisons unreliable.

However, this should not devalue these approaches but rather encourage us to reevaluate the approaches with more specific definitions of complete and partial remissions that encompass longer-term follow-up periods that are more appropriate for our current practice such as published by Klubo et al. [55].

In summary, many problems exist regarding any dosimetric approach, but physicians and patients should not see these problems as deterrents in using the Maxon and/or Benua approach when appropriate. In addition, third-party insurance payers should not interpret these problematic issues with dosimetric approaches to therapy as their rationale to declare them experimental and thereby deny reimbursement. Rather, dosimetric approaches have been in use as long as empiric approaches, and although no prospective studies assessing outcomes have been reported for dosimetric approaches, neither has prospective studies assessing outcomes have been reported for empiric approaches. Accordingly, we believe any additional cost of these dosimetric approaches over empiric fixed prescribed activity is warranted, at least in patients with metastatic disease (see Chap. 56). The remaining questions or issues regarding dosimetric approaches must be studied and resolved, and then we can move forward and hopefully achieve greater benefit for our patients.

Selecting Empiric vs Dosimetrically Determined Prescribed Activity

Of course, one of the more controversial areas in the management of metastatic DTC is that of using dosimetrically determined vs empirically selected prescribed activities of ^{131}I for the treatment of metastatic DTC. Those who favor an empiric rather than a dosimetric method may argue that until prospective data are published demonstrating that the outcomes of ^{131}I treatments based on dosimetric methods are superior to that using the empiric methods, one should use empiric methods. We agree with empiric methods for the selection of the prescribed activity of ^{131}I for remnant ablation and adjuvant treatment. However, we do not agree with this position when selecting the prescribed activity of ^{131}I for the treatment of known metastases. Rather, we submit that until further data are published demonstrating that the outcomes of ^{131}I treatment with the empiric selected prescribed activities are equal or superior to the dosimetric methods, one should use dosimetric methods. Dosimetric methods are based on—or at least are an attempt to be based on—one or both of the two fundamental principles of radiation therapy planning, namely, "… determining and delivering radiation absorbed dose to the tumor for control as well as determining and minimizing the radiation absorbed dose to the normal tissues." None of the various empiric selected prescribed activities are based on either one of these fundamental principles of radiation therapy planning. Instead, empiric selected prescribed activities are typically based on an initial proposal by one individual at one facility (see Chap. 56), and ironically no prospective outcome studies are available comparing the many different approaches of empiric selected prescribed activities of ^{131}I for the treatment of metastases of DTC. Further, if one does accept the argument that until additional data are available to demonstrate that dosimetrically determined prescribed activity yields outcomes superior to empirically selected prescribed activity, then how does one select one of the empiric prescribed activities (e.g., 3.7 GBq [100 mCi], 5.55 GBq [150 mCi], 7.4 GBq [200 mCi], or even 11.1 GBq [300 mCi]) when there is no data to demonstrate which of those empiric selected prescribed activities result in superior outcomes? This is inconsistent and illogical. Accordingly and until outcome data are published demonstrating that one empiric selected prescribed activity has any better outcomes to any other empirically selected or dosimetrically determined prescribed activity, the logical choice is to select the method that is at least based on the fundamentals—or at least one of the fundamentals—of radiation therapy planning and not on one or another's individual empiric preference(s).

In addition to the above argument and despite the frequent argument that no article has been published comparing ^{131}I treatments for metastases with empiric selected prescribed activities vs dosimetrically determined, a retrospective study has now been published by Klubo et al. [55]. This study evaluated outcomes and side effects of empirically selected prescribed activity vs dosimetrically determined prescribed activities for ^{131}I treatment of metastases. The study group consisted of 87 patients followed for 51 ± 35 months. Forty four patients were treated with an empiric prescribed activity, and 43 patients were treated with a dosimetrically determined prescribed activity of ^{131}I. By multivariate analysis, the group administered with the dosimetrically determined prescribed activity were 70 % less likely to progress (odds ratio, 0.29; 95 % confidence interval, 0.087–1.02; $p<0.052$) and more likely to obtain complete response compared to the group of patients administered with an empiric selected prescribed activity (odds ratio, 8.2; 95 % confidence interval, 1.2–53.5; $p<0.029$). The advantage of dosimetrically determined prescribed activity was more apparent in the locoregionally advanced group because complete remission was significantly higher in the dosimetrically determined group vs the empiric group (35.7 vs 3.3 %; $p<0.009$). The rates of partial response, stable disease, and progression-free survival, as well as the frequency of side effects, were not significantly different between the two groups. So, initial data, albeit retrospective, have now been published demonstrating a benefit of ^{131}I treatment for metastases when the prescribed activity has been determined by dosimetry. However, further studies are warranted.

For those who do not perform dosimetry or do not have access to a facility that performs dosimetry, simplified alternative dosimetry methods are available and can be performed in almost any nuclear medicine facility [65, 66]. Further discussion is available in Chap. 59.

Table 58.6 Recommendations for ^{131}I treatment of functioning lung metastasis of differentiated thyroid carcinoma

1. Strongly recommend referral of the patient to a site that performs dosimetry, and if that is not an option, then either perform or refer the patient to a site that performs one of the methods of percent 48 h whole-body retention. Do not exceed a prescribed activity that would either deliver more than 200 cGy (rad) to the blood or result in more than 2.96 GBq (80 mCi) whole-body retention of ^{131}I activity at 48 h[a]
2. If dosimetry or percent 48 h whole-body retention is not available, then select one of the many empiric methods from 3.7 to 11.1 GBq (100–300 mCi). However, if the patient has:
a. Macronodular pulmonary metastases, we recommend caution in exceeding 5.55 GBq (150 mCi), because as many as 10–20 % of patients may exceed 200 Gy to the blood (bone marrow) [56–59] or
b. Diffuse micronodular pulmonary metastases, we recommend caution in exceeding any prescribed activity greater than 3.7 GBq (100 mCi) because the patient is at increased risk of acute radiation pneumonitis and/or radiation pulmonary fibrosis [13]

See Chap. 56
[a]As determined by the Benua and Leeper approach

Table 58.7 Recommendations for ^{131}I treatment of functioning bone distant metastasis

1. Depending on location and number of lesions, recommend consideration of other treatment modalities such as surgical excision, external radiation therapy (e.g., CyberKnife®), radiofrequency ablation, cryotherapy, or embolization, to name several, prior to any ^{131}I treatment. However, ^{131}I treatment may be given before external radiation therapy
2. If ^{131}I treatment is to be administered, then strongly recommend referral of the patient to a site that performs dosimetry, and if that is not an option, then either perform or refer the patient to a site that performs one of the methods of percent 48 h whole-body retention
a. Do not exceed a prescribed activity that would either deliver more than 200 cGy (rad) to the blood or result in more than 4.44 GBq (120 mCi) whole-body retention of ^{131}I activity at 48 h[a]
3. If dosimetry or the simplified methods of percent 48 h whole-body retention are not available, then select one of the many empiric methods from 3.7 to 11.1 GBq (100–300 mCi). Be cautious in selecting 5.55–11.1 GBq (150–300 mCi) because as many as 10–20 % of patients may exceed 200 Gy to the blood (bone marrow) [56–59]

See Chap. 56
[a]As determined by the Benua and Leeper approach

Table 58.8 Recommendations for ^{131}I treatment of functioning brain distant metastasis

1. Depending on location and number of lesions, recommend consideration of surgical excision or external radiation therapy (e.g., gamma knife radiotherapy) prior to or in place of ^{131}I treatment
2. If ^{131}I treatment is to be administered, then strongly recommend referral of the patient to a site that performs dosimetry, and if that is not an option, then either perform or refer the patient to a site that performs one of the methods of percent 48 h whole-body retention
a. Do not exceed a prescribed activity that would either deliver more than 200 cGy (rad) to the blood or result in 4.44 GBq (120 mCi) whole-body retention of ^{131}I activity at 48 h
b. Recommend pre-treatment (i.e., steroids, glycerol, and mannitol) prior to either thyroid hormone withdrawal or administration of recombinant human thyroid stimulating hormone as well as ^{131}I treatment
3. If dosimetry or one of the simplified methods of percent 48 h whole-body retention is not available, then select one of the many empiric methods from 3.7 to 11.1 GBq (100–300 mCi). Be cautious that in selecting 5.55–11.1 GBq (150–300 mCi), as many as 10–20 % of patients may have significant bone marrow suppression [56–59]

See Chap. 56

Recommendations

Our recommendations for the use of dosimetrically determined vs empirically selected prescribed activities to help select ^{131}I prescribed activity for the treatment of metastatic thyroid carcinoma are noted in Tables 58.6, 58.7, and 58.8. Again, the selection of the amount of prescribed activity of ^{131}I is discussed further in multiple other chapters (see Chaps. 56, 59, and 65). We also recognize that many other factors such as the clinical status of the patient, the patient's location, and the patient's own desires may influence the method for the selection of the ^{131}I prescribed activity and even the final ^{131}I prescribed activity determined by any method.

Summary

^{131}I is an important option in the therapeutic armamentarium for metastatic thyroid carcinoma, and dosimetrically determined prescribed activity of ^{131}I for treatment of metastatic DTC is based on—or at least an attempt to be based—on one or both of the two fundamental principles of almost all radiation therapies. More research is needed to compare the long-term outcome and risks of the dosimetric approaches to the empiric approaches as well as to evaluate new approaches, such as patient-specific dosimetry with ^{124}I PET and the 3D internal dosimetry [67] and 3D-RD software developed by Sgouros, Hobbs, and colleagues [68]. However, until further outcome data are available, dosimetrically determined prescribed activities for the ^{131}I treatment of functioning distant metastases is a reasonable alternative, and it is our preferred method.

References

1. Beierwaltes WH, Nishiyama RH, Thompson NW, et al. Survival time and "cure" in papillary and follicular thyroid carcinoma with distant metastases: statistics following University of Michigan therapy. J Nucl Med. 1982;23:561–8.
2. Seidlin SM, Marinelli LD, Oshry E. Radioactive iodine therapy effect on functioning metastases of adenocarcinoma of the thyroid. JAMA. 1946;132:838–47.
3. Beierwaltes WH. The treatment of thyroid carcinoma with radioactive iodine. Semin Nucl Med. 1978;8:79–94.
4. Freitas JE, Gross MD, Ripley S, Shapiro B. Radionuclide diagnosis and therapy of thyroid cancer: current status report. Sem Nucl Med. 1985;15:106–31.
5. Maxon HR, Smith HS. I-131 in the diagnosis and treatment of metastatic well differentiated thyroid cancer. Endocrinol Metab Clin North Am. 1990;19:685–718.
6. Krishnamurthy GT, Blahd W. I-131 therapy in the management of thyroid cancer. Cancer. 1977;40:195–202.
7. Maheshwari YK, Hill Jr CS, Haynie III TP, et al. I-131 therapy in differentiated thyroid carcinoma. Cancer. 1981;47:664–71.
8. Edmonds CJ. Treatment of thyroid cancer. Clin Endocrinol Metab. 1979;8:223–43.
9. Tubiana M. Thyroid cancer. In: Beckers C, editor. Thyroid disease. France: Pergamon; 1982. p. 187–227.
10. Robbins J. The role of TRH and lithium in the management of thyroid cancer. In: Andreoli M, Monaco F, Robbins J, editors. Advances in thyroid neoplasia. Rome: Field Educational Italia; 1981. p. 233–44.
11. Schlumberger M, Tubiana M, DeVathaire F, et al. Long-term results of treatment of 283 patients with lung and bone metastases from differentiated thyroid carcinoma. J Clin Endocrinol Metab. 1986;63:960–7.
12. Menzel C, Grunwald A, Palmedo H, et al. "High-dose" ^{131}I therapy in advanced differentiated thyroid carcinoma. J Nucl Med. 1996;37:1496–503.
13. Benua RS, Cicale NR, Sonenberg M, Rawson RW. The relation of ^{131}I dosimetry to results and complications in the treatment of metastatic thyroid cancer. Am J Roentgenol Radium Ther Nucl Med. 1962;87:171–82.
14. Thomas SR, Maxon HR, Kereiakes JG. In vivo quantitation of lesion radioactivity using external counting methods. Med Phys. 1976;3:253–5.
15. International Commission on Radiological Protection. Radionuclide transformations. Energy and intensity of emissions. ICRP Publication 38. Ann ICRP 1983;11–13.
16. Marinelli LD, Quimby EH, Hine GJ. Prescribed activity determination with radioactive isotopes. II. Practical considerations in therapy and protection. Am J Roentgenol. 1948;59:260–81.
17. Loevinger R, Holt JG, Hine JG. Internally administered radioisotopes. In: Attix F, Roesch W, Tochlin E, editors. Radiation dosimetry. New York: Academic; 1956. p. 803–75.
18. Quimby EH. In radionuclides in medicine and biology. Philadelphia: Lea & Febiger; 1970.
19. Howell RW, Dandamudi VR, Sastry KS. Macroscopic dosimetry for radioimmunotherapy: nonuniform activity distribution in solid tumors. Med Phys. 1989;16:66–74.
20. Snyder WS, Ford MR, Warner GG, et al. "S" absorbed dose per unit cumulated activity for selected radionuclides and organs, MIRD Pamphlet, vol. 11. Reston: Society of Nuclear Medicine; 1975.

21. Zanzonico PB. Internal radionuclide radiation dosimetry: a review of basic concepts and recent developments. J Nucl Med. 2000;41:297–308.
22. Van Nostrand D, Atkins F, Yeganeh F, Acio E, Bursaw R, Wartofsky L. Dosimetrically determined doses of radioiodine for the treatment of metastatic thyroid carcinoma. Thyroid. 2002;12:121–34.
23. Lassmann M, Händscheid H, Verburg FA, Luster M. The use of dosimetry in the treatment of differentiated thyroid cancer. Q J Nucl Med Mol Imaging. 2011;55:107–25.
24. Verburg FA, Reinmers C, Hänscheid H. Approach to the patient: role of dosimetric RAI Rx in children with DTC. J Clin Endocrinol Metab. 2013;98:3912–9.
25. Keldsen N, Mortensen BT, Hansen HS. Bone marrow depression due to ^{131}I treatment of thyroid cancer. Ugeskr Laeger. 1988;150: 2817–9.
26. Benua RS, Leeper RD. A method and rationale for treating metastatic thyroid carcinoma with the largest safe prescribed activity of I-131. In: Medeiros-Neto G, Gaitan E, editors. Frontiers in thyroidology, vol. 2. New York: Plenum Medical Book Co; 1986. p. 1317–21.
27. Leeper RD, Shimaoka K. Treatment of metastatic thyroid cancer. Clin Endocrinol Metab. 1980;9:383–404.
28. Thomas SR, Maxon HR, Fritz KM, et al. A comparison of methods for assessing patient body burden following I-131 therapy for thyroid cancer. Radiology. 1980;137:839–42.
29. Thomas SR, Maxon HR, Kereiakes JG, Saenger EL. Quantitative external counting techniques enabling improved diagnostic and therapeutic decisions in patients with differentiated thyroid cancer. Radiology. 1977;122:731–7.
30. Erwin W, Groch M. Quantitative radioimmunoimaging for radioimmunotherapy treatment planning: effect of reduction in data sampling on dosimetric estimates. Cancer Biother Radiopharm. 2002; 17:699–711.
31. Wahl RL, Kroll S, Zasadny KR. Patient-specific whole-body dosimetry: principles and a simplified method for clinical implementation. J Nucl Med. 1998;39(Suppl):14S–20.
32. Zasadny KR, Gates VL, Moon S, et al. Comparison of total body dosimetry predicted with gamma-camera whole-body scans versus collimated probe for patients receiving I-131 anti-B1 antibody. Radiology. 1996;201:300P.
33. Furhang EE, Larson SM, Buranapong P, Humm JL. Thyroid cancer dosimetry using clearance fitting. J Nucl Med. 1999;40:131–6.
34. Thomas SR, Samaratunga RS, Sperling M, Maxon HR. Predictive estimate of blood dose from external counting data preceding radioiodine therapy for thyroid cancer. Nucl Med Biol. 1993;20: 157–62.
35. Robeson W, Zanzi I, Yoshida M, et al. Validation study to determine if accurate dosimetry for 131I therapy for thyroid cancer can be performed using only external counting data. J Nucl Med. 1994;15S:112P (abstract).
36. McEwan AC. Absorbed doses in the marrow during I-131 therapy. Br J Radiol. 1997;50:329–31.
37. Sgouros G. Bone marrow dosimetry for radioimmunotherapy: theoretical considerations. J Nucl Med. 1993;34:689–94.
38. Hermanska J, Karny M, Zimak J, et al. Improved prediction of therapeutic absorbed doses of ^{131}I in the treatment of thyroid carcinoma. J Nucl Med. 2001;42:1084–90.
39. Sisson JC, Carey JE. Thyroid carcinoma with high levels of function: treatment with I-131. J Nucl Med. 2001;42:975–83.
40. Eschmann S, Reischl G, Bilger K, et al. Evaluation of dosimetry of ^{131}I therapy in benign and malignant thyroid disorders by means of ^{124}I and PET. Eur J Nucl Med. 2002;29:760–7.
41. Maxon HR. Quantitative ^{131}I therapy in the treatment of differentiated thyroid cancer. Q J Nucl Med. 1999;43:313–23.
42. Koral KF, Adler RS, Carey JE, Beierwaltes WH. Iodine-131 treatment of thyroid cancer: absorbed dose calculated from post-therapy scans. J Nucl Med. 1986;27:1207–11.
43. Kimmig B, Hermann HJ. Measurement of dose during ^{131}I treatment of thyroid cancer. Acta Endocrinol. 1983;S252:72.
44. Champion C, Zanotti-Fregonara P, Hindie E. CELLDOSE: a Monte Carlo code to assess electron dose distribution – S values for I-131 in spheres of various sizes. J Nucl Med. 2008;49:151–7.
45. Leichner PK. A unified approach to photon and beta particle dosimetry. J Nucl Med. 1994;35:1721–9.
46. Hall JH. Radiation dose rate: a factor of importance in radiobiology and radiotherapy. Br J Radiol. 1972;45:81–97.
47. Schlesinger T, Flower M, McCready V. Radiation dose assessments in 131I (I-131) therapy. The necessity for in-vivo quantitation and dosimetry in the treatment of carcinoma of the thyroid. Radiother Oncol. 1989;14:35–41.
48. Dorn R, Kopp J, Vogt H, et al. Dosimetry-guided radioactive iodine treatment in patients with metastatic differentiated thyroid cancer: largest safe dose using a risk-based approach. J Nucl Med. 2003;44: 451–6.
49. Pochin EE. ^{131}I therapy of thyroid cancer. Semin Nucl Med. 1971;1:503–15.
50. Varma VM, Beierwaltes WH, Nofal MM, et al. Treatment of thyroid cancer: death rates after surgery and after surgery followed by sodium iodides I-131. JAMA. 1970;214:1437–42.
51. Nemec J, Zamrazil V, Pohunkova D, et al. Bone metastases of thyroid cancer, biological behavior and therapeutic possibilities. Acta Univ Carol Med Monogr. 1978;83:1–106.
52. Pochin EE. Prospects from the treatment of thyroid carcinoma with 131I. Clin Radiol. 1967;18:113–35.
53. Maxon HR, Thomas SR, Hertzbert VS, et al. Relation between effective radiation dose and outcome of ^{131}I therapy for thyroid cancer. N Engl J Med. 1983;309:937–41.
54. Maxon HR, Englaro EE, Thomas SR, et al. ^{131}I therapy for well differentiated thyroid cancer—a quantitative radiation dosimetric approach: outcome and validation in 85 patients. J Nucl Med. 1992;33:1132–6.
55. Klubo-Gwiezdzinska J, Van Nostrand D, Atkins F, Burman K, Jonklaas J, Mete M, Wartofsky L. Efficacy of dosimetric versus empiric prescribed activity of 131I for therapy of differentiated thyroid cancer. Thyroid. 2011;96:3217–25.
56. Leeper RD. Thyroid cancer. Med Clin North Am. 1985;69:1079–96.
57. Tuttle RM, Leboeuf R, Robbins RJ, Qualey R, Pentlow K, Larson SM, Chan CY. Empiric radioactive iodine dosing regimens frequently exceed maximum tolerated activity levels in elderly patients with thyroid cancer. J Nucl Med. 2006;47:1587–91.
58. Kulkarni K, Van Nostrand D, Atkins FB, Aiken MJ, Burman K, Wartofsky L. The frequency with which empiric amounts of radioiodine "over-" or "under-" treat patients with metastatic well-differentiated thyroid cancer. Thyroid 2006;16:1019–23.
59. Esposito G, Van Nostrand D, Atkins F, Burman K, Wartofsky L, Kulkarni K. Frequency of "Over" And "Under" treatment with empiric prescribed activity of I-131 in patients with and without lung metastasis secondary to well-differentiated thyroid cancer. J Nucl Med. 2006;47(1):238P (abstract).
60. Thomas SR, Maxon HR, Kereiakes JG, Saenger EL. Quantitative external counting techniques enabling improved diagnostic and therapeutic decisions in patients with well differentiated thyroid cancer. Radiology. 1997;122:731–7.
61. Leeper RR. Thyroid cancer. Med Clin North Am. 1985;69: 1079–96.
62. Schlumberger M, Challeton C, De Vathaire F, et al. Radioactive iodine treatment and external radiotherapy for lung and bone metastases from thyroid carcinoma. J Nucl Med. 1996;37:598–605.

63. Dinneen SF, Valimaki MJ, Bergstralh EJ, et al. Distant metastases in papillary thyroid carcinoma: 100 cases observed at one institution during 5 decades. J Clin Endocrinol Metab. 1995;80:2041–5.
64. Arnstein NB, Carey JE, Spaulding SA, et al. Determination of iodine131 diagnostic dose for imaging metastatic thyroid cancer. J Nucl Med. 1986;27:1764–9.
65. Van Nostrand D, Atkins F, Moreau S, Aiken M, Kulkarni K, Wu JS, Burman K, Wartofsky L. Utility of the radioiodine whole body retention at 48 hours for modifying empiric activity of 131-iodine for the treatment of metastatic well-differentiated thyroid carcinoma. Thyroid. 2009;1(9):1093–8.
66. Hanscheid H, Lassmann M, Luster M, et al. Blood Dosimetry from a single measurement of the whole body radioiodine retention in patients with differentiated thyroid carcinoma. Endocr Relat Cancer. 2009;16:1283–9.
67. Sgouros G, Kolbert KS, Sheikh A, et al. Patient-specific dosimetry for I-131 thyroid cancer therapy using I-124 PET and 3-dimensional internal dosimetry (3D-ID) software. J Nucl Med. 2004;45:1366–72.
68. Sgouros G, Hobbs RF, Atkins FB, Van Nostrand D, Ladenson PW, Wahl R. Three-dimensional radiobiological dosimetry (3D-RD) with ^{124}I PET for ^{131}I therapy of thyroid cancer. Eur J Nucl Med Mol Imaging. 2011;38:S41–7.

Simplified Methods of Dosimetry

59

Frank B. Atkins and Douglas Van Nostrand

Introduction

The objectives of any radiation therapy, including an ^{131}I therapy for differentiated thyroid cancer (DTC), are the same: (1) to deliver a sufficient radiation absorbed dose to the target in order to achieve the desired effect, whether it is for cure, stabilization, or palliation, and (2) to eliminate, or at least limit, the radiation absorbed dose to normal tissues so as to reduce or avoid side effects. In order to accomplish the above objectives, the radiation absorbed dose to the target (e.g., tumor) and normal tissues should be calculated. However, for ^{131}I therapy for differentiated thyroid cancer, this is difficult, and the fundamentals and controversies associated with such methods to calculate the radiation absorbed dose of ^{131}I to tumors and normal tissues have been presented earlier in Chap. 58.

Although the calculation of the radiation absorbed dose to the tumor and normal tissues is the standard practice in radiation oncology using external radiation sources, the calculation of the radiation absorbed dose to tumors and normal tissues for ^{131}I therapies is problematic for several reasons. First and as cited by Thierens et al. [1], these measurements are difficult to perform and possibly subject to large errors. Second, full dosimetry such as described by Benua and Leeper [2] (see Chap. 75) can be demanding for both the patient and personnel, and they can be outside of the capability and/or desires of many nuclear medicine facilities to perform. As a result, alternative procedures to simplify the Benua and Leeper dosimetric approach in order to help determine patient-specific prescribed activities of ^{131}I for treatment of DTC would be valuable, and a number of alternative approaches have been suggested. The objective of this chapter is to discuss several simplified dosimetric methods that have been proposed for calculating the maximum tolerated activity to the blood (or bone marrow). This chapter will not repeat the fundamentals and controversies of various dosimetric methods, and again the reader is encouraged to review Chap. 58, which also includes the restrictions recommended by Benua and Leeper. This chapter will also not discuss any simplified dosimetric methods for the calculation of the radiation absorbed dose to a tumor per administered GBq (mCi).

F.B. Atkins, PhD
Division of Nuclear Medicine, MedStar Washington Hospital Center, Georgetown University School of Medicine, Washington, DC, USA
e-mail: atkinsfb@gmail.com

D. Van Nostrand, MD, FACP, FACNM (✉)
Nuclear Medicine Research, MedStar Research Institute and Washington Hospital Center, Georgetown University School of Medicine, Washington Hospital Center,
110 Irving Street, N.W., Suite GB 60F, Washington, DC 20010, USA
e-mail: douglasvannostrand@gmail.com

Developing Simplified Patient-Specific Options

Single Blood Sampling: "The Traino Approach"

Since the majority of the radiation absorbed dose to the blood or the bone marrow is contributed by the short-range beta particles emitted from the decay of ^{131}I, information about the concentration of the radioiodine in the blood as a function of time is critical to the dosimetry analysis. However, this also represents one of the more tedious and time-consuming (albeit minimally invasive) aspects of any of the rigorous dosimetry methodology. For this reason, a few approaches have been proposed in an effort to simplify this aspect of the data collection and analysis.

Traino et al. [3] presented a method in which only a *single* blood sample might be used, instead of the typical five or more. In this study, blood samples were collected in a small group of patients ($n=4$) at four time points, namely, 3, 24, 48, and 72 h post-diagnostic administration of a capsule containing 18.5–37 MBq (0.5–1.0 mCi) of ^{131}I. At the same time

L. Wartofsky, D. Van Nostrand (eds.), *Thyroid Cancer*, DOI 10.1007/978-1-4939-3314-3_59

points, a shielded, collimated NaI (Tl) scintillation detector (the same device typically found in nuclear medicine facilities for performing thyroid uptake measurements) was positioned in a reproducible location and distance (approximately 20 cm) over the patient's thigh above the knee. This location was considered to represent an anatomical region of the patient in which the only radioiodine present was that contained in the blood pool – the volume of which in the field of view of the detector should remain constant over this time period. Therefore, it might be reasonable to assume that the general shape of the curve represented by the counts per unit time from this detector would be the same as the ^{131}I activity per ml of blood collected at the same time points. The thigh time-activity curve was normalized to the first time point and then scaled by the measured activity concentration that was measured in the first blood sample (although any time point could be used), to yield the estimated blood curve relationship given below in Eq. 59.1:

$$A_{blood}(t) = A'_{blood}(\tau)[C(t)/C(\tau)] \qquad (59.1)$$

C(t) is the measured counts per minute over the thigh at time t. τ is the time at which the reference blood sample was obtained, and A′ is the measured activity of ^{131}I per ml at time τ.

These curves were compared to the actual blood time-activity measurements at the other three time points. Visually the difference between the two curves for each patient was almost imperceptible. Using an approach such as this would improve the patient tolerance for dosimetry and reduce data processing time by eliminating all but one of the blood samples from the protocol. However, this approach would still require the patient to return on multiple occasions for the thigh counting measurements. Also drawing blood at the early time point, namely, 2–4 h post-dosing, to obtain the scaling factor for the thigh counts could introduce a large error if the patient had delayed gastric function and the blood concentration had therefore not reached its peak value. However, this method has only been demonstrated in a very small number of patients, and further validation is needed.

No Blood Samples with Multiple Whole-Body Measurements

The Thomas Approach

Since most of the radioiodine circulating in the post-thyroidectomy patient, especially when there is minimal residual normal tissue and/or metastatic disease, is confined to the intravascular compartment, there tends to be a strong correlation between the blood and whole-body time-activity curves. If there is rapid clearance of the radioiodine from the blood, then the whole-body curve likewise clears rapidly and vice versa. Recognizing the possible correlation between the whole-body and blood time-activity curves, Thomas et al. [4] evaluated a methodology which might provide a first-order approximation of the hematopoietic radiation absorbed dose based solely on the whole-body data. In this investigation, they examined the relationship between the whole-body retention and the activity in the blood following the oral administration of 74 MBq (2 mCi) of ^{131}I in 49 studies involving 46 patients. All patients were hypothyroid at the time of administration. Whole-body measurements were obtained using a calibrated probe and conjugate views at 2, 24, 48, 72, and 96 h post-administration along with blood samples collected nominally at 24, 48, and 72 h. The patient's whole blood volumes were estimated based on gender, height, and weight using Retzlaff's formulas [5]. The objective was to determine if the activity in the blood at each of the time points could be represented as a constant fraction, "f," of the whole-body activity for a given patient. More importantly, was this fraction, "f," similar enough between patients that a single value could be used for all patients? Since the extent of disease might affect these results, the patients were subdivided for analysis into three smaller groups based on the pretherapy diagnostic scan: those with (1) metastatic thyroid cancer, (2) residual thyroid tissue in the neck, and (3) no evidence of tumor or residual thyroid tissue. The mean "f" ratio for these three groups was reported to be 0.14, 0.14, and 0.17, respectively. Also, importantly, the standard deviation was similar for all three groups and approximately 0.05. Therefore, it might be possible not only to reduce the number of blood samples as in the previous section but also to eliminate them entirely from the dosimetry (blood) analysis.

The Sisson Approach

Sisson et al. [6] proposed using just a single, simple to perform, measurement of the relative whole-body retention (WBR) of ^{131}I performed 48 h after administration of the diagnostic prescribed activity. This value was subsequently used to adjust the empiric prescribed activity of ^{131}I. In this study the WBR, expressed as a percentage of the administered activity, was measured in 87 patients following thyroid hormone withdrawal. A one standard deviation region about the median value was 9–24.8 %. Sisson et al. then proposed several criteria (see Table 59.1) for increasing or decreasing the standard, empiric activity of ^{131}I based on these observa-

Table 59.1 Thresholds for modification of empiric activities of ^{131}I based on the percent whole-body retention at 48 h

WBR retention (%)	Action
>9 % and <24.8 %	No change
<9 %	Increase empiric activity
<5 %	Increase empiric activity by 50–100 %
>24.8 %	Decrease empiric activity
>40 %	Substantially decrease empiric activity

tions. Unfortunately these guidelines are neither quantitative nor objective, but the concept laid the foundation to pursue other options utilizing the percent 48-h whole-body retention.

The Hanscheid Approach

Hanscheid et al. [7] incorporated Thomas' approach into an analysis based on the formalism adopted by the Medical Internal Radiation Dose Committee [8]. These authors found in an assessment of 49 dosimetry studies a relationship between the blood and whole-body activity curves similar to that observed by Thomas et al. [4] whereby 14–17 % of the whole-body residence time could be attributed to the blood. Based on an analysis of the data from another study, [9] a value of 14 ± 3 % was deduced. Therefore, the radiation dose delivered to the blood per unit administered activity could be *estimated* using the following equation, which only uses the whole-body retention data:

$$D_{blood} / A_0 = (\frac{15.12}{BLV(ml)} + \frac{0.0188}{Wt(kg)2/3}) x \tau_{total\,body}(h) \quad (59.2)$$

BLV is the estimated patient's blood volume based on Retzlaff et al. [5], and $\tau_{total\ body}$ is the residence time for the whole-body retention derived from the whole-body counts measured at multiple time points over a time period of 4 or more days. For a given target dose to the blood, e.g., 2 Gy, one can calculate from this relationship the administered activity, A_0, that would deliver this radiation dose.

Having formulated an approach that could simplify the dosimetry by eliminating the need for blood samples, perhaps it is possible to simplify the methodology even further. As previously stated, rapid clearance of the radioiodine would likewise correlate with a rapid clearance from the blood. Since the mean effective half-life of ^{131}I in patients with DTC post-thyroidectomy or post-ablation has been reported to be in the range of 10.5–15.7 h, [10, 11] then perhaps a single assessment of the whole-body retention after only 24–48 h might provide a reasonable patient-specific estimate of the biokinetics. This was the approach adopted by Hanscheid et al. [7] in which they further simplified Eq. 59.2 as shown below:

$$D_{blood} / A_0 = (\frac{15.12}{BLV(ml)} + \frac{0.0188}{Wt(kg)2/3}) x\, t(h) / \ln(R(t)) \quad (59.3)$$

In this equation, R(t) represents the whole-body retention as a fraction of the administered dose at any time "t" expressed in units of hours. They measured the retention by normalizing the geometric mean of background-corrected anterior and posterior counts obtained from whole-body scans using a scintillation camera observed at time "t" post-administration to the value obtained at 2 h. This initial time point reflects the total prescribed activity used in the diagnostic study since the patient was not allowed to micturate during the intervening time interval. This method was evaluated in 29 patients in which the whole-body measurements and blood samples were both collected nominally at 2, 6, 24, 48, and 72 h and 4–6 days. Comparison was performed between the blood dose estimates using a standard blood dosimetry protocol and the values obtained from Eq. 59.3 using a single time point for the whole-body retention. Several time points were chosen for analysis, namely, 6, 24, and 48 h. The 6-h time point produced the greatest inter-patient variability in the estimates compared to either the 24- or 48-h retention value. An additional analysis of 59 patients was also performed using the data extracted from Hanscheid et al. [9], for which the 48-h retention could be obtained. Once again they observed a good correlation between the actual and estimated values of the blood dose per unit administered activity.

As noted by these investigators, discrepancies between the actual and estimated blood dose can be substantial if the patient deviates significantly from the assumptions employed, principally that 14 % of the total body activity can be attributed to the activity in the blood. Furthermore, as stated by the authors, this method has not been validated for patients with large tumor volumes and/or residual normal thyroid tissue with high uptake, and consequently the methods may not be applicable under these circumstances. While the median of the absolute deviations between the actual and estimated blood dose values using the 48-h retention value is relatively small (<11 %), underestimation of the actual dose by >25 % occurred in 2 of 29 assessments. Consequently, these authors recommend using a more conservative target radiation absorbed dose to the blood of 1.3 Gy (130 rad) in order to avoid accidentally exceeding the generally accepted limit of 2 Gy (200 rad). Therefore, this methodology may not be applicable for high-risk patients in which the objective is to deliver the maximum radiation absorbed dose to the metastases since on the average the calculated prescribed activity would be about 35 % less than what would be calculated using a standard dosimetry protocol.

The Atkins Approach

A similar approach to the previous one was also developed and evaluated by Van Nostrand et al. [12, 13]. This method also uses the whole-body retention (WBR) at 48 h after administration of the radioiodine to estimate the maximum tolerated activity (MTA), namely, that which would deliver 2 Gy to the blood. However, their approach does not make any implicit assumptions about the relative contribution of the blood activity as was the case for Thomas et al. [4] and Hanscheid et al. [7]. Instead a regression analysis was performed between the MTA based on the Benua-Leeper protocol (see Chap. 58) derived from Benua et al. and the patient's

WBR. In order to minimize gender differences due to blood volumes and geometric factors, the regression was performed using the calculated MTA normalized to the patient's body surface area based on the formulation of Mosteller [14]. A retrospective review was conducted in this study of patients with differentiated thyroid cancer, total thyroidectomy, suspected metastatic disease, and ^{131}I dosimetry. All patients were prepared for their dosimetry and anticipated radioiodine therapy by thyroid hormone withdrawal. Patients who received recombinant human TSH injections were excluded. The objectives of this study were [1] to assess the utility of the whole-body retention expressed as a percentage of the administered activity of ^{131}I at 48 h (%WBR_{48h}) in identifying patients for whom the standard empiric prescribed activity of 3.7 GBq (200 mCi) should be modified either up or down in the context of the various thresholds originally suggested by Sisson et al. [6] (see Table 59.1) and [2] to evaluate a quantitative relationship based on the WBR that would provide more objective information regarding the magnitude of such adjustments to the standard empiric prescribed activity. From dosimetries performed on 142 patients, data regarding the first objective were noted and published in the original article, but more importantly was the establishment of a quantitative relationship between the MTA normalized to the body surface area and the %WBR_{48h} based on a bi-exponential regression as shown in Eq. 59.4:

$$\frac{MTA(mCi)}{BSA(m^2)} = 376.3 * e^{(-0.0387*R)} + 1144.4 * e^{(-0.8522*R)} \quad (59.4)$$

where R = %$WBR_{48h.}$

Results from this study are shown in Fig. 59.1a. As noted in this figure, the normalization to the body surface area effectively eliminated any gender differences. However, just as in the approach proposed by Hanscheid et al. [7], there are individual patient variations about the predicted MTA such that the model will underestimate the radiation absorbed dose to the blood in 50 % of the patients. For this reason the authors recommended using a value that is less than that predicted by the model. As shown in Fig. 59.1b, all of the patients included in their investigation lie at or above the curve which represents a threshold at 70 % of the value determined from Eq. 59.4, which is similar to the 65 % factor recommended by Hanscheid et al. [7].

Subsequently, Atkins et al. [15] evaluated the effect of rhTSH stimulation versus thyroid hormone withdrawal on the bi-exponential dosimetry model discussed above. In 26 patients who were prepared with injection of recombinant human thyroid-stimulating hormone (rhTSH), the bi-exponential function was very similar to the bi-exponential function for the 142 patients prepared with thyroid hormone withdrawal (THW) (p<0.01) with a mean percent deviation of 3.5 % with a range of −6.6 to +7.6%. Although the % WBRs for those patients prepared with rhTSH were lower (8.8 %) than the % WBRs for patients prepared with THW, the same bi-exponential function can be used to estimate the prescribed activity of ^{131}I for the treatment of DTC using either rhTSH or THW.

Subsequently, Atkins et al. [16] reported the validation of the model based on the fractional whole-body retention at 48 hours after ^{131}I administration. In 191 dosimetries performed in 170 patients, the correlation of predicted maximum tolerated activity using the bi-exponential function to the maximum tolerated activity measure by the full Benua-Leeper dosimetry protocol was excellent (r=0.96) with an average deviation of only +/-1.2 %. However, as previously noted and to avoid overdosing of a patient on the basis of the predicted maximum tolerated activity from the bi-exponential function, no more than 70 % of the predicted value based on Eq. 59.4 should be administered.

Finally, initial evaluations of additional simplified dosimetry alternatives have been published by Jentzen et al. [17], which warrant further evaluation and validation.

Conclusion

In summary, simplified dosimetric methods have been proposed that could be useful in identifying patients whose therapeutic prescribed activity of ^{131}I should either be reduced or could be increased, and these simplified dosimetric methods may be performed in almost all nuclear medicine facilities.

However, the user needs to be mindful that the application of any of these proposed models needs to be tempered with a reduction factor of about 65–70 % in order to avoid accidentally exceeding the generally accepted maximum blood dose of 2 Gy (200 rad). In addition, although the determination of the prescribed activity using methods described in this chapter may represent an acceptable alternative for those facilities that either will not or cannot perform a more comprehensive dosimetry protocol, it is paramount to remember that in many cases this value is based on just one measurement in time in the average patients in the population studied by these investigators. Consequently, when one is trying to determine the prescribed activity for ^{131}I treatment of patients with metastatic DTC, the preferred method is a comprehensive whole-body and blood dosimetry protocol (Chap. 58), rather than one of these simplified methods. A more comprehensive dosimetry protocol provides not only a more accurate and clinically accepted estimate of the MTA (based on a limit of 200 cGy [rad] along with empiric restrictions of the whole-body retention at 48 h) but also provides the potential for a higher prescribed activity of ^{131}I to be safely administered, thereby potentially delivering a higher radiation absorbed dose to the metastases.

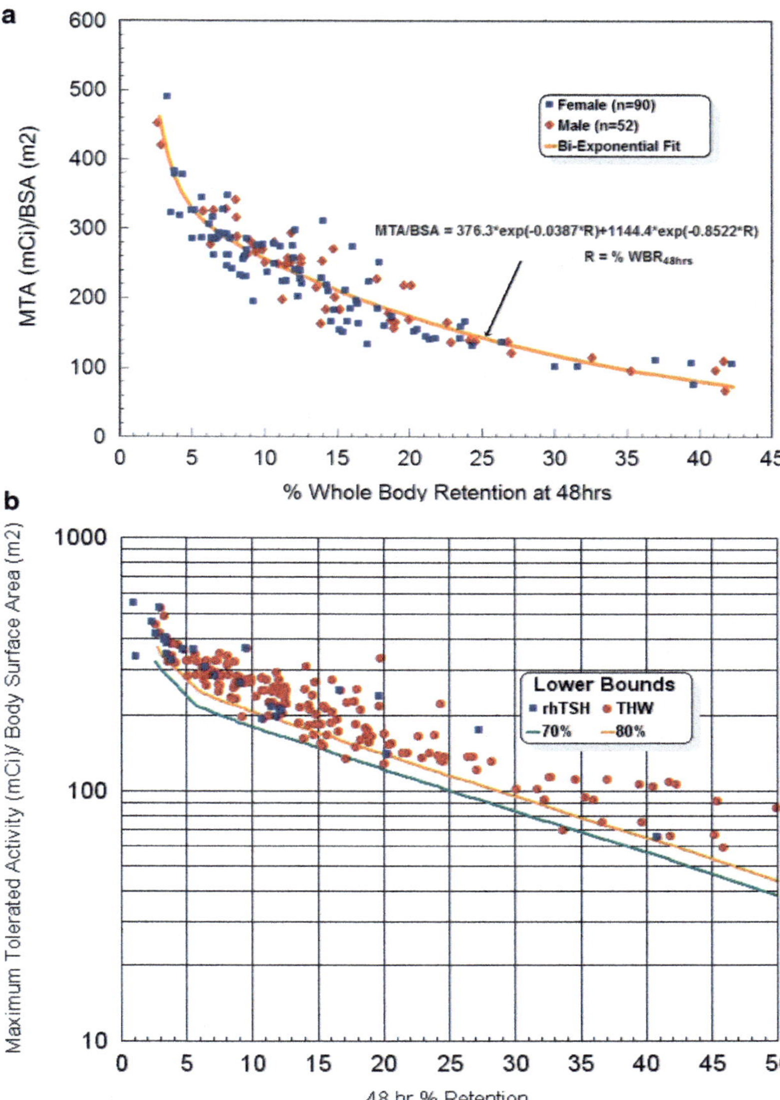

Fig. 59.1 MTA distribution for 48-h whole-body retention model normalized to the patient's body surface area. (**a**) demonstrates the results of the bi-exponential regression function of the normalized MTA versus the $\%WBR_{48h}$. (**b**) demonstrates the same data as in 59.1a with the addition of reference curves at the 70 % (*blue*) and 80 % (*orange*) thresholds demonstrating how the patient data are bounded by a fixed fraction of the predicted MTA/BSA over a broad range of WBR values

References

1. Thierens HM, Monsieurs MA, Bacher K. Patient dosimetry in radionuclide therapy: the whys and the wherefores. Nucl Med Commun. 2005;26:593–9.
2. Benua RS, Cicale NR, Sonenberg M, et al. The relation of radioiodine dosimetry to results and complications in the treatment of metastatic thyroid cancer. AJR. 1962;87:171–82.
3. Traino AC, DiMartino F, Boni G, et al. A minimally invasive method to evaluate ^{131}I kinetics in the blood. Radiat Prot Dosim. 2004;109:249–52.
4. Thomas S, Samaratunga R, Sperling M, Maxon H. Predictive estimate of blood dose from external counting data preceding radioiodine therapy for thyroid cancer. Nucl Med Biol. 1993;20:157–62.
5. Retzlaff J, Tauxe W, Kiely J, Stroebel C. Erythrocyte volume, plasma volume, and lean body mass in adult men and women. Blood. 1969;33:649–67.
6. Sisson J, Shulkin B, Lawson S. Increasing efficacy and safety of treatments of patients with well-differentiated thyroid carcinoma by measuring body retentions of ^{131}I. J Nucl Med. 2003;44:898–903.
7. Hanscheid H, Lassmann M, Luster M, et al. Blood dosimetry from a single measurement of the whole body radioiodine retention in patients with differentiated thyroid carcinoma. Endocr Relat Cancer. 2009;16:1283–9.
8. Stabin MG. MIRDOSE – the personal computer software for use in internal dose assessment in nuclear medicine. J Nucl Med. 1996;37:538–46.
9. Hanscheid H, Lassmann M, Luster M, et al. Iodine biokinetics and dosimetry in radioiodine therapy of thyroid cancer: procedures and results of a prospective international controlled study of ablation after rhTSH or hormone withdrawal. J Nucl Med. 2006;47:648–54.
10. Remy H, Borget I, Leboulleux S, et al. ^{131}I effective half-life and dosimetry in thyroid cancer patients. J Nucl Med. 2008;49:1445–50.
11. Willegaignon J, Malvestiti L, Guimaraes M, et al. ^{131}I effective half-life (T_{eff}) for patients with thyroid cancer. Health Phys. 2006;91:119–22.

12. Van Nostrand D, Atkins F, Kulkarni K, Burman K, Wartofsky L. The utility of percent 48-hour whole body retention for modifying empiric amounts of I-131 for the treatment of thyroid carcinoma. J Nucl Med. 2006;47 Suppl 1:324P (abstract).
13. Van Nostrand D, Atkins F, Moreau S, et al. Utility of the radioiodine whole-body retention at 48 hours for modifying empiric activity of 131-iodine for the treatment of metastatic well-differentiated thyroid carcinoma. Thyroid. 2009;10:1093–8.
14. Mosteller R. Simplified calculation of body surface area. N Engl J Med. 1987;17:1098.
15. Atkins F, Van Nostrand D, Moreau SL, Burman K, Wartofsky L. Percent 48-hr whole body retention for estimating maximum tolerated activity of ^{131}I for the treatment of well-differentiated thyroid cancer: the effect of rhTSH stimulation vs thyroid hormone withdrawal on a bi-exponential dosimetry model. J Nucl Med. 2007;48(2):268P (abstract).
16. Atkins F, Van Nostrand D, Moreau S, Burman K, Wartofsky L. Validation of a simple thyroid cancer dosimetry model based on the fractional whole-body retention at 48 hours post-administration of ^{131}I. Thyroid. 2015;25:1347–50.
17. Jentzen W, Bockisch A, Ruhlmann M. Assessment of simplified blood dose protocols for the estimation of the maximum tolerable activity in thyroid cancer patients undergoing radioiodine therapy using ^{124}I. J Nucl Med. 2015;56:832–83.

Radioiodine Dosimetry with Recombinant Human Thyrotropin

60

Robert Michael Tuttle, Ravinder K. Grewal, and Richard J. Robbins

Introduction

Although radioactive iodine (RAI) has been an essential tool in the management of thyroid cancer for more than 60 years, there continues to be a lack of scientific rigor regarding the optimal choice of administered activity for individual patients. Often, activities of 30–75 mCi are administered for RAI remnant ablation, 100–150 mCi for adjuvant therapy in patients at significant risk of having microscopic residual disease, while activities ranging from 150 to 250 mCi are usually reserved for treatment of known metastatic disease. In most cases, the activity selected is based on an empiric regimen without knowledge of the rate of RAI clearance or specific lesional dosimetry for that individual patient.

In the 1950s, methods were established to calculate the maximal tolerable activity (MTA) of RAI, based principally on the rate of clearance of "tracer" doses of 131I from the blood and entire body in patients undergoing traditional thyroid hormone withdrawal preparation [1–4]. In these early studies, administered activities that resulted in more than 2 Gy to the blood were associated with significant bone marrow depression. Additionally, whole-body retention of more than 80 mCi of 131I at 48 h in patients with diffuse lung metastases was linked with subsequent pulmonary fibrosis [2, 5]. More recent studies have suggested that doses as high as 3 Gy to the bone marrow may be well tolerated [6]. Using these parameters, it is often possible to safely administer activities of 500–600 mCi in selected patients with metastatic thyroid carcinoma.

The advent of recombinant human thyrotropin (rhTSH) has sparked a reevaluation of the approach to RAI scanning, remnant ablation, and therapy [7–11]. As reviewed in other sections, rhTSH is now approved in the United States, Europe, and many other countries for use both as a diagnostic aid for whole body radioactive iodine scanning, stimulated thyroglobulin measurements, and remnant ablation in differentiated thyroid cancer patients without distant metastases. Low rates of disease persistence and recurrence reported following radioactive iodine remnant ablation also demonstrate the effectiveness of radioactive iodine as adjuvant therapy given the following either rhTSH or thyroid hormone withdrawal in both low-risk and high-risk patients [12–15]. Additionally, while not approved as an adjunct to radioactive iodine therapy in patients with distant metastasis, retrospective studies demonstrate similar response to therapy and short-term overall survival in patients prepared using either rhTSH or traditional thyroid hormone withdrawal [14, 16–18].

While these clinical findings are promising, it is important to recognize that whole-body radioactive iodine clearance is significantly more rapid in patients prepared for RAI studies using rhTSH. Because iodine is principally excreted by the kidney, and hypothyroidism is associated with a significant decrease in renal glomerular filtration rate, thyroid hormone withdrawal is associated with a marked increase in whole-body RAI retention times. Patients prepared with rhTSH are either euthyroid or mildly thyrotoxic and would be expected to have a more rapid renal clearance of RAI, shorter RAI retention times, and, hence, lower whole-body radiation exposure for a given administered activity of RAI. Over the last several years, improvements in the ability

R.M. Tuttle, MD (✉)
Department of Medicine, Memorial Sloan Kettering Cancer Center, 1275 York Ave, New York, NY 10021, USA
e-mail: tuttlem@mskcc.org

R.K. Grewal, MD
Nuclear Medicine Service, Department of Radiology, Memorial Sloan Kettering Cancer Center, New York, NY 10065, USA
e-mail: grewalr@mskcc.org

R.J. Robbins, MD
Chairman, Department of Medicine, The Methodist Hospital, 6550 Fannin Street Suite SM 1001, Houston, TX 77030, USA
e-mail: rjrobbins@tmhs.org

L. Wartofsky, D. Van Nostrand (eds.), *Thyroid Cancer*, DOI 10.1007/978-1-4939-3314-3_60

to accurately determine lesional dosimetry have led to a better understanding of the iodine kinetics within individual metastatic lesions [19–21].

This chapter reviews the available data on whole-body RAI clearance and lesional dosimetry to determine the magnitude and clinical significance of the enhanced clearance of RAI in patients prepared for RAI studies with rhTSH.

Whole-Body and Blood Clearance of RAI

Whole-body retention was established in both the hypothyroid state and rhTSH preparation in 7 patients studied at the National Cancer Institute, part of the phase I/II multicenter study examining the diagnostic use of rhTSH in thyroid cancer [22]. In these patients, thyroid hormone withdrawal resulted in a 24-h whole-body retention of 16.8±7 % of the administered activity compared to 7.4±5 % in those prepared with rhTSH.

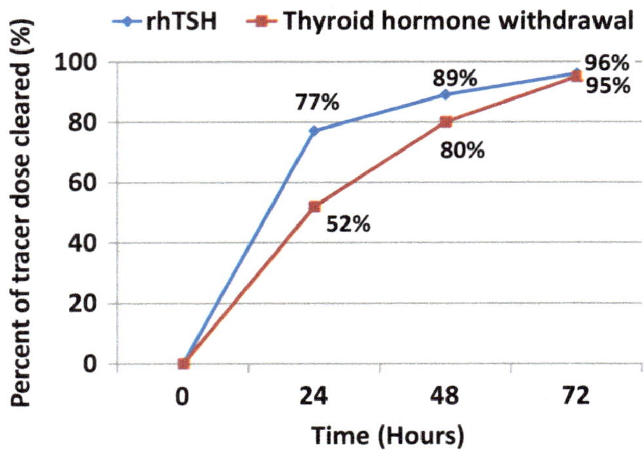

Fig. 60.1 Whole-body RAI clearance curves in 97 patients following rhTSH preparation and 52 patients following thyroid hormone withdrawal expressed as the percent of tracer dose cleared at each time point

These findings are consistent with our initial observations, which determined RAI clearance based on multiple blood and whole-body measurements over 72 h following a tracer dose of 131I [4] in patients undergoing rhTSH stimulation. In most patients, the radioactive iodine clearance is faster after rhTSH than when the RAI clearance was determined in the same patient during thyroid hormone withdrawal. As part of our routine clinical care, we performed standard RAI clearance studies in our first 97 patients following rhTSH preparation and a comparison group of 52 patients during thyroid hormone withdrawal. In these cohorts, traditional thyroid hormone withdrawal was associated with an MTA of 462±33 mCi. Preparation with rhTSH was linked with a significantly higher MTA (640±26 mCi), consistent with more rapid RAI clearance and decreased whole-body retention (see Fig. 60.1). Our studies suggest that whole-body RAI clearance is approximately 30 % faster after rhTSH preparation vs. traditional thyroid hormone withdrawal.

Consistent with these findings, Remy et al. reported a 31 % lower mean whole-body effect of half-life in 36 patients receiving rhTSH preparation compared with 218 patients who underwent thyroid hormone withdrawal (10.5 h vs. 15.7 h) [23]. Furthermore the residence times in the whole body and stomach were also significantly shorter following rhTSH, while residence times in the colon and bladder did not differ between groups.

Luster et al. studied RAI blood and whole-body clearance in nine subjects during both thyroid hormone withdrawal and rhTSH preparation using multiple blood and whole-body counts at several time points over 48 h [24]. The effective half-time of RAI in the blood was 9.7±2 h following rhTSH preparation in comparison to 11.7±2 h after thyroid hormone withdrawal. The effective half-time of RAI in the remaining whole body (not counting the thyroid remnant) was also shorter following rhTSH preparation (9.4±1.5 h) than thyroid hormone withdrawal (12.4±2.5 h).

Chiesa et al. also confirmed more rapid whole-body radioactive iodine clearance following rhTSH-stimulated radioactive iodine therapy than when dosimetry had previously been done in a single patient following thyroid hormone withdrawal [25].

Similarly, Hanscheid et al. [26] demonstrated that the absorbed dose to the blood was significantly lower following rhTSH preparation than after thyroid hormone withdrawal (mean, 0.109 +/− 0.028 mGy/MBq; maximum, 0.18 mGy/MBq with rhTSH; mean, 0.167 +/− 0.061 mGy/MBq; maximum, 0.35 mGy/MBq with thyroid hormone withdrawal). Likewise, Hartung-Knemeyer et al. demonstrated that the blood dose per administered activity was significantly higher in 100 thyroid cancer patients receiving RAI after thyroid hormone withdrawal than in 24 patients prepared with rhTSH (0.08 Gy/GBq vs. 0.06 Gy/GBq, respectively) [27]. Therefore, the same administered activity would result in lower whole-body radiation exposure in rhTSH-prepared patients when compared to hypothyroid patients after thyroid hormone withdrawal.

Bianchi et al. evaluated red marrow absorbed dose in a cohort of 27 patients with RAI-avid distant metastasis (11 prepared with rhTSH, 16 prepared with thyroid hormone withdrawal) [28]. Because of the wide distribution with respect to red marrow dosimetry and the lack of within-patient comparisons, no clear differences could be demonstrated with respect to the method of preparation.

Red marrow absorbed dose was calculated after rhTSH preparation for high-dose radioactive iodine therapy in 14 patients with metastatic thyroid cancer [29]. Clinical correlates included platelet counts prior to and 3 months after treatment.

The mean absorbed dose was 0.16 mGy/MBq corresponding to a total red marrow absorbed dose of 1.15 Gy (range 0.28–1.91 Gy). No hematologic toxicity was observed. Even though dose selection was not guided by pre-therapy dosimetry studies, the bone marrow absorbed dose in each case was below the standard accepted maximal tolerable dose of 2 Gy.

From the information above, radioactive iodine clearance from the blood and whole body can be estimated as about 25–30 % faster in euthyroid patients prepared with rhTSH than with thyroid hormone withdrawal (Fig. 60.1). The apparent benefit of lower total-body radiation exposure for a specific administered RAI activity needs to be balanced by the risk that RAI clearance is too rapid to allow adequate uptake of RAI for effective treatment of thyroid remnants or metastatic lesions.

Dosimetry in Thyroid Remnants

RAI uptake in thyroid remnants (after total thyroidectomy) was carefully examined in a phase I/II multicenter study in patients prepared with either thyroid hormone withdrawal or a wide range of rhTSH doses [22]. When all rhTSH dosing regimens were analyzed together, the uptake in the thyroid remnant was higher after thyroid hormone withdrawal in 72 % (13 of 18) of patients (2 % uptake following thyroid hormone withdrawal and 1.2 % uptake following rhTSH; $p<0.05$). However, rhTSH in doses of 10 U/day for two consecutive days (similar to 0.9 mg intramuscularly for 2 days as currently used for diagnostic scanning preparation), or 20 U of rhTSH as a single dose, resulted in uptake in the thyroid remnant that was not significantly different than thyroid hormone withdrawal. As described above, the effective half-time of RAI was significantly shortened with rhTSH preparation; thus, that part of the decreased uptake by the thyroid remnant could be likely explained by the more rapid clearance of RAI from the blood. Indeed, in a subgroup analysis of the seven subjects that had both thyroid remnant dosimetry and whole-body/blood dosimetry, no difference was seen in RAI uptake into the thyroid remnant when uptake values were corrected for RAI whole-body retention. Therefore, the percentage uptake into thyroid remnants appears to be very comparable between the preparation methods, but hypothyroidism was associated with a greater radiation delivered to the thyroid because of the slower RAI clearance from the blood.

Pacini et al. examined 24-h RAI uptake in thyroid remnants and the initial dose rate (IDR) (amount of radiation delivered to the thyroid remnant in the first hour after dosing) in three patient cohorts undergoing RAI remnant ablation [30]. Thyroid hormone withdrawal was related to a significantly higher 24-h uptake value and IDR, compared to rhTSH preparation. Interestingly, the highest uptake values and IDR were seen in patients prepared with traditional thyroid hormone withdrawal who then received rhTSH injections just prior to RAI dosing. The 24-h thyroid remnant uptake was higher in this group of Italian patients vs. the patients studied by Meier et al. within the United States [22]. This difference may be because of the difference in dietary iodine intake between the two countries. As would be expected, the lower RAI uptake in the thyroid remnants, combined with an administered activity of only 30 mCi given 48 h after the second rhTSH dose, led to successful remnant ablation in only 54 % of the patients prepared with rhTSH, compared to an 84 % success rate when 30 mCi was used after thyroid hormone withdrawal. (For additional information on rhTSH in remnant ablation, see Chaps. 10, 34, and 57.)

In a prospective randomized trial, 63 patients were randomized after total thyroidectomy to radioactive iodine remnant ablation following preparation with either thyroid hormone withdrawal or rhTSH [26]. While there were no differences in the mean 48-h radioactive iodine thyroid bed uptake and residence times, the effective half-time in the remnant thyroid tissue was significantly longer after rhTSH than thyroid hormone withdrawal (67.6 +/− 48.8 vs. 48.0 +/− 52.6, $p<0.01$).

In addition to evaluating whole-body and blood RAI clearance, Luster et al. also carefully examined 24-h uptake, effective half-life, and residence times within the thyroid remnants [24]. In eight of nine patients, rhTSH preparation was associated with a higher 24-h uptake, a longer effective half-life, and a longer residence time in the thyroid remnant, compared with the same values determined while hypothyroid. These findings vary with the reports above. The authors hypothesized that stunning could have had a major role in the findings, as all patients served as their own controls, with the rhTSH preparation evaluations conducted before the hypothyroid withdrawal studies. This sequential effect could have artificially decreased the RAI uptakes in the second scans (all done while hypothyroid), causing the uptake measured during thyroid hormone withdrawal to appear lower than it would have been if studied without the prior rhTSH scan. In support of this hypothesis, Lassmann et al. reported that thyroid remnant dosimetry with rhTSH stimulation following a thyroid hormone withdrawal scan was associated with a decrease in 24-h uptake, a reduction in effective half- life, and shorter residence time [31].

Because of the potential effect of stunning, it is difficult to compare uptake of RAI into thyroid remnants in individual patients. For practical and logistical reasons, it would be challenging to enroll patients into a study in which the order of the rhTSH scan and thyroid hormone withdrawal scan is randomized. Therefore, the current published literature cannot accurately determine the differences in RAI uptake into thyroid remnants. However, the reported clinical success of rhTSH-assisted RAI remnant ablation certainly verifies that adequate doses of radiation are being delivered to the thyroid remnants of most patients.

Tumor Dosimetry

Although the data presented above provides much information on whole-body and blood clearance rates, as well as effective half-times and residence rates within presumably "normal" thyroid remnants following total thyroidectomy, much less is known about radiation doses that can be achieved within metastatic deposits of thyroid cancer cells (lesional dosimetry). Several small series and anecdotal cases have been reported in which rhTSH stimulation prior to RAI therapy has resulted in tumoricidal effects in metastatic lesions, as evidenced by follow-up RAI imaging and cross-sectional imaging studies and short-term overall survival (see Chap. 57 on the use of rhTSH in RAI therapy).

Other reports suggest that metastatic lesions are less likely to be identified on diagnostic or post-therapy RAI scans following rhTSH preparation when compared with thyroid hormone withdrawal [32–34] suggesting that rhTSH preparation is associated with lower RAI avidity in metastatic lesions. This has been more carefully quantified in a study by Van Nostrand et al. in which the ability to detect metastatic foci on 124I PET scanning was prospectively evaluated in 24 patients following rhTSH preparation and 16 patients following thyroid hormone withdrawal [35]. More metastatic foci were detected using 124I PET following thyroid hormone withdrawal than with rhTSH preparation both in terms of the percentage of patients having positive foci and the number of positive foci detected.

A precise estimate of lesional dosimetry can be obtained when images are acquired with positron emission tomography (PET) scanners following tracer doses of the positron emitter 124I [21, 36, 37]. Recently, a pilot study evaluating the impact of an MEK inhibitor (selumetinib) on lesional dosimetry in metastatic thyroid cancers has confirmed the dose-response relationship between lesional dosimetry estimated by 124I PET scanning and subsequent response to therapy as determined by decrease in the size of the metastatic lesions on follow-up cross-sectional imaging [19].

Figure 60.2 demonstrates RAI-avid distant metastatic disease on a 2-mCi 131I rhTSH-stimulated diagnostic scan in an elderly male with recurrent, widespread metastatic follicular thyroid cancer [38]. The results of whole-body and blood 131I dosimetry and 124I PET lesional imaging after rhTSH stimulation are shown in Fig. 60.3. Despite what appears to be a markedly positive diagnostic whole-body scan, the lesion dosimetry analysis shows that the individual metastatic lesions are receiving far less than adequate tumoricidal doses (see Fig. 60.4).

In other cases, rhTSH stimulation leads to more than adequate lesional dosimetry and documented regression of metastatic lesions, as demonstrated in an elderly female with recurrent papillary thyroid cancer (see Figs. 60.5 and 60.6).

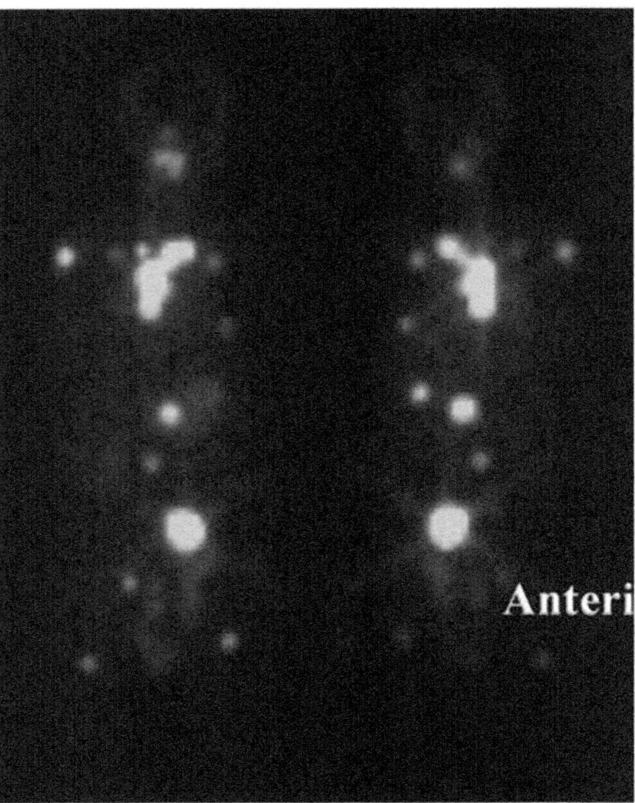

Fig. 60.2 A 2-mCi diagnostic 131I scan in an elderly male with widespread RAI-avid metastatic follicular cancer

In this patient, serial structural imaging after two rhTSH-assisted RAI therapies 6 months apart confirmed that tumoricidal doses were achieved by showing a marked decrease in the size of her mediastinal recurrence and pulmonary metastases. These anecdotal cases suggest that rhTSH stimulation can achieve tumoricidal doses of RAI within metastatic lesions in some patients.

Bianchi et al. reported lesional dosimetry findings using 124I PET in a cohort of 27 patients with RAI-avid distant metastasis (11 prepared with rhTSH, 16 prepared with thyroid hormone withdrawal) [28]. Both thyroid hormone withdrawal and rhTSH stimulation preparations were associated with a wide spectrum of lesional absorbed dose ranging from 1 to 778 Gy indicating that many lesions could be expected to achieve a tumoricidal dose using either approach.

Freudenberg studied lesional dosimetry using 124 I PET scanning by comparing the lesional dose per administered activity of RAI in a cohort of 27 patients after rhTSH with 36 patients prepared for scanning with thyroid hormone withdrawal [39]. While no statistically significant difference was detected in the mean lesional dose per administered activity between the cohorts, a subgroup analysis evaluating the lesional dosimetry obtained using the two preparation

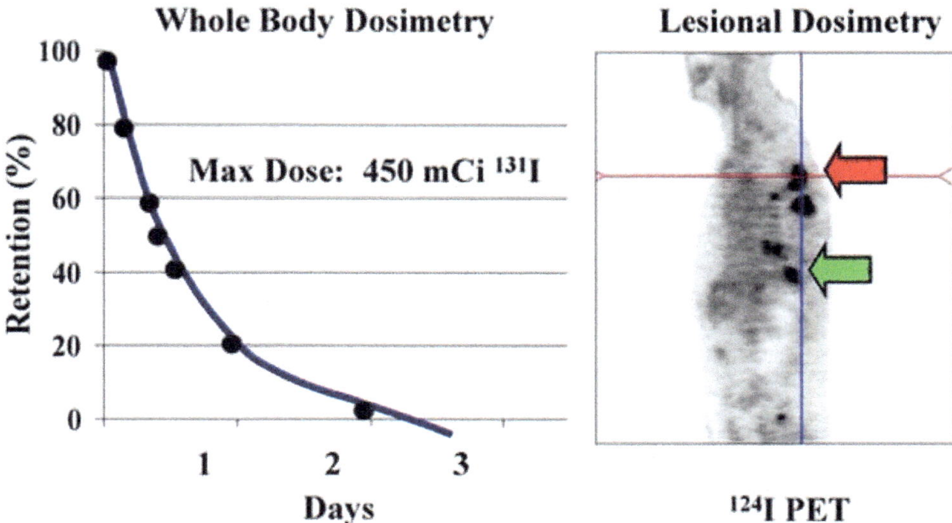

Fig. 60.3 Results of whole-body dosimetry (RAI clearance) presented on the left panel and a 124I PET scan image in the right panel, showing spinal and paraspinal metastatic lesions

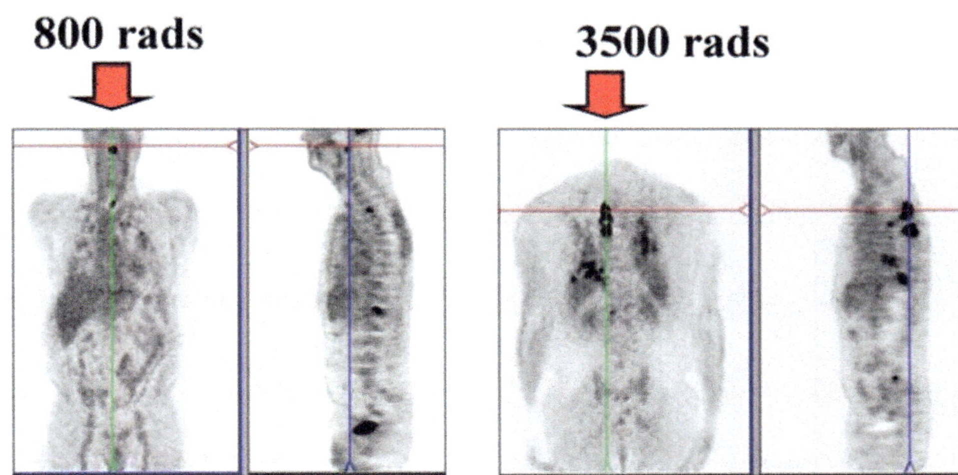

Fig. 60.4 Lesional dosimetry calculations based on a 400-mCi administered activity. Predicted lesional dosimetry is far below expected tumoricidal doses in most of his lesions

methods within the same patient suggested that the lesional dose was often higher following rhTSH preparation than thyroid hormone withdrawal).

Potzi et al. evaluated four patients with distant metastasis by performing lesional dosimetry in each patient, first following rhTSH stimulation and then 6 weeks later following thyroid hormone withdrawal [40]. The cumulative activity in the metastatic lesions was lower after rhTSH than during thyroid hormone withdrawal, although there was considerable variation between individual lesions. The median half-life in tumor tissue was 40 h during thyroid hormone withdrawal compared with 22 h following rhTSH stimulation.

De Keizer et al. reported the results of classical lesional dosimetry studies using rhTSH-assisted 131I tumor uptake measurements from post-therapy RAI scans and tumor volume estimates from structural imaging studies in 16 patients with recurrent or metastatic differentiated thyroid cancer [41]. The median lesional radiation dose was 26.3 Gy (range 1.3–368 Gy), with a median effective half-time of 2.7 days (range 0.5–6.4 days). Even within the multiple pulmonary metastatic lesions studied in an individual patient, estimated radiation doses to individual lesions ranged from 19.5 to 87.1 Gy. Although similar data on thyroid hormone withdrawal patients was not available in this study, the

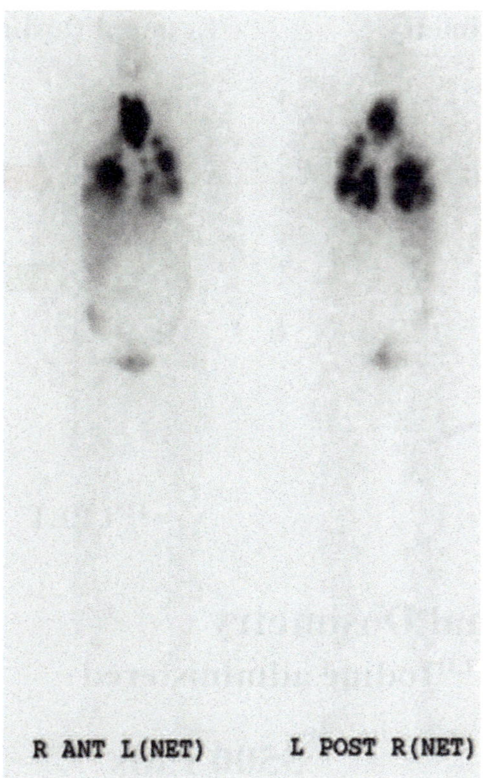

Fig. 60.5 A 2-mCi 131I scan in an elderly female with recurrent metastatic papillary thyroid cancer, showing RAI-avid disease in the mediastinum and lungs

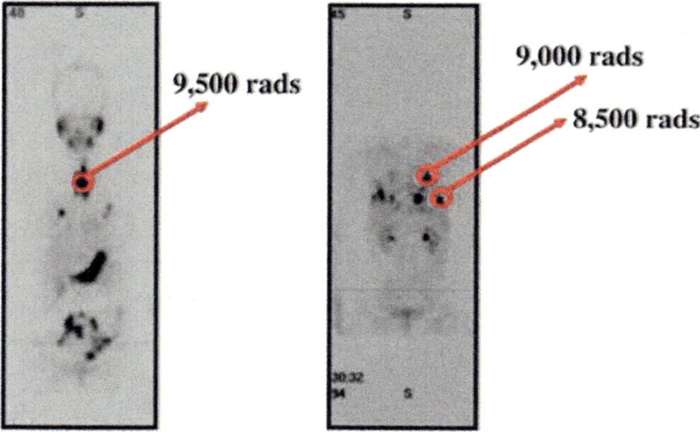

Fig. 60.6 124I PET lesional dosimetry that shows predicted lesional doses following administration of 120 mCi of 131I

authors did note that the iodine kinetics within metastatic lesions was quite similar to that reported by Maxon et al. in previously published detailed lesional dosimetry studies in hypothyroid patients [42].

Based on the data above, it is clear that rhTSH preparation can induce sufficient 131I uptake to result in tumoricidal doses of RAI in many patients with metastatic thyroid cancer, although the lesional dosimetry data suggests that a higher lesional dosimetry may be obtained in some patients using thyroid hormone withdrawal in non-randomized retrospective clinical series. Prospective randomized trials are needed to truly define the potential difference in lesional dosimetry between these two preparation methods. It will be important to define specific clinical scenarios in which an improvement in lesional dosimetry is likely to lead to a better therapeutic response. For example, even though some lesions had 50–100-fold increases in estimated lesional dose in response to selumetinib redifferentiation therapy, this dramatic increase still resulted in lesional doses that were far below the minimal therapeutically effective 2-Gy dose [19]. Furthermore, the heterogeneous nature of RAI avidity of metastatic lesions within an individual patient also needs to be considered (see Fig. 60.7). Clinical outcomes are likely to be very similar in cohorts of metastatic thyroid cancer patients treated with radioactive iodine following either method of preparation if the differences in lesional dosimetry do not cross this therapeutic boundary. Therefore, additional studies are needed to evaluate the percentage of patients likely to achieve a therapeutic lesional dose following preparation with either rhTSH or thyroid hormone withdrawal, rather than just studies comparing relative lesion doses.

Impact of Iodine Contamination on Dosimetry Studies

When comparing radioiodine kinetics in patients prepared with rhTSH to those prepared with traditional thyroid hormone withdrawal, it is important to consider the impact of the stable iodine contamination at the time of each study. As approx. 65 % of the molecular weight of levothyroxine derives from iodine, continued thyroid hormone replacement therapy during rhTSH, by necessity, adds unwanted iodine to the diet. Loffler et al. examined urinary iodine excretion in 85 patients undergoing thyroid hormone withdrawal and 61 patients undergoing rhTSH while continuing levothyroxine replacement before diagnostic RAI scanning [43]. Whereas the urinary iodine excretion was quite low in both groups of patients, the median iodine excretion rate was lower in hypothyroid withdrawal (50 μg/L) than in the rhTSH stimulation group (75 μg/L). However, the range of urinary iodine excretion rates was identical in both groups (25–600 μg/L).

In a cohort of patients in the United States, the mean urinary iodine (+/− standard deviation) measured while patients continued levothyroxine in preparation for rhTSH scanning

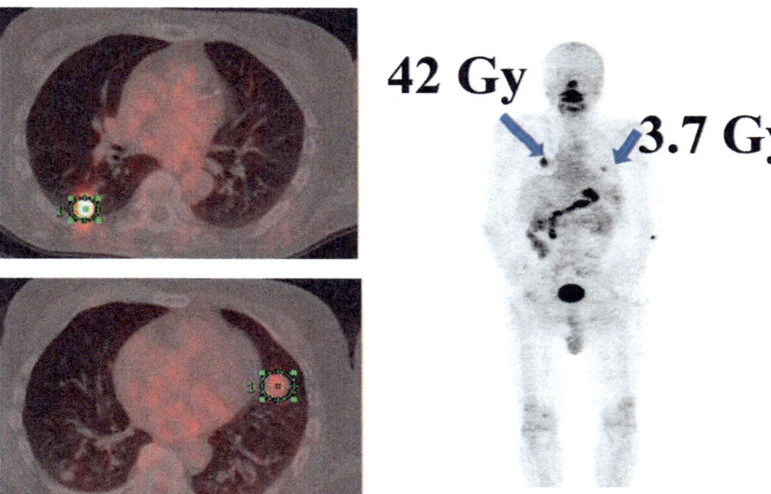

Fig. 60.7 124I PET/CT demonstrating a broad range of RAI avidity (3.7 Gy vs. 42 Gy with an administered activity of 437 mCi) between individual metastatic lesions within the same patient

was 85 +/− 44 mcg/g (urine iodine/creatinine) compared with 60 +/− 76 mcg/g in patients undergoing thyroid hormone withdrawal [44]. A 2-week low-iodine diet achieved adequate iodine deficiency in 71 % of patients continuing to take levothyroxine.

In a major thyroid cancer center in Italy, the urinary iodine at the time of RAI remnant ablation was very similar in 76 patients prepared with rhTSH (139 +/− 99 mcg/L) and in 125 patients prepared with thyroid hormone withdrawal (128 +/− 187 mcg/L) [45]. Furthermore, there was no correlation between urinary iodine levels and ablation success rates in either the patients prepared with rhTSH or thyroid hormone withdrawal.

From these data, it is clear that adequate levels of iodine depletion can be achieved with either preparation method following an adequate low-iodine diet; very similar remnant ablation rates and lesional radiation doses can be expected. It seems unlikely that the small amount of obligatory iodine contained with levothyroxine preparation would significantly impact the results of diagnostic whole-body scans or RAI therapies as used in clinical practice. However, a small effect on the precise measures of lesional dosimetry studies cannot be ruled out and needs to be considered when rhTSH dosimetry is compared with thyroid hormone withdrawal dosimetry studies.

References

1. Benua RS, Cicale NR, Sonenberg M, Rawson RW. The relation of radioiodine dosimetry to results and complications in the treatment of metastatic thyroid cancer. Am J Roentgenol Radium Ther Nucl Med. 1962;87:171–82.
2. Furhang EE, Larson SM, Buranapong P, Humm JL. Thyroid cancer dosimetry using clearance fitting. J Nucl Med. 1999;40(1):131–6.
3. Leeper RD. The effect of 131 I therapy on survival of patients with metastatic papillary or follicular thyroid carcinoma. J Clin Endocrinol Metab. 1973;36(6):1143–52.
4. Robbins RJ, Larson SM, Sinha N, et al. A retrospective review of the effectiveness of recombinant human TSH as a preparation for radioiodine thyroid remnant ablation. J Nucl Med. 2002;43(11): 1482–8.
5. Rall JE, Alpers JB, Lewallen CG, Sonenberg M, Berman M, Rawson RW. Radiation pneumonitis and fibrosis: a complication of radioiodine treatment of pulmonary metastases from cancer of the thyroid. J Clin Endocrinol Metab. 1957;17(11):1263–76.
6. Dorn R, Kopp J, Vogt H, Heidenreich P, Carroll RG, Gulec SA. Dosimetry-guided radioactive iodine treatment in patients with metastatic differentiated thyroid cancer: largest safe dose using a risk-adapted approach. J Nucl Med. 2003;44(3):451–6.
7. Duntas LH, Cooper DS. Review on the occasion of a decade of recombinant human TSH: prospects and novel uses. Thyroid. 2008;18(5):509–16.
8. Klubo-Gwiezdzinska J, Burman KD, Van Nostrand D, Mete M, Jonklaas J, Wartofsky L. Potential use of recombinant human thyrotropin in the treatment of distant metastases in patients with differentiated thyroid cancer. Endocr Pract. 2012;27:1–26.
9. Luster M, Lippi F, Jarzab B, et al. rhTSH-aided radioiodine ablation and treatment of differentiated thyroid carcinoma: a comprehensive review. Endocr Relat Cancer. 2005;12(1):49–64.
10. Robbins RJ, Robbins AK. Clinical review 156: recombinant human thyrotropin and thyroid cancer management. J Clin Endocrinol Metab. 2003;88(5):1933–8.
11. Sabra M, Tuttle RM. Recombinant human TSH to stimulate 131I uptake for remnant ablation and adjuvant therapy. Endocr Pract. 2012;27:1–25.
12. Hugo J, Robenshtok E, Grewal R, Larson S, Tuttle RM. Recombinant human thyroid stimulating hormone-assisted radioactive iodine remnant ablation in thyroid cancer patients at intermediate to high risk of recurrence. Thyroid. 2012;22:1007–15.
13. Tuttle RM, Brokhin M, Omry G, et al. Recombinant human TSH-assisted radioactive iodine remnant ablation achieves short-term clinical recurrence rates similar to those of traditional thyroid hormone withdrawal. J Nucl Med. 2008;49(5):764–70.
14. Tuttle RM, Lopez N, Leboeuf R, et al. Radioactive iodine administered for thyroid remnant ablation following recombinant human thyroid stimulating hormone preparation also has an important adjuvant therapy function. Thyroid. 2010;20(3):257–63.

15. Tuttle RM, Tala H, Shah J, et al. Estimating risk of recurrence in differentiated thyroid cancer after total thyroidectomy and radioactive iodine remnant ablation: using response to therapy variables to modify the initial risk estimates predicted by the new american thyroid association staging system. Thyroid. 2010;20(12):1341–9.
16. Klubo-Gwiezdzinska J, Burman KD, Van Nostrand D, Mete M, Jonklaas J, Wartofsky L. Radioiodine treatment of metastatic thyroid cancer: relative efficacy and side effect profile of preparation by thyroid hormone withdrawal versus recombinant human thyrotropin. Thyroid. 2012;22:310–7.
17. Robbins RJ, Driedger A, Magner J. Recombinant human thyrotropin-assisted radioiodine therapy for patients with metastatic thyroid cancer who could not elevate endogenous thyrotropin or be withdrawn from thyroxine. Thyroid. 2006;16(11):1121–30.
18. Tala H, Robbins R, Fagin JA, Larson SM, Tuttle RM. Five-year survival is similar in thyroid cancer patients with distant metastases prepared for radioactive iodine therapy with either thyroid hormone withdrawal or recombinant human TSH. J Clin Endocrinol Metab. 2011;96(7):2105–11.
19. Ho AL, Grewal RK, Leboeuf R, et al. Selumetinib-enhanced radioiodine uptake in advanced thyroid cancer. N Engl J Med. 2013; 368(7):623–32.
20. Luster M, Hanscheid H, Freudenberg LS, Verburg FA. Radioiodine therapy of metastatic lesions of differentiated thyroid cancer. J Endocrinol Invest. 2012;35(6 Suppl):21–9.
21. Sgouros G, Kolbert KS, Sheikh A, et al. Patient-specific dosimetry for 131I thyroid cancer therapy using 124I PET and 3-dimensional-internal dosimetry (3D-ID) software. J Nucl Med. 2004;45(8):1366–72.
22. Meier CA, Braverman LE, Ebner SA, et al. Diagnostic use of recombinant human thyrotropin in patients with thyroid carcinoma (phase I/II study). J Clin Endocrinol Metab. 1994;78(1):188–96.
23. Remy H, Borget I, Leboulleux S, et al. 131I effective half-life and dosimetry in thyroid cancer patients. J Nucl Med. 2008;49(9): 1445–50.
24. Luster M, Sherman SI, Skarulis MC, et al. Comparison of radioiodine biokinetics following the administration of recombinant human thyroid stimulating hormone and after thyroid hormone withdrawal in thyroid carcinoma. Eur J Nucl Med Mol Imaging. 2003;30(10):1371–7.
25. Chiesa C, Castellani MR, Vellani C, et al. Individualized dosimetry in the management of metastatic differentiated thyroid cancer. Q J Nucl Med Mol Imaging. 2009;53(5):546–61.
26. Hanscheid H, Lassmann M, Luster M, et al. Iodine biokinetics and dosimetry in radioiodine therapy of thyroid cancer: procedures and results of a prospective international controlled study of ablation after rhTSH or hormone withdrawal. J Nucl Med. 2006;47(4):648–54.
27. Hartung-Knemeyer V, Nagarajah J, Jentzen W, et al. Pre-therapeutic blood dosimetry in patients with differentiated thyroid carcinoma using 124-iodine: predicted blood doses correlate with changes in blood cell counts after radioiodine therapy and depend on modes of TSH stimulation and number of preceding radioiodine therapies. Ann Nucl Med. 2012;26(9):723–9.
28. Bianchi L, Baroli A, Lomuscio G, et al. Dosimetry in the therapy of metastatic differentiated thyroid cancer administering high 131I activity: the experience of Busto Arsizio Hospital (Italy). Q J Nucl Med Mol Imaging. 2012;56(6):515–21.
29. de Keizer B, Hoekstra A, Konijnenberg MW, et al. Bone marrow dosimetry and safety of high 131I activities given after recombinant human thyroid-stimulating hormone to treat metastatic differentiated thyroid cancer. J Nucl Med. 2004;45(9):1549–54.
30. Pacini F, Molinaro E, Castagna MG, et al. Ablation of thyroid residues with 30 mCi (131)I: a comparison in thyroid cancer patients prepared with recombinant human TSH or thyroid hormone withdrawal. J Clin Endocrinol Metab. 2002;87(9):4063–8.
31. Lassmann M, Luster M, Hanscheid H, Reiners C. Impact of 131I diagnostic activities on the biokinetics of thyroid remnants. J Nucl Med. 2004;45(4):619–25.
32. Haugen BR, Pacini F, Reiners C, et al. A comparison of recombinant human thyrotropin and thyroid hormone withdrawal for the detection of thyroid remnant or cancer. J Clin Endocrinol Metab. 1999;84(11):3877–85.
33. Hung GU, Ho M, Kao CH. Faster radioiodine washout in the treatment of pulmonary metastases of papillary thyroid cancer prepared with recombinant human thyroid-stimulating hormone. Clin Nucl Med. 2009;34(5):316–7.
34. Taieb D, Jacob T, Zotian E, Mundler O. Lack of efficacy of recombinant human thyrotropin versus thyroid hormone withdrawal for radioiodine therapy imaging in a patient with differentiated thyroid carcinoma lung metastases. Thyroid. 2004;14(6):465–7.
35. Van Nostrand D, Khorjekar GR, O'Neil J, et al. Recombinant human thyroid-stimulating hormone versus thyroid hormone withdrawal in the identification of metastasis in differentiated thyroid cancer with 131I planar whole-body imaging and 124I PET. J Nucl Med. 2012;53(3):359–62.
36. Erdi YE, Macapinlac H, Larson SM, et al. Radiation dose assessment for I-131 therapy of thyroid cancer using I-124 PET imaging. Clin Positron Imaging Off J Ins Clin PET. 1999;2(1):41–6.
37. Pettinato C, Monari F, Nanni C, et al. Usefulness of 124I PET/CT imaging to predict absorbed doses in patients affected by metastatic thyroid cancer and treated with 131I. Q J Nucl Med Mol Imaging. 2012;56(6):509–14.
38. Tuttle M, Robbins R, Larson SM, Strauss HW. Challenging cases in thyroid cancer: a multidisciplinary approach. Eur J Nucl Med Mol Imaging. 2004;31(4):605–12.
39. Freudenberg LS, Jentzen W, Petrich T, et al. Lesion dose in differentiated thyroid carcinoma metastases after rhTSH or thyroid hormone withdrawal: 124I PET/CT dosimetric comparisons. Eur J Nucl Med Mol Imaging. 2010;37(12):2267–76.
40. Potzi C, Moameni A, Karanikas G, et al. Comparison of iodine uptake in tumour and nontumour tissue under thyroid hormone deprivation and with recombinant human thyrotropin in thyroid cancer patients. Clin Endocrinol (Oxf). 2006;65(4):519–23.
41. de Keizer B, Brans B, Hoekstra A, et al. Tumour dosimetry and response in patients with metastatic differentiated thyroid cancer using recombinant human thyrotropin before radioiodine therapy. Eur J Nucl Med Mol Imaging. 2003;30(3):367–73.
42. Maxon HR, Thomas SR, Hertzberg VS, et al. Relation between effective radiation dose and outcome of radioiodine therapy for thyroid cancer. N Engl J Med. 1983;309(16):937–41.
43. Loffler M, Weckesser M, Franzius C, Kies P, Schober O. Iodine excretion during stimulation with rhTSH in differentiated thyroid carcinoma. Nuklearmedizin. 2003;42(6):240–3.
44. Park 2nd JT, Hennessey JV. Two-week low iodine diet is necessary for adequate outpatient preparation for radioiodine rhTSH scanning in patients taking levothyroxine. Thyroid. 2004; 14(1):57–63.
45. Tala Jury HP, Castagna MG, Fioravanti C, Cipri C, Brianzoni E, Pacini F. Lack of association between urinary iodine excretion and successful thyroid ablation in thyroid cancer patients. J Clin Endocrinol Metab. 2010;95(1):230–7.

The Use of Lithium as an Adjuvant to Radioiodine in the Treatment of Thyroid Cancer

61

Marina S. Zemskova and Monica C. Skarulis

Radioactive iodine (^{131}I) is the most effective medical therapy for metastatic thyroid cancer. Eradication of persistent or recurrent cancer with radioiodine is dependent on successful uptake and adequate retention of ^{131}I in tumor deposits. To optimize uptake of the radionuclide, dietary depletion of iodide and thyrotropin-secreting hormone (TSH)-induced sodium-iodide symporter activity are required. Methods to enhance the half-time of ^{131}I in the tumor tissue are limited. Iodine clearance is prolonged by alterations of renal function that occur in the hypothyroid state or by drugs such as diuretics. Hydrochlorothiazide, furosemide, and salt loading enhance renal sodium excretion leading to iodide depletion. Unfortunately, the reduced blood volume resulting from the associated loss of water ultimately diminishes iodine clearance and thus increases radiation to tumor and whole body proportionately [1]. High iodide concentrations can also inhibit proteolytic enzymes and release of ^{131}I incorporated into thyroid hormone; however, this effect cannot be exploited to advantage in the treatment of thyroid cancer because it also diminishes uptake. Lithium ion, administered as the carbonate salt, blocks thyrocyte release of ^{131}I incorporated in thyroid hormone. Unlike iodide, lithium does not affect ^{131}I uptake and is the most promising method to enhance the radiation dose to tumors and improve the therapeutic effectiveness of radioiodine.

The chapter is dedicated to the memory of our mentor, colleague, and friend, Jack Robbins (1922–2008).

M.S. Zemskova, MD
Diabetes, Obesity and Endocrinology Branch, National Institutes of Health, National Institute of Diabetes, Digestive and Kidney Diseases, Bethesda, MD, USA
e-mail: marina.zemskova@nih.gov

M.C. Skarulis, MD (✉)
National Institute of Diabetes, Digestive and Kidney Diseases, NIH Clinical Center, 10 Center Drive, CRC, Building 10 Room 6w-3940, Bethesda, MD 20892, USA
e-mail: monica_skarulis@nih.gov

The Effect of Lithium on the Thyroid

In the mid-nineteenth century, the alkaline properties of lithium salts were widely used to treat various uric acid diatheses which included the many manifestations of "brain gout" including headache, epilepsy, mania, and depression [2]. During the 1950s, the modern use of lithium in the management of mania and bipolar disease was established, and its association with goiter and thyroid dysfunction was reported by several investigators [3–5]. Subsequently, investigations commenced to discover the full effects of lithium on thyroid function [6, 7].

Early studies in humans by Sedvall demonstrated that lithium decreased serum protein-bound iodine (PBI) and increased thyroidal radioiodine uptake after 7–20 days of lithium treatment [8]. The effect was transient and both PBI and uptake returned to baseline after several months of continued lithium therapy [9, 10]. Although a direct lithium effect on the hypothalamus and/or pituitary has been proposed, observed elevations in basal TSH [11] and enhanced response to thyrotropin-releasing hormone (TSH) [12] during lithium therapy are most likely compensatory and secondary to the sometimes subtle diminished thyroid hormone feedback that occurs.

Lithium interferes with thyroid hormone synthesis and secretion and its perturbations are dose dependent. Lithium is concentrated in the thyroid, achieving levels three to four times that of the serum [5]. Iodide enters the thyrocyte through an active sodium-dependent iodide transport system known as the Na^+/I^- symporter (NIS). NIS activity occurs in a 2 Na^+:1 anion stoichiometry and is not restricted to sodium as the driving cation [13, 14]. Lithium can drive iodide transport at approximately 10–20 % of the level achieved by sodium [14]. The exact role that NIS plays in achieving the high concentrations in thyrocytes has yet to be examined. Studies of the inhibitory effect of lithium on rat thyroid demonstrated that doses above 2 mEq per liter interfered with

L. Wartofsky, D. Van Nostrand (eds.), *Thyroid Cancer*, DOI 10.1007/978-1-4939-3314-3_61

multiple steps in iodine metabolism including iodide trapping [15]; however, at therapeutic concentrations, TSH-induced iodine accumulation persisted, while TSH-induced endocytosis of colloid and release of thyroid hormone were reduced [16]. Lithium reduces TSH-induced adenyl cyclase activity through competition with magnesium at binding sites essential for enzyme activity and cAMP generation [16, 17]. Additional data suggest that lithium may also act in steps subsequent to cAMP formation [16, 18]. Effects of lithium on colloid droplet formation, microtubule function [19], and thyroglobulin hydrolysis [20] have been observed. The least understood effect of lithium is on peripheral thyroxine degradation which appears to be decreased in both euthyroid and hyperthyroid subjects [21, 22].

The Use of Lithium in Hyperthyroidism

Recognition of lithium's ability to inhibit thyroid hormone release [15, 23] inspired several small clinical studies in the early 1970s to study its efficacy either alone or in combination with thionamides or with radioiodine, in the management of hyperthyroid patients [24]. Used as a single agent, lithium quickly decreased serum thyroxine levels by approximately 30 % [24–26] and achieved a euthyroid state after 2–6 weeks of therapy in 11 of 12 patients in an observational intervention trial [27]. Several studies using lithium combined with a thionamide resulted in greater reductions of T4 and T3 levels compared to thionamide alone [28–30]. Boehm et al. [31] studied the combination of lithium and iodide noting an additive inhibition on thyroid hormone release only when lithium preceded the administration of iodide.

Importantly, several studies demonstrated that lithium prolonged the half-life of radioiodine within the thyroid gland [15, 23, 32]. It is proposed that retention of iodine within the thyroid gland maximizes the local radiation effect and minimizes total body exposure [28, 33] particularly in patients with rapid thyroidal turnover [28]. Bogazzi and coworkers demonstrated that the addition of lithium to radioactive iodine is associated with a blunted post-^{131}I hormone peak, a shorter time to euthyroidism, and increased overall cure rate in patients with Graves-induced thyrotoxicosis only [34]. However, other studies have demonstrated no improvement in the cure rate with adjuvant lithium [33, 35, 36]. Overall, lithium is rarely used to treat hyperthyroidism and is generally restricted to patients in whom the conventional therapeutic options are associated with dose-limiting adverse effects.

Demonstration of Lithium Action in Thyroid Cancer

Malignant thyroid cells are less efficient in transporting and retaining ^{131}I than normal thyroid cells. The biological half-time of ^{131}I is shorter in malignant thyroid tumors (less than 10 days) than in normal thyroid gland (approximately 60 days) [37] which limits the efficacy of therapeutic radioiodine. Using quantitative radiation dosimetry, Maxon and coworkers showed that among metastatic deposits, there is variability in iodine turnover that modifies the effect of therapy [38]. Comparing the iodine kinetics in metastases that were successfully eradicated with radioactive iodine to those that were not, the effective half-time and thereby the radiation dose (rads) were significantly lower in unresponsive tumors (2.5 days) versus responsive tumors (5.5 days), although the percent uptake of radiation was similar between the groups. The estimated lethal dose for metastases was greater than 8,000 rads, and subsequent studies demonstrated that a quantitative dosimetry strategy to achieve this dose was associated with a high cure rate [39]. In addition to the total amount of radioiodine given, the duration of its residence in metastatic lesions is a critically important factor in achieving a successful therapeutic outcome, thus providing the rationale for adjuvant lithium therapy.

The first published studies of the effect of lithium in thyroid cancer patients were a small case series by Briere [40] and a case study by Gershengorn [41]. In both of these studies, lithium increased the dose of radiation delivered to well-differentiated thyroid cancer as shown by measuring the rate of radioiodine release after a tracer dose of ^{131}I. The pre-lithium half-time ranged from 3 to 11 days (mean 6.6 days). Lithium slowed the release of radioiodine in each case but was most effective when the pre-lithium half-time of ^{131}I was less than 6 days.

Movius and coworkers showed that in the majority of metastases examined before and after lithium in a small series of patients with well-differentiated thyroid cancer, the biological half-time of ^{131}I in the individual lesions was increased 20–770 % over baseline [42]. Whole body radiation was not significantly altered except in a single patient with highly functional, bulky metastases [41, 42]. Lithium appeared to have its greatest effect in tumors with rapid turnover; on average, the calculated radiation dose to all tumors was increased by 30 %, and those that had at least a 25 % increase in tumor radiation dose had pre-lithium biological half-times less than 6 days [42].

Additional studies at NIH by Koong [43] further confirmed the inverse relationship between the beneficial lithium effect and the baseline half-time values. Lithium prolonged the effective half-time in 77 % of metastases studied, and an increase of more than 50 % was observed when the control biological half-time was less than 3 days. As lithium treatment also resulted in increased ^{131}I accumulation in tumor, the average tumor radiation dose increased twofold. No significant lithium effect could be seen if the half-time was greater than 6 days. In six of seven thyroid remnants studied, a similar positive effect was noted. However, preliminary results from a recent NIH placebo-controlled study demonstrated that a combination of lithium with 30 mCi ^{131}I and rhTSH for postsurgical ablation of thyroid remnant in low-risk patients with thyroid cancer did not improve the overall success of ablation (MS Zemskova, MC Skarulis, unpublished data, 2011).

Patient Selection

Although the effect of lithium to enhance radioiodine retention in metastatic lesions has been known for several decades, there are no well-designed clinical studies demonstrating improved outcome such as survival or disease-free survival associated with its use as an adjuvant. Lack of practice guidelines derived from clinical trials, limited availability of ^{131}I dosimetry to identify patients likely to benefit from lithium therapy, and inexperience prescribing this psychotherapeutic agent with a narrow therapeutic range to hypothyroid patients are some factors that have curtailed its use. Despite these concerns, lithium therapy should be considered in high-risk patients with demonstrated uptake of radioiodine in metastatic deposits to augment the radiation dose, particularly if there has been minimal response to prior therapy. Even when lesional dosimetry cannot be performed to identify those with rapid turnover and potential benefit, lithium can be used as an adjunct to optimize the radiation dose delivered by standard fixed quantities of ^{131}I typically given in practice.

Protocol for Lithium Use

Patients receiving adjuvant lithium should be rigorously prepared for radioiodine therapy to assure adequate TSH levels and iodine deficiency achieved by dietary restriction. Lithium is administered as lithium carbonate 2–5 days prior to the tracer dose for dosimetry and prior to ^{131}I therapy. All studies in the literature have been performed with the short-acting lithium carbonate preparation. No experience with the long-acting lithium salt has been reported but it should be avoided because of the short duration of therapy. Blockade of thyroidal iodine release occurs at serum lithium levels between 0.6 and 1.2 meq/L which is the same therapeutic target concentrations for manic depressive disorder [32]. The target concentration of lithium is generally achieved in 2–3 days if a loading dose of 600 mg is given followed by 300 mg three times daily [43]. Lithium is measured by atomic absorption spectrophotometry in serum obtained 8–12 h after the previous dose, and the administered dose is adjusted accordingly. The total daily dose required is generally 900–1,600 mg/day. Lithium carbonate is continued for 5–7 days after the therapeutic radioiodine dose is administered. During this period, toxicity must be assessed clinically because serum levels cannot be measured due to the radioactivity of the specimen, and lithium should be stopped if toxicity is suspected.

Risks of Therapy

Although lithium carbonate is associated with many side effects (Table 61.1), short-term therapy is well tolerated by most individuals. No serious toxicity was observed with lithium administration in any patients with thyroid cancer reported in the literature. Mild gastrointestinal disturbances such as nausea, vomiting, or diarrhea were reported in 10–20 % [44] of patients. In all cases in which symptoms occurred, none were severe enough to require discontinuation of the drug.

To avoid toxicity, patients must be closely monitored at the initiation of therapy. Levels are measured daily in the morning and the dosage is adjusted to achieve the therapeutic range. Gastrointestinal side effects generally occur when serum concentrations are greater than 1.5 meq/l, and central nervous system effects (confusion, somnolence, seizures) occur when levels approach 2.0 meq/l. Lethal toxicity is associated with levels greater than 2.5 meq/l.

Lithium is excreted almost entirely in the urine and is associated with diminished renal concentrating ability and nephrogenic diabetes insipidus that improves when lithium is discontinued. Patients should be counseled to avoid dehydration while on lithium. Reversible, mild elevations in serum creatinine concentrations are frequently observed in hypothyroid patients due to reduction of the glomerular filtration rate. These expected changes in renal function should not preclude the use of lithium. However, extreme caution should be exercised in patients with renal impairment. A 25–50 % reduction of lithium dose is recommended if the creatinine clearance is 10–50 ml/min and a 50–75 % reduction if the creatinine clearance is less than 10 ml/min.

The mean whole body radiation dose is usually not significantly altered by lithium despite its effect to increase the retention in tumor deposits [42–44]. However, in a single patient treated with lithium, an unexpected increase in whole body radiation was attributed to ^{131}I-labeled thyroglobulin release from bulky metastases [41], and transient leukopenia and thrombocytopenia were noted. Quantitative whole body dosimetry is recommended in all patients receiving radioiodine therapy doses of 200 mCi or greater regardless of whether adjuvant lithium carbonate is used. Close monitoring of blood counts for 6–10 weeks after high-dose ^{131}I therapy is advised to determine the effect on hematopoiesis.

Table 61.1 Adverse effects and toxicities of lithium administration

Mild	Dry mouth, polyuria, polydipsia, mild nausea
Moderate	Drowsiness, muscular weakness, diarrhea, vomiting
Severe	Vomiting, dehydration, high urine output, tinnitus, blurred vision, pseudotumor cerebri, ataxia, seizure, coma, bradycardia, hypotension

Summary

There is sufficient scientific evidence demonstrating the effects of lithium carbonate on thyrocyte function that result in an increase in the dose of radiation delivered to thyroid cancer from a given amount of ^{131}I. The patients most likely to benefit from adjuvant lithium are those who have tumors unresponsive to previous therapy and whose tumors have a short biological ^{131}I half-time retention. Lithium can be administered safely to hypothyroid patients during preparation for ^{131}I therapy but must be monitored carefully to achieve therapeutic levels and avoid toxicity. If quantitative lesional dosimetry is employed, lithium can achieve effective therapy with a lower administered dose of radioiodine and lower whole body radiation. Studies of the use of adjuvant lithium for the eradication of metastatic disease are needed to evaluate its ability to reduce the cumulative dose of radioiodine needed to successfully treat thyroid cancer and its impact on the ultimate outcome – disease-free survival.

References

1. Maruca J, Santner S, Miller K, Santen RJ. Prolonged iodine clearance with a depletion regimen for thyroid carcinoma: concise communication. J Nucl Med. 1984;25:1089–93.
2. Amdisen A, Hildebrandt J. Use of lithium in the medically ill. Psychother Psychosom. 1988;49:103–19.
3. Fieve RR, Platman S. Lithium and thyroid function in manic-depressive psychosis. Am J Psychiatry. 1968;125:527–30.
4. Gonzales R, Lauter H. On the therapy of manic-depressive psychoses with lithium salts. Nervenarzt. 1968;39:11–6.
5. Schou M, Amdisen A, Eskjaer Jensen S, Olsen T. Occurrence of goitre during lithium treatment. Br Med J. 1968;3:710–3.
6. Robbins J. Perturbations of iodine metabolism by lithium. Math Biosci. 1984;72:337–47.
7. Kushner J, Wartofsky L. Lithium-thyroid interactions. In: Neil Johnson F, editor. Lithium therapy monographs, vol. 2. Basel: S. Karger; 1988. p. 74–98.
8. Sedvall G, Jonsson B, Pettersson U, Levin K. Effects of lithium salts on plasma protein bound iodine and uptake of 131I in thyroid gland of man and rat. Life Sci. 1968;7:1257–64.
9. Cooper TB, Simpson GM. Preliminary report of a longitudinal study of the effects of lithium on iodine metabolism. Curr Ther Res Clin Exp. 1969;11:603–8.
10. Fyro B, Petterson U, Sedvall G. Time course for the effect of lithium on thyroid function in men and women. Acta Psychiatr Scand. 1973;49:230–6.
11. Emerson CH, Dysno WL, Utiger RD. Serum thyrotropin and thyroxine concentrations in patients receiving lithium carbonate. J Clin Endocrinol Metab. 1973;36:338–46.
12. Lauridsen UB, Kirkegaard C, Nerup J. Lithium and the pituitary-thyroid axis in normal subjects. J Clin Endocrinol Metab. 1974;39:383–5.
13. O'Neill B, Magnolato D, Semenza G. The electrogenic, Na+-dependent I- transport system in plasma membrane vesicles from thyroid glands. Biochim Biophys Acta. 1987;896:263–74.
14. Eskandari S, Loo DD, Dai G, Levy O, Wright EM, Carrasco N. Thyroid Na+/I- symporter. Mechanism, stoichiometry, and specificity. J Biol Chem. 1997;272:27230–8.
15. Berens SC, Bernstein RS, Robbins J, Wolff J. Antithyroid effects of lithium. J Clin Invest. 1970;49:1357–67.
16. Williams JA, Berens SC, Wolff J. Thyroid secretion in vitro: inhibition of TSH and dibutyryl cyclic-AMP stimulated 131-I release by Li+1. Endocrinology. 1971;88:1385–8.
17. Burke G. Effects of cations and ouabain on thyroid adenyl cyclase. Biochim Biophys Acta. 1970;220:30–41.
18. Mori M, Tajima K, Oda Y, Matsui I, Mashita K, Tarui S. Inhibitory effect of lithium on the release of thyroid hormones from thyrotropin-stimulated mouse thyroids in a perifusion system. Endocrinology. 1989;124:1365–9.
19. Bhattacharyya B, Wolff J. Stabilization of microtubules by lithium ion. Biochem Biophys Res Commun. 1976;73:383–90.
20. Bagchi N, Brown T, Mack R. Studies on the mechanism of inhibition of thyroid function by lithium. Biochim Biophys Acta. 1978;542:163–9.
21. Spaulding SW, Burrow GN, Bermudez F, Himmelhoch JM. The inhibitory effect of lithium on thyroid hormone release in both euthyroid and thyrotoxic patients. J Clin Endocrinol Metab. 1972;35:905–11.
22. Carlson HE, Tample R, Robbins J. Effect of lithium on thyroxine disappearance in man. J Clin Endocrinol Metab. 1973;36:1251–4.
23. Sedvall G, Jonsson B, Pettersson V. Evidence of an altered thyroid function in man during treatment with lithium carbonate. Acta psychiat Scand. 1969;207(suppl):59–67.
24. Temple R, Berman M, Wolff J. Reduction of thyroid hormone release by lithium in thyrotoxicosis. J Clin Invest. 1971;50:91a.
25. Gerdes H, Littmann KP, Joseph K, Mahlstedt J, Neugebauer R. Successful treatment of thyrotoxicosis by lithium. Acta Endocrinol Suppl (Copenh). 1973;173:23.
26. Kristensen O, Andersen HH, Pallisgaard G. Lithium carbonate in the treatment of thyrotoxicosis. A controlled trial. Lancet. 1976;1:603–5.
27. Lazarus JH, Richards AR, Addison GM, Owen GM. Treatment of thyrotoxicosis with lithium carbonate. Lancet. 1974;2:1160–3.
28. Turner JG, Brownlie BE, Rogers TG. Lithium as an adjunct to radioiodine therapy for thyrotoxicosis. Lancet. 1976;1:614–5.
29. Hedley JM, Turner JG, Brownlie BE, Sadler WA. Low dose lithium-carbimazole in the treatment of thyrotoxicosis. Aust N Z J Med. 1978;8:628–30.
30. Turner JB. Use of lithium in the treatment of thyrotoxicosis. Aust N Z J Med. 1978;8:628–30.
31. Boehm TM, Burman KD, Barnes S, Wartofsky L. Lithium and iodine combination therapy for thyrotoxicosis. Acta Endocrinol (Copenh). 1980;94:174–83.
32. Temple R, Berman M, Robbins J, Wolff J. The use of lithium in the treatment of thyrotoxicosis. J Clin Invest. 1972;51:2746–56.
33. Bogazzi F, Bartalena L, Brogioni S, et al. Comparison of radioiodine with radioiodine plus lithium in the treatment of Graves' hyperthyroidism. J Clin Endocrinol Metab. 1999;84:499–503.
34. Bogazzi F, Giovannetti C, Fessehatsion R, Tanda ML, Campomori A, Compri E, Rossi G, Ceccarelli C, Vitti P, Pinchera A, Bartalena L, Martino E. Impact of lithium on efficacy of radioactive iodine therapy for Graves' disease: a cohort study on cure rate, time to cure, and frequency of increased serum thyroxine after antithyroid drug withdrawal. J Clin Endocrinol Metab. 2010;95(1):201–8.
35. Brownlie BE, Turner JG, Millner GM, Perry EG, Ding L. Lithium associated thyroid cancer. Aust N Z J Med. 1980;10:62–3.
36. Bal CS, Kumar A, Pandey RM. A randomized controlled trial to evaluate the adjuvant effect of lithium on radioiodine treatment of hyperthyroidism. Thyroid. 2002;12:399–405.
37. Berman M, Hoff E, Barandes M, et al. Iodine kinetics in man – a model. J Clin Endocrinol Metab. 1968;28:1–14.
38. Maxon HR, Thomas SR, Hertzberg VS, et al. Relation between effective radiation dose and outcome of radioiodine therapy for thyroid cancer. N Engl J Med. 1983;309:937–41.

39. Maxon 3rd HR, Englaro EE, Thomas SR, et al. Radioiodine-131 therapy for well-differentiated thyroid cancer – a quantitative radiation dosimetric approach: outcome and validation in 85 patients. J Nucl Med. 1992;33:1132–6.
40. Briere J, Pousset G, Darsy P. The advantage of lithium in association with iodine 131 in the treatment of functioning metastasis of the thyroid cancer (author's transl). Ann Endocrinol (Paris). 1974;35:281–2.
41. Gershengorn MC, Izumi M, Robbins J. Use of lithium as an adjunct to radioiodine therapy of thyroid carcinoma. J Clin Endocrinol Metab. 1976;42:105–11.
42. Movius EG, Robbins J, Pierce LR, Reynolds JC, et al. The value of lithium in radioiodine therapy of thyroid carcinoma. In: Medeiros-Neto G, Gaitan E, editors. Frontiers in thyroidology. New York: Plenum; 1986. p. 1269–72.
43. Koong SS, Reynolds JC, Movius EG, et al. Lithium as a potential adjuvant to 131I therapy of metastatic, well differentiated thyroid carcinoma. J Clin Endocrinol Metab. 1999;84:912–6.
44. Pons F, Carrio I, Estorch M, Ginjaume M, Pons J, Milian R. Lithium as an adjuvant of iodine-131 uptake when treating patients with well-differentiated thyroid carcinoma. Clin Nucl Med. 1987;12: 644–7.

Side Effects of ^{131}I for Therapy of Differentiated Thyroid Carcinoma

62

Douglas Van Nostrand, John E. Freitas, Anna M. Sawka, and Richard W. Tsang

Introduction

The use of radioactive iodine (^{131}I) for remnant ablation, adjuvant treatment, and treatment of metastases from differentiated thyroid carcinoma may be associated with side effects in numerous organ systems (Table 62.1). Although many articles address the side effects of ^{131}I, the characterizations of these effects vary widely because of a host of different factors (Table 62.2). This chapter attempts to consolidate the literature by presenting, where appropriate, (1) the spectrum of signs and symptoms, as well as the frequency and severity of side effects; (2) a review of selected articles; (3) a discussion of preventive measures to reduce the frequency and severity of side effects; and (4) a discussion of the medical management when selected side effects do occur.

D. Van Nostrand, MD, FACP, FACNM (✉)
Nuclear Medicine Research, MedStar Research Institute and Washington Hospital Center, Georgetown University School of Medicine, Washington Hospital Center, 110 Irving Street, N.W., Suite GB 60F, Washington, DC 20010, USA
e-mail: douglasvannostrand@gmail.com

J.E. Freitas, MD
Department of Radiology, St. Joseph Mercy Health System, Ypsilanti, MI, USA
e-mail: freitasj@trinity-health.org

A.M. Sawka, MD, PhD
Division of Endocrinology and Metabolism, Department of Medicine, University Health Network – University of Toronto/Toronto General Hospital, Toronto, ON, Canada
e-mail: Anna.sawka@uhn.on.ca

R.W. Tsang, MD, FRCP(C)
Department of Radiation Oncology, Princess Margaret Hospital, University of Toronto, Toronto, ON, Canada
e-mail: Richard.tsang@rmp.uhn.on.ca

Hair

The loss of hair secondary to ^{131}I treatment is an infrequent complication and has been reported in a patient with an underlying skull metastasis [1]. Although Alexander et al. [2] found transient episodes of more generalized alopecia in 28 % (57 of 203) of patients that occurred one to several weeks after discharge from ^{131}I therapy, this side effect was not dependent on ^{131}I dosage administered. Because hypothyroid patients suffer from hair loss and cancer patients had been traditionally hypothyroid when ^{131}I is administered, hair loss has been generally considered due to the hypothyroidism, not ^{131}I per se. As more ^{131}I therapies are performed after preparation with recombinant human thyrotropin (rhTSH) with patients euthyroid, it will be of interest to determine whether there is any associated hair loss.

Brain

Brain metastases diagnosed premortem are rare in patients with thyroid cancer and most thyroid cancer brain metastases are not iodine avid as determined on diagnostic whole-body scans (17 % in one series) [3]. Although surgical resection or stereotactic radiosurgery should be strongly considered first for the treatment (even if iodine avid) (see Chap. 56), [3] ^{131}I therapy may be considered in selected patients. If ^{131}I is used, then patients with ^{131}I-avid brain metastases can experience abrupt and marked deterioration or death secondary to brain metastases swelling, hemorrhage, and/or cerebral edema in response to ^{131}I therapy [4–6].

Prior to ^{131}I therapy, such patients should be pretreated with oral steroids. One approach was the pretreatment for several hours with 16–32 mg of oral dexamethasone, which was continued in divided dosages for 5–7 days following ^{131}I

L. Wartofsky, D. Van Nostrand (eds.), *Thyroid Cancer*, DOI 10.1007/978-1-4939-3314-3_62

Table 62.1 Various sites of side effects associated with ^{131}I therapy

Hair
Brain
Spinal cord
Eye
Salivary glands
Taste and smell
Nose
Facial nerve
Vocal cord
Thyroid
Parathyroid
Pulmonary
Gastrointestinal system
Urinary bladder
Bone marrow
Fertility
Second primary neoplasms

Table 62.2 Various factors causing variability of characterizations of side effects secondary to ^{131}I therapy

Criteria for the presence of side effects
Thoroughness in the search for signs and symptoms of side effects
Various criteria for the grading of severity of side effects
Length of follow-up
Prescribed activities of ^{131}I for remnant ablation, adjuvant treatment, or treatment of known local regional or distant metastases
Total cumulative prescribed activities of ^{131}I
Time intervals between ^{131}I therapies
Methods implemented or not implemented to prevent side effects

therapy [3]. Of note, elevated thyroid-stimulating hormone (TSH) from either thyroid hormone withdrawal or injections of recombinant human TSH may also increase the potential for enlargement of the metastasis(es), hemorrhage, and/or cerebral edema, and earlier pretreatment with glucocorticoids should again be considered. Although glucocorticoids have been identified as a cause of reduced ^{131}I uptake in benign thyroid tissue in euthyroid patients, the rapidity at which this effect occurs is probably over several days (not hours) and may not be as marked in hypothyroid individuals [7]. If an alternative to glucocorticoids is required, 50 % oral glycerol (1.2–2.0 g/kg) daily has been shown as effective to reduce cerebral edema in patients undergoing external-beam therapy of brain metastases and may have similar efficacy in ^{131}I-treated patients [8].

Spinal Cord

Myelopathy after acute swelling of cord lesions has been seen after rhTSH-stimulated ^{131}I therapy, but it is difficult to distinguish whether the etiologic factor was TSH or ^{131}I [9]. In general, the same precautions for spinal cord metastases apply for brain metastases. Yevgeniya et al. [10] evaluated 202 patients with spinal metastases, and neural structure compression (e.g., myelopathy/radiculopathy) was present in 36 % and 72 % of patients with papillary and follicular thyroid cancer, respectively.

Eye

The three most important side effects involving the eye area are inflammation of the lacrimal gland, inflammation and/or obstruction of the lacrimal duct, and conjunctivitis.

Lacrimal Gland

The proposed mechanism for lacrimal gland inflammation is similar to sialoadenitis of the salivary glands with uptake of ^{131}I in the lacrimal gland resulting in radiation damage and subsequent reduction in the production of tears. However, the underlying mechanism remains controversial. Although Spitzweg et al. [11] have reported the presence of the sodium-iodide symporter in lacrimal ductules and glands, Morgenstern et al. [12] were unable to demonstrate the presence of the sodium-iodide symporter in the lacrimal gland, Wolfring and Krause glands (accessory lacrimal glands), conjunctiva, or the canaliculus.

Nevertheless, the reduction of tear production has been studied by Zettinig et al. [13] and appears to occur frequently after ^{131}I therapy. In the evaluation of 88 patients, 81 patients had at least one abnormal result out of a set of three tests used to assess the quality and quantity of tears. The Schirmer tear test, which measures the quantity of aqueous tear production, was positive (decreased tears) in 40 % of patients in one eye and 20 % in both eyes. The tear film breakup time (BUT), which measures the tear film's stability, was abnormal in 71 % of patients in at least one eye and in 57 % of patients in both eyes. The lacrimal lipid layer that thickens, stabilizes, and retards evaporation of the aqueous layer underneath was abnormal in 49 % of patients in at least one eye and in 34 % of patients in both eyes. The lipid layer is produced by the sebaceous meibomian glands in the lids as well as by the Zeis and Moll glands along the eyelid margin and lashes.

Fard-Esfahni et al. [14] evaluated 50 patients treated with ^{131}I and 50 control patients. In comparing the two groups, no significant differences in symptoms of xerophthalmia were observed. However, a lower Schirmer test value was present in the eyes of patients treated with ^{131}I (14.5 ± 10.8 mm) relative to the control group (18.2 ± 11.0 mm [$p<0.016$]).

The clinical presentation of lacrimal inflammation is xerophthalmia. Typically, the patient has no initial symptoms of pain or swelling but subsequently develops reduced production of tears, resulting in dry eyes (xerophthalmia). The frequency of xerophthalmia was 16 % (14 of 88) in patients studied. Seven patients had xerophthalmia and xerostomia, and seven had only xerophthalmia [13]. Solans et al. [15] reported xerophthalmia in 33 % (26 of 79), which persisted for 1 year in 25 %, for 2 years in 17 %, and into the third year in 14 % of patients. Keratoconjunctivitis sicca persisted in 14 % (11 of 88) of patients into the second year and in 8 % (6 of 88) after the third year. No significant relationship of xerophthalmia was found with cumulative prescribed activity of ^{131}I. However, changes in tear function tests can be seen with lower amounts of therapeutic ^{131}I prescribed activity. Koca et al. [16] reported decreased values of Schirmer test and the tear breakup time (BUT) in patients receiving prescribed activities of ^{131}I of ≤30 mCi in patients treated for hyperthyroidism. Although one may have expected a significant decrease in the frequency of xerophthalmia in patients receiving the lower recommended amounts of 30 mCi of ^{131}I for remnant ablation for differentiated thyroid cancer, Koca et al.'s study suggested that significant radiation of the lacrimal glands may still occur.

Obstruction of Lacrimal Duct

The mechanism of the obstruction of the lacrimal duct, which drains the tears to the nasal cavity, is hypothesized to be the effects of radiation exposure to the duct lining from ^{131}I in the tears and/or possibly in the cells of the duct lining, leading to subsequent inflammation, fibrosis, and narrowing. ^{131}I activity in the tears has been well described with as much as 0.01 % of the administered ^{131}I dosage secreted in tears in each eye during the first 4 h after ^{131}I administration [17]. However, an additional and potentially more important mechanism may be present. Morgenstern et al. [12] have demonstrated the presence of the Na+/I symporter (NIS) in the stratified columnar and epithelial cells of the lacrimal sac and nasolacrimal duct of humans.

The clinical presentation of nasolacrimal duct obstruction is epiphora (excessive tearing). Zettinig et al. [13] reported epiphora in 11 % (10 of 88) of patients and epiphora with photophobia in 1 % of patients. The mechanism of photophobia was not discussed. The exact mechanism of epiphora was also not discussed but must again relate to the failure of normal tear drainage to the nasal cavity. Kloos et al. [18] reported a 2.6 % incidence of epiphora (10 of 390), with symptoms appearing a mean of 6.5 months after the last ^{131}I dose (range of 3–16 months). Subsequently, Burns et al. [19] described a suspected incidence of obstructed nasolacrimal drainage of 3.4 % and 4.6 %. Fard-Esfahani et al. [20] evaluated 81 patients with dacryoscintigraphy and demonstrated findings indicative of nasolacrimal obstruction in 18 % (29/162) of the eyes in patients treated with ^{131}1 relative to 9 % (3/34) in the eyes in patients who were not treated with ^{131}I. The frequency of complete nasolacrimal obstruction increased when the cumulative dose of ^{131}I exceed 11.1 GBq (300 mCi). Orquiza et al. [21] in a prospective survey reported that epiphora was reported on the first day of ^{131}I treatment in 6 % (5/78) of patients. Between 1 and 10 days after ^{131}I treatment, 8 % (6/78) of patients reported epiphora. However, when the frequency of epiphora was adjusted for patients who reported this symptom within 30 days prior to ^{131}I treatment, the frequency of epiphora after ^{131}I therapy was not statistically increased.

Finally, nasolacrimal duct obstruction may not only be suspected only when the patient complains of epiphora but it may also be suspected when radioiodine uptake is noted on radioiodine SPECT-CT images medially in the area of the lacrimal duct and/or lacrimal sac [22].

Conjunctivitis

The mechanism of conjunctivitis is not well understood but is most likely the result, at least in part, of documented changes in the tear quality and quantity. Zettinig et al. [13] showed changes in the external eye morphology, demonstrating corneal staining with fluorescein in 42 % (37 of 88) of patients, and 35 % of patients had abnormal conjunctival findings on visual inspection. Conjunctivitis typically presents with pain and erythema. Alexander et al. [2] indicated a frequency of chronic or recurrent conjunctivitis in 23 % (46 of 203) of patients.

Preventive Management

Currently, no proven method in humans is available to reduce the radiation exposure to the lacrimal glands, sacs, or ducts; however, several potential protective options need further evaluation. Beutel et al. [23] evaluated the protective effects of amifostine, lidocaine, and pilocarpine on the lacrimal glands in 25 rabbits. Pre ^{131}I treatment with amifostine appeared to reduce functional and structural impairment of the lacrimal glands after exposure to radiation, and lidocaine had the potential for significant radioprotection. Pilocarpine had no evidence of radioprotection of the lacrimal glands. Acar et al. [24] evaluated vitamin E in 24 rats and compared one group of rats treated with 3 mCi of ^{131}I by gastric lavage and 1 ml of physiological saline injected intraperitoneally to a second group of rats that were administered with ^{131}I through the same route and with the same amount but were not injected peritoneally with vitamin E (α-tocopherol acetate). Vitamin E was initiated 2 days before and continued 5 days after the administration of ^{131}I. Twenty four hours after the last dose of vitamin E, the animals were sacrificed. Histological examination of the rats' lacrimal glands demonstrated statistically less frequent periductal and/or periacinar fibrosis in all lacrimal glands in the rats that received vitamin E. Koca et al. [25] recently reported histological changes in the lacrimal glands secondary to ^{131}I therapy and that montelukast (Singular®, Montelo-10®, Monteflo®, Likotas®) effectively protected against that damage to the lacrimal glands. Montelukast is a leukotriene D4 receptor antagonist that is administered for the treatment of asthma and relief of symptoms of seasonal allergies. In the lungs, montelukast reduces bronchoconstriction otherwise caused by the leukotriene and results in less inflammation, and the dose for such patients is one 10 mg tablet orally per day. However, the efficacy of montelukast in reducing the radiation dose to the lacrimal glands, sacs, and ducts needs to be further evaluated.

Management of Xerophthalmia, Lacrimal Duct Obstruction, Epiphora, and Conjunctivitis

The first and most important aspect regarding the management of xerophthalmia, obstruction of the nasolacrimal duct, or conjunctivitis is for the physician and patient to be aware of these potential side effects and their presenting signs and symptoms. Thus, when they do occur, the physician can implement treatment and/or refer the patient to an ophthalmologist. Depending on the severity, the patient may be simply observed without treatment, treated with artificial tears, or referred to an ophthalmologist for additional treatments, such as a dacryocystorhinostomy (surgical creation of communication between the lacrimal sac and nasal cavity) for patients with severe epiphora. Alexander et al. [2] found that four of 46 patients underwent dacryocystorhinostomy. More recently, Ramakrishnan et al. [26] reported on the use of endoscopic management of nasolacrimal duct obstruction secondary to ^{131}I treatment in five patients using silicone lacrimal stents. Out of ten stents placed, two had to be removed because of patient discomfort; however, the remaining eight had resolution or improvement of drainage with no major intraoperative or postoperative complications.

In summary, side effects of ^{131}I therapy on the lacrimal glands, lacrimal ducts, and conjunctivae occur frequently, are often overlooked, may require referral to an ophthalmologist, and need further study.

Salivary Gland

Significant amounts of ^{131}I can accumulate in the salivary glands; therefore, ^{131}I therapy can result in significant radiation exposure to the salivary glands that are manifested by both early and late untoward effects. These have been previously reviewed, [27] and the untoward effects include sialoadenitis, xerostomia, salivary duct obstruction, and tumors of the salivary gland. The latter are discussed below in this chapter in a section entitled "Second primary malignancies." The terms "sialadenitis" and "sialoadenitis" have been used interchangeably in the medical literature, and the usage of either is correct and signifies inflammation of the salivary gland. For this chapter, "sialoadenitis" will be used.

Anatomy and Physiology

To discuss the anatomy and physiology of the salivary glands in depth is beyond the scope of this chapter. However, the major pairs of salivary glands—the parotid, submandibular, and sublingual glands—can concentrate iodine as high as 7–700 times the plasma levels [28–31]. The salivary glands are composed of serous cells and mucous cells. The parotid glands have predominately serous cells, and its saliva is predominately serous secretion. The submandibular glands have a mixture of serous and mucinous cells, and its saliva is predominately mucinous secretion. The sublingual glands also have a mixture of cells and make only a small contribution in volume but affect the viscosity of saliva. The parotid glands demonstrate a higher frequency of radiation sialoadenitis than submandibular and sublingual salivary glands, the hypothetical basis for which is that the serous cells have a greater ability to concentrate ^{131}I than the mucous cells [32]. An important mechanism of salivary iodide transport is the same as in the thyroid gland, which is the sodium-iodide symporter (NIS) in salivary ductal cells. However, despite the presence of NIS, the salivary accumulation of ^{131}I does not appear to be affected by the TSH level or the state of thyroid function [30, 31, 33]. Relating to this, the histopathologic studies of Rice et al. [29] indicate that the parotid acini and serous cells are severely injured after external radiotherapy with little discernible change in the mucous cells. The salivary glands are controlled by the autonomic nervous system. The parasympathetic system apparently has a more significant impact on saliva production than the sympathetic system, but the latter still has a role [34].

Radiation-Absorbed Dose

The radiation exposure to the salivary glands has not been well studied. Donachi et al. [35] reported approximately 250 cGy (250 rad) to the salivary gland from a 185 MBq (5 mCi) dosagee, and Goolden et al. [36] demonstrated 700 cGy (rad) during the first 24 h. Liu et al. [37] reported radiation-absorbed doses of 0.20 ± 0.10 mGy/MBq (range 0.01–0.92 mGy/MBq) and 0.25 ± 0.09 mGy/MBq (range 0.01–1.52 mGy/MBq) for the parotid and submandibular glands, respectively. However, as noted by Jentzen et al. [38], the calculated radiation-absorbed doses do not correspond to the degree of radiation damage, and further investigation is under way to attempt to take into account the nonuniform distribution as La Perle et al. has demonstrated that the sodium-iodide symporter, hence ^{131}I uptake, is located in the salivary striated ductal cells [39].

Salivary Side Effects

Frequency

The most frequently reported side effect is acute radiation sialoadenitis, which has an incidence ranging from 10 to 67 % (see Table 62.3) [1, 2, 40–47, 59–62, 70, 198]. As noted earlier, the variability in frequency and severity are multifactorial (see Table 62.4), and correlations with both individual prescribed activity and cumulative prescribed activity of ^{131}I have been reported. Grewal et al. [47] showed a statistically significant dose response between administered radioactivity and salivary gland swelling but not xerostomia, altered taste, or salivary gland pain.

Signs and Symptoms

Early Presentation

The spectrum of the signs and symptoms of sialoadenitis range from an asymptomatic sialoadenitis to a very painful, tender, and swollen salivary gland, which may persist for many months. After employing the usual salivary gland-protective precautions, the glands of a patient treated for the first time with a prescribed activity of 5.55 GBq (150 mCi) or less of ^{131}I will most likely be asymptomatic, but this does not negate the presence of sialoadenitis. Although an asymptomatic form of sialoadenitis is difficult to confirm histopathologically, a "silent" sialoadenitis is indirectly or retrospectively implicated if there is subsequent development of xerostomia. Alexander et al. [2] reported that 56 % of patients with xerostomia had no prior symptoms of sialoadenitis. However, many patients do develop symptoms. As many as one third of patients will report at least mild pain, with or without tenderness and swelling of the salivary glands. This pain may begin as early as 6 h or as late as several days to even several weeks after ^{131}I treatment. The pain, tenderness, swelling, or all three signs and symptoms may be unilateral or bilateral and are more common in the parotid glands. However, the submandibular and lingual glands are still often involved. Alexander et al. [2] found that in the group of patients with sialoadenitis (67 of 203), 80.6 % (54 of 67) involved the parotids, and 14 of these were unilateral, and 40 were bilateral. Signs and symptoms of sialoadenitis in the submandibular glands were seen in 46 % (31 of 67); eight were unilateral and 23 bilateral. Albrecht et al. [42] found 59 % (30 of 51) of patients had parotid gland involvement, with 25 bilateral and five unilateral, whereas 16 % (8 of 51) had involvement of the submandibular glands. The signs and symptoms may last several weeks and occasionally as long as 1 year. However, Grewal et al. [47] reported persistent salivary side effects in 5 % or less of patients after a median follow-up of 7 years. Nevertheless, most signs and symptoms resolve spontaneously within several hours to several days with no specific treatment. When treatment was necessary, symptoms were usually easily controlled with hydration, anti-inflammatory agents (e.g., aspirin and ibuprofen), or an analgesic (e.g., acetaminophen; see discussion below for more details). Sometimes, the symptoms may be more severe and chronic, and steroids may be required. If there is a suppurative parotitis, antibiotics may be required. In three patients, Allweiss reported a suppurative sialoadenitis that needed antibiotic treatment [43].

Table 62.3 Incidence of sialoadenitis

Author (ref.)	Incidence (no. of patients)
Alexander [2]	33 % (67/203)
Albrecht [42]	59 % (30/51) (parotid)
Alweiss [43]	12 % (10/87)
Benua [1]	2 % (3/122)
Edmonds [198]	10 % (26/258)
Grewal [47]	39 % (102 /262)
Kahn [41]	34 % (17/50)
Kharazi [46] (ThyCa survey)	40 % (640/742)
Kita [200]	50 % (46/96)
Maier [45]	8 % (3/37)
Nakada [62]	37 % (46/125) to 64 % (67/105)
Pan [44]	4.6 % (16/342)
Silberstein [70]	5 % (3/60)
Van Nostrand [40]	67 % (9/15)
Walters [59]	24 % (43/176)

Table 62.4 Multiple factors affecting the frequency and severity of sialoadenitis and xerostomia

Diligence in looking for signs and symptoms of sialoadenitis or xerostomia
Individual prescribed activity of ^{131}I
Cumulative prescribed activity of ^{131}I
Interval and frequency of ^{131}I
Amount of ^{131}I uptake in the salivary glands
Previous history of other salivary gland diseases
Administration of drugs that cause xerostomia
Diligence of the patient and physician in reducing the radiation exposure to the salivary gland during ^{131}I therapy

Late Presentation

Obstruction

Although patients may present with the early signs and symptoms of an acute radiation sialoadenitis, some patients may initially present 1–12 months after ^{131}I therapy or after initial signs of an acute radiation sialoadenitis with new and different pain, tenderness, and swelling. The process of eating or just the sight of appetizing foods often evokes these symptoms, which may resolve within minutes to hours but are typically recurrent. The pathogenesis is different from inflammation of the initial acute radiation sialoadenitis and is most likely a combination of (1) narrowing of the salivary ducts secondary to scarring from inflammation and (2) altered quality and/or quantity of saliva. With normal saliva, there may be ductal narrowing with acute partial obstruction upon salivation. With reduced flow and thicker saliva, there may be stagnation and mucus precipitation, resulting in a plug (or calculus) with obstruction. Nevertheless, the pathogenesis is probably a combination of both reduced flow and narrowing of the duct to varying degrees. Although the natural history of this side effect has not been well described, in the experience of one of the authors (dvn), these symptoms usually, but not always, slowly resolve over several months, but intermittent signs and symptoms can be persistent.

Xerostomia

Xerostomia (dry mouth) is an important complication of radiation sialoadenitis. In addition, xerostomia may also be accompanied by burning oral discomfort, difficulty in eating dry foods, decreased taste sensitivity, increased production of viscous mucus or morning expectoration, and mucosal ulcerations. The reported frequency of xerostomia ranges from 2 to 55 % (see Table 62.5) [1, 2, 15, 40–43, 48–50, 59, 62, 70, 198], and the frequency and severity are again multifactorial. If xerostomia occurs, it may begin within several weeks after ^{131}I therapy and usually resolves within 3 months [2, 40, 51]. For the condition to last greater than 1 year is infrequent but does occur in 4.4–7 % of patients [2, 40, 44, 50]. Xerostomia may even be permanent [52, 53]. Interestingly, Alexander et al. [2] reported one patient whose xerostomia resolved 7 years after the last ^{131}I therapy.

Currently, there does not appear to be a demonstrable relationship of xerostomia to an earlier clinically evident presentation of sialoadenitis. As noted above, Alexander et al. [2] showed that more than half patients (56.1 %; 63 of 96) who were diagnosed with xerostomia did not have clinically evident sialoadenitis, and Malpani et al. [54] also found no link between significant reduction in the function of the salivary glands and the symptoms of sialoadenitis.

Regarding the prescribed activity of ^{131}I, Spiegel et al. [55] evaluated 20 patients with thyroid cancer and reported a dose-dependent decrease in salivary gland function. The same group specifically described a 40 % reduction of parotid gland function after prescribed activities of 9.99 GBq (270 mCi) [56]. Solans et al. [15] demonstrated no association between xerostomia and cumulative prescribed activity.

Table 62.5 Incidence of xerostomia

Author (ref.)	Incidence (no. of patients)
Albrecht [42]	22 % (11/51)
Alexander [2]	43 % (87/203)
Alweiss [43]	30 % (3/10)
Benua [1]	2 % (3/122)
Edmonds [198]	10 % (26[a]/258)
Hall [48]	53 % (1363/2573)
Kahn [41]	18 % (10/55)
Leeper [49]	Common
Lin [50]	5.4 % (3/56)
Nakaka [62]	11 % (14/125) to 24 % (25/105)
Silberstein [70]	0 % (0/60)
Solans [15]	33 % (26/79)
Van Nostrand [40]	13 % (2/15)
Walters [59]	44 % (78/176)

[a]Calculated

Complications of Xerostomia

Salivary gland dysfunction after ^{131}I therapy has been reviewed previously [57]. A major complication of xerostomia is significantly increased frequency of dental problems [57, 58]. Walters et al. [59] performed a longitudinal cohort study of 176 patients evaluating the dental safety profile after treatment with high-dose ^{131}I. The caries risk increased by 99 % with the presence of xerostomia, and the risk of required tooth extraction increased 8.14 % per gigabecquerel with increasing cumulative prescribed activity. They also suggested that salivary gland uptake after ^{131}I therapy predicted the development of sialoadenitis and xerostomia with an odds ratio of 1.31 ([1.05–1.63], $p<0.015$) and 1.58 ([1.16–2.16], $p<0.004$), respectively. Laupa et al. [58] found that despite the lower salivary flow rates after ^{131}I therapy, the frequency of widespread dental caries and demineralization, similar to that observed in externally irradiated patients, was not evident. Candidiasis is a rare but possible side effect of xerostomia, which may be severe enough to require treatment (e.g., nystatin and clotrimazole) [60]. Recommendations for xerostomia management and preventive care to minimize dental caries are noted in Table 62.6 [61–64].

Although xerostomia is a major complication of radiation sialoadenitis, it is important to note that xerostomia is a reported side effect of over 500 medications [65], and the temporal relationship of ^{131}I ablation or treatment to xerostomia does not prove that the condition is because of prior radiation. Similarly, in a study of 65-year-old residents in Maryland, an epidemiological study indicated a 17 % prevalence of dry mouth [66]. In a case report, Mandel et al. [67] further warned against assuming that the presence of xerostomia after ^{131}I therapy is secondary to that therapy. Radiation sialoadenitis may be the most likely cause, but a thorough evaluation is recommended.

Stomatitis

Stomatitis is rare, but if it occurs, it may be very painful [54]. Its mechanism has not been clarified. If severe, stomatitis may require treatment with dexamethasone elixir mouthwash

Table 62.6 Recommendations for the management of xerostomia and dental caries

Referral to a dental hygienist, dentist, otolaryngologist, or oral surgeon
Treatment of causes other than radiation sialoadenitis, such as changing a drug or drug dosage that is causing xerostomia
Adequate hydration
Impeccable dental hygiene
Artificial saliva swirled in the mouth and swallowed every 3–4 h
Repeated massages of the gland as necessary
Avoidance of anticholinergics
Administration of sialagogues [61]
Pilocarpine (Salagen®), 5–10 mg postoperatively t.i.d. Oral tablet may need to be taken for 6–12 weeks before full benefit is realized
Cevimeline [62] (Evoxac®), cholinesterase inhibitor, 30 mg postoperatively TID
Anethole trithione (Hepasulfol®, Mucinol®, Sialor®, Sonicur®, and Sufralem®). The standard dose is 37.5–75 mg typically in divided doses before meals. Doses of up to 150 mg daily have been used
Chewing gum
Trial of saliva-stimulating tablets [63], including such potential agents as disaccharides and low-dose interferon-α lozenges
Acupuncture [64]
Fluoride therapy in the form of topical fluoride applications, fluoride mouthwashes, and fluoride toothpastes
Hydrogen peroxide mouthwash diluted with mouthwash (e.g., Listerine®) Antibiotics for suppurative sialoadenitis

Table 62.7 Approaches to minimize radiation sialoadenitis and its consequences

Pre-therapy
• Assessment of salivary glands on pre therapy radioiodine whole-body scans
• Patient education about prevention
• Patient participation in implementing the preventive measures
• Pretherapy visit and management by dental hygienist or dentist
• Hydration
• Suspension of anticholinergic medications
• Consideration of use of radioprotectants (e.g., amifostine, reserpine)
Immediately posttherapy
• Hydration
• Sialagogues (see text for discussion)
• Parotid gland massage
Posttherapy
• Anti-inflammatory agents
• Steroids

or mouthwash containing viscous lidocaine, diphenhydramine and aluminum, and magnesium hydroxides [54]. Referral to an otolaryngologist is advised.

Prevention

Although Grewal et al. [47] reported that after a median of 7 years only 5 % or less of 262 patients had persistent salivary side effects, the prevention and the management of salivary complications are very important.

Prevention Prior to ^{131}I Therapy

The most important aspect of treatment to prevent or minimize sialoadenitis is to begin with preventive measure prior to the first therapy. However, three factors often undermine our preventive efforts to aggressively reduce radiation exposure to the salivary glands on the first therapy. First, the initial signs or symptoms of radiation sialoadenitis are either silent or mild and transient after the first ^{131}I therapy, which in turn discourages future aggressive preventive management with the first therapy. Second, most patients will never require another ^{131}I therapy. Third, staging helps predict which group of patients is at risk for metastasis and thus for additional ^{131}I therapies. However, neither the relative minor initial signs and symptoms, the likelihood of not needing another ^{131}I therapy, nor the implication of staging helps the individual patient who does need additional ^{131}I therapies and is at risk for sialoadenitis and its associated consequences. Thus, because the patient always has the potential of additional ^{131}I therapies and to reduce the severity and frequency of subsequent sialoadenitis and its associated consequences, one author (dvn) strongly recommends aggressive measures to minimize the radiation-absorbed dose to the salivary gland beginning with the *first* ^{131}I therapy. This will serve to reduce the severity and frequency of subsequent sialoadenitis and its associated consequences (see Table 62.7).

Assessment of the Salivary Glands

Kulkarni et al. [68] demonstrated that although there was no significantly statistical difference, the incidence of salivary gland dysfunction appeared to be higher in patients who showed moderate and marked salivary uptake of radioiodine on the diagnostic scans than those patients who had none or mild salivary gland uptake. Although these preliminary data should not alter the aggressive management to minimize radiation dose to the salivary glands, assessment of the uptake in the salivary glands on such scans still may be predictive. For example, asymmetric, persistent, relatively increased uptake in one parotid gland may forewarn of a problem in that gland. Alternatively, minimal or no radioactivity in any of the salivary glands may suggest a lower radiation dose to the salivary glands from ^{131}I and thus a lower chance of radiation sialoadenitis in that patient. In patients considered for high empiric or dosimetrically determined ^{131}I prescribed activities, marked salivary gland uptake may indicate the need to consider a reduction in prescribed activity to minimize sialoadenitis. However, as discussed below, the time of imaging after the administration of food or other sialagogues may affect the uptake of radioiodine in the salivary glands on the diagnostic study. Further research is warranted to evaluate the utility of the salivary gland uptake on pretherapy ^{131}I scans, yet until those data are available, a general assessment of salivary gland uptake may be useful.

Patient Education

Two crucial factors to reducing the radiation-absorbed dose to the salivary gland are (1) educating the patient about the importance of minimizing the radiation-absorbed dose to the salivary gland, along with the techniques to do so, and (2) encouraging the patient to be part of the treatment team, thereby promoting compliance with preventive measures.

Prophylactic Dental Hygiene

An important recommendation for the preventive management of patients who are going to receive high prescribed activity of ^{131}I is to see a dental hygienist or dentist prior to their ^{131}I therapy with proper assessment and, if necessary, treatment of the patient with preexisting conditions such as periodontal disease, caries, broken teeth, ill-fitting bridges, partials, and dentures. The dental hygienist will help ensure an optimal environment for radiation therapy [69], and dental hygienists are an important part of the treatment team.

Because of the special needs of the thyroid cancer patient, it is important that dental care is performed in a timely fashion. As already discussed in more detail above, ^{131}I therapy may result in sialoadenitis and subsequent xerostomia. In addition to dysgeusia and sialoadenitis, the lack of salivary flow allows both the oral environment to become more acidic and oral biofilm to grow out of control, making these patients more susceptible to periodontal disease, rampant caries, tooth hypersensitivity, or the worsening of a preexisting condition.

For the pretreatment stage, the dental hygienist will educate the patient and reinforce the need for proper oral hygiene during ALL phases of treatment. The hygienist will instruct daily brushing, flossing, and rinsing techniques. He/she will perform scaling and prophylaxis procedures to ensure a healthy environment and administer a fluoride varnish to help prevent tooth decay. The fluoride varnish is of particular importance because it makes the oral cavity less hospitable to bacteria by making the tooth surface more difficult to attach to. At a minimum, during the pretreatment stage, a varnish is suggested because fluoride is only available on the outer 6 μm of tooth enamel and is quickly eroded in an acidic environment. Nutritional counseling will typically be offered and includes recommendations of reducing sugar and refined carbohydrates in the diet that could augment tooth decay. Emphasis will be on the use of saliva-stimulating foods such as sugar-free gum containing xylitol and sugar-free lemon drops. Chewing hard cheese has been found to raise the pH level in the mouth and to increase bioavailable calcium in saliva to bond to and strengthen the enamel. Home fluoride treatments have been shown to reduce tooth decay. Custom trays can even be fabricated for home use to be worn 5–10 min per day.

During the pretreatment stage, the dental hygienist will also give valuable recommendations to be implemented during treatment. The dental hygienist will instruct patients to continue with optimal oral hygiene. The hygienist will educate the patient on the possible side effects such as mucositis, stomatitis, and xerostomia and recommend avoiding dentifrices containing sodium lauryl sulfates (SLS) and mouthwashes containing alcohol, which may cause irritation and dryness of the oral mucosa. To ensure sufficient lubrication of the lips and mouth, certain products will be recommended. Over-the-counter mouthwashes containing enzymes and proteins found naturally in saliva provide temporary relief for dry mouth. Xylitol-containing products draw moisture into the mouth naturally, though they should be tried by the patient prior to the treatment phase. Excessive use of xylitol-containing products can result in unwanted digestive side effects. If mucositis occurs, the dentist can prescribe one of various magic mouthwash mixtures such as mouthwash solution containing benadryl, bismuth subsalicylate (Kaopectate®), and lidocaine (Xylocaine®) for short-term use. The dental hygienist is also valuable in the management of long-term xerostomia, which is discussed in the section on the management of xerostomia.

If the patient already has an existing hygienist or dentist for his or her dental care, the physician administering ^{131}I may wish to inquire about the patient's dental health with the treating hygienist or dentist. The hygienist or dentist can advise regarding not only how long it has been since dental treatment has occurred but also if there is current disease that needs to be addressed prior to ^{131}I therapy or if there are existing conditions that may worsen after ^{131}I therapy. If the patient does not have an existing hygienist or dentist, several resources can be used to help facilitate the patient's access to dental care. The American Academy for Oral Systemic Health (www.aaosh.com) will allow the patient to search by location for either a dentist or dental hygienist with a special interest in oral systemic health. If none is available, the American Dental Hygienists Association (www.adha.org) is a national organization with state and local chapters. Searching and contacting officers via the Internet at the state and local level is recommended to the patient to use as a valuable resource. The American Dental Association (www.ada.org) is a national organization for dentists, which also has state and local chapters that may help. If cost is an issue, other options are available including public health dental clinics, dental hygiene schools, and dental schools. Some of these facilities treat patients at reduced or no cost. Nevertheless, good dental hygiene from a qualified dental hygienist or dentist is important care prior to and during ^{131}I therapy. After ^{131}I therapy and the radiation safety precautions have been terminated, the patient should discard any radioiodine-contaminated toothbrush, toothpaste tubes, and floss. The recommendation is for a dental follow-up visit 3 months posttreatment for consideration of prophylaxis and fluoride varnish application. At this visit, effects of ^{131}I treatment can be assessed and a treatment plan, if necessary, developed for the patient.

Hydration

Although there is no direct evidence to demonstrate the value of hydration to reduce the radiation dose to the salivary glands, hydration is recommended on an intuitive basis. Dehydration is known to lower saliva production, thereby increasing stasis of saliva, potentially increasing stasis of ^{131}I in the salivary glands, and potentially increasing the radiation-absorbed dose to the salivary glands. Hydration is also important for renal clearance of ^{131}I circulating in the blood, thus reducing the amount and duration of ^{131}I available in the blood for the salivary gland to take up.

Cholinergic and Anticholinergic Medications

Although anticholinergic drugs may decrease the initial ^{131}I uptake in the salivary glands in some patients, as a general rule, all anticholinergic medications should be discontinued.

Cholinergics (e.g., pilocarpine, cevimeline, anetholetrithione, and bromhexine) may be useful to stimulate salivation and hopefully increase ^{131}I turnover or throughput in the salivary gland. An empiric treatment plan based on a 5-day regimen, beginning 2 days prior to ^{131}I treatment, has been proposed [54]. However, the utility of cholinergic drugs remains controversial. Alexander et al. [2] and Silberstein [70] showed no difference in the frequency and severity of sialoadenitis in those who received pilocarpine compared to those who did not.

Amifostine

Amifostine (WR-2721, Ethyol) has been shown to protect the salivary gland from the damaging effects of ionizing radiation of external radiotherapy for head and neck tumors [71–73]. Amifostine is an organic thiophosphate and is dephosphorylated to its active metabolite WR-1065. The latter is a scavenger of oxygen-free radicals, which are the primary cause of radiation-induced tissue damage. Amifostine concentration can be 100 times greater in normal tissue than tumor tissue [74], and the conversion of amifostine to WR-1065 is more effective in an alkaline environment. Normal tissue is more alkaline than tumor tissue. One side effect of amifostine was a temporary drop in blood pressure that required temporary suspension of the infusion. However, this is usually not a problem; if it occurs, it is manageable.

Because of its value for external radiotherapy for head and neck tumors, amifostine has been proposed for use in patients with thyroid cancer [75]. With salivary gland scintigraphy, Bohuslavizki et al. [76] assessed the influence of amifostine on the adverse effects of ^{131}I therapies on salivary gland function and demonstrated that parotid and submandibular function was reduced by approximately 40 % in the placebo group and remained unchanged in the amifostine group. However, Kim et al. [77] was unable to demonstrate any cytoprotective effects of amifostine on the salivary glands in 42 patients. Nevertheless, even if amifostine has a protective effect on the salivary glands, amifostine is presently not widely used in patients receiving ^{131}I therapy because of concern that amifostine may protect tumors from the effects of radiation therapy [78].

Reserpine

In addition to the innervation of the salivary glands by the parasympathetic system, the salivary glands are also innervated by the sympathetic system. Therefore, antisympathomimetic agents may have utility. Levy et al. [79] evaluated 12 patients: nine received reserpine and three did not. Based on ^{131}I uptake on whole-body images relative to patients not given reserpine, their data suggested that patients taking reserpine had a significant decrease in the ratio of parotid-to-background counts. However, it is uncertain whether the reduced salivary gland uptake was secondary either to the reserpine or stunning from a 370 MBq (10 mCi) diagnostic prescribed activity of ^{131}I or partial treatment of the salivary gland from the 3.7–5.55 GBq (100–150 mCi) ablative prescribed activities of ^{131}I.

Vitamin E (α-Tocopherol Acetate)

As vitamin E has been evaluated as a radioprotective agent for the lacrimal glands, it has been evaluated by Bhatriya et al. [80] as a radioprotective agent for the salivary glands demonstrating a pronounced decrease in lipid peroxidation and an increase in endogenous enzymes. Human studies with vitamin E are warranted.

Ocimum sanctum

Ocimum sanctum (*O. sanctum*) is a medicinal plant used in India and is reported to have beneficial effects including radioprotection against ^{60}Co gamma radiation [81]. Leban et al. evaluated rats that were presupplemented with *O. sanctum* or amifostine and then exposed to ^{131}I exposure [81]. Subsequent histology of the parotid glands of the rats presupplemented with *O. sanctum* or amifostine was comparable to control rats that were not exposed to ^{131}I. However, the histology of the parotid glands of those rats exposed to ^{131}I without presupplemented *O. sanctum* or amifostine demonstrated multifocal areas of lipomatosis and atrophy. Further evaluation of this plant extract is warranted.

Montelukast Sodium

Koca et al. [82] evaluated montelukast administration as a potential preventive agent to reduce the radiation effects of ^{131}I in the salivary glands. The proposed mechanism of montelukast was discussed earlier in the section on preventing side effects of the lacrimal glands. They evaluated ^{99m}technetium pertechnetate scintigraphy and histopathological examinations in 50 rats after ^{131}I therapy with and without montelukast administration in various groups. The pathological changes were more significant in the groups treated with ^{131}I without montelukast than in the groups prophylactically treated with montelukast. Additional potential agents have been evaluated including zinc and turmeric extract (*Curcuma longa*), which is a member of the Zingiberaceae family. An excellent review is available by Noaparast et al. [83].

Immediate Posttherapy

Hydration

On the day of therapy and immediately afterward, hydration is again thought to be indicated and valuable. This additional fluid intake may also be valuable to increase urine flow and reduce radiation dose to the urinary bladder, the latter discussed later in this chapter. An alternative to oral intake of fluid would be continuous intravenous hydration; however, if the intravenous line is placed after therapy, this may raise radiation safety issues for the phlebotomist.

Massage

Massage of the parotid glands may also be beneficial, especially if there is initial partial-flow obstruction (see Fig. 62.1) [53]. Kim et al. [84] evaluated the effectiveness of parotid massage. Thirty patients had parotid massage performed 20 times over 1 min, and a Tc-99 m pertechnetate salivary scans were performed immediately prior to and after the parotid massage. During the massage, patients contracted their jaw and masticator muscles. The control group had the same two salivary scans performed with no parotid massage between the salivary scans. While patients who received the parotid massage demonstrated no differences in the mean parotid gland counts on the pre- and post-massaging images, the group that had no massage had significantly higher mean counts (6 %) on the second salivary scan. They concluded that parotid gland massage could help prevent salivary damage secondary to ^{131}I therapy. Although this study does not prove that one can reduce damage to the parotid glands secondary to ^{131}I I therapy and although the authors did not evaluate the effectiveness of massage with and without the use of sialagogues, anything that is easy and can potentially reduce the residence time of ^{131}I activity in the salivary glands should be considered.

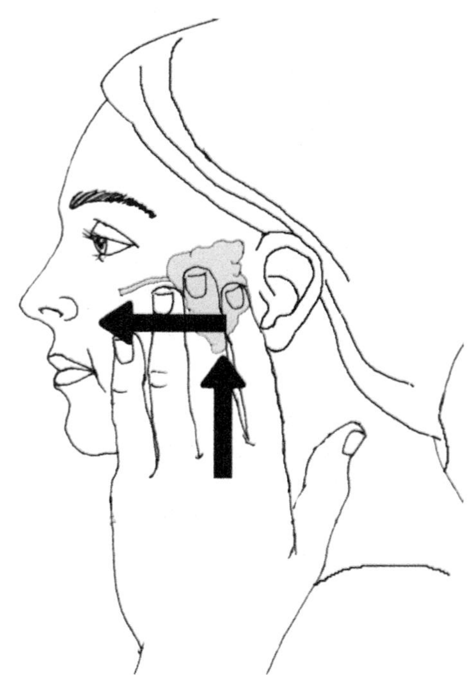

Fig. 62.1 For antegrade massage, push with the fingers mildly on the parotid gland cephalad and then anteriorly (Concept from Mandel and Mandel [57]. Reproduced with permission from Keystone Press from the book entitled "Thyroid Cancer: A Guide for Patients.")

Sialagogues

Despite their generally accepted empiric use, some authors have questioned the utility of sialagogues, and specifically, the use of sialagogues within the first 24 h after ^{131}I therapy remains controversial [70, 85–90].

Nakada et al. [86] reported that postponing the use of sialagogues until 24 h after the administration of ^{131}I therapeutic dosage reduced sialoadenitis from 63.8 % (67 of 105) to 36.8 % (46 of 125), hypogeusia (abnormally diminished acuteness of the sense of taste) or taste loss from 39 % to 25.6 %, and dry mouth from 23.8 % to 11.2 %. Permanent xerostomia decreased from 14.3 % to 5.6 %. Based on this data, Nakada et al. recommended that sialagogues should not be administered during the first 24-h period after ^{131}I therapy. As the proposed mechanism for increased radiation-absorbed dose to the salivary glands with sialagogues, they report using Doppler flow assessment in several patients demonstrating that salivation increased blood flow to the salivary glands. They hypothesized that this increased flow increased delivery and uptake of ^{131}I to the salivary glands, which in turn increased the radiation-absorbed dose to the salivary glands. Van Nostrand et al. [27] have referred to this proposed mechanism as a "rebound effect."

Liu et al. [87] evaluated 75 patients of which four groups of patients were administered 100 mg of vitamin C orally at one hr (18 pts), 5 h (18 pts), 13 h (19 pts), and 25 h (17 pts) after ^{131}I therapy, and patients received additional vitamin C every 4 h thereafter for the next 6 days, excluding the hours between 2 a.m. and 6 a.m. They concluded that "… salivary stimulation with vitamin C at any time has only a limited effect on salivary absorbed dose in thyroid cancer patients."

Jentzen et al. [88] calculated the salivary radiation-absorbed doses per administered ^{131}I activity in ten patients based on ^{124}I PET-CT. Patients began chewing lemon slices 20 min after the administration of the ^{124}I. Reportedly, these patients continuously chewed lemon slice over the first day. Ten minutes elapsed between stimulation with the lemon slices and ^{124}I scans. The stimulated patients subsequently ate lunch 2–4 h later, a snack after 6–7 h, and dinner 9–10 h later. No comment was stated about continued sialagogues during the night. The nonstimulated group "… did not chew lemon slices during the ^{124}I pre-therapy procedure and were not allowed to have food or drink until after the completion of the last PET scan on the first day, approximately 4 h after ^{124}I administration." Thereafter, patients had lunch after the first 4-h ^{124}I PET scan and then followed eating a snack and dinner as the other group. Imaging was performed 0.5, 1, 2, 4, 48, and >96 h after the administration of ^{124}I. They concluded that the radiation-absorbed dose to the salivary glands was higher when sialagogues were administered. However and as subsequently discussed below, patients with lemon stimulation had 10 min to reaccumulate the ^{124}I before imaging, and patients who were nonstimulated had no lemon or food for only the first approximately 4 h. In addition, the calculation of the monoexponential function determined from the average salivary gland ^{124}I uptake curve only used the data points from the 4 h time point and later with extrapolation of the data back to time zero. Thus, no data points were obtained prior to 4 h with the time between the successive data points having durations of 20, 24, and 48 h.

Several reports have been published suggested that sialagogues do decrease sialoadenitis and/or the radiation-absorbed dose [70, 89].

Silberstein [70] evaluated 60 patients for the effects of pilocarpine in reducing sialoadenitis. Although he concluded that pilocarpine was not effective in altering the frequency or severity of sialoadenitis, his frequency for acute sialoadenitis was 5 % (3/60), chronic sialoadenitis 1.7 % (1/60), subjective xerostomia 0 % (0/60), and dysgeusia 5 % (3/60). These frequencies were significantly less than Nakada et al.'s reported responses, regardless of whether sialagogues were used or not (see Table 62.8). Silberstein not only used continuous sialagogues while awake for a week but also every 3 h throughout the night for three nights. These data strongly indicated that the continuous use of sialagogues significantly reduces radiation sialoadenitis. However, of note, Silberstein also administered dexamethasone to all his patients, and thus, one cannot determine how much of the lower incidence of ^{131}I-induced sialoadenitis might have been due to the continuous administration of sialagogues or the use of steroids.

Van Nostrand et al. [89] evaluated the radiopharmacokinetics of radioiodine in 26 patients with preablation salivary gland scans with the administration of ^{123}I. One-minute images were obtain every minute for two consecutive phases of 1 h each with RealLemon® juice administered 5 min into each phase. These images were initiated 2 h after the administration of the ^{123}I. A typical time activity curve is shown in Figure 62.2, and the time activity curves demonstrated that indeed lemon juice is effective in stimulating the salivary gland to secrete radioiodine rapidly (mean time to nadir = ~4 min) and effectively (mean washout = ~84 %); however, the reaccumulation of radioiodine was rapid requiring a mean time to reaccumulate back to pre-lemon juice radioactivity of only 21 and 40 min during the first hour and second hour of the time activity curves, respectively. By analyzing the area under the time activity curves of all of patients and conservatively assuming that there would have been no further radioiodine accumulation had the lemon juice not initially been given, Van Nostrand et al. [89] calculated that if lemon juice was readministered at the time the radioactivity had returned to baseline (i.e., the level prior to the administration of the RealLemon® juice), one would have potentially reduced the relative radiation-absorbed dose to the parotid glands by 37–47 %, at least for these two 1-h periods.

In order to determine whether or not a "rebound" effect may exist, Kulkarni et al. [90] evaluated nine patients who had both a radioiodine salivary gland performed with and without the administration of RealLemon® juice on two different days, thereby allowing the patient to act as his/her own con-

Table 62.8 Comparison of the data from Nakada et al [86] versus Silberstein [70]

	Nakada et al. [86]		Silberstein [70]
	SG every 2–3 h while awake	No SG for the first 24 h	SG continuously during the day and q3 h during the night
Acute sialoadenitis	63.8 % (67/105)	36.8 % (46/125)	5 % (3/60)
Chronic sialoadenitis	Not separated out	Not separated out	1.7 % (1/60)
Subjective xerostomia	23.8 % (25/105)	11.2 % (14/125)	0 % (0/60)
Dysgeusia	39.0 % (41/105)	25.6 % (32/125)	5 % (3/60)

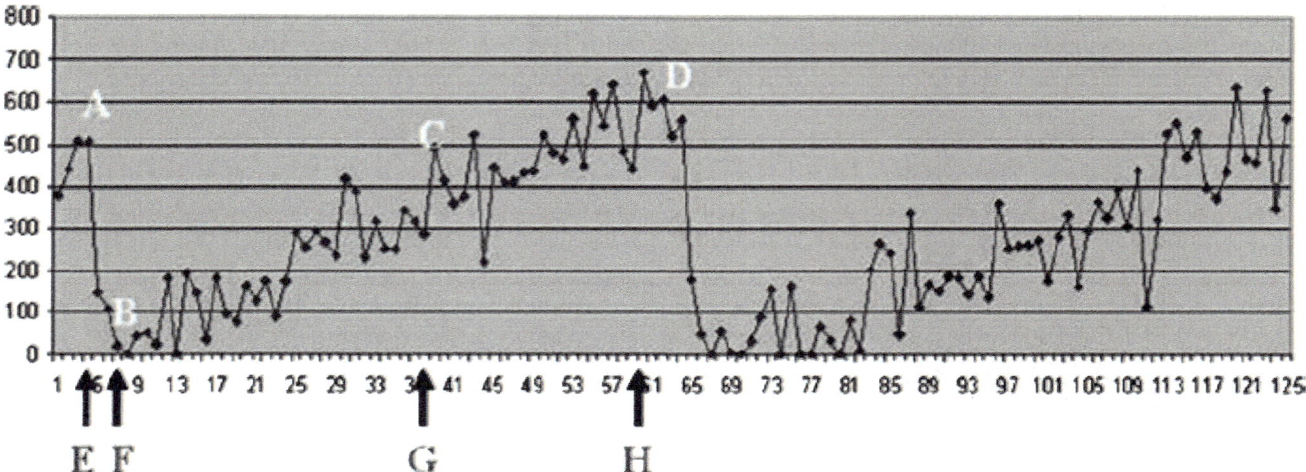

Fig. 62.2 A typical background-corrected time activity curve (TAC) demonstrating the response to the oral administration of lemon juice. The numbers on the X-axis are minutes, and the numbers on the Y-axis are counts/minute. This figure demonstrates the time points used for the calculation of the radiopharmacokinetic parameters. A: The peak activity (counts/min) when lemon juice was administered. B: The nadir (counts/min) after lemon juice administration. C: The point where activity returned to activity approximately equal to activity at point A. D: The maximum activity (counts/min) during the 1 h of imaging. E: The time after the start of imaging (min) to point A. F: The time after start of imaging (min) to point B. G: The time after start of imaging (min) to point C. H: The time after start of imaging (min) to point D. Note the prompt response to lemon juice with subsequent reaccumulation and the similar response following the second administration of lemon juice at 65 min into the acquisition. These two phases were initiated 2 h after the administration of ^{131}I (This figure was originally published in Van Nostrand et al. [89]. Reproduced with permission from Mary Ann Liebert, Inc. Publishers)

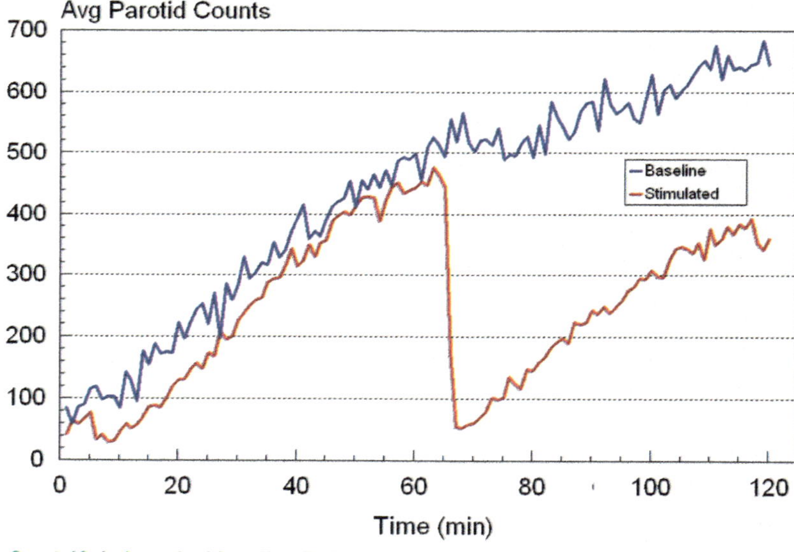

Fig. 62.3 This graph demonstrates two curves, which represent two time activity curves obtain over the parotid glands on two different days after the administration of ^{123}I. The blue (darker or upper curve) curve represents the time activity curve obtained 2 h after the administration of ^{123}I without the administration of any sialagogues. The red (lighter or lower curve) curve represents the time activity curve that was obtained in the same patient also 2 h after the administration of ^{123}I, and RealLemon® juice was administrated 5 min and 65 min after the initiation of the images. The images demonstrate that there is no "rebound effect" (e.g., the radioactivity becoming even greater than if lemon juice had not been administered) after either the first or second administration of lemon juice. These images also demonstrate that the percent washout of radioiodine was even greater after the second administration of lemon juice. Finally, even if continued imaging had demonstrated that the reaccumulation of radioiodine may have exceeded the radioiodine accumulation had a sialagogue not been administer (e.g., the "rebound effect"), these images suggest that readministration of lemon juice would have aborted any "rebound effect" (The above figure is reproduced with permission from Kulkarni [90] and the publishers, Wolters Kluwer)

trol. No rebound effect was observed in any of the nine patients during the time period imaged (see Fig. 62.3) and the mean percent reduction in radiation-absorbed dose was 34±17 %. Kulkarni et al. also observed that spontaneous salivation occurred 20 times in seven salivary scans that were performed without the administration of sialagogues.

The reports by Van Nostrand et al. and Kulkarni et al. raise questions that the time frame of administration of sialogogues of 2-3h and 4h in Nakada et al.'s and Liu et al's report, respectively, are too long. Indeed, avoidance of sialagogues for the first 24 h may be superior to sialagogues given every 2–3 h. However, from the reports of Silberstein, Van Nostrand et al., and Kulkarni et al., the sialagogues need to be administered more frequently and preferably continuously. In addition, the sialagogues may need to be administered not only during the day but frequently during the night. Although Jentzen et al. reported administering sialagogues continuously, this was only for 4 h before both groups were eating, snacking, and having dinner. However, more importantly, calculating the radiation-absorbed dose based on measurements of only four time points beginning at 4 h with periods of 20–48 h between subsequent time points does not capture what the continuous lemon slices had achieved during the short 4-h period prior to the first data point. The radiopharmacokinetics of iodine in the salivary gland are in fact "minute by minute" and are not reflected accurately when measured by periods of "4 to 24 hours."

Finally, the recommendation of avoiding sialagogues during the first 24 h to avoid salivation is not possible when patients are eating and drink lunches, snacks, and dinners, which patients of both Nakada et al. and Jentzen et al. apparently did. Thus, those patients could not avoid salivation within the first 24 h period. Further, even if one was on NPO for 24 h, it would appear based on Kulkarni's preliminary work—and we would submit based on everyone's personal experience - that spontaneous salivation cannot be avoided during a 24-h period [90]. As a result, spontaneous salivation defeats, at least in part, the proposed objective of avoidance of sialagogues for 24 h.

The controversy regarding the use of sialagogues will continue, but future studies must consider the dynamic *minute-by -minute* radiopharmacokinetics of iodine in the salivary gland.

Anti-inflammatory Agents

Whether patients should *prophylactically* take anti-inflammatory agents to reduce the inflammation and/or the signs and symptoms of sialoadenitis is not known. However, Silberstein has report prophylactic use of steroids in all patients [70]. His reported frequency of sialoadenitis and/or xerostomia was low and already noted in Table 62.8, but he also administered continuous sialagogues as discussed above.

Management of Complications

Sialoadenitis

If signs and symptoms indicating acute sialoadenitis occur, no guidelines have been evaluated to one author's (dvn) knowledge regarding when to begin anti-inflammatory agents, which anti-inflammatory agents are to be used, and/or for how long. Van Nostrand [27] has previously proposed an algorithm based on the National Cancer Institute's classification for salivary gland side effects (see Table 62.9), but as noted by Van Nostrand, no data are available to demonstrate that these guidelines are any better than any other proposal or even any better than not administering anti-inflammatory drugs. Further study is needed.

Xerostomia

Multiple recommendations have been proposed for the management of xerostomia, and a compilation of these recommendations appears in Table 62.10. One caveat regarding xerostomia is that one should not assume that the presence of xerostomia is the result of a prior radioiodine therapy. Many etiologies and combinations of etiologies may exist. However, a good history of the presence or absence of xerostomia prior to ^{131}I therapy and, if present, the severity of the patient's xerostomia prior to ^{131}I therapy will be helpful. If one does not wish to manage persistent xerostomia, then the patient should be referred to a dentist, oral surgeon, or otolaryngologist who does manage such.

Stomatitis

Stomatitis may be treated with dexamethasone elixir mouthwash or mouthwash that contains viscous lidocaine, diphenhydramine and aluminum, and magnesium hydroxides [53]. Referral of the patient to a dental hygienist, dentist, oral surgeon, or otolaryngologist is highly recommended.

Salivary Duct Obstruction

The symptoms of obstruction (as described earlier) should neither be mistaken as acute or chronic sialoadenitis nor treated as acute or chronic sialoadenitis. Although a component of chronic sialoadenitis may be present and warrant treatment, ductal obstruction should be considered because the management is different. If the pain and swelling is mild owing to mild obstruction from a mucous plug and/or radiation fibrosis, then increased retrograde or antegrade pressure with massage may resolve the symptoms by helping the normal or thickened saliva pass the ductal narrowing or help spontaneously extrude a mucous plug (see Fig. 62.1). If the symptoms are not mild or

Table 62.9 Proposed guidelines for the management of sialoadenitis, based on the severity of the signs and symptoms[1,2]

Category	Description	Treatment
Mild	Mild pain (NCI grade I = mild pain not interfering with function with a duration of <1 h)	Nonsteroidal, anti-inflammatory medication for 3 days
	No swelling	
	No tenderness to the touch	
Moderate (one or more of the following)	Moderate pain (NCI grade II = moderate pain or analgesics for pain interfering with function, but not interfering with activities of daily living of ≥1 h of duration)	Anti-inflammatory medication for 7 days
	Any swelling	
	Any tenderness to the touch	
Severe (one or more of the following)	Severe pain (NCI grade III = pain or analgesics severely interfering with activities of daily living of any duration)	Anti-inflammatory medication for 7 days,
	Moderate to severe swelling (very subjective)	
	Moderate to severe tenderness to the touch (very subjective)	Methylprednisolone dose pack or equivalent and
		Referral to dental hygienist, dentist, oral surgeon, or otolaryngologist
Extreme	Suppurative sialoadenitis	Emergency referral to otolaryngologist, oral surgeon, and/or dentist with special expertise in salivary gland management

Hydration is not listed, because this should already be encouraged and continued

No data are available to suggest that these guidelines are any more or less effective than any other guidelines or even no treatment at all

Table 62.10 Options for the management of xerostomia and dental caries

Maintain good hydration
Refer patient to a dental hygienist, dentist, oral surgeon, or otolaryngologist
Treat causes other than radiation-induced xerostomia such as reducing the dose of a drug or changing a drug that is causing xerostomia
Take frequent sips of sugar-free water or drinks
Drink frequently while eating
Keep a glass of water by one's bedside for dryness during the night or on awakening
Pause often while speaking to sip some liquids
Avoid coffee, tea, and soft drinks
Chew sugarless gum
Suck sugarless mints or hard sugarless candy allowing them to dissolve in your mouth (cinnamon and mint are often more effective)
Avoid tobacco and alcohol
Avoid spicy, salty, and highly acidic foods that may irritate the mouth
Use a humidifier, particularly at night
Maintain impeccable dental hygiene with regular checkups (3–6 months)
Use fluoride toothpaste routinely
Use nonalcoholic mouth washout such as a nonalcoholic mouthwash mixed with hydrogen peroxide
Consider fluoride therapy in the form of topical fluoride applications, fluoride mouthwashes, and fluoride toothpastes
Artificial saliva swirled in the mouth and swallowed every 3–4 h
Avoidance of anticholinergic medications
Administration of sialagogues [61]
Pilocarpine (Salagen®), 5–10 mg p.o. t.i.d. Oral tablet may need to be taken for 6–12 weeks before full benefit realized
Cevimeline (Evoxac®), cholinesterase inhibitor, 30 mg p.o. t.i.d.
Anethole trithione (Hepasulfol®, Mucinol®, Sialor®, Sonicur®, Sufralem®). The standard dose is 37.5–75 mg typically in divided doses before meals. Doses of up to 150 mg daily have been used
Trial of saliva-stimulating tablets (SST) [63] including potential agents as disaccharides and low-dose interferon-α lozenges
Acupuncture [64]
Antibiotics for suppurative sialoadenitis

Reproduced with permission from Blackwell Munksgaard

transient, then referral to otolaryngologist is strongly recommended. The otolaryngologist can then evaluate for other, albeit unlikely, etiologies of obstruction, consider ductal dilation of Stensen's duct with sialoendoscopy, and, in rare cases, consider tympanic neurectomy or ligation of the duct. Nahlieli and Nazarian evaluated 15 patients with sialoadenitis after ^{131}I therapy with sialoendoscopy under local anesthesia. All patients were reported to be free of swelling and pain in the parotid glands after one sialoendoscopy for a follow-up period of 1–4 years. Except for immediate swelling after sialoendoscopy of the affected salivary gland in all patients, there were no other complications observed. The swelling resolved spontaneously after 12 h [91]. Bomeli et al. [92] have reported on the use of interventional sialoendoscopy in 32 salivary glands in 12 patients. They were successful in 27 glands (84.4 %) with ductal stenosis in 30 % and mucus plugs removed in 44 %. Sialoendoscopy improved symptoms in 75 % (9/12) of patients with no serious complications. Allweiss et al. [43] reported one patient who required parotidectomy because of intractable salivary gland pain and discomfort, but excision of the gland should obviously be avoided. Finally, a secondary infection can occur that may require antibiotics.

In summary, sialoadenitis is an important side effect of ^{131}I therapy. Awareness of this side effect, its subsequent complications, and appropriate preventive care and treatment can be very important.

Taste and Smell

Alteration of taste and smell is well documented after ^{131}I therapy [2, 40, 41, 93] and may be described as simply a loss of taste, loss of smell (2), metallic taste, or chemical taste [93]. Occasionally, these patients may describe a salty taste that may be secondary to inadequately absorbed sodium and chloride ions in the saliva [45]. The frequency varies from 2 to 58 % of patients as noted in Table 62.11 [1, 2, 40, 42, 50, 93, 94]. The loss or change in taste or smell may occur as early as 24 h after ^{131}I ablation and was reported to occur within 168 h [93]. Although transient, the change in taste may persist from 4 weeks to as long as 52 weeks in 37 % of those patients [45]. Alexander et al. [2] found that it occurred up to several weeks after discharge and persisted for 1–12 weeks. The mechanism is most likely ^{131}I uptake in von Ebner's serous gland, located in the vicinity of the taste buds containing circumvallate papilla [53, 93]. Albrecht et al. [42] demonstrated a dependence or direct relationship on administered activity of ^{131}I.

Nasal Effects

Pain in the tip of the nose and epistaxis are rare but real side effects of ^{131}I. Van Nostrand et al. [40] described two of 15 patients who had received prescribed ^{131}I activities greater than 7.4 GBq (200 mCi) who had nasal complaints. One patient had dry nasal mucosa at 1 week, followed by easily controlled epistaxis, and a tender nose with clots and scabs during the second week. The lining of the nose has mucous cells that can accumulate ^{131}I. This accumulation can be most prominent in the tip of the nose, which is frequently seen and confirmed on ^{131}I whole-body scans (see Chap. 12) [95]. At the present time, little is known regarding methods to reduce this infrequent side effect of ^{131}I. However, if performing dosimetry and planning to administer prescribed ^{131}I activity higher than 7.4 GBq (200 mCi), the pretherapy scan for nasal uptake can be assessed to anticipate this potential complication. If there is facial activity with focal uptake in the nose area, consider a lateral view with appropriate markers. If there is marked uptake in the tip of the nose and if a high prescribed activity of ^{131}I is being considered, then the prescribed activity can be reduced. Further research is warranted evaluating drugs that may reduce this nasal uptake.

Facial Nerve

^{131}I has been associated as a rare cause of transient facial nerve paralysis. Levinson et al. [96] reported two patients who rapidly developed transient facial paralysis after ^{131}I therapy. The proposed mechanism was the passage of the affected nerve through the parotid gland, and the paralysis was attributed to the gland swelling secondary to radiation sialoadenitis with ischemia of the nerve. After resolution of the sialoadenitis, the facial nerve palsies resolved.

Thyroid Tissue

Radiation Thyroiditis

Radiation thyroiditis posttherapy is commonly seen in patients with large benign thyroid remnants (≥10 % neck uptake), especially when treated with >2.8–3.7 GBq (≥75–100 mCi) or more of ^{131}I, delivering radiation doses more than 50,000 rad (cGy). In ten patients studied retrospectively after lobectomy only, more patients demonstrated neck pain or tenderness (60 %) with ^{131}I ablation of the residual lobe than with ^{131}I ablation after more extensive excision (6 %) [97]. Neck and ear pain, dysphagia, painful swallowing, thyroid tenderness, and even airway compromise requiring intubation can be seen beginning 2–4 days posttherapy. With more extensive surgery, such as total or near-total thyroidectomy (<5 % neck uptake), radiation thyroiditis is infrequently seen. Cherk et al. [98] demonstrated that the acute thyroiditis was related to ^{131}I *uptake* and not the *amount* of prescribed activity of ^{131}I.

Table 62.11 Incidence of change in taste and/or smell

Author (ref.)	Incidence (no. of patients)
Albrecht [42]	58 % (30/51)
Alexander [2]	27 % (55/203)
Benua [1]	2 % (3/122)
Kahn [41]	16 % (8/50)
Kita [200]	9.8 % (9 /92)
Lin [50]	1.8 % (1/56)
Orquiza [94]	44 % (34/78)
Van Nostrand [40]	33 % (5/15)
Varma [93]	48 % (41/85)

However, with extensive neck metastases that are ^{131}I avid, patients may also demonstrate marked pain and swelling and even hemorrhage following ^{131}I therapy, particularly if the radiation-absorbed doses exceed 40,000 cGy (rad). Strong consideration should be given to surgical removal of all palpable neck metastatic disease to prevent such sequelae. A less common phenomenon is painless neck swelling that is manifested by edematous and firm induration of the neck, typically seen within 1–2 days of ^{131}I therapy of more than 10–15 g of thyroid tissue [99]. This is frequently associated with a neck-tightening sensation that can be very alarming to some patients. Although mild symptoms often recede with just analgesics, an oral prednisone burst and taper may be both necessary and beneficial in some patients with painful radiation thyroiditis and most patients with painless neck edema, using 30–60 mg daily for 3–5 days initially, followed by a gradual taper over 7–10 days.

Thyrotoxicosis

Thyrotoxicosis has been well documented in patients with functioning differentiated thyroid carcinoma after ^{131}I therapy [100–103]. Although rare, this is most typical of widespread metastatic follicular thyroid carcinoma. Trunnel et al. [103] reported that the signs and symptoms of hyperthyroidism appeared within 2 weeks of therapy. Cerletty et al. [104] described two cases in which the failure to control the thyrotoxic state led to thyroid storm and death.

Hypoparathyroidism

Therapeutic prescribed activity of ^{131}I can easily deliver greater than 10,000 cGy (rad) to the thyroid bed with lesser radiation to adjacent parathyroid tissue at 5–6 weeks post-thyroidectomy when surgically induced parathyroid injury may still be present. However, ^{131}I β particles (electrons) have a range of only 2.5 mm in soft tissue, and parathyroid irradiation would only be significant for intrathyroidal or closely adherent parathyroid glands. Only two cases of permanent hypoparathyroidism after ^{131}I therapy of thyroid cancer have been reported to our knowledge in patients known to be normocalcemic prior to treatment [105, 106]. Glazebrook et al. [106] have postulated that many thyroid cancer patients treated with ^{131}I exhibit diminished parathyroid reserve, as shown by stress testing in 53 patients post-thyroidectomy. When salt and water loaded prior to forced diuresis, 58 % of the 53 patients treated with 2.96–5.55 GBq (80–150 mCi) demonstrated transient hypocalcemia. In this prospective study, affected patients were more likely to have lower prestress serum calcium levels than unaffected patients. In the absence of symptoms, routine monitoring of calcemic status does not appear to be warranted.

Zhu et al. [107] reported in 58 patients that the blood parathyroid hormone (PTH), blood calcium, and blood phosphorus were not significantly affected by ^{131}I therapy with 1.48–3.70 GBq (40–102 mCi). However, in five patients, PTH levels transiently decreased to below normal levels returning to normal 4 months after ^{131}I therapy.

Carotid Artery

Cunha et al. [108] have reported a case of a rupture of a carotid artery following ^{131}I therapy in a patient with differentiated thyroid carcinoma. This patient had a large expansive solid mass with radioiodine uptake that was located at the base of the skull with tumor invasion of the left masticatory muscle and adjacent subcutaneous tissue. However, there was no invasion of the carotid space. As the authors pointed out, one should be cautious with masses that have good radioiodine uptake and are adjacent to important structures.

Vocal Cords

Recurrent laryngeal nerve injury or direct trauma from endotracheal tube placement during thyroidectomy can induce transient or permanent vocal cord paralysis, manifested by stridor or hoarseness. In symptomatic patients seen prior to anticipated ^{131}I therapy, direct laryngoscopy can document vocal cord dysfunction and should be performed. ^{131}I treatment of residual thyroid bed tissue can cause significant thyroid tissue swelling that is associated with laryngeal nerve compression and dysfunction [109, 110]. As reported by Lee et al. [109], 5.55 GBq (150 mCi) prescribed activity of ^{131}I given to treat residual right thyroid bed tissue in a patient with papillary thyroid cancer was followed by the gradual development of bilateral vocal cord paresis within 72 h. As only right thyroid bed irradiation occurred (no significant left-lobe uptake present), it was believed that a partial left recurrent laryngeal nerve injury had been present since the surgery, necessitating an emergent tracheostomy. Fortunately, the bilateral vocal cord dysfunction resolved after 8 weeks.

Pulmonary Effects

Acute radiation pneumonitis (ARP) and pulmonary fibrosis (PF) are potentially serious complications of ^{131}I treatment in patients who have pulmonary metastasis from differentiated thyroid carcinoma. Fortunately, this is very rare; however, because it is rare, most of the information regarding ARP and PF secondary to ^{131}I comes from (1) radiation pathology from external radiotherapy [111, 112], (2) two important case reports described in 1957 by Rall et al. [113], and (3) several additional reports in the literature [41, 50, 51, 114–116, 198]. The occurrence of ARP, PF, or both is directly related to the extent of pulmonary metastasis, the prescribed activity of ^{131}I, and its uptake and retention in the lung lesions. However, based on the information derived from these resources, radiation pneumonitis and pulmonary fibrosis are expected to be infrequent and rare complications of ^{131}I treatment.

Presentation

Based upon radiation pathology from external radiotherapy [111, 112], the time of ARP onset is usually 1–20 weeks after initial therapy. Its clinical presentation includes dyspnea, nonproductive cough, possible pleuritic pain, malaise, occasional fever, and rales. Radiographic changes are similar to other pneumonitis secondary to other causes, and computer tomography is more sensitive than chest X-ray in identifying the radiographic changes. The initial findings are typically perivascular haziness, which is followed by alveolar filling densities. Although these changes from external radiation therapy are typically confined to the field of irradiation, they may occur outside the field, known as *abscopal effects* [117–119]. Morgan et al. [120] suggested that these changes outside the irradiation field are from other mechanisms, such as generalized immunologically mediated lung damage.

The pathologic changes include congestion and intra-alveolar edema with alveolar macrophages, and the initial lesions probably occur in the endothelial cells of alveolar wall capillaries. Protein-rich fluid then leaks through the damaged capillary wall into the interstitium and alveolar lumen, with resultant edema in the alveolar septa and hyperplasia of the alveolar-lining cells. A hyaline membrane may occur, comparable to the pathogenesis of other etiologies of acute respiratory distress syndromes (ARDS); however, if formed, the hyaline membrane is more prominent in ARP. This description is similar to the autopsy reports of the two patients with ARP and PF, as reported by Rall et al. [113].

PF is a late clinical sequela of ARP. Although PF is typically present in most individuals who recover from ARP, PF can develop in patients who never had an initial acute illness. Most patients who develop PF are symptomatic 1 year later. If PF does occur, it is usually established and stable by 1 year after exposure and is irreversible. However, Delanian et al. [121] reported a decrease in fibrosis with treatment with a combination of pentoxifylline and tocopherol, but again, these data involved external radiation therapy. PF can also be chronic and progressive. The pathophysiology of PF involves progressive fibrosis of the alveolar septa. The laboratory changes include mildly reduced pulmonary functions, such as decreased vital capacity, decreased forced expiratory volume (FEV_1), decreased carbon monoxide diffusing capacity (DLCO), mild arterial hypoxia, decreased compliance, and reduced alveolar-capillary membrane integrity. Radiographically, computed tomography (CT) is again a more sensitive test than chest radiography and can demonstrate a progressive decrease in lung volumes, a reduction of pulmonary blood flow, and the fibrotic changes associated with PF. The pathophysiology may be the result of multiple agents including transforming growth factor-beta, interleukins, KL-6, surfactant proteins, and adhesion molecules [112].

Risk factors for clinical radiation pneumonitis are controversial. Monson [119] demonstrated an increase in clinical radiation pneumonitis in patients with a low Karnofsky performance status, a history of smoking, comorbid lung disease, or low pulmonary function tests (PFTs). In those patients with an FEV_1 of two or less, 24 % (16 of 66) of patients developed clinical radiation pneumonitis, whereas in patients with an FEV_1 above two, only 6 % (1 of 17) developed clinical radiation pneumonitis. In those patients with a forced vital capacity (FVC) of 3 liters or less, 31 % (17 of 54) developed clinical radiation pneumonitis, but no patient with an FVC more than 3 liters developed clinical radiation pneumonitis. These patients had received external radiotherapy for lung carcinoma [119]. However, there is a diversity of opinions regarding these risk factors such as pulmonary function [122].

As noted previously, limited reports exist in the literature regarding ARP and PF secondary to ^{131}I treatment in patients who have differentiated thyroid carcinoma with pulmonary metastasis. One of the most detailed reports provides valuable descriptions of two patients with documented fatal ARP and PF. Several salient features about these two patients are summarized here [113]. First, the initial respiratory symptoms occurred approximately 60 and 61 days after their ^{131}I treatments. For one patient, the presenting symptoms were shortness of breath and substernal pressure during exertion. For the other patient, symptoms were coldness, fatigue, shortness of breath, and a slightly nonproductive cough. The time interval from the initially reported respiratory symptoms to death from respiratory failure was 48 and 49 days, respectively. Rapid deterioration appeared to occur over the last 23 and 38 days. Steroids were used in one patient, which produced a significant but only transient improvement. Although other reports of ARP and PF are noted, no other significant information is available regarding time until symptoms, course of respiratory failure, the use of steroids, and so on.

Although these are only two cases and little additional information is available in the literature, several warnings appear to be appropriate and prudent. First, the signs or symptoms of ARP and/or its sequelae do not necessarily occur immediately after treatment but can be delayed as long as 8 weeks and possibly longer. Second, the initial symptoms may appear to be minor and nonspecific but should not be dismissed as unimportant or owing to other causes. Third, there may be an initial symptomatic period where *early* treatment with steroids may possibly alter the patient's course before progressive, irreversible respiratory failure begins.

Table 62.12 Fractionated radiation dose and side effects on the lung

34.9 Gy (3490 rad), 15 fractions over 19 days = 50 % developed radiographic evidence of lung damage [123]
40 Gy (4000 rad), 20–30 fractions = 8–15 % severe ARP clinically [117, 124]
54 Gy (5400 rad; fractionation N/A) = 20 % developed clinical ARP [119]
Occasionally severe lesions have occurred with lower doses
Of 377 patients treated to the mantle for Hodgkin's disease, 20 developed ARP; three died with less than 600 cGy (600 rad) to one whole lung. Five died after 600–1500 cGy (600–1500 rad) [125]

N/A = not available

Table 62.13 Single radiation dose (SD) and side effects on the lung

After 600–1000 cGy (rad) single dose, 17.5 % developed ARP 100 days later and 15 % died of ARP within 2 weeks [126]
820 cGy (rad) for 5 % incidence of ARP
930 cGy (rad) for 50 % incidence of ARP
1100 cGy (rad) for 90 % incidence of ARP [127]
700 cGy (rad) for SD to both lungs is currently proposed limit [127–129]

Table 62.14 Pulmonary fibrosis

Difficult to establish because it is typically asymptomatic but probably very frequent [130]
After 3000 cGy over 10–15 days, 30 % had radiographic changes [123, 127]
After 5000 cGy (rad) over 25 days, 90 % had radiographic changes [123, 127]

Radiation Dose to the Lung

Estimating the radiation dose to the lung from ^{131}I treatment is problematic on several counts. There are challenges in estimating ^{131}I uptake in a pulmonary lesion, inhomogeneous ^{131}I uptake within the lesion, lesion depth, attenuation of the radioactivity, radioactivity clearance from the lesion, lesion volume, and the radiation exposure to adjacent normal pulmonary tissue. Consequently, the radiation exposure to the lungs or even a portion of the lungs from ^{131}I is difficult to accurately determine. Additional studies are underway using ^{124}I, which are discussed further in Chap. 103. However, more specific data are available from external radiotherapy on the relationship between radiation dose and side effects on the lung (see Tables 62.12, 62.13, and 62.14) [112, 117, 119, 123–130]. The data from external radiotherapy are useful for an overall perspective, but extrapolation of the data to ^{131}I therapy is again difficult. Similarly, although dosimetric analysis of radiation exposure to the lungs from ^{131}I with phantoms has been reported, the information is limited [131]. However, several groups have attempted to define dose-volume histograms to help predict radiation-induced lung disease [132, 133]. Gopal et al. [132] demonstrated a significant decrease in DLCO with the local lung dose exceeding 13 Gy, but interestingly, the threshold was increased to 36 Gy when the patient was treated with amifostine. Emami et al. [134] attempted to compile tolerance for normal lung tissue with estimates of tolerance doses resulting in a 5 % complication rate and a 50 % complication rate, and Burman et al. [135] further used this model to interpolate clinical data to provide estimates of radiation pneumonitis to normal lung tissue based on dose and irradiated volume. Graham et al. [136] evaluated clinical dose-volume histograms for pneumonitis for 3D radiotherapy for non-small cell lung cancer. They reported that the total lung volume exceeding 20 Gy (2000 rad), larger effective volume, higher total lung volume mean dose, and location of the tumor (lower lung) to be statistically significant for the development of ARP. Wilner et al. [133] evaluated the relationship of ARP to "a little (dose) to a lot (of volume) or a lot to a little," and the risk of ARP increased significantly with increasing levels of high radiation dose volume. Reducing high-dose volumes reduced ARP more than reducing the low-dose volumes. Although these data are again based on external radiation therapy and a full discussion is beyond the scope of this chapter, these data raise the possibility that ARP may be more likely after ^{131}I therapy in patients with diffuse pulmonary metastases versus individual areas of pulmonary macronodular disease.

In the literature on ARP and PF secondary to ^{131}I treatment, the most valuable data are again from Rall et al. [113]

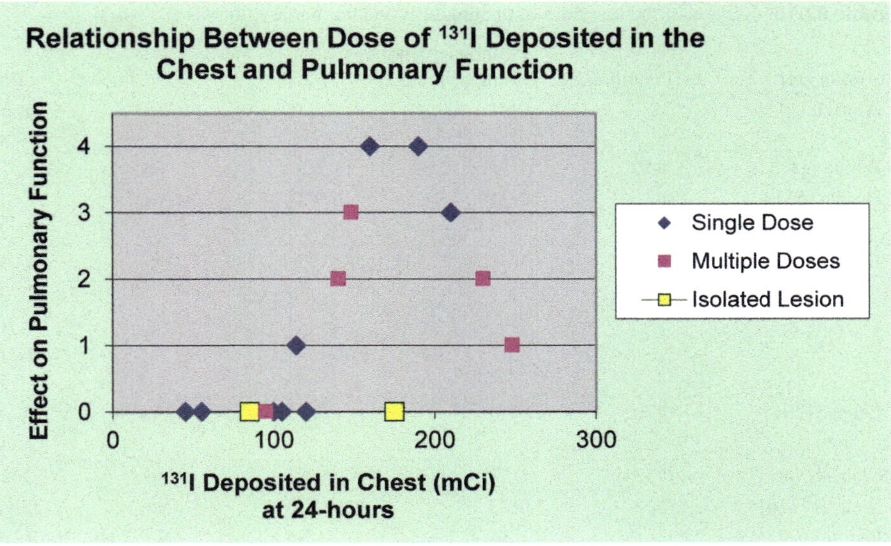

Fig. 62.4 These data were compiled from Rall's original article by one author (dvn). Changes in pulmonary function begin to appear after ^{131}I deposited in the chest at 24 h exceeded 125 mCi. The effect of pulmonary function was graded as follows: 0 = none, 1 = minimal X-ray reaction, 2 = moderate X-ray reaction, 3 = moderate X-ray reaction + symptoms, 4 = death from pulmonary insufficiency

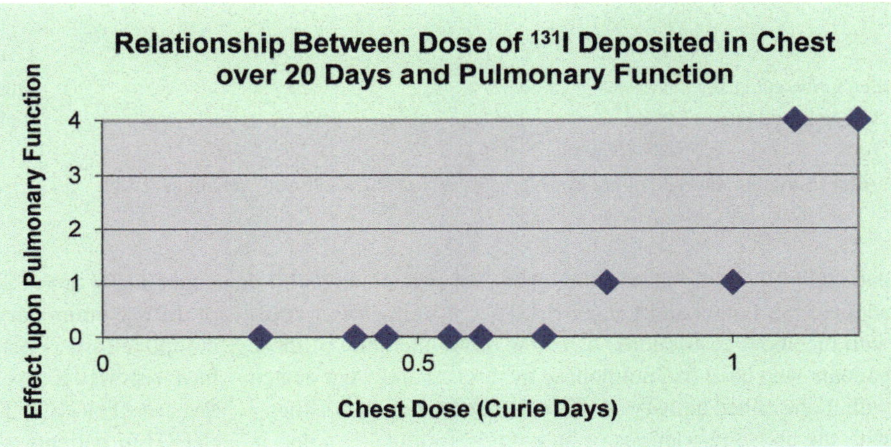

Fig. 62.5 The two fatalities from radiation pneumonitis reported by Rall et al. each had over 1 Ci-day of ^{131}I retention in the lung. This was calculated by summing the calculated lung retention for each day over 20 days. The *amount* of ^{131}I uptake and the *amount and duration* of ^{131}I *retention* appear important, which is what one would expect. The effect of pulmonary function was graded as follows: 0 = none, 1 = minimal X-ray reaction, 2 = moderate X-ray reaction, 3 = moderate X-ray reaction + symptoms, 4 = death from pulmonary insufficiency

and Benua et al. [1]. Rall et al. observed 15 patients with pulmonary metastasis from differentiated thyroid carcinoma who were treated with ^{131}I. Four of these patients developed pulmonary changes, and two subsequently died from the pulmonary changes as already noted. Figure 62.4 demonstrates the relationship between the amount of prescribed ^{131}I activity deposited in the chest and the pulmonary assessment. When the study was reported in 1957, the pulmonary assessment was made by X-ray and evaluation of symptoms. No patient who retained less than 4.63 GBq (125 mCi) in the chest at 24 h developed radiographic changes or symptoms to suggest pulmonary changes secondary to radiation effects. In Fig. 62.5, Rall's data demonstrate an association between pulmonary assessment and the quantity of ^{131}I deposited in the chest over the first 20 days following treatment. The quantity of ^{131}I deposited was expressed in units of "curie-day," which represents the sum for each of the 20 days of ^{131}I estimated quantity deposited in the lungs. Both fatalities had the highest estimates of ^{131}I exposure to the chest with over 1 Ci-day. Furthermore, no patient with approximately 0.75 Ci-day of ^{131}I deposited in the chest developed radiographic changes or symptoms to suggest any pulmonary changes secondary to radiation. In 1961, Benua et al. [1] reported on an expanded group of patients at Memorial Sloan Kettering Cancer Center (MSKCC), which included patients of Rall et al.; 59 patients were treated with 122 doses of ^{131}I. Radiation pneumonitis occurred in five of these patients. However, radiation pneumonitis did not occur when the calculated radiation dose to the blood was less than or equal to 200 cGy (rad) and the whole-body retention of ^{131}I at 48 h was less than or equal to 2.96 GBq (80 mCi) (see Chap. 58).

Based on their early experience, Benua and Leeper proposed and implemented the above restrictions for patients with pulmonary metastasis. In 1982, Leeper reported that no subsequent radiation pneumonitis had been observed at MSKCC over approximately 20 years since the original group of five

Table 62.15 Review of the literature of pneumonitis and pulmonary fibrosis

Author (ref.)	Pneumonitis	Pulmonary fibrosis or impairment	Fatal	Dosimetry	Comments
Aldrich [115]		7/35	2/35	No	Impairment may have been part of thyroid cancer or concomitant lung disease
Benua [1]	5/59	1/59	2/59	Yes	
Brown [51]	0/31	0/31	0/31	No	1. Dosage typically 150 mCi
					2. Maximum dosage 680 mCi
Edmonds [198]	0/5	1/5	0/5	No	1. Dosage typically 150 mCi
					2. Range 378–973 mCi
					3. Follow-up 8–17 years
					4. Progressive impairment, which may have been part of disease itself
Leeper [201]	0/70	0/70*	0/70*	Yes	1. Average dosage of 309 mCi
					2. Range 70–654 mCi
Maheshwari [140]	0/53	1/53	0/53	No	Dosage typically 50–200 mCi
Menzel [116]	0/23	0/23	0/23	No	Used empiric dosages as high as 300 mCi
Pacini [139]		1/86	1/86	No	Respiratory failure from thyroid cancer and ^{131}I therapy, or both could not be differentiated
Samuel [137]	1/35	1/35	0/35	No	1. Highest dosage 270 mCi
					2. Highest total dosage 1194 mCi
					3. Data based on 99mTc-DTPA clearance
Schlumberger [138]	0/23	0/23	0/23	No	Administer repeated dosages of 100 mCi
Van Nostrand [40]	0/6*	0/6*	0/6*	Yes	Highest dosage 450 mCi
Total	2 % (6/305)	2.8 % (12/426)	1.2 % (5/426)		

*After restriction imposed of not exceeding 80 mCi of ^{131}I whole body retention at 48 h

patients [48]. In the intervening years, other institutions have adopted the Benua and Leeper (MSKCC) dosimetry protocol with the above restrictions. A review of the literature of those patients who have had pulmonary metastases and were treated with a prescribed activity of ^{131}I, either according to dosimetry with the above restrictions or an empiric formula, is noted in Table 62.15 [1, 40, 51, 115, 116, 137–140, 198, 201]. The frequency of observed radiation pneumonitis in the pooled group of patients was 2 %, PF was 2.8 %, and death secondary to radiation effects to the lung was 1.2 %.

Thus, despite the absence of prospective data in the literature and the inability to extrapolate the data from external radiation therapy, significant empirical data has been accumulated over the last 60 years. These data allow at least one approach that has a reasonably acceptable risk of ARP and PF complications.

Thyroid Hormone Withdrawal Versus Recombinant Human Thyroid-Stimulating Hormone

The use of thyroid hormone withdrawal (THW) versus recombinant human thyroid-stimulating hormone (rhTSH) for the preparation of patients with distant metastases for ^{131}I has been discussed elsewhere in Chaps. 10, 60 and 103. However, whether or not the preparation of patient with either THW or rhTSH for ^{131}I therapies in patients with focal or diffuse pulmonary metastases could have greater or lesser complications is not known. However, Goffman et al. [141] have reported a case with near-lethal respiratory failure after the use of rhTSH. This case report is a caveat in the use of rhTSH in patients with pulmonary metastases and indicates that further study is warranted to evaluate whether or not the side effects are due to the rapid increase of TSH from the injection of rhTSH, ^{131}I therapy, or a combination of both and whether or not pretreatment with steroids is warranted.

Appropriate Time Interval between ^{131}I Treatments

It is also problematic to determine the appropriate time interval between ^{131}I treatments to minimize the patient's chance of developing ARP and PF. Schlumberger et al. [138] found no ARP or PF in a patient group with pulmonary metastases who were treated with ^{131}I every 4–6 months, but the prescribed activity used was only ~3.7 GBq (100 mCi). Hindié et al. [142] also reported no ARP or PF with treatments every 6 months until a cumulative prescribed activity of 18.5 GBq (500 mCi), at which time the interval was increased to 1 or 2 years. However, Hindié et al. [142] also treated patients with prescribed activities of 3.7–5.55 GBq (100–150 mCi). Rall et al. suggested that the recovery from ARP was exponential and that multiple doses should be separated by intervals of 6 months or more [113]. Leeper, who administered much higher prescribed activities of ^{131}I, empirically recommended extending the time between treatments to approximately 1 year [48]. Although further study is needed, these studies will be difficult to perform.

Existence of Prior Pulmonary Disease

Aldrich et al. [115] evaluated pulmonary function in 12 of 35 patients with differentiated thyroid carcinoma metastatic to the lung. Five patients had other known causes for lung disease, but no distinctive type of abnormal pulmonary function (e.g., obstructive, restrictive, or mixed) was identified with pulmonary metastases. Interestingly, no patient died from pulmonary complications of ^{131}I treatment if the pretherapy pulmonary functions tests were normal.

Recommended Pretherapy Management of Pulmonary Metastases To Minimize Complications

If a patient has known pulmonary metastases secondary to differentiated thyroid carcinoma, one author (dvn) recommends the following approach.

1. Obtain a history of any pulmonary disease and the results of all previous pulmonary function tests, if any.
2. Assess the extent of pulmonary metastases based on chest X-ray and chest computer tomography (CT) with or without contrast. If CT was performed with contrast, then ^{131}I therapy can be delayed until the iodine has cleared as measured by spot urine iodine/creatinine measurements.
3. Examine present pulmonary function using PFTs and diffuse capacity for the lung to clear carbon monoxide (DLCO) [143]. (Note: Hughes et al. [143] have suggested that these studies may overestimate the diffusion limitation by 30 %.)
4. If the patient has a single pulmonary metastasis with no evidence of distant metastases elsewhere by a thorough evaluation, consider a pulmonary metastasectomy [144, 145]. Although the report of Liu et al. report did not include thyroid cancer, metastasectomy of a solid pulmonary metastasis may be a reasonable option to consider [145].
5. Assess the pattern of metastases on chest X-ray, chest CT scan, and ^{131}I scan. According to the limited literature (and intuitively), the risk of ARP and PF appears to be lower when:
   (a) The radioactive uptake in the lungs is lower.
   (b) The radioactivity in the lungs clears faster.
   (c) The disease is a single focus, rather than multiple foci.
   (d) The disease pattern is more regional than diffuse, such as one or two macronodular areas of disease in one lobe instead of diffuse micronodular or miliary disease throughout both lungs. (However, note that patients with a micronodular or miliary pattern of metastases with good ^{131}I uptake may have an improved response and prognosis after treatment with ^{131}I) [1, 146, 147].
6. Determine the response on clinical exam, chest X-ray, CT, PFT with DLCOs, ^{131}I scans, and blood thyroglobulin levels after all previous ^{131}I therapies.
7. Recommend dosimetry, and follow the restrictions for pulmonary metastases as described by Benua and Leeper.
   (a) Do not exceed an amount of ^{131}I prescribed activity that would result in whole-body retention at 48 h of more than 2.96 GBq (80 mCi).
   (b) Do not exceed an amount of ^{131}I prescribed activity that would result in greater than 200 cGy (rad) to the blood (bone marrow).
8. If an empiric prescribed activity of 7.4 GBq (200 mCi) or more is going to be used and the patient has a diffuse micronodular or miliary pattern of metastases in the lung, we strongly recommend that a reliable effort be made to estimate the whole-body retention at 48 h (or the whole lung retention at 24 h) and adjust the prescribed activity based on Benua's recommendation of whole-body retention when lung metastasis are present. Of note, Esposito et al. [148] reported in 53 patients with lung metastases that the percentage (number) of patients who would have received more than 200 cGy (rad) to the blood (e.g., surrogate for bone marrow) if empiric dosages of ^{131}I of 100 mCi (3.7 GBq), 150 mCi (5.55 GBq), 200 mCi (7.4 GBq), 250 mCi (9.25 GBq), and 300 mCi (11.1 GBq) had been administered would have been 0 %(0), 7 %(4), 17 %(9), 24 %(13), and 30 %(16), respectively. For all patients, regardless if lung metastases are present or not, Leeper [49] reported that 19 % of ^{131}I prescribed activities that delivered 200 cGy (rad) to the blood were below 7.4 GBq (200 mCi). Tuttle et al. [149] reported that 5 % of patients receiving 200 mCi (7.5 GBq) of ^{131}I would have received 200 rad (cGy) or more to the blood. In 127 patients, Kulkarni et al. [150] reported that if 3.7 GBq (150 mCi), 7.4 GBq (200 mCi), and 5.55 GBq (300 mCi) of ^{131}I had been administered, 5 %, 11 %, and 17 % of the patient, respectively, would have received 200 cGy (rad) to the blood (e.g., bone marrow). This is discussed further later in this chapter.
9. Reduce the amount of prescribed activity of ^{131}I in the presence of impaired pretherapy PFTs.
10. With higher empiric or dosimetrically determined prescribed activity, retreat with ^{131}I no sooner than 1 year from the last ^{131}I therapy.
11. For patients with changes indicating PF from previous ^{131}I therapy, consider pulmonary biopsy to assess the degree of PF.

Recommended Posttherapy Management

In follow-up for ^{131}I treatment of patients who have functioning pulmonary metastases from well-differentiated thyroid carcinoma, one author (dvn) recommends the following:

- Educate the patient regarding the signs and symptoms to carefully monitor, including any cough or shortness of breath, which may be the initial warning of pulmonary complications.
- Encourage the patient to seek *early* evaluation for any respiratory symptoms.
- Schedule routine follow-up evaluations at 1 and 2 months posttherapy.
- Recommend PFTs at 1 and/or 2 months. (Until data is available to demonstrate that there is no value of PFTs at these time points, one author (dvn) believes these should be performed as part of the assessment for early pulmonary changes, to assess for both decreases in PFTs that may be a complication of ^{131}1 or improvement as a therapeutic benefit secondary to ^{131}I.
- Repeat PFTs at periodic intervals such as 6 and/or 12 months.

For those patients with possible ARP and PF, we recommend the following:

- Begin treatment as soon as possible. Don't wait.
- Consider initial therapy with nonsteroidal anti-inflammatory agents or inhaled steroids, but:
- Consider the *early* use of oral or intravenous steroids and antibiotics. For the treatment of ARP secondary to external radiation therapy to the lungs, Gomez and Rosenzweig recommend treatment with at least 60 mg/day of prednisone for 2 weeks and then gradually decreasing the dose over 3–12 weeks [112]. However, no data are available regarding whether or not this schedule is effective for ARP secondary to ^{131}I therapy.
- For patients who develop end-stage lung disease due to ^{131}I-induced pulmonary fibrosis, lung transplantation is often the only subsequent option.

Summary

In summary, ARP and PF can be serious conditions of ^{131}I treatment in patients who have functioning pulmonary metastases from differentiated thyroid cancer. Although scientific data are still limited, evidence is available based on approximately 60 years of clinical experience that suggests empiric and dosimetric approaches for ^{131}I treatment of pulmonary metastases are associated with a minimal risk of complications of ARP and PF. When the percent 48-h whole-body retention is obtain and one does not exceed the recommendations of Benua et al. regarding such, this may help reduce the risk even further. Nevertheless, additional research is needed in this area. If ARP does occur, early detection and treatment are strongly recommended.

Gastrointestinal Effects

^{131}I ingestion is followed by rapid absorption through the stomach and small bowel wall into the systemic circulation, with subsequent active gastric mucosa concentration and secretion. This direct stomach irradiation engenders no symptoms in most patients at ingested dosages below 1.11 GBq (30 mCi). However, as the administered ^{131}I dosage escalates, nausea is experienced by more patients; 5.35 % of patients complain of this side effect at a standard dose of 1.48 GBq (40 mCi) [32]. In 78 patients treated with a standard ablation prescribed activity of 2.78 GBq (75 mCi) for residual thyroid bed activity, nausea was reported in 12 % of patients when questioned at 4–5 days post-ablation (jf, unpublished data). The majority of patients (50–67 %) treated with prescribed activity of 5.55 GBq (150 mCi) of ^{131}I will complain of nausea that usually develops after 18–24 h but can be seen within 2–4 h of therapy and persists for 24–48 h [40, 41. Khorjekar et al. [151] evaluated the responses of patients to a national survey offered through the Thyroid Cancer Survivors' Association, Inc. (ThyCa) regarding the patient's last ^{131}I outpatient therapy and vomiting. Out of 801 patients responding, 10 % (81) had vomiting of which vomiting was described as mild in 25 % (19), moderate in 42 % (32), and severe in 32 % (24) in 75 respondents. In addition, patients were statistically more likely to vomit if they were younger and female and/or had a higher level of anxiety to radiation. Khorjekar et al. [152] reported vomiting with or without preceding nausea in 7.6 % [30/397] of patients receiving a prescribed activity of less than 5.55 GBq (<150 mCi) and 15 % [41/274] with amounts of ^{131}I prescribed activity greater than 5.55 GBq (150 mCi). Whether the frequency of ^{131}I associated nausea is accentuated by the concomitant use of sialagogues is not known.

Prior to May 29, 1997, the Nuclear Regulatory Commission (NRC) guidelines mandated inpatient hospitalization for any patient whose whole-body retention exceeded 1.11 GBq (30 mCi) of ^{131}I (equivalent to ≥5 mR at 1 m). If vomiting occurred in the inpatient setting, ^{131}I in gastric contents was contained within a controlled area [153]. New NRC guidelines, the so-called Patient Discharge Rules, are "exposure" based, rather than patient "activity" based. Patients receiving up to 7.4 GBq (200 mCi) of ^{131}I are now routinely released by many licensees when the total effective dose equivalent of a member of the public exposed to the patient is not likely to exceed 5 mSv (0.5 rem) [154]. Patients treated with more than 3.7 GBq (>100 mCi) of ^{131}I have returned to a medical facility after vomiting unknown quantities of ^{131}I in an uncontrolled location. The possibility of an outpatient vomiting over 1.85 GBq (>50 mCi) of ^{131}I in the home environment (or local motel), significantly contaminating family members or the general public, has greatly heightened the awareness of this issue. Patients with a multiplicity of disease processes are at increased risk of vomiting ingested ^{131}I, including anxiety disorder, cerebral palsy, any pharyngeal or esophageal motility disorder, gastroesophageal reflux disease, gastroparesis, gastric outlet obstruction, and other similar entities. To lessen the chance of dealing with a large quantity of vomited ^{131}I, one patient with a prior vomiting history shortly after diagnostic ^{131}I ingestion and another patient with marked diabetic gastroparesis received their therapy intravenously by sterilization of the commercially available oral formulation with no subsequent nausea, vomiting, or other sequelae. However, intravenous ^{131}I does not eliminate the possibility of vomiting ^{131}I entirely because blood clearance curves of oral and intravenous ^{131}I are similar and nausea and vomiting may originate centrally rather than locally in the stomach. Additionally and as noted above, a significant percentage of the intravenously administered ^{131}I will be secreted into the stomach within the next 24 h resulting in a local stimulus of nausea and vomiting.

For most patients, nausea and vomiting can usually be averted or ameliorated by premedication with antiemetic preparations, such as ondansetron (Zofran®), prochlorperazine (Compazine®), or triethylperazine (Torecan®). Emphasizing the possible side effects of nausea and vomiting seems to help precipitate their occurrence, especially in anxious patients. Our current practice is to provide the patient with a prescription for six ondansetron 8 mg tablets, taking one tablet three times daily beginning 30 min prior to ^{131}I therapy. If necessary, the first 8 mg dose of ondansetron can be administered intravenously if the patient neglects to take the medication as prescribed.

Finally, Kinuya et al. [155] reported a Mallory-Weiss syndrome caused by ^{131}I therapy for metastatic thyroid carcinoma. The patient had massive hematemesis secondary to a tear at the gastroesophageal junction, with only mild nausea and no initial vomiting.

Radiation Cystitis

Balan et al. [156] and Dobyns et al. [157] each reported one case of cystitis.

Bone Marrow

Bone marrow suppression, aplastic anemia, and leukemia are some of the most serious potential untoward affects of ^{131}I therapy. This section discusses bone marrow suppression and aplastic anemia. Leukemia is discussed later in this chapter in section "Secondary primary malignancies risk in thyroid cancer survivors".

Review of the Literature

Like all side effects of ^{131}I therapy, the variability in the reported frequency and severity of bone marrow suppression is multifactorial, and some of these factors are noted in Table 62.16. A summary of the frequency of occurrence of bone marrow suppression based on a review of the literature is presented in Table 62.17 [1, 40, 44, 48, 103, 116, 158–166, 198]. To demonstrate examples of the severity of bone marrow suppression according to National Cancer Institute (NCI) criteria and the typical time courses, two hypothetical cases are shown in Figs. 62.6 and 62.7. The Common Terminology Criteria for Adverse Events for hematologic toxicities are noted in Table 62.18. A review of the literature on the frequency of reported aplastic anemia or death due to bone marrow suppression is noted in Table 62.19 [1, 2, 40, 48, 114, 116, 158, 160, 163, 166, 167, 198]. The specifics of selected articles are subsequently discussed.

Alexander et al. [2] reported that nine out of 203 patients treated with between 3.7 and 7.4 GBq (100–200 mCi) of ^{131}I demonstrated hematological abnormalities involving moderate reduction of their leukocytes that ranged from 3200 to 4200 per μL (normal range 4300–10,000/μL). They also reported no signs of thrombocytopenia or aplastic anemia, and the total cumulative prescribed activity ranged from 0.1 to 1.9 Ci (3.7–70.3 GBq).

Benua et al. [1] reported bone marrow suppression in 38 of 59 patients who received 122 treatments. Serious bone marrow depression was observed following these treatments in eight patients; two patients subsequently died of bone marrow suppression. Benua has suggested a relationship of significant bone marrow suppression when the total radiation

Table 62.16 Variability of frequency and severity of bone marrow suppression

Individual prescribed activity of ^{131}I
Patient's rate of ^{131}I clearance
Frequency of ^{131}I therapies
Interval between ^{131}I therapies
Total cumulative prescribed activities of ^{131}I
Frequency of prescribed activities delivering greater than 200 or 300 cGy (rad) to the bone marrow determined empirically
Performance of Benua and Leeper dosimetry
Variability in the definition of bone marrow suppression
Variability in the diligence in evaluating bone marrow suppression
Patient bone marrow reserve
Extensive bone metastases
Prior or concomitant radiation therapy to the bone

Table 62.17 Summary of bone marrow suppression

Author (ref.)	Year	Total	Abnormality	Hemoglobin	WBC	Platelets
Alexander [2]	1998	203	4.4 % (9)	0 % (0)	4.4 % (9)	No evidence
Benua [1]	1962	122	31 % (38)[a]	–	–	–
Dorn [158]	2003	25	100 % (25)	–	–	–
Leeper [49]	1982		No permanent bone marrow suppression			
Edmonds [198]	1986	258	1.1 % (3)*b*	–	–	–
Grunwald [159]	1994	567	1.4 % (8)	–	–	–
Haynie [160]	1963	159	–	34 % (54)	10 %	8.4 % (5)
Keldsen [161]	1988	27	26 % (15)	–	33 % in female (and increased in male)	30 % in female and 17 in male
Matthies [162]	2004	68			22 % (15)	12 % (8)
Menzel [116] (low prescribed activity; see text)	1996	84	3.6 % (3)[c]	0 % (0)	3.6 % (3)	0 % (0)
Menzel [116] (high prescribed activity; see text)	1996	78	50 % (29)[d]	–	–	–
Molinaro [163]	2009	206		No change	9.7 % decrease from baseline at 1 year	5.8 % decrease from baseline at 1 year
Pan [44]	2004	–	–	–	4.00 %	10.40 %
Petrich [164]	2001	107	37.4 % (40/107)	–	–	–
Robeson [165]	2002	12	42 % (5/12)	25 % (3/12)	42 % (5/12)	17 % (2)
Schober [166]	1987	296		24 % (71)	11 % (33)	35 % (104)
Trunnell [103]	1949	9	100 % (9)	–	–	–
Van Nostrand [40]	1986	10	90 % (9)	–	–	–

[a]Total of 59 patients and 122 doses. Six of the 122 treatments produced severe bone marrow suppression, with two resulting in death.
[b]It isunclear from the article if the asuthor looked for bone marrow suppression other than when it as fatal.
[c]Prescribed activites of radioiodine were 1.8-5.5 GBq (49-200 mCi).
[d]Prescribed activities of radioiodine were greater than 7.4 GBq (200mCi). Bone marrow suppression was mild in thiryy, grade II in three patients, and severe in one patient. The data were not fully described.

dose to the blood exceeded 200 cGy (rad). Serious complications, including bone marrow suppression, were observed in 21 % when total radiation to the blood exceeded 200 cGy (rad) but in only 3 % when the total radiation to the blood was less than 200 cGy (rad). Furthermore, bone marrow suppression was also increased when the whole-body retention at 48 h exceeded 4.44 GBq (120 mCi). Initially, Benua reported severe and permanent bone marrow suppression in eight of 59 patients. However, after Benua imposed the restrictions of (1) a maximum of 200 cGy (rad) to the blood and (2) 4.44 GBq (120 mCi) whole-body retention at 48 h, no subsequent cases of permanent bone marrow suppression have occurred as reported by Leeper [49].

Benua further reported that the mean whole blood radiation dose from ^{131}I therapies in the 59 patients was 267 cGy (rad), with a range of 45–740 cGy (rad). For the eight patients with severe bone marrow suppression, the calculated total radiation dose to the blood from the last ^{131}I therapy ranged from 170 cGy (rad) to 582 cGy (rad). However, all had been previously treated. For six of the eight patients with severe bone marrow suppression in whom total blood radiation dose could be calculated for the cumulative ^{131}I administered, the total radiation dose to the blood ranged from 300 to 1100 cGy (rad). Severe bone marrow suppression was not observed if the total cumulative radiation dose to the blood was less than 300 cGy (rad).

Dobyns et al. [157] noted that the most likely change in the blood is a decline in the lymphocytes.

Dorn et al. [158] performed 104 therapies with prescribed activities determined by a dosimetric MIRD methodology (see Chap. 59). In 100 % (25/25) of patients who received absorbed doses of lower than 300 cGy (rad) to the bone marrow, transient bone marrow suppression was present. However, no permanent bone marrow suppression was observed. The maximum single administered dose was 38.5 GBq (1040 mCi).

Fig. 62.6 Hypothetical course of National Cancer Institute (NCI) grade I mild to moderate bone marrow suppression

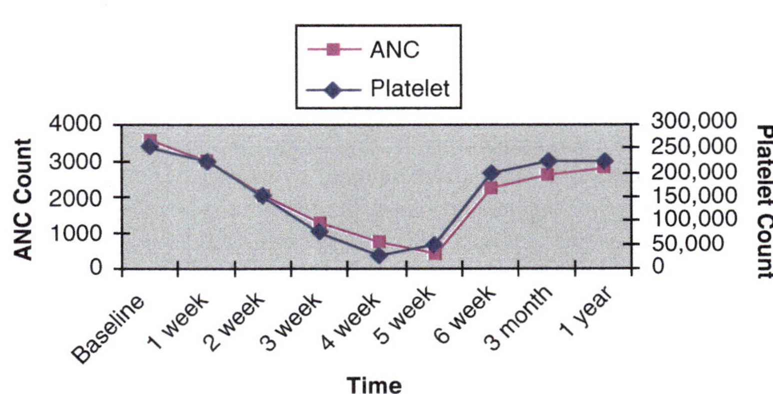

Fig. 62.7 Hypothetical course of National Cancer Institute (NCI) grade IV severe bone marrow suppression

Table 62.18 The NCI[a] common terminology criteria for adverse events

Adverse event	Grade 1	Grade 2	Grade 3	Grade 4	Grade 5
Hemoglobin	<LLN–10.0 g/dL	<10.0–8.0 g/dL	<8.0–6.5 g/dL	<6.5 g/dL	Death
Leukocytes (total WBCs)	<LLN–3000 mm^3	<3000–2000 mm^3	<2000–1000 mm^3	<1000 mm^3	Death
Neurtophilis/gran/ganluocytes	<LLN–1500 mm^3	<1500–1000 mm^3	<1000–500 mm^3	<500 mm^3	Death
Platelets	<LLN–75,000 mm^3	<75,000–50,000 mm^3	<50,000–25,000 mm^3	<25,000 mm^3	Death

<LLN, less than the lower limits of normal for that particular laboratory. Criteria are from v 3.0, December 12, 2003
[a]*NCI* National Cancer Institute

Table 62.19 Aplastic anemia or death attributed to bone marrow suppression

Author (ref.)	Year	Aplastic anemia or death
Alexander [2]	1998	0 % (0/203)
Benua [1]	1962	1.6 % (2/122)
Dorn [158]	2003	0 % (25/25)
Edmonds [198]	1986	1.2 % (3/258)
Haynie [160]	1963	0 % (0/159)
Leeper [49]	1982	0 % (0/70)
Menzel [116]	1996	0.5 % (1/167)[a]
Petrich [164]	2001	3.7 % (4/107)
Schober [166]	1987	1.0 % (3/296)
Schumichen [167]	1983	0.75 % (3/400)
Tollefson [114]	1964	0 % (0/70)[b]
Van Nostrand [40]	1986	0 % (0/10)

[a]Patient rejected for additional treatments because of persistent severe bone marrow suppression
[b]In the evaluation of 70 fatalities in patients with thyroid cancer, none were because of bone marrow suppression

Edmonds and Smith found that three patients from a group of 258 developed aplastic anemia and died within 4 years; they had extensive metastases and were treated multiple times [198]. The total radioactivity was 63 GBq (1700 mCi), 40 GBq (1080 mCi), and 31 GBq (850 mCi). In this study, patients were initially treated with 2.9 GBq (80 mCi) for ablation and, when additional therapies were necessary, with 5.5 GBq (150 mCi) every few months.

Grunwald et al. [159] indicated that 1 % (7 of 567) of patients who had ^{131}I therapies had persistent changes in blood counts. In patients who received prescribed cumulative activities of less than 18.5 GBq (500 mCi), only five of 469 had a hemoglobin less than or equal to 9.0, white blood cell count (WBC) 2500 or less, and/or platelets 50,000 or less. For prescribed activities of 18.5 GBq (500 mCi) to less than 37 GBq (<1000 mCi), one of 77 patients had changes, and with prescribed activities of 37 GBq (≥1000 mCi), six of 21 patients had blood changes, and four of these patients had pancytopenia.

Haynie and Beierwaltes reported their observations in 159 patients who received ^{131}I for the treatment of thyroid cancer at 3-month intervals (if needed) between 1947 and 1960. Evaluation of these patients included a baseline and at least one posttherapy complete blood count (CBC). Patients received prescribed activities of usually 3.7–11.1 GBq (100–300 mCi) of ^{131}I with follow-up CBC at 3-month and 1-year intervals for 10 years after completion of therapy. The most frequently observed abnormality was a subnormal hemoglobin concentration, which occurred in 34 % (54 of 159). However, only five of 159 developed a significant anemia less than 10 g percent. The hemoglobin concentration returned to the normal range in all but eight patients by 1 year. Subnormal WBC was observed in about 10 % of these patients, and the lowest value was 2000 per mm^3. No leukopenia persisted beyond 1 year. Thrombocytopenia was seen in only five (3 %) patients, whose levels were only slightly decreased below the normal limits. If it did occur, thrombocytopenia was always transient and returned to normal by 1 year. The degree of suppressed blood counts did appear to correlate with several factors: total ^{131}I dosage, prior radiation therapy, and the presence of widely disseminated metastases. Nevertheless, the authors reported that the suppressed blood count duration was brief and not associated with symptoms. They also reported no incidence of aplastic anemia.

Keldsen et al. [161] reported that 26 % (15 of 27) of their patients' WBC count dropped below 2500 and/or platelet count fell less than 150,000 at some point after treatment. The drop in platelet count was 30 % (305,000–212,000) in females and 17 % (271,000–224,000) in males. The WBC decreased 33 % (6000–4400) in women and increased in men.

In a group of 70 patients treated from 1973 to 1982, Leeper observed no permanent bone marrow suppression [48]. As previously noted, the average single therapeutic dose was 11.4 GBq (309 mCi), with a range of 2.59–24.2 GBq (70–654 mCi). No additional data was reported pertaining to the extent of reversible bone marrow suppression.

Matthias et al. [162] reported on the hematologic toxicity in 68 patients who received cumulative ^{131}I prescribed activities that ranged from 18.5 to 153.5 GBq (500–4150 mCi). Thrombocytopenia occurred in five patients with grade I or II and in three patients with grade III or IV. Grade I comprises anemia of 9.5–10.0 g Hgb/100/mL, thrombocytopenia of 75,000–99,000/mm^3, or leukopenia of 3000–3900 mm^3. Grade II is anemia of 8.0–9.4 g Hgb/100 mL, thrombocytopenia of 50,000–74,000/mm^3, or leukopenia of 2000–2900/mm^3. Grade III is classified as persistent and distinct anemia of less than 7.9 g Hgb/100 mL, thrombocytopenia of less than 49,000/mm^3, or leukopenia below 1900/mm^3. Leukopenia was observed in 14 patients with grade I or II and one patient with grade IV. The specific-grading scale used was not noted.

Menzel et al. [116] evaluated a group of 26 patients with 167 therapies. He reported that only three of 84 therapies with a low-^{131}I prescribed activity of less than 1.8–5.55 GBq (<49–150 mCi) resulted in mild hematological toxicity (leukocytes <3000/nL and/or thrombocytes <75,000/nL). For patients who received high prescribed activities of 11.1 GBq [300 mCi] or higher, 38 % (30 of 78) of therapies caused a mild decline of leukocyte count. Three patients developed World Health Organization (WHO) grade II hematotoxicity. One patient had four therapies totaling 44.4 GBq (1200 mCi); one had two therapies that totaled 22.2 GBq (600 mCi), and one patient developed severe leucopenia and thrombocytopenia (WHO grade III) after three high prescribed activity therapies. Patients in this study were typically treated at 3-month intervals.

Molinaro et al. [163] evaluated 206 consecutive patients who had a complete blood count (CBC) before and after ^{131}I therapy. The median prescribed activity of ^{131}I was 3.7 GBq (100 mCi) with the CBC performed 1 year later. The total white blood cell count dropped from $6.7 \pm 2.1 \times 10^9$ to $6.0 \pm 1.8 \times 10^9$, which was a decrease of 9.7 % ($p<0.001$). The platelet count drop from 272 ± 67 to $250 \pm 655 \times 10^9$, which was a decrease of 5.8 % ($p<0.001$).

Pan et al. [44] evaluated 342 patients over approximately 10 years. Transient platelet reduction was noted in 10.4 %, and transient leukopenia was found in 4 % of patients. The frequency of abnormalities was higher with cumulative ^{131}I prescribed activities greater than 18.5 GBq (500 mCi).

Petrich et al. [164] described the side effects of ^{131}I in the treatment of 107 patients who had bone metastases secondary to well-differentiated thyroid carcinoma. Of 107 patients, 40 (37.4 %) had a change in their blood counts. Most of the changes were WHO grade I or grade II. A total of ten patients had grade III and four patients had bone marrow aplasia.

With prescribed activities of ^{131}I equal to or exceeding 80 % of the dosimetrically determined dosage, Robeson et al. [165] found that 42 % (5 of 12) of patients had mild leukopenia, 17 % (2 of 12) had mild thrombocytopenia, and 25 % (3 of 12) had anemia. Hypocellular bone marrow biopsy was noted in one patient. They reported no difference in the average cumulative prescribed activity in patients with and without bone marrow suppression.

Schober et al. [166] reported on 296 patients who were treated with an average cumulative prescribed activity of 19.8 GBq (535 mCi). The observation period was a median of 65 months. The most frequently observed hematologic change was thrombocytopenia, occurring in 35 % of patients. Erythrocytopenia occurred in 24 %, and the leukocytes decreased in 11 % but increased in 23 %, with a median decrease of 7 %. The most severe decreased counts occurred after a high dose of 37 GBq or more (≥1000 mCi). Pancytopenia was present in 4.4 % of all patients and was probably a contributing cause of death in three patients.

Tollefsen et al. [114] examined the cause of fatalities in 70 patients who had thyroid carcinoma. None of these deaths were attributed to bone marrow suppression. Notably, some of these patients were included in earlier reports from Memorial Sloan Kettering Cancer Center.

Trunnell et al. [103] reported that all patients (nine of nine) treated for metastatic thyroid cancer had depression of one or more peripheral blood elements. The greatest drop occurred in lymphocytes from a level of one third to one fourth of baseline. They reported one fatality from pancytopenia that occurred 1 months after the last treatment, which was 9.25 GBq (250 mCi) and a total prescribed activity of 638 mCi (23.6 GBq). Bone marrow aspiration biopsies were performed in seven patients, demonstrating a uniform drop in total cell count and reversal of the erythroid myeloid ratio. With the exception of the fatality noted above, peripheral blood counts recovered in 4–6 months.

Van Nostrand et al. [40] described nine of ten patients who had bone marrow suppression that was transient and never required any transfusions. The most severe bone marrow suppression was <NCI grade I for hemoglobin, NCI grade II for leukocytes, and NCI grade I for platelets. ^{131}I prescribed activities ranged from 1.9 to 16.7 GBq (51–450 mCi), and the total previous cumulative prescribed activity was 0–25 GBq (0–665 mCi).

Recommendations for Pretherapy and Posttherapy Management

The difficulty with suggesting recommendations for the pre- and posttherapy management of possible bone marrow suppression secondary to ^{131}I therapy is that there are no good studies that have evaluated the efficacy of any specific pre- or posttherapy plan. However, the physician must still act. In the absence of good prospective data, the recommendations must be made upon incomplete retrospective data. Various suggestions have been proposed by different workers in the field, but a discussion of all these approaches is beyond the scope of this chapter. Instead, one proposed set of recommendations is presented below by one author (dvn). These recommendations should be appropriately modified according to the specific clinical situation unique to each patient, the objectives of the physician, the potential clinical benefit versus the risk of irreversible bone marrow suppression, and any new reports in the literature.

General Recommendations for All Patients

Several key methods are proposed for all patients regarding the pretherapy and posttherapy management of potential bone marrow suppression:

1. Obtain baseline complete blood counts (CBC) with differential. If the patient is undergoing thyroid hormone withdrawal, the baseline CBC with differential should be obtained when the patient is in both a euthyroid and hypothyroid state. Because the absolute neutrophil count (ANC) may be reduced in the hypothyroid state [168, 169], a baseline CBC with differentiated obtained under this condition may not be appropriate to use for long-term follow-up. However, an additional baseline CBC with differential when the patient is hypothyroid just before therapy may be useful for the short-term follow-up. This information might help identify any initial decline in blood counts relative to the baseline euthyroid CBC as secondary to the hypothyroidism and not due to ^{131}I.
2. For any reduction of the baseline CBC values, evaluate and correct any other cause for the reduced baseline CBC.
3. If the pretherapy scan demonstrates significant ^{131}I uptake in the bone, lung, and/or other distant metastases, consider dosimetric modification of the prescribed ^{131}I activity.
4. If distant metastases and "high" prescribed activity of ^{131}I is selected, recommend CBC with differential at 3, 4, 5, and 6 weeks after ^{131}I therapy. This is true whether or not the patient was administered an empirically chosen or dosimetrically determined prescribed activity. If the patient has no decrease in any blood counts after therapy, then discontinue CBCs after 5–6 weeks. If the patient has a significant drop in blood counts that may place the patient at risk for infection or bleeding within the first 6 weeks, then continue weekly blood counts until the patient clearly has a rising ANC and rising platelet count and is no longer at risk for infection or bleeding.
5. For significant bone marrow suppression, administer colony-stimulating factor(s) or transfusion as may be clinically warranted. An oncologist should be part of the treating team in determining when the bone marrow suppression is significant.
6. Finally, obtain CBC with differential at 1 year after ^{131}I therapy. Although sequential CBCs with differential after initial ^{131}I therapy will most likely not affect the clinical management of these patients at that time because the counts most likely will not drop significantly enough to require intervention, one author (dvn) believes these are prudent to track. These data, and specifically the amount of suppression, may be important information if a subsequent therapy is considered for the treatment of bone metastases. Sequential CBCs with differential counts obtained after the initial ^{131}I therapy for bone metastases may be the only information regarding the response of the patient's bone marrow to previous therapeutic prescribed activities of ^{131}I. Because of the potential value of this information, and because four to six CBCs are relatively inexpensive and usually associated with minor inconve-

nience, one author (dvn) again recommends that this be obtained in every patient treated for distant metastases.

Specific Recommendations for Selected Patients with Bone Metastases

In selecting the prescribed activity of ^{131}I for a patient with bone metastases and if the patient's CBC and differential counts are abnormal and cannot be corrected, then full or simplified ^{131}I dosimetry is recommended. However, if an empiric prescribed activity of 5.55–7.4 GBq (150–200 mCi) of ^{131}I is to be selected, then reduction of the amount of prescribed activity of ^{131}I should be considered. Unfortunately, no data are available regarding how much the empirically chosen or dosimetrically determined prescribed activity of ^{131}I should be reduced. However, despite the lack of information, the physician must again still make a decision, and one author (dvn) proposes the following guidelines. If the euthyroid baseline CBC is reduced to NCI grade I (see Table 62.18) and the planned prescribed activity of ^{131}I was 5.55–7.4 GBq (150–200 mCi), then consider a reduction of the prescribed activity by 15–20 %. For these patients, one author (dvn) would not recommend an empiric prescribed activity of ^{131}I of 11.1 GBq (300 mCi). If the prescribed activity of ^{131}I is determined by dosimetry, then reduction of that calculated prescribed activity may not be necessary. If the euthyroid baseline CBC is reduced to NCI grade II (see Table 62.18) and the planned prescribed activity was again 5.55–7.4 GBq (150–200 mCi), then consider a reduction of the prescribed activity by 20–30 %. For patients with NCI grade III, the benefits and risk should be discussed among the treating medical team and patients (see Table 62.20). For patients with NCI grade IV, the benefits and risks must again be discussed among the treating medical team and patient

Table 62.20 Recommendations for the evaluation of patients with bone marrow suppression if ^{131}I therapy is being considered

Obtain unilateral or bilateral bone marrow biopsy to assess the bone marrow cellularity and degree of adipose tissue
o Unless the purpose of bone marrow biopsy is to assess a specific area for the presence of metastatic differentiated thyroid carcinoma, bone marrow biopsy should not be obtained from a bone that is su spected to have metastasis or has had previous external radiotherapy
o Fibrosis of the marrow is not a manifestation of delayed radiation injury of the bone marrow
Assess for the presence and extent of bone metastases such as with a combination of radioiodine whole-body scan, radiographic bone survey, magnetic resonance, ^{18}F FDG positron emission tomography scan (^{18}F FDG PET), and/or ^{99m}Tc MDP or ^{18}F NaF PET-CT bone scan
Review the baseline and subsequent CBCs with differential after previous ^{131}I therapies with specific attention to the nadirs and subsequent recovery or reduce recovery to baseline
Review the history for extent of any external radiation therapy to the bone marrow
Review the response to previous ^{131}I therapy, such as change in scan, change in thyroglobulin level, and change in size of masses on clinical exam and/or on other imaging studies
Recommend blood and whole-body dosimetry:
o Do not exceed the prescribed activity calculated by dosimetry
o Do not exceed 4.44 GBq (120 mCi) of ^{131}I whole-body retention at 48 h (In the presence of pulmonary metastases, whole-body retention at 48 h should not exceed 2.96 GBq [80 mCi]. See section on acute radiation pneumonitis and pulmonary fibrosis in this chapter and Chap. 58 on dosimetry)
o If only % 48 h whole-body retention is performed(see Chapter 59), do not exceed 70 % of the maximum tolerated prescribed activity calculated by this method, and follow the other restrictions noted above
If the bone marrow aspiration/biopsy is normal:
o Weigh the potential benefit of ^{131}I therapy vs. other treatments, which will depend on such factors as the degree of radioiodine uptake, size of tumor, patient desires, etc.
o Consider reduction of the prescribed activity below the maximum tolerated dosimetrically determined prescribed activity as discussed in the text
o Consider pretreatment with the appropriate colony-stimulating factor(s)
If bone marrow biopsy is abnormal:
o Weigh the potential benefit of ^{131}I therapy vs. other therapies, which will depend on such factors as the bone marrow cellularity and degree of fat on bone marrow biopsy, degree of radioiodine uptake in the metastases, tumor size, patient desires, and so forth. "Blind treatments" (treatment when no uptake is seen on radioiodine scan) are not encouraged in these patients
o Prophylactic treatment with granulocyte- or platelet-stimulating factor
o Consider stem cell harvest for rescue bone marrow transplantation. No data are available regarding this option
o If possible, avoid treating within 1 year from previous ^{131}I therapy
o Consider amifostine treatment. Amifostine has been proposed to help protect the bone marrow; however, no data is available regarding whether the amifostine also protects thyroid cancer. Amifostine has been discussed elsewhere (see section on "Salivary gland side effects" in this chapter)

(see Table 62.20), and additional hematological support must be strongly considered prior to, during, and after ^{131}I treatment. Of note, no prospective data are available evaluating the utility or safety of these guidelines, but the most important message is consideration of reduction of empirically chosen or dosimetrically determined prescribed activity in patients with reduced CBCs and differentials.

For *subsequent* treatments for metastases in patients whose baseline CBC, ANC, and platelet count have remained normal, the empiric prescribed activity should not exceed 7.4 GBq (200 mCi). If the prescribed activity is based on dosimetry, then one may consider administering as much ^{131}I as one's facility allows up to the dosimetrically determined maximum tolerated activity. If the percent 48-h whole-body retention is calculated (see Chap. 59), then no more than 70 % of the calculated maximum tolerated activity should be administered. A minimum of 6 months and preferably 1 year is recommended between therapies in which the patient received a dosimetrically determined prescribed activity of ^{131}I [170]. At the present time, there is no evidence whether the total cumulative estimated radiation dose to the blood (not the total cumulative ^{131}I prescribed activity) should influence any reduction in dosimetrically determined prescribed activity. For subsequent therapies of metastases in patients who had previous ^{131}I treatments with an uncorrectable abnormal CBC, then again the suggestions in Table 62.20 should be considered.

Summary

Bone marrow suppression is an important untoward effect of ^{131}I therapy. Clinically significant bone marrow suppression as a result of a first ^{131}I therapy is unlikely, especially if ^{131}I therapy is for remnant ablation with prescribed activities of 1.1–1.85 GBq (30–50 mCi). However, the overall data indicate that the frequency and severity of bone marrow suppression increases when (1) the individual prescribed activity of ^{131}I increases, (2) the individual radiation-absorbed dose to the blood exceeds 200 or 300 cGy (rad), (3) the frequency of therapies increases, (4) the interval between therapies decreases, (5) the total cumulative prescribed activity of ^{131}I increases, (6) the total cumulative radiation dose to the blood increases, and (7) bone marrow metastases are more extensive.

Routine CBCs with differential counts prior to and at least 1 year after all ^{131}I remnant ablations, ^{131}I adjuvant treatments are encouraged, with more frequent CBCs with differential counts within the first 3–6 weeks after ^{131}I treatment of distant metastases. The latter may be especially helpful in those patients with distant metastases who may require additional ^{131}I therapies with high prescribed activity. If bone marrow suppression does occur, good follow-up, the availability of colony-stimulating factors, and blood transfusions should be sufficient. Infection and hemorrhage are rare.

Fertility

Gonads

^{131}I therapy irradiates the gonads to a variable extent depending on the relative radiation contributions received from multiple sources such as circulating blood, bladder, gut, and adjacent functioning soft tissue or bone metastases. Such irradiation raises concerns in regard to transient or permanent gonadal damage that could be manifest subsequently as decreased fertility or congenital anomalies in offspring.

Female

Transient ovarian failure following a single ^{131}I therapy (mean dose 9.99 GBq [270 mCi]) occurred during the first year posttherapy in 18 of 66 (27 %) older women (mean age 34 years) with regular menstrual cycles prior to therapy [171]. In this retrospective study, 18 women treated during thyroid hormone withdrawal demonstrated temporary amenorrhea with concomitant "hot flashes" that was delayed for at least one menstrual cycle posttherapy when patients were not euthyroid. The amenorrhea persisted for less than 6 months in 14 of the 18 women. In 23 women with repeatedly measured serum follicle-stimulating hormone (FSH), luteinizing hormone (LH), and serum estradiol (E) values, only the nine amenorrheic women showed elevated serum FSH and LH with low E levels. No significant differences were noted in ^{131}I prescribed activity administered, thyroidal uptake, calculated ovarian doses, or thyroid autoimmunity between the amenorrheic and non-amenorrheic patients. The estimated mean ovarian dose in the amenorrheic women was 176 versus 156 cGy (rad) ($p>0.5$) in the menstruating women, but the amenorrheic group was significantly older (median age 40 vs. 32 years [$p<0.001$]). In another retrospective study, transient ovarian failure occurred in 34 of 409 (8 %) women (median age 31) and lasted for 4–10 month. The amenorrhea developed at 1–3 months post ^{131}I therapy associated with elevated serum FSH and LH levels and was transient in all. The group of women who developed transient ovarian failure was older (mean age 36) than their normal menstruating cohort (mean age 31) [172]. In a prospective study of 50 normally menstruating women (mean age 29.8 years) treated with a single dose of ^{131}I (mean dose 4.2 GBq [114 mCi]), ten (20 %) of the women developed amenorrhea with elevated serum FSH levels that remitted by 1 year [173]. These studies consistently demonstrate that the onset of transient amenorrhea following ^{131}I therapy is typically delayed for one to three menstrual cycles, suggesting that the radiation effect predominates in developing oocytes and not on the maturing follicle. Such ovarian radiation exposure can be reduced by forced hydration for 24–48 h after ^{131}I administration, frequent urination during the day and night, and laxatives to prevent constipation and ^{131}I colonic retention.

A few retrospective controlled studies have evaluated the effect of ^{131}I therapy on the onset of menopause. Ceccarelli et al. [174] studied 257 women (130 patients, 127 controls younger than 45 years) to determine age of onset of menopause in 130 women treated with ^{131}I and suppressive doses of thyroid hormone and 127 control goitrous patients treated with suppressive doses of thyroid hormone only. ^{131}I-treated group (median dose 3.7 GBq [100 mCi]) developed menopause (mean age 49.5 years) earlier than the control group (mean age 51.0 years). In a similar fashion, Rosario et al. [175] studied 114 women (74 patients, 40 controls) and found that the onset of menopause occurred earlier in ^{131}I-treated group than the controls (mean age 46 vs. 50.4 years). The mean radioiodine dose for the 74 patients was 4.8 GBq [130 mCi] with menopause occurring at a younger age in the women treated with >3.7 GBq [100 mCi] (mean age 45) than in those women treated with ≤3.7 GBq (mean age 48). Thus, subclinical persistent ovarian damage induced by radioiodine therapy appears to manifest itself years later in a dose-related fashion by the earlier onset of menopause in treated patients versus controls.

Male

Similarly, transient testicular failure due to germinal cell injury ensues in male patients treated with even a single dose of ^{131}I. Wichers et al. [176] studied 25 men prospectively who were treated with a single or sequential doses of ^{131}I (mean dose 9.8 GBq [270 mCi]) and then followed over 18 months by serum FSH, LH, inhibin B, and free testosterone levels. At 6 months, all men demonstrated elevated serum FSH concentrations and depressed inhibin B levels, the best markers of germinal cell injury, but these values returned to normal by 18 months [176]. In a larger group (52 men, mean age 45 years) treated with a single dose of ^{131}I (mean dose 4.25 GBq [115 mCi]), testicular function was assessed by serum FSH, LH, and testosterone levels at baseline and 6, 12, and 18 months after therapy [177]. At 6 months, serum FSH values were markedly elevated in all patients, but 71 % of patients showed normal values at 12 months, and all patients had returned to basal values by 18 months. The mean serum LH concentration was significantly elevated at 6 months but normalized subsequently with no significant change in free testosterone values at any time interval consistent with compensated Leydig cell function. Employing thermoluminescent dosimetry in 14 patients, the testicular radiation-absorbed dose was shown prospectively to be approximately 2.3 cGy/GBq/testis (0.085 rad/mCi/testis), which should be insufficient to induce infertility with typical single therapies of prescribed activity 2.8–5.55 GBq (75–150 mCi) delivering 6.3–12.6 cGy (rad) [177]. Previously, a threshold prescribed activity of administered ^{131}I of 3.7 GBq (100 mCi) has been suggested since testicular damage manifested as serum FSH elevation was not seen at such prescribed activity [178]. As the mean administered cumulative prescribed activity of ^{131}I increases, there is a corresponding posttherapy rise in mean peak serum FSH values reflecting progressively greater germinal cell damage [139]. At the same time, there was no significant change in mean serum testosterone levels in men grouped by increasing cumulative administered ^{131}I thresholds. Repetitive semen analysis has confirmed a decreased sperm count from baseline in 35.8 % of men (19/53) 2–6 months after ^{131}I therapy that persisted in 36.8 % (7/19) at 1 year [179]. Moreover, studies have shown that each subsequent ^{131}I therapy magnifies the initial germinal cell insult and leads to a gradual persistent elevation of baseline serum FSH levels (measured prior to subsequent ^{131}I therapy). In 22 men with lung metastases treated with mean cumulative ^{131}I dose of 20.3 GBq (548 mCi), serum FSH values were persistently high in 12 of the 22 (54.5 %) men who received a cumulative prescribed activity of ≥13 GBq (≥351 mCi), and oligospermia (on repeated posttherapy sperm analysis) was present in 36.3 % [179]. Similarly, in four patients treated with repetitive doses of 3.7–5.55 GBq (100–150 mCi) for resistant functioning metastatic disease, serum FSH values progressively peaked at higher values and became persistently elevated indicating permanent germinal cell damage.

Infertility

Fertility of the patient and health of subsequent offspring remains a concern, expressed by patients referred for ^{131}I therapy following appropriate surgery for differentiated thyroid cancer. This concern has been addressed in several recent studies. In 1126 women treated surgically for thyroid cancer, a total of 2673 pregnancies had occurred: 2078 pregnancies prior to thyroid cancer therapy, 112 pregnancies following surgery alone, and 483 pregnancies following surgery and ^{131}I therapy [180]. In pregnancies that occurred prior to thyroid cancer therapy, 10.4 % of these pregnancies resulted in miscarriage as compared to 19 % pregnancies after surgery alone and 20.7 % of pregnancies that occurred after surgery and ^{131}I therapy. The incidence of stillbirths, preterm births, and congenital malformations was not different prior to or following ^{131}I therapy. Forty-three percent of the post ^{131}I therapy cohort of patients received ≥3.7 GBq (100 mCi) of ^{131}I for metastatic disease with estimated radiation-absorbed dose to the ovaries of up to 1 Gy (100 rad). Two subsequent reviews including other smaller patient groups confirmed these findings [181, 182]. Similarly, in 224 men treated surgically for thyroid cancer, a total of 493 pregnancies had occurred: 356 pregnancies prior to thyroid cancer therapy, 23 pregnancies following surgery only, and 114 pregnancies following surgery and ^{131}I therapy [183]. Miscarriages occurred in 7.5 % of pregnancies fathered, and this was not statistically different in frequency prior to or following ^{131}I therapy. In those pregnancies conceived after paternal exposure to ^{131}I, the estimated average radiation-absorbed dose to the testis was 9.2 cGy (rad). There was no increase in untoward events in offspring fathered after ^{131}I therapy than prior to ^{131}I therapy. This study was underpowered to determine if there was a decrease in male fertility in those fathers receiving >3.7 GBq (100 mCi) of ^{131}I, who are most likely at risk for decreasing fertility with increasing cumulative ^{131}I exposure. A review of available studies demonstrated that the evidence of permanent germinal cell injury manifested by decreased sperm count and elevated serum FSH levels is common as cumulative doses of ^{131}I exceed 13 GBq (350 mCi), and the majority of men receiving >22 GBq (>593 mCi) show persistent serum FSH levels [184]. There are no prospective studies that compare fertility rates and clinical outcomes in men with thyroid cancer treated with ^{131}I versus men treated surgically only.

When Should a Pregnancy Be Conceived?

Following ^{131}I therapy for differentiated thyroid cancer, when should a pregnancy be conceived? Clinical practice guidelines recommend that prospective parents should wait until their thyroid hormone status is stable and women should delay conception until 6–12 months and men should delay fathering a child for 3–4 months following ^{131}I therapy [185–187]. In males with extensive or resistant thyroid cancer likely to receive cumulative prescribed ^{131}I therapy of >14.8 GBq (400 mCi), family planning should be addressed. The possibility of storage of sperm or fertilized ova should be discussed if future offspring are desired. Reducing testicular radiation exposure from each ^{131}I therapy should be encouraged by optimizing ^{131}I clearance through forced hydration, frequent urination, and prevention of constipation.

Second Primary Malignancies

Second primary malignancies due to radiation therapy for cancer have been a major concern for cancers that have a high survival rate such as differentiated thyroid cancer. Second primary malignancies may include solid cancers or hematologic malignancies such as leukemia. Solid cancers have long latency periods of development, typically in excess of 10 years and often over 20 years, whereas myeloid leukemias secondary to radiation have shorter latency periods [188]. Ionizing radiation is carcinogenic chiefly through its damaging effects on cellular DNA. Experimental data would suggest a “two-step” process with radiation producing DNA breaks causing chromosomal aberrations and genomic instability of the exposed cells, and this can be passed onto many cell divisions [188]. Much later, a second step occurs that usually involves a mutation that may result in the activation of an oncogene or deactivation of a tumor suppressor gene, which in turn may result in the second malignancy. Radiation carcinogenesis is a stochastic effect [188]. This means that there is no threshold radiation-absorbed dose, and the probability of developing a second malignancy depends on the radiation-absorbed dose, either in a linear or linear quadratic relationship, down to zero radiation-absorbed dose. The carcinogenic risk of very low radiation-absorbed dose exposure (<1 cGy [10 mGy]) is controversial, but in general, ^{131}I therapy for thyroid cancer results in radiation-absorbed doses to many tissues and organs that are significant such as in the 10 cGy to 10 Gy range and not considered to be in the very low range [188]. The main beta component of ^{131}I has an energy of 0.6 MeV with a maximum range in tissue of approximate 2.5 mm, and thus through physiological distribution of ^{131}I, the beta component exposes the salivary gland, gastrointestinal tract, and urinary epithelium as well as the bone marrow to significant radiation-absorbed doses [188]. Thus, theoretically, such organs would be at especially high risk for development of ^{131}I treatment-associated second primary malignancies. Furthermore, the gamma component exposure of all bodily tissues could pose additional general carcinogenic risks.

Second Primary Malignancy Risk in Thyroid Cancer Survivors

It is important to consider epidemiologic studies examining second primary malignancy risk in thyroid cancer survivors. It is known that thyroid cancer survivors compared to the general population are at increased risk of developing a second primary malignancy [189]. In a recent meta-analysis based on pooled data from six studies of 70,844 thyroid cancer survivors, the incidence of second primary malignancies in thyroid cancer survivors was increased compared to the general population with an age-standardized incidence ratio of 1.20 (95 % confidence interval [CI] 1.17–1.24) [189]. The risk of the following second primary malignancies was significantly increased in thyroid cancer survivors compared to the general population: salivary gland, stomach, colon/colorectal, breast, prostate, kidney, brain/central nervous system, bone/joints, and adrenal cancer; soft tissue sarcoma; non-Hodgkin's lymphoma; multiple myeloma; and leukemia [189]. Conversely, significantly reduced risks of lung and cervical cancers were observed in thyroid cancer survivors compared to the general population [189]. The observed elevated second primary malignancy risk in thyroid cancer survivors could be explained by a number of factors including genetic predisposition, environmental exposures, surveillance bias, or thyroid cancer therapy (such as ^{131}I therapy or external-beam radiation therapy). In determining whether ^{131}I therapy may be associated with an increased risk of second primary malignancies in thyroid cancer survivors, Brown et al. examined data from the cancer registry records of the Surveillance, Epidemiology, and End Results (SEER) program of the National Cancer Institute in North America

[190]. Brown et al. reported that the risk of second primary malignancies was significantly higher for irradiated thyroid cancer survivors versus nonirradiated patients (relative risk 1.16, 95 % CI 1.05–1.27, $p<0.05$) [190]. In this study, 7.1 % of thyroid cancer survivors developed a second primary malignancy at a median of 8.1 years after their initial thyroid cancer diagnosis [190]. Furthermore, the rate of observed/expected (O/E) second primary cancers was significantly elevated at 1.23 (95 % CI 1.04–1.45) in thyroid cancer survivors treated with ^{131}I compared to thyroid cancer patients not treated with ^{131}I. Of note, this study had a 36-month latency exclusion in order to exclude cancers that may have been unrelated to the therapy [190]. Brown et al. reported that the risk of the following types of second primary malignancies was significantly elevated in ^{131}I-treated patients compared to those who did not receive iodine: second cancers at all sites, all solid tumors, stomach, prostate, lymphatic and hematopoietic diseases, and leukemia [190]. In a European cohort study including data from clinical centers in France, Italy, and Sweden, Rubino et al. [191] reported that the relative risk of second primary malignancy was significantly elevated at 1.2 (95 % CI 1.0–1.4) in patients treated with ^{131}I compared to those not treated with ^{131}I with a 2-year latency exclusion. In the European study, 8.4 % of individuals developed one or more second primary malignancies, and the mean time from diagnosis of thyroid cancer to second primary malignancy was 15 years [191]. Rubino et al. [191] further reported that the risk of the following types of second primary malignancies was significantly elevated in ^{131}I-treated patients compared to those thyroid cancer patients who did not receive ^{131}I: cancer at all sites, salivary glands, bone and soft tissue, uterus, female genital organs, and leukemia. Data from the SEER study [190] and the European cohort study [191] were pooled in a meta-analysis, and the overall relative risk of second primary malignancies in thyroid cancer survivors treated with ^{131}I was found to be significantly elevated at 1.19 (95 % CI 1.04–1.36, $p=0.010$), relative to thyroid cancer survivors not treated with ^{131}I. These data were from 16,502 individuals using a minimum latency period of 2 years after thyroid cancer diagnosis [192]. The pooled risk of leukemia was also significantly increased in thyroid cancer survivors treated with ^{131}I with a relative risk of 2.5 (95 % CI 1.13–5.53, $p=0.024$) [192]. Pooling of data on respective types of malignancies was limited in this meta-analysis due to differences in categorization of some malignancies between SEER and European studies [192]. However, a recent report by Gandhi et al. [193] suggested that no significant risk for second primary malignancy occurs after radioactive iodine treatment in patients with differentiated thyroid cancer.

In summary, the controversy continues, but thyroid cancer survivors appear to have an increased risk of developing second primary malignancies compared to the general population, and thyroid cancer patients treated with ^{131}I appear to have an increased risk of second primary cancer compared to thyroid cancer survivors not exposed to ^{131}I.

Factors That May Modulate Second Primary Malignancy Risk in Patients Treated with ^{131}I

It is important to consider factors that may modulate second primary malignancy risk in thyroid cancer survivors treated with ^{131}I. In considering the impact of cumulative prescribed activity of ^{131}I, Rubino et al. [191] reported that the risk of both solid tumors and leukemia significantly increased in a linear fashion with increasing cumulative prescribed activity. An excess absolute risk of 14.4 solid cancers and 0.8 leukemias per GBq (i.e., 27 mCi) of ^{131}I and 10^5 person-years of follow-up were reported in this study [191]. Furthermore, in a recent study of 1106 thyroid cancer survivors from China, a cumulative ^{131}I prescribed activity of 3.0–8.9 GBq (81–240 mCi) was independently associated with an increased risk of developing a nonsynchronous second primary malignancy (relative risk 2.38, 95 % CI 1.04–5.26, $p=0.040$) [194]. A retrospective study from Iran suggested that the risk of second primary malignancy was dramatically increased after a cumulative prescribed activity of 40 GBq (1081 mCi) [195]; however this study was limited by a very low number of observed second primary malignancies, so it may have been underpowered for meaningful prescribed activity analysis. A recent reanalysis of SEER data suggested that age may modulate the risk of second primary malignancy because individuals younger than 45 years who were treated with ^{131}I were more likely to develop a second cancer compared to older individuals [196]. However, this observation needs further validation. There is some recent evidence that the total body effective half-life and radiation-absorbed dose of ^{131}I in the large intestine, breasts, ovaries, and bone marrow may be lower in individuals pretreated with recombinant human thyrotropin compared to preparation with thyroid hormone withdrawal prior to ^{131}I therapy [197]. Although such data are relevant to consider, it is currently not known whether the preparation with recombinant human thyrotropin rather than preparation with thyroid hormone withdrawal may significantly impact the risk of second primary malignancies after ^{131}I therapy. In summary, there appears to be a relationship between cumulative prescribed activity of ^{131}I and second primary malignancy risk, but there are some conflicting findings in the literature as to an exact threshold at which the risk significantly escalates. More research is needed to validate whether young age is associated with an increased risk of second primary malignancy after ^{131}I therapy. Also, the impact of the preparation using recombinant human thyrotropin prior to ^{131}I therapy on second primary malignancy risk deserves careful study.

The Risk of Dying from a Second Primary Malignancy after ^{131}I Therapy for Thyroid Cancer

Another important consideration is whether or not ^{131}I therapy of thyroid cancer increases the risk of dying of a second primary malignancy. Currently, there is a paucity of studies examining the risk of mortality due to second primary cancer in thyroid cancer survivors, and the available studies have relatively small sample sizes, potentially underpowering their analyses. Edmonds et al. [199] reported that the standardized mortality risk was significantly elevated for leukemia ($p=0.0013$) and bladder cancer ($p=0.024$) in thyroid cancer survivors treated with ^{131}I compared to the general population. This relatively small study was limited by the lack of a thyroid cancer control group that was not treated with ^{131}I. Ishikawa et al. [199] reported that the standardized mortality risk due to second primary malignancies was significantly elevated in thyroid cancer survivors compared to the general population but that the risk did not appear to be attributed to radiotherapy. More recently, Lang et al. [194] reported that the risk of death due to nonsynchronous second primary cancer did not appear to be significantly impacted by cumulative prescribed activity of ^{131}I. To summarize, there is currently insufficient evidence to know whether ^{131}I therapy increases the risk of death due to second primary malignancy, and this is a result of the limited number and size of studies examining this topic.

Summary

In summary, thyroid cancer survivors appear to have an increased risk of developing second primary malignancies compared to the general population. Moreover, thyroid cancer patients treated with ^{131}I may have an increased risk of second primary cancers compared to those not exposed to ^{131}I. The risk of second primary cancer appears to be related to cumulative prescribed activity of ^{131}I. It is important to note that the excess risk of second cancers attributable to ^{131}I is not sufficient to warrant special screening procedures for second cancers, and established age-appropriate cancer screening programs are recommended for all thyroid cancer survivors.

Acknowledgments My deepest thanks go to the many patients who have given generous donation to help underwrite the research studies that have been performed at the MedStar Washington Hospital Center regarding the side effects of ^{131}I therapy.

In addition, my personal gratitude also goes to Kristen L. Blair, RDH (Registered Dental Hygienist), and Janice Falvo, BS, RDH (Registered Dental Hygienist), for not only their input to this chapter regarding the value of a dental hygienist but also for managing some of my post ^{131}I therapy patients.

References

1. Benua RS, Cicale NR, Sonenberg M, Rawson RW. The relation of ^{131}I dosimetry to results and complications in the treatment of metastatic thyroid cancer. Am J Roentgenol Radium Ther Nucl Med. 1962;87:171–82.
2. Alexander C, Bader JB, Schaefer A, et al. Intermediate and long-term side effects of high-dose ^{131}I therapy for thyroid carcinoma. J Nucl Med. 1998;39:1551–4.
3. Chiu AC, Delpass ES, Sherman SI. Prognosis and treatment of brain metastases in thyroid carcinoma. J Clin Endocrinol Metab. 1997;82:3637–42.
4. Holmquest DL, Lake P. Sudden hemorrhage in metastatic thyroid carcinoma of the brain during treatment with iodine-I31. J Nucl Med. 1976;17:307–9.
5. Datz FL. Cerebral edema following iodine-131 therapy for thyroid carcinoma metastatic to the brain. J Nucl Med. 1986;27:637–40.
6. Hurley JR, Becker DV. The use of ^{131}I in the management of thyroid cancer. In: Freeman LM, Weissman HS, editors. Nuclear medicine annual 1983. New York: Raven Press; 1983. p. 329–84.
7. Grayson RR. Factors which influence the radioactive iodine thyroidal uptake test. Am J Med. 1960;24:397–415.
8. Bedikian AY, Valdivieso M, Heilbrun LK, et al. Glycerol: a successful alternative to dexamethasone for patients receiving brain irradiation for metastatic disease. Cancer Treat Rep. 1978;62:1081–3.
9. Murakami H, Kawahara N, Yahata T, et al. Radiation myelopathy after radioactive iodine therapy for spine metastasis. Br J Radiol. 2008;79:e45–9.
10. Yevgeniya SK, Sergiy VK, Caroll NM, Felger E, Links TP, Bonichon F, Preul MC, Sonntag VKH, Van Nostrand D, Burman KD, Boyle LM. Spinal metastases due to thyroid carcinoma: an analysis of 202 patients. Thyroid. 2014;24:1443-55.
11. Spitzweg C, Joba W, Schriever IK, Goellner JR, Morris JC, Heufelder AE. Analysis of human sodium iodide symporter immunoreactivity in human exocrine glands. J Clin Endocrinol Metab. 1999;84:4178–84.
12. Morgenstern KE, Vadysirisack DD, Zhang Z, et al. Express of sodium iodide symporter in the lacrimal drainage system: implication for the mechanism underlying nasolacrimal duct obstruction in ^{131}I treated patients. Ophthalmic Plast Reconstr Surg. 2005;21:337–44.
13. Zettinig G, Hanselmayer G, Fueger B, et al. Long-term impairment of the lacrimal glands after ^{131}I therapy: a cross-sectional study. Eur J Nucl Med. 2002;29:1428–32.
14. Fard-Esfahni A, Mirshekarpour H, Fallahi B, et al. The effect of high-dose radioiodine treatment on lacrimal gland function in patients with differentiated thyroid carcinoma. Clin Nucl Med. 2007;32:696–9.
15. Solans R, Bosch JA, Galofre P, et al. Salivary and lacrimal gland dysfunction (sicca syndrome) after ^{131}I therapy. J Nucl Med. 2001;42:738–43.
16. Koca G, Acar U, Atilgan HI, Acar DE, Altiparmak UE, Demirel K, Yalnizi-Akkay Z, Ustun H, Korkmas M, Ornek F. Changes in conjunctival cytology and tear function tests with radioiodine treatment for hyperthyroidism. Ann Nucl Med. 2013;27:694–9.
17. Bakheet SMB, Hammami MM, Hemidan A, et al. ^{131}I secretion in tears. J Nucl Med. 1998;39:1452–4.

18. Kloos RT, Duvuri V, Jhiang SM, et al. Nasolacrimal drainage system obstruction from radioactive iodine therapy for thyroid carcinoma. J Clin Endocrinol Metab. 2002;87:5817–20.
19. Burns JA, Morgenstern KE, Cahill KV, et al. Nasolacrimal obstruction secondary to I-131 therapy. Ophthal Plast Reconstr Surg. 2004;20:1126–9.
20. Fard-Esfahani A, Farzanefar S, Fallahi B, Beiki D, Saghari M, Emami-Ardekani A, Majdi M, Eftekhari M. Nasolacrimal duct obstruction as a complication of iodine-131 therapy in patients with thyroid cancer. Nucl Med Commun. 2012;33:1077–80.
21. Orquiza M, Khorjekar G, Schneider M, Kulkarni K, Garcia C, Acio E, Burman K, Wartofsky L, Van Nostrand D. Epiphora and xerophthalmia after ^{131}I therapy: the frequency, time of onset, severity, and duration. J Nucl Med. 2014;55:1933 (abstract).
22. Yuoness S, Rachinsky I, Driedger AA, et al. Differentiated thyroid cancer with epiphora: detection of nasolacrimal duct obstruction on I-131 SPECT/CT. Clin Nucl Med. 2011;36:1149–50.
23. Beutel J, Schroder C, von Hof K, Rades D, et al. Pharmacological prevention of radiation-induced dry eye: an experimental study in a rabbit model. Arch Clin Exp Ophthalmol. 2007;245:1347–55.
24. Acar U, Atilgan HI, Acar DE, Yalniz-Akkaya Z, Yumusak N, Korkmaz M, Koca G. The effect of short-term vitamin E against radioiodine-induced early lacrimal gland damage. Ann Nucl Med. 2013;27:886–91.
25. Koca G, Yalniz-Akkaya Z, Gultekin SS, Yumuksak N, Demirel K, Korkmas M, et al. Radioprotective effect of montelukast sodium in rat lacrimal glands after radioiodine treatment. Rev Esp Med Nucl Imagen Mol. 2013;32:294–300.
26. Ramakrishnan VR, Durairaj VD, Kingdom TT. Endoscopic management of acquired nasolacrimal duct obstruction secondary to radioactive radioiodine treatment for thyroid malignancy. J Allergy Ther. 2011;2:2–6.
27. Van Nostrand D. Sialoadenitis secondary to ^{131}I therapy for well-differentiated thyroid cancer. Oral Dis. 2011;17:154–61.
28. Schiff L, Stevens CD, Molle WE, et al. Gastric (and salivary) excretion of ^{131}I in man (preliminary report). J Natl Cancer Inst. 1947;7:349–54.
29. Rice DH. Advances in diagnosis and management of salivary gland diseases. West J Med. 1984;140:238–49.
30. Myant NB. Iodine metabolism of salivary glands. Ann N Y Acad Sci. 1960;85:208.
31. Freinkel N, Ingbar SH. Concentration gradients for inorganic I-131 and chloride in mixed human saliva. J Clin Invest. 1953;32:1077–84.
32. Honour AJ, Myant NB, Rowlands EN. Secretion of ^{131}I in digestive juices and milk in man. Clin Sci. 1952;11:449–62.
33. Jhiang SM, Cho JY, Ryu KY, et al. An immunohistochemical study of Na+/I–symporter in human thyroid tissues and salivary gland tissues. Endocrinology. 1998;139:4416–9.
34. Batsakis JG. Physiology. In: Cummings CW, Schuller DE, editors. Otolaryngology-head and neck surgery, vol. 2. St. Louis: Mosby-Year Book; 1998. p. 1210–22.
35. Donachi I. Biologic effects of radiation on the thyroid. In: Werner SC, Ingbar SH, editors. The thyroid. New York: Harper & Row; 1978. p. 274–83.
36. Goolden AWG, Mallard JR, Farran HEA. Radiation sialitis following ^{131}I therapy. Br J Radiol. 1957;30:210–2.
37. Liu B, Huang R, Kuang A, Zhao Z, Zeng Y, Wang J, Tian R. Iodine kinetics and dosimetry in the salivary glands during repeated courses of radioiodine therapy for thyroid cancer. Med Phys. 2011;38:5412–9.
38. Jentzen W, Hobbs RF, Stahl A, Knust J, Sgouros G, Bockisch A. Pre-therapeutic ^{124}I PET(/CT) dosimetry confirms low average absorbed doses per administered ^{131}I activity to the salivary glands in radioiodine therapy of differentiated thyroid cancer. Eur J Nucl Med Mol Imaging. 2010;37:884–95.
39. La Perle KMD, Kim DC, Hall NC, Bobbey A, Shen DH, Nagy RS, Wakely PE, Lehman A, Jarjoura D, Jhiang SM. Modulation of sodium/iodide symporter expression in the salivary gland. Thyroid. 2001;23:1029–35.
40. Van Nostrand DV, Neutze J, Atkins F. Side effects of "rational dose" iodine-131 therapy for metastatic well differentiated thyroid carcinoma. J Nucl Med. 1986;27:1519–27.
41. Kahn S, Waxman A, Ramanna L, et al. Transient radiation effects following high dose I-131 therapy for differentiated thyroid cancer (DTC). J Nucl Med. 1994;35:15P.
42. Albrecht HH, Creutzig H. Salivary gland scintigraphy after radioiodine therapy. Functional scintigraphy of the salivary gland after high dose ^{131}I therapy. Fortschr Rontgenstr. 1976;125:546–51.
43. Allweiss P, Braunstein GD, Katz A, Waxman A. Sialoadenitis following I-131 therapy for thyroid carcinoma: concise communication. J Nucl Med. 1984;25:755–8.
44. Pan MS. Follow-up study of side effects for iodine-131 treatment in patients with differentiated thyroid cancer. J Nucl Med. 2004;5S:386P.
45. Maier H, Bihl H. Effect of radioactive iodine therapy on parotid gland function. Acta Otolaryngol. 1987;103:318–24.
46. Kharazi P, Van Nostrand D, Khorjekar G, Brennan M, McIver G, Mete M, Bloom G. Characterization of salivary gland side effects secondary to ^{131}I therapy in patients with differentiated thyroid cancer: a national ThyCa: Thyroid Cancer Survivors' Association, Inc. Survey. J Nucl Med. 2011;52S:1759 (abstract).
47. Grewal RK, Larson SM, Pentlow CE, et al. Salivary gland side effects commonly develop several weeks after initial radioactive iodine ablation. J Nucl Med. 2009;50:1605–10.
48. Hall J, Kharazi P, Van Nostrand D, Khorjekar G, Brennan M, McIver B, Mete M, Bloom G. Characterization of salivary gland side effects Up to 7 days after 131I therapy: updated report of the Thyroid Cancer Survivors' Association, Inc. (ThyCa) National Survey. J Nucl Med. 2012;53(Suppl1):306.
49. Leeper R. Controversies in the treatment of thyroid carcinoma: the New York Memorial Hospital approach. Thyroid Today. 1982;4:1–6.
50. Lin WY, Shen YY, Wang SJ. Short-term hazards of low-dose ^{131}I ablation therapy in postsurgical thyroid cancer patients. Clin Nucl Med. 1996;21:780–2.
51. Brown AP, Greening WP, McCready VR, et al. ^{131}I treatment of metastatic thyroid carcinoma: the Royal Marsden hospital experience. Br J Radiol. 1984;57:323–7.
52. Schneyer LH, Tanchester D. Some oral aspects of radioactive iodine therapy for thyroid disease. N Y J Dent. 1954;24:308–9.
53. Mandel S, Mandel L. Persistent sialoadenitis after radioactive iodine therapy: report of two cases. J Oral Maxillofac Surg. 1999;57:738–41.
54. Malpani BL, Samuel AM, Ray S. Quantification of salivary gland function in thyroid cancer patients treated with ^{131}I. Int J Radiat Oncol Biol Phys. 1996;35:535–40.
55. Spiegel W, Reiners C, Borner W. Sialoadenitis following iodine-131 therapy for thyroid carcinoma. J Nucl Med. 1985;26:816.
56. Reiners C, Eichner R, Eilles C, et al. Kamera-funktionsszintigraphie der kopfspeicheldrusen nach hoch-dosierter radiojodtherapie bei schilddrusenkarzinoma patienten. In: Nuklearmedizin, Schmidt HAE, Riccabona G, editors. Stuttgart: Schattauer 1980. p. 477–81.
57. Mandel SJ, Mandel L. Radioactive iodine and the salivary glands. Thyroid. 2003;13:265–71.
58. Laupa MS, Toth BB, Keene HJ. Effect of radioactive iodine therapy on salivary flow rates and oral streptococcus mutants prevalence in patients with thyroid cancer. Oral Surg Oral Med Oral Pathol. 1993;75:312–7.
59. Walters MA, Turtschi CP, Schindler C. The dental safety profile of high-dose radioiodine therapy for thyroid cancer: long-term results of a longitudinal cohort study. J Nucl Med. 2007;48:1620–5.

60. Busnell DL, Boles MA, Kaufman GE, et al. Complications, sequela and dosimetry of iodine-131 therapy for thyroid carcinoma. J Nucl Med. 1992;33:2214–21.
61. Davies AN. The management of xerostomia: a review. Eur J Cancer Care. 1997;6:209–14.
62. Nakada K, Hirata K, Ishibashi T, et al. Cevimeline hydrochloride hydrate in treating salivary gland dysfunction following ^{131}I therapy for thyroid cancer. J Nucl Med. 2004;45S:17P.
63. Ericson T, Lindberg A. Clinical trial of a saliva stimulating tablet SST. Tandjakartidningen. 1982;74:713–6.
64. Blom M, Lunderberg T. Long term follow up of patients treated with acupuncture for xerostomia and the influence of additional treatment. Oral Dis. 2000;6:15–24.
65. Sreebny LM, Schwartz SS. A reference guide to drugs and dry mouth. Gerodontology. 1986;5:75–99.
66. Hochberg MC, Tielsch J, Munoz B, et al. Prevalence of symptoms of dry mouth and their relationship to saliva production in community dwelling elderly; the SEE project. J Rheumatol. 1998;25:486–91.
67. Mandel SJ, Mandel L. False-positive xerostomia following radioactive iodine treatment: case report. Oral Surg Oral Med Oral Pathol Oral Radiol Endod. 2007;103:e43–7.
68. Kulkarni K, Kim SM, Intenzo C. Can salivary gland uptakes on a diagnostic I-131 scan predict acute salivary gland dysfunction in patients receiving ^{131}I therapy for thyroid cancer? J Nucl Med. 2004;5S:291P.
69. Personal communications with Kristen L. Blair, Registered Dental Hygienist (RDH) and Janice Falvo, RDH, BS.
70. Silberstein E. Reducing the incidence of ^{131}I-induced sialadenitis: the role of pilocarpine. J Nucl Med. 2008;49:546–9.
71. Shaw LM, Bonner HS, Schuchter L, et al. Pharmacokinetics of amifostine: effects of dose and method of administration. Semin Oncol. 1999;26:34–6.
72. Werner-Wasik M. Future development of amifostine as a radioprotectant. Semin Oncol. 1999;26:129–1234.
73. Dorr RT, Holmes BC. Dosing considerations with amifostine: a review of the literature and clinical experience. Semin Oncol. 1999;26:108–19.
74. Hall P, Holm LE, Lundell G, Ruden BI. Tumors after radiotherapy for thyroid cancer. Acta Oncol. 1992;31:403–7.
75. Sasse AD, Clark LG, Sasse EC, et al. Amifostine reduced side effects and improves complete response rate during radiotherapy: results of a meta-analysis. Int J Radiat Oncol Biol Phys. 2006;64:784–91.
76. Bohuslavizki KH, Klutmann S, Jenicke L, et al. Salivary gland protection by S-2-(3-amiopropylamino)-ethylphosphorothioic acid (amifostine) in high-dose ^{131}I treatment: results obtained in a rabbit animal model and in a double blind multi-arm trial. Cancer Biother Radiopharm. 1999;13:337–47.
77. Kim SJ, Choi HY, Kim IJ, et al. Limited cytoprotective effects of amifostine in high-dose radioactive iodine ^{131}I-treated well-differentiated thyroid cancer patients: analysis of quantitative salivary scan. Thyroid. 2008;18:325–31.
78. Schuchter L, Meropol NJ, Winer EP, et al. Amifostine and chemoradiation therapy: ASCO responds. Lancet Oncol. 2003;4:593.
79. Levy HA, Park CH. Effect of reserpine on salivary gland ^{131}I uptake in thyroid cancer. Clin Nucl Med. 1987;12:303–7.
80. Bhartiya US, Raut YS, Joseph LJ, Hawaldar RW, Rao BS. Evaluation of the radioprotective effect of turmeric extract and vitamin E in mice exposed to therapeutic dose of radioiodine. Indian J Clin Biochem. 2008;23:382–6.
81. Leban JJ, Bhartiya U, Raut YS, et al. Radioprotective effect of Ocimum sanctum and amifostine on the salivary gland of rats after therapeutic radioiodine exposure. Cancer Biother Radiopharm. 2011;26:737–43.
82. Koca G, Gültekin SS, Han Ü, Kuru S, Demirel K, Korkmaz M. The efficacy of montelukast as a protective agent against 131I-induced salivary gland damage in rats: scintigraphic and histopathological findings. Nucl Med Commun. 2013;34:507–17.
83. Noaparast Z, Hosseinimehr J. Radioprotective agents for the prevention of side effects induced by radioiodine-131 therapy. Futur Oncol. 2013;9:1145–59.
84. Kim HW, Ahn BY, Lee SW, Lee J. Effect of parotid gland massage on parotid gland Tc-99m pertechnetate uptake. Thyroid. 2012;22:611–6.
85. Freitas JE, Gross MD, Ripley S, Shapiro B. Radionuclide diagnosis and therapy of thyroid cancer; current status report. Semin Nucl Med. 1985;15:106–31.
86. Nakada K, Ishibashi T, Takei K, et al. Does lemon candy decrease salivary gland damage following ^{131}I therapy for thyroid cancer? J Nucl Med. 2005;46:261–6.
87. Liu B, Kuang A, Huang R, et al. Influence of vitamin C on salivary absorbed dose of ^{131}I in thyroid cancer patients; a prospective, randomized, single-blind, controlled trial. J Nucl Med. 2010;51:618–23.
88. Jentzen W, Balschuweit D, Schmitz J, et al. The influence of salivary flow stimulation on the absorbed radiation dose to the salivary glands during radioiodine therapy of thyroid cancer using ^{124}I PET/CT imaging. Eur J Nucl Med Mol Imaging. 2010;37:2298–306.
89. Van Nostrand D, Bandaru V, Chennupati V, Kulkarni K, Wexler J, Atkins F, Mete M, Gadwale G. Radiopharmacokinetics of radioiodine in the parotid glands after the administration of lemon juice. Thyroid. 2010;20:1113–9.
90. Kulkarni K, Van Nostrand D, Atkins F, Mete M, Wexler J, Wartofsky L. Does lemon juice increase radioiodine reaccumulation within the parotid glands more than if lemon juice is not administered? Nucl Med Commun. 2014;35:210–6.
91. Nahlieli O, Nazarian Y. Sialadenitis following radioiodine therapy—a new diagnostic and treatment modality. Oral Dis. 2006;12:476–9.
92. Bomeli ST, Schaitkin B, Carrau RL, et al. Interventional sialendoscopy for treatment of radioiodine-induced sialadenitis. Laryngoscope. 2009;119:864–7.
93. Varma VM, Dai WL, Henkin RI. Taste dysfunction in patients with thyroid cancer following treat with I-131. J Nucl Med. 1992;33:996.
94. Orquiza M, Khorjekar G, Schneider M, Kulkarni K, Garcia C, Acio E, Burman K, Wartofsky L, Van Nostrand D. Altered and/or loss of taste after 131I therapy: the frequency, time of onset, severity, and duration. J Nucl Med. 2014;55:1933.
95. Norby EH, Neutze JH, Van Nostrand D, et al. Nasal radioactive iodine uptake: a prospective study of frequency, intensity and pattern. J Nucl Med. 1990;31:52–4.
96. Levenson D, Coulec S, Sonnenberg M, et al. Peripheral facial nerve palsy after high-dose ^{131}I therapy in patients with papillary thyroid carcinoma. Ann Intern Med. 1994;120:576–8.
97. Burmeister LA, du Cret RP, Mariash CN. Local reaction to ^{131}I in the treatment of thyroid cancer. Am J Med. 1991;90:217–22.
98. Cherk MH, Yap KV, Topliss BM, et al. Acute radiation thyroiditis that sometimes occurs with post-thyroidectomy remnant ablation is directly related to thyroidal ^{131}I uptake and not to the amount of ^{131}I used for ablation. Clin Thyroidology. 2009;21:24–6.
99. Goolden AWG, Kam KC, Fitzpatrick ML, Munro AJ. Oedema of the neck after ablation of the thyroid with radioactive iodine. Br J Radiol. 1986;59:583–6.
100. Cooper DS, Ridgway EC, Maloof F. Unusual types of hyperthyroidism. Clin Endocrinol Metab. 1978;7:199–220.
101. Smith R, Blum C, Benua RS, Fawwaz R. Radioactive iodine treatment of metastatic thyroid carcinoma with clinical thyrotoxicosis. Clin Nucl Med. 1985;10:874–5.

102. Ikejiri K, Furuyama M, Muranaka T, et al. Carcinoma of the thyroid manifested as hyperthyroidism caused by functional bone metastasis. Clin Nucl Med. 1997;22:227–30.
103. Trunnell JB, Marinelli LD, Duffy Jr BJ, et al. The treatment of metastatic thyroid cancer with radioactive iodine: credits and debits. J Clin Endocrinol. 1949;9:1138–52.
104. Cerletty JM, Listwan WJ. Hyperthyroidism due to functioning metastatic thyroid carcinoma. Precipitation of thyroid storm with therapeutic radioactive iodine. JAMA. 1979;242:269–70.
105. Winslow CP, Meyers AD. Hypocalcemia as a complication of ^{131}I therapy. Am J Otolaryngol. 1998;19:401–3.
106. Glazebrook GA. Effect of decicurie prescribed activity of radioactive I-131 on parathyroid function. Am J Surg. 1987;154:368–73.
107. Zhu R, Yu Y, Lu H. Clinical study of 312 cases with metastatic differentiated thyroid cancer treated with large doses of ^{131}I. Chin Med J. 2005;118:425–8.
108. Cunha DDS, Izilda MI, Simões P, et al. Carotid artery rupture following radioiodine therapy for differentiated thyroid carcinoma. Arq Bras Endocrinol Metab. 2011;55:419–25.
109. Lee TC, Harbert JC, Dejter SW, et al. Vocal cord paralysis following I-131 ablation of a postthyroidectomy remnant. J Nucl Med. 1985;26:49–50.
110. Pochin EE. ^{131}I treatment of thyroid cancer. In: Hahn PF, editor. Therapeutic use of artificial radioisotopes. New York: Wiley; 1956. p. 195.
111. Fajardo L-GLF, Berthrong M, Anderson RE, editors. Radiation pathology. Oxford: University Press; 2001.
112. Gomez D, Rosenzweig KE. Lung. In: Shrieve DC, Loeffler JS, editors. Human radiation injury. Philadelphia: Wolters Kluwer; 2011. p. 306–15.
113. Rall JE, Alpers JB, Lewallen CG, et al. Radiation pneumonitis and fibrosis: a complication of ^{131}I treatment of pulmonary metastases from cancer of the thyroid. J Clin Endocrinol Metab. 1957;17:1263–76.
114. Tollefsen HR, DeCosse JJ, Hutter RVP. Papillary carcinoma of the thyroid. A clinical and pathological study of 70 fatal cases. Cancer. 1964;17:1035–43.
115. Aldrich LB, Sisson JC, Grum CM. Pulmonary function in thyroid carcinoma metastatic to the lung. J Endocrinol Invest. 1987;10:111–6.
116. Menzel C, Grunwald F, Schomburg A, et al. "High-dose" ^{131}I therapy in advanced differentiated thyroid carcinoma. J Nucl Med. 1996;37:1496–503.
117. Bennett DE, Million RR, Ackerman LV. Bilateral radiation pneumonitis. A complication of the radiotherapy of bronchogenic carcinoma. Cancer. 1969;23:1001–18.
118. Fulkerson WJ, McLendon RE, Prosnitz LR. Adult respiratory distress syndrome after limited radiotherapy. Cancer. 1986;57:1941–6.
119. Monson JM, Stark P, Reily JJ, et al. Clinical radiation pneumonitis and radiographic changes after thoracic radiation therapy for lung carcinoma. Cancer. 1998;82:842–50.
120. Morgan GW, Pharm B, Breit SN. Radiation and the lung. Int J Radiat Oncol Biol Phys. 1995;31:361–9.
121. Delanian S, Porcher R, Rudant J, et al. Kinetics of response to long-term treatments combining pentoxifylline, and tocopherol in patients with superficial radiation-induced fibrosis. J Clin Oncol. 2005;23:8570–9.
122. Choi NC, Kanarek DJ, Kazemi H. Physiologic changes in pulmonary function after thoracic radiotherapy for patients with lung cancer and role of regional pulmonary function studies predicting postradio-therapy pulmonary function before radiotherapy. Cancer Treat Symp. 1985;2:119–30.
123. Mah K, Van Dyk J, Keane T, Poon PY. Acute radiation-induced pulmonary damage: a clinical study on the response to fractionated radiation therapy. Int J Radiat Oncol Biol Phys. 1987;13:179–88.
124. Smith JC. Radiation pneumonitis. A review. Am Rev Respir Dis. 1963;87:647–65.
125. Carmel RJ, Kaplan HS. Mantle irradiation for Hodgkin's disease. An analysis of technique, tumor eradication and complications. Cancer. 1976;37:2813–25.
126. Fryer CJH, Fitzpatrick PJ, Rider WD, et al. Radiation pneumonitis: experience following a large single dose of radiation. Int J Radiat Oncol Biol Phys. 1978;4:931–6.
127. McDonald S, Rubin P, Philips TL, Marks LB. Injury to the lung from cancer therapy: clinical syndromes, measurable endpoints, and potential scoring systems. Int J Radiat Oncol Biol Phys. 1995;31:1187–203.
128. Fowler JF, Travis EL. The radiation pneumonitis syndrome in half-body radiation therapy. Int J Radiat Oncol Biol Phys. 1978;4:1111–3.
129. Keane T, Van Dyk J, Rider WD. Idiopathic interstitial pneumonia following bone marrow transplantation. The relationship with total body irradiation. Int J Radiat Oncol Biol Phys. 1981;7:1365–70.
130. Gross NJ. Pulmonary effects of radiation therapy. Ann Intern Med. 1977;86:81–92.
131. Samaan NA, Schultz PN, Haynie TP, Ordonez NG. Pulmonary metastasis of differentiated thyroid carcinoma: treatment results in 101 patients. J Clin Endocrinol Metab. 1985;60:376–80.
132. Gopal R, Tucker SI, Komaki R, et al. The relationship between local dose and loss of function for irradiated lung. Int J Radiat Oncol Biol Phys. 2003;56:106–13.
133. Wilner J, Jost A, Baier K, et al. A little to a lot or a lot to a little? An analysis of pneumonitis risk from dose-volume histogram parameter. Strahlenther Onkol. 2003;179:548–56.
134. Emami B, Lyman J, Brown A, Coia L, Goitein M, Munzenrider JE, Shank B, Solin LJ, Wesson M. Tolerance of normal tissue to therapeutic irradiation. Int J Radiat Oncol Biol Phys. 1991;21:109–22.
135. Burman C, Kutcher GJ, Emami B, Goitein M. Fitting of normal tissue tolerance data to an analytic function. Int J Radiat Oncol Biol Phys. 1991;21:123–35.
136. Graham MV, Purdy JA, Emami B, Harms W, Bosch W, Lockett MA, Perez CA. Clinical dose-volume histogram analysis for pneumonitis after 3D treatment for non-small cell lung cancer. J Radiat Oncol Biol Phys. 1999;45:323–9.
137. Samuel AM, Unnikrishnan TP, Baghel NS, Rajashekharrao B. Effect of ^{131}I therapy on pulmonary alveolar-capillary membrane integrity. J Nucl Med. 1995;36:783–7.
138. Schlumberger M, Arcangioli O, Piekarski JD, et al. Detection of and treatment of lung metastases of differentiated thyroid carcinoma in patients with normal chest x-rays. J Nucl Med. 1988;29:1790–4.
139. Pacini F, Gasperi M, Fugazzola L, et al. Testicular function in patients with differentiated thyroid carcinoma treated with ^{131}I. J Nucl Med. 1994;35:1418–22.
140. Maheshwari YK, Strattton Hill C, Haynie TP, et al. Iodine-131 therapy in differentiated thyroid carcinoma: M.D. Anderson Hospital experience. Cancer. 1981;47:664–71.
141. Goffman T, Loff V, Tuttle M, et al. Near-lethal respiratory failure after recombinant human thyroid-stimulation hormone use in a patient with metastatic thyroid carcinoma. Thyroid. 2003;13:827–30.
142. Hindiè E, Melliere D, Lange F, et al. Functioning pulmonary metastases of thyroid cancer: does ^{131}I influence the prognosis? J Nucl Med. 2003;30:974–81.
143. Hughes JM, Lockwood DN, Jones HA, et al. DLCO/Q and diffusion limitation at rest and on exercise in patients with interstitial fibrosis. Respir Physiol. 1991;83:155–66.
144. Khan JH, McElhinney DB, Rahman SB, et al. Pulmonary metastases of endocrine origin: the role of surgery. Chest. 1998;114:526–34.

145. Liu D, Labow D, Dang N, et al. Pulmonary metastasectomy for head and neck cancers. Ann Surg Oncol. 1999;6:572–8.
146. Nemec J, Zamrazil V, Pohunkova D, Roohling S. Radioiodide treatment of pulmonary metastases of differentiated thyroid cancer; results and prognostic factors. Nuklearmedizin. 1979;18:86–90.
147. Massin JP, Savoie JC, Garnier H, et al. Pulmonary metastases in differentiated thyroid carcinoma: study of 58 cases with implications for the primary tumor treatment. Cancer. 1984;53:982–92.
148. Esposito G, Van Nostrand D, Atkins F, Burman K, Wartofsky L, Kulkarni K. Frequency of "over" and "under" treatment with empiric dosage of I-131 in patients with and without lung metastasis secondary to well-differentiated thyroid cancer. J Nucl Med. 2006;47(1):238P. abstract.
149. Tuttle RM, Leboeuf R, Robbins RJ, Qualey R, Pentlow K, Larson SM, Chan CY. Empiric radioactive iodine dosing regimens frequently exceed maximum tolerated activity levels in elderly patients with thyroid cancer. J Nucl Med. 2006;47:1587–91.
150. Kulkarni K, Van Nostrand D, Atkins F, Aiken M, Burman K, Wartofsky L. The relative frequency in which empiric dosages of radioiodine would potentially overtreat or undertreat patients who have metastatic well-differentiated thyroid cancer. Thyroid. 2006;16:1019–23.
151. Khorjekar G, Van Nostrand D, Vetter R, Ringel M, Carter E, Bloom G. The frequency of vomiting after outpatient I-131 therapy in patients with well-differentiated thyroid cancer. J Nucl Med. 2010;51S:1580. abstract.
152. Khorjekar G, Van Nostrand D, Vetter R, Ringel M, Carter E, Bloom G. The relationship of several factors and vomiting after outpatient I-131 treatment in pts with well-differentiated thyroid cancer. J Nucl Med. 2010;51S:1570. abstract.
153. Quimby ES, Feitelberg S, Laughlin JS, et al. NCRP report 37: precautions in the management of patients who have received therapeutic amounts of radionuclides. Washington, DC: National Council on Radiation Protection; 1970.
154. US Nuclear Regulatory Commission. Criteria for release of individuals administered radioactive materials. Fed Regist. 1997;62:4120.
155. Kinuya S, Hwang E, Ikeda E, et al. Mallory-Weiss Syndrome caused by iodine-131 therapy for metastatic thyroid carcinoma. J Nucl Med. 1997;38:1831–2.
156. Balan KK, Raouf AH, Critchley M. Outcome of 249 patients attending a nuclear medicine department with well-differentiated thyroid cancer; a 23 year review. Br J Radiol. 1994;67:283–91.
157. Dobyns BM, Maloof F. The study and treatment of 119 cases of carcinoma of the thyroid with radioactive iodine. J Clin Endocrinol. 1951;11:1323–60.
158. Dorn R, Kopp J, Vogt H, et al. Dosimetry-guided radioactive iodine treatment in patients with metastatic differentiated thyroid cancer: largest safe dose using a risk—adapted approach. J Nucl Med. 2003;44:451–6.
159. Grunwald F, Schomburg A, Menzel C, et al. Blood count changes after ^{131}I treatment in thyroid carcinoma. Med Klin. 1994;89:522–8.
160. Haynie T, Beierwaltes W. Hematologic changes observed following therapy for thyroid carcinoma. J Nucl Med. 1963;4:85–91.
161. Keldsen N, Mortensen BT, Hansen HS. Bone marrow depression due to I-131 treatment of thyroid cancer. Ugeskr Laeger. 1988;50:2817–9.
162. Matthies A, Bender H, Distelmaier M, et al. Efficacy and side effects of high dose iodine-131 therapy in metastatic thyroid carcinoma. Eur J Nucl Med. 2004;45S:189P.
163. Molinaro E, Leboeuf R, Shue B, et al. Mild decreases in white blood cell and platelet counts are present one year after radioactive iodine remnant ablation. Thyroid. 2009;19:1035–41.
164. Petrich T, Widjaja A, Musholt TJ, et al. Outcome after ^{131}I therapy in 107 patients with differentiated thyroid carcinoma and initial bone metastases: side effects and influence of age. Eur J Nucl Med. 2001;28:203–8.
165. Robeson WR, Ellwood JE, Margulies P, Margouleff D. Outcome and toxicity associated with maximum safe dose ^{131}I treatment of metastatic thyroid cancer. Clin Nucl Med. 2002;27:556–666.
166. Schober O, Gunter HH, Schwarzrock R, Hundeshagen H. Hamatologische langzeitveranderungen bei der Radiojodtherapie des Schilddrusenkarzinoms. Strahlenther Onkol. 1987;163:464–74.
167. Schumichen C, Schmitt E, Scheuffele C. Influence of the therapy concept onto the prognosis of thyroid carcinoma. Nuklearmedizin. 1983;22:97–105.
168. Kuhn JM, Rieu M, Wolf LM, et al. Hematologic repercussions of disorders of thyroid secretion. Presse Med. 1984;13:421–5.
169. Donate RM, Gallagher NI. Hematologic alteration associated with endocrine disease. MedClin N Am. 1968;52:231–41.
170. Leeper 1980. Personal communication.
171. Raymond JP, Izembart M, Marliac V, et al. Temporary ovarian failure in thyroid cancer patients after thyroid remnant ablation with radioactive iodine. J Clin Endocrinol Metab. 1989;69:186–90.
172. Vini L, Hyer S, Al-Saadi A, et al. Prognosis for fertility and ovarian function after treatment with ^{131}I for thyroid cancer. Postgrad Med J. 2002;78:92–3.
173. Souza Rosario PW, Alvarenga Fagundes T, Villa-Boas Fagundes AS, et al. Ovarian function after ^{131}I therapy in patients with thyroid cancer. Exp Clin Endocrinol Diabetes. 2005;113:331–3.
174. Ceccarelli C, Bencivelli W, Morciano D, et al. I-131 therapy for differentiated thyroid cancer leads to an earlier onset of menopause; results of a retrospective study. J Clin Endocrinol Metab. 2001;86:3512–5.
175. Rosario PW, Fagundes TA, Fagundes AV, et al. ^{131}I therapy and age at menopause in patients with thyroid cancer. Clin Endocrinol (Oxf). 2006;64:225–6.
176. Wichers M, Benz E, Palmedo H, et al. Testicular function after ^{131}I therapy for thyroid carcinoma. Eur J Nucl Med. 2000;27:503–7.
177. Hyer S, Vini L, O'Connell M, et al. Testicular dose and fertility in mean following I-131 therapy for thyroid can. Clin Endocrinol. 2002;56:755–8.
178. Handelsman DJ, Turtle JR. Testicular damage after radioactive iodine therapy for thyroid cancer. Clin Endocrinol. 1983;18:465–72.
179. Rosario PW, Barroso AL, Rezende LL, et al. Testicular function after ^{131}I therapy in patients with thyroid cancer. Thyroid. 2006;16:667–70.
180. Esfahani AF, Eftekhari M, Zenooz N, et al. Gonadal function in patients with differentiated thyroid cancer treated with I-131. Hell J Nucl Med. 2004;7:52–5.
181. Garsi J-P, Schlumberger M, Rubino C, et al. Therapeutic administration of I-131 for differentiated thyroid cancer: radiation dose to ovaries and outcome of pregnancies. J Nucl Med. 2008;49:845–52.
182. Sawka AM, Lakra DC, Lea J, et al. A systematic review examining the effects of therapeutic radioactive iodine on ovarian function and future pregnancies in female cancer survivors. Clin Endocrinol. 2008;69:479–90.
183. Sioka C, Fotopoulos A. Effects of I-131 therapy on gonads and pregnancy outcome in patients with thyroid cancer. Fertil Steril. 2011;95:1552–9.
184. Garsi J-P, Schlumberger M, Ricard M, et al. Health outcomes of children fathered by patients treated with ^{131}I for thyroid cancer. Clin Endocrinol. 2009;71:880–3.
185. Sawka AM, Lea J, Alshehri B, et al. A systematic review of the gonadal effects of therapeutic radioactive iodine in male thyroid cancer survivors. Clin Endocrinol. 2008;68:610–7.
186. Cooper DS, Doherty GM, Haugen BR, et al. Revised American Thyroid Association management guidelines for patients with

thyroid nodules and differentiated thyroid cancer. Thyroid. 2009;19:1167–214.

187. Sisson JC, Freitas J, McDougall IR, et al. Radiation safety in the treatment of patients with thyroid diseases by ^{131}I I-131: practice recommendations of the American Thyroid Association. Thyroid. 2011;21:335–46.

188. Hall EJ, Giaccia AJ. Radiobiology for the radiologist. 6th ed. Philadelphia: Lippincott William & Wilkins; 2006.

189. Subramanian S, Goldstein DP, Parlea L, et al. Second primary malignancy risk in thyroid cancer survivors: a systematic review and meta-analysis. Thyroid. 2007;17:1277–88.

190. Brown AP, Chen J, Hitchcock YJ, Szabo A, Shrieve DC, Tward JD. The risk of second primary malignancies up to three decades after the treatment of differentiated thyroid cancer. J Clin Endocrinol Metab. 2008;93:504–15.

191. Rubino C, de Vathaire F, Dottorini ME, et al. Second primary malignancies in thyroid cancer patients. Br J Cancer. 2003;89:1638–44.

192. Sawka AM, Thabane L, Parlea L, et al. Second primary malignancy risk after ^{131}I treatment for thyroid cancer: a systematic review and meta-analysis. Thyroid. 2009;19:451–7.

193. Gandhi S, Abhyankar A, Basu S. Dual malignancies in the setting of differentiated thyroid carcinoma: their synchronous or metachronous nature, impact of radioiodine treatment on occurrence of second malignancy and other associated variables. Nucl Med Commun. 2014;35:205–9.

194. Lang BH, Wong KP. Risk factors for nonsynchronous second primary malignancy and related death in patients with differentiated thyroid carcinoma. Ann Surg Oncol. 2011;18:3559–65.

195. Fallahi B, Adabi K, Majidi M, et al. Incidence of second primary malignancies during a long-term surveillance of patients with differentiated thyroid carcinoma in relation to ^{131}I treatment. Clin Nucl Med. 2011;36:277–82.

196. Iyer NG, Morris LG, Tuttle RM, Shaha AR, Ganly I. Rising incidence of second cancers in patients with low-risk (T1N0) thyroid cancer who receive 131I therapy. Cancer. 2011;117:4439–46.

197. Taïeb D, Sebag F, Farman-Ara B, et al. Iodine biokinetics and ^{131}I exposure after recombinant human thyrotropin-assisted remnant ablation in comparison with thyroid hormone withdrawal. J Clin Endocrinol Metab. 2010;95:3283–90.

198. Edmonds CJ, Smith T. The long-term hazards of the treatment of thyroid cancer with ^{131}I. Br J Radiol. 1986;59(697):45–51.

199. Ishikawa K, Noguchi S, Tanaka K, Fukuda A, Hirohata T. Second primary neoplasms in thyroid cancer patients. Jpn J Cancer Res. 1996;87:232–9.

200. Kita T, Yokoyama K, Higuchi T, Kinuya S, Taki J, Nakajima K, Michigishi T, Tonami N. Multifactorial analysis on the short-term side effects occurring within 96 hours after radioiodine-131 for differentiated thyroid carcinoma. Ann Nucl Med. 2004;18:345–9.

201. Leeper RD. The effect of I-131 therapy on survival of patients with metastatic papillary or follicular thyroid carcinoma. J Clin Endocrinol Metab. 1973;36:1143–52.

External Radiation Therapy for Papillary Carcinoma

63

James D. Brierley and Richard W. Tsang

Introduction

The role of external beam radiotherapy (RT) in the management of papillary thyroid cancer can be subdivided into adjuvant, radical, and palliative. The intent of adjuvant therapy is to improve the results of standard therapy consisting of surgery and radioactive iodine; however, the exact role of RT is controversial. Unlike radioactive iodine, external beam radiotherapy is a local therapy; therefore, its role is confined to situations where treatment is required to maximize locoregional control of the disease, beyond what can be achieved with optimal surgery and radioactive iodine alone. Its role is generally limited to patients deemed to have a high risk of locoregional recurrence, e.g., older patients with extensive extrathyroidal extension (ETE) of disease, residual disease following surgery, or extensive lymphatic spread.

Radical External Beam Radiotherapy (RT) for Gross Disease

For patients with residual tumor following attempted surgical resection, ^{131}I is unlikely to eradicate such disease unless a high absorbed dose of radiation is achieved. O'Connell et al. [1] suggested that an absorbed dose of 100 Gy is required to destroy small remnants of tumor, while Maxon et al. [2] have shown that a single radioiodine administration resulting in an absorbed dose of greater than 80 Gy achieved destruction of neck nodes in only 74 % of patients with small-volume disease of less than 2 g. Therefore, in the presence of gross residual disease following excision, ^{131}I therapy is likely to be insufficient to achieve local control of the tumor.

The effectiveness of external beam radiation in controlling gross residual papillary cancer has been known at least since 1966 when Sheline et al. [3] reported their experience of external radiotherapy in 58 patients treated between 1935 and 1964. Although the radiation given would not now be considered adequate in many cases, they reported a good response rate for patients with palpable disease with a complete response (CR) rate of 78 %. Chow et al. [4] reported their experience with 124 patients with gross residual locoregional disease after surgery for papillary thyroid cancer. Patients were stratified by whether they also received RT after surgery. Those patients who received radiation had a significantly greater locoregional control rate at 5 years (67 % vs. 38 % $p=0.001$). Other studies have reported a similar result with approximately 40 % complete CR of gross disease after RT [5, 6] and local control rates of about 60 % at 5 years [7, 8]. There have been other retrospective series that reported good local control of gross disease with RT [4, 9, 10]. Our own most recent data from Princess Margaret Hospital [11] showed that the 10-year Cause Specific Survival (CSS) and Local Recurrence Free Period (LRFR) were 48 % and 90 % for patients with postoperative gross residual disease treated with radiation therapy. The CSS of only 48 % reveals that although radiation therapy can achieve local control, distant metastatic disease remains a major problem and is the cause of death in the majority of patients with ETE. Most of these studies including our own did not separate the results of treatment of follicular and papillary tumors although it can be assumed that the majority of patients had papillary thyroid cancer.

These reports suggest that long-term control is possible in patients with thyroid cancer in whom there is gross residual disease after attempted resection or if no resection is possible. This does not mean to say that all attempts to resect gross disease should not be made but situations still exist where surgery is not possible. These include invasion of prevertebral fascia or carotid artery and situations in which resection

J.D. Brierley, MBBS, FRCP, FRCR, FRCPC (✉)
R.W. Tsang, MD, FRCP(C)
Department of Radiation Oncology, University of Toronto, Princess Margaret Hospital,
610 University Ave, Toronto, ON M5G 2M9, Canada
e-mail: james.brierley@rmp.uhn.on.ca; Richard.tsang@rmp.uhn.on.ca

L. Wartofsky, D. Van Nostrand (eds.), *Thyroid Cancer*, DOI 10.1007/978-1-4939-3314-3_63

would result in loss of function, for instance, if laryngectomy is required. Also, if the patient is elderly or has a poor performance status and extensive surgery is not deemed appropriate or possible, leaving gross residual disease may be appropriate, to be followed by RT. Such scenarios resulting in gross disease after resection should be followed by ^{131}I and radical external RT and may result in long-term local control.

External Beam Radiotherapy as Adjuvant Therapy

One of the reasons that the adjuvant role of external RT remains uncertain and controversial is that studies reporting on its use are all retrospective and have included many patients who either have not been adequately treated with standard therapy (total/near total thyroidectomy and radioactive iodine) and also patients who may not be expected to benefit from external RT because they are not at high risk from local recurrence. Hence, it is important to identify patients who are at high risk of local recurrence and therefore may benefit from adjuvant radiation in addition to radioactive iodine. The prognostic factors for differentiated thyroid cancer are well known and have been described in detail earlier, but both extrathyroidal extension and age are major factors in predicting risk of recurrence. Mazzaferri and Jhiang [12] reported that 8 % of a series of 1,355 patients with differentiated thyroid cancer (of whom 1,077 had papillary cancer) had extrathyroidal extension. The local recurrence rate was 38 % in patients with extrathyroidal extension compared to 25 % in patients without extrathyroidal extension ($p=0.001$). Similarly, these patients were at higher risk of death from their cancer (20 % compared to 9 % if there was no extrathyroid extension, $p=0.001$). Further evidence that these patients are at high risk can be appreciated from the series of patients reported by Vassilopoulou-Selin et al. who studied 65 patients with recurrent papillary thyroid cancer, all of whom had had prior surgery and radioactive iodine [13]. Patients with recurrences in lymph nodes were far more likely to respond to further radioactive iodine and far less likely to die from their disease. In contrast, the patients who recurred in the thyroid bed most (14 out of 15 patients) failed to take up radioactive iodine. That this deleterious effect is more marked in older patients was demonstrated in a study from Memorial Sloan Kettering Cancer Center, showing a 30-year disease-free survival for patients without ETE of 87 %, but only 29 % with ETE ($p<0.0001$). This negative effect of ETE on outcome was only seen in patients over the age of 45 [14].

It may be concluded that especially older patients with extrathyroidal extension such as shown in Fig. 63.1 are at higher risk of local recurrence and are more likely to die from their disease. This is the group of patients that may benefit from intensifying their locoregional therapy with the addition of external beam RT to surgery and radioactive iodine to reduce the risk of recurrence in the thyroid bed.

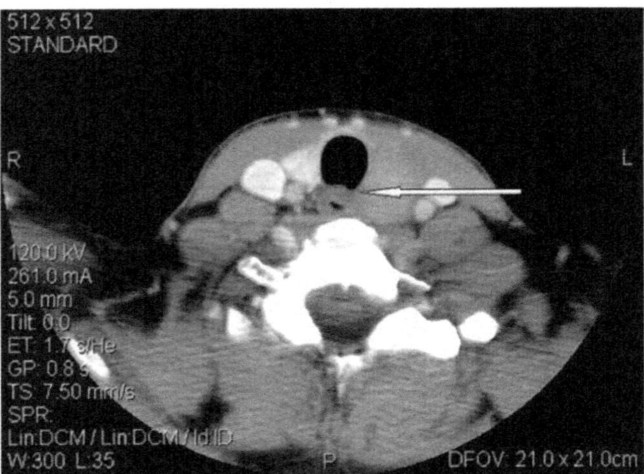

Fig. 63.1 A CT scan slice showing extrathyroid extension and invasion into tracheoesophageal groove (arrow). The scan is from a 64-year-old woman who presented with an asymptomatic 3 cm mass in the left lobe of the thyroid. Fiber-optic laryngoscopy was normal; FNA was consistent with papillary thyroid cancer. At surgery there was gross extrathyroid extension into strap muscles, the tracheoesophageal groove, and recurrent laryngeal nerve. Tumor was resected off the recurrent laryngeal nerve. There was no evidence of gross residual disease. Bilateral paratracheal nodes were resected. The final pathology confirmed a 4 cm papillary thyroid carcinoma with extrathyroid extension, positive surgical margin, and two nodes that contained metastatic tumor. Radioactive iodine was given; the post-therapy scan demonstrated minimal uptake in the thyroid bed with a TSH of 147 and a thyroglobulin of 5.7. External beam radiation: 50 Gy in 20 fractions was given to the thyroid bed

In an analysis from Princess Margaret Hospital, it was shown that in patients with papillary histology and microscopic residual disease after surgical resection, defined as tumor at or within 2 mm from the resection margin, those who received additional adjuvant external RT to the neck benefited from this treatment with an increased CSS and LRFR [7]. This analysis has been updated with a longer follow-up period. There were 154 patients, 90 of whom received RT, and 64 did not. The CSS was 100 % at 10 years in patients given RT compared to 95.3 % if RT was not prescribed ($p=0.01$); similarly the LRFR was greater in patients given RT (94.2 %) compared to those who did not receive RT (83.9 %, $p=0.02$) [15]. For those 60 years of age or less, there was a benefit in local relapse-free rate but not survival (CSS 98.2 % no RT vs. 100 % RT $p=0.09$, LRFR 85.4 % no RT vs. 95.9 % RT, $p=0.03$) (Fig. 63.2).

A different analysis was also performed in patients with papillary or follicular carcinoma. A subgroup was identified which was considered to be at high risk of relapse in the thyroid bed. These were older patients over the age of 60 years with extrathyroid extension and no gross residual disease. Seventy patients were identified who fell into this

Fig. 63.2 Effect of the use of external beam radiotherapy on cause-specific survival and local relapse-free rate in patients with papillary thyroid cancer and microscopic residual disease defined as tumor at or within 2 mm of the resection margin [15]

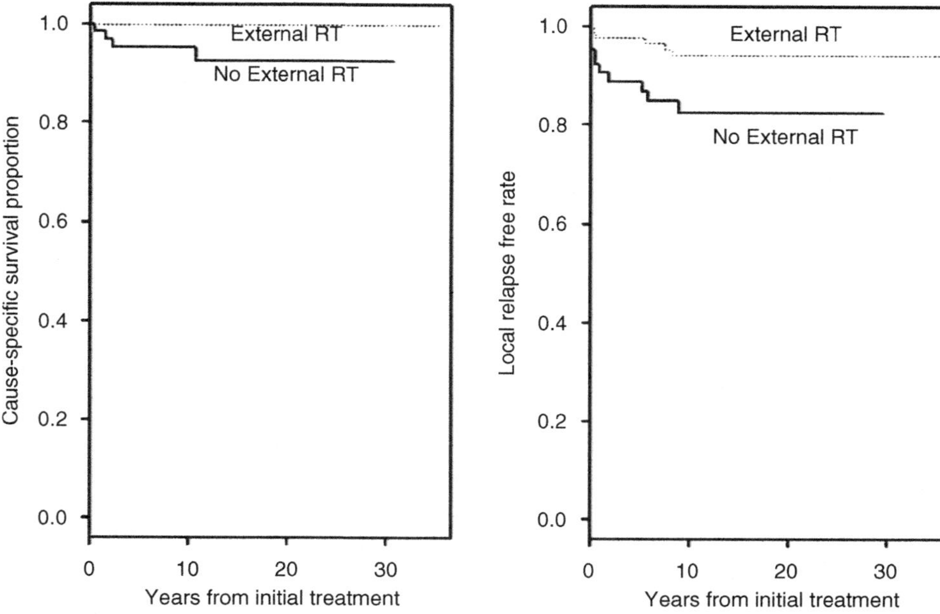

high-risk group: 47 received RT and 23 did not. There was a higher CSS (81.0 % and 64.6 % $p=0.04$) and LRFR (86.4 % and 65.7 % $p=0.01$) in patients who received RT [15].

These data suggest that external beam radiation improves both local control and survival in patients at high risk of recurrence in the thyroid bed. Unfortunately, like all studies of the role of external RT, these data have limitations as they are retrospective and unknown selection factors may produce bias in how patients were chosen for external beam radiation, which may have influenced the results. In addition, although these patients were considered to be at high risk, not all received what would now be considered standard therapy with total thyroidectomy and radioactive iodine, especially those in the earlier time period of the study.

The most convincing data in support of the adjuvant use of external radiation comes from Essen in Germany [16]. They reported an increased freedom from locoregional and distant failure in patients over the age of 40 with differentiated thyroid cancer and extrathyroidal extension and lymph node involvement, when treated with adjuvant RT. All patients had standard therapy of total thyroidectomy, ^{131}I, and TSH suppression in addition to RT. RT was a predictive factor for improvement in regard to time to locoregional recurrence ($p=0.004$) and time to distant failure ($p=0.0003$). This benefit was only seen in papillary thyroid cancer ($p=0.0001$) but not follicular thyroid cancer ($p=0.38$). Other retrospective studies (Table 63.2) have suggested a role for adjuvant external beam radiation and have led both the American (ATA) [17] and British (BTA) [18] Thyroid Associations to recommend external radiation in selected cases (Table 63.1).

These recommendations are based on retrospective series. The only way to prove a role of external radiation

Table 63.1 American Thyroid Association Guideline and British Thyroid Association Guideline on the use of external beam radiotherapy in differentiated thyroid cancer

American Thyroid Association Guideline [17]
The use of external beam irradiation to treat the primary tumor should be considered in patients over age 45 with grossly visible extrathyroidal extension at the time of surgery and a high likelihood of microscopic residual disease and for those patients with gross residual tumor in whom further surgery or RAI would likely be ineffective. The sequence of external beam irradiation and RAI therapy depends on the volume of gross residual disease and the likelihood of the tumor being RAI responsive
British Thyroid Association Guideline [18]
Gross evidence of local tumor invasion at surgery, presumed to have significant macro- or microscopic residual disease, particularly if the residual tumor fails to concentrate sufficient amounts of radioiodine. Extensive pT4 disease in patients over 60 years of age with extensive extranodal spread after optimal surgery, even in the absence of evident residual disease

would be from a randomized controlled study. Unfortunately, attempts in North America to perform such a study have been unsuccessful. A European study based in Germany was started but closed because of poor accrual [19]. Although conceived as a randomized study, only 47 patients out of a potential 311 patients consented to randomization and therefore the study changed to a prospective cohort study. Twenty-six of the randomized patients received radiation. In the radiation arm, there were no recurrences. In the nonirradiated cohort only 3 % recurred. There was one serious complication from radiation, and the study concluded that routine radiotherapy in locally invasive DTC cannot be recommended. Patients had to be only older than 18 to be included and have local extension beyond the thyroid cap-

Table 63.2 Results of adjuvant external radiotherapy in high-risk disease papillary thyroid cancer from retrospective studies: 10-year local recurrence

	Surgery with and without ^{131}I	Surgery, RT with and without ^{131}I
Esik [33]	80 %[a]	37 %[a]
Farahati [16]	56 %[b]	10 %[b]
Ford [34]	63 %[a]	18 %[a]
Keum	89 %	36 %
Kim [35][c]	37.5 %	4.8 %
Phlips [36]	21 %	3 %
Schwartz [21][d]	None reported	21 %
Simpson [9]	18 %	14 %
Terezakis [20][d]	None reported	25 %
Tsang [7]	22 %	7 %
Tubiana [8]	21 %	14 %

[a]Compares low dose vs. higher dose
[b]Local and distant failures
[c]5-year locoregional relapse rate
[d]4-year locoregional relapse rate

sule (pT3 and pT4). Of the patients who received radiation, 15 had tumors less than 1 cm and the mean age was only 47. Therefore, a significant number of patients would not have met the criteria for external radiation as recommended by the ATA and BTA. The study does not provide any convincing evidence to refute the potential benefit of external beam RT in high-risk patients. Therefore, currently at Princess Margaret Hospital, we recommend external beam RT in patients older than 50 who have gross extrathyroid extension at the time of resection (i.e., cT4) with presumed microscopic disease (i.e., gross tumor "shaved" off the larynx). There is nothing absolute about the age, as prognosis does not change dramatically at age 45 or 50 [12], and older patients may have a similar therapeutic gain from adjuvant RT with less extensive extrathyroid extension compared to younger patients with extensive extrathyroid extension. Moreover, patients less than age 45 but with T4b disease may benefit from external radiation.

Three large radiation centers have recently reported their experience with external radiation in patients with high-risk locally advanced thyroid cancers. As external radiation was standard for these patients at these centers, comparisons with nonirradiated patients were not made. The Memorial Sloan Kettering group reported a 4-year locoregional control of 72 % in 76 patients considered to be at high risk of cervical relapse (this included medullary thyroid cancer as well as papillary and follicular thyroid cancer) [20]. The 4-year overall locoregional control rate for all histologies was 72 %, and the 4-year overall survival rate was 55 %. Of the non-MTC patients, 16 (25 %) had a local failure, with more local failures in the tall cell variant cancers than in the other histologies. The MD Anderson group have reported on 131 patients with DTC, of whom 126 (96 %) had ETE [21]. Sixty-two patients (47 %) had microscopically positive surgical margins and 15 patients (11 %) had gross residual disease. The locoregional relapse-free rate was 79 % at 4 years. They concluded that external beam RT provided durable locoregional disease control in patients with high-risk DTC. The Christie Hospital, UK, reported on 19 patients with unresectable or gross residual disease and 24 patients who had microscopic residual disease [22]. The 5-year locoregional control rate for patients with macroscopic residual or inoperable disease was 69 % and 89 % for clear or macroscopically positive margins. They reported a 91 % cause-specific survival (CSS) with negative or microscopic residual disease.

Once it is decided to recommend external radiation, another controversy arises. Should all of the cervical nodes be included in the treated volume, or should only the thyroid bed and adjacent soft tissues be irradiated? The advantage of irradiating only the thyroid bed is that the volume irradiated is smaller and the side effects consequently less, especially in regard to the salivary glands which may already have reduced function following radioactive iodine. The study reported by Farahati et al. discussed above had included the cervical nodes and also included cervical node involvement as a criterion for recommending external beam radiotherapy [16]. As the majority of patients with nodal disease can be adequately treated with surgery and radioactive iodine alone, it has not been our practice to include large nodal volumes [12]. In contrast, in a study of 23 patients reported by Kim et al., there was a 55 % risk of locoregional relapse (6 out of 11 patients) treated with limited volume compared to only 8 % (1 out of 12) if an extended volume was treated [23]. In the study described above from the Christie Hospital, a high risk of failure was reported if the upper mediastinum was not treated [22]. Because these larger volumes come at the cost of higher toxicity, it is important that the volume at risk of relapse is carefully considered and cervical irradiation reserved for patients with extensive nodal involvement including gross extranodal extension and local invasion. It is also considered in patients who have relapsed in cervical nodes despite previous nodal resection and high-dose radioactive iodine who are thought to have disease that is resistant to radioactive iodine. In younger patients, RT is usually considered after their second cervical or superior mediastinal lymph node recurrence.

External Beam Radiotherapy

The thyroid bed is a technically challenging volume to treat as the thyroid bed curves around the vertebral body and includes the air column in the trachea. It can be difficult to adequately treat the thyroid bed and spare the spinal cord to

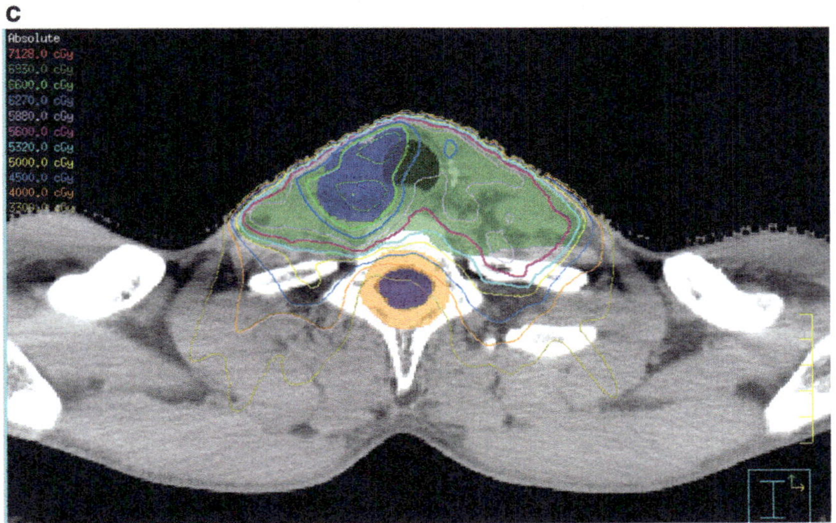

Fig. 63.3 (**a–c**) A sagittal (**a**), coronal (**b**), and axial (**c**) view of IMRT plan for a patient with papillary thyroid cancer who had significant extrathyroid extension in the tracheoesophageal grove with residual microscopic disease. The plan allows for a high dose of 66 Gy to be given to the region of greatest concern in the tracheoesophageal grove and a lower dose of 56 Gy in 33 fractions to be given to the adjacent thyroid bed and nodal region. The volume irradiated conforms to the U shape of the clinical target volume ensuring minimum radiation exposure to the normal organs such as the spinal cord. The shaded area in *green* is the volume considered at moderate risk of relapse and is prescribed 56 Gy. The crimson line is the 56 Gy isodose line, so that all the tissue within this line receives a minimum of 56 Gy. The shaded area in *blue* is at high risk and is prescribed 66 Gy. The *light green* line is the 66 Gy isodose so that all the tissue within this line receives a minimum dose of 66 Gy; other isodose lines are also included

a dose within tolerance. A variety of techniques have been described that produce adequate dose distribution [24]. Advances in radiation techniques utilizing inversed planned intensity-modulated radiation therapy (IMRT) result in better dose distribution to the areas at risk and reduce the volume of irradiated normal tissues to a minimum as described elsewhere in the book (Fig. 63.3). Well-planned external beam RT has acceptable acute toxicity and rarely produces serious complications. In patients assigned to the radiation arm of the German randomized control study in differentiated thyroid cancer that closed because of poor accrual, it was noted that the majority of patients experienced mild to moderate acute side effects only from adjuvant external beam RT [25]. At the first follow-up examination, most side effects had subsided and acute toxicity was tolerable in these patients. Late toxicity is infrequent; the most common adverse effects include skin telangiectasia, increased skin pigmentation, soft tissue fibrosis, and mild lymphedema predominantly in the submental area. Esophageal and especially tracheal stenoses are rare. Neither Tsang et al. [7] nor Farahati et al. [16] reported any RTOG grade IV late toxicity in differentiated thyroid cancer. In contrast, a more recent study using higher doses of radiation and larger volumes reported that 5 % of their patients required a percutaneous endoscopic gastrostomy tube for late esophageal stenosis [20]. It should be noted however that acute toxicity may be significant when utilizing concurrent chemoradiation and some centers recommend prophylactic enteral nutrition.

External Beam Radiotherapy for Metastases

The effectiveness of ^{131}I on metastatic disease depends greatly on the site of the metastasis. It is well known that lung metastases generally respond well to radioactive iodine. In a series of patients with distant metastases, Casara et al. reported that those over the age of 40 or with bone metastases were much less likely to concentrate radioactive iodine [26]. Only 3 % of bone metastases were considered to have achieved a complete response following radioactive iodine. Similar poor control of bone metastases has been reported by others [27–29], and therefore an aggressive surgical approach to these lesions has been recommended [29, 30]. Not all bone metastases are amenable to surgical resection, and therefore external beam radiation to a high dose such as 50 Gy in 25 fractions and radioactive iodine are appropriate and may result in long-term control [31]. External beam radiation also has an important role in palliating symptomatic bone metastases and spinal cord compression.

Brain metastases from papillary thyroid cancer are unusual. In a study of metastases to the brain of all thyroid cancer histologies (32 were differentiated), surgical resection resulted in improved survival but there was no benefit from external beam radiation. In another series, external beam radiation resulted in complete response in three out of four patients with measurable disease [32]. External beam radiotherapy should probably be offered if surgical resection is not possible, but it is uncertain if it has any additional benefit when prior complete excision of brain metastases has been performed. Single large lung metastases causing hemoptysis or bronchial obstruction may also respond to RT.

The role of RT in controlling gross residual disease after surgery and in unresectable disease was discussed above. In patients with symptomatic recurrent disease with poor performance status or widespread incurable disease in whom high-dose RT for long-term control is not thought appropriate, shorter course RT may be effective in controlling local symptoms such as pain, skin ulceration, and obstruction.

References

1. O'Connell M, Flower MA, Hinton PJ, Harmer CL, McCready VR. Radiation dose assessment in radioiodine therapy. Dose-response relationships in differentiated thyroid carcinoma using quantitative scanning and PET. Radiother Oncol. 1993;28:16–26.
2. Maxon HR, Englaro EE, Thomas SR, et al. Radioiodine-131 therapy for well-differentiated thyroid cancer – a quantitative radiation dosimetric approach: outcome and validation in 85 patients [see comments]. J Nucl Med. 1992;33:1132–6.
3. Sheline GE, Galante M, Lindsay S. Radiation therapy in the control of persistent thyroid cancer. Am J Roentgenol Radium Ther Nucl Med. 1966;97:923–30.
4. Chow S-M, Law SCK, Mendenhall WM, et al. Papillary thyroid carcinoma: prognostic factors and the role of radioiodine and external radiotherapy. Int J Radiat Oncol Biol Phys. 2002;52:784–95.
5. Glanzmann C, Lutolf UM. Long-term follow-up of 92 patients with locally advanced follicular or papillary thyroid cancer after combined treatment. Strahlenther Onkol. 1992;168:260–9.
6. O'Connell M, RP AH, Harmer CL. Results of external beam radiotherapy in differentiated thyroid carcinoma: a retrospective study from the Royal Marsden Hospital. Eur J Cancer. 1994;30A:733–9.
7. Tsang RW, Brierley JD, Simpson WJ, Panzarella T, Gospodarowicz MK, Sutcliffe SB. The effects of surgery, radioiodine and external radiation therapy on the clinical outcome of patients with differentiated thyroid cancer. Cancer. 1998;82:375–88.
8. Tubiana M, Haddad E, Schlumberger M, Hill C, Rougier P, Sarrazin D. External radiotherapy in thyroid cancers. Cancer. 1985;55:2062–71.
9. Simpson WJ, Panzarella T, Carruthers JS, Gospodarowicz MK, Sutcliffe SB. Papillary and follicular thyroid cancer: impact of treatment in 1578 patients. Int J Radiat Oncol Biol Phys. 1988;14:1063–75.
10. Wu LT, Averbuch SD, Ball DW, de Bustros A, Baylin SB, McGuire 3rd WP. Treatment of advanced medullary thyroid carcinoma with a combination of cyclophosphamide, vincristine, and dacarbazine. Cancer. 1994;73:432–6.
11. Sia MA, Tsang RW, Panzarella T, Brierley JD. Differentiated thyroid cancer with extrathyroidal extension: prognosis and the role of external beam radiotherapy. J Thyroid Res. 2010;2010:183461.
12. Mazzaferri EL, Jhiang SM. Long-term impact of initial surgical and medical therapy on papillary and follicular thyroid cancer. Am J Med. 1994;97:418–28.
13. Vassilopoulou-Sellin R, Schultz PN, Haynie TP. Clinical outcome of patients with papillary thyroid carcinoma who have recurrence after initial radioactive iodine therapy. Cancer. 1996;78:493–501.
14. Coburn MC, Wanebo HJ. Age correlates with increased frequency of high risk factors in elderly patients with thyroid cancer. Am J Surg. 1995;170:471–5.
15. Brierley JD, Tsang RW, Panzarella T. et al. Prognostic factors and the effect of treatment with radioactive iodine and external beam radiation on patients with differentiated thyroid cancer seen at a single institution over forty years. Clin Endocrinol (Oxf). 2005;63:418–27.
16. Farahati J, Reiners C, Stuschke M, et al. Differentiated thyroid cancer. Impact of adjuvant external radiotherapy in patients with perithyroidal tumor infiltration (stage pT4). Cancer. 1996;77:172–80.
17. Cooper DS, Doherty GM, Haugen BR, et al. Revised American Thyroid Association management guidelines for patients with thyroid nodules and differentiated thyroid cancer. Thyroid. 2009;19:1167–214.
18. British Thyroid Association. Guidelines for the management of thyroid cancer in adults. London: Royal College of Physicians; 2006. p. 1–70.

19. Biermann M, Pixberg M, Riemann B, et al. Clinical outcomes of adjuvant external-beam radiotherapy for differentiated thyroid cancer – results after 874 patient-years of follow-up in the MSDS-trial. Nuklearmedizin. 2009;48:89–98; quiz N15.
20. Terezakis SA, Lee KS, Ghossein RA, et al. Role of external beam radiotherapy in patients with advanced or recurrent nonanaplastic thyroid cancer: Memorial Sloan-kettering Cancer Center experience. Int J Radiat Oncol Biol Phys. 2009;73:795–801.
21. Schwartz DL, Lobo MJ, Ang KK, et al. Postoperative external beam radiotherapy for differentiated thyroid cancer: outcomes and morbidity with conformal treatment. Int J Radiat Oncol Biol Phys. 2009;74:1083–91.
22. Azrif M, Slevin NJ, Sykes AJ, Swindell R, Yap BK. Patterns of relapse following radiotherapy for differentiated thyroid cancer: implication for target volume delineation. Radiother Oncol. 2008;89:105–13.
23. Kim TH, Chung KW, Lee YJ, et al. The effect of external beam radiotherapy volume on locoregional control in patients with locoregionally advanced or recurrent nonanaplastic thyroid cancer. Radiat Oncol. 2010;5:69.
24. Tsang RW, Brierley JD. The thyroid. In: Cox JD, Kian Ang K, editors. Radiation oncology. St Louis: Mosby; 2003.
25. Schuck A, Biermann M, Pixberg MK, et al. Acute toxicity of adjuvant radiotherapy in locally advanced differentiated thyroid carcinoma. First results of the multicenter study differentiated thyroid carcinoma (MSDS). Strahlenther Onkol. 2003;179:832–9.
26. Casara D, Rubello D, Saladini G, Gallo V, Masarotto G, Busnardo B. Distant metastases in differentiated thyroid cancer: long-term results of radioiodine treatment and statistical analysis of prognostic factors in 214 patients. Tumori. 1991;77:432–6.
27. Brown AP, Greening WP, McCready VR, Shaw HJ, Harmer CL. Radioiodine treatment of metastatic thyroid carcinoma: the Royal Marsden Hospital experience. Br J Radiol. 1984;57:323–7.
28. Schlumberger M, Challeton C, De Vathaire F, et al. Radioactive iodine treatment and external radiotherapy for lung and bone metastases from thyroid carcinoma. J Nucl Med. 1996;37:598–605.
29. Proye CA, Dromer DH, Carnaille BM, et al. Is it still worthwhile to treat bone metastases from differentiated thyroid carcinoma with radioactive iodine? World J Surg. 1992;16:640–5; discussion 645–646.
30. Niederle B, Roka R, Schemper M, Fritsch A, Weissel M, Ramach W. Surgical treatment of distant metastases in differentiated thyroid cancer: indication and results. Surgery. 1986;100:1088–97.
31. Brierley JD, Tsang RW. External-beam radiation therapy in the treatment of differentiated thyroid cancer. Semin Surg Oncol. 1999;16:42–9.
32. Chiu AC, Delpassand ES, Sherman SI. Prognosis and treatment of brain metastases in thyroid carcinoma. J Clin Endocrinol Metab. 1997;82:3637–42.
33. Esik O, Nemeth G, Eller J. Prophylactic external irradiation in differentiated thyroid cancer: a retrospective study over a 30-year observation period. Oncology. 1994;51:372–9.
34. Ford D, Giridharan S, McConkey C, et al. External beam radiotherapy in the management of differentiated thyroid cancer. Clin Oncol (R Coll Radiol). 2003;15:337–41.
35. Kim TH, Yang DS, Jung KY, Kim CY, Choi MS. Value of external irradiation for locally advanced papillary thyroid cancer. Int J Radiat Oncol Biol Phys. 2003;55:1006–12.
36. Phlips P, Hanzen C, Andry G, Van Houtte P, Fruuling J. Postoperative irradiation for thyroid cancer. Eur J Surg Oncol. 1993;19:399–404.

Chemotherapy of Thyroid Cancer: General Principles

64

David A. Liebner, Sigurdis Haraldsdottir, and Manisha H. Shah

Introduction

Chemotherapy has been used as a single-modality treatment or as part of combined-modality therapy in metastatic or locally advanced thyroid cancer when other conventional treatments (e.g., surgery and radiation therapy) have failed. Recent developments in the understanding of the molecular pathogenesis of thyroid cancer have allowed for more targeted investigations, but cytotoxic chemotherapy remains an important part of the armamentarium, particularly for anaplastic and relatively undifferentiated thyroid cancers. Numerous reports on the use of chemotherapy in a variety of thyroid cancers have been published, but only a few controlled clinical trials compare the efficacy of different drug regimens. We outline both conventional cytotoxic chemotherapeutic agents and novel targeted agents below.

D.A. Liebner, MD
Division of Medical Oncology, Department of Internal Medicine, The Ohio State University, Columbus, OH USA

Department of Biomedical Informatics, The Ohio State University, Columbus, OH USA
e-mail: david.liebner@osumc.edu

S. Haraldsdottir, MD
Division of Medical Oncology, Department of Internal Medicine, The Ohio State University Comprehensive Cancer Center, Columbus, OH USA
e-mail: sigurdis.haraldsdottir@osumc.edu

M.H. Shah, MD (✉)
Division of Medical Oncology, Department of Internal Medicine, The James Cancer Hospital and Solove Research Institute, 320 West 10th Avenue, A438 Starling Loving Hall, Columbus, OH 43210, USA
e-mail: Manisha.Shah@osume.edu

Cytotoxic Chemotherapy

Prior to the early 1970s, experience with individual chemotherapeutic agents in thyroid cancer was largely limited to case reports without systematic evaluation of efficacy in clinical trials [1]. Individual cytotoxic chemotherapeutic agents with known (or proposed) antitumor activity against thyroid cancer are listed in Table 64.1. Patient nutritional status and performance statuses have been noted as important predictors of response to these agents [2, 3]. Selected agents are discussed below.

Bleomycin

Bleomycin is an antineoplastic antibiotic that impairs DNA synthesis by generating superoxide and hydroxyl radicals that cause single- and double-stranded DNA breaks. It was the first chemotherapeutic agent reported effective in thyroid cancer [4, 5]. However, due to limited activity as monotherapy with associated risk of pulmonary toxicity, subsequent study focused primarily on combination regimens. A retrospective study of doxorubicin, bleomycin, and vincristine (ABC) in thyroid cancer reported responses in 5 of 13 patients (38 %) [6], and a phase II study of ABC-melphalan reported short-term responses in 4 of 11 patients (37 %) [7]. A retrospective study of bleomycin, doxorubicin, and cis-platinum (BAP) in 21 patients noted responses in 9 patients (42 %); the best responses were seen in individuals with medullary thyroid cancer (MTC) or anaplastic thyroid cancer (ATC) [8].

Doxorubicin

Doxorubicin is an anthracycline derivative that has been the most widely used and studied cytotoxic chemotherapeutic agent in thyroid cancer. On the basis of observational experience and initial results from phase I and II studies [1, 9],

L. Wartofsky, D. Van Nostrand (eds.), *Thyroid Cancer*, DOI 10.1007/978-1-4939-3314-3_64

Table 64.1 Cytotoxic chemotherapeutic agents

Drug	Class	Toxicities
Doxorubicin	Anthracycline	Cardiotoxicity, mucositis
Epirubicin	Anthracycline	Cardiotoxicity, myelosuppression
Mitoxantrone	Anthracenedione, DNA intercalator	Myelosuppression, risk of cardiotoxicity
Bleomycin	Antitumor antibiotic	Pulmonary toxicity
Cisplatin	Heavy metal, DNA cross-linking	Nephrotoxicity
Carboplatinum	Heavy metal, DNA cross-linking	Myelosuppression
Etoposide	Topoisomerase II inhibitor	Myelosuppression
Topotecan	Topoisomerase I inhibitor	Myelosuppression, mucositis
Irinotecan	Topoisomerase I inhibitor	Myelosuppression, diarrhea
Dacarbazine	Alkylating-like agent	Myelosuppression, gastrointestinal toxicity
Cyclophosphamide	Alkylating agent	Myelosuppression, hemorrhagic cystitis
Paclitaxel	Taxane	Myelosuppression, peripheral neuropathy
Vincristine	Vinca alkaloid	Peripheral neuropathy
Methotrexate	Antimetabolite	Gastrointestinal toxicity, hepatotoxicity
Capecitabine	Oral fluoropyrimidine	Hand-foot syndrome, diarrhea
Gemcitabine	Antimetabolite	Myelosuppression

further investigation of doxorubicin monotherapy was pursued. Gottlieb and Hill enrolled patients with all histologic subtypes of thyroid cancer and reported that 11 of 30 patients treated with 45–75 mg/m^2 doxorubicin every 3 weeks had greater than 50 % reductions in the size of their metastases [10]. Responses appeared to be best in patients with pulmonary metastases followed by bone metastases, and several patients with bone metastases reported subjective improvements in bone pain with treatment. Subsequent studies of doxorubicin monotherapy were undertaken, and a summary of these early studies suggested a response rate of 38.5 % in patients with differentiated thyroid cancer (DTC) ($n=109$) and 41 % in patients with Hürthle cell carcinoma ($n=41$) [11]. However, these studies were not placebo controlled and had varying inclusion criteria and definitions of response, which limited extrapolation. A more recent retrospective study of 22 patients with progressive, metastatic, unresectable DTC or medullary thyroid cancer (MTC) treated with either doxorubicin 60 mg/m^2 every 3 weeks for 3–6 cycles or 15 mg/m^2 weekly for 8–16 cycles documented WHO partial responses (PR) in 5 % of patients and stable disease in 42 % (median 7 months) [12]. A comparison of the two dosing regimens in DTC suggested better responses with 60 mg/m^2 every 3 weeks compared to 15 mg/m^2 weekly (PR: 11 % vs. 0 %, SD: 67 % vs. 20 %, PD: 22 % vs. 80 %). Common side effects are neutropenia, nausea, emesis, and alopecia. The recommended dose is 60–75 mg/m^2 every 3 weeks, with cumulative dosing not recommended to exceed 450 mg/m^2 due to the risk of anthracycline-associated cardiomyopathy.

Epirubicin

Epirubicin is an anthracycline analog of doxorubicin, with dose-limiting myelosuppression and less cardiotoxicity than doxorubicin [13]. Santini and colleagues investigated the combination of the epirubicin with carboplatin in a small single-arm study of patients with progressive, metastatic poorly differentiated thyroid cancer [14]. A total of 14 patients were treated with carboplatin 300 mg/m^2 and epirubicin 75 mg/m^2 every 4–6 weeks. These patients also underwent TSH stimulation in an attempt to improve response to therapy. Responses were comparable to other historical regimens (CR: 6 %, PR: 31 %, SD: 44 %).

Cisplatin

Cisplatin is an inorganic platinum agent which forms intra- and interstrand DNA cross-links, leading to tumor cell death. Several early studies documented the activity of cisplatin as a single agent in advanced thyroid cancer. Hoskin and Harmer [6] reported objective responses in 5 out of 13 patients treated with cisplatin; responses were noted in all tumor histologies, including DTC, MTC, and ATC. Similar response rates were noted in subsequent studies [15], though response rates appeared lower in patients with DTC who had progressed following treatment with doxorubicin [16]. Toxicities include myelosuppression, nephrotoxicity, and ototoxicity.

Table 64.2 Selected targeted agents approved for or in development for the treatment of thyroid cancer

Drug	Target(s)	Toxicities
Axitinib	VEGFR-1–3, PDGFR, KIT	Hypertension/vascular events, fatigue, gastrointestinal toxicity
Cabozantinib (XL184)	VEGFR-2, Met, KIT, FLT3, Tie-2	Hand-foot, fatigue
Gefitinib	EGFR	Rash, gastrointestinal toxicity
Imatinib	Bcr-Abl, PDGFR, KIT, RET	Rash, gastrointestinal toxicity
Motesanib	VEGFR-1–3, PDGFR, KIT, RET	Hypertension/vascular events, fatigue, gastrointestinal toxicity
Pazopanib	VEGFR-1–3, PDGFR, KIT	Hypertension/vascular events, fatigue, gastrointestinal toxicity
Sorafenib	VEGFR-2–3, PDGFR, KIT, RET, BRAF, Raf-1, FLT3	Hand-foot, rash, fatigue, gastrointestinal toxicity
Sunitinib	VEGFR-1–2, PDGFR, KIT, RET, FLT3	Hand-foot, rash, fatigue, gastrointestinal toxicity
Tipifarnib	Farnesyltransferase	Rash, elevated lipase
Vandetanib	VEGFR-2, EGFR, RET	Hypertension/vascular events, fatigue, gastrointestinal toxicity
AZD6244	MEK	Rash, fatigue, diarrhea
Fosbretabulin	Tubulin (tumor microvasculature)	Myelosuppression, tumor pain, QTc prolongation
Plitidepsin	JNK activator (pro-apoptotic)	Anemia, thrombocytopenia, fatigue, elevated transaminases/ creatinine kinase
Vorinostat	Histone deacetylase	Thrombocytopenia, hyperglycemia, hypertension
Thalidomide	TNFα, VEGF, immunomodulator	Fatigue, peripheral neuropathy, thromboembolism
Lenalidomide	TNFα, VEGF, immunomodulator	Myelosuppression

Paclitaxel

Paclitaxel is a compound derived from the Pacific yew tree which stabilizes microtubules and inhibits cell division. Higashiyama and colleagues [17] reported objective responses in 4 out of 13 patients with anaplastic thyroid cancer treated with paclitaxel administered weekly as a 1-h infusion. A second study of paclitaxel administered as a continuous 96-h infusion in anaplastic thyroid cancer reported responses in 10 out of 20 patients [18]. Common toxicities include peripheral neuropathy and myelosuppression.

Targeted Agents

The last decade has witnessed an impressive expansion in our understanding of the disease pathobiology of advanced thyroid cancer and the advent of several novel targeted therapies. Several of these agents are summarized in Table 64.2. Selected agents are discussed below.

FDA-Approved Targeted Therapy

Vandetanib

Vandetanib (Zactima, Caprelsa) is an orally bioavailable tyrosine-kinase inhibitor of RET, VEGFR-2, and EGFR [19, 20]. The results of a randomized, double-blinded, multicenter placebo-controlled phase III trial of vandetanib in patients with locally advanced or metastatic MTC (ZETA trial) were reported in 2011 [21]. A total of 331 patients were enrolled in the trial. Progression-free survival at 6 months was 83 % in the vandetanib arm, compared to 63 % in the placebo arm (HR for progression 0.45, CI 0.30–0.69). Improvements were also noted in the overall response rate, disease control rate, and biochemical response rates. Overall survival was not significantly different between the two groups, but this was confounded in part by the crossover design of the study. Common side effects included diarrhea, rash, nausea, hypertension, and headache. It is currently one of two targeted therapies approved by the US Food and Drug Administration (FDA) for advanced, unresectable, or metastatic MTC.

Investigational Targeted Therapies

Cabozantinib

Cabozantinib (XL184) is a potent, orally bioavailable receptor tyrosine-kinase inhibitor of Met, VEGFR-2, KIT, RET, FLT3, and Tie-2. The results from a large, phase III, randomized, placebo-controlled study in patients with MTC were published in 2013 [22]. A total of 330 patients were enrolled in the trial; median PFS in patients treated with placebo was 4.0 months, compared to 11.2 months in patients receiving cabozantinib (HR 0.28, $p<0.001$). Unlike the ZETA trial, patients on this trial were not allowed to cross over on progression. Overall survival data were analyzed in an interim analysis when 44 % of 217 required events had occurred and no difference was seen between the two arms (HR 0.98; 95 % CI 0.63–1.52).

All patients were required to have evidence of disease progression within the last 14 months prior to enrollment. The most frequent grade 3 events included diarrhea (15.9 % vs. 1.8 %), hand-foot syndrome (12.6 % vs. 0 %), fatigue (9.3 % vs. 2.8 %), hypocalcemia (2.8 % vs. 0 %), and hypertension (7.9 % vs. 0 %) in the two groups, respectively. This agent was the second FDA-approved therapy for use in progressive, metastatic MTC.

Pazopanib

Pazopanib (Votrient) is an orally bioavailable inhibitor of VEGFR-1–3, PDGFR, and KIT [23] that is FDA-approved for the treatment of advanced renal cell carcinoma. Results of an NCI-sponsored multicenter, phase II trial of pazopanib in patients with locally advanced or metastatic, radioiodine-resistant DTC were reported in 2010 [24]. Despite the fact that all patients had evidence of progressive disease at enrollment, partial responses were seen in 18 of 37 patients, and there was a reported median progression-free survival of 11.7 months. Adverse events were common and similar to other VEGFR-targeted tyrosine-kinase inhibitors, including fatigue, skin and hair hypopigmentation, diarrhea, nausea, and hypertension. Two deaths occurred during treatment, including one fatal myocardial infarction and a bowel perforation following a complicated case of cholecystitis.

Sorafenib

Sorafenib (Nexavar) is a multi-kinase inhibitor with activity against VEGFR-2–3, PDGFR-β, FLT3, KIT, Raf-1, BRAF, and RET kinases and was approved by the FDA in November 2013 for use in metastatic differentiated thyroid cancer based on the results of the DECISION trial [25]. It is also approved for the treatment of hepatocellular carcinoma and renal cell carcinoma. The phase III randomized placebo-controlled DECISION trial enrolled 417 patients with radioactive iodine-refractory locally advanced or metastatic differentiated thyroid cancer that had progressed within the past 14 months and randomized them on a 1:1 basis. Median PFS was significantly longer in the sorafenib-treated group compared to the placebo-treated group (10.8 months vs. 5.8 months, HR 0.59, $p<0.0001$). Seventy-one percent of placebo-treated patients crossed over to open-label sorafenib upon disease progression. Overall survival did not differ significantly between the groups (HR 0.80, $p=0.14$), and the median survival had not been reached at the time of primary analysis data cutoff. The most frequent adverse events included hand-foot skin reaction (76.3 %), diarrhea (68.6 %), alopecia (67.1 %), and rash or desquamation (50.2 %) Five phase II clinical trials have evaluated sorafenib in patients with all histologies of thyroid cancer [26–30]. Objective response rates range from 11 to 25 % with clinical benefit rates (objective responses or stable disease of at least 6 months) of 59–74 %. Toxicities were similar in the four trials, with the most common adverse events being hand-foot syndrome, rash, fatigue, diarrhea, bloating, musculoskeletal pain, weight loss, and mucositis. Roughly one-third of patients also required adjustments in their thyroid replacement.

Sunitinib

Sunitinib (Sutent) is a multi-kinase inhibitor with activity against VEGFR-1, VEGFR-2, PDGFR, c-KIT, FLT3, and RET that is approved for treatment of renal cell carcinoma, gastrointestinal stromal tumors resistant to imatinib, and pancreatic neuroendocrine tumors. Four phase II studies have investigated sunitinib in advanced differentiated or medullary thyroid cancer [31–34]. Objective responses were seen in 13–33 % of patients. Common side effects include fatigue, lymphopenia, nausea, diarrhea, mucositis, and hand-foot syndrome.

Summary

Cytotoxic chemotherapeutic agents have historically been the backbone for treatment of advanced, unresectable thyroid cancer. Cytotoxic agents remain important as a component of multimodality therapy for anaplastic thyroid cancer. However, targeted agents have emerged as frontline therapy for the majority of patients with advanced differentiated or medullary thyroid cancers [35]. See Chaps. 71, 83, and 94 for further discussion of chemotherapy in DTC, MTC, and ATC, respectively.

References

1. Gottlieb JA, et al. Chemotherapy of thyroid cancer. An evaluation of experience with 37 patients. Cancer. 1972;30(3):848–53.
2. O'Bryan RM, et al. Dose response evaluation of adriamycin in human neoplasia. Cancer. 1977;39(5):1940–8.
3. Shimaoka K, et al. A randomized trial of doxorubicin versus doxorubicin plus cisplatin in patients with advanced thyroid carcinoma. Cancer. 1985;56(9):2155–60.
4. Harada T, et al. Bleomycin treatment for cancer of the thyroid. Am J Surg. 1971;122(1):53–7.
5. Harada T, et al. Bleomycin beneficial for thyroid cancer. Aerosp Med. 1972;43(3):330.
6. Hoskin PJ, Harmer C. Chemotherapy for thyroid cancer. Radiother Oncol. 1987;10(3):187–94.
7. Bukowski RM, et al. Combination chemotherapy of metastatic thyroid cancer. Phase II study. Am J Clin Oncol. 1983;6(5): 579–81.
8. De Besi P, et al. Combined chemotherapy with bleomycin, adriamycin, and platinum in advanced thyroid cancer. J Endocrinol Invest. 1991;14(6):475–80.
9. Bonadonna G, et al. Phase I and preliminary phase II evaluation of adriamycin (NSC 123127). Cancer Res. 1970;30(10):2572–82.
10. Gottlieb JA, Hill Jr CS. Chemotherapy of thyroid cancer with adriamycin. Experience with 30 patients. N Engl J Med. 1974;290(4): 193–7.

11. Haugen BR. Management of the patient with progressive radioiodine non-responsive disease. Semin Surg Oncol. 1999;16(1):34–41.
12. Matuszczyk A, et al. Chemotherapy with doxorubicin in progressive medullary and thyroid carcinoma of the follicular epithelium. Horm Metab Res. 2008;40(3):210–3.
13. Smith LA, et al. Cardiotoxicity of anthracycline agents for the treatment of cancer: systematic review and meta-analysis of randomised controlled trials. BMC Cancer. 2010;10:337.
14. Santini F, et al. Cytotoxic effects of carboplatinum and epirubicin in the setting of an elevated serum thyrotropin for advanced poorly differentiated thyroid cancer. J Clin Endocrinol Metab. 2002; 87(9):4160–5.
15. Droz JP, et al. Chemotherapy for medullary cancer of the thyroid. Phase II trials with adriamycin and cis-platinum administered as monochemotherapy. Bull Cancer. 1984;71(3):195–9.
16. Droz JP, et al. Phase II trials of chemotherapy with adriamycin, cisplatin, and their combination in thyroid cancers: a review of 44 cases. Int Congr Ser. 1985;684:203–8.
17. Higashiyama T, et al. Induction chemotherapy with weekly paclitaxel administration for anaplastic thyroid carcinoma. Thyroid. 2010;20(1):7–14.
18. Ain KB, Egorin MJ, DeSimone PA. Treatment of anaplastic thyroid carcinoma with paclitaxel: phase 2 trial using ninety-six-hour infusion. Collaborative Anaplastic Thyroid Cancer Health Intervention Trials (CATCHIT) Group. Thyroid. 2000;10(7):587–94.
19. Wedge SR, et al. ZD6474 inhibits vascular endothelial growth factor signaling, angiogenesis, and tumor growth following oral administration. Cancer Res. 2002;62(16):4645–55.
20. Carlomagno F, et al. ZD6474, an orally available inhibitor of KDR tyrosine kinase activity, efficiently blocks oncogenic RET kinases. Cancer Res. 2002;62(24):7284–90.
21. Wells Jr SA, et al. Vandetanib in patients with locally advanced or metastatic medullary thyroid cancer: a randomized, double-blind phase III trial. J Clin Oncol. 2012;30(2):134–41.
22. Elisei R, et al. Cabozantinib in progressive medullary thyroid cancer. J Clin Oncol. 2013;31(29):3639–46.
23. Kumar R, et al. Pharmacokinetic-pharmacodynamic correlation from mouse to human with pazopanib, a multikinase angiogenesis inhibitor with potent antitumor and antiangiogenic activity. Mol Cancer Ther. 2007;6(7):2012–21.
24. Bible KC, et al. Efficacy of pazopanib in progressive, radioiodine-refractory, metastatic differentiated thyroid cancers: results of a phase 2 consortium study. Lancet Oncol. 2010;11(10):962–72.
25. Brose MS, et al. Sorafenib in radioactive iodine-refractory, locally advanced or metastatic differentiated thyroid cancer: a randomised, double-blind, phase 3 trial. Lancet. 2014;384:319–28.
26. Gupta-Abramson V, et al. Phase II trial of sorafenib in advanced thyroid cancer. J Clin Oncol. 2008;26(29):4714–9.
27. Kloos RT, et al. Phase II trial of sorafenib in metastatic thyroid cancer. J Clin Oncol. 2009;27(10):1675–84.
28. Hoftijzer H, et al. Beneficial effects of sorafenib on tumor progression, but not on radioiodine uptake, in patients with differentiated thyroid carcinoma. Eur J Endocrinol. 2009;161(6): 923–31.
29. Lam ET, et al. Phase II clinical trial of sorafenib in metastatic medullary thyroid cancer. J Clin Oncol. 2010;28(14):2323–30.
30. Ahmed M, et al. Analysis of the efficacy and toxicity of sorafenib in thyroid cancer: a phase II study in a UK based population. Eur J Endocrinol. 2011;165(2):315–22.
31. Carr LL, et al. Phase II study of daily sunitinib in FDG-PET-positive, iodine-refractory differentiated thyroid cancer and metastatic medullary carcinoma of the thyroid with functional imaging correlation. Clin Cancer Res. 2010;16(21):5260–8.
32. Cohen E, et al. Phase 2 study of sunitinib in refractory thyroid cancer. J Clin Oncol. 2008;26(20 suppl):abstr 6025.
33. De Souza J, et al. Phase II trial of sunitinib in medullary thyroid cancer (MTC). J Clin Oncol. 2010;28(15S):abstr 5504.
34. Ravaud A, et al. Efficacy of sunitinib in advanced medullary thyroid carcinoma: intermediate results of phase II THYSU. Oncologist. 2010;15(2):212–3; author reply 214.
35. Tuttle R, et al. NCCN clinical practice guidelines in oncology (NCCN guidelines): thyroid carcinoma. 2014. www.nccn.org.

Bone Metastases from Differentiated Thyroid Carcinoma

65

Jason A. Wexler

Introduction

Thyroid cancer incidence has been increasing for decades in the United States [1, 2]. There are known risk factors for thyroid cancer including female gender, advancing age, family history, and radiation exposure, but none of these has fully explain the changing pattern of this disease over such a short period of time. Much of the rise has been attributed to increased medical surveillance, diagnostic imaging, and ultrasound-guided fine-needle aspiration, but this probably does not explain the entire observed upsurge. With increased evaluation of patients in an asymptomatic stage, it might be expected that the highest rate of increase would be seen in tumors <1.0 cm, but incidence has also been increasing for tumors of any size, especially tumors >4 cm among men and women and for distant metastases among men [3]. The more frequent diagnosis of late-stage disease has led to the rising occurrence of differentiated thyroid carcinoma and bone metastases, even as the initial presentation of disease. It is suspected that a combination of environmental factors, iodine deficiency, and genetic factors (i.e.: *BRAF mutations*) may explain the rising incidence of differentiated thyroid cancer, particularly more aggressive, late-stage disease [4, 5].

How to Make the Diagnosis of Thyroid Carcinoma

Thyroid cancer may come to clinical attention when neck nodules or lymphadenopathy are noted by the patient, are found during physical examination, or as an incidental finding during a radiological procedure. Fine-needle aspiration (FNA) biopsy, with thyroglobulin (Tg) washout in appropriate circumstances, is the standard procedure to evaluate thyroid nodules and abnormal cervical lymph nodes [6]. Thyroid ultrasonography provides excellent anatomic definition that is superior to thyroid scintigraphy and can be used in conjunction with FNA to aid in performing thyroid and/or lymph node biopsies. However, follicular and Hurthle cell cancers cannot be distinguished cytologically from follicular and Hurthle cell adenomas. Consequently, as many as 15–20 % of thyroid aspirations are classified as suspicious or indeterminate [7]. It is estimated that 10–20 % of these indeterminate lesions that are surgically resected are determined to be follicular cancers. Nevertheless, FNA is very accurate with false-negative rates ranging from 0 % to 5 % and false-positive readings in less than 5 % of patients in high-volume facilities.

How to Detect Bone Metastases

Although follicular thyroid cancer accounts for less than 15 % of all differentiated thyroid cancers, it has an incidence of bone metastases of 7–20 % [8]. Bone metastases are much less common in papillary thyroid cancer (1–7 %) [9]. Overall, bone metastases from well-differentiated thyroid cancer occur in 2–13 % of patients [10, 11].

There are many factors that can predispose certain malignancies to develop bone metastases. Blood flow is high in bone marrow, so tumors that have a tendency to spread hematogenously, such as follicular thyroid carcinoma, can arise in bone sites. Malignant cells also synthesize adhesive molecules that allow them to attach to bone matrix. Some tumor cells also secrete angiogenic compounds and factors that enhance bone resorption so tumors may find a more hospitable environment to grow and replicate in the bone. Osteolytic tumors, like thyroid carcinoma, may enhance the

J.A. Wexler, MD (✉)
Internal Medicine/Section of Endocrinology, MedStar Washington Hospital Center, Georgetown University Medical Center, 110 Irving Street, NW, Washington, DC 20010, USA
e-mail: Jason.a.wexler@medstar.net

L. Wartofsky, D. Van Nostrand (eds.), *Thyroid Cancer*, DOI 10.1007/978-1-4939-3314-3_65

production of interleukin-1, interleukin-6, and receptor activator of nuclear factor-κB ligand (RANKL) which all lead to increased osteoclastic activity and resorption of bone. This resorptive activity is thought to lead to a hospitable environment ("seed-and-soil hypothesis") for bone metastases to take root and grow [12].

Skeletal metastases of thyroid cancer can present with pain, but often are clinically silent. Pain is thought to result from tumoral release of cytokines, pressure, and mass effect within the bone [13]. Additional symptoms may include fractures and spinal cord compression that occur in 13 % and 28 % of patients, respectively [14].

It can be difficult to detect distant metastases from thyroid cancer, and diagnostic I-131 whole-body scans are notoriously insensitive for localizing bone metastases. Post-therapy I-131 whole-body scans on the other hand may be quite sensitive in detecting osseous lesions. X-rays and bone scintigraphy are used in the evaluation of osseous metastases, but even these modalities will only detect disease when more than half of an involved bone has been destroyed, and they are limited by poor specificity and lack of prospective data evaluating their utility in thyroid cancer [15]. Bone scintigraphy can detect skeletal metastases earlier than plain radiographs when there is a predominant osteoblastic component to the bone lesion. But since thyroid cancer metastases to bone are predominantly osteolytic (with secondary bone formation in response to bone destruction), bone scintigraphy may be of limited value with a high false-negative and false-positive rate [16].

MRI of the whole body or of specific bones on the other hand is superb for visualizing the medullary component of bone and detailing the intraosseous and extraskeletal extent of disease. A study of patients with a variety of different cancers showed whole-body MRI (91 % diagnostic accuracy) to be superior to PET-CT (78 % diagnostic accuracy) in detecting bone metastases [17]. CT alone can also be quite valuable in imaging cortical erosion of bone and detecting the presence of subclinical fractures in patients with bone metastases [18]. Fluorine-18 fluorodeoxyglucose (FDG) PET, whole-body scan with technetium 99m sestamibi (MIBI), and post-therapy I-131 imaging have been compared under rh-TSH stimulation for their ability to detect distant metastases [19]. Only 3 of 19 patients had follicular thyroid cancer, but FDG-PET was more sensitive than MIBI body scan and post-therapy I-131 scanning in detecting distant spread. The 19 patients had 32 isolated lesions (10 lymph node, 15 lung, 6 bone, and 1 muscle) confirmed by histopathology and/or other imaging studies (X-ray, ultrasound, CT, MRI, and bone scan). PET detected 81.3 %, MIBI 62.5 %, and radioiodine 68.8 % of the total lesions. There were no significant differences between the imaging techniques for skeletal metastases with each modality detecting about 83 % of lesions [19]. Moreover, a positive FDG-PET scan is strongly associated with a worse prognosis. In one study, patients with a positive PET scan had a median survival of only 53 months from the time of the PET scan [20].

18F-fluoride is a bone seeking, positron-emitting molecule with excellent sensitivity and specificity for detecting bone lesions, especially osteolytic metastases. When combined with PET/CT, 18F-fluroide can provide exquisite spatial resolution of osseous metastases. In one study, 18F-NaF detected 100 % of the bone metastases in thyroid cancer compared with about half of the metastases with radionuclide bone scanning [21]. A study from Japan evaluated 11 patients with well-differentiated thyroid cancer for bone metastases. Bone metastases were verified either when positive findings were obtained on both I-131 scintigraphy and CT or when MRI findings were positive. Metastases were confirmed in 9 (81.8 %) of the 11 patients. The sensitivities of 18F-fluoride PET/CT and 99mTc bone scintigraphy (SPECT) were significantly higher than those of 18F-FDG PET/CT and 99mTc bone scintigraphy (planar) ($p<0.05$). The accuracies of 18F-fluoride PET/CT and 99mTc bone scintigraphy (SPECT) were significantly higher than that of 99mTc bone scintigraphy (planar) ($p<0.05$). In this small study, the sensitivity of 18F-fluoride PET/CT was superior to 18F-FDG PET/CT [22].

Since I-131 imaging will detect some, but certainly not all bone metastases, I typically employ PET-CT in patients with extracervical metastases to proactively identify bone metastases even when patients are asymptomatic. Since 18F-fluroide PET/CT is only available on a limited basis at my institution, I generally recommend using PET-CT in these high-risk patients with either papillary or follicular thyroid cancer, even though bone metastases are more commonly linked with follicular thyroid cancer.

A potential future tool for imaging bone metastases from thyroid cancer is the positron-emitting radioisotope I-124. I-124 is taken up by the sodium iodide symporter and can produce remarkable three-dimensional imaging of tracer distribution within the tumor sites [23]. In one study of patients with thyroid cancer, CT, I-131, I-124, and I-124-PET-CT were evaluated for their effectiveness in detecting histologically proven lesions. I-124-PET-CT was superior to all the other modalities, detecting 100 % of the lesions compared to 56 % for CT, 83 % for I-131, and 87 % for I-124 [24].

When skeletal metastases are suspected, a practical approach is to obtain a skeletal survey, whole-body bone scan, or FDG-PET-CT. Whole-body MRI is particularly helpful in patients with spinal cord involvement. If a bone metastasis is discovered, then a directed MRI or CT scan should be employed to specifically define the lesion(s) of interest and aid in the planning of any surgical approaches or use of other modalities in the treatment of destructive osseous metastases.

Role of Biopsy in the Diagnosis of Bone Metastases

In most situations where the histology of a primary malignancy has been established, it is usually unnecessary to biopsy new lesions that present at distant sites. However, this recommendation does not hold for bone metastases. In those patients where the primary carcinoma is defined, it is recommended that a biopsy be obtained of a metastatic lesion to bone, especially when the skeletal metastasis represents the first manifestation of recurrent disease [25]. Bone biopsy would not be necessary in patients with thyroid carcinoma with uptake localized to bone lesions on either diagnostic or post-therapy I-131 scans. Bone biopsy is also not necessary in most patients with multiple relapses who have previously undergone a biopsy documenting bone metastases from thyroid cancer. In patients with a new osseous lesion, who have wide spread metastatic disease and who have previously undergone a biopsy of a bone lesion, clinical judgment in light of pertinent radiological studies should be used to determine if another bone biopsy is necessary.

For those patients with suspected metastases to the spine or pelvis, a needle biopsy is recommended. Other sites for bony lesions may require more intricate interventions to obtain a tumor sample. Sections of the biopsy sample should be examined carefully for histologic subtype such as papillary (classical form and variants), follicular, Hürthle cell, and poorly differentiated carcinomas. The cytologist should employ special stains for thyroid transcription factor 1 (TTF1), thyroglobulin, as well as cytokeratin and calcitonin. Supplementary immunohistochemistry such as for prostate-specific antigen (PSA) should be utilized as clinically indicated to exclude other tumor types.

Another simple technique that can be used in evaluating distant metastases is detection of thyroglobulin in the washout of fine-needle aspirates of nonthyroidal masses [26]. In this procedure, the same needle used during an FNA for cytological analysis is flushed with 1 ml of normal saline solution. The washout is centrifuged and the sample is analyzed for Tg and anti-Tg antibodies using standard lab assays. Studies of this technique in the evaluation of lymph nodes in patients with thyroid cancer have demonstrated a sensitivity and specificity approaching 100 % [27, 28]. While not specifically studied in bone metastases, the value of the technique is probably similar. Molecular profiling of primary and metastatic tumor sites may help in the future to permit more accurate diagnosis, prognosis, and personalized treatment regimens based on molecular pathophysiology rather than histology [29].

I recommend a bone biopsy for the initial presentation of a suspected skeletal metastasis even if the patient is known to have thyroid cancer since it is possible that another tumor type could be present. Once a bone biopsy has confirmed the origin of the tumor, I do not recommend biopsies of subsequent skeletal lesions except in rare circumstances. Often, the cytologic and histologic characteristics of bone metastases from thyroid cancer are significantly different from those of the original primary thyroid tumor.

Role and Efficacy of I-131 in Treating Skeletal Metastases

The overall 10-year survival rate for patients with well-differentiated thyroid cancer is 80–95 %. Once distant metastases develop, 10-year survival plummets to 40 % [30–32]. Most of the published literature on survival of patients with thyroid cancer and bone metastases is even bleaker. Several studies have measured 10-year survival of these patients in the range of 0–34 % [10, 11, 33–38]. The mean survival for patients with skeletal metastases is estimated at only 4 years [35, 39]. In these studies, nearly all patients received radioiodine and many also underwent adjuvant therapy including surgical excision of bony lesions, external beam radiotherapy, arterial embolization, or chemotherapy. While the burden of skeletal metastases and their response to I-131 are associated with survival, osteolytic metastases also significantly reduce quality of life by causing pain, fractures, and spinal cord compression [40].

In a report from Memorial Sloan Kettering Cancer Center, 52 patients with distant metastases from thyroid cancer were identified from a database. Thirty-nine patients (75 %) were diagnosed with pulmonary metastases alone and 13 (25 %) with extrapulmonary metastases (9/13 with bone metastases). After thyroid surgery, 47 patients (90 %) were treated with I-131 alone, and 2 patients had external beam radiation in addition to I-131. The 5-year overall survival and disease-specific survival were 65 % and 68 %, respectively. Extrapulmonary metastases were predictive of lower 5-year disease-specific survival (46 % vs. 75 %, $p=0.013$), and approximately half of the patients presenting with distant metastases died within 5 years of initial diagnosis [41].

Similarly, in a study of 1227 DTC patients, 51 (4.2 %) presented with distant metastases at diagnosis. All patients underwent a total thyroidectomy followed by I-131 ablation. In the multivariate analysis, osseous metastasis (RR 6.849, 95 % CI 1.495–31.250, $P=0.013$) was an independent predictor of poor cancer-specific survival [42].

But not all bone metastases are associated with a poor prognosis. In a retrospective review of medical records from Memorial Sloan-Kettering Cancer Center, 14 patients who had I-131 avid bone metastasis without structural correlate on CT or MRI were evaluated in the study. After a median follow-up period of 5 years (range 2–14 years), all patients were alive, none had evidence of structural bone metastases, and none had experienced skeletal-related events. In this select group of patients, I-131 avid bone metastases without structural correlate on cross-sectional imaging studies often resolve following RAI treatment do not cause skeletal-related complications and do not have a major prognostic significance [43].

There are no prospective, randomized, controlled clinical trials of I-131 for the treatment of bone metastases from well-differentiated thyroid cancer. Although limited due to the nature of their study design, the best available data on the efficacy of I-131 for therapy of bone metastases come from retrospective studies. One retrospective study analyzed 2,200 patients with either papillary or follicular thyroid carcinoma and identified 394 patients with lung and/or skeletal metastases [11]. Two hundred and one patients had follicular thyroid cancer. Most patients were treated with total thyroidectomy and 100 mCi I-131. One-third received external beam radiation therapy to the neck following thyroidectomy. Patients who had radioiodine activity in the lung or bone on post-therapy imaging received an additional 100 mCi I-131 3 months after the initial ablative dose of I-131. The same I-131 treatment regimen was given to patients with a detectable Tg while on levothyroxine (LT4) therapy or if the Tg was >5 ng/ml during LT4 withdrawal. Patients with radiographically confirmed skeletal metastases also received 3,000 rads of external beam radiation treatment (EBRT) to the affected region in association with I-131 therapy. Those with I-131 uptake had an improved prognosis compared to those whose I-131 scans were negative. The risk of death was highest in those with multiple bone metastases. Ten-year survival was 96 % in those <40 years old with normal chest x-rays and as low as 7 % in those >40 years old with multiple skeletal metastases. Ten-year survival for other patients was 63 %. If patients had a complete response to therapy, 5-year survival was 96 %, 10-year survival 93 %, and 15-year survival 89 %. If patients had less than a complete response, survival was 37 %, 14 %, and 8 %, respectively. The response to I-131 therapy was significantly better the earlier the disease was detected and treated. Although prolonged survival was not proven to be linked to I-131 therapy alone, those patients who lived 15 years or longer following the diagnosis of bone metastases had all been treated with I-131 alone or in combination with EBRT.

A subsequent report from the same institution investigated survival among 444 patients with distant metastases from well-differentiated thyroid cancer [9]. Of those who had radioiodine avid disease, 20-year survival was 33 % compared to only 3 % at 10 years for those without radioiodine uptake. Patients with skeletal metastases had a 20-year survival rate of only 8 %. Overall survival was not impacted by distant metastases discovered early or late in the patient's course of disease.

But some investigators have reported more successful results with I-131 in subgroups of patients with bone metastases. A retrospective review of 107 patients with an initial skeletal metastasis demonstrated significantly higher rates of total or partial remissions in patients younger than 45 years old (62.5 %) compared to patients over 45 years of age (49.5 %) [44]. In younger patients with three or fewer bone lesions, 75 % achieved complete remission, suggesting that I-131 can be used with curative intent in specific situations.

Some groups have reported survival rates far superior to historic averages for certain patients treated with I-131. In a paper published late in 2011, investigators from China published their retrospective experience investigating the clinical efficacy of I-131 therapy for bone metastases from thyroid cancer [45]. One hundred six patients were treated with I-131, and a significant decline in serum thyroglobulin was seen in nearly 35 % of the cases. Of the 61 patients with painful bone metastases, nearly two-third had significant relief of bone pain following I-131 treatment. Despite the fact that 76 % of patients had no anatomical change when imaged following I-131 therapy, the 5-year and 10-year survival rates were 86 % and 58 %, respectively. This paper adds to a growing body of evidence that supports the efficacy and potential survival benefit when patients receive I-131 treatment for bone metastases, especially for those with solitary lesions and those who underwent surgical resection bone metastases prior to receiving I-131.

Similarly, my institution has found 5-year survival rates much higher than historically reported (~78 %) with a combination of I-131 and other adjuvant treatment modalities [46]. The efficacy of I-131 in treating bone metastases may be improved in situations where dosimetry is employed rather than fixed doses of radioiodine. Several groups have demonstrated that skeletal metastases treated under a dosimetry protocol achieved greater reductions in tumor volume and thyroglobulin levels than a historical control group that was treated with a fixed dose of radioiodine [47–50]. Perhaps equally important, dosimetry may identify lesions that do not concentrate radioiodine to a degree that would allow the delivery of a therapeutic radiation dose, thus distinguishing patients who may not benefit from I-131 therapy.

Efficacy of Bisphosphonates and Monoclonal Antibodies to RANK Ligand (RANKL) in the Treatment of Bone Metastases

Bone metastases from follicular thyroid cancer, especially those that are poorly differentiated, do not respond well to I-131 and other traditional therapies for thyroid cancer. Skeletal metastases from thyroid cancer obliterate bone architecture through local osteolysis. Bisphosphonates and denosumab are approved for the treatment of bone metastases from breast cancer, prostate cancer, and other solid malignancies. Denosumab is a recently FDAapproved human monoclonal antibody that inhibits RANKL, thereby limiting osteoclast activity and reducing bone resorption.

In a retrospective review of 245 differentiated thyroid cancer patients with bone metastases, the occurrence of a skeletal-related event (SRE) was recorded from the initial diagnosis of bone metastasis until final follow-up or death. Seventy-eight percent of patients (192 of 245) either presented with or developed at least one SRE after the diagnosis of metastatic bone disease. The median time from identification of bone metastasis to first SRE was 5 months. Of the patients who sustained an initial SRE, 65 % (120 of 192) went on to sustain a second SRE at a median of 10.7 months after the first event. SREs were frequently multiple; 39 % (74 of 192) sustained three or more discrete SREs. The findings suggest that thyroid cancer bone metastases frequently cause significant and recurrent morbidity. The incidence of SREs and median time to first SRE in metastatic thyroid cancer to bone are similar to those reported in other solid tumors. This study highlights the importance of conducting prospective clinical trials to assess the efficacy of antiresorptive agents in this population [51].

Data specifically related to the use of these agents in bone metastases from thyroid cancer are lacking, but a group of investigators from Japan reported results from their experience treating bone metastases from differentiated thyroid cancer from 1976 to 2008. In their retrospective review of 50 patients [52], 28 did not receive bisphosphonate therapy, while 22 received intravenous zoledronic acid. SREs occurred in only 14 % of those who received zoledronic acid compared with 50 % of those who did not receive a bisphosphonate. Spinal cord compression was seen in 9 % of those who received zoledronic acid compared with 46 % of those who did not. Of course, these groups were treated in different eras, with those receiving bisphosphonates beginning therapy in 2006 or later. This publication is also limited by the fact that radiotherapy and surgery to the bone were not counted as skeletal-related events. Many patients in this study had already been treated with radiotherapy or surgery to painful bone metastases, skeletal fractures, and spinal cord compression prior to initiation of zoledronic acid, thereby confounding the reported efficacy of zoledronic acid in those who did see a reduction in SREs. Therefore, it cannot be known with certainty whether zoledronic acid or the other directed therapies were primarily responsible for the reduction in SREs seen in this study.

An early study of intravenous (IV) pamidronate (30 mg every 3 months for 2 years) given to patients on suppressive doses of levothyroxine (LT4) for thyroid cancer caused a suppression of bone resorption and an increase in bone mineral density (BMD) [53]. Another protocol enrolled ten patients with bone metastases from thyroid cancer and administered IV pamidronate 90 mg every month for 1 year [54]. Patients who received pamidronate reported much less bone pain by a visual analog scale, improved performance status, and a beneficial impact on quality of life assessment. Although only two of ten patients demonstrated a partial radiographic response to pamidronate, the amount of narcotic pain medication required by patients declined over time, albeit by a statistically insignificant amount. Side effects from therapy, including fever, myalgias, and electrolyte abnormalities (typically hypocalcemia), were mild and short lived.

Since there are few studies specifically employing bisphosphonates in the management of bone metastases from thyroid cancer, the potential efficacy of these agents in thyroid cancer has to be extrapolated from their use in other malignancies [55]. One study compared 4 mg zoledronic acid given intravenously every 3–4 weeks for 12 months to 90 mg of IV pamidronate given at the same frequency to breast cancer patients with at least one osteolytic lesion with skeletal-related events (SRE) as the primary outcome. SREs were defined as pathologic fracture, spinal cord compression, radiation therapy, or surgery to the bone. Zoledronic acid significantly reduced the risk of an SRE by 20 % compared to 9 % for pamidronate. Zoledronic acid was also as effective as pamidronate in reducing the proportion of patients with >1 SRE (48 % versus 58 %). In a post hoc, retrospective analysis of patients with >1 osteolytic lesion, zoledronic acid was more effective than pamidronate in delaying the time to onset of an SRE (310 days versus 174 days).

In a phase II trial, denosumab 120 mg subcutaneously every 4 weeks was associated with a significant reduction of skeletal-related events (8 %) compared to intravenous bisphosphonates (17 %) in patients with bone metastases from prostate cancer, breast cancer, and other malignancies [56]. In a phase III trial comparing denosumab with IV zoledronic acid in breast cancer patients with bone metastases, denosumab 120 mg subcutaneously every 4 weeks was found to be superior to zoledronic acid 4 mg IV monthly (adjusted for creatinine clearance) in delaying or preventing skeletal-related events [57].

Given the lack of comprehensive clinical trial data on the efficacy of intravenous bisphosphonates for patients with bone metastases from thyroid cancer, the optimal treatment regimen and duration of therapy is unknown. For those who suffer an acute pathologic fracture or have extensive, symptomatic bone metastases, or short life expectancy, I think it is reasonable to follow the prescribing information for both agents and give full doses (zoledronic acid 4 mg intravenously or denosumab 120 mg subcutaneously) every 4 weeks. In clinical trials [57, 58], zoledronic acid was given for up to 2 years and denosumab was given up to 41 months. Based on this trial data for other malignancies, I am prepared to treat severely affected patients with metastatic disease to the bone monthly for 2–4 years.

For patients who have a solitary bone metastasis or stable bone metastases, particularly if asymptomatic, and with a life expectancy more than 5 years, I think a prudent course would be to administer zoledronic acid 4 mg twice yearly and denosumab 120 mg twice yearly. For those who develop new bone metastases or progression of older metastases, I recommend treating with zoledronic acid 4 mg every 1–3 months or denosumab 120 mg every 1–3 months. If patients go on to develop stable disease, then it seems reasonable to reduce the dosing frequency of these drugs to twice yearly, especially if life expectancy is prolonged. If patients deteriorate and develop progressive or symptomatic disease from bone metastases, then it makes sense to ratchet up the dosing frequency to every 1–3 months depending on the clinical severity.

This paradigm represents my judgment and personal approach on how to manage thyroid cancer bone metastases based on an extrapolation of data derived from clinical trials of patients with breast cancer, prostate cancer, and other solid malignancies. While these recommendations differ somewhat from those with bone metastases from other solid tumors, since patients with thyroid cancer may live many years even with osseous metastases, it seems a reasonable compromise between the potential advantages bisphosphonates and denosumab may offer and the potential adverse effects that could be linked to their long-term use, specifically atypical femoral shaft fractures and osteonecrosis of the jaw.

Toxicity associated with bisphosphonates is generally mild and infrequent, but there are important adverse reactions that can occur [59, 60]. Renal toxicity, usually due to acute tubular necrosis and collapsing focal segmental glomerulosclerosis, is the main concern with intravenous bisphosphonates and is directly related to dose and infusion time (more than 90 mg over less than 2 h with pamidronate and more than 4 mg over less than 15 min with zoledronic acid) [61]. Renal failure is rare.

Adequate supplementation with calcium and vitamin D can prevent most cases of hypocalcemia. I follow the recommendations of the 2011 report on dietary reference intakes for calcium and vitamin D from the Institute of Medicine [62]. According to the new recommendations, total daily intake of calcium (from diet and supplements) should be 1,000–1,200 mg per day for most adults and total daily intake of vitamin D (from diet and supplements) should be 600–800 units per day. For those who measure 25-hydroxyvitamin D levels, the target range should be approximately >30 ng/ml to reduce the risk of hypocalcemia. It is advisable to monitor renal function and creatinine clearance with every cycle of IV bisphosphonate.

Intravenous bisphosphonates can be associated with the acute-phase response (APR) characterized by fever, myalgias, malaise, arthralgias, and bone pain in up to 30–35 % of patients receiving an initial dose [63]. APR is dose dependent and occurs mainly after the first infusion of an intravenous bisphosphonate; it is rare in subsequent infusions. Symptoms typically present within 24–36 h and subside 2–3 days later. Although the symptoms are self-limited, they can be managed with antipyretics.

Osteonecrosis of the jaw (ONJ) has been associated with IV bisphosphonates and subcutaneous denosumab. ONJ is defined as the presence of exposed bone in the maxillofacial region that does not heal within 2 months after identification. While the risk of ONJ in patients treated with bisphosphonates for osteoporosis is estimated between 1/10,000 and 1/100,000 patient-years of therapy, the risk of ONJ in cancer patients treated with high doses of IV bisphosphonates is in the range of 1–10/100 patients [64, 65]. Risk factors for ONJ include head and neck radiotherapy, periodontal disease, dental procedures involving bone surgery, edentulous regions, and trauma from poorly fitting dentures. Malignancy, chemotherapy, corticosteroids, and systemic infections are additional risk factors. The more potent IV bisphosphonates such as zoledronic acid and pamidronate and the longer the duration of treatment are also risk factors for developing ONJ.

Atypical fractures of the femoral diaphysis have been reported in patients on long-term (3–8 years) bisphosphonates [66]. Atypical fractures have also been reported in those on denosumab. Atypical femoral fractures are rare, low-energy fractures of either the subtrochanteric region of the hip or the femoral shaft. Although these fractures have been reported mostly in patients who have been treated with bisphosphonates (especially those on glucocorticoids), atypical femoral fractures have occurred in patients with no history of bisphosphonate use [67]. The American Society for Bone and Mineral Research (ASMBMR) task force on atypical femoral fractures concluded that these fractures are quite rare, but are associated with long-term use of bisphosphonates beyond 3 years, particularly in those concomitantly taking glucocorticoids [68].

Bisphosphonates can also be used as vehicles for radioisotopes. Currently available bone-specific radioisotopes for therapy of bone metastases include ^{153}Sm-EDTMP,

^{186}Re-HEDP, and ^{89}Sr chloride. These agents palliate pain from skeletal metastases and have been proposed as alternatives for patients with painful bone metastases who cannot receive external beam radiotherapy. While these agents have not been evaluated in patients with thyroid cancer and bone metastases, data from prostate and breast cancer studies suggest that pain from skeletal metastases is reduced in 40–95 % of patients and 59 % do not develop new painful metastases compared to 34 % who received placebo [69, 70].

Role of Surgery in the Treatment of Bone Metastases

Bone metastases can be treated surgically. Complete surgical resection entails removing all macroscopically identified bone tumor with pathological confirmation. Palliative surgery partially removes bone tumor or completely resects bone tumor but leaves residual tumor in other organs. In one study of 109 patients with bone metastases from thyroid cancer [33], 22 % underwent complete surgical resection of their bony lesions. Patients younger than 45 years of age were more than 2.5 times as likely to have complete resection compared to older patients. Fifty-five percent had partial resection, while 23 % did not have any surgery for their bone lesions. Complete resection of skeletal metastases was associated with a significant improvement in survival.

In a retrospective review at a single institution, 41 patients underwent surgery for thyroid carcinoma bone metastasis from 1988 to 2011. Overall patient survival probability was 72 % at 1 year, 29 % at 5 years, and 20 % at 8 years. Disease progression at the surgery site occurred more frequently with a histological diagnosis of follicular carcinoma compared with other subtypes ($p=0.023$). Patients who had their tumor excised ($p=0.001$) or presented with solitary bone involvement had a lower risk of death following surgery adjusting for age and gender [71].

Innovative Modalities in the Treatment of Bone Metastases

Percutaneous vertebroplasty and kyphoplasty are alternative modalities to surgical resection of bone metastases in patients with pathologic fractures. These procedures involve injecting bone cement called polymethylmethacrylate into buckled vertebral bodies. While few studies of these techniques for thyroid cancer patients have been published, these minimally invasive procedures have been shown to reduce the pain and deformity associated with metastatic vertebral body fractures [72, 73].

External beam radiation therapy (EBRT) is one of the main therapeutic options available to patients with skeletal metastases from thyroid cancer. The objective of EBRT is to alleviate pain and neurological complications of bone lesions. Data on the efficacy of EBRT in the management of thyroid cancer and bone metastases is lacking, but it is thought that 70 % of patients experience pain relief with palliative EBRT [74]. Patients usually report improvement in symptoms within 48–72 h, but in some cases, relief may be delayed by up to 1 month following radiotherapy. EBRT needs to be tailored to the patient's prognosis and life expectancy as well as the anatomic site of the bone metastasis and the volume of disease to be treated. EBRT is usually employed after the surgical treatment of pathologic fractures or in cases of impending fractures in order to improve the patient's functional status. Efforts are ongoing to determine if EBRT in combination with other therapies such as vertebroplasty, kyphoplasty, and radiofrequency ablation may offer further advantages to patients [75, 76]. One study of combination radiofrequency and kyphoplasty in the management of painful osteolytic metastases to the spine found a significant reduction in pain score 72 h and 6 weeks after treatment [77]. Side effects of EBRT include skin erythema, dry desquamation, and mucositis. Long-term sequelae include skin hyperpigmentation and esophageal and tracheal stenosis.

Conformal radiotherapy intensity modulation (IMRT) can allow for more precise delivery of radiation to sites outside of the thyroid bed, preserving more of the normal surrounding tissue and mitigating acute and late radiation toxicity [78]. In those with solitary bone metastases, 50 Gy is usually delivered in several fractions over 1 month. In those patients receiving radiation therapy to the spinal cord, doses should be limited to 40 Gy. A study of consecutive patients with differentiated thyroid cancer who underwent EBRT (74 patients) or IMRT (57 patients) to a median dose of 60 Gy for both groups showed similar rates of locoregional relapse-free survival, disease-specific survival, and overall survival at 4 years of 79 %, 76 %, and 73 %, respectively. IMRT did not affect overall survival, but it was associated with significantly less severe late radiation-induced morbidity (2 %) compared to EBRT (12 %) [79].

Radiofrequency ablation (RFA) is a minimally invasive technique that has been used in adjuvant fashion to treat metastatic thyroid cancer. RFA is thought to cause focal coagulative necrosis of diseased tissue within the specific region of applied therapy. RFA has predominantly been used to treat liver metastases of thyroid cancer, but RFA has also been found to reduce pain from thyroid cancer skeletal metastases [77, 80].

RFA has been studied in patients with thyroid cancer with locally recurrent as well as isolated distant metastases [81]. Three patients with well-differentiated thyroid cancer underwent RFA for solitary bone metastases. One presented 12 months later with persistent disease. This individual was retreated with RFA and I-131 and the subsequent I-131 whole-body scan was negative for iodine avid disease. A second patient had persistent disease at the treated site and developed a new bone metastasis. The third patient had no evidence for residual disease on I-131 imaging through 53 months of follow-up, and a biopsy at the previously treated bone metastasis site was negative for malignancy. In a separate study, two patients were treated with a combination of RFA and osteoplasty for skeletal metastases, noting pain relief in both patients and a reduction in the strength and amount of analgesics required to control their pain [82].

Cryotherapy is another technique for the treatment of bone metastases from thyroid cancer. Previously, cryotherapy was performed by introducing liquid nitrogen into the tumor site. Although this technique was modestly successful, nitrogen emboli, bone fractures from local necrosis of skeletal tissue, and damage to local neurovascular structures could occur. In recent years, cryotherapy has been performed using an argon-based system that allows for the controlled formation of ice around the probe [83]. One study evaluated 14 patients with metastatic osteolytic disease from various primary tumor types [83]. None of the patients treated with cryotherapy suffered neurologic injury and there were no pathologic fractures. While the data for cryotherapy of skeletal lesions from thyroid cancer are scant, this technique could be a valuable tool for the management of bone metastases from thyroid cancer with the potential of minimal risk to local surrounding structures.

Selective arterial embolization is an invasive procedure that involves visualizing the feeding arteries of tumor metastases that have been localized by cross-sectional imaging studies such as CT or MRI. In patients treated with I-131 with or without selective arterial embolization of bone metastases, thyroglobulin levels decreased by 88.7 % in the embolization group compared to 18.6 % in the I-131 alone group [84]. The procedure also offers immediate relief of pain and neurological symptoms in 59 % of patients with bone metastases from thyroid cancer [85].

In many papillary thyroid cancers, activating mutations have been discovered in genes (*RET/PTC*, *RAS*, *BRAF*) involved in the mitogen-activated protein (MAP) kinase pathway. In follicular thyroid cancer in particular, *RAS* and *PPARγ-PAX8* are thought to be the predominant mutations, though activation of the phosphatidyl 3-kinase pathway and overexpression of tyrosine kinase receptors (fibroblast growth factor, epidermal growth factor, and hepatocyte growth factor) and angiogenesis growth factors (vascular endothelial growth factors) may also occur [29].

In light of this information, various kinase inhibitors (TKIs) are being studied in patients with metastatic, progressive, radioiodine refractory well-differentiated thyroid cancer. Several phase I and II trials with motesanib, sorafenib, axitinib, sunitinib, and pazopanib have shown partial tumor response in 8–32 % and stable disease in greater than 50 % of patients with progressive disease at enrollment [29, 86–88]. The Food and Drug Administration recently approved sorafenib for use in patients with locally advanced or metastatic I-131 refractory thyroid cancer. While the general response of patients to these compounds has been encouraging with significant increases in progression-free survival, the specific value of these agents for bone metastases has not yet been elucidated. In one study, 62 patients with various subtypes of thyroid cancer were treated with sorafenib (62 %), sunitinib (22 %), and vandetanib (16 %) outside of clinical trials. Most were treated with a single TKI, but a few were exposed to several lines of TKI therapy. Of those treated with sorafenib and sunitinib, the partial response (PR) rates were 15 % and 8 %, respectively. Unfortunately, however, bone and pleural lesions were the most refractory sites to treatment, suggesting TKIs might not be an optimal therapy for those with osseous metastases as the only site of distant disease [89].

Toxicities from these therapies are an important limitation and include diarrhea, nausea, alopecia, fatigue, hypertension, leukopenia, anemia, thrombocytopenia, and a painful, blistering skin toxicity called hand-foot syndrome. Asymptomatic prolongation of the QTc interval may occur and necessitates periodic monitoring of the EKG and cardiac function.

Conclusions

Bone metastases are a relatively uncommon finding in patients with well-differentiated thyroid cancer. Comprehensive imaging studies such as whole-body bone scan, MRI, CT, and PET/CT, in addition to I-131 WBS, are indicated in these patients to fully evaluate the extent of their disease and any improvement or progression in response to therapy. Published studies demonstrate that the presence of bone metastases clearly conveys a worse prognosis for patients with thyroid cancer. Although radioactive iodine therapy remains the standard of care in patients with iodine avid tumor; its efficacy for bone metastases may be limited. Patients with skeletal metastases often require additional adjuvant therapy to alleviate symptomatic disease, prolong survival, and in some cases even render them free of disease. Surgery, EBRT, IMRT, cryotherapy, RFA, vertebroplasty, embolization, bisphosphonates, and denosumab are all important components of a comprehensive management strategy for patients with bone lesions. Tyrosine kinase inhibitors and other drugs that target molecular defects in thyroid cancer cells are undergoing clinical trials (and showing promise) in patients with progressive disease who are unresponsive to radioiodine, though their efficacy in those with bone metastases may be limited. A multidisciplinary team of experts in thyroid cancer management, including endocrinologists, surgeons, radiologists, pathologists, nuclear medicine physicians, and radiation oncologists may provide patients with the wide-ranging approach to their care that may ultimately lead to improved survival and a better quality of life. With the application of newer therapies beyond I-131 for those with bone metastases from thyroid cancer, in conjunction with ongoing research into novel targets for thyroid cancer treatment, patients may realize a dramatic improvement in their long-term survival.

References

1. Davies L, Welch HG. Increasing incidence of thyroid cancer in the United States, 1973–2002. JAMA. 2006;295:2164–7.
2. Enewold L, Zhu K, Ron E, Marrogi AJ, Stojadinovic A, Peoples GE, Devesa SS. Rising thyroid cancer incidence in the United States by demographic and tumor characteristics, 1980–2005. Cancer Epidemiol Biomarkers Prev. 2009;18:784–91.
3. Chen AY, Jemal A, Ward EM. Increasing incidence of differentiated thyroid cancer in the United States, 1988–2005. Cancer. 2009;115:3801–7.
4. Giusti F, Falchetti A, Franceschelli F, Marini F, Tanini A, Brandi ML. Thyroid cancer: current molecular perspectives. J Oncol. 2010;2010:351679.
5. McLeod DS. Current concepts and future directions in differentiated thyroid cancer. Clin Biochem Rev. 2010;31:9–19.
6. Haugen BR, Alexander EK, Bible KC, Doherty GM, Mandel SJ, Nikiforov Y, Pacini F, Randolph G, Sawka A, Shepard D, Sosa J, Tuttle RM, Wartofsky L. 2015 American Thyroid Association Management Guidelines for adult patients with thyroid nodules and differentiated thyroid cancer. Available online at Thyroid 25: DOI:10.1089/thy.2015.0020; print version in Thyroid 26:1–133, 2016.
7. Sturgeon C, Angelos P. Identification and treatment of aggressive thyroid cancers. Part 1: subtypes. Oncology (Williston Park). 2006; 20:253–60.
8. Pacini F, Schlumberger M, Dralle H, Elisei R, Smit JW, Wiersinga W, European Thyroid Cancer Taskforce. European consensus for the management of patients with differentiated thyroid carcinoma of the follicular epithelium. Eur J Endocrinol. 2006;154:787–803.
9. Durante C, Haddy N, Baudin E, Leboulleux S, Hartl D, Travagli JP, Caillou B, Ricard M, Lumbroso JD, De Vathaire F, Schlumberger M. Long-term outcome of 444 patients with distant metastases from papillary and follicular thyroid carcinoma: benefits and limits of radioiodine therapy. J Clin Endocrinol Metab. 2006;91:2892–9.
10. Fanchiang JK, Lin JD, Huang MJ, Shih HN. Papillary and follicular thyroid carcinomas with bone metastases: a series of 39 cases during a period of 18 years. Changgeng Yi Xue Za Zhi. 1998;21:377–82.
11. Schlumberger M, Challeton C, De Vathaire F, Travagli JP, Gardet P, Lumbroso JD, Francese C, Fontaine F, Ricard M, Parmentier C. Radioactive iodine treatment and external radiotherapy for lung and bone metastases from thyroid carcinoma. J Nucl Med. 1996; 37:598–605.
12. Roodman GD. Mechanisms of bone metastasis. N Engl J Med. 2004;350:1655–64.
13. Selvaggi G, Scagliotti GV. Management of bone metastases in cancer: a review. Crit Rev Oncol Hematol. 2005;56:365–78.
14. Coleman RE. Clinical features of metastatic bone disease and risk of skeletal morbidity. Clin Cancer Res. 2006;12:6243s–9.
15. Chua S, Gnanasegaran G, Cook GJ. Miscellaneous cancers (lung, thyroid, renal cancer, myeloma, and neuroendocrine tumors): role of SPECT and PET in imaging bone metastases. Semin Nucl Med. 2009;39:416–30.
16. Ito S, Kato K, Ikeda M, Iwano S, Makino N, Tadokoro M, Abe S, Nakano S, Nishino M, Ishigaki T, Naganawa S. Comparison of 18F-FDG PET and bone scintigraphy in detection of bone metastases of thyroid cancer. J Nucl Med. 2007;48:889–95.
17. Schmidt GP, Schoenberg SO, Schmid R, Stahl R, Tiling R, Becker CR, Reiser MF, Baur-Melnyk A. Screening for bone metastases: whole-body MRI using a 32-channel system versus dual-modality PET-CT. Eur Radiol. 2007;17:939–49.
18. Brage ME, Simon MA. Evaluation, prognosis, and medical treatment considerations of metastatic bone tumors. Orthopedics. 1992;15:589–96.
19. Iwata M, Kasagi K, Misaki T, Matsumoto K, Iida Y, Ishimori T, Nakamoto Y, Higashi T, Saga T, Konishi J. Comparison of whole-body 18F-FDG PET, 99mTc-MIBI SPET, and post-therapeutic 131I-Na scintigraphy in the detection of metastatic thyroid cancer. Eur J Nucl Med Mol Imaging. 2004;31:491–8.
20. Robbins RJ, Wan Q, Grewal RK, Reibke R, Gonen M, Strauss HW, Tuttle RM, Drucker W, Larson SM. Real-time prognosis for metastatic thyroid carcinoma based on 2-[18F]fluoro-2-deoxy-D-glucose-positron emission tomography scanning. J Clin Endocrinol Metab. 2006;91:498–505.
21. Schirrmeister H, Guhlmann A, Elsner K, Kotzerke J, Glatting G, Rentschler M, Neumaier B, Träger H, Nüssle K, Reske SN. Sensitivity in detecting osseous lesions depends on anatomic localization: planar bone scintigraphy versus 18F PET. J Nucl Med. 1999;40:1623–9.
22. Ota N, Kato K, Iwano S, Ito S, Abe S, Fujita N, Yamashiro K, Yamamoto S, Naganawa S. Comparison of ^{18}F-fluoride PET/CT, ^{18}F-FDG PET/CT and bone scintigraphy (planar and SPECT) in detection of bone metastases of differentiated thyroid cancer: a pilot study. Br J Radiol. 2014;87:20130444.
23. Phan HT, Jager PL, Paans AM, Plukker JT, Sturkenboom MG, Sluiter WJ, Wolffenbuttel BH, Dierckx RA, Links TP. The diagnostic value of 124I-PET in patients with differentiated thyroid cancer. Eur J Nucl Med Mol Imaging. 2008;35:958–65.
24. Freudenberg LS, Antoch G, Jentzen W, Pink R, Knust J, Görges R, Müller SP, Bockisch A, Debatin JF, Brandau W. Value of (124) I-PET/CT in staging of patients with differentiated thyroid cancer. Eur Radiol. 2004;14:2092–8.
25. Rougraff BT. Evaluation of the patient with carcinoma of unknown origin metastatic to bone. Clin Orthop Relat Res. 2003 Oct;(415 Suppl):S105–9.
26. Pacini F, Fugazzola L, Lippi F, Ceccarelli C, Centoni R, Miccoli P, Elisei R, Pinchera A. Detection of thyroglobulin in fine needle aspirates of nonthyroidal neck masses: a clue to the diagnosis of metastatic differentiated thyroid cancer. J Clin Endocrinol Metab. 1992;74:1401–4.
27. Cignarelli M, Ambrosi A, Marino A, Lamacchia O, Campo M, Picca G, Giorgino F. Diagnostic utility of thyroglobulin detection in fine-needle aspiration of cervical cystic metastatic lymph nodes from papillary thyroid cancer with negative cytology. Thyroid. 2003;13:1163–7.
28. Cunha N, Rodrigues F, Curado F, Ilhéu O, Cruz C, Naidenov P, Rascão MJ, Ganho J, Gomes I, Pereira H, Real O, Figueiredo P, Campos B, Valido F. Thyroglobulin detection in fine-needle aspirates of cervical lymph nodes: a technique for the diagnosis of metastatic differentiated thyroid cancer. Eur J Endocrinol. 2007;157:101–7.
29. Schlumberger M, Sherman SI. Clinical trials for progressive differentiated thyroid cancer: patient selection, study design, and recent advances. Thyroid. 2009;19:1393–400.
30. Hoie J, Stenwig AE, Kullmann G, Lindegaard M. Distant metastases in papillary thyroid cancer. A review of 91 patients. Cancer. 1988;61:1–6.
31. Ruegemer JJ, Hay ID, Bergstralh EJ, Ryan JJ, Offord KP, Gorman CA. Distant metastases in differentiated thyroid carcinoma: a

multivariate analysis of prognostic variables. J Clin Endocrinol Metab. 1988;67:501–8.

32. Schlumberger MJ. Papillary and follicular thyroid carcinoma. N Engl J Med. 1998;338:297–306.
33. Bernier MO, Leenhardt L, Hoang C, Aurengo A, Mary JY, Menegaux F, Enkaoua E, Turpin G, Chiras J, Saillant G, Hejblum G. Survival and therapeutic modalities in patients with bone metastases of differentiated thyroid carcinomas. J Clin Endocrinol Metab. 2001;86:1568–73.
34. Brown AP, Greening WP, McCready VR, Shaw HJ, Harmer CL. Radioiodine treatment of metastatic thyroid carcinoma: the Royal Marsden Hospital experience. Br J Radiol. 1984;57:323–7.
35. Marcocci C, Pacini F, Elisei R, Schipani E, Ceccarelli C, Miccoli P, Arganini M, Pinchera A. Clinical and biologic behavior of bone metastases from differentiated thyroid carcinoma. Surgery. 1989;106:960–6.
36. Pittas AG, Adler M, Fazzari M, Tickoo S, Rosai J, Larson SM, Robbins RJ. Bone metastases from thyroid carcinoma: clinical characteristics and prognostic variables in one hundred forty-six patients. Thyroid. 2000;10:261–8.
37. Proye CA, Dromer DH, Carnaille BM, Gontier AJ, Goropoulos A, Carpentier P, Lefebvre J, Decoulx M, Wemeau JL, Fossati P. Is it still worthwhile to treat bone metastases from differentiated thyroid carcinoma with radioactive iodine? World J Surg. 1992;16:640–5; discussion 645–6.
38. Wood WJ, Singletary SE, Hickey RC. Current results of treatment for distant metastatic well-differentiated thyroid carcinoma. Arch Surg. 1989;124:1374–7.
39. Schlumberger M, Tubiana M, De Vathaire F, Hill C, Gardet P, Travagli JP, Fragu P, Lumbroso J, Caillou B, Parmentier C. Long-term results of treatment of 283 patients with lung and bone metastases from differentiated thyroid carcinoma. J Clin Endocrinol Metab. 1986;63:960–7.
40. Lin JD, Huang MJ, Juang JH, Chao TC, Huang BY, Chen KW, Chen JY, Li KL, Chen JF, Ho YS. Factors related to the survival of papillary and follicular thyroid carcinoma patients with distant metastases. Thyroid. 1999;9:1227–35.
41. Nixon IJ, Whitcher MM, Palmer FL, Tuttle RM, Shaha AR, Shah JP, Patel SG, Ganly I. The impact of distant metastases at presentation on prognosis in patients with differentiated carcinoma of the thyroid gland. Thyroid. 2012;22:884–9.
42. Lang BH, Wong KP, Cheung CY, Wan KY, Lo CY. Evaluating the prognostic factors associated with cancer-specific survival of differentiated thyroid carcinoma presenting with distant metastasis. Ann Surg Oncol. 2013;20:1329–35.
43. Robenshtok E, Farooki A, Grewal RK, Tuttle RM. Natural history of small radioiodine-avid bone metastases that have no structural correlate on imaging studies. Endocrine. 2014 Sep;47(1):266–72. doi: 10.1007/s12020-013-0123-8. Epub 2013 Dec 24.
44. Petrich T, Widjaja A, Musholt TJ, Hofmann M, Brunkhorst T, Ehrenheim C, Oetting G, Knapp WH. Outcome after radioiodine therapy in 107 patients with differentiated thyroid carcinoma and initial bone metastases: side-effects and influence of age. Eur J Nucl Med. 2001;28:203–8.
45. Qiu ZL, Song HJ, Xu YH, Luo QY. Efficacy and survival analysis of 131I therapy for bone metastases from differentiated thyroid cancer. J Clin Endocrinol Metab. 2011;96:3078–86.
46. Khorjekar G, Van Nostrand D, Moreau S, Atkins F, Mete M, Burman K, Wartofsky L. Survival rate in patients diagnosed with well-differentiated thyroid cancer with bone metastases. J Nucl Med. 2010;51(supplement 2):1591.
47. Chiesa C, Castellani MR, Vellani C, Orunesu E, Negri A, Azzeroni R, Botta F, Maccauro M, Aliberti G, Seregni E, Lassmann M, Bombardieri E. Individualized dosimetry in the management of metastatic differentiated thyroid cancer. Q J Nucl Med Mol Imaging. 2009;53:546–61.
48. Maxon HR, Thomas SR, Hertzberg VS, Kereiakes JG, Chen IW, Sperling MI, Saenger EL. Relation between effective radiation dose and outcome of radioiodine therapy for thyroid cancer. N Engl J Med. 1983;309:937–41.
49. Maxon HR, Thomas SR, Samaratunga RC. Dosimetric considerations in the radioiodine treatment of macrometastases and micrometastases from differentiated thyroid cancer. Thyroid. 1997;7:183–7.
50. Sisson JC, Dewaraja YK, Wizauer EJ, Giordano TJ, Avram AM. Thyroid carcinoma metastasis to skull with infringement of brain: treatment with radioiodine. Thyroid. 2009;19:297–303.
51. Farooki A, Leung V, Tala H, Tuttle RM. Skeletal-related events due to bone metastases from differentiated thyroid cancer. J Clin Endocrinol Metab. 2012;97:2433–9.
52. Orita Y, Sugitani I, Toda K, Manabe J, Fujimoto Y. Zoledronic acid in the treatment of bone metastases from differentiated thyroid carcinoma. Thyroid. 2011;21:31–5.
53. Rosen HN, Moses AC, Garber J, Ross DS, Lee SL, Ferguson L, Chen V, Lee K, Greenspan SL. Randomized trial of pamidronate in patients with thyroid cancer: bone density is not reduced by suppressive doses of thyroxine, but is increased by cyclic intravenous pamidronate. J Clin Endocrinol Metab. 1998;83:2324–30.
54. Vitale G, Fonderico F, Martignetti A, Caraglia M, Ciccarelli A, Nuzzo V, Abbruzzese A, Lupoli G. Pamidronate improves the quality of life and induces clinical remission of bone metastases in patients with thyroid cancer. Br J Cancer. 2001;84:1586–90.
55. Polascik TJ. Bisphosphonates in oncology: evidence for the prevention of skeletal events in patients with bone metastases. Drug Des Dev Ther. 2009;3:27–40.
56. Fizazi K, Lipton A, Mariette X, Body JJ, Rahim Y, Gralow JR, Gao G, Wu L, Sohn W, Jun S. Randomized phase II trial of denosumab in patients with bone metastases from prostate cancer, breast cancer, or other neoplasms after intravenous bisphosphonates. J Clin Oncol. 2009;27:1564–71.
57. Stopeck AT, Lipton A, Body JJ, Steger GG, Tonkin K, de Boer RH, Lichinitser M, Fujiwara Y, Yardley DA, Viniegra M, Fan M, Jiang Q, Dansey R, Jun S, Braun A. Denosumab compared with zoledronic acid for the treatment of bone metastases in patients with advanced breast cancer: a randomized, double-blind study. J Clin Oncol. 2010;28:5132–9.
58. Rosen LS, Gordon DH, Dugan W, Major P, Eisenberg PD, Provencher L, Kaminski M, Simeone J, Seaman J, Chen BL, Coleman RE. Zoledronic acid is superior to pamidronate for the treatment of bone metastases in breast carcinoma patients with at least one osteolytic lesion. Cancer. 2004;100:36–43.
59. Pavlakis N, Schmidt R, Stockler M. Bisphosphonates for breast cancer. Cochrane Database Syst Rev. 2005 Jul 20;(3):CD003474.
60. Yuen KK, Shelley M, Sze WM, Wilt T, Mason MD. Bisphosphonates for advanced prostate cancer. Cochrane Database Syst Rev. 2006 Oct 18;(4):CD006250.
61. Perazella MA, Markowitz GS. Bisphosphonate nephrotoxicity. Kidney Int. 2008;74:1385–93.
62. Ross AC, Manson JE, Abrams SA, Aloia JF, Brannon PM, Clinton SK, Durazo-Arvizu RA, Gallagher JC, Gallo RL, Jones G, Kovacs CS, Mayne ST, Rosen CJ, Shapses SA. The 2011 report on dietary reference intakes for calcium and vitamin D from the Institute of Medicine: what clinicians need to know. J Clin Endocrinol Metab. 2011 Jan;96(1):53–8. doi: 10.1210/jc.2010-2704. Epub 2010 Nov 29.
63. Adami S, Bhalla AK, Dorizzi R, Montesanti F, Rosini S, Salvagno G, Lo Cascio V. The acute-phase response after bisphosphonate administration. Calcif Tissue Int. 1987;41:326–31.
64. Khosla S, Burr D, Cauley J, Dempster DW, Ebeling PR, Felsenberg D, Gagel RF, Gilsanz V, Guise T, Koka S, McCauley LK, McGowan J, McKee MD, Mohla S, Pendrys DG, Raisz LG, Ruggiero SL, Shafer DM, Shum L, Silverman SL, Van Poznak CH, Watts N, Woo SB, American Society for Bone and Mineral Research. Bisphosphonate-associated osteonecrosis of the jaw: report of a

task force of the American Society for Bone and Mineral Research. J Bone Miner Res. 2007;22:1479–91.
65. Woo SB, Hellstein JW, Kalmar JR. Narrative [corrected] review: bisphosphonates and osteonecrosis of the jaws. Ann Intern Med. 2006;144:753–61.
66. Visekruna M, Wilson D, McKiernan FE. Severely suppressed bone turnover and atypical skeletal fragility. J Clin Endocrinol Metab. 2008;93:2948–52.
67. Abrahamsen B, Eiken P, Eastell R. Subtrochanteric and diaphyseal femur fractures in patients treated with alendronate: a register-based national cohort study. J Bone Miner Res. 2009;24:1095–102.
68. Shane E, Burr D, Ebeling PR, Abrahamsen B, Adler RA, Brown TD, Cheung AM, Cosman F, Curtis JR, Dell R, Dempster D, Einhorn TA, Genant HK, Geusens P, Klaushofer K, Koval K, Lane JM, McKiernan F, McKinney R, Ng A, Nieves J, O'Keefe R, Papapoulos S, Sen HT, van der Meulen MC, Weinstein RS, Whyte M, American Society for Bone and Mineral Research. Atypical subtrochanteric and diaphyseal femoral fractures: report of a task force of the American Society for Bone and Mineral Research. J Bone Miner Res. 2010;25:2267–94.
69. Lam MG, de Klerk JM, van Rijk PP, Zonnenberg BA. Bone seeking radiopharmaceuticals for palliation of pain in cancer patients with osseous metastases. Anticancer Agents Med Chem. 2007;7: 381–97.
70. Storto G, Klain M, Paone G, Liuzzi R, Molino L, Marinelli A, Soricelli A, Pace L, Salvatore M. Combined therapy of Sr-89 and zoledronic acid in patients with painful bone metastases. Bone. 2006;39:35–41.
71. Satcher RL, Lin P, Harun N, Feng L, Moon BS, Lewis VO. Surgical management of appendicular skeletal metastases in thyroid carcinoma. Int J Surg Oncol. 2012;2012:417086.
72. Greenblatt DY, Chen H. Palliation of advanced thyroid malignancies. Surg Oncol. 2007;16:237–47.
73. Kushchayev S, Kushchayeva Y, Theodore N, Preul MC, Clark OH. Percutaneous vertebroplasty for thyroid cancer metastases to the spine. Thyroid. 2010;20:555–60.
74. Frassica DA. General principles of external beam radiation therapy for skeletal metastases. Clin Orthop Relat Res. 2003 Oct;(415 Suppl):S158–64.
75. Brown RL. Standard and emerging therapeutic approaches for thyroid malignancies. Semin Oncol. 2008;35:298–308.
76. O'Neill CJ, Oucharek J, Learoyd D, Sidhu SB. Standard and emerging therapies for metastatic differentiated thyroid cancer. Oncologist. 2010;15:146–56.
77. Sandri A, Carbognin G, Regis D, Gaspari D, Calciolari C, Girardi V, Mansueto G, Bartolozzi P. Combined radiofrequency and kyphoplasty in painful osteolytic metastases to vertebral bodies. Radiol Med. 2010;115:261–71.
78. Brierley JD, Tsang RW. External beam radiation therapy for thyroid cancer. Endocrinol Metab Clin N Am. 2008;37:497–509, xi.
79. Schwartz DL, Lobo MJ, Ang KK, Morrison WH, Rosenthal DI, Ahamad A, Evans DB, Clayman G, Sherman SI, Garden AS. Postoperative external beam radiotherapy for differentiated thyroid cancer: outcomes and morbidity with conformal treatment. Int J Radiat Oncol Biol Phys. 2009;74:1083–91.
80. Toyota N, Naito A, Kakizawa H, Hieda M, Hirai N, Tachikake T, Kimura T, Fukuda H, Ito K. Radiofrequency ablation therapy combined with cementoplasty for painful bone metastases: initial experience. Cardiovasc Intervent Radiol. 2005;28: 578–83.
81. Monchik JM, Donatini G, Iannuccilli J, Dupuy DE. Radiofrequency ablation and percutaneous ethanol injection treatment for recurrent local and distant well-differentiated thyroid carcinoma. Ann Surg. 2006;244:296–304.
82. Hoffmann RT, Jakobs TF, Trumm C, Weber C, Helmberger TK, Reiser MF. Radiofrequency ablation in combination with osteoplasty in the treatment of painful metastatic bone disease. J Vasc Interv Radiol. 2008;19:419–25.
83. Robinson D, Yassin M, Nevo Z. Cryotherapy of musculoskeletal tumors – from basic science to clinical results. Technol Cancer Res Treat. 2004;3:371–5.
84. Van Tol KM, Hew JM, Jager PL, Vermey A, Dullaart RP, Links TP. Embolization in combination with radioiodine therapy for bone metastases from differentiated thyroid carcinoma. Clin Endocrinol (Oxf). 2000;52:653–9.
85. Eustatia-Rutten CF, Romijn JA, Guijt MJ, Vielvoye GJ, van den Berg R, Corssmit EP, Pereira AM, Smit JW. Outcome of palliative embolization of bone metastases in differentiated thyroid carcinoma. J Clin Endocrinol Metab. 2003;88:3184–9.
86. Cohen EE, Rosen LS, Vokes EE, Kies MS, Forastiere AA, Worden FP, Kane MA, Sherman E, Kim S, Bycott P, Tortorici M, Shalinsky DR, Liau KF, Cohen RB. Axitinib is an active treatment for all histologic subtypes of advanced thyroid cancer: results from a phase II study. J Clin Oncol. 2008;26:4708–13.
87. Kloos RT, Ringel MD, Knopp MV, Hall NC, King M, Stevens R, Liang J, Wakely PE, Vasko VV, Saji M, Rittenberry J, Wei L, Arbogast D, Collamore M, Wright JJ, Grever M, Shah MH. Phase II trial of sorafenib in metastatic thyroid cancer. J Clin Oncol. 2009;27:1675–84.
88. Sherman SI, Wirth LJ, Droz JP, Hofmann M, Bastholt L, Martins RG, Licitra L, Eschenberg MJ, Sun YN, Juan T, Stepan DE, Schlumberger MJ, Motesanib Thyroid Cancer Study Group. Motesanib diphosphate in progressive differentiated thyroid cancer. N Engl J Med. 2008;359:31–42.
89. Massicotte MH, Brassard M, Claude-Desroches M, Borget I, Bonichon F, Giraudet AL, Do Cao C, Chougnet CN, Leboulleux S, Baudin E, Schlumberger M, de la Fouchardière C. Tyrosine kinase inhibitor treatments in patients with metastatic thyroid carcinomas: a retrospective study of the TUTHYREF network. Eur J Endocrinol. 2014;170:575–82.

A Summary of Rare Sites of Metastasis Secondary to Differentiated Thyroid Cancer

66

Gauri R. Khorjekar, Joanna Klubo-Gwiezdzinska, Douglas Van Nostrand, and Leonard Wartofsky

Introduction

Differentiated thyroid cancer (DTC) has a very good prognosis and good survival rates. Although most patients with DTC will never have a metastasis, the most frequent sites of metastases of DTC are the cervical lymph nodes, lung, and bone. Less frequent sites include the mediastinal lymph nodes and brain, and metastases to other sites are rare. The objectives of this chapter are to (1) list the rare sites of metastases of DTC that have been published, (2) determine the frequency of the number of reports of metastases for each rare site, and (3) describe any unique aspects of these unusual metastatic sites such as the frequency of radioiodine uptake and/or ^{18}F fluorodeoxyglucose (^{18}F-FDG) on positron emission tomography (PET).

A literature search was performed of PubMed®, Google Scholar®, and Medline® from 1966 to 2013 with keywords such as differentiated thyroid cancer, thyroid cancer metastases, struma ovarii, and organs of the body. Articles were included if DTC was histopathologically proven in the primary thyroid tumor and the metastases. Articles were excluded if the patient had poorly differentiated, medullary, or anaplastic thyroid cancers. Our review identified 264 publications, which form the basis of this chapter. Common sites of metastases in the cervical lymph nodes, lung, and bone and less frequent sites in the mediastinal lymph nodes and brain were not tabulated.

G.R. Khorjekar, MD
Division of Nuclear Medicine, Department of Medicine, MedStar Washington Hospital Center, Washington, DC, USA

J. Klubo-Gwiezdzinska, MD PhD (✉)
Combined Divisions of Endocrinology, National Institutes of Health, Bethesda, MD, USA
e-mail: joanna.klubo-gwiezdzinska@nih.gov

D. Van Nostrand, MD, FACP, FACNM
Nuclear Medicine Research, MedStar Research Institute and Washington Hospital Center, Georgetown University School of Medicine, Washington Hospital Center, 110 Irving Street, N.W., Suite GB 60F, Washington, DC 20010, USA
e-mail: douglasvannostrand@gmail.com

L. Wartofsky, MD MACP
Department of Medicine, MedStar Washington Hospital Center, Georgetown University School of Medicine, 110 Irving Street, N.W., Washington, DC 20010-2975, USA
e-mail: leonard.wartofsky@medstar.net

Rare Sites of Metastases

Sites of raremetastases were identified in 23 different areas, and these are listed in Table 66.1 from the highest to lowest number of cases reported in the literature. The most frequently reported unusual site of metastasis was the skin (82), followed by the liver (61), kidney (48), pleura (37), and eye (35). The most infrequently reported sites of metastases were the urinary bladder (3), submandibular gland (2), dura (1), and prostate (1).

Table 66.2 reflects a detailed tabulation of the rare sites of metastases. Out of all of the articles reviewed, 108 patients had radioiodine scans performed and 22 patients had PET scans performed. Radioiodine scans were positive in 53/109 patients demonstrating metastases in the skin, liver, kidney, eye, pleura, heart, adrenal, blood vessels, pericardium, soft tissue, muscle, breast, ovary, and spleen. ^{18}F-FDG activity was seen in 13/22 patients at metastatic sites such as the skin, liver, eye, pleura, blood vessels, soft tissue, muscle, and pancreas.

Sites of Metastases of DTC Originating in Struma Ovarii

DTC may also originate from struma ovarii in the ovaries. The sites of metastases from DTC originating in struma ovarii were identified in seven different areas, and these are listed in Table 66.3 from the highest to lowest number of cases reported in the literature. The most frequently reported rare

L. Wartofsky, D. Van Nostrand (eds.), *Thyroid Cancer*, DOI 10.1007/978-1-4939-3314-3_66

Table 66.1 Reported rare sites of metastases of well-differentiated thyroid cancer

Skin	82
Liver	61
Kidney	48
Pleura	37
Eye	35
Heart	32
Blood vessel	32
Adrenal	31
Pericardium	24
Parathyroid	24
Soft tissue	20
Muscle	14
Breast	10
Pancreas	8
Diaphragm	4
Gastrointestinal tract	4
Parotid gland	5
Ovary	3
Spleen	3
Urinary bladder	3
Submandibular gland	2
Dura	1
Prostate	1

sites of metastasis from struma ovarii were the contralateral peritoneum (12), ovary (10), liver (8), and diaphragm (3).

Limitation of This Literature Review

A major limitation of this review is that the frequency of rare sites of metastases reported in this chapter is not necessarily representative of the true incidence of these rate sites of metastases in patient with DTC. Rather it is representative of what has been reported in the literature. A second limitation of this study is that other case reports may have been published but were not identified to be included in this literature review. However, this review still presents a heretofore unavailable list of rare sties of metastases secondary to differentiated thyroid cancer as well as a reasonable tabulation of the frequency of those sites reported in the literature.

Conclusion

Although the common sites of metastases of differentiated thyroid cancer (DTC) include the cervical lymph nodes, lung, and bone and less frequent sites include the mediastinal

Table 66.2 Rare sites of metastases of DTC

Site of involvement	# of cases	Type of cancer	# of ^{131}I scans	# of ^{131}I pos/neg	# of ^{18}F-FDG PET scans	# of ^{18}F-FDG PET pos/neg	References
Skin	82	PTC-39, FTC-23 FVPTC-2, HCC-2, Mixed-3, NS-1	9	Pos-4 Neg-5	6	Pos-1 Neg-5	[2, 4, 8, 14, 18, 19, 31, 36, 39–42, 44, 46, 59, 60, 66, 68, 71, 85, 88, 90, 91, 94, 113, 125, 128, 130, 132, 139, 143, 146, 158, 159, 174, 177, 179–181, 186, 187, 190, 191, 194, 195, 199, 200, 213, 227, 232, 233, 236, 243, 247]
Liver	61	PTC-10, FTC-36, DTC NS-9, Mixed-4	7	Pos-5 Neg-2	1	Pos-1	[17, 22, 38, 43, 66, 73, 76, 81, 84, 88, 105, 111, 114, 115, 118, 139, 163, 202, 211, 216, 221, 239, 253, 254, 255]
Kidney	48	PTC-13, FTC-17, FVPTC-2, Mixed-2, NS-8, FTCA-1, CC-1	10	Pos-7 Neg-3	2	Neg-2	[1, 5, 27, 49, 57, 64, 73, 75, 77, 80, 88, 96, 100, 120, 122, 124, 129, 133, 136, 139, 140, 153, 156, 193, 198, 205, 206, 216, 220, 224, 239, 248, 256, 262]
Pleura	37	PTC-10, FTC-13, FVPTC-2, HCC-1, NS-8, PM-1	9	Pos-3 Neg-6	1	Pos-1	[6, 56, 86, 88, 92, 97, 98, 117, 119, 139, 145, 149, 176, 196, 214, 244, 245, 246]
Eye	35	PTC-12, FTC-12, FVPTC-1, HCC-3, PTCA-2, NS-2, CCTC-1, TCVPTC-1, SCC-1	16	Pos-9 Neg-7	2	Pos-2	[4, 13, 14, 19, 24, 28–32, 36, 39, 55, 62, 69, 73, 74, 110, 127, 134, 152, 157, 162, 168, 184, 189, 192, 207, 208, 217, 219, 234, 241, 252, 261]

(continued)

Table 66.2 (continued)

Site of involvement	# of cases	Type of cancer	# of ^{131}I scans	# of ^{131}I pos/neg	# of ^{18}F-FDG PET scans	# of ^{18}F-FDG PET pos/neg	References
Heart	32	PTC-10, FTC-12, HCC-2, Mixed-4, SCC-1, PTCA-1, NS-1	6	Pos-1 Neg-5	–	–	[11, 48, 56, 67, 70, 79, 86, 89, 95, 104, 107, 108, 123, 154, 160, 178, 183, 212, 216, 231, 237, 257]
Blood vessels	32	PTC-10, FTC-12, FVPTC-1, HCC-4, NS-1, Mixed-1	11	Pos-6 Neg-5	2	Pos-2	[3, 10, 20, 67, 83, 93, 108, 112, 121, 148, 155, 158, 160, 165, 167, 173, 176, 203, 218, 231, 235, 242, 249, 259]
Adrenal	31	PTC-17, FTC-9, Mixed-4	5	Pos-3 Neg-2	–	–	[25, 33, 66, 78, 85, 116, 120, 133, 166, 171, 216]
Pericardium	24	PTC-6, FTC-12, NS-4, PTCA-1, OPTC-1	4	Pos-2 Neg-2	1	Neg-1	[51, 76, 87, 88, 97, 117, 138, 237]
Parathyroid	24	PTC-20, FTC-3	–	–	–	–	[54, 101, 228]
Soft tissue	20	PTC-4, FTC-13, FVPTC-1, NS-1, FTCA-1	9	Pos-3 Neg-6	2	Pos-2	[6, 40, 47, 144, 147, 164, 179, 182, 188, 194, 209, 223, 230, 232, 250]
Muscle	14	PTC-7, FTC-2, FVPTC-1, NS-2, PMC-1	7	Pos-5 Neg-2	1	Pos-1	[21, 45, 56, 74, 129, 151, 169, 178, 185, 223, 238, 264]
Breast	8	PTC-2, FTC-2, FVPTC-1, HCC-2, TCVPTC-1	3	Pos-2 Neg-1	–	–	[6, 7, 12, 16, 26, 52, 58, 72, 128, 226]
Pancreas	8	PTC-4, FVPTC-1, TCVPTC-2, NS-1	5	Neg-5	3	Pos-3	[9, 12, 35, 99, 146, 215, 222]
Diaphragm	4	NS-4	–	–	–	–	[73]
GI	4	FTC-2, FVPTC-1, HCC-1	2	Neg-2	1	Neg-1	[15, 88, 111]
Parotid	5	PTC-2, FTC-1, CPTC-1	–	–	–	–	[10, 109, 137, 138, 141]
Ovary	3	PTC-2, FTC-1	1	Pos-1	–	–	[37, 126, 260]
Spleen	3	PTC-1, FTC-1, FVPTC-1	3	Pos-2 Neg-1	–	–	[102, 150, 170]
Urinary bladder	3	FTC-2, NS-1	1	Neg-1	–	–	[82, 103, 175]
Submandibular gland	2	PTC-1, PMC-1	–	–	–	–	[63, 204]
Dura	1	–	–	–	–	–	[229]
Prostate	1	PTC	1	Neg-1	1	Pos-1	[258]

PTC papillary thyroid cancer
PMC papillary microcarcinoma
FTC follicular thyroid cancer
DTC differentiated thyroid cancer
FVPTC follicular variant papillary thyroid cancer
TCVPTC tall cell variant papillary thyroid cancer
HCC Hürthle cell cancer
SCC squamous cell cancer
CC clear cell thyroid carcinoma
CPTC columnar papillary thyroid cancer
OCPTC occult papillary thyroid cancer
PMC papillary thyroid microcarcinoma
NS not specified
Neg negative
Pos positive

Table 66.3 Metastases from malignant struma ovarii

Peritoneum	12 [53, 61, 65, 135, 161, 172, 201, 225, 240, 251, 263]
Contralateral ovary	10 [34, 61, 161, 210, 251]
Liver	8 [50, 106, 114, 131, 135, 142, 197, 201]
Diaphragm	3 [106, 201, 240]
Omentum	2 [23, 172]
Pleura	1 [190]
Spleen	1 [240]

lymph nodes and brain, DTC may metastasize to many other organs. With an understanding of the different organs that DTC may metastasize to, the managing physician will be less likely to exclude DTC. Although struma ovarii is rare and the primary site of DTC is infrequent in struma ovarii, one should consider struma ovarii as the primary site of DTC when DTC is found in metastases in the abdomen such as the peritoneum, ovary, omentum, mesentery, diaphragm, and/or spleen.

References

1. Abe K, Hasegawa T, Onodera S, et al. Renal metastasis of thyroid carcinoma. Int J Urol. 2002;9:656–8.
2. Agarwal S, Rao S, Arya A, Gupta K, Rashmi A, Indrani D. Follicular thyroid carcinoma with metastasis to skin diagnosed by fine needle aspiration cytology. Int J Pathol Microbiol. 2008;51:430–1.
3. Agrawal A, Agrawal R, Asopa R. Detection of metastases to internal jugular vein and superior vena cava on 131-I scan. Clin Nucl Med. 2009;34:934–5.
4. Ahmadi MA, Nicholes D, Esmaeli B. Late choroidal metastasis secondary to papillary thyroid carcinoma. Am J Ophthalmol. 2001;132:796–8.
5. Ahmed M, Aslam M, Ahmed J, et al. Renal metastases from thyroid cancer masquerading as renal angiomyolipoma on ultrasonography. J Ultrasound Med. 2006;25:1459–64.
6. Akcay MN, Akcay G, Bilen H, Atlas E, Gundognu C. Unusual presentation of thyroid cancer four cases. Endocrinologist. 2006;16:136–9.
7. Al-Abed Y, Gray E, Wolfe K, Watters GW, Philpott JM. Metastatic Hürthle cell carcinoma of the thyroid presenting as a breast lump: a case report. Int Sem Surg Oncol. 2008;5:14.
8. Alwaheeb S, Ghazarian D, Boerner SL, Asa SL. Cutaneous manifestations of thyroid cancer: a report of 4 cases and a review of literature. J Clin Pathol. 2004;57:435–8.
9. Alzahrani AS, Al Qaraawi A, Al Sohaibani F, Almanea H, Abalkhail. Pancreatic metastasis arising from a BRAFV600E-positive papillary thyroid cancer: the role of endoscopic ultrasound-guided biopsy and response to sorafenib therapy. Thyroid. 2012;22:536–41.
10. Alzaraa A, Stone J, Williams G, Ahmed I, Quraishi M. Direct spread of thyroid follicular carcinoma to the parotid gland and the internal jugular vein: a case report. J Med Case Rep. 2008;2:297.
11. Anand KA, Manohar SRK, Harikrishnan S, Neelakandhan KS. Right ventricular mass: a histopathological surprise. Ann Thorac Surg. 2003;75:1969–71.
12. Angeles AA, Chable MF, Martinez BB, Albores S. Unusual metastases of papillary thyroid carcinoma: report of 2 cases. Ann Diagn Pathol. 2009;13:189–96.
13. Anteby I, Pe'er J, Uziely B, Krausz Y. Thyroid carcinoma metastasis to the choroid responding to systemic ^{131}I therapy. Am J Ophthalmol. 1992;113:461–2.
14. Arat YO, Boniuk M. Red lesions of the iris, choroid, and skin secondary to metastatic carcinoma of the thyroid: a review. Surv Ophthalmol. 2007;52:523–8.
15. Arnous W, Beltran S, Berger N, et al. Hürthle cell thyroid carcinoma metastatic to the sigmoid colon. Thyroid. 2007;17:169–73.
16. Ascani S, Nati S, Liberati F, Farabi R. Breast metastasis of thyroid follicular carcinoma. Acta Oncol. 1994;33:71–3.
17. Atmaran SH, Ganatra RD, Sharma SM, Ramanna L. Functioning metastases in liver from thyroid carcinoma: case report. J Nucl Med. 1975;16:919–21.
18. Auty RM. Dermal metastases from a follicular carcinoma of the thyroid. Arch Dermatol. 1977;113:675–6.
19. Avram AM, Gielczyk R, Su L, Vine AK, Sisson JC. Choroid and skin metastases from papillary thyroid cancer: case and a review of the literature. J Clin Endocrinol Metab. 2004;89:5303–7.
20. Babu S, Slih S, Kumar V, Satheesan B. Intravenous tumour thrombus from papillary carcinoma of thyroid-a case report & review of literature. Indian J Surg Oncol. 2012;3:206–7.
21. Bae SY, Lee SK, Koo MY, et al. Distant, solitary skeletal muscle metastasis in recurrent papillary thyroid carcinoma. Thyroid. 2011;21:1027–31.
22. Bakheet SM, Powe J, Muhammad M, et al. Isolated porta hepatis metastasis of papillary thyroid cancer. J Nucl Med. 1994;37:993–4.
23. Baldauf P, Koecer T. 29-jaehrige Schwangere mit uebelkeit und akutem abdomen. Der Gynaekologe. 2010;43:1028–32.
24. Basu S, Nair N, Aravind N. Unilateral proptosis with thyrotoxicosis resulting from solitary retroorbital soft tissue metastasis from follicular carcinoma thyroid. Clin Nucl Med. 2001;26:136–8.
25. Batawil N. Papillary thyroid cancer with bilateral adrenal metastases. Thyroid. 2013;23:1651–4.
26. Belous TA, Efimova O. A rare case of breast metastasis from thyroid cancer in a man. Arkh Patol. 1983;45:72–5.
27. Benchekroun A, Lachkar A, Alami M, et al. Renal metastasis from carcinoma of the thyroid. A case report. Ann Urol. 1999;33:51–4.
28. Bernstein-Lipschitz L, Lahav M, Chen V, Gutman I, Gall R, Lipschitz M. Metastatic thyroid carcinoma masquerading as lacrimal gland tumor. Graefes Arch Clin Exp Ophthalmol. 1990;228:112–5.
29. Besic N, Luznik Z. Choroidal and orbital metastases from thyroid cancer. Thyroid. 2013;23:543–51.
30. Betharia SM. Metastatic orbital carcinoma of thyroid. Indian J Ophthalmol. 1985;33:191–3.
31. Bhansali A, Dutta P, Reddy KS, et al. Unusual presentations of differentiated thyroid cancer: analysis of 55 cases from North India. Ann Saudi Med. 2005;25:428–32.
32. Biswas J, Kumar KS, Shanmugam MP, Raghavendran SR. Clear cell thyroid carcinoma metastatic to choroid: clinicopathological study of a case. Eye. 2000;14:394–5.
33. Blanchet MC, Van Box Sam P, Peix JL. Métastases surrénaliennes des cancer thyroidïens. Presse Med. 1997;26:1239–40.
34. Bolat F, Erkanli S, Kajaseselcuk F, Aslan E, Tuncer I. Malignant struma ovarii: a case report. Pathol Res Pract. 2005;201:409–12.
35. Borschitz T, Eichhorn W, Fottner C, et al. Diagnosis and treatment of pancreatic metastases of a papillary thyroid carcinoma. Thyroid. 2010;20:93–8.
36. Boughtattas S, Hassine H, Chatti K, Jomaa R, Essabbah H. Cutaneous metastasis revealing a widely disseminated follicular thyroid carcinoma. Clin Nucl Med. 2002;27:379–80.
37. Brogioni S, Viacava P, Tomisti L, Martino E, Macchia E. A special case of bilateral ovarian metastases in a woman with papillary car-

cinoma of the thyroid. Exp Clin Endocrinol Diabetes. 2007;115:397–400.
38. Brown AP, Greening WP, McCready VR, Shaw HJ, Harmer CL. Radioiodine treatment of metastatic thyroid carcinoma: the Royal Marsden Hospital experience. Brit J Rad. 1984;57:323–7.
39. Bucerius J, Meyka S, Michael B, Biersack HJ, Eter N. Papillary thyroid carcinoma with an uncommon spread of hematogenous metastases to the choroid and the skin. J Natl Med Assoc. 2008;100:104–7.
40. Califano I, Quildrian S, Coduti M, Bilbao ER, Otero J, Califano L. Soft tissue metastases from differentiated thyroid cancer diagnosed by 18F FDG PET-CT. Arq Bras Endocrinol Metab. 2013;57:317–21.
41. Caron P, Moreau-Cabarrot A, Gorguet B, Bazex J. Cutaneous metastasis from follicular carcinoma of the thyroid gland. Thyroid. 1993;3:235–7.
42. Carsuzaa F, Marlier S, de Jaureguiberry JP, Arnoux D, Jaubert D. Cutaneous metastasis diagnosed simultaneously with a vesicular carcinoma of the thyroid. (in french). Presse Med. 1992;21:1730.
43. Casara D, Busnardo B, Climitan M. Liver metastases from differentiated thyroid carcinoma. J Nucl Med Allied Sci. 1981;25:53–4.
44. Chadlou R, Beiss B, Ehring F. Klinisches bild und lokalisation hautmetastasen viszeraler karzinome. Hautartzt. 1978;29:259–65.
45. Chaffanjon PCJ, Stur N, Caravel JP, et al. Pelvic muscular metastasis of well differentiated thyroid carcinoma. Ann Chir. 2004;129:100–2.
46. Chakraborty J, Bandyopadhyay A, Choudhuri MK, Mitra K, Guha D, Mallik M. Cutaneous metastasis from follicular variant of papillary thyroid carcinoma: a case diagnosed on cytology. Indian J Pathol Microbiol. 2008;51:91–3.
47. Chaturvedy G, Kumar R, Sikka K, Karthikeyan CV, Mathur SR. An unusual site of distant metastasis in carcinoma of the thyroid. Indian J Cancer. 2010;47:479–80.
48. Chen K, Chou Y, Cheng A. Primary squamous cell carcinoma of the thyroid with cardiac metastases and right ventricle outflow tract obstruction. J Clin Oncol. 2012;30:260–3.
49. Cheon M, Choi JY, Kim HK, et al. Renal metastasis from follicular thyroid carcinoma diagnosed by I-131 whole-body scan mimicking renal cell carcinoma on contrast-enhanced computed tomography. Nucl Med Mol Imaging. 2011;45:72–5.
50. Cherng SC, Wang YF, Fan YM, et al. Malignant struma ovarii: an unusual presentation. Thyroid. 2001;11:889–92.
51. Chiewvit S, Pusuwan P, Chiewvit P, Pleehachinda R, Attanatho V, Mongkharuk J. Metastatic follicular carcinoma of thyroid to pericardium. J Med Assoc Thai. 1998;81:799–802.
52. Chisholm RC, Chung EB, Tuckson W, Khan T, White JE. Follicular carcinoma of the thyroid with metastasis to the breast. J Natl Med Assoc. 1980;72:1101–4.
53. Choi BR, Kim BW, Yoon SO, Kim YT, Lee S, Kim JH. Peritoneal dissemination of follicular carcinoma arising from struma ovarii in a pregnant woman. Korean J Obstet Gynaecol. 2012;55:1006–9.
54. Chrisoulidou A, Mandanas S, Mitsakis P, et al. Parathyroid involvement in thyroid cancer: an unforeseen event. World J Surg Oncol. 2012;10:1–5.
55. Chtourou I, Khabir A, Benzina Z, Bahri I, Hajji D, Boudawara TS. Iris metastatic thyroid follicular carcinoma: a case report. J Fr Ophthalmol. 2006;29:e21.
56. Clare-Salzler MJ, Van Herle AJ, Varki NM, Tillisch J. Endocardial metastases of follicular thyroid carcinoma: a case report and review of the literature. Eur J Surg Oncol. 1991;17:219–23.
57. Cochetti G, Puxeddu E, Del Zingaro M, et al. Laparascopic partial nephrectomy of thyroid cancer metastasis: case report and review of the literature. Oncol Targets Ther. 2013;6:355–60.
58. Cristallini EG, Ascani S, Nati S, Liberati F, Farabi R. Breast metastasis of thyroid follicular carcinoma. Acta Oncol. 1994;33:71–3.
59. Cupisti K, Ramp U, Raffel A, Krausch M, Rehders A, Knoefel WT. Multiple giant scalp metastases of a follicular thyroid carcinoma. World J Surg Oncol. 2008;6:82.
60. Dahl PR, Brodland DG, Goellner JR, Hay ID. Thyroid carcinoma metastatic to the skin: a cutaneous manifestation of widely disseminated malignancy. J Am Acad Dermatol. 1997;36:531–7.
61. Dardik RB, Dardik M, Westra W, Montz F. Malignant struma ovarii: two case reports and a review of literature. Gynecol Oncol. 1994;73:447–51.
62. Daumerie C, De Potter P, Godraind C, Rahier J, Jamar F, Squifflet JP. Orbital metastasis as primary manifestation of thyroid carcinoma. Thyroid. 2000;10:189–92.
63. Davies RJ, Pring M, Aw J, Hughes CW, Thomas SJ. Isolated submandibular metastasis from a contralateral thyroid papillary microcarcinoma: an unusual case. Dentomaxillofacial Radiol. 2009;38:546–9.
64. Davis RJ, Corson JM. Renal metastases from well-differentiated thyroid carcinoma. Cancer. 1979;43:265.
65. Devaney K, Snyder R, Norris HJ, Tavassoli FA. Proliferative and histologically malignant struma ovarii: a clinicopathologic study of 54 cases. Int J Gynecol Pathol. 1993;12:333–43.
66. Dinneen SF, Valimaki MJ, Bergstrahl EJ, Goellner JR, Gorman CA, Hay ID. Distant metastases in papillary thyroid carcinoma: 100 cases observed at one institution during 5 decades. J Clin Endocrinol Metab. 1995;80:2041–5.
67. Dogan OF, Hanci D, Sungur A, Unal OF, Demircin M. An unusual case of thyroid Hürthle cell carcinoma with direct extension to the right brachiocephalic vein, right auricle, and right atrium: case report. Heart Surg Forum. 2005;8:e114–7.
68. Doutre MS, Beylot S, Baquey A, et al. Cutaneous metastasis from papillary carcinoma of the thyroid. Dermatologica. 1988;177:241–3.
69. Dutton JJ, Barbour HL. Hürthle cell carcinoma metastatic to the uvea. Cancer. 1994;73:163–7.
70. Eichfeld U, Herrmann M, Schwarz I. Manifestation of isolated heart metastasis in follicular thyroid cancer (case report). Z Arztl Fortbild. 1994;88:55–7.
71. Elgart GW, Patterson JW, Taylor R. Cutaneous metastasis from papillary carcinoma of the thyroid gland. J Am Acad Dermatol. 1991;25:404–8.
72. Fiche M, Cassagnau E, Aillet G, et al. Breast metastasis from a "tall cell variant" of papillary thyroid carcinoma. Ann Pathol. 1998;18:130–2.
73. Filho F, Lima G, Ferrerira F, Lima M, Hissa M. Orbital metastasis as primary clinical manifestation of thyroid carcinoma: case report and literature review. Arq Bras Endocrinol Metab. 2008;52:1497–500.
74. Friedman J, Karesh J, Rodrigues M, Sun CC. Thyroid carcinoma metastatic to the medial rectus muscle. Ophthal Plast Reconstr Surg. 1990;6:122–5.
75. Gamboa-Dominguez A, Tenorico-Villarvazo A. Metastatic follicular variant of papillary thyroid carcinoma manifested as a primary renal neoplasm. Endocr Pathol. 1999;10:256–68.
76. Garcia F, Merino T, Ponce M, Pinon S. Metástasis poco habituales del carcinoma diferenciado de tiroides. (in spanish). An Med Interna. 2002;19:579–82.
77. Garcia-Sanchis L, Lopez-Aznar D, Oltra A, Rivas A, Alonso J, Montalar J, Mateo. A metastatic follicular thyroid carcinoma to the kidney: a case report. Clin Nucl Med. 1999;24:48–50.
78. Girelli ME, Casara D, Rubello D, et al. Metastatic thyroid carcinoma of the adrenal gland. J Endocrinol Invest. 1993;16:139–41.
79. Glaser M, Parry R, Davis K. Papillary carcinoma of the thyroid with cardiac metastases. Br J Clin Pract. 1981;35:52–3.

80. Graham LD, Roe SM. Metastatic papillary thyroid carcinoma presenting as a primary renal neoplasm. Am Surg. 1995;61:732–4.
81. Graves MW, Zukerberg B, Walace K, Duncan D, Scheff A. Isolated liver metastases from follicular thyroid cancer. Clin Nucl Med. 1996;21:147–8.
82. Grivas N, Housianitis Z, Doukas M, Stravropoulos NE. Follicular thyroid cancer metastasis to the urinary bladder: a report of a case and review of the literature. Case Rep Urol. 2012;2012:1–2.
83. Gross M, Mintz Y, Maly B, Pinchas R, Muggia-Sullam M. Internal jugular vein tumor thrombus associated with thyroid carcinoma. Ann Otol Rhinol Laryngol. 2003;113:738–40.
84. Guglielmi R, Pacella CM, Dottorini ME, et al. Severe thyrotoxicosis due to hyperfunctioning liver metastasis from follicular carcinoma: treatment with ^{131}I and interstitial laser ablation. Thyroid. 1999;9:173–7.
85. Hamilton D. Cutaneous metastases from follicular thyroid carcinoma. J Dermatol Surg Oncol. 1980;6:116–7.
86. Hasegawa S, Otake Y, Bando T, Cho H, Inui K, Wada H. Pulmonary dissemination of tumor cells after extended resection of thyroid carcinoma with cardiopulmonary bypass. J Thorac Cardiovasc Surg. 2002;124:635–6.
87. Haskell RJ, French WJ. Cardiac tamponade as the initial presentation of malignancy. Chest. 1985;88:70–3.
88. Heitz P, Moser H, Staub JJ. Thyroid cancer: a study of 573 thyroid tumors and 161 autopsy cases observed over a thirty-year period. Cancer. 1976;37:2329–37.
89. Hirnle T, Szymczak J, Ziółkowski P, Lenartowska L. Ectopic thyroid malignancy in the right ventricle of the heart. Eur J Cardiothorac Surg. 1997;12:147–9.
90. Hoie J, Stenwig AE, Kullmann G, Lindegard. Distant metastases in papillary thyroid cancer: a review of 91 patients. Cancer. 1988;61:1–6.
91. Horiguchi Y, Takahashi C, Mamura S. Cutaneous metastasis from papillary carcinoma of the thyroid gland: report of two cases. J Am Acad Dermatol. 1984;10:988–92.
92. Hsu KF, Hsieh CB, Duh QY, Chien CF, Li HS, Shih ML. Hürthle cell carcinoma of the thyroid with contralateral malignant pleural effusion. Onkologie. 2009;32:47–9.
93. Hyer SL, Dandekar P, Newbold K, Haq M, Wechalakar K, Harmer C. Thyroid cancer causing obstruction of the great veins in the neck. World J Surg Oncol. 2008;6:36.
94. Ibanez ML, Russell WO, Albores-Saavedra J, Lampertico P, White EC, Clark RL. Thyroid carcinoma: biologic behavior and mortality. Cancer. 1966;19:1039–52.
95. Inoue N, Takabuchi H, Tsuji T. Echocardiographic findings of metastatic thyroid cancer in the right atrial cavity originated in the right internal jugular vein. J Med Ultrason. 1984;11:605.
96. Insabato L, Di Vizio D, De Rose G, Prezioso D, Corcione F, Terracciano L. Renal metastasis from thyroid carcinoma 35 years after detection of the primary tumor. Tumori. 2003;89:99–101.
97. Jancic-Zguricas M, Jankovic R. Occult papillary carcinoma of the thyroid gland revealed by cancer pericarditis. Pathol Res Pract. 1986;181:761–4.
98. Jeon MJ, Yim JH, Kim EY, et al. Four cases of malignant pleural effusion in patients with papillary thyroid carcinoma. Endocrinol Metab. 2011;26:330–4.
99. Jobran R, Baloch ZW, Aviles V, Rosato EF, Schwartz S, LiVolsi VA. Tall cell papillary carcinoma of the thyroid: metastatic to the pancreas. Thyroid. 2000;10(2):185–7.
100. Johnson MW, Morretin LB, Sarles HE, Zaharapoulus P. Follicular carcinoma of the thyroid metastases to kidney 37 years after resection of the primary tumor. J Urol. 1982;127:114–6.
101. Kakudo K, Tang W, Ito Y, et al. Parathyroid invasion, nodal recurrence, and lung metastasis by papillary carcinoma of the thyroid. J Clin Pathol. 2004;54:245–9.
102. Kand P, Asopa R. Metastatic involvement of the spleen in differentiated carcinoma of thyroid. Indian J Nucl Med. 2010;25:171–2.
103. Kaplan AS, Van Heerden JA, McMahon MM. Follicular carcinoma of the thyroid presenting with hematuria: a case report. Surgery. 1986;100:572–5.
104. Kasprzak JD, Religa W, Krzemińska-Pakula M, Marszal-Marciniak M, Zaslonka J, Pawlowski W. Right ventricular outflow tract obstruction by cardiac metastasis as the first manifestation of follicular thyroid carcinoma. J Am Soc Echocardiogr. 1996;9:733–5.
105. Kelessis NG, Evangelos PP, Dimitra DV, Nikiforos AA, Pericles VP. Unusual metastatic spread of follicular thyroid carcinoma: report of a case. Surg Today. 2005;35:300–3.
106. Kempers RD, Dockerty MB, Hoffman DL, et al. Struma ovarii: ascetic, hyperthyroid, and asymptomatic syndromes. Ann Intern Med. 1970;72:883–93.
107. Kim G, Fallon J, Batheja N. Hürthle cell carcinoma with cardiac metastasis. Thyroid. 2000;10:443–4.
108. Kim RH, Mautner L, Henning J, Volpe R. An unusual case of thyroid carcinoma with direct extension to great veins, right heart, and pulmonary arteries. Can Med Assoc J. 1966;94:238–43.
109. Kini H, Pai R, Kalpana S. Solitary parotid metastasis from columnar cell carcinoma of the thyroid. Diagn Cytopathol. 2000;28:72–5.
110. Kiratli H, Tarlan B, Soylemezoglu F. Papillary thyroid carcinoma: bilateral choroid metastases with extrascleral extension. Korean J Ophthalmol. 2013;27:215–8.
111. Klubo-Gwiezdzinska J, Morowitz D, Van Nostrand D, et al. Metastases of well-differentiated thyroid cancer to the gastrointestinal system. Thyroid. 2010;20:381–7.
112. Koike E, Yamashita H, Watanabe S, Yamashita H, Noguchi S. Brachiocephalic vein thrombus of papillary thyroid cancer: report of a case. Surg Today. 2002;32:59–62.
113. Koller EA, Tourtelot JB, Pak HS, Cobb MW, Moad JC, Flynn EA. Papillary and follicular thyroid carcinoma metastatic to the skin: a case report and review of the literature. Thyroid. 1998;8:1045–50.
114. Konez O, Hanelin LG, Jenison EL, et al. Functioning liver metastases on an I-131 whole-body scan: a case of malignant struma ovarii. Clin Nucl Med. 2000;25:465–96.
115. Kouso H, Ikegami T, Ezaki T, et al. Liver metastases from thyroid carcinoma 32 years after resection of primary tumour: report of a case. Surg Today. 2005;35:480–2.
116. Koutkia P, Safer JD. Adrenal metastasis secondary to papillary thyroid carcinoma. Thyroid. 2001;11:1077–9.
117. Kovacs CS, Nguyen GK, Mullen JC, Crockford PM. Cardiac tamponade as the initial presentation of papillary thyroid carcinoma. Can J Cardiol. 1994;10:279–81.
118. Kraft O. Hepatic metastasis of differentiated thyroid carcinoma. Nucl Med Rev Cent East Eur. 2005;8:44–6.
119. Krishnamurthy A, Siddappa KT. Papillary thyroid carcinoma with malignant pleural effusion: dilemma of etiology. Int J Head Neck Surg. 2010;1:117–9.
120. Kumar A, Nadig M, Patra V, Srivastav DN, Verma K, Bal CS. Adrenal and renal metastases from follicular thyroid cancer. Brit J Med. 2005;78:1038–41.
121. Lalak NJ, Campbell PR. Infiltrating papillary carcinoma of the thyroid with macroscopic extension into the jugular vein. Otolaryngol Head Neck Surg. 1997;117:S228–30.
122. Lam KY, Ng WK. Follicular carcinoma of the thyroid appearing as solitary renal mass. Nephron. 1996;73:323–4.
123. Larsimont D, Renard Nm Andry G. Death from myocardial metastasis of thyroid cancers (insular, papillary with undifferentiated foci). Ann Chir. 1998;52:465–8.

124. Liou MJ, Lin JD, Chung MH, Liau CT, Hsueh C. Renal metastasis from papillary thyroid microcarcinoma. Acta Otolaryngol. 2005;125:438–42.
125. Lissak B, Vannetzel JM, Gallouedec N, Berrod JL, Rieu M. Solitary skin metastasis as the presenting feature of differentiated thyroid microcarcinoma: report of two cases. J Endocrinol Invest. 1995;18:813–6.
126. Logani S, Baloch ZW, Snyder PJ, Weinstein R, LiVolsi VA. Cystic ovarian metastasis from papillary thyroid carcinoma: a case report. Thyroid. 2001;11:1073–5.
127. Lommatzsch PK. Metastasis of differentiated follicular thyroid carcinoma to the ciliary body. Klin Monatsbl Augenheilkd. 1994;205:309–13.
128. Loureiro MM, Leite VH, Boavida JM, et al. An unusual case of papillary carcinoma of the thyroid with cutaneous and breast metastases only. Eur J Endocrinol. 1997;137:267–9.
129. Luo Q, Luo QY, Sheng SW, et al. Localization of concomitant metastases to kidney and erector spinae from papillary thyroid carcinoma using ^{131}I-SPECT and CT. Thyroid. 2008;18:663–4.
130. Luo QY, Luo Q, Chen LB, Yu YL, Lu HK, Zhu RS. Multiple subdermal metastases from papillary thyroid cancer. Thyroid. 2008;18:907–8.
131. Makni S, Bahri I, Ellouz S, et al. Malignant struma ovarii: a case report. J Gynecol Obstet Biol Reprod. 2005;34:815–8.
132. Makris A, Goepel JR. Cutaneous metastases from a thyroid carcinoma [letter]. Br J Dermatol. 1996;136:860.
133. Malhotra G, Upadhye T, Sridhar E, et al. Unusual case of adrenal and renal metastases from papillary carcinoma of thyroid. Clin Nucl Med. 2010;35:731–6.
134. Mansberg R, Son H, Kean AM. Occult carcinoma of the thyroid presenting with orbital metastasis. Clin Nucl Med. 2008;31:109–11.
135. Marcy PV, Thariat T, Benisvy D, Azuar P. Lethal malignant, metastatic struma ovarii. Thyroid. 2010;20:1037–40.
136. Marino G, Cacimano V, Taraglio S, Testori O. Metastasis of thyroid carcinoma: a case of secondary renal tumor. Minerva Urol Nefrol. 1991;43:85–8.
137. Markitziu A, Fisher D, Marmary Y. Thyroid papillary carcinoma presenting as jaw and parotid gland metastases. Int J Oral Maxillofac Surg. 1986;15:648–53.
138. Maslack M, Wilson C. ^{131}Iodine accumulation in a pericardial effusion. J Nucl Med. 1987;28:133.
139. Massin JP, Savoie JC, Garnier H, Guiraudon G, Leger FA, Bacourt F. Pulmonary metastases in differentiated thyroid carcinoma: study of 58 cases with implications for the primary tumor treatment. Cancer. 1984;53:982–92.
140. Matei DV, Verweij F, Scardino E, et al. Late solitary thyroid carcinoma metastasis to the kidney: a case report. Anticancer Res. 2003;23:561–4.
141. Mathew PC, Balagopal PG, Thomas S, Sebastian P, Preethi TR. Parotid metastasis from carcinoma of the thyroid. Int J Oral Maxillofac Surg. 2007;36:965–6.
142. McDougall IR. Metastatic struma ovarii: the burden of truth. Clin Nucl Med. 2006;31:321–4.
143. McKee PH. Cutaneous metastases. J Cutan Pathol. 1985;12:239–50.
144. McNeeley MF, Sabath A, Linnau KF. Follicular thyroid carcinoma presenting as acute cord compression due to thoracic vertebral metastasis. Radiol Case Rep. 2012;7:687.
145. Merino NJ, Kennedy SM, Nortan JA, Robbins J. Pleural involvement by metastatic thyroid carcinoma "tall cell variant": an unusual occurrence. Surg Pathol. 1990;3:59–64.
146. Meyer A, Behrend M. Is pancreatic resection justified for metastasis of papillary thyroid cancer? Anticancer Res. 2006;26: 2269–73.
147. Michal M, Chlumska A, Fakan F. Papillary carcinoma of thyroid with exuberant nodular fasciitis-like stroma. Histopathology. 1992;21:577–9.
148. Mishra A, Agarwal A, Agarwal G, Mishra S. Internal jugular vein invasion by thyroid carcinoma. Eur J Surg. 2001;167:64–7.
149. Mizukami Y, Michigishi T, Nonomura A, et al. Distant metastases in differentiated thyroid carcinomas: a clinical and pathologic study. Hum Pathol. 1990;21:283–90.
150. Mohan V, Jones RC, Drake III AJ, Daly PL, Shakir KMM. Littoral cell angioma presenting as metastatic thyroid carcinoma to the spleen. Thyroid. 2005;15:170–5.
151. Mohapatra T, Arora A, Bethune NN. Coexisting iodine avid and iodine nonconcentrating lesions with multiple distant soft tissue metastasis in papillary thyroid cancer. Indian J Nucl Med. 2012;27:38–41.
152. Moisseiev J, Gutman I, Rosen N, Blumenthal M. Orbital tumor as a presenting symptom of occult carcinoma of the thyroid. Metab Pediatr Syst Ophthalmol. 1988;11:33–4.
153. Moudouni SM, En-Nia I, Rioux-Leclerq N, Manunta A, Cullie F, Lobel B. Follicular carcinoma of the thyroid metastasis to the kidney nine years after the resection of the primary tumor. (in french). Ann Urol. 2002;36:36–7.
154. Moustafa SE, Sauve C, Amyot R. Assessment of a right ventricular metastasis using contrast echocardiography perfusion imaging. Eur J Echocardiogr. 2008;9:326–8.
155. Mruk K, Szot W, Huszno B. Pulmonary artery embolism caused by tumor mass in a case of thyroid carcinoma infiltrating the heart. Pol Tyg Lek. 1997;32:569–70.
156. Muller HJ, Weckesser M, Schober O. Bilateral renal metastasis in follicular thyroid carcinoma. Nuklearmedizin. 2000;39:45–7.
157. Munteanu M, Giuri S, Rosca C, Boruga O, Cretu O. Multifocal choroidal metastases from thyroid carcinoma: a case report. Chirurgia. 2013;108:268–72.
158. Muta N, Wada J, Kusajima K, Muroya K. A metastasis grown in the vein, from cancer of the thyroid. Nippon Igaku Hoshasen Gakkai Zasshi. 1978;38:14–22.
159. Niederkohr R, Dadras S, Leavitt M, McDougall R. F-18 FDG PET/CT imaging of a subcutaneous scalp metastasis from primary carcinoma of the thyroid. Clin Nucl Med. 2007;32:162–4.
160. Niederle B, Hausmaninger C, Kretschmer G, et al. Intraatrial extension of thyroid cancer: technique and results of a radical surgical approach. Surgery. 1990;108:951–6.
161. O'Connell ME, Fischer C, Harmer CL. Malignant struma ovarii: presentation and management. Br J Radiol. 1990;63:360–3.
162. Offret H, Saraux H, Dhermy P, Fichet D, Jagueux M. Ocular metastasis demonstrated a carcinoma of the thyroid gland. J Fr Ophthalmol. 1979;2:445–8.
163. Ohwada S, Hosomura Y, Kon Y, et al. Solitary metastasis from papillary thyroid carcinoma in cirrhotic liver with hepatocellular carcinoma. Jpn J Clin Oncol. 1993;23:309–12.
164. Okutan O, Solaroglu I, Karakus M, Saygili B, Beskonakli E. Metastatic thyroid carcinoma with initial presentation as spinal cord compression. J Neurol Sci (Turk). 2012;29:857–62.
165. Onaran Y, Terzioglu T, Oguz H, Kapran Y, Tezelman S. Great cervical vein invasion of thyroid carcinoma. Thyroid. 1988;8:59–61.
166. Orsolon P, Bagni B, Geatti O, et al. An unusual adrenal metastasis secondary to Hürthle cell carcinoma of thyroid. Clin Nucl Med. 1996;21:312–5.
167. Özülker T, Özülker F, Eker O, Özpaçaci T, Özcan D. Tumour thrombus from follicular thyroid cancer detected by 18F-FDG-PET/CT. Hell J Nucl Med. 2009;12:66–7.
168. Padma S, Tiwari A, Chaitanya R, et al. Papillary carcinoma thyroid with uveal metastases. Clin Nucl Med. 2013;38:131–4.
169. Panoussopoulos D, Theodoropoulos G, Vlahos K, Lazaris AC, Papadimitriou K. Distant solitary skeletal muscle metastasis from papillary thyroid carcinoma. Int Surg. 2007;92:226–9.

170. Paolini R, Toffoli S, Poletti A, et al. Splenomegaly as the first manifestation of thyroid cancer metastases. Tumori. 1997;83:779–82.
171. Paparel P, Tatou E, Krause D, Cognet F, Cercueil JP, Michel F. Adrenal metastasis from follicular thyroid carcinoma with intra-cardiac thrombus. Prog Urol. 2004;14:203–4.
172. Pardo-Mindan FJ, Vazquez JJ. Malignant struma ovarii: light and electron microscopic study. Cancer. 1983;51:337–43.
173. Patel PC, Millman B, Pellitteri PK, Woods EL. Papillary thyroid carcinoma presenting with massive angioinvasion of the great vessels of the neck and chest. Otolaryngol Head Neck Surg. 1997;117:S117–20.
174. Pavlidis NA, Sourla AD, Nikalaou NG, Tolis CF, Mitsi VD. Neglected cases papillary and follicular thyroid carcinoma: occurrence of subcutaneous scalp metastases. Eur J Surg Oncol. 1990;16:175–9.
175. Pepe P, Fraggettab F, Galiab A, Grassob G, Aragona F. Hematuria as the presenting symptom of a metastatic thyroid cancer. Urol Int. 2006;76:89–90.
176. Perez VC, Lecube TA, Narvaez GJ, Vilaseca MJ. Pleural metastasis as presenting form of papillary thyroid microcarcinoma: an exceptional case. Rev Clin Esp. 2003;203:217–8.
177. Pitlik S, Kitzes R, Ben-Bassat M, Rosenfeld JB. Thyroid carcinoma presenting as a solitary skin metastasis. Cutis. 1983;31:532–6.
178. Pomorski L, Bartos M. Metastasis as the first sign of thyroid cancer. Neoplasma. 1999;46:309–12.
179. Portocarrero-Ortiz L, Garcia-Lopez R, Romero-Vargas S, et al. Thyroid follicular carcinoma presenting as skull and dural metastasis mimicking a meningioma: a case report. J Neuro-Oncol. 2009;95:281–4.
180. Prasood D. Follicular carcinoma of thyroid gland presenting as scalp metastasis. Acta Cytol. 1998;42:449–51.
181. Prietzel T, Macher A, Haferkorn I, Schmitz N, Schmidt F, Aigner T. Soft tissue metastasis of thyroid carcinoma in the knee region mimicking a paraarticular inflammatory lesion. Arch Orthop Trauma Surg. 2010;130:1425–8.
182. Pucci A, Suppo M, Lucchesi G, Celeste, et al. Papillary thyroid carcinoma presenting as a solitary soft tissue arm metastasis in an elderly hyperthyroid patient. Case report and review of the literature. Virchows Arch. 2006;448:857–61.
183. Puigfel M, Falces C, Castella M, Roig E. Metastatic cardiac tamponade in a patient with papillary carcinoma of the thyroid. Med Clin (Barc). 1996;107:197–8.
184. Puri P, Motwani N, Pande M. Squamous carcinoma of the thyroid metastatic to the choroid: a report. Eur J Cancer Care (Engl). 2001;10:63–4.
185. Qui ZL, Luo QY. Erector spinae metastases from differentiated thyroid cancer identified by I-131 SPECT/CT. Clin Nucl Med. 2009;34:137–40.
186. Quinn TR, Duncan LM, Zembowicz A, Faquin WC. Cutaneous metastases of follicular thyroid carcinoma: a report of four cases and a review of the literature. Am J Dermatopathol. 2005;27:306–12.
187. Rahman GA, Abdulkadir Y, Olatoke SA, Yusuf IF, Braimoh T. Unusual cutaneous metastatic follicular thyroid carcinoma. J Surg Tech Case Rep. 2010;2:35–8.
188. Renner GJ, Davis WE, Templer JW. Metastasis of thyroid carcinoma to the paranasal sinuses. Otolaryngol Head Neck Surg. 1984;92:233–7.
189. Repanos C, Ho YM, Bird K, Coman S, Coman WB, Wallwork B. Metastatic papillary thyroid carcinoma involving orbit: a case report and review. ANZ J Surg. 2011;81:375–6.
190. Ribeiro-Silva A, Bezerra AM, Serafini LN. Malignant struma ovarii: an autopsy report of a clinically unsuspected tumor. Gynecol Oncol. 2002;87:213–5.
191. Rico MJ, Penneys NS. Metastatic follicular carcinoma of the thyroid to the skin: a case confirmed by immunohistochemistry. J Cutan Pathol. 1985;12:103–5.
192. Ritland JS, Eide N, Walaas L, Høie J. Fine-needle aspiration biopsy diagnosis of a uveal metastasis from a follicular thyroid carcinoma. Acta Ophthalmol Scand. 1999;77:594–6.
193. Ro HJ, Ha HK, Kim HS, Shinn KS. Renal metastasis from thyroid carcinoma visible as a hyperdense lesion on unenhanced CT [letter]. Am J Roentgenol. 1995;165:1018.
194. Rodrigues G, Ghosh A. Synchronous bony and soft tissue metastases from follicular carcinoma of the thyroid. J Korean Med Sci. 2003;18:914–6.
195. Ronga G, Cholandria M, Montesano T, et al. Solitary skin metastases from papillary thyroid cancer. Thyroid. 2007;17:477–8.
196. Rosenstengel A, Lim EM, Millward M, Lee YCG. A distinctive colour associated with high iodine content in malignant pleural effusion from metastatic papillary thyroid cancer: a case report. J Med Case Reports. 2013;7:147–51.
197. Rotman-Pikielny P, Reynolds JC, Barker WC, et al. Recombinant human thyrotropin for the diagnosis and treatment of a highly functional metastatic struma ovarii. J Clin Endocrinol Metab. 2000;85:237–44.
198. Ruggiero FP, Frauenhoffer EE, Stack BC. Papillary thyroid cancer with an initial presentation of abdominal and flank pain. J Otolaryngol Head Neck Med Surg. 2005;26:142–5.
199. Ruiz de Erenchun F, España A, Idoate MA, Quintanilla E. Cutaneous metastases from a follicular carcinoma of the thyroid. Acta Dermatol Venereol (Stockh). 1993;73:154–5.
200. Runne U, Modder G. Hautmetastasen drch schiddrusen-karzinome. Dtsch Med Wochenschr. 1976;101:1831–4.
201. Salvatori M, Dambra DP, D'Angelo G, et al. A case of metastatic struma ovarii treated with ^{131}I therapy: focus on preservation of fertility and selected review of the literature. Gynecol Endocrinol. 2008;24:312–9.
202. Salvatori M, Perotti G, Rufini V, et al. Solitary liver metastasis from Hürthle cell thyroid cancer: a case report and review of the literature. J Endocrinol Invest. 2004;27:52–6.
203. Sanioglu S, Sokullu O, Ozgen A, Demirci D, Sargin M, Bilgen F. Unusual metastasis of the papillary thyroid adenocarcinoma. Ann Thorac Surg. 2009;87:1928–30.
204. Sarda AK, Pandey D, Bhalla SA, Goyal A. Isolated submandibular gland metastasis from an occult papillary thyroid cancer. Indian J Cancer. 2004;41:89–91.
205. Sardi A, Agone CM, Pelegrini. A renal metastasis from papillary thyroid carcinoma. J La State Med Soc. 1992;144:416–20.
206. Sarma DP, Simmons GT. Intra glomerular metastases from papillary carcinoma of the thyroid. J La State Med Soc. 1989;141:26–8.
207. Scott AW, Cummings TJ, Kirkpatrick JP, Mruthyunjaya P. Choroidal metastasis of follicular thyroid adenocarcinoma diagnosed by 25-gauge transretinal biopsy. Ann Ophthalmol (Skokie). 2008;40:110–2.
208. Seniviratne DR, Stavrou P, Good P. Late-state metastasis to the choroid from follicular thyroid carcinoma-case report. Optometry. 2011;82:215–7.
209. Sevinc A, Buyukberber S, Sari R, Baysal T, Mizrak B. Follicular thyroid cancer presenting initially with soft tissue metastasis. Jpn J Clin Oncol. 2000;30:27–9.
210. Shaco-Levy R, Bean SM, Bentley RC, Robboy SJ. Natural history of biologically malignant struma ovarii: analysis of 27 cases with extraovarian spread. Int J Gynecol Pathol. 2010;29:212–27.
211. Shah D, Samuel A. Metastasis to the liver in well-differentiated carcinoma of the thyroid. Thyroid. 1996;6:607–11.
212. Shai SE, Hsieh SR, Song YM, Shen GH. Resection of follicular thyroid cancer metastasized to the left lower lobe of the lung

extending into the left atrium as a huge intracardial tumour. Thyroid. 2005;15:1417–8.
213. Shon W, Ferguson SB, Comfere NO. Metastatic Hürthle cell carcinoma of the thyroid presenting as ulcerated scrotum nodules. Am J Dermatopathol. 2010;32:392–4.
214. Siddaraju N, Viswanathan VK, Saka VK, Basu D, Shanmugham C. Fine needle aspiration of follicular variant of papillary thyroid carcinoma presenting with pleural effusion: a case report. Acta Cytol. 2007;51:911–5.
215. Siddiqui AA, Olansky L, Sawh RN, Tierney WM. Pancreatic metastasis of tall cell variant of papillary thyroid carcinoma: diagnosis by endoscopic ultrasound-guided fine needle aspiration. J Pancreas. 2006;7:417–22.
216. Silliphant WM, Klinck GH, Levitin MS. Thyroid carcinoma and death: a clinico-pathological study of 193 autopsies. Cancer. 1964;17:513–25.
217. Singh U, Kaushik S, Pandav SS, et al. Papillary carcinoma thyroid presenting as a choroidal metastasis. Report of a case and brief review of literature. Indian J Ophthalmol. 2003;51:81–3.
218. Sirota DK. Axillary vein thrombosis as the initial symptom in metastatic papillary carcinoma of the thyroid. Mt Sinai J Med. 1989;56:111–3.
219. Slamovits TL, Mondzelewski JP, Kennerdell JS. Thyroid carcinoma metastatic to the globe. Br J Ophthalmol. 1979;63:169–72.
220. Smallridge RC, Castro MR, Morris JC, et al. Renal metastases from thyroid papillary carcinoma: study of sodium iodide symporter expression. Thyroid. 2001;11:795–804.
221. Studer H, Veraguth P, Wyss F. Thyrotoxicosis due to a solitary hepatic metastasis of thyroid carcinoma. J Clin Endocrinol Metab. 1961;21:1334–8.
222. Sugimura H, Tamura S, Kodama T, Kakitsubata Y, Asada K, Watanabe K. Metastatic pancreas cancer from the thyroid; clinical imaging mimicking non functioning islet cell tumor. Radiat Med. 1991;9:167–9.
223. Tagore KR, Kumar RA. Unusual presentation of papillary microcarcinoma of thyroid as thigh mass. Case Rep Pathol. 2011;2011:1–2.
224. Takayasu H, Kumamoto Y, Terawaki Y, Ueno A. A case of bilateral metastasis renal tumor originating from a thyroid carcinoma. J Urol. 1968;100:717.
225. Takeuchi K, Murata K, Fujita L. Malignant struma ovarii with peritoneal metastasis: report of two cases. Eur J Gynaecol Oncol. 2000;21:260–1.
226. Tan PK, Chua CL, Poh WT. Thyroid papillary carcinoma with unusual breast metastasis. Ann Acad Med Singapore. 1991;20:801–2.
227. Tanaka N, Katsuta Y. A case of primary thyroid carcinoma with multiple skin metastases. Nippon Rinsho. 1971;29:1420–6.
228. Tang W, Kakudo K, Nakamura Y, et al. Parathyroid gland involvement by papillary carcinoma of the thyroid gland. Arch Pathol Lab Med. 2002;126:1511–4.
229. Tazi EM, Essadi I, Errihani H. Thyroid carcinoma presenting as a dural metastasis mimicking a meningioma: a case report. N Am J Med Sci. 2011;3:39–42.
230. Thomas G, Sreelatha KT, Pradeep VM, Pandey M. Follicular carcinoma of the thyroid gland with initial presentation as an oral soft tissue mass: report of a case. J Oral Maxillofac Surg. 2001;59:819–22.
231. Thompson NW, Brown J, Orringer M, Sisson J, Nishiyama R. Follicular carcinoma of the thyroid with massive angioinvasion: extension of tumor thrombus to the heart. Surgery. 1978;83:451–7.
232. Tiong H, White S, Khanna D, Furness P, Nicholson M. An unusual presentation of follicular carcinoma of the thyroid. Thyroid. 2001;11:591–3.
233. Toyota N, Asaga H, Hirokawa M, Iizkuka H. A case of skin metastasis from follicular thyroid carcinoma. Dermatology. 1994;188:69–71.
234. Tran K, Bigby KJ, Hughes BG, Lee L, Allison R. Clinicopathological report: bilateral choroidal metastases from papillary thyroid cancer. Asia Pac J Clin Oncol. 2011;7:11–4.
235. Tripathi M, Sharma R, Jaimini A, et al. Metastatic follicular carcinoma of the thyroid with tumor thrombus in the superior vena cava and right brachiocephalic and internal jugular veins: FDG-PET/CT findings. Clin Nucl Med. 2008;33:426–8.
236. Tronnier M, Winzer M, Wolff HH. Cutaneous metastases from follicular thyroid carcinoma: histology, immunohistology, and electron microscopy. Dermatologica. 1991;183:286–9.
237. Tsoukalas N, Kostakis ID, Demiri S, et al. Neoplastic pericarditis as the initial manifestation of a papillary thyroid carcinoma. Ups J Med Sci. 2013;118:196–8.
238. Tunio MA, AlAsiri M, Riaz K, AlShakwer W, AlArifi M. Skeletal muscle metastasis as an initial presentation of follicular thyroid carcinoma: a case report and review of the literature. Case Rep Endocrinol. 2013;2013:1–4.
239. Tur GE, Asanuma Y, Sato T, et al. Resection of metastatic thyroid carcinomas to the liver and the kidney: report of a case. Surg Today. 1994;24:844–8.
240. Vadmal MS, Smilari TF, Lovecchio JL, Klein IL, Hajdu SI. Diagnosis and treatment of disseminated struma ovarii with malignant transformation. Gynecol Oncol. 1997;64:541–6.
241. Vanderpump MP, Tunbridge WM. Hürthle cell carcinoma presenting with retroorbital metastasis. J R Soc Med. 1992;85:493–4.
242. Varghese BT, Sebastian P. Internal jugular vein thrombus associated with thyroid carcinoma. Ann Otol Rhinol Laryngol. 2005;114:656.
243. Varma D, Jain S, Khurana N. Papillary carcinoma of thyroid presenting with skin ulceration. Cytopathology. 2007;18:260–71.
244. Vassilopoulou-Sellin R, Sneige N. Pleural effusion in patients with differentiated papillary thyroid cancer. South Med J. 1994;87:1111–6.
245. Vega CP, Torello AL, García JN, Momplet JV. Pleural metastasis as presenting form of papillary thyroid microcarcinoma: an exceptional case. Rev Clin Esp. 2003;203:217–8.
246. Vernon AN, Sheeler LR, Biscotti CV, Stoller JK. Pleural effusion resulting from metastatic papillary carcinoma of the thyroid. Chest. 1992;101:1448–50.
247. Vives R, Valcayo A, Menendez E, Guarch R. Follicular thyroid carcinoma metastatic to the skin [letter]. J Am Acad Dermatol. 1992;27:276–7.
248. Von Falck C, Beer G, Gratz K, Galanski M. Renal metastases from follicular thyroid cancer on SPECT/CT. Clin Nucl Med. 2007;32:751–2.
249. Wada N, Masudo K, Hirakawa S, et al. Superior vena cava (SVC) reconstruction using autologous tissue in two cases of differentiated thyroid carcinoma presenting with SVC syndrome. World J Surg Oncol. 2009;7:75–83.
250. Whitaker B, Robinson K, Hewan-Lowe K, Budnick S. Thyroid metastasis to the oral soft tissues: case report of a diagnostic dilemma. J Oral Maxillofac Surg. 1993;51:588–93.
251. Willemse PHB, Oosterhuis JW, Aalders JG, et al. Malignant struma ovariectomy treated by ovariectomy, thyroidectomy, and 131I administration. Cancer. 1987;60:178–82.
252. Wirz K. Choroid metastasis of a thyroid gland cancer-a clinicopathologic case report. Fortschr Ophthalmol. 1984;81:360–2.
253. Wolfenden JM, Waxman AD, Wolfstein RS, Siemsen JK. Scintigraphic evaluation of liver metastases from thyroid carcinoma. J Nucl Med. 1975;16:669–71.
254. Wood Jr WJ, Singletary SE, Hickey RC. Current results of treatment for distant metastatic well-differentiated thyroid carcinoma. Arch Surg. 1989;124:1374–7.

255. Woodruff DJ, Rauh JT, Markley RL. Ovarian struma. Obstet Gynecol. 1966;27:194–201.
256. Xu H, Zeng W, Tang Y. Metastatic thyroid follicular carcinoma presenting as a primary renal tumor. Intern Med. 2012;51:2193–6.
257. Yamagami Y, Tori M, Sakaki M, et al. Thyroid carcinoma with extensive tumor thrombus in the atrium. Gen Thorac Cardiovasc Surg. 2008;56:555–8.
258. Personal communication: Douglas Van Nostrand 2012.
259. Yoshida T, Yokoe T, Takeshita M, et al. Thyroid carcinoma with internal jugular vein thrombus: report of a case. Kitakanto Med J. 2003;53:315–8.
260. Young RH, Jackson A, Wells M. Ovarian metastasis from thyroid carcinoma 12 years after partial thyroidectomy mimicking struma ovarii: report of a case. Int J Gynecol Pathol. 1994;13:181–5.
261. Yunta Abarca PJ, Ponce JL, Prieto M, Lopez-Aznar D, Sancho-Fornos S. Papillary thyroid carcinoma that metastasized to the choroid. Eur J Surg. 1999;165:998–9.
262. Zagrebin VM. Thyroid cancer metastasis to a clear-cell cancer of the kidney. Arkh Patol. 1984;46:76–8.
263. Zakhem A, Aftimos G, Kreidy R, Salem P. Malignant struma ovarii: report of two cases and selected review of the literature. J Surg Oncol. 1990;43:61–5.
264. Zhao LX, Li L, Li FL, Zhao Z. Rectus abdominis muscle metastasis from papillary thyroid cancer identified by I-131 SPECT/CT. Clin Nucl Med. 2010;35:360–1.

Adjunctive Local Approaches to Thyroid Nodules and Metastatic Thyroid Cancer

67

Leonard Wartofsky

Introduction

The overwhelming majority of differentiated thyroid cancers are curable, and this optimistic outlook applies particularly to stage I, II, and most stage III tumors. Stage IV tumors are typically and clearly in a different category, as the prognosis is significantly worse once distant metastases are present. In the author's view, a worse prognosis is not a justification for therapeutic nihilism but instead demands more aggressive therapy, with the hopeful expectation of improving outcome and prognosis. Not infrequently, some stage I and II patients have local disease that is resistant to ablation by conventional surgery and radioiodine.

This chapter attempts to summarize some approaches used to eradicate or at least control local foci of both distant and regional metastatic disease. In many cases, these local approaches are viewed as preferable alternatives to surgery or radioactive iodine administration. Repeat surgery may be declined by the patient or may be burdened with higher risk after multiple prior dissections or following external radiation therapy. In addition, external radiation may not be an option because of having exceeded the safe upper limits of local radiation or because of proven radioresistance of the particular cancer. (External radiation therapy is discussed in detail in Chaps. 63, 78, 88, and 101.) Radioiodine treatment may be an unappealing option when a patient may have already approached or exceeded their maximally safe cumulative dose of radioiodine or when 131I treatment is not feasible because the metastases are not iodine avid. Chemotherapeutic approaches are another option (see Chaps. 64, 99, and 105), with potential molecularly targeted therapies (see Chaps. 64, 104, 105). However, the local approaches described below may be used before or after radioiodine or external radiation or with chemotherapy or when chemotherapy is either ineffective or unacceptable to the patient.

L. Wartofsky, MD, MACP (✉)
Department of Medicine, MedStar Washington Hospital Center, Georgetown University School of Medicine,
110 Irving Street, N.W., Washington, DC 20010-2975, USA
e-mail: leonard.wartofsky@medstar.net

Ethanol Ablation

The percutaneous injection of 95 % ethanol into hyperfunctioning thyroid nodules began in Europe and has achieved only modest use in the United States ([1, 2]; see Chap. 17). Benign cysts and even "cold nodules" have been managed by ethanol injection after initially proven by fine-needle aspiration to be benign [3]. The procedure may have to be repeated several times to be effective, and the instillations of alcohol may be very painful to the patient. Much of this pain is believed to be from leakage of ethanol to surrounding soft tissues. In addition to local pain, some fever and hematoma formation are common. Perhaps the most onerous complication, albeit rare in experienced hands, is damage to the recurrent laryngeal nerve with vocal cord paralysis.

The role and safety of ethanol ablation for recurrent thyroid cancer in the neck have been reviewed recently by Shin et al. [4]. Gangi et al. [5] may have been the first to employ ethanol injection into bone metastases under computed tomography (CT) guidance to achieve pain relief. From the Mayo Clinic, Lewis et al. [6] were the first group to publish a report of percutaneous ethanol injection of thyroid cancer metastases in cervical lymph nodes. A total of 14 patients with 29 metastatic nodes were described. Twenty patients who had 23 nodes injected were reported from the same group several months later by Hay at the meetings of the American Thyroid Association [7], and it is unclear if any of these represent the same patients. In the initial analysis, the patients were not considered candidates for either surgery or further radioiodine therapy. A 25-gauge needle was used and

L. Wartofsky, D. Van Nostrand (eds.), *Thyroid Cancer*, DOI 10.1007/978-1-4939-3314-3_67

placed under sonographic guidance by a radiologist, with the needle penetrated deeply into the node. After the first injection of 0.05–0.1 mL of ethanol, the needle was repositioned, followed by an additional three to ten injections of small amounts of ethanol. A total of 0.1–0.8 mL was used with each patient undergoing up to four treatment visits. Responses to ethanol were assessed by follow-up ultrasonographic measurement at an average of 18 months posttreatment. Lymph node volumes were decreased from a mean basal value of 492–76 mm3 1 year later and lowered further to 20 mm3 after 2 years. As mentioned above, patients experienced some local pain, and a few had transient pain radiating to the jaw or chest, but they observed no major complications and achieved excellent control of metastatic lymph node disease in 12 of 14 patients. No serum thyroglobulin (Tg) data before and after the ethanol ablations were provided by the authors at that time.

In the presentation by Hay [7] of 20 patients, decreases in node size were described in all 23 nodes injected, with 6 disappearing completely. At subsequent reevaluation of 16 patients, 7 had nodes that required a second injection of ethanol. However, successful control was achieved in 15 of these 16 patients, with only 1 requiring additional surgical intervention. An average 0.7-mL dose of ethanol was injected in two occasions with no significant complications. Our own experience at the Washington Hospital Center has been similar to that of the Mayo group in a limited series of patients with local lymph node metastases. Ethanol injection has also been used for distant bone metastases by Nakada et al. [8].

In a series of 16 patients with 24 neck recurrences of papillary thyroid carcinoma (PTC) treated by Lim et al., four lesions disappeared completely and the mean reduction in lesion diameter approached 50 % [9]. No recurrence was noted after ethanol ablation in 6/6 patients treated by Monchik et al. during a follow-up averaging 18 months [10]. It has been suggested that treatments be continued until vascular flow on Doppler has disappeared [11]. In a retrospective analysis of a larger series of 47 neck recurrences of PTC in 27 patients reported by Kim et al. [12], the efficacy of ablation was based on loss of vascularity on Doppler as well as volume reduction. The average number of ethanol instillations was 2.1, with an average of 1.1 ml injected each time, and an average reduction in volume of 94 % was observed. All of these data allow us to conclude that ethanol ablation of local recurrences is certainly an option for therapy, especially for patients who are poor surgical candidates or who are strongly opposed to another surgical procedure.

Embolization of Metastases

The earliest applications of embolization therapy were for vascular malformations and hemangiomas. Materials used for embolization have included polyvinyl alcohol beads (Ivalon) and gelfoam. Embolization has been employed for such benign tumors as parathyroid adenomas and uterine fibroids. The earliest malignant tumors treated were craniofacial and head and neck tumors, with bone metastases from renal carcinoma treated shortly thereafter. Embolization is the most safe and effective when a single feeding artery to a tumor can be identified that does not also supply a more critical distal tissue. Transarterial chemoembolization has been attempted for metastatic medullary thyroid carcinoma to the liver [13], and yttrium-90 microspheres have been embolized for liver metastases of neuroendocrine tumors [14] but not to our knowledge for metastatic thyroid cancer.

Bone metastases have been particularly suitable for embolization therapy, and this approach is discussed at greater length in Chap. 65. Once bone metastases occur with thyroid cancer, prognosis is sufficiently worse [15, 16] to warrant aggressive and innovative therapeutic methods. After an analysis of prognostic factors associated with survival, Bernier et al. also recommended that this type of therapy, particularly in young patients, should be as aggressive as possible [17].

Perhaps the earliest description of embolization for thyroid cancer metastatic to bone was by Camille et al. in 1980 [18] in a report of four patients with metastases to the spine and pelvis. Smit et al. [19] studied four patients with follicular carcinoma metastases to the spine with cord compression. They postulated that they would achieve maximal tumor destruction by first administering radioiodine and then embolizing the lesions about 3–6 days later. Selective catheterization of the vessel(s) "feeding" the tumor was performed after magnetic resonance or CT imaging to identify the best vessel and determine that there was no downstream vital structure (e.g., spinal cord). Pain was the predominant symptom in their patients, and embolization was associated with significant reduction in pain. Recurrent pain or persistence of tumor based on rising serum thyroglobulin (Tg) or visible growth on imaging was an indication for repeat embolization, with or without additional radioiodine. Pain relief is observed faster than seen after radioiodine or external radiation therapy, and a reduction (but not elimination) may be seen in serum Tg. One possible complication of embolization is a "postembolization syndrome" associated with pain and fever and believed owed to acute tumor necrosis.

Smit et al. speculated that a potential negative aspect of embolization might be the creation of tumor tissue hypoxia, which might then drive angiogenesis and neovascularization. They suggested a possible role for adjunctive antiangiogenesis chemotherapy. Some benefit in this regard might also derive from bisphosphonate therapy, with reports of thyroid cancer metastases treated with both pamidronate [20, 21] and zoledronic acid [22, 23] to reduce pain and tumor growth (see Chap. 53).

The same group (Smit et al.) reported on an updated larger patient series with follow-up periods of 2 months to 8.6 years [24]. There were 16 patients treated with a total of 41 separate embolizations for pain, spinal cord compression, or both. They noted reduced or stable tumor size on CT in 18 of 22 treatments and considered the procedure successful overall in 24 of the 41 treatments. They did not confirm greater efficacy of treatment when combined with radioactive iodine therapy, but there was an apparently longer duration of benefit. Intervals of success were 6.5 months for embolization alone and 15 months for embolization coupled with either radioiodine or external radiation. Otherwise, there was no clear additional benefit in patients who had adjunctive surgery or external radiation. The patients tolerated the procedures well, and there was only one case of the postembolization syndrome.

Van Tol et al. [25] examined five patients with symptomatically painful bone metastases to determine whether there was any benefit from adjunctive radioactive iodine therapy. The patients had 5.55-GBq ablation and embolization 4–6 weeks later with polyvinyl alcohol particles, and then a second dose of 5.55 GBq of radioiodine 3 months later was administered. The response relating to tumor metastasis size and serum Tg was assessed with the latter parameter vs that in a control group of six patients relatively matched for disease who were treated without embolization. The combination therapy led to a median tumor volume reduction of 52.5 % and a significantly improved average Tg decrement of 88.7 %, in contrast to an 18.6 % reduction in the control group. Although there were pain relief and some neurologic symptoms with embolization, other than the more dramatic drop in serum Tg, the degree of improvement was probably not different from that seen with radioiodine alone. One patient developed postembolization syndrome. Early measurement of serum Tg after embolization may be misleading, as a striking rise in levels may occur shortly after therapy [26], which can be seen after radioiodine as well.

In several patients, additional radioiodine or surgery was required for recurrence, but all of the combination-treatment patients were alive at the end of the study. During the longer follow-up period of the six control patients, all eventually died after a median period of 52 months. As mentioned above, the prognosis for patients with bone metastases is not good. For both the treating clinician and the patient with extensive bone metastases, perhaps the most important issue to consider is that these therapies are only palliative and not curative. In the series by Eustatia-Rutten et al. [24], 9 of 16 patients died during the follow-up period and the other 5 had progression of their disease.

Other Palliative Approaches to Spinal Metastases

Vertebroplasty and Kyphoplasty

Back pain is the typical symptom that leads to the discovery of spinal metastases of thyroid cancer. A solitary metastatic lesion in the spine may be managed surgically by shelling out the tumor in the involved vertebral body and replacing it with bone cement, with or without reinforcement by a titanium cage or plates, as needed.

Most of the pain associated with spinal metastases is caused by compression fractures of the vertebral bodies. Both acute and chronic pain may result from these fractures, along with deformities, limitations in mobility, and a higher mortality rate. In addition to the adjunctive measures of external radiation therapy and bisphosphonates mentioned above, a benefit may be achieved by aggressive surgical approaches to the spine, especially in younger patients. An excellent overview of these procedures has appeared by Halpin et al. [27], and these techniques are also discussed by Wexler in Chap. 65.

In brief, vertebroplasty is an attempt to stabilize and strengthen bone weakened by metastatic cancer and relieve pain from compression fractures. The procedure is done by a minimally invasive percutaneous approach, injecting polymethyl methacrylate into the vertebral body. The vertebral bodies need to be incompletely compressed to technically inject the material; local infection, low platelet count, or coagulation problems are contraindications to the procedure [28].

The literature indicates excellent results in selected patients, and 90 % of subjects had pain reduction and improved mobility within 24 h of the procedure. The methacrylate cement fills the vertebral body, and the pain relief may be the result of destruction of nerve endings, stabilization, or actual tumor necrosis from ischemia. This procedure is burdened with many potential minor and major complications [27, 28] and should be reserved to centers with experienced staff and success with the technique. Nonetheless, it should be considered for the relief of symptomatic patients with spinal metastases [29].

Kyphoplasty involves the same principle as vertebroplasty—stabilizing the vertebrae by percutaneously injecting methacrylate—but the procedure differs in two ways. The vertebral body is first expanded by the insertion via cannula of a balloon that is inflated to expand the body and then deflated prior to the cement injection [30, 31]. Second, the cement is a more viscous or dense form than that used for vertebroplasty. Kyphoplasty is generally more effective than vertebroplasty in restoring greater height of the vertebral body and relieving pain and is the preferred procedure in many cases. Like vertebroplasty, kyphoplasty can predictably reduce pain and deformity and also improve mobility. Some of the same contraindications exist. In the series by Ledlie and Fenfro [31], there were only six patients with metastatic cancer, but they had an excellent result. Four indicated the disappearance of pain, and one had reduction of pain. The same caveats regarding performance by experienced operators apply to reduce the potential complication rate.

Radiofrequency Ablation

Prior to its use in the treatment of local recurrences of thyroid carcinoma, the utility and safety of radiofrequency ablation (RFA) for the treatment of benign thyroid nodules had been well demonstrated [32–37]. RFA is performed either under general anesthesia or with local anesthesia and conscious sedation. Originally, the tumor metastases that were managed by RFA included the liver and bone [27, 38–40], but it was rapidly adapted and applied to a wide variety of solid tumors, including lung metastases [41, 42] and adrenal tumors [43]. It is particularly effective in the bone and may be combined with vertebroplasty [44, 45]. The procedure is based essentially on inducing coagulation necrosis of tumor by the generation of heat from an electrode inserted percutaneously. Basically, it is similar to an electrocautery in that no heat actually flows through the device. Rather, high-frequency alternating current travels through the needle probe device, which serves as an antenna that elicits heat by friction, and then the heat denatures the protein of the tumor. Coagulation necrosis occurs when tissues reach 50–52 °C over 4–5 min. At this time, the devices are approved by the Food and Drug Administration for the treatment of bone and soft-tissue metastases. The equipment used at our medical center is provided by Rita Medical Systems and includes their Generator Model 1,500 that provides 460-kHz frequency, with a maximum power of 150 W and the StarBurst XL probe. Other workers have employed a Boston Scientific RF 3,000 Radiofrequency Generator with a LaVeen Needle Electrode system.

RFA is done as an outpatient procedure, with assistance by an anesthetist for conscious sedation and with use of computerized tomographic imaging (CT) guidance for placement of the probe. Fentanyl and Versed may be titrated to achieve adequate sedation. The lesions to be treated may have been identified by CT or 18-fluorodeoxyglucose positron emission tomography (PET) and then confirmed as malignant by FNA biopsy and, in the case of differentiated thyroid cancer, would be likely associated with high and rising serum Tg levels. The lesions should be sufficiently distant from key adjacent structures, such as the spinal cord, major blood vessels, or nerves. Halpin et al. [27] pointed out that a layer of cortical or cancellous bone between tumor in a vertebral body and the spinal cord or nerve roots can serve as a protective insulator. Specific details about how the procedure is typically done for thyroid cancer are described by Dupuy et al. [46] and for bone metastases, by Callstrom et al. [47]. The patients treated by Callstrom et al. experienced significant pain relief.

As is also done for liver metastases, especially neuroendocrine tumors [48–50], the procedure involves introduction of the electrode through a nick in the skin using guidance by ultrasound, CT, or both. The StarBurst XL described above is a 14-gauge 6.4-F needle with an active electrode trocar tip and nine electrodes that spread out into a spherical formation in the tissue being treated. This generates a necrotic core of 5-cm diameter; however, size is adjustable based on the length of the exposed electrode. The insulated needle tip is placed into the lesion, and the electrode is advanced through the soft portion of the lesion until the electrode tips butt against the interface between soft tissue and bone, precluding further advancement. The position of the needle tip is confirmed by ultrasound or CT with continuous real-time monitoring to ensure a proper electrode position. The temperature goal is 100 °C, which is variably maintained for at least 3–5 min with a range of 5–15 min.

One treatment may be sufficient for small lesions, whereas larger lesions require the patient to return for multiple therapies. After the ablative procedure, the spread electrodes are withdrawn back into the needle, and the needle is removed. With bone lesions, post-procedure pain may be a problem for several hours and can be controlled by a local injection of Marcaine and intravenous fentanyl, with or without Versed. Some patients tolerate the procedure amazingly well. In the series of 16 patients treated by Monchik et al. [10], one patient experienced a minor skin burn but one had permanent vocal cord paralysis. In their follow-up period of slightly more than 40 months, two-third patients treated for bone lesions were free of disease, and one treated for a lung metastasis was free of disease at 10 months of follow-up.

Laser Thermal Ablation

For over a decade, laser thermal ablation has been used for the treatment of various metastases and primary hepatomas [51, 52] and more recently was shown to be effective for benign thyroid nodules [53] and for thyroid malignancies [53–55]. The technique involves ultrasound-guided insertion of 21-gauge spinal needles into the lesion(s) within the sheath, of which a 300-μm diameter quartz optical fiber is threaded. The energy for the ablation is provided by a Nd: YAG laser with an output of 3–5 W. Patients described the sensation as painful but tolerable. With larger lesions, the needles are slightly withdrawn and repositioned for several additional treatments.

The procedure has been used relatively successfully for ablation of papillary microcarcinoma and would have indication in extreme elderly patients or those who could not tolerate general anesthesia and surgery [56, 57]. Details of the procedure can be reviewed in the report by Pacella et al. [58], who described the results of percutaneous laser thermal ablation of 25 patients, 16 of whom had benign "hot" nodules, 8 had "cold" nodules, and only 1 had thyroid cancer, an anaplastic carcinoma. The patients were deemed poor candidates for surgery. Nodule size was reduced by an average of 3.3 mL in the hot nodules and 7.7 mL in the cold nodules. The sole anaplastic carcinoma experienced necrosis of 32 mL of tissue. Another patient with anaplastic thyroid carcinoma has also been so treated [59].

I believe it still too early to recommend this approach to treatment of recurrent thyroid cancer. The therapy was considered relatively ineffective for the hot nodules (which would still require 131I therapy), and there are clearly insufficient data on thyroid cancer to warrant its use. Rather, controlled clinical trials should be performed to determine whether this therapeutic modality will have any future role in the management of metastatic thyroid cancer. Preliminary studies are also being done with high-intensity focused ultrasound [60–62] but it is too early to assess whether this approach might be applicable to recurrent and inoperable thyroid cancer. Any of the above local ablative techniques may be applied to the management of any type of thyroid cancer. The greatest benefit or indication for these local procedures lies in the patient who has demonstrable tumor burden and who cannot tolerate or refuses surgical approaches. Finally, it should be noted that most of these procedures will be palliative but not curative.

References

1. Bennedbaek FN, Hegedus L. Treatment of recurrent thyroid cysts with ethanol: a randomized double-blind controlled trial. J Clin Endocrinol Metab. 2003;88:5773–7.
2. Guglielmi R, Pacella CM, Bianchini A, et al. Percutaneous ethanol injection treatment in benign thyroid lesions: role and efficacy. Thyroid. 2004;14:125–31.
3. Valcalvi R, Frasoldati A. Ultrasound-guided percutaneous ethanol injection therapy in thyroid cystic nodules. Endocrinol Pract. 2004;10:269–75.
4. Shin JE, Baek JH, Lee JH. Radiofrequency and ethanol ablation for the treatment of recurrent thyroid cancers: current status and challenges. Curr Opin Oncol. 2013;25:14–9.
5. Gangi A, Kastler B, Klinkert A, Dietemann JL. Injection of alcohol into bone metastases under CT guidance. J Comput Assist Tomogr. 1994;18:932–5.
6. Lewis BD, Hay ID, Charboneau JW, et al. Percutaneous ethanol injection for treatment of cervical lymph node metastases in patients with papillary thyroid carcinoma. Am J Roentgenol. 2002;178:699–704.
7. Hay I, Charboneau W, Lewis B, et al. Successful ultrasound-guided percutaneous ethanol ablation of neck nodal metastases in 20 patients with postoperative TNM Stage I papillary thyroid carcinoma resistant to conventional therapy. Los Angeles: 74th Meeting, American Thyroid Association. 2002. Abstract 176.
8. Nakada K, Kasai K, Watanabe Y, et al. Treatment of radioiodine-negative bone metastasis from papillary thyroid carcinoma with percutaneous ethanol injection therapy. Ann Nucl Med. 1996;10:441–4.
9. Lim CY, Yun J-S, Lee J, Nam K-H, Chung WY, Park CS. Percutaneous ethanol injection therapy for locally recurrent papillary thyroid carcinoma. Thyroid. 2007;17:347–50.
10. Monchik JM, Donatini G, Iannuccilli J, Dupuy DE. Radiofrequency ablation and percutaneous ethanol injection treatment for recurrent local and distant well-differentiated thyroid carcinoma. Ann Surg. 2006;244:296–304.
11. Sohn Y-M, Hong SW, Kim E-Y, Kim MJ, Moon HJ, Kim SJ, et al. Complete eradication of metastatic lymph node after percutaneous ethanol injection therapy: pathologic correlation. Thyroid. 2009;19:317–9.
12. Kim BM, Kim MJ, Kim EK, Park SI, Park CS, Chung WY. Controlling recurrent papillary thyroid carcinoma in the neck by ultrasonography-guided percutaneous ethanol injection. Eur Radiol. 2008;18:835–42.
13. Fromigue J, DeBaere T, Baudin E, Dromain C, Leboulleux S, Schlumberger M. Chemoembolization for liver metastases from medullary thyroid carcinoma. J Clin Endocrinol Metab. 2006;91:2496–9.
14. Kalinowski M, Dressler M, Konig A, El-Sheik M, Rinke A, Hoffken H, et al. Selective internal radiotherapy with Yttrium-90 microspheres for hepatic metastatic neuroendocrine tumors: a prospective single center study. Digestion. 2009;79:137–42.
15. Schlumberger M, Challeton C, De Vathaire F, et al. Radioactive iodine treatment and external radiotherapy for lung and bone metastases from thyroid carcinoma. J Nucl Med. 1996;37:598–605.
16. Muresan MM, Olivier P, Leclere J, Sirveaux F, Brunaud L, Klein M, et al. Bone metastases from differentiated thyroid carcinoma. Endocr Relat Cancer. 2008;15:37–49.
17. Bernier M-O, Leenhardt L, Hoang C, et al. Survival and therapeutic modalities in patients with bone metastases of differentiated thyroid carcinoma. J Clin Endocrinol Metab. 2001;86:1568–73.
18. Camille RR, Leger FA, Merland JJ, et al. Recent advances in the treatment of bone metastases from cancer of the thyroid. Chirurgie. 1980;106:32–6.
19. Smit JW, Vielvoye GJ, Goslings BM. Embolization for vertebral metastases of follicular thyroid carcinoma. J Clin Endocrinol Metab. 2000;85:989–94.
20. Vitale G, Fonderico F, Martignetti A, et al. Pamidronate improves the quality of life and induces clinical remission of bone metastases in patients with thyroid cancer. Br J Cancer. 2001;84:1586–90.
21. Rosen HN, Moses AC, Garber J, et al. Randomized trial of pamidronate in patients with thyroid cancer: bone density is not reduced by suppressive doses of thyroxine, but is increased by cyclic intravenous pamidronate. J Clin Endocrinol Metab. 1998;83:2324–30.
22. Rosen LS, Gordon D, Tchekmedyian S, et al. Zoledronic acid versus placebo in the treatment of skeletal metastases in patients with lung cancer and other solid tumors: a phase III, double-blind, randomized trial—the zoledronic acid lung cancer and other solid tumors study group. J Clin Oncol. 2003;21:3150–7.
23. Rosen LS, Gordon D, Tchekmedyian NS, et al. Long-term efficacy and safety of zoledronic acid in the treatment of skeletal metastases in patients with non-small cell lung carcinoma and other solid tumors. Cancer. 2004;100:2613–21.
24. Eustatia-Rutten CF, Romijn JA, Guijt MJ, et al. Outcome of palliative embolization of bone metastases in differentiated thyroid carcinoma. J Clin Endocrinol Metab. 2003;88:3184–9.

25. Van Tol KM, Hew JM, Jager PL, et al. Embolization in combination with radioiodine therapy for bone metastases from differentiated thyroid carcinoma. Clin Endocrinol. 2000;52:653–9.
26. Elshafie O, Hussein S, Jeans WD, Woodhouse NJ. Massive rise in thyroglobulin with adult respiratory distress syndrome after embolisation of thyroid cancer metastasis. Br J Radiol. 2000;73:547–9.
27. Halpin RJ, Bendok BR, Liu JC. Minimally invasive treatments for spinal metastases: vertebroplasty, kyphoplasty, and radiofrequency ablation. J Support Oncol. 2004;2:339–55.
28. Peh WC, Gilula LA. Percutaneous vertebroplasty: indications, contraindications, and technique. Br J Radiol. 2003;76:69–75.
29. Kushchayev S, Kushchayev Y, Theodore N, Preul MC, Clark OH. Percutaneous vertebroplasty for thyroid cancer metastases to the spine. Thyroid. 2010;20:555–60.
30. Ahmad Z, Abbasi F, Mitsunaga M, Portner B. Pain reduction and functional improvement after kyphoplasty: a retrospective study of 50 patients. Archit Phys Med Rhab. 2003;84:A21.
31. Ledlie JT, Fenfro M. Balloon kyphoplasty: one-year outcomes in vertebral body height restoration, chronic pain, and activity levels. J Neurosurg. 2003;98:36–42.
32. Faggiano A, Ramundo V, Assanti AP, Fonderic PE, Macchia PE, Misso C, et al. Thyroid nodules treated with percutaneous radiofrequency thermal ablation: a comparative study. J Clin Endocrinol Metab. 2012;97:4439–45.
33. Huh JY, Baek JH, Choi H, Kim JK, Lee JH. Symptomatic benign thyroid nodules: efficacy of additional radiofrequency ablation treatment session – prospective randomized study. Radiology. 2012;263:909–16.
34. Na DG, Lee JH, Jung SL, Kim JH, Sung JY, Shin JH, et al. Radiofrequency ablation of benign thyroid nodules and recurrent thyroid cancers: consensus statement and recommendations. Kor J Radiol. 2012;13:117–25.
35. Ha JH, Baek J, Lee JH. The efficacy and complications of radiofrequency of thyroid nodules. Curr Opin Endocrinol Diabetes Obes. 2011;18:310–4.
36. Wallace LB, Berber E. Percutaneous and video-assisted ablation of endocrine tumors: liver, adrenal and thyroid. Surg Lap, Endosc Percutan Tech. 2011;21:255–9.
37. Baek JH, Lee JH, Valcavi R, Pacella CM, Rhim H, Na DG. Thermal ablation for benign thyroid nodules: radiofrequency and laser. Kor J Radiol. 2011;12:525–40.
38. McGahan JP, Dodd GD. Radiofrequency ablation of the liver: current status. Am J Roentgenol. 2001;176:3–16.
39. Dupuy DE. Minimally invasive therapies in the treatment of bone malignancies. Crit Rev. 1998;75:161–71.
40. Goetz MP, Callstrom MR, Charboneau JW, et al. Percutaneous image-guided radiofrequency ablation of painful metastases involving bone: a multicenter study. J Clin Oncol. 2004;22:300–6.
41. Schaefer O, Lohrmann C, Ghanem N, Langer M. CT-guided radiofrequency heat ablation of malignant lung tumors. Med Sci Monit. 2003;9:127–31.
42. Dupuy DE, Zagoria RJ, Akerley W, et al. Percutaneous radiofrequency ablation of malignancies in the lung. Am J Roentgenol. 2000;174:57–9.
43. Berber E, Siperstein A. Laparoscopic radiofrequency thermal ablation of adrenal tumors: technical details. Surg Laparosc Endosc Percutan Tech. 2010;20:58–62.
44. Schaefer O, Lohrmann C, Markmiller M, et al. Technical innovation: combined treatment of a spinal metastasis with radiofrequency heat ablation and vertebroplasty. Am J Roentgenol. 2003;180: 1075–7.
45. Halpin RJ, Bendok BB, Sato KT, et al. Combination treatment of vertebral metastases using image-guided percutaneous radiofrequency ablation and vertebroplasty: a case report. Surg Neurol. 2005; 63:469–74.
46. Dupuy DE, Monchik JM, Decrea C, Pisharodi L. Radiofrequency ablation of regional recurrence from well-differentiated thyroid malignancy. Surgery. 2001;130:971–7.
47. Callstrom MR, Charboneau JW, Goetz MP, et al. Painful metastases involving bone: feasibility of percutaneous CT- and US-guided radio-frequency ablation. Radiology. 2002;224:87–97.
48. Mazzaglia PJ, Berber E, Milas M, Siperstein AE. Laparoscopic radiofrequency ablation of neuroendocrine liver metastases: a 10-year experience evaluating predictors of survival. Surgery. 2007;142:10–9.
49. Akyildiz HY, Mitchell J, Milas M, Siperstein A, Berber E. Laparoscopic radiofrequency thermal ablation of neuroendocrine hepatic metastases: long-term follow-up. Surgery. 2010;148: 1288–93.
50. Berber E, Siperstein A. Local recurrence after laparoscopic radiofrequency ablation of liver tumors: an analysis of 1032 tumors. Ann Surg Oncol. 2008;15:2757–64.
51. Pacella CM, Bizzarri G, Ferrari FS, et al. Interstitial photocoagulation with laser in the treatment of liver metastases. Radiol Med. 1996;92:438–47.
52. Pacella CM, Bizzarri G, Magnolfi F, et al. Laser thermal ablation in the treatment of small hepatocellular carcinoma: results in 74 patients. Radiology. 2001;221:712–20.
53. Papini E, Bizzarri G, Pacella CM. Percutaneous laser ablation of benign and malignant thyroid nodules. Curr Opin Endocrinol Diabetes Obes. 2008;15:434–9.
54. Guglielmi R, Pacella CM, Dottorini MF, et al. Severe thyrotoxicosis due to hyperfunctioning liver metastases from follicular carcinoma treatment with 131-I and interstitial laser ablation. Thyroid. 1999;9:173–7.
55. Pacella CM, Bizzarri G, Guglielmi R, et al. Thyroid tissue: US-guided percutaneous interstitial laser ablation—a feasibility study. Radiology. 2000;217:673–7.
56. Papini E, Guglielmi R, Gharib AH, Misischi I, Graziano F, Chianelli M, et al. Ultrasound-guided laser ablation of incidental papillary thyroid microcarcinoma: a potential therapeutic approach in patients at surgical risk. Thyroid. 2011;21:917–20.
57. Valcavi R, Piana S, Bortolan GS, Lai R, Barbieri V, Negro R. Ultrasound-guided percutaneous laser ablation of papillary thyroid microcarcinoma: a feasibility study on three cases with pathological and immunohistochemical evaluation. Thyroid. 2013;23:1578–82.
58. Pacella CM, Bizzari G, Spiezia S, et al. Thyroid tissue: US-guided percutaneous laser thermal ablation. Radiology. 2004;232:272–80.
59. Cakir B, Topaloglu O, Gul K, Agac T, Aydin C, Dirikoc A, et al. Ultrasound-guided percutaneous laser ablation treatment in inoperable aggressive course anaplastic thyroid carcinoma: the introduction of a novel alternative palliative therapy-second experience in the literature. J Endocrinol Invest. 2007;30:624–5.
60. Esnault O, Franc B, Chapelon J-Y. Localized ablation of thyroid tissue by high-intensity focused ultrasound: improvement of noninvasive tissue necrosis methods. Thyroid. 2009;19:1085–91.
61. Esnault, Franc B, Menegaux F, Rouxel A, DeKerviler E, Bourrier P, Lacoste F, et al. High-intensity focused ultrasound ablation of thyroid nodules: first human feasibility study. Thyroid. 2011;21: 965–73.
62. Leenhardt L, Borson-Chazot F, Calzada B, Carnaille A, Charrie B, Cochand-Priollet CD, et al. Good practice guide for cervical ultrasound scan and echo-guided techniques in treating differentiated thyroid cancer of vesicular origin. Ann Endocrinol. 2011;72: 173–97.

68 Radioiodine-Refractory Thyroid Cancer: Restoring Response to Radioiodine Therapy

Stephanie A. Fish and James A. Fagin

Introduction

Most cases of thyroid cancer can be treated effectively with total thyroidectomy alone or combined with postoperative radioactive iodine (RAI) ablation. Iodine is concentrated in thyroid tissue in a relatively selective manner, since the ability to transport iodine is restricted to very few cell types. This explains the overall efficacy of this therapy, with few side effects and modest long-term toxicities. Unfortunately, some patients with metastatic thyroid cancer have tumors that can no longer trap iodine. This is associated with a worse prognosis. The 10-year survival of patients with metastatic thyroid cancer that retains RAI avidity is ~60 %, whereas the survival is only 10 % if the metastases do not trap iodine [1]. Identifying treatments that can restore the ability of these cancer metastases to incorporate iodine could represent a significant therapeutic advance and has been a long-standing goal of clinical investigation in this field.

Loss of Iodine Uptake

Iodine uptake by thyroid cells and its storage as thyroid hormone precursors is a complex process that requires well-controlled metabolic steps and the appropriate function of several proteins, including the sodium-iodine symporter (NIS), pendrin, thyroglobulin (Tg), and thyroid peroxidase (TPO). The first step in thyroid hormone synthesis is the uptake of iodine across the basal membrane of the thyrocytes via NIS, which cotransports two sodium ions along with one iodine ion. It has been postulated that iodine then has to efflux into the follicular lumen through the action of pendrin, which is a highly hydrophobic membrane protein located at the apical membrane of thyrocytes. Once iodine reaches the cell-colloid interface, it is oxidized and rapidly organified by incorporation into the tyrosine residues of Tg. This reaction is catalyzed by TPO in the presence of hydrogen peroxide and results in the formation of mono- and diiodotyrosines. TPO also catalyzes the coupling of two iodotyrosines to form either triiodothyronine (T3) or thyroxine (T4).

TSH is the major regulator of thyroid cell proliferation, differentiation, and function. TSH acts by binding to the TSH receptor (TSHR), which is a member of the G-protein-coupled receptor superfamily. The effects of TSH are primarily mediated through the activation of adenylyl cyclase via the GTP-binding protein Gsα (alpha), a component of a heterotrimeric G-protein complex engaged upon ligand binding to the receptor. The activated TSHR also stimulates the phosphatidylinositol-Ca2+ (PIP2) cascade with inositol 1,4,5-triphosphate (InsP3) and diacylglycerol functioning as second messengers. The two pathways, in turn, modulate numerous cellular functions, including the transcription of thyroid-specific genes, such as those coding for NIS, TG, and TPO.

In thyroid cancer, dysfunction at any stage in the process of iodine incorporation into thyroid hormone precursors can lead to a less differentiated tumor that does not respond to traditional treatments, especially to RAI. Several agents have been studied in an attempt to alter thyroid cancer cells so that they can regain these functional properties and become susceptible to radioiodine therapy.

S.A. Fish, MD
Department of Medicine, Memorial Sloan-Kettering Cancer Center and Weill Cornell Medical College, New York, NY, USA
e-mail: fishs@mskcc.org

J.A. Fagin, MD (✉)
Department of Medicine, Memorial Sloan-Kettering Cancer Center, 1275 York Avenue, Box 296, New York, NY 10065, USA
e-mail: faginj@mskcc.org

L. Wartofsky, D. Van Nostrand (eds.), *Thyroid Cancer*, DOI 10.1007/978-1-4939-3314-3_68

Retinoids

Retinoids are a group of natural and synthetic molecules that are structurally and functionally related to retinol (vitamin A) and retinoic acid (RA). Retinoids are critical for cell growth and differentiation during development. The action of retinoids is mediated by binding to specific nuclear hormone receptors, the retinoic acid (RAR), and the retinoid X receptors (RXR). These ligand-bound receptors can stimulate or suppress gene expression by interaction with the regulatory region of a diverse set of genes. RAR and RXR cooperate as heterodimers to mediate the action of retinoids on gene expression. RXR can also form heterodimers with many other nuclear hormone receptors, including the thyroid hormone receptor, to further modulate gene expression and cellular function. Since retinoids appear to induce differentiation in development, these agents have been studied as potential cancer therapies [2, 3].

Normal human thyroid cells express RARα (alpha) and RXRγ (gamma), but RARα (alpha) expression is reduced in thyroid cancer cells. Retinoids were reported to inhibit growth and induce radioiodine uptake in human thyroid cancer cell lines [4]. Additionally, retinoids induce type I iodothyronine 5′-deiodinase isoenzymes [5, 6], thyroglobulin [7], and NIS mRNA [8]. Several of these experiments were done with human thyroid cancer cell lines that were later found to be misclassified and not derived from a thyroid lineage [9], rendering some these findings difficult to interpret. However, based in part on these experiments, clinical studies of retinoids in patients with advanced thyroid cancer were initiated.

The initial clinical trials used isotretinoin (13-cis-retinoic acid). Overall, 20–40 % of patients showed a response to isotretinoin therapy including reduced tumor size, increased radioiodine uptake, changes in Tg levels, or alterations in fluorodeoxyglucose positron emission tomography (FDG-PET) uptake [10–15]. These initial studies did not include a control group which limits the interpretation of the findings. In addition, more recent clinical studies utilizing isotretinoin in patients with advanced thyroid cancer show that few patients have a clinically meaningful response [16, 17]. Based on these results, retinoid therapy alone does not appear to be an effective therapy for RAI-resistant metastatic thyroid cancer.

Thiazolidinediones

The peroxisome proliferator-activated receptor (PPAR) is also a member of the nuclear hormone receptor superfamily, which mediates pleiotropic effects on cell metabolism, differentiated properties, and cell growth [18]. Thiazolidinediones (TZD) are PPARγ (gamma) agonists that are used primarily in the treatment of type 2 diabetes mellitus due to their ability to improve insulin sensitivity [19]. However, TZDs have also been shown to prevent tumorigenesis in transgenic mouse models, to inhibit cellular proliferation by causing cell cycle arrest and apoptosis, to induce redifferentiation, and to inhibit angiogenesis [20–23].

PPARγ (gamma) expression has been reported to be dysregulated in differentiated thyroid cancer [24–26]. In addition, a chromosomal rearrangement of the *PAX8* and *PPARG* genes has been observed in about 50 % of follicular thyroid cancers and 17 % of follicular adenomas [24, 27], as well as in some follicular-variant papillary thyroid cancers. Based on this information, it was hypothesized that TZDs may be effective agents in the treatment of thyroid cancer expressing PPARγ (gamma). A recent study found that treatment of transgenic mice expressing PAX8-PPARγ (gamma) in thyroid cells with the TZD pioglitazone induced trans-differentiation into adipocyte-like cells [28].

Frohlich et al. found that the TZD troglitazone increased apoptosis and decreased DNA synthesis and cell growth in normal porcine thyrocytes and in follicular thyroid carcinoma cell lines. They also found that membrane NIS abundance was increased [22]. Ohta et al. reported antiproliferative effects in vitro and growth inhibition in vivo of troglitazone in PTC cell lines [29]. Martelli et al. reported that restoration of PPARγ (gamma) in thyroid cancer cells lacking expression of this nuclear receptor inhibited cell growth, which was further blocked by treatment with PPARγ (gamma) agonists [30].

Based on these preclinical findings, Kebebew et al. treated 20 patients with metastatic non-RAI-avid thyroid cancer with the TZD rosiglitazone [31]. Five patients had a positive RAI scan after treatment, but none of them had a clinical response by Response Evaluation Criteria in Solid Tumors (RECIST) criteria. Thus, monotherapy with TZDs does not appear to be a promising approach to increase responses to RAI in patients with advanced thyroid cancer. However, the patients in the clinical trial were not selected based on their genetic characteristics, and it remains to be seen if patients harboring tumors with *PAX8-PPARG* may respond to TZDs.

Of note, PPARγ (gamma) mediates the effects of TZDs on gene expression by forming a heterodimer with RXR. The combination of TZDs and RXR-selective retinoids has been shown to exert cooperative effects on terminal differentiation of liposarcoma cells [32]. Whether this may also be the case in cancers of the thyroid lineage remains to be conclusively established, but if this were the case, this combination treatment may be worth studying in the future.

Histone Deacetylase Inhibitors

Histone acetylation and deacetylation can modulate chromatin structure and regulate gene expression leading to DNA replication, transcription, differentiation, and apoptosis. Histone acetylation decreases the ability of the histones to bind to DNA and allows chromatin expansion, permitting genetic transcription to take place. When the acetyl groups are removed from histone, there is high-affinity binding of histone to the DNA backbone, which turns off transcription. Thus, histone deacetylase (HDAC) inhibitors decrease histone-DNA binding and induce gene transcription. Studies have looked at the effects of HDAC inhibitors on the expression of thyroid-specific genes in poorly differentiated papillary and anaplastic thyroid cancer cell lines. Kitazono et al. reported that depsipeptide markedly increased Tg and NIS mRNA as well as RAI uptake at low concentrations in poorly differentiated thyroid cancer cell lines [33]. In addition, Imanishi et al. found that depsipeptide increased apoptosis, suggesting this agent may be used for both redifferentiation and tumoricidal effects [34].

Although these agents have shown beneficial effects in thyroid cancer cell lines, the clinical data has been disappointing [35, 36]. This may be due to the fact that some of the preclinical experiments with HDAC inhibitors that provided the rationale for the clinical trials were flawed, because many of the cancer cell lines used were later found to have been misidentified and not to be of thyroid origin [9]. Moreover, the magnitude of the effects in vitro was modest when compared to the iodine uptake of well-differentiated, non-transformed, thyroid cells.

DNA-Demethylating Agents

Methylation is a key epigenetic mechanism that controls gene expression. Hypermethylation of cytosine residues is associated with decreased gene transcription. In thyroid cancer cells, TTF-1 (Nkx2.1) has been reported to be silenced through hypermethylation [37]. Nkx2.1 is a key transcription factor that regulates the expression of thyroid-specific genes such as *TG*, *TPO*, *TSHR*, *SLC26A4* (encoding Pendrin), and *NIS* [37–39]. Venkataraman et al. examined DNA methylation of the regulatory region of *NIS* in dedifferentiated thyroid carcinoma. They found hypermethylation in three regions of the *NIS* promoter in different types of thyroid cancer. There was some correlation between *NIS* promoter hypermethylation, low NIS mRNA expression, and absence of RAI uptake in tumors [40].

Given these findings, demethylating agents, such as 5-azacytidine, have been studied for effects on gene expression and differentiated function in thyroid cancer cells, with some evidence supporting increases in NIS gene expression [41, 42]. A phase 1B clinical trial of 5-azacytidine in patients with RAI-refractory thyroid cancer was performed, but not formally reported. Sixteen patients were enrolled and underwent I-131 scans under hypothyroid conditions before and after treatment with 30 or 70 mg 5-azacytidine/m2/day for 10 or 20 days. None of the patients showed evidence of restoration of iodide uptake, and the trial was discontinued (Kenneth Ain, M.D., Univ. Kentucky, personal communication).

Caveats in the Design of Clinical Trials with Agents to Sensitize Thyroid Cancers to Radioiodine

Table 68.1 summarizes the data from the clinical trials that have looked at the effectiveness of some of these agents in restoring RAI uptake in patients with RAI-refractory metastatic thyroid cancer. While there have been several clinical trials utilizing isotretinoin and two trials utilizing rosiglitazone, there have been no published clinical trials looking at the effectiveness of HDAC inhibitors or DNA-demethylating agents in restoring RAI uptake.

So far, the studies of retinoid therapy have shown modest benefit. There are several limitations related to the study methods. In general, the assessment of treatment effectiveness has been determined by visually comparing posttreatment whole body scan after retinoid treatment with a prior posttreatment scans after RAI alone. Without a quantitative measurement of uptake, it is difficult to determine if a change is clinically significant. The availability of ^{124}I PET dosimetry provides the means to overcome this drawback [43, 44]. In determining the response to treatment over time, only a few of the studies used standardized criteria, such as RECIST or WHO. In those studies that did quantify response to treatment, only 21–55 % of patients showed a partial response or stable disease.

In the two published studies with TZDs, the authors looked at iodine uptake after drug treatment, but did not follow the patients over time to assess whether there was a clinical response. This is likely because there was a very minor increase in RAI uptake after TZD therapy, making a clinical response unlikely. These agents are safe and well-tolerated; however, current evidence indicates that there is no meaningful clinical response.

Role of Oncogenic Activation of MAPK on Loss of Iodide Incorporation

While all of the agents noted above have the potential to induce redifferentiation in thyroid cancer cells, none so far has been effective in restoring RAI uptake in clinical trials (Table 68.1). It is possible that these agents are not effective

Table 68.1 Summary of clinical trials of agents used to restore RAI uptake

	Design	Pts (#)	RAI Rx	Measure of effectiveness	Biochemical response to treatment	Structural response to treatment
Retinoids-*isotretinoin* (*13-cis-RA*)						
Oh 2011 [57]	Open-label clinical trial	47	47 after THW	Post-Rx scan compared to previous post-Rx scan	Determined by Tg	WHO response criteria
				Interpreted visually	*Clinical response*: combination of serum Tg response and change in tumor size (WHO response criteria)	
				0 = no uptake	10/47 (21 %) responders	
				1 = faint uptake	37/47 (79 %) nonresponders	
				2 = definite uptake		
Coelho 2011 [17]	Open-label clinical trial	16	16 after THW	Post-Rx scan compared to previous post-Rx scan	Not assessed	RECIST criteria
				Interpreted visually		PR: 3/16
						SD: 4/16
						PD: 9/16
Kim 2009 [58]	Open-label clinical trial	11	11 after THW	Post-Rx scan compared to previous post-Rx scan	Determined by Tg	RECIST criteria
				Interpreted visually	Increased (8/11)	TgAb+ (1/11)
				No uptake (9 pts)	Stable/decrease (2/11)	SD: 6/11
				Faint uptake (2 pts)		PD:5/11
				Increased uptake (0 pts)		
Handkiewicz-Junak 2009 [16]	Open-label clinical trial	53	53 after rhTSH	Post-Rx scan compared to pre-Rx scan	Not assessed	No tumor regression in 9 responders
				Interpreted visually		Disease progression in 4/9 responders at 12 months
				(Yes/no)		
				Yes: 9/53		
				No: 44/53		
Short 2004 [59]	Open-label clinical trial	16	None	1/16 pts with increased uptake on WBS (not enough to permit a significant treatment dose of iodine)	Not assessed	Not assessed
Grüning 2003 [15]	Open-label clinical trial	25	25 after THW	Post-Rx scan compared to pre-Rx scan: semiquantitative lesional dosimetry	Tg and FDG-PET did not correlate with response to RAI	
				5/25 pts with increased uptake	Out of 5 responders, 2 are symptom-free, one is clinically well, one has deteriorated, and one is dead	

Simon 2002 [60]	Prospective multicenter study without controls	50 (75 enrolled)	50 after THW	*WBS* (interpreted visually and by dosimetry in 6 pts)	Clinical outcome: based on Tg and/or tumor size (no RECIST)	
				Increased 21/50 (marked increase in 13)	Responders 10/50 (20 %)	
				Stable 29/50	Stable dz 9/50 (18 %)	
				Structural imaging (*n*=*37*)	Dz progression 31/50 (62 %)	
				Increase 9/37	11 pts showed dz progression despite increased RAI uptake	
				Stable 22/37		
				Decrease 6/37		
Grünwald 1998 [11]	Open-label clinical trial	12	12	Post-Rx scan compared to pre-Rx scan	Tg levels increased significantly more in the responders vs nonresponders	Not assessed
				interpreted visually		
				5/12 responders (2 pts with therapeutically useful uptake, 3 pts with faint uptake)		
				7/12 nonresponders		
Simon 1998 [12]	Open-label clinical trial	20	None	*WBS*: interpreted visually	Not assessed	Not assessed
				Increased 8/16		
				Stable 8/16		
				Structural imaging:		
				Increase 9/15		
				Stable 5/15		
				Decrease 1/15		
PPAR-gamma: *rosiglitazone*						
Kebebew 2009 [31]	Open-label clinical trial	20	None	Pre-Rx WBS vs post-Rx WBS	Not assessed	Not assessed
				Positive 5/20		
				Imaging: *RECIST criteria*		
				PD: 7/13		
				CR: 0		
				PR: 0		
Tepmongkol 2008 [61]	Open-label clinical trial	23	23 after THW	Post-Rx scan compared with previous post-Rx scan	Not assessed	Not assessed
				Interpreted visually		
				6/23 positive post-Rx scan		
				17/23 negative post-Rx scan		

Abbreviations: pts patients, *RAI Rx* radioactive iodine treatment, *TWH* thyroid hormone withdrawal, *post-Rx* posttreatment, *pre-Rx* pretreatment, *Tg* thyroglobulin, *RECIST* Response Evaluation Criteria in Solid Tumors, *CR* complete response, *PR* partial response, *SD* stable disease, *PD* progressive disease, *TgAb* thyroglobulin antibodies, *rhTSH* recombinant human thyrotropin, *WBS* whole body scan, *FDG-PET* fluorodeoxyglucose positron emission tomography because they were not selected based on an understanding of the specific molecular mechanisms responsible for the loss of iodine uptake in thyroid tumors. Papillary thyroid cancers (PTC) are associated with mutually exclusive mutations of oncogenes encoding effectors of the mitogen-activated protein kinase (MAPK) signaling pathway (i.e., *RET*, *NTRK*, *RAS*, and *BRAF*). Oncogenic activation of MAPK signaling in thyroid cells leads to loss of expression of genes required for thyroid hormone biosynthesis, including NIS and TG [45, 46].

The activating $BRAF^{V600E}$ mutation is the most frequent genetic alteration in PTC and confers patients with a poor prognosis [47–50]. BRAF activation is associated with tumors with lowered expression of NIS [51], which likely explains the clinical observation that PTCs with *BRAF* mutations are often particularly resistant to RAI therapy [48]. The most likely explanation for this disruption is provided by studies in PCCL3 cells, a rat thyroid cell line that retains most of the differentiated properties of normal thyrocytes. Conditional expression of oncogenic RET/PTC, RAS, or BRAF in PCCL3 cells downregulates expression of NIS and other thyroid-specific genes [46, 52], which is partially restored by treatment with RAF or MEK inhibitors [52, 53]. Tellingly, thyroid-specific endogenous expression of $BRAF^{V600E}$ in mice leads to profound downregulation of expression of thyroid-specific genes and induction of hypothyroidism.

The mechanisms through which MAPK activation inhibits NIS expression and iodide transport are being actively investigated. BRAF markedly inhibits expression of PAX8 and induces TGFβ1 (beta) secretion in vitro and in vivo, which has been postulated to mediate the effects of BRAF through an autocrine loop. This is because TGFβ (beta) activates SMAD3, which binds to PAX8 and prevents it from binding DNA and transactivating NIS [54]. However, recent data suggest that MAPK activation may have direct effects on NIS, independent of these TGFβ (beta)-mediated pathways.

Mice with doxycycline-inducible expression of BRAF-V600E in thyroid cells have been developed to explore the biological effects of the oncoprotein and to determine whether the transformed cells are dependent on its activity for viability. One week after expression of mutant BRAF, the mice develop invasive lesions that are histologically consistent with papillary thyroid cancers. When doxycycline is discontinued, the cancers regress. Moreover, activation of BRAF leads to a profound decrease in the expression of thyroid-specific genes and of radioactive iodine uptake in vivo, which is restored when doxycycline is discontinued. When the mice are treated with inhibitors of RAF or MEK, ^{124}I uptake is partially restored [55].

Based on these results, a pilot phase 2 clinical trial with the allosteric MEK inhibitor selumetinib has been completed in patients with RAI-refractory metastatic thyroid cancer, with very promising results. In this study, ^{124}I PET scans were used to obtain quantitative lesional dosimetry before and after treatment with the compound, and 60 % of patients showed increased iodine incorporation into metastatic lesions. Moreover, the predicted dose allowed 40 % of patients to be treated productively with 131-I, with remarkable clinical responses [56].

Conclusion

The development of new treatment modalities for patients with RAI-resistant metastatic thyroid cancer is crucial because of the lack of effective therapies for this disease. The "redifferentiating" agents studied to date have not been effective in clinical trials, although the technology available at the time these studies were performed did not allow rigorous measurement of effects on iodide uptake in response to the experimental agents. Moreover, the clinical responses to 131-I therapy were not always monitored systematically.

Inhibition of MAPK signaling with MEK or RAF inhibitors has shown promising results in mouse models of thyroid cancer. An early clinical trial with one of these agents is showing significant promise, providing hope that RAI incorporation can indeed be increased to levels that will allow effective therapeutic administration of the isotope and to significant clinical benefit.

References

1. Durante C, Haddy N, Baudin E, et al. Long-term outcome of 444 patients with distant metastases from papillary and follicular thyroid carcinoma: benefits and limits of radioiodine therapy. J Clin Endocrinol Metab. 2006;91(8):2892–9.
2. Evans TR, Kaye SB. Retinoids: present role and future potential. Br J Cancer. 1999;80(1–2):1–8.
3. Smith MA, Anderson B. Where to next with retinoids for cancer therapy? Clin Cancer Res Off J Am Assoc Cancer Res. 2001; 7(10):2955–7.
4. Elisei R, Vivaldi A, Agate L, et al. All-trans-retinoic acid treatment inhibits the growth of retinoic acid receptor beta messenger ribonucleic acid expressing thyroid cancer cell lines but does not reinduce the expression of thyroid-specific genes. J Clin Endocrinol Metab. 2005;90(4):2403–11.
5. Van Herle AJ, Agatep ML, Padua 3rd DN, et al. Effects of 13 cis-retinoic acid on growth and differentiation of human follicular carcinoma cells (UCLA R0 82 W-1) in vitro. J Clin Endocrinol Metab. 1990;71(3):755–63.
6. Schreck R, Schnieders F, Schmutzler C, Kohrle J. Retinoids stimulate type I iodothyronine 5′-deiodinase activity in human follicular thyroid carcinoma cell lines. J Clin Endocrinol Metab. 1994;79(3): 791–8.
7. Kurebayashi J, Tanaka K, Otsuki T, et al. All-trans-retinoic acid modulates expression levels of thyroglobulin and cytokines in a new human poorly differentiated papillary thyroid carcinoma cell line, KTC-1. J Clin Endocrinol Metab. 2000;85(8):2889–96.
8. Schmutzler C, Winzer R, Meissner-Weigl J, Kohrle J. Retinoic acid increases sodium/iodide symporter mRNA levels in human thyroid cancer cell lines and suppresses expression of functional symporter

in nontransformed FRTL-5 rat thyroid cells. Biochem Biophys Res Commun. 1997;240(3):832–8.
9. Schweppe RE, Klopper JP, Korch C, et al. Deoxyribonucleic acid profiling analysis of 40 human thyroid cancer cell lines reveals cross-contamination resulting in cell line redundancy and misidentification. J Clin Endocrinol Metab. 2008;93(11):4331–41.
10. Grunwald F, Pakos E, Bender H, et al. Redifferentiation therapy with retinoic acid in follicular thyroid cancer. J Nucl Med Off Publ Soc Nucl Med. 1998;39(9):1555–8.
11. Grunwald F, Menzel C, Bender H, et al. Redifferentiation therapy-induced radioiodine uptake in thyroid cancer. J Nucl Med Off Publ Soc Nucl Med. 1998;39(11):1903–6.
12. Simon D, Koehrle J, Reiners C, et al. Redifferentiation therapy with retinoids: therapeutic option for advanced follicular and papillary thyroid carcinoma. World J Surg. 1998;22(6):569–74.
13. Schmutzler C, Kohrle J. Retinoic acid redifferentiation therapy for thyroid cancer. Thyroid Off J Am Thyroid Assoc. 2000;10(5): 393–406.
14. Boerner AR, Petrich T, Weckesser E, et al. Monitoring isotretinoin therapy in thyroid cancer using 18F-FDG PET. Eur J Nucl Med Mol Imaging. 2002;29(2):231–6.
15. Gruning T, Tiepolt C, Zophel K, Bredow J, Kropp J, Franke WG. Retinoic acid for redifferentiation of thyroid cancer – does it hold its promise? Eur J Endocrinol Eur Fed Endocr Soc. 2003;148(4):395–402.
16. Handkiewicz-Junak D, Roskosz J, Hasse-Lazar K, et al. 13-cis-retinoic acid re-differentiation therapy and recombinant human thyrotropin-aided radioiodine treatment of non-functional metastatic thyroid cancer: a single-center, 53-patient phase 2 study. Thyroid Res. 2009;2(1):8.
17. Coelho SM, Vaisman F, Buescu A, Mello RC, Carvalho DP, Vaisman M. Follow-up of patients treated with retinoic acid for the control of radioiodine non-responsive advanced thyroid carcinoma. Braz J Med Biol Res Rev Bras Pesquisas Med Biol Soc Bras Biofisica. 2011;44(1):73–7.
18. Corton JC, Lapinskas PJ, Gonzalez FJ. Central role of PPARalpha in the mechanism of action of hepatocarcinogenic peroxisome proliferators. Mutat Res. 2000;448(2):139–51.
19. Lebovitz HE. Rationale for and role of thiazolidinediones in type 2 diabetes mellitus. Am J Cardiol. 2002;90(5A):34G–41.
20. Koeffler HP. Peroxisome proliferator-activated receptor gamma and cancers. Clin Cancer Res Off J Am Assoc Cancer Res. 2003; 9(1):1–9.
21. Park JW, Zarnegar R, Kanauchi H, et al. Troglitazone, the peroxisome proliferator-activated receptor-gamma agonist, induces antiproliferation and redifferentiation in human thyroid cancer cell lines. Thyroid Off J Am Thyroid Assoc. 2005;15(3):222–31.
22. Frohlich E, Machicao F, Wahl R. Action of thiazolidinediones on differentiation, proliferation and apoptosis of normal and transformed thyrocytes in culture. Endocr Relat Cancer. 2005;12(2): 291–303.
23. Philips JC, Petite C, Willi JP, Buchegger F, Meier CA. Effect of peroxisome proliferator-activated receptor gamma agonist, rosiglitazone, on dedifferentiated thyroid cancers. Nucl Med Commun. 2004;25(12):1183–6.
24. Marques AR, Espadinha C, Frias MJ, et al. Underexpression of peroxisome proliferator-activated receptor (PPAR)gamma in PAX8/PPARgamma-negative thyroid tumours. Br J Cancer. 2004;91(4): 732–8.
25. Sahin M, Allard BL, Yates M, et al. PPARgamma staining as a surrogate for PAX8/PPARgamma fusion oncogene expression in follicular neoplasms: clinicopathological correlation and histopathological diagnostic value. J Clin Endocrinol Metab. 2005; 90(1):463–8.
26. Karger S, Berger K, Eszlinger M, et al. Evaluation of peroxisome proliferator-activated receptor-gamma expression in benign and malignant thyroid pathologies. Thyroid Off J Am Thyroid Assoc. 2005;15(9):997–1003.
27. Kroll TG, Sarraf P, Pecciarini L, et al. PAX8-PPARgamma1 fusion oncogene in human thyroid carcinoma [corrected]. Science. 2000;289(5483):1357–60.
28. Dobson ME, Diallo-Krou E, Grachtchouk V, et al. Pioglitazone induces a proadipogenic antitumor response in mice with PAX8-PPARgamma fusion protein thyroid carcinoma. Endocrinology. 2011;152(11):4455–65.
29. Ohta K, Endo T, Haraguchi K, Hershman JM, Onaya T. Ligands for peroxisome proliferator-activated receptor gamma inhibit growth and induce apoptosis of human papillary thyroid carcinoma cells. J Clin Endocrinol Metab. 2001;86(5):2170–7.
30. Martelli ML, Iuliano R, Le Pera I, et al. Inhibitory effects of peroxisome proliferator-activated receptor gamma on thyroid carcinoma cell growth. J Clin Endocrinol Metab. 2002;87(10): 4728–35.
31. Kebebew E, Lindsay S, Clark OH, Woeber KA, Hawkins R, Greenspan FS. Results of rosiglitazone therapy in patients with thyroglobulin-positive and radioiodine-negative advanced differentiated thyroid cancer. Thyroid Off J Am Thyroid Assoc. 2009; 19(9):953–6.
32. Tontonoz P, Singer S, Forman BM, et al. Terminal differentiation of human liposarcoma cells induced by ligands for peroxisome proliferator-activated receptor gamma and the retinoid X receptor. Proc Natl Acad Sci U S A. 1997;94(1):237–41.
33. Kitazono M, Robey R, Zhan Z, et al. Low concentrations of the histone deacetylase inhibitor, depsipeptide (FR901228), increase expression of the Na(+)/I(−) symporter and iodine accumulation in poorly differentiated thyroid carcinoma cells. J Clin Endocrinol Metab. 2001;86(7):3430–5.
34. Imanishi R, Ohtsuru A, Iwamatsu M, et al. A histone deacetylase inhibitor enhances killing of undifferentiated thyroid carcinoma cells by p53 gene therapy. J Clin Endocrinol Metab. 2002;87(10): 4821–4.
35. Schlumberger MJ, Elisei R, Bastholt L, et al. Phase II study of safety and efficacy of motesanib in patients with progressive or symptomatic, advanced or metastatic medullary thyroid cancer. J Clin Oncol Off J Am Society Clin Oncol. 2009;27(23): 3794–801.
36. Woyach JA, Kloos RT, Ringel MD, et al. Lack of therapeutic effect of the histone deacetylase inhibitor vorinostat in patients with metastatic radioiodine-refractory thyroid carcinoma. J Clin Endocrinol Metab. 2009;94(1):164–70.
37. Kondo T, Nakazawa T, Ma D, et al. Epigenetic silencing of TTF-1/NKX2-1 through DNA hypermethylation and histone H3 modulation in thyroid carcinomas. Lab Invest J Tech Methods Pathol. 2009;89(7):791–9.
38. Kusakabe T, Kawaguchi A, Hoshi N, Kawaguchi R, Hoshi S, Kimura S. Thyroid-specific enhancer-binding protein/NKX2.1 is required for the maintenance of ordered architecture and function of the differentiated thyroid. Mol Endocrinol. 2006;20(8): 1796–809.
39. Xing M, Tokumaru Y, Wu G, Westra WB, Ladenson PW, Sidransky D. Hypermethylation of the Pendred syndrome gene SLC26A4 is an early event in thyroid tumorigenesis. Cancer Res. 2003;63(9): 2312–5.
40. Venkataraman GM, Yatin M, Marcinek R, Ain KB. Restoration of iodide uptake in dedifferentiated thyroid carcinoma: relationship to human Na+/I-symporter gene methylation status. J Clin Endocrinol Metab. 1999;84(7):2449–57.
41. Li W, Venkataraman GM, Ain KB. Protein synthesis inhibitors, in synergy with 5-azacytidine, restore sodium/iodide symporter gene expression in human thyroid adenoma cell line, KAK-1, suggesting trans-active transcriptional repressor. J Clin Endocrinol Metab. 2007;92(3):1080–7.

42. Vivaldi A, Miasaki FY, Ciampi R, et al. Re-differentiation of thyroid carcinoma cell lines treated with 5-Aza-2′-deoxycytidine and retinoic acid. Mol Cell Endocrinol. 2009;307(1–2):142–8.
43. Kolbert KS, Pentlow KS, Pearson JR, et al. Prediction of absorbed dose to normal organs in thyroid cancer patients treated with 131I by use of 124I PET and 3-dimensional internal dosimetry software. J Nucl Med Off Publ Soc Nuclear Med. 2007;48(1):143–9.
44. Van Nostrand D, Khorjekar GR, O'Neil J, et al. Recombinant human thyroid-stimulating hormone versus thyroid hormone withdrawal in the identification of metastasis in differentiated thyroid cancer with 131I planar whole-body imaging and 124I PET. J Nucl Med Off Publ Soc Nucl Med. 2012;53(3):359–62.
45. Knauf JA, Kuroda H, Basu S, Fagin JA. RET/PTC-induced dedifferentiation of thyroid cells is mediated through Y1062 signaling through SHC-RAS-MAP kinase. Oncogene. 2003;22(28):4406–12.
46. Mitsutake N, Knauf JA, Mitsutake S, Mesa Jr C, Zhang L, Fagin JA. Conditional BRAFV600E expression induces DNA synthesis, apoptosis, dedifferentiation, and chromosomal instability in thyroid PCCL3 cells. Cancer Res. 2005;65(6):2465–73.
47. Nikiforova MN, Kimura ET, Gandhi M, et al. BRAF mutations in thyroid tumors are restricted to papillary carcinomas and anaplastic or poorly differentiated carcinomas arising from papillary carcinomas. J Clin Endocrinol Metab. 2003;88(11):5399–404.
48. Xing M, Westra WH, Tufano RP, et al. BRAF mutation predicts a poorer clinical prognosis for papillary thyroid cancer. J Clin Endocrinol Metab. 2005;90(12):6373–9.
49. Elisei R, Ugolini C, Viola D, et al. BRAF(V600E) mutation and outcome of patients with papillary thyroid carcinoma: a 15-year median follow-up study. J Clin Endocrinol Metab. 2008;93(10):3943–9.
50. Ricarte-Filho JC, Ryder M, Chitale DA, et al. Mutational profile of advanced primary and metastatic radioactive iodine-refractory thyroid cancers reveals distinct pathogenetic roles for BRAF, PIK3CA, and AKT1. Cancer Res. 2009;69(11):4885–93.
51. Durante C, Puxeddu E, Ferretti E, et al. BRAF mutations in papillary thyroid carcinomas inhibit genes involved in iodine metabolism. J Clin Endocrinol Metab. 2007;92(7):2840–3.
52. Knauf JA, Ouyang B, Croyle M, Kimura E, Fagin JA. Acute expression of RET/PTC induces isozyme-specific activation and subsequent downregulation of PKCepsilon in PCCL3 thyroid cells. Oncogene. 2003;22(44):6830–8.
53. Liu D, Liu Z, Jiang D, Dackiw AP, Xing M. Inhibitory effects of the mitogen-activated protein kinase kinase inhibitor CI-1040 on the proliferation and tumor growth of thyroid cancer cells with BRAF or RAS mutations. J Clin Endocrinol Metab. 2007;92(12):4686–95.
54. Costamagna E, Garcia B, Santisteban P. The functional interaction between the paired domain transcription factor Pax8 and Smad3 is involved in transforming growth factor-beta repression of the sodium/iodide symporter gene. J Biol Chem. 2004;279(5):3439–46.
55. Chakravarty D, Santos E, Ryder M, et al. Small-molecule MAPK inhibitors restore radioiodine incorporation in mouse thyroid cancers with conditional BRAF activation. J Clin Invest. 2011;121(12):4700–11.
56. Ho AL, Grewal RK, Leboeuf R, Sherman EJ, Pfister DG, Deandreis D, Pentlow KS, Zanzonico PB, Haque S, Gavane S, Ghossein RA, Ricarte-Filho JC, Dominguez JM, Shen R, Tuttle RM, Larson SM, Fagin JA. Selumetinib-Enhanced Radioiodine Uptake in Advanced Thyroid Cancer. N Engl J Med 2013;368:623–32.
57. Oh SW, Moon SH, Park do J, et al. Combined therapy with 131I and retinoic acid in Korean patients with radioiodine-refractory papillary thyroid cancer. Eur J Nucl Med Mol Imaging. 2011;38(10):1798–805.
58. Kim WG, Kim EY, Kim TY, et al. Redifferentiation therapy with 13-cis retinoic acids in radioiodine-resistant thyroid cancer. Endocr J. 2009;56(1):105–12.
59. Short SC, Suovuori A, Cook G, Vivian G, Harmer C. A phase II study using retinoids as redifferentiation agents to increase iodine uptake in metastatic thyroid cancer. Clin Oncol (R Coll Radiol). 2004;16(8):569–74.
60. Simon D, Korber C, Krausch M, et al. Clinical impact of retinoids in redifferentiation therapy of advanced thyroid cancer: final results of a pilot study. Eur J Nucl Med Mol Imaging. 2002;29(6):775–82.
61. Tepmongkol S, Keelawat S, Honsawek S, Ruangvejvorachai P. Rosiglitazone effect on radioiodine uptake in thyroid carcinoma patients with high thyroglobulin but negative total body scan: a correlation with the expression of peroxisome proliferator-activated receptor-gamma. Thyroid Off J Am Thyroid Assoc. 2008;18(7):697–704.

69 Alternative and Complementary Treatment of Thyroid Disorders

Barbara Mensah Onumah

National centers for complementary and alternative medicine (NCCAM) define complementary and alternative medicine (CAM) as a group of diverse medical and health care systems, practices, and products that are not generally considered part of conventional medicine. Complementary medicine refers to use of nonconventional medicine together with conventional medicine, while alternative medicine refers to use of nonconventional medicine instead of conventional medicine. Many Americans use a variety of different types of CAM. The 2007 National Health Interview Survey (NHIS), which included a comprehensive survey of CAM use by Americans, showed that approximately 38 % of adults use CAM [1].

Complementary and alternative medicine can be divided into some broad categories [2]. Some practices may fall into more than one category.

1. Natural products such as vitamins, minerals, and "natural products"
2. Mind and body medicine such as meditation, yoga, acupuncture, hypnotherapy, progressive relaxation, and tai chi
3. Manipulative and body-based practices such as spinal manipulation and massage
4. Movement therapies, such as pilates
5. Whole medical systems, such as Ayurvedic medicine and traditional Chinese medicine

The majority of patients use CAM in a complementary fashion rather than as an alternative to conventional medicine [3]. Various reasons exist as to why people choose CAM. CAM may be chosen to help a patient feel better, because their symptoms may not be fully controlled by conventional medicine. Sometimes, people desire to use treatments that are more natural and help them feel more in control. There may be concerns about side effects of conventional treatments and CAM may seem less toxic and natural. For others, CAM may be used largely because these health care alternatives may be more congruent with their own values, beliefs, and philosophical orientations toward health and life [4]. CAM use is more common in women and adults with higher educational attainment. Native American Indian or or Alaska Native adults and white adults are more likely to use CAM than Asian adults or black adults, but it is important to note that use of CAM is not confined to any particular ethnic background or segment of the population [1, 5].

Thyroid dysfunction is a common endocrine problem. Hypothyroidism occurs in 6–17 % of the general population with increased prevalence in women and the elderly [6]. Overall prevalence of hyperthyroidism is reported to be 1.3 %, increasing to about 4–5 % in older women [7]. The clinical manifestations of thyroid disorders can vary considerably from person to person. The symptoms of hypothyroidism include fatigue, weakness, constipation, weight gain, sluggishness, cold extremities, edema, and muscle aches. Currently levothyroxine (LT4) is the only mainstay therapy for replacement of thyroid hormone in patients with hypothyroidism (7A.). Guidelines from all professional societies recommend LT4 monotherapy as the treatment of hypothyroidism [8–11]. Symptoms of hyperthyroidism include sweating, heat intolerance, unintentional weight loss, increased heart rate, tremors, and anxiety. Conventional management of hyperthyroidism includes treatment with antithyroid drugs such as methimazole or propylthiouracil, steroids, radioactive iodine, or surgery. This chapter will outline some of the commonly used CAM for thyroid disorders.

B.M. Onumah, MD (✉)
Medicine – Section of Endocrinology, Medstar Washington Hospital Center, 110 Irving Street, NW Suite 2A 72, Washington, DC 20010, USA
e-mail: barbara.m.onumah@medstar.net

L. Wartofsky, D. Van Nostrand (eds.), *Thyroid Cancer*, DOI 10.1007/978-1-4939-3314-3_69

Natural Preparations

Natural Prescription Thyroid Medication

One of the alternative therapies used in the treatment of hypothyroidism is "natural prescription thyroid medication" or dessicated thyroid derived from porcine thyroid gland. Common brand names include Armour Thyroid, Nature-Throid, and Westhroid. These preparations are a combination of thyroxine (T4) and triiodothyronine (T3). For instance, Armour Thyroid has a ratio of approximately 4:1 of T4 to T3, and 1 grain of Armour Thyroid will provide 38 mcg of T4 and 9 mcg of T3. In general, most authorities discourage the use of T3-containing preparations for thyroid replacement therapy because T3 is rapidly absorbed and has a relatively short half-life resulting in wide fluctuations of serum T3 levels between doses. In addition, the commercially available dessicated thyroid preparations contain higher T3 concentrations as compared to normal human thyroid secretions. For instance, a person taking a T3-containing preparation might have a supra-physiological serum T3 concentration for several hours after each dose, followed by a rapid decline in the T3 levels. Several studies have evaluated the efficacy of combination T4 and T3 preparations and concluded that there are no more beneficial effects of treating hypothyroid patients with combination T4/T3 preparations as compared to T4 alone [12–16]. While other studies have shown that using combination T4/T3 therapy significantly improves measures of mood and cognitive function as well as other object measures of thyroid health [17, 18]. It is important to note that some patients may prefer combined T4/T3 therapy even though objective clinical measures show no difference between T4/T3 combination and T4 alone therapy [17, 19]. Certain genetic polymorphisms in the type 2 deiodinase (enzyme responsible for peripheral conversion of T4 to T3) gene may explain why some patients have better psychological well-being on T4/T3 combination as compared to T4 monotherapy alone [20, 20A].

Selenium

Selenium is a chemical element that was discovered by the Swedish chemist, J. J Berzelius in 1817. It has antioxidant activity and anti-inflammatory and chemopreventive and antiviral characteristics. Selenium coordinates the functioning of certain proteins designated at selenoproteins [21]. Key selenoprotein families include glutathione peroxidases (GPxs), thioredoxin reductases (TRxs), and iodothyronine deiodinases (DIs) [22–24]. GPxs possess oxidoreductase functions and protect the cell from oxidative stress. The TRxs form a cellular redox system which is essential for cell development and proliferation. Deiodinase catalyzes the conversion of T4 to T3. The major role of selenium as it pertains to the thyroid is related to its antioxidant function and its association with the function of all three thyroid deiodinases which are responsible for the conversion of T4 to T3 and reverse T3. The thyroid gland contains more selenium per gram of tissue than any other organ [25, 26]. Selenium deficiency has been implicated in the pathogenesis of thyroid autoimmunity in both Hashimoto's thyroiditis and Graves' disease. Several studies have demonstrated that selenium supplementation ranging from physiological doses of 80 ug/day to supra-physiological doses of 200 ug/day are effective in reducing antithyroid peroxidase antibodies and improve thyroid ultrasound pattern [27–30]. Additionally, it has been shown that patients with Graves' disease when treated with a mixture of antioxidants including selenium combined with methimazole achieved euthyroidism faster than those treated with methimazole alone [31]. Among patients with Graves' orbitopathy, selenium administration of 100 ug twice per day for 6 months significantly improved quality of life, reduced ocular involvement, and slowed progression of the disease [32].

The entry point of selenium in humans is via edible plants which absorb the element in its organic form. Certain foods are particularly rich in selenium such as shell fish, crabs, kidney, liver, and Brazil nuts. The recommended daily intake of dietary selenium is estimated to be about 55 ug/day (range 30–85 ug/day) [33]. Selenium supplementation is safer in the organic forms than in the inorganic forms. Dose as high as 1,600 mcg/day has been tolerated without toxicity [34, 35]. However, an increased risk of diabetes has been reported in individuals getting selenium supplementation of 200 ug/day [36]. If selenium toxicity (otherwise known as "selenosis") occurs, it is characterized by diarrhea, fatigue, hair loss, and fingernail discoloration [37].

Iodine

Iodine is a nonmetallic trace chemical element. It is necessary for the synthesis of the thyroid hormones T4 and T3. The thyroid gland actively traps iodine and incorporate it into thyroid hormones that are released into the circulation, when needed. Inadequate iodine supply leads to inadequate hormone production and then to hypothyroidism. The spectrum of iodine deficiency disorders includes mental retardation, hypothyroidism, goiter, and varying degrees of other growth and developmental abnormalities. Goiter is usually the first and most visible sign of iodine deficiency in the adults [38, 39].

Sufficiency of dietary iodine intake for the general US population has been monitored since 1971 through the

National Health and Nutrition Survey (NHANES). Iodine status is assessed using urinary iodine concentrations, as they directly reflect dietary iodine intake. The general US population in 2007–2008 was nutritionally iodine sufficient [40]. However, a good percentage of the world's population lives in areas of iodine deficiency [41]. Dietary sources of iodine include iodized salt and seafood, seaweed, dairy products, and some vegetables. Salt iodination is legally mandated in many countries. In the US, dairy and grain products are the primary sources of iodine in the American diet [42].

Because iodine plays such a paramount role in the synthesis of thyroid hormones, certain herbs with high iodine content are used as CAM treatment for hypothyroidism, even though there are no studies to support their efficacy and safety. Examples of such herbs are Kelp and bladder wrack [43, 44].

Kelp is a large type of brown seaweed belonging to the order laminariales. It is a rich source of dietary iodine. The amount and dose of kelp that has been used for the treatment of hypothyroidism depends on the individual's specific thyroid ailment.

Bladder wrack (*Fucus vesiculosus*) is another type of brown seaweed with high iodine content. The recommended dose for hypothyroidism is 600 mg one to three times daily.

Taking iodine is not without risk. Too much iodine can cause hypothyroidism, as explained by the Wolff-Chaikoff effect. The Wolff-Chaikoff effect is an autoregulatory phenomenon of the thyroid, where sudden exposure to too much iodide, inhibits organification of iodide, thereby diminishing thyroid hormone synthesis. Additionally, iodine-induced hyperthyroidism can occur in patients with iodine deficiency that is rapidly corrected corrected by the excessive administration of iodine, particularly in those patients with autonomous thyroid nodules.

Other Herbs and Supplements for Hypothyroidism

Coleus (*Coleus forskohlii*) is a plant that comes from the mountains of Asia and is related to the lavender and mint family of plants. It is a potent stimulator of adenylate cyclase (the enzyme that activates adenosine monophosphate or cyclic AMP) in many systems, including the thyroid gland. It is said to increase the release of hormones from the thyroid gland [45, 46]. The recommended dose is 50–100 mg of coleus extract two or three times each day. Doses as high as 250 mg twice a day have been used with no apparent adverse effects [47].

Guggul is a yellowish resin produced by the stem of a small thorny plant called Mukul Myrrh that is distributed throughout India. This resin has been used for centuries as part of India's traditional medicine philosophy called Ayurveda. Guggul has been shown to have a stimulatory effect on thyroid even though the exact mechanism remains unknown [48]. Dose recommended for "thyroid support" is 250–500 mg of guggul extract three times daily.

L-tyrosine is an amino acid that is essential to the thyroid gland for the manufacture of the thyroid hormones. That is essential to the thyroid gland for the manufacture of the thyroid hormones. The thyroid combines tyrosine with iodine to make T3 and T4. Tyrosine can be produced by the body from phenylalanine, another amino acid. Dietary-rich sources of phenylalanine include poultry, fish, soy dairy, some beans, nuts, and seeds. Although most people on normal diets have adequate intake of tyrosine, some patients with an underactive thyroid gland may still choose to use use supplements containing tyrosine. The generally recommended dose is 500–1000 mg daily [49].

Primrose oil is another supplement that is sometimes used as CAM for treatment of hypothyroidism. It is a high source of omega–6 fatty acids. The exact action of omega–6 fatty acids on thyroid is not well known. However, it is known that omega–6 fatty acids have potent anti-inflammatory qualities that conceivably may help with hypothyroidism that is due to autoimmune process (Hashimoto's). Exposure to high dietary omega–6 can cause increased T4 and T3 hormone levels [50].

CAM Treatments for Hyperthyroidism

As the most common cause of hyperthyroidism is Graves' disease which is an autoimmune inflammatory condition, several herbs and supplements with anti-inflammatory properties are proposed as CAM for hyperthyroidism. Examples include bugleweed, lemon balm, alpha lipoic acid, and motherwort.

Bugleweed (*Lycopus virginicus*) is a member of the mint family and inhibits thyroid-stimulating antibodies (the cause of Graves' disease) from binding to the normal thyroid and thus decreases thyroid hormone production. It has also been shown to decrease normal thyroid-stimulating hormone (TSH) secretion from the pituitary gland, resulting in low T4 and T3 levels. Bugleweed is available as a tincture, and drops are usually added to a beverage [51, 52].

Lemon balm (*Melissa officinalis*) is also a member of the mint family. Essential oils made from lemon balm leaves contain plant chemicals called terpenes, which play at least some role in the herb's relaxing and antiviral effects. Lemon balm is supposed to block TSH's ability to stimulate thyroid function, but the exact mechanism is unknown. Lemon balm is best available as a liquid extract or as fresh or dried herbs. It is best consumed as an herbal infusion or tea. The recommended dose for lemon balm is 300–500 mg, three times daily [53, 54].

Motherwort (*Leonurus cardiaca*) is another kind of herb, belonging to the mint family. It has been used under the belief that it will treat symptoms of overactive thyroid. It does not necessarily have a direct effect on thyroid hormone secretion but treats the symptoms that are associated with hyperthyroidism such as palpitations and anxiety [53].

Alpha lipoic acid has been said to decrease conversion of T4 to the active form of thyroid hormone T3, and for this reason it is sometimes used to treat hyperthyroidism [55].

Mind-Body Therapies (MBT)

Mind-body medicine is described by the National Center for Complementary and Alternative Medicine as a range of healing practices that share a common intention "to enhance the mind's capacity to affect bodily function and symptoms." MBT is one of the most commonly used categories of CAM in the United States, with nearly one in five adults using at least one form of mind-body therapy annually [56]. Mind-body therapy is used for treatment on many chronic conditions including thyroid disease. Studies looking at CAM use in thyroid patients show that, among MBT users, the most popular modes of treatment include acupuncture, yoga and meditation, relaxation techniques, and tai chi [57, 58]. Despite the popularity of MBT and the large numbers of patients engaging in MBT sessions, there is a paucity of scientific data to support efficacy and continued use. However, in one report, approximately two thirds of all patients who use MBT for a specific condition found it helpful [58].

Acupuncture is regarded as a viable option in treatment of thyroid dysfunction. A Russian study, reported females with subclinical hypothyroidism who had elevated TSH levels and symptoms of arthralgias and myalgias who completed two therapeutic courses of acupuncture with 3–4-month intervals between them and had significant improvement in their symptoms. In addition, values of TSH fell to physiologic levels, and characteristics of the quality of life became comparable with those of healthy subjects [59]. Moxibustion, a form of fire heat treatment that stimulates specific acupuncture points of the body, has been reported to reduce the thyroid antibodies in the peripheral blood of patients with hypothyroidism [60].

Various articles on the use of acupuncture and reflex therapy in management of hyperthyroidism and exophthalmos exist and report therapeutic benefits with the use of these modalities [61–63]. Increased exercise and acupuncture have helped shrink thyroid nodules [64], but results have not been proven. The exact mechanism as to how these various types of CAM achieve therapeutic benefits remains unknown. Most of the information regarding these treatment options is derived from case studies and few if any randomized studies exist on these topics.

Thyroid Cancer

Patient belief in the use of CAM for cancer is widespread. A meta-analysis, using studies from 18 countries including the United States, reported the prevalence of current use of CAM in cancer patients to be 40 %. The study also noted a continued increase in CAM since 1970 [65]. The main reasons why cancer patients use CAM are based on a belief that they will decrease or prevent the adverse effects of existing treatment and to increase the body's ability to fight cancer.

Controlled amino acid therapy (CAAT) is one such proposed alternative to cancer therapy that promises both prevention and cure of thyroid cancer. CAAT was developed by Angelo P John of the A. P John Institute for Cancer Research. It is an amino acid and carbohydrate deprivation protocol. The implied goal of this therapy is to disrupt the development of cancer cells by altering cell formation through structure, energy, blood vessels, growth hormone, and cell functions. The regimen consists of a carbohydrate- and protein-restricted diet with added supplements. The protocol is meant to be maintained for 6–9 months as an adjunct to conventional cancer treatment [66]. Whereas the Institute's website describes studies that support theories behind the protocol, no independent studies have been conducted to determine the efficacy of the regimen itself. There does not appear to be any scientific evidence that the specific controlled amino acid therapy prevents or treats cancer. There is not enough evidence to support CAAT as effective to fight against cancer, and it has not been approved by the FDA for cancer treatment [67].

Other nutritional supplements that may be advised as ostensibly effective in the management of thyroid cancer include: parsley, green tea extract, antioxidants, whey protein, calcium D-glucurate, licorice root extract, and others. These supplements are believed to restrict the growth of cancer cells and improve the body's response to conventional treatment methods. Furthermore, they are also believed to improve the general health of the individuals with thyroid cancer [68]. There are no good scientific studies supporting these claims.

Mind-body therapies involving practicing various relaxation methods such as yoga, acupuncture, meditation, biofeedback, hypnosis, music, and art have been reported to be helpful in relaxing the mind and instilling a positive attitude toward health and life in individuals affected with cancer. Randomized trials have shown hypnosis to be effective in relieving pain as well as in decreasing anxiety and depression and improving mood in newly diagnosed cancer patients [69–72]. Music therapy has also proven effective in reducing pain, anxiety, depression, and pain particularly in the palliative setting [73–79]. Evidence from clinical trials supports the use of acupuncture for nausea, vomiting, and pain [80, 81].

All of these CAM approaches for thyroid cancer may be useful in treating the symptoms associated with the cancer and its treatment, but there is no scientific evidence to support the beneficial effects of these therapies in curing thyroid cancer or any other type of cancer. As it pertains to thyroid cancer, supplements and herbs containing iodine may prevent patients from becoming adequately iodine depleted in preparation for radioactive iodine treatment. Others may have anticoagulant effects and may increase bleeding, a risk in patients receiving surgical treatment. For example, garlic and ginseng are felt to cause permanent dysfunction of circulating platelets and are recommended to be discontinued 7 days prior to any surgery [82, 83].

Conclusions

Several forms of CAM exist and have been recommended by proponents of CAM for the treatment of thyroid disorders. In spite of the absence of scientific data supporting their efficacy, the use of CAM is widespread and continues to increase. The majority of the data available on efficacy and safety are anecdotal, and there is a lack of good scientific studies in most instances. The majority of patients using CAM do not voluntarily disclose their use to their physicians. Although, CAM and its approaches can sometimes augment patient care, many supplements have potential interactions and side effects. For patients, it is important to talk to your primary care physician when considering a CAM therapy and important to gather basic information such as education and experience on the CAM practitioner that you are planning to use. Physicians should inquire specifically about CAM use in their patients. Patient-doctor communication about CAM is necessary to maintain patient safety and well-being.

References

1. Barnes PM, Bloom B, Nahin RL. Complementary and alternative medicine use among adults and children: United States, 2007. Natl Health Stat Rep. 2008(12):1–23.
2. National Institute of Complementary and Alternative Medicine website http://nccam.nih.gov/health/whatiscam.
3. Druss BG, Rosenheck RA. Association between use of unconventional therapies and conventional medical services. JAMA. 1999;282(7):651–6.
4. Astin JA. Why patients use alternative medicine: results of a national study. JAMA. 1998;279(19):1548–53.
5. Eisenberg DM, Kessler RC, Foster C, Norlock FE, Calkins DR, Delbanco TL. Unconventional medicine in the United States. Prevalence, costs, and patterns of use. N Engl J Med. 1993; 328(4):246–52.
6. Roberts CG, Ladenson PW. Hypothyroidism. Lancet. 2004; 363(9411):793–803.
7. Hollowell JG, Staehling NW, Flanders WD, et al. Serum TSH, T(4), and thyroid antibodies in the United States population (1988 to 1994): National Health and Nutrition Examination Survey (NHANES III). J Clin Endocrinol Metab. 2002;87(2):489–99.

7a. Biondi B, Wartofsky L.Treatment with Thyroid Hormone. Endocrine Reviews, published ahead of print: doi: 10/1210/er.2013-1083; 35: 433–512, June 2014.

8. Baskin HJ, Cobin RH, Duick DS, et al. American Association of Clinical Endocrinologists medical guidelines for clinical practice for the evaluation and treatment of hyperthyroidism and hypothyroidism. Endocr Pract. 2002;8(6):457–69.
9. Surks MI, Ortiz E, Daniels GH, et al. Subclinical thyroid disease: scientific review and guidelines for diagnosis and management. JAMA. 2004;291(2):228–38.
10. Singer PA, Cooper DS, Levy EG, et al. Treatment guidelines for patients with hyperthyroidism and hypothyroidism. Standards of Care Committee, American Thyroid Association. JAMA. 1995;273(10):808–12.
11. Wartofsky L. Levothyroxine therapy for hypothyroidism: should we abandon conservative dosage titration? Arch Intern Med. 2005;165(15):1683–4.
12. Clyde PW, Harari AE, Getka EJ, Shakir KM. Combined levothyroxine plus liothyronine compared with levothyroxine alone in primary hypothyroidism: a randomized controlled trial. JAMA. 2003;290(22):2952–8.
13. Sawka AM, Gerstein HC, Marriott MJ, MacQueen GM, Joffe RT. Does a combination regimen of thyroxine (T4) and 3,5,3′-triiodothyronine improve depressive symptoms better than T4 alone in patients with hypothyroidism? Results of a double-blind, randomized, controlled trial. J Clin Endocrinol Metab. 2003;88(10):4551–5.
14. Saravanan P, Simmons DJ, Greenwood R, Peters TJ, Dayan CM. Partial substitution of thyroxine (T4) with tri-iodothyronine in patients on T4 replacement therapy: results of a large community-based randomized controlled trial. J Clin Endocrinol Metab. 2005;90(2):805–12.
15. Rodriguez T, Lavis VR, Meininger JC, Kapadia AS, Stafford LF. Substitution of liothyronine at a 1:5 ratio for a portion of levothyroxine: effect on fatigue, symptoms of depression, and working memory versus treatment with levothyroxine alone. Endocr Pract. 2005;11(4):223–33.
16. Siegmund W, Spieker K, Weike AI, et al. Replacement therapy with levothyroxine plus triiodothyronine (bioavailable molar ratio 14: 1) is not superior to thyroxine alone to improve well-being and cognitive performance in hypothyroidism. Clin Endocrinol (Oxf). 2004;60(6):750–7.
17. Bunevicius R, Kazanavicius G, Zalinkevicius R, Prange Jr AJ. Effects of thyroxine as compared with thyroxine plus triiodothyronine in patients with hypothyroidism. N Engl J Med. 1999;340(6):424–9.
18. Bunevicius R, Prange AJ. Mental improvement after replacement therapy with thyroxine plus triiodothyronine: relationship to cause of hypothyroidism. Int J Neuropsychopharmacol. 2000;3(2): 167–74.
19. Appelhof BC, Fliers E, Wekking EM, et al. Combined therapy with levothyroxine and liothyronine in two ratios, compared with levothyroxine monotherapy in primary hypothyroidism: a double-blind, randomized, controlled clinical trial. J Clin Endocrinol Metab. 2005;90(5):2666–74.
20. Panicker V, Saravanan P, Vaidya B, et al. Common variation in the DIO2 gene predicts baseline psychological well-being and response to combination thyroxine plus triiodothyronine therapy in hypothyroid patients. J Clin Endocrinol Metab. 2009;94(5):1623–9.

20a. BBiondi B, Wartofsky L. Combination treatment with T4 and T3: Toward personalized replacement therapy in hypothyroidism. J Clin Endocrinol Metab 97: 2256–2271, 2012.

21. Rayman MP. The importance of selenium to human health. Lancet. 2000;356(9225):233–41.

22. Rotruck JT, Pope AL, Ganther HE, Swanson AB, Hafeman DG, Hoekstra WG. Selenium: biochemical role as a component of glutathione peroxidase. Science. 1973;179(4073):588–90.
23. Berry MJ, Banu L, Larsen PR. Type I iodothyronine deiodinase is a selenocysteine-containing enzyme. Nature. 1991;349(6308): 438–40.
24. Hill KE, McCollum GW, Boeglin ME, Burk RF. Thioredoxin reductase activity is decreased by selenium deficiency. Biochem Biophys Res Commun. 1997;234(2):293–5.
25. Dickson RC, Tomlinson RH. Selenium in blood and human tissues. Clin Chim Acta. 1967;16(2):311–21.
26. Tiran B, Karpf E, Tiran A. Age dependency of selenium and cadmium content in human liver, kidney, and thyroid. Arch Environ Health. 1995;50(3):242–6.
27. Gartner R, Gasnier BC. Selenium in the treatment of autoimmune thyroiditis. Biofactors. 2003;19(3–4):165–70.
28. Duntas LH, Mantzou E, Koutras DA. Effects of a six month treatment with selenomethionine in patients with autoimmune thyroiditis. Eur J Endocrinol. 2003;148(4):389–93.
29. Turker O, Kumanlioglu K, Karapolat I, Dogan I. Selenium treatment in autoimmune thyroiditis: 9-month follow-up with variable doses. J Endocrinol. 2006;190(1):151–6.
30. Mazokopakis EE, Papadakis JA, Papadomanolaki MG, et al. Effects of 12 months treatment with L-selenomethionine on serum anti-TPO Levels in patients with Hashimoto's thyroiditis. Thyroid. 2007;17(7):609–12.
31. Bacic Vrca V, Skreb F, Cepelak I, Mayer L. Supplementation with antioxidants in the treatment of Graves' disease: the effect on the extracellular antioxidative parameters. Acta Pharm. 2004;54(2): 79–89.
32. Marcocci C, Kahaly GJ, Krassas GE, et al. Selenium and the course of mild Graves' orbitopathy. N Engl J Med. 2011;364(20): 1920–31.
33. Rayman MP. Food-chain selenium and human health: emphasis on intake. Br J Nutr. 2008;100(2):254–68.
34. Moreno-Reyes R, Suetens C, Mathieu F, et al. Kashin-Beck osteoarthropathy in rural Tibet in relation to selenium and iodine status. N Engl J Med. 1998;339(16):1112–20.
35. Reid ME, Stratton MS, Lillico AJ, et al. A report of high-dose selenium supplementation: response and toxicities. J Trace Elem Med Biol. 2004;18(1):69–74.
36. Stranges S, Marshall JR, Natarajan R, et al. Effects of long-term selenium supplementation on the incidence of type 2 diabetes: a randomized trial. Ann Intern Med. 2007;147(4):217–23.
37. MacFarquhar JK, Broussard DL, Melstrom P, et al. Acute selenium toxicity associated with a dietary supplement. Arch Intern Med. 2010;170(3):256–61.
38. Delange F. The disorders induced by iodine deficiency. Thyroid. 1994;4(1):107–28.
39. Dunn JT. Seven deadly sins in confronting endemic iodine deficiency, and how to avoid them. J Clin Endocrinol Metab. 1996;81(4):1332–5.
40. Caldwell KL, Makhmudov A, Ely E, Jones RL, Wang RY. Iodine status of the U.S. population, National Health and Nutrition Examination Survey, 2005–2006 and 2007–2008. Thyroid. 2011; 21(4):419–27.
41. International council for the control of Iodine deficiency. http://www.iccidd.org/.
42. Murray CW, Egan SK, Kim H, Beru N, Bolger PM. US Food and Drug Administration's total diet study: dietary intake of perchlorate and iodine. J Expo Sci Environ Epidemiol. 2008;18(6):571–80.
43. Supplements for thyroid problems. http://www.livestrong.com/article/294353-supplements-for-thyroid-problems/.
44. Home Remedies for thyroid problems. http://www.livestrong.com/article/234801-home-remedies-for-thyroid-problems/.
45. Litosch I, Hudson TH, Mills I, Li SY, Fain JN. Forskolin as an activator of cyclic AMP accumulation and lipolysis in rat adipocytes. Mol Pharmacol. 1982;22(1):109–15.
46. Ealey PA, Kohn LD, Marshall NJ, Ekins RP. Forskolin stimulation of naphthylamidase in guinea pig thyroid sections detected with a cytochemical bioassay. Acta Endocrinol (Copenh). 1985;108(3): 367–71.
47. Henderson S, Magu B, Rasmussen C, et al. Effects of coleus forskohlii supplementation on body composition and hematological profiles in mildly overweight women. J Int Soc Sports Nutr. 2005;2:54–62.
48. Tripathi YB, Tripathi P, Malhotra OP, Tripathi SN. Thyroid stimulatory action of (Z)-guggulsterone: mechanism of action. Planta Med. 1988;54(4):271–7.
49. The effects of L tyrosine on the thyroid. http://www.livestrong.com/article/488548-the-effects-of-l-tyrosine-on-the-thyroid/.
50. Deshpande N, Hulbert AJ. Dietary omega 6 fatty acids and the effects of hyperthyroidism in mice. J Endocrinol. 1995;144(3):431–9.
51. Beer AM, Wiebelitz KR, Schmidt-Gayk H. Lycopus europaeus (Gypsywort): effects on the thyroidal parameters and symptoms associated with thyroid function. Phytomedicine. 2008;15(1–2): 16–22.
52. Winterhoff H, Gumbinger HG, Vahlensieck U, Kemper FH, Schmitz H, Behnke B. Endocrine effects of Lycopus europaeus L. following oral application. Arzneimittelforschung. 1994;44(1):41–5.
53. Herbal treatments for overactive thyroid. http://www.livestrong.com/article/309421-herbal-treatments-for-an-overactive-thyroid.
54. Saeed SA, Bloch RM, Antonacci DJ. Herbal and dietary supplements for treatment of anxiety disorders. Am Fam Physician. 2007;76(4):549–56.
55. Segermann J, Hotze A, Ulrich H, Rao GS. Effect of alpha-lipoic acid on the peripheral conversion of thyroxine to triiodothyronine and on serum lipid-, protein- and glucose levels. Arzneimittelforschung. 1991;41(12):1294–8.
56. Barnes PM, Powell-Griner E, McFann K, Nahin RL. Complementary and alternative medicine use among adults: United States, 2002. Adv Data. 2004(343):1–19.
57. Brake MK, Bartlett C, Hart RD, Trites JR, Taylor SM. Complementary and alternative medicine use in the thyroid patients of a head and neck practice. Otolaryngol Head Neck Surg. 2011;145(2):208–12.
58. Bertisch SM, Wee CC, Phillips RS, McCarthy EP. Alternative mind-body therapies used by adults with medical conditions. J Psychosom Res. 2009;66(6):511–9.
59. Luzina KE, Luzina LL, Vasilenko AM. The influence of acupuncture on the quality of life and the level of thyroid-stimulating hormone in patients presenting with subclinical hypothyroidism. Vopr Kurortol Fizioter Lech Fiz Kult. 2011(5):29–33.
60. Hu G, Chen H, Hou Y, He J, Cheng Z, Wang R. A study on the clinical effect and immunological mechanism in the treatment of Hashimoto's thyroiditis by moxibustion. J Tradit Chin Med. 1993;13(1):14–8.
61. Xu WM, Guo YH, Chen BX. Efficacy observation on infiltrative exophthalmos treated with acupuncture and acupoint massage. Zhongguo Zhen Jiu. 2011;31(2):101–4.
62. Xia Y, Shu S, Li Y, Liu SM, He JS. Therapeutic effect and side effect of treatment on hyperthyroid exophthalmos with the combination of acupuncture and medication. Zhongguo Zhen Jiu. 2010;30(10):806–9.
63. Yiu HH, Tam KC. Acupuncture for several functional disorders. Part I. Am J Chin Med (Gard City N Y). 1976;4(3):281–8.
64. Guo XZ, Li CJ, Gao BH, Ye MR, Zhao RW. Acupuncture treatment of benign thyroid nodules. Clinical observation of 65 cases. J Tradit Chin Med. 1984;4(4):261–4.
65. Horneber M, Bueschel G, Dennert G, Less D, Ritter E, Zwahlen M. How many cancer patients use complementary and alternative

medicine: a systematic review and metaanalysis. Integr Cancer Ther. 2012;11(3):187–203.
66. A P John Institute for Cancer Research. http://www.apjohncancer-institute.org/.
67. US Food and Drug Adminstration website. http://www.fda.gov/.
68. Alternative Treatment for Thyroid Cancer. http://www.steady-health.com/articles/Alternative_Treatments_for_Thyroid_Cancer_a917.html.
69. Sellick SM, Zaza C. Critical review of 5 nonpharmacologic strategies for managing cancer pain. Cancer Prev Control. 1998;2(1):7–14.
70. Bindemann S, Soukop M, Kaye SB. Randomised controlled study of relaxation training. Eur J Cancer. 1991;27(2):170–4.
71. Bridge LR, Benson P, Pietroni PC, Priest RG. Relaxation and imagery in the treatment of breast cancer. BMJ. 1988; 297(6657):1169–72.
72. Walker LG, Walker MB, Ogston K, et al. Psychological, clinical and pathological effects of relaxation training and guided imagery during primary chemotherapy. Br J Cancer. 1999;80(1–2):262–8.
73. Smith M, Casey L, Johnson D, Gwede C, Riggin OZ. Music as a therapeutic intervention for anxiety in patients receiving radiation therapy. Oncol Nurs Forum. 2001;28(5):855–62.
74. Wang SM, Kulkarni L, Dolev J, Kain ZN. Music and preoperative anxiety: a randomized, controlled study. Anesth Analg. 2002;94(6):1489–94, table of contents.
75. Kaempf G, Amodei ME. The effect of music on anxiety. A research study. AORN J. 1989;50(1):112–8.
76. Burns DS. The effect of the bonny method of guided imagery and music on the mood and life quality of cancer patients. J Music Ther. 2001;38(1):51–65.
77. Waldon EG. The effects of group music therapy on mood states and cohesiveness in adult oncology patients. J Music Ther. 2001; 38(3):212–38.
78. Zimmerman L, Pozehl B, Duncan K, Schmitz R. Effects of music in patients who had chronic cancer pain. West J Nurs Res. 1989;11(3):298–309.
79. Beck SL. The therapeutic use of music for cancer-related pain. Oncol Nurs Forum. 1991;18(8):1327–37.
80. Vickers AJ. Can acupuncture have specific effects on health? A systematic review of acupuncture antiemesis trials. J R Soc Med. 1996;89(6):303–11.
81. Alimi D, Rubino C, Leandri EP, Brule SF. Analgesic effects of auricular acupuncture for cancer pain. J Pain Symptom Manage. 2000;19(2):81–2.
82. Ang-Lee MK, Moss J, Yuan CS. Herbal medicines and perioperative care. JAMA. 2001;286(2):208–16.
83. Kaye AD, Clarke RC, Sabar R, et al. Herbal medicines: current trends in anesthesiology practice – a hospital survey. J Clin Anesth. 2000;12(6):468–71.

Part VIII

Well-Differentiated Thyroid Cancer: Follicular Carcinoma

70 Follicular Thyroid Carcinoma

Leonard Wartofsky

Introduction

There are several important distinctions in cytologic and histologic differential diagnosis that relate to the respective diagnoses of papillary thyroid carcinoma (PTC) versus follicular thyroid carcinoma (FTC), follicular adenoma versus FTC, and minimally invasive FTC versus widely invasive FTC. The follicular variant of papillary thyroid carcinoma (FVPTC) generally behaves clinically as a PTC [1–4] and hence is discussed in the chapters on PTC. As described in Chap. 32 (Pathology of FTC), FTC is much less often multicentric than PTC and the diagnostic distinction between FTC and PTC is based on their appearance under the microscope.

On cytologic examination, classic PTC demonstrates overlapping, crowding, or palisading nuclei, with many that show nuclear clefts and intranuclear cytoplasmic pseudoinclusions ("orphan Annie eyes") or vacuoles, whereas FTC does not exhibit the latter nuclear features. Moreover, it is extremely difficult to distinguish on the basis of cytologic findings between the follicular architecture of a benign follicular adenoma from that of follicular carcinoma. The distinction is made on the basis of demonstrating capsular and vascular invasion in carcinoma, neither of which can be seen in a fine-needle aspirate (FNA) of only cellular material, and histologic tissue sections are required, i.e., surgical pathology after thyroidectomy [5]. Based upon the Bethesda classification system [6–9], with indeterminate follicular lesions on FNA, the cytopathologist may call the lesion a follicular lesion of undetermined significance (FLUS) or a follicular neoplasm. The Bethesda guideline helps clarify the dilemma presented by the indeterminate nodule in regard to weighing the risk of cancer and relative indication for surgical thyroidectomy.

In one study of 197 patients with FNA cytology read as "follicular lesion of undetermined significance" who went to thyroidectomy, the overall incidence of malignancy was 16.2 % with 17 cases (8.6 %) that were follicular carcinoma, 6 cases (3.1 %) that were classic PTC, and 9 cases (4.6 %) that were follicular variant PTC [10]. Molecular mutational analysis is currently available to help make the distinction between benign and malignant follicular lesions (see below). When faced with an indeterminate follicular lesion, the management decision in the past often has been to perform a subtotal thyroidectomy and to subsequently perform completion thyroidectomy once the surgical pathology confirms carcinoma. The next decision for a proven FTC, i.e., whether or not to administer radioiodine for ablation, is typically linked to whether the tumor is of the minimally invasive or more advanced invasive type, although radioiodine ablation is done routinely in many centers for either variety of FTC. While tumors classified as minimally invasive can either present with or subsequently develop distant metastasis, this is considered sufficiently unusual that the American Thyroid Association (ATA) cancer guidelines indicate that radioiodine ablation is not necessary when there is only minimal microscopic capsular invasion without angioinvasion [11].

In an attempt to identify certain risk factors in minimally invasive FTC that might be associated with good or worse outcomes, Sugino et al. [12] reviewed the course of a group of 229 patients from the Ito Hospital with minimally invasive FTC at diagnosis who were followed for a median period of 7.2 years. They found that age >45 years and tumor size >4 cm were poor prognostic factors associated with subsequent metastasis, whereas patients <age 45 with tumors <4 cm had excellent prognosis with only a very rare recurrence of tumor, and hence, these authors suggested that the

L. Wartofsky, MD, MACP (✉)
Department of Medicine, MedStar Washington Hospital Center, Georgetown University School of Medicine, 110 Irving Street, N.W., Washington, DC 20010-2975, USA
e-mail: leonard.wartofsky@medstar.net

L. Wartofsky, D. Van Nostrand (eds.), *Thyroid Cancer*, DOI 10.1007/978-1-4939-3314-3_70

latter patients could be spared both completion thyroidectomy and radioiodine ablation. However, it should be noted that 54/229 (21.5 %) of their patients had distant metastases diagnosed at the time of their original thyroidectomy and yet were considered minimally invasive FTC. My concern would be that although risk of metastasis may be minimized by considering the risk factors of age and tumor size, it is not eliminated. Therefore, patients who do not undergo total thyroidectomy and radioiodine ablation still need to be followed closely for recurrence, and the usual means of doing so, i.e., measurements of serum thyroglobulin (Tg) or radioisotope scanning, are likely to be problematic in such patients due to the presence of residual functioning thyroid tissue that will both take up radioiodine and secrete Tg. On the other hand, an Armed Forces Institute of Pathology review of 95 cases of minimally invasive FTC concluded that the prognosis was so good that aggressive surgical management was not necessary for a positive outcome [13].

Prognostic factors in minimally invasive follicular carcinoma were examined in another series of 292 patients from Kuma Hospital in Japan [14]. Again age >45 and tumors >4 cm were poor prognostic features for disease-free survival, while the presence of M1 status with distant metastases discovered at initial time of diagnosis was the most important issue for cause-specific survival. While capsular invasion was not an important factor, vascular invasion determined at four separate sites was another independent prognostic factor. Thus, this degree of vascular invasion, age >45, tumor size of 4 cm or greater, and presence of distant metastases are reasonable indications for selection of patients for completion thyroidectomy followed by radioactive iodine ablation.

For FTC, the most important distinction to be made is whether the tumor is one or the other of two general types—well encapsulated and minimally invasive or more poorly differentiated, less well encapsulated, and more widely invasive. While most PTCs are not encapsulated, FTC typically is, and the pathologist's description of tumor invasion into or through the capsule is a key aspect of the histopathologic diagnosis. Thus, when managing the patient with a diagnosis of FTC, it is important to make the distinction between a minimally invasive tumor and a widely invasive tumor because the treatment imperatives in regard to both total or completion thyroidectomy and radioiodine ablation therapy likely will differ. A third potentially more invasive form of FTC, as classified by the World Health Organization [15], is the Hurthle cell (Askanazy cell or oncocytic) variant of FTC, which is described further below and in Chap. 73.

As indicated above, the distinction between a well-encapsulated, minimally invasive FTC and a benign follicular adenoma may be difficult, and not surprisingly, this type of FTC tends to have an excellent prognosis. Williams et al. [16] had proposed labeling these questionably invasive tumors as "well-differentiated follicular tumor of indeterminate malignant potential." Such a designation is clearly less helpful to the clinician, rendering the decision more difficult regarding the need for radioiodine ablation and a meaningful discussion of prognosis with the patient. Clearly, as shown in the study of Sugino et al. [12], there are patients with the so-called minimally invasive tumors who may present with distant metastases either initially or subsequently. To complicate decision making for the clinician even further, and notwithstanding the presence of characteristic features on fine-needle aspiration cytology, there can be significant variation in diagnosis, even between expert pathologists [17]. Baloch and LiVolsi [18]; and Chap. 21 have elegantly summarized the controversy in pathologic diagnosis and provided useful recommendations on the distinction between these various forms of follicular neoplasm.

Some older but still excellent general reviews regarding follicular thyroid carcinoma (FTC) can be recommended [19–21] as well as guidelines for management from both the United States [11, 22] and the United Kingdom [23]. Similar to papillary thyroid carcinoma (PTC), follicular carcinoma is also a relatively well-differentiated thyroid cancer (DTC). Together, both types of tumor represent the most common malignancy of the endocrine system [24]. Several decades ago, PTC was said to constitute approximately 80 % of all DTCs, with FTC occurring in 15 % of patients. Due to a variety of reasons described below, PTC may now comprise 90 % of these tumors, whereas FTC has progressively fallen in frequency of occurrence [25]. FTC represented 13 % of tumors that presented between 1985 and 1995 according to the National Cancer Database [26] but dropped to 6.7 % of tumors described between 2001 and 2005 in the Surveillance, Epidemiology, and End Results (SEER) database [27] and down to 2.7 % of tumors in the most recent analysis [28]. In the United States, the frequency of FTC appears to be decreasing relative to the incidence of PTC, a phenomenon that has been linked to the higher iodine content of the American diet as well as to absolute increases in PTC and perhaps to changes in the histologic classification of some follicular lesions [28]. Incidence of follicular cancer has not declined in geographic areas with relative iodine deficiency.

Controversies exist over how aggressively to approach the early management of PTC (i.e., subtotal vs. total thyroidectomy) or whether to administer radioiodine ablation, but this debate is significantly less of an issue with well-differentiated FTC but depends upon whether the tumor is classified as minimally invasive or invasive [29]. There is full recognition that the invasive variant of FTC behaves in an aggressive manner, with the propensity to invade both the thyroid capsule and blood vessels and show up as metastases in sites distant from the neck. Hence, in order to identify and treat such metastases with radioiodine, there is full justification for postoperative radioiodine ablation to ensure that there are no remaining normal thyroid follicular cells in the neck that would be competing for the tracer isotope. Thus, total thyroidectomy and radioiodine ablation may be justified by data that indicate a somewhat worse prognosis for FTC than PTC, but either tumor may be fully curable if caught at an early stage. Establishing a specific and clear distinction between the behavior of these two types of thyroid cancer from the published literature is somewhat difficult because most describe their experience with patients who have differentiated thyroid cancer (DTC), thereby grouping FTC with PTC. Some analyses of prognosis in differentiated FTC may combine outcomes of minimally invasive tumors with that of the less differentiated invasive variant of FTC, much as outcome data for PTC combines the excellent outcomes of papillary microcarcinomas with more advanced stage PTC. Thus, it is important to keep these distinctions in mind in regard to a given patient, and differences between the presentation and behavior of the various cancer types are emphasized in this chapter.

A significant problem in interpreting the literature extant on disease-free survival and outcomes with various therapeutic FTC approaches is the great variability in histologic description and classification alluded to above. Clearly there is a correlation between invasiveness and prognosis. D'Avanso et al. [30] reviewed 132 patients who were stratified into three groups: minimally invasive (only capsular invasion), moderately invasive (blood vessel invasion with or without capsular invasion), or widely invasive. The 5-year survival rates were 98 %, 80 %, and 38 %, respectively. In general, staging systems (see Chap. 9) in common usage are as valid for FTC as for PTC. Lang et al. [31] found that any of 13 different staging systems could be applied to FTC, although the most commonly employed TNM system was found to have the best predictability of outcome. In an analysis of prognostic factors in 1,227 patients with differentiated thyroid cancer, this same group of investigators [32] found that having FTC was a poor prognostic factor for cancer-specific survival (relative risk = 3.1) along with older age, presence of bone metastases, and lack of avidity for radioiodine.

Finally, the most aggressive variant of FTC has cytologic features of both a follicular tumor and an anaplastic carcinoma and has been designated as "poorly differentiated follicular thyroid carcinoma." These tumors have been variably described on the basis of their histologic features which may include elements of insular, trabecular, solid, or microfollicular growth patterns. The patients tend to be older and have larger tumors (>4 cm) with greater risk of early metastases and death. In one series of 40 patients, the 5-year survival rate was only 63 % [33]. In the latter series of patients, analysis of a wide variety of markers of cell proliferation and differentiation indicated that only high expression of dual oxidase (Duox) was associated with a better prognosis and reduced risk of death.

Clinical Presentation

FTC typically presents as a single, painless thyroid nodule in an older (age >55 years) patient. Although FTC like PTC is more common in women by twofold or more, men tend to have a worse prognosis. Because extension to local nodes typical of PTC is not a characteristic of FTC, lymphadenopathy from involved cervical nodes is uncommon, but distant metastases will be present in the lung or bone in 10–20 % of patients at the time of initial presentation [34–38]. When cervical lymph node metastases are present, the primary tumor may be a follicular variant of papillary thyroid cancer rather than a true follicular carcinoma. FTC tends to occur in endemic (iodide deficient) goiters and in preexisting adenomatous goiters. Iodide deficiency or the secondary thyrotropin (TSH) stimulation associated with it appears to be etiologically related to the development of these tumors [39]. In one recent series from Norway, decreased risk was linked with the use of iodized salt, and increased risk was shown in areas of endemic goiter [40]. In areas of iodide sufficiency in the western hemisphere, papillary carcinoma seems to be more common. The frequency of thyroid cancer in the United States has increased each year over the past two decades; it is estimated that the number of new cases will have more than doubled to 60,220 in 2013 from 25,690 new cases in 2005 with approximately 1,740 deaths [24]. Of this total number, it is predicted that a smaller proportion will be from FTC, with a higher proportion of PTC due to the increasing incidence of PTC [41]. A decline in the reported frequency of pure FTC may also be partly related to more rigid pathologic diagnostic criteria. In many hospitals, follicular tumors are more often misdiagnosed (i.e., false positive) because of confusion with other lesions, such as benign follicular adenomas, adenomatoid goiter, or the follicular variants of either papillary or medullary carcinoma [42].

In addition to iodide deficiency and endemic goiter, there are several other possible predisposing factors for FTC, including advancing age, female gender, and radiation exposure to the head and neck. The greater frequency in women and the somewhat increased presentation of thyroid cancer during pregnancy imply an association with higher endogenous estrogen levels. The high levels of human chorionic gonadotropin (hCG) that occur in early pregnancy could be another etiologic or permissive factor, as hCG binds to the TSH receptor and can constitute a stimulus to both hormone production and thyroid hypertrophy. Nevertheless, pregnancy does not appear to have an adverse impact on ultimate outcome [43]. Moreover, men with FTC have a worse prognosis for long-term survival than women [44].

Although ultrasonography cannot reliably distinguish between a follicular adenoma and a follicular cancer, there are certain ultrasonographic characteristics that are more common in a malignant follicular lesion; these include a hypoechoic appearance, the absence of a so-called halo around the nodule, and the absence of cystic change. Moreover, the malignant lesions tended to be larger and more likely to occur in male patients of more advanced age [45]. Within subtypes of FTC, older patients with heterogeneous nodules without internal calcification were somewhat more likely to have the Hurthle cell variant of FTC. Others have also found that larger nodule size was associated with a greater risk of malignancy in a follicular neoplasm [46, 47].

The not uncommon occurrence of FTC in an adenomatous goiter suggests a pathogenetic evolution of these cancers from lesions that were originally benign. Both follicular adenoma and FTC appear to have a monoclonal origin. Evolution of an adenoma into a malignant lesion could occur via mutational or translocational activation of oncogenes, particularly the RAS oncogene that has been specifically identified in follicular tumors [48, 49]. Evolution of adenoma into carcinoma could occur through the genetic loss of tumor suppressor genes that, taken together with RAS oncogene activation, would lead to clonal expansion and the growth of a malignant subclone of cells. Certain cytogenetic alterations have been linked to more aggressive tumor behavior [50]. Recent investigation has also focused on mutations of the TSH receptor in various thyroid disorders, and there may be mutations of the TSH receptor or the α subunit of the stimulatory G protein, which could also lead to tumorigenesis [48, 51]. A patient with an activating mutation of the TSH receptor in a tumor metastatic to lungs and lymph nodes sufficient to cause thyrotoxicosis has been described [52]. These tumors may be rich in the deiodinases 1 and 2 that convert thyroxine to triiodothyronine (T3) such that as many as one in five patients with metastatic FTC may have T3 toxicosis [53]. One consequence of this is that their levothyroxine dosage will need to be reduced if their tumor burden persists and continues to release T3.

Thyroid Function Tests and Imaging Evaluation

At presentation of a FTC, all routine blood thyroid function tests are likely to be within normal limits, including the serum TSH (except in the presence of severe iodine deficiency and endemic goiter). As described in Chap. 37, measurement of serum thyroglobulin (Tg) serves as the marker for residual or recurrent tumor [54]. However, preoperative measurement of Tg is not recommended in the ATA Guidelines [11]. Moreover, in the initial evaluation of a follicular neoplasm, serum Tg may be elevated, but a diagnosis of cancer should not be inferred as levels may be quite high in benign adenomata. The validity and utility of Tg measurements may vary widely between laboratories [55]. General aspects of Tg monitoring are discussed elsewhere (Chaps. 37 and 38) and may be adversely affected by interfering antithyroglobulin antibodies, which usually falsely lower serum Tg levels. This may be more problematic with immunoluminometric assays than with highly specific radioimmunoassays for Tg [54, 55]. Unfortunately, as much as 25–30 % of thyroid cancer patients may have underlying Hashimoto's disease with positive antithyroglobulin autoantibodies [56, 57]. While it has been hoped that management of such patients might be facilitated by measurement of Tg mRNA in serum [58], this method has not yet lived up to its expectations (see Chap. 39 by Ringel). Other unproven techniques have attempted to distinguish between circulating Tg derived from benign versus malignant thyroid tissue [59]. One such assay that initially showed some promise was the measurement of carcinoembryonic antigen (CEA) mRNA in blood. CEA has proven a useful tumor marker for medullary thyroid cancer and other nonthyroid tumors, and Sato et al. proposed that measurement of CEA mRNA could allow distinction between benign follicular adenomas and FTC [60].

Continuous periodic monitoring of serum Tg as the marker for residual or recurrent disease is critically essential to the basic management of patients with thyroid cancer. Patients with known metastatic or residual thyroid cancer should be followed by an endocrinologist or thyroid specialist, in addition to their primary care physician. The physician should ensure that serum Tg is measured only in a high-quality laboratory. This measurement should be in the same laboratory at each follow-up interval, and ideally the laboratory should provide companion Tg levels from remeasurement of stored serum from the prior venapuncture. In the postoperative state, a clearly measurable or rising serum Tg when the patient is TSH suppressed on levothyroxine implies residual disease and may be a definite clue to future recurrence. But an undetectable Tg when TSH is suppressed does not always imply cure, and serum Tg levels are most useful for prognosis when measured while the TSH is elevated, either when the patient is hypothyroid, e.g., during preparation for follow-up scanning, or after administration of recombinant human (rh) TSH [61–64] (see Chap. 34). The management dilemma presented by patients with negative radioiodine scan surveys but elevated serum Tg is discussed in Chap. 47.

Nuclear medicine studies are of limited use in the evaluation of patients with thyroid nodules that represent either a PTC or a FTC. The radioiodine uptake is normal, and an isotopic scan discloses a "cold" nodule that corresponds to the palpable lesion. However, a nuclear scan is indicated when the FNA cytology of a nodule is determined to be a follicular neoplasm, because such lesions may reflect benign follicular adenomata. If sufficiently hyperfunctioning, such adenomas will appear as a single "hot" nodule on the scan with uptake suppressed in the extranodular thyroid tissue. In such patients, the TSH will be very low to undetectable. In a multinodular gland, there may be other "hot" or autonomously hyperfunctioning nodules, but malignancy in the latter or in a single hyperfunctioning adenoma is very rare.

Thyroid ultrasound imaging is useful to confirm the presence of the nodule or nodules detected on physical examination and to determine the nodule size, ultrasonographic features, and multinodularity. Ultrasonography cannot reliably distinguish between benign and malignant lesions, but a purely cystic (anechoic) lesion only rarely harbors a malignancy, and a clear area around a solid (echogenic) lesion may represent an intact capsule ("halo" sign), suggesting benignancy [45].

Although the diagnostic sine qua non for evaluating thyroid nodules is usually the cytologic examination derived from fine-needle aspiration (FNA), this technique also does not reliably distinguish between benign and malignant follicular neoplasms. There is a very close similarity in the appearance of follicular cells in benign adenomata and those of follicular carcinoma, making it impossible in most cases to distinguish between the two with a cytologic examination after FNA. Some cytopathologists may detect a greater degree of nuclear "atypia" and an increased rate of mitoses in malignant lesions, but the distinction may be so difficult that it may even be treacherous. Instead, the diagnosis of FTC is based on histologic, not cytologic, criteria, including evidence for either capsular or vascular invasion. Relating to the Hurthle cell variant of FTC, Renshaw [65] has proposed that the application of specific cytologic criteria could distinguish benign Hurthle cell adenomas from carcinoma. However, this is disputed by Skoog and Tani in an accompanying editorial [66]. The authors urged caution in accepting these criteria as sufficiently accurate and expressed hope that molecular markers will soon serve this function.

A nodule with cytology that is described as "indeterminate" presents a special problem in management to the clinician. The varied cytologic diagnoses that may fall under the indeterminate group include designations such as follicular neoplasm, follicular lesion of unknown significance (FLUS), follicular tumor, atypia of unknown significance (AUS), or simply suspicious for malignancy. In the recent past, the decision has been either to repeat the FNA in 3–4 months if the nodule remains stable in size or to refer these nodules for thyroidectomy. In electing to send the patient with an indeterminate nodule on biopsy for thyroidectomy, one risks the possible morbidity of surgical complications versus failure to identify a malignancy which will be present in up to 50 % of these indeterminate nodules.

In order to attempt to resolve the dilemma of the indeterminate nodule, numerous investigators have explored different potential tumor markers and genetic analysis to distinguish benign from malignant lesions [67–69]. The many advances in the application of molecular markers to the diagnosis of malignancy in thyroid nodules are discussed at length in Chap. 20; only a few brief comments are addressed here. In one early study examining the presence of PAX8PPARγ1 in thyroid sections from adenomata and carcinomas, a greater number of the malignant lesions were found to have this fused gene [70]. However, although this finding tended to be confirmed by Marques et al. [71] in FNA aspirates of follicular neoplasms, it was not sufficiently specific to reliably separate malignant from benign lesions. Greater promise of potential utility and reliability as both a sensitive and specific presurgical marker for follicular thyroid cancer is suggested by a number of reports that have looked at the presence of polypeptide, galectin-3 [72, 73]. Prior studies had shown galectin-3 expression in other thyroid cancers. The specificity for distinguishing follicular adenoma from minimally invasive follicular carcinoma appears certain to promote growing application of other molecular approaches to both presurgical FNA aspirates and surgical pathologic tissues of controversial diagnosis.

The ATA Guidelines [11] recommend that FNA cytology results are to be reported employing the Bethesda classification [6–9]. Should the interpretation be of "atypia of uncertain significance" (AUS) or "follicular lesion of uncertain significance" (FLUS), the ATA recommendation would be to try to obtain a more specific diagnosis by repeating the FNA and doing mutational testing (see below) if the same AUS/FLUS reading is obtained or alternatively referring to a surgeon for thyroidectomy. Approximately 30–40 % of these FNAs will be AUS/FLUS on the repeat FNA [10]. No immediate further workup is warranted when the FNA cytology is benign, whereas the patient whose cytology is interpreted as indicating malignancy will be referred for thyroidectomy.

The various molecular markers that are becoming available to distinguish between benign and malignant nodule are described below in Chap. 22 by Xing and in earlier reviews [74–77], and the hope has been that better understanding of the significance of molecular markers would avoid unnecessary surgeries and the attendant potential complications [78]. The ATA 2014 Guidelines [11] have expanded on the issue of molecular testing given the more recent advances in the field. It is recommended that clinical decisions be based only on molecular analyses performed in approved CLIA or CAP certified laboratories and that these tests should be considered when the FNA results are indeterminate (e.g., atypia of uncertain significance (AUS), follicular lesion of uncertain significance (FLUS), follicular neoplasm, suspicious for follicular neoplasm).

Cytologic differentiation of follicular adenoma from carcinoma has been difficult, but frozen section analysis during the operative procedure is even worse in most [79], but not all [80], hands. An experienced pathologist should be able to diagnose the more aggressive and invasive type of follicular carcinoma, which often presents with distant metastases to the bone or lung. Although local lymph node invasion can be discovered during thyroidectomy in possibly 5–10 % of follicular cancers, it is much less common than in the papillary variety, which may present with involved cervical nodes in 35–45 % of patients. This is true as well for the Hurthle cell variant of FTC which has been found to spread locally in the neck via vascular channels and present as soft tissue nodules rather than as extension to lymph nodes [81]. In addition to the typically higher frequency of metastases to bone (spine, skull, and pelvis) and the lungs, other less common sites for distant metastases include the brain and, rarely, the liver.

The presence of bone metastases may be heralded by pain or fracture and significantly alters long-term prognosis and survival [82]. Two recent reviews summarize the typical presentation and management of the patient with bone metastases from FTC [83, 84]. The extent of disease is determined by imaging, and CT/PET scanning may be most useful employing either FDG, 124-iodine, or fluoride to identify sites of tumor, with MRI providing the most detailed imaging. MRI is particularly useful for spinal metastases to determine presence or risks of spinal cord compression [85]. In addition to local approaches to therapy, 131-iodine remains the primary therapeutic approach [86, 87] along with adjuncts such as zoledronic acid [88]. The presence of distant metastases can drop the 10-year survival rate from 85–90 % to 40 %, and bone metastases are associated with an even worse prognosis of 13–21 % [83] to as low as 14 % for those patients >40 years of age with multiple bone metastases and macronodular metastases to the lungs [89].

Possible confusion with papillary cancer could occur in tumors with the greatest degree of potential overlapping characteristics, i.e., the follicular variant of papillary carcinoma [90, 91]. However, these tumors exhibit biologic behavior much more similar to papillary than to follicular carcinoma, including a pattern of metastasis to regional nodes, rather than hematogenous spread to distant sites, as well as a better prognosis. Intraoperative frozen section or FNA cytology has been indicated to help distinguish FVPTC from a real follicular lesion and thus better guide the surgical procedure [4].

Zidan et al. [92] have proposed that the distinction between FVPTC and PTC is moot because with comparable treatment, the two have similar prognosis and survival. In their series, more advanced age was the most impressive negative prognostic factor, and the presence or degree of either distant metastases or local lymph node metastases did not significantly differ. In a subsequent communication [93], LiVolsi strongly disagreed with the interpretation of Zidan et al. Additionally, a close relationship to FTC is suggested by observations that some chromosomal aberrations in FVPTC seem to resemble FTC to a greater level than PTC [94]. However, other authors [95] have confirmed the conclusions of Zidan et al., with comparable outcome measures seen with FVPTC as with PTC but not with FTC [96]. Another study also indicated that FVPTC had an even more benign course than PTC [3].

The initial evaluation of a patient proven to have FTC should include a chest radiograph. Notably, however, even if interpreted as negative, the lungs may still demonstrate radionuclide uptake, suggesting metastases either on the postoperative diagnostic 131I scan or the post-ablation scan. If pulmonary metastases are evident, a chest computed tomography scan provides excellent anatomical imaging as a baseline study for future comparisons after therapy, and a brain MRI to rule out cerebral metastases is also recommended. Pulmonary metastases may be particularly difficult to fully eliminate, as demonstrated in children and young adults [97–101]. The mainstay of follow-up, however, is periodic serial monitoring of serum Tg levels and isotopic (131I) scans. The frequency of both depends on tumor staging and the specific clinical circumstances (e.g., low vs. intermediate or high risk) of each patient, as discussed in Chaps. 74 and 75. Cancer recurrences after initial thyroidectomy and radioiodine ablation and therapy are most likely to occur within the first 18–60 months. Patients with known tumor based on rising serum Tg levels but negative radioiodine scans may be studied with other imaging techniques, such as 201Tl, sestamibi, or 18-fluorodeoxyglucose (see Chap. 25). Hurthle cell variants often (perhaps 40 %) do not concentrate radioiodine.

Tumor staging is important to establish prognosis, but preference and application of staging methods remain somewhat controversial ([102–104]; see Chap. 9 particularly for FTC. The TNM (tumor, nodes, and metastasis) system remains the most widely applied of all staging systems for thyroid carcinoma in use [31, 105, 106]. This system allows the determination of the category of relative risk (low vs. high) and provides prognostic indicators for recurrence and death from the tumor. Prognostic indicators have been incorporated into systems that consist of a scale of risk. The AGES system, devised and advocated by the Mayo Clinic [107], incorporates the risks contributed by patient age, tumor grade, extracapsular invasion, and tumor size. Such systems provide useful parameters in the discussion of prognosis with patients in reasonably precise terms, considering the wide variability and uncertainty underlying prognosis of any malignancy. In the review of differing staging systems by DeGroot and colleagues [108], the TNM system was thought to provide the best risk stratification, at least for PTC. The practical importance and clinical relevance of risk stratification to treatment and management was carefully analyzed by Shaha in a retrospective review of more than 1,000 patients with DTC [109]. In one analysis of 13 different staging systems, the TNM system was determined to offer the best predictability as to outcome [31].

Summary

Although most primary thyroidal cancers arise from follicular epithelium, the most common type of thyroid malignancy is the well-differentiated papillary carcinoma, which accounts for about 75–85 % of thyroid tumors, with true follicular carcinomas accounting for only 10–12 % of all thyroid cancers. Follicular cancer is more common in older patients and spreads via blood vessel invasion, often presenting with metastases in the lungs or bone. Rarely, the mass of functioning metastatic cancer may be so great as to cause thyrotoxicosis. FTC may be contrasted with PTC, which occurs more frequently in younger patients, is slowly growing and less aggressive, and has a more favorable prognosis. Certain characteristics of FTC are associated with a worse prognosis, including a more invasive or metastatic tendency, male gender, and larger size, especially with lesions larger than 4 cm in diameter. Although age over 50 is generally considered to be an independent adverse risk factor, this was not found to be the only case by Besic et al. [110] who warned that younger patients with large tumors or distant metastases are also at risk of poor outcomes. Unlike papillary carcinoma, follicular carcinoma is much less likely to occur because of prior radiation exposure to the head and neck.

The management of FTC differs from that of PTC in one important way: the requirement for the early operative management of FTC to more often consist of a total, rather than subtotal, thyroidectomy [111]. This difference relates to the propensity of FTC to be angioinvasive and present with distant metastases and the need to destroy all residual thyroid tissue in the neck to visualize these distant metastases with radioiodine scanning. However, one review of 82 patients with FTC found that the extent of surgery did not affect the rate of disease-free survival, which was more directly related to radioiodine therapy [112]. The approach recommended by O'Neill et al. is predicated on the difference between the minimally invasive and invasive forms of FTC and associated risk factors. Thus, subtotal thyroidectomy would be adequate in a patient under age 45 with no vascular invasion, whereas they would perform total thyroidectomy followed by radioiodine ablation for all other patients with FTC [113].

When indicated, i.e., for an invasive FTC, thyroidectomy is then followed by radioiodine ablation of any remnant tissue. This procedure is a prerequisite to the potential need to more effectively treat distant metastases in the lung or bone with radioiodine by removing all residual thyroid tissue that might compete for radioiodine [114, 115]. Traditionally, ablation is effected postoperatively while patients are hypothyroid from levothyroxine withdrawal. However, sufficient data are now available on the efficacy of employing rhTSH for facilitating ablation (as summarized in Chap. 34) to make this the method of choice, even with low dosage activities of radioiodine [116, 117].

Depending on the surgical techniques, a considerable portion of the contralateral thyroid lobe may remain after a subtotal thyroidectomy or so-called near-total thyroidectomy [118]. Because of the need to destroy all remaining thyroid tissue to achieve satisfactory surveillance scanning, most experts would consider a completion thyroidectomy. Alternatively, other investigators have advocated radioiodine ablation of larger remnants of the thyroid, rather than introducing the risks that are inherent with a completion thyroidectomy [119, 120]. Patients with FTC are more likely to have advanced disease (stage III or IV) at presentation, placing them at a higher risk than patients with PTC [102]. One reported 10-year overall survival rate for follicular cancer was 85 % [121], whereas papillary cancers tend to have a more favorable prognosis with a 93 % 10-year survival [20, 21], especially if less than 1.5 cm in size and, if so, may not require aggressive management with radioiodine. Subsequent surveillance to determine a cancer cure or recurrence involves follow-up evaluations with 131I scanning and measurement of serum Tg as a tumor marker for recurrence. Traditionally, periodic evaluations consisted of allowing TSH to rise following discontinuation of L-thyroxine therapy. The availability of recombinant human TSH (rhTSH) [61–63] has radically altered routine follow-up evaluations for residual or recurrent disease. Several studies have examined the cutoff levels of Tg on suppression or after rhTSH stimulation that correlate with either presence of persistent disease or with cure [122, 123].

References

1. Vivero M, Kraft S, Barletta JA. Risk stratification of follicular variant of papillary thyroid carcinoma. Thyroid. 2013;23:273–9.
2. Yu X-M, Schneider DF, Leverson G, Chen H, Sippel RS. Follicular variant of papillary thyroid carcinoma is a unique clinical entity: a population-based study of 10,740 cases. Thyroid. 2013;23:1263–8.
3. Jain M, Khan A, Patwardhan N, et al. Follicular variant of papillary thyroid carcinoma: a comparative study of histopathologic features and cytology results in 141 patients. Endocr Pract. 2001;7:79–84.
4. Kesmodel SB, Terhune KP, Canter RJ, et al. The diagnostic dilemma of follicular variant of papillary thyroid carcinoma. Surgery. 2003;134:1005–12.
5. Daniels GH. What if many follicular variant papillary thyroid carcinomas are not malignant? A review of follicular variant papillary thyroid carcinoma and a proposal for a new classification. Endocr Pract. 2011;17(5):768–87.
6. Bongiovanni M, Spitale A, Faquin WC, Mazzucchelli L, Baloch ZW. The Bethesda system for reporting thyroid cytopathology: a meta-analysis. Acta Cytol. 2012;56:333–9.
7. Cibas Es, Ali SZ. The Bethesda system for reporting thyroid cytopathology. Thyroid. 2009;19:1159–65, and Am J Clin Pathol. 2009;132:658–665.

8. Theoharis CGA, Schofield KM, Hammers L, Udelsman R, Chhieng DC. The Bethesda thyroid fine-needle aspiration classification system: year 1 at an academic institution. Thyroid. 2009;19:1215–23.
9. Bose S, Walts AE. Thyroid fine needle aspirate: a post-Bethesda update. Adv Anat Pathol. 2012;19:160–9.
10. Teixeira GV, Chikota H, Teixeira T, Manfro G, Pal SI, Tufano RP. Incidence of malignancy in thyroid nodules determined to be follicular lesions of undetermined significance on fine-needle aspiration. World J Surg. 2012;36:69–74.
11. Haugen BR, Alexander EK, Bible KC, Doherty GM, Mandel SJ, Nikiforov Y, et al. 2015 American Thyroid Association Management Guidelines for patients with thyroid nodules and differentiated thyroid cancer. Thyroid 25: doi:10.1089/thy.2015.0020; print version in Thyroid 26:2016.
12. Sugino K, Kameyama K, Ito K, Nagahama M, Kitagawa W, Shibuya H, et al. Outcomes and prognostic factors of 251 patients with minimally invasive follicular thyroid carcinoma. Thyroid. 2012;22:798–804.
13. Thompson LDR, Wierneke JA, Paal E, et al. A clinicopathologic study of minimally invasive follicular carcinoma of the thyroid gland with a review of the English literature. Cancer. 2001;91:505–24.
14. Ito Y, Hirokawa M, Masuoka H, Yabuta T, Kihara M, Higashiyama T, et al. Prognostic factors of minimally invasive follicular thyroid carcinoma: extensive vascular invasion significantly affects patient prognosis. Endocr J. 2013;60:737–642.
15. Hedinger CE, Williams ED, Sobin LH. Histological typing of thyroid tumors. In: Hedinger CE, editor. International histological classification of tumors, vol. 11. Berlin: Springer; 1988.
16. Williams ED, Abrosimov A, Bogdanova TI, et al. Two proposals regarding the terminology of thyroid tumors. Int J Surg Pathol. 2000;8:181–3.
17. Elsheikh TM, Asa SL, Chan JK, et al. Interobserver and intraobserver variation among experts in the diagnosis of thyroid follicular lesions with borderline nuclear features of papillary carcinoma. Am J Clin Pathol. 2008;130:736–44.
18. Baloch AZ, LiVolsi VA. Follicular-patterned lesions of the thyroid: the bane of the pathologist. Am J Clin Pathol. 2002;117:143–50.
19. Haigh PI. Follicular thyroid carcinoma. Curr Treat Options Oncol. 2002;3:349–54.
20. Mazzaferri EL, Kloos RT. Current approaches to primary therapy for papillary and follicular thyroid cancer. J Clin Endocrinol Metab. 2001;86:1447–63.
21. Schlumberger MJ. Papillary and follicular thyroid carcinoma. N Engl J Med. 1998;338:297–306.
22. National Comprehensive Cancer Network (NCCN) Thyroid carcinoma: clinical practice guidelines 2013, J Natl Compr Cancer Netw; Version 2.2013.
23. British Thyroid Association. Guidelines for the management of differentiated thyroid cancer in adults. Available at: www.british-thyroidassociation.org/guidelines.htm, 2nd ed. 2007.
24. Siegel R, Naishadham D, Jemal A. Cancer statistics, 2013. CA Cancer J Clin. 2013;63:11–30.
25. Sobrinho-Simoes M, Eloy C, Magalhaes J, Lobo C, Amaro T. Follicular thyroid carcinoma. Mod Pathol. 2011;2:S10–8.
26. Hundahl SA, Cady B, Cunningham MP, et al. Initial results from a progressive cohort study of 5583 cases of thyroid carcinoma treated in the United States during 1996. Cancer. 2000;89:202–17.
27. National Cancer Institute Surveillance, Epidemiology and End Results Program. Available at http://www.seer.cancer.gov.
28. Otto KJ, Lam JSC, MacMilllan C, Freeman JL. Diminishing diagnosis of follicular thyroid carcinoma. Head Neck. 2010;32:1629–34.
29. Huang CC, Hsueh C, Liu FH, Chao TC, Lin JD. Diagnostic and therapeutic strategies for minimally and widely invasive follicular thyroid carcinomas. Surg Oncol. 2011;20:1–6.
30. D'Avanzo A, Treseler P, Ituarte PHG, et al. Follicular thyroid carcinoma: histology and prognosis. Cancer. 2004;100:1123–9.
31. Lang BH-H, Lo C-Y, Chan W-F, Lam K-Y, Wan K-Y. Staging systems for follicular thyroid carcinoma: application to 171 consecutive patients treated in a tertiary referral centre. Endocr-Rel Cancer. 2007;14:29–42.
32. Lang BH, Wong KP, Cheung CY, Wan KY, Lo CY. Evaluating the prognostic factors associated with cancer-specific survival of differentiated thyroid carcinoma presenting with distant metastasis. Ann Surg Oncol. 2013;20:1329–35.
33. Pulcrano M, Boukheris H, Talbot M, et al. Poorly differentiated follicular thyroid carcinoma: prognostic factors and relevance of histologic classification. Thyroid. 2007;17:639–46.
34. Jensen MH, Davis RK, Derrick L. Thyroid cancer: a computer-assisted review of 5287 cases. Otolaryngol Head Neck Surg. 1990;102:51–65.
35. Ruegemer JJ, Hay ID, Bergstralh EJ, et al. Distant metastases in differentiated thyroid carcinoma: a multivariate analysis of prognostic variables. J Clin Endocrinol Metab. 1988;67:501–8.
36. Schlumberger M, Tubiana M, de Vathaire F, et al. Long-term results of treatment of 283 patients with lung and bone metastases from differentiated thyroid carcinoma. J Clin Endocrinol Metab. 1986;63:960–6.
37. Young RL, Mazzaferri EL, Rahe AJ, Dorfman SG. Pure follicular carcinoma: impact of therapy in 214 patients. J Nucl Med. 1980;21:733–7.
38. Simpson WJ, McKinney SE, Carruthers JS, et al. Papillary and follicular thyroid cancer: prognostic factors in 1578 patients. Am J Med. 1987;83:479–88.
39. Franceschi S. Iodine intake and thyroid carcinoma—a potential risk factor. Exper Clin Endocrinol Diabetes. 1998;106 Suppl 3:S38–44.
40. Galanti MR, Hansson L, Bergstrom R, et al. Diet and the risk of papillary and follicular thyroid carcinoma: a population-based case-control study in Sweden and Norway. Cancer Causes Control. 1997;8:205–14.
41. Wartofsky L. Rising world incidence of thyroid cancer: increased detection or higher radiation exposure? Hormones. 2010;9:103–8.
42. LiVolsi VA, Asa SL. The demise of follicular carcinoma of the thyroid gland. Thyroid. 1994;4:233–6.
43. Moosa M, Mazzaferri EL. Outcome of differentiated thyroid cancer diagnosed in pregnant women. J Clin Endocrinol Metab. 1997;82:2862–6.
44. Eichhorn W, Tabler H, Lippold R, et al. Prognostic factors determining long-term survival in well-differentiated thyroid cancer: an analysis of four hundred eighty-four patients undergoing therapy and aftercare at the same institution. Thyroid. 2003;13:949–58.
45. Sillery JC, Reading CC, Charboneau JW, et al. Thyroid follicular carcinoma: sonographic features of 50 cases. AJR. 2010;194:44–54.
46. Mihai R, Parker AJ, Roskell D, Sadler GP. One in four patients with follicular thyroid cytology has a thyroid carcinoma. Thyroid. 2009;19:33–7.
47. Raparia K, Min SK, Mody DR, Anton R, Amrikachi M. Clinical outcomes for "suspicious" category in thyroid fine-needle aspiration: patient's sex and nodule size are possible predictors of malignancy. Arch Pathol Lab Med. 2009;133:787–90.
48. Challeton C, Bounacer A, DuVillard JA, et al. Pattern of ras and gsp oncogene mutations in radiation-associated human thyroid tumors. Oncogene. 1995;11:601–3.

49. Freitas BC, Cerutti JM. Genetic markers differentiating follicular thyroid carcinoma from benign lesions. Mol Cell Endocrinol. 2010;321(1):77–85.
50. Roque L, Clode A, Beige G, et al. Follicular thyroid carcinoma: chromosome analysis of 19 cases. Genes Chromosomes Cancer. 1998;21:250–5.
51. Russo D, Aruri F, Schlumberger M, et al. Activating mutations of the TSH receptor in differentiated thyroid carcinoma. Oncogene. 1995;11:1907–11.
52. Russo D, Tumino S, Arturi F, et al. Detection of an activating mutation of the thyrotropin receptor in a case of an autonomously hyperfunctioning thyroid insular carcinoma. J Clin Endocrinol Metab. 1997;82:735–8.
53. Miyauchi A, Takamura Y, Ito Y, et al. 3,5,3′-Triiodothyronine thyrotoxicosis due to increased conversiόn of administered levothyroxine in patients with metastátic follicular thyroid carcinoma. J Clin Endocrinol Metab. 2008;93:2239–42.
54. Spencer CA, Fatemi S, Singer P, Nicoloff J, LoPresti J. Serum basal thyroglobulin measured by a second-generation assay correlates with the recombinant human thyrotropin-stimulated thyroglobulin response in patients treated for differentiated thyroid cancer. Thyroid. 2010;20:587–95.
55. Schlumberger M, Hitzel A, Toubert ME, et al. Comparison of seven serum thyroglobulin assays in the follow-up of papillary and follicular thyroid cancer patients. J Clin Endocrinol Metab. 2007;92:2487–95.
56. Spencer CA. Clinical utility of thyroglobulin antibody (TgAb) measurements for patients with differentiated thyroid cancers (DTC). J Clin Endocrinol Metab. 2011;96:3615–27.
57. Spencer CA, Petrovic I, Fatemi S. Current thyroglobulin autoantibody (TgAb) assays often fail to detect interfering TgAb that ca result in the reporting of falsely low/undetectable serum Tg IMA values for patients with differentiated thyroid cancer. J Clin Endocrinol Metab. 2011;96:1283–91.
58. Ringel MD, Ladenson PW, Levine MA. Molecular diagnosis of residual and recurrent thyroid cancer by amplification of thyroglobulin messenger ribonucleic acid in peripheral blood. J Clin Endocrinol Metab. 1998; 83:4435–42. Editorial comment by Haber RS. The diagnosis of recurrent thyroid cancer—a new approach. J Clin Endocrinol Metab. 1998; 83:4189–90.
59. Maruyama M, Kato R, Kobayashi S, Kasuga Y. A method to differentiate between thyroglobulin derived from normal thyroid tissue and from thyroid carcinoma based on analysis of reactivity to lectins. Arch Pathol Lab Med. 1998;122:715–20.
60. Sato T, Harao M, Nakano S, et al. Circulating tumor cells detected by reverse transcription-polymerase chain reaction for carcinoembryonic antigen mRNA: Distinguishing follicular thyroid carcinoma from adenoma. Surgery. 2005;137:552–8.
61. Wartofsky L. Using baseline and recombinant human TSH-stimulated thyroglobulin measurements to manage thyroid cancer without diagnostic 131-I scanning. J Clin Endocrinol Metab. 2002;87:1486–9.
62. Robbins RJ, Robbins AK. Recombinant human thyrotropin and thyroid cancer management. J Clin Endocrinol Metab. 2003;88:1933–8.
63. Wartofsky L, the rhTSH-Stimulated Thyroglobulin Study Group. Management of low risk well differentiated thyroid cancer based only upon thyroglobulin measurement after recombinant human thyrotropin. Thyroid. 2002;12:583–92.
64. Mazzaferri EL, Robbins RJ, Spencer CA, et al. A consensus report on the role of serum thyroglobulin as a monitoring method for low risk patients with papillary thyroid carcinoma. J Clin Endocrinol Metab. 2003;88:1433–41.
65. Renshaw A, Gould EW. Why there is the tendency to "overdiagnose" the follicular variant of papillary thyroid carcinoma. Am J Clin Pathol. 2002;117:19–21.
66. Skoog L, Tani E. Hurthle cell carcinoma: time for a drastic change? Cancer. 2002;96:259–60.
67. Arturi F, Russo D, Giuffrida D, et al. Early diagnosis by genetic analysis of differentiated thyroid cancer metastases in small lymph nodes. J Clin Endocrinol Metab. 1997;82:1638–41.
68. Winzer R, Schmutzler C, Jakobs TC, et al. Reverse transcriptase-polymerase chain reaction analysis of thyrocyte-relevant genes in fine-needle aspiration biopsies of the human thyroid. Thyroid. 1998;8:981–7.
69. Handkiewicz-Junak D, Czarniecka A, Jarzab B. Molecular prognostic markers in papillary and follicular thyroid cancer: current status and future directions. Mol Cell Endocrinol. 2010;322(1–2):8–28.
70. Kroll TG, Sarraf P, Pecciarini L, et al. PAX8-PPARγ-1 fusion in oncogene human thyroid carcinoma. Science. 2000;289:1357–60.
71. Marques AR, Espadinha C, Catarino AL, et al. Expression of PAX8PPARγ1 rearrangements in both follicular thyroid carcinomas and adenomas. J Clin Endocrinol Metab. 2002;87:3947–52.
72. Bartolazzi A, Gasbarri A, Papotti M, et al. Application of an immunodiagnostic method for improving diagnosis of nodular thyroid lesions. Lancet. 2001;357:1644–50.
73. Saggiorato E, Cappia S, De Giuli P, et al. Galectin-3 as a presurgical immuno cytodiagnostic marker of minimally invasive follicular thyroid carcinoma. J Clin Endocrinol Metab. 2001;86:5152–8.
74. Weber F, Eng C. Update on the molecular diagnosis of endocrine tumors: toward-omics-based personalized healthcare? J Clin Endocrinol Metab. 2008;93:1097–104.
75. Nikiforov Y, Nikiforova MN. Molecular genetics and diagnosis of thyroid cancer. Nat Rev Endocrinol. 2011;7:569–80.
76. Prasad NB, Kowalski J, Tsai H-L, Talbot K, Somervell H, Kouniavsky G, et al. Three-gene molecular diagnostic model for thyroid cancer. Thyroid. 2012;22:275–84.
77. Nikiforova MN, Nikiforov YE. Molecular diagnostics and predictors in thyroid cancer. Thyroid. 2009;19:1351–61.
78. Alexander EK. Approach to the patient with a cytologically indeterminate thyroid nodule. J Clin Endocrinol Metab. 2008;93:4175–82.
79. Collins SL. Thyroid cancer: controversies and etiopathogenesis of thyroid cancer. In: Falk S, editor. Thyroid disease: endocrinology, surgery, nuclear medicine, and radiotherapy. 2nd ed. New York: Raven Press; 1997. p. 495–564.
80. Paphavasit A, Thompson GB, Hay ID, et al. Follicular and Hürthle cell thyroid neoplasms: is frozen section evaluation worthwhile? Arch Surg. 1997;132:674–8.
81. Bishop JA, Wu G, Tufano RP, Westra WH. Histological patterns of locoregional recurrence in Hurthle cell carcinoma of the thyroid gland. Thyroid. 2012;22:690–4.
82. Orita Y, Sugitani I, Matsuura M, et al. Prognostic factors and the therapeutic strategy for patients with bone metastasis from differentiated thyroid carcinoma. Surgery. 2010;147:424–31.
83. Muresan MM, Olivier P, Leclere J, et al. Bone metastases from differentiated thyroid carcinoma. Endocr Relat Cancer. 2008;15:37–49.
84. Wexler JA. Approach to the thyroid cancer patient with bone metastases. J Clin Endocrinol Metab. 2011;96:2296–3307.
85. Schmidt GP, Schoenberg SO, Schmid R, et al. Screening for bone metastases: whole body MRI using a 32-channel system versus dual modality. Eur Radiol. 2006;174:939–49.
86. Qiu Z-L, Song H-J, Xu Y-H, Luo Q-Y. Efficacy and survival analysis of ^{131}I therapy for bone metastases from differentiated thyroid cancer. J Clin Endocrinol Metab. 2011;96:3078–86.
87. Wartofsky L, Van Nostrand D. Radioiodine treatment of well-differentiated thyroid cancer. Endocrine. 2012;42:506–13.

88. Orita Y, Sugitani I, Toda K, Manabe J, Fujimoto Y. Zoledronic acid in the treatment of bone metastases from differentiated thyroid carcinoma. Thyroid. 2011;21:31–5.
89. Durante C, Haddy N, Baudin E, et al. Long-term outcome of 444 patients with distant metastases from papillary and follicular thyroid carcinoma: benefits and limits of radioiodine therapy. J Clin Endocrinol Metab. 2006;91:2892–9.
90. Tielens ET, Sherman SI, Hruban RH, Ladenson PW. Follicular variant of papillary thyroid carcinoma: a clinical pathologic study. Cancer. 1994;73:424–31.
91. Baloch ZW, Gupta PK, Yu GH, et al. Follicular variant of papillary carcinoma. Cytologic and histologic correlation. Am J Clin Pathol. 1999;111:216–22.
92. Zidan J, Karen D, Stein M, et al. Pure versus follicular variant of papillary thyroid carcinoma; clinical features, prognostic factors, treatment, and survival. Cancer. 2003;97:1181–5.
93. LiVolsi VA and reply by Zidan J. (Letters) Pure versus follicular variant of papillary thyroid carcinoma. Cancer. 2003;98:1997–8.
94. Wreesman VB, Ghossein RA, Hezel M, et al. Follicular variant of papillary thyroid carcinoma: genome-wide appraisal of a controversial entity. Genes Chromosomes Cancer. 2004;40:355–64.
95. Burningham AR, Krishnan J, Davidson BJ, Ringel MD, Burman KD. Papillary and follicular variant of papillary carcinoma of the thyroid: Initial presentation and response to therapy. Otolaryngol Head Neck Surg. 2005;132:840–4.
96. Passler C, Prager G, Scheuba C, et al. Follicular variant of papillary thyroid carcinoma: a long-term follow-up. Arch Surg. 2003;138:1362–6.
97. Vassilopoulou-Sellin R, Klein MJ, Smith TH, et al. Pulmonary metastases in children and young adults with differentiated thyroid cancer. Cancer. 1993;71:1348–52.
98. Samuel AM, Rajashekharrao B, Shah DH. Pulmonary metastases in children and adolescents with well-differentiated thyroid cancer. J Nucl Med. 1998;39:1531–6.
99. Feinmesser R, Lubin E, Segal K, Noyek A. Carcinoma of the thyroid in children—a review. J Fed Endocrinol Metab. 1997;10:561–8.
100. Poorten VV, Hens G, Delaere P. Thyroid cancer in children and adolescents. Curr Opin Otolaryngol Head Neck Surg. 2013;21:135–42.
101. Hung W, Sarlis NJ. Current controversies in the management of pediatric patients with well-differentiated nonmedullary thyroid cancer: a review. Thyroid. 2002;12:683–702.
102. Sherman SI, Brierley JD, Sperling M, et al. Prospective multicenter study of thyroid carcinoma treatment: initial analysis of staging and outcome. Cancer. 1998;83:1012–21.
103. Cady B. Staging in thyroid carcinoma. Cancer. 1998;83:844–7.
104. Sherman SI. Editorial: Staging in thyroid carcinoma—a reply. Cancer. 1998;83:848–50.
105. Brierley JD, Panzarella T, Tsang RW, et al. A comparison of different staging systems predictability of patient outcome: thyroid carcinoma as an example. Cancer. 1997;79:2414–23.
106. Loh K-C, Greenspan FS, Gee L, et al. Pathological tumor-node-metastasis (pTNM) staging for papillary and follicular thyroid carcinomas: a retrospective analysis of 700 patients. J Clin Endocrinol Metab. 1997;82:3553–62.
107. Hay ID, Bergstralh EJ, Goellner JR, et al. Predicting outcome in papillary thyroid carcinoma: development of a reliable prognostic scoring system in a cohort of 1779 patients treated surgically at one institution during 1940 through 1989. Surgery. 1993;114:1050–8.
108. DeGroot LJ, Kaplan EL, Straus FH, Shukla MS. Does the method of management of papillary thyroid carcinoma make a difference in outcome? World J Surg. 1994;18:123–30.
109. Shaha AR. Implications of prognostic factors and risk groups in the management of differentiated thyroid cancer. Laryngoscope. 2004;114:393–402.
110. Besic N, Zgajnar J, Hocevar M, Frkovic-Grazio S. Is patient's age a prognostic factor for follicular thyroid carcinoma in the TNM classification system? Thyroid. 2005;15:439–48.
111. Schwartz AE, Clark OH, Ituarte P, LoGerfo P. Thyroid surgery—the choice. J Clin Endocrinol Metab. 1998;83:1097–105.
112. Taylor T, Specker B, Robbins J, et al. Outcome after treatment of high-risk papillary and non-Hürthle cell follicular thyroid carcinoma. Ann Intern Med. 1998;129:622–7.
113. O'Neill CJ, Vaughan L, Learoyd DL, Sidhu SB, Delbridge LW, Sywak MS. Management of follicular thyroid carcinoma should be individualized based on degree of capsular and vascular invasion. Eur J Surg Oncol. 2011;37:181–5.
114. Lin JD, Kao PF, Chao TC. The effects of radioactive iodine in thyroid remnant ablation and treatment of well differentiated thyroid carcinoma. Br J Radiol. 1998;71:307–13.
115. Pelikan DM, Lion HL, Hermans J, Goslings BM. The role of radioactive iodine in the treatment of advanced differentiated thyroid carcinoma. Clin Endocrinol. 1997;47:713–20.
116. Schlumberger M, Catargi B, Borget I, Deandreis D, Zerdoud S, Bridji B, et al. Strategies of radioiodine ablation in patients with low-risk thyroid cancer. N Engl J Med. 2013;366:1663–73.
117. Mallick U, Harmer C, Yap B, Wadsley J, Clarke S, Moss L, et al. Ablation with low-dose radioiodine and thyrotropin alfa in thyroid cancer. N Engl J Med. 2013;366:1674–85.
118. Suliburk J, Delbridge L. Surgical management of well-differentiated thyroid cancer: state of the art. Surg Clin N Am. 2009;89(5):1171–91.
119. Lin JD, Chao TC, Huang MJ, et al. Use of radioactive iodine for thyroid remnant ablation in well-differentiated thyroid carcinoma to replace thyroid reoperation. Am J Clin Oncol. 1998;21:77–81.
120. Barbesino G, Goldfarb M, Parangi S, Yang J, Ross DS, Daniels GH. Thyroid lobe ablation with radioactive iodine as an alternative to completion thyroidectomy after hemithyroidectomy in patients with follicular thyroid cancer: long-term follow-up. Thyroid. 2012;22:369–76.
121. Hundahl SA, Fleming ID, Fremgen AM, Menck HR. A national cancer data base report on 53, 856 cases of thyroid carcinoma treated in the U.S., 1985–1995. Cancer. 1998;83:2638–48.
122. Brassard M, Borget I, Edet-Sanson A, Giraudet A-L, et al. Long-term follow-up of patients with papillary and follicular thyroid cancer: a prospective study of 715 patients. J Clin Endocrinol Metab. 2011;96:1352–9.
123. Klubo-Gwiezdzinska J, Burman KD, Van Nostrand D, Wartofsky L. Does an undetectable rhTSH-stimulated Tg level 12 months after initial treatment of thyroid cancer indicate remission? Clin Endocrinol. 2011;74:111–7.

Surgical Management of Follicular Cancer

71

Gerard M. Doherty

Follicular thyroid cancers are derived from follicular epithelium within the thyroid gland, accounting for about 10 % of all thyroid cancers, though the incidence seems to be decreasing [1, 2]. Follicular thyroid cancers differ from the more common follicular adenomas because the follicular cells in the cancers invade the vessels, capsule, or both. These tumors are usually unifocal and encapsulated. In contrast to papillary thyroid cancers that often metastasize to regional lymph nodes, follicular thyroid cancers infrequently involve the lymph nodes (<10 % of patients) but more frequently hematogenously metastasize to the lung and bones [3–5]. Patients with follicular thyroid cancer generally have a worse prognosis than patients with papillary thyroid cancer. However, most of the difference in prognosis is associated with patients' older age and more advanced tumor stage at presentation.

The principles of surgical management of follicular thyroid carcinomas are similar to those for papillary thyroid cancer: a thorough initial operation tailored to the patient's extent of disease and to the value of subsequent adjuvant therapy or surveillance tools (see Chap. 24). For example, patients with small minimally invasive follicular tumors rarely have extension of disease beyond the thyroid gland and are usually completely treated by thyroid lobectomy [6]. Conversely, patients with widely invasive follicular tumor may require extensive resection for local disease and to allow adjuvant radioiodine therapy and thyroglobulin measurement in follow-up.

Hürthle cell cancer behaves in a similar clinical manner as follicular cancer. They are judged malignant when angioinvasion, capsular invasion, or distant metastases occurs. Hürthle cell cancers, however, are more likely to be multifocal, to involve regional lymph nodes, to not concentrate radioiodine effectively, to recur locally, and more likely to be lethal and so are more likely to require more complete operative resection.

The problem of managing many patients with follicular or Hürthle cell cancer is that diagnosis is often not made preoperatively but only becomes clear after permanent histological sections are available. The role of reoperation to remove remaining thyroid tissue in a patient who has had less than total thyroidectomy (completion thyroidectomy) for follicular cancer is controversial [7–9]. The frequency with which this issue presents should be minimized by careful initial surgery and gross intraoperative evaluation. Patients can have very benign histologic appearance of the follicular cancer in the thyroid gland. However if the patient has metastasis to lymph nodes near the thyroid or has evidence of local soft tissue invasion outside the thyroid glands, then the patient probably would benefit from a total or near-total thyroidectomy. Frozen section analysis of the thyroid gland itself is not often helpful in making this decision; the utility of frozen section analysis of follicular thyroid lesions has been assessed by a randomized clinical trial. However, careful gross evaluation, attention to the clinical situation, and judicious use of frozen section analysis of abnormalities away from the primary tumor may make the need for total thyroidectomy apparent at the initial operation [10].

The most common indication for completion thyroidectomy is a frozen section analysis of a thyroid lesion that is interpreted as benign follicular adenoma. On subsequent permanent pathology, areas of invasion are identified and the diagnosis is changed to follicular carcinoma. In this situation the surgeon is faced with the decision of whether to go back and remove the contralateral thyroid gland for completion of the thyroidectomy or whether to leave the contralateral gland in place. Studies have demonstrated that completion thyroidectomy can be done safely by experienced surgeons and that

G.M. Doherty, MD, FACS (✉)
Department of Surgery, Boston Medical Center, Boston University, 88 East Newton Street, Collamore Building Suite 500, Boston, MA 02118, USA
e-mail: dohertyg@bu.edu

L. Wartofsky, D. Van Nostrand (eds.), *Thyroid Cancer*, DOI 10.1007/978-1-4939-3314-3_71

cancer can be found in the contralateral thyroid in a significant proportion of these patients [7, 8]. There are no data to demonstrate that the completion thyroidectomy has an effect on recurrence or survival, because no one has prospectively studied this topic. The ATA guidelines recommend consideration of completion thyroidectomy if a total thyroidectomy would have been performed initially if all of the information had been available [11]. If the patient is in a very good prognostic group, e.g., a 35-year woman with a 1 cm follicular tumor that has minimal invasion of the capsule only, then it is reasonable to maintain the patient on thyroxine suppression and not perform completion thyroidectomy. If, however, the patient has any risk factors at all that might indicate a more significant risk for tumor recurrence and mortality, then reoperation for completion of the thyroidectomy should be more strongly advised.

For those patients in the worse prognostic groups, and for those with previous neck irradiation, complete removal of the thyroid gland is more clearly indicated. Radiation exposure increases the risk of multicentric disease, and patients with follicular tumors after radiation exposure are at a particularly increased risk of recurrence [12]. Complete removal of the thyroid gland removes gross or occult contralateral disease and allows therapy with I-131 that can treat both local, regional, and distant follicular carcinoma. Most surgeons avoid procedures that might alter function for the patient in the presence of a well-differentiated follicular tumor. For example, radical neck dissection or laryngectomy would very rarely be indicated for disease that is not resectable by less mutilating means, given the efficacy of I-131 therapy and external beam radiotherapy to achieve local control.

In patients with metastases, therapy should begin with thyroidectomy. This will be the quickest way to make the patient hypothyroid and allow total body I-131 scanning and potential therapy. Patients with a single demonstrable resectable metastasis should have resection, as this may lead to cure or prolonged survival. Multiple metastases are best treated by radioactive iodine therapy and occasionally adjuvant chemotherapy or external beam irradiation. Local therapies to relieve symptoms from bone metastases generally are palliative [13].

References

1. LiVolsi VA, Baloch ZW. Follicular neoplasms of the thyroid: view, biases, and experiences. Adv Anat Pathol. 2004;11(6):279–87.
2. LiVolsi VA, Baloch ZW. Follicular-patterned tumors of the thyroid: the battle of benign vs. malignant vs. so-called uncertain. Endocr Pathol. 2011;22(4):184–9.
3. Goldstein RE, Netterville JL, Burkey B, Johnson JE. Implications of follicular neoplasms, atypia, and lesions suspicious for malignancy diagnosed by fine-needle aspiration of thyroid nodules. Ann Surg. 2002;235(5):656–62; discussion 662–654.
4. Witte J, Goretzki PE, Dieken J, Simon D, Roher HD. Importance of lymph node metastases in follicular thyroid cancer. World J Surg. 2002;26(8):1017–22.
5. Zaydfudim V, Feurer ID, Griffin MR, Phay JE. The impact of lymph node involvement on survival in patients with papillary and follicular thyroid carcinoma. Surgery. 2008;144(6):1070–7; discussion 1077–1078.
6. van Heerden JA, Hay ID, Goellner JR, et al. Follicular thyroid carcinoma with capsular invasion alone: a nonthreatening malignancy. Surgery. 1992;112:1130–8.
7. DeGroot LJ, Kaplan EL. Second operations for "completion" of thyroidectomy in treatment of differentiated thyroid cancer. Surgery. 1991;110:936–40.
8. De Jong SA, Demeter JG, Lawrence AM, Paloyan E. Necessity and safety of completion thyroidectomy for differentiated thyroid carcinoma. Surgery. 1992;112:734–9.
9. Shaha AR, Jaffe BM. Completion thyroidectomy: a critical appraisal. Surgery. 1992;112:1148–53.
10. Udelsman R, Westra WH, Donovan PI, Sohn TA, Cameron JL. Randomized prospective evaluation of frozen-section analysis for follicular neoplasms of the thyroid. Ann Surg. 2001;233(5):716–22.
11. Cooper DS, Doherty GM, Haugen BR, et al. Revised American Thyroid Association management guidelines for patients with thyroid nodules and differentiated thyroid cancer. Thyroid. 2009; 19(11):1167–214.
12. Schneider AB, Recant W, Pinsky SM, Ryo UY, Bekerman C, Shore-Freedman E. Radiation-induced thyroid carcinoma. Ann Intern Med. 1986;105:405.
13. Smit JW, Vielvoye GJ, Goslings BM. Embolization for vertebral metastases of follicular thyroid carcinoma. J Clin Endocrinol Metab. 2000;85(3):989–94.

Pathology of Follicular Cancer

72

Zubair W. Baloch and Virginia A. LiVolsi

Follicular carcinomas are rare in today's industrialized nations [1, 2]. This cancer type does not have the nuclear features of papillary carcinoma, usually has no papillae, lacks amyloid and calcitonin, and does not contain the numerous spindle cells, giant cells, and mitotic figures of undifferentiated (anaplastic) carcinoma. Most published classifications are based on the degree of cancer invasiveness, but histological patterns of the neoplasm may also provide clues to its likely behavior [3–5]. At present, evaluating the neoplasm's relationship to the surrounding tissues has proved to be the most useful guide to categorizing these tumors [5–7].

Inspection of the tissues usually reveals a single, spherical, solid, fleshy neoplasm, with pink-to-tan cut surfaces (if fresh) or pale tan-to-pale gray surfaces if fixed in formaldehyde [7–9]. Tumors composed of oncocytic/oxyphilic cells (Askanazy/Hürthle cells) are brown. If the tumor contains a considerable amount of colloid, the cut surface may appear translucent and gelatinous. Small hemorrhages may be present, along with focal scarring (especially in the center) [10]. A few cancers present as multiple neoplastic nodules, with "daughter nodules" around the nodule with the thickest capsule. Cystic change and focal necrosis sometimes occur. The tumors are usually encapsulated, but if a tumor is quite invasive, only remnants of the capsule can be detected. Capsules vary in thickness (are often thick), and when a small tumor has a thick capsule, the pathologist should suspect carcinoma, not adenoma [9, 11, 12].

Z.W. Baloch, MD, PhD (✉) • V.A. LiVolsi, MD
Department of Pathology and Laboratory Medicine, Perelman School of Medicine, University of Pennsylvania Medical Center, 6 Founders Pavilion, 3400 Spruce Street, Philadelphia, PA 19104, USA
e-mail: balocj@mail.med.upenn.edu; linus@mail.med.upenn.edu

A moderate proportion of follicular carcinomas occur in association with multiple adenomatoid nodules/multinodular goiter (or adenomas). It can be difficult to decide which tumor is malignant upon gross examination; thus, systematic sectioning of such a specimen is essential [9].

Follicular carcinomas can be considered minimally invasive, angioinvasive, or widely invasive [7, 9, 13]. Assessment is performed after surgical resection of the tumor (or occasionally at autopsy) and requires multiple sections of the periphery of the neoplasm to exclude an adenoma. A total of ten tissue blocks from the periphery of the tumor is desirable, or more if the tumor is particularly cellular or contains many mitotic figures [7, 9, 13]. For small tumors, the entire neoplasm should be embedded in such a way as to enable multiple views of its periphery to be obtained [9, 12].

Follicular carcinoma can be subdivided into encapsulated and widely invasive variants. In our practice, we further divide the encapsulated variant into minimally invasive showing only tumor capsule invasion and those with invasion of vessels within tumor capsule, i.e., angioinvasive follicular carcinoma (Figs. 72.1 and 72.2). When only capsular penetration appears to be present, the patient probably does not have distant spread [14], but the pathologist should search vigorously for vascular invasion [12]. Therefore, if a tumor is not evaluated systematically, it may be mistaken for an adenoma [12]. Differentiating capsular invasion from invasion of small vessels in the capsule can be a task. Therefore, discussion of such phenomena must be evaluated with caution and strict criteria should be applied [9, 12]. Widely invasive carcinoma is uncommon, with extensive protrusion into surrounding tissues and/or extension into multiple vessels (often large vascular spaces; Fig. 72.3).

Cells of follicular carcinoma are often small and monotonous in histological sections, with uniform round nuclei, stippled chromatin, and central nucleoli. The nucleoli vary considerably in size from one carcinoma to another. Mitotic figures range greatly in number in each tumor; atypical

L. Wartofsky, D. Van Nostrand (eds.), *Thyroid Cancer*, DOI 10.1007/978-1-4939-3314-3_72

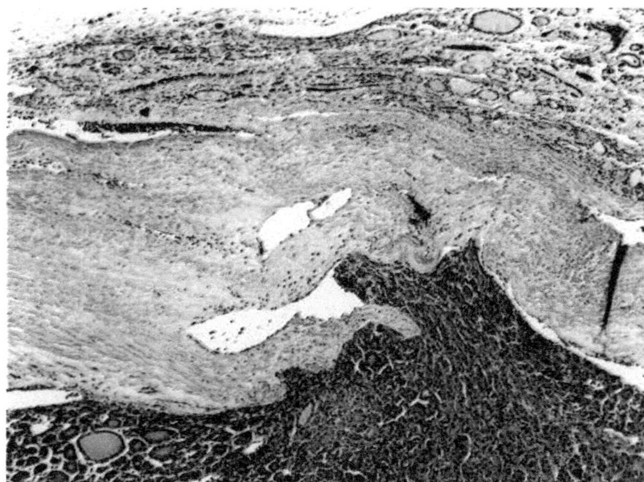

Fig. 72.1 Angioinvasive follicular carcinoma. The cancer extends into a vessel in the thick capsule (hematoxylin and eosin [H&E] stain)

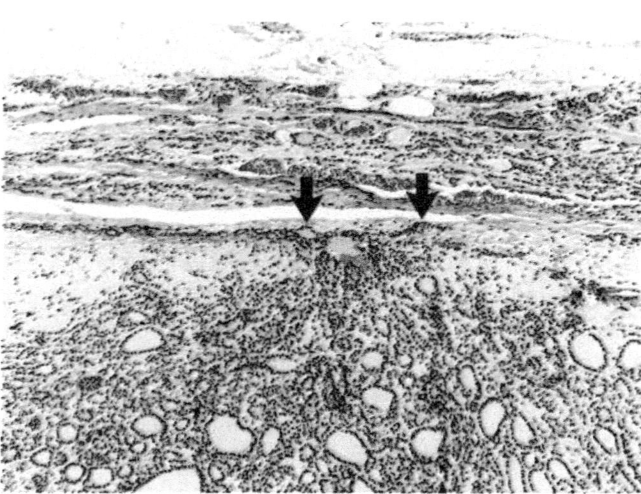

Fig. 72.2 Minimally invasive follicular carcinoma. There is subtle infiltration of the tumor capsule (*arrows*; H&E stain)

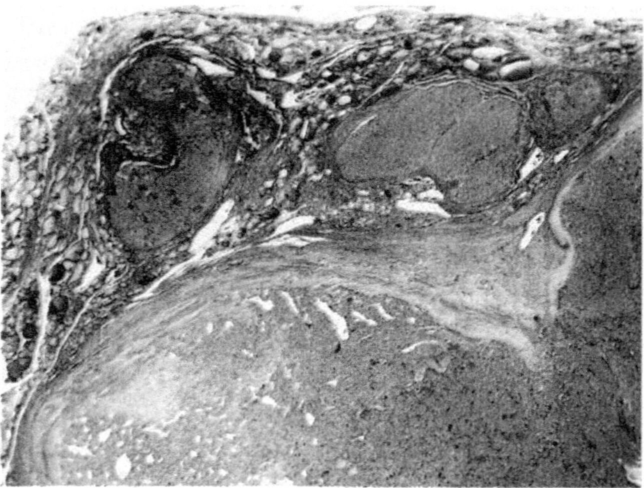

Fig. 72.3 Widely invasive follicular carcinoma. Vessels are distended by the carcinoma (superior part of the field; H&E stain)

mitoses are rare. Scattered large or bizarre nuclei may occur, but they appear in atypical adenomas, as well as in the carcinomas, and their prognostic significance is uncertain [15, 16]. Cytoplasm is lightly eosinophilic or amphophilic but rarely clear. Papillae are usually absent, but if present, they are few, small, and simple [1]. Psammoma bodies are also often nonexistent; when present, they lie in the colloid of the neoplastic follicles [1].

Assessing differentiation by examining routine histological sections can be beneficial, especially when combined with immunohistochemical staining using antithyroglobulin [15, 16]. Patterns within a neoplasm may be uniform or notably heterogeneous. Consequently, biopsies have limited value in determining the degree of differentiation. Well-differentiated follicular carcinomas are composed entirely (or almost entirely) of either empty or colloid-filled follicles [17]. These may vary from microfollicles (easily visualized with the PAS technique, showing the tiny droplets of colloid) to follicles even larger than those of normal thyroid tissue, macrofollicles [1, 18]. Most follicular carcinoma demonstrate a predominant microfollicular and solid growth pattern [18]. Large amounts of immunoreactive thyroglobulin are present in the cells and follicles of many of these tumors. Some investigators report that a predominantly follicular pattern has a more favorable prognosis [4, 7]. Follicular carcinomas with moderately differentiated architecture contain follicular elements of variable size and are mixed with solid islands of cells and/or cords of cells (trabeculae) [19]. Both the solid regions and trabeculae may contain some microfollicles. Considerable thyroglobulin is present in some areas, but it is sparse or absent in others. Some neoplastic cells may be elongated, even spindled, especially in regions where the cells form trabeculae. Such growth patterns should not be confused with poorly differentiated carcinomas due to presence of well-defined architecture, and a lack of both numerous mitotic figures and necrosis.

The term *poorly differentiated follicular carcinoma* is a heterogeneous group of malignant thyroid tumors and includes carcinomas that originate from follicular epithelium (often with evidence of coexistent papillary or follicular carcinoma). The common pathological features of poorly differentiated carcinomas are solid/trabecular/insular growth, large size, frequent extrathyroidal extension, extensive vascular invasion, presence of necrosis, and increased mitotic activity (Figs. 72.4 and 72.5). They may be associated with well-differentiated components, of either follicular or papillary type, and less frequently with anaplastic carcinoma [20, 21]. Rarely, poorly differentiated carcinoma can be seen as encapsulated tumors; in this small subset the survival is better than expected for poorly differentiated thyroid cancer.

Insular carcinoma is a hallmark lesion of poorly differentiated thyroid carcinoma. The term "insular" is used to describe the histologic growth pattern of the lesions, which is

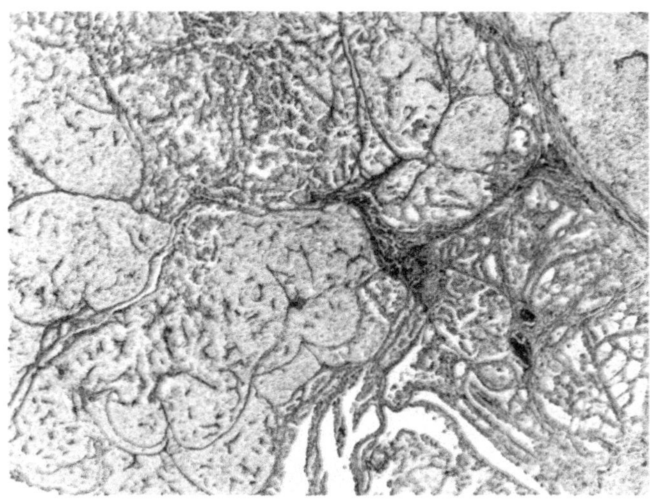

Fig. 72.4 Poorly differentiated carcinoma. Both insular and cribriform patterns are evident (hematoxylin and eosin [H&E] stain)

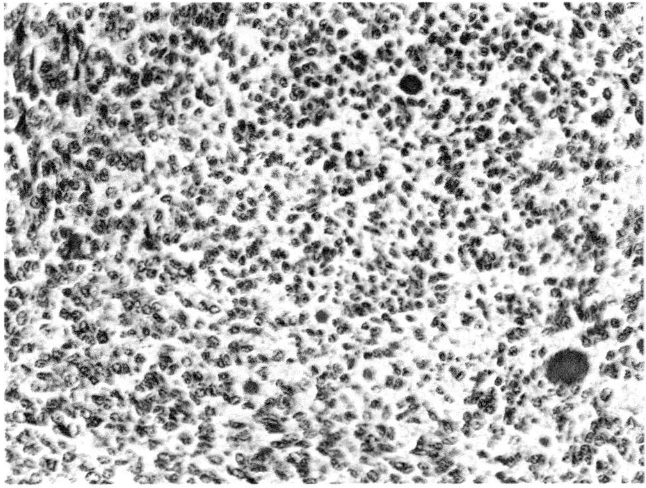

Fig. 72.5 Poorly differentiated carcinoma. The solid part has small- to medium-sized cells. Two small follicles are filled with dense colloid (H&E stain)

characterized by small nests of cells, which have a neuroendocrine growth pattern (carcinoid-like). The lesions are often large, gray white in color, and infiltrative show extensive necrosis, and vascular invasion is frequent. By immunohistochemistry the tumor cells express thyroglobulin and not calcitonin. The Turin proposal suggests that the term "insular" be used to describe a pattern of growth and not a separate diagnostic term for a particular thyroid tumor; it is not uncommon to see partly "insular" growth in an otherwise solid or trabecular poorly differentiated carcinoma [20]. A distinct molecular pathway has been reported in poorly differentiated carcinomas which almost exclusively involve RAS gene alterations [22].

Metastases to cervical lymph nodes are rare [7, 23] and often accompanied by direct extrathyroidal extension of the cancer. The presence of such nodal involvement should provoke a review of the histological features of the resected tissues to exclude follicular variant of papillary thyroid carcinoma [24, 25].

Assessing nuclear ploidy has not provided a reliable means of differentiating follicular adenomas from follicular carcinomas, and the prognostic value is uncertain [26–28]. Argyrophilic staining of nucleolar-organizing regions might be useful to recognize the malignant follicular neoplasms, but thus far, it is only one of various special techniques not yet proven sufficiently to consider its use on a routine basis [29, 30].

Aspirates from these lesions are diagnosed as follicular neoplasms, which include both follicular adenomas and carcinomas [31, 32]. Upon aspiration, these neoplasms bleed easily; therefore, many specimens are diluted by blood and may be interpreted as unsatisfactory. If the physician performing the aspiration is experienced and exceptionally careful, a specimen with adequate tumor cellularity may be obtained.

In the hypocellular smears, the presence of a few microfollicles with inspissated colloid should raise the possibility of a follicular neoplasm. Some follicular cells arranged in rosettes and tubules may also be seen. These cases should not be deemed as non-diagnostic but reported as "follicular lesion of undetermined significance" and repeat FNA can be recommended [32, 33].

The hypercellular smears contain many follicular cells set in rosettes and tubules (Fig. 72.6), microfollicles often with inspissated dark blue colloid (Fig. 72.7) and tissue fragments.

The neoplastic follicular cells are enlarged and have delicate, pale pink, or bluish cytoplasm (a scant-to-moderate amount), with poorly demarcated borders. The nuclei are enlarged, the chromatin varies in density, and it usually has a mottled appearance. The nuclear borders are slightly irregular, and nucleoli may be visible. In some tumors (both benign and malignant), the variation in nuclear size may be marked.

Colloid is usually absent, except for the droplets of inspissated colloid observed in some neoplastic microfollicles.

All follicular carcinomas express thyroglobulin and show a similar cytokeratin profile to normal thyroid parenchyma. HBME1 expression can occur in 90–100 % of follicular carcinomas and not adenomas; however, it is also expressed in adenomatoid nodules and follicular adenomas [34–37]. A specific translocation t (2;3) leads to the expression of PAX8 peroxisome proliferator-activated receptor gamma

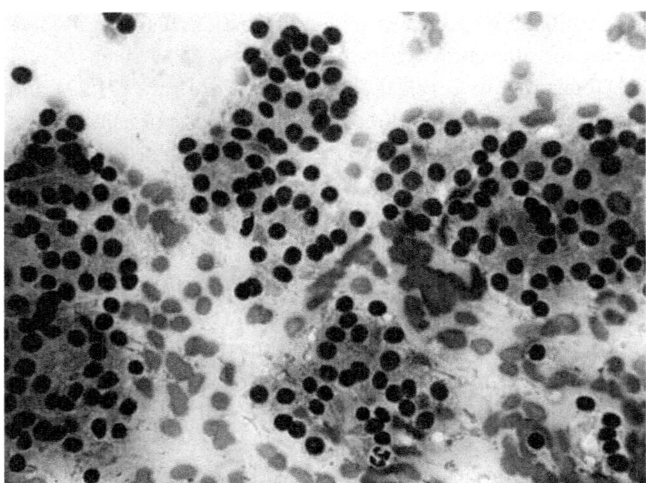

Fig. 72.6 Follicular neoplasm. Hypercellular smear with neoplastic cells arranged predominantly in rosettes. Resected specimen revealed a follicular adenoma (Diff-Quik stain)

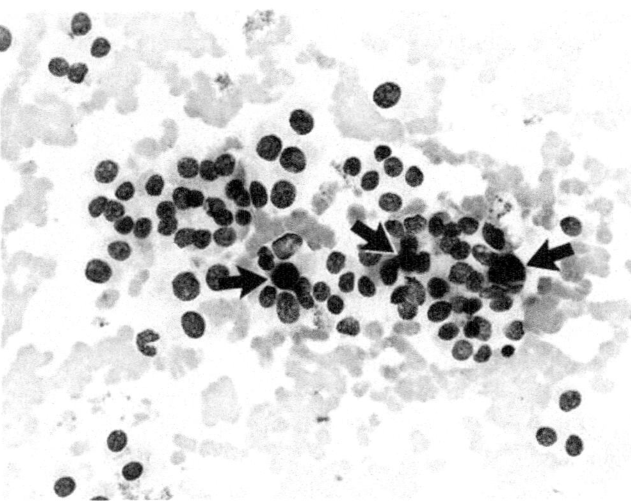

Fig. 72.7 Follicular neoplasm. Aspirate contains rosettes and three follicles with inspissated colloid (*arrows*). Resected specimen revealed a follicular adenoma (Diff-Quik stain)

(PPAR-gamma) chimeric protein. This has been reported in follicular carcinoma and is currently being used in a molecular assay panel for triaging FNA specimens diagnosed as atypia/follicular lesion of undetermined significance and follicular neoplasm [38]. However, PPAR-gamma expression can occur in some cases of follicular adenoma and adenomatoid nodules [39, 40].

Ras mutations are more frequent in follicular carcinoma as compared to follicular adenoma; some authors have found an association between *ras* mutations and clinically aggressive follicular carcinomas [41–43]. Loss of heterozygosity on chromosome 10q and 3p can be seen in follicular carcinoma suggesting a role of tumor suppressor genes in its pathogenesis [44, 45].

Well-Differentiated Follicular "Tumors of Undetermined Malignant Potential"

This designation has been proposed by some experts for follicular-patterned encapsulated tumors that have been controversial and difficult to diagnose due to questionable or minimal nuclear features of papillary thyroid carcinoma or questionable or one focus of capsular invasion that is confined to tumor capsule and does not traverse the entire thickness of capsule and lacks any nuclear features of papillary thyroid carcinoma [46]. This terminology may be extremely helpful to pathologists in the diagnoses of certain follicular-patterned lesions; however, clinicians may find it problematic to establish treatment strategies due to lack of follow-up data [47].

Follicular carcinoma with oxyphilic/oncocytic cells (Askanazy/Hürthle cells) are composed mostly or completely of these distinctive cells. Recognizing the malignant potential of a tumor depends on evidence of aggressive behavior at its periphery [10, 48, 49]. Trabecular patterns are common [48, 50]. Bizarre, large, and/or hyperchromatic nuclei may be striking histological features, but these are more common in the benign proliferations of oxyphilic cells. The proliferative cell nuclear antigen is reported to be present at higher levels in indeterminate and malignant oxyphilic cell neoplasms, compared to oxyphilic cell adenomas [51]. Metastases to cervical lymph nodes are more common than with the usual follicular carcinoma, especially after the patient has undergone surgery to treat the cancer. Some studies suggest that oxyphilic follicular carcinomas are more aggressive than typical non-oxyphilic follicular carcinomas. The presence of non-diploid cells in an oxyphilic carcinoma indicates a poorer prognosis than that with diploid nuclei [52].

The cytological smears show tumor cellularity and often a monotonous cell population. In most cases, the cells are large (but can be small) and have generous amounts of grayish-pink to grayish-blue cytoplasm, large round nuclei, and prominent nucleoli. Binucleation is common. They are arranged in large tissue fragments often with transgressing vessels, small clusters, or as scattered single cells [53, 54]. Frequently, the cellular borders are well demarcated (Fig. 72.8). The neoplastic follicles are common but appear empty (Fig. 72.9). Some follicles with inspissated blue colloid may be seen.

Oncocytic follicular tumors of the thyroid are biologically different than other follicular-derived tumors. H*ras* mutations are more frequent in Hürthle cell carcinoma than

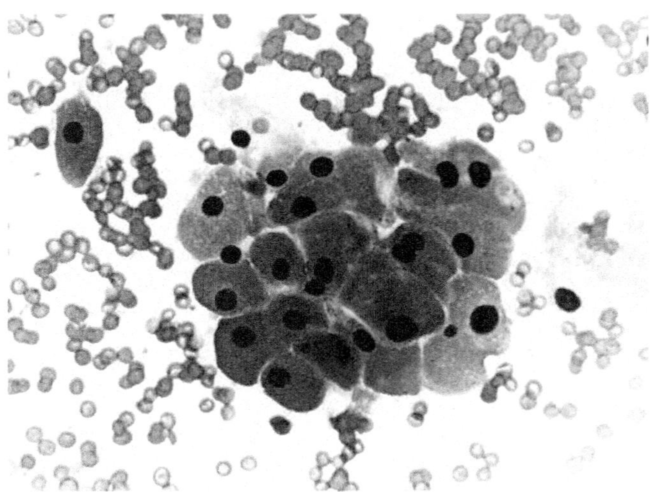

Fig. 72.8 Follicular neoplasm with oncocytic/oxyphilic cells. Smear shows neoplastic cells with abundant dense cytoplasm and well-demarcated borders (Diff-Quik stain)

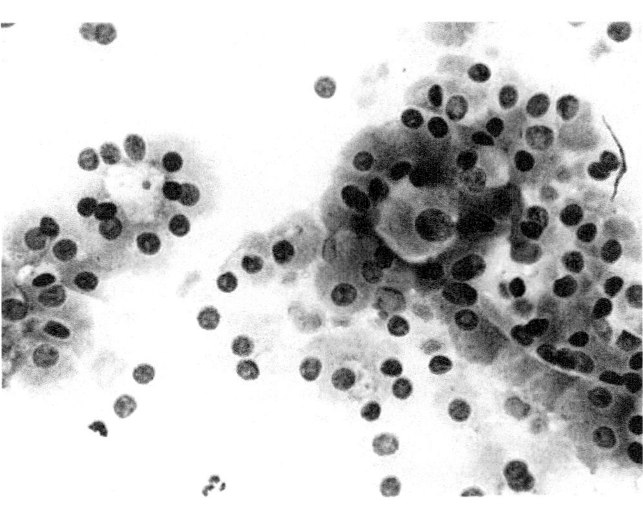

Fig. 72.9 Follicular neoplasm with oncocytic/oxyphilic cells. Smear shows large neoplastic cells with abundant cytoplasm and conspicuous nucleoli. Three empty follicles are visible in the superior half of the field (Diff-Quik stain)

follicular carcinoma [55, 56] and are marked by a high percentage of allelic alterations as compared to other follicular-derived tumors. A study by Maximo et al. showed that Hürthle cell tumors display a relatively higher percentage of common deletions of mitochondrial DNA as compared to other follicular-derived tumors. In addition, Hürthle cell tumors also showed germline polymorphisms of ATPase 6 gene, which is required for the maintenance of mitochondrial DNA [57].

References

1. Franssila KO, Ackerman LV, Brown CL, Hedinger CE. Follicular carcinoma. Semin Diagn Pathol. 1985;2:101–22.
2. Baloch ZW, Livolsi VA. Follicular-patterned lesions of the thyroid: the bane of the pathologist. Am J Clin Pathol. 2002;117:143–50.
3. D'Avanzo A, Ituarte P, Treseler P, Kebebew E, Wu J, Wong M, Duh QY, Siperstein AE, Clark OH. Prognostic scoring systems in patients with follicular thyroid cancer: a comparison of different staging systems in predicting the patient outcome. Thyroid. 2004; 14:453–8.
4. D'Avanzo A, Treseler P, Ituarte PH, Wong M, Streja L, Greenspan FS, Siperstein AE, Duh QY, Clark OH. Follicular thyroid carcinoma: histology and prognosis. Cancer. 2004;100:1123–9.
5. Franc B, de la Salmoniere P, Lange F, Hoang C, Louvel A, de Roquancourt A, Vilde F, Hejblum G, Chevret S, Chastang C. Interobserver and intraobserver reproducibility in the histopathology of follicular thyroid carcinoma. Hum Pathol. 2003;34:1092–100.
6. Shaha AR, Loree TR, Shah JP. Prognostic factors and risk group analysis in follicular carcinoma of the thyroid. Surgery. 1995; 118:1131–6. discussion 1136–1138.
7. Thompson LD, Wieneke JA, Paal E, Frommelt RA, Adair CF, Heffess CS. A clinicopathologic study of minimally invasive follicular carcinoma of the thyroid gland with a review of the English literature. Cancer. 2001;91:505–24.
8. Rosai J, Carcangui ML, DeLellis RA. Tumors of the thyroid gland. Washington, DC: Armed Forces Institute of Pathology; 1992.
9. Baloch ZW, LiVolsi VA. Our approach to follicular-patterned lesions of the thyroid. J Clin Pathol. 2007;60:244–50.
10. Baloch ZW, LiVolsi VA. Oncocytic lesions of the neuroendocrine system. Semin Diagn Pathol. 1999;16:190–9.
11. Evans HL. Follicular neoplasms of the thyroid. A study of 44 cases followed for a minimum of 10 years with emphasis on differential diagnosis. Cancer. 1984;54:535–40.
12. Yamashina M. Follicular neoplasms of the thyroid. Total circumferential evaluation of the fibrous capsule. Am J Surg Pathol. 1992; 16:392–400.
13. Sobrinho-Simoes M, Eloy C, Magalhaes J, Lobo C, Amaro T. Follicular thyroid carcinoma. Mod Pathol. 2011;24 Suppl 2:S10–8.
14. van Heerden JA, Hay ID, Goellner JR, et al. Follicular thyroid carcinoma with capsular invasion alone: a nonthreatening malignancy. Surgery. 1992;112:1130–8.
15. Hazard JB, Kenyon R. Atypical adenoma of the thyroid. Arch Pathol. 1954;58:554–63.
16. Jorda M, Gonzalez-Campora R, Mora J, Herrero-Zapatero A, Otal C, Galera H. Prognostic factors in follicular carcinoma of the thyroid. Arch Pathol Lab Med. 1993;117:631–5.
17. Harach HR, Franssila KO. Thyroglobulin immunostaining in follicular thyroid carcinoma. Histopathology. 1988;13:43–54.
18. Baloch Z, LiVolsi VA. Pathology of the thyroid gland. Philadelphia: Churchill Livingstone; 2002.
19. Akslen LA, LiVolsi VA. Poorly differentiated thyroid carcinoma – it is important. Am J Surg Pathol. 2000;24:310–3.
20. Volante M, Collini P, Nikiforov YE, Sakamoto A, Kakudo K, Katoh R, Lloyd RV, LiVolsi VA, Papotti M, Sobrinho-Simoes M, Bussolati G, Rosai J. Poorly differentiated thyroid carcinoma: the Turin proposal for the use of uniform diagnostic criteria and an algorithmic diagnostic approach. Am J Surg Pathol. 2007;31:1256–64.
21. Rivera M, Ricarte-Filho J, Tuttle RM, Ganly I, Shaha A, Knauf J, Fagin J, Ghossein R. Molecular, morphologic, and outcome analysis of thyroid carcinomas according to degree of extrathyroid extension. Thyroid. 2010;20:1085–93.

22. Nikiforov YE, Erickson LA, Nikiforova MN, Caudill CM, Lloyd RV. Solid variant of papillary thyroid carcinoma: incidence, clinical- pathologic characteristics, molecular analysis, and biologic behavior. Am J Surg Pathol. 2001;25:1478–84.
23. Schroder S, Pfannschmidt N, Dralle H, Arps H, Bocker W. The encapsulated follicular carcinoma of the thyroid. A clinicopathologic study of 35 cases. Virchows Arch A Pathol Anat Histopathol. 1984;402:259–73.
24. Baloch Z, LiVolsi VA, Henricks WH, Sebak BA. Encapsulated follicular variant of papillary thyroid carcinoma. Am J Clin Pathol. 2002;118:603–5. discussion 605–606.
25. Baloch Z, LiVolsi VA. Diagnostic dilemmas in thyroid pathology: follicular variant of papillary thyroid carcinoma and classic papillary thyroid carcinoma arising in lymphocytic thyroiditis. Pathol Case Rev. 2003;8:47–56.
26. Harlow SP, Duda RB, Bauer KD. Diagnostic utility of DNA content flow cytometry in follicular neoplasms of the thyroid. J Surg Oncol. 1992;50:1–6.
27. Castro P, Eknaes M, Teixeira MR, Danielsen HE, Soares P, Lothe RA, Sobrinho-Simoes M. Adenomas and follicular carcinomas of the thyroid display two major patterns of chromosomal changes. J Pathol. 2005;206:305–11.
28. Joensuu H, Klemi P, Eerola E. DNA aneuploidy in follicular adenomas of the thyroid gland. Am J Pathol. 1987;124:373–6.
29. Shechtman L, Koren R, Horowitz A, Shechtman I, Halpern M, Gal R. Diagnostic value of AgNOR staining in thyroid cytology. Anal Quant Cytol Histol. 1998;20:187–91.
30. Camargo RS, Shirata NK, di Loreto C, Garcia EA, Castelo A, Longatto Filho A. Significance of AgNOR measurement in thyroid lesions. Anal Quant Cytol Histol. 2006;28:188–92.
31. Baloch ZW, Fleisher S, LiVolsi VA, Gupta PK. Diagnosis of "follicular neoplasm": a gray zone in thyroid fine-needle aspiration cytology. Diagn Cytopathol. 2002;26:41–4.
32. Faquin WC, Baloch ZW. Fine-needle aspiration of follicular patterned lesions of the thyroid: diagnosis, management, and follow-up according to National Cancer Institute (NCI) recommendations. Diagn Cytopathol. 2010;38:731–9.
33. Deveci MS, Deveci G, LiVolsi VA, Baloch ZW. Fine-needle aspiration of follicular lesions of the thyroid. Diagnosis and follow-up. Cytojournal. 2006;3:9.
34. Miettinen M, Karkkainen P. Differential reactivity of HBME-1 and CD15 antibodies in benign and malignant thyroid tumours. Preferential reactivity with malignant tumours. Virchows Arch. 1996;429:213–9.
35. van Hoeven KH, Kovatich AJ, Miettinen M. Immunocytochemical evaluation of HBME-1, CA 19-9, and CD-15 (Leu-M1) in fine-needle aspirates of thyroid nodules. Diagn Cytopathol. 1998; 18:93–7.
36. Papotti M, Rodriguez J, Pompa RD, Bartolazzi A, Rosai J. Galectin-3 and HBME-1 expression in well-differentiated thyroid tumors with follicular architecture of uncertain malignant potential. Modern Pathology. 2005;18:541–546.
37. Rosai J. Immunohistochemical markers of thyroid tumors: significance and diagnostic applications. Tumori. 2003;89:517–9.
38. Kroll TG, Sarraf P, Pecciarini L, Chen CJ, Mueller E, Spiegelman BM, Fletcher JA. PAX8-PPAR[gamma] 1 fusion in oncogene human thyroid carcinoma. Science. 2000;289:1357–60.
39. Marques AR, Espadinha C, Catarino AL, Moniz S, Pereira T, Sobrinho LG, Leite V. Expression of PAX8-PPAR gamma 1 rearrangements in both follicular thyroid carcinomas and adenomas. J Clin Endocrinol Metab. 2002;87:3947–52.
40. Gustafson KS, LiVolsi VA, Furth EE, Pasha TL, Putt ME, Baloch ZW. Peroxisome proliferator-activated receptor gamma expression in follicular-patterned thyroid lesions. Caveats for the use of immunohistochemical studies. Am J Clin Pathol. 2003;120:175–81.
41. Esapa CT, Johnson SJ, Kendall-Taylor P, Lennard TW, Harris PE. Prevalence of Ras mutations in thyroid neoplasia. Clin Endocrinol. 1999;50:529–35.
42. Basolo F, Pisaturo F, Pollina LE, Fontanini G, Elisei R, Molinaro E, Iacconi P, Miccoli P, Pacini F. N-ras mutation in poorly differentiated thyroid carcinomas: correlation with bone metastases and inverse correlation to thyroglobulin expression. Thyroid. 2000; 10:19–23.
43. Capella G, Matias-Guiu X, Ampudia X, de Leiva A, Perucho M, Prat J. Ras oncogene mutations in thyroid tumors: polymerase chain reaction- restriction-fragment-length polymorphism analysis from paraffin- embedded tissues. Diagn Mol Pathol. 1996; 5:45–52.
44. Grebe SK, McIver B, Hay ID, Wu PS, Maciel LM, Drabkin HA, Goellner JR, Grant CS, Jenkins RB, Eberhardt NL. Frequent loss of heterozygosity on chromosomes 3p and 17p without VHL or p53 mutations suggests involvement of unidentified tumor suppressor genes in follicular thyroid carcinoma. J Clin Endocrinol Metab. 1997;82:3684–91.
45. Matsuo K, Tang SH, Fagin JA. Allelotype of human thyroid tumors: loss of chromosome 11q13 sequences in follicular neoplasms. Mol Endocrinol. 1991;5:1873–9.
46. Williams ED, Abrosimov A, Bogdanova TI, Rosai J, Sidorov Y, Thomas GA. Two proposals regarding the terminology of thyroid tumors. Guest editorial. Int J Surg Pathol. 2000;8:181–3.
47. LiVolsi VA, Baloch ZW. Follicular neoplasms of the thyroid: view, biases, and experiences. Adv Anat Pathol. 2004;11:279–87.
48. Asa SL. My approach to oncocytic tumours of the thyroid. J Clin Pathol. 2004;57:225–32.
49. Montone KT, Baloch ZW, LiVolsi VA. The thyroid Hurthle (oncocytic) cell and its associated pathologic conditions: a surgical pathology and cytopathology review. Arch Pathol Lab Med. 2008;132:1241–50.
50. Carcangiu ML, Bianchi S, Savino D, Voynick IM, Rosai J. Follicular Hurthle cell tumors of the thyroid gland. Cancer. 1991;68: 1944–53.
51. Vasko V, Garcia S, Henry JF, De Micco C. Expression of proliferating cell nuclear antigen in follicular thyroid tumors: correlation with clinicopathological findings. Oncol Rep. 1999;6:359–64.
52. Bronner MP, Clevenger CV, Edmonds PR, Lowell DM, McFarland MM, LiVolsi VA. Flow cytometric analysis of DNA content in Hurthle cell adenomas and carcinomas of the thyroid. Am J Clin Pathol. 1988;89:764–9.
53. Giorgadze T, Rossi ED, Fadda G, Gupta PK, Livolsi VA, Baloch Z. Does the fine-needle aspiration diagnosis of "Hurthle-cell neoplasm/follicular neoplasm with oncocytic features" denote increased risk of malignancy? Diagn Cytopathol. 2004;31:307–12.
54. Yang YJ, Khurana KK. Diagnostic utility of intracytoplasmic lumen and transgressing vessels in evaluation of Hurthle cell lesions by fine-needle aspiration. Arch Pathol Lab Med. 2001;125:1031–5.
55. Schark C, Fulton N, Yashiro T, Stanislav G, Jacoby R, Straus 2nd FH, Dytch H, Bibbo M, Kaplan EL. The value of measurement of ras oncogenes and nuclear DNA analysis in the diagnosis of Hurthle cell tumors of the thyroid. World J Surg. 1992;16:745–51. discussion 752.
56. Bouras M, Bertholon J, Dutrieux-Berger N, Parvaz P, Paulin C, Revol A. Variability of Ha-ras (codon 12) proto-oncogene mutations in diverse thyroid cancers. Eur J Endocrinol. 1998;139: 209–16.
57. Maximo V, Soares P, Lima J, Cameselle-Teijeiro J, Sobrinho-Simoes M. Mitochondrial DNA somatic mutations (point mutations and large deletions) and mitochondrial DNA variants in human thyroid pathology: a study with emphasis on Hurthle cell tumors. Am J Pathol. 2002;160:1857–65.

Hürthle Cell Carcinoma

73

Kenneth D. Burman and Leonard Wartofsky

Introduction

The Hürthle cell variant of follicular carcinoma is composed of large acidophilic, Askanazy, or oncocytic cells that are considered altered follicular cells [1–10]. For instance, Hürthle cells bind thyrotropin (TSH) and have TSH receptors, like other types of follicular thyroid cells [11, 12]. Similar to other follicular neoplasms, Hürthle cell carcinoma is more common in women than men, but the patients tend to be older than those with typical follicular thyroid carcinoma (FTC; see Chap. 70). Hürthle cells contain many mitochondria (which are the basis for the abundant, eosinophilic, and granular cytoplasm), frequently eccentric nuclei, and visible nucleoli. The Hürthle cell carcinoma variant of follicular carcinoma discussed here is to be distinguished from the variant of papillary thyroid cancer, "Hürthle cell papillary thyroid carcinoma," which also contains an abundance of oxyphilic cells [13]. The central genetic or environmental factors that allow a thyrocyte to differentiate into a Hürthle cell are unknown, and Hürthle cells may occur in a variety of thyroid disorders. Solitary thyroid nodules may have a predominance of Hürthle cells, to the exclusion of more typical thyrocytes, and these lesions are often highly cellular with minimal colloid. When such a lesion is aspirated for cytologic examination, the interpretation would likely be "suggestive of a Hürthle cell neoplasm," because as with follicular tumors, a definite diagnosis of benign or malignant would be difficult or impossible to make. Hürthle cell neoplasms may be benign or malignant, and the distinction is based on the demonstration of vascular or capsular invasion, metastatic capacity, and growth rate, similarly to other follicular neoplasms [7, 14, 15].

When patients with Hürthle cell carcinoma are stratified regarding low vs high risk, there does not appear to be a significantly worse prognosis than that for follicular carcinoma; see Chaps. 70 and 79 [16, 17]. In contrast to other follicular carcinomas, they have a higher rate of bilaterality or multi-centricity.

With the use of fine-needle aspiration (FNA) cytology, some solitary thyroid nodules may also have a more varied appearance, where Hürthle cells intermingle with thyrocytes, macrophages, and lymphocytes and have moderate amounts of colloid. In such circumstances, the cytology may be more difficult to interpret, and when insufficient Hürthle cells are present, the tumor is characterized as a Hürthle cell neoplasm. Furthermore, Hürthle cells may be found in the thyroid glands of patients with Hashimoto's thyroiditis and other benign thyroid disorders but usually in this circumstance, the Hürthle cells are scattered and are not the predominant cell type [7, 18]. In one study, age greater than 65 years and an elevated preoperative serum thyroglobulin level aided in the prediction of a follicular neoplasm being malignant [8].

The typical Hürthle cell neoplasm is composed mostly of these distinctive cells and is generally considered to be a variant of follicular carcinoma. Recognizing the malignant potential of a tumor depends on the evidence of aggressive behavior at its periphery [19–23]. Bizarre, large, and/or hyperchromatic nuclei may be a striking histological feature, and these are more common than in benign proliferations of oxyphilic cells.

Metastases to cervical lymph nodes are more frequent than with the usual follicular carcinoma, especially after the patient has undergone surgery. Notwithstanding the comments above, there are some studies that suggest oxyphilic

K.D. Burman, MD (✉)
Director, Divisions of Endocrinology, Washington Hospital Center and Georgetown University Hospital, 110 Irving Street, N.W. 2A-72, Washington, DC 20010, USA
e-mail: kenneth.d.burman@medstar.net

L. Wartofsky, MD, MACP
Department of Medicine, MedStar Washington Hospital Center, Georgetown University School of Medicine, 110 Irving Street, N.W., Washington, DC 20010-2975, USA
e-mail: leonard.wartofsky@medstar.net

L. Wartofsky, D. Van Nostrand (eds.), *Thyroid Cancer*, DOI 10.1007/978-1-4939-3314-3_73

follicular carcinomas are more aggressive than typical nonoxyphilic follicular carcinomas. Particularly, the presence of nondiploid cells in an oxyphilic carcinoma indicates a poorer prognosis than that with diploid nuclei [24]. Papillary carcinomas may also contain significant populations of these cells [13]. Whether they are more aggressive than a nonoxyphilic cancer with otherwise similar characteristics remains uncertain.

However, what does appear clear is that without specific attention to risk stratification, Hürthle cell malignancies will tend to have a worse prognosis than other follicular tumors in many [24–26], but not all, studies [27]. This may be partly because of their greater tendency to be locally invasive and propensity to concentrate radioiodine less avidly, thereby rendering them more difficult to manage with isotopic scanning and therapy [28, 29]. Yet, this is not universal, and some Hürthle cell cancers will trap iodine [30]). In a review of 89 cases of Hürthle cell carcinoma seen at the MD Anderson Cancer Center, Lopez-Penabad et al. [31] expressed a rather pessimistic assessment of the efficacy of currently available therapies for this variant of FTC. There was a 40 % cause-specific mortality over their long follow-up interval, with no improvement in mortality rates found over the past 50 years. Larger tumor size and more advanced age were negative prognostic indicators. Additionally, in the setting of metastatic disease, there was no further survival advantage seen with more extensive surgery, external radiation therapy, chemotherapy, or even radioactive iodine therapy. Mills et al. noted that the stage of disease, the existence of metastatic lesions, and the presence of cervical lymph node disease affected outcome in patients with Hürthle cell carcinoma [32].

Clinical Presentation

Hürthle cell carcinomas may represent about 3–5 % of all types of thyroid carcinomas. Most Hürthle cell carcinomas appear to be a more aggressive kind of follicular carcinoma, with more frequent recurrences, higher morbidity, and higher mortality [7, 14, 18, 24, 26, 31]. The tumors are frequently multifocal and bilateral.

Thompson and associates [14, 19, 20] suggested that it is difficult to differentiate benign from malignant Hürthle cell tumors. The implication of their studies is that even experienced pathologists may not be able to make a reliable distinction. Carcangiu and coworkers [33] and Grant and associates [22] support the concept that strict histological criteria and adequate sampling may be able to differentiate Hürthle cell carcinoma from adenoma in nearly all cases. Grant et al. [22] reviewed the world literature and observed that only 6 of 642 patients with apparent benign Hürthle cell adenomas were found to have a recurrence, thereby indicating that the tumor was a carcinoma, with an incidence of less than 1 %. Gosain and Clark [23] found no patients with Hürthle cell adenoma in whom recurrences were observed. Similarly, Bondeson and coworkers [24] studied 42 patients diagnosed with Hürthle cell adenoma over a 2–20-year period and found no recurrences.

The above reports help to support the contention that Hürthle cell adenomas can be accurately diagnosed and distinguished from carcinoma on histological examination by experienced pathologists. As with other follicular carcinomas, the major histological criteria that separate a Hürthle cell adenoma from a carcinoma are vascular and/or capsular invasion. However, subtleties do remain. For example, does the capsular invasion have to be completely through the capsule, or is invasion into, but not through, the capsule enough to make the diagnosis? It is also important to ensure that sufficient histologic sections were taken and examined. Notwithstanding these concerns, it is likely that experienced pathologists can reliably make this differential diagnosis.

The absence of radioiodine uptake by residual or metastatic follicular cancer renders management much more difficult, but not impossible. Typically, these tumors are less avid for radioactive iodine and therefore respond less often than the usual follicular carcinoma. Several groups are currently evaluating the thyroidal sodium iodide symporter (Na^+/I^- symporter function and expression in Hürthle cell carcinomas relative to FTC [11, 12, 18]. These studies are exploring methods for the management of follicular cancers that have lost their ability to either trap iodide (and be treatable with radioiodine) or to synthesize and release thyroglobulin. The ability of both normal and malignant thyroid cells to concentrate iodide is dependent on expression of the *NIS* gene [34–36]. The loss of this gene during tumor dedifferentiation can account for the tumor's failure to concentrate iodide. Gene therapy or redifferentiation therapy with retinoic acid, depsipeptide, and other agents had been thought to hold promise for the restoration of both radioiodine uptake for potential treatment and thyroglobulin production for monitoring recurrence [37–41]. However, further analysis of results with retinoic acid was less than optimistic [42].

It is reasonable to assume that one major reason why these tumors do not respond as well to therapy is because they do not concentrate radioiodine as well as usual follicular carcinomas. It may be appropriate to approach Hürthle cell carcinomas as if they were medullary carcinomas, i.e., with more aggressive diagnostic procedures and treatment [23, 43].

In most clinical circumstances, patients diagnosed with a Hürthle cell neoplasm by FNA should undergo surgery somewhat promptly. We recommend a near-total to total thyroidectomy by an experienced thyroid surgeon. It is important to discuss with the patient the alternative approaches of a near-total thyroidectomy compared to a lobectomy with isthmusectomy [44]. If only a lobectomy and isthmusectomy are performed, and if the lesion is found to be cancerous, then a subsequent completion thyroidectomy must be performed. This completion thyroidectomy frequently causes mental and psychosocial distress to the patient, especially if the requirement for this procedure is not expected by the patient. However, only about 20 % of Hürthle cell neoplasms diagnosed by FNA are found to be malignant. If a total thyroidectomy is conducted initially, then in 80 % of cases, this procedure would be unnecessarily aggressive and exposes the patient to a higher risk of temporary and permanent hypocalcemia, along with recurrent laryngeal nerve paralysis.

The decision regarding which operation is needed for a patient with a solitary thyroid nodule and an FNA consistent with Hürthle cell neoplasm is difficult. A frozen-section interpretation is often problematic and therefore not helpful [45]. It is important to candidly discuss the advantages and disadvantages of each approach with the patient and family and arrive at a mutual decision. The initial operation should include an ipsilateral central node dissection. Obviously, the surgeon must be allowed to exercise judgment at the time of surgery about the precise operative procedures. It has been suggested [11] that a routine modified radical neck dissection be performed when the tumor is found in the central compartment or cervical nodes or, alternatively, a total thyroidectomy [44].

Because these tumors are somewhat less differentiated than most papillary thyroid cancers and FTCs, there is a reasonable chance that they can be detected by 18-fluorodeoxyglucose positron emission tomography (FDG-PET) when they do not concentrate radioiodine. Lowe et al. [46] found PET scanning to be useful to identify both local and metastatic disease, thereby facilitating disease management. Growth of Hürthle cell tumors has been described to reflect the net of proliferative vs apoptotic indices, and it may become feasible to exploit these characteristics to distinguish benign from malignant lesions [47].

McDonald and coworkers [48] reviewed 40 cases of Hürthle cell carcinoma, noting that this number represented 4 % of all thyroid cancers in their experience. Their median follow-up interval after thyroidectomy was 8.5 years. Vascular or capsular invasion was observed in 32 patients, extrathyroidal invasion in 11, and regional lymph node involvement in 2. One patient had distant metastases at presentation, and only nine patients received ^{131}I. Of 34 subjects analyzed, 5 died of thyroid cancer, 9 died of nonthyroidal causes, 4 were alive with existing disease, and 16 were alive without evidence of disease. At about an average of 4 years, nine patients had recurrences and five had distant disease. Recurrent disease was associated with mortality in half of these patients. Risk factors assessed at initial presentation were useful to help predict recurrence. Low-risk tumors did not recur (e.g., tumors less than 5-cm diameter, lack of distant metastases, men younger than 41 year, and women younger than 51 year). Tumor size and the presence of distant metastases were more important prognostic indicators than age in one recent series of patients [49].

Bhattacharyya [50] performed a retrospective review of the Surveillance, Epidemiology, and End Results (SEER) database for cases between 1973 and 1998, finding that 3 % of cases represented Hürthle cell carcinoma, and 555 of the patients (377 women, 178 men) were analyzed. Outcomes in 411 were compared to outcomes in 411 matched patients with follicular carcinoma; 5- and 10-year mortality rates were 15 % and 29 % vs 11 % and 45 %, respectively. The survival time was also not different, with an average of 109 months for Hürthle cell carcinoma and 113 months for follicular cancer. For the patients with Hürthle cell carcinoma, increased mortality was associated with larger tumor size and male gender, but not the presence of local invasion. In a small patient series, Lopez-Penabad et al. [31] observed the worst prognosis in older patients with larger tumors and local extension. Similar findings were reported by Kushchayeva et al. in a series of 33 patients [51].

Because some Hürthle cell carcinomas were found to have *ret/PTC* gene rearrangements similar to papillary thyroid cancers [52], as well as a propensity to spread to local lymph nodes like papillary cancers, it may be that there can be subspecies of what we have presumed to be classic Hürthle cell carcinoma that represent variants of either follicular or papillary thyroid cancer [13]. Such differences might account for our difficulty in comparing individual reports in the literature with mortality and morbidity rates, of which some but not all support the view that Hürthle cell carcinoma is linked with a poorer prognosis than the usual FTC or papillary thyroid cancer.

Following appropriate surgery for Hürthle cell carcinoma, radioiodine scanning and therapy is recommended. Scan preparation would be routine and is usually performed about 6 weeks after surgery. Preparation by the use of levothyroxine withdrawal or stimulation by the use of rhTSH can be utilized. A diagnostic radioiodine scan is important before therapy to help determine the avidity of the remaining thyroid cells for radioiodine and to define the nature and extent of remaining thyroid tissue or disease. Assuming that there is visible uptake, the diagnostic scan is then followed by radioiodine therapy, usually with 100–150 mCi ^{131}I. A post-treatment scan is performed approx 7–10 day after treatment. (These protocols are detailed in Chaps. 11, 19, 33 and 34) rhTSH stimulation is not presently approved by the FDA for use in patients with metastatic thyroid cancer, although two recent studies have suggested it may be as effective as levothyroxine withdrawal [53, 54].

As described above, many Hürthle cell cancers will not trap radioiodine, and sometimes only as little as 10 % of Hürthle cell cancers will trap and respond to radioiodine. This number seems low in our experience and, of course, somewhat depends on the dose of ^{131}I used for scanning, the length of time that the patient did not receive thyroid hormone, the extent of TSH elevation, and possibly the assiduous adherence to a low-iodine diet. Based on published reports, it may be difficult to adequately assess these factors. Perhaps in some cases, lack of apparent iodine avidity by the tumor may not be an accurate representation of the tumor's true properties.

For surveillance over the subsequent 5 years after initial surgery and ablation, we recommend following the patient with physical examinations, thyroid function tests, and thyroglobulin monitoring about every 3–6 months for the first several years, and possibly every 4–6 months for the next several years if there has been no evidence of disease recurrence. Our approach of utilizing radioiodine scans is consistent with that of Besic et al. [30]. In the initial year or two of surveillance, levothyroxine therapy is used in a dosage designed to achieve suppressed TSH in most patients (0.1 μU/mL or lower), depending on the clinical context. Thyroglobulin levels are analyzed at the same time as thyroid function tests, and the thyroglobulin level during L-thyroxine suppression must be less than 2 ng/mL (according to the assay). rhTSH stimulation testing may be employed as outlined by a consensus group of thyroid cancer investigators [55] The latter follow-up would generally include a repeat whole-body ^{131}I scan in 1 year, then again 3–5 years later. Given the aggressive nature of this tumor, we may also obtain occasional radiographs of the chest. An imaging study of the neck, such as a magnetic resonance image or sonogram, is routinely performed, especially if the tumor is not iodine-avid, if the thyroglobulin level is increasing, or if palpable cervical abnormalities become manifest. In women, particularly those who are postmenopausal, suppressive doses of levothyroxine therapy should be accompanied by measures to prevent osteoporosis (daily oral ingestion of 1–1.5 g of calcium, 400 U of vitamin D, exercise against gravity, and the possible addition of a bisphosphonate as appropriate.

Other scanning agents may have reasonably good utility for the detection of Hürthle cell carcinoma. In a study comparing radioiodine and thallium scanning to that with ^{99m}Tc-MIBI, Yen et al. [56] reported a 100 % specificity and an 82 % sensitivity for ^{99m}Tc-MIBI in patients with Hürthle cell carcinoma. The utility of FDG-PET scanning has already been mentioned [46] and was also reported earlier [57] to have an 80 % specificity and a 92 % sensitivity for this tumor. The issue of which scanning agent to employ arises when serum thyroglobulin levels indicate residual or recurrent disease. Despite the proven value of PET scanning, because of its cost and lack of widespread availability, we believe that radioiodine scanning should be attempted first, followed by ^{99m}Tc-MIBI, before utilizing FDG-PET.

Hürthle cell cancer is discussed further in Chaps. 55, 56, and 57. These and other follicular cancers that do not concentrate radioiodine may be treated with chemotherapy (see Chaps. 64 and 99), external radiation therapy [58–61]; see Chaps. 63, 78, 88 and 101, or redifferentiation therapy with retinoic acid or other agents could be attempted [37–39, 62]. However, although external radiation therapy may cause apparent tumor regression and provide palliation and reduced recurrence rate, even in Hürthle cell carcinoma [63], the effect may be transitory with little improvement in survival rate [64].

Recent advances in molecular analysis of thyroid FNA samples and thyroid histopathology samples hold promise of improved ability to predict the presence of thyroid cancer as well as its potential aggressiveness [3, 65–67].

References

1. Mete O, Asa SL. Oncocytes, oxyphils, Hurthle, and Askanazy cells: morphological and molecular features of oncocytic thyroid nodules. Endocr Pathol. 2010;21(1):16–24.
2. Parameswaran R, Brooks S, Sadler GP. Molecular pathogenesis of follicular cell derived thyroid cancers. Int J Surg. 2010;8(3): 186–93.
3. Vriens MR, et al. MicroRNA expression profiling is a potential diagnostic tool for thyroid cancer. Cancer. 2012;118:3426–3432.
4. Umbricht CB, et al. Telomerase activity: a marker to distinguish follicular thyroid adenoma from carcinoma. Cancer Res. 1997; 57(11):2144–7.
5. Cochand-Priollet B, et al. The Bethesda terminology for reporting thyroid cytopathology: from theory to practice in Europe. Acta Cytol. 2011;55(6):507–11.
6. Watson RG, et al. Invasive Hurthle cell carcinoma of the thyroid: natural history and management. Mayo Clin Proc. 1984;59(12): 851–5.
7. Haugen BR, Alexander EK, Bible KC, Doherty GM, Mandel SJ, Nikiforov Y, Pacini F, Randolph G, Sawka A, Shepard D, Sosa J, Tuttle RM, Wartofsky L. 2015 American Thyroid Association Management Guidelines for adult patients with thyroid nodules and differentiated thyroid cancer. Available online at Thyroid 25: DOI:10.1089/ thy.2015.0020; print version in Thyroid 26:1–133, 2016.
8. Strazisar B, et al. Predictive factors of carcinoma in 279 patients with Hurthle cell neoplasm of the thyroid gland. J Surg Oncol. 2010;101(7):582–6.
9. Guerrero MA, et al. Age and tumor size predicts lymph node involvement in Hurthle cell carcinoma. J Cancer. 2010;1:23–6.
10. Troncone G, et al. Accumulation of p27(kip1) is associated with cyclin D3 overexpression in the oxyphilic (Hurthle cell) variant of follicular thyroid carcinoma. J Clin Pathol. 2007;60(4):377–81.
11. Soh EY, Clark OH. Surgical considerations and approach to thyroid cancer. Endocrinol Metab Clin North Am. 1996;25(1):115–39.
12. Cooper DS, Schneyer CR. Follicular and Hurthle cell carcinoma of the thyroid. Endocrinol Metab Clin North Am. 1990;19(3): 577–91.
13. Beckner ME, Heffess CS, Oertel JE. Oxyphilic papillary thyroid carcinomas. Am J Clin Pathol. 1995;103(3):280–7.
14. Gundry SR, et al. Total thyroidectomy for Hurthle cell neoplasm of the thyroid. Arch Surg. 1983;118(5):529–32.
15. Cannon J. The significance of hurthle cells in thyroid disease. Oncologist. 2011;16(10):1380–7.
16. Kutun S, et al. The predicting factors for clinical outcomes in patients with Hurthle cell carcinoma: how we do it. Clin Otolaryngol. 2011;36(1):73–7.
17. Kushchayeva Y, et al. Comparison of clinical characteristics at diagnosis and during follow-up in 118 patients with Hurthle cell or follicular thyroid cancer. Am J Surg. 2008;195(4):457–62.
18. Azadian A, et al. Management considerations in Hurthle cell carcinoma. Surgery. 1995;118(4):711–4. discussion 714–5.

19. Thompson NW, et al. Hurthle cell lesions of the thyroid gland. Surg Gynecol Obstet. 1974;139(4):555–60.
20. McLeod MK, Thompson NW. Hurthle cell neoplasms of the thyroid. Otolaryngol Clin North Am. 1990;23(3):441–52.
21. Carangiu M. Hurthle cell carcinoma: clinic-pathologic and biological aspects. Tumori. 2003;89:529–32.
22. Grant CS, et al. Benign Hurthle cell tumors of the thyroid: a diagnosis to be trusted? World J Surg. 1988;12(4):488–95.
23. Gosain AK, Clark OH. Hurthle cell neoplasms. Malignant potential. Arch Surg. 1984;119(5):515–9.
24. Bondeson L, et al. Oxyphil tumors of the thyroid: follow-up of 42 surgical cases. Ann Surg. 1981;194(6):677–80.
25. Samaan NA, et al. The results of various modalities of treatment of well differentiated thyroid carcinomas: a retrospective review of 1599 patients. J Clin Endocrinol Metab. 1992;75(3):714–20.
26. Samaan NA, et al. Pulmonary metastasis of differentiated thyroid carcinoma: treatment results in 101 patients. J Clin Endocrinol Metab. 1985;60(2):376–80.
27. Har-El G, et al. Hurthle cell carcinoma of the thyroid gland. A tumor of moderate malignancy. Cancer. 1986;57(8):1613–7.
28. Thoresen SO, et al. Survival and prognostic factors in differentiated thyroid cancer – a multivariate analysis of 1,055 cases. Br J Cancer. 1989;59(2):231–5.
29. Sugino K, et al. Hurthle cell tumor of the thyroid: analysis of 188 cases. World J Surg. 2001;25(9):1160–3.
30. Besic N, et al. The role of radioactive iodine in the treatment of Hurthle cell carcinoma of the thyroid. Thyroid. 2003;13(6):577–84.
31. Lopez-Penabad L, et al. Prognostic factors in patients with Hurthle cell neoplasms of the thyroid. Cancer. 2003;97(5):1186–94.
32. Mills SC, et al. Hurthle cell carcinoma of the thyroid: retrospective review of 62 patients treated at the Royal Marsden Hospital between 1946 and 2003. Eur J Surg Oncol. 2009;35(3):230–4.
33. Carcangiu ML, et al. Follicular Hurthle cell tumors of the thyroid gland. Cancer. 1991;68(9):1944–53.
34. Arturi F, et al. Iodide symporter gene expression in human thyroid tumors. J Clin Endocrinol Metab. 1998;83(7):2493–6.
35. Dohan O, et al. The sodium/iodide symporter (NIS): characterization, regulation, and medical significance. Endocr Rev. 2003;24(1): 48–77.
36. Dadachova E, Carrasco N. The Na/I symporter (NIS): imaging and therapeutic applications. Semin Nucl Med. 2004;34(1):23–31.
37. Grunwald F, et al. Redifferentiation therapy-induced radioiodine uptake in thyroid cancer. J Nucl Med. 1998;39(11):1903–6.
38. Schmutzler C, et al. Retinoic acid increases sodium/iodide symporter mRNA levels in human thyroid cancer cell lines and suppresses expression of functional symporter in nontransformed FRTL-5 rat thyroid cells. Biochem Biophys Res Commun. 1997; 240(3):832–8.
39. Park JW, Clark OH. Redifferentiation therapy for thyroid cancer. Surg Clin North Am. 2004;84(3):921–43.
40. Braga-Basaria M, Ringel MD. Clinical review 158: beyond radioiodine: a review of potential new therapeutic approaches for thyroid cancer. J Clin Endocrinol Metab. 2003;88(5):1947–60.
41. Spitzweg C, Morris JC. Gene therapy for thyroid cancer: current status and future prospects. Thyroid. 2004;14(6):424–34.
42. Gruning T, et al. Retinoic acid for redifferentiation of thyroid cancer – does it hold its promise? Eur J Endocrinol. 2003;148(4):395–402.
43. Clark OH, Hoelting T. Management of patients with differentiated thyroid cancer who have positive serum thyroglobulin levels and negative radioiodine scans. Thyroid. 1994;4(4):501–5.
44. Chao TC, Lin JD, Chen MF. Surgical treatment of Hurthle cell tumors of the thyroid. World J Surg. 2005;29(2):164–8.
45. Chen H, Nicol TL, Udelsman R. Follicular lesions of the thyroid. Does frozen section evaluation alter operative management? Ann Surg. 1995;222(1):101–6.
46. Lowe VJ, et al. 18F-FDG PET of patients with Hurthle cell carcinoma. J Nucl Med. 2003;44(9):1402–6.
47. Lazzi S, et al. Oncocytic (Hurthle cell) tumors of the thyroid: distinct growth patterns compared with clinicopathological features. Thyroid. 1999;9(2):97–103.
48. McDonald MP, et al. Hurthle cell carcinoma of the thyroid gland: prognostic factors and results of surgical treatment. Surgery. 1996; 120(6):1000–4. discussion 1004–5.
49. Besic N, et al. Is patient's age a prognostic factor for follicular thyroid carcinoma in the TNM classification system? Thyroid. 2005; 15(5):439–48.
50. Bhattacharyya N. Survival and prognosis in Hurthle cell carcinoma of the thyroid gland. Arch Otolaryngol Head Neck Surg. 2003; 129(2):207–10.
51. Kushchayeva Y, et al. Prognostic indications for Hurthle cell cancer. World J Surg. 2004;28(12):1266–70.
52. Belchetz G, et al. Hurthle cell tumors: using molecular techniques to define a novel classification system. Arch Otolaryngol Head Neck Surg. 2002;128(3):237–40.
53. Tala H, et al. Five-year survival is similar in thyroid cancer patients with distant metastases prepared for radioactive iodine therapy with either thyroid hormone withdrawal or recombinant human TSH. J Clin Endocrinol Metab. 2011;96:2105–11.
54. Klubo-Gwiezdzinska J, Burman KD, Van Nostrand D, Mete M, Jonklaas J, Wartofsky L. Thyroid. radioiodine treatment of metastatic thyroid cancer: relative efficacy and side effect profile of preparation by thyroid hormone withdrawal versus recombinant human thyrotropin. Thyroid. 2012;22(3):310–7.
55. Mazzaferri EL, et al. A consensus report of the role of serum thyroglobulin as a monitoring method for low-risk patients with papillary thyroid carcinoma. J Clin Endocrinol Metab. 2003;88(4): 1433–41.
56. Yen TC, et al. The role of technetium-99m sestamibi whole-body scans in diagnosing metastatic Hurthle cell carcinoma of the thyroid gland after total thyroidectomy: a comparison with iodine-131 and thallium-201 whole-body scans. Eur J Nucl Med. 1994; 21(9):980–3.
57. Plotkin M, et al. Implication of 2-18fluor-2-deoxyglucose positron emission tomography in the follow-up of Hurthle cell thyroid cancer. Thyroid. 2002;12(2):155–61.
58. Simpson WJ, et al. Papillary and follicular thyroid cancer: impact of treatment in 1578 patients. Int J Radiat Oncol Biol Phys. 1988;14(6):1063–75.
59. Brierley JD, Tsang RW. External-beam radiation therapy in the treatment of differentiated thyroid cancer. Semin Surg Oncol. 1999;16(1):42–9.
60. Ford D, et al. External beam radiotherapy in the management of differentiated thyroid cancer. Clin Oncol (R Coll Radiol). 2003; 15(6):337–41.
61. Schuck A, et al. Acute toxicity of adjuvant radiotherapy in locally advanced differentiated thyroid carcinoma. First results of the multicenter study differentiated thyroid carcinoma (MSDS). Strahlenther Onkol. 2003;179(12):832–9.
62. Grunwald F, et al. Redifferentiation therapy with retinoic acid in follicular thyroid cancer. J Nucl Med. 1998;39(9):1555–8.
63. Foote RL, et al. Is there a role for radiation therapy in the management of Hurthle cell carcinoma? Int J Radiat Oncol Biol Phys. 2003;56(4):1067–72.
64. Lin JD, et al. Results of external beam radiotherapy in patients with well differentiated thyroid carcinoma. Jpn J Clin Oncol. 1997; 27(4):244–7.
65. Nikiforov YE. Thyroid carcinoma: molecular pathways and therapeutic targets. Mod Pathol. 2008;21 Suppl 2:S37–43.
66. Nikiforova MN, Nikiforov YE. Molecular genetics of thyroid cancer: implications for diagnosis, treatment and prognosis. Expert Rev Mol Diagn. 2008;8(1):83–95.
67. Li H, et al. Cost-effectiveness of a novel molecular test for cytologically indeterminate thyroid nodules. J Clin Endocrinol Metab. 2011;96(11):E1719–26.

Follow-Up Strategy in Follicular Thyroid Cancer

74

Merica Shrestha and Henry B. Burch

Introduction

As with papillary thyroid cancer (PTC), the effort applied to the search for recurrent follicular thyroid cancer (FTC) is determined by an estimate of the likelihood risk of tumor recurrence and death from disease. The presence or absence of certain poor prognostic indicators is used to tailor the frequency and intensity of surveillance for tumor recurrence. Many of the same determinants of prognosis in PTC (see Chap. 48) are applicable to patients with FTC. Based largely on tumor histology and findings at the time of surgery, patients with FTC may be divided into two nonoverlapping subtypes: minimally invasive (MI-FTC), representing 80–90 % of cases, and widely invasive (WI-FTC) tumors (10–20 %) [1–3]. Patients with WI-FTC have a higher risk of distant (and, rarely, regional) metastases at diagnosis when compared to MI-FTC [4], as well as a higher incidence of cancer-related death and decreased survival than patients with PTC [1, 5, 6]. Conversely, patients with MI-FTC are at a relatively low risk for recurrence and cancer-related death [7–11]. Although current guidelines tend to group surveillance strategies of PTC and FTC together, as noted above, biological differences are apparent [12]. This chapter reviews the rationale used to determine appropriate follow-up for patients with FTC and provides a current overview of the tools available to assist in this objective.

Disclaimer: The opinions expressed in this paper reflect the personal views of the authors and not the official views of the United States Army or the Department of Defense.

M. Shrestha, MD
Endocrinology Service, Dwight David Eisenhower Army Medical Center, Ft. Gordon, GA, USA

H.B. Burch, MD, FACE (✉)
Endocrine Division, Uniformed Services University of the Health Sciences, Walter Reed National Military Medical Center, 8901 Wisconsin Avenue, American Building, Room 5053, Bethesda, MD 20889, USA
e-mail: Henry.burch@med.navy.mil

Surveillance Level

The higher rate of cancer-related death associated with WI-FTC mandates a higher index of suspicion for recurrent disease than with PTC. The propensity for early hematogenous spread also directs attention to distant sites, such as the lungs, bones, brain, and liver, in cases of suspected persistent or recurrent disease. Numerous unusual patterns of hematogenous metastasis have been described in patients with follicular thyroid cancer, including the skin, iris, pericardium, kidney, adrenal gland, and paranasal sinuses [13–18]. Hürthle cell carcinoma is considered a variant of follicular cancer and a more aggressive histologic type. Risk factors for recurrence and decreased survival such as extrathyroidal invasion, presence of metastases at diagnosis, male gender, and less than total thyroidectomy have been described and should tailor a more stringent surveillance strategy [19, 20].

Adverse events appear to occur earlier in patients with FTC compared to those with PTC [1, 8, 11, 19, 21, 22]. An extensive literature review for FTC found that most recurrences and cancer-related deaths occur in the first 5 years after diagnosis. In fact, 50–80 % of adverse events took place in the first 2 years after diagnosis [1]. A study involving 49 patients with follicular and Hürthle cell thyroid cancer found that all recurrences and deaths occurred within 13 years of diagnosis, whereas PTC patients at the same institution continued to experience adverse events throughout 40 year of observation [22].

At the authors' medical center, the approach to patients with WI-FTC is total thyroidectomy, followed by radioiodine ablation with 100–150 mCi of ^{131}I. While a great deal of provider and medical center-specific variability exists in early management [23] and subsequent follow-up regimens, the following approach seems reasonable based on current evidence and practice (Fig. 74.1). Patients with WI-FTC undergo whole-body scanning (WBS) and TSH-stimulated serum thyroglobulin (TSH-Tg) every 6 months for the first 18 months and then TSH-Tg annually (without WBS if prior results were negative) until the fifth year of follow-up. Thereafter, if there

L. Wartofsky, D. Van Nostrand (eds.), *Thyroid Cancer*, DOI 10.1007/978-1-4939-3314-3_74

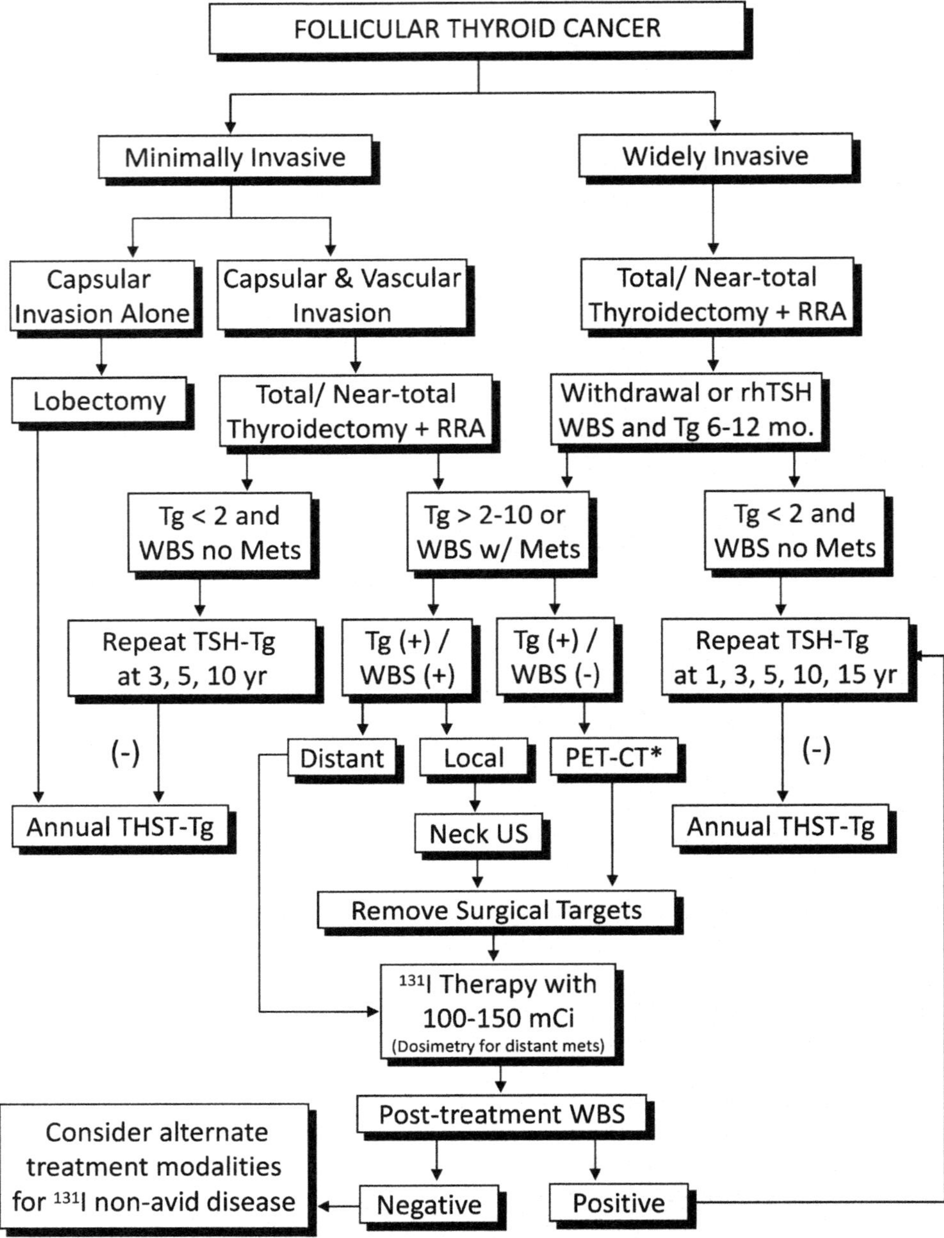

Fig. 74.1 An algorithmic approach to the follow-up of FTC. Following initial thyroid surgery, patients are classified as minimally invasive (MI-FTC) or widely invasive (WI-FTC), based on a minimum of ten sections through the nodule capsule. MI-FTC is further classified into cases with capsular invasion alone and those with both capsular and vascular invasion. Following thyroidectomy and RRA, patients undergo surveillance testing at intervals determined by their histological category. Patients with persistent or recurrent disease are assessed for surgical targets and generally treated with radioiodine therapy. Patients with progressive, non-radioiodine-avid disease are considered for additional treatment modalities. *rhTSH* recombinant human thyrotropin, *Tg* thyroglobulin, *WBS* whole-body scan, *US* ultrasound, *PET-CT* fluorodeoxyglucose positron emission tomography-computed tomography

is no evidence of residual disease, TSH-Tg is generally obtained at 3–5 year intervals until approximately 15 years after diagnosis, after which annual neck exam and thyroglobulin (Tg) testing on thyroid hormone suppressive therapy (THST-Tg) is performed. Many patients with minimally invasive disease are also treated initially with total thyroidectomy and radioiodine ablation. Following treatment, they undergo WBS and TSH-Tg at 12 months, and if results are negative, TSH-Tg testing alone is performed at 3–5-year intervals for the first 10 years after surgery, after which they are followed using THST-Tg. Patients with MI-FTC and capsular invasion alone (no vascular invasion) represent a particularly low-risk group. These patients have a particularly indolent course with normal disease-specific survival [3, 9], and the above surveillance approach may therefore be too aggressive for this particular subset.

The revised American Thyroid Association guidelines for the long-term management of FTC are similar to those for PTC [24]. Since follicular and Hurthle cell histologies are considered higher-risk tumors, radioactive iodine remnant ablation (RRA) is recommended in most cases. As noted above, in patients with MI-FTC, surgical resection generally yields an excellent prognosis and RRA may not be necessary, particularly in those with capsular invasion alone. RRA dose should be dependent on risk category (30–100 mCi for low risk vs 100–200 mCi for higher risk). WBS following withdrawal or rhTSH 6–12 months after RRA is recommended along with cervical neck ultrasound. The subsequent rate of follow-up is based on response to therapy and risk of recurrence.

The National Comprehensive Cancer Network (NCCN) practice guidelines [25] recommend that patients with FTC who have no gross residual disease receive a WBS and TSH-Tg measurement at 4–6 weeks postoperatively, which determines subsequent management. Patients with a negative WBS in the thyroid bed and an undetectable TSH-Tg (with negative antithyroglobulin antibodies) are not given RRA. Conversely, patients with positive thyroid bed uptake or TSH-Tg >10 ng/mL are treated with RRA, and larger, treatment doses of radioiodine are used in patients with known metastatic disease on WBS. For follow-up of FTC patients, a TSH-Tg is recommended in patients with negative THST-Tg and anti-Tg antibody. WBS should be considered in patients with T3–T4 lesions or M1 at initial staging, elevated THST-Tg levels, positive antithyroglobulin antibodies (TgAbs), or abnormal neck US. If there is suspicion for recurrence based on these tests, therapy is generally rendered and repeat WBS performed every 12–24 months until negative. Additional imaging (e.g., 18-FDG-PET/CT) is recommended in the NCCN guidelines if TSH-Tg is elevated and WBS is negative. In patients believed free of disease, NCCN guidelines advise annual neck exam, THST-Tg, and anti-Tg antibody measurement.

Serum TG and Antithyroglobulin Antibody Measurement

Patients with WI-FTC generally have higher levels of TSH-Tg than those with papillary carcinoma [26]. In a retrospective study, 214 follicular cancer patients were divided into low-, moderate-, and high-risk groups based on American Joint Cancer Committee/Union Internationale Contre le Cancer (AJCC/UICC) staging [27, 28]. Postoperative serum Tg values were found to be significantly higher in higher-risk groups, and this translated into a significant association with persistent/recurrent disease, decreased survival, and increased mortality during a mean follow-up of 9.6 years.

TgAb, present in up to 25 % of patients with DTC [29], tend to decrease following thyroidectomy and complete remnant ablation, disappearing at a median of 3 years in one study [30]. Persistent or increasing TgAb may serve as a serum marker for persistent thyroid cancer [31–34]. A study of 51 patients with differentiated thyroid cancer and undetectable serum Tg but positive TgAbs found a higher incidence of recurrent disease (49 % vs 3.4 %) than in a group of patients with negative Tg and TgAbs [31]. Another study examining 43 thyroid cancer patients with positive TgAbs found that 5 of 19 (26 %) patients with persistent TgAbs had residual disease, compared to 0 of 23 patients whose TgAbs decreased after therapy [35]. Finally, in a recent study of 56 thyroid cancer patients with positive TgAbs at 6–12 months post-remnant ablation, 10 of 56 (18 %) patients had recurrence, whereas only 10 of 768 (1 %) patients with negative TgAbs had recurrence during a 73.6 months follow-up. The magnitude of TgAb elevation correlated with recurrence rates [36]. Apparently, the presence of functioning thyroid tissue – metastatic or otherwise – is necessary to perpetuate Tg antibody synthesis.

References

1. Grebe SK, Hay ID. Follicular thyroid cancer. Endocrinol Metab Clin North Am. 1995;24:761–801.
2. Brassard M, Borget I, Edet-Sanson A, et al. Long-term follow-up of patients with papillary and follicular thyroid cancer: a prospective study on 715 patients. J Clin Endocrinol Metab. 2011;96(5):1352–9. Epub 2011 Mar 9.
3. O'Neill CJ, Vaughan L, Learoyd DL, Sidhu SB, Delbridge LW, Sywak MS. Management of follicular thyroid carcinoma should be individualised based on degree of capsular and vascular invasion. Eur J Surg Oncol. 2011;37(2):181–5. Epub 2010 Dec 8.
4. Asari R, Koperek O, Scheuba C, et al. Follicular thyroid carcinoma in an iodine-replete endemic goiter region: a prospectively collected, retrospectively analyzed clinical trial. Ann Surg. 2009;249:1023–31.
5. Chow SM, Law SC, Au SK, et al. Differentiated thyroid carcinoma: comparison between papillary and follicular carcinoma in a single institute. Head Neck. 2002;24:670–7.
6. Mazzaferri EL, Kloos RT. Current approaches to primary therapy for papillary and follicular thyroid cancer. J Clin Endocrinol Metab. 2001;86:1447–63.
7. Davis NL, Bugis SP, McGregor GI, Germann E. An evaluation of prognostic scoring systems in patients with follicular thyroid cancer. Am J Surg. 1995;170:476–80.
8. Jorda M, Gonzalez-Campora R, Mora J, et al. Prognostic factors in follicular carcinoma of the thyroid. Arch Pathol Lab Med. 1993;117:631–5.
9. van Heerden JA, Hay ID, Goellner JR, et al. Follicular thyroid carcinoma with capsular invasion alone: a nonthreatening malignancy. Surgery. 1992;112:1130–6.
10. Thompson LD, Wieneke JA, Paal E, et al. A clinicopathologic study of minimally invasive follicular carcinoma of the thyroid gland with a review of the English literature. Cancer. 2001;91:505–24.
11. D'Avanzo A, Treseler P, Ituarte PH, et al. Follicular thyroid carcinoma: histology and prognosis. Cancer. 2004;100:1123–9.
12. Lang BH, Lo C-Y, Chan W-F, et al. Prognostic factors in papillary and follicular thyroid carcinoma: their implications for cancer staging. Ann Surg Oncol. 2006;14:730–8.
13. Koller EA, Tourtelot JB, Pak HS, et al. Papillary and follicular thyroid carcinoma metastatic to the skin: a case report and review of the literature. Thyroid. 1998;8:1045–50.
14. Ainsworth JR, Damato BE, Lee WR, Alexander WD. Follicular thyroid carcinoma metastatic to the iris: a solitary lesion treated with iridocyclectomy. Arch Ophthalmol. 1992;110:19–20.
15. Chiewvit S, Pusuwan P, Chiewvit P, et al. Metastatic follicular carcinoma of thyroid to pericardium. J Med Assoc Thai. 1998;81:799–802.

16. Lam KY, Ng WK. Follicular carcinoma of the thyroid appearing as a solitary renal mass. Nephron. 1996;73:323–4.
17. Altman KW, Mirza N, Philippe L. Metastatic follicular thyroid carcinoma to the paranasal sinuses: a case report and review. J Laryngol Otol. 1997;111:647–51.
18. Kumar A, Nadig M, Patra V, et al. Adrenal and renal metastases from follicular thyroid cancer. Br J Radiol. 2005;78:1038–41.
19. Kushchayeva Y, Duh Q-Y, Kebebew E, et al. Comparison of clinical characteristics at diagnosis and during follow-up in 118 patients with hurthle cell or follicular thyroid cancer. Am J Surg. 2008;195:457–62.
20. Carcangiu ML, Bianchi S, Savino D, et al. Follicular hurthle cell tumors of the thyroid gland. Cancer. 1991;68:1944–53.
21. Zidan J, Kassem S, Kuten A. Follicular carcinoma of the thyroid gland: prognostic factors, treatment, and survival. Am J Clin Oncol. 2000;23:1–5.
22. DeGroot LJ, Kaplan EL, Shukla MS, et al. Morbidity and mortality in follicular thyroid cancer. J Clin Endocrinol Metab. 1995;80: 2946–53.
23. Haymart MR, Banerjee M, Stewart AK, Koenig RJ, Birkmeyer JD, Griggs JJ. Use of radioactive iodine for thyroid cancer. JAMA. 2011;306(7):721–8.
24. Haugen BR, Alexander EK, Bible KC, Doherty GM, Mandel SJ, Nikiforov YE, Pacini F, Randolph GW, Sawka AM, Schlumberger M, Schuff KG, Sherman SI, Sosa JA, Steward DL, Tuttle RM, Wartofsky L. 2015 American Thyroid Association Management Guidelines for Adult Patients with Thyroid Nodules and Differentiated Thyroid Cancer: American Thyroid Association Guidelines Task Force on Thyroid Nodules and Differentiated Thyroid Cancer. Thyroid. 2016;26:1–133.
25. Tuttle RM, Ball DW, Byrd D, et al. Thyroid carcinoma. J Natl Compr Canc Netw. 2010;8:1228–74.
26. Torrens JI, Burch HB. Serum thyroglobulin measurement. Utility in clinical practice. Endocrinol Metab Clin North Am. 2001;30:429–67.
27. Lin J-D, Chao T-C, Chen S-T, et al. Operative strategy for FTC in risk groups stratified by pTNM staging. Surg Oncol. 2007;16:107–13.
28. Edge SB, Byrd DR, Compton CC, et al. AJCC cancer staging manual. 7th ed. New York: Springer; 2009.
29. Spencer CA, Takeuchi M, Kazarosyan M, et al. Serum thyroglobulin autoantibodies: prevalence, influence on serum thyroglobulin measurement, and prognostic significance in patients with differentiated thyroid carcinoma. J Clin Endocrinol Metab. 1998;83: 1121–7.
30. Chiovato L, Latrofa F, Braverman LE, et al. Disappearance of humoral thyroid autoimmunity after complete removal of thyroid antigens. Ann Intern Med. 2003;139:346–51.
31. Chung JK, Park YJ, Kim TY, et al. Clinical significance of elevated level of serum antithyroglobulin antibody in patients with differentiated thyroid cancer after thyroid ablation. Clin Endocrinol. 2002;57:215–21.
32. Kumar A, Shah DH, Shrihari U, et al. Significance of antithyroglobulin autoantibodies in differentiated thyroid carcinoma. Thyroid. 1994;4:199–202.
33. Rubello D, Girelli ME, Casara D, et al. Usefulness of the combined antithyroglobulin antibodies and thyroglobulin assay in the follow-up of patients with differentiated thyroid cancer. J Endocrinol Invest. 1990;13:737–42.
34. Phan HT, Jager PL, van der Wal JE, et al. The follow-up of patients with differentiated thyroid cancer and undetectable thyroglobulin (Tg) and Tg antibodies during ablation. Eur J Endocrinol. 2008;158:77–83.
35. Rubello D, Casara D, Girelli ME, et al. Clinical meaning of circulating antithyroglobulin antibodies in differentiated thyroid cancer: a prospective study. J Nucl Med. 1992;33:1478–80.
36. Kim WG, Yoon JH, Kim WB, et al. Change of serum antithyroglobulin antibody levels is useful for prediction of clinical recurrence in thyroglobulin-negative patients with differentiated thyroid carcinoma. J Clin Endocrinol Metab. 2008;93:4683–9.

Radionuclide Imaging and ^{131}I Therapy in Follicular Thyroid Carcinoma

75

Douglas Van Nostrand

Introduction

Radionuclide imaging and ^{131}I therapy including dosimetry are addressed in multiple separate chapters. This brief chapter addresses the relation of special aspects of radionuclide imaging and ^{131}I therapy to follicular thyroid cancer (FTC). Although papillary and follicular differentiated thyroid cancers are histologically different, their biological behaviors are similar. As a result, most published reports do not differentiate between the two, describing outcomes for "differentiated thyroid carcinoma," and this is especially true for the literature involving radionuclide imaging and ^{131}I therapy. Accordingly, the other chapters discussing various issues for papillary carcinoma are for the most part also applicable to patients with follicular carcinoma. However, several distinctions between these two types of thyroid malignancy are noteworthy.

First, FTC is significantly less likely to metastasize to local cervical lymph nodes than is PTC. For example, whereas PTC may metastasize to cervical lymph nodes in as many as 35–45 % of patients, metastases to cervical lymph nodes are found in patients with FTC in only 5–17 % of patients [1–5]. Consequently, radioiodine uptake in lymph node metastases is much less likely to be visualized on imaging studies in patients with FTC than is typically observed in papillary carcinoma. Histologically, FTC typically demonstrates a microfollicular pattern, but follicular tumors with less radioiodine uptake tend to show more solid growth with macrofollicles and high levels of cellular atypia. FTC is also more likely to be unifocal, whereas papillary cancers are often multicentric, particularly with several satellite microcarcinomata.

D. Van Nostrand, MD, FACP, FACNM (✉)
Nuclear Medicine Research, MedStar Research Institute and Washington Hospital Center, Georgetown University School of Medicine, Washington Hospital Center, 110 Irving Street, N.W., Suite GB 60F, Washington, DC 20010, USA
e-mail: douglasvannostrand@gmail.com

Secondly, FTC is angioinvasive and may metastasize hematogenously to the lung, bone, liver, brain, and kidney [2]. Thus, distant metastases in these various sites are visualized more frequently on radionuclide imaging in patients with FTC relative to PTC.

One variant of FTC, Hürthle cell carcinoma (see Chap. 73), is frequently less differentiated than FTC with reduced ability to transport iodide via the sodium/iodide symporter (NIS) and little if any radioiodine uptake [3–7]. Papillary and non-Hürthle cell follicular carcinoma may have radioiodine uptake in 60 and 64 % of patients, respectively, whereas Hürthle cell carcinomas may take up radioiodine in only 36 % of patients [3]. This may make both imaging and therapy with ^{131}I more problematic in these patients. However, because of variability in patient populations, patient age, sample size, and possibly the diagnostic criteria for Hürthle cell carcinoma, the frequency of radioiodine uptake in Hürthle cell carcinoma will be variable. For example, Besic et al. [4] reported uptake in 69 % (11 of 16) of patients with Hürthle cell carcinoma and concluded that ^{131}I therapy may be effective in a significant number of these patients.

While both PTC and FTC are often considered as differentiated thyroid cancer (DTC), the biological behavior of FTC often differs from PTC regarding prognostic factors associated with tumor recurrence [5] and survival [6]. In one large follow-up series of 1578 patients, thyroid cancer was the cause of death in just over half of the PTC deaths and in two thirds of FTC deaths [7]. The follicular variant of papillary carcinoma is discussed in Chaps. 29 and 32 and is generally considered to behave more like PTC [8] although multicentricity, lymph node metastases, and local soft tissue invasion may be seen less often than in PTC [9].

Nevertheless, and despite the above clear differences between PTC and FTC, for all practical purposes they are similarly regarded in terms of radionuclide imaging, ^{131}I ablation, ^{131}I adjuvant treatment, and ^{131}I treatment for distant

L. Wartofsky, D. Van Nostrand (eds.), *Thyroid Cancer*, DOI 10.1007/978-1-4939-3314-3_75

metastases. In addition to the chapters cited in this text, excellent general reviews on FTC are available [10, 11], and the most recently published guidelines from the American Thyroid Association, European Consensus, National Comprehensive Cancer Network, and British Thyroid Association on radioisotopic scanning and treatment are valuable resources [12–15].

References

1. Wartofsky L. Follicular thyroid carcinoma, clinical aspects. In: Wartofsky L, editor. Thyroid cancer: a comprehensive guide to clinical management. Totowa: Humana Press; 2000.
2. Mazzaferri EL. Radioiodine and other treatments and outcomes. In: Braverman LE, Utiger RD, editors. Werner and Ingbar's the thyroid: a fundamental and clinical text. Philadelphia: Lippincott-Raven Press; 1996.
3. Samaan NA, Schultz PN, Haynie TP, Ordonez NG. Pulmonary metastasis of differentiated thyroid carcinoma: treatment results in 101 patients. J Clin Endocrinol Metab. 1985;60:376–80.
4. Besic N, Vidergar-Kralj B, Frkovic-Grazio S, et al. The role of radioactive iodine in the treatment of Hurthle cell carcinoma of the thyroid. Thyroid. 2003;13:577–84.
5. Simpson WJ, McKinney SE, Carruthers JS, et al. Papillary and follicular thyroid cancer. Prognostic factors in 1,578 patients. Am J Med. 1987;83:479–88.
6. Eichhorn W, Tabler H, Lippold R, et al. Prognostic factors determining long-term survival in well-differentiated thyroid cancer. An analysis of 484 patients undergoing therapy and aftercare at the same institution. Thyroid. 2003;13:949–58.
7. Simpson WJ, Panzarella T, Carruthers JS, et al. Papillary and follicular thyroid cancer; impact of treatment in 1578 patients. Int J Radiat Oncol Biol Phys. 1988;14:1063–75.
8. Zidan J, Karen D, Stein M, et al. Pure versus follicular variant of papillary thyroid carcinoma. Cancer. 2003;97:1181–5.
9. Jain M, Khan A, Patwardhan N, et al. Follicular variant of papillary thyroid carcinoma: a comparative study of histopathologic features and cytology results in 141 patients. Endocr Pract. 2001;7:79–84.
10. Kinder BK. Well differentiated thyroid cancer. Curr Opin Oncol. 2003;15:71–7.
11. Haigh PI. Follicular thyroid carcinoma. Curr Treat Options Oncol. 2002;3:349–54.
12. Cooper DS, Doherty GM, Haugen BR, Kloos RT, Lee SL, Mandel SJ, Mazzaferri EL, McIver B, Pacini F, Schlumberger M, Sherman SI, Steward DL, Tuttle RM. Revised American Thyroid Association management guidelines for patients with thyroid nodules and differentiated thyroid cancer. Thyroid. 2009;19:1167–214.
13. Pacini F, Schlumberger M, Dralle H, Elisei R, Smit JWA, Wiersinga W, European Thyroid Cancer Taskforce. European consensus for the management of patients with differentiated thyroid carcinoma of the follicular epithelium. Eur J Endocrinol. 2006;154:787–803.
14. National Comprehensive Cancer Network (NCCN). Clinical practice guidelines in oncology. Thyroid carcinoma. Follicular thyroid carcinoma. Version 2.2015. Available at: http://www.nccn.org/professionals/physician_gls/pdf/thyroid.pdf.
15. British Thyroid Association and Royal College of Physicians. Guidelines for the management of thyroid cancer. 2nd ed. Available at: http://www.british-thyroid-ssociation.org/news/Docs/Thyroid_cancer_guidelines_2007.pdf.

PET/CT in Follicular Cancer Including Hürthle Cell Cancer

76

Iain Ross McDougall and Andrei Iagaru

Introduction

The role of positron emission tomography (PET) and computer tomography (CT) using ^{18}F-fluorodeoxyglucose (^{18}F-FDG) was reviewed in depth in the Chap. 43 on differentiated thyroid cancer. The main role of ^{18}F-FDG PET-CT is in helping to identify the source of thyroglobulin (Tg) production in a patient whose cancer does not take up radioiodine. Most of the references cited in the earlier chapter included patients with both papillary and follicular cancers, and in most cases, it is not possible to separate these two cancer types and analyze the results. For example, Dietlein et al. presented results in 58 patients, 38 of whom had papillary cancer, 15 had follicular cancer, and 5 had variants of follicular cancer [1]. In another paper there were 11 follicular and 3 Hürthle cell cancers out of a total of 51 patients [2]. Some of the reports simply state that patients had papillary or follicular cancer [3]. Some studies even include patients with anaplastic cancer as well as differentiated cancer [4].

The multicenter report by Grunwald et al. does allow the results of ^{18}F-FDG PET-CT PET in different tumor types to be calculated [5]. There were 80 patients with follicular cancer and of these 52 had a negative scan with radioiodine. The sensitivity, specificity, and positive predictive value were 78, 100, and 100 %, respectively. In 28 patients with well-differentiated cancer that was capable of taking up iodine, the ^{18}F-FDG PET-CT scan was negative in 8 (29 %). A detailed meta-analysis in differentiated thyroid cancer that includes several of the papers discussed above and does not separate follicular from papillary cancers is nevertheless representative. Overall, sensitivity in patients with measurable Tg and a negative ^{131}I scan was 0.885 (95 % CI: 0.828–0.929) and specificity 0.847 (95 % CI: 0.715–0.934). In the six investigations dealing with ^{18}F-FDG PET-CT sensitivity and specificity were 0.935 (95 % CI: 0.870–0.973) and 0.839 (95 % CI: 0.723–0.920), respectively [6].

I.R. McDougall, MD, PhD, FRCP
Department of Radiology, Nuclear Medicine, Stanford University Hospital and Clinics, Stanford, CA, USA

A. Iagaru, MD (✉)
Department of Radiology, Nuclear Medicine, Stanford University Medical Center, Stanford School of Medicine,
300 Pasteur Dr, H2230 MC 5281, Stanford, CA 94305, USA
e-mail: aiagaru@stanford.edu

^{18}F-FDG-PET/CT in Hürthle Cell Cancer

Hürthle cell cancer is more aggressive than standard follicular cancer, but some authorities classify it as a variant of follicular carcinoma. The 5- and 20-year survival for follicular cancer are 87 % and 81 %, respectively. This falls to 81 % and 65 % for Hürthle cell cancer. The management of Hürthle cell cancer that has metastasized is difficult. The lesions frequently do not take up iodine and therefore are a classic example of iodine-negative Tg-positive lesions. As a consequence, therapy with high-dose ^{131}I is usually ineffective. The results of ^{18}F-FDG PET and ^{18}F-FDG PET-CT can be useful. Case reports indicate that ^{18}F-FDG uptake was effective in identifying iodine-negative metastases [7, 8]. Of 17 patients with Hürthle cell cancer evaluated by ^{18}F-FDG PET [9], 13 had an elevated Tg, and ^{18}F-FDG PET was positive in all cases. Additional testing confirmed metastases in 10 of the 13 patients with no confirmation in 2 patients and a false positive in 1. In four patients, there was suspicion of cancer but a low Tg. The ^{18}F-FDG PET scan was a true negative in three and a false positive in the fourth patient. In the multicenter study presented above, 20 patients had Hürthle cell cancer. The sensitivity of ^{18}F-FDG PET was 87 % and the specificity and positive predictive values were both 100 % [5]. Lowe et al. used ^{18}F-FDG PET in 12 patients with Hürthle cell cancer, and a total of 14 scans were obtained [10]. ^{18}F-FDG PET identified sites of disease that was not detected by any other test in seven of the scans. In another seven the extent of local and distant metastases was greater on ^{18}F-FDG PET scan.

L. Wartofsky, D. Van Nostrand (eds.), *Thyroid Cancer*, DOI 10.1007/978-1-4939-3314-3_76

The management was altered in seven patients on the basis of the scan results. A report of ^{18}F-FDG PET in 44 patients demonstrated a sensitivity of 96 % and a specificity of 95 %. The authors recommend PET as the principal investigation after surgery [11]. A recent review of ^{18}F-FDG PET/CT in aggressive thyroid cancer including Hürthle cell type by Tregli et al. confirms the value of this imaging test [12].

Summary

In summary, the role of ^{18}F-FDG PET-CT in differentiated follicular cancer that does not take up iodine is the same as for papillary cancer. In patients with metastatic Hürthle cell cancer, which has poor uptake of radioiodine, ^{18}F-FDG PET-CT is extremely valuable in identifying sites of disease.

References

1. Dietlein M, Scheidhauer K, Voth E, Theissen P, Schicha H. Fluorine-18 fluorodeoxyglucose positron emission tomography and iodine-131 whole-body scintigraphy in the follow-up of differentiated thyroid cancer. Eur J Nucl Med. 1997;24:1342–8.
2. Giammarile F, Hafdi Z, Bournaud C, et al. Is [18F]-2-fluoro-2-deoxy-d-glucose (FDG) scintigraphy with non-dedicated positron emission tomography useful in the diagnostic management of suspected metastatic thyroid carcinoma in patients with no detectable radioiodine uptake? Eur J Endocrinol. 2003;149:293–300.
3. Conti PS, Durski JM, Bacqai F, Grafton ST, Singer PA. Imaging of locally recurrent and metastatic thyroid cancer with positron emission tomography. Thyroid. 1999;9:797–804.
4. Fridrich L, Messa C, Landoni C, et al. Whole-body scintigraphy with 99mTc-MIBI, ^{18}F-FDG-PET and ^{131}I in patients with metastatic thyroid carcinoma. Nucl Med Commun. 1997;18:3–9.
5. Grunwald F, Kalicke T, Feine U, et al. Fluorine-18 fluorodeoxyglucose positron emission tomography in thyroid cancer: results of a multicentre study. Eur J Nucl Med. 1999;26:1547–52.
6. Dong MJ, Liu ZF, Zhao K, Ruan LX, Wang GL, Yang SY, Sun F, Luo XG. Value of 18F-FDG PET/PET-CT in differentiated thyroid carcinoma with radioiodine-negative whole-body scan: a meta-analysis. Nucl Med Commun. 2009;30:639–50.
7. Blount CL, Dworkin HJ. F-18 FDG uptake by recurrent Hürthle cell carcinoma of the thyroid using high-energy planar scintigraphy. Clin Nucl Med. 1996;21:831–3.
8. Wiesner W, Engel H, von Schulthess GK, Krestin GP, Bicik I. FDG PET-negative liver metastases of a malignant melanoma and F-FDG PET-positive Hürthle cell tumor of the thyroid. Eur Radiol. 1999;9:975–8.
9. Plotkin M, Hautzel H, Krause BJ, et al. Implication of 2-^{18}fluor-2-deoxyglucose positron emission tomography in the follow-up of Hurthle cell thyroid cancer. Thyroid. 2002;12:155–61.
10. Lowe VJ, Mullan BP, Hay ID, McIver B, Kasperbauer JL. ^{18}F-FDG PET of patients with Hurthle cell carcinoma. J Nucl Med. 2003;44:1402–6.
11. Pryma DA, Schöder H, Gönen M, Robbins RJ, Larson SM, Yeung HWD. Diagnostic accuracy and prognostic value of ^{18}F-FDG PET in Hürthle cell thyroid cancer patients. J Nucl Med. 2006;47:1260–6.
12. Treglia G, Annunziata S, Muoio B, Salvatori M, Ceriani L, Giovanella L. The role of fluorine-18-fluorodeoxyglucose positron emission tomography in aggressive histological subtypes of thyroid cancer: an overview. Int J Endocrinol. 2013;2013:856189.

77 Follicular Thyroid Cancer: Special Aspects in Children and Adolescents

Steven G. Waguespack and Andrew J. Bauer

With an age-adjusted annual incidence of 0.5 cases per million [1], follicular thyroid cancer (FTC) in children is a very rare malignancy that has received very little specific scrutiny in regard to surgical or medical management in the pediatric population. Recent studies and clinical experience from iodine-sufficient regions suggest that FTC currently represents around 10 % or less of thyroid cancer cases diagnosed during childhood and young adulthood [1–4]. More often than not, FTC has been grouped with papillary thyroid cancer (PTC) in previous studies and large pediatric thyroid carcinoma case series, which makes it difficult to study the unique aspects of FTC in this age group. Furthermore, distinguishing true FTC from follicular-variant PTC in the older medical literature is difficult, and the prevalence of true FTC appears to be decreasing over time [5]. Thus, the prevalence and clinical phenotype of pediatric FTC is evolving.

While we will attempt to draw conclusions on the clinical nature and management of FTC in children, we caution that these observations are drawn from a small number of cases and from medical centers in geographically diverse areas of the world. Furthermore, recommendations for the appropriate medical and surgical treatment are even more limited as no single study to date has evaluated the treatment and long-term outcome of a large cohort of pediatric FTC. As with any pediatric thyroid malignancy, treatment at a tertiary center with multidisciplinary experience in thyroid cancer treatment should optimize outcomes and facilitate future research into these rare malignancies.

S.G. Waguespack, MD
Endocrine Neoplasia and Hormonal Disorders, The University of Texas MD Anderson Cancer Center, Houston, TX, USA

A.J. Bauer, MD (✉)
Division of Endocrinology and Diabetes, Department of Pediatrics, The Children's Hospital of Philadelphia, The Perelman School of Medicine, The University of Pennsylvania,
34th Street and Civic Center Boulevard, Suite 11 NW30, Philadelphia, PA 19014, USA
e-mail: bauera@chop.edu

Pathology and Subtypes of FTC

Follicular carcinoma is defined by the World Health Organization (WHO) as a malignancy of thyroid follicular cell differentiation that lacks the characteristic nuclear changes of papillary carcinoma [6]. Most follicular tumors are encapsulated lesions, and the diagnosis of FTC is based on the pathologic identification of capsular and/or vascular invasion in the resected tumor [7, 8] distinguishing FTC from a benign follicular adenoma. FTC is currently subdivided into two major groups depending on the extent of invasion: minimally invasive and widely invasive FTC [9]. Historically, tumors with capsular and/or very limited vascular invasion are classified as minimally invasive carcinomas, whereas those with significant transcapsular and vascular invasion are deemed widely invasive FTC. This distinction is important because the extent of disease and prognosis directly relate to the degree of invasion [7–12].

The major histopathologic variants of FTC are the oncocytic (Hürthle cell) and clear cell variants [6]. Hürthle cell carcinomas (HCC) are follicular carcinomas that are composed of >75 % oncocytes, mitochondria-rich cells with abundant granular eosinophilic cytoplasm [9, 13]. Poorly differentiated thyroid carcinomas are defined by the WHO as follicular cell malignancies with limited evidence of follicular cell differentiation [6]. Such cancers represent an intermediate tumor between the well-differentiated PTC/FTC and the undifferentiated (anaplastic) thyroid carcinomas. These tumors may have insular, trabecular, or solid growth patterns with evidence of mitotic activity, necrosis, and vascular invasion. They can arise de novo or from a preexisting PTC/FTC. Such tumors are exceedingly rare in the pediatric population [14, 15], and they will not be discussed in detail.

L. Wartofsky, D. Van Nostrand (eds.), *Thyroid Cancer*, DOI 10.1007/978-1-4939-3314-3_77

Etiology and Clinical Behavior

The exact etiology of pediatric FTC remains unknown in most cases. One clear risk factor for the development of FTC is iodine deficiency, and iodine-deficient countries have a higher prevalence of FTC compared with PTC [8, 16–18]. Unlike PTC, ionizing radiation has a less clear role in FTC pathogenesis [19, 20].

Several nonoverlapping somatic genetic events have been reported in adult FTC, primarily mutations in *RAS* (40–50 %) and the PAX8/PPARγ rearrangement (30–35 %), but also rarely mutations in the *PTEN* and *PIK3CA* genes [9, 21–27]. The prevalence of these mutations in pediatric FTC remains unstudied. In adults, the presence of a *RAS* mutation may identify carcinomas that are more prone to dedifferentiation and metastatic spread, but it is not a universal indicator of prognosis in all cases [28]. FTCs that have the PAX8/PPARγ rearrangement may be more common in younger patients, be of smaller size, and have a propensity to more vascular invasion [25, 27].

In contrast to conventional FTC, HCC have a very low frequency of RAS mutations or PAX8/PPARγ rearrangements, suggesting that HCC develop along a separate molecular pathway [9]. Somatic mutations of the *GRIM-19* gene, which is involved in mitochondrial metabolism and apoptosis, have been implicated in the pathogenesis of oncocytic thyroid tumors [29]. Poorly differentiated carcinomas have been most commonly associated with mutations in *RAS*, *TP53*, *BRAF*, *CTNNB1*, *PIK3CA*, and *AKT1* [9, 28].

Rarely, FTC is a component of the PTEN hamartoma tumor syndrome, primarily Cowden syndrome, due to germline mutations in the *PTEN* gene [30–33]. Therefore, in children with FTC, a detailed family history should be undertaken to identify tumors that are associated with Cowden syndrome (chiefly breast cancer and genitourinary neoplasia). In children with a suggestive family history, characteristic mucocutaneous lesions, and/or macrocephaly, genetic counseling and germline testing for a *PTEN* mutation is warranted [31, 33]. FTC may also rarely develop as part of the Carney complex, Pendred syndrome, and Werner syndrome [34].

FTC is more commonly diagnosed in adolescents and, unlike PTC, there is also less of a female to male preponderance [2, 16, 35–37]. In addition, FTC differs from PTC in that it is typically a unifocal tumor that rarely spreads to regional lymph nodes [2, 6–8, 36, 38–41], unless it is one of the more aggressive FTC variants. However, FTC is prone to early hematogenous metastases, usually to the lungs and bone, which occurs even in the absence of cervical node involvement [42, 43]. The highest-risk patients appear to be those >45 years of age with larger tumors and more widespread angioinvasion [7, 9, 11, 42, 44]. Compared with the adult experience, pediatric FTC may be less aggressive than PTC, being associated with less advanced disease, fewer distant metastases, and a lower rate of relapse [2, 35, 37, 38, 45]. Similar to PTC, conventional FTC has an excellent prognosis when diagnosed during childhood, with long-term survival being the norm [1, 46, 47]. Those children presenting with distant metastases, however, may ultimately succumb to their disease [37].

Minimally invasive FTC has the lowest risk for recurrence and/or metastases, whereas widely invasive FTC is associated with significant morbidity and mortality [7, 9–12, 40, 42, 44, 48]. The most important clinical determinant appears to be vascular invasion, and any degree of vascular invasion may portend more advanced disease and a worse prognosis [7, 10–12, 44, 49]. However, other studies have not clearly demonstrated a negative impact of vascular invasion [42, 50]. Size of the primary tumor also appears to be an important factor, with metastases less likely to occur in smaller malignancies [39, 42, 43, 48, 49].

HCC are an aggressive malignancy that is more prone to direct soft tissue invasion, lymph node involvement, and distant metastases compared with conventional FTC [9, 51, 52]. HCC are also less likely to concentrate radioactive iodine, making this treatment modality less effective in the treatment of distant metastases [51, 52].

Evaluation and Treatment

The child with nonsyndromic FTC usually presents with a solitary thyroid mass [2, 35], which may rarely be an autonomous nodule [53–55]. Presentation due to a symptomatic bone metastasis is not uncommon in older adults, but can very rarely be the presenting symptom in younger individuals [56].

Ultrasonography (US) and fine-needle aspiration biopsy (FNAB) are the initial steps in the evaluation of any child with a nonfunctioning thyroid nodule. There are no consistently reliable US features that can distinguish FTC from a benign follicular adenoma [57, 58], but the absence of intra-nodular blood flow in a follicular neoplasm suggests a low probability of FTC [59]. FNAB of a FTC is characterized by abundant follicular epithelial cells in sheets with crowding and overlapping of cells, microfollicle formation, and scant or no colloid [8]. Cytology is usually classified as an indeterminate lesion: "atypia of undetermined significance," "follicular lesion of undetermined significance," "follicular neoplasm," or "suspicious for follicular neoplasm" [60]. If oncocytic cells are identified, the diagnosis of "Hürthle cell neoplasm" will be rendered. Recently, there has been the increasing use of adjunctive molecular testing of the FNA specimen to identify those indeterminate lesions that are more likely to be malignant [61–64]. In addition, one study measuring thyrotropin receptor (TSHR) mRNA in peripheral blood suggests that a TSHR mRNA >1 ng/μg has a high predictive value for the presence of carcinoma in indeterminate nodules [65]. Unfortunately, none of these novel approaches has been extensively validated in the adult population or tested in children.

In clinical practice, the initial evaluation and treatment of FTC in children is generally the same as for PTC [66–68]. Surgery by a high-volume thyroid surgeon is the definite therapy for pediatric FTC. At a minimum, the child with a FNAB that documents a follicular neoplasm should undergo an ipsilateral thyroid lobectomy and isthmusectomy. In children with previous radiation exposure to the thyroid, primary tumor size >4 cm, and/or significant contralateral thyroid nodularity, total thyroidectomy may be preferred. Total thyroidectomy is indicated for any child with known distant metastases. Lymph node dissection is rarely required, but in poorly differentiated tumors and HCC, tumors >4 cm, or in the rare case of the preoperative identification of malignant lymphadenopathy, the surgical management should be similar to PTC [69]. Intraoperative frozen section can be considered, specifically to assess for PTC, but frozen section cannot reliably distinguish FTC from benign disease and is not routinely recommended [70].

With a small minimally invasive FTC, lobectomy alone may be an adequate treatment [40], but with angioinvasive FTC or minimally invasive tumors >4 cm, completion thyroidectomy is typically considered. Completion thyroidectomy would also be advised for poorly differentiated tumors and HCC.

Once the diagnosis of FTC is made, imaging of the chest can be considered to assess for distant metastases, although the role of routine chest CT in the initial evaluation of children with FTC remains undetermined. In those children who have had thyroidectomy, a postoperative radioactive iodine (RAI) scan and a stimulated thyroglobulin level can help to stage the pediatric FTC patient and determine who may benefit from routine RAI treatment [66]. The universal prescription of RAI may not be warranted in low-risk FTC [40], but there is a paucity of data regarding the optimal treatment and outcomes of this disease when diagnosed during childhood. RAI should be given to treat known or suspected iodine-avid distant metastases and strongly considered in all children with widely invasive FTC.

The routine follow-up of children with FTC is similar to PTC, with monitoring of the thyroglobulin level while maintaining mild TSH suppression over the short term. One notable difference is that neck US is not as relevant for the pediatric FTC patient, particularly for conventional FTC, when there is no evidence of disease based upon the thyroglobulin data.

Conclusion

Pediatric FTC is a rare thyroid malignancy with a good prognosis. Although generally evaluated and treated similar to PTC, FTC is a distinct thyroid malignancy with different clinical behavior and pathophysiology. Further studies are needed to determine how best to identify children at high risk for FTC prior to surgery, to understand better long-term outcomes, and to better risk stratify those children who would benefit from more extensive thyroid surgery and RAI therapy. As with all thyroid tumors, children with FTC should be cared for at tertiary referral centers with expertise in pediatric thyroid cancer in order to optimize outcomes and facilitate research.

References

1. Hogan AR, Zhuge Y, Perez EA, Koniaris LG, Lew JI, Sola JE. Pediatric thyroid carcinoma: incidence and outcomes in 1753 patients. J Surg Res. 2009;156:167–72.
2. O'Gorman CS, Hamilton J, Rachmiel M, Gupta A, Ngan BY, Daneman D. Thyroid cancer in childhood: a retrospective review of childhood course. Thyroid. 2010;20:375–80.
3. Raval MV, Bentrem DJ, Stewart AK, Ko CY, Reynolds M. Utilization of total thyroidectomy for differentiated thyroid cancer in children. Ann Surg Oncol. 2010;17:2545–53.
4. Roy R, Kouniavsky G, Schneider E, et al. Predictive factors of malignancy in pediatric thyroid nodules. Surgery. 2011;150:1228–33.
5. Otto KJ, Lam JS, MacMillan C, Freeman JL. Diminishing diagnosis of follicular thyroid carcinoma. Head Neck. 2010;32:1629–34.
6. DeLellis RA, Lloyd RV, Heitz PU, Eng C, editors. Pathology and genetics of tumours of endocrine organs, World Health Organization Classification of Tumours, vol. 8. Lyon: IARC Press; 2004.
7. Sobrinho-Simoes M, Eloy C, Magalhaes J, Lobo C, Amaro T. Follicular thyroid carcinoma. Mod Pathol. 2011;24 Suppl 2:S10–8.
8. McHenry CR, Phitayakorn R. Follicular adenoma and carcinoma of the thyroid gland. Oncologist. 2011;16:585–93.
9. DeLellis RA. Pathology and genetics of thyroid carcinoma. J Surg Oncol. 2006;94:662–9.
10. Lo CY, Chan WF, Lam KY, Wan KY. Follicular thyroid carcinoma: the role of histology and staging systems in predicting survival. Ann Surg. 2005;242:708–15.
11. Lang W, Choritz H, Hundeshagen H. Risk factors in follicular thyroid carcinomas. A retrospective follow-up study covering a 14-year period with emphasis on morphological findings. Am J Surg Pathol. 1986;10:246–55.
12. D'Avanzo A, Treseler P, Ituarte PH, et al. Follicular thyroid carcinoma: histology and prognosis. Cancer. 2004;100:1123–9.
13. Sobrinho-Simoes M, Maximo V, Castro IV, et al. Hurthle (oncocytic) cell tumors of thyroid: etiopathogenesis, diagnosis and clinical significance. Int J Surg Pathol. 2005;13:29–35.
14. Lo CY, Lam KY, Wan KY. Insular thyroid carcinoma in adolescents. Eur J Surg. 2000;166:585–8.
15. Yusuf K, Reyes-Mugica M, Carpenter TO. Insular carcinoma of the thyroid in an adolescent: a case report and review of the literature. Curr Opin Pediatr. 2003;15:512–5.
16. Kumar A, Bal CS. Differentiated thyroid cancer. Indian J Pediatr. 2003;70:707–13.
17. Woodruff SL, Arowolo OA, Akute OO, Afolabi AO, Nwariaku F. Global variation in the pattern of differentiated thyroid cancer. Am J Surg. 2010;200:462–6.
18. Mishra A, Mishra SK, Agarwal A, Das BK, Agarwal G, Gambhir S. Metastatic differentiated thyroid carcinoma: clinicopathological profile and outcome in an iodine deficient area. World J Surg. 2002;26:153–7.
19. Demidchik YE, Saenko VA, Yamashita S. Childhood thyroid cancer in Belarus, Russia, and Ukraine after Chernobyl and at present. Arq Bras Endocrinol Metabol. 2007;51:748–62.

20. LiVolsi VA, Abrosimov AA, Bogdanova T, et al. The Chernobyl thyroid cancer experience: pathology. Clin Oncol R Coll Radiol Great Brit. 2011;23:261–7.
21. Nikiforov YE, Nikiforova MN. Molecular genetics and diagnosis of thyroid cancer. Nat Rev Endocrinol. 2011;7:569–80.
22. Esapa CT, Johnson SJ, Kendall-Taylor P, Lennard TW, Harris PE. Prevalence of Ras mutations in thyroid neoplasia. Clin Endocrinol (Oxf). 1999;50:529–35.
23. Manenti G, Pilotti S, Re FC, Della Porta G, Pierotti MA. Selective activation of ras oncogenes in follicular and undifferentiated thyroid carcinomas. Eur J Cancer. 1994;30A:987–93.
24. Kroll TG, Sarraf P, Pecciarini L, et al. PAX8-PPARgamma1 fusion oncogene in human thyroid carcinoma [corrected]. Science. 2000;289:1357–60.
25. Nikiforova MN, Lynch RA, Biddinger PW, et al. RAS point mutations and PAX8-PPAR gamma rearrangement in thyroid tumors: evidence for distinct molecular pathways in thyroid follicular carcinoma. J Clin Endocrinol Metab. 2003;88:2318–26.
26. Eberhardt NL, Grebe SK, McIver B, Reddi HV. The role of the PAX8/PPARgamma fusion oncogene in the pathogenesis of follicular thyroid cancer. Mol Cell Endocrinol. 2010;321:50–6.
27. French CA, Alexander EK, Cibas ES, et al. Genetic and biological subgroups of low-stage follicular thyroid cancer. Am J Pathol. 2003;162:1053–60.
28. Nikiforov YE. Molecular diagnostics of thyroid tumors. Arch Pathol Lab Med. 2011;135:569–77.
29. Maximo V, Botelho T, Capela J, et al. Somatic and germline mutation in GRIM-19, a dual function gene involved in mitochondrial metabolism and cell death, is linked to mitochondrion-rich (Hurthle cell) tumours of the thyroid. Br J Cancer. 2005;92:1892–8.
30. Liaw D, Marsh DJ, Li J, et al. Germline mutations of the PTEN gene in Cowden disease, an inherited breast and thyroid cancer syndrome. Nat Genet. 1997;16:64–7.
31. Nagy R, Ganapathi S, Comeras I, et al. Frequency of germline PTEN mutations in differentiated thyroid cancer. Thyroid. 2011;21:505–10.
32. Smith JR, Marqusee E, Webb S, et al. Thyroid nodules and cancer in children with PTEN hamartoma tumor syndrome. J Clin Endocrinol Metab. 2011;96:34–7.
33. Ngeow J, Mester J, Rybicki LA, Ni Y, Milas M, Eng C. Incidence and clinical characteristics of thyroid cancer in prospective series of individuals with Cowden and Cowden-like syndrome characterized by germline PTEN, SDH, or KLLN alterations. J Clin Endocrinol Metab. 2011;96:E2063–71.
34. Nose V. Thyroid cancer of follicular cell origin in inherited tumor syndromes. Adv Anat Pathol. 2010;17:428–36.
35. Welch Dinauer CA, Tuttle RM, Robie DK, et al. Clinical features associated with metastasis and recurrence of differentiated thyroid cancer in children, adolescents and young adults. Clin Endocrinol (Oxf). 1998;49:619–28.
36. Giuffrida D, Scollo C, Pellegriti G, et al. Differentiated thyroid cancer in children and adolescents. J Endocrinol Invest. 2002;25:18–24.
37. Chow SM, Law SC, Mendenhall WM, et al. Differentiated thyroid carcinoma in childhood and adolescence-clinical course and role of radioiodine. Pediatr Blood Cancer. 2004;42:176–83.
38. Farahati J, Bucsky P, Parlowsky T, Mader U, Reiners C. Characteristics of differentiated thyroid carcinoma in children and adolescents with respect to age, gender, and histology. Cancer. 1997;80:2156–62.
39. Machens A, Holzhausen HJ, Dralle H. The prognostic value of primary tumor size in papillary and follicular thyroid carcinoma. Cancer. 2005;103:2269–73.
40. Thompson LD, Wieneke JA, Paal E, Frommelt RA, Adair CF, Heffess CS. A clinicopathologic study of minimally invasive follicular carcinoma of the thyroid gland with a review of the English literature. Cancer. 2001;91:505–24.
41. Alfalah H, Cranshaw I, Jany T, et al. Risk factors for lateral cervical lymph node involvement in follicular thyroid carcinoma. World J Surg. 2008;32:2623–6.
42. Sugino K, Ito K, Nagahama M, et al. Prognosis and prognostic factors for distant metastases and tumor mortality in follicular thyroid carcinoma. Thyroid. 2011;21:751–7.
43. Lin JD, Chao TC, Chen ST, Huang YY, Liou MJ, Hsueh C. Operative strategy for follicular thyroid cancer in risk groups stratified by pTNM staging. Surg Oncol. 2007;16:107–13.
44. van Heerden JA, Hay ID, Goellner JR, et al. Follicular thyroid carcinoma with capsular invasion alone: a nonthreatening malignancy. Surgery. 1992;112:1130–6. discussion 1136–1138.
45. La Quaglia MP, Corbally MT, Heller G, Exelby PR, Brennan MF. Recurrence and morbidity in differentiated thyroid carcinoma in children. Surgery. 1988;104:1149–56.
46. Kowalski LP, Goncalves Filho J, Pinto CA, Carvalho AL, de Camargo B. Long-term survival rates in young patients with thyroid carcinoma. Arch Otolaryngol Head Neck Surg. 2003;129:746–9.
47. Lee YM, Lo CY, Lam KY, Wan KY, Tam PK. Well-differentiated thyroid carcinoma in Hong Kong Chinese patients under 21 years of age: a 35-year experience. J Am Coll Surg. 2002;194:711–6.
48. Asari R, Koperek O, Scheuba C, et al. Follicular thyroid carcinoma in an iodine-replete endemic goiter region: a prospectively collected, retrospectively analyzed clinical trial. Ann Surg. 2009;249:1023–31.
49. Mai KT, Khanna P, Yazdi HM, et al. Differentiated thyroid carcinomas with vascular invasion: a comparative study of follicular, Hurthle cell and papillary thyroid carcinoma. Pathology. 2002;34:239–44.
50. Furlan JC, Bedard YC, Rosen IB. Clinicopathologic significance of histologic vascular invasion in papillary and follicular thyroid carcinomas. J Am Coll Surg. 2004;198:341–8.
51. Lopez-Penabad L, Chiu AC, Hoff AO, et al. Prognostic factors in patients with Hurthle cell neoplasms of the thyroid. Cancer. 2003;97:1186–94.
52. Stojadinovic A, Hoos A, Ghossein RA, et al. Hurthle cell carcinoma: a 60-year experience. Ann Surg Oncol. 2002;9:197–203.
53. Tan C, Sidhu S, Sywak M, Delbridge L. Management of hyperfunctioning single thyroid nodules in the era of minimally invasive thyroid surgery. ANZ J Surg. 2009;79:386–9.
54. Yalla NM, Reynolds LR. Hurthle cell thyroid carcinoma presenting as a "hot" nodule. Endocr Pract. 2011;17:e68–72.
55. Croom 3rd RD, Thomas Jr CG, Reddick RL, Tawil MT. Autonomously functioning thyroid nodules in childhood and adolescence. Surgery. 1987;102:1101–8.
56. Ying AK, Huh W, Bottomley S, Evans DB, Waguespack SG. Thyroid cancer in young adults. Semin Oncol. 2009;36:258–74.
57. Sillery JC, Reading CC, Charboneau JW, Henrichsen TL, Hay ID, Mandrekar JN. Thyroid follicular carcinoma: sonographic features of 50 cases. AJR. 2010;194:44–54.
58. Seo HS, Lee DH, Park SH, Min HS, Na DG. Thyroid follicular neoplasms: can sonography distinguish between adenomas and carcinomas? J Clin Ultrasound. 2009;37:493–500.
59. Iared W, Shigueoka DC, Cristofoli JC, et al. Use of color Doppler ultrasonography for the prediction of malignancy in follicular thyroid neoplasms: systematic review and meta-analysis. J Ultrasound Med. 2010;29:419–25.
60. Cibas ES, Ali SZ. The Bethesda system for reporting thyroid cytopathology. Am J Clin Pathol. 2009;132:658–65.
61. Nikiforov YE, Ohori NP, Hodak SP, et al. Impact of mutational testing on the diagnosis and management of patients with cytologically indeterminate thyroid nodules: a prospective analysis of 1056 FNA samples. J Clin Endocrinol Metab. 2011;96:3390–7.
62. Vriens MR, Weng J, Suh I, et al. MicroRNA expression profiling is a potential diagnostic tool for thyroid cancer. Cancer. 2012;118:3426–32.

63. Melck AL, Yip L. Predicting malignancy in thyroid nodules: molecular advances. Head Neck. 2012;34:1355–61.
64. Ferraz C, Eszlinger M, Paschke R. Current state and future perspective of molecular diagnosis of fine-needle aspiration biopsy of thyroid nodules. J Clin Endocrinol Metab. 2011;96:2016–26.
65. Milas M, Shin J, Gupta M, et al. Circulating thyrotropin receptor mRNA as a novel marker of thyroid cancer: clinical applications learned from 1758 samples. Ann Surg. 2010;252:643–51.
66. Waguespack SG, Francis G. Initial management and follow-up of differentiated thyroid cancer in children. J Natl Compr Canc Netw. 2010;8:1289–300.
67. Tuttle RM, Ball DW, Byrd D, et al. Thyroid carcinoma. J Natl Compr Canc Netw. 2010;8:1228–74.
68. Haugen BR, Alexander EK, Bible KC, Doherty GM, Mandel SJ, Nikiforov YE, Pacini F, Randolph GW, Sawka AM, Schlumberger M, Schuff KG, Sherman SI, Sosa JA, Steward DL, Tuttle RM, Wartofsky L. 2015 American Thyroid Association Management Guidelines for Adult Patients with Thyroid Nodules and Differentiated Thyroid Cancer: American Thyroid Association Guidelines Task Force on Thyroid Nodules and Differentiated Thyroid Cancer. Thyroid. 2016;26:1–133.
69. Grubbs EG, Rich TA, Li G, et al. Recent advances in thyroid cancer. Curr Probl Surg. 2008;45:156–250.
70. Udelsman R, Westra WH, Donovan PI, Sohn TA, Cameron JL. Randomized prospective evaluation of frozen-section analysis for follicular neoplasms of the thyroid. Ann Surg. 2001;233:716–22.

External Radiation Therapy for Follicular Carcinoma

78

James D. Brierley and Richard W. Tsang

Introduction

The role of external beam radiation therapy (RT) in the management of follicular thyroid cancer can be subdivided into adjuvant, radical, and palliative. The intent of adjuvant therapy is to improve the results of standard therapy consisting surgery and radioactive iodine; however, the exact role is controversial. Unlike radioactive iodine, external beam RT is a local therapy; therefore, its role is confined to situations where a local therapy is required to maximize local regional control of the disease, beyond what can be achieved with optimal surgery and radioactive iodine. Therefore its role is generally limited to patients deemed to have unresectable or residual disease after surgery, or patients at high risk of locoregional recurrence, e.g., older patients with extensive extrathyroidal extension of disease, residual disease following surgery, or extensive lymphatic spread.

Radical External Beam Radiotherapy for Gross Disease

In Sheline et al.'s report from 1966 on their experience of RT in 58 patients treated between 1935 and 1964, they described the use of RT in a variety of thyroid histologies and clinical situations [1]. Despite the limitations of the radiation during this time period, the paper described the effectiveness of RT in controlling gross residual disease. Nine patients had follicular tumors and four with gross disease, and one died from progressive tumor growth 3 years later, but three were free of disease 2–16 years after radiation. Five other patients had infiltration of the trachea but no gross disease; two died of local disease and three had no evidence of disease 5–18 years after treatment. This data although old suggests that external beam RT can control gross follicular thyroid cancer and may have a role in patients with microscopic residual disease. Other studies have reported a complete clinical response rate for gross disease ranging from 40 % [2, 3] to 60 % at 5 years [4, 5]. However these studies did not separate the results of treatment of follicular and papillary tumors.

J.D. Brierley, MBBS, FRCP, FRCR, FRCPC (✉)
R.W. Tsang, MD, FRCP(C)
Department of Radiation Oncology, Princess Margaret Hospital, University of Toronto, 610 University Ave., Toronto, ON M5G 2M9, Canada
e-mail: james.brierley@rmp.uhn.on.ca

External Beam Radiotherapy as Adjuvant Therapy

As discussed in the section on papillary thyroid cancer, external beam RT is a local therapy and would only be expected to be beneficial when there is a high risk of local recurrence. This usually means when there is residual disease after surgical resection in patients with extrathyroidal extension. Mazzaferri and Jhiang reported 278 patients with follicular thyroid cancer among 1,355 patients with differentiated thyroid cancer, 12 % of which had extrathyroid extension, compared with 8 % in patients with papillary thyroid cancer [6]. The local recurrence rate was 38 % in patients with extrathyroidal extension compared to 25 % in patients without extrathyroidal extension ($p=0.001$), although this difference was observed in papillary thyroid cancer and not follicular. However, for both histologies there was a higher risk of death from cancer in patients with extrathyroidal extension ($p=0.001$). Given the higher risk of extrathyroidal extension in follicular compared to papillary thyroid cancer, it might be thought that it would be easier to demonstrate a benefit from RT in patients with follicular thyroid cancer. However as discussed below, the evidence for a benefit in follicular thyroid cancer is less strong than in papillary thyroid cancer (Table 78.1). This might be because of the smaller number of patients but also because of the natural history of high-risk follicular thyroid cancer in which there is

L. Wartofsky, D. Van Nostrand (eds.), *Thyroid Cancer*, DOI 10.1007/978-1-4939-3314-3_78

a greater risk of distant metastases resulting in tumor-related death. Therefore, it may be more difficult to demonstrate improved local control, and local issues may be less important to the patient if the predominant problem is that of distant spread of disease causing death.

Simpson et al. in the transCanada study suggested that patients with microscopic residual follicular cancer following resection may benefit from RT. The local control rates in patients treated by surgery and radioactive iodine were similar to those treated with the addition of external beam radiation, despite that patients who had additional external beam radiation tended to have more extensive disease. In the two studies which demonstrated a benefit to adjuvant external beam radiation in papillary thyroid cancer, neither showed a benefit in follicular thyroid cancer [4, 12]. In contrast Esik et al. reported on a series of 56 patients with follicular cancer of whom 43 patients had no gross residual disease [7]. Patients treated with radiation had a significantly better local regional relapse-free rate when the dose was considered to be adequate, compared to those given an inadequate dose, but none of the patients received radioactive iodine [7]. Most reports that suggest a role for adjuvant external beam radiation do not separate differentiated cancers into papillary or follicular [5, 13, 14]. An analysis of patients with papillary or follicular carcinoma identified a high-risk subgroup who were older (age of 60 year or older) with extrathyroid extension and no gross residual disease. Among the 70 patients with these features, 47 received RT and 23 did not. There was a higher CSS (78 % versus 59 % $p=0.04$) and LRFR (84 % versus 57 % $p=0.01$) in patients who received RT (Fig. 78.1).

The group from MD Anderson has reported on their experience in treating locally advanced differentiated thyroid carcinoma with external beam radiotherapy [10]. As RT was standard in their institution for these patients, there was no comparison with patients who did not receive radiation therapy. They reported an overall 4-year local regional relapse-free rate of 79 % in these high-risk patients and concluded that postoperative conformal RT provides durable locoregional disease control for patients with high-risk differentiated thyroid cancer. There were 104 papillary thyroid cancers and 21 follicular cancers in the cohort. In a univariate analysis, follicular histology was associated with a significantly poorer local regional control and survival than papillary thyroid cancer, but there was no difference by multivariate analysis.

Despite the differing conclusions and a lack of definitive data specific to follicular thyroid cancer, we believe that in patients at high risk of recurrence in the thyroid bed (older patients with gross extrathyroid extension and gross or microscopic residual disease without metastatic disease), it is logical to assume that they may benefit from intensifying

Table 78.1 Results of adjuvant external beam radiotherapy in high-risk disease follicular thyroid cancer from retrospective studies: 10-year local recurrence

	Surgery with and without ^{131}I	Surgery, RT, and with and without ^{131}I
Esik [7]	42 %[a]	2 %[a]
Ford[b] [8]	63 %[a]	18 %[a]
Phlips [9]	21 %	3 %
Schwartz[c] [10]		21 %
Tubiana[b] [11]	21 %	14 %

[a]Compares low dose vs. higher dose
[b]Papillary and follicular histologies combined
[c]At 4 years, papillary and follicular combined, no RT arm

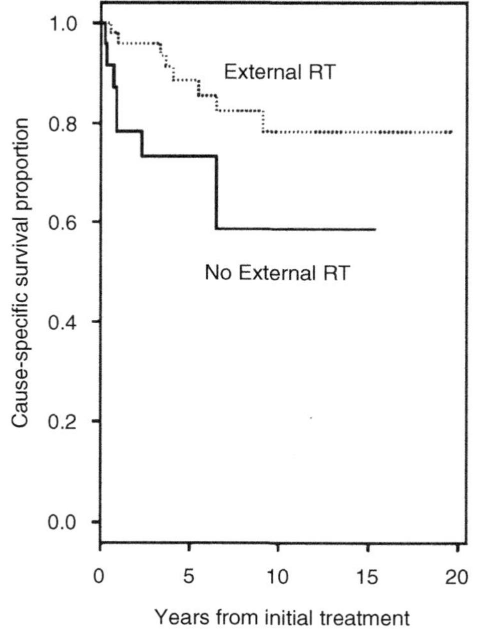

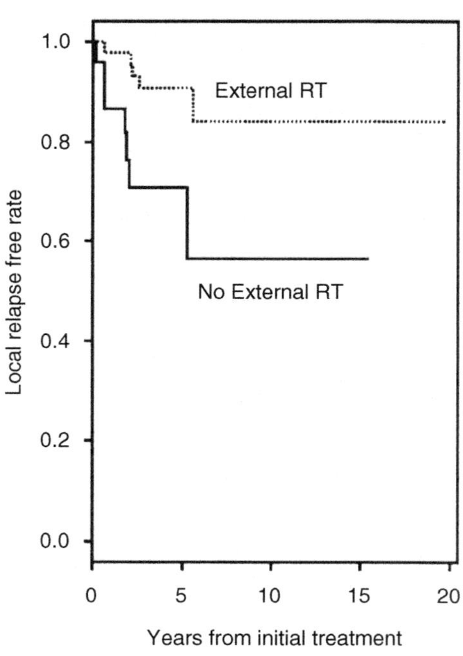

Fig. 78.1 Effect of the use of beam radiotherapy on cause specific survival and local relapse-free rate in patients over the age of 60 with differentiated thyroid cancer (papillary and follicular combined) with extrathyroid extension and no evidence of gross residual disease by Kaplan Meier analysis [13]

local regional therapy with the addition of external beam radiation, in addition to radioactive iodine. The thyroid bed alone is irradiated in patients at high risk of recurrence in the thyroid bed. The cervical lymph nodes are included in patients with extensive nodal involvement with extranodal extension and soft tissue invasion. RT to the cervical lymph nodes is also considered in patients with nodal disease that does not take up radioactive iodine such as Hürthle cell tumors as discussed below.

Hürthle Cell Carcinoma

In an analysis of 18 patients with Hürthle cell carcinoma treated at a single institution over a 50-year period, a role for external beam radiation was suggested in a variety of situations. In nine patients treated either adjuvantly or for salvage following recurrence, there was a 50 % local regional control rate at 5 years; however, all ten patients who died succumbed from metastatic disease. All patients who received palliative radiation experienced relief of pain or similar symptoms for a median of 12 months. It was concluded that Hürthle cell carcinoma is a radiosensitive tumor, and patients with large invasive tumors, particularly when other adverse features are present such as nodal metastases and vascular or extrathyroidal extension, may benefit from adjuvant external beam radiation [15].

External Beam Radiotherapy

The thyroid bed is a technically challenging volume to treat as the thyroid bed curves around the vertebral body and includes the air column in the trachea. It can be difficult to adequately treat the thyroid bed and spares the spinal cord to a dose within tolerance. A variety of techniques have been described that produce adequate dose distribution [16]. Advances in radiation techniques utilizing inversed planned intensity-modulated radiation therapy (IMRT) that result in better dose distribution to the areas at risk and reduce the volume of normal tissues to a minimum are described elsewhere in the book. Well-planned external beam RT has acceptable acute toxicity and rarely produces serious complications. In patients assigned to the radiation arm of the German randomized control study in differentiated thyroid cancer that closed because of poor accrual, it was noted that the majority of patients experience mild to moderate acute side effects only from adjuvant external beam radiotherapy [17]. At the first follow-up examination, most side effects had subsided, and acute toxicity was tolerable in these patients. Late toxicity is infrequent, and the most common is skin telangiectasia, increased skin pigmentation, soft tissue fibrosis, and mild lymphedema predominantly in the submental area. Esophageal and especially tracheal stenosis is rare. Neither Tsang et al. [4] nor Farahati et al. [12] reported any RTOG grade IV late toxicity in differentiated thyroid cancer. In contrast a more recent study using higher doses of radiation and larger volumes reported that 5 % of their patients required percutaneous endoscopic gastrostomy tube for late esophageal stenosis [18]. It should be noted however that when utilizing concurrent chemoradiation, acute toxicity may be significant and some centers recommend prophylactic enteral nutrition.

Palliation

The effectiveness of ^{131}I for metastatic disease depends greatly on the site of the metastasis. It is well known that as a generalization, lung metastases respond well to radioactive iodine. Although it has been noted that the outcome of patients with metastases from follicular histology is worse than for papillary thyroid histology, most studies on the management of metastases do not analyze the clinical outcome by histology. Casara et al. in a series of patients with distant metastases reported that those aged 40 or older or those with bone metastases were much less likely to concentrate radioactive iodine and achieve a complete response [19]. Only 3 % of bone metastases were considered to have achieved a complete response following radioactive iodine. Similar poor control of bone metastases have been reported by others [20–22], and therefore an aggressive surgical approach has been recommended [22, 23]. Not all bone secondaries, however, are amenable to surgical resection, and therefore external beam radiation in addition to radioactive iodine is appropriate and may result in long-term control [24]. External beam radiation also has an important role in palliating symptomatic bone pain or spinal cord compression.

Brain metastases from thyroid cancer are unusual. In a study of metastases from the brain of all histologies, 32 were treated with surgical excision and had a better median disease-specific survival (16.7 months) than those that did not underwent surgery (median survival 3.4 months), and there was no apparent benefit from external beam radiation [25]. In another series external beam radiation resulted in complete response in three out of four patients with measurable disease [26]. External beam radiotherapy should probably be offered if surgical resection is not possible; however, it is uncertain if it has any benefit after complete excision of brain metastases. Single large lung metastases causing hemoptysis or obstruction may also respond to RT.

The role of RT in controlling gross residual disease after surgery and in unresectable disease was discussed above. In patients with symptomatic recurrent disease and poor performance status or widespread incurable disease in whom high-dose RT for long-term control is not appropriate, shorter-course RT may be effective in controlling local symptoms such as pain, skin ulceration, and obstruction.

References

1. Sheline GE, Galante M, Lindsay S. Radiation therapy in the control of persistent thyroid cancer. Am J Roentgenol Radium Ther Nucl Med. 1966;97:923–30.
2. Glanzmann C, Lutolf UM. Long-term follow-up of 92 patients with locally advanced follicular or papillary thyroid cancer after combined treatment. Strahlenther Onkol. 1992;168:260–9.
3. O' Connell M, A'Hern RP, Harmer CL. Results of external beam radiotherapy in differentiated thyroid carcinoma: a retrospective study from the Royal Marsden Hospital. Eur J Cancer. 1994;30A: 733–9.
4. Tsang RW, Brierley JD, Simpson WJ, Panzarella T, Gospodarowicz MK, Sutcliffe SB. The effects of surgery, radioiodine and external radiation therapy on the clinical outcome of patients with differentiated thyroid cancer. Cancer. 1998;82:375–88.
5. Tubiana M, Haddad E, Schlumberger M, Hill C, Rougier P, Sarrazin D. External radiotherapy in thyroid cancers. Cancer. 1985;55: 2062–71.
6. Mazzaferri EL, Jhiang SM. Long-term impact of initial surgical and medical therapy on papillary and follicular thyroid cancer. Am J Med. 1994;97:418–28.
7. Esik O, Nemeth G, Eller J. Prophylactic external irradiation in differentiated thyroid cancer: a retrospective study over a 30-year observation period. Oncology. 1994;51:372–9.
8. Ford D, Giridharan S, McConkey C, et al. External beam radiotherapy in the management of differentiated thyroid cancer. Clin Oncol (R Coll Radiol). 2003;15:337–41.
9. Phlips P, Hanzen C, Andry G, Van Houtte P, Fruuling J. Postoperative irradiation for thyroid cancer. Eur J Surg Oncol. 1993;19:399–404.
10. Schwartz DL, Lobo MJ, Ang KK, et al. Postoperative external beam radiotherapy for differentiated thyroid cancer: outcomes and morbidity with conformal treatment. Int J Radiat Oncol Biol Phys. 2009;74:1083–91.
11. Tubiana M, Schlumberger M, Rougier P, et al. Long-term results and prognostic factors in patients with differentiated thyroid carcinoma. Cancer. 1985;55:794–804.
12. Farahati J, Reiners C, Stuschke M, et al. Differentiated thyroid cancer. Impact of adjuvant external radiotherapy in patients with perithyroidal tumor infiltration (stage pT4). Cancer. 1996;77: 172–80.
13. Brierley JD, Tsang RW, Panzarella T. et al. Prognostic factors and the effect of treatment with radioactive iodine ane external beam radiation on patient with differentiated thyroid cancer seen at a single institution over forty years. Clin Endocrinol (Oxf) 2005;63:418–27.
14. Sautter-Bihl ML, Raub J, Hetzel-Sesterheim M, Heinze HG. Differentiated thyroid cancer: prognostic factors and influence of treatment on the outcome in 441 patients. Strahlenther Onkol. 2001;177:125–31.
15. Foote RL, Brown PD, Garces YI, McIver B, Kasperbauer JL. Is there a role for radiation therapy in the management of Hurthle cell carcinoma? Int J Radiat Oncol Biol Phys. 2003;56:1067–72.
16. Tsang RW, Brierley JD. The thyroid. In: Cox JD, Kian Ang K, editors. Radiation oncology. St Louis: Mosby; 2003.
17. Schuck A, Biermann M, Pixberg MK, et al. Acute toxicity of adjuvant radiotherapy in locally advanced differentiated thyroid carcinoma. First results of the multicenter study differentiated thyroid carcinoma (MSDS). Strahlenther Onkol. 2003;179:832–9.
18. Terezakis SA, Lee KS, Ghossein RA, et al. Role of external beam radiotherapy in patients with advanced or recurrent nonanaplastic thyroid cancer: memorial Sloan-Kettering Cancer Center experience. Int J Radiat Oncol Biol Phys. 2009;73:795–801.
19. Casara D, Rubello D, Saladini G, Gallo V, Masarotto G, Busnardo B. Distant metastases in differentiated thyroid cancer: long-term results of radioiodine treatment and statistical analysis of prognostic factors in 214 patients. Tumori. 1991;77:432–6.
20. Brown AP, Greening WP, McCready VR, Shaw HJ, Harmer CL. Radioiodine treatment of metastatic thyroid carcinoma: the Royal Marsden Hospital experience. Br J Radiol. 1984;57:323–7.
21. Schlumberger M, Challeton C, De Vathaire F, et al. Radioactive iodine treatment and external radiotherapy for lung and bone metastases from thyroid carcinoma. J Nucl Med. 1996;37:598–605.
22. Proye CA, Dromer DH, Carnaille BM, et al. Is it still worthwhile to treat bone metastases from differentiated thyroid carcinoma with radioactive iodine? World J Surg. 1992;16:640–5; discussion 5–6.
23. Niederle B, Roka R, Schemper M, Fritsch A, Weissel M, Ramach W. Surgical treatment of distant metastases in differentiated thyroid cancer: indication and results. Surgery. 1986;100:1088–97.
24. Brierley JD, Tsang RW. External-beam radiation therapy in the treatment of differentiated thyroid cancer. Semin Surg Oncol. 1999;16:42–9.
25. Chiu AC, Delpassand ES, Sherman SI. Prognosis and treatment of brain metastases in thyroid carcinoma. J Clin Endocrinol Metab. 1997;82:3637–42.
26. McWilliams RR, Giannini C, Hay ID, Atkinson JL, Stafford SL, Buckner JC. Management of brain metastases from thyroid carcinoma: a study of 16 pathologically confirmed cases over 25 years. Cancer. 2003;98:356–62.

Determinants of Prognosis of Follicular Thyroid Carcinoma

79

Henry B. Burch

Determinants of Prognosis in Follicular Thyroid Cancer

A large number of retrospective analyses have examined patient and tumor characteristics associated with a poor prognosis in patients with follicular thyroid cancer (FTC) [1–6]. Compared to patients with papillary thyroid cancer (PTC), follicular thyroid cancer (FTC) patients are more likely to be older, more likely to be male (although the male-to-female ratio remains less than one), more likely to have unifocal disease, less likely to have direct tumor extension or cervical lymph nodes, and more likely to have distant metastases [7]. Factors consistently found to negatively impact prognosis in follicular thyroid cancer include patient age greater than 45, tumor size larger than 4 cm, local tumor extension beyond the thyroid, extensive capsular and vascular invasion, and the presence of distant metastases (Table 79.1). In addition, certain variants of follicular thyroid cancer, including oxyphilic (Hürthle cell) carcinomas (HCC) and insular carcinomas, are associated with a generally worse prognosis [8, 9].

The impact of clinical factors on survival is illustrated in an early series of 100 patients with pure follicular thyroid cancer receiving treatment at the Mayo Clinic over a 35-year period [10]. The overall cancer-related mortality was 29 % at 20 years. However, patients with only one negative prognostic indicator had a 20-year mortality of only 14 %, while those patients with two or more predictors had a 92 % likelihood of having died from thyroid cancer at 20 years. A study from the University of San Francisco found that patients with tumor-specific deaths were older (66±9.3 years) at the time of diagnosis, compared to those with recurrence (59±10 years) and those remaining disease-free (42±17 years) [2]. Similarly, these authors found that disease-free patients had initial tumor sizes of 3.0±2.0 cm, compared to 4.8±4.0 in those dying from their disease. Another study, including 198 cases with follicular and oxyphilic (Hürthle cell) thyroid cancer, found that patients aged less than 40 years, with tumors smaller than 5 cm and no local extension or distant metastases, had a 100 % 15-year survival, compared to 40 % survival in older patients, those with larger tumors, or those with disease outside the thyroid [3]. A 2002 study, including 215 patients with follicular thyroid cancer, found that factors negatively influencing disease-specific survival included the presence of known postoperative residual macroscopic disease, extrathyroidal extension, distant metastases, or failure to treat with postoperative radioiodine therapy [6]. An Austrian study in 2004 compared prognostic factors in 435 patients with PTC to those in 168 patients with FTC [11]. Disease-specific mortality at 20 years was 28 % in FTC patients, compared to 9 % in PTC patients. FTC patients were older and more likely to present with distant metastases than PTC patients. By multivariate analysis, only tumor size and the presence of distant metastases were associated with decreased survival in FTC patients, compared to PTC patients in whom age ≥45 and lymph node involvement were also associated with worse survival.

As noted above, patients with the Hürthle cell carcinoma (HCC) variant of FTC tend to have a worse prognosis. A study comparing 89 HCC patients to 38 patients with Hürthle cell adenomas (HCA) found that HCC patients were older and had larger tumors than HCA patients [9]. Local invasion was noted in 39 % of patients, distant metastases in 18 %, and lymph node metastases in 25 %, and foci of anaplastic transformation were found in 8 % of patients. Forty percent of HCC patients died from thyroid carcinoma or complications of treatment during an average follow-up period of 10.7 years.

Two recent studies have examined prognosis in FTC patients with distant metastases [12, 13]. One study of 233 FTC patients receiving care at a single medical center compared prognosis in 70 patients with lung metastases to

H.B. Burch, MD, FACE (✉)
Endocrinology Division, Uniformed Services University of the Health Sciences, Walter Reed National Military Medical Center, 8901 Wisconsin Avenue, American Building, Room 5053, Bethesda, MD 20889, USA
e-mail: Henry.burch@med.navy.mil

L. Wartofsky, D. Van Nostrand (eds.), *Thyroid Cancer*, DOI 10.1007/978-1-4939-3314-3_79

Table 79.1 Poor prognostic factors for differentiated thyroid cancer

Large tumors (>4. 0 cm)
Male sex
Advanced tumor grade
Tumors with local extension
Distant metastases
Extensive vascular and capsular invasion

163 patients without distant metastases [12]. Patients with lung metastases were older (55.6 vs. 40.1 years), had larger tumors (6.1 cm vs. 3.6 cm), were less likely to be disease-free on subsequent follow-up (5.7 % vs. 98 %), and more likely to die of their disease (42.9 % vs. 4.3 %). A second study compared prognosis in FTC and PTC patients with distant metastases [13]. Three-year survival was significantly lower (62 % vs. 75 %) in FTC than in PTC patients with distant metastases, and both FTC histology and iodine non-avidity were associated by multivariate analysis with decreased survival.

Minimally Invasive Follicular Thyroid Cancer (MI-FTC)

An important prognostic consideration in patients with follicular thyroid carcinoma is the degree of capsular and vascular invasion. FTC patients may be divided into a minimally invasive (MI-FTC) group, representing 80–90 % of cases, and widely invasive (WI-FTC) group, representing 10–20 % of cases in modern series [1, 14, 15]. MI-FTC patients are further categorized into those with capsular invasion alone and those with both capsular and vascular invasion. Patients with WI-FTC have a higher risk of distant metastases at diagnosis [16] and higher risk for recurrence and cancer-related death compared to patients with MI-FTC [17–21]. Patients with capsular invasion alone have a particularly indolent disease and a survival rate which approximates that of the general population [15, 19]. A study published in 2011 examined outcomes in 124 patients with FTC, classified by degree of invasion into three groups, including capsular invasion alone (Group 1), minimally invasive with both capsular and vascular invasion (Group 2), and widely invasive (Group 3) [15]. Disease-free survival was 97 % in Group 1, 81 % in Group 2, and 45 % in Group 3, respectively. Another study, examining disease-specific survival in 156 FTC patients followed an average of 14.4 years, found mortality rates of 20.2 % in patients with widely invasive FTC compared to 0 % in patients with minimally invasive disease [20].

Effect of Therapy on Prognosis

As is the case with papillary thyroid cancer, retrospective assessment of the effect of therapy on prognosis is hampered by the fact that patients selected to receive more extensive therapy are likely to have more advanced disease. Therefore, a finding of no difference in survival between patients receiving or not receiving a therapy, such as radioiodine ablation, might actually indicate a beneficial effect since these patients would have been expected to have a shorter survival than those with less advanced disease. Looking at the effect of the extent of surgery on survival, one study found that among 214 patients operated upon for follicular thyroid cancer, those treated with total thyroidectomy had survival rates similar to patients receiving less extensive procedures [22]. Another study, after adjusting for other risk factors in a multivariate analysis, found no difference in survival between 19 patients undergoing lobectomy and 81 patients treated with a bilateral procedure [10]. Finally, an analysis of 215 patients with follicular thyroid cancer treated at a single institution found no difference in local-regional control or survival in patients undergoing lobectomy compared to those treated with total or near-total thyroidectomy [6]. Conversely, most studies have shown that patients with incomplete removal of their tumor (generally due to non-resectability) have worse survival than those with no known residual macroscopic or microscopic disease after surgery [1, 20]. The use of radioiodine for remnant ablation after thyroidectomy for FTC has been found to have variable effects on survival, with a definite beneficial effect found in some studies [6, 22, 23], a marginal effect in one study [24], and no effect in still another study [25]. Surveillance for recurrence is generally facilitated by remnant ablation [26].

References

1. Grebe SK, Hay ID. Follicular thyroid cancer. Endocrinol Metab Clin North Am. 1995;24(4):761–801.
2. Emerick GT, Duh QY, Siperstein AE, Burrow GN, Clark OH. Diagnosis, treatment, and outcome of follicular thyroid carcinoma. Cancer. 1993;72(11):3287–95.
3. Rao RS, Parikh HK, Deshmane VH, Parikh DM, Shrikhande SS, Havaldar R. Prognostic factors in follicular carcinoma of the thyroid: a study of 198 cases. Head Neck. 1996;18(2):118–24.
4. Lin JD, Huang MJ, Juang JH, et al. Factors related to the survival of papillary and follicular thyroid carcinoma patients with distant metastases. Thyroid. 1999;9(12):1227–35.
5. Zidan J, Kassem S, Kuten A. Follicular carcinoma of the thyroid gland: prognostic factors, treatment, and survival. Am J Clin Oncol. 2000;23(1):1–5.
6. Chow SM, Law SC, Mendenhall WM, et al. Follicular thyroid carcinoma: prognostic factors and the role of radioiodine. Cancer. 2002;95(3):488–98.

7. Chow SM, Law SC, Au SK, et al. Differentiated thyroid carcinoma: comparison between papillary and follicular carcinoma in a single institute. Head Neck. 2002;24(7):670–7.
8. Baloch ZW, LiVolsi VA. Unusual tumors of the thyroid gland. Endocrinol Metab Clin North Am. 2008;37(2):297–310, vii.
9. Lopez-Penabad L, Chiu AC, Hoff AO, et al. Prognostic factors in patients with hürthle cell neoplasms of the thyroid. Cancer. 2003;97:1186–94.
10. Brennan MD, Bergstralh EJ, van Heerden JA, McConahey WM. Follicular thyroid cancer treated at the Mayo Clinic, 1946 through 1970: initial manifestations, pathologic findings, therapy, and outcome. Mayo Clin Proc. 1991;66(1):11–22.
11. Passler C, Scheuba C, Prager G, et al. Prognostic factors of papillary and follicular thyroid cancer: differences in an iodine-replete endemic goiter region. Endocr Relat Cancer. 2004;11(1):131–9.
12. Lin JD, Chao TC, Hsueh C. Follicular thyroid carcinomas with lung metastases: a 23-year retrospective study. Endocr J. 2004;51(2): 219–25.
13. Sampson E, Brierley JD, Le LW, et al. Clinical management and outcome of papillary and follicular (differentiated) thyroid cancer presenting with distant metastasis at diagnosis. Cancer. 2007;110(7):1451–6.
14. Brassard M, Borget I, Edet-Sanson A, et al. Long-term follow-up of patients with papillary and follicular thyroid cancer: a prospective study on 715 patients. J Clin Endocrinol Metab. 2011;96(5): 1352–9. Epub 2011 Mar 9.
15. O'Neill CJ, Vaughan L, Learoyd DL, et al. Management of follicular thyroid carcinoma should be individualised based on degree of capsular and vascular invasion. Eur J Surg Oncol. 2011;37(2):181–5. Epub 2010 Dec 8.
16. Asari R, Koperek O, Scheuba C, et al. Follicular thyroid carcinoma in an iodine-replete endemic goiter region: a prospectively collected, retrospectively analyzed clinical trial. Ann Surg. 2009;249:1023–31.
17. Davis NL, Bugis SP, McGregor GI, Germann E. An evaluation of prognostic scoring systems in patients with follicular thyroid cancer. Am J Surg. 1995;170(5):476–80.
18. Jorda M, Gonzalez-Campora R, Mora J, Herrero-Zapatero A, Otal C, Galera H. Prognostic factors in follicular carcinoma of the thyroid. Arch Pathol Lab Med. 1993;117(6):631–5.
19. van Heerden JA, Hay ID, Goellner JR, et al. Follicular thyroid carcinoma with capsular invasion alone: a nonthreatening malignancy. Surgery. 1992;112(6):1130–6.
20. Lo CY, Chan WF, Lam KY, Wan KY. Follicular thyroid carcinoma. The role of histology and staging systems in predicting survival. Ann Surg. 2005;22:708–15.
21. Thompson LD, Wieneke JA, Paal E, Frommelt RA, Adair CF, Heffess CS. A clinicopathologic study of minimally invasive follicular carcinoma of the thyroid gland with a review of the English literature. Cancer. 2001;91(3):505–24.
22. Young RL, Mazzaferri EL, Rahe AJ, Dorfman SG. Pure follicular thyroid carcinoma: impact of therapy in 214 patients. J Nucl Med. 1980;21(8):733–7.
23. Samaan NA, Schultz PN, Hickey RC, et al. The results of various modalities of treatment of well differentiated thyroid carcinomas: a retrospective review of 1599 patients. J Clin Endocrinol Metab. 1992;75(3):714–20.
24. DeGroot LJ, Kaplan EL, Shukla MS, Salti G, Straus FH. Morbidity and mortality in follicular thyroid cancer. J Clin Endocrinol Metab. 1995;80(10):2946–53.
25. Jensen MH, Davis RK, Derrick L. Thyroid cancer: a computer-assisted review of 5287 cases. Otolaryngol Head Neck Surg. 1990;102(1):51–65.
26. Mazzaferri EL, Kloos RT. Clinical review 128: current approaches to primary therapy for papillary and follicular thyroid cancer. J Clin Endocrinol Metab. 2001;86(4):1447–63.

Part IX

Variants of Thyroid Cancer

Aggressive Variants of Papillary Thyroid Carcinoma and Poorly Differentiated Carcinoma

80

Zubair W. Baloch and Virginia A. LiVolsi

This chapter will discuss the salient pathologic features of aggressive variants of papillary thyroid carcinoma and poorly differentiated thyroid carcinoma. Thyroid papillary carcinoma, the most common endocrine malignancy, is a tumor of such indolent biological and clinical behavior that the survival rate for patients with this tumor is equal or almost equal to that of individuals who never had cancer. Only a small percentage of patients with papillary carcinoma of the thyroid are affected by tumors of considerable clinical aggressiveness. Some experts have referred to these papillary carcinoma variants as "real carcinomas" of the thyroid [1]. These include tall-cell, columnar-cell, and diffuse sclerosing variants and the hobnail variant.

Tall-Cell Variant

The tall-cell variant (TCV) was initially defined as an aggressive lesion by Hawk and Hazard in 1976 [2]. The definition they proposed was the presence of a papillary tumor whose cells are at least twice as long (tall) as they are wide; however, recently this has been modified to tumor cells being three times their width [3]. These tumors show complex papillary architecture and the papillae are elongated. The papillae may coalesce, and the low-power appearance may simulate a trabecular and/or solid growth pattern in parts of the tumor. The cells are large and often eosinophilic without cytoplasmic granularity, features which distinguish them from true oncocytic/Hürthle cells [3, 4] (Fig. 80.1). The nuclei are elongated and sometimes conform to the elongated cell in which they are contained and have prominent intranuclear grooves, clearing, and intranuclear inclusions [4, 5]. Multiple intranuclear inclusions (aka soap bubble inclusions) may be seen, and these can be especially helpful in fine-needle aspiration preparations in diagnosing this tumor as a tall-cell variant of papillary carcinoma [6].

Many clinicians feel that there are significant clinical consequences to the pathologic diagnosis of TCV [7, 8]. However, according to the literature there appears to be confusion on the part of pathologists in recognizing this tumor or alternatively in overdiagnosing the TCV. In our experience, the pathology review of these cases often raises the following questions: How much of a tumor needs to show the features of TCV to be diagnosed as such? What is not a TCV? What are the consequences of a diagnosis of TCV? And finally, what are the molecular features of this group of tumors, and how can they be helpful in understanding the pathogenesis and behavior of this subtype of papillary carcinoma of the thyroid.

A tall-cell variant of papillary thyroid carcinoma should be comprised of at least 50 % TCV morphology [5, 9, 10]. The literature is problematic in this regard with TCV being diagnosed in tumors having anywhere from 10 to 70 % of TCV morphology in a particular tumor [10]. To further complicate this issue, some early publications have included tall-cell variant under the heading of poorly differentiated thyroid carcinoma [11]. It is of particular importance to note that many classic variant of PTC, especially the Warthin-like variant, will show a minor component of TCV (usually 5–10 %) [9]. These are not to be diagnosed as a TCV papillary carcinoma, but the finding should be mentioned in the pathology report. In our experience, metastases or recurrences of these cases may show a higher percentage of TCV.

In order to isolate true examples of TCV, it is necessary to not include other neoplasms that may superficially resemble that tumor but do not have its prognostic implications. These include Warthin-like papillary carcinoma, oncocytic papillary carcinoma or its follicular variant, Hürthle cell

Z.W. Baloch, MD, PhD (✉) • V.A. LiVolsi, MD
Department of Pathology and Laboratory Medicine, Perelman School of Medicine, University of Pennsylvania Medical Center, 6 Founders Pavilion, 3400 Spruce Street, Philadelphia, PA 19104, USA
e-mail: balocj@mail.med.upenn.edu; linus@mail.med.upenn.edu

L. Wartofsky, D. Van Nostrand (eds.), *Thyroid Cancer*, DOI 10.1007/978-1-4939-3314-3_80

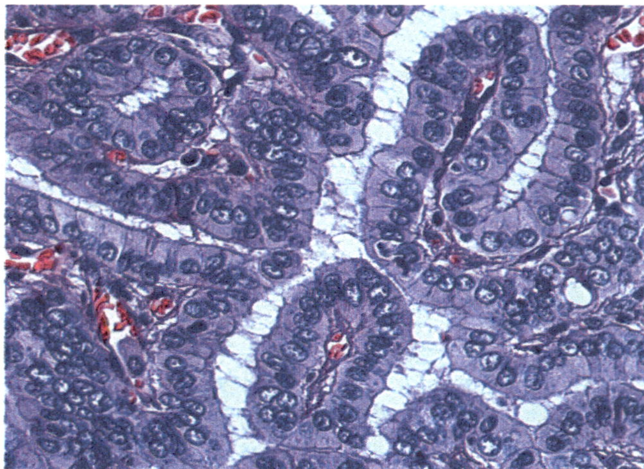

Fig. 80.1 Tall-cell variant. Papillary formations are lined by tumor cells with eosinophilic cytoplasm and cell height two to three times the width

tumor, or nodule with papillary growth pattern [4]. There is a general consensus that as a group, the TCV has both a higher likelihood of recurrence and a higher death rate than classical PTC. Initially, this was attributed to the fact that TCV presented as large tumors with extrathyroidal extension (ETE) in older patients [5]. However, Ghossein et al. have reported their experience indicating that gland-confined TCV without ETE has followed a more aggressive clinical course as compared to conventional intrathyroidal PTC [7].

It has been suggested that the aggressive behavior of TCV-PTC is associated with the molecular profile of these tumors [12]. The aggressive behavior of TCV could be related to certain factors elaborated by the tumor. The high expression of Muc1 and type IV collagenase (matrix metalloproteinase-2) in TCV tumors may allow for degradation of stroma and greater invasive properties [13, 14]. The aggressive behavior of TCV may also be related to the higher prevalence of activating point mutations of the BRAF, as these mutations in PTC have been associated with higher frequency of extra-glandular extension and nodal metastases. Finally, another important clinical aspect of TCV-PTC is the fact that it is overrepresented in those thyroid carcinomas that are refractory to radioactive iodine (RAI) therapy [5, 12].

In summary, the clinicopathologic data available on TCV clearly demonstrate that this is a biologically and clinically aggressive form of papillary thyroid carcinoma. Therefore, it is prudent that the presence of any foci of tall cells should be mentioned in a pathology report regardless of the percentage of tall-cell cytology that is found. This information then should prompt the clinician to fully treat and more carefully monitor the patient for recurrence, distant metastasis, and transformation to anaplastic carcinoma.

Columnar-Cell Variant (CCV)

The identification of this particular thyroid tumor was initially made by Evans in 1986, who described two cases of this clinically aggressive thyroid tumor with unique histologic features of papillary formation, hyperchromatic elongated nuclei, and prominent nuclear pseudostratification [15] (Fig. 80.2). LiVolsi later described an additional feature of prominent subnuclear vacuolation resembling early secretory endometrium in cases of columnar-cell carcinoma [16]. This peculiar morphology is also reminiscent of colonic adenomas/adenocarcinomas [17]. CDX2, a nuclear transcription factor important in intestinal development, has been shown to be selectively expressed in 50 % of cases of CCV [18, 19]. In the past, some authors have lumped these tumors with TCV-PTC; however, most experts believe the tumor to be a distinct variant of papillary thyroid carcinoma. It has been proposed that a diagnosis of CCV should only be rendered when a thoroughly sampled tumor contains at least 30 % columnar cells [3]. It is not unusual to see papillary, follicular, trabecular, and solid patterns in CCV. Clinically, it has been observed that CCV is aggressive, due to its rapid growth, high local recurrence rate, and frequent lung, brain, and bone metastases. As a consequence, aggressive surgical and medical management are recommended for these tumors [20].

The encapsulated variant of CCV also reported by Evans [21] is a thickly encapsulated tumor, which may only show capsular invasion and behave in a more indolent fashion. Wenig et al. [22] have reported similar observations. In this study the cases of CCV, which were encapsulated or limited to the thyroid, had favorable clinical course as compared to two cases with extensive extrathyroidal extension. Thus, the spectrum of CCV has been broadened; when one includes

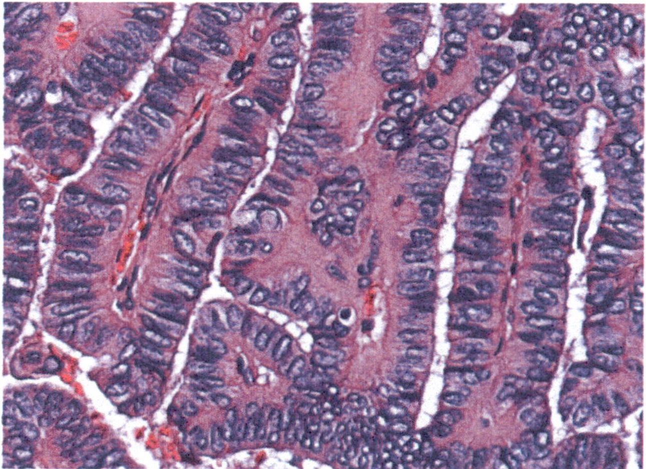

Fig. 80.2 Columnar-cell variant. Papillary formation, hyperchromatic elongated nuclei, and prominent nuclear pseudostratification

tumors that are predominantly encapsulated and are confined within the thyroid, the adverse prognosis originally reported does not appear to be present [21]. BRAF mutations can be seen in approximately 33 % of CCV-PTC similar to conventional PTC [23].

Diffuse Sclerosis Variant (DSV)

The diffuse sclerosis variant is a rare subtype of PTC which was first described by Vickery et al. in 1985 [24]. It represents only about 1.8 % of all papillary carcinomas in large series. This tumor, which most often affects children and young adults, may present as bilateral goiter [25, 26]. It is histologically characterized by dense sclerosis, extensive squamous metaplasia, focal to diffuse lymphocytic infiltration, numerous psammoma bodies, and small papillary to solid tumor deposits within intraglandular lymphatics (Fig. 80.3). The squamous metaplasia of the tumor papillae resembles "morular" metaplasia of the endometrium [1].

Due to presence of numerous psammoma bodies, an ultrasound of the thyroid will show lymphatics outlined by calcium sometimes referred to as a "snow-storm appearance" [27]. Grossly, the tumor is extremely hard reflecting the extensive calcification [28, 29]. As stated above, the lymphocytic infiltrates are found around the tumor foci; indeed, the background thyroid shows well-developed chronic lymphocytic thyroiditis [30]. Both the histology and immunoprofile of the background thyroid are identical to Hashimoto's disease. It is unclear if the thyroiditis precedes the tumor or develops as a reaction to the neoplasm [29]. The lesions are virtually all associated with regional nodal metastases at diagnosis. They often show extracapsular extension, distant, and nodal metastases (almost 100 % will have regional node involvement at presentation) and recur in the neck. Earlier studies have shown that these tumors have a somewhat more serious prognosis than usual childhood/adolescent papillary cancer and a decreased disease-free survival when compared with the usual-type papillary carcinoma [28, 30, 31]. However, the overall survival is not significantly different. The recent reports and case series have shown that the prognosis of this DSV-PTC is as good as that of classic PTC after complete surgical treatment and postoperative radioiodine ablation [26].

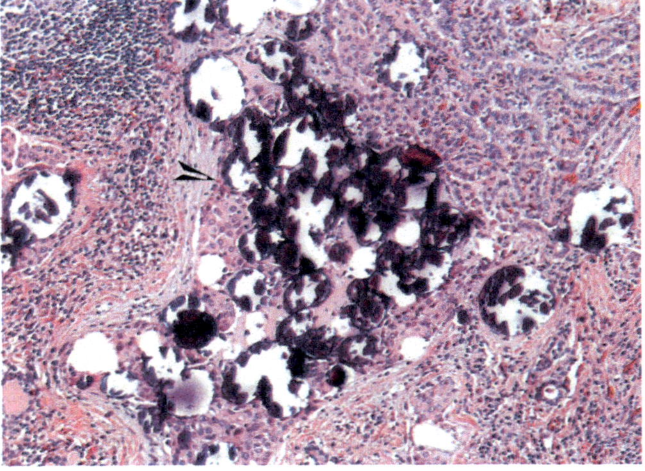

Fig. 80.3 Diffuse sclerosis variant. Nests of tumor cells (*arrowhead*) containing numerous psammoma bodies in a background of chronic lymphocytic thyroiditis

In a study of the genetic alterations in the DSV, no BRAF (V600) mutations were found, but all the cases showed RET proto-oncogene (RET)/PTC rearrangements [32]. These rearrangements, especially RET/PTC1, are more common in tumors seen in children and young adults, especially those associated with a history of radiation exposure. The morphologic features of DSV have been described in some of the thyroid tumors from children exposed to radiation after the Chernobyl accident [33, 34]. Therefore, it is not surprising that the presence of RET/PTC is a prominent genetic event that may render DSV-PTC susceptible to RET-directed therapy.

Solid Variant (SV)

A solid growth pattern is noted focally in many papillary carcinomas. When the solid growth represents >50 % of the tumor mass, a diagnosis of the solid variant of papillary carcinoma may be made [1]. The solid variant is most commonly seen in children and has been reported in >30 % of patients with papillary carcinoma after the Chernobyl nuclear accident [35]. It usually presents as a solid nodule with infiltration into the surrounding thyroid parenchyma. By light microscopy the tumor shows solid nests of tumor cells with nuclear features of papillary carcinoma, separated by delicate to broad collagenous bands (Fig. 80.4). Some tumors may show focal areas of follicular and papillary architecture. The nuclear features are those of papillary carcinoma, although the nuclei tend to be more rounded than oval. About 40 % of these tumors show vascular invasion and extrathyroidal extension [35].

Although some studies, particularly those from Japan, have considered the solid papillary carcinoma as a poorly differentiated tumor with a guarded prognosis; this has not been found in North America and Europe. It is important to recognize that these lesions are papillary carcinomas and to not overdiagnose them as more aggressive tumors such as poorly differentiated (insular) carcinoma [36]. Both papillary and non-papillary cancers of the thyroid can demonstrate areas of solid growth and/or insular growth patterns. We believe that these two should be morphologically separated; the areas of insular carcinoma usually show well-defined nests of monotonous tumor cells with round nuclei and scant cytoplasm. Loose connective tissue stroma and prominent vascularity separate the tumor nests from each other. Occasionally these areas may show foci of tumor necrosis [37]. Albores-Saavedra et al. described five cases of macrofollicular variant of papillary carcinoma that exhibited a minor insular transformation. All these patients survived albeit with metastasis in 40 %, and these authors believed that the presence of insular component did not alter the excellent prognosis associated with papillary carcinoma [38]. Similar findings were reported by Ashfaq et al. who found that the aggressive clinical behavior of tumors with focal insular change is more dependent on the age of the patient and tumor stage rather than the presence of an insular growth pattern [39].

Solid variant does occur in adults, and in our experience, over one-third of these arise in patients with systemic autoimmune disease. The interrelationship of these disorders is unknown. The prognosis of solid variant of papillary cancer is almost as good as classic papillary carcinoma, both in children and in adults. They do not have the guarded prognosis of poorly differentiated carcinoma, even in the presence of necrosis [1, 35].

On molecular analysis, cases of SV-PTC arising in association with radiation exposure have shown RET/PTC rearrangements. Interestingly, a triplet deletion of the BRAF gene leading to the replacement of a valine and a lysine by a glutamate (BRAF V600E + K601) was first reported only in the solid variant of PTC by Trovisco et al. [40] and has been confirmed by other investigators [41].

Hobnail Variant

This rare variant of papillary thyroid carcinoma was described by Asioli et al. [42]. These tumors commonly occur in women and are associated with significant mortality as was seen in 50 % of the eight reported cases. The tumors in the reported series usually had more than 30 % of the tumor with hobnail features. This peculiar feature is characterized by tumor cell nuclei located in the middle or in the apex of the cytoplasm, i.e., bulging of the nuclei at the tip of the cell imparting the so-called "hobnail" appearance to the cells (Fig. 80.5). This morphology is also encountered in serous papillary carcinoma of the ovary, primary serous carcinoma of the peritoneum, breast micropapillary carcinoma, and bladder, kidney, and lung adenocarcinomas with hobnail features [42]. In a short communication Albores-Saavedra [43] elegantly explained that these cases represent the rare oncocytic variant of papillary carcinoma based on the fact that similar cell morphology can be seen in oncocytic tumors as originally described by Rosai et al. [44]. In addition, these tumors demonstrate eosinophilic cytoplasm, and electron microscopic studies will show mitochondrial-rich cytoplasm further supporting an oncocytic lineage. BRAF (V600E) mutations have been detected in >50 % of these tumors confirming the classification of these tumors as variants of PTC [42].

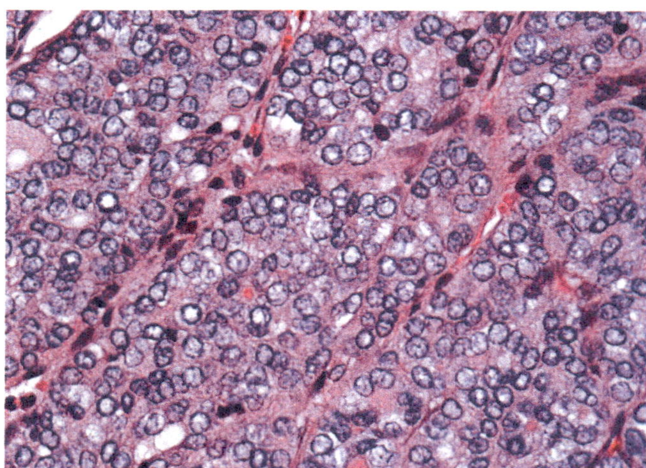

Fig. 80.4 Solid variant: solid nests of tumor cells showing nuclear features of papillary thyroid carcinoma

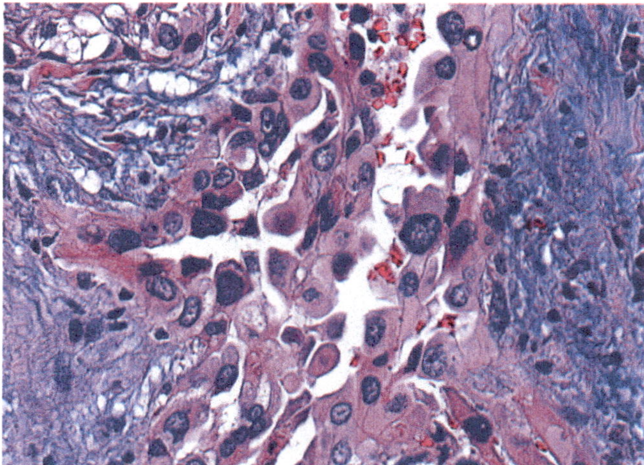

Fig. 80.5 Hobnail variant. Tumor cell with oncocytic cytoplasm and nuclei located in the middle or in the apex of the cytoplasm

Poorly Differentiated Thyroid Carcinoma (PDTC)

The term poorly differentiated thyroid carcinoma (PDTC) was first introduced by Granner and Buckwalter in 1963 [45] and then again defined in the 1980s by two different groups using two very different sets of criteria [11, 37]. The World Health Organization (WHO) finally acknowledged the entity of PDTC in 2004 as a follicular cell-derived neoplasm that shows limited evidence of structural follicular cell architecture and occupies both morphologically and behaviorally an intermediate position between differentiated and undifferentiated (anaplastic) carcinoma [3]. Because the insular growth pattern is considered to be one of the hallmark features of PDTC, it is prudent for the present discussion to further describe "insular carcinoma" of the thyroid.

In 1984 Carcangiu and colleagues described insular carcinoma as a tumor characterized by solid nests or islands ("insulae") of small and uniform tumor cells containing a variable number of microfollicles surrounded by thin-walled vessels (Fig. 80.6). The aggressive nature of this tumor was evident by the presence of mitotic figures, foci of necrosis, and frequently by lymphovascular invasion. Metastases to regional lymph nodes, lung, and bones were commonly seen with a high mortality rate as compared to conventional papillary and follicular carcinoma. These authors described the biologic behavior of this tumor as intermediate between well-differentiated and anaplastic thyroid carcinoma [37]. However, Sakamoto and colleagues proposed that the term poorly differentiated carcinoma should be applied to the tumors that are solid or trabecular and have loss of follicular and/or papillary architecture [11]. These variable definitions have led many authors to classify as PDTC even some of the aggressive variants of papillary carcinoma such as tall-cell and columnar-cell variants [46–49].

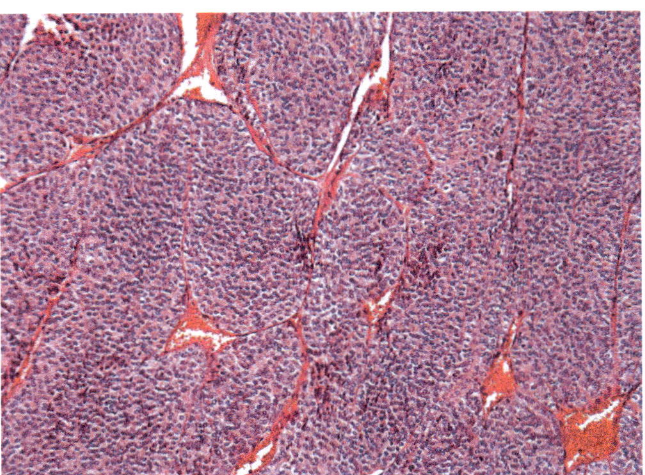

Fig. 80.6 Poorly differentiated carcinoma. Solid nests or islands ("insulae") of small and uniform tumor cells surrounded by thin-walled vessels

In 2006, a meeting was held in Turin to standardize the diagnostic criteria for PDTC. According to a consensus derived from that meeting, the poorly differentiated carcinoma is defined as a tumor with solid/trabecular/insular growth pattern, absence of classic nuclear features of papillary carcinoma, and presence of either convoluted nuclei, necrosis, or mitotic activity. This consensus was in accordance with the WHO definition of PDTC [50]. However, the Turin recommendations fell short of defining the amount of poorly differentiated areas within a thyroid carcinoma required to render a diagnosis of PDTC. Some authors have shown that a minor insular component within a well-differentiated carcinoma does not affect the prognosis, while others have shown that prognosis is altered adversely by the presence of a major insular component. In a study by Dettmer et al., even a minor component of PD (10–50 %) could adversely affect the prognosis [51].

Many PDTC will show a relationship to a well-differentiated carcinoma. This may be identified in the lesion at diagnosis of PDTC or may be found in previously resected tumors (i.e., the patient has a history of a thyroid carcinoma, and the poorly differentiated component is found in a recurrence or metastatic site). The well-differentiated tumor may be papillary carcinoma or a variant thereof (often follicular variant) or true follicular carcinoma [37, 52, 53].

Molecular profiling of PDTC reveals extremely heterogeneous findings with different studies describing BRAF, KRAS, and RET/PTC rearrangements. However, in a report describing molecular analysis of 65 cases of PDTC, RAS mutations in codon 61 were by far the most common genetic alteration in poorly differentiated carcinomas (23 % of cases), with all mutations in NRAS except one in the HRAS gene. No KRAS, RET/PTC, or PAX8/PPAR gamma genetic alteration was detected, and only a single BRAF mutation was found in a poorly differentiated carcinoma with a residual component of a TCV of papillary carcinoma [54, 55].

References

1. LiVolsi VA. Papillary thyroid carcinoma: an update. Mod Pathol. 2011;24 Suppl 2:S1–9.
2. Hawk WA, Hazard J. The many appearances of papillary carcinoma of the thyroid. Cleve Clin Q. 1976;43:207–16.
3. DeLellis RA, Lloyd RD, Heitz PU, Eng C, editors. WHO: pathology and genetics. Tumours of endocrine organs. Lyon: IARC Press; 2004.
4. LiVolsi VA. Papillary carcinoma tall cell variant (TCV): a review. Endocr Pathol. 2010;21:12–5.
5. Ghossein R, Livolsi VA. Papillary thyroid carcinoma tall cell variant. Thyroid. 2008;18:1179–81.
6. Solomon A, Gupta PK, LiVolsi VA, Baloch ZW. Distinguishing tall cell variant of papillary thyroid carcinoma from usual variant of

papillary thyroid carcinoma in cytologic specimens. Diagn Cytopathol. 2002;27:143–8.
7. Ghossein RA, Leboeuf R, Patel KN, Rivera M, Katabi N, Carlson DL, Tallini G, Shaha A, Singh B, Tuttle RM. Tall cell variant of papillary thyroid carcinoma without extrathyroid extension: biologic behavior and clinical implications. Thyroid. 2007;17:655–61.
8. Rivera M, Ghossein RA, Schoder H, Gomez D, Larson SM, Tuttle RM. Histopathologic characterization of radioactive iodine-refractory fluorodeoxyglucose-positron emission tomography-positive thyroid carcinoma. Cancer. 2008;113:48–56.
9. Akslen LA, LiVolsi VA. Prognostic significance of histologic grading compared with subclassification of papillary thyroid carcinoma. Cancer. 2000;88:1902–8.
10. Johnson TH, Lloyd R, Thompson NW, Beierwalters WH, Sisson JC. Prognostic implications of the tall cell variant of papillary carcinoma. Am J Surg Pathol. 1988;12:22–7.
11. Sakamoto A, Kasai N, Sugano H. Poorly differentiated carcinoma of the thyroid. Cancer. 1983;52:1849–55.
12. Rivera M, Ricarte-Filho J, Tuttle RM, Ganly I, Shaha A, Knauf J, Fagin J, Ghossein R. Molecular, morphologic, and outcome analysis of thyroid carcinomas according to degree of extrathyroid extension. Thyroid. 2010;20:1085–93.
13. Wreesmann VB, Sieczka EM, Socci ND, Hezel M, Belbin TJ, Childs G, Patel SG, Patel KN, Tallini G, Prystowsky M, Shaha AR, Kraus D, Shah JP, Rao PH, Ghossein R, Singh B. Genome-wide profiling of papillary thyroid cancer identifies MUC1 as an independent prognostic marker. Cancer Res. 2004;64:3780–9.
14. Chen Y, Zhu M, Zhou X, Lin W, Ni C, Li F, Zhang S, Gong Z. Expression of TTF-1 in thyroid tumors originating from follicular epithelium and its correlation with expression of RET, Galectin-3 and Mucin-1 genes. Zhonghua Yi Xue Za Zhi. 2002;82:257–61.
15. Evans HL. Columnar-cell carcinoma of the thyroid. A report of two cases of an aggressive variant of thyroid carcinoma. Am J Clin Pathol. 1986;85:77–80.
16. LiVolsi VA. Surgical pathology of the thyroid. Philadelphia: WB. Saunders; 1990.
17. LiVolsi VA. Unusual variants of papillary thyroid carcinoma. Adv Endocrinol Metab. 1995;6:39–54.
18. Sujoy V, Pinto A, Kovacs CM, et al. CDX2 is rarely expressed in columnar cell variant of papillary thyroid carcinoma: a study of ten cases. Mod Pathol. 2011;24:142A.
19. Enriquez ML, Baloch Z, Montone KT, Zhang PJ, LiVolsi V. CDX2 expression in columnar cell variant of papillary thyroid carcinoma. Am J Clin Pathol. 2012;137(5):722–6.
20. Silver CE, Owen RP, Rodrigo JP, Rinaldo A, Devaney KO, Ferlito A. Aggressive variants of papillary thyroid carcinoma. Head Neck. 2011;33:1052–9.
21. Evans HL. Encapsulated columnar-cell carcinoma of the thyroid. A report of four cases suggesting a favorable outcome. Am J Surg Pathol. 1996;20:1205–11.
22. Wenig BM, Thompson LD, Adair CF, Shmookler B, Heffess CS. Thyroid papillary carcinoma of columnar cell type: a clinicopathologic study of 16 cases. Cancer. 1998;82:740–53.
23. Chen JH, Faquin WC, Lloyd RV, Nose V. Clinicopathological and molecular characterization of nine cases of columnar cell variant of papillary thyroid carcinoma. Mod Pathol. 2011;24:739–49.
24. Vickery Jr AL, Carcangiu ML, Johannessen JV, Sobrinho-Simoes M. Papillary carcinoma. Semin Diagn Pathol. 1985;2:90–100.
25. McElvanna K, McCusker G, Stirling I. Diffuse sclerosing variant of papillary thyroid carcinoma – a rare cause of goitre in a young patient. Ulster Med J. 2007;76:113–4.
26. Lam AK, Lo CY. Diffuse sclerosing variant of papillary carcinoma of the thyroid: a 35-year comparative study at a single institution. Ann Surg Oncol. 2006;13:176–81.
27. Zhang Y, Xia D, Lin P, Gao L, Li G, Zhang W. Sonographic findings of the diffuse sclerosing variant of papillary carcinoma of the thyroid. J Ultrasound Med. 2010;29:1223–6.
28. Carcangiu ML, Bianchi S. Diffuse sclerosing variant of papillary thyroid carcinoma. Clinicopathologic study of 15 cases. Am J Surg Pathol. 1989;13:1041–9.
29. Soares J, Limbert E, Sobrinho-Simoes M. Diffuse sclerosing variant of papillary thyroid carcinoma. A clinicopathologic study of 10 cases. Pathol Res Pract. 1989;185:200–6.
30. Siegal A, Mimouni M, Kovalivker M, Griffel B. Latent childhood thyroid carcinoma in diffuse lymphocytic thyroiditis. J Surg Oncol. 1983;23:155–7.
31. Matias-Guiu X, Esquius J. Aberrant expression of HLA-DR antigen in diffuse sclerosing variant of papillary carcinoma of thyroid. J Clin Pathol. 1989;42:1309.
32. Sheu SY, Schwertheim S, Worm K, Grabellus F, Schmid KW. Diffuse sclerosing variant of papillary thyroid carcinoma: lack of BRAF mutation but occurrence of RET/PTC rearrangements. Mod Pathol. 2007;20:779–87.
33. Nikiforov YE, Rowland JM, Bove KE, Monforte-Munoz H, Fagin JA. Distinct pattern of ret oncogene rearrangements in morphological variants of radiation-induced and sporadic thyroid papillary carcinomas in children. Cancer Res. 1997;57:1690–4.
34. Nikiforov YE. Molecular diagnostics of thyroid tumors. Arch Pathol Lab Med. 2011;135:569–77.
35. LiVolsi VA, Abrosimov AA, Bogdanova T, Fadda G, Hunt JL, Ito M, Rosai J, Thomas GA, Williams ED. The Chernobyl thyroid cancer experience: pathology. Clin Oncol (R Coll Radiol). 2011;23:261–7.
36. Nikiforov YE, Erickson LA, Nikiforova MN, Caudill CM, Lloyd RV. Solid variant of papillary thyroid carcinoma: incidence, clinical- pathologic characteristics, molecular analysis, and biologic behavior. Am J Surg Pathol. 2001;25:1478–84.
37. Carcangiu ML, Zampi G, Rosai J. Poorly differentiated ("insular") thyroid carcinoma. A reinterpretation of Langhans' "wuchernde Struma". Am J Surg Pathol. 1984;8:655–68.
38. Albores-Saavedra J, Housini I, Vuitch F, Snyder 3rd WH. Macrofollicular variant of papillary thyroid carcinoma with minor insular component. Cancer. 1997;80:1110–6.
39. Ashfaq R, Vuitch F, Delgado R, Albores-Saavedra J. Papillary and follicular thyroid carcinomas with an insular component. Cancer. 1994;73:416–23.
40. Trovisco V, Soares P, Soares R, Magalhaes J, Sa-Couto P, Sobrinho-Simoes M. A new BRAF gene mutation detected in a case of a solid variant of papillary thyroid carcinoma. Hum Pathol. 2005;36:694–7.
41. Chiosea S, Nikiforova M, Zuo H, Ogilvie J, Gandhi M, Seethala RR, Ohori NP, Nikiforov Y. A novel complex BRAF mutation detected in a solid variant of papillary thyroid carcinoma. Endocr Pathol. 2009;20:122–6.
42. Asioli S, Erickson LA, Sebo TJ, Zhang J, Jin L, Thompson GB, Lloyd RV. Papillary thyroid carcinoma with prominent hobnail features: a new aggressive variant of moderately differentiated papillary carcinoma. A clinicopathologic, immunohistochemical, and molecular study of eight cases. Am J Surg Pathol. 2010;34:44–52.
43. Albores-Saavedra J. Papillary thyroid carcinoma with prominent hobnail features: a new aggressive variant of moderately differentiated papillary carcinoma. A clinicopathologic, immunohistochemical, and molecular study of 8 cases. Am J Surg Pathol. 2010;34:913. author reply 914.
44. Rosai J, Carcangui ML, DeLellis RA. Tumors of the thyroid gland. Washington, DC: Armed Forces Institute of Pathology; 1992.
45. Granner DK, Buckwalter JA. Poorly differentiated carcinoma of the thyroid gland. Surg Gynecol Obstet. 1963;116:650–6.

46. Sobrinho-Simoes M, Nesland JM, Johannessen JV. Columnar-cell carcinoma. Another variant of poorly differentiated carcinoma of the thyroid. Am J Clin Pathol. 1988;89:264–7.
47. Habib K, Auriol M, Sarfati E, de Roquancourt A, Wann AR, Brocheriou C, Chomette G. Undifferentiated carcinomas of the thyroid corpus. Apropos of 10 cases. Arch Anat Cytol Pathol. 1993;41:129–39.
48. Fonseca E, Sobrinho-Simoes M. Diagnostic problems in differentiated carcinomas of the thyroid. Pathol Res Pract. 1995;191:318–31.
49. Papotti M, Torchio B, Grassi L, et al. Poorly differentiated oxyphilic (Hurthle cell) carcinomas of the thyroid. Am J Surg Pathol. 1996;20:686–94.
50. Volante M, Landolfi S, Chiusa L, Palestini N, Motta M, Codegone A, Torchio B, Papotti MG. Poorly differentiated carcinomas of the thyroid with trabecular, insular, and solid patterns: a clinicopathologic study of 183 patients. Cancer. 2004;100:950–7.
51. Dettmer M, Schmitt A, Steinert H, Haldemann A, Meili A, Moch H, Komminoth P, Perren A. Poorly differentiated thyroid carcinomas: how much poorly differentiated is needed? Am J Surg Pathol. 2011;35:1866–72.
52. Basolo F, Pisaturo F, Pollina LE, Fontanini G, Elisei R, Molinaro E, Iacconi P, Miccoli P, Pacini F. N-ras mutation in poorly differentiated thyroid carcinomas: correlation with bone metastases and inverse correlation to thyroglobulin expression. Thyroid. 2000;10:19–23.
53. Tallini G. Poorly differentiated thyroid carcinoma. Are we there yet? Endocr Pathol. 2011;22:190–4.
54. Volante M, Rapa I, Gandhi M, Bussolati G, Giachino D, Papotti M, Nikiforov YE. RAS mutations are the predominant molecular alteration in poorly differentiated thyroid carcinomas and bear prognostic impact. J Clin Endocrinol Metab. 2009;94:4735–41.
55. Soares P, Trovisco V, Rocha AS, Feijao T, Rebocho AP, Fonseca E, Vieira de Castro I, Cameselle-Teijeiro J, Cardoso-Oliveira M, Sobrinho-Simoes M. BRAF mutations typical of papillary thyroid carcinoma are more frequently detected in undifferentiated than in insular and insular-like poorly differentiated carcinomas. Virchows Arch. 2004;444:572–6.

81 Miscellaneous and Unusual Tumors of the Thyroid Gland

Kenneth D. Burman, Matthew D. Ringel, and Barry M. Shmookler

Introduction

The majority of epithelial thyroid tumors maintain some degree of thyroid follicular cell function, as shown by thyroglobulin production and the ability to concentrate iodine. They also have typical histological appearances, such as those seen in papillary and follicular carcinomas. This chapter discusses a group of unusual primary thyroid neoplasms characterized by limited, or the absence of, differentiated thyroid cellular function and structure. In general, these tumors have more aggressive clinical courses than differentiated carcinomas. The term "poorly differentiated" is relatively nonspecific. To a pathologist, it might refer to the cellular architecture, whereas a clinician might believe a tumor is "poorly differentiated" when it traps radioiodine poorly. To both groups, however, the implication of more aggressive disease and poorer prognosis applies. This chapter also reviews tumors that metastasize to the thyroid gland. The thyroid tumors discussed in this chapter have been classified by the World Health Organization (WHO) under the category of "other" thyroid carcinomas, nonepithelial tumors, and, in the case of several histological types to be discussed, variants of papillary and follicular carcinoma [1, 2].

Most thyroid neoplasms originate from thyroid follicular epithelium, and poorly differentiated thyroid neoplasms represent 5–15 % of all thyroid tumors [3, 4] where the most common is probably anaplastic carcinoma. Based on the WHO recommendation, the previously described variants of spindle cell and giant cell carcinoma are now included under anaplastic carcinoma, whereas the small cell carcinoma variant is not included because nearly all these tumors have been reclassified as non-Hodgkin's lymphomas [5–7]. In addition, many tumors classified in the past as sarcomas have been reclassified as anaplastic carcinomas, but some sarcomas of the thyroid clearly exist. The important clinical and histological diagnostic features of these rare, often aggressive, tumors are discussed as well as the therapeutic options. Similar to the diagnosis and management of most cancers, the importance of approaching these patients in an organized multidisciplinary manner should be emphasized.

Squamous Cell Carcinoma of the Thyroid

Demographics

Primary squamous cell carcinoma of the thyroid is a rare disorder, containing cells of uncertain origin. The WHO classification defines squamous cell carcinoma as a tumor comprised entirely of cells that demonstrate intercellular bridges and/or form keratin [1]. This definition of squamous cell carcinoma is quite important, as up to 43 % of papillary carcinomas contain regions of squamous cell metaplasia, and many anaplastic carcinomas are partly comprised of squamoid regions (see Chap. 96). Adenosquamous cell carcinomas and adenoacanthomas, tumors containing regions of squamous cell carcinoma and adenocarcinoma (usually papillary), are also excluded by this WHO definition. Using these strict criteria, the incidence of squamous cell carcinoma of the thyroid is less than 1 % of all thyroid malignancies [8–11]. Squamous cell carcinoma appears to have a predilection to develop in thyroglossal duct remnants, accounting for an estimated 1 % of thyroglossal duct tumors

K.D. Burman, MD (✉)
Director, Divisions of Endocrinology, Washington Hospital Center and Georgetown University Hospital, 110 Irving Street NW 2A-72, Washington, DC 20010, USA
e-mail: kenneth.d.burman@medstar.net

M.D. Ringel, MD
Division of Endocrinology, Diabetes and Metabolism, Department of Internal Medicine, Wexner Medical Center, The Ohio State University, Columbus, OH, USA

B.M. Shmookler, MD
Department of Pathology, Washington Hospital Center and Medlantic Research Institute, Washington, DC, USA

L. Wartofsky, D. Van Nostrand (eds.), *Thyroid Cancer*, DOI 10.1007/978-1-4939-3314-3_81

(see Chap. 53). The vast majority of thyroglossal duct neoplasms are papillary thyroid cancer, and approximately 6 % have squamous cell origin [12]. Care must be taken to exclude local extension or metastasis from a laryngeal or other head and neck carcinoma. Squamous cell carcinoma of the lung can also metastasize to the thyroid gland.

The demographics of this tumor are difficult to determine because of the rarity of pure squamous cell thyroid carcinomas. We have reviewed recent case reports of pure squamous cell carcinoma published in the English literature since 1970 [8–11, 13–35] (Table 81.1). Similar to anaplastic carcinoma, the tumors usually present in the fifth, sixth, or seventh decades of life, but cases have been described in patients as young as 35 years of age. The female/male ratio is approximately 1.7:1.

Clinical Characteristics

Several cases of squamous cell carcinoma have been associated with thyroiditis and squamous cell metaplasia, but the etiology of this rare variant remains obscure. One patient with adenosquamous thyroid carcinoma has been described after radiation therapy [36], but thus far, no cases have been described in several large cohorts of patients with Hodgkin's disease who were followed longitudinally, making a relationship with prior radiation therapy unlikely.

The origin of squamous cells within the thyroid remains controversial, and several hypotheses have been proposed. Squamous cell carcinoma has been found within thyroglossal duct remnants and lingual thyroid glands and in association with lymphoma [16, 36–38]. These tumors were believed to derive from squamous epithelial cells in the walls of these cell rests. A few cases of pure squamous cell carcinoma appear to have developed from squamous metaplasia. However, as Klinck and Menk observed [39], this pattern of squamous metaplasia, leading to squamous cell carcinoma, has not been identified in other organs. Moreover, Harada and colleagues [11] did not identify any areas of squamous metaplasia in their series of squamous cell carcinomas. If squamous cell carcinoma commonly arose from squamous metaplasia, a higher occurrence of these cancers would be expected in clinical conditions associated with squamous metaplasia (e.g., thyroiditis, papillary thyroid carcinoma, and adenomatoid nodules), but this has not been reported.

Bond and colleagues [40] reported a variant thyroid epithelial cell population characterized by a squamoid appearance, the absence of thyroglobulin staining, and positive immunostaining for cytokeratin and vimentin. These cells had a higher proliferative capacity than the follicular cells in primary culture. The authors suggest that these cells may represent areas of squamous metaplasia within the thyroid gland; yet, they might also represent a small population of normal

Table 81.1 Demographics of patients with squamous cell carcinoma of the thyroid

First author	Number (n)	Age (years, mean)	Female (n)	Male (n)
Prakash	1	38	1	0
Bahuleyan	1	35	1	0
Harada	2	71 (at death)	2	0
White[a]	1	61	0	1
Kapoor	1	45	1	0
Misonou	1	61	1	0
Tsuchiya	3	63	2	1
Kampsen	2	65	2	0
Sarda	7	46	5	2
Theander	1	72	1	0
Chaudhary	1	76	1	0
Budd	2	59	1	1
Simpson	8	60	3	5
Huang	4	58	2	2
Bukachevsky[b]	1	73	1	0
Korvonin	4	62	3	1
Riddle	1	66	0	1
Shimaoka	3	60	1	2
Saito	1	71	1	0
Zimmer	1	64	1	0
Zhou	4			
Total	50	59	30	16

[a]Thyroglossal duct tumor
[b]Lingual thyroid cancer

squamoid thyroid cells that grow well in the cell culture environment.

Zimmer et al. [32] described a 64-year-old woman with an asymptomatic nodule who was determined to have squamous cell carcinoma of the thyroid gland as confirmed by cytokeratin staining and transmission electron microscopy. The patient developed local recurrence and expired 7 months after resection from local invasion and airway obstruction. Zhou [33] reviewed the clinical records of four patients with squamous cell thyroid cancer. Two of the four patients had surgical excision plus radiotherapy but died of local tumor recurrence at 6 and 13 months. One patient had surgery alone and died 4 months later of respiratory distress. The fourth patient had radical surgery coupled with radiotherapy and chemotherapy and was disease-free at 26-month follow-up. Squamous cell thyroid carcinoma may also occur in association with a well-differentiated carcinoma (particularly papillary carcinoma), an adenoma, a multinodular goiter, or (occasionally) chronic autoimmune thyroiditis [1, 2, 4]. Because of the intimate relationship to neoplastic glandular elements, some squamous cancers have been called "adenosquamous carcinomas." Undifferentiated carcinoma may be evident, along with the predominant squamous carcinoma [5]. Squamous carcinoma with extensive spindle cell change has been reported in association with tall-cell papillary carcinoma [6]. Mucin-producing carcinoma has been linked with squamous carcinoma [2, 41]. The presence of mucosubstances in the thyroid presents a complex diagnostic problem, and uncertainty about such neoplasms continues [42, 43]. Bland focal squamous metaplasia may occur in both follicular and papillary carcinomas, but this does not usually behave as squamous carcinoma.

Most patients with squamous cell carcinoma of the thyroid present with the rapid growth of a firm mass in a previously existing multinodular goiter. Symptoms generally begin over several weeks to months. The quick growth is often associated with pain, weight loss, night sweats, and local symptoms, e.g., dysphagia and dysphonia. Similar to some cases of anaplastic carcinoma, a syndrome of leukocytosis and non-parathyroid hormone-mediated hypercalcemia has been described [29, 31, 44, 45]. At least one cell line derived from a patient with squamous cell thyroid carcinoma has been characterized to make an interleukin la-like factor and a colony-stimulating factor [31]. Although many patients develop distant metastases during the course of their illness, the majority of patients present with only local neck complaints.

The diagnosis of squamous cell carcinoma is usually made on fine-needle aspiration (FNA) cytology or at the time of surgery for progressive local symptoms. These lesions do not typically concentrate radioiodine and are "cold" on radionuclide scanning. Care must be taken to exclude the possibility of metastases from local head and neck tumors or lung carcinoma. Appropriate radiological studies should be performed, such as neck and chest computed tomographic (CT), or magnetic resonance imaging (MRI) scans, bronchoscopy, endoscopy, and an otolaryngologic examination should be performed preoperatively to ensure that the tumor originated from the thyroid.

Treatment and Clinical Course

Squamous cell carcinoma of the thyroid has a clinical course that resembles anaplastic carcinoma. Complete surgical resection is the primary curative therapy, in combination with postoperative external beam radiation therapy. Radioiodine scanning and treatment have limited value, as nearly all these tumors are not iodine avid. A variety of chemotherapeutic regimens have been attempted to cure individual cases, including bleomycin, doxorubicin, and cisplatin, all with disappointing results. Thyroid hormone suppression is usually initiated, but the clinical utility of this treatment has not been documented well. These cancers, similar to anaplastic cancers, have likely sustained sufficient genetic alterations to lead to thyrotropin-independent growth. Palliative surgery and radiation therapy are appropriate in selected patients to avoid airway compromise and the inability to swallow.

Nearly all the patients reported with squamous cell carcinoma died within 16 months of diagnosis. These deaths were caused by distant metastases or local complications of disease. The rare long-term survivors of these tumors are those who presented with earlier stage disease who had a near-complete or complete surgical resection. After surgery, these patients were generally treated with external beam radiation.

Summary

Pure squamous cell carcinoma is a rare thyroid cancer with an extremely poor prognosis. Like anaplastic carcinoma, these tumors present as rapidly enlarging masses in older patients and are generally not responsive to radioiodine or conventional chemotherapy. Direct extension or metastases from other squamous cell carcinomas of the head, neck, and lungs must be ruled out before choosing a treatment plan. A cure seems possible only in those rare patients who present with surgically resectable disease. Generally, postoperative radiation therapy should be prescribed in these patients. Radioiodine and thyroid hormone suppression therapy have limited utility in this disease; however, thyroid hormone replacement is obviously required after thyroidectomy. Control of local disease is important to preserve the quality of life in patients with squamous cell carcinoma.

Poorly Differentiated ("Insular") Carcinoma

Demographics

Insular thyroid carcinoma was originally described by Langhans in 1907 [46] and termed "Wuchernde Struma." Subsequently, in 1984, Carcangiu and colleagues [47] renamed this variant, poorly differentiated carcinoma (insular carcinoma), because of the solid clusters of polygonal cells characteristic of this tumor and resembling pancreatic islet cells. Insular carcinoma is included as a variant of follicular carcinoma by the WHO [2] and generally appears to be more aggressive than well-differentiated follicular carcinoma but less aggressive than anaplastic carcinoma. From a histological standpoint, poorly differentiated carcinoma defines a group of follicular thyroid epithelium that retain sufficient differentiation to produce scattered small follicular structures and some thyroglobulin but that generally lack the typical morphological characteristics of papillary and follicular carcinoma [48, 49]. Instead, the histological patterns are described as solid, insular (islands of cells separated by connective tissue and artifactual spaces), trabecular, and alveolar, with tiny scattered follicles containing colloid within the solid, insular, and trabecular regions. These patterns may mix with each other, and small foci of characteristic follicular and papillary carcinoma may also be found, even both within the same neoplasm. The Bcl-2 protein (a suppressor of apoptosis) has been described in a large proportion of these tumors, in contrast to undifferentiated carcinoma [50].

We have reviewed the literature concerning well-documented cases of insular carcinoma [47, 48, 51–56]. The median age at presentation for the group is approx 54 years, with a range of 12–78 years. The incidence of this histological variant appears low. Mizukami and associates [57] identified only three cases of insular carcinoma of 800 thyroid tumors resected at their institution during 20 years. Machens et al. [52] found that 14 of 127 differentiated thyroid cancers were the insular subtype. Higher rates have been described in other populations; however, many of these groups included tumors with other "poorly differentiated" appearances, such as solid, trabecular, and alveolar patterns. It remains unclear whether this group of tumors described as "poorly differentiated" is a spectrum of one tumor type identified during the dedifferentiating process or whether each histological type represents a specific entity.

Clinical Characteristics

The prognosis of insular carcinoma has been controversial because of the varied histological pattern and the evidence of well-differentiated papillary or follicular carcinoma that can be found within most of these neoplasms. Although the controversy is understandable, the presence of the "primordial cells" in these neoplasms must be taken into account and the fact that they display many characteristics differing from well-differentiated cancers [58–61].

We have compared the presenting characteristics and clinical outcomes of patients with insular carcinoma reported in the literature by Mazzaferri and Jhiang [62] who studied 1,355 patients with well-differentiated thyroid cancer (Table 81.1).

Many larger patient series are summarized in detail below. Patients with insular carcinoma tended to be older, had larger primary tumors, and were more likely to present with metastases, compared to patients with differentiated carcinoma. Often, there is a preceding history of goiter in adults with insular carcinoma. The male/female ratio is similar to well-differentiated carcinoma. In the three largest series, the female/male ratio was 2.1:1. The most common complaint was an enlarging mass, but metastases in the neck, mediastinum, and femur have been reported. The duration of enlargement appears variable, but most of these tumors are slow-growing nodules that often enlarge for months or years before clinical diagnosis. These lesions are not typically iodine or technetium avid relative to normal thyroid tissue, and FNA biopsy is usually suggestive of malignancy. Children with this entity tend to present with early nodal metastases, either in the neck or mediastinum [57, 63, 64]. As with anaplastic and squamous cell carcinomas, insular carcinoma frequently develops in the setting of prior multinodular goiter, underscoring the importance of both long-term follow-up and the rapid recognition of changes in growth pattern.

Treatment and Clinical Course

The clinical course of insular thyroid carcinoma was initially described by Carcangiu in 1984 [47]. In their series of 25 patients, 11 (44 %) presented with intrathyroidal disease, 11 (44 %) with neck metastases or invasion of local neck structures, and 4 (12 %) with metastatic disease. With a mean follow-up of 3.5 years (range of 1–8 years), 11 (44 %) died of disease and 7 (28 %) were alive with disease. Of the four patients presenting with distant metastases, three died of disease during follow-up. The authors concluded that insular carcinoma was more aggressive than well-differentiated carcinoma but less aggressive than anaplastic carcinoma.

Falvo et al. [65] assessed 9 patients with insular thyroid cancer and compared their clinical characteristics to 27 patients of similar age and tumor size who had follicular and papillary cancer (follow-up range of 24–72 months). All the patients underwent total thyroidectomy. Vascular invasion was observed in 44 % of insular carcinomas ($p<0.05$ vs.

papillary carcinomas). No significant differences were observed relating to multifocality, lymph node metastases, or TNM (tumor, nodes, metastasis) tumor stage. The death rate of patients with insular carcinoma (33.3 %) was higher than that of patients with follicular ($p<0.05$) and papillary carcinoma ($p<0.01$). Distant metastases were observed in 66 % of insular carcinomas ($p<0.005$ vs. follicular carcinoma and $p<0.001$ vs. papillary carcinoma). Two patients (22.2 %) with insular carcinoma have remained disease-free ($p<0.001$ vs. those with follicular and papillary carcinomas). This study emphasized the poor prognostic features of insular thyroid cancer. Luna-Ortiz [66] have also concluded that insular thyroid cancer is generally aggressive, typically occurs later in life, and is frequently accompanied by a history of a chronic goiter. Ashfaq and colleagues [67] examined 41 patients who had insular carcinoma with a mean follow-up of 4 years (range, 1 month to 12 years). Clinical outcome information was available on 28 patients: 18 % died of disease, 21 % were alive with disease at the time of the study, 50 % were alive with no evidence of disease, and 11 % died of other causes but had known disease. Similar to the findings by Carcangiu and colleagues, only 41 % of patients presented with intrathyroidal lesions. They reported no difference in clinical outcome between patients with a minor (10–40 %) or predominant (50–90 %) histological component of insular carcinoma. The majority of these patients were treated with thyroidectomy followed by radioiodine.

Papotti and coworkers [58] addressed the treatment of thyroid cancers containing a "primordial cell" component by considering two tumor groups: those comprised predominantly of insular carcinoma ($n=31$) and those with predominant trabecular or solid patterns and a minor component of insular carcinoma ($n=32$). The only presentation or outcome difference between the two groups was a higher recurrence rate among tumors with a predominant insular histology, with a mean follow-up of 4.6 years. After surgery, 46 (72 %) of the patients were free of disease, whereas 16 (28 %) had evidence of metastases or invasion of local structures at presentation. Other than those with incidentally discovered malignancies at thyroidectomy, all patients received near-total thyroidectomy, followed by ^{131}I and subsequent L-thyroxine suppression therapy. Of the 46 patients initially rendered disease-free at surgery, 27 were free of disease at follow-up; 83 % of the tumors were iodine avid and produced measurable serum levels of thyroglobulin, which indicated differentiated follicular cell function. Of the total 63 patients in the study, 35 had persistent or recurrent disease. Of these 35 with recurrence, 30 had evidence of iodine uptake on diagnostic scan and were treated with ^{131}I. Iodine scanning and measurements of serum thyroglobulin showed 17 % of those patients as cured, 27 % were alive with disease, and 56 % died of disease. Five patients with noniodine-avid recurrence or metastases were treated with chemotherapy and/or external beam radiation therapy, three of whom were alive with disease 1–15 years after presentation.

Chao et al. [68] have emphasized the aggressive clinical course of these patients. They studied eight patients with insular cancer and observed that local invasion into the strap muscles, pulmonary metastases, and local cervical nodes metastases were frequent. Four patients died of their disease. Machens et al. [52] retrospectively analyzed 127 patients with differentiated thyroid cancer and identified 14 with the insular subtype. Greater tumor size (>4 cm) and the presence of distant metastasis correlated with this subtype.

Similar data were reported by Sasaki and colleagues [69], who identified 44 cases of papillary or follicular carcinoma with an insular component. For the time period reviewed, this number represented 1.8 % of thyroid carcinomas. Although the follow-up was variable, 17 patients died of their disease, 18 patients were free of disease, and 2 were alive with disease. Multivariate analysis revealed that the presence of insular carcinoma as well as tumor size, the absence of a tumor capsule, vascular invasion, and necrosis within the tumor were all independently associated with a worse prognosis. Many other groups have reported successful ^{131}I therapy in patients with metastatic disease. Metastatic insular carcinoma has been detected utilizing ^{99}Tc [51, 70], and levels of serum thyroglobulin are also useful in monitoring patients for tumor recurrence. Table 81.2 compares the outcome of patients with insular carcinoma to the outcome of those with well-differentiated carcinoma, as reported by Mazzaferri and Jhiang [62]. The follow-up related to insular carcinoma was shorter, and the treatment modalities were variable, compared to the cohort with well-differentiated tumors. Among patients presenting with metastatic insular thyroid carcinoma with relatively short follow-up periods (several years), 60 % died of disease and 20 % were alive with disease. The remaining 20 % were believed to be cured from their metastatic carcinoma following treatment with ^{131}I.

Therapy with L-thyroxine is prudent in patients with insular thyroid carcinoma. Because many of these patients have tumors that display differentiated epithelial function, doses of L-thyroxine to fully suppress pituitary production of thyrotropin (TSH) are recommended. We believe that the target TSH level in these patients is a value less than 0.01 μU/mL, if tolerated and if the patient has no contraindications to such therapy related to age and cardiovascular status. This TSH level should be achieved relatively gradually with the levothyroxine dose sufficient to just suppress the TSH level to this range. The average daily dose of exogenous L-thyroxine required to suppress TSH in thyroid cancer patients is approx 2.1 μg/kg of body weight. Because the recurrence and mortality rates for this tumor are higher than for differentiated carcinoma, and as these carcinomas generally remain iodine avid, aggressive surgical and ^{131}I therapy are appropriate. This should be followed by frequent monitoring for tumor

Table 81.2 Clinical presentation and outcome of insular thyroid cancer compared with differentiated thyroid carcinoma

Characteristics	Insular	Differentiated[a]	Outcome	Insular (%)	Differentiated (%)
Age (year)	54	36	Died of disease	20	8
Size (cm)	4.7	2.5	Alive with disease	30	29
Intrathyroidal Regional distant	34 %	48 %	No disease	44	63
	36 %	50 %	Died with disease	6	0
	30 %	2 %			

[a]Data on differentiated cancer reported by Mazzaferri and Jhiang [62] (Adapted from Ref. [71] with permission of W. B. Saunders Co)

recurrence with radioiodine scanning and measurements of serum thyroglobulin. We also believe that the adjunctive use of radiological procedures, e.g., neck sonogram, CT, and/or MRI, may be useful in diagnosing recurrent disease as early as possible. 18-Fluorodeoxyglucose positron emission tomography (FDG-PET) scans are often useful in detecting disease, especially in poorly differentiated thyroid cancers, such as the insular variety [72].

Summary

Insular thyroid carcinoma is a histological variant with a clinical course more aggressive than well-differentiated carcinoma but less aggressive than anaplastic thyroid carcinoma. Therefore, insular carcinoma may represent an important intermediate stage in the dedifferentiation of thyroid carcinoma. Patients with insular carcinoma are more likely to present with metastases and to develop tumor recurrence than those with well-differentiated tumors, but the majority present with either intrathyroidal lesions or regional disease. These tumors generally maintain differentiated thyroid follicular cell function, allowing for ^{131}I therapy and scanning and measurement of serum thyroglobulin levels.

Most patients with local disease are successfully treated surgically and with ^{131}I therapy, followed by L-thyroxine suppression. Tumor recurrence rates appear to be higher among patients with local or regional disease than seen with more well-differentiated tumors. Patients with distant metastases treated with ^{131}I and thyroid hormone suppression appear to have a cure rate of approximately 20 %, justifying aggressive treatment with surgery, ^{131}I, and thyroid hormone suppression.

Tall-Cell Variant of Papillary Carcinoma

Demographics

The tall-cell variant of papillary carcinoma (TCV) was initially reported by Hazard in 1964 [73], who defined a group of papillary tumors with certain characteristics in at least 30 % of the tumor. These included papillary structures, epithelial cell height at least twice the cellular width, oxyphilic cytoplasm, and hyperchromic basilar nuclei. Hawk and Hazard [74] found that 9 % of their papillary tumors met this definition. They also described these tumors as being grossly larger and more locally invasive than non-tall-cell papillary carcinoma, affecting an older group of patients (mean age of 57 years). Most studies report that TCV represents approximately 5–10 % of thyroid carcinomas. The female predominance typically linked with other forms of thyroid cancer remains. The literature on TCV has been reviewed [11, 74–92].

Clinical Characteristics

At least 30 % of the tumor must be composed of tall cells to be considered a TCV tumor (see Chap. 80). However, the inherent subjectivity involved in this diagnosis is of concern. For example, no studies have been published in which identical slides were sent in a blinded manner to multiple pathologists to determine the frequency of a TCV diagnosis. TCV must be differentiated from the less common columnar cell variant, which is characterized by "tall" cells but with nuclear stratification, as opposed to basilar nuclei and scant, nonoxyphilic, but often vacuolated, cytoplasm. These two closely related variants of papillary carcinoma were recently described in the same patient, suggesting a similar pathogenesis [93].

TCV has been found in combination with cell types other than the usual forms of papillary carcinoma. A recent report describes five TCV cases in tumors with regions of a variant of anaplastic carcinoma, described as spindle cell squamous carcinoma [94]. These cases, in addition to the general occurrence of TCV within tumors containing usual papillary carcinoma and a high incidence of *p53* mutations [95], suggest that this lesion might represent a transition between papillary and anaplastic carcinoma, similar to the intermediate stage assigned to insular carcinoma. The similarities between TCV and the columnar cell variant have been described above. These two variants have been classified separately but may represent similar "transition" tumors. The consistency and reliability in diagnosing TCV requires further study. The interobserver variability is unknown but may be quite important when attempting to compare published data on the frequency and clinical course of TCV.

Table 81.3 compares the presenting characteristics of 163 patients with TCV compiled from the literature to the patient cohort with typically differentiated papillary carcinoma, as reported by Mazzaferri and Jhiang [62]. Patients with TCV tend to be older, have larger lesions, and are more likely to have metastases outside of the neck than patients with well-differentiated tumors.

The aggressiveness of TCV has been debated in the literature since its initial description, particularly in younger patients (see below; [80, 84]). The mechanism for this aggressive behavior is not known. However, *RET* rearrangements were recently identified in about 36 % of TCV (14 of 39 cases). Interestingly, the prevalence of *RET/PTC1* and *RET/PTC3* abnormalities was almost equal in classic papillary and follicular thyroid cancer, whereas all the TCV-positive cases expressed the *RET/PTC3* rearrangement [96].

Treatment and Clinical Course

Johnson and associates [84] attempted to define TCV prognosis by comparing 12 patients with TCV to a similar group of age- and gender-matched patients with typical papillary thyroid carcinomas. The groups were different in the extent of disease at presentation. All patients with usual papillary carcinoma had either intrathyroidal (58 %) or regional lymphatic spread (42 %). Of the patients with TCV, 25 % had intrathyroidal disease, 33 % had cervical lymphatic spread, and 42 % had invasion into cervical soft tissue or distant metastases. Tumor size correlated with recurrence and tumor-related mortality. Clinical outcome was different between the TCV and usual papillary thyroid carcinoma only among patients older than 50 years, but the authors concluded that TCV was more aggressive than typical papillary thyroid carcinoma.

Terry and colleagues [80] compared 19 patients with TCV to those with usual papillary carcinoma. The follow-up times were similar for both groups (62 and 93 months, respectively). Patients with TCV had larger tumors than those with papillary carcinoma (4.2 vs. 2.8 cm). Patients older than 50 years with TCV had larger tumors than younger patients with TCV (5.6 vs. 2.7 cm) and had a higher incidence of distant metastases and locally invasive disease. The authors performed a multivariate analysis on their data, comparing TCV to usual papillary carcinoma, and found that patients older than 50 with tumor size larger than 4 cm had an increased risk of tumor recurrence, but not mortality. Similar to Johnson and colleagues [84], they could find no difference in the prognosis of patients younger than 50 with TCV versus usual papillary carcinoma.

Moreno Egea and colleagues [97] reported a series of five patients with TCV ages 58–73 years. All these patients presented with large tumors and extrathyroidal disease.

When compared to 85 patients with typical papillary carcinoma, a statistically significant increase in tumor recurrence and mortality was reported. The patients in these series were treated with a variety of protocols; nearly all included thyroidectomy and ^{131}I therapy. Some patients received palliative external beam radiation therapy to control local recurrence. When compared to the large cohort of Mazzaferri and Jhiang (Table 81.4), the clinical outcomes of patients under the age of 50 were indistinguishable from those with the usual forms of papillary carcinoma. Yet, older patients were more likely to have recurrence of their tumors. The patients with TCV were followed for a shorter time period, and treatment may have been more variable than in this reference group. Mortality and recurrence rates may rise as the follow-up period lengthens. The data suggest a poor prognosis for older patients with TCV that present with larger primary tumors. This tumor variant most commonly occurs in patients older than 50, but the distinction between younger and older patients may be important when determining the prognosis of younger patients with a small TCV tumor.

Sywak et al. [99] have also reviewed the literature and conclude (in a summary of 209 cases) that TCV is generally a more aggressive tumor, associated with distant metastases in 22 % of cases and had a mean tumor-related mortality of 16 %. They concluded that the histological diagnosis of TCV was a poor prognostic factor, regardless of patient age or tumor size. Further studies in this area are required, especially to examine this tumor in younger patients with smaller sized tumors, a group for whom the literature is less clear

Table 81.3 Clinical presentation of TCV compared with differentiated thyroid cancer

Characteristic	TCV ($n = 163$)	Differentiated thyroid carcinoma[a] ($n = 1,355$)
Age (yr)	51.8	36
Size (cm)	3.2	2.5
Intrathyroid	33 %	48 %
Regional (neck)	19 %	50 %
Distant metastases	19 %	2 %
Female	74 %	67 %

[a]Data on differentiated cancer reported by Mazzaferri and Jhiang [62] (Adapted from ref. [72] with permission of W. B. Saunders Co)

Table 81.4 Clinical outcomes of TCV compared with differentiated thyroid cancer

Miscellaneous thyroid tumors						
All patients (%)			Patients over age 50 (%)		Patients under age 50 (%)	
	Tall cell[a]	Differentiated[b]	Tall cell	Differentiated[b]	Tall cell	Differentiated[b]
Outcomes	(*n* = *148*)	(*n* = *1355*)	(*n* = *41*)	(*n* = *222*)	(*n* = *35*)	(*n* = *1133*)
Died of disease	19	8	21	19	6	2
Alive with disease	26	29	27	23	17	21
No disease	55	63	32	58	77	77

[a]Follow-up data included on 148 of 163 patients with TCV; presenting age included on 76 of 163
[b]Data on differentiated cancer by Mazzaferri and Jhiang [62] (Adapted from Ref. [98] with permission of W. B. Saunders Co)

whether this tumor may frequently exhibit a more aggressive nature. Morris et al. [75] analyzed the National Cancer Institute's Surveillance, Epidemiology, and End Results database in which 278 patients with the tall-cell variant were compared to 2,522 patients with classical papillary thyroid cancer. Patients in these two groups were matched for multiple factors, including age, gender, extrathyroidal invasion, metastases, and surgical and adjuvant therapy. The patients with tall-cell variant papillary thyroid carcinoma were older (54.3 years vs. 46.3 years, $p<0.0001$) and had decreased disease-related survival at 5 years (81.9 % vs. 91.3 %, $p=0.049$).

Surgical therapy followed by ^{131}I and L-thyroxine suppression is appropriate. These tumors typically produce thyroglobulin and are iodine avid. Loss of these characteristics of differentiation should be taken as further dedifferentiation of the tumor.

TCV typically presents in older patients with a higher frequency of local adenopathy or invasion and distant metastases. It has been linked with well-differentiated papillary carcinoma and anaplastic carcinoma, suggesting that it may represent a "transition" histology between these two types. These tumors generally maintain thyroglobulin production and iodine avidity. Among older patients with thyroid cancer, TCV appears to have a higher recurrence rate and possibly a higher mortality than the usual form of papillary thyroid carcinoma. In the unusual younger patient who presents with a small locally confined TCV tumor, the prognosis appears similar to usual papillary carcinoma. Patients with TCV, probably regardless of size or invasive features, should be treated aggressively with thyroidectomy, ^{131}I, and long-term L-thyroxine suppression. Follow-up should include periodic ^{131}I scanning and determinations of serum thyroglobulin levels. Routine cervical sonogram, CT scans, and/or MRI can also help detect evidence of recurrence as soon as possible. When there are suggestive changes with these techniques, guided biopsies can be performed to confirm recurrent cancer and distinguish it from a benign reactive process.

Columnar Cell Variant of Papillary Carcinoma

Demographics

The columnar cell variant of papillary carcinoma is a rare tumor ([49, 93–95, 100–106] see Chap. 80). Patients with columnar cell carcinoma had a mean age of 45 years, with a range of 16–76 years and a female/male ratio of 1.4:1. As described above, the pathology is similar to that of TCV, as the height of the cells should be at least three times the width to qualify for diagnosis. The nuclei are stratified, not basilar, and the cytoplasm is clear, as opposed to pink [93, 95, 101, 102, 105]. These tumors form large distinct papillae, and the follicular cells are immunoreactive for thyroglobulin. The tumors are typically large, with a mean longest dimension of 5.4 cm. Cytopathology is most commonly consistent with papillary carcinoma.

Columnar cell carcinoma has been described in an otherwise unremarkable well-differentiated papillary carcinoma [102], along with anaplastic carcinoma [95, 105], or in combination with tall-cell carcinoma [93]. Initial reports of the columnar cell variant of papillary cancer suggested a highly aggressive neoplasm. However, Gaertner et al. [103] analyzed 16 cases of this rare tumor and concluded that extrathyroidal extension at the time of presentation, rather than cell type, was predictive of a more aggressive clinical course. Chen et al. [100] analyzed nine patients with the columnar variant of papillary thyroid cancer. In general, older patients had larger size tumors with more aggressive features, such as local and distant metastasis. Of the nine patients, a V660E BRAF oncogene mutation was identified in three, two of whom were considered aggressive tumors.

Clinical Characteristics

Neoplasms have been described where the columnar cell pattern was mixed with tall-cell papillary carcinoma [102, 106] as well as with solid regions of typical papillary carcinoma) [102, 103]. Also, extensive insular and trabecular patterns have been seen adjacent to the columnar cell pattern.

Research suggests that the locally infiltrative tumors are usually fatal [93, 95, 101, 102, 105], but those that are encapsulated may be successfully resected [96, 97].

Treatment and Clinical Course

In patients with large tumor masses, metastatic disease was present in 29 %, including six to the lungs, one to the adrenal glands, one to the brain, and two to the bone. Patients were treated with thyroidectomy and radioactive iodine. Of the 24 patients described, 58 % were free of disease at follow-up. Recurrences typically occurred within 2 years of the initial surgery. In all, 38 % (9 of 24) of the patients died of their columnar cell carcinoma.

Treatment should be directed at early diagnosis by FNA cytology, followed by a complete surgical resection when possible. Treatment with ^{131}I is appropriate, along with subsequent L-thyroxine suppression. If the primary tumor is large, and a complete surgical resection is not possible, local palliative control with external beam therapy has been utilized.

Swyak et al. [99] also reviewed the literature relating to columnar cell thyroid cancer (41 cases). They confirmed a significant mortality rate of 32 %. However, they also concluded that when the tumor was encapsulated at the original surgery, the prognosis was comparable to typical papillary thyroid cancer. However, patients with tumors that were not encapsulated had extrathyroidal spread in 67 % and had distant metastases in 87 %.

Summary

Columnar cell carcinoma is a rare variant of papillary thyroid carcinoma that appears to have a course similar to TCV, consistent with dedifferentiation in comparison to well-differentiated papillary thyroid carcinoma. Early metastases and local tumor invasion are common; the key to curative therapy is early diagnosis followed by complete surgical resection.

Diffuse Sclerosing Variant of Papillary Carcinoma

Diffuse sclerosing variant of papillary thyroid cancer is rare and tends to occur in younger patients, with a mean age of approximately 31 years [97, 107–118]. There were 13 patients (21 %) younger than 20 years old. Pathologically, diffuse sclerosing papillary carcinoma is characterized by pronounced fibrosis, numerous psammoma bodies, and extensive lymphocytic infiltrates. Mucin may be present; thus, these tumors may be misclassified as mucoepidermoid or anaplastic carcinomas. Although the prognostic significance of this variant is not clear, these tumors most commonly present as diffuse enlarging lobes or entire thyroid glands. Their clinical course is not yet well characterized, but it appears that they behave similarly to well-differentiated papillary carcinomas [101] and should be treated with surgery, radioiodine, and thyroxine suppression.

Swyak et al. [99] suggested that diffuse sclerosing variant of papillary thyroid cancer ($n=65$) had a tendency for intrathyroidal extension (40 %) and a high propensity for nodal metastases (68 %). However, tumor-related mortality was similar to that of well-differentiated thyroid cancer: 2 % at 8-year follow-up.

Regalbuto [109] studied 34 patients with diffuse sclerosing variant of papillary thyroid cancer and compared their clinical features to 245 patients with classical papillary thyroid cancer. The patients with the diffuse sclerosing variant presented with higher stage disease, and these patients were relatively similar to patients with high-risk classical variant of papillary carcinoma. Koo et al. [111] studied 28 cases of diffuse sclerosing variant papillary thyroid cancer in individuals less than 20 years old. They noted that a surprising 41.2 % of these young patients had the sclerosing variant and that it was associated with more frequent extrathyroidal extension and more frequent recurrences.

Solid Variant of Papillary Thyroid Carcinoma

Until recently, this variant was poorly described in the literature; however, the apparent unique association between the solid variant of papillary carcinoma and the Chernobyl nuclear accident in 1986 has stimulated renewed interest in its pathogenesis and prognosis [119–122]. Although rare in adults, this histological pattern is frequently identified in tumors in children but usually comprises a small amount of an otherwise well-differentiated tumor. The prognostic significance of these small regions is unclear but is not reported to impact survival.

The role of radiation exposure and the high prevalence of *ret/PTC3* gene rearrangements in solid variant tumors support the notion that this tumor type is a unique thyroid malignancy. Nikiforov and colleagues [120, 122] compared the histologies of thyroid tumors removed from children who were exposed to the Chernobyl accident versus a control group of sporadic thyroid tumors removed from children from the United States. These investigators found that 37 % of the "radiation-induced" tumors had solid variant as the predominant growth pattern compared to 4 % of the "sporadic" tumors. About 79 % of the solid variant tumors had *ret/PTC3* gene rearrangements. These data support the hypothesis that rearrangements of this gene occurred in response to the radiation exposure and may be involved in the tumorigenesis. Increased p53 immunohistochemical staining has been reported in some solid regions of these tumors, raising the concern of more aggressive clinical behavior [120, 122].

Sywak et al. [99] also found that the solid variant of papillary thyroid cancer (in Chernobyl victims) had cervical lymph node metastases in 83 % of patients. Long-term follow-up studies of these children are required. The impact of the solid variant histology in adults may differ from the impact in children as well, and it is unknown if patients with this disorder who had radiation-induced tumors from the Chernobyl accident have the same clinical course as those who develop it spontaneously.

Mixed Medullary-Follicular Cell Carcinoma

These variants of medullary thyroid carcinoma (MTC) display the microscopic features of both MTC and carcinomas of follicular cells [1, 2]. The tumor regions are immunoreactive with calcitonin, whereas other regions have thyroglobulin production. Normal follicles may be "trapped" within any MTC and seemingly cause thyroglobulin immunoreactivity in MTC. This pattern differs from the mixed variants that have regions of follicular or papillary cancer adjacent to MTC regions [123–130]. Similar medullary-papillary cancers have been reported [131, 132]. Occasionally, these mixed tumors can be suspected even on cytological FNA samples [133].

The pathogenesis of these tumors is uncertain. Care must be taken to exclude insular thyroid carcinoma, which may have a similar histological appearance to MTC but expresses only thyroglobulin. Paragangliomas may also present like MTC but are rare in the thyroid. The appearance of these mixed tumors suggests the presence of a progenitor thyroid cell that differentiates into follicular or C-cell lineages; yet, most researchers believe these cell types are derived from separate lineages. Pappoti and associates [123] identified rare cells expressing both thyroglobulin and calcitonin in 2 of 11 cases. However, in some instances, the medullary-follicular cell carcinoma may represent a "collision tumor" of the thyroid.

Clinical recommendations are difficult to formulate for such rare tumors. As with most cases of MTC, aggressive surgical therapy is appropriate. Treatment with ^{131}I and L-thyroxine suppression, not performed for usual forms of MTC, are recommended for these rare lesions. Serum calcitonin and thyroglobulin measurements are helpful. The prevalence of mutations in the *ret* gene is not known, but familial occurrences of the medullary-follicular and medullary-papillary variants have been reported [127, 131]. It would seem reasonable to examine the white blood cells of a patient with mixed medullary-follicular carcinoma for mutations in the *ret* oncogene and to ensure (to the extent possible) that this entity is not part of a familial syndrome. However, there are no specific studies addressing this issue.

Mucoepidermoid Carcinoma

Demographics

Mucoepidermoid carcinoma is a rare variant of thyroid carcinoma of uncertain cell lineage. A report of 6 new cases of mucoepidermoid carcinoma also identified 31 cases in the literature [134]. This type is more common in women than men (2.9:1), with the majority of patients presenting with a solitary "cold" nodule. There is no clear relationship with risk factors, such as a prior history of radiation therapy or a family history of thyroid cancer. The mean presenting age of patients with mucoepidermoid carcinoma is 42 years (range, 10–71 years) with four patients younger than 20 years old. These neoplasms are usually a low grade of malignancy, and their histogenesis is uncertain. Sometimes the tumor is associated with papillary carcinoma (or even present as a metastatic focus in a papillary carcinoma; [134–142]). An adjacent undifferentiated (anaplastic) carcinoma has been reported [139]. The tumors are typically solid, firm, light-colored masses, not encapsulated, and sometimes cystic and can have mucus visible on the cut surfaces. Various sizes (1–8 cm) have been documented. A rare variant, sclerosing mucoepidermoid cancer with eosinophils, has also been described [141]. This tumor usually occurs in patients with Hashimoto's thyroiditis, potentially representing metaplastic changes. Extensive eosinophil infiltration is noted in the stroma and tumor nests. The natural history of this variant needs to be further defined.

Prichard et al. [143] recently reported three patients with mucoepidermoid carcinoma (two women, ages 22 and 52; one man, age 58) in whom the tumor was thought to arise from well-differentiated thyroid cancer that had dedifferentiated. They observed a continued transition between well-differentiated thyroid cancer and the mucoepidermoid component with concomitant loss of well-differentiated markers such as thyroid transcription factor-1 and thyroglobulin.

Clinical Presentation and Diagnosis

Most of the 31 patients presented with a painless neck mass or a slowly growing thyroid nodule [60, 101]. When obtained, radioiodine scanning revealed a photopenic region corresponding to the nodule. FNA cytology has been diagnostic of carcinoma but is not specific for mucoepidermoid carcinoma [140]. The diagnosis is usually made or confirmed histologically at the time of thyroidectomy. Both partial and near-total thyroidectomies have been performed, the former only for small, well-circumscribed tumors. At presentation, 17 of 31 (55 %) had extrathyroidal disease, and all but one patient had disease confined to the neck. Patients with cervical node metastases or invasion of local structures were treated with surgery, followed by external beam radiation therapy. There have been no reports of postoperative ^{131}I scanning after the usual preparation with thyroid hormone withdrawal.

Clinical Course and Treatment

Among patients with local adenopathy, complete remission rates are quite high, but the duration of follow-up is variable. These tumors appear to be more indolent than many other forms of dedifferentiating thyroid carcinoma. Similar to most other forms of thyroid cancer, cure depends on early diagnosis and surgical intervention. Patients with small primary tumors (<2 cm) confined to the thyroid appear to do well [134]. Therapy for those patients with locally advanced disease (utilizing surgery and external beam radiation) appears to induce remission in most patients. Several patients have either presented with or developed distant metastases. Treatment has not been reported; however, the lesions tend to be indolent, similar to well-differentiated thyroid carcinoma. The utility of thyroid hormone therapy and radioiodine scanning and treatment have not yet been evaluated in these tumors.

Summary

Mucoepidermoid thyroid carcinoma is a rare tumor that affects adults. It is commonly coincident with lymphocytic thyroiditis and shares some features with papillary thyroid carcinoma. It has been identified adjacent to well-differentiated papillary carcinoma and anaplastic carcinoma. The so-called adenosquamous carcinoma could represent an aggressive variant of mucoepidermoid carcinoma. These factors raise the possibility that this tumor represents a slowly growing variant of papillary carcinoma, but this is an unproven hypothesis. A cure seems possible with a complete surgical resection (when feasible) and external beam radiation therapy for residual local disease. The role of ^{131}I therapy in mucoepidermoid carcinoma requires further evaluation.

Sarcomas of the Thyroid

True primary sarcomas of the thyroid gland are exceedingly rare. Some cases of sarcoma have been reclassified as anaplastic carcinoma and, in a few cells, display mixed immunohistochemical markers of epithelial and mesenchymal lineages (so-called carcinosarcomas). Careful ultrastructural and immunohistochemical analyses have convincingly described several cases of leiomyosarcoma [144–147], osteosarcoma [148, 149], chondrosarcoma [147], fibrosarcomas [147], liposarcomas [150], and, most commonly, angiosarcomas [147, 151–154]. Angiosarcomas (malignant hemangioepitheliomas) have been found mostly in European Alpine regions known to be iodine deficient.

In general, sarcomas often present in older patients with a long-standing history of a goiter. Three thyroid sarcomas have been described in those with a prior history of external beam radiation therapy, including in a 23-year-old patient, but no cases were reported among a large group of previously irradiated patients with Hodgkin's disease [150].

These tumors resemble sarcomas arising in other locations. Angiosarcomas typically have features of endothelial differentiation with immunoreactivity for factor VIII-related antigens, CD34 and CD31. Keratin immunoreactivity has been indicated in some cases. Because of this characteristic, some authors prefer to consider these neoplasms as angiomatoid carcinomas [151, 155]. There may be little importance in differentiating sarcomas from anaplastic carcinomas. Most patients presented with large primary tumors that invaded local structures and had lymphatic spread. The majority of these patients die from aggressive local or metastatic disease. Similar to anaplastic carcinoma, a cure seems possible only with complete surgical resection. Local control with radiation therapy seems advisable if the patient is clinically stable following surgical resection. The utility of chemotherapy for thyroid sarcomas has not been described.

Sarcomas may rarely metastasize to the thyroid gland. A primary originating organ, other than the thyroid, should be excluded in any patient presenting with thyroid sarcoma, as primary thyroid sarcomas are identical to sarcomas in other organs. Kaposi's sarcoma, a well-recognized secondary disease in patients with AIDS, has been found to infiltrate the thyroid. A case of thyroid infiltration by KS-causing hypothyroidism has been reported [154]. An interesting association exists between systemic sarcomas and thyroid abnormalities. Of 610 patients with sarcoma, 28 (4.6 %) had related significant thyroid disorder. The interval between the diagnosis of the thyroid disorder and the sarcoma varied as long as 10–15 years with thyroid disorders, including goiter, thyroiditis, and carcinoma [156].

Spindle Epithelial Tumor with Thymus-Like Differentiation of the Thyroid (SETTLE)

Spindle cell epithelial tumors to the thyroid with thymus-like differentiation (SETTLE) are extremely rare and may arise from thymus tissue ectopically located within the thyroid gland or from branchial pouch remnants [157–163]. This tumor most frequently occurs in children (reported as young as 2 years old) or adolescents, but may also occur in adults [157–163]. Given the few patients that have been reported, there are not controlled studies assessing treatment. Most reports performed a thyroidectomy and then monitored the patients closely as local recurrence and distant metastases can occur. Chemotherapy does not seem to be particularly effective. Given the thymic origin of the tumor, it is not expected that radioactive iodine treatment would be effective.

Teratomas of the Thyroid

The diagnosis of teratoma, whether benign or malignant, requires demonstration of various cells with characteristics of the three germ cell layers. Teratomas of the thyroid are rare, usually occur in childhood, and are most often benign. Most benign teratomas are found in infancy and are generally quite large, often greater than 10 cm. Buckley and colleagues [164] identified 139 cases of childhood thyroid teratoma, nearly all of which were benign, usually presenting as a mass causing local compressive symptoms. Thyroidal origin is inferred by identifying the blood supply as arising from the thyroidal vessels.

Among adults, teratomas are even more unusual than in children but are more commonly malignant. Bowker and Whittaker [165] recently reported a case of malignant teratoma in a 17-year-old patient and reviewed nine other cases reported in the literature [164–170]. Adults with malignant thyroid teratoma had a mean age of 31.2 years, with a range of 17–68 years. There were no specific risk factors linked with malignant teratoma. The majority were quite large (up to 17 cm in diameter). Patients were treated with thyroidectomy, radiation, and chemotherapy. Cervical and/or distant metastases were found in all patients. No cases of long-term survival have been reported, and response to radiation therapy and chemotherapy appears to be transient. Only the patient described by Bowker and Whitaker was disease-free at 7-month follow-up [165]. The remaining patients died within 22 months of diagnosis. Children with rare malignant thyroid teratomas have a similarly poor prognosis.

Rare, Mostly Benign Thyroid Tumors

There are case reports of rare histological types of benign tumors involving the thyroid; we will mention a few nonepithelial varieties. Benign leiomyomas [144, 171, 172] and neurilemomas [171–174] have presented as slowly growing, palpable masses that were "cold" on radioiodine imaging. They were composed of spindle cells with abundant eosinophilic cytoplasm, but no atypia or evidence of increased mitotic activity. Immunoperoxidase staining confirmed the neural or smooth muscle nature of these tumors. The lack of extrathyroidal invasion and absence of recurrent disease after 1–6 years of follow-up support a benign diagnosis. There has been one case of granulosa cell tumor of the thyroid in a girl treated for short stature with relatively high doses of ethinyl estradiol (0.1 mg daily) and medroxyprogesterone (10 mg) for several years [175]. This patient has also done well after surgical resection. Microscopically, this tumor resembled Hurthle cell adenoma because of the abundant eosinophilic cytoplasm.

Hyalinizing Trabecular Neoplasms, Usually Adenomas

These rare neoplasms are solid masses and often less than 3.0 cm in diameter and are well circumscribed (usually encapsulated; [176–180]). Psammoma bodies may be scattered through the tumor. Most cells contain immunoreactive thyroglobulin and keratin. Calcitonin has never been demonstrated. Colloid is not present, but irregular masses of hyaline material are adjacent to the cell clusters. Nuclei often contain grooves and cytoplasmic inclusions that, in addition to the psammoma bodies, are reminiscent of papillary thyroid carcinoma. Thus, aspirates of these lesions have been confused with papillary neoplasms. Rarely, the tumors have been invasive, involving cervical lymph nodes, and have been termed the "cribriform variant of papillary carcinoma" [181]. An alteration resembling this hyalinizing tumor has been described in adenomatoid nodules in multinodular goiter [180].

Thymic and Related Neoplasms

Thymic, parathyroid, and salivary gland tissues may be found in the thyroid [182–184]. Therefore, it is not surprising that occasional neoplasms occur in the thyroid and inferior part of the neck that resemble the thymus [185–187]. Such tumors may be benign or malignant.

Embryologic Thyroid Remnants

Thyroglossal Duct Cysts (See Also Chap. 53)

A recent review [188] observed that ectopic thyroid tissue most frequently occurs in the lingual, sublingual, laryngotracheal, thyroglossal, or lateral cervical areas. More rarely, ectopic thyroid tissue may occur in distant structures such as esophagus, mediastinum, heart, skin, and abdominal structure. Thyroid cancer can be found in any site of ectopic tissue but is most frequent in the thyroglossal duct tract. The thyroglossal tract in adults may be a vestigial remnant or may be a more fully developed structure, composed of thyroid follicles, a duct (usually lined by ciliated pseudostratified columnar epithelium), connective tissue, and lymphoid tissue. The thyroid follicles in this tract may undergo any of the changes that occur in the gland proper, even papillary or follicular thyroid cancer [189, 190]. When thyroid cancer occurs at the more proximal portion of this duct, it may actually involve the base of the tongue. Generally, the thyroglossal tract resides in the midline, and a thyroglossal tumor may move cephalad when the tongue is protruded because of the persistent connection between the mass and the tongue. When a tumor is present in the thyroglossal tract, it may be associated with a similar tumor within the thyroid gland itself. Thyroglossal tumors must be differentiated from thyroglossal cysts, branchial cleft cysts, and cystic hygromas (fluid-filled multiloculated lymphangiomas present at birth). Thyroid cancers that arise exclusively in the thyroglossal tract are rare and discussed at greater length in this chapter.

Clinical Presentation

The proper approach to thyroglossal duct tumors is largely unknown, but our approach is to perform FNA and base our therapeutic decision largely on the cytological findings [176–178, 188, 189, 191]. If the FNA is positive or suspicious for thyroid cancer, we generally recommend removal of the entire thyroglossal tract from the base of the tongue to the thyroid gland. If the FNA is diagnostic of thyroid cancer, the thyroid gland may be removed at the initial surgery. If the FNA is suspicious for thyroid cancer, we may recommend, in conjunction with discussions with the patient, the removal of the thyroid gland at the initial operation. Some prefer a subsequent thyroidectomy when the diagnosis of thyroid cancer in the thyroglossal tract has been confirmed. Carcinoma that resides within the thyroglossal tract may emanate from the thyroid epithelium in this area or, alternatively, could arise within the thyroid gland and (rarely) metastasize to the thyroglossal tract. The diagnostic and therapeutic approach to thyroglossal duct tumors is controversial, as long-term controlled studies assessing various options have not been performed. The natural history of thyroid carcinomas derived from the thyroglossal duct tract is poorly understood. Heshmati and coworkers [192] retrospectively reviewed thyroglossal carcinoma in 12 patients seen over a 44-year period at the Mayo Clinic. Age at presentation ranged from 17 to 60 years, with a mean of 40 years. The patients were equally divided between men and women. The most common complaint was a midline neck mass. In all 12 cases, papillary thyroid cancer was found, and three patients also had involvement of the thyroid gland. Nine patients had a subtotal or near-total thyroidectomy. Despite that only three patients received postoperative radioactive iodine therapy, no patient had recurrence, distant metastases, or disease-specific mortality during a mean follow-up period of 13 years.

The usual surgical approach included a Sistrunk procedure in combination with a thyroidectomy. Because these patients were reviewed over a long time period, especially before our improved understanding of thyroid cancer, we do not necessarily concur with their recommendations that radioactive iodine is not necessary and that these patients have an excellent prognosis. Tew and coworkers [193] found 90 thyroglossal duct cysts or nodules over a 30-year period. Four patients had thyroid cancer in the thyroglossal duct cyst, an incidence similar to that of carcinoma arising in an intrathyroidal location. Mahnke and colleagues [194] estimate that approximately 150 cases of thyroid carcinoma from a thyroglossal tract have been reported. We tend to treat patients who have thyroglossal papillary thyroid cancer with a Sistrunk procedure, a total or near-total thyroidectomy, and, most frequently, radioiodine therapy, based on the clinical findings. At present, there is no reason to expect these tumors will behave differently than an intrathyroidal papillary cancer. Size, capsular invasion, soft tissue invasion, and vascular or nodal invasion should be considered in the decision on how to treat a patient with thyroglossal papillary thyroid cancer.

In addition to papillary thyroid cancer, squamous cell carcinoma and lymphoma may arise within this tissue [195, 196].

Deshpande and Bobhate [197] believed that only nine cases of squamous cell carcinoma from a thyroglossal tract have been reported. This tumor is difficult to diagnose; we suggest that a Sistrunk procedure, along with a total or near-total thyroidectomy, be performed for these rare tumors.

Metastatic Cancers to the Thyroid Gland

Metastatic tumors in the thyroid gland in patients with separate primary cancers can occur when examined at autopsy, but the clinical manifestations of these metastases certainly are uncommon. Generally, a metastatic tumor in the thyroid gland presents as a solitary nodule, which is usually hypofunctioning on radioisotope scans. Involvement of an existing adenomatoid nodule or adenoma is likely, thereby complicating the morphological features. The most common primary sites of such tumors are the breast, kidney, lung, and skin (malignant melanoma; [198–201]). There is often widespread metastatic disease present, and the manifestations in the thyroid gland are clinically unimportant. Nevertheless, solitary thyroid metastasis to the thyroid gland may be the initial evidence of disease or the first presentation of recurrent disease. For example, we have seen a patient with acute myelogenous leukemia who had been treated earlier, and the first evidence of recurrent disease was in the thyroid gland.

Nakhjavani and colleagues [199] reported a total of 43 patients (23 women, 20 men) with tumors metastatic to the thyroid gland. Solitary thyroid nodules or a multinodular gland was the presentation in 40 patients, whereas the remaining three had tracheal compression, necessitating thyroid surgery. Renal cell carcinoma was found in 14 patients, lung cancer in 7, and breast cancer in 7. More rarely, parathyroid cancer, salivary gland tumors, ovarian or uterine cancer, skin cancer, and esophageal cancer were found. In some instances, the source of the tumor was identified concurrently with the thyroid gland metastases. However, renal cell carcinoma within the thyroid gland was found as long as 26 years after the original tumor diagnosis; 15 % of subjects had evidence of thyroidal involvement before the diagnosis of metastasis to other sites. Although the investigators suggest that a thyroidectomy was associated with enhanced survival, compared to a nonsurgical approach (to the thyroid gland), we believe that more information is required to adequately address this issue.

The diagnostic evaluation revolves around the FNA and examination of the cytological sample. In most cases, there is abundant cellularity, and the cells may be typical of the original site, especially when specific immunohistochemical stains are performed. Obviously, diagnostic evaluation for the original tumor site and for the presence of other metastatic sites is important before approaching management. Occasionally, it may be difficult to determine if the cytological specimen represents metastatic disease or if it is originating from the thyroid gland, such as an anaplastic thyroid carcinoma or the unusual clear cell variant of follicular carcinoma. The therapeutic approach depends on the clinical context and cytological examination. For example, if there is widespread metastasis from an obvious extrathyroidal site, and the thyroid nodule cytology examination suggests metastasis from the same site, it may not be appropriate to remove the thyroid gland. Alternatively, if the patient had renal cell carcinoma that was treated successfully several years earlier, and now the patient presents with a thyroid nodule, cytologically appearing to resemble renal cell carcinoma, it might be useful to perform a lobectomy for diagnostic reasons. In fact, if an evaluation confirms that this single thyroid nodule might be the only evidence of metastatic disease, some clinicians might approach the thyroid lesion for diagnostic and even therapeutic reasons. Our general opinion is that it is desirable to obtain as much information as possible from the thyroid cytological specimen, including specific staining, and that radiological evaluation for other sites of metastasis for staging will be useful. Once as much information as reasonably possible is obtained, a frank discussion of the prognosis should take place with the patient and their family. In general, the outlook of patients with metastasis to the thyroid gland is poor, but individual tumors or circumstances may require a different method of treatment [202].

Tumors may also invade the thyroid gland by local extension. This mostly occurs with laryngeal, pharyngeal, and esophageal tumors, and such invasion may present as a neck mass in or around the thyroid gland. Cervical lymph node enlargement may also be noted. Radiological studies, e.g., CT (generally without contrast to avoid the iodine load), MRI, and direct visualization of the larynx or esophagus, may be useful. On thyroid isotope scanning, this invasion may present as a hypofunctioning area.

Occasionally, metastatic disease to the thyroid gland may cause destruction of the thyroid gland, with resultant leakage of iodothyronines into the circulation and hyperthyroidism [203]. This hyperthyroidism is thought to be a type of carcinoma-induced thyroiditis and may be associated with a low radioiodine uptake, but it has not been adequately studied using modern techniques.

Summary

This chapter has reviewed various types of unusual thyroid tumors and discussed their general pattern of clinical presentation and progression. Several general points should be made. There are no relevant controlled prospective studies assessing treatment modalities in any of these tumors; thus, we have to rely on clinical reports and experience. Furthermore, different institutions follow patients with any thyroid tumor, much less these relatively unusual disorders, in a variety of ways. After thyroidectomy, in addition to radioiodine scans and monitoring serum thyroglobulin levels, we think it is appropriate to clinically stage and monitor most patients with periodic radiological studies, such as neck MRI or sonogram and chest CT (without contrast when ^{131}I scanning or treatment is being considered). In selected circumstances, tumor assessment at other distant locations, e.g., brain, liver, kidneys, and bone, may also be needed. FDG-PET scans can help identify and/or follow sites of disease activity, especially if the PET activity can be fused digitally with a CT scan or MRI. In certain patients, it may also be beneficial to search for osseous metastases. TSH suppression by exogenous L-thyroxine therapy seems reasonable, based on the clinical context. When TSH is suppressed, preventative measures for osteoporosis should be undertaken, such as the ingestion of calcium and vitamin D and periodic bone mineral densities, as necessary. Some patients should receive treatment with a bisphosphonate with the proper prescribing precautions. It is also extremely important that these patients be addressed in a multidisciplinary manner, with necessary involvement of the patient in clinical decisions.

References

1. Hedinger C, Williams E, Sobin L. Histological typing of thyroid tumors. Berlin: Springer; 1988.
2. Hedinger C, Williams ED, Sobin LH. The WHO histological classification of thyroid tumors: a commentary on the second edition. Cancer. 1989;63(5):908–11.
3. Mazzaferri E. Undifferentiated thyroid carcinomas and unusual thyroid malignancies. In: Mazzaferri E, Samaan N, editors. Endocrine tumors. Boston: Blackwell Scientific Publications; 1993. p. 378–98.
4. Samaan NA, Ordonez NG. Uncommon types of thyroid cancer. Endocrinol Metab Clin N Am. 1990;19(3):637–48.
5. Holting T, et al. Immunohistochemical reclassification of anaplastic carcinoma reveals small and giant cell lymphoma. World J Surg. 1990;14(3):291–4. discussion 295.
6. Schmid KW, et al. Small cell carcinoma of the thyroid. A reclassification of cases originally diagnosed as small cell carcinomas of the thyroid. Pathol Res Pract. 1986;181(5):540–3.
7. Wolf BC, et al. Immunohistochemical analysis of small cell tumors of the thyroid gland: an Eastern Cooperative Oncology Group study. Hum Pathol. 1992;23(11):1252–61.
8. Prakash A, Kukreti SC, Sharma MP. Primary squamous cell carcinoma of the thyroid gland. Int Surg. 1968;50(6):538–41.
9. Bahuleyan CK, Ramachandran P. Primary squamous cell carcinoma of thyroid. Indian J Cancer. 1972;9(1):89–91.
10. Harada T, et al. Squamous cell carcinoma with cyst of the thyroid. J Surg Oncol. 1989;42(2):136–43.
11. Harada T, et al. Rarity of squamous cell carcinoma of the thyroid: autopsy review. World J Surg. 1994;18(4):542–6.
12. Motamed M, McGlashan JA. Thyroglossal duct carcinoma. Curr Opin Otolaryngol Head Neck Surg. 2004;12(2):106–9.
13. Mercante G, et al. Mixed squamous cell carcinoma and follicular carcinoma of the thyroid gland. Auris Nasus Larynx. 2011;8:1–5.
14. Chen CY, et al. Primary squamous cell carcinoma of the thyroid gland with eggshell calcification: sonographic and computed tomographic findings. J Ultrasound Med. 2010;29(11):1667–70.
15. Yucel H, et al. Primary squamous cell carcinoma of the thyroid years after radioactive iodine treatment. Neth J Med. 2010;68(5):224–6.
16. White IL, Talbert WM. Squamous cell carcinoma arising in thyroglossal duct remnant cyst epithelium. Otolaryngol Head Neck Surg. 1982;90(1):25–31.
17. Kapoor VK, et al. Primary squamous cell carcinoma of the thyroid gland – a case report. Jpn J Surg. 1985;15(1):60–2.
18. Misonou J, et al. Pure squamous cell carcinoma of the thyroid gland – report of an autopsy case and review of the literature. Jpn J Surg. 1988;18(4):469–74.
19. Tsuchiya A, et al. Squamous cell carcinoma of the thyroid – a report of three cases. Jpn J Surg. 1990;20(3):341–5.
20. Kampsen EB, Jager N, Max MH. Squamous cell carcinoma of the thyroid: a report of two cases. J Surg Oncol. 1977;9(6):567–78.
21. Sarda AK, et al. Squamous cell carcinoma of the thyroid. J Surg Oncol. 1988;39(3):175–8.
22. Theander C, et al. Primary squamous carcinoma of the thyroid – a case report. J Laryngol Otol. 1993;107(12):1155–8.
23. Chaudhary RK, Barnes EL, Myers EN. Squamous cell carcinoma arising in Hashimoto's thyroiditis. Head Neck. 1994;16(6):582–5.
24. Budd DC, et al. Squamous cell carcinoma of the thyroid. J Med Soc N J. 1982;79(11):838–40.
25. Simpson WJ, Carruthers J. Squamous cell carcinoma of the thyroid gland. Am J Surg. 1988;156(1):44–6.
26. Huang TY, Assor D. Primary squamous cell carcinoma of the thyroid gland: a report of four cases. Am J Clin Pathol. 1970;55:93–8.
27. Bukachevsky RP, et al. Squamous cell carcinoma and lingual thyroid. Ear Nose Throat J. 1991;70(8):505–7.
28. Korovin GS, et al. Squamous cell carcinoma of the thyroid: a diagnostic dilemma. Ann Otol Rhinol Laryngol. 1989;98(1 Pt 1):59–65.
29. Riddle PE, Dincsoy HP. Primary squamous cell carcinoma of the thyroid associated with leukocytosis and hypercalcemia. Arch Pathol Lab Med. 1987;111(4):373–4.
30. Shimaoka K, Tsukada Y. Squamous cell carcinomas and adenosquamous carcinomas originating from the thyroid gland. Cancer. 1980;46(8):1833–42.
31. Saito K, et al. Primary squamous cell carcinoma of the thyroid associated with marked leukocytosis and hypercalcemia. Cancer. 1981;48(9):2080–3.
32. Zimmer PW, Wilson D, Bell N. Primary squamous cell carcinoma of the thyroid gland. Mil Med. 2003;168(2):124–5.
33. Zhou XH. Primary squamous cell carcinoma of the thyroid. Eur J Surg Oncol. 2002;28(1):42–5.
34. LiVolsi VA, Merino MJ. Squamous cells in the human thyroid gland. Am J Surg Pathol. 1978;2(2):133–40.
35. Katoh R, et al. Squamous differentiation in thyroid carcinoma with special reference to histogenesis of squamous cell carcinoma of the thyroid. Acta Pathol Jpn. 1980;39:306–12.
36. Bakri K, et al. Adenosquamous carcinoma of the thyroid after radiotherapy for Hodgkin's disease. A case report and review. Cancer. 1983;52(3):465–70.
37. Bakri KM, et al. Association of thyroid carcinoma with malignant lymphoma. Jpn J Clin Oncol. 1983;13(4):645–55.
38. Renard TH, et al. Carcinoma of the thyroglossal duct. Surg Gynecol Obstet. 1990;171(4):305–8.
39. Klinck GH, Menk KF. Squamous cells in the human thyroid. Mil Surg. 1951;109(4):406–14.
40. Bond JA, et al. A variant epithelial sub-population in normal thyroid with high proliferative capacity in vitro. Mol Cell Endocrinol. 1993;93(2):175–83.
41. Carcangiu ML, et al. Anaplastic thyroid carcinoma. A study of 70 cases. Am J Clin Pathol. 1985;83(2):135–58.
42. Hadar T, et al. Anaplastic carcinoma of the thyroid. Eur J Surg Oncol. 1993;19(6):511–6.
43. Tan RK, et al. Anaplastic carcinoma of the thyroid: a 24-year experience. Head Neck. 1995;17(1):41–7. discussion 47–8.
44. Sato K, et al. Production of interleukin 1 alpha-like factor and colony-stimulating factor by a squamous cell carcinoma of the thyroid (T3M-5) derived from a patient with hypercalcemia and leukocytosis. Cancer Res. 1987;47(24 Pt 1):6474–80.
45. Okabe T, Nomura H, Oshawa N. Establishment and characterization of a human colony-stimulating factor-producing cell line from a squamous cell carcinoma of the thyroid gland. J Natl Cancer Inst. 1982;69(6):1235–43.
46. Langhans T. Uber die epithelialen formen der malignen struma. Virchows Arch Pathol Anat. 1907;385:125–41.
47. Carcangiu ML, Zampi G, Rosai J. Poorly differentiated ("insular") thyroid carcinoma. A reinterpretation of Langhans' "wuchernde Struma". Am J Surg Pathol. 1984;8(9):655–68.
48. Sakamoto A, Kasai N, Sugano H. Poorly differentiated carcinoma of the thyroid. A clinicopathologic entity for a high-risk group of papillary and follicular carcinomas. Cancer. 1983;52(10):1849–55.
49. Hwang TS, et al. Poorly differentiated carcinoma of the thyroid retrospective clinical and morphologic evaluation. J Korean Med Sci. 1990;5(1):47–52.

50. Pilotti S, et al. A novel panel of antibodies that segregates immunocytochemically poorly differentiated carcinoma from undifferentiated carcinoma of the thyroid gland. Am J Surg Pathol. 1994;18(10):1054–64.
51. Yen TC, et al. Comparative radionuclide imaging of metastatic insular carcinoma of the thyroid: value of technetium-99m-(V) DMSA. J Nucl Med. 1996;37(1):78–80.
52. Machens A, et al. Multivariate analysis of clinicopathologic parameters for the insular subtype of differentiated thyroid carcinoma. Arch Surg. 2001;136(8):941–4.
53. Fat I, et al. Insular variant of poorly differentiated thyroid carcinoma. Endocr Pract. 2011;17(1):115–21.
54. Diggelmann HR, et al. Insular thyroid carcinoma in a patient with Cowden syndrome. Laryngoscope. 2010;120(3):454–7.
55. Donnellan KA, et al. Metastatic insular thyroid carcinoma in the pediatric patient. Am J Otolaryngol. 2009;30(1):61–4.
56. Meyer-Rochow GY, et al. Intra-abdominal insular thyroid carcinoma metastasis. Thyroid. 2009;19(5):527–30.
57. Mizukami Y, et al. Poorly differentiated ('insular') carcinoma of the thyroid. Pathol Int. 1995;45(9):663–8.
58. Papotti M, et al. Poorly differentiated thyroid carcinomas with primordial cell component. A group of aggressive lesions sharing insular, trabecular, and solid patterns. Am J Surg Pathol. 1993;17(3):291–301.
59. Papotti M, et al. Poorly differentiated oxyphilic (Hurthle cell) carcinomas of the thyroid. Am J Surg Pathol. 1996;20(6):686–94.
60. Sobrinho-Simoes M, et al. Poorly differentiated carcinomas of the thyroid gland: a review of the clinicopathologic features of a series of 28 cases of a heterogeneous, clinically aggressive group of thyroid tumors. Int J Surg Pathol. 2002;10(2):123–31.
61. Sironi M, Collini P, Cantaboni A. Fine needle aspiration cytology of insular thyroid carcinoma. A report of four cases. Acta Cytol. 1992;36(3):435–9.
62. Mazzaferri EL, Jhiang SM. Long-term impact of initial surgical and medical therapy on papillary and follicular thyroid cancer. Am J Med. 1994;97(5):418–28.
63. Kotiloglu E, Kale G, Senocak ME. Follicular thyroid carcinoma with a predominant insular component in a child: a case report. Tumori. 1995;81(4):296–8.
64. Justin EP, et al. Insular carcinoma: a distinct thyroid carcinoma with associated iodine-131 localization. J Nucl Med. 1991;32(7):1358–63.
65. Falvo L, et al. Prognostic factors of insular versus papillary/follicular thyroid carcinoma. Am Surg. 2004;70(5):461–6.
66. Luna-Ortiz K, et al. Clinical course of insular thyroid carcinoma. Med Sci Monit. 2004;10(3):CR108–11.
67. Ashfaq R, et al. Papillary and follicular thyroid carcinomas with an insular component. Cancer. 1994;73(2):416–23.
68. Chao TC, Lin JD, Chen MF. Insular carcinoma: infrequent subtype of thyroid cancer with aggressive clinical course. World J Surg. 2004;28(4):393–6.
69. Sasaki A, et al. Insular component as a risk factor of thyroid carcinoma. Pathol Int. 1996;46(12):939–46.
70. Zak IT, Seabold JE, Gurll NJ. Tc-99m MIBI scintigraphic detection of metastatic insular thyroid carcinoma. Clin Nucl Med. 1995;20(1):31–6.
71. Burman KD, Ringel MD, Wartofsky L. Unusual types of thyroid neoplasms. Endocrinol Metab Clin N Am. 1996;25(1):49–68.
72. Diehl M, et al. F-18 FDG PET in insular thyroid cancer. Clin Nucl Med. 2003;28(9):728–31.
73. Hazard JB. Classification and staging of thyroid cancer. J Surg Oncol. 1981;16(3):255–7.
74. Hawk WA, Hazard JB. The many appearances of papillary carcinoma of the thyroid. Cleve Clin Q. 1976;43(4):207–15.
75. Morris LG, et al. Tall-cell variant of papillary thyroid carcinoma: a matched-pair analysis of survival. Thyroid. 2010;20(2):153–8.
76. Choi YJ, et al. Tall cell variant of papillary thyroid carcinoma: sonographic and clinical findings. J Ultrasound Med. 2011;30(6):853–8.
77. Lloyd RV, Buehler D, Khanafshar E. Papillary thyroid carcinoma variants. Head Neck Pathol. 2011;5(1):51–6.
78. Silver CE, et al. Aggressive variants of papillary thyroid carcinoma. Head Neck. 2011;33(7):1052–9.
79. Urano M, et al. Tall cell variant of papillary thyroid carcinoma: its characteristic features demonstrated by fine-needle aspiration cytology and immunohistochemical study. Diagn Cytopathol. 2009;37(10):732–7.
80. Terry JH, et al. Tall cell papillary thyroid cancer: incidence and prognosis. Am J Surg. 1994;168(5):459–61.
81. Harach HR, Zusman SB. Cytopathology of the tall cell variant of thyroid papillary carcinoma. Acta Cytol. 1992;36(6):895–9.
82. Hicks MJ, Batsakis JG. Tall cell carcinoma of the thyroid gland. Ann Otol Rhinol Laryngol. 1993;102(5):402–3.
83. Robbins J, et al. Thyroid cancer: a lethal endocrine neoplasm. Ann Intern Med. 1991;115(2):133–47.
84. Johnson TL, et al. Prognostic implications of the tall cell variant of papillary thyroid carcinoma. Am J Surg Pathol. 1988;12(1):22–7.
85. Ain KB. Papillary thyroid carcinoma. Etiology, assessment, and therapy. Endocrinol Metab Clin N Am. 1995;24(4):711–60.
86. Ostrowski ML, Merino MJ. Tall cell variant of papillary thyroid carcinoma: a reassessment and immunohistochemical study with comparison to the usual type of papillary carcinoma of the thyroid. Am J Surg Pathol. 1996;20(8):964–74.
87. Ozaki O, et al. Papillary carcinoma of the thyroid. Tall-cell variant with extensive lymphocyte infiltration. Am J Surg Pathol. 1996;20(6):695–8.
88. Segal K, et al. Papillary carcinoma of the thyroid. Otolaryngol Head Neck Surg. 1995;113(4):356–63.
89. Ruter A, Nishiyama R, Lennquist S. Tall-cell variant of papillary thyroid cancer: disregarded entity? World J Surg. 1997;21(1):15–20. discussion 20–1.
90. van den Brekel MW, et al. Prognostic features in tall cell papillary carcinoma and insular thyroid carcinoma. Laryngoscope. 1997;107(2):254–9.
91. Gamboa-Dominguez A, et al. Tall cell variant of papillary thyroid carcinoma. A cytohistologic correlation. Acta Cytol. 1997;41(3):672–6.
92. Bocklage T, et al. Tall cell variant of papillary thyroid carcinoma: cytologic features and differential diagnostic considerations. Diagn Cytopathol. 1997;17(1):25–9.
93. Asklen L, Verhaug J. Thyroid carcinoma with mixed tall-cell and columnar-cell carcinoma: another variant of poorly differentiated carcinoma of the thyroid. Am J Clin Pathol. 1990;94:442–5.
94. Bronner MP, LiVolsi VA. Spindle cell squamous carcinoma of the thyroid: an unusual anaplastic tumor associated with tall cell papillary cancer. Mod Pathol. 1991;4(5):637–43.
95. Evans HL. Columnar-cell carcinoma of the thyroid. A report of two cases of an aggressive variant of thyroid carcinoma. Am J Clin Pathol. 1986;85(1):77–80.
96. Basolo F, et al. Potent mitogenicity of the RET/PTC3 oncogene correlates with its prevalence in tall-cell variant of papillary thyroid carcinoma. Am J Pathol. 2002;160(1):247–54.
97. Moreno Egea A, et al. Prognostic value of the tall cell variety of papillary cancer of the thyroid. Eur J Surg Oncol. 1993;19(6):517–21.
98. Ringel MD, Burman KD, Shmookler BM. Unusual types of thyroid cancer. In: Wartofsky L, editor. Thyroid cancer: a comprehensive guide to clinical management. Totowa: Humana Press; 1999. p. 421–51.
99. Sywak M, Pasieka JL, Ogilvie T. A review of thyroid cancer with intermediate differentiation. J Surg Oncol. 2004;86(1):44–54.

100. Chen JH, et al. Clinicopathological and molecular characterization of nine cases of columnar cell variant of papillary thyroid carcinoma. Mod Pathol. 2011;24(5):739–49.
101. Sobrinho-Simoes M, Nesland JM, Johannessen JV. Columnar-cell carcinoma. Another variant of poorly differentiated carcinoma of the thyroid. Am J Clin Pathol. 1988;89(2):264–7.
102. Mizukami Y, et al. Columnar cell carcinoma of the thyroid gland: a case report and review of the literature. Hum Pathol. 1994;25(10):1098–101.
103. Gaertner EM, Davidson M, Wenig BM. The columnar cell variant of thyroid papillary carcinoma. Case report and discussion of an unusually aggressive thyroid papillary carcinoma. Am J Surg Pathol. 1995;19(8):940–7.
104. Ferreiro JA, Hay ID, Lloyd RV. Columnar cell carcinoma of the thyroid: report of three additional cases. Hum Pathol. 1996;27(11):1156–60.
105. Evans HL. Encapsulated columnar-cell neoplasms of the thyroid. A report of four cases suggesting a favorable prognosis. Am J Surg Pathol. 1996;20(10):1205–11.
106. Hui PK, et al. Columnar cell carcinoma of the thyroid. Fine needle aspiration findings in a case. Acta Cytol. 1990;34(3):355–8.
107. Mizukami Y, et al. Diffuse sclerosing variant of papillary carcinoma of the thyroid. Report of three cases. Acta Pathol Jpn. 1990;40(9):676–82.
108. Caplan R, Wester K, Kisken W. Diffuse sclerosing variant of papillary thyroid carcinoma of the thyroid: fine needle aspiration findings in a case. Endocr Pract. 1997;3:287–92.
109. Regalbuto C, et al. A diffuse sclerosing variant of papillary thyroid carcinoma: clinical and pathologic features and outcomes of 34 consecutive cases. Thyroid. 2011;21(4):383–9.
110. Calo PG, et al. Sclerosing mucoepidermoid thyroid carcinoma requiring cervical reconstruction: a case report and review of the literature. Am Surg. 2010;76(8):918–9.
111. Koo JS, Hong S, Park CS. Diffuse sclerosing variant is a major subtype of papillary thyroid carcinoma in the young. Thyroid. 2009;19(11):1225–31.
112. Kwak JY, et al. Diffuse sclerosing variant of papillary carcinoma of the thyroid gland: specimen radiographic features with histopathological correlation. J Clin Endocrinol Metab. 2009;94(5):1491–2.
113. Chan JK, Tsui MS, Tse CH. Diffuse sclerosing variant of papillary carcinoma of the thyroid: a histological and immunohistochemical study of three cases. Histopathology. 1987;11(2):191–201.
114. Soares J, Limbert E, Sobrinho-Simoes M. Diffuse sclerosing variant of papillary thyroid carcinoma. A clinicopathologic study of 10 cases. Pathol Res Pract. 1989;185(2):200–6.
115. Wu PS, et al. Diffuse sclerosing papillary carcinoma of thyroid: a wolf in sheep's clothing. Clin Endocrinol (Oxf). 1989;31(5):535–40.
116. Carcangiu ML, Bianchi S. Diffuse sclerosing variant of papillary thyroid carcinoma. Clinicopathologic study of 15 cases. Am J Surg Pathol. 1989;13(12):1041–9.
117. Fujimoto Y, et al. Diffuse sclerosing variant of papillary carcinoma of the thyroid. Clinical importance, surgical treatment, and follow-up study. Cancer. 1990;66(11):2306–12.
118. Hayashi Y, et al. Diffuse sclerosing variant of papillary carcinoma of the thyroid. A histopathological study of four cases. Acta Pathol Jpn. 1990;40(3):193–8.
119. Furmanchuk AW, et al. Pathomorphological findings in thyroid cancers of children from the Republic of Belarus: a study of 86 cases occurring between 1986 ('post-Chernobyl') and 1991. Histopathology. 1992;21(5):401–8.
120. Nikiforov YE, et al. Solid variant of papillary thyroid carcinoma: incidence, clinical-pathologic characteristics, molecular analysis, and biologic behavior. Am J Surg Pathol. 2001;25(12):1478–84.
121. Klugbauer S, et al. High prevalence of RET rearrangement in thyroid tumors of children from Belarus after the Chernobyl reactor accident. Oncogene. 1995;11(12):2459–67.
122. Nikiforov YE, et al. Distinct pattern of ret oncogene rearrangements in morphological variants of radiation-induced and sporadic thyroid papillary carcinomas in children. Cancer Res. 1997;57(9):1690–4.
123. Papotti M, et al. Mixed medullary-follicular carcinoma of the thyroid. A morphological, immunohistochemical and in situ hybridization analysis of 11 cases. Virchows Arch. 1997;430(5):397–405.
124. Hales M, et al. Carcinoma of the thyroid with a mixed medullary and follicular pattern: morphologic, immunohistochemical, and clinical laboratory studies. Cancer. 1982;50(7):1352–9.
125. Kashima K, et al. Mixed medullary and follicular carcinoma of the thyroid: report of two cases with an immunohistochemical study. Acta Pathol Jpn. 1993;43(7–8):428–33.
126. Ljungberg O, et al. A compound follicular-parafollicular cell carcinoma of the thyroid: a new tumor entity? Cancer. 1983;52(6):1053–61.
127. Mizukami Y, et al. Mixed medullary-follicular carcinoma of the thyroid occurring in familial form. Histopathology. 1993;22(3):284–7.
128. Tanaka T, et al. Simultaneous occurrence of medullary and follicular carcinoma in the same thyroid lobe. Hum Pathol. 1989;20(1):83–6.
129. Tanda F, et al. Mixed follicular-parafollicular carcinoma of the thyroid: a light, electron microscopic and histoimmunologic study. Surg Pathol. 1990;3:65–74.
130. Papotti M, et al. Thyroid carcinomas with mixed follicular and C-cell differentiation patterns. Semin Diagn Pathol. 2000;17(2):109–19.
131. Lamberg BA, et al. Concurrent medullary and papillary thyroid carcinoma in the same thyroid lobe and in siblings. Acta Med Scand. 1981;209(5):421–4.
132. Lax SF, et al. Coexistence of papillary and medullary carcinoma of the thyroid gland-mixed or collision tumour? Clinicopathological analysis of three cases. Virchows Arch. 1994;424(4):441–7.
133. Duskova J, et al. Fine needle aspiration biopsy of mixed medullary-follicular thyroid carcinoma. A report of two cases. Acta Cytol. 2003;47(1):71–7.
134. Wenig BM, Adair CF, Heffess CS. Primary mucoepidermoid carcinoma of the thyroid gland: a report of six cases and a review of the literature of a follicular epithelial-derived tumor. Hum Pathol. 1995;26(10):1099–108.
135. Rhatigan RM, Roque JL, Bucher RL. Mucoepidermoid carcinoma of the thyroid gland. Cancer. 1977;39(1):210–4.
136. Rocha AS, et al. Mucoepidermoid carcinoma of the thyroid: a tumour histotype characterised by P-cadherin neoexpression and marked abnormalities of E-cadherin/catenins complex. Virchows Arch. 2002;440(5):498–504.
137. Cameselle-Teijeiro J, Febles-Perez C, Sobrinho-Simoes M. Cytologic features of fine needle aspirates of papillary and mucoepidermoid carcinoma of the thyroid with anaplastic transformation. A case report. Acta Cytol. 1997;41(4 Suppl):1356–60.
138. Cameselle-Teijeiro J, Chan JK. Cribriform-morular variant of papillary carcinoma: a distinctive variant representing the sporadic counterpart of familial adenomatous polyposis-associated thyroid carcinoma? Mod Pathol. 1999;12(4):400–11.
139. Cameselle-Teijeiro J, Febles-Perez C, Sobrinho-Simoes M. Papillary and mucoepidermoid carcinoma of the thyroid with anaplastic transformation: a case report with histologic and immunohistochemical findings that support a provocative histogenetic hypothesis. Pathol Res Pract. 1995;191(12):1214–21.
140. Franssila KO, Harach HR, Wasenius VM. Mucoepidermoid carcinoma of the thyroid. Histopathology. 1984;8(5):847–60.

141. Chan JK, et al. Sclerosing mucoepidermoid thyroid carcinoma with eosinophilia. A distinctive low-grade malignancy arising from the metaplastic follicles of Hashimoto's thyroiditis. Am J Surg Pathol. 1991;15(5):438–48.
142. Katoh R, et al. Mucoepidermoid carcinoma of the thyroid gland. Cancer. 1990;65(9):2020–7.
143. Prichard RS, et al. Mucoepidermoid carcinoma of the thyroid: a report of three cases and postulated histogenesis. Thyroid. 2012;22(2):205–9.
144. Thompson LD, et al. Primary smooth muscle tumors of the thyroid gland. Cancer. 1997;79(3):579–87.
145. Kawahara E, et al. Leiomyosarcoma of the thyroid gland. A case report with a comparative study of five cases of anaplastic carcinoma. Cancer. 1988;62(12):2558–63.
146. Chetty R, Clark SP, Dowling JP. Leiomyosarcoma of the thyroid: immunohistochemical and ultrastructural study. Pathology. 1993;25(2):203–5.
147. Iida Y, et al. Primary leiomyosarcoma of the thyroid gland. Acta Pathol Jpn. 1993;43(1–2):71–5.
148. Lindahl F. Sarcoma of the thyroid gland: twenty-two cases in Denmark 1943–1968. Dan Med Bull. 1976;23(3):103–7.
149. Syrjanen KJ. An osteogenic sarcoma of the thyroid gland (report of a case and survey of the literature). Neoplasma. 1979;26(5):623–8.
150. Griem KL, et al. Radiation-induced sarcoma of the thyroid. Arch Otolaryngol Head Neck Surg. 1989;115(8):991–3.
151. Mills SE, et al. Angiomatoid carcinoma and 'angiosarcoma' of the thyroid gland. A spectrum of endothelial differentiation. Am J Clin Pathol. 1994;102(3):322–30.
152. Lamovec J, Zidar A, Zidanik B. Epithelioid angiosarcoma of the thyroid gland. Report of two cases. Arch Pathol Lab Med. 1994;118(6):642–6.
153. Chan YF, et al. Angiosarcoma of the thyroid. An immunohistochemical and ultrastructural study of a case in a Chinese patient. Cancer. 1986;57(12):2381–8.
154. Mollison LC, et al. Hypothyroidism due to destruction of the thyroid by Kaposi's sarcoma. Rev Infect Dis. 1991;13(5):826–7.
155. Mills SE, Stallings RG, Austin MB. Angiomatoid carcinoma of the thyroid gland. Anaplastic carcinoma with follicular and medullary features mimicking angiosarcoma. Am J Clin Pathol. 1986;86(5):674–8.
156. Merimsky O, et al. Sarcoma and thyroid disorders: a common etiology? Oncol Rep. 2002;9(4):863–9.
157. Erickson ML, McKee M, Reyes-Mugica M. Rapid progression of SETTLE tumor with micrometastasis. Pediatr Dev Pathol. 2008;11(1):68.
158. Haberal AN, et al. Unusual spindle cell tumor of thyroid (SETTLE). Thyroid. 2008;18(1):85–7.
159. Folpe AL, et al. Spindle epithelial tumor with thymus-like differentiation: a morphologic, immunohistochemical, and molecular genetic study of 11 cases. Am J Surg Pathol. 2009;33(8):1179–86.
160. Ajmi S, et al. Spindle epithelial tumor with thymus-like differentiation of the thyroid. Clin Nucl Med. 2008;33(12):887–8.
161. Grushka JR, et al. Spindle epithelial tumor with thymus-like elements of the thyroid: a multi-institutional case series and review of the literature. J Pediatr Surg. 2009;44(5):944–8.
162. Magnata Filho LA, et al. Thyroid spindle epithelial tumor with thymus-like differentiation (SETTLE): case report and review. Arq Bras Endocrinol Metabol. 2010;54(7):657–62.
163. Llamas-Gutierrez FJ, et al. Spindle epithelial tumor with thymus-like differentiation of the thyroid (SETTLE): Report of two cases (one associated with a parathyroid adenoma). Ann Diagn Pathol. 2013;17:217–21.
164. Buckley NJ, Burch WM, Leight GS. Malignant teratoma in the thyroid gland of an adult: a case report and a review of the literature. Surgery. 1986;100(5):932–7.
165. Bowker CM, Whittaker RS. Malignant teratoma of the thyroid: case report and literature review of thyroid teratoma in adults. Histopathology. 1992;21(1):81–3.
166. Stone HH, Henderson WD, Guidio FA. Teratomas of the neck. Am J Dis Child. 1967;113(2):222–4.
167. Buckwalter JA, Layton JM. Malignant teratoma in the thyroid gland of an adult. Ann Surg. 1954;139(2):218–23.
168. Kimler SC, Muth WF. Primary malignant teratoma of the thyroid: case report and literature review of cervical teratomas in adults. Cancer. 1978;42(1):311–7.
169. Hajdu SI, Hajdu EO. Malignant teratoma of the neck. Arch Pathol. 1967;83(6):567–70.
170. O'Higgins N, Taylor S. Malignant teratoma in the adult thyroid gland. Br J Clin Pract. 1975;29(9):237–8.
171. Andrion A, et al. Leiomyoma and neurilemoma: report of two unusual non-epithelial tumours of the thyroid gland. Virchows Arch A Pathol Anat Histopathol. 1988;413(4):367–72.
172. Hendrick JW. Leiomyoma of thyroid gland; report of case. Surgery. 1957;42(3):597–9.
173. Delaney WE, Fry KE. Neurilemoma of the thyroid gland. Ann Surg. 1964;160:1014–7.
174. Goldstein J, Tovi F, Sidi J. Primary Schwannoma of the thyroid gland. Int Surg. 1982;67(4 Suppl):433–4.
175. Mahoney CP, Patterson SD, Ryan J. Granular cell tumor of the thyroid gland in a girl receiving high-dose estrogen therapy. Pediatr Pathol Lab Med. 1995;15(5):791–5.
176. Carney JA, Ryan J, Goellner JR. Hyalinizing trabecular adenoma of the thyroid gland. Am J Surg Pathol. 1987;11(8):583–91.
177. Sambade C, et al. Hyalinizing trabecular adenoma: a misnomer for a peculiar tumor of the thyroid gland. Endocr Pathol. 1991;2:83–91.
178. Goellner JR, Carney JA. Cytologic features of fine-needle aspirates of hyalinizing trabecular adenoma of the thyroid. Am J Clin Pathol. 1989;91(2):115–9.
179. Bondeson L, Bondeson AG. Clue helping to distinguish hyalinizing trabecular adenoma from carcinoma of the thyroid in fine-needle aspirates. Diagn Cytopathol. 1994;10(1):25–9.
180. Chan JK, Tse CC, Chiu HS. Hyalinizing trabecular adenoma-like lesion in multinodular goitre. Histopathology. 1990;16(6):611–4.
181. Chan JK, Loo KT. Cribriform variant of papillary thyroid carcinoma. Arch Pathol Lab Med. 1990;114(6):622–4.
182. Mizukami Y, et al. Ectopic thymic tissue in the thyroid gland. Endocr Pathol. 1993;4:162–4.
183. LiVolsi V. Branchial and thymic remnants in the thyroid gland and cervical region: an explanation for unusual tumors and microscopic curiosities. Endocr Pathol. 1993;4:115–9.
184. Russell WO, et al. Thyroid carcinoma. Classification, intraglandular dissemination, and clinicopathological study based upon whole organ sections of 80 glands. Cancer. 1963;16:1425–60.
185. Mizukami Y, et al. Thymic carcinoma involving the thyroid gland: report of two cases. Hum Pathol. 1995;26(5):576–9.
186. Chan JK, Rosai J. Tumors of the neck showing thymic or related branchial pouch differentiation: a unifying concept. Hum Pathol. 1991;22(4):349–67.
187. Harach HR, Saravia Day E, Franssila KO. Thyroid spindle-cell tumor with mucous cysts. An intrathyroid thymoma? Am J Surg Pathol. 1985;9(7):525–30.
188. Klubo-Gwiezdzinska J, et al. Clinical review: ectopic cervical thyroid carcinoma – review of the literature with illustrative case series. J Clin Endocrinol Metab. 2011;96(9):2684–91.
189. Pollock WF, Stevenson EO. Cysts and sinuses of the thyroglossal duct. Am J Surg. 1966;112(2):225–32.
190. Jaques DA, Chambers RG, Oertel JE. Thyroglossal tract carcinoma. A review of the literature and addition of eighteen cases. Am J Surg. 1970;120(4):439–46.

191. LiVolsi VA, Perzin KH, Savetsky L. Carcinoma arising in median ectopic thyroid (including thyroglossal duct tissue). Cancer. 1974;34(4):1303–15.
192. Heshmati HM, et al. Thyroglossal duct carcinoma: report of 12 cases. Mayo Clin Proc. 1997;72(4):315–9.
193. Tew S, et al. Papillary thyroid carcinoma arising in thyroglossal duct cysts: incidence and management. Aust N Z J Surg. 1995;65(10):717–8.
194. Mahnke CG, et al. Primary papillary carcinoma of the thyroglossal duct: case report and review of the literature. Auris Nasus Larynx. 1994;21(4):258–63.
195. Kwan WB, et al. Concurrent papillary and squamous carcinoma in a thyroglossal duct cyst: a case report. Can J Surg. 1996;39(4):328–32.
196. Udoji WC. Thyroglossal duct cyst mass with Hashimoto's disease and non-Hodgkin's lymphoma. J Tenn Med Assoc. 1996;89(4):113–4.
197. Deshpande A, Bobhate SK. Squamous cell carcinoma in thyroglossal duct cyst. J Laryngol Otol. 1995;109(10):1001–4.
198. Czech JM, et al. Neoplasms metastatic to the thyroid gland. Surg Gynecol Obstet. 1982;155(4):503–5.
199. Nakhjavani MK, et al. Metastasis to the thyroid gland. A report of 43 cases. Cancer. 1997;79(3):574–8.
200. Giuffrida D, et al. Metastasis to the thyroid gland: a case report and review of the literature. J Endocrinol Invest. 2003;26(6):560–3.
201. Chung AY, Tran TB, Brumund KT, Weisman RA, Bouvet M. Metastases to the thyroid: a review of the literature from the last decade. Thyroid. 2012;22:258–68.
202. Mirallie E, et al. Management and prognosis of metastases to the thyroid gland. J Am Coll Surg. 2005;200(2):203–7.
203. Miyakawa M, et al. Severe thyrotoxicosis induced by thyroid metastasis of lung adenocarcinoma: a case report and review of the literature. Thyroid. 2001;11(9):883–8.

82 Pathology of Miscellaneous and Unusual Cancers of the Thyroid

Zubair W. Baloch and Virginia A. LiVolsi

Hyalinizing Trabecular Neoplasms

These rare neoplasms are solid masses, often less than 3 cm in diameter, and are well circumscribed (usually encapsulated). The cut surfaces are light colored, and vessels and small foci of fibrosis may be visible. Microscopically, the tumors consist of trabeculae and lobules of elongated, oval, or polygonal cells, usually medium sized and with poorly defined borders. The groups of cells are surrounded by capillaries and variable amounts of eosinophilic, hyalinized material, which consists of clumps of type IV collagen and laminin [1]. The numerous cytoplasmic microfilaments (presumably keratin) present in many of the epithelial cells also contribute to the eosinophilic zones [2, 3].

The neoplastic cells have been described as eosinophilic, amphophilic, or clear with fine granules apparent in the cytoplasm. Nuclei appear rounded, oval, or elongated and often grooved (Fig. 82.1). They may contain cytoplasmic inclusions and clear zones; in turn, these zones contain tiny rods composed of bundles of minute filaments (visible on electron microscopy) [2]. Variable numbers of small follicles occur in the trabeculae, some with colloid and some empty. Electron microscopy shows intercellular spaces surrounded by microvilli, presumably representing developing follicles [4]. Psammoma bodies may be scattered throughout the tumor. Most cells show immunoreactivity for TTF-1, thyroglobulin, and keratin; calcitonin has never been demonstrated [4, 5]. An alteration similar to that of this hyalinizing tumor has been described in the adenomatoid nodules of a nodular goiter [6].

It has been proposed that hyalinizing trabecular adenomas actually represent an encapsulated variant of papillary carcinoma. This is due to the similar nuclear cytology, immunoprofile, and RET-oncogene rearrangements in both tumors [7]. However, a benign behavior has so far been described in all cases of hyalinizing trabecular neoplasm, and none of these tumors have been shown to harbor BRAF mutations [8].

Aspirates of these lesions have been misinterpreted as follicular neoplasms, papillary carcinomas, and medullary carcinomas [9]. Moderate-to-marked cellularity is evident, with the cells forming clusters and follicles. Colloid is not present, but irregular masses of hyaline material are adjacent to the cell clusters. This material has been described with fringed or granular margins and a suggestion of a fibrillary structure. It is purple red or magenta with May-Grunwald-Giemsa stain [9, 10] and pink to gray blue with Papanicolaou stain [10]. Cells are rounded, polygonal, or elongated with cytoplasm of diverse density. Nuclei often contain grooves (in Papanicolaou-stained material) and cytoplasmic inclusions. Small psammoma bodies have been seen in some cases.

Metastatic (Secondary) Neoplasms

The most common metastatic neoplasms in the gland that may mimic primary tumors are those from the lung, breast, and kidney. These neoplasms have the usual range of histological patterns, depending on the primary sites. Involvement of an existing adenomatoid nodule, adenoma and rarely carcinoma may occur, thereby complicating the morphological features. Immunohistochemical procedures are helpful in separating metastatic lesions from primary thyroid neoplasms when uncertainty exists with the interpretation. Data and

Z.W. Baloch, MD, PhD (✉) • V.A. LiVolsi, MD
Department of Pathology and Laboratory Medicine, Perelman School of Medicine, University of Pennsylvania Medical Center, 6 Founders Pavilion 3400 Spruce Street, Philadelphia, PA 19104, USA
e-mail: balocj@mail.med.upenn.edu; linus@mail.med.upenn.edu

L. Wartofsky, D. Van Nostrand (eds.), *Thyroid Cancer*, DOI 10.1007/978-1-4939-3314-3_82

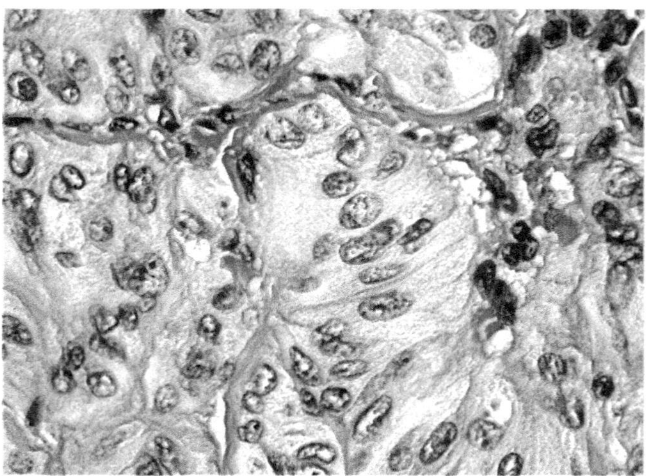

Fig. 82.1 Hyalinizing trabecular neoplasm. Elongated tumor cells with intranuclear grooves and nuclear chromatin clearing (H&E stain)

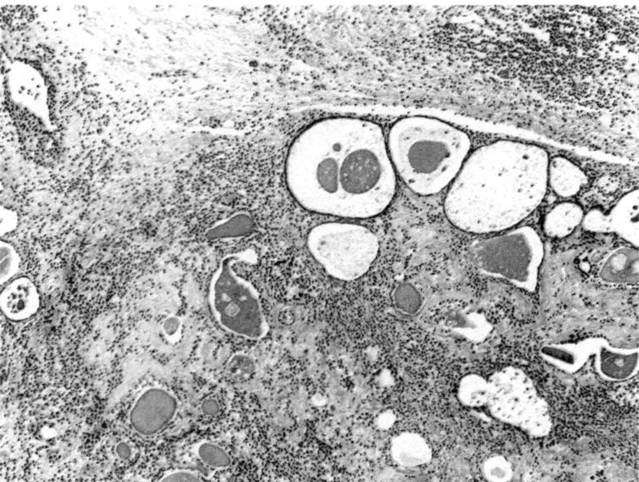

Fig. 82.2 Mucoepidermoid carcinoma. Dilated cystic spaces are visible (H&E stain)

materials must be evaluated carefully, however, because some nonspecific uptake of thyroglobulin may occur by the metastatic cells. Malignant melanoma involves the thyroid with moderate frequency, but the patient's clinical history allows this metastasis to be somewhat easy to diagnose [11, 12].

Squamous Cell Carcinoma

This rare aggressive neoplasm usually occur in middle-aged or elderly patients, often in glands containing a well-differentiated carcinoma (especially papillary carcinoma), an adenoma, a multinodular goiter, or occasionally, chronic autoimmune thyroiditis [13–15]. Because of the intimate relationship to neoplastic glandular elements, some squamous cancers have been called "adenosquamous carcinomas." Undifferentiated carcinoma may be evident, along with the predominant squamous carcinoma. Squamous carcinoma with extensive spindled cell change has been reported in association with tall-cell papillary carcinoma [16]. An occasional squamous carcinoma of the thyroid has been linked with hypercalcemia and leukocytosis [17].

Mucoepidermoid Carcinoma

This category consists of two rare and distinct neoplasms: mucoepidermoid carcinoma and sclerosing mucoepidermoid carcinoma [18–20]. *Mucoepidermoid carcinoma* is a distinctive variant of thyroid carcinoma. It is composed of solid masses of squamoid cells and mucin-producing cells, sometimes forming glands (Figs. 82.2 and 82.3). Because all cases show thyroglobulin expression, some authors consider that it is a variant of papillary carcinoma; lesions may metastasize to regional nodes and rarely distantly. Death from disease is rare [21–23]. *Sclerosing mucoepidermoid carcinoma with eosinophilia* is usually seen in a background of lymphocytic thyroiditis and is characterized by tumor cells arranged in small sheets, anastomosing trabeculae and narrow strands associated with dense fibrosis and numerous eosinophils. While these lesions may metastasize to lymph nodes and show extracapsular spread, vascular invasion, and perineural invasion, death due to disease is uncommon [20, 23]. The tumor cells usually stain negative for thyroglobulin and calcitonin and positive for cytokeratin and p63 [24]. In lieu of their immunoprofile, it is believed that these tumors are derived from ultimobranchial body rests/solid cell nests [24].

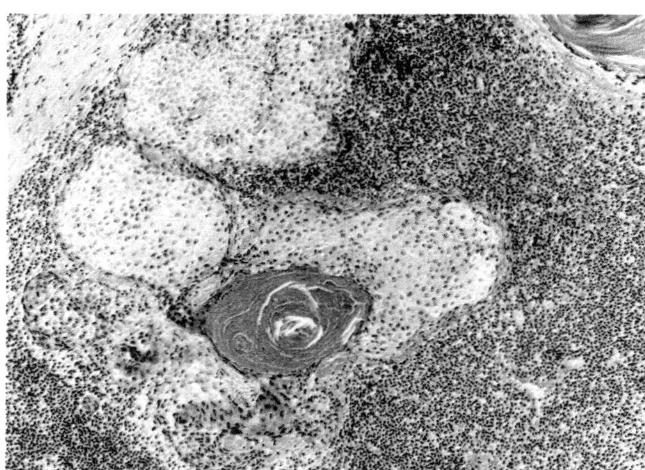

Fig. 82.3 Mucoepidermoid carcinoma. Nests of squamous cells and two keratin pearls lie in a heavy infiltrate of lymphocytes (H&E stain)

Intrathyroidal Thymoma-Like Neoplasms

This group represents rare thyroid tumors which include *spindled and epithelial tumor with thymus-like differentiation (SETTLE)* [25, 26] *and carcinoma with thymus-like differentiation (CASTLE)* [27]. These lesions originate from branchial pouch remnants within and adjacent to the thyroid [28].

Follicular-Derived Familial Tumors

The frequency of follicular cell-derived tumors as familial events is estimated to be between 1 % and 5 % of all thyroid tumors [29]. This group comprises of familial non-medullary thyroid carcinoma (FNMTC) as the predominant lesion of a familial tumor syndrome or associated with syndromes having extrathyroidal manifestations [30].

PTC may occur in multiple family members. In order to be considered familial cancer, at least three first-degree relatives should be affected. The histology of these tumors is not different from nonfamilial although multifocal and bilateral lesions are found. Some series indicate that these tumors clinically behave more aggressively than sporadic tumors [31]. Though chromosomal abnormalities have been detected in these tumors, specific associated genes are yet to be identified [29].

PTC and other follicular-derived thyroid tumors can be seen in association with PTEN hamartoma syndrome, McCune-Albright syndrome, Carney complex, Peutz-Jeghers syndrome, Werner syndrome, and MEN syndromes [29, 30, 32–34].

Neoplasms Associated with Familial Intestinal Adenomatous Polyposis

These rare neoplasms have trabecular, solid, papillary, and cribriform patterns that are formed by spindled, polygonal, and tall columnar cells and are different from the usual papillary and follicular carcinomas. Small whorls of cells may be found, but these are not squamous foci. Cytoplasm is oxyphilic to amphophilic, sometimes clear. Nuclei are hyperchromatic, slightly irregular, and medium sized; nucleoli vary in size and visibility. Cytoplasmic inclusions in the nuclei vary in number and size, and some nuclear grooves may be seen. Focal positivity for thyroglobulin can be found, but colloid is present in minimal amounts or absent.

These neoplasms are usually small and multiple, and the majority have occurred in girls and young women [35–38].

Angiosarcoma

This neoplasm has been regarded as rare, even in endemic goiter regions [39–41]; several tumors with histological features consistent with angiosarcoma have expressed immunoreactive keratins, as well as endothelial features (e.g., factor VIII-associated antigens and Weibel-Palade bodies). Authors have suggested that some of these neoplasms might be considered as angiomatoid carcinomas (a form of undifferentiated or anaplastic carcinoma [42, 43], expressing epithelial markers and endothelial characteristics). Most patients are middle aged or elderly, and most tumors are extremely aggressive, similar to typical anaplastic carcinomas.

Leiomyosarcoma

Leiomyosarcoma has been reported but is extremely rare. A characteristic histological pattern is not only required, but immunohistochemical techniques are often needed to separate leiomyosarcoma from anaplastic carcinoma [44, 45].

Thyroglossal Duct Cancer

Thyroglossal duct extends in the midline from the foramen cecum at the base of the tongue to the isthmus of the normal gland [46]. It is usually attached to and may extend through the center of the hyoid bone and is intimately related to the surrounding skeletal muscle. By light microscopy, it consists of connective tissue, the thyroglossal duct, lymphoid tissue, and thyroid follicles. The thyroglossal duct is typically lined by ciliated pseudostratified epithelium. In case of trauma or infection, the epithelium may undergo transitional or squamous metaplasia or may be totally replaced by fibrous tissue. Fluid accumulation in the duct can lead to development of a thyroglossal cyst [47, 48].

In rare instances, portions of thyroglossal duct are embedded within the thyroid gland proper and can give rise to an intrathyroidal cyst [46]. Nearly all of the tumors that arise in the thyroid tissue that accompanies the duct or cyst are papillary carcinomas [46, 49, 50], a few are follicular carcinomas [46, 49], and rarely anaplastic carcinoma has been reported [51]. Squamous carcinoma has been documented [52], presumably arising from the respiratory epithelium of the thyroglossal duct or cyst. Fine-needle aspiration is useful in diagnosing thyroglossal abnormalities. If the aspirate consists of more than the usual hypocellular specimen from a cyst, then the standard criteria are applied for recognizing thyroid tumors [52, 53].

Teratoma

Benign teratomas in newborns and infants may cause various obstructive phenomena, especially when cystic, and must be resected promptly. They do not recur or spread [54]. Malignant teratomas have been seen in adults, most commonly in women, and are composed of primitive epithelial, mesenchymal, and neuroectodermal elements [54–56]. They spread locally and may have regional and distant metastases [54].

References

1. Carney JA, Ryan J, Goellner JR. Hyalinizing trabecular adenoma of the thyroid gland. Am J Surg Pathol. 1987;11:583–91.
2. Katoh R, Jasani B, Williams ED. Hyalinizing trabecular adenoma of the thyroid. A report of three cases with immunohistochemical and ultrastructural studies. Histopathology. 1989;15:211–24.
3. Fornes P, Lesourd A, Dupuis G, Merceron RE, Sarfati E, Guettier C, Brocheriou C. Hyalinizing trabecular adenoma of the thyroid gland. Histologic and immunohistochemical study. Report of 2 cases. Arch Anat Cytol Pathol. 1990;38:203–7.
4. Chetty R, Beydoun R, LiVolsi VA. Paraganglioma-like (hyalinizing trabecular) adenoma of the thyroid revisited. Pathology. 1994;26: 429–31.
5. Fonseca E, Nesland J, Sobrinho-Simoes M. Expression of stratified epithelial type cytokeratins in hyalinizing trabecular adenoma supports their relationship with papillary carcinoma of the thyroid. Histopathology. 1997;31:330–5.
6. Chan JK, Tse CC, Chiu HS. Hyalinizing trabecular adenoma-like lesion in multinodular goitre. Histopathology. 1990;16:611–4.
7. Papotti M, Volante M, Giuliano A, Fassina A, Fusco A, Bussolati G, Santoro M, Chiappetta G. RET/PTC activation in hyalinizing trabecular tumors of the thyroid. Am J Surg Pathol. 2000;24:1615–21.
8. Nakamura N, Carney JA, Jin L, Kajita S, Pallares J, Zhang H, Qian X, Sebo TJ, Erickson LA, Lloyd RV. RASSF1A and NORE1A methylation and BRAFV600E mutations in thyroid tumors. Lab Invest. 2005;85:1065–75.
9. Strong CJ, Garcia BM. Fine needle aspiration cytologic characteristics of hyalinizing trabecular adenoma of the thyroid. Acta Cytol. 1990;34:359–62.
10. Bondeson L, Bondeson AG. Clue helping to distinguish hyalinizing trabecular adenoma from carcinoma of the thyroid in fine-needle aspirates. Diagn Cytopathol. 1994;10:25–9.
11. Lam KY, Lo CY. Metastatic tumors of the thyroid gland: a study of 79 cases in Chinese patients. Arch Pathol Lab Med. 1998;122:37–41.
12. Baloch ZW, LiVolsi VA. Tumor-to-tumor metastasis to follicular variant of papillary carcinoma of thyroid. Arch Pathol Lab Med. 1999;123:703–6.
13. Motoyama T, Watanabe H. Simultaneous squamous cell carcinoma and papillary adenocarcinoma of the thyroid gland. Hum Pathol. 1983;14:1009–10.
14. Morikawa Y, Ishihara Y, Kawano I, Matsuura N, Kaname A, Kakudo K. Cystic squamous cell carcinoma of the thyroid a possible new subgroup of intrathyroidal epithelial thymoma. Endocr Pathol. 1995;6:77–81.
15. Syed MI, Stewart M, Syed S, Dahill S, Adams C, McLellan DR, Clark LJ. Squamous cell carcinoma of the thyroid gland: primary or secondary disease? J Laryngol Otol. 2011;125:3–9.
16. Gopal PP, Montone KT, Baloch Z, Tuluc M, Livolsi V. The variable presentations of anaplastic spindle cell squamous carcinoma associated with tall cell variant of papillary thyroid carcinoma. Thyroid. 2011;21:493–9.
17. Sato K, Fujii Y, Ono M, Nomura H, Shizume K. Production of interleukin 1 alpha-like factor and colony-stimulating factor by a squamous cell carcinoma of the thyroid (T3M-5) derived from a patient with hypercalcemia and leukocytosis. Cancer Res. 1987; 47:6474–80.
18. Rhatigan RM, Roque JL, Bucher RL. Mucoepidermoid carcinoma of the thyroid gland. Cancer. 1977;39:210–4.
19. Franssila KO, Harach HR, Wasenius VM. Mucoepidermoid carcinoma of the thyroid. Histopathology. 1984;8:847–60.
20. Chan JK, Albores-Saavedra J, Battifora H, Carcangiu ML, Rosai J. Sclerosing mucoepidermoid thyroid carcinoma with eosinophilia. A distinctive low-grade malignancy arising from the metaplastic follicles of Hashimoto's thyroiditis. Am J Surg Pathol. 1991; 15:438–48.
21. Katoh R, Sugai T, Ono S, Takayama K, Tomichi N, Kurihara H, Takamatsu M. Mucoepidermoid carcinoma of the thyroid gland. Cancer. 1990;65:2020–7.
22. Wenig BM, Adair CF, Heffess CS. Primary mucoepidermoid carcinoma of the thyroid gland: a report of six cases and a review of the literature of a follicular epithelial-derived tumor. Hum Pathol. 1995;26:1099–108.
23. Baloch ZW, Solomon AC, LiVolsi VA. Primary mucoepidermoid carcinoma and sclerosing mucoepidermoid carcinoma with eosinophilia of the thyroid gland: a report of nine cases. Mod Pathol. 2000;13:802–7.
24. Hunt JL, LiVolsi VA, Barnes EL. p63 expression in sclerosing mucoepidermoid carcinomas with eosinophilia arising in the thyroid. Mod Pathol. 2004;17:526–9.
25. Hofman P, Mainguene C, Michiels JF, Pages A, Thyss A. Thyroid spindle epithelial tumor with thymus-like differentiation (the "SETTLE" tumor). An immunohistochemical and electron microscopic study. Eur Arch Otorhinolaryngol. 1995;252:316–20.
26. Chetty R, Goetsch S, Nayler S, Cooper K. Spindle epithelial tumour with thymus-like element (SETTLE): the predominantly monophasic variant. Histopathology. 1998;33:71–4.
27. Roka S, Kornek G, Schuller J, Ortmann E, Feichtinger J, Armbruster C. Carcinoma showing thymic-like elements – a rare malignancy of the thyroid gland. Br J Surg. 2004;91:142–5.
28. Chan JK, Rosai J. Tumors of the neck showing thymic or related branchial pouch differentiation: a unifying concept. Hum Pathol. 1991;22:349–67.
29. Nose V. Familial non-medullary thyroid carcinoma: an update. Endocr Pathol. 2008;19:226–40.
30. Dotto J, Nose V. Familial thyroid carcinoma: a diagnostic algorithm. Adv Anat Pathol. 2008;15:332–49.
31. Kraimps JL, Bouin-Pineau MH, Amati P, Mothes D, Bonneau D, Marechaud R, Barbier J. Familial papillary carcinoma of the thyroid. Surgery. 1997;121:715–8.
32. Fenton PA, Clarke SE, Owen W, Hibbert J, Hodgson SV. Cribriform variant papillary thyroid cancer: a characteristic of familial adenomatous polyposis. Thyroid. 2001;11:193–7.
33. Goto M, Miller RW, Ishikawa Y, Sugano H. Excess of rare cancers in Werner syndrome (adult progeria). Cancer Epidemiol Biomarkers Prev. 1996;5:239–46.
34. Blumenthal GM, Dennis PA. PTEN hamartoma tumor syndromes. Eur J Hum Genet. 2008;16:1289–300.
35. Cameselle-Teijeiro J, Chan JK. Cribriform-morular variant of papillary carcinoma: a distinctive variant representing the sporadic counterpart of familial adenomatous polyposis-associated thyroid carcinoma? Mod Pathol. 1999;12:400–11.
36. Hirokawa M, Kuma S, Miyauchi A, Qian ZR, Nakasono M, Sano T, Kakudo K. Morules in cribriform-morular variant of papillary thyroid carcinoma: immunohistochemical characteristics and distinction from squamous metaplasia. APMIS. 2004;112:275–82.
37. Uchino S, Noguchi S, Yamashita H, Yamashita H, Watanabe S, Ogawa T, Tsuno A, Murakami A, Miyauchi A. Mutational analysis of the APC gene in cribriform-morula variant of papillary thyroid carcinoma. World J Surg. 2006;30:775–9.
38. Abrosimov A. Thyroid cancer with cribriform-morular structures: the problems of morphology and classification. Arkh Patol. 2008;70:18–21.
39. Maiorana A, Collina G, Cesinaro AM, Fano RA, Eusebi V. Epithelioid angiosarcoma of the thyroid. Clinicopathological analysis of seven cases from non-alpine areas. Virchows Arch. 1996; 429:131–7.
40. Chan YF, Ma L, Boey JH, Yeung HY. Angiosarcoma of the thyroid. An immunohistochemical and ultrastructural study of a case in a Chinese patient. Cancer. 1986;57:2381–8.

41. Lamovec J, Zidar A, Zidanik B. Epithelioid angiosarcoma of the thyroid gland. Report of two cases. Arch Pathol Lab Med. 1994; 118:642–6.
42. Mills SE, Stallings RG, Austin MB. Angiomatoid carcinoma of the thyroid gland. Anaplastic carcinoma with follicular and medullary features mimicking angiosarcoma. Am J Clin Pathol. 1986;86: 674–8.
43. Mills SE, Gaffey MJ, Watts JC, Swanson PE, Wick MR, LiVolsi VA, Nappi O, Weiss LM. Angiomatoid carcinoma and 'angiosarcoma' of the thyroid gland. A spectrum of endothelial differentiation. Am J Clin Pathol. 1994;102:322–30.
44. Iida Y, Katoh R, Yoshioka M, Oyama T, Kawaoi A. Primary leiomyosarcoma of the thyroid gland. Acta Pathol Jpn. 1993;43:71–5.
45. Kawahara E, Nakanishi I, Terahata S, Ikegaki S. Leiomyosarcoma of the thyroid gland. A case report with a comparative study of five cases of anaplastic carcinoma. Cancer. 1988;62:2558–63.
46. Katz AD, Hachigian M. Thyroglossal duct cysts. A thirty year experience with emphasis on occurrence in older patients. Am J Surg. 1988;155:741–4.
47. Topf P, Fried MP, Strome M. Vagaries of thyroglossal duct cysts. Laryngoscope. 1988;98:740–2.
48. Mansberger Jr AR, Wei JP. Surgical embryology and anatomy of the thyroid and parathyroid glands. Surg Clin North Am. 1993; 73:727–46.
49. Page CP, Kemmerer WT, Haff RC, Mazzaferri EL. Thyroid carcinomas arising in thyroglossal ducts. Ann Surg. 1974;180: 799–803.
50. Maziak D, Borowy ZJ, Deitel M, Jaksic T, Ralph-Edwards A. Management of papillary carcinoma arising in thyroglossal-duct anlage. Can J Surg. 1992;35:522–5.
51. Woods RH, Saunders Jr JR, Pearlman S, Hirata RM, Jaques DA. Anaplastic carcinoma arising in a thyroglossal duct tract. Otolaryngol Head Neck Surg. 1993;109:945–9.
52. Ranieri E, D'Andrea MR, Vecchione A. Fine needle aspiration cytology of squamous cell carcinoma arising in a thyroglossal duct cyst. A case report. Acta Cytol. 1996;40:747–50.
53. Pitts WC, Tani EM, Skoog L. Papillary carcinoma in fine needle aspiration smears of a thyroglossal duct lesion. Acta Cytol. 1988; 32:599–601.
54. Thompson LD, Rosai J, Heffess CS. Primary thyroid teratomas: a clinicopathologic study of 30 cases. Cancer. 2000;88: 1149–58.
55. Perez-Mies B, Regojo Zapata RM, Garcia-Fernandez E, Serrano MN. Malignant teratoma of the thyroid in a pregnant woman. Ann Diagn Pathol. 2010;14:264–7.
56. Chen JS, Lai GM, Hsueh S. Malignant thyroid teratoma of an adult: a long-term survival after chemotherapy. Am J Clin Oncol. 1998;21:212–4.

Part X

Undifferentiated Tumors: Medullary Thyroid Carcinoma

Clinical Aspects of Medullary Thyroid Carcinoma

83

Douglas W. Ball and Leonard Wartofsky

Introduction

Medullary thyroid cancer (MTC), an uncommon neoplasm stemming from the calcitonin-producing thyroid parafollicular C cells, accounts for approximately 5 % of cases of thyroid cancer. It exists in both sporadic and hereditary forms but is unique among all types of thyroid cancer because of the tight association of MTC with inherited tumor syndromes in approximately 20 % of patients. Activating mutations in the *ret* proto-oncogene account for the hereditary basis of MTC and contribute significantly to sporadic tumor development as well. These findings have a major impact on the diagnosis and therapy of MTC. The tumor was only first reported in 1959 [1]. MTC does not produce thyroglobulin and hence the latter protein does not serve as a tumor marker for residual or recurrent disease, but the neuropeptides, calcitonin, and carcinoembryonic antigen (CEA) are produced by C cell and do serve this function. The American Thyroid Association has published guidelines for the diagnosis and management of MTC [2] along with commentary relevant to application of the guidelines for the care of adults [3] and children [4].

D.W. Ball, MD (✉)
Departments of Medicine, Oncology, and Radiology, Johns Hopkins University School of Medicine, 1650 Orleans Street, Bunting Blaustein Cancer Research Building 553, Baltimore, MD 21231, USA
e-mail: dball@jhmi.edu

L. Wartofsky, MD, MACP
Department of Medicine, MedStar Washington Hospital Center, Georgetown University School of Medicine, 110 Irving Street, N.W., Washington, DC 20010-2975, USA
e-mail: leonard.wartofsky@medstar.net

Genetics

MTC is traditionally classified as sporadic versus hereditary. The three autosomal dominant hereditary MTC syndromes, collectively referred to as MEN 2, are described in Table 83.1. Multiple endocrine neoplasia type 2A (*MEN2A*) comprising MTC in 95 % of affected individuals, pheochromocytoma in approximately 50 %, and hyperparathyroidism in 10–15 % is the most common MEN2 syndrome. *MEN2B* comprises MTC (often with early onset), pheochromocytoma, ganglioneuromas of the oral mucosa and gastrointestinal tract, a characteristic elongated facies, a marfanoid body habitus, and no increase in hyperparathyroidism. The MTC in MEN 2B tends to be more aggressive and has presented earlier in life than MEN 2A tumors. *FMTC* (familial medullary thyroid cancer) is a term used to describe families with MTC but no other associated manifestations as are seen in MEN2A or MEN2B (see [5] for review). There is substantial overlap between ret mutations associated with MEN2A and FMTC. Two minor variants of MEN2A have been described: MEN2A associated with Hirschsprung's disease (hypoplasia of intestinal myenteric plexus) and MEN2A associated with the skin disorder cutaneous lichen amyloidosis [6, 7].

The ret proto-oncogene encodes a receptor tyrosine kinase most closely related to the fibroblast growth factor receptor family. The physiologic role of ret is to activate growth-related signaling pathways in a limited range of neural crest-derived tissues that express the receptor. Downstream signaling pathways activated by ret include ras-MAPK and PI-3K/Akt [8]. Activating point mutations in ret lead to constitutive activity of the receptor, sometimes with altered substrate specificity. In the thyroid, these mutations lead to C-cell hyperplasia (CCH) and emergence of multiple foci of MTC that start as medullary microcarcinomata and eventually progress to larger tumors [9].

L. Wartofsky, D. Van Nostrand (eds.), *Thyroid Cancer*, DOI 10.1007/978-1-4939-3314-3_83

Table 83.1 Classification of medullary thyroid carcinoma

Type	Associated lesion	Ret gene mutation (codon)	Clinical behavior
Sporadic	None	Somatic (esp 918)	Intermediate
FMTC	None	Germline (609, 611, 618, 620, 634, 768, 790 791, 804, 891)	Variable, less aggressive
MEN2A	Pheochromocytoma Hyperparathyroidism	Germline (609, 611, 618, 620, 630, 634, 790 791, 804)	Intermediate
MEN2B	Pheochromocytoma Ganglioneuromatosis Marfanoid habitus	Germline (918, rarely 883)	More aggressive

The range of ret codon mutations seen in the various forms of hereditary and sporadic MTC is listed in Table 83.1. Molecular screening for the ret proto-oncogene is more sensitive for the detection of subjects at risk for MTC than provocative testing, e.g., with calcium infusion. Ultimate clinical outcomes in patients at risk can be significantly enhanced after detection by screening and earlier treatment. From the standpoint of genetic testing, it is fortunate that >97 % of MEN2 families can be identified by analysis of six exons of the ret gene, including all of the mutant codons listed in Table 83.1 [5]. Exons 10 and 11 include mutation sites at codons 609, 611, 618, 620, 630, and 634 which are associated with both MEN2A and FMTC. Each of these codons encodes a cysteine residue in the extracellular domain of ret involved in the three-dimensional ligand binding pocket. Disruption of this pocket through mutation of any of these cysteine residues leads to ligand-independent dimerization and receptor activation. Exons 13–16 include intracellular domain mutation sites associated primarily with FMTC and in the case of exon 16 (codon 918), MEN 2B. The relatively limited variety of ret gene mutations within these six exons has facilitated genetic testing. Although a small percentage of MEN2 families have had no ret gene mutation detected, apparently all affected families studied to date exhibit genetic linkage to the ret gene locus [5].

Specific germline ret mutations carry important implications regarding the penetrance of MTC and associated lesions. For example, the most common germline ret mutation site, codon 634 (exon 11), accounts for approximately 60 % of all MEN2 families [9]. The majority of these families are classified as MEN2A rather than FMTC. Approximately 20 % of individuals with a codon 634 mutation develop hyperparathyroidism, whereas this manifestation is otherwise uncommon with other ret mutations [10]. Patients with codon 634 mutations have significantly earlier progression from CCH to MTC and earlier lymph node involvement than do patients with most other mutations associated with MEN2A and FMTC. A large European consortium study reported by Machens and colleagues offers detailed clinical penetrance data, analyzed according to individual mutations [9].

In MEN 2B, the great majority of patients exhibit a single mutation at codon 918 (methionine to threonine), resulting in an alteration of the substrate recognition pocket of the tyrosine kinase enzyme [11]. Unlike MEN2A, MEN2B germline mutations frequently arise de novo in the presenting individual, e.g., are not detectable in either parent. The de novo mutation is noted at a much higher frequency in the allele inherited from the patient's father [12]. An alternate mutation at codon 883 in exon 15 has been found in a small number of MEN2B families [13].

When MTC patients with a negative family history are investigated with germline ret testing, approximately 3–6 % are found to harbor such mutations [14]. The ret mutations linked with cryptic heritable MTC tend to be disproportionately clustered in the intracellular domain (exons 13–15), associated with reduced MTC penetrance compared to the more classic familial patterns associated with extracellular mutations in exons 10–11. Based on this relatively high frequency of detection in family history-negative patients and the important "multiplier effect" of identifying other family members at risk, germline ret testing is currently recommended in all MTC patients, even in the absence of family history. Currently, a "complete" ret mutation test should include exons 10, 11, 13, 14, 15, and 16.

As many as 80 % of all MTCs are of the sporadic form [15] and acquired or somatic ret gene mutations (occurring in the tumor DNA only) also may be critical to pathogenesis in these tumors. Approximately 50 % of specimens contain ret mutations [16], most frequently the codon 918 mutation seen in MEN2B [17]. However, the discovery that mutation-positive and mutation-negative regions coexist in MTC tumors suggests that these mutations may not always be initiating or essential [18]. To further assess this tumor heterogeneity phenomenon, Schilling and colleagues examined multiple lymph nodes from sporadic MTC patients for somatic codon 918 mutations. Seventy-six percent of patients had concordant mutation results in all lymph nodes tested (43 % all positive, 33 % all negative) [19]. Patients with somatic codon 918 mutations had a significantly increased rate of metastases to the lung, bone, or liver and reduced overall survival. Greater understanding of the molecular genetics of MTC is leading to identification of molecular targets for new therapies [20]. Although the clinical utility of somatic ret mutation analysis is currently undefined, clinical trials are starting to correlate somatic ret mutation status with response to therapy.

Biochemistry

The characteristic secreted product of thyroid C cells and the most useful circulating marker for MTC is the polypeptide hormone calcitonin. The mature 32-amino acid polypeptide is synthesized as a large 135-amino acid precursor, which is processed by prohormone convertases in the C cell. Calcitonin is encoded by a multi-exon gene which produces two principal messenger RNA species. In addition to calcitonin itself, alternative splicing of the primary calcitonin transcript yields calcitonin gene-related peptide (CGRP). The resulting polypeptide hormones are unique and interact with distinct receptors. Calcitonin secretion predominates in normal thyroid C cells whereas CGRP predominates in neural tissue [21]. In MTC, abnormal RNA splicing permits an approximately equal ratio of calcitonin to CGRP, although CGRP measurement is not employed clinically. Whereas substantial elevations of calcitonin (>100 pg/ml) are usually diagnostic for MTC, modest elevations can be seen from extrathyroidal disorders including pulmonary inflammatory diseases, small-cell lung cancer, gastrinoma, carcinoid tumors, and renal failure [22]. An important thyroidal cause of calcitonin hypersecretion is C-cell hyperplasia (CCH). CCH may be genetic – as a precursor lesion in the three hereditary MTC disorders – or sporadic, either idiopathic or associated with such conditions as autoimmune thyroiditis, papillary thyroid cancer, or primary hyperparathyroidism [23]. At low levels of calcitonin excess, CCH can be very difficult to distinguish from microscopic MTC. In otherwise healthy individuals, extrathyroidal sources of calcitonin are usually undetectable in serum, using a specific, highly sensitive assay. Thus patients in remission following successful thyroidectomy characteristically have serum calcitonin values <1 pg/ml.

Current-generation calcitonin immunoradiometric assays (IRMA) with a detection limit of approximately 1 pg/ml are significantly more sensitive and specific than older calcitonin radioimmunoassays. Use of the calcitonin IRMA has coincided with reduced use of provocative testing with the calcitonin secretagogues calcium and pentagastrin in the USA, although several large European centers continue routine provocative testing. In normal adults given a pentagastrin infusion of 0.5 mcg/kg, normal peak values are less than 30 pg/ml. Pentagastrin is not available in the USA and will soon no longer be available in Europe as well.

In addition to calcitonin, MTC cells express biochemical markers typifying secretory cells of the diffuse neuroendocrine system. Polypeptide hormones produced by MTC cells include somatostatin [24], ACTH [25], gastrin-releasing peptide [26], substance P [27], and vasoactive intestinal peptide [28]. Other neuroendocrine markers include neuron specific enolase, NCAM, chromogranin A, prohormone convertases, synaptophysin, and the amine synthetic enzyme L-dopa decarboxylase [29]. Approximately 80 % of MTCs express the thyroid and lung-related foregut transcription factor TTF-1 [30]. In addition, many MTC tumors express two surface markers that have been exploited for diagnostic and therapeutic purposes, carcinoembryonic antigen (CEA) and somatostatin receptor.

Diagnosis

The clinical diagnosis of MTC can be challenging, due to a potential for misdiagnosis as a more common form of thyroid cancer or metastatic tumor from another site. Early accurate diagnosis is critical, to avoid the possibility of undiagnosed pheochromocytoma and to allow for an appropriate surgical approach. The important differences in surgical approach to MTC versus papillary and follicular cancer are detailed in Chap. 85.

Sporadic MTC: Clinical Presentation

Outside of the 20 % of cases where there is known heritable disease, the diagnosis of MTC most commonly begins with the palpation of an asymptomatic thyroid nodule. Because the majority of C cells are located in the upper lobes of the thyroid, most MTC will present in these locations. The nodule as well as any lymph nodes harboring tumor metastases may contain calcifications that will be identified on CT scan or ultrasound examination. The calcifications tend to be more dense than the speckling seen with papillary thyroid carcinoma. Sporadic cases present typically in the third to seventh decades of life with a nearly equal prevalence in males and females with a slight preponderance in women. In most instances, the history and physical exam do not offer any distinctive information compared to typical patients with thyroid nodules. A sufficiently detailed family history is warranted to detect the presence of thyroid cancer, pheochromocytoma, or hyperparathyroidism in first-degree relatives. Fine-needle aspiration cytology will allow a diagnosis of MTC in a thyroid nodule in perhaps 60–70 % of these tumors. Positive cytologic diagnosis may be aided by specific staining for calcitonin. Ultrasonography or CT scanning of the neck for detection of lymph nodes suspicious for metastasis should follow a positive FNA diagnosis. As many as half the patients will have lymph node metastases at presentation, and approximately 20 % of patients present with locally advanced disease with dysphagia, painful lymph node metastases, or recurrent laryngeal nerve invasion and about 5 % will have distant metastases. Uncommon individuals may present with a chief complaint related to paraneoplastic manifestation of MTC, such as flushing, secretory diarrhea, or symptoms of hypercortisolism and the ectopic ACTH syndrome. If prominent, such paraneoplastic manifestations usually indicate a significant tumor burden.

An increasing number of patients with sporadic MTC are now being identified with primary tumors that are incidentally discovered by imaging directed at another condition, such as carotid ultrasonography or staging of an unrelated tumor. Although the appearance of incidentally discovered MTC on ultrasound, CT or FDG-PET is not sufficiently distinctive to provide a radiologic diagnosis, MTC lesions (like PTC) may contain calcifications [31]. Even clinically unapparent sub-centimeter MTC lesions have a potential for metastasis and warrant appropriate surgical intervention. A MTC may also be incidentally discovered in the thyroid surgical specimen after thyroidectomy performed for another indication or for a nodule with a false-negative fine-needle aspiration cytology [32]. These circumstances of missed preoperative diagnosis are potentially hazardous insofar as they may miss coexisting hyperparathyroidism or pheochromocytoma the identification of which would have altered the surgical management.

All patients suspected of having MTC should have blood tested for calcitonin, CEA, calcium, and RET analysis. A controversial approach to MTC diagnosis is the routine use of calcitonin testing in patients with nodular goiter. Two large European studies found significantly elevated calcitonin levels and MTC in a combined 0.6 % of patients undergoing surgery for multinodular goiter. According to these authors, only one third of these MTC cases were diagnosed independently by fine-needle aspiration biopsy [33, 34]. A follow-up Italian study found a prevalence of 0.4 % of significant hypercalcitoninemia and MTC in over 10,000 patients undergoing thyroidectomy for nodular thyroid disease (basal calcitonin range 20–6,200 pg/ml). In this subset of patients, 65 % of individuals had an FNA result that was positive for MTC or other cancer [35]. The 2014 Guidelines of the American Thyroid Association [36] do not recommend either for or against calcitonin assay as part of the routine evaluation of a thyroid nodule or a nodular goiter, although some endocrinologists add this to standard assessment using FNA and TSH, especially if any clinical features suggest MTC. The 2014 guidelines do recommend ultrasonographic imaging of the neck for lymph node mapping although some workers have reported that preoperative levels of calcitonin may be more predictive of lymph node metastases than ultrasound findings [37]. The degree of calcitonin elevation correlates with tumor size and metastases for both familial and sporadic forms of MTC.

Sporadic MTC: Biopsy

The standard diagnostic procedure of choice for sporadic MTC is thyroid fine-needle aspiration biopsy for cytologic examination, either with direct palpation or ultrasound guidance. The sensitivity of thyroid cytopathology for MTC is theoretically equivalent to that in papillary cancer. In practice, the cytopathologist needs an adequate index of suspicion for atypical, cellular, colloid-poor specimens, in order to employ the diagnostic calcitonin immunostaining. In cases where there is clinical suspicion but insufficient cytologic material, a serum calcitonin level can help confirm or rule out the diagnosis. Occasionally specimens are misdiagnosed as atypical follicular neoplasms, or poorly differentiated/anaplastic cancers. The practice of referring patients directly to thyroidectomy without preceding biopsy is especially discouraged. Where lymph node enlargement is first identified rather than a thyroid nodule, fine-needle aspiration biopsy is favored over lymph node excisional biopsy, in order to preserve the lymph node compartment for subsequent comprehensive neck dissection.

Calcitonin Testing

Virtually all patients with clinically evident MTC have elevated basal levels of calcitonin. For clinically occult early MTC, basal calcitonin values may merge with the upper limit of the normal range, which is typically 8 pg/ml in men and 4 pg/ml in women. Although very rare, medullary microcarcinomas have been reported in patients with a normal basal calcitonin level [38]. At what calcitonin level is the presence of MTC confirmed and in what range is CCH or nonspecific elevation more likely? This question cannot be answered precisely owing to conflicting results in multiple studies [39]. A reasonable generalization is that basal calcitonin IRMA values between 10 and 100 pg (prior to thyroidectomy) include both early MTC and CCH, with an overall prevalence of MTC in the 15–30 % range [39]. Above 100 pg/ml, the prevalence of MTC rises substantially although rare CCH cases can still be observed in this range.

Preoperative calcitonin levels correlate generally with tumor size. In a large French series, a calcitonin level above 1,000 pg/ml corresponded to a median tumor diameter of 2.5 cm, whereas calcitonin levels below 1,000 pg/ml corresponded to a median tumor size of 0.7 cm and levels below 100 pg/ml to 0.3 cm. A calcitonin level greater than 1,000 pg/ml was associated with a 10 % risk of distant metastases versus 3 % for levels less than 1,000 [40]. Similarly, the degree of preoperative calcitonin elevation is an important predictor of the chances of normalizing the serum calcitonin with surgery. The chance of postop normalization falls from 97 % (if the preop level is less than 50 pg/ml) to 42 % (preop greater than 50 pg/ml) and 8 % (preop greater than 4,000 pg/ml) [40].

Sporadic MTC: Other Preop Testing

In our institutions, individuals with newly diagnosed MTC, even in the absence of a family history of MTC, are evaluated with ret proto-oncogene DNA testing, 24 h urine metanephrines or plasma fractionated metanephrines, serum calcium, and CEA, in addition to calcitonin. The objective is to detect those cases of MTC that may represent MEN2 and have associated hyperparathyroidism or pheochromocytoma.

Sporadic MTC: Preoperative Imaging

The preoperative imaging workup varies from patient to patient. Differences in the application of optimal imaging modalities for sporadic and hereditary MTC, including PET-CT, have been reviewed recently [41]. At a minimum, a high-quality thyroid and neck ultrasound is useful to detect multifocal thyroid involvement and metastasis to central compartment and jugular chain nodes. False-negative neck ultrasound has been reported in approximately one third of patients with MTC [37]. The absence of abnormal lymph nodes on palpation or ultrasound does not obviate the need for lymph nodal dissection however. Lymph node prevalence in sporadic MTC can be estimated from the surgical-pathological data analyzed by Scollo et al. Both central compartment and ipsilateral jugular chain node involvement occurred in more than 50 % of patients, whereas contralateral jugular chain nodes had a 25–30 % prevalence [42]. Even in the absence of central compartment lymph node involvement, positive node metastases may be found in the lateral neck in 10 % of patients and will be found with virtually 100 % of patients when there is involvement of four or more central compartment nodes [43]. Chapter 85 provides a detailed description of operative management for MTC. The ATA Guidelines [2] recommend total thyroidectomy with both central and lateral compartment dissection in patients with ultrasonographic evidence of lateral regional node involvement. Dralle and Machens [44] have urged caution for lateral neck dissection to balance potential benefit vs. risk of nerve damage. Less aggressive surgery is warranted when distant metastases are present. In our institutions, the choice of additional imaging modalities is guided by the degree of calcitonin elevation. Very high levels may indicate metastatic disease with the most frequent sites being to the lungs, liver, and bones. Neck and chest CT with contrast and dual-phase (early and late) contrast scan of the abdomen are most commonly employed in preoperative staging. Postoperatively, a neck ultrasound should be obtained when calcitonin levels are detectable but <150 pg/ml [2], and CT or MRI is recommended when calcitonin is >150 pg/ml or when calcitonin levels are noted to be rising. MRI may be most useful for bone metastases and FDG-PET may be more useful than CT for lower neck or mediastinal metastases [45]. FDG-PET has been found to be less sensitive than other imaging modalities [46] especially when serum calcitonin levels are less 500 pg/ml [47].

Diagnosis of Hereditary MTC

Since the late 1990s, a consensus has emerged that ret proto-oncogene testing, rather than calcitonin provocative testing, is the preferred method for diagnosis of hereditary MEN2. The sensitivity of ret testing is excellent, currently estimated at approximately 98 % for known families [5]. The test is widely available through commercial laboratories. Efficient family testing focuses on identifying the mutation in a known affected individual and then proceeding systematically through first-degree relatives. The primary goal of this testing is to identify presymptomatic young individuals at risk for MTC and allow for appropriate prophylactic thyroidectomy. Additional goals are identification of subjects with existing MTC needing treatment, as well as subjects at risk for pheochromocytoma and hyperparathyroidism. Prophylactic thyroidectomy, at the stage of CCH or microscopic MTC, is associated with marked improvements in morbidity and mortality, compared with historical patterns of tumor detection later in life [5]. Earlier stage disease will be found with prophylactic thyroidectomy resulting in less need for subsequent aggressive node dissections and in higher cure rates [48]. Indeed, most individuals with FMTC and MEN2A have normal life expectancy after undergoing childhood prophylactic thyroidectomy.

The optimal timing of genetic testing (and prophylactic surgery) is somewhat controversial. These decisions are predicated on data for the earliest onset of MTC and nodal metastases for a particular ret mutation site. The most complete data currently available, from Machens et al., indicate that for the most common mutation at codon 634, microscopic MTC can occur as early as age 15 months and lymph nodal metastases can begin as early as age 6, although ages 14–20 are more common [9]. For other extracellular codons including 609, 611, 618, and 620, no patients have been reported to develop MTC prior to age 6 [9]. Smaller numbers of patients have been studied for the intracellular mutant codons 768, 790, 791,804, and 891, associated predominantly

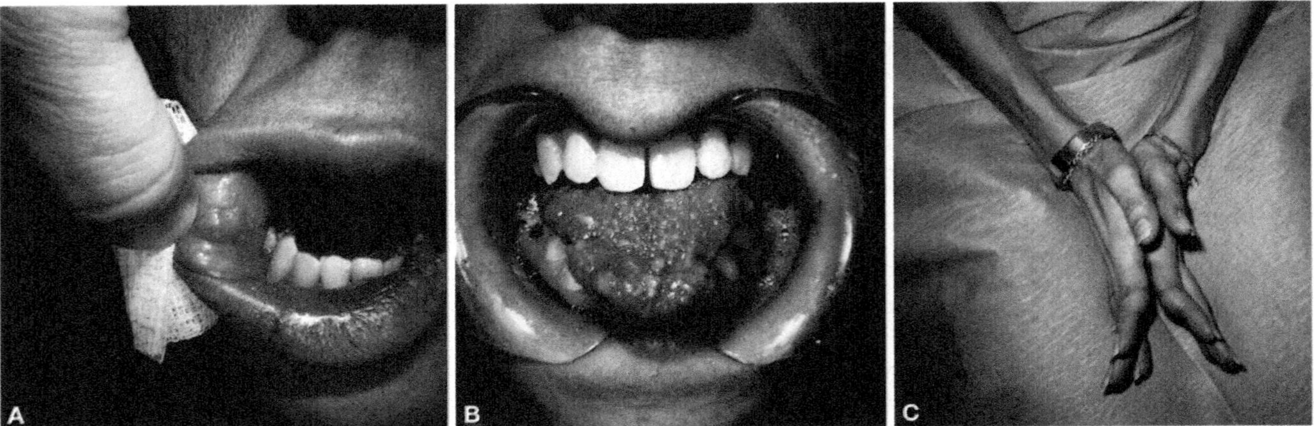

Fig. 83.1 Photograph of a patient with MEN2B showing the typical mucosal neuromas associated with a marfanoid habitus. **a** Lips; **b** tongue; **c** hyperextensibility of the hands

with FMTC. With the exception of patients with codon 804 mutations that may variably develop cancer at an earlier age, few patients with these intracellular codon lesions have developed MTC prior to age 20. For individuals with a 918 mutation and the MEN2B phenotype, metastatic MTC has been reported in the first year of life. Thyroidectomy should be considered as early as the first month of life in those infants with high-risk mutations in 883, 918, and 922 [45].

Based on data for MTC onset and metastasis, an international consensus panel has recommended prophylactic thyroidectomy by age 5 for subjects harboring mutations in codon 611, 618, 620, or 634 [45, 49]. For codons 609, 768, 790, 791, 804, and 891, no consensus was reached, with either a range of 5–10 years chosen [5] or ongoing close monitoring with serum calcitonin and CEA levels [45]. Because of frequent de novo mutations, patients with MEN2B are often first suspected not on the basis of family history but because of a characteristic elongated facies and oral ganglioneuromas involving the lips and tongue (see Fig. 83.1). DNA diagnosis then provides confirmation. Clearly identification of MEN2B should be as early as possible, with surgical cure increasingly unlikely after the first 5 years of life.

Hereditary MTC: Preoperative Studies

All patients diagnosed with hereditary MEN 2 should have an assessment of catecholamine secretion prior to surgical procedures, as well as a basal calcitonin determination, CEA, and serum calcium. For young patients undergoing prophylactic thyroidectomy, no imaging studies are usually employed. Patients in their teens and beyond or patients with significant calcitonin elevations are considered for imaging studies, as described above for sporadic disease. The choice of operation, particularly the extent of lymph nodal dissection and prophylactic parathyroid resection, depends on a knowledge of natural history of inherited MTC and the impact of different ret mutations. In general, this surgery should be performed in a specialized center by surgeons familiar with these issues, as discussed in Chap. 85.

Tumor Progression and Complications

Of typical patients with a palpable sporadic MTC who have undergone thyroidectomy and neck exploration, the majority will have persistent elevations of calcitonin [50]. Those patients who prove to be node negative with appropriate comprehensive lymph nodal exploration have a 95 % chance of an undetectable basal calcitonin level [42]. On the other hand, the presence of lymphadenopathy reduces the likelihood of calcitonin normalization to 32 % [42]. Even patients considered to have undergone complete resection at the time of surgery have a strong likelihood of persistent hypercalcitoninemia. In the absence of overt adenopathy or extensive distant metastases, the clinical course is usually characterized by slow disease progression. Patients with minimal calcitonin elevations and no radiologically detectable metastasis after primary surgery have an 86 % 10-year survival rate and relatively little tumor-associated morbidity [51]. Similarly a Memorial Sloan-Kettering series reported 94 % 5-year survival in patients with nodal disease alone versus 41 % in patients with Stage IV disease [52] (see Table 83.2). Thus, Stage III or IV disease is associated with a significant reduction in disease-specific survival.

In addition to regional lymphadenopathy, the most common metastatic sites include lung and hilar or mediastinal lymph nodes, liver and abdominal lymph nodes, and bone. Lung and liver metastases occur in a diffuse, hematogenous

Table 83.2 Clinical staging of medullary thyroid cancer*

Stage I	C-cell hyperplasia
Stage II	Tumors less than 1 cm and negative lymph nodes
Stage III	Tumors 1 cm or more or tumor of any size with positive nodes
Stage IV	Tumors of any size with metastases outside the neck or with extrathyroidal extension

*Clinical Tumor Staging, National Thyroid Cancer Treatment Cooperative Study

pattern, usually with slow growth. Fortunately, modest metastatic burdens in the lung, and to a lesser extent liver, can be compatible with lengthy survival. Standard imaging modalities including contrast CT, MRI, and PET are quite insensitive for detecting early liver metastases [53]. The inclusion of an arterial phase-contrast protocol with MRI apparently improves sensitivity for liver metastasis detection [45]. Laparoscopic liver visualization and biopsy or hepatic venous sampling are more invasive approaches to this diagnosis. Occasionally, liver metastases can become bulky and painful. Extensive liver metastases are also frequently associated with diarrhea. Although liver resection is not routinely advocated for MTC liver metastases because of the multifocality of the process, surgical debulking of symptomatic masses can provide useful palliation [54].

The most frequent serious complications observed in advanced MTC relate to local tumor invasion into the thyroid bed, trachea, carotid sheath, and brachial plexus or progressive metastasis in the upper mediastinum, lung, or pericardium. Recurrent laryngeal nerve paresis, tracheal and esophageal invasion, superior vena cava syndrome, aspiration-related and post-obstructive pneumonia, and hemoptysis all may be seen in patients with advanced disease and contribute to disease mortality. Another significant cause of morbidity is lytic bone metastasis. Although MTC lesions are not generally considered radiation sensitive, external beam radiation is a useful palliative measure for painful bone lesions or lytic metastases in weight-bearing sites.

The principal paraneoplastic humoral complications of MTC are flushing, diarrhea, and the ectopic ACTH syndrome. The etiology of flushing in MTC patients is still a cause of some debate. One likely mediator is CGRP, a potent vasodilator capable of inducing prolonged cutaneous erythema with intradermal administration [55]. Symptomatic flushing sometimes can be improved by subcutaneous octreotide injection [56]. Unfortunately, octreotide has little efficacy in MTC-associated diarrhea; some patients paradoxically worsen.

Like flushing, the pathophysiology of diarrhea in MTC requires further clarification. The small minority of MEN2A patients with Hirschsprung's disease, as well as MEN2B patients, have well-characterized abnormalities in enteric nerve development with resulting obstruction and megacolon [57]. In contrast, there are no reproducible structural abnormalities in most MTC patients with diarrhea. Functional studies have shown no consistent evidence for either malabsorption or a secretory abnormality in the small intestine. Instead, patients exhibit colonic hypermotility and a decreased ability to absorb water [58]. Intravenous CGRP can increase colonic output of water and electrolytes [59], although the relative importance of other mediators including vasoactive intestinal peptide, histamine, and prostaglandins remains unclear. ATA Guidelines recommend use of antimotility agents such as loperamide and diphenoxylate to lengthen colonic transit time and provide symptomatic relief [2]. Calcitonin excess, per se, is not associated with any clinically significant changes in bone or mineral metabolism.

Prognosis

Medullary thyroid cancer occupies an intermediate position among thyroid cancer histologic types with respect to biologic behavior and long-term prognosis. Although there is intrinsic variability in patients' clinical course, prognostic factors apparent at the time of diagnosis and initial surgery have important utility in predicting long-term outcomes of MTC. An accurate understanding of the influence of prognostic factors in both sporadic and hereditary contexts is essential for selecting appropriate levels of therapeutic intervention.

Sporadic MTC

The most comprehensive reviews of prognostic factors in MTC to date are based on nationwide cancer surveillance in Sweden, with follow-up to 30 years [60, 61]. These studies have revealed several important predictors of survival. Among all sporadic MTC patients, relative survival (the ratio between observed and expected survival) was 63 % at 10 years and 50 % at 20 years. The most important prognostic factor was initial clinical stage (see Table 83.2). Stage III (nodal disease) and Stage IV (distant metastases) were associated with relative hazards of 3.3 and 4.1 compared to patients with no nodal or distant disease. Similarly, a French study including 79 patients with Stage IV disease and a US study found a 5-year survival of 35–40 % [52, 56]. Initial clinical stage remains highly predictive of future mortality even up to 20 years after diagnosis [61]. Other important negative prognostic indicators include tumor size >3 cm, capsular invasion, weak or heterogeneous calcitonin staining, male gender, and older age. By contrast, patients with a tumor measuring <1 cm without known metastases do not differ in survival from the general population [61, 62]. The impact of new molecular markers on MTC prognostic assessment is still unclear. Although somatic mutations in ret at codon 918 appear to be associated with an adverse prognosis, the impact in a large multivariate analysis is unknown. Patients with codons 918, 883, and 992 mutations will have the highest likelihood of persistent residual disease after initial therapy and the highest mortality rates [63]. It is likely, though unproven, that different ret gene mutations will impact on response to tyrosine kinase inhibitors and other experimental therapies.

Hereditary MTC

The significant improvement in outcome seen over the last three decades for patients with heritable MTC can be attributed to the success of presymptomatic screening programs, first with calcitonin secretagogues and more recently with genetic testing. Survival rates of MEN 2A subjects identified in early childhood are projected to be indistinguishable from the general population [61, 62]. An unsettled question is whether the MTC in MEN2A behaves intrinsically less aggressively than sporadic tumors when matched for clinical stage. Swedish MTC registry data suggest statistically similar outcomes for non-screened MEN2A and sporadic patients [62]. At either extremes of the hereditary MTC spectrum, FMTC associated with some intracellular codons appears significantly less aggressive than classic MEN2A in terms of disease latency and survival [64]. MEN2B is generally more aggressive [5, 9].

The age-specific likelihood that a MEN2A gene carrier would present with detectable calcitonin hypersecretion or with symptomatic MTC has been studied by Ponder and colleagues [65]. Approximately 65 % of obligate gene carriers exhibit calcitonin hypersecretion at age 20 years. By age 35, fully 95 % of gene carriers have a positive provocative test. In contrast, the likelihood of a clinical presentation with MTC is only 25 % at age 35 and only approximately 60 % at age 70 [65]. These data cannot be extrapolated to less penetrant hereditary MTC associated with intracellular domain mutations however.

Clinical Surveillance

Goals of clinical surveillance in MTC are to detect recurrences in patients in surgical remission and especially to prevent morbidity from cancer progression in patients with persistent disease. It is reasonable to restage patients prior to performing neck reoperation, for the purpose of excluding Stage IV, inoperable disease. An emerging aim is to select patients who could potentially benefit from clinical trials of systemic therapies for MTC. The intensity of clinical surveillance depends on the risk of death and morbidity and the likelihood of a beneficial intervention.

For patients with modest calcitonin elevations after primary surgery, follow-up testing utilizes a combination of biochemical tumor markers and radiologic studies to screen for disease progression. In one commonly used scheme, serum calcitonin, CEA, and thyroid function tests are obtained 6 weeks after surgery and then at approximately 6-month intervals. The timing of the postoperative calcitonin nadir may be variable [66] and calcitonin levels may vary considerably from measurement to measurement. This variability likely stems from variable secretion by tumors rather than assay variability. In contrast to calcitonin, CEA levels exhibit less inconsistency and, if elevated at baseline, are useful to detect disease progression. Measurements of a combination of calcitonin and CEA every 6 months, with repeated testing for outlying results, will allow estimation of doubling times and identify most patients with progressive disease [67]. A particularly worrisome pattern over time is a flat calcitonin level coupled with rapid doubling in CEA. Overall, the most typical doubling time for calcitonin and CEA is approximately 18 months, reflecting the generally indolent course of this disease. The ATA Guidelines recommend initiation of treatment, perhaps in a clinical trial, when the doubling time is less than 2 years [2]. Certainly, imaging studies such as FDG-PET/CT should be considered to attempt to identify the source of the calcitonin or CEA in order to rule in or out other therapeutic interventions such as surgery, radiation, or local ablative techniques.

Of the available imaging modalities, high-quality neck ultrasound appears to have greatest sensitivity for lymphadenopathy in the central compartment and jugular chains [68]. Because of variability in imaging protocols and interpretation, high-quality neck ultrasound imaging is not available in all centers. Distinct advantages of ultrasound compared to CT/MRI are precise lesional measurements, assessment of the presence of a fatty hilum (characteristic of reactive nodes), and especially the ability to perform ultrasound-guided FNA of lymph nodes if needed. Neck CT and MRI are complementary to ultrasound by providing wider coverage in the neck and more detailed anatomic localization of lymph nodes, once they are detected. Patients with small elevations of calcitonin (<50 pg/ml) frequently do not have disease detectable by imaging. Patients with more significant calcitonin elevations (>500 pg/ml) are frequently followed with periodic whole-body imaging in addition to ultrasound, including either CT (neck, chest, dual-phase abdomen) or FDG-PET [47].

In spite of the wide range of imaging options now available, a vexing problem for clinicians and patients is the issue of occult residual MTC, i.e., elevated calcitonin and negative imaging studies. At low levels of calcitonin, this problem generally reflects low disease burden, below threshold sensitivities of even sensitive techniques such as neck ultrasound. Even with higher levels of calcitonin and ostensibly greater disease burdens, patients may undergo frustrating and expensive rounds of unproductive imaging. The issue of which whole-body modality is best for imaging occult disease remains unsettled. There is general consensus that octreotide, DMSA (dimercaptosuccinic acid), and 131-MIBG scintigraphy have lower overall sensitivity, whereas CT and FDG-PET have greater sensitivity overall [69]. The choice between CT and FDG-PET is not clear-cut, with advantages at different metastatic sites for both modalities, as discussed in Chap. 87. In patients in whom baseline calcitonin levels are undetectable but levels rise minimally after stimulation, identification of the source of the calcitonin is unlikely and such follow-up retesting is not recommended [2].

Therapeutic Choice in Residual MTC

Faced with a rising calcitonin level and/or metastatic lesions seen on imaging studies, patients and clinicians can choose between a course of watchful waiting or intervention with surgery, radiotherapy, or systemic therapy. Specific surgical, radiation, and chemotherapeutic approaches to MTC are discussed elsewhere in this text. The decision to undertake these interventions presupposes an understanding of MTC natural history and appropriate use of biochemical and imaging data, as well as an effective treatment option.

Patients with only biochemical evidence of persistent MTC and negative imaging studies are frequently managed expectantly. In patients with mild hypercalcitoninemia and negative imaging, an excellent overall prognosis supports such a conservative approach [51, 52]. A more aggressive approach with neck reoperation with a potential curative intent seems justified in some patients who have not had recommended primary surgery, as described in Chap. 85. On the other hand, the low to moderate success rates in normalizing the calcitonin level following repeat lymph nodal dissection suggest that this approach be used highly selectively [70–72].

Radioactive iodine is ineffective for patients with MTC as are somatostatin analogues. Cytotoxic chemotherapy is not routinely recommended [2] but may be attempted for recurrent metastatic disease in patients who are ineligible for clinical trials with targeted molecular therapy. Locoregional recurrence is frequently managed surgically. In the presence of Stage IV disease, especially with distant progression, the goals of such neck surgery become focused on symptom palliation and to a lesser extent on the prevention of anticipated complications. The importance of locoregional control, even in patients with Stage IV disease, has been emphasized [73]. The limited potential role of adjuvant neck radiation following surgery is discussed in Chap. 88 and has been reviewed [74]. ATA Guidelines [2] note that radiation is not a substitute for surgery for patients with neck involvement and recommend consideration of postoperative radiation for incompletely resected disease in the neck or in bones, for brain metastases not amenable to surgical excision, and for painful bone metastases. There was no recommendation either for or against the use of bisphosphonates in patients with bone metastases.

Patients with distant metastases should be considered as potential candidates for investigational systemic therapy or clinical trials, as no currently available regimen produces frequent, durable responses. The decision to undertake such a therapy rests on a variety of factors including the rate of metastatic progression on interval scanning, study availability, comorbidities, and patient preference. At this writing, a variety of experimental therapies have been under active investigation for MTC including sunitinib, sorafenib, motesanib, axitinib, cabozantinib, and vandetanib [75]. These therapies are targeted at ret kinase inhibition, additional cellular kinases, tumor angiogenesis, and protein chaperone function. One of the more promising tyrosine kinase inhibitors is vandetanib [76–80] which has been effective in stabilizing disease although worrisome side effects like QTc prolongation are a concern. Conceivably, combinations of targeted therapies or targeted plus cytotoxic therapies will prove most effective.

References

1. Hazard JB, Crile Jr G. Medullary (solid) carcinoma of the thyroid: a clinic-pathologic entity. J Clin Endocrinol Metab. 1959;19: 152–61.
2. Wells SA, et al., Revised American Thyroid Association Guidelines for the Management of Medullary Thyroid Carcinoma prepared by the American Thyroid Association Guidelines Task Force on Medullary Thyroid Carcinoma. Thyroid. 2015; 25: 567–610.
3. Ball DW. American Thyroid Association guidelines for management of medullary thyroid cancer: an adult endocrinology perspective. Thyroid. 2009;19:547–50.
4. Waguespack SG, Rich TA, Perrier ND, Jimenez C, Cote GJ. Management of medullary thyroid carcinoma and MEN2 syndromes in childhood. Nature Reviews Endocrinology. 2011;7(10):596–607.
5. Brandi ML, Gagel RF, Angeli A, Bilezikian JP, et al. Guidelines for diagnosis and therapy of MEN type 1 and type 2. J Clin Endocrinol Metab. 2001;86:5658–71.
6. Frilling A, Becker H, Roehr H-D. Unusual features of multiple endocrine neoplasia. Henry Ford Hosp Med J. 1992;40: 233–5.
7. Gagel RF, Levy ML, Donovan DT, et al. Multiple endocrine neoplasia type 2a associated with cutaneous lichen amyloidosis. Ann Intern Med. 1989;111:802–6.
8. De Vita G, Melillo RM, Carlomagno F, et al. Tyrosine 1062 of RET-MEN2A mediates activation of Akt (protein kinase B) and mitogen-activated protein kinase pathways leading to PC12 cell survival. Cancer Res. 2000;60:3727–31.

9. Machens A, Niccoli-Sire P, Hoegel J, et al. Early malignant progression of hereditary medullary thyroid cancer. N Engl J Med. 2003;349:1517–25.
10. Schuffenecker I, Virally-Monod M, Brohet R, et al. Risk and penetrance of primary hyperparathyroidism in multiple endocrine neoplasia type 2A families with mutations at codon 634 of the RET proto-oncogene. J Clin Endocrinol Metab. 1998;83:487–91.
11. Santoro M, Carlomagno F, Romano A, Bottaro DP, et al. Activation of RET as a dominant transforming gene by germline mutations of MEN2A and MEN2B. Science. 1995;267:381–3.
12. Carlson KM, Bracamontes J, Jackson CE, Clark R, et al. Parent-of-origin effects in multiple endocrine neoplasia type 2B. Am J Hum Genet. 1994;5:1076–82.
13. Gimm O, Marsh DJ, Andrew SD, Frilling A, et al. Germline dinucleotide mutation in codon 883 of the RET proto-oncogene in multiple endocrine neoplasia type 2B without codon 918 mutation. J Clin Endocrinol Metab. 1997;82:3902–4.
14. Wohllk N, Cote GJ, Bugalho MM, et al. Relevance of RET proto-oncogene mutations in sporadic medullary thyroid carcinoma. J Clin Endocrinol Metab. 1996;81:3740–5.
15. Pitman MB, Oertel YC, Geisinger KR. Medullary thyroid carcinoma. In: Ali SZ, Cibas ES, editors. The Bethesda system for reporting thyroid cytopathology. 1st ed. New York: Springer; 2010. p. 117–28.
16. Elisei R, Cosci B, Romei C, et al. Prognostic significance of somatic RET oncogene mutations in sporadic medullary thyroid cancer: a 10-year follow-up study. J Clin Endocrinol Metab. 2008;93:682–7.
17. Blaugrund JE, Johns Jr MM, Eby YJ, Ball DW, et al. RET proto-oncogene mutations in inherited and sporadic medullary thyroid cancer. Hum Mol Genet. 1994;3:1895–7.
18. Eng C, Mulligan LM, Healey CS, et al. Heterogeneous mutation of the RET proto-oncogene in subpopulations of medullary thyroid carcinoma. Cancer Res. 1996;56:2167–70.
19. Schilling T, Burck J, Sinn HP, Clemens A, et al. Prognostic value of codon 918 (ATG-->ACG) RET proto-oncogene mutations in sporadic medullary thyroid carcinoma. Int J Cancer. 2001;95:62–6.
20. Cerrato A, De Falco V, Santoro M. Molecular genetics of medullary thyroid carcinoma: the quest for novel therapeutic agents. J Mol Endocrinol. 2009;43:143–55.
21. Amara SG, Jonas V, Rosenfeld MG, Ong ES, Evans RM. Alternative RNA processing in calcitonin gene expression generates mRNAs encoding different polypeptide products. Nature. 1982;298:240–4.
22. Becker KL, Nash D, Silva OL, et al. Increased serum and urinary calcitonin in patients with pulmonary disease. Chest. 1981;79: 211–6.
23. Perry A, Molberg K, Albores-Saavedra J. Physiologic versus neoplastic C-cell hyperplasia of the thyroid: separation of distinct histologic and biologic entities. Cancer. 1996;77:750–6.
24. Roos BA, Lindall AW, Ells J, et al. Increased plasma and tumor somatostatin-like immuno reactivity in medullary thyroid carcinoma and small cell lung cancer. J Clin Endocrinol Metab. 1981;52:187–94.
25. Melvin KE, Tashjian Jr AH, Cassidy CE, Givens JR. Cushing's syndrome caused by ACTH and calcitonin-secreting medullary carcinoma of the thyroid. Metabolism. 1970;19:831–8.
26. Kameya T, Bessho T, Tsumuraya M, et al. Production of gastrin-releasing peptide in medullary carcinoma of the thyroid. Virchows Arch [A]. 1983;401:99–107.
27. Skrabanek P, Cannon D, Dempsey J, et al. Substance P in medullary carcinoma of the thyroid. Experientia. 1979;35:1259–60.
28. Said SI. Evidence for secretion of vasoactive intestinal peptide by tumours of pancreas, adrenal medulla, thyroid and lung. Clin Endocrinol (Oxf). 1976;5(Suppl):201S–4.
29. Baylin SB, Mendelsohn G. Medullary thyroid carcinoma: a model for the study of human tumor progression and cell heterogeneity. In: Owens Jr AH, Coffey DS, Baylin SB, editors. Tumor cell heterogeneity, origins and implications. New York: Academic; 1982. p. 12.
30. Katoh R, Miyagi E, Nakamura N, Li X, et al. Expression of thyroid transcription factor-1 (TTF-1) in human C cells and medullary thyroid carcinomas. Hum Pathol. 2000;31:386–93.
31. McDonnell 3rd CH, Fishman EK, Zerhouni EA. CT demonstration of calcified liver metastases in medullary thyroid carcinoma. J Comput Assist Tomogr. 1986;10:976–8.
32. Ahmed SR, Ball DW. Incidentally discovered medullary thyroid cancer: diagnostic strategies and treatment. J Clin Endocrinol Metab. 2011;96:1237–45.
33. Pacini F, Fontanelli M, Fugazzola L, et al. Routine measurement of serum calcitonin in nodular thyroid diseases allows the preoperative diagnosis of unsuspected sporadic medullary thyroid carcinoma. J Clin Endocrinol Metab. 1994;78:826–9.
34. Rieu M, Lame MC, Richard A, et al. Prevalence of sporadic medullary thyroid carcinoma: the importance of routine measurement of serum calcitonin in the diagnostic evaluation of thyroid nodules. Clin Endocrinol (Oxf). 1995;42:453–60.
35. Elisei R, Bottici V, Luchetti F, Di Coscio G, et al. Impact of routine measurement of serum calcitonin on the diagnosis and outcome of medullary thyroid cancer: experience in 10,864 patients with nodular thyroid disorders. J Clin Endocrinol Metab. 2004;89: 163–8.
36. Haugen BR, Alexander EK, Bible KC, Doherty GM, Mandel SJ, Nikiforov YE, Pacini F, Randolph GW, Sawka AM, Schlumberger M, Schuff KG, Sherman SI, Sosa JA, Steward DL, Tuttle RM, Wartofsky L. 2015 American Thyroid Association Management Guidelines for Adult Patients with Thyroid Nodules and Differentiated Thyroid Cancer: American Thyroid Association Guidelines Task Force on Thyroid Nodules and Differentiated Thyroid Cancer. Thyroid. 2016;26:1–133.
37. Machens A, Dralle H. Biomarker-based risk stratification for previously untreated medullary thyroid cancer. J Clin Endocrinol Metab. 2010;95:2655–63.
38. Niccoli P, Wion-Barbot N, Caron P, Henry JF, et al. Interest of routine measurement of serum calcitonin: study in a large series of thyroidectomized patients. J Clin Endocrinol Metab. 1997;82: 338–41.
39. Hodak SP, Burman KD. The calcitonin conundrum – is it time for routine measurement of serum calcitonin in patients with thyroid nodules? J Clin Endocrinol Metab. 2004;89:511–4.
40. Cohen R, Campos JM, Salaun C, Heshmati HM, et al. Preoperative calcitonin levels are predictive of tumor size and postoperative calcitonin normalization in medullary thyroid carcinoma. J Clin Endocrinol Metab. 2000;85:919–22.
41. Ganeshan D, Paulson E, Duran C, Cabanillas ME, Busaidy NL, Charnsangavej C. Current update on medullary thyroid carcinoma. AJR. 2013;201:W867–76.
42. Scollo C, Baudin E, Travagli JP, Caillou B, et al. Rationale for central and bilateral lymph node dissection in sporadic and hereditary medullary thyroid cancer. J Clin Endocrinol Metab. 2003;88: 2070–5.
43. Machens A, Hauptmann S, Dralle H. Prediction of lateral lymph node metastases in medullary thyroid cancer. Br J Surg. 2008; 95:586–91.
44. Dralle H, Machens A. Surgical management of the lateral neck compartment for metastatic thyroid cancer. Curr Opin Oncol. 2013;25:20–6.
45. Roman S, Mehta P, Sosa JA. Medullary thyroid cancer: early detection and novel treatments. Curr Opin Oncol. 2008;21:5–10.
46. Giraudet AL, Vanel D, Leboulleux S, Auperin A, Dromain C, et al. Imaging medullary thyroid carcinoma with persistent elevated calcitonin levels. J Clin Endocrinol Metab. 2007;92:4185–90.
47. Ong SC, Schoder H, Patel SG, Tabangay-Lim IM, Doddamane I, et al. Diagnostic accuracy of 18F-FDG-PET in restaging patients with medullary thyroid carcinoma and elevated calcitonin levels. J Nucl Med. 2007;48:501–7.
48. Castellone MD, Santoro M. Dysregulated RET signaling in thyroid cancer. Endocrinol Metab Clin N Am. 2008;37:363–74.

49. Zenaty D, Aigrain Y, Peuchmaur M, et al. Medullary thyroid carcinoma identified within the first year of life in children with hereditary multiple endocrine neoplasia type 2A (codon 634) and 2B. Eur J Endocrinol. 2009;160:807–13.
50. Wells Jr SA, Dilley WG, Farndon JA, Leight GS, Baylin SB. Early diagnosis and treatment of medullary thyroid carcinoma. Arch Intern Med. 1995;145:1248–52.
51. van Heerden JA, Grant CS, Gharib H, et al. Long-term course of patients with persistent hypercalcitoninemia after apparent curative primary surgery for medullary thyroid carcinoma. Ann Surg. 1990;212:395–400.
52. Ellenhorn JD, Shah JP, Brennan MF. Impact of therapeutic regional lymph node dissection for medullary carcinoma of the thyroid gland. Surgery. 1993;114:1078–81.
53. Tung WS, Vesely TM, Moley JF. Laparoscopic detection of hepatic metastases in patients with residual or recurrent medullary thyroid cancer. Surgery. 1995;118:1024–9.
54. Chen H, Roberts JR, Ball DW, Eisele DW, et al. Effective long-term palliation of symptomatic, incurable metastatic medullary thyroid cancer by operative resection. Ann Surg. 1998;227:887–95.
55. Brain SD, Williams TJ, Tippins JR. Calcitonin gene-related peptide is a potent vasodilator. Nature. 1985;313:54–6.
56. Modigliani E, Cohen R, Joannidis S, Siame-Mourot C, et al. Results of long-term continuous subcutaneous octreotide administration in 14 patients with medullary thyroid carcinoma. Clin Endocrinol (Oxf). 1992;36:183–6.
57. Cohen MS, Phay JE, Albinson C, DeBenedetti MK, et al. Gastrointestinal manifestations of multiple endocrine neoplasia type 2. Ann Surg. 2002;235:648–54.
58. Rambaud JC, Jian R, Flourie B, et al. Pathophysiological study of diarrhoea in a patient with medullary thyroid carcinoma: evidence against a secretory mechanism and for the role of shortened colonic transit time. Gut. 1988;29:537–43.
59. Rolston RK, Ghatei MA, Mulderry PK, Bloom SR. Intravenous calcitonin gene-related peptide stimulates net water secretion in rat colon in vivo. Dig Dis Sci. 1989;34:612–6.
60. Bergholm U, Adami HO, Auer G, et al. Histopathologic characteristics and nuclear DNA content as prognostic factors in medullary thyroid carcinoma: a nationwide study in Sweden. The Swedish MTC Study Group. Cancer. 1989;64:135–42.
61. Bergholm U, Bergstrom R, Ekbom A. Long-term follow-up of patients with medullary carcinoma of the thyroid. Cancer. 1997;79:132–8.
62. Modigliani E, Cohen R, Campos JM, Conte-Devolx B, et al. Prognostic factors for survival and for biochemical cure in medullary thyroid carcinoma: results in 899 patients. Clin Endocrinol (Oxf). 1998;48:265–73.
63. Pelizzo MR, Boschin IM, Bernante P, Toniato A, Piotto A, et al. Natural history, diagnosis, treatment and outcome of medullary thyroid cancer: 37 years experience on 157 patients. Eur J Surg Oncol. 2007;33:493–7.
64. Farndon JR, Leight GS, Dilley WG, et al. Familial medullary thyroid carcinoma without associated endocrinopathies: a distinct clinical entity. Br J Surg. 1986;73:278–81.
65. Ponder BA, Ponder MA, Coffey R, et al. Risk estimation and screening in families of patients with medullary thyroid carcinoma. Lancet. 1989;1:397–401.
66. Stepanas AV, Samaan NA, Hill Jr CS, Hickey RC. Medullary thyroid carcinoma: importance of serial serum calcitonin measurement. Cancer. 1979;43:825–37.
67. Barbet J, Campion L, Kraeber-Bodere F, Chatal J-F, et al. Prognostic impact of serum calcitonin and carcinoembryonic antigen doubling-times in patients with medullary thyroid carcinoma. J Clin Endocrinol Metab. 2005;90:6077–84.
68. Kouvaraki MA, Shapiro SE, Fornage BD, et al. Role of preoperative ultrasonography in the surgical management of patients with thyroid cancer. Surgery. 2003;134:946–54.
69. Gotthardt M, Battmann A, Hoffken H, et al. 18F-FDG PET, somatostatin receptor scintigraphy, and CT in metastatic medullary thyroid carcinoma: a clinical study and an analysis of the literature. Nucl Med Commun. 2004;25:439–43.
70. Kebebew E, Kikuchi S, Duh QY, Clark OH. Long-term results of reoperation and localizing studies in patients with persistent or recurrent medullary thyroid cancer. Arch Surg. 2000;135: 895–901.
71. Fleming JB, Lee JE, Bouvet M, Schultz PN, et al. Surgical strategy for the treatment of medullary thyroid carcinoma. Ann Surg. 1999; 230:697–707.
72. Moley JF, Dilley WG, DeBenedetti MK. Improved results of cervical reoperation for medullary thyroid carcinoma. Ann Surg. 1997;225:734–40.
73. Yen TW, Shapiro SE, Gagel RF, Sherman SI, Lee JE, Evans DB. Medullary thyroid carcinoma: results of a standardized surgical approach in a contemporary series of 80 consecutive patients. Surgery. 2003;134:890–9.
74. Brierley JD. Update on external beam radiation therapy in thyroid cancer. J Clin Endocrinol Metab. 2011;96:2289–95.
75. Sugawara M, Geffner DL, Martinez D, Hershman JM. Novel treatment of medullary thyroid cancer. Curr Opin Endocrinol Diabetes Obes. 2009;16:367–72.
76. Campbell MJ, Seib CD, Gosnell J. Vandetanib and the management of advanced medullary thyroid cancer. Curr Opin Oncol. 2013;25: 39–43.
77. Solomon B, Rischin D. Progress in molecular targeted therapy for thyroid cancer: vandetanib in medullary thyroid cancer. J Clin Oncol. 2012;30:119–21.
78. Wells SA, Robinson BG, Gagel RF, et al. Vandetanib in patients with locally advanced or metastatic medullary thyroid cancer: a randomized double-blind phase III trial. J Clin Oncol. 2012;30: 134–41.
79. Robinson BG, Paz-Ares L, Krebs A, et al. Vandetanib (100 mg) in patients with locally advanced or metastatic hereditary medullary thyroid cancer. J Clin Endocrinol Metab. 2010;95: 2664–71.
80. Wells SA, Gosnell JE, Gagel RF, et al. Vandetanib for the treatment of patients with locally advanced or metastatic hereditary medullary thyroid cancer. J Clin Oncol. 2010;28:767–72.

Cytology and Pathology of Medullary Thyroid Cancer

84

Zubair W. Baloch and Virginia A. LiVolsi

First defined in the 1950s [1, 2], medullary carcinoma of the thyroid is a tumor derived from the non-follicular C cell in the gland. The origin of this tumor was first proposed in the mid-1960s by ED Williams, who postulated (based on a few cases) that this unusual thyroid tumor, medullary carcinoma, might indeed be derived from non-follicular thyroid cells, i.e., the C cells, and that a new hormone might be produced by these cells in the thyroid. If so, he theorized that medullary carcinoma could produce calcitonin, and this could become a diagnostic and prognostic marker for this neoplasm [3]. Most importantly the precursor lesion known as C-cell hyperplasia was identified [4].

In a short period of time, the clinical and pathological features of the lesion were described, and familial forms were defined. In addition medullary carcinoma was noted to be an integral part of two multiple endocrine neoplasia syndromes (MEN 2A (Sipple syndrome) and MEN 2B) [5, 6]. The latter is associated with other endocrine neoplasms, most frequently, pheochromocytoma (Fig. 84.1).

Based upon investigations at the more basic level in many laboratories around the world and by linkage analysis, the "hot spot" on chromosome 10 was implicated in tumorigenesis of medullary carcinoma. These studies led to the discovery of ***ret*** mutations in the germline of these familial cases as well as in the tumors [7]. The elegance of germline genetic testing with essentially no false-positive tests has been a major advance in oncology and has served as the model to be found for many common cancers (unfortunately the genetics of common cancers has proven to be quite complex and not as easily followed as medullary carcinoma cases). Multiple point mutations in *ret* can give rise to medullary carcinoma, and there have now been studies that show the specific mutations can be correlated with distinct pathologic features, specific patterns of organ involvement, clinical features and prognostic outcomes [8, 9].

Pathologically, sporadic tumors are solitary and not associated with other lesions in the thyroid or in other endocrine organs; familial cases showed multifocal bilateral tumors and both diffuse and nodular C-cell hyperplasia [4, 10]. Characteristically the tumors are located in the lateral lobes of the thyroid (never in the isthmus); this reflects the normal distribution of the C cells in human thyroids [11].

Grossly in the common sporadic case, the tumor is circumscribed (rarely infiltrative) and yellow tan in color. In familial cases there may be numerous subcentimeter firm white-tan nodules usually in the upper lateral aspects of the gland [12].

Histologically, the most interesting feature of medullary carcinoma is the variability of patterns it can show: the tumors may grow in nests or as spindle cells (or a combination of the two), and they may show glands, papillae, follicles, trabeculae, or islands. The cells may be bland or pleomorphic with multiple nuclei; in many cases the cells assume a plasmacytoid appearance. The cytoplasm may be basophilic or rarely eosinophilic and granular. The nuclei share the characteristic "salt and pepper pattern" of neuroendocrine cells. In about 75 % of cases, stromal amyloid is found [12–15] (Fig. 84.2). This represents precipitation of the prohormone of calcitonin. Stromal collagen is seen in many cases, while rare examples show small cell cytology "oat cell" (some of these may not demonstrate immunostaining for calcitonin) [16–18]. Occasional examples of this tumor demonstrate oncocytic features and may be misdiagnosed as Hurthle cell neoplasms [19–21]. Clear cell and squamous cell patterns have also been described. Some tumors produce mucin [22], and rarely a few form melanin granules [23, 24]. Amyloid deposits may be accompanied by giant cells of the foreign body type [16, 25, 26]. Because of

Z.W. Baloch, MD, PhD (✉) • V.A. LiVolsi, MD
Department of Pathology and Laboratory Medicine, University of Pennsylvania Medical Center, Perelman School of Medicine, 6 Founders Pavilion, 3400 Spruce Street, Philadelphia, PA 19104, USA
e-mail: balocj@mail.med.upenn.edu; linus@mail.med.upenn.edu

L. Wartofsky, D. Van Nostrand (eds.), *Thyroid Cancer*, DOI 10.1007/978-1-4939-3314-3_84

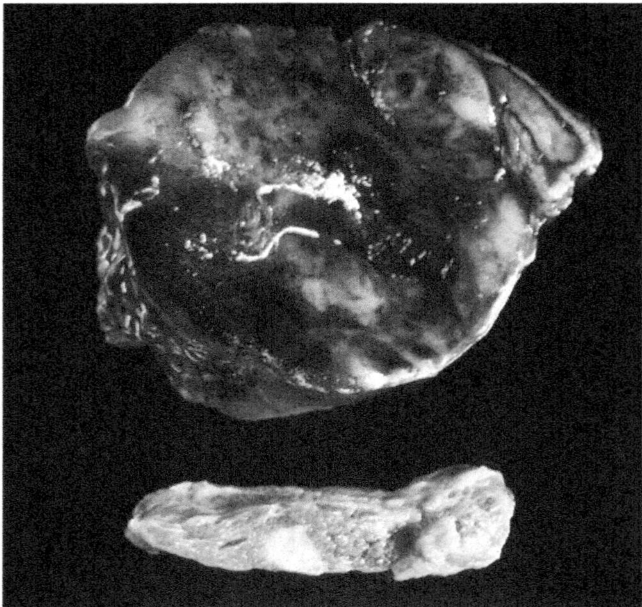

Fig. 84.1 A small medullary carcinoma lies in part of the thyroid lobe cut in cross-section. In the upper part, a pheochromocytoma replaces most of the adrenal gland. Hemorrhages are visible in the pheochromocytoma

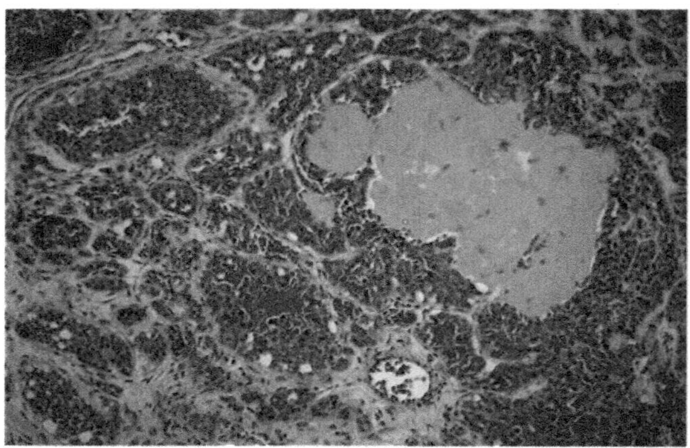

Fig. 84.2 Medullary carcinoma from a 47-year-old woman. Note the deposit of amyloid (hematoxylin and eosin [H&E stain])

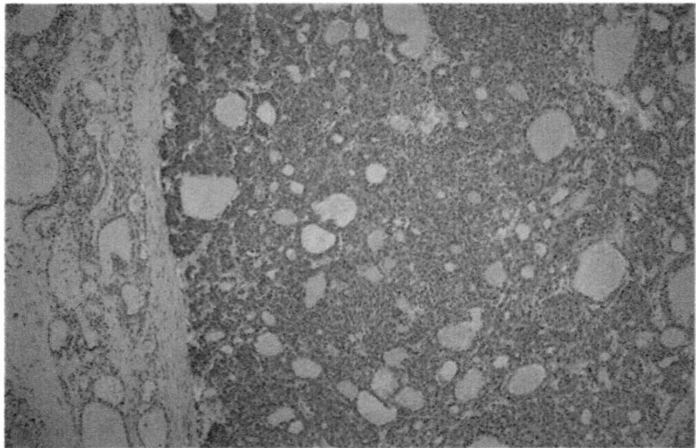

Fig. 84.3 Medullary carcinoma has trapped several normal thyroid follicles. The anticalcitonin procedure has stained the neoplastic cells

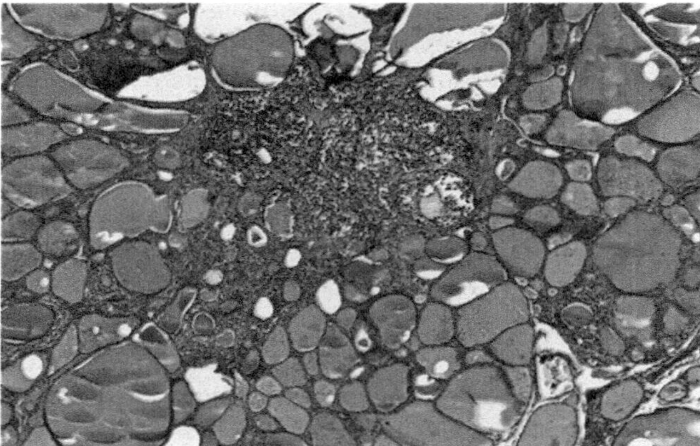

Fig. 84.4 A tiny medullary carcinoma was discovered incidentally in this thyroid of a 62-year-old man (H&E stain)

the numerous patterns that medullary carcinoma can present, it is recommended that any unusual thyroid neoplasm be immunostained for calcitonin to assess the possibility of medullary carcinoma (Fig. 84.3).

Although most tumors freely invade the surrounding thyroid parenchyma, they may grossly appear encapsulated. Lymphatic and vascular invasion are very common. Over 80 % of clinically identified medullary carcinomas will have lymph node metastases in the central and/or lateral neck compartments. These may be clinically or radiologically obvious or may represent only micrometastases. Within carcinomas, there may be focal necrosis, cystic change, desmoplastic stroma, irregular calcification, and psammoma bodies [12]. Histological features which have been associated with a poor prognosis include foci of necrosis, numerous mitoses, cellular pleomorphism small cell cytology, and absence of amyloid [27–29].

The associated thyroid lesions of medullary carcinoma include lymphocytic thyroiditis, adenomatous goiter, and other malignancies especially papillary carcinoma [30–33]. In syndromic cases, lesions in parathyroids, adrenal medulla, and neuronal or ganglioneuronal tissues (especially of the GI tract) are found [6, 34–36].

Most medullary carcinomas are discovered as clinical nodules. In genetically based cases, wherein the patients with known mutations undergo prophylactic thyroidectomy, subcentimeter tumors are found [37]. In some thyroid glands removed for adenomas, papillary carcinoma, or goiter, incidental subcentimeter micro-medullary carcinomas may be seen [38] (Fig. 84.4). These are not unlike papillary incidentalomas and if solitary are probably cured by the lobectomy [39].

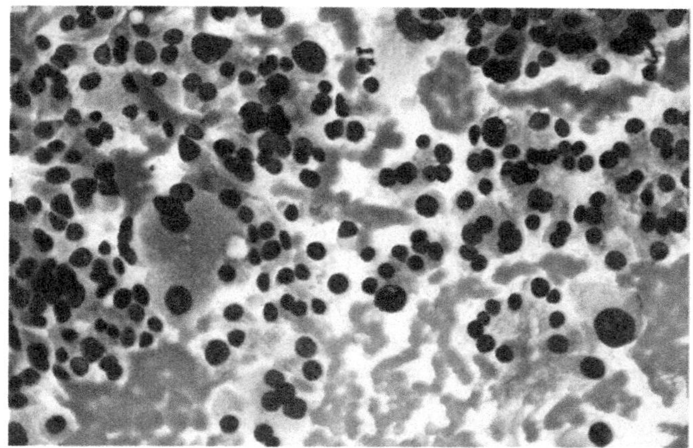

Fig. 84.5 Medullary carcinoma. Smear shows "tumor cellularity." Note loosely cohesive cells and the variation in nuclear size (Diff-Quik stain)

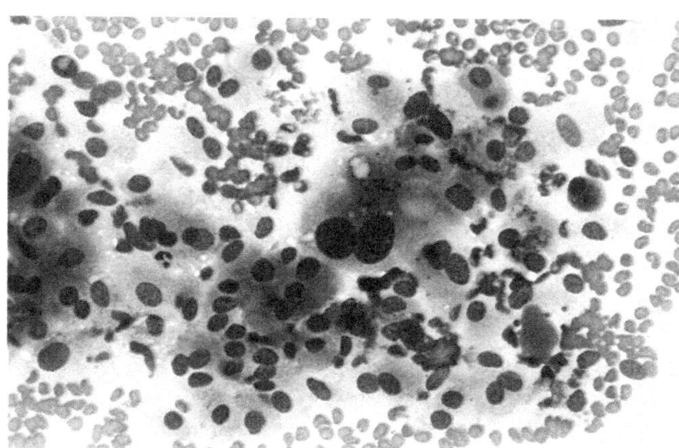

Fig. 84.7 Medullary carcinoma. Smear shows large binucleated cell with cytoplasmic vacuoles (Diff-Quik stain)

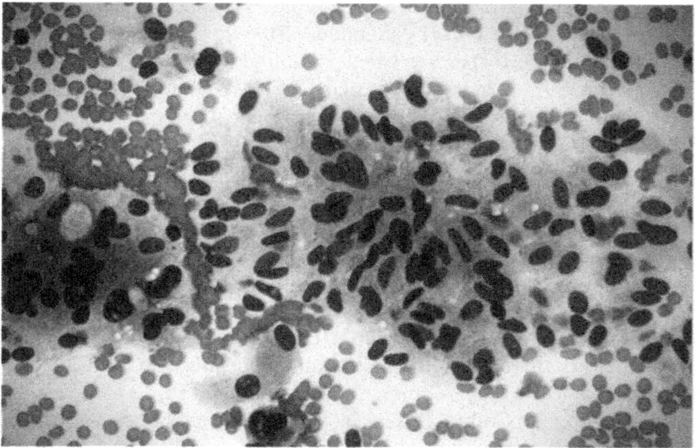

Fig. 84.6 Medullary carcinoma. Smear shows spindled cells with tenuous cytoplasm (Diff-Quik stain)

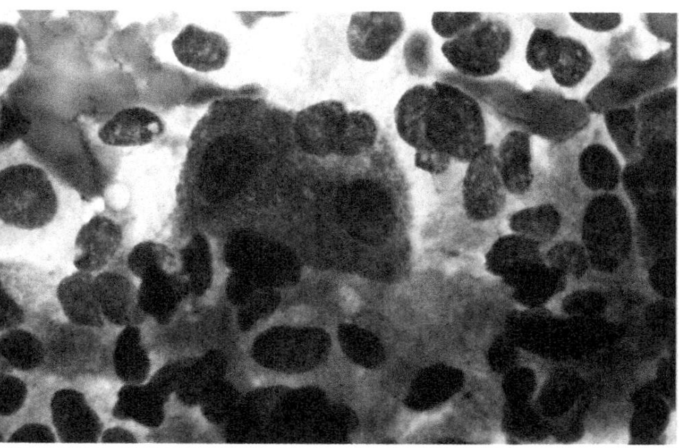

Fig. 84.8 Medullary carcinoma. Two of the neoplastic cells (with *pink*-staining cytoplasm) show calcitonin granules (Diff-Quik stain)

Recent evidence from the SEER database however indicates that some of these tiny lesions may be associated with a poor prognosis (especially if serum calcitonin is elevated and if there are multiple lesions [40].

A cytological diagnosis of medullary carcinoma is possible, but the pathologist must always consider this entity in the differential diagnosis [15, 41, 42]. The most commonly encountered cytologic features of aspirates from medullary carcinoma include significant lack of cellular cohesiveness, pleomorphic multinucleated neoplastic cells scattered among the predominant cell population (Fig. 84.5), lack of prominent nucleoli, cells with plasmacytoid features, spindled cells (Fig. 84.6), and frequent binucleation (Fig. 84.7). Multinucleated histiocytes (usually associated with the presence of amyloid) are seen rarely. Calcitonin cytoplasmic granules (that stain pink if hematological stains are used) are found in approximately 30 % of cases (Fig. 84.8). In patients with known family history or a known germline mutation, the pathologist thinking along the C-cell tumor lines will be able to strongly suggest or definitively diagnose medullary carcinoma. In sporadic cases this cytodiagnosis can be challenging. The smears show a cellular specimen with absent colloid, stromal amyloid, and neuroendocrine nuclei; in such cases the diagnosis can be highly probable or definite [42]. However, many thyroid cytopathologists would diagnose such a case as neoplasm that presents and suggests serum calcitonin studies to confirm the cytomorphologic impression [43, 44]. Some authors have recommended measuring calcitonin in washouts of the fine-needle aspiration needle to confirm the morphologic impression of medullary carcinoma [45]. A note of caution: the pathologist must be aware that calcitonin antibodies used for immunostaining can be "sticky," i.e., demonstrate aberrant staining on cell block material, and false-positive diagnoses of medullary carcinoma may be rendered on such cases.

Very rare neoplasms have been reported in the literature which demonstrate dual differentiation toward C cells (calcitonin production) and follicular cells (thyroglobulin production) [46–48]. The follicular elements have been described as similar to follicular and papillary carcinoma. Critical examination of such a neoplasm is needed to exclude collision tumors and nonspecific uptake of thyroglobulin by medullary carcinoma.

References

1. Horn RC. Carcinoma of the thyroid: description of a distinctive morphologic variant and report of seven cases. Cancer. 1951;4: 697–707.
2. Hazard JB, Hawk WA, Crile G. Medullary (solid) carcinoma of the thyroid. A clinicopathologic entity. J Clin Endocrinol Metab. 1959;19:152–61.
3. Williams ED. Histogenesis of medullary carcinoma of the thyroid. J Clin Pathol. 1966;19:114–8.
4. Wolfe HJ, Melvin KE, Cervi-Skinner SJ, Saadi AA, Juliar JF, Jackson CE, Tashjian Jr AH. C-cell hyperplasia preceding medullary thyroid carcinoma. N Engl J Med. 1973;289:437–41.
5. Sipple JH. The association of pheochromocytoma with carcinoma of the thyroid gland. Am J Med. 1961;31:163–6.
6. Skinner MA, Wells Jr SA. Medullary carcinoma of the thyroid gland and the MEN 2 syndromes. Semin Pediatr Surg. 1997; 6:134–40.
7. Mulligan LM, Eng C, Attie T, Lyonnet S, Marsh DJ, Hyland VJ, Robinson BG, Frilling A, Verellen-Dumoulin C, Safar A, et al. Diverse phenotypes associated with exon 10 mutations of the RET proto-oncogene. Hum Mol Genet. 1994;3:2163–7.
8. Massoll N, Mazzaferri EL. Diagnosis and management of medullary thyroid carcinoma. Clin Lab Med. 2004;24:49–83.
9. Asa SL. How familial cancer genes and environmentally induced oncogenes have changed the endocrine landscape. Mod Pathol. 2001;14:246–53.
10. Wolfe HJ, Delellis RA. Familial medullary thyroid carcinoma and C cell hyperplasia. Clin Endocrinol Metab. 1981;10:351–65.
11. DeLellis RA, Nunnemacher G, Bitman WR, Gagel RF, Tashjian Jr AH, Blount M, Wolfe HJ. C-cell hyperplasia and medullary thyroid carcinoma in the rat. An immunohistochemical and ultrastructural analysis. Lab Invest. 1979;40:140–54.
12. Albores-Saavedra J, LiVolsi VA, Williams ED. Medullary carcinoma. Semin Diagn Pathol. 1985;2:137–46.
13. Holm R, Sobrinho Simoes M, Nesland JM, Gould VE, Johannessen JV. Medullary carcinoma of the thyroid gland: an immunocytochemical study. Ultrastruct Pathol. 1985;8:25.
14. Ho C, Lin JD, Huang YY, Huang HS, Huang BY, Hsueh C. Clinical experience of medullary thyroid carcinoma in Chang Gung Memorial Hospital. Chang Keng I Hsueh. 1996;19:142–8.
15. Forrest CH, Frost FA, de Boer WB, Spagnolo DV, Whitaker D, Sterrett BF. Medullary carcinoma of the thyroid: accuracy of diagnosis of fine-needle aspiration cytology. Cancer. 1998;84:295–302.
16. Kaushal S, Iyer VK, Mathur SR, Ray R. Fine needle aspiration cytology of medullary carcinoma of the thyroid with a focus on rare variants: a review of 78 cases. Cytopathology. 2010.
17. Mendelsohn G, Baylin SB, Bigner SH, Wells Jr SA, Eggleston JC. Anaplastic variants of medullary thyroid carcinoma: a light-microscopic and immunohistochemical study. Am J Surg Pathol. 1980;4:333–41.
18. Yerly S, Triponez F, Meyer P, Kumar N, Bongiovanni M. Medullary thyroid carcinoma, small cell variant, as a diagnostic challenge on fine needle aspiration: a case report. Acta Cytol. 2010;54:911–7.
19. Harach HR, Bergholm U. Medullary (C cell) carcinoma of the thyroid with features of follicular oxyphilic cell tumours. Histopathology. 1988;13:645–56.
20. Dedivitis RA, Di Giovanni JH, Silva GF, Marinho LC, Guimaraes AV. Oncocytic variant of medullary thyroid carcinoma: case report. Arq Bras Endocrinol Metabol. 2004;48:315–7.
21. Tranchida P, Estigarribia J, Sethi S, Giorgadze T. Cytologic diagnosis of recurrent medullary thyroid carcinoma with oncocytic change twenty-one years post-thyroidectomy: case report and review of the literature. Diagn Cytopathol. 2011;39:641–6.
22. Zaatari GS, Saigo PE, Huvos AG. Mucin production in medullary carcinoma of the thyroid. Arch Pathol Lab Med. 1983;107:70–4.
23. Singh K, Sharma MC, Jain D, Kumar R. Melanotic medullary carcinoma of thyroid – report of a rare case with brief review of literature. Diagn Pathol. 2008;3:2.
24. Ben Romdhane K, Khattech R, Ben Othman M, Gamoudi A, Ammar A, Cammoun M. Melanin production in medullary thyroid carcinoma. Histopathology. 1995;27:569–71.
25. Khurana R, Agarwal A, Bajpai VK, Verma N, Sharma AK, Gupta RP, Madhusudan KP. Unraveling the amyloid associated with human medullary thyroid carcinoma. Endocrinology. 2004;145: 5465–70.
26. Us-Krasovec M, Auersperg M, Bergant D, Golouh R, Kloboves-Prevodnik V. Medullary carcinoma of the thyroid glad: diagnostic cytopathological characteristics. Pathologica. 1998;90:5–13.
27. Samaan NA, Schultz PN, Hickey RC. Medullary thyroid carcinoma: prognosis of familial versus sporadic disease and the role of radiotherapy. J Clin Endocrinol Metab. 1988;67:801–5.
28. Schroder S, Bocker W, Baisch H, Burk CG, Arps H, Meiners I, Kastendieck H, Heitz PU, Kloppel G. Prognostic factors in medullary thyroid carcinomas. Survival in relation to age, sex, stage, histology, immunocytochemistry, and DNA content. Cancer. 1988;61:806–16.
29. Bergholm U, Adami HO, Auer G, Bergstrom R, Backdahl M, Grimelius L, Hansson G, Ljungberg O, Wilander E. Histopathologic characteristics and nuclear DNA content as prognostic factors in medullary thyroid carcinoma. A nationwide study in Sweden. The Swedish MTC Study Group. Cancer. 1989;64:135–42.
30. Pastolero GC, Coire CI, Asa SL. Concurrent medullary and papillary carcinomas of thyroid with lymph node metastases. A collision phenomenon. Am J Surg Pathol. 1996;20:245–50.
31. Oertel YC, Oertel JE. Diagnosis of malignant epithelial thyroid lesions: fine needle aspiration and histopathologic correlation. Ann Diagn Pathol. 1998;2:377–400.
32. Zeppa P, Benincasa G, Lucariello A, Palombini L. Association of different pathologic processes of the thyroid gland in fine needle aspiration samples. Acta Cytol. 2001;45:347–52.
33. Costanzo M, Marziani A, Papa V, Arcerito MC, Cannizzaro MA. Simultaneous medullary carcinoma and differentiated thyroid cancer. Case report. Ann Ital Chir. 2010;81:357–60.
34. Randolph GW. Medullary carcinoma of the thyroid: subtypes and current management. Compr Ther. 1996;22:203–10.
35. Heptulla RA, Schwartz RP, Bale AE, Flynn S, Genel M. Familial medullary thyroid carcinoma: presymptomatic diagnosis and management in children. J Pediatr. 1999;135:327–31.
36. Wu LS, Roman SA, Sosa JA. Medullary thyroid cancer: an update of new guidelines and recent developments. Curr Opin Oncol. 2011;23:22–7.
37. Albores-Saavedra JA, Krueger JE. C-cell hyperplasia and medullary thyroid microcarcinoma. Endocr Pathol. 2001;12:365–77.
38. Mizukami Y, Kurumaya H, Nonomura A, Michigishi T, Terahata S, Noguchi M, Hashimoto T, Matsubara F. Sporadic medullary microcarcinoma of the thyroid. Histopathology. 1992;21:375–7.
39. Etit D, Faquin WC, Gaz R, Randolph G, DeLellis RA, Pilch BZ. Histopathologic and clinical features of medullary microcarcinoma and C-cell hyperplasia in prophylactic thyroidectomies for medullary carcinoma: a study of 42 cases. Arch Pathol Lab Med. 2008;132:1767–73.

40. Kazaure HS, Roman SA, Sosa JA. Medullary thyroid microcarcinoma: a population-level analysis of 310 patients. Cancer. 2011.
41. Collins BT, Cramer HM, Tabatowski K, Hearn S, Raminhos A, Lampe H. Fine needle aspiration of medullary carcinoma of the thyroid. Cytomorphology, immunocytochemistry and electron microscopy. Acta Cytol. 1995;39:920–30.
42. Papaparaskeva K, Nagel H, Droese M. Cytologic diagnosis of medullary carcinoma of the thyroid gland. Diagn Cytopathol. 2000;22:351–8.
43. Boyd LA, Earnhardt RC, Dunn JT, Frierson HF, Hanks JB. Preoperative evaluation and predictive value of fine-needle aspiration and frozen section of thyroid nodules. J Am Coll Surg. 1998;187:494–502.
44. Ozgen AG, Hamulu F, Bayraktar F, Yilmaz C, Tuzun M, Yetkin E, Tuncyurek M, Kabalak T. Evaluation of routine basal serum calcitonin measurement for early diagnosis of medullary thyroid carcinoma in seven hundred seventy-three patients with nodular goiter. Thyroid. 1999;9:579–82.
45. Trimboli P, Rossi F, Baldelli R, Laurenti O, Nigri G, Ventura C, Appetecchia M, Attanasio D, Romanelli F, Guidobaldi L, Guarino M, Crescenzi A, Valabrega S. Measuring calcitonin in washout of the needle in patients undergoing fine needle aspiration with suspicious medullary thyroid cancer. Diagn Cytopathol. 2011.
46. Parker LN, Kollin J, Wu SY, Rypins EB, Juler GL. Carcinoma of the thyroid with a mixed medullary, papillary, follicular, and undifferentiated pattern. Arch Intern Med. 1985;145:1507–9.
47. Albores-Saavedra J, Gorraez de la Mora T, de la Torre-Rendon F, Gould E. Mixed medullary-papillary carcinoma of the thyroid: a previously unrecognized variant of thyroid carcinoma. Hum Pathol. 1990;21:1151–5.
48. Sobrinho-Simoes M. Mixed medullary and follicular carcinoma of the thyroid. Histopathology. 1993;23:287–9.

Medullary Carcinoma of the Thyroid: Surgical Management

85

Gerard M. Doherty

Medullary thyroid cancer (MTC) accounts for less than 10 % of all thyroid malignancies [1]. About 75 % of patients with MTC have sporadic disease, and 25 % have disease based upon *Ret* proto-oncogene mutation. Management for presymptomatic genetically affected patients, and for patients with clinically evident disease, requires separate consideration [2].

Most patients with clinically evident MTC are first detected by fine-needle aspiration of a thyroid nodule. When suspected by cytological examination, the diagnosis of MTC should be further assessed by testing blood calcitonin levels and with histochemical stains for calcitonin on the cytological specimen. Because of possible unrecognized MEN-2 syndrome, all patients with suspected MTC by cytological examination should have their serum calcium levels tested to determine whether hyperparathyroidism is present and plasma tests for fractionated metanephrine levels to rule out a pheochromocytoma. If present, surgical management of pheochromocytoma takes precedence over an initial surgical approach to the medullary cancer. All patients with MTC require direct genetic testing for *Ret* proto-oncogene mutations.

Surgical Approach

Patients with clinically evident MTC have operation based upon their extent of disease. Medullary cancer cells do not trap iodine, and so in contrast to the management of papillary thyroid cancer, there is no value to radioiodine therapy and no other effective adjuvant therapy for MTC, so effective treatment is based entirely upon operative resection.

Recommendations for operative management are based upon the extent of evident disease [2]:

1. Patients with known or highly suspected MTC with no evidence of advanced local invasion by the primary tumor, no evidence of cervical lymph node metastases on physical examination and cervical US, and no evidence of distant metastases should undergo total thyroidectomy and prophylactic central compartment (level VI) neck dissection.
2. Patients with suspected limited local metastatic disease to regional lymph nodes in the central compartment (with a normal US examination of the lateral neck compartments) in the setting of no distant (extracervical) metastases or limited distant metastases should typically undergo a total thyroidectomy and level VI compartmental dissection.
3. Patients with suspected limited local metastatic disease to regional lymph nodes in the central and lateral neck compartments (with US-visible lymph node metastases in the lateral neck compartments) in the setting of no distant metastases or limited distant metastases should typically undergo a total thyroidectomy, central (level VI), and lateral neck (levels IIA, III, IV, V) dissection.
4. In the presence of distant metastatic disease, less aggressive neck surgery may be appropriate to preserve speech, swallowing, and parathyroid function while maintaining locoregional disease control to prevent central neck morbidity.

Presymptomatic genetically affected patients are managed based upon the defined risk of MTC associated with their specific mutation [2]. The greatest risk mutation status is in MEN-2B patients, who should have prophylactic thyroidectomy before age 2; if thyroidectomy is accomplished before age 1 year, then no central neck dissection is necessary. Patients who have non-MEN-2B mutations are separated into high-, higher-, and highest-risk groups [3]. Highest-risk patients should have prophylactic thyroidectomy

G.M. Doherty, MD, FACS (✉)
Department of Surgery, Boston Medical Center, Boston University, 88 East Newton Street Collamore Building Suite 500, Boston, MA 02118, USA
e-mail: dohertyg@bu.edu

L. Wartofsky, D. Van Nostrand (eds.), *Thyroid Cancer*, DOI 10.1007/978-1-4939-3314-3_85

before age 5 years. Those in the high-risk group can delay thyroidectomy until older age, as long as their annual calcitonin and surveillance ultrasound remain normal, if the family prefers. Patients in the higher-risk group should consider thyroidectomy prior to age 5 years but may also reasonably delay if asymptomatic, with normal calcitonin levels and cervical ultrasound examinations, and if there has not been aggressive behavior of MTC in other family members [2].

Operative results including complication rates are best among surgeons who regularly perform thyroidectomy [4].

References

1. Tuttle RM, Ball DW, Byrd D, et al. Medullary carcinoma. J Natl Compr Canc Netw. 2010;8(5):512–30.
2. American Thyroid Association Guidelines Task F, Kloos RT, Eng C, et al. Medullary thyroid cancer: management guidelines of the American Thyroid Association. Thyroid. 2009;19(6):565–612.
3. Brandi ML, Gagel RF, Angeli A, et al. Guidelines for diagnosis and therapy of MEN type 1 and type 2 [see comment]. J Clin Endocrinol Metab. 2001;86(12):5658–71.
4. Tuggle CT, Roman SA, Wang TS, et al. Pediatric endocrine surgery: who is operating on our children? Surgery. 2008;144(6):869–77; discussion 877.

86 Radionuclide Imaging of Medullary Carcinoma

Giuseppe Esposito

Introduction

Medullary thyroid cancer (MTC) has a favorable prognosis if locally confined at diagnosis, whereas survival rates decline in patients with more advanced disease that involves the lateral cervical lymph nodes and in patients with distant metastases. In most of the cases, total thyroidectomy and lymph node dissection represent the main treatment for MTC. In selected patients being evaluated for thyroid nodules and with low thyroid stimulating hormone (TSH), thyroid scan with ^{123}I or ^{99m}Tc may be helpful to decide whether fine needle biopsy is warranted (see the American Thyroid Association (ATA) guidelines on thyroid cancer [1]). For the initial presurgical evaluation of patients with a new diagnosis of MTC, nuclear medicine studies are generally less accurate in detecting lymph node metastases when compared to other imaging modalities and are not recommended as first-line investigation at this stage of patient management. Neck ultrasound (US) is the imaging modality of choice for the initial exploration of the cervical lymph nodes. If lymph node metastases are detected by neck US or suspected from high presurgical serum calcitonin levels (>400 pg/ml), then, according to ATA and National Comprehensive Cancer Network (NCCN) guidelines [2, 3], additional imaging evaluation is warranted to search for sites of more distant metastases and to guide the surgical approach and possible adjuvant treatments. Contrast computed tomography (CT) or magnetic resonance imaging (MRI) of the neck, chest CT, and contrast CT or MRI of the liver are the first-line imaging studies to evaluate whether or not metastatic disease has involved the mediastinal lymph nodes, lungs, bones, or liver. In patients in whom advanced disease is suspected, bone scintigraphy is a first-line imaging modality for the evaluation of skeletal metastases. In fact, bone scans have demonstrated similar overall sensitivity when compared to MRI but appear more accurate to detect lesions in the extra-axial skeleton (e.g., ribs and skull) [4]. Other nuclear medicine studies can be helpful when other imaging modalities have not been able to fully characterize disease extension. Radiolabeled somatostatin analogs (RSAs), pentavalent ^{99m}Tc-dimercaptosuccinic acid (DMSA), and metaiodobenzylguanidine (MIBG) are some of the radiotracers that have been used for the initial imaging evaluation and in the follow-up of patients suspected of having residual disease or metastases after the initial surgery. ^{18}F-fluoro-2-deoxyglucose (^{18}F-FDG) PET can be helpful for the evaluation of more advanced lymph node and distant metastases, particularly when more aggressive disease is suspected based on a rapid doubling time of the tumoral markers, calcitonin and carcinoembryonic antigen (CEA). Other PET tracers of amino acid metabolism such as ^{18}fluorine-dihydroxyphenylalanine (^{18}F-DOPA) or of somatostatin receptors (SRs) such as ^{68}Ga-DOTA-TOC have a very promising role in the evaluation of patients with neuroendocrine tumors (NETs), including MTC. The role of PET in MTC is discussed in detail in Chap. 87.

Nuclear medicine studies are most useful in the follow-up of patients after the initial surgery when residual disease is suspected on the basis of a persistently elevated calcitonin level. In these patients, a thorough search for sites of residual or metastatic disease using imaging is important as some cases may benefit from the early recognition of lesions that potentially can be removed surgically with curative intent. Both the ATA and NCCN guidelines recommend neck US as a first-line evaluation of patients with residual elevation of calcitonin levels 2–3 months after surgery. This is so because residual disease is localized to cervical lymph nodes in a large proportion of these cases. However, higher postsurgical calcitonin levels (>150 pg/ml) are associated with a greater

G. Esposito, MD (✉)
Division of Nuclear Medicine, MedStar Georgetown University Hospital, 3800 Reservoir Road, NW, Washington, DC 20818, USA
e-mail: exg11@gunet.georgetown.edu

L. Wartofsky, D. Van Nostrand (eds.), *Thyroid Cancer*, DOI 10.1007/978-1-4939-3314-3_86

likelihood that disease extends beyond the cervical lymph nodes, and additional imaging evaluation is therefore needed. In such cases, and particularly when extensive metastatic disease is suspected from very high postsurgical calcitonin levels (>1000 pg/ml), nuclear medicine studies such as bone scan, RSA imaging, and ^{18}F-FDG PET can be most valuable as adjunctive imaging modalities to identify sites of metastases when CT and MRI of the neck, chest, and abdomen have not achieved conclusive results. When incurable disseminated disease is present, palliative treatment of the symptomatic metastases with local interventions (e.g., surgery, embolization, and radiation) or systemic therapy within clinical trials should be considered. In such patients, the nuclear medicine studies can provide important functional information on aspects of tumor biology that can be potential targets or indicators of response for therapeutic trials. For example, nuclear medicine studies with ^{111}In-octreotide can assess the degree of expression of somatostatin receptors and predict the potential efficacy of pharmaceutical treatment with somatostatin analogs or of combined pharmaceutical and radiation treatment using somatostatin analogs labeled with emitters of beta radiation such as ^{90}Y or ^{177}Lu. Treatments with ^{131}I-MIBG or with anti-CEA antibodies labeled with ^{131}I are other examples of imaging agents and therapeutic tools that are being evaluated in preclinical investigations and/or in clinical trials for their potential use in patients with MTC and NETs. A detailed discussion of the available nuclear medicine agents follows below.

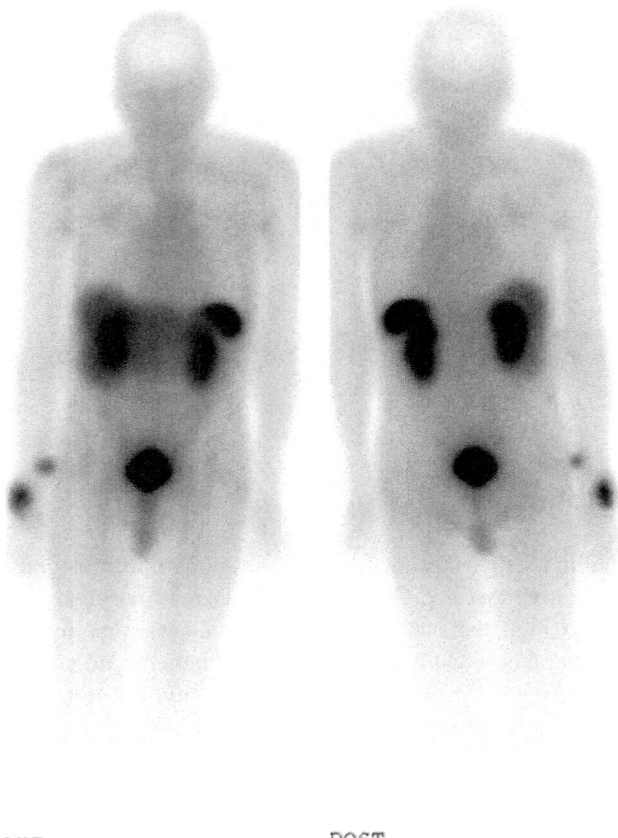

Fig. 86.1 Normal distribution of ^{111}In-pentetreotide. The normal distribution of ^{111}In-pentetreotide is shown in this figure with normal uptake in the kidneys, spleen, liver, and urinary bladder. Faint uptake is seen in the large bowel, which is also normal. Focal uptake in the right hand and wrist is the site of intravenous injection

Radiolabeled Somatostatin Analogs (RSAs)

^{111}In-pentetreotide (OctreoScan®) is among the first and the most commonly used of the RSAs [5]. Pentetreotide is a synthetic analog of somatostatin that binds with higher affinity to the subtype 2 somatostatin receptors. Somatostatin receptors are present on a number of tumor cells that can be visualized with ^{111}In-pentetreotide including: pituitary adenomas, meningiomas, pancreatic islet cell tumors, lung cancer particularly small cell lung cancer, carcinoids, and other neuroendocrine cancers, including medullary thyroid cancer and pheochromocytomas [6, 7]. Lymphocytes are also rich in somatostatin receptors, and this explains the uptake of ^{111}In-pentetreotide in granulomas, lymphomas, autoimmune disorders such as Graves' disease, and Graves' ophthalmopathy in particular [8].

Dose and Normal Body Distribution

For diagnostic applications, ^{111}In-pentetreotide is administered intravenously in a dose of approximately 222 MBq (6 mCi). It is preferable to discontinue any therapy with cold octreotide for 2 days before administration of the radiotracer because it will interfere with the radiolabeled ^{111}In-pentetreotide uptake. Whole-body planar and SPECT images are usually performed at 4 and 24 h after administration to allow clearance of background activity. Figure 86.1 shows the normal distribution of OctreoScan® (^{111}In-pentetreotide) in the body.

^{111}In-pentetreotide is mainly excreted through the kidneys via glomerular filtration. Some degree of excretion occurs through the hepatobiliary route. The spleen and kidneys represent the dose-limiting organs [9].

Normal uptake is visualized in the pituitary gland, thyroid gland, spleen, liver, kidneys, and urinary bladder. Activity in the gallbladder and bowel is sometimes visualized, particularly on images acquired at 24 h due to biliary excretion. In the normal thyroid, pituitary gland, and spleen, the uptake is due to interaction with specific somatostatin receptors [5]. Diffuse breast uptake can be seen normally in young women. Uptake has been described in the nose and lung hila in

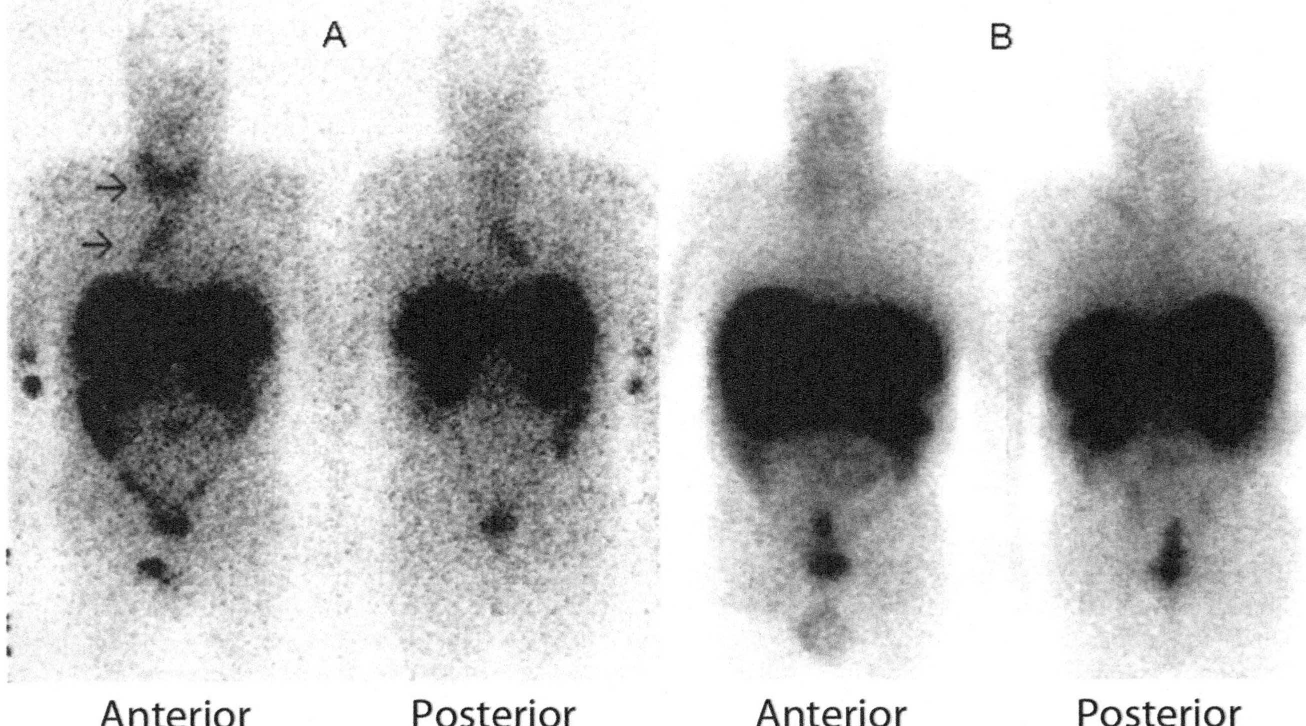

Fig. 86.2 Medullary thyroid cancer. In this patient with medullary thyroid cancer, the left image (**a**) was performed before any treatment and demonstrates multiple areas of abnormal uptake in the neck, chest, and abdomen (*arrows*) secondary to metastases. The right image (**b**) was performed after three treatments with high amount of ^{111}In-pentetreotide and 9 months after the first image. Complete resolution of the previous abnormal uptake is noted suggesting a complete response. The colonic uptake is physiologic (Reprinted by permission of the Society of Nuclear Medicine from: Buscombe et al. [42])

conjunction with cold/flu symptoms and is due to activated lymphocytes. After surgery or external radiation therapy, uptake of ^{111}In-pentetreotide has been described and is related to the concomitant inflammatory/reactive changes [5].

Indications

The reported sensitivity of ^{111}In-pentetreotide for detection of MTC varies widely across studies from 65 % to 100 % [9–13]. Sensitivity is lower for detection of primary tumor localizations in the thyroid gland and of metastatic disease in the liver [14], probably because of the higher background activity present in the surrounding tissues of these organs. Figure 86.2 shows visualization of metastatic disease from medullary thyroid cancer by whole-body octreotide scan.

The ability to detect foci of metastatic disease strongly depends, however, on the expression of somatostatin receptors on the tumor cells. ^{111}In-pentetreotide appears less sensitive for less differentiated medullary cancers that present with a lower calcitonin/CEA plasma ratio [15] and express fewer somatostatin receptors. Sensitivities are in general lower for MTC compared to other neuroendocrine tumors probably because MTC expresses lower densities of SRs and has greater variability in SSTR subtypes with a lower rate of expression of the subtypes 2 and 5 that bind octreotide with higher affinity [16, 17].

Because of the relatively lower sensitivity, ^{111}In-pentetreotide and other RSAs are not usually recommended as first-line imaging agents, but they may play a well-defined role as an adjunct to conventional imaging for the evaluation of metastatic MTC. ^{111}In-pentetreotide may detect additional lesions compared to conventional imaging. Krauz et al. reported that pathological uptake was detected in nine of ten patients with persistent or recurrent MTC with five of these foci not seen by other diagnostic modalities (CT or MRI) [18]. In another series, tumor localization was demonstrated by pentetreotide scanning in 11 of 17 patients [9]. In a prospective study of 18 patients with MTC, ^{111}In-pentetreotide outperformed MRI in some of the patients with minimal residual disease diagnosed by persistent elevation of calcitonin [19]. The adjunctive role of ^{111}In-pentetreotide in cases not clarified by conventional imaging was evaluated by Baudin et al. in patients in whom metastatic disease was suspected on the basis of an elevated calcitonin level [12]. In 12 patients with metastatic disease that were identified by conventional imaging, ^{111}In-pentetreotide imaging did not add additional clinically relevant information even though some smaller lesions were identified by ^{111}In-pentetreotide, and not by conventional imaging. In 12 patients with negative or indeterminate results on conventional imaging, ^{111}In-pentetreotide was negative in ten patients but correctly identified disease in two patients. Accuracy of ^{111}In-pentetreotide imaging was worse than conventional imaging particularly for lesions less than 1 cm in size. In a series of 20 patients with elevated calcitonin levels after initial surgery, ^{111}In-pentetreotide detected 15 pathological uptake foci in 11 patients, and CT detected 17 foci in 11 patients [20]. A false-positive scan occurred in a patient with sarcoidosis. The patients with true-positive ^{111}In-pentetreotide studies had significantly higher basal calcitonin and CEA levels than the patients with negative isotopic studies. The authors concluded that the sensitivity of ^{111}In-pentetreotide imaging for detection of metastatic disease is in general lower than conventional imaging but is more favorable in patients with high calcitonin serum levels. They also concluded that ^{111}In-pentetreotide should be used when conventional imaging is negative or ambiguous or when treatment with somatostatin analogs is being considered. Lower sensitivity of ^{111}In-pentetreotide compared to conventional imaging was also found in a group of 11 children and adolescents [21]. In a retrospective study on 14 patients with recurrent metastatic MTC, Arslan et al. compared ^{111}In-pentetreotide imaging with conventional imaging including CT, MRI, and US and found that the 78.5 % sensitivity of ^{111}In-pentetreotide to detect disease on a patient basis was comparable to that of conventional imaging. But ^{111}In-pentetreotide detected fewer lesions in those patients compared to conventional imaging (81.3 % vs. 44 %) [22]. As seen in other studies, ^{111}In-pentetreotide was able to detect few lesions that were not revealed by conventional imaging, and the highest sensitivities for lesion detection were reached with the combination of conventional and radionuclide imaging (85.7 %).

To increase the ability to detect disease and improve the yield of surgical approach, handheld intraoperative probes have been used to search for removable tumors that express somatostatin receptors [23]. The use of combined SPECT/CT acquisition can also increase accuracy of ^{111}In-pentetreotide. In a series of 72 patients, the combined acquisition affected the diagnostic interpretation in 32 % of the patients and changed clinical management in 14 % of the patients compared to routine acquisition protocols [18].

Other Diagnostic Imaging Agents

Pentavalent ^{99m}Tc-dimercaptosuccinic acid (DMSA) appears to localize in MTC due to increased turnover of calcium and phosphate ions and has shown satisfactory tumor/background ratios to permit good scintigraphic images [24]. However, experience with DMSA has been limited by difficulties in the preparation and storage of the radioisotope [25]. Guerra et al. found an overall 84 % sensitivity of ^{99m}Tc (V) DMSA in 26 patients with MTC [26]. Clarke et al. found an even higher sensitivity of 95 % for ^{99m}Tc (V) DMSA for detection of bone and soft tissue metastases [27]. The use of ^{99m}Tc (V) DMSA is limited by the fact that it is not available commercially in the United States but must be prepared in each laboratory by adding sodium bicarbonate to standard DMSA kits. However, small inaccuracies in the preparation can cause dramatic decrease in the quality of images as well as sensitivity of the scan. DMSA is overall less accurate than ^{111}In-pentetreotide to detect metastatic MTC [22], although the two methods combined may sometimes show additive value in the visualization of metastatic lesions.

Metaiodobenzylguanidine (MIBG) is a radiolabeled norepinephrine analog taken up by cells through a specific, energy-dependent transport mechanism in which the tracer competes with norepinephrine. Sensitivities for ^{131}I MIBG imaging are highest for detection of pheochromocytoma and less satisfactory for MTC [28]. Several case reports confirm accurate localization of primary and recurrent MTC in sporadic and familial cases using ^{131}I MIBG with the advantage of potentially detecting concurrent pheochromocytomas in familial syndromes [29, 30]. In a larger series, the diagnostic accuracy of MIBG was found to be limited by low overall sensitivity to detect metastatic MTC [23]. In a direct comparison study, ^{111}In-pentetreotide imaging was more sensitive than MIBG in the detection of metastatic disease across different neuroendocrine tumors, including MTC [31].

^{99m}Tc-methylene diphosphonate (MDP) has been used for years for nonspecific but extremely sensitive detection of bone metastases of a variety of tumors, including MTC [27]. Bone imaging is recommended as a first-line study to evaluate for bone metastases in patients with MTC because the scan sensitivity is similar to that of MRI and better than other imaging modalities [4]. ^{18}F-sodium fluoride PET bone imaging is now being performed and may be superior to ^{99m}Tc-MDP.

Other radiopharmaceutical agents such ^{201}Thallium (^{201}T1) [32] or ^{99m}Tc-sestamibi [33, 34] have been used in metastatic MTC, but they have not proven to be more accurate compared to imaging with DMSA or RSA [35].

Evaluation of Treatment with Somatostatin Analogs (SAs)

Although somatostatin analogs have a role in the treatment of NETs, their role in MTC is controversial with regard to the ability to induce a therapeutic response [36–38]. Because the degree of RSA uptake is directly related to the number of somatostatin receptors expressed in the tumor, nuclear medicine imaging offers the possibility to specifically select or stratify patients being evaluated for treatment with SAs based on the degree of uptake. This can prove useful in experimental protocols that wish to explore the effectiveness of somatostatin analogs.

Treatment with RSAs and Radioimmunotherapy (RIT)

The success of radioimmunotherapy in the treatment of B-cell lymphomas that are refractory to conventional chemotherapy or radiation therapy has drawn scientific and commercial interest in the use of radiolabeled peptides for therapeutic applications. ^{111}In-pentetreotide at high doses (from a minimum of 20 GBq to a maximum acceptable for bone marrow toxicity of 100 GBq [corresponding to 540–2,700 mCi]) [39] has been among the first peptides used for therapeutic applications in oncology. It combines the pharmacologic action of the somatostatin analog octreotide and the radiotoxic effect of ^{111}In [39]. The radioactive ligand-somatostatin receptor complex is internalized into the cells and transported into the nucleus so that the radioactive ^{111}In can exert its action into the nucleus [40]. Several phase I/II studies of radionuclide treatment with ^{111}In-pentetreotide in neuroendocrine tumors have showed variable response rates (as high as ~60 %) in patients refractory to other treatment modalities with limited side effects [41, 42]. Somatostatin analogs labeled with other radionuclides such as ^{90}Y and ^{177}Lu have been used for the treatment of NETs and MTC [43–47]. These radionuclides have a theoretical therapeutic advantage because they emit beta radiation that has a longer range of action compared to the Auger electrons emitted by ^{111}In, thus extending their effectiveness to nearby cells that do not internalize the receptor-radioligand complex, the latter known as a *cross-fire* effect. This represents a theoretical advantage in larger tumors where the nonuniform vascularization leaves some of the tumor cells out of the reach of the radioligand.

A phase IIa clinical trial in Europe used a different somatostatin analog, lanreotide labeled with ^{90}Y, and administered doses of up to 8.6 GBq (232 mCi) in 154 different tumor patients [43]. In 63 of 154 patients (41 %), disease remained stable, while regression was observed in 14 % of the patients. Quantitative assessment of uptake from the different tumors showed that NETs accumulate pentetreotide more that lanreotide and that lanreotide accumulated better in radioiodine-negative thyroid cancer, hepatocellular cancer, lung cancers, and brain tumors. A more recent phase II clinical trial used median doses of 12.6 GBq (340 mCi) of ^{90}Y-DOTA-TOC in 31 patients with progressive metastatic MTC and achieved a significant longer survival in responders experiencing a reduction in calcitonin levels [48].

Metastatic MTC may be visualized with anti-CEA monoclonal antibodies labeled with ^{99m}Tc, ^{131}I, or ^{111}In, particularly in tumors that have a higher CEA/calcitonin plasma ratio [49]. Phase I and II clinical trials have tested the efficacy of radioimmunotherapy (RIT) with ^{131}I- or ^{90}Y-labeled anti-CEA monoclonal antibodies alone or in association with different chemotherapeutic regimens [50, 51]. Partial responses were achieved only at myeloablative doses. Trials conducted in France [52, 53] using pre-targeted anti-CEA RIT with ^{131}I in patients with metastatic MTC have resulted in disease stabilization in a significant portion of the patients. The outcome of the trials indicated that this treatment was more beneficial for high-risk patients who were defined as having a calcitonin doubling time of less than 2 years. In general, better tumor/background ratios, better antitumor effect, and the possibility for outpatient treatment favor labeling with ^{90}Y compared to ^{131}I. A subsequent phase II pRAIT study in 45 patients with progressive MTC with calcitonin doubling time (DT) shorter than 5 years used 1.8 GBq/m 2 of bivalent indium-DTPA hapten labeled with ^{131}I. Disease control was achieved in 76 % of patients, and 57 % of patients showed a significant impact of the doubling time of calcitonin or CEA or a prolonged decrease of the biomarker concentrations [54]. Subacute toxicity was mainly hematological, requiring careful post-RAIT blood monitoring. Response, pre-RAIT biomarker DT, and impact on DT were predictors of survival, confirming the value of serum biomarkers in selecting patients and monitoring therapy. Interestingly, these authors found that ^{18}F-FDG PET was more sensitive than CT to detect metastatic disease in cervical and mediastinal lymph nodes and that the tumor metabolic activity expressed as SUVmax correlated significantly with calcitonin doubling time. In addition, posttreatment imaging of the ^{131}I-labeled anti-CEA monoclonal antibody was highly accurate to detect metastatic disease.

Somatostatin Analogs in Differentiated Thyroid Cancer

Several reports have shown that imaging with RSA may be useful to detect metastatic thyroid cancer that has lost the ability to concentrate radioiodine and has become unresponsive to ^{131}I treatment [55–58], suggesting that somatostatin receptor expression may occur in differentiated cancer that has lost the ability to take up iodine [58]. However, in iodine-negative patients ^{18}F-FDG PET/CT has become the imaging modality of choice and is superior to imaging with RSA [59, 60].

It has been hypothesized that thyroid cancers that have lost the ability to take up iodine but express somatostatin receptors could benefit from treatment with radiolabeled somatostatin analogs [57]. Based upon very limited data, there is uncertainty that any therapeutic benefit can be achieved with RSAs as Gorges et al. failed to obtain response in three patients treated with ^{90}Y-DOTA-TOC [55]. New agents, refinement of treatment protocols, and better selection of patients may improve the outcome of these novel therapeutic strategies.

Summary and Future Directions

For the diagnostic evaluation of medullary thyroid cancer, nuclear medicine techniques are most useful when used as an adjunct to conventional radiologic imaging (i.e., neck US, CT, and MRI) to evaluate suspected metastatic disease. Radiolabeled somatostatin analogs offer a more favorable combination of diagnostic accuracy, technical flexibility, and availability compared to other nuclear medicine radiotracers. Conventional imaging has an overall better diagnostic accuracy for the evaluation of metastatic disease and should always represent the first line in the diagnostic process. Somatostatin analogs however may detect disease not identified by conventional imaging, particularly in cases of still well-differentiated disease that maintains high calcitonin/CEA plasma values. The accuracy of imaging with somatostatin analogs is reduced when less well-differentiated disease is suspected, for example, when there are relatively greater serum levels of CEA compared to calcitonin. In these cases, ^{18}F-FDG PET imaging may have better accuracy, as discussed elsewhere in this book (Chap. 87). The unique contribution of the radiolabeled somatostatin analogs is based on the ability to assess the expression of somatostatin receptors on foci of metastatic disease that constitutes targets for possible treatment with either cold or radiolabeled somatostatin analogs that combine pharmacologic and radiotoxic actions on the tumor cells. The introduction of new somatostatin analogs that have either a wider spectrum of action across the different subtypes of somatostatin receptors or greater specificity for single subtypes may improve treatment and visualization of disease that expresses different subtypes. This is particularly true for MTC. Progress in the radiochemistry of somatostatin analogs now offers the flexibility to label them to different radionuclides (^{111}In, ^{90}Y, ^{177}Lu). It is conceivable that different somatostatin analogs may be used for different tumors according to the specific receptor subtype profiles. Technical advancement in hardware (e.g., PET, PET/CT, and SPECT/CT) has already made an impact in the management of different tumors. The role of ^{18}F-FDG PET in MTC and other NETs has been explored in Chap. 87. Somatostatin analogs labeled with positron emission emitters have been synthesized already which may bring new exciting advances in the diagnostic and therapeutic management of patients with neuroendocrine and other tumors [61, see also Ref. 36 for review].

References

1. Haugen BR, Alexander EK, Bible KC, Doherty GM, Mandel SJ, Nikiforov YE, Pacini F, Randolph GW, Sawka AM, Schlumberger M, Schuff KG, Sherman SI, Sosa JA, Steward DL, Tuttle RM, Wartofsky L. 2015 American Thyroid Association Management Guidelines for Adult Patients with Thyroid Nodules and Differentiated Thyroid Cancer: American Thyroid Association Guidelines Task Force on Thyroid Nodules and Differentiated Thyroid Cancer. Thyroid. 2016;26:1–133.
2. Wells SA, et al., Revised American Thyroid Association Guidelines for the Management of Medullary Thyroid Carcinoma prepared by the American Thyroid Association Guidelines Task Force on Medullary Thyroid Carcinoma. Thyroid 2015;25:567–610.
3. NCCN Clinical Practice Guidelines in Oncology: Thyroid carcinoma. Version 3.2011.
4. Giraudet AL, Vanel D, Leboulleux S, et al. Imaging medullary thyroid carcinoma with persistent elevated calcitonin levels. J Clin Endocrinol Metab. 2007;92:4185–90.
5. Krenning EP, Kwekkeboom DJ, Bakker WH, Breeman WA, Kooij PP, Oei HY, van Hagen M, Postema PT, de Jong M, Reubi JC, et al. Somatostatin receptor scintigraphy with [^{111}In-DTPA-D-Phe1]- and [^{123}I-Tyr3]-octreotide: the Rotterdam experience with more than 1000 patients. Eur J Nucl Med. 1993;20:716–31.
6. Reubi JC, Laissue J, Krenning E, Lamberts SW. Somatostatin receptors in human cancer: incidence, characteristics, functional correlates and clinical implications. J Steroid Biochem Mol Biol. 1992;43:27–35.
7. Reubi JC, Chayvialle JA, Franc B, Cohen R, Calmettes C, Modigliani E. Somatostatin receptors and somatostatin content in medullary thyroid carcinomas. Lab Invest. 1991;64:567–73.
8. Krenning EP, Bakker WH, Kooij PP, Breeman WA, Oei HY, de Jong M, et al. Somatostatin receptor scintigraphy with indium-111-DTPA-D-Phe-1-octreotide in man: metabolism, dosimetry and comparison with iodine-123-Tyr-3-octreotide. J Nucl Med. 1992; 33:652–8.
9. Kwekkeboom DJ, Reubi JC, Lamberts SW, Bruining HA, Mulder AH, Oei HY, Krenning EP. In vivo somatostatin receptor imaging in medullary thyroid carcinoma. J Clin Endocrinol Metab. 1993; 76:1413–7.
10. Tisell LE, Ahlman H, Wangberg B, Hansson G, Molne J, Nilsson O, Lindstedt G, Fjalling M, Forssell-Aronsson E. Somatostatin receptor scintigraphy in medullary thyroid carcinoma. Br J Surg. 1997;84:543–7.
11. Adams S, Baum RP, Hertel A, Schumm-Draeger PM, Usadel KH, Hor G. Comparison of metabolic and receptor imaging in recurrent medullary thyroid carcinoma with histopathological findings. Eur J Nucl Med. 1998;25:1277–83.
12. Baudin E, Lumbroso J, Schlumberger M, Leclere J, Giammarile F, Gardet P, Roche A, Travagli JP, Parmentier C. Comparison of octreotide scintigraphy and conventional imaging in medullary thyroid carcinoma. J Nucl Med. 1996;37:912–6.
13. Kurtaran A, Scheuba C, Kaserer K, Schima W, Czerny C, Angelberger P, Niederle B, Virgolini I. Indium-111-DTPA-D-Phe-1-octreotide and technetium-99m-(V)-dimercaptosuccinic acid scanning in the preoperative staging of medullary thyroid carcinoma. J Nucl Med. 1998;39:1907–9.
14. Frank-Rave K, Bihl H, Dorr, Buhr H, Ziegler R, Rave F. Somatostatin receptor imaging in persistent medullary thyroid carcinoma. Clin Endocrinol. 1995;42:31–7.
15. Rougier P, Calmettes C, Laplanche A, Travagli JP, Lefevre M, Parmentier C, Milhaud G, Tubiana M. The values of calcitonin and carcinoembryonic antigen in the treatment and management of non-familial medullary thyroid carcinoma. Cancer. 1983;51:855–62.

16. Papotti M, Kumar U, Volante M, Pecchioni C, Patel YC. Immunohistochemical detection of somatostatin receptor types 1–5 in medullary carcinoma of the thyroid. Clin Endocrinol (Oxf). 2001;54:641–9.
17. Pacini F, Elisei R, Anelli S, Basolo F, Cola A, Pinchera A. Somatostatin in medullary thyroid cancer. In vitro and in vivo studies. Cancer. 1989;63:1189–95.
18. Krausz Y, Keidar Z, Kogan I, Even-Sapir E, Bar-Shalom R, Engel A, Rubinstein R, Sachs J, Bocher M, Agranovicz S, Chisin R, Israel O. SPECT/CT hybrid imaging with ^{111}In-pentetreotide in assessment of neuroendocrine tumours. Clin Endocrinol (Oxf). 2003;59: 565–73.
19. Dorr U, Wurstlin S, Frank-Raue K, Raue F, Hehrmann R, Iser G, Scholz M, Guhl L, Buhr HJ, Bihl H. Somatostatin receptor scintigraphy and magnetic resonance imaging in recurrent medullary thyroid carcinoma: a comparative study. Horm Metab Res Suppl. 1993;27:48–55.
20. Berna L, Chico A, Matias-Guiu X, Mato E, Catafau A, Alonso C, Mora J, Mauricio D, Rodriguez-Espinosa J, Mari C, Flotats A, Martin JC, Estorch M, Carrio I. Use of somatostatin analogue scintigraphy in the localization of recurrent medullary thyroid carcinoma. Eur J Nucl Med. 1998;25:1482–8.
21. Lodish M, Dagalakis U, Chen CC, Sinaii N, Whitcomb P, Aikin A, Dombi E, Marcus L, Widemann B, Fox E, Chuk M, Balis F, Wells Jr S, Stratakis CA. ^{111}In-octreotide scintigraphy for identification of metastatic medullary thyroid carcinoma in children and adolescents. J Clin Endocrinol Metab. 2012;97:E207–12.
22. Arslan N, Ilgan S, Yuksel D, Serdengecti M, Bulakbasi N, Ugur O, Ozguven MA. Comparison of In-111 octreotide and Tc-99m (V) DMSA scintigraphy in the detection of medullary thyroid tumor foci in patients with elevated levels of tumor markers after surgery. Clin Nucl Med. 2001;26:683–8.
23. Benjegard SA, Forssell-Aronsson E, Wangberg B, Skanberg J, Nilsson O, Ahlman H. Intraoperative tumour detection using ^{111}In-DTPA-D-Phe1-octreotide and a scintillation detector. Eur J Nucl Med. 2001;28:1456–62.
24. Miyauchi A, Endo K, Ohta H, Torizuka K, Matsuzuka F, Kobayashi A, Kuma K, Maeda M. 99mTc(V)-dimercaptosuccinic acid scintigraphy for medullary thyroid carcinoma. World J Surg. 1986;10: 640–5.
25. Skowsky WR, Wilf LH. Iodine-131 metaiodobenzylguanidine scintigraphy of medullary carcinoma of the thyroid. South Med J. 1991;84:636–41.
26. Guerra UP, Pizzocaro C, Terzi A, Giubbini R, Maira G, Pagliaini R, Bestagno M. New tracers for the imaging of the medullary thyroid carcinoma. Nucl Med Commun. 1989;10:285–95.
27. Clarke SE, Lazarus CR, Wraight P, Sampson C, Maisey MN. Pentavalent ^{99m}Tc DMSA, ^{131}I MIBG, and ^{99m}Tc MDP – an evaluation of three imaging techniques in patients with medullary carcinoma of the thyroid. J Nucl Med. 1988;29:33–8.
28. Shapiro B, Copp JE, Sisson JC, Eyre PL, Wallis J, Beierwaltes WH. Iodine-131 metaiodobenzylguanidine for the locating of suspected pheochromocytoma: experience in 400 cases. J Nucl Med. 1985;26:576–85.
29. Sone T, Fukunaga M, Otsuka N, Morita R, Muranaka A, Yanagimoto S, Tomomitsu T, Nakayama H, Harada T. Metastatic medullary thyroid cancer: localization with iodine-131 metaiodobenzylguanidine. J Nucl Med. 1985;26:604–8.
30. Ansari AN, Siegel ME, DeQuattro V, Gazarian LH. Imaging of medullary thyroid carcinoma and hyperfunctioning adrenal medulla using iodine-131 metaiodobenzylguanidine. J Nucl Med. 1986;27: 1858–60.
31. Kaltsas G, Korbonits M, Heintz E, Mukherjee JJ, Jenkins PJ, Chew SL, Reznek R, Monson JP, Besser GM, Foley R, Britton KE, Grossman AB. Comparison of somatostatin analog and meta-iodobenzylguanidine radionuclides in the diagnosis and localization of advanced neuroendocrine tumors. J Clin Endocrinol Metab. 2001;86:895–902.
32. Koizumi M, Yamada Y, Nomura E, Amano M, Okajima Y, Okizuka H, Yamada K, Sawano S, Kitahara T, Yamashita T, et al. Scintigraphic detection of recurrence of medullary thyroid cancer. Ann Nucl Med. 1995;9:101–4.
33. Learoyd DL, Roach PJ, Briggs GM, Delbridge LW, Wilmshurst EG, Robinson BG. Technetium-99m-sestamibi scanning in recurrent medullary thyroid carcinoma. J Nucl Med. 1997;38:227–30.
34. Lebouthillier G, Morais J, Picard M, Picard D, Chartrand R, D'Amour P. Tc-99m sestamibi and other agents in the detection of metastatic medullary carcinoma of the thyroid. Clin Nucl Med. 1993;18:657–61.
35. Adalet I, Kocak M, Oguz H, Alagol F, Cantez S. Determination of medullary thyroid carcinoma metastases by ^{201}Tl, ^{99m}Tc(V)DMSA, ^{99m}Tc-MIBI and ^{99m}Tc-tetrofosmin. Nucl Med Commun. 1999;20:353–9.
36. Modigliani E, Cohen R, Joannidis S, Siame-Mourot C, Guliana JM, Charpentier G, Cassuto D, Bentata Pessayre M, Tabarin A, Roger P, et al. Results of long-term continuous subcutaneous octreotide administration in 14 patients with medullary thyroid carcinoma. Clin Endocrinol (Oxf). 1992;36:183–6.
37. Janson ET, Westlin JE, Eriksson B, Ahlstrom H, Nilsson S, Oberg K. [^{111}In-DTPA-D-Phe1] octreotide scintigraphy in patients with carcinoid tumours: the predictive value for somatostatin analogue treatment. Eur J Endocrinol. 1994;131:577–81.
38. Vainas I, Koussis C, Pazaitou-Panaylotou K, et al. Somatostatin receptor expression in vivo and response to somatostatin analog therapy with or without other neoplastic treatments in advanced medullary thyroid carcinoma. J Exp Clin Cancer Res. 2004; 23:549–59.
39. Valkema R, De Jong M, Bakker WH, Breeman WA, Kooij PP, Lugtenburg PJ, De Jong FH, Christiansen A, Kam BL, De Herder WW, Stridsberg M, Lindemans J, Ensing G, Krenning EP. Phase I study of peptide receptor radionuclide therapy with [In-DTPA] octreotide: the Rotterdam experience. Semin Nucl Med. 2002; 32:110–22.
40. Hofland LJ, Lamberts SW. The pathophysiological consequences of somatostatin receptor internalization and resistance. Endocr Rev. 2003;24:28–47.
41. De Jong M, Breeman WA, Bernard HF, Kooij PP, Slooter GD, Van Eijck CH, Kwekkeboom DJ, Valkema R, Macke HR, Krenning EP. Therapy of neuroendocrine tumors with radiolabeled somatostatin-analogues. Q J Nucl Med. 1999;43:356–66.
42. Buscombe JR, Caplin ME, Hilson AJW. Long-term efficacy of high-activity ^{111}In-pentreotide therapy in patients with disseminated neuroendocrine tumors. J Nucl Med. 2003;44:1–6.
43. Virgolini I, Britton K, Buscombe J, Moncayo R, Paganelli G, Riva P. In- and Y-DOTA-lanreotide: results and implications of the MAURITIUS trial. Semin Nucl Med. 2002;32:148–55.
44. Virgolini I, Traub T, Novotny C, Leimer M, Fuger B, Li SR, Patri P, Pangerl T, Angelberger P, Raderer M, Burggasser G, Andreae F, Kurtaran A, Dudczak R. Experience with indium-111 and yttrium-90-labeled somatostatin analogs. Curr Pharm Des. 2002;8: 1781–807.
45. de Jong M, Breeman WA, Bernard BF, et al. [^{177}Lu-DOTA(0), Tyr3] octretate for somatostatin receptor-targeted radionuclide therapy. Int J Cancer. 2001;92:628–33.
46. Bodei L, Handkiewicz-Junak D, Grana C, et al. Receptor radionuclide therapy with ^{90}Y-DOTA-TOC in patients with medullary thyroid carcinomas. Cancer Biother Radiopharm. 2004;19: 65–71.
47. Gao Z, Biersack HJ, Ezziddin S, et al. The role of combined imaging in metastatic medullary thyroid carcinoma: ^{111}In-DTPA-octreotide and ^{131}I/^{123}I-MIBG as predictors for radionuclide therapy. J Cancer Res Clin Oncol. 2004;130:649–56.

48. Iten F, Müller B, Schindler C, et al. Response to [^{90}Yttrium–dota]-toc treatment is associated with long-term survival benefit in metastasized medullary thyroid cancer: a phase II clinical trial. Clin Cancer Res. 2007;13:6696–702.
49. Behr TM, Sharkey RM, Juweid ME, Blumenthal RD, Dunn RM, Griffiths GL, Bair HJ, Wolf FG, Becker WS, Goldenberg DM. Reduction of the renal uptake of radiolabeled monoclonal antibody fragments by cationic amino acids and their derivatives. Cancer Res. 1995;55:3825–34.
50. Stein R, Chen S, Reed L, Richel H, Goldenberg DM. Combining radioimmunotherapy and chemotherapy for treatment of medullary thyroid carcinoma: effectiveness of dacarbazine. Cancer. 2002; 94:51–61.
51. Stein R, Govindan SV, Mattes MJ, Shih LB, Griffiths GL, Hansen HJ, Goldenberg DM. Targeting human cancer xenografts with monoclonal antibodies labeled using radioiodinated, diethylenetriaminepentaacetic acid-appended peptides. Clin Cancer Res. 1999; 5(10 Suppl):3079s–87.
52. Chatal JF, Campion L, Kraeber–Bodéré F, et al. On behalf of the French Endocrine Tumor Group. Survival improvement in patients with medullary thyroid carcinoma who undergo pretargeted anti-carcinoembryonic-antigen radioimmunotherapy: a collaborative study with the French Endocrine Tumor Group. J Clin Oncol. 2006;24:1705–11.
53. Oudoux A, Salaun PY, Bournaud C, et al. Sensitivity and prognostic value of positron emission tomography with F-18–fluorodeoxyglucose and sensitivity of immunoscintigraphy in patients with medullary thyroid carcinoma treated with anticarcinoembryonic antigen-targeted radioimmunotherapy. J Clin Endocrinol Metab. 2007;92:4590–7.
54. Salaun PY, Campion L, Bournaud C, Faivre-Chauvet A, Vuillez JP, Taieb D, Ansquer C, Rousseau C, Borson-Chazot F, Bardet S, Oudoux A, Cariou B, Mirallié E, Chang CH, Sharkey RM, Goldenberg DM, Chatal JF, Barbet J, Kraeber-Bodéré F. Phase II trial of anticarcinoembryonic antigen pretargeted radioimmunotherapy in progressive metastatic medullary thyroid carcinoma: biomarker response and survival improvement. J Nucl Med. 2012;53:1185–92.
55. Gorges R, Kahaly G, Muller-Brand J, Macke H, Roser HW, Bockisch A. Radionuclide-labeled somatostatin analogues for diagnostic and therapeutic purposes in nonmedullary thyroid cancer. Thyroid. 2001;11:647–59.
56. Stokkel MP, Reigman HI, Verkooijen RB, Smit JW. Indium-111-octreotide scintigraphy in differentiated thyroid carcinoma metastases that do not respond to treatment with high-dose I-131. J Cancer Res Clin Oncol. 2003;129:287–94.
57. Christian JA, Cook GJ, Harmer C. Indium-111-labelled octreotide scintigraphy in the diagnosis and management of non-iodine avid metastatic carcinoma of the thyroid. Br J Cancer. 2003;89: 258–61.
58. Haslinghuis LM, Krenning EP, De Herder WW, Reijs AE, Kwekkeboom DJ. Somatostatin receptor scintigraphy in the follow-up of patients with differentiated thyroid cancer. J Endocrinol Invest. 2001;24:415–22.
59. Gabriel M, Froehlich F, Decristoforo C, Ensinger C, Donnemiller E, von Guggenberg E, Heute D, Moncayo R. ^{99m}Tc-EDDA/HYNIC-TOC and ^{18}F-FDG in thyroid cancer patients with negative ^{131}I whole body scans. Eur J Nucl Med Mol Imaging. 2004;31: 330–41.
60. Sarlis NJ, Gourgiotis L, Guthrie LC, Galen B, Skarulis MC, Shawker TH, Patronas NJ, Reynolds JC. In-111 DTPA-octreotide scintigraphy for disease detection in metastatic thyroid cancer: comparison with F-18 FDG positron emission tomography and extensive conventional radiographic imaging. Clin Nucl Med. 2003;28:208–17.
61. Virgolini I, Patri P, Novotny C, Traub T, Leimer M, Fuger B, Li SR, Angelberger P, Raderer M, Wogritsch S, Kurtaran A, Kletter K, Dudczak R. Comparative somatostatin receptor scintigraphy using In-111-DOTA-lanreotide and In-111-DOTA-Tyr3-octreotide versus F-18-FDG-PET for evaluation of somatostatin receptor-mediated radionuclide therapy. Ann Oncol. 2001;12 Suppl 2:S41–5.

PET/CT in Medullary Thyroid Cancer

87

Iain Ross McDougall and Andrei Iagaru

Introduction

The optimal treatment for medullary cancer of the thyroid is total thyroidectomy and central nodal lymphadenectomy at a time the primary cancer is small and has not spread [1]. In the three phenotypes of familial medullary cancer, namely, familial medullary cancer and MEN 2A and 2B, screening of families for patients with a mutation in the RET proto-oncogene and a genetic predisposition for the diseases allows surgery at an even earlier stage [2–4]. Unfortunately, not all patients are treated at the optimal time. Patients with sporadic medullary cancer frequently have extensive local and distant metastases at the time of diagnosis. It is important to define the extent of disease when planning treatment.

The management guidelines of the American Thyroid Association do not favor an extensive battery of imaging at the time of presentation [5]. Postoperatively a basal calcitonin and CEA are recommended, and when these are undetectable calcitonin should be measured at intervals of 6–12 months and then annually. In patients who have undergone appropriate surgery and are found to have a measurable calcitonin after the operation, it is optimal when the site or sites of calcitonin production can be identified when they are small and amenable to reoperation. When a decision is reached to identify the sites of residual or recurrent cancer, there should be an organized approach starting with a careful clinical examination. The surgical and pathological reports should be reviewed since they can provide clues to the most likely site of cancer. The management guidelines recommend stratification into those with values <150 pg/ml and those with values >150 pg/ml. Some investigators have found ^{18}FDG PET has a low sensitivity even when the calcitonin is between 150 and 500 pg/ml. However, the identification of serum calcitonin after total thyroidectomy implies there is residual disease in the thyroid bed or lymph nodes or distant sites, but in the first setting the disease can be microscopic and difficult to find and in the latter neck US, chest CT, neck CT, three-phase contrast-enhanced multidetector liver CT, contrast-enhanced MRI, bone MRI of the spine, and pelvis and bone scan are recommended. These investigations are of no use when they do not include the anatomic region of the metastases and even when they do, the low sensitivities mean that the cancer is not identified in many patients. Scintigraphic investigations to increase the diagnosis in the past include thallium-201 (^{201}Tl) and technetium-99m (^{99m}Tc)-sestamibi or technetium-99m (^{99m}Tc)-tetrofosmin or technetium-99m (^{99m}Tc)-pentavalent dimercaptosuccinic acid (DMSA) [6–8]. Metaiodobenzylguanidine (MIBG) labeled with either ^{131}I or ^{123}I can sometimes identify sites of medullary cancer [9]. Antibodies against antigens from medullary cancer cells and CEA have been labeled with radiotracers and tested for imaging, and all of the above are discussed further in Chap. 86 [10]. More recently PET after intravenous injection of fluorine-18 (^{18}F) deoxyglucose (^{18}FDG) has been investigated for this purpose. Since the last edition of this textbook, the combination of ^{18}FDG PET and CT has become standard. The CT provides anatomic correlation plus attenuation correction of ^{18}F, and we include newer studies using PET/CT. The fused images allow the nuclear medicine physician to determine whether abnormal sites of ^{18}FDG are pathological or in physiological sites such as muscles of speech, salivary glands, or brown fat [11]. An example of ^{18}FDG PET/CT in a patient with medullary thyroid cancer is shown in Fig. 87.1. The number of patients with

I.R. McDougall, MD, PhD, FRCP
Department of Radiology, Nuclear Medicine, Stanford University Hospital and Clinics, Stanford, CA, USA
e-mail: Ressmedouglall@stanford.edu

A. Iagaru, MD (✉)
Department of Radiology, Nuclear Medicine, Stanford University Medical Center, Stanford School of Medicine, 300 Pasteur Dr H2230 MC 5281, Stanford, CA 94305, USA
e-mail: aiagaru@stanford.edu

L. Wartofsky, D. Van Nostrand (eds.), *Thyroid Cancer*, DOI 10.1007/978-1-4939-3314-3_87

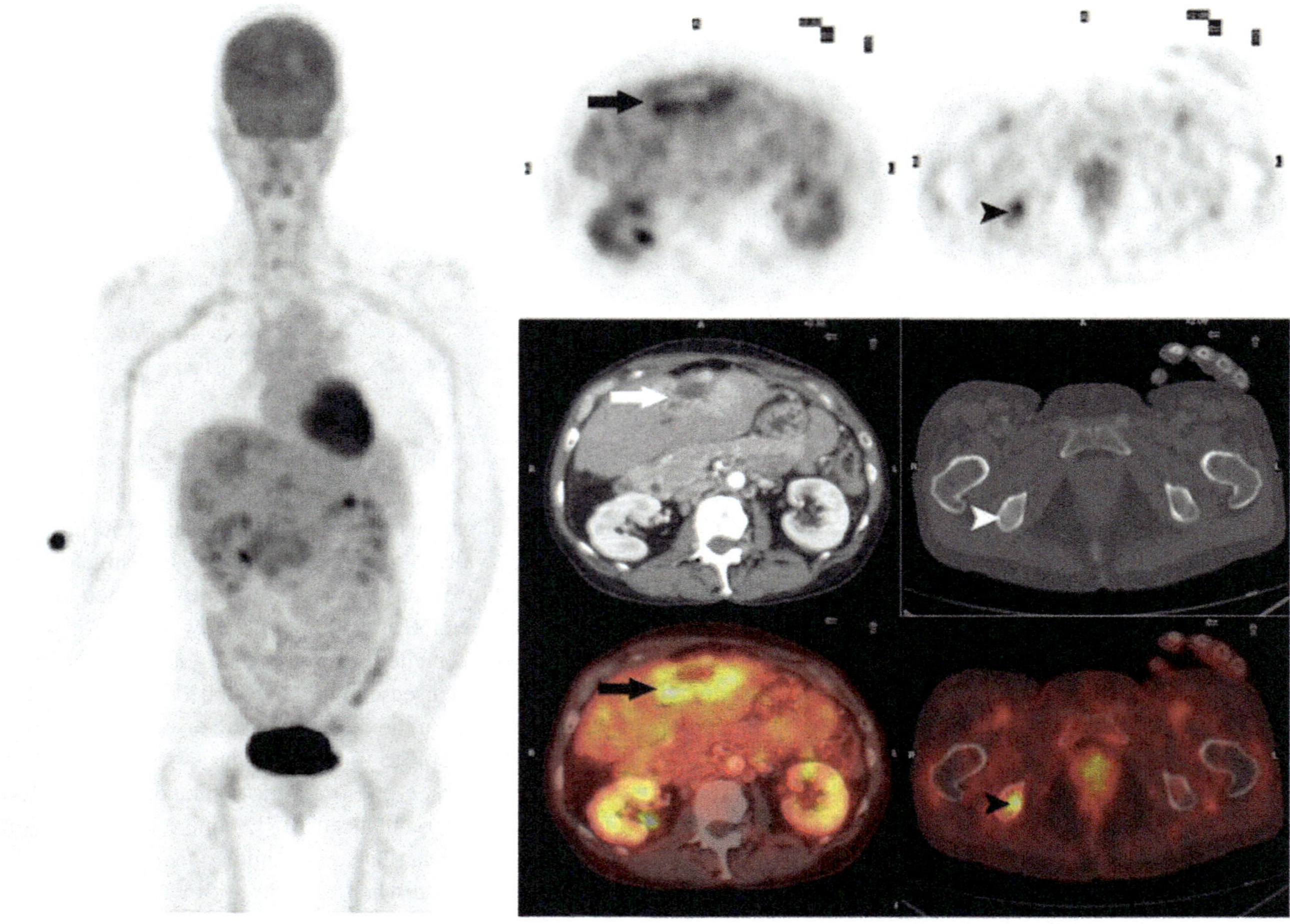

Fig. 87.1 Whole-body anterior and transaxial views in a 54-year-old woman who had thyroidectomy for medullary cancer. Images made 1 h after injection of 12 mCi ^{18}FDG (444 MBq). On left whole-body anterior projection, *upper right* (two images) shows transaxial PET images at the level of the liver and lower pelvis. *Lower right* (four images) shows CT and fused CT and PET at the same levels in color. There is normal uptake of FDG in the brain, heart, and urinary tract. There are no areas of abnormal uptake in the neck. There are metastases in the liver anteriorly and right ischium

medullary cancer who have been studied using PET and PET/CT has increased over 6 years but is considerably less than those with differentiated thyroid cancer. In addition other radiopharmaceuticals apart from ^{18}FDG have been employed. Information related to these alternative PET radiopharmaceuticals including ^{18}F-fluorodopamine, ^{18}F-dihydroxyphenylalanine, ^{68}Ga-DOTA-TOC and ^{68}Ga-DOTA-TATE is presented after ^{18}FDG [12, 13].

^{18}FDG PET/CT and PET in Identifying Medullary Cancer

In the last edition of this textbook, we reported that Bockisch et al. found ^{18}FDG PET is the most sensitive investigation with a sensitivity and specificity of approximately 80 % [14]. In another early study seven patients with recurrent medullary thyroid cancer and rapidly increasing CEA levels were evaluated using ^{18}FDG PET and ^{99m}Tc-DMSA [15]. DMSA identified only 3 lesions in 2 patients; PET found abnormalities in all 7 patients including 1 pulmonary, 3 skeletal, 20 mediastinal, 10 cervical, and 4 liver metastases. Twenty-nine of these cancer sites were confirmed and nine lymph node metastases were removed by operation.

In a report from different investigators, 20 patients were studied using ^{18}FDG PET [16]. Some of the patients had abnormal ultrasound findings in the neck and all had elevated calcitonin. ^{18}FDG PET identified the cancer in 13/17 patients that were confirmed by other imaging tests or biopsies. Five patients had negative PET scans and four of these were judged to be false negatives. ^{18}FDG PET detected 12/14 sites of cancer in the neck, 6/7 in the mediastinum, and both pulmonary and bone metastases. In two patients with elevated calcitonin levels, no site of cancer was found by any test. The sensitivity of ^{18}FDG PET was 76 % (95 % confidence interval 53–94 %). A multi-institutional study reported on 100

^{18}FDG PET scans in 85 patients with elevated calcitonin or CEA, and several had abnormal ultrasound findings [17]. Several of the authors of this paper have published independent reports, and therefore some of the patients might be included in more than one article. One hundred and eighty-one lesions were identified by one imaging test and 55 sites were confirmed pathologically. ^{18}FDG PET detected 123 of the lesions (68 %). In patients with proven sites of medullary cancer, the investigators identified 32 true-positive, 3 false-positive, 11 true-negative, and 9 false-negative lesions. The sensitivity for proven cancers was 78 % and the specificity was 79 %. In comparison the sensitivities were 25 % for ^{111}In-OctreoScan, 33 % for ^{99m}Tc-DMSA, 25 % for ^{99m}Tc-sestamibi, 50 % for CT, and 82 % for MRI.

In a separate investigation in 40 patients with elevated calcitonin values after thyroidectomy, ^{18}FDG detected 270 foci, MRI identified 116 lesions, and CT 141 [18]. For lesions in the neck, PET, MRI, and CT found 98, 34, and 34 lesions, respectively. PET was also superior in the mediastinum.

Iagaru et al. evaluated 13 patients with MTC and increased serum calcitonin levels using ^{18}FDG PET and PET/CT. Conventional imaging was negative. They found a sensitivity of 85.7 % and specificity of 83.3 % for detection of MTC recurrence [19].

Rubello et al. evaluated 19 patients with MTC with ^{111}In (DTPA)-pentetreotide, contrast-enhanced CT, and ^{18}FDG PET/CT: the last was the most sensitive (79 % compared to 58 % for CT and 42 % for pentetreotide) in detecting metastases of recurrent MTC in patients with increased serum calcitonin levels and was useful to plan a more accurate reoperation [20].

In contrast in a study of 55 patients with elevated calcitonin, the authors concluded that ^{18}FDG PET had a low sensitivity [21]. They compared PET with ultrasound and CT for regional disease, and lesions were identified in 32 %, 56 %, and 42 %, respectively, using these investigations. Bone scan and MRI found skeletal metastases in 40 % compared to 35 % for PET. MRI and CT were superior for liver metastases.

False-Positive and False-Negative ^{18}FDG PET Results

False-positive ^{18}FDG PET was discussed in detail in the section in differentiated thyroid cancer (see Chap. 43) and includes inflammatory diseases such as TB, sarcoidosis, and histoplasmosis. Abnormal uptake of ^{18}FDG in muscles of the neck and in brown fat can be misinterpreted as nodal metastases. These are best correctly recognized by fused PET/CT that increases the specificity of the investigation [11, 22]. Several investigators have studied precursors of calcitonin now called procalcitonin as a serum marker for MTC [23–25]. However this serum test is also used to diagnose bacterial infection. Although the test is negative in aseptic patients with carcinoma, it is possible that a rare patient with MTC could have a bacterial infection [26]. Since ^{18}F-FDG scan is often positive in bacterial infection, this could be false positive. Cook et al. have summarized a comprehensive list of potential false positives; however an experienced nuclear medicine physician using current instrumentation should recognize these [27, 28].

False-negative results are usually due to inability to identify small cancers that secrete calcitonin but are below the resolution of current PET/CT cameras. This is variably reported at about 6–8 mm for PET, hence the importance of the level of calcitonin. When this is $<$150 pg/ml ^{18}FDG PET/CT is unlikely to identify disease and is not recommended. In addition, very well-differentiated cancers are likely to trap less ^{18}FDG.

In summary, in a meta-analysis ^{18}FDG PET or PET/CT had a sensitivity of 59 % when patients were considered. As expected this increased in those with calcitonin values greater than 1,000 pg/ml (75 %) or doubling times of less than a year (76 %). When CEA doubling time was less than 24 months, the sensitivity was 91 % [45].

^{18}F-Fluorodihydroxyphenylalanine (^{18}F-DOPA)

^{18}F-DOPA an analog of dopamine is transported into cells such as adrenal cells by the norepinephrine membrane transporters, decarboxylated, and stored. Several studies have shown it is superior to MIBG for identifying pheochromocytoma. ^{18}F-DOPA PET has been used as an alternative to ^{18}FDG in patients with pheochromocytoma, neuroblastoma, and malignant paraganglioma. In patients with MEN 2 who were investigated for pheochromocytoma, lesions caused by medullary cancer were identified, and as a result ^{18}F-DOPA has been used mostly in Europe in patients with high calcitonin postoperatively to identify sites of cancer [29]. This PET radiopharmaceutical is not available commercially in the USA or Canada, but because it is widely used in Europe, some animal and clinical data are presented.

Animal Data

A study was designed to compare ^{18}F-DOPA and ^{18}FDG in identifying medullary cancer in mice with a MEN 2 genotype [30]. ^{18}F-DOPA was superior. It could identify cancers 1.8 mm in diameter; the SUV increased with the size of the cancer and with the age of the mice. ^{18}FDG did not identify many of the lesions most likely due to the relatively well-differentiated nature of the cancers and the higher background activity.

Clinical Studies

There are clinical reports of the value of ^{18}F-DOPA in detecting recurrent medullary cancer [30–32]. Kauhanen et al. studied 82 patients with neuroendocrine cancers including 12 patients with medullary cancer. The accuracy of PET was determined by pathology and clinical follow-up. The overall accuracy of ^{18}F-DOPA PET was 90 %, and the sensitivity in 12 cases of recurrent medullary thyroid cancer was 90 % [32].

Hoergerle et al. used several imaging tests including ^{18}F-DOPA and ^{18}FDG, ^{111}In-OctreoScan, CT, and MRI to calculate sensitivity and specificity in detecting 27 known lesions [33]. Three were in the thyroid region, 16 in lymph nodes, and 8 were distant metastases. The tests were complementary. The sensitivity of ^{18}F-DOPA PET was 63 % compared to 44 % for ^{18}FDG PET and 52 % for ^{111}In-OctreoScan. Morphological procedures had the highest sensitivity at 81 % but their specificities were lowest. The same authors reported a 100 % sensitivity for ^{18}F-DOPA PET in 17 pheochromocytomas [34]. This was superior to MIBG. This has been confirmed by other investigators [35].

Recently ^{18}F-DOPA has been evaluated more fully using current technology. Luster et al. compared interpretation of combined PET/CT with PET alone and CT alone [36]. There were 28 sets of images from 26 patients. In each case the images were obtained at the same time and interpreted by a nuclear medicine physician and a radiologist at intervals of a week with no identifying data. Combined PET/CT identified 51 lesions compared to 33 by CT and 30 by PET alone. The site of all 51 lesions was defined using PET/CT and 33 with CT. In contrast only 7 of 30 were localized anatomically with precision. This study shows ^{18}F-DOPA works and the sensitivity was 100 % when the calcitonin value was >150 pg/ml, and it confirms PET/CT is superior to either PET or CT, but it does not prove ^{18}F-DOPA is necessarily the agent of choice.

In a study with 21 patients with recurrent or residual MTC, Koopmans et al. compared ^{18}F-DOPA PET, ^{18}FDG PET, DMSA-V scintigraphy, MRI, and CT. They found a sensitivity of 62 % for ^{18}F-DOPA PET, 37 % for morphological imaging, 28 % for DMSA-V, and 24 % for ^{18}FDG PET [37]. ^{18}F-DOPA was more sensitive in patients with calcitonin values >500 pg/ml, but ^{18}FDG was superior when calcitonin doubling times were less than 12 months.

The data presented by Marzola et al. infers that in aggressive MTC, ^{18}F-DOPA PET/CT is characterized by moderately higher sensitivity than ^{18}FDG PET/CT [38]. However, in some patients, ^{18}FDG PET/CT was superior to ^{18}F-DOPA imaging, and the intensity of uptake was significantly higher in ^{18}FDG-positive lesions than in ^{18}F-DOPA-positive lesions. These investigators promote ^{18}F-DOPA and ^{18}FDG as complementary. Beuthien-Baumann et al. also indicate these two PET procedures have a complementary role; when both were used in 15 patients, the sensitivity was increased [39]. The investigators also noted that ^{18}F-DOPA PET had more specific uptake than ^{18}FDG PET for metastatic disease. They used a third PET agent 3-O-methyl-6-[(18)F]fluoro-DOPA but this was inferior to ^{18}F-DOPA and ^{18}F-FDG.

The timing of imaging is usually 60–90 min after injection of ^{18}F-DOPA. A case report of a patient with a metastasis to the right ventricle illustrated that ^{18}F-DOPA was positive (SUV 3.6) at 15 min, but by 75 min the lesion was difficult to identify [40]. So early and late images could be valuable.

Somatostatin Analogs, ^{68}Ga-DOTA-TATE, ^{68}Ga-DOTA-TOC, and Others

Medullary cancer cells express somatostatin receptors (SSR types 2 and 5). Other PET radiopharmaceuticals based on somatostatin receptor analogs have demonstrated clinical value. Koukouraki et al. scanned 15 subjects with 63 lesions from neuroendocrine tumors (NETs) with ^{68}Ga-DOTA-TOC PET and ^{18}FDG [41]. They found a sensitivity of 90 % (57/63 lesions) that was superior to ^{18}FDG, although the results were complementary. In contrast, in another study although ^{68}Ga-DOTA-TOC was inferior to ^{18}FDG PET, it was useful to determine which patients would be suitable for radionuclide therapy with ^{90}Y-DOTA-TOC or ^{177}Lu-DOTA-TATE, something confirmed by other investigators [42–44]. In a comparison of ^{68}Ga-DOTA-TATE and ^{68}Ga-DOTA-TOC in 40 patients with neuroendocrine cancers, ^{68}Ga-DOTA-TOC had advantages of identifying more lesions (262 vs. 254) and having a higher lesion SUV (20.4 ± 14.7 vs. 16.0 ± 10.8 $P<0.01$) [45, 46].

Summary

PET/CT has a definite role in staging medullary cancer in a patient who has a large primary cancer and a very high level of calcitonin. However, the main role of PET/CT is to identify the site or sites of calcitonin production in a patient who has had surgery and continues to have a measurable calcitonin. ^{18}FDG is the preferred radiopharmaceutical because it is widely available. As indicated above combined PET/CT has the advantage of demonstrating the exact anatomic position of abnormal accumulation of ^{18}FDG. The results with ^{18}F-DOPA and ^{68}Ga-DOTA-TOC are encouraging, and these might prove to be clinically valuable radiopharmaceuticals when they are approved and available for routine use. Sadly no single radiopharmaceutical will identify all sites of residual or metastatic medullary thyroid cancer.

References

1. Kebebew E, Ituarte PHG, Siperstein AE, Duh Q-Y, Clark OH. Medullary thyroid carcinoma. Clinical characteristics, treatment, prognostic factors, and a comparison of staging systems. Cancer. 2000;88:1139–48.
2. Machens A, Niccoli-Sire P, Hoegel J, Frank-Raue K, van Vroonhoven TJ, Roeher HD, Wahl RA, Lamesch P, Raue F, Conte-Devolx B, Dralle H. Early malignant progression of hereditary medullary thyroid cancer. N Engl J Med. 2003;349:1517–25.
3. Eng C, Clayton D, Schuffenecker I, Lenoir G, Cote G, Gagel RF, van Amstel HK, Lips CJ, Nishisho I, Takai SI, Marsh DJ, Robinson BG, Frank-Raue K, Raue F, Xue F, Noll WW, Romei C, Pacini F, Fink M, Niederle B, Zedenius J, Nordenskjold M, Komminoth P, Hendy GN, Mulligan LM, et al. The relationship between specific RET proto-oncogene mutations and disease phenotype in multiple endocrine neoplasia type 2. International RET mutation consortium analysis. JAMA. 1996;276:1575–9.
4. Cote GJ, Gagel RF. Lessons learned from the management of a rare genetic cancer. N Engl J Med. 2003;349:1566–8.
5. Wells SA, et al., Revised American Thyroid Association Guidelines for the Management of Medullary Thyroid Carcinoma prepared by the American Thyroid Association Guidelines Task Force on Medullary Thyroid Carcinoma. Thyroid 2015;25:567–610.
6. Forssell-Aronsson EB, Nilsson O, Bejegard SA, Kolby L, Bernhardt P, Molne J, Hashemi SH, Wangberg B, Tisell LE, Ahlman H. ^{111}In-DTPA-D-Phe1-octreotide binding and somatostatin receptor subtypes in thyroid tumors. J Nucl Med. 2000;41:636–42.
7. Adalet I, Demirkale P, Unal S, Ouz H, Alagol F, Cantez S. Disappointing results with Tc-99m tetrofosmin for detecting medullary thyroid carcinoma metastases comparison with Tc-99m VDMSA and TI-201. Clin Nucl Med. 1999;24:678–83.
8. Adams BK, Fataar A, Byrne MJ, Levitt NS, Matley PJ. Pentavalent technetium-99m (V)-DMSA uptake in a pheochromocytoma in a patient with Sipple's syndrome. J Nucl Med. 1990;31:106–8.
9. Baulieu JL, Guilloteau D, Delisle MJ, Perdrisot R, Gardet P, Delepine N, Baulieu F, Dupont JL, Talbot JN, Coutris G, et al. Radioiodinated meta-iodobenzylguanidine uptake in medullary thyroid cancer. A French cooperative study. Cancer. 1987;60:2189–94.
10. Sharkey RM, Hajjar G, Yeldell D, et al. A phase I trial combining high-dose 90Y-labeled humanized anti-CEA monoclonal antibody with doxorubicin and peripheral blood stem cell rescue in advanced medullary thyroid cancer. J Nucl Med. 2005;46:620–33.
11. Cohade C, Mourtzikos KA, Wahl RL. "USA-Fat": prevalence is related to ambient outdoor temperature-evaluation with ^{18}F-FDG PET/CT. J Nucl Med. 2003;44:1267–70.
12. Ambrosini V; Campana D; Tomassetti P; Grassetto G; Rubello D; Fanti S. PET/CT with ^{68}Gallium-DOTA-peptides in NET: an overview. European J Radiology. 2011;80:e116–9.
13. Ambrosini V, Marzola MC, Rubello D, Fanti S. ^{68}Ga-somatostatin analogues PET and ^{18}F-DOPA PET in medullary thyroid carcinoma. Eur J Nucl Med Mol Imaging. 2010;37:46–8.
14. Bockisch A, Brandt-Mainz K, Gorges R, Muller S, Stattaus J, Antoch G. Diagnosis in medullary thyroid cancer with [18F]FDG-PET and improvement using a combined PET/CT scanner. Acta Med Austriaca. 2003;30:22–5.
15. Adams S, Baum R, Rink T, Schumm-Drager PM, Usadel KH, Hor G. Limited value of fluorine-18 fluorodeoxyglucose positron emission tomography for the imaging of neuroendocrine tumours. Eur J Nucl Med. 1998;25:79–83.
16. Brandt-Mainz K, Muller SP, Gorges R, Saller B, Bockisch A. The value of fluorine-18 fluorodeoxyglucose PET in patients with medullary thyroid cancer. Eur J Nucl Med. 2000;27:490–6.
17. Diehl M, Risse JH, Brandt-Mainz K, Dietlein M, Bohuslavizki KH, Matheja P, Lange H, Bredow J, Korber C, Grunwald F. Fluorine-18 fluorodeoxyglucose positron emission tomography in medullary thyroid cancer: results of a multicentre study. Eur J Nucl Med. 2001;28:1671–6.
18. Szakall Jr S, Esik O, Bajzik G, Repa I, Dabasi G, Sinkovics I, Agoston P, Tron L. ^{18}F-FDG PET detection of lymph node metastases in medullary thyroid carcinoma. J Nucl Med. 2002;43:66–71.
19. Iagaru A, Masamed R, Singer PA, Conti PS. Detection of occult medullary thyroid cancer recurrence with 2-deoxy-2-[F-18]fluoro-D: -glucose-PET and PET/CT. Mol Imaging Biol. 2007;9:72–7.
20. Rubello D, Rampin L, Nanni C, et al. The role of ^{18}F-FDG PET/CT in detecting metastatic deposits of recurrent medullary thyroid carcinoma: a prospective study. Eur J Surg Oncol. 2008;34:581–6.
21. Giraudet AL, Vanel D, Leboulleux S, et al. Imaging medullary thyroid carcinoma with persistent elevated calcitonin levels. J Clin Endocrinol Metab. 2007;92:4185–90.
22. Barrington S, Maisey MN. Skeletal muscle uptake of fluorine-18 FDG: effect of oral diazepam. J Nucl Med. 1996;37:1127–9.
23. Bihan H, Becker KL, Snider RH, et al. Calcitonin precursor levels in human medullary thyroid carcinoma. Thyroid. 2003;13:819–22.
24. Algeciras-Schimnich A, Preissner CM, Theobald JP, Finseth MS, Grebe SK. Procalcitonin: a marker for the diagnosis and follow-up of patients with medullary thyroid carcinoma. J Clin Endocrinol Metab. 2009;94:861–8.
25. Kratzsch J, Petzold A, Raue F, et al. Basal and stimulated calcitonin and procalcitonin by various assays in patients with and without medullary thyroid cancer. Clin Chem. 2011;57:467–74.
26. Giovanella L, Suriano S, Ricci R, Ravani P, Ceriani L. Circulating procalcitonin in aseptic carcinoma patients: a specificity study with ^{18}F-fluorodeoxyglucose positron-emission tomography/computed tomography as benchmark. Clin Chem Lab Med. 2010;48:1163–5.
27. Cook G, Maisey MN, Fogelman I. Normal variants, artefacts and interpretative pitfalls in PET with 18-fluoro-2-deoxyglucose and carbon-11 methionine. Normal variants, artefacts and interpretative pitfalls in PET with 18-fluoro-2-deoxyglucose and carbon-11 methionine. Eur J Nucl Med. 1999;26:1363–78.
28. Cook G, Wegner EA, Fogelman I. Pitfalls and artifacts in ^{18}FDG PET and PET/CT oncologic imaging. Semin Nucl Med. 2004; XXXIV:122–33.
29. Jager PL, Chirakal R, Marriott CJ, Brouwers AH, Koopmans KP, Gulenchyn KY. 6-L-18F-fluorodihydroxyphenylalanine PET in neuroendocrine tumors: basic aspects and emerging clinical applications. J Nucl Med. 2008;49:573–86.
30. Pestourie CT, Kuhnast B, Le Helleix B, Gombert S, Dolle KF, et al. PET imaging of medullary thyroid carcinoma in MEN2A transgenic mice using 6-[(18)F]F-L-DOPA. Eur J Nucl Med Mol Imaging. 2010;37:58–66.
31. Gourgiotis L, Sarlis NJ, Reynolds JC, VanWaes C, Merino MJ, Pacak K. Localization of medullary thyroid carcinoma metastasis in a multiple endocrine neoplasia type 2A patient by 6-[18F]-fluorodopamine positron emission tomography. J Clin Endocrinol Metab. 2003;88:637–41.
32. Kauhanen S, Seppanen M, Ovaska J, et al. The clinical value of [18F]fluoro-dihydroxyphenylalanine positron emission tomography in primary diagnosis, staging, and restaging of neuroendocrine tumors. Endocr Relat Cancer. 2009;16:255–65.
33. Hoegerle S, Altehoefer C, Ghanem N, Brink I, Moser E, Nitzsche E. ^{18}F-DOPA positron emission tomography for tumour detection in patients with medullary thyroid carcinoma and elevated calcitonin levels. Eur J Nucl Med. 2001;28:64–71.
34. Hoegerle S, Nitzsche E, Altehoefer C, Ghanem N, Manz T, Brink I, Reincke M, Moser E, Neumann HP. Pheochromocytomas: detection with ^{18}F DOPA whole body PET – initial results. Radiology. 2002;222:507–12.
35. Ilias I, Yu J, Carrasquillo JA, Chen CC, Eisenhofer G, Whatley M, McElroy B, Pacak K. Superiority of 6-[18F]-fluorodopamine posi-

tron emission tomography versus [131I]-metaiodobenzylguanidine scintigraphy in the localization of metastatic pheochromocytoma. J Clin Endocrinol Metab. 2003;88:4083–7.
36. Luster M, Karges W, Zeich K, Pauls S, Verburg FA, Dralle H, et al. Clinical value of 18-fluorine-fluorodihydroxyphenylalanine positron emission tomography/computed tomography in the follow-up of medullary thyroid carcinoma. Thyroid. 2010;20:527–33.
37. Koopmans KP, de Groot JW, Plukker JT, et al. ^{18}F-dihydroxy-phenylalanine PET in patients with biochemical evidence of medullary thyroid cancer: relation to tumor differentiation. J Nucl Med. 2008;49:524–31.
38. Marzola MC, Pelizzo MR, Ferdeghini M, et al. Dual PET/CT with ^{18}F-DOPA and ^{18}F-FDG in metastatic medullary thyroid carcinoma and rapidly increasing calcitonin levels: comparison with conventional imaging. Eur J Surg Oncol. 2010;36:414–21.
39. Beuthien-Baumann B, Strumpf A, Zessin J, Bredow J, Kotzerke J. Diagnostic impact of PET with ^{18}F-FDG, ^{18}F-DOPA and 3-O-methyl-6-[18F]fluoro-DOPA in recurrent or metastatic medullary thyroid carcinoma. Eur J Nucl Med Mol Imaging. 2007;34:1604–9.
40. Morel O, Giraud P, Cahouet A, Lacoeuille F, Girault S. Visualization of cardiac metastasis from medullary thyroid carcinoma on F-18 DOPA PET/CT scan. Clin Nucl Med. 2010;35:253–5.
41. Koukouraki S, Strauss LG, Georgoulias V, Eisenhut M, Haberkorn U, Dimitrakopoulou-Strauss A. Comparison of the pharmacokinetics of ^{68}Ga-DOTATOC and ^{18}F-FDG in patients with metastatic neuroendocrine tumours scheduled for ^{90}Y-DOTATOC therapy. Eur J Nucl Med Mol Imaging. 2006;33:1115–22.
42. Conry BG, Papathanasiou ND, Prakash V, Kayani I, Caplin M, Mahmood S, Bomanji JB. Comparison of ^{68}Ga-DOTATATE and ^{18}F-fluorodeoxyglucose PET/CT in the detection of recurrent medullary thyroid carcinoma. Eur J Nucl Med Mol Imaging. 2010;37:49–57.
43. Bodei L, Handkiewicz-Junak D, Grana C, Mazzetta C, Rocca P, Bartolomei M, Lopera Sierra M, et al. Receptor radionuclide therapy with ^{90}Y-DOTATOC in patients with medullary thyroid carcinomas. Cancer Biother Radiopharm. 2004;19:65–71.
44. Turker O, Dogan I. The clinical role of molecular imaging: positron emission tomography/computed tomography and (90)yttrium-DOTATOC in the management of medullary thyroid cancer. Thyroid. 2010;20:233–4.
45. Treglia G, Villani MF, Giordano A, Rufini V. Detection rate of recurrent medullary thyroid carcinoma using fluorine-18 fluorodeoxyglucose positron emission tomography: a meta-analysis. Endocrine. 2012;42:535–45.
46. Poeppel TD, Binse I, Petersenn S, Lahner H, Schott M, Antoch G, Brandau W, Bockisch A, Boy C. ^{68}Ga-DOTATOC versus ^{68}Ga-DOTATATE PET/CT in functional imaging of neuroendocrine tumors. J Nucl Med. 2011;52:1864–70.

External Radiation Therapy for Medullary Cancer

88

James D. Brierley and Richard W. Tsang

Introduction

Surgical management is the main definitive treatment for nonmetastatic medullary thyroid cancer (MTC). External beam radiation therapy (RT) to the neck has no role in postsurgical management of MTC patients with small, intrathyroidal primary tumors where regional spread is absent. For those with a high risk of residual disease in the neck (extrathyroidal extension, extensive nodal involvement, or persistent tumor markers postop with no overt metastatic disease), adjuvant RT may be considered for locoregional control of disease but does not improve survival. Functional imaging is often helpful in detecting subclinical sites of disease, whether regional or metastatic. RT doses of 50–70 Gy in conventional fractionation result in significant acute toxicity but late sequela is usually mild. Technological advances in RT have made it possible to give higher doses more safely. External beam RT is often beneficial for unresectable gross local disease and for palliation of bone metastasis. Somatostatin analogues may reduce symptoms (e.g., diarrhea) due to high calcitonin levels and can be used in combination with RT.

Gross Residual Disease

For patients with gross residual disease after surgery, the local control rate after RT is unsatisfactorily low (20–25 %) [1, 2]. Therefore, every attempt should be made to diagnose MTC at an early stage and then a surgical management plan to achieve complete excision of the disease. When this is not possible, external RT may result in long-term local control in only a few patients. Innovative approaches with novel systemic agents [3–6] or radioimmunotherapy [7] continue to be investigated.

Adjuvant Therapy

External beam RT has no role in postsurgical management of MTC patients with small, intrathyroidal primary lesions where spread to regional lymph nodes is absent. However, for patients with high-risk features such as gross or microscopic residual disease, extrathyroidal invasion, or extensive regional lymph node involvement, postoperative adjuvant external RT to the thyroid bed and regional lymph nodes may be considered. In a Surveillance, Epidemiology, and End Results (SEER) database review between 1988 and 2004, only 12 % of patients (among 534 patients with MTC) were treated with RT [8]. The American Thyroid Association guidelines suggested adjuvant RT to be considered for T4 lesions [9]. With surgery alone, approximately half of high-risk patients may recur in the neck. Radiation doses of 4,000 cGy in 2 Gy fractions to the cervical and superior mediastinal lymph nodes followed by a boost to the thyroid bed to a total dose of 5,000 cGy have been associated with a 10-year local regional control rate of 86 % [2]. External beam RT does not impact overall survival [8], but optimal local regional control is important because a relapse in neck tissues after prior extensive neck surgery may be difficult to treat and has a deleterious impact on the patient's quality of life. However, it is important to remember that patients at high risk of local regional relapse are also at high risk of distant metastases. Other investigators have confirmed similar results of improved local regional control in high-risk patients following radiation and are summarized in Table 88.1 [1, 10–13].

Following standard surgical therapy generally involving total thyroidectomy and central and bilateral cervical lymph node dissection, a patient may continue to have high levels of calcitonin with no detectable metastasis clinically. Imaging

J.D. Brierley, MBBS, FRCP, FRCR, FRCPC (✉)
R.W. Tsang, MD, FRCP(C)
Department of Radiation Oncology, University of Toronto, Princess Margaret Hospital, 610 University Ave, Toronto, Ontario M5G 2M9, Canada
e-mail: james.brierley@rmp.uhn.on.ca; Richard.tsang@rmp.uhn.on.ca

L. Wartofsky, D. Van Nostrand (eds.), *Thyroid Cancer*, DOI 10.1007/978-1-4939-3314-3_88

Table 88.1 Results of adjuvant external radiotherapy in high-risk medullary thyroid cancer from retrospective studies: 10-year local recurrence

	Surgery alone	Surgery and RT
	10 year local/regional recurrence	10 year local/regional recurrence
Brierley [2]	86 %	52 %
Fersht [12]	59 %	29 %
Mak [10]	76 %	16 %
Schwartz [13]	N/A	13 %
Nguyen [11]	N/A	30 %

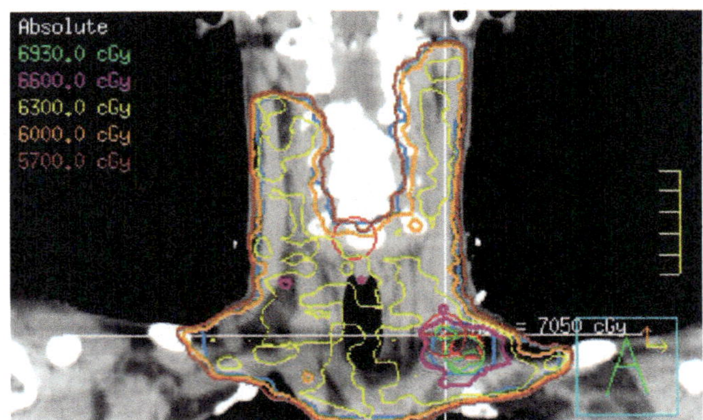

Fig. 88.1 An IMRT plan for a patient with medullary thyroid cancer who had a thyroidectomy and bilateral neck dissection. She had extrathyroidal extension. There was nodal disease adherent to the left supraclavicular artery and gross disease was left behind. 56 Gy in 33 fractions was given to the thyroid bed and regional nodal volume and 66 Gy to the gross residual disease. The maximum point dose was 70 Gy. The volume irradiated conforms to the U shape of the clinical target volume ensuring minimum radiation exposure to the normal organs such as the spinal cord

with radionuclides (e.g., metaiodobenzyl-guanidine, or MIBG) or somatostatin analogues (e.g., octreotide) may show abnormalities and may help direct therapy [14–16]. If there is no evidence of disease below the clavicles, a decision to offer local regional neck radiation may be considered as an alternative to reoperation and meticulous neck dissection. Selective venous catheterization may occasionally locate the main source of calcitonin [17, 18]. More recently ^{18}F fluorodeoxyglucose positron emission tomography (^{18}F-FDG PET) has shown promise in locating small tumor volumes and assisted in the overall management of the patient [19–22]. The levels of calcitonin and CEA in the blood correlate with tumor bulk, and patients with high levels of calcitonin may be symptomatic of watery diarrhea. It is not unusual to see elevated but stable calcitonin/CEA levels for a long period of time (e.g., 5–10 years), without obvious progression of disease [23]. Because of this, the presence of asymptomatic subclinical metastatic disease is not an absolute contraindication to adjunctive local regional RT to the neck. However, any consideration of cytotoxic treatment for an asymptomatic patient should be viewed with some trepidation since the patient may have indolent disease [12]. Symptoms of diarrhea can be palliated with antidiarrheal drugs (e.g., diphenoxylate, loperamide) or somatostatin analogue [24] with or without interferon [25, 26]. A drop in the calcitonin level may not necessarily be a reflection of tumor regression, as it can be secondary to dedifferentiation and heralds a more aggressive clinical course [27]. Therefore RT for hypercalcitoninemia should only be considered in the adjuvant setting when there is a high risk of recurrence in the neck because of extensive extrathyroid extension, extensive nodal disease, or both.

External Beam Radiotherapy

The thyroid bed is a technically challenging volume to treat as the thyroid bed curves around the vertebral body and includes the air column in the trachea. It can be difficult to adequately treat the thyroid bed and spares the spinal cord to a dose within tolerance. A variety of techniques have been described that produce adequate dose distribution [28–30]. Advances in radiation techniques utilizing inverse-planned intensity-modulated radiation therapy (IMRT) (Fig. 88.1) result in better dose distribution to the areas at risk and reduce the volume of normal tissues to a minimum and are described elsewhere in the book. Well-planned external-beam RT has acceptable acute toxicity and rarely produces serious complications. In patients assigned to the radiation arm of the German randomized control study in differentiated thyroid cancer that closed because of poor accrual, it was noted that the majority of patients experience mild to moderate acute side effects only from adjuvant external-beam radiotherapy [31]. At the first follow-up examination, most side effects had subsided and acute toxicity was tolerable in these patients. Late toxicity is infrequent, and the most common toxicities are skin telangiectasia, increased skin pigmentation, soft tissue fibrosis, and mild lymphedema predominantly in the submental area. Esophageal and especially tracheal stenosis is rare. Neither Tsang et al. [28] nor Farahati et al. [32] reported any RTOG grade IV late toxicity in differentiated thyroid cancer. In contrast a more recent study using higher doses of radiation and larger volumes reported that 5 % of their patients required percutaneous endoscopic gastrostomy tube for late esophageal stenosis [33].

Metastatic Disease

Metastasis is unfortunately common in sporadic MTC, and the most frequently involved organs are the liver, lung, and bone. The treatment is palliative and includes supportive measures, analgesic drugs, and considerations of potential benefits of hormonal therapy, chemotherapy, and local radiation. Hormonal therapy consists of somatostatin analogue (e.g., octreotide), which have been reported to lessen symptoms and reduce calcitonin levels, but generally does not induce tumor responses [24, 26, 34–36]. A combination of octreotide and interferon alpha may result in a higher response rate [24–26]. Compared with hormones, chemotherapy is associated with more toxicity but is documented to have a tumor response rate of only 15–30 %. Active drugs include doxorubicin either as single agent or with cisplatin [37], 5-FU-containing combinations [38–41], and others [3, 42, 43].

Drugs targeting the tyrosine kinase receptors inhibiting tumor angiogenesis (e.g. vandetanib) have response rates of approximately 15–20 % and disease stabilization rates of 50–60 % [4–6, 44]

For locally symptomatic metastatic disease, local radiation should be considered. Unfortunately neither the liver nor large volumes of lung tolerate RT well. Thus, RT is usually reserved for painful osseous metastases typically a dose of 2,000 cGy in 5 daily fractions or 3,000 cGy in 10 fractions, which should result in pain relief. Single large lung metastases causing hemoptysis or obstruction may also respond to RT. Experimental therapy with targeted radiation by monoclonal antibodies (e.g., anti-CEA or ^{111}indium-octreotide) conjugated to radionuclides is being investigated [45–50].

References

1. Fife KM, Bower M, Harmer CL. Medullary thyroid cancer: the role of radiotherapy in local control. Eur J Surg Oncol. 1996;22: 588–91.
2. Brierley JD, Tsang RW, Gospodarowicz MK, Sutcliffe SB, Simpson WJ, Panzarella T. Medullary thyroid cancer – analyses of survival and prognostic factors and the role of radiation therapy in local control. Thyroid. 1996;6:305–10.
3. Kaczirek K, Schindl M, Weinhausel A, et al. Cytotoxic activity of camptothecin and paclitaxel in newly established continuous human medullary thyroid carcinoma cell lines. J Clin Endocrinol Metab. 2004;89:2397–401.
4. Lam ET, Ringel MD, Kloos RT, et al. Phase II clinical trial of sorafenib in metastatic medullary thyroid cancer. J Clin Oncol. 2010;28:2323–30.
5. Wells Jr SA, Gosnell JE, Gagel RF, et al. Vandetanib for the treatment of patients with locally advanced or metastatic hereditary medullary thyroid cancer. J Clin Oncol. 2010;28:767–72.
6. Wells SA, Jr., Robinson BG, Gagel RF, et al. Vandetanib in patients with locally advanced or metastatic medullary thyroid cancer: a randomized, double-blind phase III Trial. J Clin Oncol. 2012; 30:134-41.
7. Kraeber-Bodere F, Salaun PY, Oudoux A, Goldenberg DM, Chatal JF, Barbet J. Pretargeted radioimmunotherapy in rapidly progressing, metastatic, medullary thyroid cancer. Cancer. 2010; 116(4 Suppl):1118–25.
8. Martinez SR, Beal SH, Chen A, Chen SL, Schneider PD. Adjuvant external beam radiation for medullary thyroid carcinoma. J Surg Oncol. 2010;102:175–8.
9. Kloos RT, Eng C, Evans DB, et al. Medullary thyroid cancer: management guidelines of the American Thyroid Association. Thyroid. 2009;19:565–612.
10. Mak A, Morrison W, Garden A, Ordonez N, Weber R, Peters L. The value of postoperative radiotherapy for regional medullary carcinoma of the thyroid. Int J Radiat Oncol Biol Phys. 1994;30:234.
11. Nguyen TD, Chassard JL, Lagarde P, et al. Results of postoperative radiation therapy in medullary carcinoma of the thyroid: a retrospective study by the French Federation of Cancer Institutes – the Radiotherapy Cooperative Group. Radiother Oncol. 1992; 23:1–5.
12. Fersht N, Vini L, A'Hern R, Harmer C. The role of radiotherapy in the management of elevated calcitonin after surgery for medullary thyroid cancer. Thyroid. 2001;11:1161–8.
13. Schwartz DL, Rana V, Shaw S, et al. Postoperative radiotherapy for advanced medullary thyroid cancer – local disease control in the modern era. Head Neck. 2008;30:883–8.
14. Baudin E, Lumbroso J, Schlumberger M, et al. Comparison of octreotide scintigraphy and conventional imaging in medullary thyroid carcinoma. J Nucl Med. 1996;37:912–6.
15. Tisell LE, Ahlman H, Wangberg B, et al. Somatostatin receptor scintigraphy in medullary thyroid carcinoma. Br J Surg. 1997;84:543–7.
16. Parisella M, D'Alessandria C, van de Bossche B, et al. ^{99m}Tc-EDDA/HYNIC-TOC in the management of medullary thyroid carcinoma. Cancer Biother Radiopharm. 2004;19:211–7.
17. Abdelmoumene N, Schlumberger M, Gardet P, et al. Selective venous sampling catheterisation for localisation of persisting medullary thyroid carcinoma. Br J Cancer. 1994;69:1141–4.
18. Ben Mrad MD, Gardet P, Roche A, et al. Value of venous catheterization and calcitonin studies in the treatment and management of clinically inapparent medullary thyroid carcinoma. Cancer. 1989;63:133–8.
19. Schoder H, Yeung HW. Positron emission imaging of head and neck cancer, including thyroid carcinoma. Semin Nucl Med. 2004;34:180–97.
20. Gotthardt M, Battmann A, Hoffken H, et al. ^{18}F-FDG PET, somatostatin receptor scintigraphy, and CT in metastatic medullary thyroid carcinoma: a clinical study and an analysis of the literature. Nucl Med Commun. 2004;25:439–43.
21. Bockisch A, Brandt-Mainz K, Gorges R, Muller S, Stattaus J, Antoch G. Diagnosis in medullary thyroid cancer with ^{18}F-FDG-PET and improvement using a combined PET/CT scanner. Acta Med Austriaca. 2003;30:22–5.
22. Skoura E, Rondogianni P, Alevizaki M, et al. Role of ^{18}F-FDG-PET/CT in the detection of occult recurrent medullary thyroid cancer. Nucl Med Commun. 2010;31:567–75.
23. Girelli ME, Nacamulli D, Pelizzo MR, et al. Medullary thyroid carcinoma: clinical features and long-term follow-up of seventy-eight patients treated between 1969 and 1986. Thyroid. 1998;8: 517–23.
24. di Bartolomeo M, Bajetta E, Buzzoni R, et al. Clinical efficacy of octreotide in the treatment of metastatic neuroendocrine tumors. A study by the Italian Trials in Medical Oncology Group. Cancer. 1996;77:402–8.
25. Lupoli G, Cascone E, Arlotta F, et al. Treatment of advanced medullary thyroid carcinoma with a combination of recombinant interferon alpha-2b and octreotide. Cancer. 1996;78:1114–8.
26. Vitale G, Tagliaferri P, Caraglia M, et al. Slow release lanreotide in combination with interferon-alpha2b in the treatment of symptomatic advanced medullary thyroid carcinoma. J Clin Endocrinol Metab. 2000;85:983–8.
27. Saad M, Orddonez N, Rashid R, et al. Medullary carcinoma: prognostic factors and treatment. Int J Radiat Oncol Biol Phys. 1984;9:161–9.

28. Tsang RW, Brierley JD, Simpson WJ, Panzarella T, Gospodarowicz MK, Sutcliffe SB. The effects of surgery, radioiodine and external radiation therapy on the clinical outcome of patients with differentiated thyroid cancer. Cancer. 1998;82:375–88.
29. Nutting CM, Convery DJ, Cosgrove VP, et al. Improvements in target coverage and reduced spinal cord irradiation using intensity-modulated radiotherapy (IMRT) in patients with carcinoma of the thyroid gland. Radiother Oncol. 2001;60:173–80.
30. Schwartz DL, Lobo MJ, Ang KK, et al. Postoperative external beam radiotherapy for differentiated thyroid cancer: outcomes and morbidity with conformal treatment. Int J Radiat Oncol Biol Phys. 2009;74:1083–91.
31. Schuck A, Biermann M, Pixberg MK, et al. Acute toxicity of adjuvant radiotherapy in locally advanced differentiated thyroid carcinoma. First results of the multicenter study differentiated thyroid carcinoma (MSDS). Strahlenther Onkol. 2003;179:832–9.
32. Farahati J, Reiners C, Stuschke M, et al. Differentiated thyroid cancer. Impact of adjuvant external radiotherapy in patients with perithyroidal tumor infiltration (stage pT4). Cancer. 1996;77:172–80.
33. Terezakis SA, Lee KS, Ghossein RA, et al. Role of external beam radiotherapy in patients with advanced or recurrent nonanaplastic thyroid cancer: Memorial Sloan-Kettering Cancer Center experience. Int J Radiat Oncol Biol Phys. 2009;73:795–801.
34. Frank-Raue K, Ziegler R, Raue F. The use of octreotide in the treatment of medullary thyroid carcinoma. Horm Metab Res Suppl. 1993;27:44–7.
35. Mahler C, Verhelst J, de Longueville M, Harris A. Long-term treatment of metastatic medullary thyroid carcinoma with the somatostatin analogue octreotide. Clin Endocrinol (Oxf). 1990;33:261–9.
36. Modigliani E, Cohen R, Joannidis S, et al. Results of long-term continuous subcutaneous octreotide administration in 14 patients with medullary thyroid carcinoma. Clin Endocrinol (Oxf). 1992;36:183–6.
37. Shimaoka K, Schoenfeld DA, DeWys WD, Creech RH, DeConti R. A randomized trial of doxorubicin versus doxorubicin plus cisplatin in patients with advanced thyroid carcinoma. Cancer. 1985;56:2155–60.
38. Schlumberger M, Abdelmoumene N, Delisle MJ, Couette JE. Treatment of advanced medullary thyroid cancer with an alternating combination of 5 FU-streptozocin and 5 FU-dacarbazine. The Groupe d'Etude des Tumeurs a Calcitonine (GETC). Br J Cancer. 1995;71:363–5.
39. Orlandi F, Caraci P, Berruti A, et al. Chemotherapy with dacarbazine and 5-fluorouracil in advanced medullary thyroid cancer. Ann Oncol. 1994;5:763–5.
40. Bajetta E, Rimassa L, Carnaghi C, et al. 5-Fluorouracil, dacarbazine, and epirubicin in the treatment of patients with neuroendocrine tumors. Cancer. 1998;83:372–8.
41. Di Bartolomeo M, Bajetta E, Bochicchio AM, et al. A phase II trial of dacarbazine, fluorouracil and epirubicin in patients with neuroendocrine tumours. A study by the Italian Trials in Medical Oncology (I.T.M.O.) Group. Ann Oncol. 1995;6:77–9.
42. Wu LT, Averbuch SD, Ball DW, de Bustros A, Baylin SB, McGuire 3rd WP. Treatment of advanced medullary thyroid carcinoma with a combination of cyclophosphamide, vincristine, and dacarbazine. Cancer. 1994;73:432–6.
43. Ekman ET, Lundell G, Tennvall J, Wallin G. Chemotherapy and multimodality treatment in thyroid carcinoma. Otolaryngol Clin N Am. 1990;23:523–7.
44. Wells Jr SA, Santoro M. Targeting the RET pathway in thyroid cancer. Clin Cancer Res. 2009;15:7119–23.
45. Behr TM, Sharkey RM, Juweid ME, et al. Phase I/II clinical radioimmunotherapy with an iodine-131-labeled anti- carcinoembryonic antigen murine monoclonal antibody IgG. J Nucl Med. 1997;38:858–70.
46. Juweid M, Sharkey RM, Behr T, et al. Radioimmunotherapy of medullary thyroid cancer with iodine-131-labeled anti-CEA antibodies. J Nucl Med. 1996;37:905–11.
47. Stein R, Juweid M, Zhang CH, Goldenberg DM. Assessment of combined radioimmunotherapy and chemotherapy for treatment of medullary thyroid cancer. Clin Cancer Res. 1999;5(10 Suppl):3199s–206.
48. Juweid ME, Hajjar G, Stein R, et al. Initial experience with high-dose radioimmunotherapy of metastatic medullary thyroid cancer using ^{131}I-MN-14 F(ab)2 anti-carcinoembryonic antigen MAb and AHSCR. J Nucl Med. 2000;41:93–103.
49. Monsieurs M, Brans B, Bacher K, Dierckx R, Thierens H. Patient dosimetry for ^{131}I-MIBG therapy for neuroendocrine tumours based on ^{123}I-MIBG scans. Eur J Nucl Med Mol Imaging. 2002;29:1581–7.
50. Buscombe JR, Caplin ME, Hilson AJ. Long-term efficacy of high-activity ^{111}in-pentetreotide therapy in patients with disseminated neuroendocrine tumors. J Nucl Med. 2003;44:1–6.

Medullary Carcinoma of the Thyroid: Chemotherapy

89

David A. Liebner, Sigurdis Haraldsdottir,
and Manisha H. Shah

Introduction

Medullary thyroid cancer is a malignancy of the parafollicular thyroid C cells, accounting for 2–8% of all thyroid cancers [1, 2]. Early detection and surgery offer the only possibility of cure, and patients with localized disease are typically treated with surgical resection with or without adjuvant external beam radiation therapy. However, despite aggressive surgical therapy, nearly 50 % of patients with a palpable neck mass who are diagnosed with localized medullary thyroid cancer will subsequently recur [3]. In patients with unresectable disease, the clinical course is often protracted. Chemotherapeutic options for the patient with unresectable or metastatic disease are discussed below.

D.A. Liebner, MD
Division of Medical Oncology, Department of Internal Medicine, The Ohio State University, Columbus, OH, USA

Department of Biomedical Informatics, The Ohio State University, Columbus, OH, USA
e-mail: david.liebner@osumc.edu

S. Haraldsdottir, MD
Division of Medical Oncology, Department of Internal Medicine, The Ohio State University Comprehensive Cancer Center, Columbus, OH, USA
e-mail: sigurdis.haraldsdottir@osumc.edu

M.H. Shah, MD (✉)
Department of Internal Medicine, The James Cancer Hospital and Solove Research Institute, 320 West 10th Avenue, A438 Starling Loving Hall, Columbus, OH 43210, USA
e-mail: Manisha.Shah@osume.edu

Cytotoxic Chemotherapy

Doxorubicin-Based Regimens

Doxorubicin is an anthracycline antibiotic which induces tumor cell death through DNA intercalation, inhibition of topoisomerase II, and generation of free oxide radicals. Gottlieb and Hill published their original results with doxorubicin monotherapy in 30 patients with advanced thyroid carcinoma, including a subset of 5 patients with MTC [4]. Responses were seen in three of these five patients. Objective responses in subsequent reports of doxorubicin monotherapy ranged from 14 to 40 % [5–8]. The major dose-limiting toxicity in these studies was cumulative doxorubicin-mediated cardiomyopathy, necessitating lifetime dose ceilings to allow safe administration. Given these early results with doxorubicin monotherapy in thyroid cancer, further investigation utilizing doxorubicin as the backbone of multidrug combination regimens was pursued. Drugs included in these regimens included cisplatin, vindesine, bleomycin, 5-fluorouracil, and streptozocin [5, 9–14]. Response rates in MTC ranged from 0 to 33 %, but the small number of patients with MTC in these studies precludes direct comparison with doxorubicin monotherapy.

Other Regimens

Several alternative chemotherapeutic agents have been proposed and investigated either alone or in combination, including cisplatin, carboplatin, etoposide, methotrexate, dacarbazine (DTIC), 5-fluorouracil (5-FU), cyclophosphamide, vincristine, epirubicin, streptozocin, paclitaxel, and gemcitabine [7, 15–20]. Direct comparisons with doxorubicin-based regimens have not been performed, but response rates are similar. Selected studies are summarized in Table 89.1.

L. Wartofsky, D. Van Nostrand (eds.), *Thyroid Cancer*, DOI 10.1007/978-1-4939-3314-3_89

Table 89.1 Selected studies of cytotoxic chemotherapy in medullary thyroid cancer

Regimen	Ref	Treatment plan	N	Responses
Doxorubicin-based regimens				
Doxorubicin	[4]	Doxorubicin: 45–75 mg/m² q3 weeks	5	3
	[6]	Doxorubicin: various dose schedules	20	8
	[7]	Doxorubicin: 60 mg/m² q4 weeks	14	2
	[5]	Doxorubicin: 60 mg/m² q3 weeks	4	1
	[8]	Doxorubicin: 15 mg/m² qwk or 60 mg/m² q3 weeks	9	1
Doxorubicin, cisplatin	[5]	Doxorubicin, 60 mg/m²; cisplatin, 40 mg/m² q3 weeks	6	2
	[13]	Doxorubicin, 60–75 mg/m²; cisplatin, 60–75 mg/m² q3 weeks	6	0
	[10]	Doxorubicin, 50 mg/m²; cisplatin, 70 mg/m² q3 weeks	6	0
Doxorubicin, streptozocin	[11]	Doxorubicin, 20 mg/m²; streptozocin, 1000 mg/m²	5	1
Doxorubicin, cisplatin, vindesine	[9]	Doxorubicin, 50 mg/m²; cisplatin, 60 mg/m²; vindesine, 3 mg/m²	10	1
Bleomycin, doxorubicin, cisplatin (BAP)	[12]	Bleomycin, 30 U days 1–3; doxorubicin, 60 mg/m² day 5; cisplatin, 60 mg/m² day 5	9	3
Doxorubicin, streptozocin/DTIC, 5-FU	[14]	Doxorubicin, 60 mg/m² day 1; streptozocin, 500 mg/m² days 1–5 alternating with DTIC, 200 mg/m² day 1–5; 5-FU, 400 mg/m² days 1–5 q4 weeks	20	3
DTIC-based regimens				
DTIC, 5-FU	[16]	DTIC, 250 mg/m² days 1–5; 5-FU, 450 mg/m² q4 weeks	5	3
DTIC, cyclophosphamide, vincristine	[17]	DTIC, 600 mg/m² days 1–2; cyclophosphamide, 750 mg/m² day 1; vincristine, 1.4 mg/m² day 1 every 3–4 weeks	7	2
DTIC, 5-FU, epirubicin	[18]	DTIC, 200 mg/m² days 1–3; 5-FU, 250 mg/m² days 1–3; epirubicin, 25 mg/m² day 1–3 q3 weeks	7	1
	[20]	DTIC, 200 mg/m² days 1–3; 5-FU, 500 mg/m² days 1–3; epirubicin, 30 mg/m² days 1–3 q3 weeks	1	1
DTIC, 5-FU/5-FU, streptozocin	[19]	DTIC, 200 mg/m² days 1–5; 5-FU, 500 mg/m² days 1–5 alternating with 5-FU, 400 mg/m² days 1–5; streptozocin, 500 mg/m² days 1–5 q3 weeks	20	3
Other regimens				
Cisplatin	[7]	Cisplatin: 90 mg/m² q4 weeks	14	3
Paclitaxel, gemcitabine	[8]	Paclitaxel, 90–100 mg/m²; gemcitabine, 1000 mg/m² q3 weeks	2	0

Targeted Therapies

Given the limitations of standard, cytotoxic chemotherapy, there has been an emphasis on the development of novel targeted therapies in medullary thyroid cancer. Mutations in RET have long been recognized as the dominant pathogenetic abnormality in almost all forms of MTC, occurring in nearly 96 % of hereditary cases [21] and up to 65 % of individuals with sporadic MTC [22], making RET inhibition conceptually appealing. RAS appears to be important in patients with sporadic MTC and can be seen in up to 68 % of patients without coexisting mutations in RET [23]. Tumor neovascularization is also important to the development and progression of MTC [24], and several agents with antiangiogenic properties have been evaluated recently in the treatment of MTC. Clinical trials with selected targeted therapies are summarized in Table 89.2.

Vandetanib

Vandetanib (AZD6474/ZD6474, Caprelsa, Zactima) is an orally bioavailable inhibitor of mutant and wild-type RET, VEGFR-2, and EGFR [25–28]. Preclinical studies have demonstrated activity in vitro against TT and MZ-CRC-1 RET-mutant MTC cell lines, and two recent phase 2 trials showed promising results for patients with hereditary MTC [29, 30]. In the phase 2 studies, objective responses were confirmed in 18 % of patients, all of whom had radiographic partial response (PR); an additional 53 % of patients had stable disease (SD) for at least 24 weeks. Treatment was generally well tolerated, with the most common adverse events being diarrhea, rash, fatigue, and nausea. The results of a randomized, double-blinded, multicenter placebo-controlled phase 3 trial of vandetanib in patients with locally advanced or metastatic MTC (ZETA trial) were recently reported [31]. Between 2006 and 2007, 331 patients with advanced MTC (hereditary MTC, 10 %; sporadic or unknown MTC, 90 %) were randomized in a 2:1 ratio to vandetanib 300 mg daily or placebo. The primary endpoint was PFS. Patients were unblinded at the time of progression, and patients on the placebo arm could receive vandetanib on an open-label follow-up trial. Progression-free survival at 6 months was 83 % in the vandetanib arm, compared to 63 % in the placebo arm (HR for progression 0.45, CI 0.30–0.69). Median progression-free survival was not reached in the vandetanib arm, compared to 19.3 months in the placebo arm. Statistically significant improvements were also noted in the objective response rate (43 % vs. 13 %) and disease control rate (87 % vs. 71 %). Overall survival was not significantly different between the two groups (HR 0.89, CI 0.28–2.85), though this was confounded by the crossover design. Adverse events were similar to those reported in the phase 2 trials, with diarrhea (11 %), hypertension (9 %), QTc prolongation (8 %), and fatigue (6 %) being the most common grade 3+ toxicities. Dose reductions were more common in the vandetanib arm (35 % vs. 3 %). After review of the phase 3 trial, the Food and Drug Administration (FDA) approved vandetanib for advanced, symptomatic, or progressive MTC in April 2011, making it the first FDA-approved targeted therapy for advanced thyroid cancer. Due to concerns about potential toxicities, including QTc prolongation and the risk of sudden death, vandetanib should only be prescribed by experts familiar with its toxicity profile and only to patients who can be monitored closely. All prescribers are currently required to enroll in the Caprelsa Risk Evaluation and Mitigation Strategy (REMS) program.

Cabozantinib

Cabozantinib (XL-184) is a potent, orally bioavailable receptor tyrosine kinase inhibitor with activity against Met, VEGFR-2, KIT, RET, FLT3, and Tie-2. An initial phase 1 trial enrolled 85 patients with advanced malignancies, with an expansion cohort to include a total of 37 patients with advanced MTC [32]. Dose-limiting grade 3+ adverse events included hand-foot syndrome (10 %), fatigue (10 %), elevated lipase (9 %), diarrhea (7 %), elevated amylase (5 %), weight loss (3 %), and elevated AST and ALT (3 %). 34 patients with advanced MTC were assessable for response: 10 patients had a partial response (27 %) with an additional 15 patients (41 %) having stable disease for at least 6 months. Given the early phase 1 results, a large multicenter, international, phase 3, placebo-controlled study of XL-184 in medullary thyroid cancer (Efficacy of XL-184 in Advanced MTC, EXAM) was undertaken. All patients were required to have evidence of disease progression in the 14 months prior to enrollment. Patients were randomized 2:1 to cabozantinib 140 mg orally daily vs. placebo and crossover to open-label cabozantinib was not allowed for patients who progressed on the placebo arm. Median PFS in patients treated with placebo was 4.0 months, compared to 11.2 months in patients receiving cabozantinib (HR 0.28, $p<0.001$). This was observed across all subgroups including prior TKI treatment and RET mutation status. Partial responses were observed in 28 % vs. 0 % with a median duration of response of 14.6 months in the cabozantinib arm. An interim analysis of overall survival with 44 % of 217 required events did not show a difference between the two arms (HR 0.98; 95 % CI 0.63–1.52). The most frequent grade 3 events included diarrhea (15.9 % vs. 1.8 %), hand-foot syndrome (12.6 % vs. 0 %), fatigue (9.3 % vs. 2.8 %), hypocalcemia (2.8 % vs. 0 %), and hypertension (7.9 % vs. 0 %). Adverse events leading to treatment discontinuation were seen in 16 % of cabozantinib-treated patients vs. 8 % of placebo-treated patients [33]. An analysis of RET and RAS mutations was presented at ASCO in 2013. While patients with

Table 89.2 Selected clinical trials of targeted agents in medullary thyroid cancer

Regimen	Target(s)	Ref	Study	Treatment plan	N	Responses		Median PFS
						CR, PR	SD ≥6 months	
FDA-approved therapies								
Vandetanib	VEGFR2, EGFR, RET	[29]	Phase 2	300 mg daily	30	20 %	53 %	27.9 months
		[30]	Phase 2	100 mg daily	19	16 %	53 %	NR
		[31]	Phase 3	300 mg daily	331	45 %	≥38 %	NR[a]
Cabozantinib (XL184)	VEGFR2, Met, KIT, RET, FLT3, Tie-2	[32]	Phase 1	MTD 175 mg daily	37	27 %	41 %	NR
		[33]	Phase 3	140 mg daily	330	28 %	NR	11.2 months[b]
Investigational therapies								
Receptor kinase inhibitors								
Axitinib	VEGFR1-3, PDGFR, KIT	[45]	Phase 2	5 mg bid	11	18 %	NR	NR
Gefitinib	EGFR	[47]	Phase 2	250 mg daily	4	0 %	0 %	NR
Imatinib	Bcr-Abl, PDGFR, KIT, RET	[48]	Phase 2	600 mg daily	15	0 %	>27 %	NR
		[49]	Phase 2	600 mg daily	9	0 %	56 %	NR
Lenvatinib	VEGFR1-3, FGFR1-4, RET, KIT, PDGFR	[35]	Phase 2	24 mg daily	59	36 %	NR	9.0 months
Motesanib	VEGFR1-3, PDGFR, KIT, RET	[38]	Phase 2	125 mg daily	91	2 %[c]	48 %[c]	12 months
Sorafenib	VEGFR2-3, PDGFRβ, KIT, RET, BRAF, Raf-1, FLT3	[53]	Phase 2	400 mg bid	1	0 %	NR	NR
		[40]	Phase 2	400 mg bid	21	21 %	53 %	NR[d]
Sunitinib	VEGFR1-2, PDGFR, KIT, RET, FLT3	[43]	Phase 2	37.5 mg daily	7	43 %	37 %	NR
		[42]	Phase 2	50 mg days 1–28 q6 weeks	25	32 %	NR	NR[e]
		[41]	Phase 2	50 mg days 1–28 q6 weeks	15	33 %	NR	NR
Ras-MAPK inhibitors								
Tipifarnib (+ sorafenib)	Farnesyl-transferase	[46]	Phase 1/2	MTD 200 mg (+600 mg) daily	13	38 %	31 %	NR
Other agents								
Plitidepsin	JNK activation (proapoptotic), VEGF inhibition	[50]	Phase 2	5 mg/m^2 every 2 weeks	16	0 %	38 %	5.3 months
Vorinostat	HDAC	[51]	Phase 2	200 mg daily, 2 weeks every 3 weeks	3	0 %	33 %	NR

[a]PFS significantly improved with vandetanib vs. placebo (HR 0.45, 95 % CI 0.30–0.69)
[b]Median PFS on placebo arm 4.0 months (HR 0.28, $p<0.001$)
[c]Rates of PR + SD were 69 % in RET mutant ($n=33$) vs. 42 % in RET wild type ($n=13$)
[d]Median PFS in sporadic MTC, 17.9 months; median PFS not reached in hereditary MTC
[e]1-year PFS among patients with RET-activating mutations was 88 %

RET-mutated, RET wild-type, and RET unknown tumors all had prolonged PFS on cabozantinib, the RET mutational subgroup had longer median PFS (60 weeks) than patients with RET wild-type tumors (25 weeks, PFS difference $p=0.0001$) [34]. The FDA approved cabozantinib for progressive, metastatic MTC in November 2012.

Lenvatinib

Lenvatinib is an oral multi-kinase inhibitor of VEGFR1-3, FGFR1-4, RET, KIT, and PDGFR which was tested in a phase 2 trial enrolling 59 patients. Preliminary results, presented at ASCO in 2012, showed an overall response rate of 35 % for patients who had received prior VEGFR-directed treatment and 36 % for patients without prior VEGFR-directed treatment. The median PFS was 9.0 months with only 46 % of events observed at the time of presentation. The most frequent grade 3 adverse events included hypertension (7 %), fatigue (5 %), diarrhea (5 %), weight loss (3 %), and proteinuria (2 %) [35].

Motesanib

Motesanib (AMG-706) is an orally bioavailable inhibitor of VEGFR-1-3, PDGFR, and KIT [36], which showed promising results against thyroid cancer in the initial phase 1 study [37]. Schlumberger and colleagues [38] outlined the results of a large phase 2 study of motesanib in patients with advanced MTC who had progressed in the 6 months prior to study enrollment. A total of 91 patients were enrolled (sporadic MT, 84 %; hereditary MTC, 14 %; unknown, 2 %) and were treated with motesanib 125 mg daily until progression or intolerable side effects. Objective responses were seen in only two patients, both of whom had partial responses (2 %). However, stable disease was seen in an additional 74 patients (81 %), of whom 44 (48 %) had durable stable disease lasting at least 24 weeks. The median progression-free survival was 48 weeks, with 1-year survival of 75 %. Adverse events were similar to those seen with other multi-kinase and anti-VEGF therapies, with 88 % of patients experiencing at least one drug-related adverse event. The most common adverse events were diarrhea, fatigue, hypothyroidism, hypertension, nausea, anorexia, and abdominal pain. Retrospective analysis of this trial and a companion trial in differentiated thyroid cancer suggested that increases in serum placental growth factor (PIGF) after 1 week of treatment and decreases in soluble VEGFR-2 after 3 weeks of treatment correlated with a favorable response to therapy [39].

Sorafenib

Sorafenib (Nexavar) is a multi-kinase inhibitor with activity against VEGFR-2-3, PDGFR-β, FLT3, KIT, Raf-1, BRAF, and RET kinases that is approved for the treatment of hepatocellular carcinoma, renal cell carcinoma, and differentiated thyroid cancer. Our group reported the results of an NCI-sponsored multicenter phase 2 trial of sorafenib in patients with advanced MTC in 2010 [40]. A total of 21 patients were accrued to the trial, including 16 patients with sporadic MTC and 5 patients with hereditary MTC. All patients with hereditary MTC had germline *RET* mutations; *RET* mutations were seen in 10 of the 12 patients with sporadic MTC who could be evaluated. Response rates were consistent with other clinical trials of sorafenib, with partial responses seen in 2 patients (10 %) and durable stable disease lasting at least 6 months in 11 patients (53 %). Nine patients (43 %) had stable disease lasting at least 15 months. The median progression-free survival in patients with sporadic MTC was 17.9 months; it was not reached in hereditary MTC. The median overall survival was not reached during the study. Of note, patients were not required to have evidence of progressive disease prior to study enrollment. However, a post hoc analysis noted that ten patients with sporadic MTC had progressive disease within 12 months prior to study. Five of these patients (50 %) demonstrated clinical benefit to therapy (partial responses or stable disease of at least 6-month duration).

Sunitinib

Sunitinib (Sutent) is a multi-kinase inhibitor with activity against VEGFR-1, VEGFR-2, PDGFR, KIT, FLT3, and RET. It is approved for treatment of renal cell carcinoma, gastrointestinal stromal tumors resistant to imatinib, and pancreatic neuroendocrine tumors. Three small studies, encompassing 47 patients with advanced medullary thyroid cancer, have investigated the activity of sunitinib in this disease [41–43]. Objective responses were seen in 16 patients (34 %, range of 32–43 %). Rates of durable stable disease were not reported in all trials. Common side effects of sunitinib include fatigue, lymphopenia, nausea, diarrhea, mucositis, and hand-foot syndrome [42, 44].

Axitinib

Axitinib is a small molecule tyrosine kinase inhibitor of VEGFR1-3, PDGFR, and KIT. A recent phase 2 study of axitinib in advanced thyroid cancer included 11 patients with medullary thyroid cancer [45]. Objective responses were seen in two patients (18 %); rates of durable stable disease in this subpopulation were not reported.

Tipifarnib

Farnesylation is required to anchor the Ras family of proteins to the inner cell membrane where they function in signal transduction. Tipifarnib is a farnesyltransferase inhibitor that was studied in combination with sorafenib in a phase 1/2 trial that included 13 patients with medullary thyroid cancer [46]. Five patients (38 %) had objective responses to therapy with an additional four patients (31 %) demonstrating durable stable disease. The most common adverse events were fatigue, rash, neuropathy, diarrhea, and elevations in serum lipase.

Other Agents

Other agents that have been studied include gefitinib [47], imatinib [48, 49], plitidepsin [50], and vorinostat [51]. No objective responses were observed in the small number of patients with medullary thyroid cancer included in the above clinical trials, though disease stabilization has been reported in some patients. Further research is ongoing.

Summary

MTC has historically been viewed as relatively chemoresistant disease, with reported objective response rates to traditional cytotoxic chemotherapy in the range of 0–30 %. Improvements in the understanding of the underlying disease pathobiology and development of RET- and angiogenesis-targeted therapies, however, have allowed for a better therapeutic approach. Vandetanib (2011) and cabozantinib (2012) are the first agents to be FDA approved for the treatment of advanced MTC. While such drugs are simple to administer, patients must be closely monitored for early recognition and treatment of drug-associated side effects. Cytotoxic chemotherapy should no longer be considered first-line therapy for patients with advanced MTC [52].

References

1. Ball DW, et al. Selective growth inhibition in BRAF mutant thyroid cancer by the mitogen-activated protein kinase kinase 1/2 inhibitor AZD6244. J Clin Endocrinol Metab. 2007;92(12):4712–8.
2. Pacini F, et al. Medullary thyroid carcinoma. Clin Oncol (R Coll Radiol). 2010;22(6):475–85.
3. Moo-Young TA, Traugott AL, Moley JF. Sporadic and familial medullary thyroid carcinoma: state of the art. Surg Clin N Am. 2009;89(5):1193–204.
4. Gottlieb JA, Hill Jr CS. Chemotherapy of thyroid cancer with adriamycin. Experience with 30 patients. N Engl J Med. 1974;290(4):193–7.
5. Shimaoka K, et al. A randomized trial of doxorubicin versus doxorubicin plus cisplatin in patients with advanced thyroid carcinoma. Cancer. 1985;56(9):2155–60.
6. Benker G, Reinwein D. Results of chemotherapy in thyroid cancer. Dtsch Med Wochenschr. 1983;108(11):403–6.
7. Droz JP, et al. Chemotherapy for medullary cancer of the thyroid. Phase II trials with adriamycin and cis-platinum administered as monochemotherapy. Bull Cancer. 1984;71(3):195–9.
8. Matuszczyk A, et al. Chemotherapy with doxorubicin in progressive medullary and thyroid carcinoma of the follicular epithelium. Horm Metab Res. 2008;40(3):210–3.
9. Scherubl H, Raue F, Ziegler R. Combination chemotherapy of advanced medullary and differentiated thyroid cancer. Phase II study. J Cancer Res Clin Oncol. 1990;116(1):21–3.
10. Athanassiades P, et al. Serial serum calcitonin concentrations to evaluate response to therapy of patients with medullary thyroid carcinoma. Chemioterapia. 1988;7(3):195–7.
11. Frame J, et al. A phase II trial of streptozotocin and adriamycin in advanced APUD tumors. Am J Clin Oncol. 1988;11(4):490–5.
12. De Besi P, et al. Combined chemotherapy with bleomycin, adriamycin, and platinum in advanced thyroid cancer. J Endocrinol Invest. 1991;14(6):475–80.
13. Williams SD, Birch R, Einhorn LH. Phase II evaluation of doxorubicin plus cisplatin in advanced thyroid cancer: a Southeastern Cancer Study Group Trial. Cancer Treat Rev. 1986;70(3):405–7.
14. Nocera M, et al. Treatment of advanced medullary thyroid cancer with an alternating combination of doxorubicin-streptozocin and 5 FU-dacarbazine. Groupe d'Etude des Tumeurs a Calcitonine (GETC). Br J Cancer. 2000;83(6):715–8.
15. Hoskin PJ, Harmer C. Chemotherapy for thyroid cancer. Radiother Oncol. 1987;10(3):187–94.
16. Orlandi F, et al. Chemotherapy with dacarbazine and 5-fluorouracil in advanced medullary thyroid cancer. Ann Oncol. 1994;5(8):763–5.
17. Wu LT, et al. Treatment of advanced medullary thyroid carcinoma with a combination of cyclophosphamide, vincristine, and dacarbazine. Cancer. 1994;73(2):432–6.
18. Di Bartolomeo M, et al. A phase II trial of dacarbazine, fluorouracil and epirubicin in patients with neuroendocrine tumours. A study by the Italian Trials in Medical Oncology (I.T.M.O.) Group. Ann Oncol. 1995;6(1):77–9.
19. Schlumberger M, et al. Treatment of advanced medullary thyroid cancer with an alternating combination of 5 FU-streptozocin and 5 FU-dacarbazine. The Groupe d'Etude des Tumeurs a Calcitonine (GETC). Br J Cancer. 1995;71(2):363–5.
20. Bajetta E, et al. 5-Fluorouracil, dacarbazine, and epirubicin in the treatment of patients with neuroendocrine tumors. Cancer. 1998;83(2):372–8.
21. Eng C, et al. The relationship between specific RET proto-oncogene mutations and disease phenotype in multiple endocrine neoplasia type 2. International RET mutation consortium analysis. JAMA. 1996;276(19):1575–9.
22. Moura MM, et al. Correlation of RET somatic mutations with clinicopathological features in sporadic medullary thyroid carcinomas. Br J Cancer. 2009;100(11):1777–83.
23. Moura MM, et al. High prevalence of RAS mutations in RET-negative sporadic medullary thyroid carcinomas. J Clin Endocrinol Metab. 2011;96(5):E863–8.
24. Capp C, et al. Increased expression of vascular endothelial growth factor and its receptors, VEGFR-1 and VEGFR-2, in medullary thyroid carcinoma. Thyroid. 2010;20(8):863–71.
25. Wedge SR, et al. ZD6474 inhibits vascular endothelial growth factor signaling, angiogenesis, and tumor growth following oral administration. Cancer Res. 2002;62(16):4645–55.

26. Carlomagno F, et al. ZD6474, an orally available inhibitor of KDR tyrosine kinase activity, efficiently blocks oncogenic RET kinases. Cancer Res. 2002;62(24):7284–90.
27. Vidal M, et al. ZD6474 suppresses oncogenic RET isoforms in a Drosophila model for type 2 multiple endocrine neoplasia syndromes and papillary thyroid carcinoma. Cancer Res. 2005;65(9): 3538–41.
28. Vitagliano D, et al. The tyrosine kinase inhibitor ZD6474 blocks proliferation of RET mutant medullary thyroid carcinoma cells. Endocr Relat Cancer. 2010;18(1):1–11.
29. Wells Jr SA, et al. Vandetanib for the treatment of patients with locally advanced or metastatic hereditary medullary thyroid cancer. J Clin Oncol. 2010;28(5):767–72.
30. Robinson BG, et al. Vandetanib (100 mg) in patients with locally advanced or metastatic hereditary medullary thyroid cancer. J Clin Endocrinol Metab. 2010;95(6):2664–71.
31. Wells Jr SA, et al. Vandetanib in patients with locally advanced or metastatic medullary thyroid cancer: a randomized, double-blind phase III trial. J Clin Oncol. 2012;30(2):134–41.
32. Kurzrock R, et al. Long-term results in a cohort of medullary thyroid cancer (MTC) patients (pts) in a phase I study of XL184 (BMS 907351), an oral inhibitor of MET, VEGFR2, and RET. J Clin Oncol. 2010;28((15S)):abstr 5502.
33. Elisei R, et al. Cabozantinib in progressive medullary thyroid cancer. J Clin Oncol. 2013;31(29):3639–46.
34. Sherman S, et al. Efficacy of cabozantinib (Cabo) in medullary thyroid cancer (MTC) patients with RAS or RET mutations: results from a phase III study. J Clin Oncol. 2013;31(suppl):abstr 6000.
35. Schlumberger M, et al. A phase II trial of the multitargeted kinase inhibitor lenvatinib (E7080) in advanced medullary thyroid cancer (MTC). J Clin Oncol. 2012;30(suppl):abstr 5591.
36. Polverino A, et al. AMG 706, an oral, multikinase inhibitor that selectively targets vascular endothelial growth factor, platelet-derived growth factor, and kit receptors, potently inhibits angiogenesis and induces regression in tumor xenografts. Cancer Res. 2006;66(17):8715–21.
37. Rosen LS, et al. Safety, pharmacokinetics, and efficacy of AMG 706, an oral multikinase inhibitor, in patients with advanced solid tumors. J Clin Oncol. 2007;25(17):2369–76.
38. Schlumberger MJ, et al. Phase II study of safety and efficacy of motesanib in patients with progressive or symptomatic, advanced or metastatic medullary thyroid cancer. J Clin Oncol. 2009; 27(23):3794–801.
39. Bass MB, et al. Biomarkers as predictors of response to treatment with motesanib in patients with progressive advanced thyroid cancer. J Clin Endocrinol Metab. 2010;95(11):5018–27.
40. Lam ET, et al. Phase II clinical trial of sorafenib in metastatic medullary thyroid cancer. J Clin Oncol. 2010;28(14):2323–30.
41. Ravaud A, et al. Efficacy of sunitinib in advanced medullary thyroid carcinoma: intermediate results of phase II THYSU. Oncologist. 2010;15(2):212–3, author reply 214.
42. De Souza J, et al. Phase II trial of sunitinib in medullary thyroid cancer (MTC). J Clin Oncol. 2010;28(15S):abstr 5504.
43. Carr LL, et al. Phase II study of daily sunitinib in FDG-PET-positive, iodine-refractory differentiated thyroid cancer and metastatic medullary carcinoma of the thyroid with functional imaging correlation. Clin Cancer Res. 2010;16(21):5260–8.
44. Cohen E, et al. Phase 2 study of sunitinib in refractory thyroid cancer. J Clin Oncol. 2008;26:May 20 suppl:abstr 6025.
45. Cohen EE, et al. Axitinib is an active treatment for all histologic subtypes of advanced thyroid cancer: results from a phase II study. J Clin Oncol. 2008;26(29):4708–13.
46. Hong DS, et al. Inhibition of the Ras/Raf/MEK/ERK and RET kinase pathways with the combination of the multikinase inhibitor sorafenib and the farnesyltransferase inhibitor tipifarnib in medullary and differentiated thyroid malignancies. J Clin Endocrinol Metab. 2011;96(4):997–1005.
47. Pennell NA, et al. A phase II study of Gefitinib in patients with advanced thyroid cancer. Thyroid. 2008;18(3):317–23.
48. de Groot JW, et al. A phase II trial of imatinib therapy for metastatic medullary thyroid carcinoma. J Clin Endocrinol Metab. 2007; 92(9):3466–9.
49. Frank-Raue K, et al. Efficacy of imatinib mesylate in advanced medullary thyroid carcinoma. Eur J Endocrinol. 2007;157(2): 215–20.
50. Baudin E, et al. Phase II study of plitidepsin 3-hour infusion every 2 weeks in patients with unresectable advanced medullary thyroid carcinoma. Am J Clin Oncol. 2010;33(1):83–8.
51. Woyach JA, et al. Lack of therapeutic effect of the histone deacetylase inhibitor vorinostat in patients with metastatic radioiodine-refractory thyroid carcinoma. J Clin Endocrinol Metab. 2009; 94(1):164–70.
52. Tuttle R, et al. NCCN clinical practice guidelines in oncology (NCCN guidelines): thyroid carcinoma. www.nccn.org, 2012.
53. Gupta-Abramson V, et al. Phase II trial of sorafenib in advanced thyroid cancer. J Clin Oncol. 2008;26(29):4714–9.

A Comparison of the ATA, NCCN, ETA, and BTA Guidelines for the Management of Medullary Thyroid Cancer

90

Rossella Elisei

Introduction

Medullary thyroid carcinoma (MTC) is a well-differentiated thyroid tumor that derives from the parafollicular or calcitonin-producing C cells, of which it maintains the biochemical and physiological features [1–3]. The overall frequency of MTC is not well established, but it accounts for 5–10 % of all thyroid malignancies and 0.4–1.4 % of all thyroid nodules and is present in less than 1 % of the thyroids of subjects submitted to autopsy [4–7].

Two different forms of MTC are recognized: the sporadic form, which accounts for approximately 75 % of cases, and the hereditary or familial form, which accounts for the remaining 25 %. The familial form can be classified into three different syndromes depending on the presence of other endocrine neoplasias, such as pheochromocytoma or parathyroid hyperplasia/adenomas (i.e., multiple endocrine neoplasia [MEN 2 syndromes] type 2A and/or the absence of any other associated disease (i.e., familial medullary thyroid cancer [FMTC]). The hereditary form can affect children, and more aggressive syndromes generally produce clinical symptoms in younger children [8–10].

The biological behavior of MTC is much less favorable than that of the other well-differentiated thyroid carcinomas, although it is not as unfavorable as that of anaplastic carcinoma [11]. A 10-year survival of approximately 50 % has been reported for MTC patients in several series [12–14]. Both the cure and survival of these patients are positively impacted by an early diagnosis [14–16]; however, only patients with intrathyroidal tumor with no lymph node metastases or few micrometastases of the central compartment can achieve a full clinical and biochemical cure [13, 17, 18].

Calcitonin (Ct) is a small polypeptide hormone of 32 amino acids that is normally produced almost exclusively by C cells. It is the most specific and sensitive serum marker of MTC, both before and after thyroidectomy [19, 20], and, with few exceptions, elevated basal levels of serum Ct are diagnostic of MTC [21].

Because of these unique features and especially because of the rarity of the disease, MTC patients should be referred to tertiary cancer centers with experienced multidisciplinary teams to receive the best care. Several guidelines for the management of MTC patients have been developed by groups of experts to facilitate the clinical decisions that the patient management team must make at both the diagnostic and therapeutic levels. At present, there are several published guidelines for the management of thyroid cancer and/or of thyroid nodules. The guidelines that are most focused on MTC management are those published in 2009 by the American Thyroid Association (ATA) Task Force [22]. This 47-page document was developed by a group of experts, including two of the major European experts in this field, and has been endorsed by several other societies, including the European Thyroid Association; and, for this reason, here following they will be indicated as ATA/ETA guidelines. Separate documents were produced by ATA and ETA for the management of patients with thyroid nodules and differentiated thyroid cancer in 2009 and 2006, respectively [23, 24]. These guidelines are important for the management of MTC, especially for diagnostic procedures, because both sporadic and familial MTCs usually appear initially as thyroid nodules. Other relevant guidelines for the management of MTC are those published by the British Thyroid Association (BTA) [25] and the National Comprehensive Cancer Network (NCCN) [26], which are devoted to the general management of all types of thyroid cancer patients.

The aim of this chapter is to compare the BTA, NCCN, and ATA/ETA guidelines and to highlight areas of consensus

R. Elisei, MD (✉)
Endocrine Unit, Department of Clinical and Experimental Medicine, University Hospital of Pisa, Via Paradisa, 2, Pisa, Italy 56124
e-mail: rossella.elisei@med.unipi.it

L. Wartofsky, D. Van Nostrand (eds.), *Thyroid Cancer*, DOI 10.1007/978-1-4939-3314-3_90

Table 90.1 Major shared indications among different guidelines

1. Serum Ct measurement at least when a presurgical suspicious of MTC is present
2. Presurgical evaluation of the presence of pheochromocytoma and/or hyperparathyroidism even in apparently sporadic MTC
3. Total thyroidectomy and, at least, central node neck dissection by principle when a presurgical MTC diagnosis has already done
4. External radiation therapy on the neck if a gross unresectable disease is already present at the first surgical treatment
5. Measurement of both basal serum Ct and CEA during follow-up with particular regard to the DT
6. Imaging procedures should be performed when postoperative serum Ct is >150 pg/ml
7. Surgical treatment for local disease and TKI for advanced and aggressive disease as further treatments for persistent or recurrent MTC
8. Germline RET genetic screening in all MTC patients
9. At the present, no need to search for somatic RET mutation in sporadic MTC

Ct serum calcitonin, *MTC* medullary thyroid cancer, *CEA* carcinoembryonic antigen, *DT* doubling time, *TKI* tyrosine kinase inhibitors, *RET* rearranged during transfection (oncogene)

Table 90.2 Major controversial issues among different guidelines

1. Routine measurement of serum Ct in the workup of thyroid nodules
2. Indications for neck ultrasound and other imaging procedures before surgery
3. Completion thyroidectomy in case of microMTC incidentally found after hemithyroidectomy
4. Timing for prophylactic thyroidectomy in gene carriers
5. Extension of lymph node dissection at the time of thyroidectomy
6. Appropriate time for the first control after surgical treatment
7. Postoperative Ct stimulation test in patients with normal/undetectable basal serum Ct levels

Ct serum calcitonin, *MTC* medullary thyroid cancer

(Table 90.1) and disagreement (Table 90.2). The different reasons for consensus or disagreement are discussed, with reference to the evidence published by other experts in the field.

The Diagnosis

The most common clinical presentation of sporadic MTC is a thyroid nodule, either single or belonging to a series of nodules in the context of a multinodular goiter. With the exception of the simultaneous presence of diarrhea and/or flushing syndrome, which is rare and usually related to an advanced metastatic disease, patients do not exhibit any specific symptoms. The association of thyroid nodular disease with a lump in the neck may lead the clinician to suspect a thyroid malignancy, though usually not an MTC specifically. Furthermore, hereditary MTC in the context of MEN 2 syndrome has the clinical appearance of a thyroid nodular disease, similar to that of the sporadic form but with the exception that it is usually bilateral, multicentric, and almost invariably associated with C-cell hyperplasia (CCH) [27–29].

All guidelines agree that a patient with a thyroid nodule >1 cm should undergo a workup including neck ultrasound, the evaluation of thyroid function by measuring free thyroxine (FT4) and thyrotropin-stimulating hormone (TSH), thyroid scintigraphy if TSH levels are low, and fine-needle aspiration for cytology. Differing opinions are expressed in the different guidelines regarding the routine measurement of serum Ct in all patients with thyroid nodule(s). BTA and NCCN share the view that serum Ct should be measured anytime a presurgical diagnosis of MTC is suspected either due to positive fine-needle aspiration cytology or familial history or to the simultaneous presence of other endocrine neoplasia. In this case, serum Ct measurement is performed not for diagnostic purposes but to provide a baseline value of serum Ct to be compared with measurements obtained after surgery. ATA guidelines for the management of thyroid nodules [23] do not recommend for or against routine serum Ct testing. In contrast, the ETA consensus [24] clearly states that this procedure should be applied in the workup of all thyroid nodules because it is more sensitive than fine-needle aspiration cytology. In 2010, a new document signed by the American Association of Clinical Endocrinologists (AACE), the Associazione Medici Endocrinologici (AME), and the European Thyroid Association (ETA) was published, declaring that routine serum Ct may be useful, especially before surgery, and strongly recommending its measurement in certain high-risk groups [30].

This controversial issue is often debated among experts, and both those in favor and those against have valuable arguments in their favor. Several studies have demonstrated that the routine measurement of serum Ct is the most accurate diagnostic tool for the detection of MTC in patients with thyroid nodules [31–37]. However, low-mild elevated values of serum Ct can be falsely positive for technical reasons [38–40] or due to the presence of other rare pathological conditions (e.g., other neuroendocrine tumors, hyperparathyroidism, renal failure, etc.) [41]. To distinguish among these situations, subjects with a low-mild elevated basal serum Ct

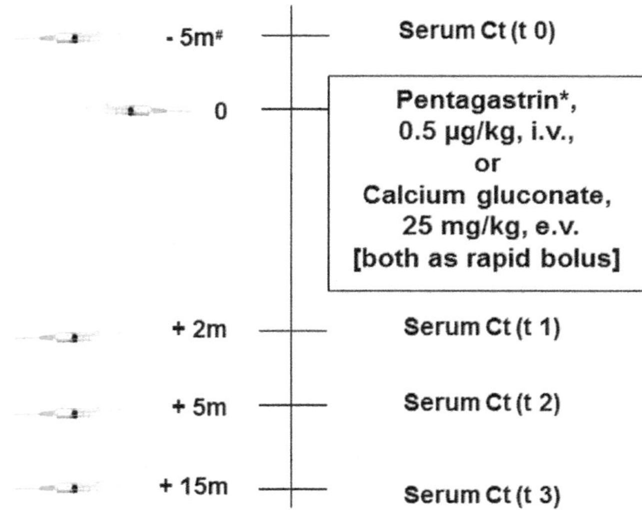

Fig. 90.1 Schematic representation of both pentagastrin and calcium stimulation test: dose of the two drugs and times for blood taken are indicated. The two tests have been demonstrated to be comparable [45]

should be subjected to a stimulation test with either calcium (2.3 mg/Kg of calcium ion or 25 mg/Kg of calcium gluconate) or pentagastrin (0.5 mg/kg iv) [42–45] (Fig. 90.1). Although the routine measurement of serum Ct in all subjects with thyroid nodules is still controversial [46, 47], there is evidence to suggest that this approach allows early diagnosis and treatment, thus significantly improving the outcome of this potentially lethal disease [15, 16].

Dedicated thyroid and neck bilateral ultrasonography is recommended by ATA/ETA and NCCN guidelines before thyroidectomy. This is relevant for planning the surgical strategy; a total thyroidectomy and central neck dissection should be performed by principle, whereas the lateral neck dissection is elective and should only be performed when neck lymph node metastases are documented. Whenever lymph node metastasis is suspected, ATA/ETA guidelines recommend ultrasound-guided fine-needle aspiration cytology and a measurement of Ct in the washout of the needle [48]. In contrast, the BTA guidelines do not mention dedicated presurgical neck ultrasound.

Cytology represents the gold standard diagnostic tool in the workup of thyroid nodules. However, although the cytological pattern of MTC is generally distinctive, several series have shown a high rate of failure in presurgical diagnosis [31–33, 49]. Among other explanations, the negative results might arise because MTC may be present in a nodule that was not submitted to FNAC, especially in cases of multinodular goiter. In this context, serum Ct measurement is more reliable because it is elevated even in the presence of microfocal MTC [31, 34].

BTA guidelines clearly state that preoperative staging of MTC with computerized tomography (CT scan) or magnetic resonance imaging (MRI) is not essential before the first intervention and does not alter the need for neck surgery. Both ATA/ETA and NCCN guidelines share this view, but they also recommend that total body imaging procedures be performed in MTC cases with highly elevated presurgical serum levels of Ct (i.e., >400 pg/ml), especially when it is associated with elevated serum levels of CEA.

Concomitant hyperparathyroidism and/or pheochromocytoma is unlikely in the absence of MEN 2A or 2B. However, 5–10 % of familial cases are discovered by *RET* genetic testing [50], which can require several weeks and generally does not produce results prior to surgery. Because the presence of a pheochromocytoma can introduce severe complications during thyroidectomy, it is important to exclude the presence of this tumor before surgical treatment for MTC. Meanwhile, calcium measurement, which should be associated with parathyroid hormone and vitamin D measurement, is indicated to evaluate hyperparathyroidism. These recommendations are made in both the NCCN and ATA/ETA guidelines.

Unsuspected MTC can also be unexpectedly found at histology, after an hemithyroidectomy. In this case, the NCCN guidelines suggest that *RET* germline mutation, familial history of MEN 2, histological evidence of C-cell hyperplasia, and serum Ct levels be evaluated and to consider proceeding to a complete thyroidectomy and central neck dissection if there is a high probability of hereditary disease. The ATA/ETA guidelines also consider the possibility of an MTC diagnosis after hemithyroidectomy, but they suggest that the serum Ct levels be considered and recommend long-term surveillance if the serum Ct value is <150 pg/ml or further imaging procedures and surgical treatment if serum Ct is >150 pg/ml [51, 52]. This situation is virtually never encountered in countries in which the routine serum Ct measurement of all thyroid nodules is performed because this can detect even small foci of MTC that are not visible at neck ultrasound [31–34].

Initial Treatment

All MTC guidelines agree that the minimal standard initial therapeutic procedure for both sporadic and familial forms is total (or near total) thyroidectomy with central neck lymph node dissection. The need for total thyroidectomy is supported by the multicentricity and bilaterality of the MTC that occurs in approximately 100 % of hereditary cases and 30 % of sporadic cases [27]. Furthermore, CCH, which is considered a preneoplastic lesion, is almost invariably associated with the hereditary form of MTC and, to a lesser extent, with the sporadic form [29]. An additional reason in favor of total thyroidectomy is that 5–7 % of apparently sporadic cases are in fact hereditary forms, which almost invariably cause bilateral disease [53, 54].

The central node compartment is the primary lymphatic drainage site of the thyroid, and 50–60 % of MTCs show node metastases in this area at the time of presentation [55, 56]. The removal of the central compartment also has prophylactic significance and must be performed regardless of the size of the primary tumor and the presurgical evidence of lymph node involvement. However, despite a general agreement that total thyroidectomy and central neck dissection should be performed as the initial treatment, the NCCN guidelines include a note of caution for MTCs ≤1 cm in diameter and suggest that central neck dissection may not be necessary in cases of microMTC, especially if presented as unilateral micronodule at neck ultrasound.

This approach is also suggested in *RET* gene carriers (GC) without clinical evidence of disease, which can be completely cured by total thyroidectomy, especially if performed prophylactically. It remains controversial whether central node dissection should be performed in *RET* GC [57, 58]. In this regard, the NCCN guidelines strongly suggest that neck dissection be considered in all MEN 2B gene carriers, whereas the ATA/ETA guidelines maintain that prophylactic neck dissection is not necessary in MEN 2B patients treated within the first year of age. Both guidelines agree that this procedure can be avoided in MEN 2A and FMTC GC, independent of age, if serum Ct is less than 40 pg/ml. This suggestion is based on several lines of evidence, including very recently published data, that a preoperative basal serum Ct below the institutional cutoff (generally 30–60 pg/ml) is almost invariably associated with the absence of lymph node metastasis [59, 60]. In contrast, BTA guidelines do not consider the serum Ct but rather suggest that central neck dissection be performed (or not performed) along with total thyroidectomy according to the age of the gene carrier. In particular, they recommend that this procedure be avoided in MEN 2A GC younger than 10 years of age and in FMTC GC younger than 20 years of age at the time of surgery, whereas the central compartment should be always removed in MEN 2B GC. The reason for this important distinction is related to the higher risk of permanent hypoparathyroidism when total thyroidectomy is associated with central neck dissection, especially in young children [61]. Given the relevant risks of thyroidectomy in very young children, all guidelines suggest that these children should be referred to a surgical team with extensive experience in thyroid surgery, not necessarily a pediatric team, but certainly a group working in a tertiary care setting.

It is still debated whether a modified radical neck dissection with the removal of the nodes in the ipsilateral or bilateral compartment should be performed in any situation. Because uni- or bilateral cervical nodal metastases occur in up to 90 % of patients with MTC, especially when the primary tumor is palpable [34, 62], several authors strongly suggest an “en bloc” dissection of both the central and bilateral neck compartments, along with the thyroid gland [63]. This is of great clinical significance because adequate initial surgical treatment is a prerequisite for the effective cure of the MTC. Thus, the choice of the most appropriate initial procedure is fundamental. However, it is worth considering that radical neck dissection may result in significant morbidity but has not been clearly shown to improve the prognosis of the disease; the prognosis is instead dependent on other factors such as the local extension of the disease at the time of diagnosis, the presence or absence of other endocrine neoplasia, and the presence of cervical lymph node metastases. ATA/ETA, NCCN, and BTA guidelines agree that whenever a presurgical clinical diagnosis of node metastasis is achieved, the surgical dissection of the corresponding lateral node compartment should be included, but they do not indicate this procedure as standard treatment for all MTC cases. It is important to note that whereas the BTA guidelines do not suggest performing a neck ultrasound as a standard preoperative investigation, which means that the presence of lymph node metastasis can be determined only by clinical examination, both ATA/ETA and NCCN suggest performing a preoperative neck ultrasound which, if followed by fine-needle aspiration of a suspicious lymph node, can unequivocally detect lymph node metastases. Indeed, neck ultrasound can easily reveal metastatic lymph nodes that are not palpable and not clinically suspected, thus allowing an earlier diagnosis of lymph node metastases. However, when lateral node metastases are present at diagnosis, a definitive cure is rarely achieved with the initial treatment, regardless of the extension of the surgical procedure [64–66].

In MTC patients with gross local disease, especially that associated with distant metastasis, neck surgery is still recommended by all guidelines to prevent the subsequent compromise of the trachea, esophagus, and recurrent laryngeal nerves. However, if these structures are already involved by the tumor, less aggressive surgery may be appropriate to preserve speech and swallowing while maintaining locoregional disease.

All guidelines suggest that patients with aggressive local disease that is not completely removed by primary resection should be treated by external beam radiotherapy after surgery. Although bulky MTC deposits are consistently resistant to external radiotherapy, there is evidence that radiotherapy is associated with a decreased risk (from two to fourfold) of local recurrence in patients with residual disease [67, 68]. This procedure should be reserved for patients who have undergone complete central compartment and lateral neck dissection and postponed a second surgical treatment or those who have received a less aggressive primary resection.

Hormone replacement therapy with L-thyroxine (LT4) should be started immediately after thyroidectomy.

Because MTC is not dependent on TSH for growth or function, there is no need to treat patients with LT4 suppressive therapy; the daily dose should be tailored by measuring serum FT4 and TSH, aiming to keep their values within the normal range. These indications are clearly given by the ATA/ETA, only mentioned in the NCCN guidelines and completely omitted from the BTA guidelines.

Follow-Up and Diagnosis of Persistent Disease

After the initial therapy is performed, both serum Ct and carcinoembryonic antigen (CEA), which is another MTC marker [69], should be measured to verify the completeness of the treatment. Both the ATA/ETA and NCCN guidelines suggest performing the first control 2–3 months after the surgical treatment, whereas the BTA guidelines indicate that the most informative serum Ct levels are obtained 6 months after thyroidectomy and clearly state not to measure serum Ct until at least 10 days after surgical treatment. This particular point is related to the fact that Ct has a relatively long half-life; thus, if performed too early, measurements of serum Ct may be misleading, especially if a high serum concentration was present preoperatively [70]. Of course, this first follow-up visit must include a physical examination, neck ultrasound, and the measurement of serum FT4 and TSH, which are requested for monitoring the progress of LT4 replacement therapy.

It is still debated whether a stimulation test with either pentagastrin or calcium is indicated in these cases. ATA/ETA guidelines do not clearly recommend this procedure, but they report that this issue is controversial and that there were differences in opinions among the task force members. Neither the BTA nor NCCN guidelines mention this specific issue because they maintain that the likelihood of significant residual disease with an undetectable basal level of serum Ct is very low. It is true that an undetectable level of basal Ct following thyroidectomy is predictive of clinical remission within 10 years in 90 % of cases [71]. If serum Ct remains undetectable even after stimulation with either pentagastrin or calcium, the likelihood of recurrence in long-term follow-up is reduced to only 3 % [64]. These data indicate that the information derived from a negative stimulation test is substantially important to reassure the patient about his/her clinical remission status and to better plan the subsequent follow-up. Whether the stimulation test is performed or not, all guidelines agree that MTC patients with undetectable basal serum Ct and CEA should be retested on an annual basis, and if both markers remain undetectable, no additional imaging or more frequent testing is required.

Frequently, basal and/or stimulated serum Ct remains elevated after the initial surgery. Because serum Ct is a very sensitive and specific tumor marker, the finding of detectable serum levels of basal or stimulated Ct is an indication of persistent disease. The basal levels of serum Ct seem to play a role in the follow-up strategy for both NCCN and ATA/ETA guidelines. When postoperative serum Ct levels are <150 pg/ml, only locoregional disease is expected; distant metastases, if present, are usually small or limited in number and thus very difficult to be detected [72–74]. For these reasons, both the NCCN and ATA/ETA guidelines suggest a less stringent follow-up for these patients. In particular, NCCN suggests clinical and biochemical evaluation but no imaging if the serum values are stable, whereas ATA/ETA recommends a careful neck ultrasound and additional imaging to serve as a baseline for comparisons in the event of a future increase in serum Ct levels. These imaging procedures are strongly recommended by all guidelines when serum Ct is elevated and particularly in cases when it is >150 pg/ml. According to all guidelines, neck ultrasound, chest and neck CT scan, liver CT or liver magnetic resonance imaging (MRI), bone MRI of the spine and pelvis, and bone scan should be performed to identify the source of serum Ct production. NCCN guidelines suggest that bone MRI of the spine and pelvis and bone scans be performed only in MTC patients with highly elevated serum levels of Ct. Other imaging techniques, such as octreoscan, 123MIBG, and PET, may be useful, although at present they do not appear to be particularly sensitive, especially in cases of micrometastases [75–77]. The most accurate technique for the localization of occult metastases is most likely the measurement of serum Ct after selective venous sampling catheterization: the presence of a gradient in the neck, mediastinum, or suprahepatic veins suggests the presence of a metastatic disease in the region in which the higher levels of serum Ct were found. It should be taken into account that this method is rather invasive and does not significantly improve the curative rate [78–80]. Although discussed, no specific recommendations are given by guidelines for these imaging procedures.

Approximately 50 % of patients who are not cured by surgery have no evidence of metastatic disease when studied with traditional imaging techniques (i.e., CT, MRI, and PET). In this condition of "biochemical disease," characterized by the persistence of detectable levels of basal and/or stimulated serum Ct but absence of evidence of metastatic lesions, the most widely accepted therapeutic strategy is a "wait and see" approach. Detectable serum Ct is in fact compatible with long-term survival, during which Ct may remain stable or increase slowly over time. All guidelines agree that these MTC patients should be periodically monitored at intervals of 6 months to 1 year.

Both NCCN and ATA/ETA guidelines recommend that patients with high levels of serum Ct and CEA, with known or unknown metastases, must be checked according to the doubling time (DT) of the serum levels of these markers;

more aggressive disease is characterized by a more rapid increase in serum Ct. Although the BTA guidelines do not specifically mention the DT of serum markers, they recommend 6-month intervals for biochemical and imaging follow-up in MTC patients with progressively increasing Ct levels. The DT of Ct levels is an important prognostic factor related to the proliferative activity of tumor cells [81, 82]. Patients with a serum Ct DT <6 months have the poorest prognosis and must be strictly monitored to plan adequate therapeutic strategies. Because the rate of increase is an important prognostic parameter, serial serum Ct determinations should be performed in the same laboratory with the same assay to ensure comparability, as is clearly stated by the ATA/ETA guidelines and thyroid laboratory guidelines [83, 84].

Further Treatments

Further treatments should be taken into account for MTC patients with metastatic disease. The recommendations given by the guidelines are very similar. If a well-defined local disease is present, reoperative surgery in the neck and mediastinum should be considered to prevent complications related to the infiltration or compression of the trachea, esophagus, or laryngeal nerves. Several studies have reported experiences with repeat neck surgery for MTC, but no randomized studies demonstrating an advantage in progression-free survival or overall survival in reoperated vs non-reoperated patients have been performed to date. However, according to the published series, approximately 30 % of reoperated patients show low or undetectable serum Ct levels [85–91].

With respect to the treatment of distant metastases, all guidelines share the same view and indicate the same strategy, which depends on the localization, symptoms, and rate of growth. Asymptomatic and stable distant metastases can be observed without any active therapy, whereas symptomatic lesions should be treated with palliative resection, radiofrequency ablation, or embolization. Patients with disseminated symptomatic disease should be included in clinical trials for tyrosine kinase inhibitors (TKI). In the USA and several European countries in which Caprelsa (previously known as Zactima or ZD6474) is already approved and available, treatment with this TKI should be considered in MTC patients with aggressive and advanced disease [92]. Because some studies have shown a relatively high clinical benefit from treatment with sorafenib or sutent, the "off-label" use of these drugs is suggested by both NCCN and ATA/ETA guidelines as an alternative for patients who do not have access to Caprelsa [93]. According to the ATA/ETA guidelines, the use of standard chemotherapeutic agents should not be considered as first-line therapy given their low response rates [94]. This treatment remains an option for BTA and NCCN guidelines, especially for those patients who, for any reason, cannot enter clinical trials and cannot receive TKI.

Genetic Tests

Screening for RET Gene Mutations

RET mutation analysis represents one of the most useful genetic screening tools in clinical practice [95]. The mutation is inherited as an autosomal and dominant trait; because the penetrance of *RET* mutations is almost 100 %, with few exceptions [96], virtually all gene heterozygous GC will develop MTC. Furthermore, no evidence of false-positive *RET* mutation diagnosis has been described, and all patients who underwent thyroidectomy on the basis of the genetic screening were found to have an MTC or at least CCH, which is considered a preneoplastic disease [97] (Fig. 90.2).

In approximately 4–10 % of MEN 2A or FMTC patients and approximately 95 % of those with MEN 2B, the germline *RET* mutation is a "de novo" mutation, as demonstrated by negative findings of *RET* genetic analysis in the patients' parents [98]. For this reason, between 5 % and 10 % of apparently sporadic MTC cases found to harbor a germline *RET* mutation are "de novo" or misdiagnosed familial cases [50].

Based on these lines of evidence, all guidelines recommend that all patients with MTC, regardless of their apparent sporadic origin, should be submitted to a blood test as a genetic screen for *RET* gene mutation. This procedure is of great relevance for the early diagnosis of gene carrier status in family members who are unaware of their condition [99].

All guidelines indicate that *RET* screening should begin with the analysis of the exons that are most likely to be involved according to the phenotype, if any, and then continue with the other more frequently involved exons. Sequencing of the entire coding region of the *RET* oncogene is not recommended as an initial testing method. However, ATA/ETA guidelines recommend whole-gene analysis when exons 10, 11, 13, 14, 14, 15, and 16 are negative for mutations despite a clinical presentation of MEN 2 or an unequivocal familial history (Fig. 90.3).

Screening for RET Gene Mutations in MEN 2 Family Members

Screening for *RET* gene mutations allows the early discovery of GC who can be treated with precocious or even prophylactic thyroidectomy, which may provide a definitive cure for this potentially lethal thyroid disease [100]. For this reason, family members of an MTC patient who harbors a germline

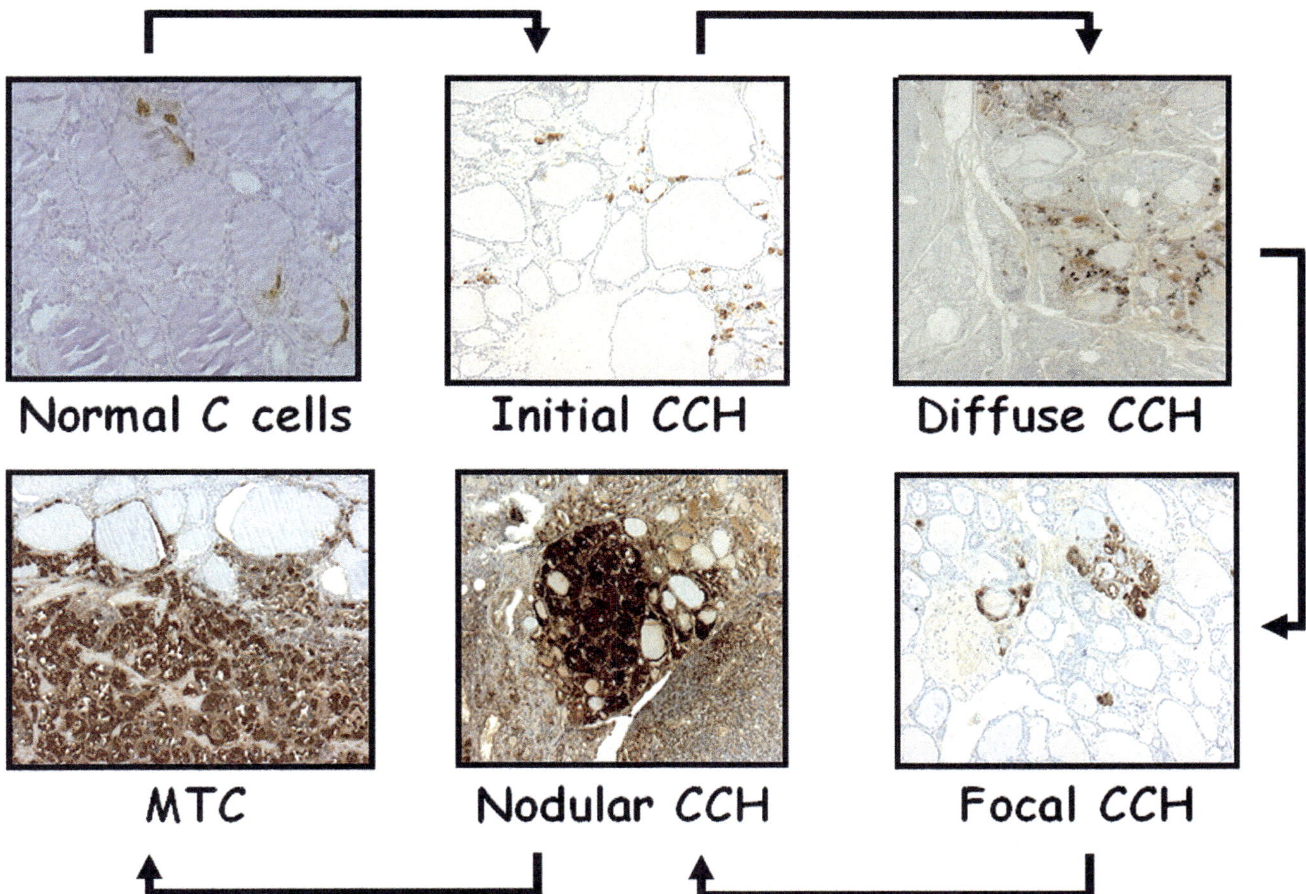

Fig. 90.2 Progression from normal C cells to medullary thyroid cancer (MTC) occurs through the development of C-cell hyperplasia (CCH) that is considered a preneoplastic lesion [97]

RET mutation (i.e., the index case) should be screened for the same *RET* mutation. This allows the early identification of GCs who are still clinically unaffected. It has also the advantage of exempting non-GC from further testing for the rest of their lives. All guidelines recommend that the genetic screening of family members be performed by qualified professional staff in close liaison with a genetic counselor, when possible.

Once the presence of a germline *RET* mutation has been established, the diagnosis of MEN 2/FMTC syndrome is unequivocal, but GC must undergo further clinical and biochemical evaluation to ascertain the actual development of the MTC and its extension, if already present. The question of when the GC should receive total thyroidectomy remains a matter of debate. ATA/ETA guidelines classify GC into four different risk levels for *RET* mutations (A, the lowest, to D, the highest) according to the aggressiveness and age of onset of MTC. This classification is suggested as a guide to plan surgical treatment of GC while the relationship between serum Ct levels and MTC development has been almost completely disregarded. Based on this classification ATA/ETA guidelines indicate that GC with ATA-D mutations should undergo prophylactic thyroidectomy as soon as possible, within the first year of age if already recognized; GC with ATA-C mutations should be submitted to prophylactic thyroidectomy before 5 years of age; GC with ATA-B and A mutations can be treated beyond age 5 years if serum Ct and neck ultrasound are negative and the familial history suggests a less aggressive MTC. Although neither BTA nor NCCA guidelines adopted any kind of *RET* mutation classification, both of them share the view of ATA/ETA guidelines about an early prophylactic thyroidectomy for GC who harbor *RET* mutations related to MEN 2B (i.e., ATA-D mutations). At variance, NCCN guidelines suggest to perform prophylactic thyroidectomy before 5 years of age in all GCs other than MEN 2B GC (i.e., ATA-C, ATA-B, and ATA-A mutations) but they specify that among these GCs the timing of prophylactic thyroidectomy should be better suggested by the aggressiveness of the inherited *RET* mutations. BTA guidelines suggest prophylactic thyroidectomy before 5 years of age for GC with mutations mainly related to MEN 2A (i.e, ATA-C and some ATA-B mutations) and after

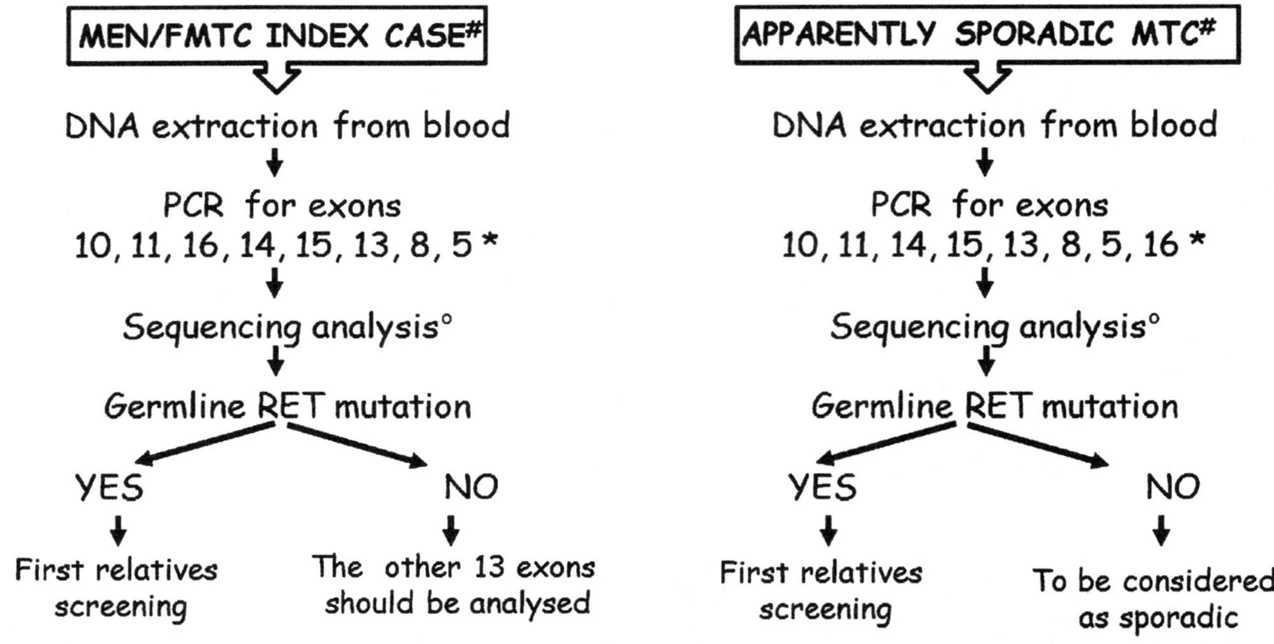

Fig. 90.3 Algorithm for germline *RET* mutations screening in patients with either a familial or an apparently sporadic MTC

10 years of age in GC with *RET* mutations related to FMTC (i.e, ATA-A and some ATA-B mutations). Recently, several evidences have been reported which show that the serum Ct levels, both basal or stimulated, can represent the best parameter to plan the timing and the extension of thyroidectomy (i.e., plus or minus central neck dissection) [59, 60].

The search for the involvement of other endocrine organs [101, 102] is recommended by all guidelines. Because of the strong genotype-phenotype correlation, screening for pheochromocytoma (MEN 2B or 2A) and hyperparathyroidism (MEN 2A) should be performed annually, whereas less frequent screening may be appropriate for patients with hereditary cases involving *RET* mutations at codons 768, 790, 804, and 891 or others that are frequently associated with FMTC. This is very clearly stated by the NCCN and, to a lesser extent, BTA guidelines. The ATA/ETA guidelines also provide an indication of the minimal age at which this screening should be performed: 8 years for MEN 2B and MEN 2A GC harboring a *RET* 634 or 630 mutation and 20 years of age for all FMTC GC and MEN 2A GC with other *RET* mutations. Again, this discussion is related to the evidence of a strong correlation between genotype and phenotype as well as the evidence that some *RET* mutations have less transforming potential and lower penetrance [103, 104].

Screening for Somatic RET Gene Mutations in Sporadic Cases

At present, the question of whether *RET* gene analysis should be performed to look for somatic mutations in sporadic MTC cases is not considered by either the BTA or NCCN guidelines. Conversely, this issue is discussed in the ATA/ETA guidelines; they ultimately do not recommend the routine evaluation of somatic mutation in sporadic MTC, although the opinion of the task force members was not unanimous. As reported in the ATA/ETA guidelines, there are at least three reasons for which the *RET* gene analysis should also be performed in frozen or paraffin-embedded tumoral tissue: (a) the discovery of a somatic mutation, which occurs in 45 % of cases, strongly supports the sporadic nature of the tumor [50]; (b) the presence/absence of the somatic mutation has prognostic value [105, 106]; (c) *RET* mutated patients may be able to be treated with drugs specifically aimed at inhibiting the altered *RET* gene in the future [92]. Considering all these observations, it appears that this information may have an important role in the planning of appropriate therapeutic and follow-up strategies.

Although current guidelines do not recommend a routine evaluation of somatic oncogene mutations in thyroid tumors, it could be useful to obtain it immediately after surgery on fresh tumor tissue as part of the pathological description because it is relatively difficult to get this information from paraffin-embedded tissue at a later date [107].

Conclusions

All MTC patients should be referred to a tertiary cancer center because MTC is a rare disease that requires an experienced multidisciplinary team to provide the best care. Nevertheless, even experienced specialists need guidelines, and these guidelines should be revised continuously. At present, there are several guidelines, but the BTA, NCCN, and ATA/ETA, each of which has its own unique recommendations, are the most up to date. Although the BTA and NCCN guidelines are relatively straightforward and focus immediately on the recommendations, the ATA/ETA guidelines cover the comprehensive management of MTC and addresses in detail the diagnosis and treatment of different types of MTC cases, from advanced disease to GC who have not yet developed a tumor. Despite these structural differences, a general consensus exists for the most important topics among these guidelines.

Some discordances may be related to differences in local standards of care; for example, in some countries, neck ultrasound is widely applied as a diagnostic tool by many specialists, including endocrinologists, oncologists and surgeons, and radiologists, whereas in other countries, its use is still restricted to a small number of specialists, making its use less friendly. Similarly, the controversy surrounding the issue of routine serum Ct measurement in all patients with thyroid nodules is, at least in part, related to the difficulty of obtaining pentagastrin in some countries, which is fundamental to confirm the suspicion of MTC based on relatively high serum levels of Ct. Furthermore, the problem of cost-effectiveness remains unresolved. These types of inconsistencies will be settled only by further studies.

Other still-debated issues, such as the ideal time to perform thyroidectomy in GC, require studies with long-term follow-up and a better characterization of the different *RET* germline mutations and their transforming activity. A novel area of research is represented by the tumor tissue molecular analysis, which is a common practice in some countries but completely ignored in others. Also, in this case, only the results of clinical trials with TKI and the relationship between the presence of *RET* somatic mutations and drug response will clarify the real need to perform *RET* molecular analysis in sporadic MTC.

While we await further studies that can improve our knowledge of the best management practices for this disease, the available guidelines represent an important reference point for multidisciplinary teams that must manage MTC patients in all their disease complexity.

References

1. Hazard JB, Hawk WA, Crile Jr G. Medullary (solid) carcinoma of the thyroid; a clinicopathologic entity. J Clin Endocrinol Metab. 1959;19:152–61.
2. Melvin KE, Tashjian Jr AH. The syndrome of excessive thyrocalcitonin produced by medullary carcinoma of the thyroid. Proc Natl Acad Sci U S A. 1968;59:1216–22.
3. Dube WJ, Bell GO, Aliapoulios MA. Thyrocalcitonin activity in metastatic medullary thyroid carcinoma. Further evidence for its parafollicular cell origin. Arch Intern Med. 1969;123:423–7.
4. Bergholm U, Adami HO, Telenius-Berg M, Johansson H, Wilander E. Incidence of sporadic and familial medullary thyroid carcinoma in Sweden 1959 through 1981. A nationwide study in 126 patients. Swedish MCT Study Group. Acta Oncol (Stockholm, Sweden). 1990;29:9–15.
5. Christensen SB, Ljungberg O, Tibblin S. A clinical epidemiologic study of thyroid carcinoma in Malmo, Sweden. Curr Probl Cancer. 1984;8:1–49.
6. Bondeson L, Ljungberg O. Occult thyroid carcinoma at autopsy in Malmo, Sweden. Cancer. 1981;47:319–23.
7. Bhattacharyya N. A population-based analysis of survival factors in differentiated and medullary thyroid carcinoma. Otolaryngol Head Neck Surg. 2003;128:115–23.
8. Machens A, Niccoli-Sire P, Hoegel J, et al. Early malignant progression of hereditary medullary thyroid cancer. N Engl J Med. 2003;349:1517–25.
9. Niccoli-Sire P, Murat A, Baudin E, et al. Early or prophylactic thyroidectomy in MEN 2/FMTC gene carriers: results in 71 thyroidectomized patients. The French Calcitonin Tumours Study Group (GETC). Eur J Endocrinol/Eur Fed Endocr Soc. 1999; 141:468–74.
10. Sanso GE, Domene HM, Garcia R, et al. Very early detection of RET proto-oncogene mutation is crucial for preventive thyroidectomy in multiple endocrine neoplasia type 2 children: presence of C-cell malignant disease in asymptomatic carriers. Cancer. 2002;94:323–30.
11. Christensen SB, Ljungberg O. Mortality from thyroid carcinoma in Malmo, Sweden 1960–1977. A clinical and pathologic study of 38 fatal cases. Cancer. 1984;54:1629–34.
12. Kebebew E, Ituarte PH, Siperstein AE, Duh QY, Clark OH. Medullary thyroid carcinoma: clinical characteristics, treatment, prognostic factors, and a comparison of staging systems. Cancer. 2000;88:1139–48.
13. Pelizzo MR, Boschin IM, Bernante P, et al. Natural history, diagnosis, treatment and outcome of medullary thyroid cancer: 37 years experience on 157 patients. Eur J Surg Oncol. 2007; 33:493–7.
14. Gharib H, McConahey WM, Tiegs RD, et al. Medullary thyroid carcinoma: clinicopathologic features and long-term follow-up of 65 patients treated during 1946 through 1970. Mayo Clin Proc. 1992;67:934–40.
15. Elisei R, Bottici V, Luchetti F, et al. Impact of routine measurement of serum calcitonin on the diagnosis and outcome of medullary thyroid cancer: experience in 10,864 patients with nodular thyroid disorders. J Clin Endocrinol Metab. 2004;89:163–8.
16. Vierhapper H, Niederle B, Bieglmayer C, Kaserer K, Baumgartner-Parzer S. Early diagnosis and curative therapy of medullary thyroid carcinoma by routine measurement of serum calcitonin in patients with thyroid disorders. Thyroid. 2005;15:1267–72.
17. Miccoli P, Minuto MN, Ugolini C, et al. Clinically unpredictable prognostic factors in the outcome of medullary thyroid cancer. Endocr Relat Cancer. 2007;14:1099–105.
18. Machens A, Frank-Raue K, Lorenz K, Rondot S, Raue F, Dralle H. Clinical relevance of RET variants G691S, L769L, S836S and

S904S to sporadic medullary thyroid cancer. Clin Endocrinol (Oxf). 2012;76:691–7.
19. Tashjian Jr AH, Melvin EW. Medullary carcinoma of the thyroid gland. Studies of thyrocalcitonin in plasma and tumor extracts. N Engl J Med. 1968;279:279–83.
20. Tubiana M, Milhaud G, Coutris G, Lacour J, Parmentier C, Bok B. Medullary carcinoma and thyrocalcitonin. Br Med J. 1968; 4:87–9.
21. Elisei R. Routine serum calcitonin measurement in the evaluation of thyroid nodules. Best Pract Res Clin Endocrinol Metab. 2008;22:941–53.
22. Kloos RT, Eng C, Evans DB, et al. Medullary thyroid cancer: management guidelines of the American Thyroid Association. Thyroid. 2009;19:565–612.
23. Cooper DS, Doherty GM, Haugen BR, et al. Revised American Thyroid Association management guidelines for patients with thyroid nodules and differentiated thyroid cancer. Thyroid. 2009;19:1167–214.
24. Pacini F, Schlumberger M, Dralle H, Elisei R, Smit JW, Wiersinga W. European consensus for the management of patients with differentiated thyroid carcinoma of the follicular epithelium. Eur J Endocrinol. 2006;154:787–803.
25. British Thyoid Association RCoPRottcgug. Management of medullary thyroid cancer. In: Perros P, editor. Guidelines for the management of thyroid cancer. London: Royal College of Physician; 2007. p. 41–8.
26. Tuttle RM BD, Byrd D, Dilawari RA, Doerthy GM, Duh Q, Ehya H, Farrar WB, Haddad RI, Gallagher L, Hunt JP, Kandeel F, Kloos RT, Kopp P, Lamonica DM, Loree TR, Lydiatt WM, McCaffrey J, Moley JF, Olson JA, Parks l, Ridge JA, Shah JP, Sherman SI, Sturgeon C, Waguespack SG, Wang TN, Wirth J. National Comprehensive Cancer Network (NCCN) guidelines on thyroid carcinoma. 2012. http://www.nccn.org/index.asp.
27. Block MA, Jackson CE, Greenawald KA, Yott JB, Tashjian Jr AH. Clinical characteristics distinguishing hereditary from sporadic medullary thyroid carcinoma. Treatment implications. Arch Surg. 1980;115:142–8.
28. Baylin SB, Gann DS, Hsu SH. Clonal origin of inherited medullary thyroid carcinoma and pheochromocytoma. Science (New York, NY). 1976;193:321–3.
29. Wolfe HJ, Delellis RA. Familial medullary thyroid carcinoma and C cell hyperplasia. Clin Endocrinol Metab. 1981;10:351–65.
30. Gharib H, Papini E, Paschke R, et al. American Association of Clinical Endocrinologists, Associazione Medici Endocrinologi, and European Thyroid Association medical guidelines for clinical practice for the diagnosis and management of thyroid nodules: executive summary of recommendations. J Endocrinol Invest. 2010;33:51–6.
31. Pacini F, Fontanelli M, Fugazzola L, et al. Routine measurement of serum calcitonin in nodular thyroid diseases allows the preoperative diagnosis of unsuspected sporadic medullary thyroid carcinoma. J Clin Endocrinol Metab. 1994;78:826–9.
32. Rieu M, Lame MC, Richard A, et al. Prevalence of sporadic medullary thyroid carcinoma: the importance of routine measurement of serum calcitonin in the diagnostic evaluation of thyroid nodules. Clin Endocrinol (Oxf). 1995;42:453–60.
33. Niccoli P, Wion-Barbot N, Caron P, et al. Interest of routine measurement of serum calcitonin: study in a large series of thyroidectomized patients. The French Medullary Study Group. J Clin Endocrinol Metab. 1997;82:338–41.
34. Vierhapper H, Raber W, Bieglmayer C, Kaserer K, Weinhausl A, Niederle B. Routine measurement of plasma calcitonin in nodular thyroid diseases. J Clin Endocrinol Metab. 1997;82:1589–93.
35. Kaserer K, Scheuba C, Neuhold N, et al. C-cell hyperplasia and medullary thyroid carcinoma in patients routinely screened for serum calcitonin. Am J Surg Pathol. 1998;22:722–8.
36. Ozgen AG, Hamulu F, Bayraktar F, et al. Evaluation of routine basal serum calcitonin measurement for early diagnosis of medullary thyroid carcinoma in seven hundred seventy-three patients with nodular goiter. Thyroid. 1999;9:579–82.
37. Hahm JR, Lee MS, Min YK, et al. Routine measurement of serum calcitonin is useful for early detection of medullary thyroid carcinoma in patients with nodular thyroid diseases. Thyroid. 2001; 11:73–80.
38. Bieglmayer C, Scheuba C, Niederle B, Flores J, Vierhapper H. Screening for medullary thyroid carcinoma: experience with different immunoassays for human calcitonin. Wien Klin Wochenschr. 2002;114:267–73.
39. Tommasi M, Brocchi A, Cappellini A, Raspanti S, Mannelli M. False serum calcitonin high levels using a non-competitive two-site IRMA. J Endocrinol Invest. 2001;24:356–60.
40. Giovanella L, Suriano S. Spurious hypercalcitoninemia and heterophilic antibodies in patients with thyroid nodules. Head Neck. 2011;33:95–7.
41. Toledo SP, Lourenco Jr DM, Santos MA, Tavares MR, Toledo RA, Correia-Deur JE. Hypercalcitoninemia is not pathognomonic of medullary thyroid carcinoma. Clinics (Sao Paulo). 2009;64: 699–706.
42. Doyle P, Duren C, Nerlich K, et al. Potency and tolerance of calcitonin stimulation with high-dose calcium versus pentagastrin in normal adults. J Clin Endocrinol Metab. 2009;94:2970–4.
43. Barbot N, Calmettes C, Schuffenecker I, et al. Pentagastrin stimulation test and early diagnosis of medullary thyroid carcinoma using an immunoradiometric assay of calcitonin: comparison with genetic screening in hereditary medullary thyroid carcinoma. J Clin Endocrinol Metab. 1994;78:114–20.
44. Samaan NA, Castillo S, Schultz PN, Khalil KG, Johnston DA. Serum calcitonin after pentagastrin stimulation in patients with bronchogenic and breast cancer compared to that in patients with medullary thyroid carcinoma. J Clin Endocrinol Metab. 1980;51: 237–41.
45. Colombo C, Verga U, Mian C, et al. Comparison of calcium and pentagastrin tests for the diagnosis and follow-up of medullary thyroid cancer. J Clin Endocrinol Metab. 2012;97:905–13.
46. Hodak SP, Burman KD. The calcitonin conundrum – is it time for routine measurement of serum calcitonin in patients with thyroid nodules? J Clin Endocrinol Metab. 2004;89:511–4.
47. Deftos LJ. Should serum calcitonin be routinely measured in patients with thyroid nodules – will the law answer before endocrinologists do? J Clin Endocrinol Metab. 2004;89:4768–9; author reply 9–70.
48. Boi F, Maurelli I, Pinna G, et al. Calcitonin measurement in washout fluid from fine needle aspiration of neck masses in patients with primary and metastatic medullary thyroid carcinoma. J Clin Endocrinol Metab. 2007;92:2115–8.
49. Forrest CH, Frost FA, de Boer WB, Spagnolo DV, Whitaker D, Sterrett BF. Medullary carcinoma of the thyroid: accuracy of diagnosis of fine-needle aspiration cytology. Cancer. 1998;84:295–302.
50. Elisei R, Romei C, Cosci B, et al. RET genetic screening in patients with medullary thyroid cancer and their relatives: experience with 807 individuals at one center. J Clin Endocrinol Metab. 2007;92:4725–9.
51. Ahmed SR, Ball DW. Clinical review: incidentally discovered medullary thyroid cancer: diagnostic strategies and treatment. J Clin Endocrinol Metab. 2011;96:1237–45.
52. Raffel A, Cupisti K, Krausch M, Wolf A, Schulte KM, Roher HD. Incidentally found medullary thyroid cancer: treatment rationale for small tumors. World J Surg. 2004;28:397–401.
53. Eng C, Mulligan LM, Smith DP, et al. Low frequency of germline mutations in the RET proto-oncogene in patients with apparently sporadic medullary thyroid carcinoma. Clin Endocrinol (Oxf). 1995;43:123–7.

54. Wiench M, Wygoda Z, Gubala E, et al. Estimation of risk of inherited medullary thyroid carcinoma in apparent sporadic patients. J Clin Oncol. 2001;19:1374–80.
55. Ukkat J, Gimm O, Brauckhoff M, Bilkenroth U, Dralle H. Single center experience in primary surgery for medullary thyroid carcinoma. World J Surg. 2004;28:1271–4.
56. Moley JF, DeBenedetti MK. Patterns of nodal metastases in palpable medullary thyroid carcinoma: recommendations for extent of node dissection. Ann Surg. 1999;229:880–7; discussion 7–8.
57. Fleming JB, Lee JE, Bouvet M, et al. Surgical strategy for the treatment of medullary thyroid carcinoma. Ann Surg. 1999;230: 697–707.
58. Dralle H, Gimm O, Simon D, et al. Prophylactic thyroidectomy in 75 children and adolescents with hereditary medullary thyroid carcinoma: German and Austrian experience. World J Surg. 1998;22:744–50; discussion 50–1.
59. Rohmer V, Vidal-Trecan G, Bourdelot A, et al. Prognostic factors of disease-free survival after thyroidectomy in 170 young patients with a RET germline mutation: a multicenter study of the Groupe Francais d'Etude des Tumeurs Endocrines. J Clin Endocrinol Metab. 2011;96:E509–18.
60. Elisei R, Romei C, Renzini G, et al. The timing of total thyroidectomy in RET gene mutation carriers could be personalized and safely planned on the basis of serum calcitonin: 18 years experience at one single center. J Clin Endocrinol Metab. 2012; 97:426–35.
61. Kahraman T, de Groot JW, Rouwe C, et al. Acceptable age for prophylactic surgery in children with multiple endocrine neoplasia type 2a. Eur J Surg Oncol. 2003;29:331–5.
62. Jadoul M, Leo JR, Berends MJ, et al. Pheochromocytoma-induced hypertensive encephalopathy revealing MEN-IIa syndrome in a 13-year old boy. Implications for screening procedures and surgery. Horm Metab Res. 1989;21:46–9.
63. Scollo C, Baudin E, Travagli JP, et al. Rationale for central and bilateral lymph node dissection in sporadic and hereditary medullary thyroid cancer. J Clin Endocrinol Metab. 2003;88:2070–5.
64. Franc S, Niccoli-Sire P, Cohen R, et al. Complete surgical lymph node resection does not prevent authentic recurrences of medullary thyroid carcinoma. Clin Endocrinol (Oxf). 2001;55:403–9.
65. Dralle H, Damm I, Scheumann GF, Kotzerke J, Kupsch E. Frequency and significance of cervicomediastinal lymph node metastases in medullary thyroid carcinoma: results of a compartment-oriented microdissection method. Henry Ford Hosp Med J. 1992;40:264–7.
66. Gimm O, Ukkat J, Dralle H. Determinative factors of biochemical cure after primary and reoperative surgery for sporadic medullary thyroid carcinoma. World J Surg. 1998;22:562–7; discussion 7–8.
67. Brierley J, Tsang R, Simpson WJ, Gospodarowicz M, Sutcliffe S, Panzarella T. Medullary thyroid cancer: analyses of survival and prognostic factors and the role of radiation therapy in local control. Thyroid. 1996;6:305–10.
68. Fersht N, Vini L, A'Hern R, Harmer C. The role of radiotherapy in the management of elevated calcitonin after surgery for medullary thyroid cancer. Thyroid. 2001;11:1161–8.
69. Wells Jr SA, Haagensen Jr DE, Linehan WM, Farrell RE, Dilley WG. The detection of elevated plasma levels of carcinoembryonic antigen in patients with suspected or established medullary thyroid carcinoma. Cancer. 1978;42:1498–503.
70. Fugazzola L, Pinchera A, Luchetti F, et al. Disappearance rate of serum calcitonin after total thyroidectomy for medullary thyroid carcinoma. Int J Biol Markers. 1994;9:21–4.
71. Pellegriti G, Leboulleux S, Baudin E, et al. Long-term outcome of medullary thyroid carcinoma in patients with normal postoperative medical imaging. Br J Cancer. 2003;88:1537–42.
72. Faggiano A, Grimaldi F, Pezzullo L, et al. Secretive and proliferative tumor profile helps to select the best imaging technique to identify postoperative persistent or relapsing medullary thyroid cancer. Endocr Relat Cancer. 2009;16:225–31.
73. Giraudet AL, Vanel D, Leboulleux S, et al. Imaging medullary thyroid carcinoma with persistent elevated calcitonin levels. J Clin Endocrinol Metab. 2007;92:4185–90.
74. Koopmans KP, de Groot JW, Plukker JT, et al. 18F-dihydroxyphenylalanine PET in patients with biochemical evidence of medullary thyroid cancer: relation to tumor differentiation. J Nucl Med. 2008;49:524–31.
75. Baudin E, Lumbroso J, Schlumberger M, et al. Comparison of octreotide scintigraphy and conventional imaging in medullary thyroid carcinoma. J Nucl Med. 1996;37:912–6.
76. Szakall Jr S, Esik O, Bajzik G, et al. 18F-FDG PET detection of lymph node metastases in medullary thyroid carcinoma. J Nucl Med. 2002;43:66–71.
77. Arslan N, Ilgan S, Yuksel D, et al. Comparison of In-111 octreotide and Tc-99m (V) DMSA scintigraphy in the detection of medullary thyroid tumor foci in patients with elevated levels of tumor markers after surgery. Clin Nucl Med. 2001;26: 683–8.
78. Abdelmoumene N, Schlumberger M, Gardet P, et al. Selective venous sampling catheterisation for localisation of persisting medullary thyroid carcinoma. Br J Cancer. 1994;69:1141–4.
79. Frank-Raue K, Raue F, Buhr HJ, Baldauf G, Lorenz D, Ziegler R. Localization of occult persisting medullary thyroid carcinoma before microsurgical reoperation: high sensitivity of selective venous catheterization. Thyroid. 1992;2:113–7.
80. Ben Mrad MD, Gardet P, Roche A, et al. Value of venous catheterization and calcitonin studies in the treatment and management of clinically inapparent medullary thyroid carcinoma. Cancer. 1989;63:133–8.
81. Meijer JA, le Cessie S, van den Hout WB, et al. Calcitonin and carcinoembryonic antigen doubling times as prognostic factors in medullary thyroid carcinoma: a structured meta-analysis. Clin Endocrinol (Oxf). 2010;72:534–42.
82. Barbet J, Campion L, Kraeber-Bodere F, Chatal JF. Prognostic impact of serum calcitonin and carcinoembryonic antigen doubling-times in patients with medullary thyroid carcinoma. J Clin Endocrinol Metab. 2005;90:6077–84.
83. Baloch Z, Carayon P, Conte-Devolx B, et al. Laboratory medicine practice guidelines. Laboratory support for the diagnosis and monitoring of thyroid disease. Thyroid. 2003;13:3–126.
84. Demers LM, Spencer CA. Laboratory medicine practice guidelines: laboratory support for the diagnosis and monitoring of thyroid disease. Clin Endocrinol (Oxf). 2003;58:138–40.
85. Tamagnini P, Bernante P, Piotto A, Toniato A, Pelizzo MR. Reoperation of medullary thyroid carcinoma: long-term results. Ann Chir. 2001;126:762–7.
86. Kebebew E, Kikuchi S, Duh QY, Clark OH. Long-term results of reoperation and localizing studies in patients with persistent or recurrent medullary thyroid cancer. Arch Surg. 2000;135: 895–901.
87. Tisell LE, Jansson S. Recent results of reoperative surgery in medullary carcinoma of the thyroid. Wien Klin Wochenschr. 1988; 100:347–8.
88. Tisell LE, Hansson G, Jansson S, Salander H. Reoperation in the treatment of asymptomatic metastasizing medullary thyroid carcinoma. Surgery. 1986;99:60–6.
89. Moley JF, Debenedetti MK, Dilley WG, Tisell LE, Wells SA. Surgical management of patients with persistent or recurrent medullary thyroid cancer. J Intern Med. 1998;243:521–6.
90. Dralle H. Lymph node dissection and medullary thyroid carcinoma. Br J Surg. 2002;89:1073–5.
91. Fialkowski E, DeBenedetti M, Moley J. Long-term outcome of reoperations for medullary thyroid carcinoma. World J Surg. 2008;32:754–65.

92. Wells Jr SA, Robinson BG, Gagel RF, et al. Vandetanib in patients with locally advanced or metastatic medullary thyroid cancer: a randomized, double-blind phase III trial. J Clin Oncol. 2012; 30:134–41.
93. Schlumberger M, Carlomagno F, Baudin E, Bidart JM, Santoro M. New therapeutic approaches to treat medullary thyroid carcinoma. Nat Clin Pract Endocrinol Metab. 2008;4:22–32.
94. Orlandi F, Caraci P, Mussa A, Saggiorato E, Pancani G, Angeli A. Treatment of medullary thyroid carcinoma: an update. Endocr Relat Cancer. 2001;8:135–47.
95. Eng C, Clayton D, Schuffenecker I, et al. The relationship between specific RET proto-oncogene mutations and disease phenotype in multiple endocrine neoplasia type 2. International RET mutation consortium analysis. Jama. 1996;276:1575–9.
96. Elisei R, Cosci B, Romei C, et al. Identification of a novel point mutation in the RET gene (Ala883Thr), which is associated with medullary thyroid carcinoma phenotype only in homozygous condition. J Clin Endocrinol Metab. 2004;89:5823–7.
97. LiVolsi VA. C cell hyperplasia/neoplasia. J Clin Endocrinol Metab. 1997;82:39–41.
98. Schuffenecker I, Ginet N, Goldgar D, et al. Prevalence and parental origin of de novo RET mutations in multiple endocrine neoplasia type 2A and familial medullary thyroid carcinoma. Le Groupe d'Etude des Tumeurs a Calcitonine. Am J Hum Genet. 1997;60:233–7.
99. Romei C, Cosci B, Renzini G, et al. RET genetic screening of sporadic medullary thyroid cancer (MTC) allows the preclinical diagnosis of unsuspected gene carriers and the identification of a relevant percentage of hidden familial MTC (FMTC). Clin Endocrinol (Oxf). 2011;74:241–7.
100. Pacini F, Romei C, Miccoli P, et al. Early treatment of hereditary medullary thyroid carcinoma after attribution of multiple endocrine neoplasia type 2 gene carrier status by screening for ret gene mutations. Surgery. 1995;118:1031–5.
101. Jimenez C, Gagel RF. Genetic testing in endocrinology: lessons learned from experience with multiple endocrine neoplasia type 2 (MEN2). Growth Horm IGF Res. 2004;14(Suppl A): S150–7.
102. Brandi ML, Gagel RF, Angeli A, et al. Guidelines for diagnosis and therapy of MEN type 1 and type 2. J Clin Endocrinol Metab. 2001;86:5658–71.
103. Cosci B, Vivaldi A, Romei C, et al. In silico and in vitro analysis of rare germline allelic variants of RET oncogene associated with medullary thyroid cancer. Endocr Relat Cancer. 2011;18:603.
104. Erlic Z, Hoffmann MM, Sullivan M, et al. Pathogenicity of DNA variants and double mutations in multiple endocrine neoplasia type 2 and von Hippel-Lindau syndrome. J Clin Endocrinol Metab. 2010;95:308–13.
105. Elisei R, Cosci B, Romei C, et al. Prognostic significance of somatic RET oncogene mutations in sporadic medullary thyroid cancer: a 10-year follow-up study. J Clin Endocrinol Metab. 2008;93:682–7.
106. Moura MM, Cavaco BM, Pinto AE, et al. Correlation of RET somatic mutations with clinicopathological features in sporadic medullary thyroid carcinomas. Br J Cancer. 2009;100:1777–83.
107. Tang W, David FB, Wilson MM, Barwick BG, Leyland-Jones BR, Bouzyk MM. DNA extraction from formalin-fixed, paraffin-embedded tissue. Cold Spring Harb Protoc. 2009;2009:pdb prot5138.

Part XI

Undifferentiated Tumors: Thyroid Lymphoma

Thyroid Lymphoma

91

Robert C. Smallridge

Epidemiology

Thyroid lymphomas (TLs) [1–68] represent but a small fraction of thyroid malignancies. Unlike differentiated thyroid cancers (DTCs) which are associated in some instances with environmental radioiodine exposure, the principal risk factor for primary thyroid lymphoma is preexisting chronic lymphocytic thyroiditis (Hashimoto's disease) [5, 10, 33, 69]. In fact, the risk of TL has been reported as increased more than 60-fold by thyroiditis [2, 60]. The thyroid gland is normally devoid of lymphocytes, and it has been proposed that their infiltration can initiate the process of lymphomagenesis [33, 70, 71]. However, the efficiency of such an evolution is weak, as chronic thyroiditis affects millions of patients worldwide. In contrast, thyroid cancer comprises no more than a small percentage of all malignancies. Furthermore, thyroid lymphomas are even rarer. Geographic distributions have reported that TLs represent 3.4 % of thyroid malignancies at Mayo Clinic in the United States [50], 2.9 % in Italy [67], 1.3 % in Turkey [20], 1.2 % in the SEER database [72], 1.1 % in Saudi Arabia [47], and 0.6 % in Greece [48]. The frequency may be higher in areas where iodine prophylaxis increases the incidence of thyroiditis [61].

Histopathology

Thyroid lymphoma is almost always due to a monoclonal population of B cells, with T-cell TLs occurring infrequently [3, 12, 39, 49, 52, 56, 59, 62, 66, 73]. The most common and aggressive histologic subtype is the diffuse large B-cell lymphoma (DLBCL), seen in a median of 67 % of patients (range: 40–100 %) [11–13, 17, 24, 30, 38, 39, 52, 56, 59, 72], followed by the mucosa-associated lymphoid tissue (MALT) lymphoma in a median of 28 % [4, 8, 11, 12, 17, 18, 24, 38, 39, 52, 56, 59, 63, 72]. Follicular lymphomas have been described in 5.5 % [11, 12, 17, 38, 39, 52, 56, 59, 72], with the exception of a report by Bacon et al. [35] containing only follicular cell lymphomas. Hodgkin's thyroid lymphomas are also uncommon [5, 17, 25, 38, 41, 65]. Differentiated thyroid cancer is observed rarely as a second malignancy associated with thyroid lymphomas [58].

Clinical Characteristics

Thyroid lymphoma has a similar presentation to anaplastic thyroid carcinoma in that it occurs primarily in women (3:1) in their mid-60s (Table 91.1) with a chief complaint of a rapidly expanding neck mass in almost all cases [1, 5, 6, 8, 10–13, 15, 17, 22, 23, 25, 32, 39, 41, 49, 52, 55–57, 59, 64, 65, 74, 75]. Other symptoms noted due to the tumor include hoarseness [6, 10–13, 23, 25, 41, 49, 52, 55, 57, 59, 64–66], dysphagia [6, 10–13, 23, 25, 41, 49, 52, 55, 57, 63–66, 74, 75], dyspnea [11, 13, 23, 25, 49, 52, 55, 57, 59, 63–66, 75], and on occasion, the superior vena cava syndrome [57, 65] (Table 91.2). Systemic, or "B" symptoms (e.g., night sweats, fever, weight loss) [8, 10, 13, 23, 25, 38, 41, 49, 52, 55, 59, 74, 75] occur in 10 %, and hypothyroidism due to chronic thyroiditis is present in one-third of patients [5, 6, 10, 22, 25, 39, 41, 49, 52, 64, 65, 74].

Staging is according to the Ann Arbor staging classification [76], and defines whether the lymphoma is confined to the thyroid gland (stage IE), is restricted to the thyroid and locoregional sites (IIE) or is disseminated (stage IIIE involves more distant lymph nodes and/or the spleen, while IVE involves additional non-lymphatic organs). Unlike differentiated thyroid cancers, which usually are

R.C. Smallridge, MD (✉)
Division of Endocrinology & Metabolism, Mayo Clinic, Jacksonville, FL, USA

Department of Medicine, Mayo Clinic, Jacksonville, FL, USA

Department of Cancer Biology, Mayo Clinic, Jacksonville, FL, USA
e-mail: smallridge.robert@mayo.edu

L. Wartofsky, D. Van Nostrand (eds.), *Thyroid Cancer*, DOI 10.1007/978-1-4939-3314-3_91

Table 91.1 Clinical characteristics of patients with thyroid lymphoma

Gender	3219
Female	2420
Male	799
Age (year)	
Median (range) (n=26)	66 (9–95)
Mean (n=21)	64.4
Chronic thyroiditis (n=27)	60 % (14–100)
Stage, median	
IE (n=32)	54 % (8–82)
IIE (n=33)	34 % (5–76)
III-IVE (n=18)	9 % (4–46)

n number of reports

Table 91.2 Frequency of symptoms at presentation of thyroid lymphoma

Symptoms (n)	Frequency (median)
Neck mass (n=27)	98 % (30–100)
Hoarse/dysphonia (n=17)	30 % (2–58)
Dysphagia (n=19)	30 % (7–33)
Dyspnea (n=15)	28 % (6–65)
SVC syndrome	7 % (4–10)
B symptoms (n=13)	10 % (2–35 %)
Hypothyroid (n=12)	32 % (23–56)

SVC superior vena cava syndrome, *n* number of reports

not extensively staged prior to surgery, accurate anatomic (and histologic) staging of thyroid lymphomas plays an important role in guiding initial therapy.

Diagnosis

Papillary thyroid cancers are diagnosed with high success by fine-needle aspiration (FNA), while follicular and Hürthle cell cancers require surgical resection for adequate tissue sample. FNA also has a variable success rate for diagnosing thyroid lymphomas. Sun et al. [52] reported a low yield of 5 % with FNA, while others have reported a median positivity for FNA of 59 % (range: 25–90 %) [4, 6, 16, 22, 26, 39, 41, 46, 49]. Diffuse large B-cell lymphomas are relatively easy to recognize, while MALT lymphomas, with their small cells, are difficult to distinguish from lymphocytic thyroiditis [22, 29]. At Mayo Clinic, 1,945 thyroid FNAs were reviewed, and the sensitivity/specificity was 0.73/0.99 for suspicious and 0.25/0.99 for positive lymphoma [50]. Light chain restriction can aid in distinguishing chronic thyroiditis from lymphoma [3, 10]. When suspected, a core tissue or open biopsy is often required [70], and the diagnosis is confirmed by flow cytometry and immunophenotyping [46, 68, 70, 77]. B-cell phenotype can be recognized by having CD20(+) cells on immunocytochemistry [11, 22, 30], and some lymphomas have been distinguished from anaplastic thyroid cancer when IgM, IgG, or IgA was demonstrated by IHC [78]. Other test strategies have included an IHC algorithm (GCETI; CD10; Bcl6; MUM1; FOXP1) [40] and vectorette PCR detection of (IgH) heavy chain rearrangement [26, 79]. One T-cell lymphoma was recognized by ICC as CD20 and CD30 (–) and CD40RO and CD43(+) [62]. Molecular genetic abnormalities have been reported [80]. Streubel et al. [81] detected a t(3:14)(p14.1q32) translocation in three of six thyroidal MALT lymphomas. Takakuwa et al. [14] found Fas gene mutations in 17/26 (65.4 %) of thyroid lymphomas, but also in 3 of 11 (27.3 %) cases of Hashimoto's disease, suggesting this could be an early event. These authors more recently described aberrant somatic hypermutations (ASHM) of several proto-oncogenes, with the highest frequency in thyroid follicular lymphomas [43], while hypermethylation of p73 has also been noted [28]. Aggarwal et al. [82] examined 33 thyroid lymphoma patients for mutations seen in thyroid carcinoma. BRAF mutations were detected in six cases of DLBCL (only one was the V600E mutation), and NRAS mutations were found in two cases.

Imaging

Patients with thyroid lymphoma should have extensive imaging for proper staging. No single technique is specific, but FDG-PET [31, 83], PET/CT [36, 44, 53], ^{67}Gallium [22], and MRI [9] have all been utilized. Thyroid lymphoma has a higher SUVmax and lower CT density than does chronic thyroiditis on 18 FDG-PET/CT imaging [84]. Kim et al. [18] described three types of CT findings in the thyroid in a small number of patients: type 1 = solitary nodule; type 2 = multinodular goiter; type 3 = homogenous, bilateral enlargement. The latter finding occurred most commonly and in the setting of rapid development should suggest lymphoma (or anaplastic cancer). An illustrative case is seen in Fig. 91.1.

Therapy

Therapeutic options include surgery, radiotherapy, and chemotherapy. When it was determined that thyroid lymphomas were sensitive to chemo- and radiotherapy, surgery was no longer recommended except for biopsy and acute airway compromise. Nevertheless, surgery (including lobectomy and subtotal and total thyroidectomy) was employed in a median of 54 % of patients (range: 10–100 %) [1, 4, 5, 8, 13, 15, 18, 19, 23–25, 35, 39, 49, 52, 55–57, 59, 63, 74, 75], usually in

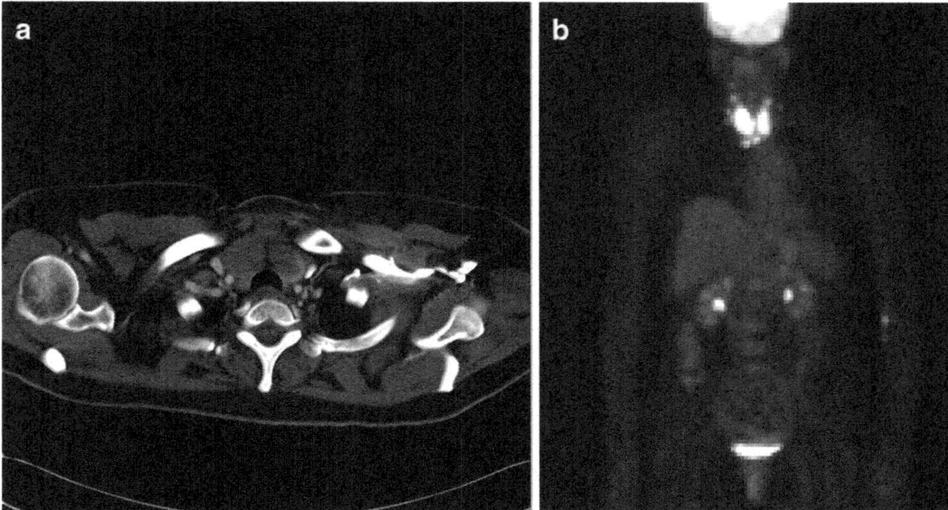

Fig. 91.1 A 66-year-old woman presented with a 6-week history of a choking sensation, cough, hoarseness, and enlarging neck mass. Neck symptoms improved after thyroid isthmusectomy. Pathology confirmed a low-grade thyroid MALT lymphoma, CD20+. No fusions of API2 or MALT1 gene loci were detected. Thyroid peroxidase and thyroglobulin antibodies were positive. Bone marrow exam was negative. (**a**) CT scan 8 days post-op showed bilateral thyroid enlargement and a hypodense lesion and bilateral lymph nodes. (**b**) A PET scan showed intense hypermetabolic activity within the thyroid gland and cervical lymph nodes

conjunction with radiation and/or chemotherapy. Tracheostomy has also been needed at times [5, 13, 41, 52, 56, 57, 63, 75] (Table 91.3).

Radiation therapy is effective for local neck disease, particularly for MALT lymphoma, with a median dose of 40 Gy commonly reported [8, 23, 52, 65]. Chemotherapy is also effective, with the usual regimen being CHOP (cyclophosphamide, doxorubicin, vincristine, and prednisone). In recent years, rituximab, an anti-CD 20 monoclonal antibody, has been added to the regimen for B-cell lymphomas [85], but most series reviewed have not included this addition for thyroid lymphoma except in a few patients [17, 37, 45, 54]. There are no prospective trials demonstrating a superior treatment paradigm, although randomized trials of nodal and extranodal non-Hodgkin's lymphoma showed CHOP + radiotherapy was more effective than chemotherapy alone [86, 87], and Table 91.3 illustrates that many combinations involving monotherapy and combination multimodal therapy (CMT) have been used. CMT is employed most commonly, and Mian et al. [55] reported a higher complete response rate (90 vs. 76 %) using CMT, and Matsuzuka et al. [6] found that radiotherapy + CHOP (6 courses) was associated with a higher survival (100 vs. 75 %) than radiotherapy + MOPP (1–2 courses). In an evidence-based review, chemoradiation was recommended in all but stage IE thyroid MALT lymphomas [29]. A phase II prospective study of local radiation for extranodal stage IE MALT lymphomas showed a high CR rate, but only 11 % of patients have thyroid lymphomas [88]. Another general review on thyroid lymphoma has appeared recently [89].

Response Rates

Doria et al. [7] reviewed 211 patients and noted a relapse rate of 43 % after chemotherapy and 37.1 % after radiation therapy but only 7.7 % after combined modality treatment. Table 91.4 depicts the complete response (CR) and relapse rates and some possible predictive factors. A variety of factors may contribute to the percentage of patients achieving a CR including histologic type, stage at presentation, and treatment modality. In the study by Laing et al. [8], the high response rate of 96 % might be expected, as 82 % of patients had stage IE disease (and none were stage III-IVE), and 69 % have MALT lymphomas, which generally are more indolent. However, only 9 % of the patients received combined modality therapy, which may explain the 26 % recurrence rate. There are few studies with sufficiently comparable data, however, which makes comparisons across series difficult (Table 91.4).

Survival

Survival has been reported in several ways. Some authors have provided 5-year progression-free survivals (PFS), with a range of 57–84 % (Table 91.5). Only one study showed PFS for stage IE vs. IIE patients (91 and 59 %, respectively) [13]. Several studies provide 5-year disease (or cause-)-specific survival (DSS), with a range of 46–100 %. The most commonly available metric is 5-year overall survival data with a median of 70 % (Table 91.5).

Table 91.3 Treatment modalities in primary thyroid lymphoma

Ref.	No.	Surg	Trach	RT	ChemoRx	Surg+RT	Surg+Ch	RT+chemo (±surg)
Alzouebi [74]	70	4 %	–	41 %	26 %	24 %	3 %	[a]
Aozasa [1]	79	3 %	–	[a]	[a]	[a]	[a]	24 %
Bacon [35]	22[b]	9 %	–	–	–	18 %	9 %	32 %
Belal [13]	52	6 %	17 %	4 %	25 %	–	–	65 %
Derringer [11]	108	25 %	–	–	–	18 %	15 %	42 %
DiBiase [19]	27	–	–	22 %	–	48 %	–	30 %
Doria [7]	211	[a]	–	75 %	6 %	[a]	[a]	19 %
Gupta [22]	10	–	–	–	–	–	–	100 %
Harrington [23]	91	–	–	–	2 %	68 %	–	30 %
Hwang [39]	44	12 %	–	2 %	25 %	18 %	20 %	23 %
Joshi [41]	9	Limited role	11 %	–	–	–	–	100 %
Katna [75]	64	[a]	3 %	[a]	[a]	[a]	[a]	44 %
Kuper-Hommel [24]	38	11 %	–	16 %	13 %	24 %	13 %	18 %
Laing [8]	45	2 %	–	87 %	2 %	–	–	9 %
Mian [55]	48	–	–	6 %	27 %	2 %	15 %	50 %
Onal [56]	87	–	9 %	6 %	14 %	19 %	19 %	42 %
Penney [57]	63	[a]	21 %	[a]	[a]	[a]	[a]	49 %
Pyke [4]	62	10 %	–	–	–	68 %	16 %	6 %
Rasbach [64]	20	Limited role	–	40 %	5 %	15 %	–	40 %
Sasai [66]	22	[a]	–	[a]	[a]	[a]	[a]	86 %
Scholefield [5]	22	4 %	9 %[c]	23 %	14 %	41 %	–	14 %
Sippel [63]	27	11 %	18 %	–	–	37 %	15 %	37 %
Skacel [12]	42	–	–	26 %	29 %	5 %	2 %	38 %
Sun [52]	40	[a]	5 %	[a]	[a]	[a]	[a]	70 %
Watanabe [59]	161	[a]	–	[a]	[a]	[a]	[a]	59 %
Wirtzfeld [15]	10	10 %	–	–	–	40 %	30 %	20 %
Median		9.5 %	10 %	22.5 %	14 %	24 %	15 %	38 %

Surg surgery, *Trach* tracheostomy, *RT* radiation therapy, *ChemoRx* chemotherapy
– Information not mentioned
[a]Unable to determine percentage
[b]Information not available in 7
[c]One patient had tracheostomy only

Table 91.4 Response and relapse rates: effects of histology, stage, and multimodal therapy (percentages)

			Histology		Stage			
References	Complete response	Relapse	DLBCL	MALT	IE	IIE	III-IVE	Multimodal therapy
Pyke [4]	74	19	–	16	63	16	8	6
Laing [8]	96	26	–	69	82	18	0	9
Belal [13]	81 (IE); 89 (IIE)	6 (IE); 22(IIE)	85	–	31	69	0	65
Thieblemont [17]	76	12	50	23	–	–	46	–
Kuper-Hommel [24]	64	11	63	29	37	34	29	18
Niitsu [30]	94	–	100	–	56	44	0	NA
Hwang [39]	78	–	48	39	50	30	20	23
Joshi [41]	67	–	78	–	100	–	–	100
Mian [55]	85	10	100	–	–	55	–	50
Onal [56]	–	17/10[a]	64	21	61	39	0	42
Penney [57]	–	14	83	–	56	36	8	49
Wirtzfeld [15]	100	–	50	–	80	20	–	20
Alzouebi [74]	60	10	–	–	83	17	–	27
Katna[b] [75]	81	0	87	3	–	–	–	42

– Information not available
[a]Local/distant relapses
[b]2 each: Hodgkin's; Burkitt's; T-cell lymphoma

Table 91.5 Five-year survival rates in primary thyroid lymphoma

Refs	DSS (IE/IIE/III-IVE)	OS (IE/IIE/III-IVE)	PFS
Alzouebi [74]		45 % (DLBCL); 62 % (MALT)	
Aozasa [1]		74 %	
Belal [13]		88 % (100/81/–)	72 % (91/59/–)
Derringer [11]	79 %		
DiBiase [19]		56 %	57 %
Graff-Baker [38]	79 % (86/81/64)	66 %	
Harrington [23]		48 %	
Kuper-Hommel [24]		43 % (IE-IIE = 47 %)	57 %
Mian [55]	89 %	52 %	
Mizukami		70 %	
Niitsu [30]		90 %	84 %
Onal [56]		74 %	68 %
Pedersen [10]	46 % (57/50/17)	34 % (41/40/17)	
Penney [57]		62 % (73/48/–)	
Pyke [4]		53 % (80/50/36)	
Rasbach [64]		42 %	
Ruggiero [68]		61 % (42/100/50)	
Sasai [66]		85 % (100/63/–)	
Scholefield [5]		57 %	
Sippel [63]		77 %	
Skacel [12]		75 %	
Sun [52]		82 %	74 %
Thieblemont [17]		77 %	
Tupchong [65]		40 %	
Wirtzfeld [15]	100 %	80 % (8.6 year)	
Watanabe [59]		85 % (89/83/–)	
Laing [8]	79 %	77 %	

DSS disease-specific survival, *OS* overall survival, *PFS* progression-free survival
– No information available

Survival Predictors

Table 91.6 depicts the number of studies that either did or did not statistically influence survivals. Few predictors were unanimous, although neither gender [1, 10, 11, 13, 38, 39, 52, 55, 56, 59, 64–66, 75] nor serum LDH [10, 13, 30, 39, 66, 75] had any predictive power, while better performance status [13, 17, 55] was always associated with improved survival. Patient age was as likely [1, 10, 17, 19, 23, 24, 38, 55, 59] as not [8, 11–13, 30, 39, 52, 56, 64, 65, 75] to influence survival. Perhaps surprisingly, several factors—histology [1, 8, 11, 12, 38, 39]-yes, [4, 10, 13, 17, 24, 52, 59]-no; tumor stage [10–12, 23, 32, 38, 39, 52, 66]-yes, [1, 4, 8, 13, 19, 24, 30, 55–57, 59, 65, 75]-no; and treatment modality [23, 38, 55–57, 75]-yes, [11–13, 52, 59]-no—were predictive in only about half the studies, and tumor bulk predicted survival in only two [1, 56] studies but not in others [11, 13, 24, 30, 39, 55, 64, 66].

There are numerous factors contributing to these findings. All studies were retrospective and nonrandomized and, given the rarity of thyroid lymphomas, extended over many years or decades, during which treatments varied. In general, DLBCL is felt to be more aggressive. However, the distribution of histologic types varied across reports. Similarly, staging was not uniform, with stage III-IVE patients excluded from some series. Further, with all these factors, the descriptions were not uniform among studies and data were often incomplete.

Table 91.6 Predictors of survival in patients with thyroid lymphoma (no. studies)

	Yes	No
Age	9	11
Gender	0	14
Stage	9	13
Histology	6	7
Tumor bulk	2	8
Performance status	3	0
Treatment modality	6	5
Mediastinum involved	4	1
LDH	0	6

Future Directions

Optimal therapy for primary thyroid lymphoma is hampered by the lack of any prospective clinical trials. Despite the rarity of patients with advanced differentiated, medullary, and anaplastic thyroid cancers, there have been a number of recent successful multicenter phase 2 and 3 clinical trials. The time is appropriate to propose such trials for thyroid lymphomas. Two important unanswered questions are (a) is radiotherapy alone sufficient for first-line treatment of stage IE MALT lymphoma, and (b) does immunotherapy added to chemoradiation improve outcomes in thyroid B-cell lymphomas? Standardized imaging and appropriate control of stage and histological types are essential to properly resolve the uncertainties that currently exist.

References

1. Aozasa K, Inoue A, Tajima K, et al. Malignant lymphomas of the thyroid gland. Analysis of 79 patients with emphasis on histologic prognostic factors. Cancer. 1986;58:100–4.
2. Hyjek E, Isaacson PG. Primary B cell lymphoma of the thyroid and its relationship to Hashimoto's thyroiditis. Hum Pathol. 1988;19:1315–26.
3. Mizukami Y, Michigishi T, Nonomura A, et al. Primary lymphoma of the thyroid: a clinical, histological and immunohistochemical study of 20 cases. Histopathology. 1990;17:201–9.
4. Pyke CM, Grant CS, Habermann TM, et al. Non-Hodgkin's lymphoma of the thyroid: is more than biopsy necessary? World J Surg. 1992;16:604–9. discussion 609–10.
5. Scholefield JH, Quayle AR, Harris SC, et al. Primary lymphoma of the thyroid, the association with Hashimoto's thyroiditis. Eur J Surg Oncol. 1992;18:89–92.
6. Matsuzuka F, Miyauchi A, Katayama S, et al. Clinical aspects of primary thyroid lymphoma: diagnosis and treatment based on our experience of 119 cases. Thyroid. 1993;3:93–9.
7. Doria R, Jekel JF, Cooper DL. Thyroid lymphoma. The case for combined modality therapy. Cancer. 1994;73:200–6.
8. Laing RW, Hoskin P, Hudson BV, et al. The significance of MALT histology in thyroid lymphoma: a review of patients from the BNLI and Royal Marsden Hospital. Clin Oncol (R Coll Radiol). 1994;6:300–4.
9. Takashima S, Nomura N, Noguchi Y, et al. Primary thyroid lymphoma: evaluation with US, CT, and MRI. J Comput Assist Tomogr. 1995;19:282–8.
10. Pedersen RK, Pedersen NT. Primary non-Hodgkin's lymphoma of the thyroid gland: a population based study. Histopathology. 1996;28:25–32.
11. Derringer GA, Thompson LD, Frommelt RA, et al. Malignant lymphoma of the thyroid gland: a clinicopathologic study of 108 cases. Am J Surg Pathol. 2000;24:623–39.
12. Skacel M, Ross CW, Hsi ED. A reassessment of primary thyroid lymphoma: high-grade MALT-type lymphoma as a distinct subtype of diffuse large B-cell lymphoma. Histopathology. 2000;37:10–8.
13. Belal AA, Allam A, Kandil A, et al. Primary thyroid lymphoma: a retrospective analysis of prognostic factors and treatment outcome for localized intermediate and high grade lymphoma. Am J Clin Oncol. 2001;24:299–305.
14. Takakuwa T, Dong Z, Takayama H, et al. Frequent mutations of Fas gene in thyroid lymphoma. Cancer Res. 2001;61:1382–5.
15. Wirtzfeld DA, Winston JS, Hicks Jr WL, et al. Clinical presentation and treatment of non-Hodgkin's lymphoma of the thyroid gland. Ann Surg Oncol. 2001;8:338–41.
16. Cha C, Chen H, Westra WH, et al. Primary thyroid lymphoma: can the diagnosis be made solely by fine-needle aspiration? Ann Surg Oncol. 2002;9:298–302.
17. Thieblemont C, Mayer A, Dumontet C, et al. Primary thyroid lymphoma is a heterogeneous disease. J Clin Endocrinol Metab. 2002;87:105–11.
18. Kim HC, Han MH, Kim KH, et al. Primary thyroid lymphoma: CT findings. Eur J Radiol. 2003;46:233–9.
19. DiBiase SJ, Grigsby PW, Guo C, et al. Outcome analysis for stage IE and IIE thyroid lymphoma. Am J Clin Oncol. 2004;27:178–84.
20. Coskun H, Bozbora A, Kapran Y, et al. The incidence of primary thyroid lymphoma in thyroid malignancies. Kulak Burun Bogaz Ihtis Derg. 2004;12:11–5.
21. Widder S, Pasieka JL. Primary thyroid lymphomas. Curr Treat Options Oncol. 2004;5:307–13.
22. Gupta N, Nijhawan R, Srinivasan R, et al. Fine needle aspiration cytology of primary thyroid lymphoma: a report of ten cases. Cytojournal. 2005;2:21.
23. Harrington KJ, Michalaki VJ, Vini L, et al. Management of non-Hodgkin's lymphoma of the thyroid: the Royal Marsden Hospital experience. Br J Radiol. 2005;78:405–10.
24. Kuper-Hommel MJ, Snijder S, Jansen-Heijnen ML, et al. Treatment and survival of patients with thyroid lymphoma: a population-based study with clinical and pathologic reviews. Clin Lymphoma Myeloma. 2005;6:240–7.
25. Wang SA, Rahemtullah A, Faquin WC, et al. Hodgkin's lymphoma of the thyroid: a clinicopathologic study of five cases and review of the literature. Mod Pathol. 2005;18:1577–84.
26. Takano T, Miyauchi A, Matsuzuka F, et al. Detection of monoclonality of the immunoglobulin heavy chain gene in thyroid malignant lymphoma by vectorette polymerase chain reaction. J Clin Endocrinol Metab. 2005;90:720–3.
27. Green LD, Mack L, Pasieka JL. Anaplastic thyroid cancer and primary thyroid lymphoma: a review of these rare thyroid malignancies. J Surg Oncol. 2006;94:725–36.
28. Au WY, Fung A, Ma ES, et al. HLA associations, microsatellite instability and epigenetic changes in thyroid lymphoma in Chinese. Leuk Lymphoma. 2007;48:531–4.
29. Mack LA, Pasieka JL. An evidence-based approach to the treatment of thyroid lymphoma. World J Surg. 2007;31:978–86.
30. Niitsu N, Okamoto M, Nakamura N, et al. Clinicopathologic correlations of stage IE/IIE primary thyroid diffuse large B-cell lymphoma. Ann Oncol. 2007;18:1203–8.
31. Lee CJ, Hsu CH, Tai CJ, et al. FDG-PET for a thyroid MALT lymphoma. Acta Oncol. 2008;47:1165–7.
32. Meyer-Rochow GY, Sywak MS, Reeve TS, et al. Surgical trends in the management of thyroid lymphoma. Eur J Surg Oncol. 2008;34:576–80.
33. Moshynska OV, Saxena A. Clonal relationship between Hashimoto thyroiditis and thyroid lymphoma. J Clin Pathol. 2008;61:438–44.
34. Yang H, Li J, Shen T. Primary T-cell lymphoma of the thyroid: case report and review of the literature. Med Oncol. 2008;25:462–6.
35. Bacon CM, Diss TC, Ye H, et al. Follicular lymphoma of the thyroid gland. Am J Surg Pathol. 2009;33:22–34.
36. Basu S, Li G, Bural G, et al. Fluorodeoxyglucose positron emission tomography (FDG-PET) and PET/computed tomography imaging characteristics of thyroid lymphoma and their potential clinical utility. Acta Radiol. 2009;50:201–4.
37. Foppiani L, Secondo V, Arlandini A, et al. Thyroid lymphoma: a rare tumor requiring combined management. Hormones (Athens). 2009;8:214–8.

38. Graff-Baker A, Roman SA, Thomas DC, et al. Prognosis of primary thyroid lymphoma: demographic, clinical, and pathologic predictors of survival in 1,408 cases. Surgery. 2009;146:1105–15.
39. Hwang YC, Kim TY, Kim WB, et al. Clinical characteristics of primary thyroid lymphoma in Koreans. Endocr J. 2009;56: 399–405.
40. Choi WW, Weisenburger DD, Greiner TC, et al. A new immunostain algorithm classifies diffuse large B-cell lymphoma into molecular subtypes with high accuracy. Clin Cancer Res. 2009;15:5 494–502.
41. Joshi A, Chan J, Bruch G, et al. Thyroid lymphoma and airway obstruction – is there a rationale for surgical management? Int J Clin Pract. 2009;63:1647–52.
42. Lee J, Won JH, Kim HC, et al. Emergency dilation by self-expandable tracheal stent for upper airway obstruction in a patient with a giant primary thyroid lymphoma. Thyroid. 2009;19:193–5.
43. Takakuwa T, Miyauchi A, Aozasa K. Aberrant somatic hypermutations in thyroid lymphomas. Leuk Res. 2009;33:649–54.
44. Graff-Baker A, Sosa JA, Roman SA. Primary thyroid lymphoma: a review of recent developments in diagnosis and histology-driven treatment. Curr Opin Oncol. 2010;22:17–22.
45. Jonak C, Troch M, Mullauer L, et al. Rituximab plus dose-reduced cyclophosphamide, mitoxantrone, vincristine, and prednisolone are effective in elderly patients with diffuse large B-cell lymphoma of the thyroid. Thyroid. 2010;20:425–7.
46. Morgen EK, Geddie W, Boerner S, et al. The role of fine-needle aspiration in the diagnosis of thyroid lymphoma: a retrospective study of nine cases and review of published series. J Clin Pathol. 2010;63:129–33.
47. Refeidi AA, Al-Shehri GY, Al-Ahmary AM, et al. Patterns of thyroid cancer in Southwestern Saudi Arabia. Saudi Med J. 2010;31:1238–41.
48. Gkountouvas A, Nikas M, Chatjimarkou F, et al. Thyroid cancer in Greece. A tertiary center experience. J Buon. 2010;15:674–8.
49. Sarinah B, Hisham AN. Primary lymphoma of the thyroid: diagnostic and therapeutic considerations. Asian J Surg. 2010;33:20–4.
50. Seningen JL, Nassar A, Henry MR. Correlation of thyroid nodule fine-needle aspiration cytology with corresponding histology at Mayo Clinic, 2001–2007: an institutional experience of 1,945 cases. Diagn Cytopathol. 2010;40 Suppl 1:E27-32.
51. Straus DJ. Primary thyroid lymphoma, a rare disease with a good treatment outcome. J Surg Oncol. 2010;101:543–4.
52. Sun TQ, Zhu XL, Wang ZY, et al. Characteristics and prognosis of primary thyroid non-Hodgkin's lymphoma in Chinese patients. J Surg Oncol. 2010;101:545–50.
53. Arabi M, Dvorak R, Smith LB, et al. Fluorodeoxyglucose positron emission tomography in primary thyroid lymphoma with coexisting lymphocytic thyroiditis. Thyroid. 2011;21:1153–6.
54. Kahara T, Iwaki N, Kaya H, et al. Transition of thyroid autoantibodies by rituximab treatment for thyroid MALT lymphoma. Endocr J. 2011;58:7–12.
55. Mian M, Gaidano G, Conconi A, et al. High response rate and improvement of long-term survival with combined treatment modalities in patients with poor-risk primary thyroid diffuse large B-cell lymphoma: an International Extranodal Lymphoma Study Group and Intergruppo Italiano Linfomi study. Leuk Lymphoma. 2011;52:823–32.
56. Onal C, Li YX, Miller RC, et al. Treatment results and prognostic factors in primary thyroid lymphoma patients: a rare cancer network study. Ann Oncol. 2011;22:156–64.
57. Penney SE, Homer JJ. Thyroid lymphoma: acute presentation and long-term outcome. J Laryngol Otol 2011;125:1256-62.
58. Vassilatou E, Economopoulos T, Tzanela M, et al. Coexistence of differentiated thyroid carcinoma with primary thyroid lymphoma in a background of Hashimoto's thyroiditis. J Clin Oncol. 2011;29:e709–12.
59. Watanabe N, Noh JY, Narimatsu H, et al. Clinicopathological features of 171 cases of primary thyroid lymphoma: a long-term study involving 24 553 patients with Hashimoto's disease. Br J Haematol. 2011;153:236-43.
60. Holm LE, Blomgren H, Lowhagen T. Cancer risks in patients with chronic lymphocytic thyroiditis. N Engl J Med. 1985;312:601–4.
61. Harach HR, Williams ED. Thyroid cancer and thyroiditis in the goitrous region of Salta, Argentina, before and after iodine prophylaxis. Clin Endocrinol (Oxf). 1995;43:701–6.
62. Coltrera MD. Primary T-cell lymphoma of the thyroid. Head Neck. 1999;21:160–3.
63. Sippel RS, Gauger PG, Angelos P, et al. Palliative thyroidectomy for malignant lymphoma of the thyroid. Ann Surg Oncol. 2002;9:907–11.
64. Rasbach DA, Mondschein MS, Harris NL, et al. Malignant lymphoma of the thyroid gland: a clinical and pathologic study of twenty cases. Surgery. 1985;98:1166–70.
65. Tupchong L, Hughes F, Harmer CL. Primary lymphoma of the thyroid: clinical features, prognostic factors, and results of treatment. Int J Radiat Oncol Biol Phys. 1986;12:1813–21.
66. Sasai K, Yamabe H, Haga H, et al. Non-Hodgkin's lymphoma of the thyroid. A clinical study of twenty-two cases. Acta Oncol. 1996;35:457–62.
67. Sangalli G, Serio G, Zampatti C, et al. Fine needle aspiration cytology of primary lymphoma of the thyroid: a report of 17 cases. Cytopathology. 2001;12:257–63.
68. Ruggiero FP, Frauenhoffer E, Stack Jr BC. Thyroid lymphoma: a single institution's experience. Otolaryngol Head Neck Surg. 2005;133:888–96.
69. Kato I, Tajima K, Suchi T, et al. Chronic thyroiditis as a risk factor of B-cell lymphoma in the thyroid gland. Jpn J Cancer Res. 1985;76:1085–90.
70. Kossev P, Livolsi V. Lymphoid lesions of the thyroid: review in light of the revised European-American lymphoma classification and upcoming World Health Organization classification. Thyroid. 1999;9:1273–80.
71. Zeppa P, Cozzolino I, Peluso AL, et al. Cytologic, flow cytometry, and molecular assessment of lymphoid infiltrate in fine-needle cytology samples of Hashimoto thyroiditis. Cancer. 2009;117:174–84.
72. Costa LJ, Xavier AC. Features and outcomes of diffuse large B-cell lymphoma of the thyroid in a large contemporary cohort. Leuk Lymphoma. 2014;55:283-7.
73. Motoi N, Ozawa Y. Malignant T-cell lymphoma of the thyroid gland associated with Hashimoto's thyroiditis. Pathol Int. 2005;55:425–30.
74. Alzouebi M, Goepel JR, Horsman JM, et al. Primary thyroid lymphoma: the 40 year experience of a UK lymphoma treatment centre. Int J Oncol. 2012;40:2075–80.
75. Katna R, Shet T, Sengar M, et al. Clinicopathologic study and outcome analysis of thyroid lymphomas: experience from a tertiary cancer center. Head Neck. 2013;35:165–71.
76. Carbone PP, Kaplan HS, Musshoff K, et al. Report of the committee on Hodgkin's disease staging classification. Cancer Res. 1971;31:1860–1.
77. Filie AC, Asa SL, Geisinger KR, et al. Utilization of ancillary studies in thyroid fine needle aspirates: a synopsis of the National Cancer Institute Thyroid Fine Needle Aspiration State of the Science Conference. Diagn Cytopathol. 2008;36:438–41.
78. Holting T, Moller P, Tschahargane C, et al. Immunohistochemical reclassification of anaplastic carcinoma reveals small and giant cell lymphoma. World J Surg. 1990;14:291–4. discussion 295.
79. Takano T, Asahi S, Matsuzuka F, et al. Aspiration biopsy-nucleic acid diagnosis of thyroid malignant lymphoma by vectorette PCR: experience of eight cases. Leuk Res. 2008;32:151–4.
80. Rossi D. Thyroid lymphoma: beyond antigen stimulation. Leuk Res. 2009;33:607–9.

81. Streubel B, Simonitsch-Klupp I, Mullauer L, et al. Variable frequencies of MALT lymphoma-associated genetic aberrations in MALT lymphomas of different sites. Leukemia. 2004;18:1722–6.
82. Aggarwal N, Swerdlow SH, Kelly LM, et al. Thyroid carcinoma-associated genetic mutations also occur in thyroid lymphomas. Mod Pathol. 2012;25:1203–11.
83. Chander S, Zingas AP, Bloom DA, et al. Positron emission tomography in primary thyroid lymphoma. Clin Nucl Med. 2004;29:572–3.
84. Nakadate M, Yoshida K, Ishii A, et al. Is 18F-FDG PET/CT useful for distinguishing between primary thyroid lymphoma and chronic thyroiditis? Clin Nucl Med. 2013;38:709–14.
85. Motta G, Cea M, Moran E, et al. Monoclonal antibodies for non-Hodgkin's lymphoma: state of the art and perspectives. Clin Dev Immunol. 2010;2010:428253.
86. Miller TP, Dahlberg S, Cassady JR, et al. Chemotherapy alone compared with chemotherapy plus radiotherapy for localized intermediate- and high-grade non-Hodgkin's lymphoma. N Engl J Med. 1998;339:21–6.
87. Horning SJ, Weller E, Kim K, et al. Chemotherapy with or without radiotherapy in limited-stage diffuse aggressive non-Hodgkin's lymphoma: Eastern Cooperative Oncology Group study 1484. J Clin Oncol. 2004;22:3032–8.
88. Isobe K, Kagami Y, Higuchi K, et al. A multicenter phase II study of local radiation therapy for stage IEA mucosa-associated lymphoid tissue lymphomas: a preliminary report from the Japan Radiation Oncology Group (JAROG). Int J Radiat Oncol Biol Phys. 2007;69:1181–6.
89. Stein SA, Wartofsky L. Primary thyroid lymphoma: a clinical review. J Clin Endocrinol Metab. 2013;98:3131–8.

Pathology of Lymphoma of the Thyroid

92

Zubair W. Baloch and Virginia A. LiVolsi

The thyroid may be involved secondarily by lymphoma from other sites in the body or by leukemic infiltrates [1–3]. Most primary thyroidal lymphomas are B-cell types, but both Hodgkin's lymphoma [1, 3] and T-cell lymphoma [4] may occur.

From an epidemiologic viewpoint, almost all primary thyroid lymphomas arise on a background of severe chronic lymphocytic thyroiditis [1–3]. Clinically, women are more commonly affected. These patients often have a history of a goiter with hypothyroidism. Rapid growth of a mass lesion is noted.

Gross examination reveals homogeneous, pale, and firm tissue that has replaced the thyroid irregularly. If advanced autoimmune thyroiditis is also present, the lymphoma probably cannot be distinguished from the inflammatory infiltrate without histologic examination. Microscopically, the regions of autoimmune thyroiditis reveal either the usual benign lymphoplasmacytic infiltrates or the common alterations of the follicular epithelial cells (e.g., oxyphilic cell metaplasia) [1, 5].

The lymphoma usually consists of a monotonous infiltrate of abnormal lymphoid cells which replace the thyroid parenchyma, fill and distend some thyroid follicles (Figs. 92.1 and 92.2), and permeate the walls of some of the larger vessels [1]. Extra-glandular extension into perithyroidal fat and skeletal muscle is very often present [1, 6]. Cytokeratin antibodies can demonstrate displaced and distorted follicular epithelium; lymphoepithelial lesions characteristic of so-called mucosa-associated lymphoid tissue (MALT) lymphoma are seen [6–8]. Cervical lymph nodes may be involved.

Smears from the aspirates may show predominantly chronic lymphocytic thyroiditis, and it is necessary to perform multiple aspirates until the lymphomatous regions are sampled [9, 10]. The latter show a monotonous lymphoid population, readily observed mitotic figures, and a conspicuous absence of follicular epithelial cells. There is controversy about the wisdom of making a primary cytological diagnosis of malignant lymphoma without addition of ancillary techniques such as flow cytometry or gene rearrangement studies [11, 12].

Sometimes in order to make a diagnosis of a specific subtype of lymphoma, an open surgical wedge biopsy of the mass may be needed.

The lymphoma may be diffuse or follicular (nodular). Separating the lymphoma from an adjacent infiltrate of autoimmune thyroiditis requires careful appraisal of the abnormal cells in the routine histologic sections and the use of immunohistochemical stains. In large cell malignant lymphoma, this is usually confirmatory and the histologic diagnosis is obvious; in cases of small cell lymphoma, special studies are warranted and needed to make the diagnosis [13].

Some thyroid lymphomas present as aggressive neoplasms, often in the elderly. A considerable number of thyroid lymphomas are of intermediate or low grade. Cases of this type have led to the concept that a thyroid involved with autoimmune disease is comparable to mucosa-associated lymphoid tissue (MALT), such as the Peyer's patches of the intestine [13, 14]. Thus, it has been suggested that the majority of thyroidal lymphomas are MALT lymphomas [14]. These lymphomas may tend to be localized for extended periods of time, possibly explaining why some thyroid lymphomas have been cured by surgery alone. Thyroid lymphomas may spread to other sites of MALT (e.g., small bowel); in some patients, extranodal MALT lymphoma of the lung or bowel may precede the development of thyroid lymphoma. Some of these tumors may show plasmacytic differentiation [1, 3]. Such

Z.W. Baloch, MD, PhD (✉) • V.A. LiVolsi, MD
Department of Pathology and Laboratory Medicine, University of Pennsylvania Medical Center, Perelman School of Medicine, 6 Founders Pavilion, 3400 Spruce Street, Philadelphia, PA 19104, USA
e-mail: balocj@mail.med.upenn.edu; linus@mail.med.upenn.edu

L. Wartofsky, D. Van Nostrand (eds.), *Thyroid Cancer*, DOI 10.1007/978-1-4939-3314-3_92

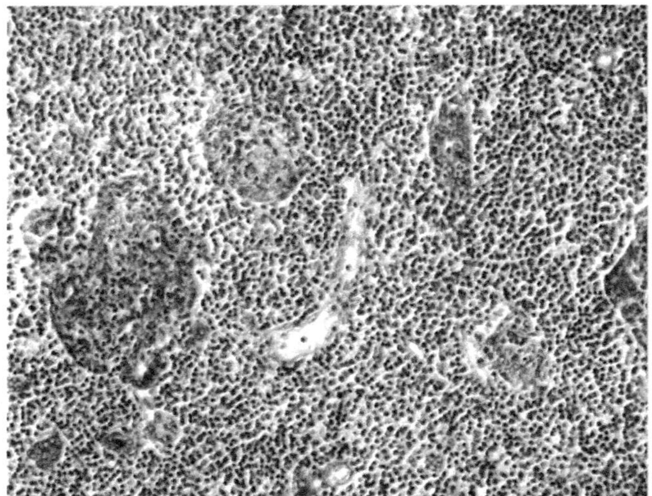

Fig. 92.1 Malignant lymphoma. A number of thyroid follicles are formed by metaplastic epithelial cells, presumably because of previous Hashimoto's thyroiditis. Both the interstitial tissue and the altered follicles are extensively infiltrated by the lymphoma (H&E stain)

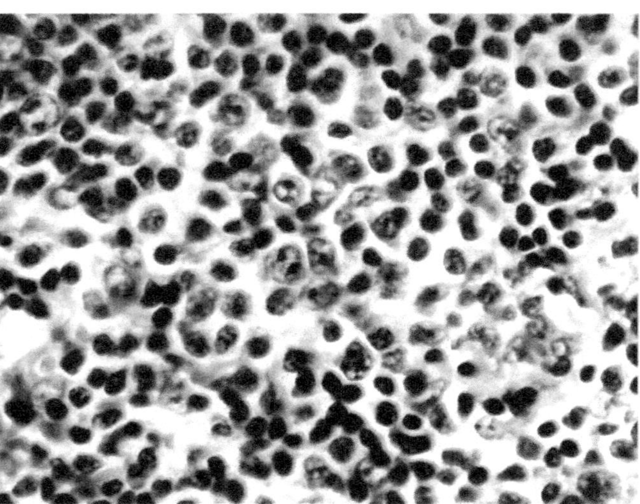

Fig. 92.2 Malignant lymphoma. Many abnormal lymphoid cells are visible. The smallest cells are likely normal lymphocytes that accompany the malignant infiltrate (H&E stain)

cells are usually monotypic with immunoglobulin light-chain restriction. The lymphoma cells may extend into the reactive lymphoid follicles of the autoimmune thyroiditis, thereby explaining the follicular (nodular) pattern of some lymphomas [15]. Also, persisting lymphoid follicles have been reported in the rare plasmacytomas of the thyroid [16], possibly supporting the theory that plasmacytomas of the thyroid are mature MALT lymphomas. When a high-grade lymphoma is present, there is often evidence that it has arisen from a low-grade MALT lymphoma [17].

References

1. Kossev P, Livolsi V. Lymphoid lesions of the thyroid: review in light of the revised European-American lymphoma classification and upcoming World Health Organization classification. Thyroid. 1999;9:1273–80.
2. Kebapcilar L, Alacacioglu I, Comlekci A, Ozcan MA, Piskin O, Kargi A, Undar B, Yesil S. Primary thyroid lymphoma: case series with literature review. J BUON. 2009;14:295–9.
3. Lam KY, Lo CY, Kwong DL, Lee J, Srivastava G. Malignant lymphoma of the thyroid. A 30-year clinicopathologic experience and an evaluation of the presence of Epstein-Barr virus. Am J Clin Pathol. 1999;112:263–70.
4. Kim NR, Ko YH, Lee YD. Primary T-cell lymphoma of the thyroid associated with Hashimoto's thyroiditis, histologically mimicking MALT-lymphoma. J Korean Med Sci. 2010;25:481–4.
5. Hamburger JI, Miller JM, Kini SR. Lymphoma of the thyroid. Ann Intern Med. 1983;99:685–93.
6. Derringer GA, Thompson LD, Frommelt RA, Bijwaard KE, Heffess CS, Abbondanzo SL. Malignant lymphoma of the thyroid gland: a clinicopathologic study of 108 cases. Am J Surg Pathol. 2000;24:623–39.
7. Sun TQ, Zhu XL, Wang ZY, Wang CF, Zhou XY, Ji QH, Wu Y. Characteristics and prognosis of primary thyroid non-Hodgkin's lymphoma in Chinese patients. J Surg Oncol. 2010;101:545–50.
8. Thieblemont C, Mayer A, Dumontet C, Barbier Y, Callet-Bauchu E, Felman P, Berger F, Ducottet X, Martin C, Salles G, Orgiazzi J, Coiffier B. Primary thyroid lymphoma is a heterogeneous disease. J Clin Endocrinol Metab. 2002;87:105–11.
9. Babu N, Dey P. Fine needle aspiration cytology of non-Hodgkin's lymphoma of thyroid. Cytopathology. 2002;13:188.
10. Lu JY, Lin CW, Chang TC, Chen YC. Diagnostic pitfalls of fine-needle aspiration cytology and prognostic impact of chemotherapy in thyroid lymphoma. J Formos Med Assoc. 2001;100:519–25.
11. Cha C, Chen H, Westra WH, Udelsman R. Primary thyroid lymphoma: can the diagnosis be made solely by fine- needle aspiration? Ann Surg Oncol. 2002;9:298–302.
12. Takano T, Miyauchi A, Matsuzuka F, Yoshida H, Kuma K, Amino N. Diagnosis of thyroid malignant lymphoma by reverse transcription- polymerase chain reaction detecting the monoclonality of immunoglobulin heavy chain messenger ribonucleic acid. J Clin Endocrinol Metab. 2000;85:671–5.
13. Straus DJ. Primary thyroid lymphoma, a rare disease with a good treatment outcome. J Surg Oncol. 2010;101:543–4.
14. Sarinah B, Hisham AN. Primary lymphoma of the thyroid: diagnostic and therapeutic considerations. Asian J Surg. 2010;33:20–4.
15. Isaacson PG, Androulakis-Papachristou A, Diss TC, Pan L, Wright DH. Follicular colonization in thyroid lymphoma. Am J Pathol. 1992;141:43–52.
16. Ohshima M, Momiyama T, Souda S, Kuratani T, Toda K, Hiasa Y. Primary plasmacytoma of the thyroid: a case report and comparative literature study between western nations and Japan. Pathol Int. 1994;44:645–51.
17. Pedersen RK, Pedersen NT. Primary non-Hodgkin's lymphoma of the thyroid gland: a population based study. Histopathology. 1996;28:25–32.

PET/CT in Lymphoma and Lymphoma of the Thyroid

93

Iain Ross McDougall and Andrei Iagaru

Introduction

Primary thyroid lymphomas (PTLs) are uncommon, accounting for approximately 1–5 % of thyroid cancers and 2 % of all extranodal lymphomas [1]. Most are non-Hodgkin lymphoma. The incidence is higher in older women and many of them have previously been diagnosed with Hashimoto's thyroiditis. It typically presents as a rapidly enlarging, painless thyroid mass, which may cause dyspnea, dysphagia, and hoarseness.

Systemic disease is common in lymphomas, and a contrast-enhanced CT of the chest, abdomen, and pelvis, PET/CT, and bone marrow biopsy are required for staging [1]. Besides detecting thyroidal involvement, ^{18}F-FDG PET may also be positive in autoimmune thyroiditis. Therefore, PET should not be used to make a diagnosis, but for staging by identifying sites of disease outside of the thyroid. Buchmann et al. found that ^{18}F-FDG PET was significantly superior to CT, except in infradiaphragmatic regions, in which two methods produced equivalent results. In detecting bone marrow infiltration, ^{18}F-FDG PET was superior to CT and was equivalent to bone marrow biopsy. Indeed, in 8 % of the patients, ^{18}F-FDG PET led to an upstaging and a change therapy [2].

I.R. McDougall, MD, PhD, FRCP (✉)
Department of Radiology, Nuclear Medicine, Stanford University Hospital and Clinics, 300 Pasteur Drive, Stanford, CA 94305, USA
e-mail: RossMcDougall@Stanford.edu

A. Iagaru, MD
Department of Radiology, Nuclear Medicine, Stanford University Medical Center, Stanford School of Medicine, Stanford, CA, USA
e-mail: aiagaru@stanford.edu

^{18}F-FDG PET/CT in Management of Lymphoma

Using the radiopharmaceutical 2-(fluorine-18) fluoro-2-deoxy-D-glucose (^{18}F-FDG), the most common indications for PET/CT at Stanford are for staging, following the response to therapy and for surveillance of patients with lymphoma. However, primary lymphoma of the thyroid is rare accounting for about 2 % of patients with extranodal lymphoma and a similar proportion of patients with cancer of the thyroid. The role of PET/CT in lymphoma will be discussed first and then specifically primary lymphoma of the thyroid.

PET using the radiopharmaceutical ^{18}F-FDG has been approved for imaging patients who have lymphoma. The instruments and methods are as described in the section on well-differentiated cancer (see Chap. 43) recognizing that combined PET/CT is now the standard imaging method rather than PET alone. In brief, the patient is fasted for 6 h and injected intravenously with 370–550 MBq ^{18}F-FDG. After a rest in a quiet warm environment, the patient is imaged from the base of the skull to the mid-thighs. The use of combined PET/CT improves the diagnostic accuracy and reduces the number of false-positive results and also increases the throughput of patients. This test is important in the staging of disease, in determining the response to therapy and in making a decision to stop or continue chemotherapy or to change to a different regime and in the detection of recurrence. There are comprehensive reviews of the topic [3,4].

^{18}F-FDG PET/CT and PET have been shown to be better than CT or Gallium-67 citrate (^{67}Ga) for staging both Hodgkin disease and non-Hodgkin lymphoma. In an investigation on cost-effectiveness, $30,000 was saved in 18 patients when PET was the first test and additional work-up based on that [5]. PET can change the management by increasing the stage of disease in some patients and decreasing the stage in others. There are several reports where the

L. Wartofsky, D. Van Nostrand (eds.), *Thyroid Cancer*, DOI 10.1007/978-1-4939-3314-3_93

sensitivities range from 85 % to 90 % and the specificities are greater than 90 % [2,6–8]. ^{18}F-FDG PET/CT at the end of treatment is predictive of how the patient will do. There is a high probability of recurrence when there is persistent uptake of ^{18}F-FDG in a lesion. This contrasts with anatomic imaging such as CT, which can show a residual mass but that could be cancer or scarring. PET was conducted 1–3 months after completion of chemotherapy in 93 patients with non-Hodgkin lymphoma [9]. In those with negative scans, there was an 85 % progression-free survival. This contrasted with 4 % for those with a positive scan. There is development of data showing that PET can be used in the middle of therapy to determine the response to treatment and to decide on a change in management. Relapse occurred in all 33 patients with a positive PET in mid-treatment compared with 7 of 37 in whom the test was negative [10]. PET was used after one cycle of chemotherapy in 30 patients [11]. Thirteen of 15 patients with a positive scan relapsed compared with 2 of 15 where the scan was negative [12]. ^{18}F-FDG PET has a high sensitivity for the early detection of recurrent disease and it is superior to CT [13,14].

There are studies that demonstrate the superiority of ^{18}F-FDG PET over ^{67}Ga. In a comparison in 51 patients, PET increased the stage of disease in 13 patients [15]. In a similar study in 50 patients, PET identified more lesions in 19 patients [8].

^{18}F-FDG PET/CT in Management of Primary Lymphoma of the Thyroid

Lymphoma of the thyroid is uncommon. The typical patient is an older woman (ratio of approximately 4/1) with the median age in the seventh decade, and generally, a history or clinical or immunological evidence of preexisting chronic lymphocytic thyroiditis is present [16–19]. The gland enlarges rapidly, and evidence of pressure on the trachea and esophagus may be present in addition to patient hoarseness [20–22]. The differential diagnosis is a rapidly growing primary cancer of the thyroid, anaplastic cancer, Reidel's thyroiditis, and, when there is pain, subacute thyroiditis. Most of the lymphomas arising in the thyroid are giant B-cell lymphoma. That diagnosis can usually be made by FNA using modern methods. A smaller proportion of primary thyroid lymphomas ranging from 10 % to 30 % in several series are mucosa-associated lymphoid tissue (MALT). These are more difficult to diagnose using FNA and open biopsy can be required. There are very rare reports of Hodgkin disease, T-cell lymphoma, Burkitt lymphoma, and small lymphocytic lymphoma (chronic lymphatic leukemia) arising in the thyroid [23]. A proportion of patients have the disease confined to the thyroid (stage I_E), and they have an excellent prognosis.

^{18}F-FDG PET is positive in the primary lesion, but it is also positive in uncomplicated autoimmune thyroiditis and that can be confused as a cancer [24–26]. However, Nakadate et al. [27] evaluated ^{18}F-FDG PET/CT scans in 10 patients with primary thyroid lymphoma and 51 patients with chronic thyroiditis. The standardized uptake value (SUV max) was significantly higher, and the CT density was significantly lower in patients with primary thyroid lymphoma relative to those patients with chronic thyroiditis. They suggested a potential role of ^{18}F-FDG PET scans in differentiating primary thyroid lymphoma from chronic thyroiditis. Nevertheless, at the time of diagnosis, the main role of ^{18}F-FDG PET is to identify sites of disease outside of the thyroid and thus accurately stage the disease (Fig. 93.1).

A meta-analysis of outcome demonstrated that patients treated with local external radiation fared worse than those treated with a combination of radiation and chemotherapy [28] – the implication being that some patients had disease outside the radiotherapy port. The extrathyroidal disease would have been identified in most patients using PET/CT. However, the article cited predated the use of PET or PET/CT, and these tests are sensitive for detecting lymphoma at all sites thus accurately staging most patients.

Basu et al. compared ^{18}F-FDG PET, PET/CT, CT, and MRI in primary lymphoma of the thyroid and indicated a potential role of ^{18}F-FDG PET at initial diagnosis, following therapeutic intervention and post-remission surveillance [29]. In their analysis, recurrence was detected earlier with ^{18}F-FDG PET compared to CT. However, this report, although specifically related to lymphoma originating in the thyroid, is restricted to 20 scans (14 PET, 6 PET/CT) in six patients with primary lymphoma of the thyroid. The results are similar to the larger experience in lymphoma arising in lymph nodes referred above. The test predicts the extent of disease and helps tailor treatment for the individual patient and is valuable for determining the response to treatment. However, Nakada et al. [30] evaluated 36 patients with primary thyroid lymphoma to determine whether ^{18}F-FDG PET/CT was valuable in assessing therapy response. Both visual evaluation and semiquantitative analysis of ^{18}F-FDG had limited value. They believed that this was most likely due to coexisting Hashimoto's thyroiditis. Persistent thyroidal ^{18}F-FDG uptake after therapy must be interpreted with caution.

Of note, one case report of the use of PET for follow-up of lymphoma of the thyroid raises a concern [31]. The patient had Hashimoto's and 4 years later developed a thyroid mass. She had an operative biopsy but not thyroidectomy. The pathology was diffuse large B-cell lymphoma. She was treated with cyclophosphamide, doxorubicine, vincristine, and prednisone. PET scan was obtained 4 months after therapy and it showed intense uptake in the left lower lobe of the thyroid. This was excised and showed only necrosis. There is evidence that uptake of ^{18}F-FDG can be seen up to 6 weeks after radiation therapy or surgery, whereas this false positive was after a longer delay. Therefore, some caution needs to be taken in the interpretation of PET of the thyroid. The test

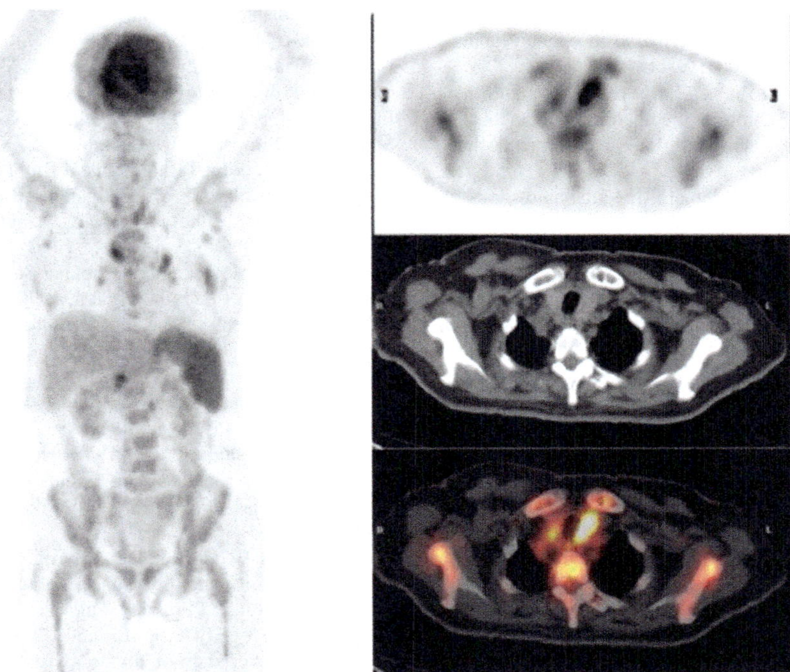

Fig. 93.1 A 76-year-old woman with non-Hodgkin lymphoma. Staging ^{18}F-FDG PET/CT demonstrates intense uptake in the left thyroid lobe (*arrowhead*), as well as additional lesions in the thorax and axillae. The increased uptake of ^{18}F-FDG in the spleen is most likely due to lymphoma

does provide useful information of the response of lesions outside of the thyroid. However, there are reports of increased focal uptake of ^{18}F-FDG in the thyroid after systemic therapy of lymphoma where other sites of disease had responded well. These hot spots turned out to be primary thyroid cancer; hence the general advice is to obtain an ultrasound-guided fine-needle aspiration of focal hot spots (^{18}F-FDG) in the thyroid.

Historically, there is a report of the utility of ^{67}Ga in diagnosing lymphoma of the thyroid in eight patients with a prior diagnosis of Hashimoto's thyroiditis [32]. Seven of the eight patients had "strong or very strong" uptake in the thyroid. Unfortunately, there can also be uptake of ^{67}Ga in benign chronic lymphocytic thyroiditis [33]. Therefore, the specificity of that test is poor.

In summary, there is an abundance of information of the use of ^{18}F-FDG PET and PET/CT in lymphoma. There is little data published on the specific use in primary lymphoma of the thyroid due to the rarity of this presentation. Because PET is positive in chronic lymphocytic thyroiditis, further study is warranted to evaluate its utility in differentiating primary thyroid lymphoma from chronic lymphocytic thyroiditis. Its main roles are staging the disease, prognostication, follow-up after radiochemotherapy, and for long-term surveillance. The use of ^{67}Ga as an alternative to ^{18}F-FDG PET/CT is not advised.

References

1. Straus D. Primary thyroid lymphoma, a rare disease with a good treatment outcome. J Surg Oncol. 2010;101:543–4.
2. Buchmann I, Reinhardt M, Elsner K, et al. 2-(fluorine-18)fluoro-2-deoxy-D-glucose positron emission tomography in the detection and staging of malignant lymphoma. A bicenter trial. Cancer. 2001;91:889–99.
3. Schiepers C, Filmont JE, Czernin J. PET for staging of Hodgkin's disease and non-Hodgkin's lymphoma. Eur J Nucl Med Mol Imaging. 2003;30 Suppl 1:S82–8.
4. Israel O, Keidar Z, Bar-Shalom R. Positron emission tomography in the evaluation of lymphoma. Semin Nucl Med. 2004;34:166–79.
5. Hoh CK, Glaspy J, Rosen P, et al. Whole-body FDG-PET imaging for staging of Hodgkin's disease and lymphoma. J Nucl Med. 1997;38:343–8.
6. Stumpe KD, Urbinelli M, Steinert HC, Glanzmann C, Buck A, von Schulthess GK. Whole-body positron emission tomography using fluorodeoxyglucose for staging of lymphoma: effectiveness and comparison with computed tomography. Eur J Nucl Med. 1998;25:721–8.
7. Najjar F, Hustinx R, Jerusalem G, Fillet G, Rigo P. Positron emission tomography (PET) for staging low-grade non-Hodgkin's lymphomas (NHL). Cancer Biother Radiopharm. 2001;16:297–304.
8. Wirth A, Seymour JF, Hicks RJ, et al. Fluorine-18 fluorodeoxyglucose positron emission tomography, gallium-67 scintigraphy, and conventional staging for Hodgkin's disease and non-Hodgkin's lymphoma. Am J Med. 2002;112:262–8.
9. Spaepen K, Stroobants S, Dupont P, et al. Prognostic value of positron emission tomography (PET) with fluorine-18 fluorodeoxyglu-

cose ([18F]FDG) after first-line chemotherapy in non-Hodgkin's lymphoma: is [18F]FDG-PET a valid alternative to conventional diagnostic methods? J Clin Oncol. 2001;19:414–9.
10. Spaepen K, Stroobants S, Dupont P, et al. Early restaging positron emission tomography with ^{18}F-fluorodeoxyglucose predicts outcome in patients with aggressive non-Hodgkin's lymphoma. Ann Oncol. 2002;13:1356–63.
11. Kostakoglu L, Leonard JP, Kuji I, Coleman M, Vallabhajosula S, Goldsmith SJ. Comparison of fluorine-18 fluorodeoxyglucose positron emission tomography and Ga-67 scintigraphy in evaluation of lymphoma. Cancer. 2002;94:879–88.
12. Kostakoglu L, Coleman M, Leonard JP, Kuji I, Zoe H, Goldsmith SJ. PET predicts prognosis after 1 cycle of chemotherapy in aggressive lymphoma and Hodgkin's disease. J Nucl Med. 2002;43: 1018–27.
13. Dittmann H, Sokler M, Kollmannsberger C, et al. Comparison of FDG-PET with CT scans in the evaluation of patients with residual and recurrent Hodgkin's lymphoma. Oncol Rep. 2001;8:1393–9.
14. Bangerter M, Kotzerke J, Griesshammer M, Elsner K, Reske SN, Bergmann L. Positron emission tomography with 18-fluorodeoxyglucose in the staging and follow-up of lymphoma in the chest. Acta Oncol. 1999;38:799–804.
15. Kostakoglu L, Goldsmith SJ. Positron emission tomography in lymphoma: comparison with computed tomography and gallium-67 single photon emission computed tomography. Clin Lymphoma. 2000;1:67–74; discussion 5–6.
16. Anscombe AM, Wright DH. Primary malignant lymphoma of the thyroid – a tumour of mucosa-associated lymphoid tissue: review of seventy-six cases. Histopathology. 1985;9:81–97.
17. Burke J, Butler JJ, Fuller LM. Malignant lymphomas of the thyroid. A clinical pathologic study of 35 patients including ultrastructure observations. Cancer. 1977;39:1587–602.
18. Compagno J, Oertel JE. Malignant lymphoma and other lymphoproliferative disorders of the thyroid gland. A clinicopathologic study of 245 cases. Am J Clin Pathol. 1980;74:1–11.
19. Matsuzuka F, Miyauchi A, Katayama S, et al. Clinical aspects of primary thyroid lymphoma: diagnosis and treatment based on our experience of 119 cases. Thyroid. 1993;3:93–9.
20. Belal AA, Allam A, Kandil A, et al. Primary thyroid lymphoma: a retrospective analysis of prognostic factors and treatment outcome for localized intermediate and high grade lymphoma. Am J Clin Oncol. 2001;24:299–305.
21. Logue JP, Hale RJ, Stewart AL, Duthie MB, Banerjee SS. Primary malignant lymphoma of the thyroid: a clinicopathological analysis. Int J Radiat Oncol Biol Phys. 1992;22:929–33.
22. Souhami L, Simpson WJ, Carruthers JS. Malignant lymphoma of the thyroid gland. Int J Radiat Oncol Biol Phys. 1980;6:1143–7.
23. Kalinyak JE, Kong CS, McDougall IR. Burkitt's lymphoma presenting as a rapidly growing thyroid mass. Thyroid. 2006;16:1053–7.
24. Yasuda S, Ide M, Takagi S, Shohtsu A. Cancer screening with whole-body FDG PET. Kaku Igaku. 1996;33:1065–71.
25. Schmid DT, Kneifel S, Stoeckli SJ, Padberg BC, Merrill G, Goerres GW. Increased ^{18}F-FDG uptake mimicking thyroid cancer in a patient with Hashimoto's thyroiditis. Eur Radiol. 2003;13:2119–21.
26. Yasuda S, Shohtsu A, Ide M, et al. Chronic thyroiditis: diffuse uptake of FDG at PET. Radiology. 1998;207:775–8.
27. Nakadate M, Yoshida K, Ishii A, Koizumi M, Tochigi N, et al. Is ^{18}F-FDG PET/CT useful for distinguishing between primary thyroid lymphoma and chronic thyroiditis? Clin Nucl Med. 2013;38:709–14.
28. Doria R, Jekel JF, Cooper DL. Thyroid lymphoma. The case for combined modality therapy. Cancer. 1994;73:200–6.
29. Basu S, Li G, Bural G, Alavi A. Fluorodeoxyglucose positron emission tomography (FDG-PET) and PET/computed tomography imaging characteristics of thyroid lymphoma and their potential clinical utility. Acta Radiol. 2009;50:201–4.
30. Nakada K, Kamijo K, Fujimoto N, Sugie H, Sakurai M. Clinical value of FDG PET/CT in response assessment of primary thyroid lymphoma. J Nucl Med. 2014;55 Suppl 1:667.
31. Marchesi M, Biffoni M, Biancari F. False-positive finding on ^{18}F-FDG PET after chemotherapy for primary diffuse large B-cell lymphoma of the thyroid: a case report. Jpn J Clin Oncol. 2004;34:280–1.
32. Higashi T, Itoh K, Ozaki O, Yashiro T, Momotani N, Mimura T. Ga-67 scintigram in evaluation of malignant lymphoma of the thyroid originating from chronic thyroiditis. Rinsho Hoshasen. 1989;34:977–81.
33. Nishiyama Y, Yamamoto Y, Yokoe K, Satoh K, Ohkawa M. Diagnosis of thyroid lymphoma and follow-up evaluation using Ga-67 scintigraphy. Ann Nucl Med. 2003;17:351–7.

Part XII

Undifferentiated Tumors: Anaplastic Thyroid Cancer

Anaplastic Thyroid Carcinoma: Clinical Aspects

94

Robert C. Smallridge and Ejigayehu G. Abate

Anaplastic thyroid carcinoma (ATC), like differentiated thyroid cancers (DTC), is more prevalent in women than men (Table 94.1), with a ratio of 1.9:1 [1–44]. Unlike DTC, however, ATC presents much more commonly in older individuals. The mean age is 66.5 years and the median is 69 years, with an age range of 15–98 years (Table 94.1) [1–44]. Onset below age 50 is uncommon. It is believed that ATC dedifferentiates from DTC, at least in some cases, and patients may have either a prior history of DTC or coexisting DTC and ATC in the same tumor (Table 94.1) [4, 5, 9–11, 14, 17–21, 23, 24, 27, 33, 34, 41, 45].

ATC fortunately is an uncommon form of thyroid cancer but occurs worldwide. Table 94.2 defines the reported frequency of ATC as a percentage of all thyroid cancers in geographically diverse locations, with a median of 3.8 % of cancer cases but ranging from 0.6 % to 9.8 %. Of interest is that in several countries, the frequency of ATC as a percentage of total thyroid cancer cases decreased dramatically as iodine intake increased, with an 80 % reduction in Germany [14] and 60 % decrease in Ireland [46]. While the percentage of cases was not given, in Slovenia, the mean number of patients was reduced from 6.2 to 4/year ($p=0.049$) after salt iodinization [47]. In the US SEER database, the frequency of ATC varied among race/ethnic groups as follows: Hispanic White (0.6 %), Asian/Pacific Islander (1.0 %), non-Hispanic White (1.1 %), American Indian native (1.3 %), and Black (1.8 %) [48].

R.C. Smallridge, MD (✉)
Division of Endocrinology & Metabolism, Mayo Clinic, Jacksonville, FL, USA

Department of Medicine, Mayo Clinic, Jacksonville, FL, USA

Department of Cancer Biology, Mayo Clinic, Jacksonville, FL, USA
e-mail: smallridge.robert@mayo.edu

E.G. Abate, MD
Division of Endocrinology & Metabolism, Mayo Clinic, Jacksonville, FL, USA

Department of Medicine, Mayo Clinic, Jacksonville, FL, USA

The clinical presentation of anaplastic thyroid carcinoma is notable for its explosive onset and rapid progression to death. While patients with differentiated thyroid cancer usually have limited preoperative staging, patients with ATC should be comprehensively assessed and quickly. Imaging techniques commonly employed include CT scans, PET/CT, and/or MRI, with FDG-PET having excellent sensitivity [44, 49]. The initial management plan should be developed after determining the extent of locoregional neck disease, the presence or absence of distant metastases (and their locations), and the patient's performance status. Once obtained, this information will permit the patient's medical team to provide a realistic determination as to whether the patient would possibly benefit from aggressive multimodal therapy or whether palliative care would be more appropriate. This information then should be discussed with the patient and his/her family or caregiver to arrive at an action plan according to the wishes of the patient. Unfortunately, in some instances, patients present with advanced disease, and urgent management of airway compromise takes precedence [50].

Most patients present with a neck mass, usually of recent origin (Table 94.3) [3–5, 7–9, 11, 17–19, 21–27, 29, 33, 39, 41, 42]. The mass is of sufficient size to cause a variety of symptoms due to encroachment upon vital locoregional structures. The median tumor size is 6.8 cm (range: 0.5–25 cm) [5, 11, 18, 21, 28, 30–32, 41]. Damage to the recurrent laryngeal nerve produces hoarseness or dysphonia in a third of cases [3, 5, 8, 9, 11, 19, 21, 23–25, 27, 39], and airway compromise with dyspnea develops in about one fourth of patients [3, 5, 8, 9, 11, 19, 21, 23–25, 27, 39, 42]. Associated respiratory symptoms of cough and hemoptysis were reported in 10 % of cases [11]. Elective tracheostomy is not recommended, but tracheostomy or cricothyrotomy is necessary when the airway is impaired [50].

Esophageal impingement and dysphagia are reported in 37.5 % of patients [3, 5, 8, 9, 11, 19, 21, 23, 24, 27, 39, 42]. If needed, enteral nutrition can be provided with a PEG tube, but placement may be difficult due to tumor encroachment.

L. Wartofsky, D. Van Nostrand (eds.), *Thyroid Cancer*, DOI 10.1007/978-1-4939-3314-3_94

Table 94.1 Clinical characteristics of patients with anaplastic thyroid carcinoma

Gender	2881
Female	1898
Male	983
Age (yr) (range: 15–98)	
Median (range) ($n=26$)	69 (58–76)
Mean ($n=19$)	66.5
Tumor size, median (range)	6.8 cm (0.5–25)
Associated DTC ($n=18$)	27 % (3–52)
Distant metastasis	
At presentation ($n=30$)	42 % (11–90)
Causes of death ($n=5$)	
Local	15.5 % (5–37)
Distant metastases	59 % (12–68)
Both	26.2 % (25–51)

DTC differentiated thyroid carcinoma, *N* number of reports

Table 94.2 Geographic variations in frequency of anaplastic thyroid cancer as a percentage of all thyroid cancers

Country (Refs.)	%
Germany[a] [14]	35/19/7
Ireland[a] [46]	24.3/18.3/9.8
The Netherlands [52]	7.9
Israel [9]	7.5
India [53]	4.7
New Zealand [54]	4.2
Jordan [55]	3.6
Japan [24, 40]	3.6–4.1
Romania [56]	3.4
Italy [32, 57]	0.7–2.9
Austria [58]	2.0
Luxembourg [59]	1.9
The United States [48, 60]	1.1–1.7
Australia [61]	1.3
Greece [62]	0.6

Refs. references
[a]Before and after increase in dietary iodide

Table 94.3 Frequency of symptoms at presentation of anaplastic thyroid carcinoma

Symptoms	Frequency
Neck mass	86.5 % (46–100)
Hoarseness/dysphonia	33 % (16–58)
Dysphagia	37.5 % (1–58)
Dyspnea	27 % (4–44)
Pain	15.5 % (8.9–32)
Cough	10 %
Hemoptysis	10 %
SVC syndrome	8.5 % (5–12)

SVC superior vena cava syndrome

Table 94.4 Distant metastasis locations in anaplastic thyroid carcinoma

Location	Frequency
Lung	37.2 % (14.3–60)
Mediastinum	25 %
Bone	6.4 % (2.5–30)
Liver	10.1 % (5–15)
Brain	4.4 % (0.7–6.8)
Heart	5.2 % (2.8–7.7)
Adrenals	5.2 % (5–5.3)
Kidney	5.3 %

One case each involving the stomach, skin, pancreas, spleen, salivary gland, and tonsil

On occasion, the tumor is sufficiently bulky to produce the superior vena cava syndrome (Table 94.3) [5, 21].

Distant metastases are common when patients are initially seen, with lung lesions being the leading location (Table 94.4) [1, 4, 6, 9, 13–15, 18, 21, 23, 26, 38, 40, 41, 44]. Next in frequency are the mediastinum [44] followed by liver [18, 38, 44] and bone [1, 4, 6, 9, 14, 18, 38, 40, 41, 44], with heart [18, 38], adrenals [18, 44], and kidney [18] reported less frequently. Tan et al. [11] found in 12 ATC patients at autopsy metastases in cervical lymph nodes (83 %), lung (75 %), esophagus/mediastinum (50 %), trachea (42 %), adrenals (33 %), supraclavicular nodes (25 %), mesenteric and pelvic nodes (17 %), bone (8 %), and brain (8 %). An autopsy study of 45 patients with ATC showed a similar organ distribution, but a frequency two to four times the percentages noted during life [51]. Death is most often attributed to either locoregional complications, distant metastases, or both (Table 94.1) [15, 23, 26, 38, 45]. Once initial stabilization (if required), staging, and development of management goals are achieved, then therapy should begin promptly. After the planned course of therapy, many patients will have persistent disease, but some will be in apparent remission. It is then appropriate to reassess for continued or adjuvant therapy, based on the initial response and patient wishes, and to then design a surveillance/monitoring plan. This may be a more intensive imaging and follow-up for those patients who have good performance status, have responded well, and desire continued aggressive therapy or it may be palliative care.

References

1. Carcangiu ML, Steeper T, Zampi G, et al. Anaplastic thyroid carcinoma. A study of 70 cases. Am J Clin Pathol. 1985;83:135–58.
2. Kim JH, Leeper RD. Treatment of locally advanced thyroid carcinoma with combination doxorubicin and radiation therapy. Cancer. 1987;60:2372–5.
3. Tennvall J, Tallroth E, el Hassan A, et al. Anaplastic thyroid carcinoma. Doxorubicin, hyperfractionated radiotherapy and surgery. Acta Oncol. 1990;29:1025–8.
4. Venkatesh YS, Ordonez NG, Schultz PN, et al. Anaplastic carcinoma of the thyroid. A clinicopathologic study of 121 cases. Cancer. 1990;66:321–30.

5. Demeter JG, De Jong SA, Lawrence AM, et al. Anaplastic thyroid carcinoma: risk factors and outcome. Surgery. 1991;110:956–61; discussion 961–3.
6. Schlumberger M, Parmentier C, Delisle MJ, et al. Combination therapy for anaplastic giant cell thyroid carcinoma. Cancer. 1991;67:564–6.
7. Wong CS, Van Dyk J, Simpson WJ. Myelopathy following hyperfractionated accelerated radiotherapy for anaplastic thyroid carcinoma. Radiother Oncol. 1991;20:3–9.
8. Junor EJ, Paul J, Reed NS. Anaplastic thyroid carcinoma: 91 patients treated by surgery and radiotherapy. Eur J Surg Oncol. 1992;18:83–8.
9. Hadar T, Mor C, Shvero J, et al. Anaplastic carcinoma of the thyroid. Eur J Surg Oncol. 1993;19:511–6.
10. Levendag PC, De Porre PM, van Putten WL. Anaplastic carcinoma of the thyroid gland treated by radiation therapy. Int J Radiat Oncol Biol Phys. 1993;26:125–8.
11. Tan RK, Finley 3rd RK, Driscoll D, et al. Anaplastic carcinoma of the thyroid: a 24-year experience. Head Neck. 1995;17:41–7; discussion 47–8.
12. Chemotherapy Committee The Japanese Society of Thyroid Surgery. Intensive chemotherapy for anaplastic thyroid carcinoma: combination of cisplatin, doxorubicin, etoposide and peplomycin with granulocyte colony-stimulating factor support. Jpn J Clin Oncol. 1995;25:203–7.
13. Kobayashi T, Asakawa H, Umeshita K, et al. Treatment of 37 patients with anaplastic carcinoma of the thyroid. Head Neck. 1996;18:36–41.
14. Passler C, Scheuba C, Prager G, et al. Anaplastic (undifferentiated) thyroid carcinoma (ATC). A retrospective analysis. Langenbecks Arch Surg. 1999;384:284–93.
15. Voutilainen PE, Multanen M, Haapiainen RK, et al. Anaplastic thyroid carcinoma survival. World J Surg. 1999;23:975–8; discussion 978–9.
16. Ain KB. Anaplastic thyroid carcinoma: behavior, biology, and therapeutic approaches. Thyroid. 1998;8:715–26.
17. Busnardo B, Daniele O, Pelizzo MR, et al. A multimodality therapeutic approach in anaplastic thyroid carcinoma: study on 39 patients. J Endocrinol Invest. 2000;23:755–61.
18. Lam KY, Lo CY, Chan KW, et al. Insular and anaplastic carcinoma of the thyroid: a 45-year comparative study at a single institution and a review of the significance of p53 and p21. Ann Surg. 2000;231:329–38.
19. Rodriguez JM, Pinero A, Ortiz S, et al. Clinical and histological differences in anaplastic thyroid carcinoma. Eur J Surg. 2000;166:34–8.
20. Haigh PI, Ituarte PH, Wu HS, et al. Completely resected anaplastic thyroid carcinoma combined with adjuvant chemotherapy and irradiation is associated with prolonged survival. Cancer. 2001;91:2335–42.
21. Pierie JP, Muzikansky A, Gaz RD, et al. The effect of surgery and radiotherapy on outcome of anaplastic thyroid carcinoma. Ann Surg Oncol. 2002;9:57–64.
22. Sugino K, Ito K, Mimura T, et al. The important role of operations in the management of anaplastic thyroid carcinoma. Surgery. 2002;131:245–8.
23. De Crevoisier R, Baudin E, Bachelot A, et al. Combined treatment of anaplastic thyroid carcinoma with surgery, chemotherapy, and hyperfractionated accelerated external radiotherapy. Int J Radiat Oncol Biol Phys. 2004;60:1137–43.
24. Kihara M, Miyauchi A, Yamauchi A, et al. Prognostic factors of anaplastic thyroid carcinoma. Surg Today. 2004;34:394–8.
25. Veness MJ, Porter GS, Morgan GJ. Anaplastic thyroid carcinoma: dismal outcome despite current treatment approach. ANZ J Surg. 2004;74:559–62.
26. Besic N, Hocevar M, Zgajnar J, et al. Prognostic factors in anaplastic carcinoma of the thyroid-a multivariate survival analysis of 188 patients. Langenbecks Arch Surg. 2005;390:203–8.
27. Goutsouliak V, Hay JH. Anaplastic thyroid cancer in British Columbia 1985–1999: a population-based study. Clin Oncol (R Coll Radiol). 2005;17:75–8.
28. Kebebew E, Greenspan FS, Clark OH, et al. Anaplastic thyroid carcinoma. Treatment outcome and prognostic factors. Cancer. 2005;103:1330–5.
29. Wang Y, Tsang R, Asa S, et al. Clinical outcome of anaplastic thyroid carcinoma treated with radiotherapy of once- and twice-daily fractionation regimens. Cancer. 2006;107:1786–92.
30. Brignardello E, Gallo M, Baldi I, et al. Anaplastic thyroid carcinoma: clinical outcome of 30 consecutive patients referred to a single institution in the past 5 years. Eur J Endocrinol. 2007;156: 425–30.
31. Kim TY, Kim KW, Jung TS, et al. Prognostic factors for Korean patients with anaplastic thyroid carcinoma. Head Neck. 2007;29:765–72.
32. Miccoli P, Materazzi G, Antonelli A, et al. New trends in the treatment of undifferentiated carcinomas of the thyroid. Langenbecks Arch Surg. 2007;392:397–404.
33. Yau T, Lo CY, Epstein RJ, et al. Treatment outcomes in anaplastic thyroid carcinoma: survival improvement in young patients with localized disease treated by combination of surgery and radiotherapy. Ann Surg Oncol. 2008;15:2500–5.
34. Bhatia A, Rao A, Ang KK, et al. Anaplastic thyroid cancer: clinical outcomes with conformal radiotherapy. Head Neck. 2010;32:829–36.
35. Dandekar P, Harmer C, Barbachano Y, et al. Hyperfractionated accelerated radiotherapy (HART) for anaplastic thyroid carcinoma: toxicity and survival analysis. Int J Radiat Oncol Biol Phys. 2009;74:518–21.
36. Swaak-Kragten AT, de Wilt JH, Schmitz PI, et al. Multimodality treatment for anaplastic thyroid carcinoma – treatment outcome in 75 patients. Radiother Oncol. 2009;92:100–4.
37. Vrbic S, Pejcic I, Vrbic M, et al. Therapy of stage IV B anaplastic thyroid carcinoma: single institution experience. J BUON. 2009;14:41–4.
38. Siironen P, Hagstrom J, Maenpaa HO, et al. Anaplastic and poorly differentiated thyroid carcinoma: therapeutic strategies and treatment outcome of 52 consecutive patients. Oncology. 2010;79:400–8.
39. Akaishi J, Sugino K, Kitagawa W, et al. Prognostic factors and treatment outcomes of 100 cases of anaplastic thyroid carcinoma. Thyroid. 2011;21:1183–9.
40. Ito KI, Hanamura T, Murayama K, et al. Multimodality therapeutic outcomes in anaplastic thyroid carcinoma: improved survival in subgroups of patients with localized primary tumors. Head Neck. 2012;34:230–7.
41. McIver B, Hay ID, Giuffrida DF, et al. Anaplastic thyroid carcinoma: a 50-year experience at a single institution. Surgery. 2001;130:1028–34.
42. Tashima L, Mitzner R, Durvesh S, et al. Dyspnea as a prognostic factor in anaplastic thyroid carcinoma. Eur Arch Otorhinolaryngol. 2012;269:1251–5.
43. Sherman EJ, Lim SH, Ho AL, et al. Concurrent doxorubicin and radiotherapy for anaplastic thyroid cancer: a critical re-evaluation including uniform pathologic review. Radiother Oncol. 2011;101:425–30.
44. Poisson T, Deandreis D, Leboulleux S, et al. 18F-fluorodeoxyglucose positron emission tomography and computed tomography in anaplastic thyroid cancer. Eur J Nucl Med Mol Imaging. 2010;37:2277–85.
45. Segerhammar I, Larsson C, Nilsson IL, et al. Anaplastic carcinoma of the thyroid gland: treatment and outcome over 13 years at one institution. J Surg Oncol. 2012;106:981–6.
46. Dijkstra B, Prichard RS, Lee A, et al. Changing patterns of thyroid carcinoma. Ir J Med Sci. 2007;176:87–90.
47. Besic N, Hocevar M, Zgajnar J. Lower incidence of anaplastic carcinoma after higher iodination of salt in Slovenia. Thyroid. 2010;20:623–6.

48. Yu GP, Li JC, Branovan D, et al. Thyroid cancer incidence and survival in the national cancer institute surveillance, epidemiology, and end results race/ethnicity groups. Thyroid. 2010;20:465–73.
49. Bogsrud TV, Karantanis D, Nathan MA, et al. 18F-FDG PET in the management of patients with anaplastic thyroid carcinoma. Thyroid. 2008;18:713–9.
50. Shaha AR. Airway management in anaplastic thyroid carcinoma. Laryngoscope. 2008;118:1195–8.
51. Besic N, Gazic B. Sites of metastases of anaplastic thyroid carcinoma: autopsy findings in 45 cases from a single institution. Thyroid. 2013;23:709–13.
52. Netea-Maier RT, Aben KK, Casparie MK, et al. Trends in incidence and mortality of thyroid carcinoma in The Netherlands between 1989 and 2003: correlation with thyroid fine-needle aspiration cytology and thyroid surgery. Int J Cancer. 2008;123:1681–4.
53. Agrawal S, Rao RS, Parikh DM, et al. Histologic trends in thyroid cancer 1969–1993: a clinico-pathologic analysis of the relative proportion of anaplastic carcinoma of the thyroid. J Surg Oncol. 1996;63:251–5.
54. Brownlie B, Mercer P, Turner J, et al. Thyroid malignancies: a New Zealand South Island thyroid clinic experience 1995–2006. N Z Med J. 2008;121:36–45.
55. Shomaf MS, Younes NA, Albsoul NM, et al. New trends in the clinicopathological features of differentiated thyroid cancer in Central Jordan. Saudi Med J. 2006;27:185–90.
56. Catana R, Boila A, Borda A. Thyroid cancer profile in Mures County (Romania): a 20 years study. Rom J Morphol Embryol. 2012;53:1007–12.
57. Pingitore R, Vignati S, Bigini D, et al. Post-operative examination of 2930 thyroid glands: observations on primary carcinoma. Incidental carcinoma and the preoperative diagnostic assessment of thyroidectomy for cancer. Pathologica. 1993;85:591–605.
58. Gomez Segovia I, Gallowitsch HJ, Kresnik E, et al. Descriptive epidemiology of thyroid carcinoma in Carinthia, Austria: 1984–2001. Histopathologic features and tumor classification of 734 cases under elevated general iodination of table salt since 1990: population-based age-stratified analysis on thyroid carcinoma incidence. Thyroid. 2004;14:277–86.
59. Scheiden R, Keipes M, Bock C, et al. Thyroid cancer in Luxembourg: a national population-based data report (1983–1999). BMC Cancer. 2006;6:102.
60. Hundahl SA, Fleming ID, Fremgen AM, et al. A National Cancer Data Base report on 53,856 cases of thyroid carcinoma treated in the U.S., 1985–1995. Cancer. 1998;83:2638–48.
61. Burgess JR. Temporal trends for thyroid carcinoma in Australia: an increasing incidence of papillary thyroid carcinoma (1982–1997). Thyroid. 2002;12:141–9.
62. Gkountouvas A, Nikas M, Chatjimarkou F, et al. Thyroid cancer in Greece. A tertiary center experience. J Buon. 2010;15:674–8.

Surgical Management of Anaplastic Thyroid Carcinoma

95

Gerard M. Doherty

Anaplastic carcinoma is one of the most aggressive malignancies and is usually deadly. Most patients with anaplastic thyroid cancer do poorly regardless of treatment. They typically die of either distant metastatic disease or from the effects of local tumor invasion; the median survival time is about 6 months, and the overall mortality rate is nearly 100 % [1]. At initial examination, patients usually have a large (5–10 cm) fixed mass, and about 30 % already have distant metastases, often in the lungs. Many patients with anaplastic thyroid cancer also have coexistent well-differentiated thyroid cancer. Some of these tumors demonstrate progression from well-differentiated papillary cancers through the insular variant then into anaplastic cancer. Anaplastic thyroid cancers are more likely to have *p53* and platelet-derived growth factor mutations than differentiated thyroid cancers [2].

Anaplastic thyroid cancers occur most often in older patients, especially in areas of endemic goiter. Iodine deficiency appears to be an important factor, and the incidence of anaplastic cancer has decreased in some areas with the improvement in dietary iodine [3]. Even when anaplastic thyroid cancers are found incidentally when removing a differentiated thyroid cancer, the outcome is guarded. However, patients who have tumors that can be completely resected and are younger have a slightly better prognosis [4]. An updated analysis of the SEER database indicated that age less than 60 years, tumor confined to the thyroid, female sex, surgical resection, and external beam radiotherapy or combination surgical resection with radiotherapy were favorable prognostic factors [5].

G.M. Doherty, MD, FACS (✉)
Department of Surgery, Boston Medical Center, Boston University, 88 East Newton Street Collamore Building Suite 500, Boston, MA 02118, USA
e-mail: dohertyg@bu.edu

Most patients with anaplastic thyroid cancer are not difficult to diagnose. They are usually older patients, and 80 % report a long history of goiter or a thyroid nodule. A typical history is that the thyroid goiter or nodule suddenly begins to grow rapidly, and patients develop pain, dysphagia, and/or hoarseness. Some patients may be misdiagnosed with subacute thyroiditis. Fine needle aspiration cytology is usually definitive, but tumor cells may be scant in large tumors because of hemorrhagic necrosis, requiring core needle or incisional biopsy.

Based on the large size of these tumors at presentation, cross-sectional imaging is recommended to document the extent of the disease. It can also determine if there is intratracheal growth or invasion. Although most of these tumors do not have thyrotropin receptors, take up radioiodine, or make thyroglobulin, some of these tumors do, as they have originated from more differentiated tumors. Therefore, documenting thyroid function and serum thyroglobulin levels is also recommended.

There are three basic roles for operative intervention. Occasionally, a diagnostic incisional or core biopsy is necessary to definitively make the diagnosis; often the issue is to exclude lymphoma. Secondly, there is sometimes the necessity to secure the airway with a tracheostomy in order to prolong the patient's life and to provide comfort. Finally, there are some patients for whom complete operative resection is feasible. This appears to be helpful for those patients for whom locoregional control of the disease in the neck can prevent death from this miserable aspect of the disease. From a technical point of view, when conducting thyroidectomy in these patients, in contrast to other patients with thyroid cancer, it may be helpful to remove the least involved lobe first, so as to orient the surgeon to the trachea. Once this portion of the thyroid gland has been taken away, removing the side that is more involved with tumor may become easier.

L. Wartofsky, D. Van Nostrand (eds.), *Thyroid Cancer*, DOI 10.1007/978-1-4939-3314-3_95

Once the diagnosis has been made by cytological examination or open biopsy, treatment with multimodality therapy seems necessary because the results of other treatments are dismal. The eventual outcome of patients with anaplastic thyroid cancer is dictated by local progression and distant disease. While operative management may be an important component for some patients, and may contribute to long-term disease control in a few patients, the need in the therapeutic strategy is for more effective systemic agents [6]. Adjuvant therapy for locally resected disease with external beam radiotherapy and systemic chemotherapy is typically recommended but is rarely definitive. Best supportive care with early involvement of palliative care services is often the best available management [7].

References

1. Smallridge RC, Copland JA. Anaplastic thyroid carcinoma: pathogenesis and emerging therapies. Clin Oncol (R Coll Radiol). 2010;22(6):486–97.
2. Nikiforov YE, Nikiforova MN. Molecular genetics and diagnosis of thyroid cancer. Nat Rev Endocrinol. 2011;7(10):569–80.
3. Dijkstra B, et al. Changing patterns of thyroid carcinoma. Ir J Med Sci. 2007;176(2):87–90.
4. McIver B, et al. Anaplastic thyroid carcinoma: a 50-year experience at a single institution. Surgery. 2001;130(6):1028–34.
5. Kebebew E, et al. Anaplastic thyroid carcinoma. Treatment outcome and prognostic factors. Cancer. 2005;103(7):1330–5.
6. Smallridge RC. Approach to the patient with anaplastic thyroid carcinoma. J Clin Endocrinol Metab. 2012;97(8):2566–72.
7. Smallridge RC, et al. American Thyroid Association guidelines for management of patients with anaplastic thyroid cancer. Thyroid. 2012;22(11):1104–39.

Pathology of Anaplastic Carcinoma

96

Zubair W. Baloch and Virginia A. LiVolsi

Anaplastic carcinoma (undifferentiated carcinoma) is a rare extremely malignant neoplasm and is usually fatal (mortality rate at 1 year 90 %) [1–3]. From a clinical standpoint, the thyroid gland in these patients has often been enlarged for years, containing multiple nodules or a low-grade, well-differentiated carcinoma that has grown slowly. Recent rapid growth with tracheal compromise is often noted. Clinically and surgically these cancers usually infiltrate and replace the thyroid parenchyma and the juxtathyroidal tissues. Metastases to the regional lymph nodes and lungs are common [1, 4].

Grossly, the neoplastic tissue is pale, firm or hard, and opaque. Foci of hemorrhage and necrosis are frequent. Foci of calcification are rare, and occasionally, there are regions of metaplastic cartilage and/or bone [4, 5]. Varied histological patterns are present including: (1) rounded to irregular medium- to giant-sized cells with eosinophilic cytoplasm and large or giant nuclei (often bizarre), (2) fusiform (spindle) cells in a fascicular or storiform pattern (Fig. 96.1), and (3) medium- to large-sized cells with squamoid characteristics (Fig. 96.2). Some of these cells may have clear cytoplasm. The neoplastic giant cells may have a single nucleus or may be multinucleated. These various cellular types can be mixed together, and transitional forms can be seen. Bizarre nuclei, often vesicular, are common; large nucleoli may be present. There are numerous mitotic figures, and some are atypical. "Osteoclast-type" giant cells of histiocytic origin exist in a few tumors [6] (Fig. 96.1).

Neoplastic cells may replace some portions of vessel walls, and small clusters of neoplastic cells may extend into individual thyroid follicles. Polymorphonuclear leukocytes can infiltrate the tumor and can be great in number near the necrotic regions [4]; some tumors have a prominent eosinophilic leukocytic infiltrate in areas that are not necrotic; tissue culture studies indicate that these types of anaplastic carcinoma can secrete eosinophil chemotactic factor [7].

A paucicellular variant has been reported *and* must be distinguished from Riedel's disease and fibromatosis of the neck. Clues to this distinction include foci of hypercellularity, necrosis, and abnormal mitoses. The sparse neoplastic cells have atypical nuclei [8].

In all types of anaplastic carcinoma, immunoreactive thyroglobulin is typically absent; when present, it is evident only in some larger "epithelioid" cells. Often it is only noted at the invasive edges of the tumor which indicates false positivity due to diffusion from destroyed thyroid follicles. Immunoreactive keratin may be demonstrated and is the most common marker that suggests epithelial characteristics; however, different cytokeratins (by molecular weights) are expressed in some tumors, and on the other hand, many examples show no cytokeratin immunoreactivity [2, 9, 10]. Approximately 30 % of anaplastic carcinomas express thyroid transcription factor-1 (TTF-1); this marker if positive is extremely helpful in diagnosis of anaplastic carcinoma especially in small biopsies [11]. Interpretation of immunostains must be done with caution because both normal thyroid epithelium and remnants of well-differentiated carcinoma (or a benign nodule) may be trapped within the aggressive neoplasm.

Evidence of a previous nodular goiter or a follicular, Hurthle, or papillary carcinoma may be often found if multiple sections of the neoplasm are taken. The tumors with substantial spindle cell or giant and spindle cell components may be mistaken for soft tissue neoplasms, but they are usually not recognizable as one of the well-characterized sarcomas [1, 4, 12, 13]. Most so-called small-cell anaplastic carcinomas diagnosed in the past were malignant lymphomas. Small-cell carcinoma does exist, but it is usually a medullary or poorly differentiated carcinoma and can be appropriately diagnosed with judicious use of immunostains [2, 5, 14].

Z.W. Baloch, MD, PhD (✉) • V.A. LiVolsi, MD
Department of Pathology and Laboratory Medicine, University of Pennsylvania Medical Center, Perelman School of Medicine, 6 Founders Pavilion 3400 Spruce Street, Philadelphia, PA 19104, USA
e-mail: balocj@mail.med.upenn.edu; linus@mail.med.upenn.edu

L. Wartofsky, D. Van Nostrand (eds.), *Thyroid Cancer*, DOI 10.1007/978-1-4939-3314-3_96

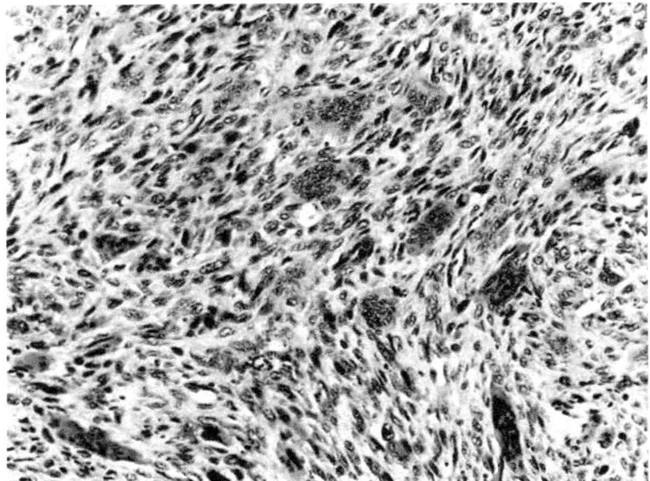

Fig. 96.1 Undifferentiated carcinoma. Spindle cells and osteoclast-type giant cells are present (hematoxylin and eosin [H&E] stain)

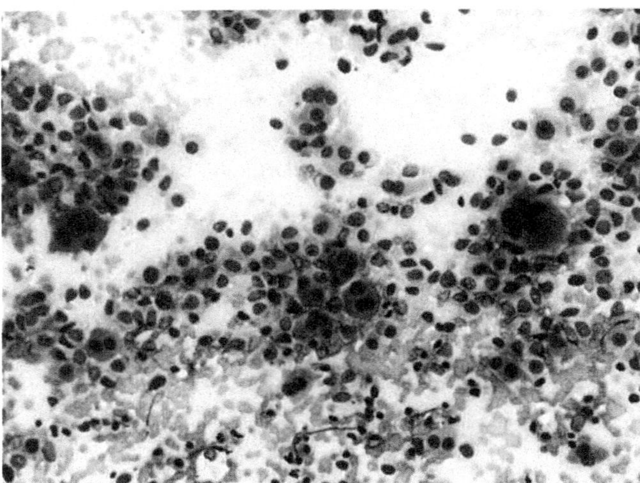

Fig. 96.3 Undifferentiated carcinoma. Hypercellular aspirate with marked variation in the size of the neoplastic cells. Multinucleated cells are evident (Diff-Quik® stain)

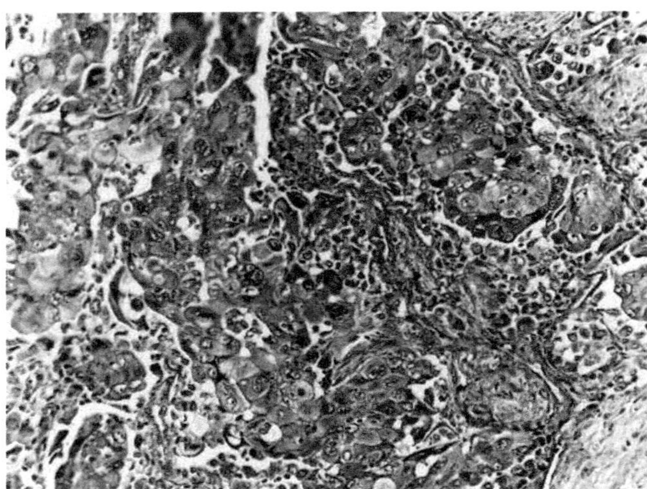

Fig. 96.2 Undifferentiated carcinoma. Part of the neoplasm has a "squamoid" appearance (H&E stain)

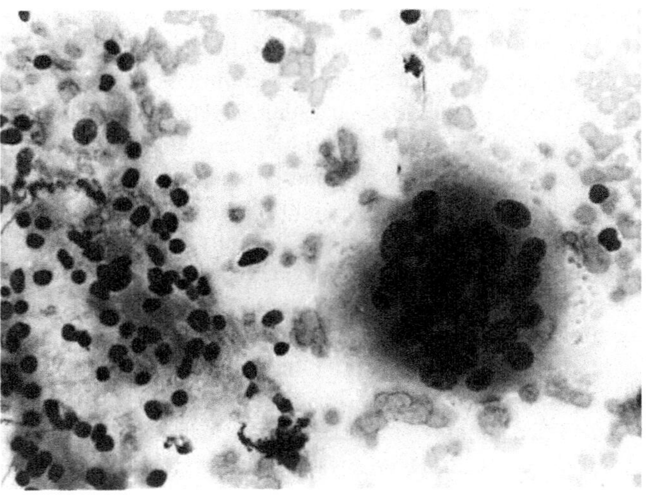

Fig. 96.4 Undifferentiated carcinoma. Hypercellular aspirate with an osteoclast-type cell on the right (Diff-Quik® stain)

In middle-aged or elderly patients, a portion of an otherwise well-differentiated carcinoma may be anaplastic carcinoma, which has grave prognostic implications. If such a focus is only a few millimeters in diameter, it may have little effect on the patient's long-term survival, but in some patients, this is unfortunately not true [15–17]. The same concept applies for a tiny anaplastic carcinoma discovered in a thyroid that was removed for multinodular goiter.

The cytology of anaplastic carcinoma shows marked cellularity or necrosis and hemorrhage (Fig. 96.3), depending on the part of the mass sampled [18, 19]. Leukocytes can be numerous. Spindle and giant cells are present [20] with bizarre neoplastic cells with one or several nuclei (Fig. 96.4). Abnormal mitotic figures may be seen. The smears may show cells from a follicular neoplasm or papillary carcinoma if one coexists with the anaplastic carcinoma [21]. Therefore, this possibility illustrates the requirement that several aspirations should be performed when a fast-growing mass is present. Also, these neoplasms may be hemorrhagic or fibrotic; thus, the epithelial cells may be sparse or diluted by blood.

References

1. Carcangiu ML, Steeper T, Zampi G, Rosai J. Anaplastic thyroid carcinoma. A study of 70 cases. Am J Clin Pathol. 1985;83:135–58.
2. LiVolsi VA, Brooks JJ, Arendash-Durand B. Anaplastic thyroid tumors. Immunohistology. Am J Clin Pathol. 1987;87:434–42.

3. Shvero J, Gal R, Avidor I, Hadar T, Kessler E. Anaplastic thyroid carcinoma. A clinical, histologic, and immunohistochemical study. Cancer. 1988;62:319–25.
4. Chang TC, Liaw KY, Kuo SH, Chang CC, Chen FW. Anaplastic thyroid carcinoma: review of 24 cases, with emphasis on cytodiagnosis and leukocytosis. Taiwan Yi Xue Hui Za Zhi. 1989;88:551–6.
5. Venkatesh YS, Ordonez NG, Schultz PN, Hickey RC, Goepfert H, Samaan NA. Anaplastic carcinoma of the thyroid. A clinicopathologic study of 121 cases. Cancer. 1990;66:321–30.
6. Kobayashi S, Yamadori I, Ohmori M, Kurokawa T, Umeda M. Anaplastic carcinoma of the thyroid with osteoclast-like giant cells. An ultrastructural and immunohistochemical study. Acta Pathol Jpn. 1987;37:807–15.
7. Vassilatou E, Fisfis M, Morphopoulos G, Savva S, Voucouti E, Stefanoudaki K, Tzavara I. Papillary thyroid carcinoma producing granulocyte-macrophage colony-stimulating factor is associated with neutrophilia and eosinophilia. Hormones (Athens). 2006;5:303–9.
8. Wan SK, Chan JK, Tang SK. Paucicellular variant of anaplastic thyroid carcinoma. A mimic of Reidel's thyroiditis. Am J Clin Pathol. 1996;105:388–93.
9. Beltrami CA, Criante P, Di Loreto C. Immunocytochemistry of anaplastic carcinoma of thyroid gland. Appl Pathol. 1989;7:122–33.
10. Miettinen M, Franssila KO. Variable expression of keratins and nearly uniform lack of thyroid transcription factor 1 in thyroid anaplastic carcinoma. Hum Pathol. 2000;31:1139–45.
11. Gopal PP, Montone KT, Baloch Z, Tuluc M, Livolsi V. The variable presentations of anaplastic spindle cell squamous carcinoma associated with tall cell variant of papillary thyroid carcinoma. Thyroid. 2011;21:493–9.
12. Casterline PF, Jaques DA, Blom H, Wartofsky L. Anaplastic giant and spindle-cell carcinoma of the thyroid: a different therapeutic approach. Cancer. 1980;45:1689–92.
13. Kapp DS, LiVolsi VA, Sanders MM. Anaplastic carcinoma following well-differentiated thyroid cancer: etiological considerations. Yale J Biol Med. 1982;55:521–8.
14. Wolf BC, Sheahan K, DeCoste D, Variakojis D, Alpern HD, Haselow RE. Immunohistochemical analysis of small cell tumors of the thyroid gland: an Eastern Cooperative Oncology Group study. Hum Pathol. 1992;23:1252–61.
15. Perri F, Lorenzo GD, Scarpati GD, Buonerba C. Anaplastic thyroid carcinoma: a comprehensive review of current and future therapeutic options. World J Clin Oncol. 2011;2:150–7.
16. Foote RL, Molina JR, Kasperbauer JL, Lloyd RV, McIver B, Morris JC, Grant CS, Thompson GB, Richards ML, Hay ID, Smallridge RC, Bible KC. Enhanced survival in locoregionally confined anaplastic thyroid carcinoma: a single-institution experience using aggressive multimodal therapy. Thyroid. 2011;21:25–30.
17. Rapkiewicz A, Roses D, Goldenberg A, Levine P, Bannan M, Simsir A. Encapsulated anaplastic thyroid carcinoma transformed from follicular carcinoma: a case report. Acta Cytol. 2009; 53:332–6.
18. Luze T, Totsch M, Bangerl I, Hittmair A, Sandbichler P, Ladurner D, Schmid KW. Fine needle aspiration cytodiagnosis of anaplastic carcinoma and malignant haemangioendothelioma of the thyroid in an endemic goitre area. Cytopathology. 1990;1:305–10.
19. Saunders CA, Nayar R. Anaplastic spindle-cell squamous carcinoma arising in association with tall-cell papillary cancer of the thyroid: a potential pitfall. Diagn Cytopathol. 1999;21:413–8.
20. Schneider V, Frable WJ. Spindle and giant cell carcinoma of the thyroid: cytologic diagnosis by fine needle aspiration. Acta Cytol. 1980;24:184–9.
21. Vinette DS, MacDonald LL, Yazdi HM. Papillary carcinoma of the thyroid with anaplastic transformation: diagnostic pitfalls in fine-needle aspiration biopsy. Diagn Cytopathol. 1991;7:75–8.

PET/CT in Anaplastic Cancer of the Thyroid

97

Iain Ross McDougall and Andrei Iagaru

PET/CT in Anaplastic Cancer

Anaplastic thyroid carcinoma (ATC) is the most aggressive solid cancer in man, with a median survival of 3 months. Because of the rapid onset and relentless progression of the disease and its dismal prognosis, early diagnosis is important. Scintigraphy or ultrasound does not help in the diagnosis and can delay management. ^{18}F-FDG PET/CT has been found helpful in selected patients to define the local extent of disease and presence of metastases.

The role of ^{18}F-FDG PET/CT scan in well-differentiated carcinoma has been presented in a prior chapter. That section contains methods and the basics are repeated here. The patient should be fasted for 6–8 h and have a normal fasting serum glucose value. 10–15 mCi (370–555) MBq ^{18}F-fluorine-deoxyglucose (^{18}F-FDG) is injected intravenously and scanning commenced after a delay of 60 min, although some authorities prefer a delay of 90–120 min. It is important that the patient is resting in a quiet environment and not speaking or chewing over the hour between the administration of FDG and scanning. Usually the scan should be from the base of the skull to the upper thighs, although when widespread metastases are judged to be likely, the whole body can be scanned. Combined PET/CT that includes attenuation correction and anatomic correlation is now routine.

From the original descriptions of the value of ^{18}F-FDG PET in differentiated thyroid cancer, it became apparent that there was a reciprocal relationship between the uptake of ^{18}F-FDG and radioiodine seen on conventional nuclear medicine studies. The difference depended on the degree of differentiation of the cancer [1]. Well-differentiated cancers trap radioiodine, but not ^{18}F-FDG, and poorly differentiated cancers show avid uptake of ^{18}F-FDG, but they are likely to not trap iodine [1, 2]. Iodine is concentrated by the sodium-iodide symporter (NIS) [3]. Glucose is taken into cells by glucose transporters including GLUT 1–5 and GLUT 7. As cancers become more dedifferentiated, the quantity of NIS at the latero-basal membrane of follicular cells decreases, and its appropriate cellular positioning can be lost [4, 5]. Anaplastic cancers have basically forgotten that they are thyroidal in origin and lose the ability to trap iodine. However, as cancers become more anaplastic, there is increased expression of glucose transporters. In one study, the quantity of GLUT 1 was studied in 45 thyroid cancers [6]. Five of the cancers were anaplastic and the remaining 40 were graded for the degree of aggressiveness. All anaplastic cancers demonstrated more membranous and cytoplasmic GLUT 1, and the quantity of GLUT 1 in differentiated cancer cells was linearly but inversely related to the grade of malignancy. A different investigation demonstrated that GLUT 3 is the most prevalent transporter in differentiated thyroid cancers. However, in anaplastic cancers there was an increase in both GLUT 1 and GLUT 3. These data indicated that ^{18}F-FDG PET/CT should be a powerful and accurate imaging test in patients with anaplastic cancer. There are only a few reports on ^{18}F-FDG PET/CT in anaplastic thyroid cancer related to the fact that the cancer is relatively rare accounting for 1–3 % of thyroid cancers, and PET/CT scan is a relatively new investigative tool [7, 8]. However, these cancers show intense trapping and concentration of ^{18}F-FDG, and the standardized uptake values (SUV) are among the highest measured for solid cancers (Fig. 97.1).

As stated, anaplastic cancer is an extremely fast-growing cancer that is locally invasive and usually causes a rapid death by local compressive effects. It is estimated that about 80 % of patients have regional nodal metastases and 50 %

I.R. McDougall, MD, PhD, FRCP
Department of Radiology, Nuclear Medicine, Stanford University Hospital and Clinics, Stanford, CA, USA

A. Iagaru, MD (✉)
Department of Radiology, Nuclear Medicine, Stanford University Medical Center, Stanford School of Medicine,
300 Pasteur Dr H2230 MC 5281, Stanford, CA 94305, USA
e-mail: aiagaru@stanford.edu

L. Wartofsky, D. Van Nostrand (eds.), *Thyroid Cancer*, DOI 10.1007/978-1-4939-3314-3_97

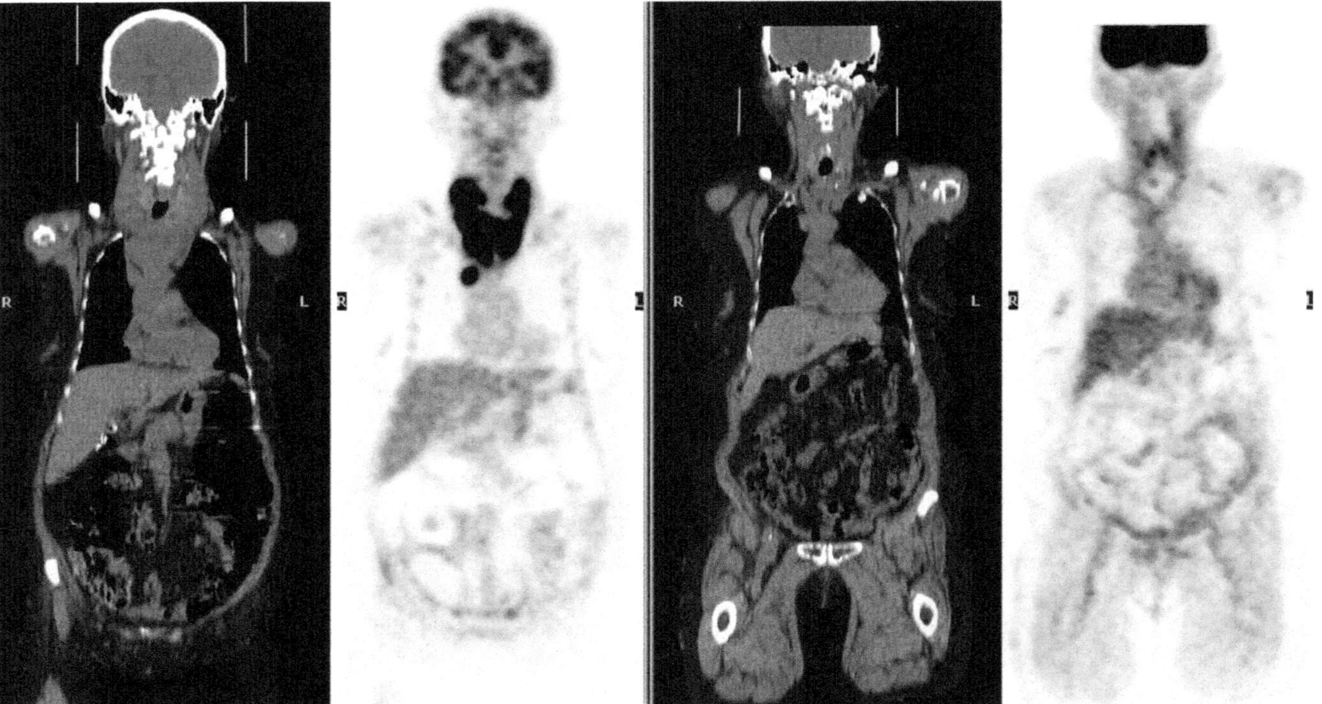

Fig. 97.1 The illustration shows ^{18}F-FDG PET scan in an elderly woman with a rapidly growing thyroid mass. The patient had difficulty breathing and swallowing. FNA demonstrated anaplastic thyroid cancer. The two figures on the *left* are at presentation and show a large mediastinal mass on CT, and there is intense uptake of ^{18}F-FDG with irregular edges in the cancer, and the inferior extension is most likely a tumor thrombus. The two figures on the *right* show CT and PET after chemotherapy demonstrating a remarkably good response

distant metastases at presentation. PET/CT can be used to stage the disease [9, 10]. This staging can help make a decision whether to operate first or to treat with systemic chemotherapy and/or radiotherapy. For example, when distant lesions are found, it is not appropriate to conduct extensive surgery on the primary lesion. Several case reports attest to the value of ^{18}F-FDG PET [12–14]. Now there are a few series, although the number of patients studied is not large. In a study by Bogsrud et al., PET altered management in 50 % of patients [11]. In this investigation, 16 patients were studied, and the primary cancer was detected in every patient and in all 9 patients who had regional nodal metastases. The sensitivity for pulmonary metastases was lower at 62 % (5/8) confirming a general finding that PET alone is inferior to CT for small lung lesions. However, when combined PET/CT is conducted, there is the benefit of identifying lesions by abnormal function on PET and by anatomy on CT.

Poisson et al. recently published their findings using PET/CT in 20 patients, 18 with metastases. PET/CT identified 62 of 63 organs involved with cancer and 264 of 265 separate metastases. Thirty-five percent of the lesions were only identified by PET/CT. Therapy was altered in about a quarter of the patients. The investigators determined the volume of disease, and prognosis was poor when the volume was >300 mls. Similarly, an SUV >18 was statistically associated with a worse outcome. These investigators demonstrated that the high FDG uptake in the lesions on PET/CT provides a better staging than CT and/or bone scintigraphy and should be routinely performed during initial staging. PET/CT was also useful in following the response to therapy recognizing that most patients with this disease have a dismal prognosis (Fig. 97.1). Other investigators have demonstrated that the prognosis in thyroid cancer can be related to the uptake of ^{18}F-FDG, and lesions showing a high uptake usually do not trap iodine and they portend a sinister outcome [15, 16].

We have reported metastasis from anaplastic cancer to unusual sites such as the adrenal gland (also reported by other investigators in Hürthle cell cancer) [17, 18]. Malignant thrombus extending from the primary cancer has been identified using combined PET/CT [19]. PET has also been valuable in cancers that fall on the interface between differentiated and anaplastic such as insular thyroid carcinoma [20, 21].

^{18}F-FDG PET/CT scanning has a role in defining the local, regional, and distant sites of metastases in patients with poorly differentiated (insular) cancer and anaplastic cancer and is important in staging; it helps define prognosis and is valuable in determining the response to treatment.

References

1. Joensuu H, Ahonen A. Imaging of metastases of thyroid carcinoma with fluorine-18 fluorodeoxyglucose. J Nucl Med. 1987;28: 910–4.
2. Feine U. Fluor-18-deoxyglucose positron emission tomography in differentiated thyroid cancer. Eur J Endocrinol. 1998;138:492–6.
3. Dai G, Levy O, Carrasco N. Cloning and characterization of the thyroid iodide transporter. Nature. 1996;379:458–60.
4. Min JJ, Chung JK, Lee YJ, Jeong JM, Lee DS, Jang JJ, Lee MC, Cho BY. Relationship between expression of the sodium/iodide symporter and ^{131}I uptake in recurrent lesions of differentiated thyroid carcinoma. Eur J Nucl Med. 2001;28:639–45.
5. Lazar V, Bidart JM, Caillou B, Mahe C, Lacroix L, Filetti S, Schlumberger M. Expression of the Na+/I- symporter gene in human thyroid tumors: a comparison study with other thyroid-specific genes. J Clin Endocrinol Metab. 1999;84:3228–34.
6. Schonberger J, Ruschoff J, Grimm D, Marienhagen J, Rummele P, Meyringer R, Kossmehl P, Hofstaedter F, Eilles C. Glucose transporter 1 gene expression is related to thyroid neoplasms with an unfavorable prognosis: an immunohistochemical study. Thyroid. 2002;12:747–54.
7. Hundahl SA, Fleming ID, Fremgen AM, Menck HR. A National Cancer Data Base report on 53,856 cases of thyroid carcinoma treated in the U.S., 1985–1995. Cancer. 1998;83:2638–48.
8. Kitagawa W, Shimizu K, Akasu H, Tanaka S. Endocrine surgery. The ninth report: the latest data on and clinical characteristics of the epidemiology of thyroid carcinoma. J Nippon Med Sch. 2003;70:57–61.
9. Lind P, Kresnik E, Kumnig G, Gallowitsch HJ, Igerc I, Matschnig S, Gomez I. F-FDG-PET in the follow-up of thyroid cancer. Acta Med Austriaca. 2003;30:17–21.
10. Kumnig G. Value of F-18 fluorodeoxyglucose positron emission tomography in thyroid carcinoma. Wien Med Wochenschr. 2002;152:280–5.
11. Bogsrud TV, Karantanis D, Nathan MA, et al. ^{18}F-FDG PET in the management of patients with anaplastic thyroid carcinoma. Thyroid. 2008;18:713–9.
12. Jadvar H, Fischman AJ. Evaluation of rare tumors with [F-18]fluorodeoxyglucose positron emission tomography. Clin Positron Imaging. 1999;2:153–8.
13. Kresnik E, Gallowitsch HJ, Mikosch P, Stettner H, Igerc I, Gomez I, Kumnig G, Lind P. Fluorine-18-fluorodeoxyglucose positron emission tomography in the preoperative assessment of thyroid nodules in an endemic goiter area. Surgery. 2003;133:294–9.
14. McDougall IR, Davidson J, Segall GM. Positron emission tomography of the thyroid, with an emphasis on thyroid cancer. Nucl Med Commun. 2001;22:485–92.
15. Wang W, Larson SM, Fazzari M, Tickoo SK, Kolbert K, Sgouros G, Yeung H, Macapinlac H, Rosai J, Robbins RJ. Prognostic value of [18F]fluorodeoxyglucose positron emission tomographic scanning in patients with thyroid cancer. J Clin Endocrinol Metab. 2000;85:1107–13.
16. Wang W, Larson SM, Tuttle RM, Kalaigian H, Kolbert K, Sonenberg M, Robbins RJ. Resistance of ^{18}F-fluorodeoxyglucose-avid metastatic thyroid cancer lesions to treatment with high-dose radioactive iodine. Thyroid. 2001;11:1169–75.
17. Iagaru A, McDougall IR. F-18 FDG PET/CT demonstration of an adrenal metastasis in a patient with anaplastic thyroid cancer. Clin Nucl Med. 2007;32:13–5.
18. Namwongprom S, Nunez RF, Yeung HW, Kim EE, Macapinlac HA. Unusual adrenal metastasis and abdominal carcinomatosis secondary to Hurthle cell carcinoma of the thyroid. Exp Clin Endocrinol Diabetes. 2007;115:694–6.
19. Strobel K, Steinert HC, Bhure U, Koma AY, Gassmann N, Stockli SJ. Tumour thrombus in the superior vena cava from anaplastic carcinoma of the thyroid: FDG-PET/CT imaging findings. Eur J Nucl Med Mol Imaging. 2007;34:813.
20. Diehl M, Graichen S, Menzel C, Lindhorst E, Grunwald F. F-18 FDG PET in insular thyroid cancer. Clin Nucl Med. 2003;28: 728–31.
21. Zettinig G, Leitha T, Niederle B, Kaserer K, Becherer A, Kletter K, Dudczak R. FDG positron emission tomographic, radioiodine, and MIBI imaging in a patient with poorly differentiated insular thyroid carcinoma. Clin Nucl Med. 2001;26:599–601.

External Radiation Therapy for Anaplastic Thyroid Cancer

98

James D. Brierley and Richard W. Tsang

As discussed elsewhere complete surgical resection gives the best chance of cure; however, this is only possible in a few patients. As ATC does not concentrate ^{131}I, external beam RT is the mainstay treatment for local control and palliation of symptoms to maintain quality of life. In a series of 91 patients, with an overall survival of 11 % at 3 years, 95 % had external beam radiation [1]. There was complete response to RT in 40 %, but 10 % progressed locally during their radiation. Although there was a trend to improved survival with increase in radiation dose, this was not statistically significant. Of the 70 patients on whom information was available, 36 % relapsed locally, 29 % at distant sites, and 36 % both locally and at distant sites. This study demonstrated that although radiation alone can result in a complete response, long-term local control remains a problem, and even if this is achieved, distant metastases almost invariably result in death. In a phase 2 study of hyperfractionated radiotherapy without chemotherapy in 17 patients (60.8 Gy in 32 fractions 2 fractions a day over 20–24 days), complete response was reported in 3 (17.6 %) patients and a partial response in 7 (41.2 %) [2]. Despite this response rate the median survival was only 10 weeks and the toxicity was unacceptable. The majority of patients developed grade 3 or 4 toxicity, and in 5, death occurred before the toxicity resolved.

The ineffectiveness of radiation alone has led to the development of both novel fractionation schedules and concurrent chemotherapy regimens. Because anaplastic thyroid cancer grows rapidly, hyperfractionated and accelerated radiation regimens have been used, sometimes in combination with chemotherapy and surgical resection. The rationale for altered fractionation is that in rapidly growing tumors giving the radiation in as short a time as possible counteracts any repopulation of the tumor by the rapidly multiplying cancer cells. The results of published studies on altered fractionation with and without chemotherapy are summarized in Table 98.1. The most successful regimen in obtaining local control is that described in a series of publications from Sweden. Combined hyperfractionated radiation and concurrent chemotherapy often with doxorubicin are given preoperatively followed by surgical resection. In the first two of three consecutive series, after surgical resection, further radiation and chemotherapy were given. In the third series a higher dose of preoperative treatment was given and there was no post-resection therapy. In a total of 55 patients treated between 1985 and 1999, surgery was possible in 40 patients. Although this aggressive approach resulted in an impressive local recurrence-free rate of 60 %, the median survival was still only 3.5 months with a 9 % survival at 2 years [8].

In a series of 33 patients with an overall median survival of 3.8 months, Haigh et al. identified a small and highly selected subgroup of 8 patients with anaplastic thyroid cancer [3], who had an estimated 5-year survival of 50 %. These eight patients underwent surgical resection with no residual disease or only microscopic residual disease and subsequently had combined chemotherapy and radiotherapy. In another recent report of 32 patients, 82 % had tumors less than 4 cm and 31 % were able to undergo a total thyroidectomy [4]. Twenty-three patients were treated between 1981 and 1999, most of whom had twice daily radiation and concurrent chemotherapy with a 2-year survival rate of 52 %. In contrast to these two small studies, a large series of 134 patients treated at the Mayo Clinic with [6] multimodality therapy did not improve survival as compared with standard care, although there was a small nonsignificant improvement in median survival in patients who received radiation compared to those who did not (3 vs. 5 months, $p=0.08$). However in a small number of patients (13 out of 134) who were able to receive debulking surgery, radiation, and

J.D. Brierley, MBBS, FRCP, FRCR, FRCPC (✉)
R.W. Tsang, MD, FRCP(C)
Department of Radiation Oncology, University of Toronto, Princess Margaret Hospital, 610 University Ave., Toronto, ON M5G 2M9, Canada
e-mail: james.brierley@rmp.uhn.on.ca; Richard.tsang@rmp.uhn.on.ca

L. Wartofsky, D. Van Nostrand (eds.), *Thyroid Cancer*, DOI 10.1007/978-1-4939-3314-3_98

Table 98.1 Local control and survival following fractionated radiation and concurrent chemotherapy in anaplastic thyroid cancer

	Patients	Local control	Median survival (months)	2-year survival	Fractionation	Concurrent chemotherapy
Haigh [3]	33	n/s	3.8	20 %	Not stated	Yes
Heron [4]	32			48 %[a]	Daily	In 15
Juror [1]	91		5	11 %[b]	Daily	In 18
Kim [5]	19	68 %	6	20 %	Hyperfractionated	Yes
McIver [6]	29	n/s	5	9 %[a]	Daily[c]	In 13
Mitchell [2]	17	76 %	2.5	n/s	Accelerated	No
Schlumberger [7]	20	n/s	n/s	15 %[d]	Hypofractionated	Yes
Tennvall [8]	55	60 %	2–4.5	9 %	Hyperfractionated	Yes
Wong [9]	32	22 %	6	18 %	Accelerated/hyperfractionated	Yes

n/s not specified
[a]At 1 year
[b]At 3 years
[c]For the group as a whole (134 patient), median survival was 3 months
[d]At 20 months

chemotherapy, the 1-year survival was 23 % compared to 9 % overall ($p=019$). These studies suggest that hyperfractionated radiation and chemotherapy may result in a better outcome but only in a select series of patients with small tumors amenable to surgical resection with minimal residual disease.

In general, patients with good performance status and no evidence of distant metastatic disease may benefit from an aggressive approach with high-dose altered fractionated radiotherapy with or without concurrent chemotherapy. Currently at Princess Margaret Hospital, where we rarely see patients who have potentially resectable disease, patients with good performance status are considered for accelerated hyperfractionated radiation without chemotherapy, 60 Gy in 40 fractions over 4 weeks, with 2 fractions of 1.5 Gy per day. The rationale for this is that anaplastic thyroid cancer has a very low response rate to chemotherapy (86), and combining hyperfractionated radiation with chemotherapy results in moderately severe toxicity. Therefore by not giving concurrent chemotherapy, a higher dose of radiation can be given more safely without the risk of interruption and intensive support measures. For patients with poor performance status, lower dose palliative radiation (e.g., 2000 cGy in five daily fractions) is given.

External Beam Radiotherapy

The thyroid bed is a technically challenging volume to treat as the thyroid bed curves around the vertebral body and includes the air column in the trachea. It can be difficult to adequately treat the thyroid bed and spare the spinal cord to a dose within tolerance. A variety of techniques have been described that produce adequate dose distribution [10]. Advances in radiation techniques that result in better dose distribution to the areas at risk and reduce the volume of normal tissues to a minimum are described elsewhere in the book. Well-planned external beam RT has acceptable acute toxicity and rarely produces serious complications. In patients assigned to the radiation arm of the German randomized control study in differentiated thyroid cancer that closed because of poor accrual, it was noted that the majority of patients experience mild to moderate side effects from adjuvant external beam radiotherapy [11]. At the first follow-up examination, most side effects had subsided and acute toxicity was tolerable in these patients. Late toxicity is infrequent; the most common is skin telangiectasia, increased skin pigmentation, soft tissue fibrosis, and mild lymphedema predominantly in the submental area. Esophageal and tracheal stenosis is extremely rare. Neither Tsang et al. [12] nor Farahati et al. [13] reported any RTOG grade IV late toxicity in differentiated thyroid cancer.

Metastases

Unlike papillary and follicular carcinoma, the prognosis of patients who have developed distant metastasesfrom anaplastic thyroid cancer has an extremely poor prognosis. The surgical resection of bone metastases even if the lesion is apparently solitary is not warranted, unless there is a significant risk of a pathological fracture. Therefore external beam radiation has an important role in palliation of bone metastases.

Similarly in patients with brain metastases, whole-brain radiation should be considered except in the elderly who do not tolerate whole-brain radiation well.

References

1. Junor E, Paul J, Reed N. Anaplastic thyroid carcinoma: 91 patients treated by surgery and radiotherapy. Eur J Surg. 1992;18:83–8.
2. Mitchell G, Huddart R, Harmer C. Phase II evaluation of high dose accelerated radiotherapy for anaplastic thyroid carcinoma. Radiother Oncol. 1999;50:33–8.

3. Haigh PI, Ituarte PH, Wu HS, et al. Completely resected anaplastic thyroid carcinoma combined with adjuvant chemotherapy and irradiation is associated with prolonged survival. Cancer. 2001;91:2335–42.
4. Heron DE, Karimpour S, Grigsby PW. Anaplastic thyroid carcinoma: comparison of conventional radiotherapy and hyperfractionation chemoradiotherapy in two groups. Am J Clin Oncol. 2002;25:442–6.
5. Kim JH, Leeper RD. Treatment of locally advanced thyroid carcinoma with combination doxorubicin and radiation therapy. Cancer. 1987;60:2372–5.
6. McIver B, Hay ID, Giuffrida DF, et al. Anaplastic thyroid carcinoma: a 50-year experience at a single institution. Surgery. 2001;130:1028–34.
7. Schlumberger M, Parmentier C, Delisle MJ, Couette JE, Droz JP, Sarrazin D. Combination therapy for anaplastic giant cell thyroid carcinoma. Cancer. 1991;67:564–6.
8. Tennvall J, Lundell G, Wahlberg P, et al. Anaplastic thyroid carcinoma: three protocols combining doxorubicin, hyperfractionated radiotherapy and surgery. Br J Cancer. 2002;86:1848–53.
9. Wong CS, Van Dyk J, Simpson WJ. Myelopathy following hyperfractionated accelerated radiotherapy for anaplastic thyroid carcinoma. Radiother Oncol. 1991;20:3–9.
10. Tsang RW, Brierley JD. The thyroid. In: Cox JD, Kian Ang K, editors. Radiation oncology. St Louis: Mosby; 2003.
11. Schuck A, Biermann M, Pixberg MK, et al. Acute toxicity of adjuvant radiotherapy in locally advanced differentiated thyroid carcinoma. First results of the multicenter study differentiated thyroid carcinoma (MSDS). Strahlenther Onkol. 2003;179: 832–9.
12. Tsang RW, Brierley JD, Simpson WJ, Panzarella T, Gospodarowicz MK, Sutcliffe SB. The effects of surgery, radioiodine and external radiation therapy on the clinical outcome of patients with differentiated thyroid cancer. Cancer. 1998;82: 375–88.
13. Farahati J, Reiners C, Stuschke M, et al. Differentiated thyroid cancer. Impact of adjuvant external radiotherapy in patients with perithyroidal tumor infiltration (stage pT4). Cancer. 1996;77:172–80.

Chemotherapy for Anaplastic Thyroid Cancer

99

David A. Liebner, Sigurdis Haraldsdottir, and Manisha H. Shah

Introduction

Anaplastic thyroid cancers (ATC) account for roughly 2.2 % of all thyroid cancers in the USA [1] and are believed to arise from differentiated thyroid cancers (DTC) via the accumulation of genetic abnormalities that result in dedifferentiation and an aggressive phenotype [2]. Unfortunately, ATC is usually advanced at the time of diagnosis, with approximately 76–79 % of all patients having disease extending beyond the thyroid/neck at the time of presentation [1, 3]. In the vast majority of patients, surgery alone has been associated with poor outcomes, leading to investigation into additional therapeutic options.

Cytotoxic Chemotherapy

Early chemotherapy regimens were not associated with improvements in patient survival [4], though there were occasional reports of clinical complete responses and prolonged remission [5]. Selected chemotherapy regimens are summarized in Table 99.1. Gottlieb and Hill [6] reported on their initial experience in 1974 with the anthracycline antibiotic, doxorubicin, in thyroid cancer, noting that two of nine patients with ATC had a greater than 50 % decrease in the size of metastatic lesions following treatment. Several subsequent studies attempted to improve on this result.

Shimaoka and colleagues [7] reported the results of a large randomized study conducted by the Eastern Cooperative Oncology Group (ECOG) of doxorubicin alone versus doxorubicin plus cisplatin administered every 3 weeks in patients with advanced thyroid cancer. Among 39 patients with ATC enrolled in the study, there was a single partial response among the 21 patients treated with doxorubicin alone, compared to 6 responses, including 3 complete responses, among 18 patients treated with the combination chemotherapy (5 % versus 33 %, $p=0.03$). Among all patients treated in the study, response to therapy was associated with improved overall survival, but the difference in overall survival was not statistically significant between the two groups. Toxicities, specifically nausea and hematologic toxicity, were greater in the combination arm. De Besi and colleagues [8] investigated the addition of bleomycin to doxorubicin and cisplatin in a small study of 22 patients with advanced thyroid cancer of all histologies. Two of five patients with ATC had complete responses.

The Japanese Society of Thyroid Surgery [9] completed a prospective study in ATC using an intensified regimen consisting of doxorubicin, cisplatin, etoposide, and peplomycin administered every 3 weeks. Granulocyte colony-stimulating factors were given in an attempt to mitigate chemotherapy-induced neutropenia. Patients were allowed to receive local radiation therapy if it was deemed to be indicated. Responses were limited, with only two of ten patients with measurable disease having partial responses and these lasting on average 2–3 months. Despite growth factor support, all patients experienced major neutropenia.

D.A. Liebner, MD
Division of Medical Oncology, Department of Internal Medicine, The Ohio State University, Columbus, OH, USA

Department of Biomedical Informatics, The Ohio State University, Columbus, OH, USA
e-mail: david.liebner@osumc.edu

S. Haraldsdottir, MD
Division of Medical Oncology, Department of Internal Medicine, The Ohio State University Comprehensive Cancer Center, Columbus, OH, USA
e-mail: sigurdis.haraldsdottir@osumc.edu

M.H. Shah, MD (✉)
Division of Medical Oncology, Department of Internal Medicine, The James Cancer Hospital and Solove Research Institute, 320 West 10th Avenue, A438 Starling Loving Hall, Columbus, OH 43210, USA
e-mail: Manisha.Shah@osumc.edu

L. Wartofsky, D. Van Nostrand (eds.), *Thyroid Cancer*, DOI 10.1007/978-1-4939-3314-3_99

Table 99.1 Selected studies of chemotherapy and targeted agents in anaplastic thyroid cancer

Chemotherapy	Ref.	Treatment plan	N	Responses
Doxorubicin-based regimens				
Doxorubicin	[6]	Doxorubicin: 45–75 mg/m² q 3 weeks	9	2
	[7]	Doxorubicin: 60 mg/m² q 3 weeks	21	1
Doxorubicin, cisplatin	[7]	Doxorubicin: 60 mg/m²; cisplatin: 40 mg/m² q 3 weeks	18	6
Bleomycin, doxorubicin, cisplatin	[8]	Bleomycin: 30 mg/day day 1–3; doxorubicin: 60 mg/m² day 5; cisplatin: 60 mg/m² day 5	5	2 CR
Doxorubicin, cisplatin, etoposide, peplomycin	[9]	Doxorubicin: 60 mg/m² day 1; cisplatin: 40 mg/m² day 1; etoposide: 100 mg/m²/day day 1–5; peplomycin: 5 mg/day day 1–5 q 3 weeks	10[a]	2
Other cytotoxic chemotherapy regimens				
Paclitaxel	[11]	Paclitaxel: 120–140 mg/m² as a 96-h infusion weekly	20	10
	[12]	Paclitaxel: 80 mg/m² day 1, 8, 15 q 3–4 weeks	13	4
Docetaxel	[13]	Doxorubicin: 60 mg/m² q 3 weeks	7	1
Carboplatin, paclitaxel	[16]	Carboplatin: AUC 6 d1; paclitaxel: 200 mg/m² day 1	NR[b]	NR[c]
Vasculature-targeting agents				
Fosbretabulin	[15]	Fosbretabulin: 45 mg/m² IV, day 1, 8, 15 q 4 weeks	26	0[d]
Fosbretabulin, carboplatin, paclitaxel	[16]	Fosbretabulin: 60 mg/m² day 1, 8, 15; carboplatin: AUC 6 day 1; paclitaxel: 200 mg/m² day 1	NR[b]	NR[c]
Receptor kinase inhibitors				
Axitinib	[24]	Axitinib: 5 mg bid	2	1
Sorafenib	[22]	Sorafenib: 400 mg bid	2	0
	[23]	Sorafenib: 400 mg bid	4	0
Gefitinib	[21]	Gefitinib: 250 mg daily	5	0
Imatinib	[18]	Imatinib: 400 mg bid	11	2[e]
mTOR inhibitors				
Everolimus	[24]	Everolimus: 10 mg daily	5	1

[a]An additional six patients were treated adjuvantly, with 3 pts NED (3–11 months)
[b]75 patients received treatment and were randomized 2:1 to fosbretabulin combination arm versus carboplatin, paclitaxel alone
[c]Median OS 5.2 months in fosbretabulin combination arm versus 4.0 months in carboplatin, paclitaxel only arm ($p = 0.065$)
[d]Median OS, 4.7 months; 6-month OS, 34 %; 12-month OS, 23 %
[e]All tumors overexpressed PDGFR by immunohistochemistry. 6-month PFS (27 %), OS (46 %)

Several alternative, non-anthracycline regimens have also been explored [10]. In 2000, the Collaborative Anaplastic Thyroid Cancer Health Intervention Trials Group reported the results of a phase 2 study of paclitaxel, administered as a 96-h continuous intravenous infusion to 20 patients with ATC [11]. Doses of paclitaxel were increased from 120 mg/m²/week (7 patients) to 140 mg/m²/week (13 patients). The authors used a modified WHO classification system to describe responses to therapy, requiring that optimal responses last for at least 2 weeks instead of the typical 4 weeks in an attempt to account for rapid tumor doubling time. Ten responses were reported, with one complete response and nine partial responses. At the time of progression, nine of these patients were treated off protocol with a 1-h weekly infusion of high-dose paclitaxel 225 mg/m². Among seven patients who had had a prior response to the 96-h infusion, there were two partial responses; among the two patients who had not responded to the 96-h infusion, there was one partial response. The 96-h continuous intravenous infusion was well tolerated, with no toxicities greater than grade 2. Five of nine patients given the 1-h weekly infusion of paclitaxel developed grade 2–3 neuropathy.

Higashiyama and colleagues [12] evaluated paclitaxel as induction therapy prior to surgery in 13 patients with stage IVB or IVC ATC between 2005 and 2008. Patients were treated with weekly paclitaxel 80 mg/m² as a 1-h infusion given on days 1, 8, and 15 every 3–4 weeks. Four patients had a response to chemotherapy (one complete response, three partial responses) with an additional four patients having stable disease at 8 weeks after initiating therapy. Therapy was generally well tolerated with only one patient having a grade 3 drug-related adverse event (reversible pulmonary toxicity). Retrospective comparison of outcomes with ATC patients who had not received paclitaxel induction suggested a possible benefit in patients with stage IVB, but not stage IVC disease.

A recent publication from Kawada and associates [13] investigated the second-generation taxane, docetaxel, in ATC. Seven chemotherapy-naive patients with good performance status and measurable disease were treated with docetaxel 60 mg/m² as a 1-h infusion every 3 weeks. One patient had a complete response, and two patients had stable disease. The median time to progression was 6 weeks. The authors recommended further investigation into docetaxel in ATC.

Targeted Therapy

As more is known about the molecular underpinnings of this disease, there has been increased interest in developing targeted therapies for ATC (see Table 99.1).

Antiangiogenic approaches have been conceptually appealing, given the highly vascular nature of ATC. Fosbretabulin (combretastatin A4 phosphate) is a novel chemotherapeutic agent which disrupts endothelial cell function leading to occlusion of vessels. Tumor microvasculature is more sensitive to the effects of fosbretabulin than normal vessels, and blood flow reduction in the phase 1 study was noted to be the greatest in highly vascular tumors, such as thyroid cancer [14]. Twenty-six patients with advanced ATC who had failed multimodality therapy were enrolled on a phase 2 trial of fosbretabulin administered at a dose of 45 mg/m^2 weekly for 3 weeks every 28 days [15]. Treatment was well tolerated. No objective responses were noted, and stable disease was seen in 27 % of patients. Median survival was 4.7 months, with a 1-year survival of 23 %. The results of a phase 2/3 randomized comparison of fosbretabulin plus paclitaxel and carboplatin versus paclitaxel and carboplatin alone have been reported [16]. Only 80 out of the intended 180 patients were enrolled to the trial due to slow accrual. Median survival in the combination arm was 5.2 months compared to 4 months in the control arm (HR 0.65 [0.38–1.1]). One-year survival was improved in the combination arm though it did not reach statistical significance (27 % versus 9 %, $p=0.065$). Treatment was generally well tolerated, with hypertension and neutropenia more common in patients receiving fosbretabulin. This agent has been moved into a phase 3 trial which is in development. Crolibulin, a microtubule-destabilizing agent which disrupts vascular endothelial cells and, in turn, blood flow to the tumor was combined with cisplatin in a phase 1 trial. Eight patients with ATC were treated at dose level 3, and one had a complete response and remained on study with single-agent crolibulin. One additional patient had stable disease [17].

Given that ATC cell lines and tissues have been reported to overexpress PDGFR, Ha and colleagues [18] investigated the use of imatinib (Glivec, Gleevec), a tyrosine-kinase inhibitor with activity against several targets including Bcr-Abl, PDGFR-α/β, c-KIT, and RET, in patients with ATC. Eleven patients were enrolled, all of whom had immunohistochemical evidence of PDGFR overexpression. Two patients had a partial response, with an additional four patients demonstrating stable disease at 2 months. At 6 months, overall survival was estimated at 46 %, with 27 % of patients free of progression. Further investigation is of interest, particularly in patients with evidence of overexpression of PDGFR.

EGFR has also been a target of interest in ATC. Evidence of EGFR overexpression has been documented in ATC cell lines and selected cases of ATC [19], and case reports have suggested occasional clinical response to EGFR inhibitors [20]. Response, however, may be limited in an unselected population. Of five patients with ATC enrolled in a phase 2 study of the EGFR inhibitor gefitinib, no patient had an objective response [21]. However, one patient did demonstrate stable disease of at least 12 months.

Two studies investigating the multikinase inhibitor sorafenib in advanced thyroid cancer have included patients with ATC [22, 23]. Sorafenib is approved for treatment of metastatic differentiated thyroid cancer, advanced hepatocellular carcinoma, and renal carcinoma and has activity against VEGFR, PDGFR, FLT3, KIT, Raf-1, BRAF, and RET kinases. Much of its activity is believed to be mediated via the antiangiogenic effect of VEGFR blockade, though additional signaling pathways are likely important as well. A total of six patients were enrolled on the two studies: no patient had a response to therapy, though one patient did have stable disease lasting at least 6 months. Axitinib is a second small-molecule tyrosine-kinase inhibitor with activity against VEGFR, PDGFR, and KIT. Two patients with ATC were enrolled on a phase 2 study investigating the activity of axitinib in advanced thyroid cancer: one patient had a partial response to therapy [24].

A phase 2 trial with the mTOR inhibitor everolimus included five patients with ATC and results were presented in 2013 [25]. One complete response was seen in a patient with ATC and was sustained for 18 months. Whole-exome sequencing of the tumor revealed a somatic loss of function mutation affecting the tuberous sclerosis 2 (TSC2) protein, a negative regulator of mTOR activity.

Multimodality Therapy

Unfortunately, as outlined above, overall response rates to cytotoxic chemotherapy alone are poor, and there have been no studies that have been able to demonstrate a survival benefit in patients treated with chemotherapy alone. Retrospective studies have suggested the importance of a multimodality approach in the treatment of ATC, and patients who receive all three modalities, including surgery, radiation therapy, and chemotherapy, have improved outcomes [26]. Selection of patients who will benefit most from multimodality therapy has been an area of active research [27]. Selected reports of multimodality approaches are summarized in Table 99.2.

The Swedish experience at Lund University and Karolinska University Hospital has provided important insights into the benefits and limitations of chemoradiation with or without surgery in patients with advanced ATC [28–36]. From 1971 to 1973, patients at these institutes were treated with methotrexate 5 mg daily plus external beam radiation therapy daily for 3–4 weeks to a cumulative dose of 30–40 Gy [29]. Of the initial eight patients, responses were seen in seven patients, but the majority of patients subsequently progressed locally (six of eight patients). Though median survival was 9 months, toxicity was felt to be considerable (severe mucositis, gastrointestinal bleeding, hepatotoxicity), and given the palliative aim of the therapy, the protocol was subsequently amended.

Table 99.2 Selected studies of multimodality therapy in anaplastic thyroid cancer

Treatment	Ref.	Treatment plan	N	Local control	Median survival	Comments
Doxorubicin-based regimens						
Doxorubicin + radiation + surgery[a]	[37]	Doxorubicin: 10 mg/m^2 weekly; HART: 57.6 Gy	9	13	NR	
		Above plus surgery	10			
	[31]	Doxorubicin: 20 mg weekly; HART (30 Gy pre-op, 16 Gy post-op, 1 Gyx2/day)	7	0	3.5 months	Treatment period 1984–1988
		Above plus surgery	9	5		
		Doxorubicin: 20 mg weekly + HART (30 Gy pre-op, 16 Gy post-op, 1.3 Gyx2/day)	3	0	4.5 months	Treatment period 1989–1992
		Above plus surgery	14	11		
	[33]	Doxorubicin: 20 mg weekly + HART (46 Gy pre-op, 1.6 Gyx2/day)	5	0	2 months	Treatment period 1993–1999
		Above plus surgery	17	17		
Doxorubicin, cisplatin + radiation + surgery[a]	[38]	Doxorubicin: 60 mg/m^2; cisplatin: 90 mg/m^2 q 4 weeks × 4 cycles; RT (70 Gy)	3	1	NR	Patients <65 years
		Above plus surgery	9	7		
Doxorubicin, docetaxel + radiation + surgery[a]	[40]	Doxorubicin: 60 mg/m^2; docetaxel 60 mg/m^2 × 4 cycles‡; IMRT (57.6–70 Gy)	1	7	36 months	All patients had stage IVA or IVB disease
		Above plus surgery	9			
Other regimens						
Methotrexate + radiation	[29]	MTX: 5 mg/day; RT (30–40 Gy)	8	2	9 months	Severe toxicity noted in all patients
Bleomycin, cyclophosphamide, 5-FU + radiation + surgery[a]	[35]	Bleomycin: 5 mg/day; cyclophosphamide: 200 mg/day; 5-FU 500 mg q od × 10 day; RT (30–40 Gy)	8	NR	3 months	Patient treated with surgery alive and disease-free 12+ years
		Above plus surgery	1	1		
	[28]	Bleomycin: (none); cyclophosphamide: 200 mg/day; 5-FU 500 mg q od × 10 day; RT (48 Gy)	8	1	3 months	1 long-term CR 59+ months
		Above plus surgery	5	3	5 months	
Mitoxantrone + radiation	[38]	Mitoxantrone: 14 mg/m^2 q 4 weeks × 4 cycles; RT (70 Gy)	5	2	NR	Patients >65 years
		Above plus surgery	3	3		

[a]If feasible

Between 1973 and 1979, 22 patients were recruited to a study of 5-fluorouracil (5-FU) and cyclophosphamide administered concurrently with daily radiation therapy (48 Gy over 4 weeks) [28, 29, 32]. One patient treated with chemoradiation alone had a complete response and was disease-free after 59 months, but all other patients treated with chemoradiation alone (seven of eight patients) died of progressive local disease. Local control rates were improved in patients treated with surgery in addition to chemoradiation, with only two of five patients experiencing local failure; two of these patients died of metastatic disease, and one patient was a long-term survivor. Addition of bleomycin to the above regimen (BCF) was evaluated in nine patients during the same period [35]. Objective responses were seen in seven of nine patients. Surgery was performed on a single patient at the peak of remission; this patient was the only long-term survivor (12+ years).

Subsequent protocols were amended to include surgery whenever possible, and radiation therapy was modified to include hyperfractionated regimens. From 1975 to 1980, 19 patients were treated with BCF plus ≤30 Gy neoadjuvant hyperfractionated radiation therapy, followed by surgery and followed by postoperative concurrent chemoradiation (15 Gy) [36]. Patients could then receive additional 5-FU and cyclophosphamide every other month for an additional five cycles. Median survival in patients with more advanced disease was 7 months, and there were no long-term survivors; median survival in ten patients with less advanced disease was 12 months, and three patients were deemed long-term survivors with no evidence of disease at 31+, 61+, and 80+ months. Local failure rates were not reported, but no patients required tracheostomy.

Between 1984 and 1992, 33 consecutive patients with cytologically verified ATC were treated with a regimen of doxorubicin 20 mg weekly given concurrently with 30 Gy preoperative and 16 Gy postoperative hyperfractionated radiation therapy [31]. Radiation was given as 1 Gy twice daily prior to 1988 and 1.3 Gy twice daily after 1988, but the total dose of radiation did not differ between cohorts. The majority of patients were able to proceed to surgery. Local recurrences occurred in 17 patients (52 %) and 8 patients (24 %) died of local disease. Four patients were considered long-term disease-free survivors. All radiation was subsequently given in a neoadjuvant fashion from 1993 to 1999 as 1.6 Gy twice daily to a cumulative dose of 46 Gy [33]. All 17 patients who are able to proceed to surgery had local control, though the majority subsequently died of metastatic disease (15 of 17). Median survival remained suboptimal at 3 months. Similar results have been reported in other studies [37–39].

More recently, Foote and colleagues [40] summarized their experience at the Mayo Clinic between 2003 and 2007 with aggressive, multimodal therapy in a subset of patients with regionally advanced ATC (stages IVA and IVB). Planned therapy included surgery when feasible, four cycles of docetaxel and doxorubicin with growth factor support, and intensity-modulated radiation therapy (IMRT) initiated with the first cycle of chemotherapy. Actual chemotherapy regimens were modified based on underlying patient comorbidities, and total radiation doses ranged from 57.6 to 70 Gy. Results were encouraging, with 1-year overall survival of 70 % and five of ten patients disease-free at 32+, 40+, 44+, 52+, and 89+ months. These compared favorably to historical experience with stage IVA and IVB disease. The authors noted that the advent of IMRT, the addition of taxane therapy to anthracycline-based regimens, and the administration of adjuvant chemotherapy in addition to radiosensitizing doses of chemotherapy may have contributed to the improved outcomes. Further validation was recommended.

Summary

ATC is an aggressive, relatively chemoresistant subtype of thyroid cancer, with limited response to conventional treatment regimens. Mechanisms of chemoresistance remain poorly understood but may include overexpression of the multidrug resistance-associated protein (MRP) and mutations in p53 and other cell-cycle regulatory proteins [41, 42]. Aggressive, multimodality therapy currently provides the best opportunity for clinical response and can provide a small subset of patients with long-term disease-free survival. Additionally, even in patients with distant metastases, local control with combined treatment may prevent distressing upper airway obstruction and improve quality of life. There remains a great need for improvement in current treatment regimens, and targeted therapies have the potential to revolutionize the treatment of this disease in the future. Clinical trials open to patients with ATC are summarized in Table 99.3. Additional novel approaches to therapy are discussed in Chap. 98.

Table 99.3 Ongoing clinical trials open to patients with anaplastic thyroid cancer

Investigational therapy	Selected mechanisms	Title	Phase	Lead institution
Clinical trials with a focus on anaplastic thyroid cancer				
EPC2407 (crolibulin) ± cisplatin	Microtubule inhibitor, DNA cross-linking	A phase 1/2 trial of crolibulin (EPC2407) plus cisplatin in adults with solid tumors with a focus on anaplastic thyroid cancer (ATC)	Phase 1/2	NCI (USA)
Bevacizumab + doxorubicin	VEGF inhibitor, topoisomerase II inhibitor	Avastin and doxorubicin postoperatively for patients with anaplastic thyroid cancer	Phase 2	Lund University Hospital (Sweden)
Other clinical trials open to patients with anaplastic thyroid cancer				
Pemetrexed + paclitaxel	Antifolate, microtubule inhibitor	Pemetrexed + paclitaxel in patients with recurrent/advanced thyroid cancer	Phase 2	University of Kiel (Germany)
Pazopanib	VEGFR1–3, PDGFR, KIT inhibitor	Pazopanib in treating patients with advanced thyroid cancer	Phase 2	Mayo Clinic (USA)
PLX108-01 (PLX3397)	FMS, KIT, FLT3 inhibitor	Safety study of PLX108-01 in patients with solid tumors	Phase 1	Plexxikon (USA)
Everolimus	mTOR inhibitor	Everolimus in treating patients with progressive or recurrent, unresectable, or metastatic thyroid cancer	Phase 2	Leiden University Medical Center (Netherlands)
		Everolimus in treating patients with locally advanced or metastatic thyroid cancer	Phase 2	Yonsei University (Korea)
Dabrafenib and trametinib	BRAF inhibitor and MEK inhibitor	Efficacy and safety of the combination therapy of dabrafenib and trametinib in subjects with BRAF V600E-mutated rare cancers	Phase 2	GSK (USA)

References

1. Hossain A, et al. Epidemiology, treatment outcome, and survival of anaplastic thyroid cancer (ATC) in the United States: a period prevalence SEER database study 1973–2006. J Clin Oncol. 2010; 28(15s):abstr 5588.
2. Wiseman S, et al. Derangement of p53 and MDM2 is involved in transformation of differentiated into anaplastic thyroid cancer. J Clin Oncol. 2006;24(18s):abstr 5556.
3. Chen J, et al. Surgery and radiotherapy improves survival in patients with anaplastic thyroid carcinoma: analysis of the surveillance, epidemiology, and end results 1983–2002. Am J Clin Oncol. 2008; 31(5):460–4.
4. Schoumacher P, et al. Anaplastic carcinoma of the thyroid gland. Eur J Cancer. 1977;13(4–5):381–3.
5. Simpson WJ. Anaplastic thyroid carcinoma: a new approach. Can J Surg. 1980;23(1):25–7.
6. Gottlieb JA, Hill Jr CS. Chemotherapy of thyroid cancer with adriamycin. Experience with 30 patients. N Engl J Med. 1974;290(4):193–7.
7. Shimaoka K, et al. A randomized trial of doxorubicin versus doxorubicin plus cisplatin in patients with advanced thyroid carcinoma. Cancer. 1985;56(9):2155–60.
8. De Besi P, et al. Combined chemotherapy with bleomycin, adriamycin, and platinum in advanced thyroid cancer. J Endocrinol Invest. 1991;14(6):475–80.
9. Tamura K, et al. Intensive chemotherapy for anaplastic thyroid carcinoma: combination of cisplatin, doxorubicin, etoposide and peplomycin with granulocyte granulocyte colony-stimulating factor support. Chemotherapy Committee, The Japanese Society of Thyroid Surgery. Jpn J Clin Oncol. 1995;25(5):203–7.
10. Gottlieb JA, et al. Chemotherapy of thyroid cancer. An evaluation of experience with 37 patients. Cancer. 1972;30(3):848–53.
11. Ain KB, Egorin MJ, DeSimone PA. Treatment of anaplastic thyroid carcinoma with paclitaxel: phase 2 trial using ninety-six-hour infusion. Collaborative Anaplastic Thyroid Cancer Health Intervention Trials (CATCHIT) Group. Thyroid. 2000;10(7):587–94.
12. Higashiyama T, et al. Induction chemotherapy with weekly paclitaxel administration for anaplastic thyroid carcinoma. Thyroid. 2010;20(1):7–14.
13. Kawada K, et al. The feasibility study of docetaxel in patients with anaplastic thyroid cancer. Jpn J Clin Oncol. 2010;40(6):596–9.
14. Stevenson JP, et al. Phase I trial of the antivascular agent combretastatin A4 phosphate on a 5-day schedule to patients with cancer: magnetic resonance imaging evidence for altered tumor blood flow. J Clin Oncol. 2003;21(23):4428–38.
15. Mooney CJ, et al. A phase II trial of fosbretabulin in advanced anaplastic thyroid carcinoma and correlation of baseline serum-soluble intracellular adhesion molecule-1 with outcome. Thyroid. 2009; 19(3):233–40.
16. Sosa JA, et al. A randomized phase II/III trial of a tumor vascular disrupting agent fosbretabulin tromethamine (CA4P) with carboplatin (C) and paclitaxel (P) in anaplastic thyroid cancer (ATC): final survival analysis for the FACT trial. J Clin Oncol. 2011;29(15s):abstr 5502.
17. Gramza A, et al. Phase I/II trial of crolibulin and cisplatin in solid tumors with a focus on anaplastic thyroid cancer: phase I results. J Clin Oncol. 2013;31(suppl):abstr 6074.
18. Ha HT, et al. A phase II study of imatinib in patients with advanced anaplastic thyroid cancer. Thyroid. 2010;20(9):975–80.
19. Schiff BA, et al. Epidermal growth factor receptor (EGFR) is overexpressed in anaplastic thyroid cancer, and the EGFR inhibitor gefitinib inhibits the growth of anaplastic thyroid cancer. Clin Cancer Res. 2004;10(24):8594–602.
20. Hogan T, et al. Oncocytic, focally anaplastic, thyroid cancer responding to erlotinib. J Oncol Pharm Pract. 2009;15(2): 111–7.
21. Pennell NA, et al. A phase II study of gefitinib in patients with advanced thyroid cancer. Thyroid. 2008;18(3):317–23.
22. Gupta-Abramson V, et al. Phase II trial of sorafenib in advanced thyroid cancer. J Clin Oncol. 2008;26(29):4714–9.
23. Kloos RT, et al. Phase II trial of sorafenib in metastatic thyroid cancer. J Clin Oncol. 2009;27(10):1675–84.
24. Cohen EE, et al. Axitinib is an active treatment for all histologic subtypes of advanced thyroid cancer: results from a phase II study. J Clin Oncol. 2008;26(29):4708–13.
25. Lorch J, et al. A phase II study of everolimus in patients with aggressive RAI refractory (RAIR) thyroid cancer (TC). J Clin Oncol. 2013;31(suppl):abstr 6023.
26. Lee Y, et al. Multimodal therapeutic approach in anaplastic thyroid cancer. J Clin Oncol. 2006;24(18s):abstr 15533.
27. Orita Y, et al. Prospective application of our novel prognostic index in the treatment of anaplastic thyroid carcinoma. Surgery. 2011; 150(6):1212–9.
28. Tennvall J, et al. Undifferentiated giant and spindle cell carcinoma of the thyroid. Report on two combined treatment modalities. Acta Radiol Oncol Radiat Phys Biol. 1979;18(5):408–16.
29. Tallroth E, et al. Multimodality treatment in anaplastic giant cell thyroid carcinoma. Cancer. 1987;60(7):1428–31.
30. Tennvall J, et al. Anaplastic thyroid carcinoma. Doxorubicin, hyperfractionated radiotherapy and surgery. Acta Oncol. 1990; 29(8):1025–8.
31. Tennvall J, et al. Combined doxorubicin, hyperfractionated radiotherapy, and surgery in anaplastic thyroid carcinoma. Report on two protocols. The Swedish Anaplastic Thyroid Cancer Group. Cancer. 1994;74(4):1348–54.
32. Nilsson O, et al. Anaplastic giant cell carcinoma of the thyroid gland: treatment and survival over a 25-year period. World J Surg. 1998;22(7):725–30.
33. Tennvall J, et al. Anaplastic thyroid carcinoma: three protocols combining doxorubicin, hyperfractionated radiotherapy and surgery. Br J Cancer. 2002;86(12):1848–53.
34. Wallin G, Lundell G, Tennvall J. Anaplastic giant cell thyroid carcinoma. Scand J Surg. 2004;93(4):272–7.
35. Andersson T, et al. Combined therapy for undifferentiated giant and spindle cell carcinoma of the thyroid. Acta Otolaryngol. 1977; 83(3–4):372–7.
36. Werner B, et al. Multimodal therapy in anaplastic giant cell thyroid carcinoma. World J Surg. 1984;8(1):64–70.
37. Kim JH, Leeper RD. Treatment of locally advanced thyroid carcinoma with combination doxorubicin and radiation therapy. Cancer. 1987;60(10):2372–5.
38. Schlumberger M, et al. Combination therapy for anaplastic giant cell thyroid carcinoma. Cancer. 1991;67(3):564–6.
39. Tanaka K, Sugitani I, Fujimoto Y. A novel chemo-radiotherapy with low-dose daily cisplatin, 5-fluorouracil and doxorubicin for anaplastic thyroid carcinoma: a preliminary report. Jpn J Clin Oncol. 2011;41(9):1074–8.
40. Foote RL, et al. Enhanced survival in locoregionally confined anaplastic thyroid carcinoma: a single-institution experience using aggressive multimodal therapy. Thyroid. 2011;21(1):25–30.
41. Sugawara I, et al. Expression of multidrug resistance-associated protein (MRP) in anaplastic carcinoma of the thyroid. Cancer Lett. 1994;82(2):185–8.
42. Lavra L, et al. Gal-3 is stimulated by gain-of-function p53 mutations and modulates chemoresistance in anaplastic thyroid carcinomas. J Pathol. 2009;218(1):66–75.

100 Anaplastic Thyroid Carcinoma: Prognosis

Robert C. Smallridge and Ejigayehu G. Abate

The prognosis for anaplastic thyroid cancer (ATC) is dismal, with survival usually but a few months, unlike that of differentiated thyroid cancers in which patients often live years even with distant metastases. The median overall survival for ATC is only 4.9 months, with a 1-year survival of 20 % [1–44]. All ATC patients are stage IV by American Joint Committee on Cancer (AJCC) criteria. Stage IVA encompasses patients with intrathyroidal ATC and carries the best prognosis but represents a minority of patients at presentation. Stage IVB patients have disease confined to the neck, while IVC requires distant metastases.

Table 100.1 illustrates the frequencies of stage IVA–C disease according to TNM classification. Stage IVA disease is, unfortunately, the least common presentation, with a median of only 10%. The median frequencies of stage IVB and IVC disease are similar, at 40.1 % and 45.8 %, respectively. As expected, the survival rates are highest for stage IVA patients (Table 100.2). Nevertheless, the 2-year survival for intrathyroidal disease is only 62 %. And no one with stage IVC disease lived 2 years [39]. Chen et al. [45] reported similar results when analyzing the Surveillance, Epidemiology, and End Results (SEER) database. They examined outcomes in 241 patients who had surgery performed or recommended and who survived a month or longer. If disease was confined to the thyroid, median survival was 50 % longer (9 vs. 6 months) than if adjacent tissues were involved and three times longer than if the tumor was more advanced (Table 100.3). However, even patients with stage IVA disease had only a 23 % 5-year survival. These findings emphasize that patients with disease seemingly confined to the thyroid also have a high mortality rate. Thus, microscopic metastases are present frequently, and aggressive systemic adjuvant therapy will be required to improve outcomes. The most favorable prognosis is seen when an incidental focus of ATC is identified in a thyroid specimen resected for goiter or differentiated cancer. Akaishi et al. [39] had six such cases; all were alive at 1 year, but one died 9 years later with pulmonary metastases. Pierie et al. [21] reported a 3-year survival of 90 % if ATC was discovered incidentally, while Sugino et al. [22] found 1- and 2-year survivals of 73 % and 46 %, respectively, with incidental ATC. Choi et al. [46] identified microscopic anaplastic foci (MAF) in 0.4 % of 3,587 PTC cases; 5-year cause-specific survival was 64 % in the MAF group and 98 % in the pure PTC cases.

Predictors of survival have been examined in many studies, using both univariate and multivariate analyses. The most obvious candidates would be size of the tumor, completeness of surgical resection, and lack of distant metastases, and this is borne out in Fig. 100.1 which illustrates the longest survival for patients with stage IVA cancer and shortest with IVC, as well as in Tables 100.2 and 100.3. What remains unexplained is why some patients are more fortunate and their cancer is detected at stage IVA, rather than IVB or IVC. It is recognized that all ATCs contain a plethora of genetic abnormalities responsible for the remarkable aggressiveness of the tumor [47–49]. It will be important to better understand the molecular derangements that contribute to the pathogenesis and progression at each stage of ATC, in order to develop more accurate predictive and therapeutic strategies.

The prognostic factors most commonly evaluated are listed in Table 100.4. Younger patients (<70, 65, or 60 years) have longer survival times in some studies [4, 18, 21, 26, 28,

R.C. Smallridge, MD (✉)
Division of Endocrinology & Metabolism, Mayo Clinic, Jacksonville, FL, USA

Department of Medicine, Mayo Clinic, Jacksonville, FL, USA

Department of Cancer Biology, Mayo Clinic, Jacksonville, FL, USA
e-mail: smallridge.robert@mayo.edu

E.G. Abate
Division of Endocrinology & Metabolism, Mayo Clinic, Jacksonville, FL, USA

Department of Medicine, Mayo Clinic, Jacksonville, FL, USA

L. Wartofsky, D. Van Nostrand (eds.), *Thyroid Cancer*, DOI 10.1007/978-1-4939-3314-3_100

Table 100.1 Staging distribution in anaplastic thyroid carcinoma

		Stage (%)		
Ref.	No.	IVA	IVB	IVC
Passler et al. [14]	120	19	36	45
McIver [41][a]	122	15.6	37.7	46.7
Kebebew [28]	455	8.6	42.6	48.8
Kim [31]	121	9	–	–
Swaak-Kragten [36]	75	9	51	40
Ito [40]	40	0	62.5	37.5
Akaishi [39]	100	11	31	58
De Crevoisier [23]	30	10	70	20
Poisson [44]	19	10.5	15.8	73.7

[a]Personal communication

Table 100.2 Survival according to TNM stage in anaplastic thyroid carcinoma [39]

Survival	IVA	IVB	IVC
Median (months)	33.5 m	6.1 m	2.5 m
6 months (%)	100	49.6	22.4
1 year (%)	72.7	24.8	8.2
2 years (%)	62.3	10.6	0

Table 100.3 Overall survival according to tumor extent in 241 patients with anaplastic thyroid cancer [45]

Survival	Confined (15 %)	Adjacent structures invaded (46 %)	Further extension; distant metastases (39 %)
Median (months)	9 m	6 m	3 m
1 year (%)	50.0	27.6	7.4
2 years (%)	32.7	16.2	2.1
5 years (%)	22.9	10.1	–

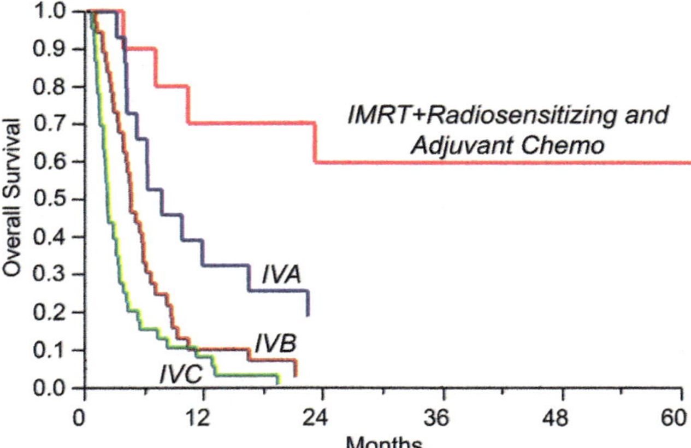

Fig. 100.1 Overall Kaplan-Meier survival in months. Data for historical 50-year Mayo Clinic outcomes for stage IVA, IVB, and IVC anaplastic thyroid cancer are compared to outcomes resulting from our recent practice change combining intensity-modulated radiation therapy with adjuvant and radiosensitizing chemotherapy. *IMRT* intensity-modulated radiation therapy (Reprinted with permission from Foote et al. [54])

Table 100.4 Predictors of survival in patients with anaplastic thyroid carcinoma (no. studies)

	Yes	No
Age	10	8
Gender	1	8
Tumor size	8	4
Surgery extent	18	5
Radiotherapy	14	5
Combination therapy	6	11
Distant metastases	12	2
Associated DTC	4	4
WBC >10,000	3	1
Dyspnea	3	0
Dysphagia	1	0
FDG-PET activity	1	0

DTC differentiated thyroid carcinoma

31, 33, 39, 43, 50], but not in all [13, 15, 24, 30, 32, 34, 35, 42]. Gender, on the other hand, did not influence survival in most studies [15, 24, 28, 31, 42, 43, 50, 51], but did in one [21]. Smaller primary tumors (<5, 6, or 7 cm) portend a more favorable outcome in eight reports [11, 13, 18, 21, 24, 31, 50, 51], but not in four others [28, 32, 39, 43]. The most striking, but not unexpected, predictor is extent of surgical resection, with longer survival observed in 81 % of studies [6, 8, 11, 13–15, 20–24, 27, 28, 30, 36, 39, 41, 50], but not in a minority [29, 31, 32, 43, 51]. Patients with a microscopic focus of ATC have the highest chance of survival, followed by patients with intrathyroidal stage IVA disease and R0 (negative margins) resections. Ito et al. [40] recently reported that stage IVB patients could be subdivided with IVB-a tumors involving the soft tissue, trachea, larynx, recurrent laryngeal nerve, or esophagus and IVB-b tumors which encased the carotid artery or mediastinal vessels or invaded the prevertebral fascia. Median survival was improved from 4.0 to 9.6 months in the IVB-a vs. IVB-b patients. Super-radical resection (trachea/larynx, esophagus/pharynx, major cervical arteries) in stage IVB patients improves survival compared to palliative but not restricted radical surgery [52].

Radiotherapy improved outcomes in 72 % of studies [10, 11, 13, 15, 21, 27–29, 34, 36, 39, 41, 43, 50], particularly in obtaining locoregional control of tumor and reducing death from airway and esophageal complications, but failed to improve survival in others [8, 24, 31, 35, 42]. Distant metastases, as one would predict, carried the worst prognosis in most [4, 6, 15, 26, 28–30, 33, 34, 39, 50, 51] but not all [24, 32] reports. Prior or concurrent differentiated thyroid cancer had an inconsistent effect on survival with a better prognosis in four reports [15, 19, 22, 23], but not in others [4, 14, 31, 51]. Leukocytosis carried a worse prognosis in several [39, 50, 53] but not all [24] studies, and dyspnea [8, 21, 42] and dysphagia [21] at presentation also are worrisome. FDG-PET uptake and intensity are inversely related to survival [44].

The causes of death are generally related to locoregional complications (asphyxia, pneumonia) or distant metastases. As radiotherapy techniques were modified to better accommodate the rapid doubling time of ATC, death rates from airway complications were reduced [3, 10, 13, 15, 27]. In one study, death was attributed to local complications in 37 %, distant metastases in 12 %, and both in 57 % of patients [38].

No single therapy has been optimal for ATC. While combination therapy has not improved survival in most studies [3, 8, 10, 21, 22, 24, 31–33, 41, 42] (Table 100.4), this reflects series spanning many decades during which the surgical, radiation, and chemotherapy approaches have evolved. Several studies of aggressive multimodal therapy [4, 17, 34, 40, 43, 50, 54] have shown some promise, at least in stage IVA and IVB ATC. Further experience and refinement of these strategies, and testing of newer agents with benefits demonstrated in preclinical studies [48, 49], will hopefully improve outcome in patients with all stages of ATC.

References

1. Carcangiu ML, Steeper T, Zampi G, et al. Anaplastic thyroid carcinoma. A study of 70 cases. Am J Clin Pathol. 1985;83:135–58.
2. Kim JH, Leeper RD. Treatment of locally advanced thyroid carcinoma with combination doxorubicin and radiation therapy. Cancer. 1987;60:2372–5.
3. Tennvall J, Tallroth E, el Hassan A, et al. Anaplastic thyroid carcinoma. Doxorubicin, hyperfractionated radiotherapy and surgery. Acta Oncol. 1990;29:1025–8.
4. Venkatesh YS, Ordonez NG, Schultz PN, et al. Anaplastic carcinoma of the thyroid. A clinicopathologic study of 121 cases. Cancer. 1990;66:321–30.
5. Demeter JG, De Jong SA, Lawrence AM, et al. Anaplastic thyroid carcinoma: risk factors and outcome. Surgery. 1991;110:956–61; discussion 961–3.
6. Schlumberger M, Parmentier C, Delisle MJ, et al. Combination therapy for anaplastic giant cell thyroid carcinoma. Cancer. 1991;67:564–6.
7. Wong CS, Van Dyk J, Simpson WJ. Myelopathy following hyperfractionated accelerated radiotherapy for anaplastic thyroid carcinoma. Radiother Oncol. 1991;20:3–9.
8. Junor EJ, Paul J, Reed NS. Anaplastic thyroid carcinoma: 91 patients treated by surgery and radiotherapy. Eur J Surg Oncol. 1992;18:83–8.
9. Hadar T, Mor C, Shvero J, et al. Anaplastic carcinoma of the thyroid. Eur J Surg Oncol. 1993;19:511–6.
10. Levendag PC, De Porre PM, van Putten WL. Anaplastic carcinoma of the thyroid gland treated by radiation therapy. Int J Radiat Oncol Biol Phys. 1993;26:125–8.
11. Tan RK, Finley 3rd RK, Driscoll D, et al. Anaplastic carcinoma of the thyroid: a 24-year experience. Head Neck. 1995;17:41–7; discussion 47–8.
12. Chemotherapy Committee, The Japanese Society of Thyroid Surgery. Intensive chemotherapy for anaplastic thyroid carcinoma: combination of cisplatin, doxorubicin, etoposide and peplomycin with granulocyte colony-stimulating factor support. Jpn J Clin Oncol. 1995;25:203–7.
13. Kobayashi T, Asakawa H, Umeshita K, et al. Treatment of 37 patients with anaplastic carcinoma of the thyroid. Head Neck. 1996;18:36–41.
14. Passler C, Scheuba C, Prager G, et al. Anaplastic (undifferentiated) thyroid carcinoma (ATC). A retrospective analysis. Langenbecks Arch Surg. 1999;384:284–93.
15. Voutilainen PE, Multanen M, Haapiainen RK, et al. Anaplastic thyroid carcinoma survival. World J Surg. 1999;23:975–8; discussion 978–9.
16. Ain KB. Anaplastic thyroid carcinoma: behavior, biology, and therapeutic approaches. Thyroid. 1998;8:715–26.
17. Busnardo B, Daniele O, Pelizzo MR, et al. A multimodality therapeutic approach in anaplastic thyroid carcinoma: study on 39 patients. J Endocrinol Invest. 2000;23:755–61.
18. Lam KY, Lo CY, Chan KW, et al. Insular and anaplastic carcinoma of the thyroid: a 45-year comparative study at a single institution and a review of the significance of p53 and p21. Ann Surg. 2000;231:329–38.
19. Rodriguez JM, Pinero A, Ortiz S, et al. Clinical and histological differences in anaplastic thyroid carcinoma. Eur J Surg. 2000; 166:34–8.
20. Haigh PI, Ituarte PH, Wu HS, et al. Completely resected anaplastic thyroid carcinoma combined with adjuvant chemotherapy and irradiation is associated with prolonged survival. Cancer. 2001;91: 2335–42.
21. Pierie JP, Muzikansky A, Gaz RD, et al. The effect of surgery and radiotherapy on outcome of anaplastic thyroid carcinoma. Ann Surg Oncol. 2002;9:57–64.
22. Sugino K, Ito K, Mimura T, et al. The important role of operations in the management of anaplastic thyroid carcinoma. Surgery. 2002;131:245–8.
23. De Crevoisier R, Baudin E, Bachelot A, et al. Combined treatment of anaplastic thyroid carcinoma with surgery, chemotherapy, and hyperfractionated accelerated external radiotherapy. Int J Radiat Oncol Biol Phys. 2004;60:1137–43.
24. Kihara M, Miyauchi A, Yamauchi A, et al. Prognostic factors of anaplastic thyroid carcinoma. Surg Today. 2004;34:394–8.
25. Veness MJ, Porter GS, Morgan GJ. Anaplastic thyroid carcinoma: dismal outcome despite current treatment approach. ANZ J Surg. 2004;74:559–62.
26. Besic N, Hocevar M, Zgajnar J, et al. Prognostic factors in anaplastic carcinoma of the thyroid-a multivariate survival analysis of 188 patients. Langenbecks Arch Surg. 2005;390:203–8.
27. Goutsouliak V, Hay JH. Anaplastic thyroid cancer in British Columbia 1985–1999: a population-based study. Clin Oncol (R Coll Radiol). 2005;17:75–8.
28. Kebebew E, Greenspan FS, Clark OH, et al. Anaplastic thyroid carcinoma. Treatment outcome and prognostic factors. Cancer. 2005;103:1330–5.
29. Wang Y, Tsang R, Asa S, et al. Clinical outcome of anaplastic thyroid carcinoma treated with radiotherapy of once- and twice-daily fractionation regimens. Cancer. 2006;107:1786–92.
30. Brignardello E, Gallo M, Baldi I, et al. Anaplastic thyroid carcinoma: clinical outcome of 30 consecutive patients referred to a single institution in the past 5 years. Eur J Endocrinol. 2007; 156:425–30.
31. Kim TY, Kim KW, Jung TS, et al. Prognostic factors for Korean patients with anaplastic thyroid carcinoma. Head Neck. 2007;29: 765–72.
32. Miccoli P, Materazzi G, Antonelli A, et al. New trends in the treatment of undifferentiated carcinomas of the thyroid. Langenbecks Arch Surg. 2007;392:397–404.
33. Yau T, Lo CY, Epstein RJ, et al. Treatment outcomes in anaplastic thyroid carcinoma: survival improvement in young patients with localized disease treated by combination of surgery and radiotherapy. Ann Surg Oncol. 2008;15:2500–5.
34. Bhatia A, Rao A, Ang KK, et al. Anaplastic thyroid cancer: clinical outcomes with conformal radiotherapy. Head Neck. 2010;32: 829–36.

35. Dandekar P, Harmer C, Barbachano Y, et al. Hyperfractionated accelerated radiotherapy (HART) for anaplastic thyroid carcinoma: toxicity and survival analysis. Int J Radiat Oncol Biol Phys. 2009;74:518–21.
36. Swaak-Kragten AT, de Wilt JH, Schmitz PI, et al. Multimodality treatment for anaplastic thyroid carcinoma – treatment outcome in 75 patients. Radiother Oncol. 2009;92:100–4.
37. Vrbic S, Pejcic I, Vrbic M, et al. Therapy of stage IV B anaplastic thyroid carcinoma: single institution experience. J BUON. 2009;14:41–4.
38. Siironen P, Hagstrom J, Maenpaa HO, et al. Anaplastic and poorly differentiated thyroid carcinoma: therapeutic strategies and treatment outcome of 52 consecutive patients. Oncology. 2010;79:400–8.
39. Akaishi J, Sugino K, Kitagawa W, et al. Prognostic factors and treatment outcomes of 100 cases of anaplastic thyroid carcinoma. Thyroid. 2011;21:1183–9.
40. Ito KI, Hanamura T, Murayama K, et al. Multimodality therapeutic outcomes in anaplastic thyroid carcinoma: improved survival in subgroups of patients with localized primary tumors. Head Neck. 2012;34:230–7.
41. McIver B, Hay ID, Giuffrida DF, et al. Anaplastic thyroid carcinoma: a 50-year experience at a single institution. Surgery. 2001;130:1028–34.
42. Tashima L, Mitzner R, Durvesh S, et al. Dyspnea as a prognostic factor in anaplastic thyroid carcinoma. Eur Arch Otorhinolaryngol. 2012;269:1251–5.
43. Sherman EJ, Lim SH, Ho AL, et al. Concurrent doxorubicin and radiotherapy for anaplastic thyroid cancer: a critical re-evaluation including uniform pathologic review. Radiother Oncol. 2011; 101:425–30.
44. Poisson T, Deandreis D, Leboulleux S, et al. 18F-fluorodeoxyglucose positron emission tomography and computed tomography in anaplastic thyroid cancer. Eur J Nucl Med Mol Imaging. 2010;37:2277–85.
45. Chen J, Tward JD, Shrieve DC, et al. Surgery and radiotherapy improves survival in patients with anaplastic thyroid carcinoma: analysis of the surveillance, epidemiology, and end results 1983–2002. Am J Clin Oncol. 2008;31:460–4.
46. Choi JY, Hwang BH, Jung KC, et al. Clinical significance of microscopic anaplastic focus in papillary thyroid carcinoma. Surgery. 2013;154:106–10.
47. Smallridge RC, Copland JA. Anaplastic thyroid carcinoma: pathogenesis and emerging therapies. Clin Oncol. 2010;22: 486–97.
48. Smallridge RC, Marlow LA, Copland JA. Anaplastic thyroid cancer: molecular pathogenesis and emerging therapies. Endocr Relat Cancer. 2009;16:17–44.
49. Abate E, Smallridge R. Managing anaplastic thyroid cancer. Expert Rev Endocrinol Metab. 2011;6:793–809.
50. Sugitani I, Miyauchi A, Sugino K, et al. Prognostic factors and treatment outcomes for anaplastic thyroid carcinoma: ATC research consortium of Japan cohort study of 677 patients. World J Surg. 2012;36:1247–54.
51. Segerhammar I, Larsson C, Nilsson IL, et al. Anaplastic carcinoma of the thyroid gland: treatment and outcome over 13 years at one institution. J Surg Oncol. 2012;106:981–6.
52. Sugitani I, Hasegawa Y, Sugasawa M, et al. Super-radical surgery for anaplastic thyroid carcinoma: a large cohort study using the anaplastic thyroid carcinoma research consortium of Japan database. Head Neck. 2014;36:328–33.
53. Sugitani I, Kasai N, Fujimoto Y, et al. Prognostic factors and therapeutic strategy for anaplastic carcinoma of the thyroid. World J Surg. 2001;25:617–22.
54. Foote RL, Molina JR, Kasperbauer JL, et al. Enhanced survival in locoregionally confined anaplastic thyroid carcinoma: a single-institution experience using aggressive multimodal therapy. Thyroid. 2011;21:25–30.

Part XIII

New Frontiers and Future Directions

Advances in Radiation Therapy

101

James D. Brierley and Richard W. Tsang

Introduction

Before discussing the recent advances in radiation therapy, it is important to consider the basic principles. The design for a proper course of radiation therapy (RT) must take into account the extent of extrathyroidal disease and the location of lymph node disease, as well as the radiation tolerance of normal tissues and organs. The accepted terminology to describe radiation dose and target volume in the planning of radiotherapy is summarized in Table 101.1. The principle is to deliver the prescribed dose to the entire clinical target volume (CTV) with reasonable dose uniformity (+/– 5 %). Custom-designed fields should be used to conform to the target volume while keeping the volume of irradiated normal tissues to a minimum. In general the aim should be to deliver 50–60 Gy to the CTV and 60–70 Gy to the gross tumor volume (GTV, in 1.8–2.0 Gy fractions, over 5–7 weeks [1–6]. External beam RT is delivered with linear accelerators generating X-ray beams in the megavoltage range of 4–25 MV (photons).

Radiation Treatment Planning

The process of planning radiation treatment requires simulation in the desired treatment position with an appropriate immobilization mask to ensure day-to-day reproducibility. Simulation is performed with a CT simulator, which simulates the actual geometric characteristics of the linear accelerator while imaging the area of interest. At simulation, reference marks are placed on the patient's mask in order to reproduce and align the beam profiles accurately. CT simulation allows the planning of treatment in three dimensions (3D), performed on the computer (therefore "virtual simulation"). The process involves designation of the various target volumes (Table 101.1), critical structures and normal organs of interest, beam profiles, and other modifying devices and then displaying these outlines in different 3D perspectives (axial, coronal, and sagittal). Dose distributions of the treatment plan can be displayed in isodose lines and dose-volume histograms for both the target volume and normal organ(s) of interest. The most common method of planning RT is based on the CT simulator, although other imaging modalities such as MRI and functional imaging (e.g. ^{18}F-deoxyglucose positron emission tomography and functional MRI) can be imported and fused with the CT images to more accurately determine the extent of any gross residual disease.

Treatment Volumes

The typical thyroid bed clinical target volume (CTV) is an inverse "U"-shaped volume on an axial image, with the spinal cord being the critical dose-limiting normal organ [1, 3]. Lymph nodes immediately adjacent to the thyroid bed (including zone 6, central compartment; zone 3, mid-jugular; and zone 4, supraclavicular) are generally included into the CTV. At the Princess Margaret Hospital, the current technique involves inverse planning intensity-modulated radiation therapy (IMRT) as discussed below. If IMRT is not available, planning a conformal set of multiple photon beams may be used. When there is no significant posterior extension of disease, lateral beams angled caudally to avoid the shoulders may produce an acceptable distribution. Additional established methods and techniques are well described by other investigators [1–3].

Advances in RT Planning and Delivery

IMRT refers to a planning and delivery process that attempts to achieve better conformation of the high-dose region to the target by additionally varying the fluence intensity within

J.D. Brierley, MBBS, FRCP, FRCR, FRCPC (✉)
R.W. Tsang, MD, FRCP(C)
Department of Radiation Oncology,
Princess Margaret Hospital, University of Toronto,
610 University Ave., Toronto, Ontario M5G 2M9, Canada
e-mail: james.brierley@rmp.uhn.on.ca;
Richard.tsang@rmp.uhn.on.ca

L. Wartofsky, D. Van Nostrand (eds.), *Thyroid Cancer*, DOI 10.1007/978-1-4939-3314-3_101

Table 101.1 Definition of radiation therapy terms

Term	Definition[a]	Comment
Absorbed dose	The energy deposited by ionizing radiation per unit mass of material (J/kg), expressed in the SI unit, the gray (Gy)	1 Gy = 100 centigray (cGy) 1 Gy = 100 rads
Gross tumor volume (GTV)	The gross demonstrable extent and location of the malignant growth	Includes the extrathyroidal disease and any involved regional nodes Determined by clinical examination and imaging tests
Clinical target volume (CTV)	A tissue volume that contains a demonstrable GTV and/or subclinical malignant disease that must be eliminated. This volume must be treated adequately in order to achieve the aim of radical therapy	Includes the thyroid bed and any extrathyroidal tissues and lymph nodes with suspected involvement or at high risk of subclinical involvement
Image-guided radiotherapy (IGRT)	Images taken during or just before the radiation is delivered enable changes to be made ensuring the correct volume is treated	Enables a smaller volume to be treated and thereby reduce toxicity
Intensity-modulated radiotherapy (IMRT)	By modulating the intensity and shape of the radiation fields, the radiation can be made more conformal (tailored)	IMRT has the potential to reduce toxicity to normal structures further and potentially enabling a higher radiation dose to be given
Planning target volume (PTV)	PTV is a geometric concept used for treatment planning, and it is defined to select appropriate beam sizes and beam arrangements, to ensure that the prescribed dose is actually delivered to the CTV	Includes internal margin (e.g., to account for organ motion) and setup margin (e.g., uncertainties in patient positioning and beam alignment)

[a]As defined in Report 62 of the ICRU (International Commission on Radiation Units and Measurements)

each beam [1, 7]. By setting the target dose(s) to the various tumor target volume(s) and the dose limits to the designated normal organs at risk, the computer performs iterations to arrive at the optimal beam arrangement and individual beam intensity profile. This is termed inverse planning, in contrast to forward planning in which the radiation dosimetrist places fields and the computer calculates the resulting dose and fields are adjusted by the dosimetrists to achieve the intended dose distribution. IMRT is capable of further reducing the spinal cord dose as compared with 3D conformal radiotherapy [1, 7]. IMRT is especially suitable for treating complex treatment volumes and avoiding dose-limiting normal structures and by enabling different doses of radiation to be given to volumes of differing risk of recurrence (Fig. 101.1). By using IMRT we can ensure that the appropriate dose is given to the volume at risk of recurrence without the compromises that were previously required that almost invariably resulted in a degree of underdosing, thus potentially resulting in a greater therapeutic gain from RT. IMRT is becoming increasing available [1, 7]. Cancer Care Ontario's Program of Evidence-Based Care has recently reviewed the evidence in support of IMRT for thyroid cancer. Although insufficient evidence was obtained in a systematic review to propose evidence-based recommendations in support of the use of IMRT in thyroid cancer, by extension from other head and neck cancers in which IMRT reduces toxicity and improves local control, it was concluded that there are compelling reasons why IMRT should be offered to patients with thyroid cancer as an alternative to conventional treatment planning [8].

Another significant advance in the delivery of radiation therapy involves image-guided radiotherapy (IGRT) whereby images are taken during the radiation treatment on a daily basis and ensure accurate day-to-day setup. In the past radiation volumes were increased to allow for uncertainties caused by patient movement during and between treatments. IGRT enables the radiation oncologist to treat a smaller volume of normal tissue and should further reduce potential toxicity.

Toxicity of External Beam RT

Well-planned external beam RT has moderate yet acceptable acute toxicity and rarely produces serious complications [3, 6, 9]. It does not preclude future surgical intervention if required. During the course of radiation, moderate skin erythema will develop, and dry desquamation or occasionally patchy moist desquamation of the skin occurs. Mucositis of the esophagus, trachea, and larynx, giving rise to dysphagia of solid foods, dryness, pain and irritation, and dysphonia usually occur toward the end of the course and will require symptomatic management with soft diet and analgesics. In patients assigned to the radiation arm of the German randomized control study that closed because of poor accrual, it was noted that the majority of patients experience mild to moderate side effects from adjuvant external beam radiotherapy [10]. At the first follow-up examination, most side effects had subsided and acute toxicity was tolerable in these patients; however in one patient who had preexisting laryn-

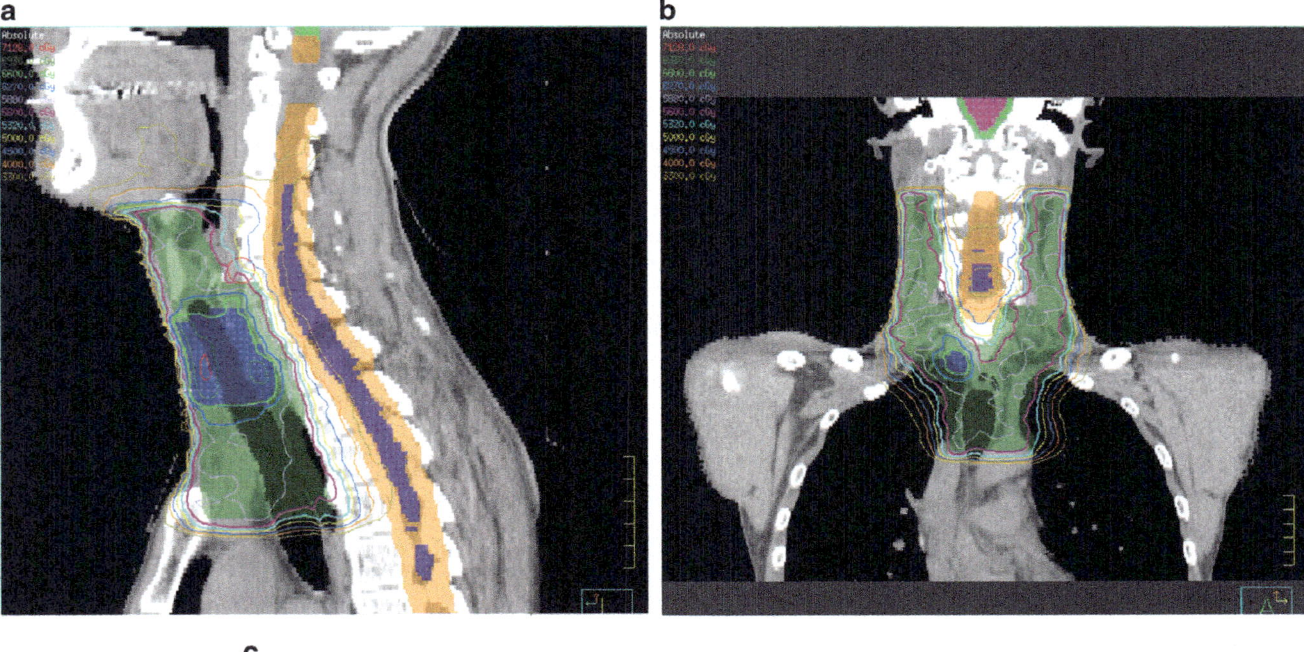

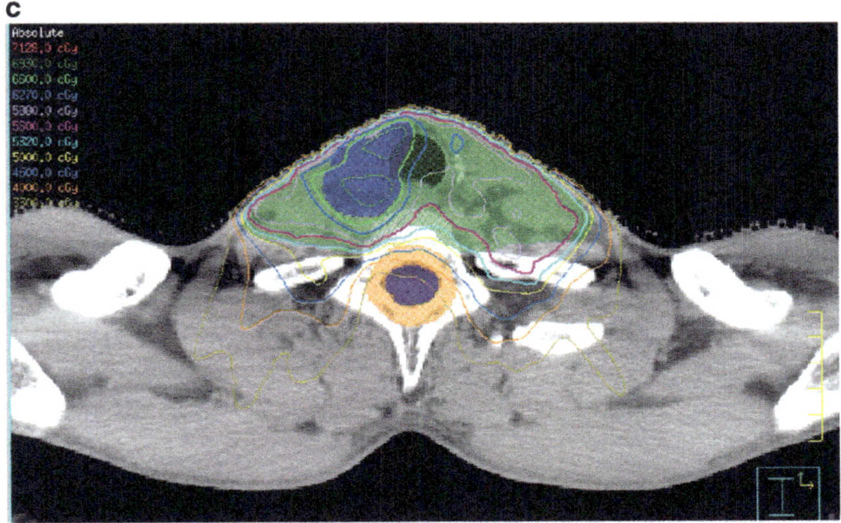

Fig. 101.1 Sagittal (**a**), coronal (**b**), and axial (**c**) views of IMRT plan for a patient with papillary thyroid cancer who had significant extrathyroid extension in the tracheoesophageal grove with residual microscopic disease. The plan allows for a high-dose 66 Gy to be given to the region of greatest concern in the tracheoesophageal grove and a lower dose of 56 Gy in 33 fractions to be given to the adjacent thyroid bed and nodal regions. The volume irradiated conforms to the U shape of the clinical target volume, ensuring minimum radiation exposure to the normal organs such as the spinal cord. The shaded area in *green* is the volume considered at moderate risk of relapse and is prescribed 56 Gy. The *crimson line* is the 56 Gy isodose line so that all the tissue within this line receives a minimum of 56 Gy. The shaded area in blue is at high risk and is prescribed 66 Gy. The light *green line* is the 66 Gy isodose so that all the tissue within this line receives a minimum dose of 66 Gy; other isodose lines are also included.

geal polypoid degeneration, laryngeal edema occurred. Depending on the superior extent of the fields, change of taste and xerostomia may occur. Late toxicity is dose dependent and generally infrequent, the most common is mild lymphedema usually seen just below the chin, skin telangiectasias, skin pigmentation, and soft tissue fibrosis, particularly in patients treated with cervical lymph node dissections [11]. Esophageal and tracheal stenosis is rare with conventional fractionation. Tsang et al. [6] found no RTOG grade IV toxicity in patients given 40–50 Gy in 2–2.5 Gy fractions to the neck and superior mediastinum. Farahati et al. [9] observed no irreversible late toxicity in 99 patients given 50–60 Gy in 1.8–2.0 Gy fractions to a large volume. In contrast a study from New York reported grade 3 acute mucositis in 14 (18 %) and grade 3 dysphagia in 24 (32 %) patients with a variety of thyroid histologies. Four patients (5 %) required percutaneous endoscopic gastrostomy tube for late esophageal stenosis [12]. Asymptomatic pulmonary fibrosis at the lung apices is expected and will be commonly visible on CT scan in subsequent follow-up and should not be mistaken for lung metastasis.

Summary

Advance radiation techniques including IMRT and IGRT which have the potential to improve target coverage and reduce toxicity should ideally be employed when treating thyroid cancer with RT.

References

1. Nutting CM, Convery DJ, Cosgrove VP, et al. Improvements in target coverage and reduced spinal cord irradiation using intensity-modulated radiotherapy (IMRT) in patients with carcinoma of the thyroid gland. Radiother Oncol. 2001;60:173–80.
2. O' Connell M, A'Hern RP, Harmer CL. Results of external beam radiotherapy in differentiated thyroid carcinoma: a retrospective study from the Royal Marsden Hospital. Eur J Cancer. 1994;30A:733–9.
3. Harmer C, Bidmead M, Shepherd S, Sharpe A, Vini L. Radiotherapy planning techniques for thyroid cancer. Br J Radiol. 1998;71:1069–75.
4. Brierley JD, Tsang RW. External-beam radiation therapy in the treatment of differentiated thyroid cancer. Semin Surg Oncol. 1999;16:42–9.
5. Brierley JD, Tsang RW. External radiation therapy in the treatment of thyroid cancer. In: Burman KD, editor. Thyroid cancer II, Endocrinol Metab Clin North America. Philadelphia: W. B. Saunders Co; 1996. p. 141–57.
6. Tsang RW, Brierley JD, Simpson WJ, Panzarella T, Gospodarowicz MK, Sutcliffe SB. The effects of surgery, radioiodine and external radiation therapy on the clinical outcome of patients with differentiated thyroid cancer. Cancer. 1998;82:375–88.
7. Posner MD, Quivey JM, Akazawa PF, Xia P, Akazawa C, Verhey LJ. Dose optimization for the treatment of anaplastic thyroid carcinoma: a comparison of treatment planning techniques. Int J Radiat Oncol Biol Phys. 2000;48:475–83.
8. Brierley J, Rumble R, Warde P, Panel IIE. The role of IMRT in thyroid cancers. http://www.cancercare.on.ca/toolbox/qualityguidelines/clin-program/radther/: Cancer Care Ontario. 2011.
9. Farahati J, Reiners C, Stuschke M, et al. Differentiated thyroid cancer. Impact of adjuvant external radiotherapy in patients with perithyroidal tumor infiltration (stage pT4). Cancer. 1996;77:172–80.
10. Schuck A, Biermann M, Pixberg MK, et al. Acute toxicity of adjuvant radiotherapy in locally advanced differentiated thyroid carcinoma. First results of the multicenter study differentiated thyroid carcinoma (MSDS). Strahlenther Onkol. 2003;179:832–9.
11. Biermann M, Pixberg M, Riemann B, et al. Clinical outcomes of adjuvant external-beam radiotherapy for differentiated thyroid cancer – results after 874 patient-years of follow-up in the MSDS-trial. Nuklearmedizin. 2009;48:89–98; quiz N15.
12. Terezakis SA, Lee KS, Ghossein RA, et al. Role of external beam radiotherapy in patients with advanced or recurrent nonanaplastic thyroid cancer: Memorial Sloan-kettering Cancer Center experience. Int J Radiat Oncol Biol Phys. 2009;73:795–801.

102 New Approaches in Nuclear Medicine for Thyroid Cancer

Douglas Van Nostrand

Prologue to the Third Edition

When I wrote this chapter for the second edition of this textbook in 2006 [1], I was not necessarily writing about the future developments of nuclear medicine in thyroid cancer within the next 6 years. Rather, I was attempting to communicate the spectrum of potential changes that might develop not only in the near future but also the distant future. Accordingly, the concepts that were the basis for my previous chapter in the second edition of this textbook have not changed significantly, and I have retained that chapter for this edition.

However, there have been many significant changes since writing the previous chapter, and accordingly, the introduction for this chapter in the third edition of this textbook presents an overview of the progress in the last 6 years in nuclear medicine equipment, radiotracers, and radiotherapy as they relate to thyroid cancer. For such a short period of time, I believe the accomplishments are impressive.

Developments in Imaging Equipment

Several major developments in nuclear medicine imaging equipment have been achieved over the last 6 years.

Single-photon emission tomography (SPECT) gamma cameras combined with computer tomography (CT) scanners have become more widespread and been used more frequently in the pretherapy and post-therapy evaluation of patients with differentiated thyroid cancer. In addition, multiple authors have published numerous articles in the last 6 years demonstrating the utility of SPECT-CT in altering the management of patients with differentiated thyroid cancer, again not only for post-therapy scans but also pretherapy scans. These publications are discussed in further detail by Kulkarni et al. in Chap.14.

Advances in positron emission tomography (PET) scanners now include new "time-of-flight" technology and the first commercially available digital PET scans. The new "time-of-flight" technology of PET harnesses a slight difference in the arrival time between the two 511 keV coincidence gamma rays on the detectors of the PET scanner to more precisely localize within the body the origin of the two 511 keV gamma rays. Specifically, when a radioisotope "decays" by the emission of a position (i.e., a positively charged electron), the positron will travel a short distance and then collide with an electron, resulting in the two particles destroying each other (i.e., annihilation) with the emission of two 511 keV gamma rays that travel away in the opposite direction of each other (i.e., 180°) from the point of annihilation. A standard PET scanner harnesses these two gamma rays by collecting only those gamma rays that arrive "simultaneously" (i.e., coincidence) on the two detectors of the PET scanner 180° apart. However, unless the two coincidence gamma rays originate an equal distance from the two PET detectors, they do not arrive at precisely the same time. Rather, one ray will typically have to travel slightly farther through the body to hit the detector than the other ray, and this slightly longer distance results in a slightly different arrival time. Since gamma rays are traveling at the speed of light and the difference in the distance traveled by the two gamma rays is very small, the differences in the arrival time is measured in picoseconds, and 1 ps is 1 trillionth of a second. Until recently, we did not have the capability to accurately measure these very small time differences. However, with the "time-of-flight" technology, several PET scanners now can measure these time differences, and these scanners can now more precisely localize where the two coincident 511 keV gamma rays originated from within the body.

D. Van Nostrand, MD, FACP, FACNM (✉)
Nuclear Medicine Research, MedStar Research Institute and Washington Hospital Center, Georgetown University School of Medicine, Washington Hospital Center, 110 Irving Street, N.W., Suite GB 60F, Washington, DC 20010, USA
e-mail: douglasvannostrand@gmail.com

L. Wartofsky, D. Van Nostrand (eds.), *Thyroid Cancer*, DOI 10.1007/978-1-4939-3314-3_102

The development of the first digital PET-CT scanner also takes PET imaging to a whole new level. The advantages of digital PET-CT include (1) solid state instead of analog technology, (2) improved time resolution (e.g., measuring differences of time of <325 ps) resulting in improved spatial resolution, (3) reduced signal-to-noise ratios resulting in improved contrast resolution, and (4) increased count rates resulting in faster acquisition time, increased throughput, and/or lower prescribed activity reducing radiation exposure, to name several.

The other advancement in the development of PET scanners is the combining of a PET scanner and a MR scanner, and several hybrid PET-MR scanners are now commercially available. This has required the development of technology that allows the significant reduction of the effects of a PET scanner on the MR scanner and vice versa. An initial pilot study by Millo et al. evaluating the quality of a PET scan performed on a dedicated PET scanner to a PET scan performed in the same patient on a hybrid PET-MR has demonstrated that the overall quality of the PET images are comparable [2]. Although one might predict that hybrid PET-MR scanners would be widely implemented based on the rapid and widespread implementation of hybrid PET-CT, this is yet to be determined. PET images and MR images typically require a significant amount of time, and a hybrid machine that obtains the two images *sequentially* means that the PET scanner will not be imaging whenever the MR scanner is imaging and vice versa. This means that the number of scans performed on a hybrid PET-MR scanner will be significantly less than the number of scans that could be performed on dedicated stand-alone PET scanner and a dedicated stand-alone MR scanner. However, hybrid PET-MR scanners have been developed to obtain both PET and MR images *simultaneously* rather than sequentially, and these scanners offer potential savings in time for the patient and technologists as well as potential reduction in space requirements. However, will a PET-MR offer savings or increase revenues for the imaging facility? If a PET-MR is not replacing an existing PET as well as an existing MR, then will an additional PET-MR be cost-effective? Again, we will have to await further evaluation.

Developments in Radiopharmaceuticals

Multiple articles have been published and have advanced our knowledge regarding the use of ^{18}F fluorodeoxyglucose (^{18} F FDG) not only in the evaluation of thyroid cancer but also regarding the significance of serendipitous uptake of ^{18}F FDG uptake in thyroid nodules, and these reports are discussed further in Chaps. 25, 43, 76, 87, 93, and 97. I anticipate that ^{18}F-FDG PET and PET-CT imaging will remain an important diagnostic modality for the evaluation of patients with thyroid cancer for many years to come or at least until more specific molecular imaging PET radiopharmaceutical agents are developed.

Likewise, multiple articles have been published predominantly in Europe regarding imaging somatostatin receptors, which has been discussed further by Dr. Avram et al. in Chap. 44 and Dr. Esposito in Chap. 86.

A radiopharmaceutical with great promise is ^{124}I, which emits a positron and has been more extensively reviewed in Chap. 103. With the confirmation that high-quality PET images can be obtained, multiple authors in Europe have published articles evaluating lesion detection of differentiated thyroid cancer, and with the commercial availability of ^{124}I by several companies in the United States, additional publications have further validated that ^{124}I can detect significantly more lesions than planar imaging performed with ^{131}I or ^{123}I. Further study is warranted comparing detection of lesions with ^{131}I and ^{123}I SPECT-CT and ^{124}I PET-CT.

Finally, with the combination of events over the last year including the development of the commercial availability of ^{18}F sodium fluoride (^{18}F NaF), the recent 2011 worldwide shortages of ^{99m}Tc pertechnetate, and the reimbursement for ^{18}F NaF by Medicare for patients participating in the National Oncologic PET Registry (NOPR) in the United States, ^{18}F NaF PET and PET-CT imaging have become available for the evaluation of patients with thyroid cancer who are insured by Medicare. Initial data demonstrate the superiority of ^{18}F NaF PET and PET-CT relative to standard bone scans performed with ^{99m}Tc radiolabeled phosphate compounds [3], and Schneider et al. in a pilot study of nine patients reported data suggesting that ^{18}F NaF PET bone scans may eliminate additional noninvasive diagnostic testing in as many as 78 % of pts, avoid invasive procedure in 56 % of pts, and alter management in as many as 67 % of pts with thyroid cancer [4]. Although I anticipate that these numbers will decrease in future studies with less pre-selection of patients, I still anticipate that ^{18}F NaF PET-CT will be confirmed as superior to and may potentially replace ^{99m}Tc radiolabeled phosphate compounds for evaluation of bone metastases. However, the complimentary and competitive roles of ^{18}F-FDG PET-CT and ^{18}F NaF PET-CT are more difficult to predict in regard to the evaluation of bone metastases secondary to thyroid cancer. In the end, the choice of either ^{18}F-FDG PET-CT or ^{18}F NaF PET-CT may be based on patient-specific indications. However, the renewal of ^{18}F NaF PET-CT for evaluating bone metastases in thyroid cancer has been an important development in the last 6 years.

Developments in Nuclear Medicine Radiotherapy

Initial progress is finally being achieved with studies evaluating the amount of ^{131}I prescribed activity for remnant ablation, adjuvant treatment, and treatment of distant metastases (see Chaps. 33 and 57) with examples such as Mallick et al. [5], Schlumberger et al. [6], and Klubo et al.'s publication on dosimetric vs empiric determined prescribed activity of ^{131}I [7]. Likewise, additional progress involving the treatment of selected thyroid cancers with somatostatin receptor agents continues, which is again achieved predominantly in Europe (see Chaps. 44 and 86).

In regard to dosimetry to help select the prescribed activity of ^{131}I for treatment of differentiated thyroid carcinoma based on calculation of radiation absorbed dose to lesions and/or to calculate the radiation absorbed dose to other organs such as the salivary glands, Hobbs et al. and Sgouros et al. (see Chap. 103) have improved on their 3D-ID® dosimetry with 3D-RD® dosimetry. Khorjekar et al. have also evaluated the 3D-RD® dosimetry in further evaluating lesional dosimetry (see Chap. 103).

In order to offer simplified methods to estimate radiation absorbed dose per mCi to the blood as a surrogate for the bone marrow and thus estimates of maximum tolerated prescribed activity of ^{131}I for therapy of metastatic disease, Van Nostrand et al. and Hanscheid et al. have independently published two approaches (see Chap. 59). These methods allow an estimation of the maximum tolerated prescribed activity of ^{131}I for therapy with as little as one measurement of the retention of radioiodine in the whole body at 48 h.

Another exciting area in radioisotope therapy is radium-233 chloride (Xofigo®). Xofigo® is an alpha particle that was recently approved by the Food and Drug Administration (FDA) for the treatment of bone metastases. Although Xofigo® is presently approved only for the treatment of patients with castration-resistant prostate cancer metastatic to the bone, this radioisotope hopefully represents the first of many indications for alpha particle radiotherapy and the first of many alpha particles to become available in the future, which may have potential benefit for patients with metastatic thyroid cancer.

Redifferentiation

In regard to ^{131}I therapy and thyroid cancers that have lost their ability to take up iodine, Ho et al. [8] have published initial results using selumetinib to "redifferentiate" thyroid cancer to re-take up radioiodine, and their data are very encouraging (See Chapt. 68).

Summary

In the short time span of only 6 years, many accomplishments have been achieved in nuclear medicine equipment, radiotracers, and radiotherapies as they relate to the diagnosis and management of thyroid cancer. However, as equally important as these accomplishments are, our failures are also important. Although these are rarely recognized or published, they are paradoxically also "accomplishments." When Thomas Edison was asked about his failures, he stated, "I have not failed. I've just found 10,000 ways that won't work" [9]. Accordingly, we have made significant progress through not only our successes but also our failures, and for the next 6 years, I believe we can be equally optimistic about our future successes and failures.

Prologue to Second Edition 2010

In 1899, Charles Duell, Director of the United States Patent and Trademark Office, stated: "Everything that can be invented has been invented." In terms of a complete listing of specific potential advances in nuclear medicine, I am certain to miss the target as much as Mr. Duell did, but I will not miss the target regarding the general potential for advancements in nuclear medicine for the diagnosis and treatment of thyroid cancer. In Chap. 12 of the 2nd edition of this textbook [10], Henry Wagner quoted the president and CEO of General Electric Medical Systems, Joseph M. Hogan, who stated, "In the years to come, we envision a health care system that uses molecular medicine to diagnose and treat patients before symptoms appear and treatments that are tailored to an individual based on his or her genetic makeup." Indeed, molecular approaches to medicine are being applied now and will be an important part of the future, and nuclear medicine using radiotracers will play a major role in molecular medicine.

This chapter briefly reviews only a few of the many exciting areas of research and development underway in nuclear medicine relating to equipment, imaging, and therapy. The role of nuclear medicine in the diagnosis, evaluation, and treatment of patients who have thyroid cancer has never been more exciting.

Equipment

The major advancements in equipment in the near future will be in positron emission tomography (PET) scanners and single-photon emission computer tomography (SPECT) cameras.

The equipment employed for PET will continue to improve rapidly, and some advancement will likely include integration of different imaging modalities, expanding capabilities, increasing software speed, development of specialized scanners, design of better detectors, implementation of respiratory gating, and development of time-of-flight scanners. The benefits of both PET and CT scanners into a single unit have already been proven; this is not just a convenience to the patient but is also a major advancement that improves the sensitivity and specificity of the PET and CT findings. Although combining a PET and magnetic resonance imaging (MRI) is more difficult, such a scanner has already been achieved for small-scale animal research with a single slice system [11]. The utility of PET will increase to include the ability to perform a biopsy or fine-needle aspiration of a nodule or a suspected metastasis that is localized only by a PET scanner. This will be very important to help in the management of "PET-positive CT-negative" or "PET-positive MRI-negative" abnormalities. PET-CT capabilities will also continue to expand in the planning of external radiation therapy for cancers (including thyroid cancer). PET-CT scanners will improve the delineation of tumor treatment target volumes by combining anatomic localization and volumes with heretofore unavailable functional volumes. PET software will have better and faster processing algorithms. As a result, acquisition times and processing times will be reduced.

Scanners will also be developed with specialized functions. Micro-PET scanners with exquisite resolution are already available for imaging small animals (e.g., rodents) for research. Naviscan has already developed a PET scanner, which is approximately the size of a mammography unit and images the breast and other areas of the body, such as joints in humans. The Food and Drug Administration has already approved this unit, and other specialized PET scanners will be developed. Conceivably, a specialized PET scanner could be designed to maximize the imaging of a nodule within the thyroid with a positron-emitting radionuclide labeled to a peptide, an antibody, or a reporter probe unique to thyroid cancer cells, resulting in "hot-spot" imaging.

Detectors will also improve. Although it is beyond the scope of this chapter, new designs of detectors are already underway. For the past 15 years, the block-type detector for the organization of the crystals has dominated [12]. With new variants of the block design such as quadrant sharing and high-resolution research tomography [13], improved positional information may be obtained without loss in energy resolution. This can also enable the simultaneous acquisition of emission and transmission data, which then may decrease the whole-body acquisition times to 5 or 10 min, with minimal or no compromise in image quality [14]. This will not only lower imaging time for the patient but can also help to reduce the cost of a PET exam.

Respiratory motion has been a major problem for PET-CT imaging of the chest, creating artifacts on the fusion of PET and CT images of the lung. This may be important in the evaluation of thyroid cancer metastases in these areas. New respiratory gating techniques may reduce respiratory artifacts.

Finally, perhaps "time-of-flight" PET scanners may become a reality. These imaging systems, which Ter-Pogossian et al. [15] first considered in 1980, would harness the difference in the arrival times of the two 180° annihilation photons from the positron emitter. This difference in time would allow the localization of the annihilation site along the path of the two photons.

Equipment development will not be limited just to PET scanners but will also involve SPECT cameras. SPECT-CT scanners have already been introduced and will develop in many of the same areas as PET-CT. This will then allow the further expansion of single-photon emission radiotracers.

Imaging

Regarding nuclear medicine imaging for patients who have thyroid cancer, the potential is unlimited. The future includes the development of numerous molecular imaging probes and additional positron emitters.

Molecular Imaging

With the dawn of molecular imaging, an ever-increasing array of molecular probes will be developed to image such processes as tumor metabolism, cellular proliferation, specific cell surface receptors, inflammation, angiogenesis, tumor hypoxia, and apoptosis. Receptor-targeted radiopeptide imaging, bispecific antibodies, and PET reporter-gene reporter-probe imaging represent three promising areas.

Receptor-Targeted Radiopeptide Imaging

Receptor-targeted radiopeptides have already been used and hold great promise not only for imaging but also for therapy [16]. Peptides are molecules that are derived from amino acids and have typically 2–50 amino acids linked together. Peptides have many important functions, such as modulating and regulating cellular function and intracellular communication. Table 102.1 lists many receptors expressed on human tumors. Some advantages of radiolabeled peptides include (1) rapid diffusion and localization, (2) quick clearance from the body, (3) rapid internalization, (4) potentially long residence time, (5) possibly easy chemical synthesis, (6) lack of immunogenicity, and (7) metabolic stability.

To date, one of the best examples of the future use of receptor-targeted radiopeptides for imaging and treatment of cancers, specifically thyroid cancer, involves the somatostatin receptors. The prototype of the somatostatin receptor-targeted radiopeptide is ^{111}In-DTPA octreotide (^{111}In-pentetreotide), OctreoScan®, which has been used in medullary thyroid carcinoma and even well-differentiated thyroid carcinoma (see Chaps. 44 and 86). Radiolabeled octreotide has also been used by harnessing the therapeutic benefits of the auger electrons from ^{111}In and the β-emission from ^{90}Yttrium. The therapeutic benefits of auger electrons are discussed further below. Another radiolabeled somatostatin analog, ^{177}Lu-1,4,7,10-tetra-azacyclododecane-

Table 102.1 Examples of expression of various peptide receptors in various tumors

Peptide	Tumors
Somatostatin	Neuroendocrine tumors, thyroid cancer
VIP/PACAP	Adenocarcinomas
CCK/gastrin	Medullary thyroid cancer
LHRH	Breast and prostate cancer
α-MSH	Melanoma
Bombesin/GRP	Medullary thyroid cancer
Neurotensin	Ewing sarcoma, medullary thyroid cancer
Opioid	Breast cancer
Substance P	Medullary thyroid cancer
GLIP-1	Insulinoma
Oxytocin	Endometrium, breast cancer
Neuropeptide Y	Breast cancer

N,*N′*,*N″*,*N‴*-tetra-acetic acid^0 (DOTA), Tyr^3-octreotate (^{177}Lu-DOTATATE), has been used to treat five patients with nonradioiodine-avid well-differentiated thyroid cancer with some success [17]. We are only beginning to address the potential application of receptor-targeted radiopeptides for imaging and treatment.

Bispecific Antibodies

The use of antibodies for diagnosis and therapy had been significantly improved because of monoclonal antibody technology. However, the percent of injected dose of the monoclonal antibody that targets a gram of tumor is low and ranges from 0.001 to 0.01 % of injected activity per gram of tumor [18]. Multiple strategies have been evaluated to improve target-organ activity and to decrease background activity. One such strategy is bispecific antibodies, which has been reported by Reardon et al. [19] and modified by Khaw et al. [20]. The goal with bispecific antibodies is that two antibodies are linked with one of the antibodies specific for the target and the other for radiolabeled chelates. This can significantly increase the sensitivity for detection and localization of specific antigens.

Reporter Gene Imaging

Reporter gene imaging is one of the most exciting areas for future research and development for thyroid cancer [21]. In brief, the concept is the placement of a gene (the reporter gene) into the nucleus of a cell, and the DNA of that gene is transcribed into its corresponding mRNA, which then makes its specific protein (the reporter protein). A radiolabeled chemical (the reporter probe), specifically designed to metabolize or bind to the reporter protein, is administered and metabolized or bound to the reporter protein. Then a PET scanner or SPECT camera images the radiolabeled emissions.

Specifically, genetic material may be placed into cells directly (in vivo) or indirectly (in vitro) by gene therapy vectors, which are the delivery systems. The gene therapy vectors may be generally classified as nonviral or viral vectors. Nonviral vectors may include a broad spectrum of methods, including DNA-protein complexes, liposomes, and naked DNA. Viral vectors use the gene-delivery mechanisms of various viruses and are efficient delivery systems. Once delivered, the DNA reporter gene is then transcribed with the production of the corresponding mRNA, which makes one of three broad categories of reporter proteins: enzymes, receptors, or transporters. A radiolabeled reporter probe is then administered and depending on the type of reporter protein is (1) enzymatically metabolized within the cell, (2) attached to a receptor (e.g., on the cell wall), or (3) transported across the cell wall into the cytoplasm of the cell.

The prototype for the "enzyme" reporter gene is the herpes simplex type 1 virus thymidine kinase (HSV1-tk) and has been used as a therapeutic gene. After gene expression within the cell and after the administration of an acycloguanosine (e.g., ganciclovir), the ganciclovir enters the cell. It is monophosphorylated by the HSV1-tk enzyme to ganciclovir triphosphate, which kills the cell. Derivatives of acycloguanosine can also be radiolabeled with positron emitters that allow PET imaging of the reporter protein of the HSV1-tk.

The prototype for the "receptor" reporter gene is SSTr2, an analog of somatostatin (i.e., octreotide). As already noted above, imaging with somatostatin analogs has potential application for various types of thyroid cancers, and the SSTr2 as part of a PET reporter-gene reporter-probe system has already been labeled with the positron emitters of ^{64}Cu and ^{68}Ga [22, 23], as well as ^{99m}Tc for SPECT imaging [24].

The prototype for a gene to transport a protein is the sodium-iodide symporter (NIS). This is one of the most interesting genes for thyroid cancer, with possible application to thyroid cancer cells that do not organify iodine. For example, NIS incorporation into medullary carcinoma could allow a method for visualization and treatment of this tumor. Indeed, Chen et al. [25] have reported preliminary data indicating that the transduction of the NIS gene is sufficient to induce iodide transport in medullary thyroid carcinoma cells both in vitro and in vivo. A more in-depth discussion of the role of NIS in nuclear medicine is available [26].

The potential clinical utility of PET reporter genes and PET reporter probes will be in imaging and therapy. Relevant areas include (1) avoidance of invasive procedures for gene therapy monitoring, (2) pretherapy diagnosis, (3) treatment evaluation of other gene therapies at the biochemical level, (4) patient follow-up, and (5) prognostic indicators [21].

Although promising and exciting, molecular imaging, such as for tumor metabolism, cellular proliferation, specific cell surface receptors, inflammation, angiogenesis, tumor hypoxia, apoptosis, receptor-targeted radiopeptides, bispecific antibodies, and gene expression, is complicated, and there are many hurdles still to overcome. The combination of radioisotopes with chemicals is complex; the molecular targeting is difficult; increasing specificity and reducing nonspecific binding is problematic; and a radioconjugate can even irradiate itself and decompose. The important difference is that unlike the initial years of the development of radiotracers, when nuclear medicine was the only imaging modality that imaged physiologic processes, these newer imaging modalities can image molecular processes. These include targeted MRI imaging, targeted echocardiographic nanotechnology, optical coherence imaging, and optical imaging. While each new approach has its limitations, the future for radiotracers in molecular imaging is extremely exciting and is only in its infancy.

PET Radiotracers

^{18}F is the most widely used positron emitter and has the most extensive database on targetry, target chemistry, and radiochemistry available [27]. ^{18}F will continue to be evaluated and used with many new carriers, of which several have already been discussed. However, PET radiotracers are not limited to ^{18}F. Pagani et al. [28] have reviewed alternative positron emitters and the effects of their physical properties on image quality and potential clinical applications.

Glaser et al. [29] have recently reviewed the potential role of the positron-emitting halogens of ^{75}Br, ^{76}Br, and ^{124}I. Bromines have two advantages over other halogenation reactions. First, the chemistry of bromine is easier for synthesis than fluorine. Second, bromine radiotracers are anticipated to be much more stable in vivo, owing to the higher binding energy of bromine-carbon. However, there are always trade-offs. The targetry and target chemistry of bromine is more difficult, requiring relatively higher beam energy for production, which is available in only a few centers. For imaging thyroid cancer, ^{124}I holds the most exciting promise. Although the first scan with ^{124}I in an animal was performed in 1959 [30], and the first treatment in a thyroid cancer patient was performed with ^{124}I in 1960 [31], the use and availability of ^{124}I has been limited. Yet, at the time of this book's publication, ^{124}I is now routinely produced commercially by one company: Eastern Isotopes, Inc. This should significantly increase the availability of ^{124}I, the breadth and extent of ^{124}I research, and the clinical utility of ^{124}I. Relative to ^{123}I and ^{131}I, the imaging of the positron emitter ^{124}I with a PET scanner will have several advantages. These include superior sensitivity, the ability to estimate "functional volume" of thyroid tissue [29], and the ability to perform lesional and whole-body dosimetry [32]. ^{124}I will also have the advantages of excellent tomographic images and the ability to fuse with CT and MRI.

In addition to the use of ^{124}I as a radioiodine element for imaging itself, ^{124}I has also been labeled to other carriers, including antibodies, reporter genes, peptides, and amino acids. Examples include 5-{^{124}I}iodo-2′-deoxyurindine (^{124}I-IUdR), which is a thymidine analog, and 1-{2-fluoro-2-deoxy-B-D-arabinofuranosyl}-5-[^{124}I} iodouracil (^{124}IFIAU), used for reporter gene imaging with HSV1-tk expression as discussed above. Additional examples include ^{124}I-metaiodobenzylguanidine (^{124}I MIBG) for possibly imaging medullary thyroid carcinoma and ^{124}I annexin-V for imaging apoptosis during oncolytic therapy. ^{124}I will likely be labeled to other carriers as yet unreported, and it holds great promise for the imaging of thyroid cancer.

In addition to the development of areas noted above, many other areas involving nuclear medicine imaging of thyroid cancer, albeit perhaps less glamorous, will be evaluated with future resolution of many questions and problems. Some of these are listed in Table 102.2.

Table 102.2 Additional examples of future nuclear medicine research and development for thyroid cancer

Further evaluation of the utility of ^{123}I for surveillance scans for metastatic well-differentiated thyroid cancer
Further clarification of the role of alternative imaging modalities, such as ^{18}F fluorodeoxyglucose and other radioisotopes
Further evaluation and implementation of mechanisms to improve radioiodine uptake and retention time in metastasis
Better identification of patients for radioiodine treatment
Evaluation of the best radioisotope for the treatment of thyroid cancer
Evaluation of the clinical effectiveness of "blind treatments" (thyroglobulin-positive radioiodine-negative) and if so, better identification of those patients who will benefit
Evaluation of the efficacy of fractionated prescribed activity
Evaluation of methods to reduce side effects secondary to radioiodine treatments
Development of better methods to assess bone marrow reserve after previous radioiodine treatments
Evaluation of the relationship of total bone marrow accumulative radiation-absorbed dose relative to time
Further comparisons of outcome and side effects of radioiodine treatments with prescribed activities determined by various approaches (e.g., empiric fixed, Benua-Leeper, MIRD, Thomas-Maxon, and combinations of each)

Therapy

The most exciting aspect of nuclear medicine is radiotherapy and specifically "FedEx'ing" radiation to the cell for more localized radiation therapy. A limitation of external-beam radiotherapy is that it is "external" and thus must also pass through and irradiate normal tissue. Significant advancements, such as intensity-modulated radiation therapy, γ-knife, and CyberKnife, have reduced the radiation exposure to the normal tissue; however, the ideal is to deliver the radiation by a carrier directly to the cell. In other words, the ideal is to "FedEx" the package by a vehicle to a specific address, with minimal travel time and minimal errors in

Table 102.3 Potential radioisotopes for therapeutic application

α	β (mean range of <200 μm)	β (mean range of >200 μm to <1 mm)	β (mean range of > 1 mm)	
^{211}At	^{33}P	^{47}Sc	^{32}P	^{67}Ga
^{212}Bi(^{212}Pb)	^{121}Sn	^{67}Cu	^{89}Sr	^{71}Ge
^{223}Ra	^{177}Lu	^{77}As	^{90}Y	^{77}Br
	^{191}Os	^{105}Rh	^{114}mIn	^{103}Pd
^{225}Ac	^{199}Au	^{109}Pb	^{188}Ret	^{119}Sb
		^{111}Ag		^{123}I
		^{131}I		^{125}I
		^{143}Pr		^{131}Cs
		^{153}Sm		^{193}mPt
		^{161}Te		^{197}Hg
		^{186}Re		

Ac actinium, *Ag* silver, *At* astatine, *Au* gold, *Bi* bismuth, *Br* bromine, *Cs* cesium, *Cu* copper, *Ga* gallium, *Ge* germanium, *Hg* mercury, *I* iodine, *In* indium, *Lu* lutetium, *Os* osmium, *P* phosphorus, *Pd* palladium, *Pr* praseodymium, *Pt* platinum, *Ra* radium, *Re* rhenium, *Rh* rhodium, *Sb* antimony, *Sm* samarium, *Sn* tin, *Sr* strontium, *Te* tellurium

delivery. The "package" is the radiation. The "vehicles" are carriers, such as peptides, antibodies, and receptor probes, and the "addresses" are receptors, antigens, or reporter genes. Improvements in specifically delivering or "FedEx'ing" radiation to the cell will come at many different points in the transportation and delivery process. Some developments in the "vehicles" and "addresses" have already been discussed above, and what is in the "packages" is discussed below.

"The Radiation Package" to "FedEx" to the Cell

Theradioisotopes predominately used for therapy have been ^{131}I and ^{90}Y, but the options are far more extensive. Humm [32] classified many potential radioisotopes for therapy by the distance of the principal radiation emitted, and Ackery tabulated them (see Table 102.3; [25]). Humm restricted the list to radioisotopes with half-lives that are most valuable for therapy, i.e., 6 h to 4 weeks.

It is important to have an armamentarium of different therapeutic radioisotopes because one will want to package different radioisotopes, depending on the therapeutic objectives and the address to which the package is being sent. Sisson et al. [36] noted that as a tumor becomes smaller and smaller, the β- and γ-energy from ^{131}I deposited within the actual tumor decreases. For a sphere of 0.5 mm in diameter, less than 40 % of the energy of ^{131}I is deposited within that sphere [36]. Accordingly, one may wish to use a different radionuclide or even a combination of radioisotopes based on the tumor size. For smaller tumors, one may wish the principal radiation emitted to travel and deposit most of its energy over a short distance. For large bulky tumors, one may wish to use a radioisotope that deposits its energy over a longer distance, which would also harness the crossfire effect. This effect is the deposit in one cancer cell of the energy of a β- or γ-ray originating from another cancer cell.

One type of radioisotope that deposits significant amounts of energy over short distances is the α-emitter [37]. Typically, α-emitters travel a short distance of 50–90 μm (1 μm is 1/1,000 of 1 mm) and may deposit as much as 800 keV or approx 0.25 Gy in a distance of 10 μm. A nucleus may measure in the order of 10 μm. For certain cells, this may require only approx 3–6 α-"hits" per nucleus to reduce the fraction of surviving cells by an average of 37 %. In addition, this is enough energy to give multiple double-strand breaks in DNA, which may result in irreparable radiation damage [33]. To appreciate the potential benefit of α-emitters, it would require up to 400 β-particles to deposit the same energy in a nucleus as 1 α-particle. As Kassis et al. [38] have stated, it may take up to 20,000 β-particles to traverse a cell nucleus to sterilize that cell, whereas it may take only 1–4 α-emitters to traverse a cell nucleus to kill that cell. One of the α-emitters that has excellent potential is ^{211}At and has been used in a human [39].

At the other end of the spectrum of radionuclides are those that decay by electron capture, such as ^{123}I. Although ^{123}I is not typically associated with therapeutic potential, ^{123}I can have a significant therapeutic effect if it is packaged into a carrier and "FedEx'ed" to the nucleus of a cell to be treated. When a radioisotope such as ^{123}I decays by electron capture, a low-energy characteristic X-ray is emitted as the electrons are rearranged in their orbits to replace the electron that was just absorbed into the nucleus. For heavy elements, the energy of this X-ray could be sufficient to be used for medical imaging. However, for ^{123}I, the energies of the characteristic X-rays are too small (maximum of about 30 keV) for conventional devices, such as the γ-camera. Yet, in many of the decays, and especially for those originating from beyond the L electron orbit, the expected characteristic X-ray never makes it out of the atom. Instead, its energy interacts with another electron from that same atom and "ejects" that electron out of the atom entirely. This ejected electron is called an "Auger electron." In fact, there is a cascade of Auger electrons of progressively lower energy that are emitted following each decay. Although most Auger electrons have very low energy (typically about 15 eV to several keV), they also travel only a short range over which they deposit their energy, typically less than 1 nm or about the diameter of the DNA helix. Consequently, the cytotoxic effect of ^{123}I can be significantly enhanced if it can be concentrated in proximity to the DNA relative to other cellular locations. The killing effects of Auger electrons from ^{123}I have been confirmed with the conjugation of ^{123}I with deoxyuridine [40], and significant damage can be potentially achieved if the "package" is delivered close to the cellular DNA.

Thus, with more radioisotopes available and with better selection of the isotope based on the objectives and the "address" of the thyroid cancer, a greater therapeutic potential with less untoward effects is possible. Of course, "FedEx'ing" radiation to the cell is complicated, and there are many major foreseen and unforeseen problems to be solved. The process of combining elements with chemicals is complex; molecular targeting is difficult; nonspecific binding is problematic; and as mentioned earlier, the radiochemical or conjugate can even irradiate itself and decompose. But with a firm faith in the ingenuity of man, this author believes that these hurdles will be overcome. If not, then different and even better approaches will be identified and successfully implemented.

Redifferentiation

Well-differentiated thyroid cancer may dedifferentiate and lose its ability to take up radioiodine, and future efforts will be made to redifferentiate these cells to take up radioiodine. Initial success of redifferentiation has already been achieved and is reviewed in Chap.68. In brief, Grunwald et al. [41] administered retinoic acid to 12 patients, of which 4 had improved radioiodine uptake, and 2 patients had radioiodine uptake reestablished to allow radioiodine therapy. Schmutzler has extensively reviewed the use of retinoids [42]. In addition to retinoic acid, many other approaches have been evaluated. Furuya et al. [43] demonstrated accumulation of ^{125}I in poorly differentiated papillary and anaplastic thyroid cancer cells after reexpression of thyroid-specific genes by mRNA-induced histone deacetylase inhibitors. Chen et al. [44] were able to create iodide uptake in medullary thyroid carcinoma cells after transfer of the NIS gene. Misaki et al. [45] showed that tumoricidal cytokines may enhance radioiodine uptake, but this occurred in cultured thyroid cancer cells.

Enhancers

In addition to the mechanisms to restore radioiodine uptake, the future is bright regarding potential mechanisms to enhance radioiodine retention. For example, Koong et al. [46] have demonstrated the utility of lithium in enhancing the efficacy of increasing the retention of radioiodine. Zarnegar et al. [47] demonstrated that an increase in NIS and a decrease in pendrin activity may be associated with increased radioactive iodine effectiveness and could make radioiodine therapy more beneficial in patients with thyroid cancer.

Radiosensitizers

Radiosensitizers act to accentuate the effects of radiation, and several hold great potential. Kvols has selectively reviewed radiosensitizers (e.g., chemotherapeutic agents) that could increase the impact of radiotherapy [48].

Miscellaneous

As noted in the imaging section, many other less dramatic but equally important clinical questions and problems involving therapy in nuclear medicine will be evaluated in the future and hopefully solved (see Table 102.2).

Summary

The future of nuclear medicine in the diagnosis, management, and treatment of thyroid cancer is bright and exciting; this promise is also true for nuclear medicine innovations that will be applied to other realms of medicine. Indeed, the overall future of medicine warrants the cliché: It will be beyond our wildest imagination. Who thought: We would communicate in a way similar to Dick Tracy's two-way wrist radio? We could visit the Titanic in a Jules Verne-like vessel? We could go to the moon as H.G. Wells described? We could sweep over the outside of our patients with an imaging scanner like Dr. McCoy on the Starship Enterprise and give Captain Kirk the diagnosis in a matter of minutes or even seconds? It is only a matter of time before patients in a remote location will be able to test or image themselves for a specific molecular or bodily function by an implanted device or by sweeping a scanner over the outside of their body, with the data transmitted halfway around the world to a computer. In fact, it is already being done. Charles Duell could not have been more wrong.

References

1. Van Nostrand D. New approaches in nuclear medicine for thyroid cancer. In: Wartofsky L, Van Nostrand D, editors. Thyroid cancer a comprehensive guide to clinical management. New York: Springer; 2006.
2. Millo C, Khorjekar G, Maass-Moreno R, Neumann R, Bluemke D. Comparison of PET images obtained with PET-CT vs PET-MR: a pilot study. J Nucl Med. 2012;53:551. abstract.
3. Grant FD, Fahey FH, Packard AB, Davis RT, Alavi A, Treves ST. Skeletal PET with ^{18}F Fluoride: applying new technology to an old tracer. J Nucl Med. 2008;49:68–78. 4.
4. Schneider MT, Garcia C, O'Neil J, Van Nostrand D, Wexler J, Burman K, Wartofsky L. Retrospective study of the utility of ^{18}F sodium fluoride PET bone scans in patients with thyroid cancer. J Nucl Med (abstract) 2012;53(S):2067.
5. Mallick U, Harmer C, Yap B, Wadsley J, Clarke S, Moss L, Nicole A, Clarke PM, Franell K, McCready R, Smellie J, Frankly JA, John R, Nutting CM, Newbold K, Lemon C, Gerard G, Abdel-Hamid A, Hardman J, Macias E, Roques T, Whitaker S, Vijayn R, Alvarez P, Beare S, Forsyth S, Kadalayil L, Hackshaw A. Ablation with low-dose radioiodine and thyrotopin alfa in thyroid cancer. NEJM. 2012;366:1674–85.
6. Schlumberger M, Catargi B, Borget I, Deandreis D, Zerdoud S, Bridji B, Bardet S, Leenhardt L, Bastie D, Schvartz C, Vera P, Morel O, Benisvy D, Bournaud C, Bonichon F, Dejax C, Toubert ME, Leboulleux S, Ricard M, Benhamou E. Strategies of radioio-

dine ablation in patients with low-risk thyroid cancer. NEJM. 2012;366:1663–73.
7. Klubo-Gwiezdzinska J, Van Nostrand D, Atkins F, Burman K, Jonklaas J, Mete M, Wartofsky L. Efficacy of dosimetric versus empiric prescribed activity of ^{131}I for therapy of differentiated thyroid cancer. Thyroid. 2011;96:3217–25.
8. Ho AL, Grewal RK, Leboeuf R, Sherman EJ, et al. Selumetinib-enhanced radioiodine uptake in advanced thyroid cancer. NEJM. 2013;368:623–32.
9. Randall ES, editor. The Wizard of Menlo Park: how Thomas Alva Edison invented the modern world. New York: Broadway Publishers; 2008.
10. Wagner H. History of the role of nuclear medicine in the thyroid gland and its diseases: a personal perspective. In: Wartofsky L, Van Nostrand D, editors. Thyroid cancer: a comprehensive guide to clinical management. New York: Springer; 2006. Shao Y, Cherry SR, Farahani K. Simultaneous PET and MR imaging. Phys Med Biol. 1997;42:1965–1970.
11. Guy MJ, Castellano-Smith IA, Flower MA, et al. DETECT—dual energy transmission estimation CT—for improved attenuation correction in SPECT and PET. IEEE Trans Nucl Sci. 1998;45: 1261–7.
12. Wong WH, Uribe J, Hicks K, Hu G. An analog decoding GBO block detector using circular photomultipliers. IEEE Trans Nucl Sci. 1997;42:1095–101.
13. Nahmias C, Nutt R, Hichwa RD, et al. PET tomograph designed for five minute routine whole-body studies. J Nucl Med. 2002;43:S36.
14. Ter-Pogossian MM, Mullani NA, Ficke DC, et al. Photon time of flight assisted positron emission tomography. J Comput Assist Tomogr. 1981;5:227–39.
15. Mäcke HR, Muller-Brand J. Receptor-targeted radiopeptide therapy. In: Ell PJ, Gambhir SS, editors. Nuclear medicine in clinical diagnosis and treatment, vol. 1. 3rd ed. New York: Churchill Livingstone; 2004. p. 459–72.
16. Teunissen JJM, Kwekkeboom DJ, Kooij PPM, et al. Peptide receptor radionuclide therapy for non-radioiodine-avid differentiated thyroid carcinoma. J Nucl Med. 2005;46:107S–14.
17. Chang CH, Sharkey RM, Rossi EA, et al. Molecular advances in pre-targeting radioimmunotherapy with bispecific antibodies. Mol Cancer Ther. 2002;1:530–63.
18. Reardon DT, Meares CF, Goodwin DA, et al. Antibodies against metal chelated. Nature. 1985;316:265–8.
19. Khaw BA, Kilbanov A, O'Donnell SM, et al. Gamma imaging with negatively charge-modified monoclonal antibody; modification with synthetic polymers. J Nucl Med. 1991;32:1742–51.
20. Peñuelas I, Boán JF, Martí-Climent MJ, et al. Positron emission tomography and gene therapy: basic concepts and experimental approaches for in vivo gene expression imaging. Mol Imaging Biol. 2004;6:225–38.
21. Anderson CJ, Dehdashti F, Cutler PD, et al. 64 Cu-TETA-octreotide as a PET imaging agent for patients with neuroendocrine tumors. J Nucl Med. 2001;42:213–21.
22. Henze M, Schuhmacher J, Hipp P, et al. PET imaging of somatostatin receptors using 68Ga-DOTA-D-Phel-Tyr3-octreotide: first results in patients with meningiomas. J Nucl Med. 2001;42:1053–6.
23. Zinn KR, Chaudhuri TR. The type 2 human somatostatin receptor as a platform for reporter gene imaging. Eur J Nucl Med. 2002;29:388–99.
24. Chen LB, Zhu RS, Lu HK, et al. Iodide uptake in medullary thyroid carcinoma cells after transfer of human sodium/iodide symporter gene. J Nucl Med. 2004; 5S:337P.
25. Chung JK. Sodium iodide symporter: its role in nuclear medicine. J Nucl Med. 2002;43:1188–200.
26. Pike VW SG. Radiopharmaceuticals for positron emission tomography. In: Cox P, editor. Methodological aspects. Developments in nuclear medicine. Dordrecht: Kluwer Academic Publishers; 1993. p. 24.
27. Pagani M, Stone-Elander S, Larsson SA. Alternative positron emission tomography with non-conventional positron emitters: effects of their physical properties on image quality and potential clinical applications. Eur J Nucl Med. 1997;24:1031–327.
28. Glaser M, Luthra M, Brady F. Applications of positron-emitting halogens in PET oncology (review). Int J Oncol. 2003;22:253–67.
29. Newery GR. Cyclotron-produced isotopes in clinical and experimental medicine. Br J Radiol. 1959;32:633–41.
30. Phillips AF, Haybittle JL, Newbery GR. Use of iodine-124 for the treatment of carcinoma of the thyroid. Acta Union Intern Contra Cancrum. 1960;16:1434–8.
31. Sgouros G, Kolbert KS, Sheikh A, et al. Patient-specific dosimetry for I-131 thyroid cancer therapy using I-124 PET and 3-dimensional internal dosimetry (3D-ID) software. J Nucl Med. 2004;45:1366–72.
32. Humm JL. Dosimetric aspects of radiolabeled antibodies for tumor therapy. J Nucl Med. 1986;27:1490–7.
33. Ackery D. Principles of radionuclide therapy. In: Ell PJ, Gambhir SS, editors. Nuclear medicine in clinical diagnosis and treatment, vol. 1. 3rd ed. New York: Churchill Livingstone; 2004. p. 359–62.
34. Sisson JC, Jamadar DDA, Kazerooni EA, et al. Treatment of micronodular lung metastases of papillary thyroid cancer: are the tumors too small for effective irradiation from radioiodine? Thyroid. 1998;8:215–21.
35. Couturier O, Supiot S, Degraef-Mougin M, et al. Cancer radioimmunotherapy with alpha-emitting nuclides. Eur J Nucl Med Mol Imaging. 2005;32:601–14.
36. Kassis AI, Adelstein SJ. Radiobiologic principles of radionuclide therapy. J Nucl Med. 2005;46:4S–12.
37. Brown I. Astatine-211: its possible applications in cancer therapy. Appl Radiat Isot. 1986;37:789–98.
38. Makrigiorgos GM, Kassis AI, Baranowska-Kortylewicz J, et al. Radiotoxicity of 5-{^{123}I}iodo-2′-deoxyuridine in V79 cells: a comparison with 5-{^{125}I}iodo-2′-deoxyuridine. Radiat Res. 1989;118: 532–44.
39. Grunwald F, Pakos E, Bender H, et al. Redifferentiation therapy with retinoic acid in follicular thyroid cancer. J Nucl Med. 1998;39:1555–8.
40. Schmutzler C. Regulation of the sodium/iodide symporter by retinoids: a review. Exp Clin Endocrinol Diabetes. 2001;109:41–4.
41. Furuya F, Shimura H, Suzuki H, et al. Histone deacetylase inhibitors restore radioiodide uptake and retention in poorly differentiated and anaplastic thyroid cancer cells by expression of the sodium/iodide symporter thyroperoxidase and thyroglobulin. Endocrinology. 2004;145:2865–75.
42. Chen LB, Zhu RS, Lu HK, et al. Iodide uptake in medullary thyroid carcinoma cells after transfer of human sodium/iodide symporter gene. J Nucl Med. 2004;5S:337P.
43. Misaki T, Miyamoto S, Alam MS, et al. Tumoricidal cytokines enhance radioiodine uptake in cultured thyroid cancer cells. J Nucl Med. 1996;37:646–8.
44. Koong SS, Reynolds JC, Movius EG, et al. Lithium as a potential adjuvant to 131-I therapy of metastatic, well differentiated thyroid carcinoma. J Clin Endocrinol Metab. 1999;84:912–6.
45. Zarnegar R, Brunaud L, Kanauchi H, et al. Increasing the effectiveness of radioactive iodine therapy in the treatment of thyroid cancer using Trichostatin A, a histone deacetylase inhibitor. Surgery. 2002;132:984–90.
46. Kvols LK. Radiation sensitizers: a selective review of molecules targeting DNA and non-DNA targets. J Nucl Med. 2005;46: 187S–90190.

^{124}I in Differentiated Thyroid Cancer

103

Douglas Van Nostrand, Robert Hobbs, Frank B. Atkins, and George Sgouros

Introduction

^{124}I was first used in 1960 by Phillips et al. [1] for the treatment of differentiated thyroid carcinoma (DTC). However, because the decay of ^{131}I was more suited for therapy and its production was easier and less expensive than ^{124}I, ^{131}I has remained the most frequently used radioiodine isotope for the treatment of DTC. Likewise, because the decay characteristics of ^{131}I were more suitable for the imaging equipment at that time, ^{131}I became the most frequently used radioiodine isotope for diagnostic imaging of the thyroid. Subsequently, ^{123}I became available in the mid-1960s [2], and in the United States ^{123}I is now the most frequently used radioisotope of iodine for diagnostic imaging in differentiated thyroid carcinoma (DTC).

However, with the increased availability of cyclotrons, a few medical facilities in several countries and several commercial companies in the United States have begun producing ^{124}I, and with the availability of positron emission tomography (PET) scanners, which are the preferred imaging devices, several of these facilities have initiated studies to evaluate ^{124}I for both imaging and dosimetry in DTC.

Initial results suggest significant potential of ^{124}I for imaging and dosimetry, and this chapter reviews the production, decay, radiopharmacokinetics, advantages, disadvantages, lesion detection, dosimetry, and other studies using ^{124}I. The chapter concludes with a discussion of the future utility of ^{124}I imaging in DTC.

Production, Decay, and Radiopharmacokinetics of Radioiodine: The Basics

Isotopes of Iodine

Iodine is the 53rd element in the periodic table, which means that every atom of the element iodine contains 53 protons. However, there are a number of isotopes of iodine, which differ from each other only in the number of neutrons within the nucleus. Although their atomic masses (i.e., sum of the protons and neutrons) are different, biochemically all of these various isotopes of iodine behave identically. In fact, over 35 different isotopes of iodine have been identified, and their physical properties have been well characterized. However, among all of these isotopes, only one isotope of iodine, namely, ^{127}I, is stable. Consequently, this is the only form of iodine that can be found to occur naturally in our environment. All of the other isotopes of iodine undergo a nuclear transformation over some time interval and in the process convert into an isotope of a different element, which in turn may or may not be stable.

The number (mass number) that is associated with the chemical symbol "*I*" represents the number of neutrons in the nucleus of that particular isotope of iodine plus the element number (i.e., 53). Any isotope of iodine with a value less than 127 would therefore have fewer neutrons than the

D. Van Nostrand, MD, FACP, FACNM (✉)
Nuclear Medicine Research, MedStar Research Institute and Washington Hospital Center, Georgetown University School of Medicine, Washington Hospital Center, 110 Irving Street, N.W., Suite GB 60F, Washington, DC 20010, USA
e-mail: douglasvannostrand@gmail.com

R. Hobbs, PhD
Department of Radiation Oncology, Johns Hopkins University, School of Medicine, Baltimore, MD, USA

F.B. Atkins, PhD
Division of Nuclear Medicine, MedStar Washington Hospital Center, Georgetown University School of Medicine, Washington, DC, USA

G. Sgouros, PhD
Department of Radiology and Radiological Science, Johns Hopkins University, School of Medicine, Baltimore, MD, USA

L. Wartofsky, D. Van Nostrand (eds.), *Thyroid Cancer*, DOI 10.1007/978-1-4939-3314-3_103

stable form of iodine. Likewise, higher values would indicate more neutrons.

Half-Life

One way of expressing the instability of any radioactive isotope (radionuclide) is in terms of its physical half-life ($T_{1/2}$). This represents the average time interval required for half of the atoms of that radionuclide present at any instant in time to undergo a nuclear transformation into another element and is independent of the chemical and physical environment containing these radionuclides. More importantly, not only does the number of unstable atoms diminish over time at this rate but so does the *activity*, a quantity defined as the number of nuclear transformations per second. This is typically expressed in units of megabecquerels [MBq] or millicuries [mCi] and is proportional to the number of radioactive atoms present at that instant of time. After an elapsed time equal to $7 \times T_{1/2}$ (the half-life), less than 1 % of the initial activity will remain. The 35 known isotopes of iodine range from the lightest (^{108}I) to the heaviest (^{144}I). In general, the farther away the atomic number is from the value for the stable form of that element, the shorter is its half-life. As a consequence, all of the radioisotopes of iodine lighter than ^{120}I have half-lives <20 min, while those heavier than ^{133}I have half-lives <60 min with ^{135}I being an exception at $T_{1/2}=6.6$ h. There is one radioactive isotope of iodine, namely, ^{129}I, which has a very long half-life (15.7 million years). With a few exceptions, those radioisotopes of iodine lighter than ^{127}I will transform into the preceding element in the periodic table (tellurium) while the heavier radioisotopes of iodine transform into the next higher element (xenon).

Radioactive Decay

In general, the most common mechanisms by which these unstable radionuclides transform (i.e., *decay*) depend on their weight relative to the stable configuration. In the case of radioisotopes of iodine, those isotopes that are lighter than ^{127}I decay by either *electron capture* (ec) or *positron* emission (β^+) and those that are heavier decay by electron (better known as beta) emission (β^-). Positrons (β^+) are special particles that are created during the nuclear transformation by some radionuclides. They have characteristics that are similar to the electrons found in all atoms with one main exception, namely, they carry a positive rather than a negative charge. As such, positrons are not a normal constituent of matter and in fact belong to a group referred to as "antimatter." The ultimate fate of this antiparticle after it is ejected from the nucleus is to slow down as it loses energy until it eventually can combine with its corresponding particle, namely, the electron. At this point in time, the antiparticle-particle combination cannot coexist and the two particles destroy (i.e., *annihilate*) each other with the simultaneous formation of two high-energy photons (511 keV gamma rays) that travel away from the point of annihilation in nearly opposite directions (opposite from the center of mass reference frame). It is this unique feature of all positron emitting radionuclides, including ^{124}I, that is exploited in PET imaging systems – namely, the simultaneous detection (coincidence) of two gamma rays of very specific energy originating from the same location that results in superior imaging capability over conventional gamma camera imaging. However, a discussion of ec, β^+, and $\beta-$ is beyond the scope of this chapter.

Choice of Radioiodine for Imaging, Dosimetry, and Therapy

Due to the preferential uptake of iodide (I^-) into thyroid epithelial cells by the sodium-iodide symporter (NIS), radioisotopes of iodine have played an important role in the diagnosis and treatment of benign and malignant thyroid diseases. The temporal aspects of the uptake and clearance of iodine within normal and metastatic thyroid tissue can be quite variable. Nevertheless, it is a relatively slow process in which the maximum concentration of an orally administered quantity of any of the radioisotopes of iodine may take 24 h or longer to achieve. Likewise, the release of the iodine from these cells occurs gradually over the course of several or more days. As a result of the relatively slow iodine biokinetics, (1) diagnostic imaging is generally more optimal when performed ~24–72 h after administration of the radioiodine, and (2) dosimetry studies to determine patient-specific prescribed activities of ^{131}I for therapeutic purposes typically require measurements to be performed over a minimum of 4 days. Consequently, short-lived (half-life <12 h) radioisotopes of iodine are not practical for the diagnosis and treatment of thyroid disease since very little radioactivity would still be present in the patient after a few days. Of all of the radioisotopes of iodine potentially available, only four meet the above characteristics and have been used as tracers and therapeutic agents in medicine (see Table 103.1). However, depending on its intended purpose, other characteristics of the radioiodine may either be a benefit or a detriment. For diagnostic imaging and dosimetry, a nuclear transformation that results in the production of gamma rays is beneficial because it is this form of radiation that allows localization, quantification, and subsequent kinetic analysis of the distribution of iodine within the patient. Two of these

Table 103.1 Physical decay characteristics of common radioisotopes of iodine used for medical applications

Radionuclide	Half-life	Decay mechanism
^{123}I	13.2 h	ec (100 %)
^{124}I	4.18 days	ec (76 %); β^+ (24 %)
^{125}I	59.4 days	ec (100 %)
^{131}I	8.02 days	β^-

radioiodines, namely, ^{123}I and ^{131}I, have gamma rays that can be imaged using conventional gamma cameras. The gamma rays that result from the annihilation of the positron emitted from ^{124}I also allows ^{124}I to be used for both imaging and dosimetry, but in this case a PET scanner is preferred. However, unless the energy of the gamma ray is sufficiently high enough to allow it to escape from the patient, it would not be useful for in vivo imaging, which is the case for ^{125}I. For therapy purposes, a nuclear transformation resulting in the release of a β particle is beneficial because the β particles may deposit a significant amount of energy, i.e., radiation absorbed dose, in the tissue that "takes up" and stores the radioiodine. This in turn results in a potential therapeutic effect. ^{131}I is typically used for therapies, but ^{124}I has also been considered for this application.

Iodine-124 (^{124}I)

^{124}I is a very promising radioisotope. It has a half-life of 4.18 days, which is sufficiently long enough to allow dosimetry to be performed. This radioisotope is also different from the other longer-lived isotopes of iodine in that it is a positron emitter (β^+), which means that diagnostic imaging can be performed using a PET scanner rather than a gamma camera. As a result there is a significant improvement in the overall quality of these images when compared to those of ^{131}I, as well as a more accurate, quantitative assessment of the uptake and clearance of iodine within both normal and metastatic tissues. The latter can then be used to predict the radiation absorbed dose to individual lesions that would be delivered from a subsequent therapeutic treatment of ^{131}I. Furthermore, most of the PET imaging devices today are hybrid PET/CT systems so that precise anatomical localization of the regions of radioiodine uptake can also be determined.

Unfortunately, some of the characteristics of the decay scheme of ^{124}I (Fig. 103.1) are less than ideal. To begin with, ^{124}I is not a pure β^+ emitter. Only 23.5 % of the decays actually result in positron emission, which means fewer annihilation photons that can be used for imaging. In addition, there is an abundance of high-energy gamma rays, which can potentially interfere with the imaging process. This is especially true for the 603 keV gamma rays that are emitted in cascade with the β^+ positrons. Fortunately, these can be

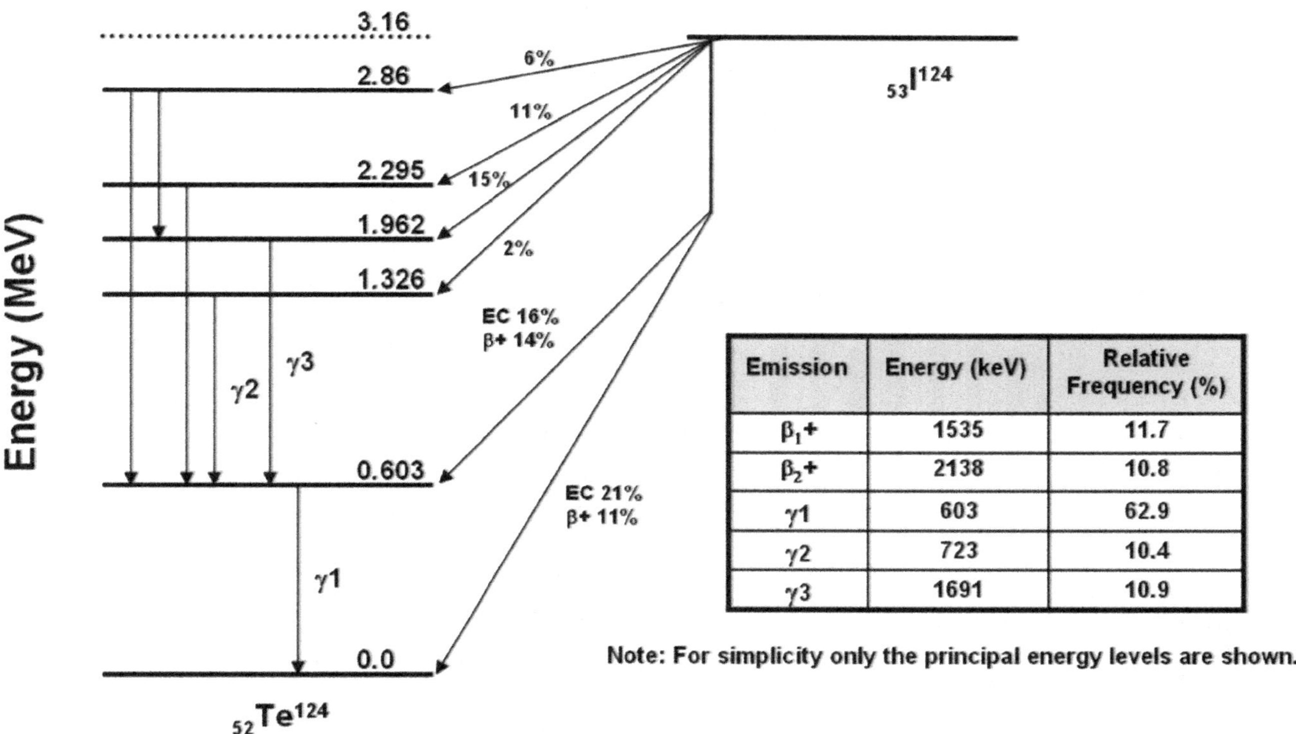

Emission	Energy (keV)	Relative Frequency (%)
β_1+	1535	11.7
β_2+	2138	10.8
γ1	603	62.9
γ2	723	10.4
γ3	1691	10.9

Fig. 103.1 This is a simplified decay scheme for ^{124}I listing the principal pathways for positron emission and electron capture and the nuclear energy levels for ^{124}Te

eliminated to a large extent by energy discrimination from the 511 keV annihilation photons, although a non-negligible fraction of 603 keV photons that have scattered and subsequently lost energy will still be detected in a narrow 511 keV window. Finally, the positrons themselves are ejected with a relatively high energy, which can also result in a degradation of image quality since the annihilation photons used to form the image will originate from a location a short distance away from the actual location of the ^{124}I atom – the higher the β^+ energy, the greater this distance. Despite these limitations, ^{124}I has been shown to produce high-quality, quantitative images using a PET imaging system at an acceptable radiation dose to a patient [3–8]. ^{124}I also has potential for its use as a therapeutic radionuclide, although cost and availability would be issues.

Radiopharmacokinetics

It is generally assumed that ^{124}I and ^{131}I are equivalent biokinetically, and this was confirmed in a study by Atkins et al. [9] who examined the clearance of oral administration in capsular form of both ^{131}I and ^{124}I from the blood compartment in a group of 22 patients with DTC (see Graph 103.1). In this study an effective half-life was determined for each patient based on a mono-exponential regression to both sets of clearance data. The average effective half-life in the blood compartment for the group (excluding the one patient noted) was 14.4 ± 5.0 h for ^{124}I and 13.7 ± 4.5 h for ^{131}I, which were not statistically different.

Production of ^{124}I

Due to the short half-life of ^{124}I, this is not a radionuclide that is found naturally occurring within the environment. Therefore, it must be artificially produced [10–12]. One common way in which a variety of medically useful radionuclides are produced, especially those that decay by positron emission, utilizes a cyclotron, an example of which is shown in Fig. 103.2.

This device is used to accelerate projectiles such as a beam of protons or deuterons (the name given to the bound state of a proton and a neutron) to sufficiently high energies such that they can enter the nucleus of a target atom at which they are directed. Often these collisions cause one or more constituents of the nucleus (i.e., protons and/or neutrons) to be ejected. As a result, the final nucleus could be a different element than that of the target. This process is often expressed using the following format: Target Nucleus (Incident

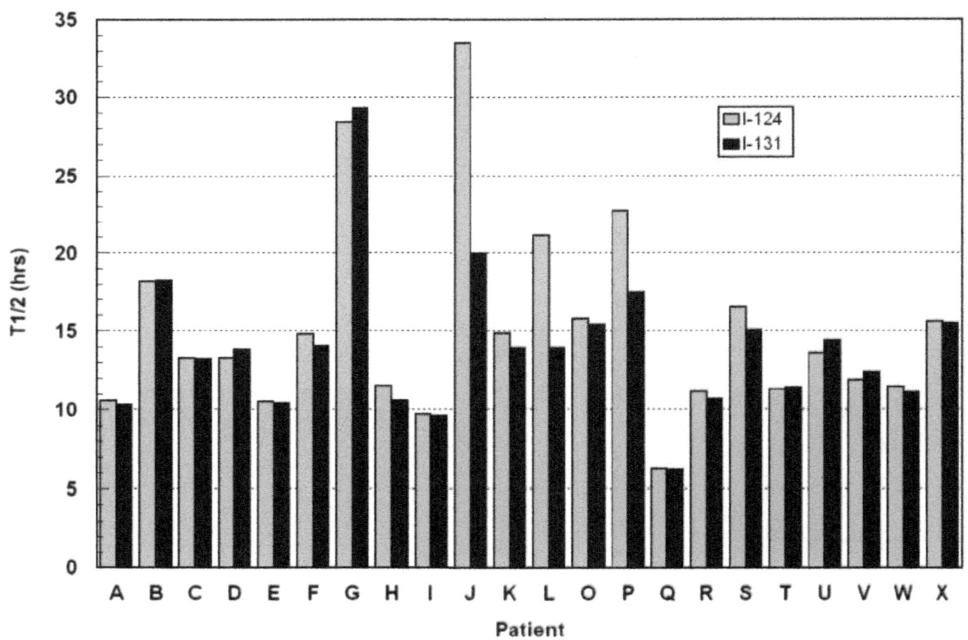

Graph 103.1 Effective half-life of ^{131}I in group of patients (N=22) with metastatic well-differentiated thyroid cancer who were studied using both ^{131}I and ^{124}I. The clearance data for ^{124}I was corrected for the different half-lives of the two radioisotopes of iodine. One patient (J) experienced complications due to his hypothyroid state and required admission to the hospital during the study. This probably accounts for the large discrepancy in this case, and this patient was excluded from the final analysis. Three other patients (not shown) were either for preablation therapy or had extensive metastatic disease which resulted in an increasing or relatively flat clearance due to protein-bound radioiodine, which is not removed by renal excretion and hence could not be represented by a simple effective half-life measurement

Projectile, Ejected particles) Resulting Nucleus. For example, ^{111}In can be produced from the interaction ^{112}Cd (p,2n)^{111}In. In this case, high-energy protons bombard ^{112}Cd and remain in the nucleus while knocking out two neutrons. This results in the production of ^{111}In, the next element in the periodic table. Likewise, ^{124}I is a cyclotron-produced radionuclide. Various methods have been used to produce ^{124}I that employ different target materials, projectiles, and energies, some of which are listed in Table 103.2. The method highlighted in the table, namely, the (p,n) reaction on a $^{124}TeO_2$ target, is the approach used by IBA Molecular in the commercial production of ^{124}I. This method, while not providing the highest yield, does give the best radioiodine purity such that their Na^{124}I capsules contain <0.1 % impurities (unwanted radionuclides) of ^{125}I, ^{126}I, ^{130}I, and ^{131}I and <3 % impurities of ^{123}I. However, unlike iodine, which has only one stable isotope, Te (tellurium) has effectively eight stable isotopes, six of which are truly stable and the other two that have half-lives that are so long (>10^{18} years) that for practical purposes they can be considered as stable. Consequently, Te exists in nature in all of these elemental forms. If ^{130}Te, which is the most abundant isotope of tellurium, were to be bombarded by the same protons in the cyclotron, then ^{130}I could also be produced in the target along with ^{124}I. This would result in an unnecessary radiation dose to the patient. In order to minimize the production of other radioactive impurities, it is then necessary to first process the tellurium such that the amount of ^{124}Te present in the target has been substantially increased from its natural abundance of only 4.75 % to approximately 99.8 %. When used in this *highly enriched* ^{124}Te oxide form, the production of other radioisotopes of iodine can be kept at an acceptable level.

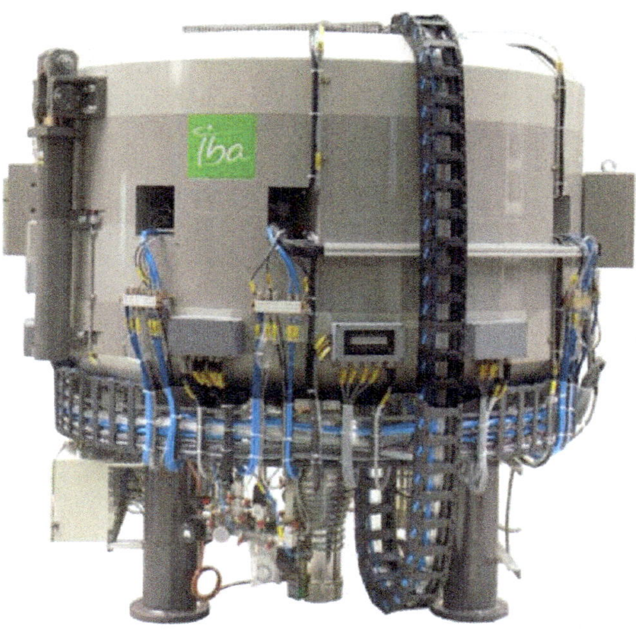

Fig. 103.2 Medical cyclotron *Cyclone 18/9* from IBA (Ion Beam Applications) capable of accelerating protons to 18 MeV in energy. Using a highly enriched (>99.9 %) $^{124}TeO_2$ target, a recovered activity of 50 mCi ^{124}I is possible after a 5 h irradiation (This image has been reproduced with permission from IBA (Ion Beam Applications)

Imaging Technique

When radionuclides, such as ^{123}I and ^{131}I, are imaged using gamma cameras (see Chap. 11), it requires collimators, image uniformity corrections, and window settings that are appropriate to the energy of the gamma ray(s) emitted by the particular radionuclide be used. Although the energy and relative abundance of the positrons that are emitted by β^+ radionuclides might be very different, they have a commonality in terms of the imaging. The photons used to generate these images are always the same, namely, the pair of 511 keV photons that are formed simultaneously by the annihilation of the positron with the electron and then travel in nearly opposite directions. However, the abundance and energy of prompt photons (gamma rays) that might accompany the β^+ decay do indeed depend on the particular isotope. From that standpoint, the decay scheme of ^{124}I includes a number of high-energy photons, unlike ^{18}F. The consequence of these extra photons is that they could in principal increase the number of false coincidences as measured by the detector; however, in practice, choosing a narrower rather than a wider energy range around the 511-keV photopeak decreases these false coincidences to near background level.

Table 103.2 Common methods of cyclotron production of ^{124}I [65]

Nuclear reaction	Effective energy (MeV)	Target material	Enrichment (%)	Yield (MBq/μAh)	Radioiodine impurities (%)
^{124}Te(p,n)^{124}I	13→9	Te	99.51	20	^{123}I(41)
	12.9→0	TeO_2	99.8	13	^{123}I(10.039), ^{125}I(0.018), ^{126}I(0.041), ^{130}I(0.379)
^{125}Te(p,2n)^{124}I	20.1→10.5	TeO_2	93	43.3	^{123}I(8), ^{125}I(5)
^{123}Te(d,n)^{124}I	15→8	Te	91.7	18.9	^{125}I(0.35), ^{126}I(0.39),^{131}I(0.08)

Advantages and Disadvantages

The advantages and disadvantages of ^{124}I are several as listed in Table 103.3. First, ^{124}I decays by positron emission. This, of course, allows ^{124}I to be imaged using a PET scanner resulting in (1) better contrast and spatial resolution, (2) 3D tomographic images, and (3) fusion of the tomographic images with computer tomographic images (CT) and/or magnetic resonance images (MRI). The capability to superimpose or fuse the PET images with the CT or MRI images is very important in helping to determine whether a region concentrating ^{124}I is located within a physiological structure, such as the salivary glands, gastrointestinal tract, and/or residual functioning thyroid tissue remnant or in a structure where iodine is not normally found, the latter suggesting metastatic thyroid cancer. ^{124}I PET imaging also allows superior lesion, organ, and whole-body dosimetry, which will be discussed in more detail later in this chapter. An additional advantage is that ^{124}I is relatively easy to produce in adequate quantities from available small medical cyclotrons, and finally, the radiochemistry of iodine is well established.

However, ^{124}I also has disadvantages (see Table 103.3). Until recently, the availability of ^{124}I was limited to only university-affiliated or research facilities that had a cyclotron and the resources to produce ^{124}I. At the time of the publication of this textbook, IBA Molecular Imaging is commercially manufacturing and distributing ^{124}I from a cyclotron in Richmond, Virginia. Unfortunately, ^{124}I is still not widely available, not approved by the Food and Drug Administration (FDA), expensive, and not approved for reimbursement by third-party payers in the United States. In addition, because the positron emitted from ^{124}I travels a slightly longer distance than a positron emitted from ^{18}F before colliding with an electron, the spatial resolution of ^{124}I is slightly worse than that of ^{18}F.

Table 103.3 Advantages and disadvantages of ^{124}I

Advantages
• Favorable half-life of 4.2 days
• As a result of coincidence PET imaging, improved special and contrast resolution relative to planar imaging
• Additional improved spatial resolution because of "time-of-flight" technology
• Tomographic images instead of planar images
• Fusion of PET tomographic images with CT and MR tomographic images resulting in improved specificity
• Lesion, organ, and whole-body dosimetry
• Easier production from small medical cyclotrons [66], which are becoming more widely available
• Established iodine radiochemistry
Disadvantages
• Availability
• Cost
• Not approved by the Food and Drug Administration
• Not reimbursed by third-party payers
• Slightly lower spatial resolution than ^{18}F

Lesion Detection

^{124}I may be used for superior detection and localization of sites of normal residual and/or functioning metastatic DTC.

Lesion Detection and Comparison with ^{131}I Planar Imaging

An excellent review was published by Freudenberg et al. [5] in 2011, and Freudenberg et al. [3], Phan et al. [6], Capocetti et al. [7], Van Nostrand et al. [8], and Khorjekar et al. [13] have reported the detection of sites of functioning normal residual thyroid tissue and/or metastases from differentiated thyroid cancer (see Graph 103.2). Each of these studies demonstrated overall better detection of functioning areas of normal thyroid tissue and/or metastatic disease secondary to differentiated thyroid cancer using ^{124}I PET and/or PET-CT compared to ^{131}I radioiodine planar scans, and the improved detection of metastases can be dramatic (see Figs. 103.3 and 103.4). Of note, the ^{131}I radioiodine planar scans performed by Freudenberg et al. [3], Phan et al. [6], and Capocetti et al. [7] were post-therapy ^{131}I scans. The reason for the variance in the number of patients with more lesions detected (not

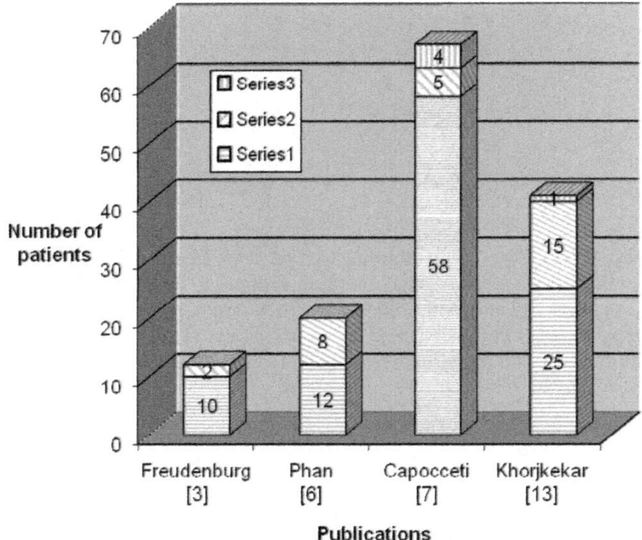

Graph 103.2 The *horizontal line* areas represent patients whose ^{124}I PET images were similar to the ^{131}I planar images. The *diagonal line* areas represents patients whose ^{124}I PET images detected more lesions than the ^{131}I planar images, and the *vertical line* areas represent patients whose ^{131}I planar images detected more lesions than ^{124}I PET images [3, 6, 7, 13]

Fig. 103.3 Both of the above images were obtained in the same patient. The image on the *left* is a pre-therapy posterior planar ^{131}I whole body image demonstrating approximately 18 foci of ^{131}I uptake indicative of metastatic differentiated thyroid cancer. Although modest diffuse liver activity is present, this is not a post-therapy scan and this is not diffuse metastases. The image on the *right* is the posterior ^{124}I PET image from the maximum intensity projection (MIPS) demonstrating multiple additional foci of ^{124}I uptake suggesting metastatic differentiated thyroid cancer that were not detected on the ^{131}I images (This figure was originally published in Van Nostrand et al. [8]. Reproduced with permission from Mary Ann Liebert, Inc. Publishers)

shown) as well as the actual numbers of additional lesions detected most likely represents the different patient populations studied having higher and lower incidences of metastatic disease.

However, despite the improved detection of metastatic foci of DTC by ^{124}I PET scans, a new artifact has already been described. Fatah et al. [14] reported that areas of ^{124}I uptake near the trachea may result in annihilations of the positron occurring in the opposite wall of the trachea resulting in false-positive uptake of ^{124}I in that area. As noted earlier, the PET scanner does not image the positron; instead it forms an image using both of the 511 keV gamma rays that result from the annihilation of the positron with an electron. As a result, the annihilation may actually occur a small distance away from where the positron was actually emitted. In 17 % of the 29 patients that Fatah et al. [14] evaluated with ^{124}I PET/CT, this artifact, a so-called shine-through artifact, was observed with a relative intensity between 0.7 % and 14 % (see Fig. 103.5). Phantom experiments by this group also demonstrated the artifact nicely and showed that the effect decreases sharply as the thickness of the material between the activity and air cavity increases.

Comparison with SPECT-CT

To our knowledge, no data have been published comparing the lesion detection of ^{124}I PET scans to SPECT-CT scans using either ^{123}I or ^{131}I. Such a comparison is certainly warranted and encouraged. However, in addition to evaluating lesion detection, one must also consider cost, potential alteration of management, and if possible the impact on patient outcome. Although one might anticipate that the cost would be less for the ^{123}I or ^{131}I SPECT-CT scans, this may not be the case. A radioiodine SPECT-CT scan for one area of the body may take more time that an ^{124}I PET scan of the entire whole body. In addition, SPECT-CT scans of the entire whole body may be prohibitive from a time standpoint.

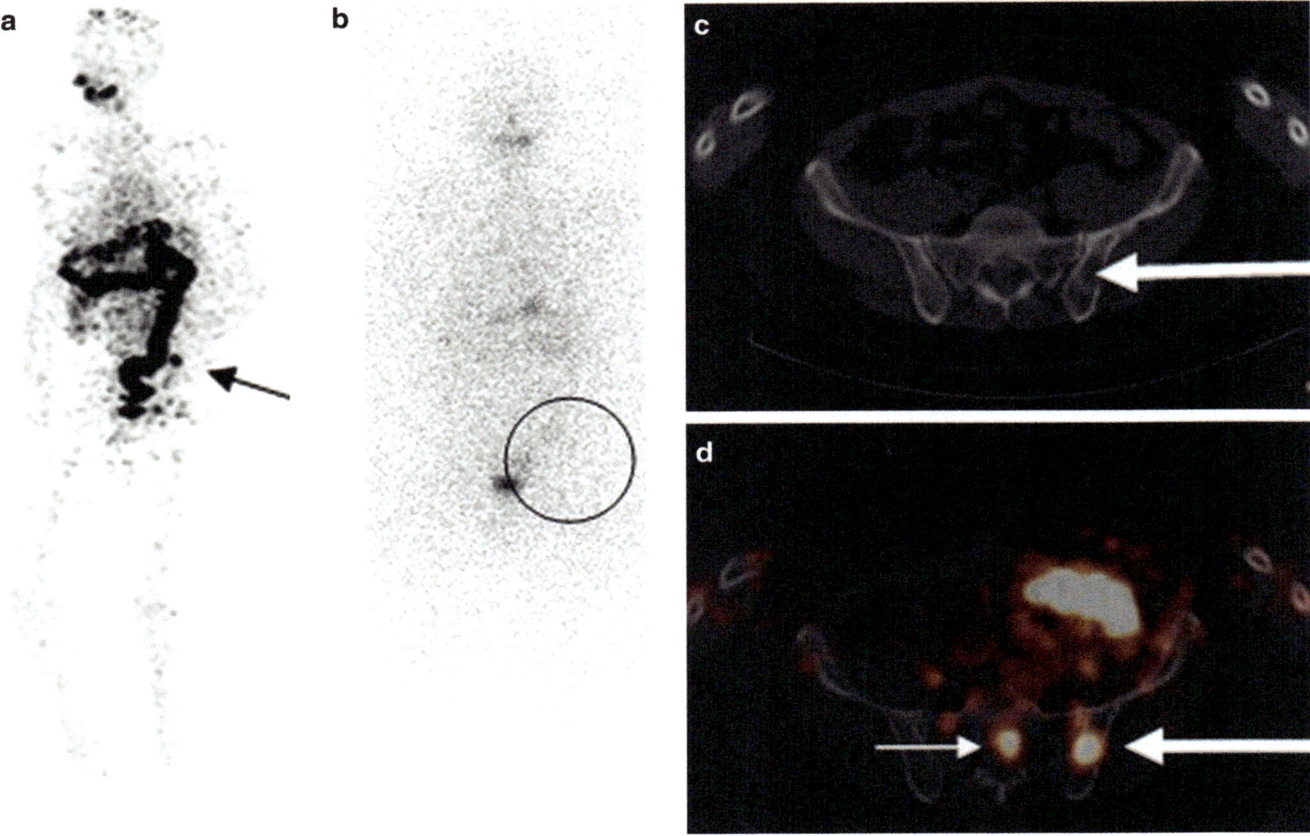

Fig. 103.4 The first image, (**a**), demonstrates a single projection of the ^{124}I PET MIPS image in the left anterior oblique position with an abnormal focus of uptake (*arrow*), and (**b**) demonstrates an anterior ^{131}I image in the same patient, which is completely normal. The posterior image was also normal. No planar LAO image was obtained. In image (**b**), a focus has been *circled* where the abnormality noted on the ^{124}I PET image should have been seen on the ^{131}I image. Image (**c**) is a transverse CT image of the pelvis demonstrating an abnormal lytic finding in the patient's left pelvic bone (*arrow*), which corresponds to the abnormal focus of uptake on the ^{124}I PET image noted in (**a**). Image (**d**) is the fusion of the transverse CT image of the pelvis with the corresponding transverse ^{124}I PET image (*color*), which demonstrates the utility of fusing the ^{124}I PET image with the CT image. The fused images demonstrate that the ^{124}I abnormal uptake (*reddish-yellow-white area*) corresponds precisely to the abnormality on the CT scan (*large white arrow*). In addition to the identification of this abnormality, the ^{124}I images demonstrate a second focus of abnormal ^{124}I uptake, which correlates with another abnormality in the sacrum on the CT image suggesting metastatic disease (*small white arrow*). In this patient, the ^{124}I PET scan identified at least three and possible four foci of radioiodine uptake that were not identified on the ^{131}I images. All these additional foci were suggestive of metastatic thyroid cancer (This figure was originally published in Van Nostrand et al. [8]. Reproduced with permission from Mary Ann Liebert, Inc. Publishers)

Comparison of ^{124}I PET-CT and ^{124}I PET-MR

Nagaraha et al. [15] compared the utility of intrinsically co-registered ^{124}I positron emission tomography (^{124}I PET) and computer tomography (CT) together designated as ^{124}I PET-CT with software co-registered ^{124}I PET and magnetic resonance imaging (MRI) together designated as ^{124}I PET-MR in 33 patients evaluated for thyroid remnant tissue and lymph node metastases in the neck. Patient-based analysis demonstrated that 26 of the 33 (79 %) patients had at least 1 lesion classified as thyroid tissue remnant based on the PET images only, but only 11 (42 %) and 16 (62 %) had any morphological correlation on CT and MRI, respectively. Twelve (36 %) patients had at least 1 lesion classified as lymph node on PET images alone, of which 9 (75 %) had a morphological correlation on both CT and MRI. For lesion-based analysis, ^{124}I PET identified a total of 61 lesions as thyroid remnant tissue, of which 16 (26 %) correlated with morphological findings on CT and 33 (54 %) on MRI, and a total of 29 (27 %) lesions as lymph nodes, of which 18 (62 %) correlated with morphological findings on CT and 24 (83 %) on MRI. A change of diagnosis using the combined ^{124}I PET-CT data occurred in eight patients and with ^{124}I PET-MRI in 10 patients. They concluded that ^{124}I PET-MRI was superior to ^{124}I PET-CT in the neck.

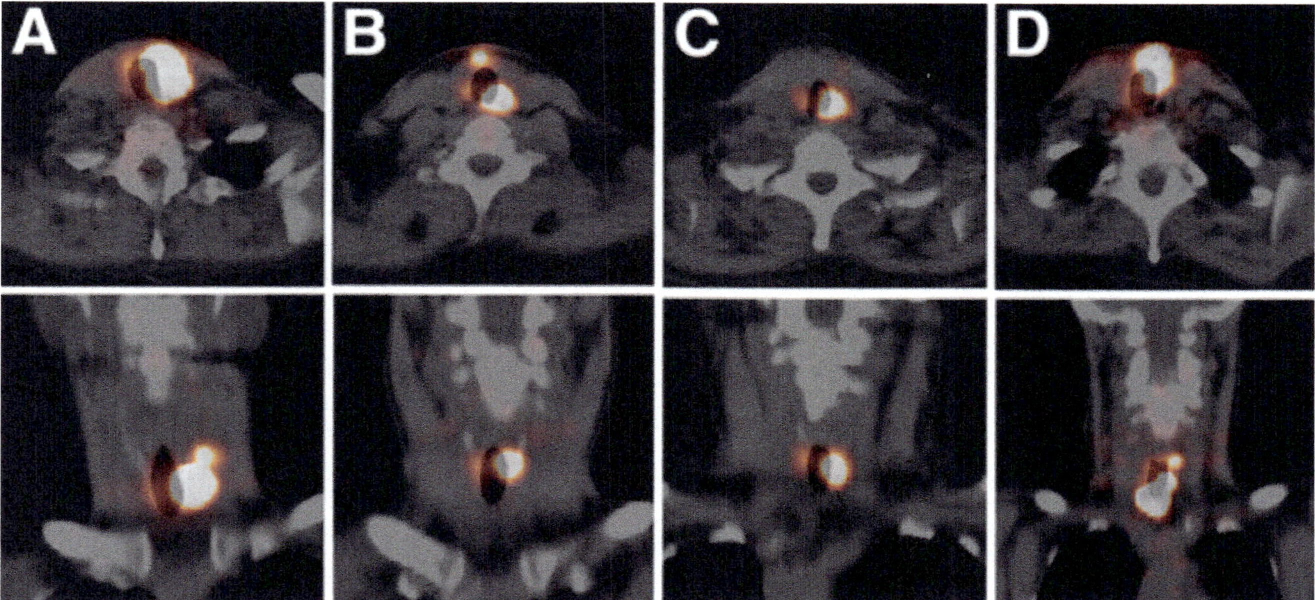

Fig. 103.5 These images from Fatah et al. [14] demonstrate shine-through in four patient studies at 96 h after oral intake of 20–25 MBq of ^{124}I. *Top row* shows transaxial PET/CT images; *bottom row*, coronal images. (**a–d**) represent four different patients with *top* level of viewing windows of 29 %, 4 %, 24 %, and 2 % of image maximum (This figure was originally published in *JNM*. Abdul-Fatah et al. [14]. © by the Society of Nuclear Medicine and Molecular Imaging, Inc.)

The Frequency of Positive ^{131}I Post-Therapy Scans in Patients Who Had a Negative ^{124}I Pre-Therapy Pet Scans and Were Treated with ^{131}I

In patients with a negative pre-therapy radioiodine scan and an elevated serum thyroglobulin level, treatment with ^{131}I is frequently referred to as a "blind treatment," and "blind treatments" are very controversial. One may argue that if one cannot visualize uptake on the pre-therapy scan, there will be no significant therapeutic effect. Alternatively, with decreasing amounts of prescribed activity used for the pre-therapy scan, a negative diagnostic radioiodine scan does not necessarily mean that a metastatic focus is non-radioiodine avid and that a therapeutic radiation absorbed dose cannot be delivered to that metastatic focus. In support of the potential beneficial effect from a "blind treatment," many authors have evaluated the frequency of positive post-therapy ^{131}I scans in this group of patients. Wells et al. [16] reviewed 13 studies that evaluated the frequency of positive ^{131}I post-therapy scans in patients who had negative pre-therapy radioiodine scans. The frequency of positive ^{131}I post-therapy scans ranged from 25 to 94 %, and for the composite results of all these articles, 61 % (200/329) of the patients had a positive ^{131}I post-therapy scan.

With the initial data indicating that ^{124}I PET scans are superior to ^{131}I planar scans, the question is whether or not ^{124}I PET scans could better differentiate which patients would have uptake on the post-therapy ^{131}I scan, thereby providing a potentially better prediction of those patients who may benefit from a "blind treatment." Unfortunately, preliminary data from Freudenberg et al. [17] and Chennupati et al. [18] might suggest otherwise. In six of seven patients with disseminated iodine-avid lung metastases, Freudenberg et al. [17] reported that the ^{131}I post-therapy scan was positive despite the ^{124}I PET scan being negative. However, Freudenberg et al. used a prescribed activity of ^{124}I of only 24 ± 2 MBq (0.65 mCi). In five of seven patients, Chennupati et al. [18] reported that the ^{131}I post-therapy scan was positive despite the ^{124}I PET scan being negative. In this study the prescribed activity of ^{124}I was only 63 MBq (1.7 mCi). An update by Khorjekar et al. [19] reported that in 12 patients with negative diagnostic ^{124}I PET scan, 10 patients had positive post-^{131}I therapy scans. This report suggests that a negative ^{124}I PET scan will not be any better than ^{131}I imaging in determining (1) if metastatic differentiated thyroid cancer foci are radioiodine avid, (2) whether or not a post-therapy scan after an ^{131}I "blind treatment" will be positive, or (3) whether or not a therapy with ^{131}I will alter patient . However, higher prescribed actitivies of ^{124}I may be necessary.

^{124}I PET Lesion Detection to Evaluate Patient Preparation

^{124}I PET scans have already been used to evaluate other issues involving DTC and one example is the evaluation of the effectiveness of patient preparation (e.g., THW versus

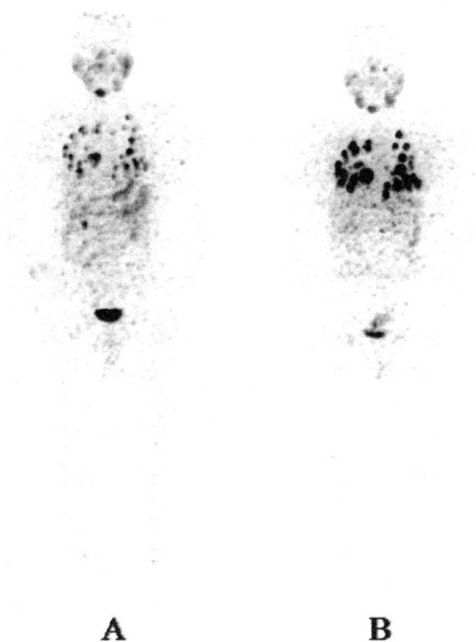

Fig. 103.6 This is a 47-year-old male with metastatic thyroid carcinoma. Image (**a**) is the maximum intensity projection image obtained 48 h after the administration of ~33.3 MBq (0.9 mCi) of ^{124}I after the patient was prepared with two intramuscular injections of 0.9 mg of recombinant human thyroid-stimulating hormone. Image (**b**) is also the anterior maximum intensity projection image obtained 48 h after the administration of ~33.3 MBq (0.9 mCi) of ^{124}I after the patient was prepared with thyroid hormone withdrawal. This image was obtained 1 week after image (**a**). All imaging parameters were the same. More intense foci of ^{124}I are observed in this patient after preparation with thyroid hormone withdrawal. However, further evaluation is warranted (Images reproduced with permission from Keystone Press, Inc)

rhTSH injection) in the detection of metastatic foci in patients in whom metastatic DTC is suspected. Freudenberg et al. [20] using ^{124}I PET-CT scans retrospectively evaluated 63 patients, of whom 27 were prepared using recombinant human thyroid-stimulating hormone (rhTSH) and 36 by thyroid hormone withdrawal (THW). Their data suggested that preparation with rhTSH resulted in a lower radiation absorbed dose to DTC metastases than preparation with THW, but their data was not statistically significant. In 40 patients of whom 24 patients were prepared with rhTSH injections and 16 were prepared with THW, Van Nostrand et al. [21] using ^{124}I PET scans reported data favoring THW relative to rhTSH injection. Two patients had ^{124}I PET imaging performed after preparation with both THW and rhTSH injections. For both of these patients, the THW preparation demonstrated more metastatic lesions (see Fig. 103.6). A full discussion of which method of preparation is superior in the management of patients with metastatic DTC is beyond the scope of this chapter, but rather these studies demonstrate the potential use of ^{124}I PET scans in the evaluation of other controversial aspects of the management of DTC.

Dosimetry

Overview

Dosimetry is essentially the calculation of radiation absorbed dose, which is defined in terms of the energy imparted by radioactive substances divided by the mass of the target tissue and can be used to help determine the likely damage to tissue. More specifically, absorbed dose has been shown to correlate to damage in normal organs [22, 23], which is the main reason that accurate calculation of absorbed dose is fundamentally important in therapeutic nuclear medicine. Used prospectively, dosimetry can enable the optimization of treatment by maximizing the amount of radioactive substance to administer to a patient while still adhering to constraints of toxicity. Used retrospectively, dosimetry can establish tumor dose-response relationships [24–26].

^{124}I-based dosimetry does not differ from dosimetry for any other radiopharmaceutical. That is, the same principles still apply and the different techniques are the same. The two most common methods are (a) the absorbed fraction methodology and (b) three-dimensional personalized dosimetry. A brief review of these two methods follows.

In therapeutic nuclear medicine, in the ubiquitous classic "absorbed fraction" paradigm, the dose to a target region (typically an organ), used to ascertain likely toxicity to that organ, consists of dose contributions from all organs in the body, which take up activity and whose emissions may deposit energy in the target organ. The basic equation that describes this approach is the following [MIRD] (Medical Internal Radiation Dose) (http://www.nndc.bnl.gov/mird/):

$$D_t = \sum_s \frac{A_s \cdot \Delta \cdot \phi_{t \leftarrow s}}{m_t}$$

That is, the absorbed dose in a target region (usually an organ) is equal to the sum of the dose contributions from all source organs in the body, where the major source organ contributor is usually the target organ itself (self-dose contribution). Each contribution is equal to the time-integrated activity (TIA, or number of decays), $\tilde{A}s$, in the source multiplied by the energy per decay, Δ, (isotope dependent) multiplied by the absorbed fraction of emitted energy, ϕ, that originates in the source organ and is deposited in the target organ and divided by the target mass mt. In order to facilitate the application of this formula, a first-order anthropomorphic phantom model was developed by Cristy and Eckerman [27], and a library of results were generated by the MIRD committee which incorporates the mass, absorbed fraction, and energy per decay parameters into a single parameter referred to as the S-factor that simplifies the equation above:

$$D_t = \sum_s \tilde{A}_s \cdot S_{t \leftarrow s}$$

This phantom model allowed the creation of a library of data from which dosimetric calculations could be made simply by knowing the number of decays (TIA) in each organ ($\tilde{A}s$). A software program which exploits this library and is the most common means for estimating dose is OLINDA/EXM [28]. Note that typically for DTC, the therapeutic isotope is ^{131}I; therefore, the S-values, ϕ and Δ, pertain to that isotope.

The number of decays, or time-integrated activity, is determined by integrating the activity in an organ over time, as the name implies. Practically, this is realized by (a) imaging, (b) quantifying the activity in a particular region (organ) at several time points, (c) adjusting the activity to account for the half-life difference between ^{124}I and ^{131}I, (d) graphing the activity as a function of time, and (e) integrating the activity by computing the area under the curve fit to an a priori function (or the area under the curve formed by linearly connecting the different points followed by an exponentially decaying tail). That several time points are necessary follows from the fact that the activity is redistributing between organs over time as it decays. This redistribution occurs predominantly at earlier time points, although these can still be on the order of days as is the case for radioiodine. Clearly, more time points will provide a more accurate fit for the integration; however, the time and cost of imaging limit the number of sessions. The typical range for radioiodine dosimetry is three to five images, but a method exists that uses only two time points, which is relatively reliable [29].

Just as clearly, accurate quantification of the activity is essential for reliable dosimetry. From this standpoint, the advantage of ^{124}I PET imaging over ^{131}I planar or even SPECT imaging is unequivocal. As a rule of thumb, the relative merits of the imaging modalities vis-à-vis detection discussed in the previous section translate to an even greater degree for quantification. In particular, the issues with quantitation derived from planar imaging have been discussed at length [30, 31], and no matter the various scatter and attenuation corrections, two-dimensional dosimetry is approximate at best and subject to large errors. Consequently, results published using absorbed dose values derived from two-dimensional dosimetry have arguably done more harm than good in establishing confidence in dosimetry-based treatment planning.

Once the TIAs for the different organs have been established, it becomes a simple matter of converting the TIAs to absorbed dose either by using the OLINDA/EXM software or by applying the S-values directly. The advantage of such a method is its ease of use; the disadvantages lie in that the phantoms used for deriving the S-values may differ significantly in anatomy from the individual patients. Moreover, the S-values only exist for normal organs, not tumors. A spherical tumor model does exist within OLINDA/EXM, but it does not allow for tumor heterogeneity of shape or uptake and only calculates dose from the activity within the tumor, neglecting the contribution from activity in the surrounding tissues. As our understanding of dosimetry evolves, the disadvantage of the lack of versatility in the tumor model becomes increasingly clear; it is becoming more apparent that tumor response to dose depends on a variety of different factors and parameters, including dose rate and heterogeneity of dose, which are not accounted for in an absorbed fraction method which only provides the mean absorbed dose.

The alternative to the absorbed fraction method is personalized three-dimensional dosimetry, either using Monte Carlo simulations directly or via point kernel methods. These simulate the decay of activity in the patient's body using the patient's own CT and emission (PET or SPECT) images by tracking each decaying particle according to the probabilities that it will interact in a variety of different possible ways with the matter it is traversing. The Monte Carlo programs are so named because they figuratively "roll the dice" to determine the direction, energy deposition, and secondary particle creation that each decaying radionuclide will take. While this method is not accurate for individual particles, given a statistically large number of events as is the case for the number of decaying radionuclides in therapeutic nuclear medicine, the macroscopic results are accurate to within a few percentage points. Several points are worthy of note regarding these computer models: (1) while the number of events simulated is generally fairly large (one to ten million is a typical range), it is still small compared to the number of decaying particles in a patient (up to 10^{12}–10^{15} for a whole-body radioiodine treatment) and (2) such simulations are the basis for establishing the S-values used in the absorbed fraction methodology.

The energy deposited by the various decaying particles is collected in a three-dimensional matrix of voxels (volume elements) in which the patient has been segmented using the CT images and then converted to radiation dose on a voxel as well as an organ level. Several such personalized dosimetry codes exist including 3D-ID [32], 3D-RD [33], RMDP [34], Oedipe [35], FLUKA [36], and VoxelDose [37], among others. The advantages of Monte Carlo are obvious: a greater personal accuracy and the ability to incorporate tumor dosimetry and heterogeneities at the voxel level into the calculations as well as display result in a more elaborate manner such as with dose-volume histograms, for example. One disadvantage lies in the time necessary to perform the Monte Carlo analysis, on the order of hours for each simulation depending on the computer hardware.

3D-ID

3D-ID (3D internal dosimetry), the earliest 3D imaging-based targeted radionuclide dosimetry package described in the literature, was heavily influenced by treatment planning techniques developed for external radiotherapy treatment planning [32]. It has been used to examine the impact of different radionuclides on the dose distribution, given a fixed cumulated activity distribution. In particular, 3D-ID has been used in thyroid cancer patients using ^{124}I PET imaging data along with CT images for radioiodine tumor dosimetry [38]; this study demonstrated use of sequential PET image studies that were co-registered across time and integrated, voxel-by-voxel, to provide a 3-D cumulated activity image used in the tumor dosimetry calculation. The same data set and general approach were also used to perform normal organ dosimetry [39]. A next-generation version of 3D-ID, named 3D-RD, has been developed that incorporates radiobiological modeling, i.e., not just simply the radiation dose or energy deposition but also the response of the tissue to this insult.

Radiobiological Modeling

Radiobiological modeling was introduced into the 3D-ID (which subsequently became known as 3D-RD) analysis by incorporating models derived from the linear-quadratic model of cell response to radiation. Specifically, the surviving fraction of cells (SF) measured in vitro in response to varying quantities of single fractions of external radiation, D, is given by the equation:

$$\mathrm{SF} = e^{-\alpha D - \beta D^2}$$

where α and β are the linear and quadratic radiobiological coefficients, respectively. The biological effective dose (BED) is the equivalent absorbed dose delivered at a low dose rate; [40] this concept is given mathematically by

$$\alpha \mathrm{BED} = \alpha D + \beta D^2$$

Thus for low dose rates, the BED and the absorbed dose are similar, while for higher dose rates, the BED grows much larger than the absorbed dose. That this is a relevant biological quantity has been justified by the BED-response correlations established for normal organs [19, 20]. Note that according to the linear-quadratic model, cell death is associated with double-strand DNA breaking. The quadratic term relates to a double-strand break brought about by two different events separated in time as opposed to the single-event double-strand break represented by the linear term. Therefore, a repair mechanism was modeled into the BED formulation, the so-called Lea-Catcheside factor G [41], such that the equation for the BED becomes

$$\mathrm{BED} = D(1 + \frac{G(\infty)}{\alpha / \beta} \cdot D)$$

The equivalent uniform dose (EUD) is an attempt to give a representative single dose value for a heterogeneous region or organ. This concept is also based on the linear-quadratic response and is formulated thusly

$$e^{-\alpha EUD} = \frac{1}{N} \sum_{N}^{i=1} e^{-\alpha D_i - \beta D_i^2}$$

That is, the EUD is the single BED value which every voxel in a region would have in order to have the same surviving fraction of cells as the measured heterogeneous dose distribution [42]:

$$EUD = -\frac{1}{\alpha} \ln \left(\sum_{N}^{i=1} \frac{e^{-\alpha BED_i}}{N} \right)$$

To implement these models, absorbed dose rate images are calculated for each time point rather than the integrated absorbed dose from a cumulated activity map.

Assuming an exponential repair process, a BED value can be generated for each voxel, either by using a formula derived for a specific exponential functional fit [43, 44] or numerically using an algorithm [45]; subsequently, an EUD value for a particular user-defined volume can also be calculated [33].

Real-Time 3D-RD Calculation and Comparison with Conventional Dosimetry

As an example, 3D-RD was used prospectively for the planning of an ^{131}I therapy for an 11-year-old girl, who presented post-thyroidectomy with metastatic papillary carcinoma based on ^{124}I imaging [46]. In this case ^{124}I was chosen since a diagnostic quantity of ^{131}I had been administered at a different institution a week prior, of which the patient still retained a significant quantity. As previously discussed, PET utilizes coincidence photons from the positron-electron annihilation event, which are essentially unaffected by the additional emissions from ^{131}I. More precisely, the false coincidence rate from single scattered photons from the 637-keV gamma emission that occurs in about 7 % of the ^{131}I decays combining with one of the two 511-keV photons from ^{124}I decay was assumed to be negligible. The patient presented with radioiodine-avid bilateral temporal lobe lesions along with diffuse lung metastases and a serum thyroglobulin concentration of 9,553 ng/ml. Pulmonary function tests indicated both obstructive and restrictive lung defects. The real-time aspect of the 3D-RD calculations took advantage of the 3D-RD software package design that allows dose calculations to start without the need for the complete temporal data set. This was accomplished by calculating the dose rate obtained from each scan at each time point and then integrating these over time after the last scan had been collected and processed. In this way, the time-intensive Monte Carlo calculations were performed during the interval between image acquisitions and the more rapid integration over time was performed on the dose rate images. The disease-laden lungs were dose limiting in this case and treatment planning was designed to identify the administered activity that would deliver no more than 27 Gy to the entire lungs (including tumor). The administered activity corresponding to this limit was 5.11 GBq.

Recognizing that most voxels are likely a combination of tumor and normal lung tissue due to the disseminated nature of the metastases, an effort was made to identify "tumor" vs "normal lung" voxels. Segmentation based on activity uptake at 24 h was applied; voxels with activity >30 mBq/voxel were considered tumor, the rest normal lung tissue. Discrimination by density, determined by converting CT values as used in a previous 3D-RD calculation, and clearance rate did not provide as good and consistent a tumor delineation although there was a great degree of overlap between all the approaches considered.

The voxel-averaged BED to lung voxels identified as tumor was 43.2 Gy. Accounting for the spatial non-uniformity of the absorbed dose to tumor gave an EUD of 23 Gy. The BED values for the brain lesions were 1,220 and 142 Gy; the corresponding EUD values were 89.1 and 55.9 Gy. The administered activity determined using OLINDA/EXM to deliver 27 Gy to the lungs was 3.14 GBq. Retrospective analyses revealed that the difference was due to the assumption of disease-free lungs and a reference lung mass in the OLINDA/EXM calculation. No lung mass assumption was needed in the 3D-RD calculation because the density as obtained from CT is applied to the calculation which inherently accounts for target voxel mass. When the reference lung mass used in the OLINDA/EXM calculation was adjusted for the patient's total lung mass (as determined from the CT image using 3D-RD), an administered activity of 5.17 GBq was obtained.

The patient experienced no pulmonary, neurological, or other adverse clinical response to ^{131}I treatment. At 12 and 24 months of follow-up, the patient's serum thyroglobulin after comparable thyroid hormone withdrawal had declined from its pretreatment level of 9,553 ng/ml to 777 and 130 ng/ml, respectively. The patient's metastatic lesions in the left and right lobes of the brain, which initially measured 24 and 9 mm, respectively, were both undetectable on cranial MRI at 26 months after initial radioiodine therapy.

This example highlights the importance of accurate dosimetry to avoid over- or underdosing patients. The move to greater accessibility to personalized three-dimensional dosimetry falls in line with one of the stated "pillars" of the NIH mission. In this case, the ability to move to a diagnostic imaging agent with a different, more specific, imaging modality was critical to the quick implementation of the diagnostic dosing. Waiting for the previously administered diagnostic ^{131}I to clear would have delayed treatment or necessitated a more ad hoc determination of therapeutic administered activity.

More recently, Khorjekar et al. [47] used ^{124}I and the 3DRD software discussed above to calculate the radiation absorbed dose to metastatic foci and compared the change in size of pulmonary metastases on computer tomography to the calculated radiation dose delivered in 15 pulmonary lesions in 3 patients. The calculated EUD in Gy correlated with the clinical response. Based on a logistic regression model, an EUD score of >8 predicted a combined outcome of stable disease, partial response, and clinical response versus progression. The preliminary data suggest that the calculated EUD has potential for helping to determine which lesions may respond to various amounts of prescribed activity of ^{131}I.

Utility of Organ Dosimetry: Salivary Gland Toxicity

Radiopharmaceutical therapy using ^{131}I is the treatment of choice for differentiated thyroid carcinoma of papillary and follicular origin because the ^{131}I naturally targets the thyroid tumors and thyroid remnants through the sodium-iodine symporter mechanism. However, radioiodine can also concentrate in the parotid and submandibular salivary glands, although not to any noticeable extent in the sublingual salivary glands [48]. Radioiodine activity dependent damage to the salivary parenchyma as a result of ^{131}I radiation has been reported, consequently resulting in, *inter alia*, sialadenitis and xerostomia. These conditions in turn can induce dysphagia, infectious diseases of the oral and pharyngeal mucosa, and dental and periodontal diseases. Radiation-induced salivary gland toxicity is a serious issue that affects the patients' health-related quality of life significantly [49, 50].

Normal organ toxicity from radiopharmaceutical therapy has been traditionally correlated with absorbed dose, most often in the form of a maximum tolerated dose. However, to date, no correlation between any dosimetric quantity and clinically observed toxicity has been established for the salivary gland toxicity resulting from ^{131}I therapy for thyroid cancer [51]. In particular, a study using ^{131}I, gamma camera imaging, and volume estimations primarily from ultrasound imaging resulted in absorbed dose values five to ten times too low to satisfactorily explain the observed glandular radiation damages in radioiodine therapy [52]. The dosimetry in this case was based on standard MIRD methodology of absorbed fractions and, therefore, assumed homogenous distribution of activity in the salivary glands.

An ^{124}I PET-based salivary gland dosimetry study was undertaken with the goal of reconciling dosimetry and observed clinical toxicities; however, that study also calculated low absorbed dose results comparable to those from the previous study, and the discrepancy between absorbed and observed toxicity remained unresolved [53]. In a further study, the salivary gland dosimetry was performed using 3D-RD on a similar patient data set using ^{124}I with the idea that (a) the BED may correlate better with toxicity, (b) external factors such as thyroid remnants and lymph node metastases with high uptake proximal to the salivary glands may have a significant contribution to the absorbed dose of the salivary glands, or (c) voxelized results may lead to improved identification of the local distribution of the absorbed dose [54]. The results to date have shown that regions of high uptake external to the salivary gland can increase the total absorbed dose by a factor of two; however the contribution from this effect and the dose rate effect modeled by the BED are insufficient to explain the observed clinical toxicities. This suggests that the third proposed possibility, a more accurate voxelized analysis may be necessary; this corresponds to a localization of the activity within the gland itself, thus resulting in regions of higher uptake and dose, so-called hot spots. Previously published results have established that iodine is concentrated into the epithelium of the salivary glands' intralobular ducts before being released into the saliva, which provide the anatomical reference for the region of higher uptake [55, 56]. However, there are technical difficulties associated with voxelized quantification of salivary gland uptake, which must be taken into account. One is common to all small volumes, including small tumors and the salivary glands as a whole: the partial volume effect (PVE), also known as the "spill-out" effect, which is essentially the accuracy at which the activity can be localized in a volume. For all volumes containing activity, a certain quantity of activity at the edge of the volume will be measured outside of the volume. As the size of the VOIs decrease, the ratio of surface to volume decreases resulting in a proportionately larger amount of activity, which is mislocated. This effect has been quantified for volumes the size of salivary glands by Jentzen et al. [57, 58] and Teo et al. [59]; however, these adjustments (known as recovery coefficients) assume a homogenous distribution of activity, which enables accurate whole gland (or tumor) dosimetry, but defeats the objective of accurate voxelized dosimetry.

A second issue more specific to the salivary glands, and another controversial one, is the effect of sialogogues, including the use of lemon candies, on the uptake and retention of activity in the salivary glands. Nakada et al. [60] and Jentzen et al. [61] have claimed that the use of lemon juice increases absorbed dose to the salivary glands due to the increased salivary flow, while Van Nostrand et al. [62] demonstrated that if sialogogues are given as frequently as 20–40 min rather than every 2–3 h as evaluated by Nakada et al., the radiation absorbed dose to the salivary glands may potentially be significantly reduced. Two possible reasons for these different results may have to do with the frequency of administration of sialogogues and the measurements of radioactivity in the salivary glands at periodic intervals of hours vs minutes. What is known is that there is a great deal of uncertainty in the absorbed dose and activity uptake measurements due to the rapid and extreme fluctuations in the quantity of radioiodine in the salivary glands from salivation and uptake. From this standpoint the approach by van Nostrand et al. [60] which monitors the activity on a much shorter time scale (minute-by-minute) appears to be more reliable and may prove to be necessary for dosimetry as well.

Therapy

^{124}I as an alternative to ^{131}I for therapy of DTC was first proposed in 1954 by Philips et al. [63]. They argued that the uptake of iodine in sites of thyroid cancer is nonuniform with reduced uptake of radioiodine in areas as large as 1–5 mm. The β particles from ^{131}I have a maximum range of only about 2 mm with about half of them traveling only about 0.2 mm. By comparison, the β particles from ^{124}I are not only more energetic and therefore more penetrating, but the decay is also accompanied by a greater abundance of x-rays and higher energy γ-rays (see Fig. 103.1). Furthermore, ^{124}I has a reasonable physical half-life, namely, 4.18 days (see Table 103.1), and all of these factors may result in ^{124}I being a superior radioisotope for therapy in selected situations. In 1960, Phillips et al. [1] reported the first patient treated with ^{124}I, and they reported a partial response. Goolden et al. [64] treated three patients with thyroid cancer with ^{124}I to ablate residual thyroid tissue remaining after a hemithyroidectomy. The prescribed activities were 1.11 GBq (30 mCi) for the first two patients and 0.72 GBq (19.5) mCi for the third patient. Successful ablation was achieved in the first two patients. However, it was most likely that ^{124}I as a therapeutic radioisotope of iodine for the therapy of DTC did not become routine because of availability, cost, and little initial data to support a significant advantage over ^{131}I. Although it may be time to reconsider ^{124}I as a therapeutic radioisotope of iodine, perhaps even as a "cocktail" along with ^{131}I, for DTC, the three original limitations remain – availability, cost, and a lack of documentation of a significant advantage over ^{131}I.

Future

For differentiated thyroid cancer, ^{124}I holds significant promise for lesion detection as well as lesion, organ, and whole-body dosimetry, and ^{124}I PET-CT may one day be available for routine clinical imaging and dosimetry. However, it is difficult to predict when that will occur in the United States and whether or not ^{124}I PET will completely replace ^{131}I and/or ^{123}I for either imaging or dosimetry for one major reason. To our knowledge, ^{124}I cannot be patented, which is a major obstacle for funding the clinical studies and other regulatory requirements needed to obtain approval by the Food and Drug Administration (FDA) in the United States. Thus, there is little incentive for any company to invest the time, money, and resources to develop and submit a new drug application (NDA) to the FDA when upon that NDA's approval any company would be able to market ^{124}I without having shared in any of the development costs.

Although cost and availability are two disadvantages of ^{124}I as noted above, one author (dvn) believes that once ^{124}I is approved by the FDA, third-party payers will begin to reimburse for ^{124}I PET-CT scan in selected patients, and then as volumes increase, availability will increase, and the cost will decrease.

Summary

In summary, ^{124}I is a promising isotope of radioiodine that will improve the diagnostic imaging of differentiated thyroid cancer by allowing PET-CT imaging, which in turn will improve resolution, offer tomographic images, and permit fusing of the PET images with CT and/or MR images. In addition, ^{124}I will help determine more accurately and reproducibly estimates of radiation absorbed doses to thyroid cancer cells and other organs of the body for ^{131}I treatments.

Acknowledgments Studies evaluating ^{124}I performed at MedStar Washington Hospital Center were supported by grants from the Latham Fund, Genzyme Corporation, IBA Corporation, and grateful patients.

References

1. Phillips A, Haybittle J, Newbery G. Use of ^{124}I for the treatment of carcinoma of the thyroid. Acta Unio Int Contra Cancrum. 1960;16:1434–8.
2. Rhodes B, Wagner H, Gerald M. Iodine-123: development and usefulness of a new radiopharmaceutical. Isot Radiat Technol. 1967;4:275–80.
3. Freudenberg LS, Antoch G, Jentzen W, et al. Value of ^{124}I-PET/CT in staging of patients with differentiated thyroid cancer. Eur Radiol. 2004;14:2092–8.
4. Rault E, Vandenberghe S, Holen R, Beenhouwer J, Staelens S, Lemahieu I. Comparison of image quality of different iodine isotopes (^{123}I, ^{124}I, and ^{131}I). Cancer Biother Radiopharm. 2007;22:423–30.
5. Freudenberg L, Jentzen W, Sahl A, Bockishc A, Rosenbaum-Krumme S. Clinical applications of ^{124}I PET-CT in patients with differentiated thyroid cancer. Eur J Nucl Med Mol Imaging. 2011;38(Suppl):S48–56.
6. Phan H, Jager P, Paans A, et al. The diagnostic value of ^{124}I-PET in patients with differentiated thyroid cancer. Eur J Nucl Med Mol Imaging. 2008;35:958–65.
7. Capoccetti F, Criscuoli B, Rossi G, Rerretti F, Manni C, Brianzoni E. The effectiveness of ^{124}I PET/CT in patients with differentiated thyroid cancer. Q J Nucl Med Mol Imaging. 2009;53:536–45.
8. Van Nostrand D, Moreau S, Bandaru V, Atkins A, Chennupati S, Mete M, Burman K, Wartofsky L. ^{124}I positron emission tomography versus ^{131}I planar imaging in the identification of residual thyroid tissue and/or metastasis in patients who have well-differentiated thyroid cancer. Thyroid. 2010;20:879–83.
9. Atkins F, Van Nostrand D, Moreau S, et al. Comparison of the blood biokinetics of ^{124}I and ^{131}I in patients with well-differentiated thyroid cancer (WDTC). J Nucl Med. 2008;49(Suppl):323.
10. Lambrecht R, Sajjad M, Qureshi M, Al-Yanbawi S. Production of iodine-124. J Radioanal Nucl Chem Lett. 1988;127:143–50.
11. Sharma H, Zweit J, Downey S, et al. Production of ^{124}I for positron emission tomography. J Label Compd Rad. 1988;26:165–7.
12. Firouzbakht M, Schlyer D, Finn R, et al. Iodine-124 production: excitation functions for the ^{124}Te(d,2n)^{124}I and ^{124}Te(d,3n)^{123}I reactions from 7 to 24 MeV. Nucl Instrum Methods B. 1993;79:909–10.
13. Khorjekar G, Van Nostrand D, Kharazi P, Moreau S, Atkins F, Chennupati S, Mete M, Burman K, Wartofsky L. ^{124}I versus ^{131}I in the identification of functioning residual thyroid tissue and/or metastases in patients with differentiated thyroid cancer: update of initial report. J Nucl Med. 2011;52(Suppl):1295.
14. Abdul-Fatah S, Zamburlini M, Halders S, Brans B, Teule G, Kemerink G. Identification of a shine-through artifact in the trachea with ^{124}I PET/CT. J Nucl Med. 2009;50:909–11.
15. Nagarajah J, Jentzen W, Hartung V, Rosenbaum-Krumme S, Mikat C, Heusner Till A, Antoch G, Bockisch A, Stahl A. Diagnosis and dosimetry in differentiated thyroid carcinoma using ^{124}I PET: comparison of PET/MRI vs PET/CT of the neck. Eur J Nucl Med Mol Imaging. 2011;38:1862–8.
16. Wells K, Moreau S, Shin YR, Van Nostrand D, Burman K, Wartofsky L. Positive (+) post-treatment (tx) scans after the radioiodine (RAI) tx of patients who have well-differentiated thyroid cancer (WDTC), positive serum thyroglobulin levels (TG+), and negative diagnostic (dx) RAI whole body scans (WBS-): predictive values and frequency. J Nucl Med. 2008;49(Suppl):238P.
17. Freudenberg L, Jentzen W, Muller S, Bockisch. Disseminated iodine-avid lung metastases in differentiated thyroid cancer: a challenge to ^{124}I PET. Eur J Nucl Med Mol Imaging. 2008;33:502–8.
18. Chennupati S, Bandaru VV, Prasad K, Van Nostrand D. Do negative diagnostic ^{131}I and ^{124}I scans exclude ^{131}I as a treatment option in patients with positive thyroglobulin levels? J Nucl Med. 2009;50(Suppl):343P.
19. Khorjekar GR, Van Nostrand D, Garcia C, O'Neil J, Moreau S, Atkins FB, Mete M, Orquiza MH, Burman K, Wartofsky L. Do Negative ^{124}I Pre-therapy Positron Emission Tomography Scans in Patients with Elevated Serum Thyroglobulin Levels Predict Negative ^{131}I Post-therapy Scans? Thyroid. 2014;24:1394–99.
20. Freudenberg LS, Jentzen W, Petrich T, et al. Lesion dose in differentiated thyroid carcinoma metastases after rhTSH or thyroid hormone withdrawal: ^{124}I PET/CT dosimetric comparisons. Eur J Nucl Med Mol Imaging. 2010;37:2264–76.
21. Van Nostrand D, Khorjekar G, O'Neil J, Moreau S, Atkins F, Kharazi P, Mete M, Chennupati S, Burman K, Wartofsky L. Recombinant human thyroid stimulating hormone versus thyroid hormone withdrawal in the identification of metastasis in differentiated thyroid cancer with ^{131}I planar whole body and ^{124}I PET. J Nucl Med. 2012;53:359–62.
22. Barone R, Borson-Chazot F, Valkema R, Walrand S, Chauvin F, Gogou L, et al. Patient-specific dosimetry in predicting renal toxicity with ^{90}Y-DOTATOC: relevance of kidney volume and dose rate

in finding a dose-effect relationship. J Nucl Med. 2005;46 Suppl 1:99S–106.
23. Wessels BW, Konijnenberg MW, Dale RG, Breitz HB, Cremonesi M, Meredith RF, et al. MIRD pamphlet No. 20: the effect of model assumptions on kidney dosimetry and response--implications for radionuclide therapy. J Nucl Med. 2008;49:1884–99.
24. Dewaraja Y, Schipper M, Roberson P, Wilderman S, Amro H, Regan D, Koral K, Kaminski M, Avram A. ^{131}I-tositumomab radioimmunotherapy: initial tumor dose-response results using 3-dimensional dosimetry including radiobiologic modeling. J Nucl Med. 2010;51:1155–62.
25. Senthamizhchelvan S, Hobbs RF, Song H, Frey EC, Zhang Z, Armour E, Wahl RL, Loeb DM, Sgouros G. Tumor dosimetry and response for ^{153}Sm-EDTMP therapy of high-risk osteosarcoma. J Nucl Med. 2012;53:215–24.
26. Maxon HR, Thomas SR, Hertzberg VS, et al. Relation between effective radiation dose and outcome of radioiodine therapy for thyroid cancer. N Engl J Med. 1983;309:937–41.
27. Cristy M, Eckerman K. Specific absorbed fractions of energy at various ages from internal photon sources. 1987 Oak Ridge National Laboratory Report ORNL/TM-8381 V1-7.
28. Stabin M, Sparks R, Crowe E. OLINDA/EXM: the second-generation personal computer software for internal dose assessment in nuclear medicine. J Nucl Med. 2005;46:1023–7.
29. Jentzen W, Freudenberg L, Eising EG, Sonnenschein W, Knust J, Bockisch A. Optimized ^{124}I PET dosimetry protocol for radioiodine therapy of differentiated thyroid cancer. J Nucl Med. 2008;49:1017–23.
30. Flux G, Bardies M, Monsieurs M, Savolainen S, Strands SE, Lassmann M. The impact of PET and SPECT on dosimetry for targeted radionuclide therapy. Z Med Phys. 2006;16:47–59.
31. He B, Frey E. Comparison of conventional, model-based quantitative planar, and quantitative SPECT image processing methods for organ activity estimation using In-111 agents. Phys Med Biol. 2006;51:3967–81.
32. Sgouros G, Kolbert K. The three-dimensional internal dosimetry software package, 3D-ID. In: Zaidi H, Sgouros G, editors. Therapeutic applications of Monte Carlo calculations in nuclear medicine. Philadelphia: Institute of Physics; 2002. p. 249–61.
33. Prideaux A, Song H, Hobbs R, He B, Frey E, Ladenson P, Wahl R, Sgouros G. Three-dimensional radiobiologic dosimetry: application of radiobiologic modeling to patient-specific 3-dimensional imaging-based internal dosimetry. J Nucl Med. 2007;48:1008–16.
34. Guy M, Flux G, Papavasileiou P, Flower M, Ott R. RMDP: a dedicated package for ^{131}I SPECT quantification, registration and patient-specific dosimetry. Cancer Biother Radiopharm. 2003;18:61–9.
35. Franck D, de Carlan L, Pierrat N, Broggio D, Lamart S. OEDIPE: a new graphical user interface for fast construction of numerical phantoms and MCNP calculations. Radiat Prot Dosimetry. 2007;127:262–5.
36. Botta F, Mairani A, Battistoni G, Cremonesi M, Di Dia A, Fassò A, Ferrari A, Ferrari M, Paganelli G, Pedroli G, Valente M. Calculation of electron and isotopes dose point kernels with FLUKA Monte Carlo code for dosimetry in nuclear medicine therapy. Med Phys. 2011;38:3944–54.
37. Dieudonné A, Hobbs R, Bolch W, Sgouros G, Gardin I. Fine resolution voxel S-values for constructing absorbed dose distributions at variable voxel size. J Nucl Med. 2010;51:1600–7.
38. Sgouros G, Kolbert K, Sheikh A, et al. Patient-specific dosimetry for ^{131}I thyroid cancer therapy using ^{124}I PET and 3-dimensional-internal dosimetry (3D-ID) software. J Nucl Med. 2004;45:1366–72.
39. Kolbert K, Pentlow K, Pearson J, et al. Prediction of absorbed dose to normal organs in thyroid cancer patients treated with ^{131}I by use of ^{124}I PET and 3-dimensional internal dosimetry software. J Nucl Med. 2007;48:143–9.
40. Dale R. Use of the linear-quadratic radiobiological model for quantifying kidney response in targeted radiotherapy. Cancer Biother Radiopharm. 2004;19:363–70.
41. Millar WT. Application of the linear-quadratic model with incomplete repair to radionuclide directed therapy. Br J Radiol. 1991;64:242–51.
42. Niemierko A. Reporting and analyzing dose distributions: a concept of equivalent uniform dose. Med Phys. 1997;24:103–10.
43. Howell RW, Goddu SM, Rao DV. Application of the linear-quadratic model to radioimmunotherapy: further support for the advantage of longer-lived radionuclides. J Nucl Med. 1994;35:1861–9.
44. Baechler S, Hobbs R, Prideaux A, Wahl R, Sgouros G. Extension of the biological effective dose to the MIRD schema and possible implications in radionuclide therapy dosimetry. Med Phys. 2008;35:1123–34.
45. Hobbs R, Sgouros G. Calculation of the biological effective dose (BED) for piecewise defined dose-rate fits. Med Phys. 2009;36:904–7.
46. Hobbs RF, Wahl RL, Lodge MA, Javadi MS, Cho S, Chien D, Ewertz ME, Esaias CE, Ladenson PW, Sgouros G. ^{124}I PET-based 3D-RD dosimetry for pediatric thyroid cancer patient: case study for real-time patient-specific dosimetry. J Nucl Med. 2009;50:1844–7.
47. Khorjekar G, Senthamizhchelvan S, Hobbs R, Orquiza M, Atkins F, Mete M, Garcia C, Wartofsky L, Sgouros G, Van Nostrand, Douglas. Correlation of ^{124}I PET dosimetry with clinical response of ^{131}I therapy for metastatic differentiated thyroid cancer. Oral presentation presented at: The Society of Nuclear Medicine annual Meeting (2013), Vancouver, British Columbia, Canada. J Nuc Med. 2013;54(Suppl):52.
48. Zanzonico PB. Radiation dose to patients and relatives incident to ^{131}I therapy. Thyroid. 1997;7:199–204.
49. Van Nostrand D. Sialoadenitis secondary to ^{131}I therapy for well-differentiated thyroid cancer. Oral Dis. 2010;17:154–61.
50. Langendijk JA, Doornaert P, Verdonck-de Leeuw IM, Leemans CR, Aaronson NK, Slotman BJ. Impact of late treatment-related toxicity on quality of life among patients with head and neck cancer treated with radiotherapy. J Clin Oncol. 2008;26:3770–6.
51. Raza H, Khan AU, Hameed A, Khan A. Quantitative evaluation of salivary gland dysfunction after radioiodine therapy using salivary gland scintigraphy. Nucl Med Commun. 2006;27:495–9.
52. Jentzen W, Schneider E, Freudenberg L, Eising EG, Gorges R, Muller SP, et al. Relationship between cumulative radiation dose and salivary gland uptake associated with radioiodine therapy of thyroid cancer. Nucl Med Commun. 2006;27:669–76.
53. Jentzen W, Hobbs RF, Stahl A, Knust J, Sgouros G, Bockisch A. Pre-therapeutic ^{124}I PET(/CT) dosimetry confirms low average absorbed doses per administered ^{131}I activity to the salivary glands in radioiodine therapy of differentiated thyroid cancer. Eur J Nucl Med Mol Imaging. 2010;37:884–95.
54. Hobbs R, Jentzen W, Bockisch A, Sgouros G. Monte Carlo-based 3-dimensional dosimetry of salivary glands in radioiodine treatment of differentiated thyroid cancer estimated using ^{124}I PET. Q J Nucl Med Mol Imaging. 2013;57:79–91.
55. Gates GA, Work WP. Radioisotope scanning of the salivary glands. A preliminary report. Laryngoscope. 1967;77:861–75.
56. Mishkin FS. Radionuclide salivary gland imaging. Semin Nucl Med. 1981;11:258–65.
57. Jentzen W. Experimental investigation of factors affecting the absolute recovery coefficients in iodine-124 PET lesion imaging. Phys Med Biol. 2010;55:2365–98.
58. Jentzen W, Weise R, Kupferschlager J, et al. Iodine-124 PET dosimetry in differentiated thyroid cancer: recovery coefficient in

2D and 3D modes for PET(/CT) systems. Eur J Nucl Med Mol Imaging. 2008;35:611–23.
59. Teo BK, Seo Y, Bacharach SL, Carrasquillo JA, Libutti SK, Shukla H, et al. Partial-volume correction in PET: validation of an iterative postreconstruction method with phantom and patient data. J Nucl Med. 2007;48:802–10.
60. Nakada K, Ishibashi T, Takei T, et al. Does lemon candy decrease salivary gland damage after radioiodine therapy for thyroid cancer? J Nucl Med. 2005;46:261–6.
61. Jentzen W, Balschuweit D, Schmitz J, et al. The influence of saliva flow stimulation on the absorbed radiation dose to the salivary glands during radioiodine therapy of thyroid cancer using ^{124}I PET/CT imaging. Eur J Nucl Med Mol Imaging. 2010;37: 2298–306.
62. Van Nostrand D, Bandaru V, Chennupati V, Kulkarni K, Wexler J, Atkins F, Mete M, Gadwale G. Radiopharmacokinetics of radioiodine in the parotid glands after the administration of lemon juice. Thyroid. 2010;20:1113–9.
63. Phillips AF. The gamma -ray dose in carcinoma of the thyroid treated by radio-iodine. Acta Radiol. 1954;41:533–44.
64. Goolden AWG, Fowler JF, Matthews CM. Comparison of iodine 124 and iodine 131 for thyroid ablation. Br J Radiol. 1963;36:346–9.
65. Koehler L, Gagnon K, McQuarrie S, Wuest F. Iodine-124: a promising positron emitter for organic PET chemistry. Molecules. 2010;15:2686–718.
66. Hall T, Siegel M, et al. Production of ^{124}I by the deuteron bombardment of tellurium. Phys Rev. 1954;95:1208.

104 Future Directions for Advanced Thyroid Cancer Therapy

Matthew D. Ringel

Introduction

The unique features of thyroid cells long have enabled clinicians to target therapy for patients with differentiated thyroid cancers. The retained expression and function of the thyrotropin receptor (TSHR) and the Na, I symporter (NIS) in most thyroid cells have allowed for the successful use of TSH-suppressive doses of levothyroxine (L-T4) and radioiodine in selected patients. These targeted treatments, in combination with surgery, have led to long-term survival rates for patients with early-stage thyroid cancers that approach 98 % at 20 years [1, 2]. However, this excellent prognosis is not shared by individuals with aggressive, metastatic thyroid cancers or those with malignancies that dedifferentiate and lose expression and function of the TSH receptor and NIS. Indeed, patients with these more aggressive thyroid cancers typically have poor responses to traditional therapies resulting in a much higher incidence of cancer-related death. Alternative therapies using nontargeted cytotoxic chemotherapeutic agents have been largely disappointing. Therefore, a major effort is ongoing to identify effective treatments for patients with aggressive thyroid cancers. Proper therapeutic targeting for these tumors requires clarification of the pathways most critical for tumor progression and tumor cell survival and the mechanisms responsible for the loss of TSHR and NIS expression (Table 104.1) [3]. As better tolerated therapies that target pathways involved in cancer have been developed, a number of teams focused on thyroid cancer clinical trials have successfully completed studies assessing efficacy in patients with progressive and metastatic thyroid cancer. This approach has resulted in the approval of three agents for treating progressive and metastatic thyroid cancer including two for medullary cancer (cabozantinib and vandetanib) and one for follicular-cell-derived thyroid cancer (sorafenib). In addition, a number of FDA-approved compounds for other malignancies have been shown to have disease-modifying activating in thyroid cancer and could be prescribed by clinicians in the United States. While these studies and subsequent approvals are a significant advance for patients with thyroid cancer, thus far all of the approvals are based on improved progression-free survival but an overall survival benefit has not been shown and durable complete remissions have not been described. Moreover, side effects are common, some of which can be severe. Thus, at this time the use of these agents is limited to patients with progressive and life-threatening forms of thyroid cancer. In this chapter, the potential targets for alternative therapies, the key data that resulted in the approvals of these compounds, future directions now that new approved therapies exist will be discussed. Specific ongoing or published clinical trials beyond those will not be reviewed in detail.

M.D. Ringel, MD (✉)
Division of Endocrinology, Diabetes and Metabolism, Department of Internal Medicine, Wexner Medical Center, The Ohio State University, 565 McCampbell Hall 1581 Dodd Drive, Columbus, OH 43210, USA
e-mail: matthew.ringel@osumc.edu

Clinical Trials for Cancer

Thyroid cancer patients are typically treated by endocrinologists and nuclear medicine physicians rather than medical and/or radiation oncologists, many of whom do not enroll patients in therapeutic cancer clinical trials frequently [4, 5]. For patients with more aggressive thyroid cancers, such as differentiated or poorly differentiated tumors with progressive metastases and anaplastic thyroid cancer, it is important that the team includes physicians and nurses who are comfortable with typical oncological practices and have access to cancer clinical trials. If a patient is not tolerant of or not appropriate for treatment with a FDA-approved kinase inhibitor, or if they have anaplastic thyroid cancer, clinical trials remain an important alternative to consider. This will give

L. Wartofsky, D. Van Nostrand (eds.), *Thyroid Cancer*, DOI 10.1007/978-1-4939-3314-3_104

Table 104.1 Targets for thyroid cancer therapies

Targets
Tyrosine kinase receptors
RET
cMET
IGF-1
VEGF
FGF
EGF
Signaling molecule inhibitors
BRAF
RAS
PI3K
mTOR
AKT
RAP1
PKC
FAK
PAK
Angiogenesis inhibition
VEGF
PDGF
FGF
Combretastatins
Thalidomide
Apoptosis sensitizers
TRAIL
BCL-2
AKT
Gene therapy
Enhancing iodine uptake
MEK
BRAF
PI3K
Hypermethylation
Histone deacetylation
Retinoids
Gene therapy
Enhanced chemotherapy effects
Drug resistance gene inhibitors
Combination therapy
Immunotherapy
Gene therapy
Tumor vaccines
BCG
Multimodality therapy including radiation therapy and I-131
BRAF inhibitor + I-131
MEK inhibitor + I-131
PI3K/Akt inhibitor + I-131
Demethylating agents + I-131

patients access to new agents with potential for activity and allow investigators to determine if a particular approach is beneficial.

Clinical trials are divided into phase 1, 2, and 3 studies. Phase 1 studies are the first human studies of an agent or combination of agents. These studies are designed primarily to assess toxicity of the new treatment. These trials are of greatest risk to the patients, but may be very appealing if the therapy has been tested against thyroid cancer cells and animal models, and if the agent, or combination of agents, has particular logic for use as thyroid cancer therapy, or if patient does not qualify for phase 2 or 3 studies. Phase 2 studies focus on particular diseases, or a particular disease-causing mutation that is being targeted by a compound, for which there were clinical responses in phase 1 studies or strong logic based on mechanism of action. Phase 3 trials are generally large, and often multi-institutional studies designed to determine if an agent or combination of agents is appropriate for FDA approval for treatment of a specific disease. All of the studies may be performed in multiple institutions through consortia agreement, improving access to patients and physicians to studies.

Several resources are available to identify clinical trials. The most common is clnicaltrials.gov through the National Institutes of Health which provides a searchable list of all registered ongoing clinical trials. Physicians who care for patients with aggressive thyroid cancers should become facile with these resources or enlist the help of an appropriate consultant involved in clinical trials to facilitate enrollments if this becomes necessary.

Approaches to Thyroid Cancer Therapeutic Targeting

Increasing Iodine Uptake in Iodine Nonresponsive Thyroid Cancer

I-131 therapy has been a mainstay of treatment for localized and metastatic thyroid cancer for decades. While some patients with metastatic thyroid cancer respond to I-131 therapy, primary resistance to therapy and/or progression after a period of stability following I-131 is common. The resistance may in part be related to reduced cellular uptake of I-131 that occurs as tumors dedifferentiate or express specific oncogenes. Thus, there has been a major interest to devise strategies to improve radioiodine uptake and retention in thyroid cancer cells. The cloning of the Na, I symporter (NIS) gene, and its promoter, and the development of reliable antibodies to allow for detection of the protein have led to the determination that abnormalities in NIS gene and protein expression, and protein localization is common in thyroid cancer [6–10]. Subsequent work identified that several mechanisms led to reduced NIS expression and that these can be exploited with therapeutic intent. One epigenetic mechanism that leads to reduced NIS expression is hypermethylation of the NIS promoter leading to reduced NIS gene transcription. Several investigators have treated thyroid cancer cell lines with demethylating agents or histone deacetylase (HDAC) inhibitors, such as 5-azacytidine and depsipeptide, respectively, and demonstrated reduced methylation of the NIS promoter, re-expression of the NIS gene, increased iodine uptake, and enhanced efficacy of radioactive iodine therapy in vitro [11, 12]. 5-Azacytidine is being used as a parent compound to develop new agents due to the rapid induction of resistance to this drug in vivo. Vorinostat, an HDAC inhibitor, is one of several agents with similar activity that has been studied in clinical trials, albeit not in combination with I-131 therapy. Only modest benefit has been reported thus far [13].

Retinoid receptor agonists also have been reported to enhance iodine uptake in vitro and in patients with thyroid cancers that do not respond to radioiodine. The initial studies appeared quite promising, both in vitro and in human studies [14, 15]. However, it has become clear that the use of more generalized retinoic acid receptor agonists appears to be limited for the majority of patients, although a subset may still respond [14, 16]. Over time, it has been recognized that thyroid cancers express a number of different retinoid receptors. The development of specific receptor subtype agonists has led to a number of studies evaluating their effect in vitro and raise potential for their use as enhancers of iodine uptake and as primary therapy for thyroid cancer [17].

More recently, it has been demonstrated that activation of the MAP kinase pathway leads to reduced expression and function of the entire thyroid differentiation cascade, including iodine uptake, through a combination of transcriptional, translation, and posttranslational mechanisms. It has been demonstrated that increased signaling through BRAF/MEK/ERK rapidly downregulates expression of the genes involved in thyroid hormone production including NIS and the TSH receptor in vitro and in vivo [18–20]. In vivo studies were performed demonstrating that treatment of mice with thyroid-specific expression of BRAF V600E with a MEK inhibitor increased iodine uptake [21]. This led to a small clinical trial in which patients with defined I-131 resistant distant metastases were treated transiently with selumetinib, a MEK inhibitor, prior to I-131 scanning to determine if it would enhance iodine uptake; and if it did, they received I-131 therapy while on the compound [22]. In this study, 12/20 patients had an increase in uptake; 8 of those 12 patients increased above the predefined limit required for treatment with I-131. Of that group of eight patients, five had a partial response by RECIST criteria (i.e., >30 % reduction in tumor volume) while three had stable disease. Unexpectedly, there was a suggestion that those with tumors harboring a mutation in NRAS (5/20) were more sensitive in comparison to patients with BRAF mutations (9/20). Larger studies using both MEK and BRAF inhibitors to enhance I-131 therapy efficacy are planned or are ongoing. This approach has the advantage of lower toxicities from the kinase inhibitors due to the short duration of treatment. Other signaling pathways have been shown to regulate NIS expression and/or function, including the PI3 kinase and others known to be involved in thyroid cancer progression [23, 24]. The impact of targeting these pathways alone or in combination with MEK inhibition is an area of ongoing research that may lead to future clinical trials.

NIS gene therapy presents another alternative approach to increase NIS expression in cancers and enhance iodine uptake. The ability to target expression of a gene in cells is determined by the specificity of the promoter that drives the gene expression in the vector that is utilized. In the case of thyroid cells, several specific promoters exist, particularly the thyroglobulin gene promoter. Numerous in vitro and transgenic animals have been created using vectors that link the thyroglobulin promoter to a gene of interest, enabling thyroid-specific expression of that gene. Gene therapy has therefore been utilized for years in the laboratory to enhance expression of proteins in thyroid cells, including NIS. By placing this thyroglobulin promoter-NIS fusion gene into a gene therapy vector (such as a virus), it is possible to enhance expression of NIS in thyroid cells in vivo. In animal models, several groups have successfully induced expression of NIS in thyroid cancer cells with low endogenous NIS levels or into non-thyroid tumors with no endogenous NIS expression by direct injection or transfection of the virus into tumors [25–27]. This approach has translational limitations as most patients with metastatic thyroid cancer have multiple small lesions that may not be amenable to direct injection. Thus, systemic therapy (inhaled or IV) is the goal. Unfortunately, the development of a systemic approach to gene therapy has been hampered thus far by the immune response triggered by the viral vector and hepatic first-pass effect. The development of non-viral gene transporters holds promise for less antigenic delivery methods for future therapy.

Therapy Targeted Against Angiogenesis

The excessive growth and metabolic activity of cancer cells create a need for access to nutrients and oxygen. Cancer cells invade and grow in regions that are not typically rich in blood vessels; thus, to maintain growth and to invade, they need to create new blood vessels (neovascularization) in order to survive and grow [28]. This process, angiogenesis, is therefore central to the ability of cancers to survive and proliferate. Disruption of angiogenesis by targeting a variety of angiogenic signals has been successfully applied to a number of cancers as both monotherapy and as part of combinatorial approaches.

Thyroid cancer metastases are often highly vascular, making it a logical approach to consider for patients with progressive metastatic disease. Key regulators of angiogenesis include a number of growth factors, including vascular endothelial growth factor (VEGF) and fibroblast growth factor (FGF) [29]. Thyroid cancers are characterized by increased expression of all of these angiogenic proteins creating interest for inhibitors of receptors for these proteins, and other angiogenic mechanisms, in thyroid cancer treatment.

Combretastatin A4 phosphate (fosbretabulin) is a vascular-targeted compound that has been reported to have activity against human poorly differentiated thyroid cancer in early clinical trials. Combretastatins are tubulin-binding proteins isolated from the African Willow. This family of compounds is vascular targeted but also had direct cellular cytotoxic effects. In a phase 1 trial, three of six thyroid cancer patients, including one with anaplastic thyroid cancer, had partial or complete responses to fosbretabulin [30, 31]. In follow-up of this study, a phase 2 trial of fosbretabulin for anaplastic thyroid cancer enrolled 26 patients, but responses were not reported [32]. The primary toxicity of this compound is cardiac, both vascular and arrhythmia. Thus, patients need to be cleared by a cardiac evaluation prior to starting this agent. Thalidomide and lenalidomide are additional vascular-targeted agents that are available for clinical use. Thalidomide has been studied in clinical trials for thyroid cancer with modest effects reported [33].

VEGF, as noted above, is an important stimulator of new blood vessel formation. Expression of VEGF and its receptors are stimulated by hypoxia through activation of a family of hypoxia-inducible transcription factors. VEGF-neutralizing antibodies, such as bevacizumab, and specific receptor blockers are either being used in clinical trials or are FDA approved. In addition, it is of interest that VEGF receptors are a common target of all of the kinase inhibitors shown to have activity in treating patients with metastatic thyroid cancer, including the three FDA-approved compounds, suggesting its inhibition is important in therapeutic activity [34]. In addition to VEGF, many of the multikinase inhibitors in both clinical trials and practice inhibit other angiogenic receptors (PDGF, FGF, cMET) as well as oncogene target kinases (such as Raf or Ret); it is likely that a major component of the clinical activity is due to angiogenesis inhibition. As a group, antiangiogenic kinase inhibitors are primarily cytostatic rather than cytotoxic, as one would predict based on their mechanisms of action. This may account for the lack of complete responses in clinical trials with these compounds.

Overall, the concept of vascular targeting for thyroid cancer is evolving. Similar to other novel therapies, predictors of response, such as the degree of tumor vascularity as identified either on pathology staining or by new imaging modalities, such as dynamic contrast enhanced MRI, may be predictive of response or lack of response to a compound in individual patients. The use of angiogenic inhibitors in combination therapy may be ultimately the best use of this class of compounds in thyroid cancer therapy. This concept is being tested in clinical trials.

Therapy Targeted against Cell Signaling Pathways

Cancer-causing genes are classically described either as oncogenes or tumor suppressor genes. Oncogenes are "positive" regulators of tumorigenesis such that gain of function mutations, overexpression, or upstream activation is sufficient to transform cells into cancer. Tumor suppressor proteins in contrast, generally slow cell growth or induce apoptosis and are therefore inhibitors of transformation. Loss of expression or loss of function mutations of one or both alleles is sufficient to transform cells. The genetic or epigenetic changes that result in tumor formation may also drive late-stage tumor progression, although this is not certain for all tumors as secondary changes can occur throughout the life of a tumor. Over the past few decades, the genetic alterations responsible for the majority of thyroid cancers have been identified and the list has been continually expanding. Overexpression or oncogenic rearrangements in tyrosine kinase receptors, such as RET, cMET, ALK, and IGF-1; activating mutations of downstream serine-threonine kinases, including RAS and BRAF; and loss of tumor suppressor expression [35–39] have all been identified and characterized. Several of these genetic abnormalities are specific for papillary thyroid cancer (e.g., BRAF mutations and RET/PTC rearrangements), while others are common in follicular forms of thyroid cancer (PTEN loss and RAS mutations). Some appear to be induced by environmental factors, such as exposure to ionizing radiation (RET rearrangements). In rare cases, germline genetic alterations have been found to confer risk to thyroid cancer in families, including loss of PTEN expression in Cowden's syndrome [40] and activating mutations of RET medullary thyroid cancer and multiple endocrine neoplasia syndromes [41].

In terms of therapeutic targeting in patients with progressive metastatic thyroid cancer, the goal is to block "driver" pathways of cancer progression. In thyroid cancer, initiating oncogenes in the primary tumors appear to be maintained in recurrent thyroid cancer tissue, suggesting that these pathways may be critical to the aggressive phenotype of some thyroid cancers [36]. BRAF V600E has been particularly scrutinized for a potential role in both papillary thyroid cancer development and progression due to its high frequency in clinical trial populations [42] and its association with more aggressive tumor behavior [43]. While alone, it may not be a strong predictor of aggressive tumor behavior, recent studies suggest that its presence in combination with other specific genetic changes may predict aggressive tumor behavior [44, 45]. Importantly, the depth of knowledge regarding driver pathways in thyroid cancer along with the development of more specific inhibitors has allowed for opportunities to develop and test targeted therapies.

Kinase inhibitors have been developed to exploit driver mutations and have led to remarkable responses when applied to some tumor types. Among the most successful has been inhibition of BCR/ABL and C-KIT in chronic myelogenous leukemia and gastrointestinal stromal tumors using imatinib a specific inhibitor of these two kinases [46, 47]}. A second example is the use of specific epidermal growth factor receptor (EGFR) inhibitors (erlotinib and gefitinib) as first-line therapy for patients with lung cancer that have EGFR mutations [48, 49]. These types of successes has resulted in FDA approval of a growing number of kinase inhibitors for specific tumors; the development of clinical trials focused on the presence of a mutation rather than organ-driven clinical trial approach and has led to the development of a large number of new kinase inhibitors. Of particular interest for thyroid cancer are compounds that inhibit the MAP kinase pathway by inhibiting either RAF or MEK or those that block activation of RET that is involved in both PTC and MTC.

Sorafenib is a multikinase inhibitor that has been approved by the FDA in the United States for several cancer types, most recently differentiated thyroid cancer. Sorafenib inhibits VEGF receptors, Ret, Raf (including BRAF), and other kinases and it is believed that the activity is most likely derived from its antiangiogenic properties. In several single-arm phase II studies in an international phase III placebo-controlled study, sorafenib was shown to have disease-modifying effects in patients with progressive metastatic differentiated thyroid cancer. In the phase III study, 417 patients with progressive thyroid cancer were randomized, 207 received sorafenib, and 210 received placebo. The patients treated with sorafenib had a 10.8-month progression-free survival vs. 5.8 months in the placebo group as assessed by RECIST criteria. Partial remissions were achieved in 12.2 % of the patients treated with sorafenib and 42 % had stable disease ≥6 months vs. 0.5 % and 33 % for the placebo group, respectively. Seventy percent of the patients treated with placebo received open-label sorafenib after progression. The presence of a BRAF V600E or RAS activating mutation was not predictive of response suggesting that the activity of sorafenib is not only related to its Raf kinase inhibitory effect. Side effects occurred including hand-foot skin reaction, diarrhea, hypertension, and fatigue and two deaths in the study were attributed to sorafenib [50]. In addition for a role for the RET kinase in PTC due to RET/PTC gene rearrangements, RET is also a target for medullary thyroid cancer (MTC) due to a high frequency of activating mutations in the germline in MEN2 or somatically in sporadic MTC. Several multikinase inhibitors in addition to sorafenib have activity against the Ret tyrosine kinase including two inhibitors, vandetanib and cabozantinib, that have achieved FDA approval for treating patients with metastatic progressive MTC. In a randomized placebo-controlled phase III study of 331 patients, vandetanib was shown to improve progression-free survival from 19.5 months in the placebo group to an estimated 30.5 months in the vandetanib group. Because patients on placebo were able to receive vandetanib after progression, overall survival was not able to be assessed. Progression defined by growth of lesion >20 % on CT scans was not required for study enrollment. Twelve percent of patients treated with vandetanib had the medication discontinued due to side effects. The most common side effects were diarrhea, rash, and hypertension which occurred in ~30 % of patients on vandetanib. Eight percent of patients had QTc prolongation requiring dose reduction and 49 % required an increase in the dose of levothyroxine [51]. The phase III study with cabozantinib was limited to patients with RECIST-defined progression over 14 months and was also placebo controlled. In this study a crossover was not allowed. Treatment with cabozantinib resulted in improved progression-free survival compared with placebo (11.2 months vs. 4.0 months) and 47.3 % of these patients who entered the study with progressive disease had stable disease still after 12 months of treatment. An overall survival benefit was not identified; however, the number of events was felt to be too small at the time of analysis so subsequent analysis is planned. Adverse events were common (79 %) and often improved with dose reductions. The most common were diarrhea, rash, and fatigue. Serious adverse events occurred in 42 % of the treated patients and included fistula formation and pulmonary embolism felt to be study compound related. Serious adverse events also occurred in 23 % of the placebo patients likely related to the extent of disease and progression required at the time of study enrollment [52]. Thus, while the side effects of the two compounds are not identical, the type of side effects may be important in selecting patients for a particular medication. Because many of the side effects are dose related, defining activity levels of the compounds started on lower dose of the medications is being assessed. There is substantial individual variability in developing side effects from these compounds. Further studies are needed to identify predictors of side effects but these data demonstrate that these compounds are appropriate at this time only for patients with progressive a life-threatening thyroid cancer.

Tyrosine kinase receptors activate numerous downstream signaling pathways. Principal among them are the RAS/MAP kinase pathway and the PI3 kinase/Akt pathway. In addition to activation from tyrosine kinase receptors, genetic abnormalities in the genes encoding the genes encoding RAS and its downstream target, BRAF, have been described in follicular and papillary thyroid cancers, respectively. Akt activation occurs as a result in loss of PTEN activity in Cowden's syndrome, and activation of this pathway is reported to have an important role in metastases and recurrence [36, 53, 54]. For these reasons, direct disruption of these signaling molecules has been utilized as an alternative targeting strategy for cancer therapy. Inhibitors of BRAF, RAS, and Akt have all been developed and are being studied in thyroid cancer alone or as part of combination strategies.

BRAF V600E is the most common gene mutation in PTC (~40 %) and has been shown to be a driver of thyroid tumorigenesis in vitro and in vivo [18]. It is typically preserved in recurrent lesions and is therefore thought to play an important role in late-stage progression., Nearly all studies associate BRAF V600E with more aggressive PTC in large populations, although its predictive power beyond clinical features in individual patients such as tumor size and patient age as a solitary predictor of cancer progression is not certain [43]. Nonetheless, the presence of BRAF V600E in the primary tumors from patients with progressive metastatic PTC makes this a promising target for individuals appropriate for this type of therapy [55]. Because BRAF V600E is also highly prevalent in other tumor types (e.g., melanoma, hairy cell leukemia, colon cancer), compounds that inhibit the mutant protein with great specificity for the BRAF V600E mutant (vemurafenib, dabrafenib) have been developed and are FDA approved for melanoma. Of interest is that the response rates of different tumor types that express BRAF V600E have not been consistent and, even in the responders, resistance is typical [56]. Thus, it is clear that while the use of BRAF inhibitors either alone or in combination requires tumor type-specific validation, and also combinatorial strategies will be needed. Combinations of either BRAF V600E inhibitors or general RAF inhibitors with MEK, Ret, mTOR, or PI3K are currently being evaluated in vitro and in vivo. Side effects of the BRAF V600E inhibitors include the development of skin tumors which require monitoring during therapy [57].

In addition to kinase inhibitors, other mechanisms that regulated signaling pathway activity, such as protein farnesylation and protein stability, have been exploited to develop treatments for cancer largely in preclinical models. These include the enzyme that mediates protein farnesylation (farnesyl transferase), protein scaffolds that facilitate signaling such as heat shock protein (HSP) 90, and proteasome activity. Farnesyl transferase inhibitors, HSP 90 blockers, and proteasome inhibitors have now been included in clinical trials as monotherapies or as part of combinatorial strategies although their role in thyroid cancer treatment remains uncertain as kinase inhibitors have evolved.

As noted above, because inhibition of these signaling pathways enhances the sensitivity of cells to cell death, it is possible that the most effect use of these drugs will be in combination with other approaches, such as radioiodine, radiation therapy, cytotoxic chemotherapy, or in combination with one another.

Therapies Designed to Induce Cell Death

Cell growth is characterized by a skew in the balance toward proliferation and away from cell death. The mechanisms that regulate cell death are manifold and include production of proteins that block external stimuli that initiate cell death pathways, expression of intracellular proteins that are anti-apoptotic, and persistent expression of proteins to maintain chromosome length. In thyroid cancer, each of these mechanisms has been described and have been shown to the functional regulators of resistance to therapy. Many of the families of agents described earlier also induce cell death, either by inducing apoptosis (programmed cell death), inhibiting antiapoptotic pathways, or causing cell necrosis. In addition to these agents, several other novel compounds have been created to design to more directly target cell survival pathways. Tumor necrosis factor (TNF) and the FAS ligand are two common initiators of apoptosis, particular when mediated by immune cells [58]. Thyroid cancer cells are remarkably resistant to these two apoptosis inducers through both intracellular mechanisms and release of inhibitory proteins. Downstream of the TNF receptors is a related effector molecule, the TNF-related apoptosis-inducing ligand (TRAIL) receptor. Direct activation of this receptor is possible using recombinant human TRAIL, and its use has been reported to induce apoptosis in a number of apoptosis-resistant cell lines, including thyroid cancer cells [59–61]. Another approach to inhibit antiapoptotic signaling molecules is to directly block endogenous inhibitors such as BCL-2. BCL-2 is upregulated by Akt and RAS and its levels can be reduced indirectly by signaling inhibitor or directly using antisense RNA. This approach has been reported in clinical trials, although not yet for thyroid cancer. Gene therapy can be utilized to carry vectors that induce cytotoxicity directly or after incubation of cancer cells with an activator of the newly expressed protein ("suicide gene therapy"). Similar to the re-expression of NIS, this model utilizes a vector that couples a "suicide gene" to the thyroglobulin gene promoter to induce thyroid-specific expression of this gene. The most commonly reported method is to induce thyroid cell expression of thymidine kinase by infecting thyroid cancer cells with a virus carrying a transgene coupling the thyroglobulin promoter to the gene encoding thymidine kinase, a protein that is not normally expressed in mammalian cells. Expression of thymidine kinase uniquely sensitizes the cancer cells to the antiviral drug, ganciclovir [26, 62]. It faces similar challenges to other forms of vector-dependent gene transfer for systemic delivery.

Other Potential Therapies for Thyroid Cancer

As noted above, thyroid cancer cells are typically resistant to cytotoxic chemotherapies. There are many potential mechanisms for this resistance including oncogene expression leading to activation of signaling pathways not altered by a particular cytotoxic agent. Another possibility is that the thyroid cancer cells express proteins specific for drug resistance. Indeed, thyroid cancer and many other malignant cells can express multiple drug resistance genes (MDR) that lead to chemotherapy resistance. Some of these proteins specifically cause resistance to cytotoxic compounds with documented activity against anaplastic thyroid cancer, including taxanes and doxorubicin. It is likely that cancer cells will develop new methods to resist the antitumor effect of the newer targeted agents as well. Thus, the use of antisense RNA and other approaches targeted against drug resistance mechanisms represents an important direction for cancer therapy. Clearly, these agents have potential to enhance the activity of chemotherapies against resistant thyroid cancer cells.

Immunotherapy has been an important line of research for thyroid cancer for decades [63–66]. The development of vaccines directed against specific antigens expressed by tumor cells to target cytotoxic immune responses has been the focus of therapy for many different types of cancer. For thyroid cancer, an important clue could be the development of thyroiditis reported in patients treated with interferon or interleukins. These reports have led to enhanced interest in this area of therapeutic research. One potential advantage of this option is to tailor therapy for a patient based on the specific antigens expressed by their specific tumor. This individualized therapy is an important concept as new therapies develop.

Other areas of focus include efforts to target signaling pathways that regulate cytoskeletal changes required for cell invasion and motility, such as focal adhesion kinase (FAK) or p21-activated kinase (PAK) [67, 68]. In addition, there have been efforts to target other potential thyroid oncogenes including PPARγ that is often involved in rearrangements in follicular thyroid tumors [69].

Future Directions

Now that three compounds are approved by the FDA in the United States for individuals with progressive metastatic thyroid cancer, a population will arise with either primary or secondary resistance to these treatments or that are intolerant or unable to take the medication. For these individuals, second-line treatments are needed and will need to be developed using appropriate models of resistance. As more knowledge grows through efforts such as The Cancer Genome Atlas and approaches are used for "precision" oncology whereby genetic profiles of individual tumors drive therapeutic choices, opportunities to improve treatments and minimize side effects for patients with these aggressive forms of thyroid cancer will continue to evolve. Importantly, predictors and mechanisms of toxicity will need to be better understood so patients at highest risk of toxicity can be identified and treated uniquely in a similar manner. By establishing these types of information, a more individualized approach to treating patients with progressive metastatic thyroid cancer can be developed.

References

1. American Thyroid Association Guidelines Task Force on Thyroid Nodules and Differentiated Thyroid Cancer. Haugen BR, Alexander EK, Bible KC, Doherty GM, Mandel SJ, Nikiforov YE, Pacini F, Randolph GW, Sawka AM, Schlumberger M, Schuff KG, Sherman SI, Sosa JA, Steward DL, Tuttle RM, Wartofsky L. 2015 American Thyroid Association Management Guidelines for Adult Patients with Thyroid Nodules and Differentiated Thyroid Cancer. Thyroid 2016; 26:1–133.
2. Pacini F, Castagna MG, Brilli L, Pentheroudakis G, Group EGW. Thyroid cancer: ESMO clinical practice guidelines for diagnosis, treatment and follow-up. Ann Oncol. 2010;21 Suppl 5:v214–9.
3. Haugen BR, Sherman SI. Evolving approaches to patients with advanced differentiated thyroid cancer. Endocr Rev. 2013;34:439–55.
4. Colevas AD, Shah MH. Evaluation of patients with disseminated or locoregionally advanced thyroid cancer: a primer for medical oncologists. Am Soc Clin Oncol Educ Book. 2012;32:384–8.
5. Haraldsdottir S, Shah MH. An update on clinical trials of targeted therapies in thyroid cancer. Curr Opin Oncol. 2014;26:36–44.
6. Dai G, Levy O, Carrasco N. Cloning and characterization of the thyroid iodide transporter. Nature. 1996;379:458–60.
7. Portulano C, Paroder-Belenitsky M, Carrasco N. The Na+/I− symporter (NIS): mechanism and medical impact. Endocr Rev. 2014;35:106–49.
8. Smanik PA, Liu Q, Furminger TL, Ryu K, Xing S, Mazzaferri EL, Jhiang SM. Cloning of the human sodium iodide symporter. Biochem Biophys Res Commun. 1996;226:339–45.
9. Vadysirisack DD, Chen ES, Zhang Z, Tsai MD, Chang GD, Jhiang SM. Identification of in vivo phosphorylation sites and their functional significance in the sodium iodide symporter. J Biol Chem. 2007;282:36820–8.
10. Ringel MD, Anderson J, Souza SL, Burch HB, Tambascia M, Shriver CD, Tuttle RM. Expression of the sodium iodide symporter and thyroglobulin genes are reduced in papillary thyroid cancer. Mod Pathol. 2001;14:289–96.
11. Furuya F, Shimura H, Suzuki H, Taki K, Ohta K, Haraguchi K, Onaya T, Endo T, Kobayashi T. Histone deacetylase inhibitors restore radioiodide uptake and retention in poorly differentiated and anaplastic thyroid cancer cells by expression of the sodium/iodide symporter thyroperoxidase and thyroglobulin. Endocrinology. 2004;145:2865–75.
12. Venkataraman GM, Yatin M, Marcinek R, Ain KB. Restoration of iodide uptake in dedifferentiated thyroid carcinoma: relationship to human Na+/I-symporter gene methylation status. J Clin Endocrinol Metab. 1999;84:2449–57.
13. Woyach JA, Kloos RT, Ringel MD, Arbogast D, Collamore M, Zwiebel JA, Grever M, Villalona-Calero M, Shah MH. Lack of therapeutic effect of the histone deacetylase inhibitor vorinostat in patients with metastatic radioiodine-refractory thyroid carcinoma. J Clin Endocrinol Metab. 2009;94:164–70.

14. Zhang Y, Jia S, Liu Y, Li B, Wang Z, Lu H, Zhu C. A clinical study of all-trans-retinoid-induced differentiation therapy of advanced thyroid cancer. Nucl Med Commun. 2007;28:251–5.
15. Grunwald F, Pakos E, Bender H, Menzel C, Otte R, Palmedo H, Pfeifer U, Biersack HJ. Redifferentiation therapy with retinoic acid in follicular thyroid cancer. J Nucl Med. 1998;39:1555–8.
16. Gruning T, Tiepolt C, Zophel K, Bredow J, Kropp J, Franke WG. Retinoic acid for redifferentiation of thyroid cancer – does it hold its promise? Eur J Endocrinol. 2003;148:395–402.
17. Haugen BR, Larson LL, Pugazhenthi U, Hays WR, Klopper JP, Kramer CA, Sharma V. Retinoic acid and retinoid X receptors are differentially expressed in thyroid cancer and thyroid carcinoma cell lines and predict response to treatment with retinoids. J Clin Endocrinol Metab. 2004;89:272–80.
18. Knauf JA, Fagin JA. Role of MAPK pathway oncoproteins in thyroid cancer pathogenesis and as drug targets. Curr Opin Cell Biol. 2009;21:296–303.
19. Knauf JA, Ma X, Smith EP, Zhang L, Mitsutake N, Liao XH, Refetoff S, Nikiforov YE, Fagin JA. Targeted expression of BRAFV600E in thyroid cells of transgenic mice results in papillary thyroid cancers that undergo dedifferentiation. Cancer Res. 2005;65:4238–45.
20. Mitsutake N, Knauf JA, Mitsutake S, Mesa Jr C, Zhang L, Fagin JA. Conditional BRAFV600E expression induces DNA synthesis, apoptosis, dedifferentiation, and chromosomal instability in thyroid PCCL3 cells. Cancer Res. 2005;65:2465–73.
21. Chakravarty D, Santos E, Ryder M, Knauf JA, Liao XH, West BL, Bollag G, Kolesnick R, Thin TH, Rosen N, Zanzonico P, Larson SM, Refetoff S, Ghossein R, Fagin JA. Small-molecule MAPK inhibitors restore radioiodine incorporation in mouse thyroid cancers with conditional BRAF activation. J Clin Invest. 2011;121:4700–11.
22. Ho AL, Grewal RK, Leboeuf R, Sherman EJ, Pfister DG, Deandreis D, Pentlow KS, Zanzonico PB, Haque S, Gavane S, Ghossein RA, Ricarte-Filho JC, Dominguez JM, Shen R, Tuttle RM, Larson SM, Fagin JA. Selumetinib-enhanced radioiodine uptake in advanced thyroid cancer. N Engl J Med. 2013;368:623–32.
23. Jhiang SM. Regulation of sodium/iodide symporter. Rev Endocr Metab Disord. 2000;1:205–15.
24. Liu YY, Zhang X, Ringel MD, Jhiang SM. Modulation of sodium iodide symporter expression and function by LY294002, Akti-1/2 and rapamycin in thyroid cells. Endocr Relat Cancer. 2012;19:291–304.
25. DeGroot LJ, Zhang R. Clinical review 131: gene therapy for thyroid cancer: where do we stand? J Clin Endocrinol Metab. 2001;86:2923–8.
26. DeGroot LJ, Zhang R. Viral mediated gene therapy for the management of metastatic thyroid carcinoma. Curr Drug Targets Immune Endocr Metabol Disord. 2004;4:235–44.
27. Schmutzler C, Koehrle J. Innovative strategies for the treatment of thyroid cancer. Eur J Endocrinol. 2000;143:15–24.
28. Folkman J. Tumor angiogenesis: therapeutic implications. N Engl J Med. 1971;285:1182–6.
29. Giatromanolaki A, Lyberakidis G, Lyratzopoulos N, Koukourakis MI, Sivridis E, Manolas C. Angiogenesis and angiogenic factor expression in thyroid cancer. J BUON. 2010;15:357–61.
30. Cooney MM, Radivoyevitch T, Dowlati A, Overmoyer B, Levitan N, Robertson K, Levine SL, DeCaro K, Buchter C, Taylor A, Stambler BS, Remick SC. Cardiovascular safety profile of combretastatin a4 phosphate in a single-dose phase I study in patients with advanced cancer. Clin Cancer Res. 2004;10:96–100.
31. Dowlati A, Robertson K, Cooney M, Petros WP, Stratford M, Jesberger J, Rafie N, Overmoyer B, Makkar V, Stambler B, Taylor A, Waas J, Lewin JS, McCrae KR, Remick SC. A phase I pharmacokinetic and translational study of the novel vascular targeting agent combretastatin a-4 phosphate on a single-dose intravenous schedule in patients with advanced cancer. Cancer Res. 2002;62:3408–16.
32. Mooney CJ, Nagaiah G, Fu P, Wasman JK, Cooney MM, Savvides PS, Bokar JA, Dowlati A, Wang D, Agarwala SS, Flick SM, Hartman PH, Ortiz JD, Lavertu PN, Remick SC. A phase II trial of fosbretabulin in advanced anaplastic thyroid carcinoma and correlation of baseline serum-soluble intracellular adhesion molecule-1 with outcome. Thyroid. 2009;19:233–40.
33. Ain KB, Lee C, Williams KD. Phase II trial of thalidomide for therapy of radioiodine-unresponsive and rapidly progressive thyroid carcinomas. Thyroid. 2007;17:663–70.
34. Sherman SI. Targeted therapies for thyroid tumors. Mod Pathol. 2011;24 Suppl 2:S44–52.
35. Nikiforova MN, Wald AI, Roy S, Durso MB, Nikiforov YE. Targeted next-generation sequencing panel (ThyroSeq) for detection of mutations in thyroid cancer. J Clin Endocrinol Metab. 2013;98:E1852–60.
36. Ricarte-Filho JC, Ryder M, Chitale DA, Rivera M, Heguy A, Ladanyi M, Janakiraman M, Solit D, Knauf JA, Tuttle RM, Ghossein RA, Fagin JA. Mutational profile of advanced primary and metastatic radioactive iodine-refractory thyroid cancers reveals distinct pathogenetic roles for BRAF, PIK3CA, and AKT1. Cancer Res. 2009;69:4885–93.
37. Xing M. Molecular pathogenesis and mechanisms of thyroid cancer. Nat Rev Cancer. 2013;13:184–99.
38. Demeure MJ, Aziz M, Rosenberg R, Gurley SD, Bussey KJ, Carpten JD. Whole-genome sequencing of an aggressive BRAF wild-type papillary thyroid cancer identified EML4-ALK translocation as a therapeutic target. World Journal of Surgery. 2014;38(6):1296–305.
39. Kelly LM, Barila G, Liu P, Evdokimova VN, Trivedi S, Panebianco F, Gandhi M, Carty SE, Hodak SP, Luo J, Dacic S, Yu YP, Nikiforova MN, Ferris RL, Altschuler DL, Nikiforov YE. Identification of the transforming STRN-ALK fusion as a potential therapeutic target in the aggressive forms of thyroid cancer. Proc Natl Acad Sci U S A. 2014;111:4233–8.
40. Kebebew E. Hereditary non-medullary thyroid cancer. World J Surg. 2008;32:678–82.
41. American Thyroid Association Guidelines Task F, Kloos RT, Eng C, Evans DB, Francis GL, Gagel RF, Gharib H, Moley JF, Pacini F, Ringel MD, Schlumberger M, Wells Jr SA. Medullary thyroid cancer: management guidelines of the American Thyroid Association. Thyroid. 2009;19:565–612.
42. Kloos RT, Ringel MD, Knopp MV, Hall NC, King M, Stevens R, Liang J, Wakely Jr PE, Vasko VV, Saji M, Rittenberry J, Wei L, Arbogast D, Collamore M, Wright JJ, Grever M, Shah MH. Phase II trial of sorafenib in metastatic thyroid cancer. J Clin Oncol. 2009;27:1675–84.
43. Xing M, Alzahrani AS, Carson KA, Viola D, Elisei R, Bendlova B, Yip L, Mian C, Vianello F, Tuttle RM, Robenshtok E, Fagin JA, Puxeddu E, Fugazzola L, Czarniecka A, Jarzab B, O'Neill CJ, Sywak MS, Lam AK, Riesco-Eizaguirre G, Santisteban P, Nakayama H, Tufano RP, Pai SI, Zeiger MA, Westra WH, Clark DP, Clifton-Bligh R, Sidransky D, Ladenson PW, Sykorova V. Association between BRAF V600E mutation and mortality in patients with papillary thyroid cancer. JAMA. 2013;309:1493–501.
44. Landa I, Ganly I, Chan TA, Mitsutake N, Matsuse M, Ibrahimpasic T, Ghossein RA, Fagin JA. Frequent somatic TERT promoter mutations in thyroid cancer: higher prevalence in advanced forms of the disease. J Clin Endocrinol Metab. 2013;98:E1562–6.
45. Liu X, Qu S, Liu R, Sheng C, Shi X, Zhu G, Murugan AK, Guan H, Yu H, Wang Y, Sun H, Shan Z, Teng W, Xing M. TERT promoter mutations and their association with BRAF V600E mutation and aggressive clinicopathological characteristics of thyroid cancer. J Clin Endocrinol Metab. 2014;99:E1130–6. jc20134048.
46. Druker BJ, Sawyers CL, Kantarjian H, Resta DJ, Reese SF, Ford JM, Capdeville R, Talpaz M. Activity of a specific inhibitor of the BCR-ABL tyrosine kinase in the blast crisis of chronic myeloid

leukemia and acute lymphoblastic leukemia with the Philadelphia chromosome. N Engl J Med. 2001;344:1038–42.
47. Heinrich MC, Corless CL, Demetri GD, Blanke CD, von Mehren M, Joensuu H, McGreevey LS, Chen CJ, Van den Abbeele AD, Druker BJ, Kiese B, Eisenberg B, Roberts PJ, Singer S, Fletcher CD, Silberman S, Dimitrijevic S, Fletcher JA. Kinase mutations and imatinib response in patients with metastatic gastrointestinal stromal tumor. J Clin Oncol. 2003;21:4342–9.
48. Paez JG, Janne PA, Lee JC, Tracy S, Greulich H, Gabriel S, Herman P, Kaye FJ, Lindeman N, Boggon TJ, Naoki K, Sasaki H, Fujii Y, Eck MJ, Sellers WR, Johnson BE, Meyerson M. EGFR mutations in lung cancer: correlation with clinical response to gefitinib therapy. Science. 2004;304:1497–500.
49. Sordella R, Bell DW, Haber DA, Settleman J. Gefitinib-sensitizing EGFR mutations in lung cancer activate anti-apoptotic pathways. Science. 2004;305:1163–7.
50. Brose MS, Nutting CM, Jarzab B, Elisei R, Siena S, Bastholt L, de la Fouchardiere C, Pacini F, Paschke R, Shong YK, Sherman SI, Smit JW, Chung J, Kappeler C, Pena C, Molnar I, Schlumberger MJ, on behalf of the Decision investigators. Sorafenib in radioactive iodine-refractory, locally advanced or metastatic differentiated thyroid cancer: a randomised, double-blind, phase 3 trial. Lancet. 2014;384:319–28.
51. Wells Jr SA, Robinson BG, Gagel RF, Dralle H, Fagin JA, Santoro M, Baudin E, Elisei R, Jarzab B, Vasselli JR, Read J, Langmuir P, Ryan AJ, Schlumberger MJ. Vandetanib in patients with locally advanced or metastatic medullary thyroid cancer: a randomized, double-blind phase III trial. J Clin Oncol. 2012;30:134–41.
52. Elisei R, Schlumberger MJ, Muller SP, Schoffski P, Brose MS, Shah MH, Licitra L, Jarzab B, Medvedev V, Kreissl MC, Niederle B, Cohen EE, Wirth LJ, Ali H, Hessel C, Yaron Y, Ball D, Nelkin B, Sherman SI. Cabozantinib in progressive medullary thyroid cancer. J Clin Oncol. 2013;31:3639–46.
53. Kim CS, Vasko VV, Kato Y, Kruhlak M, Saji M, Cheng SY, Ringel MD. AKT activation promotes metastasis in a mouse model of follicular thyroid carcinoma. Endocrinology. 2005;146:4456–63.
54. Shinohara M, Chung YJ, Saji M, Ringel MD. AKT in thyroid tumorigenesis and progression. Endocrinology. 2007;148:942–7.
55. Xing M, Haugen BR, Schlumberger M. Progress in molecular-based management of differentiated thyroid cancer. Lancet. 2013;381:1058–69.
56. Chapman PB, Hauschild A, Robert C, Haanen JB, Ascierto P, Larkin J, Dummer R, Garbe C, Testori A, Maio M, Hogg D, Lorigan P, Lebbe C, Jouary T, Schadendorf D, Ribas A, O'Day SJ, Sosman JA, Kirkwood JM, Eggermont AM, Dreno B, Nolop K, Li J, Nelson B, Hou J, Lee RJ, Flaherty KT, McArthur GA, Group B-S. Improved survival with vemurafenib in melanoma with BRAF V600E mutation. N Engl J Med. 2011;364:2507–16.
57. Lacouture ME, Duvic M, Hauschild A, Prieto VG, Robert C, Schadendorf D, Kim CC, McCormack CJ, Myskowski PL, Spleiss O, Trunzer K, Su F, Nelson B, Nolop KB, Grippo JF, Lee RJ, Klimek MJ, Troy JL, Joe AK. Analysis of dermatologic events in vemurafenib-treated patients with melanoma. Oncologist. 2013;18:314–22.
58. Palacios C, Yerbes R, Sanchez-Perez T, Martin-Perez R, Cano-Gonzalez A, Lopez-Rivas A. The long and winding road to cancer treatment: the trail system. Current Pharmaceutical Design. 2014;20(17):2819–33.
59. Ahmad M, Shi Y. TRAIL-induced apoptosis of thyroid cancer cells: potential for therapeutic intervention. Oncogene. 2000;19: 3363–71.
60. Bretz JD, Rymaszewski M, Arscott PL, Myc A, Ain KB, Thompson NW, Baker Jr JR. TRAIL death pathway expression and induction in thyroid follicular cells. J Biol Chem. 1999;274:23627–32.
61. Mitsiades N, Poulaki V, Mitsiades CS, Koutras DA, Chrousos GP. Apoptosis induced by FasL and TRAIL/Apo2L in the pathogenesis of thyroid diseases. Trends Endocrinol Metab. 2001;12:384–90.
62. Shimura H, Suzuki H, Miyazaki A, Furuya F, Ohta K, Haraguchi K, Endo T, Onaya T. Transcriptional activation of the thyroglobulin promoter directing suicide gene expression by thyroid transcription factor-1 in thyroid cancer cells. Cancer Res. 2001;61:3640–6.
63. Casterline PF, Jaques DA, Blom H, Wartofsky L. Anaplastic giant and spindle-cell carcinoma of the thyroid: a different therapeutic approach. Cancer. 1980;45:1689–92.
64. Gunda V, Cogdill AP, Bernasconi MJ, Wargo JA, Parangi S. Potential role of 5-aza-2′-deoxycytidine induced MAGE-A4 expression in immunotherapy for anaplastic thyroid cancer. Surgery. 2013;154:1456–62; discussion 1462.
65. Schott M, Feldkamp J, Klucken M, Kobbe G, Scherbaum WA, Seissler J. Calcitonin-specific antitumor immunity in medullary thyroid carcinoma following dendritic cell vaccination. Cancer Immunol Immunother. 2002;51:663–8.
66. Schott M, Scherbaum WA, Seissler J. Dendritic cell-based immunotherapy in thyroid malignancies. Curr Drug Targets Immune Endocr Metabol Disord. 2004;4:245–51.
67. Ma Y, McCarty SK, Kapuriya NP, Brendel VJ, Wang C, Zhang X, Jarjoura D, Saji M, Chen CS, Ringel MD. Development of p21 activated kinase-targeted multikinase inhibitors that inhibit thyroid cancer cell migration. J Clin Endocrinol Metab. 2013;98:E1314–22.
68. Schweppe RE, Kerege AA, French JD, Sharma V, Grzywa RL, Haugen BR. Inhibition of Src with AZD0530 reveals the Src-Focal Adhesion kinase complex as a novel therapeutic target in papillary and anaplastic thyroid cancer. J Clin Endocrinol Metab. 2009;94:2199–203.
69. Vu-Phan D, Grachtchouk V, Yu J, Colby LA, Wicha MS, Koenig RJ. The thyroid cancer PAX8-PPARG fusion protein activates Wnt/TCF-responsive cells that have a transformed phenotype. Endocr Relat Cancer. 2013;20:725–39.

Potential Approaches to Chemotherapy of Thyroid Cancer in the Future

105

David A. Liebner, Sigurdis Haraldsdottir, and Manisha H. Shah

Introduction

Molecular studies have led to an increased appreciation for the heterogeneity of thyroid neoplasms, and recent work has outlined the importance of hereditary predisposition, somatic mutation, epigenetic modulation, and tumor microenvironment and their contributions to tumor histology, clinical presentation, and prognosis. Preclinical data has supported the role of several new targets in the advanced thyroid cancer, which are summarized in Table 105.1. Clinical trials in advanced thyroid cancer are outlined in Table 105.2. Selected targets are discussed below.

D.A. Liebner, MD
Division of Medical Oncology, Department of Internal Medicine, The Ohio State University, 3186 Leesville Way, Columbus, OH, USA

Department of Biomedical Informatics, The Ohio State University, Columbus, OH, USA
e-mail: david.liebner@osumc.edu

S. Haraldsdottir, MD
Division of Medical Oncology, Department of Internal Medicine, The Ohio State University Comprehensive Cancer Center, Columbus, OH, USA
e-mail: sigurdis.haraldsdottir@osumc.edu

M.H. Shah, MD (✉)
Division of Medical Oncology, Department of Internal Medicine, The James Cancer Hospital and Solove Research Institute, 320 West 10th Avenue A438 Starling Loving Hall, Columbus, OH 43210, USA
e-mail: Manisha.Shah@osumc.edu

Novel Targets

VEGF-Mediated Neovascularization

Thyroid cancers are highly vascular tumors, and both preclinical and clinical studies have demonstrated increased expression of vascular endothelial growth factor (VEGF) [29–34], which has been correlated with clinical outcome [35,36]. Many small-molecule tyrosine kinase inhibitors that have been recently approved or are under development for advanced thyroid cancer have activity against the VEGF receptor (VEGFR), including axitinib, cabozantinib, motesanib, sorafenib, sunitinib, and vandetanib [37–43]. The humanized, anti-VEGF murine monoclonal antibody bevacizumab binds to circulating VEGF and impairs endothelial cell migration and tumor neovascularization [44]. Bevacizumab has shown activity in murine models of thyroid cancer [28] and is currently under investigation in combination with doxorubicin in anaplastic thyroid cancer (NCT00804830).

RET

Approximately 96 % of families with hereditary medullary thyroid cancer have identifiable germline mutations in the RET gene [45], and up to 65 % of individuals with sporadic medullary thyroid cancer have somatic RET mutations [46]. Vandetanib, which has recently been approved for advanced, unresectable, progressive, or symptomatic medullary thyroid cancer, has activity against both mutant and oncogenic RET [47]. Several other tyrosine kinase inhibitors in development for advanced medullary thyroid cancer also have some activity against RET, including cabozantinib (XL184), motesanib, sorafenib, and sunitinib. Additionally, oncogenic translocations of *RET* and *PTC* (*RET/PTC* rearrangements) have been documented in 3–60 % of papillary thyroid cancer

L. Wartofsky, D. Van Nostrand (eds.), *Thyroid Cancer*, DOI 10.1007/978-1-4939-3314-3_105

Table 105.1 Selected investigational therapeutic drug targets for advanced thyroid cancer

Potential target	Reference(s)
AKT	[1,2]
ALK	[3]
BRAF (V600E mutant)	[4,5]
Estrogen receptor	[6]
FOXO3a	[7]
HDAC, DAC inhibition	[8–10]
HIF-1α, HSP90	[11]
HMGA CoA reductase	[12,13]
Lithium response pathways (GSK-3ss)	[14]
MEK	[15]
microRNA (MiR-886-3p, MiR-146b-5p)	[16,17]
mTOR	[18,19]
p53	[20]
PAX8/PPARγ fusion	[21]
PI3K	[22,23]
Proteasome	[24,25]
RET/PTC fusion	[26,27]
VEGF	[28]

[48–51]. Gonçalves and colleagues [26] reported that treatment of RET/PTC mutant papillary thyroid cancer cells with orthovanadate resulted in increased phosphorylation of tyrosine 451 of RET/PTC and increased activation of the mTOR/S6R branch of AKT-associated signaling and were associated with apoptosis. The exact mechanism of action is unknown. Raouane and associates [27] showed the feasibility of downregulating the RET/PTC fusion oncogene with a conjugated siRNA, with associated inhibition of tumor growth in a mouse model.

RAF

Mutations in BRAF are seen in approximately 36–69 % of differentiated thyroid cancers and a subset of anaplastic thyroid cancers, with the BRAF V600E mutation being the most common [52–58]. Nehs and colleagues [4] reported that administration of the BRAF inhibitor PLX4720 could result in tumor regression in a murine model of BRAF V600E mutant anaplastic thyroid cancer. PLX4720 was similarly effective in a murine model of BRAF V600E mutant papillary thyroid cancer [5]. In the initial phase 1 trial of the potent BRAF inhibitor vemurafenib (PLX4032), three of five patients with papillary thyroid cancer had partial or complete responses, with the other two patients having stable disease lasting 8 and 11 months, respectively [59]. In a phase I trial with dabrafenib (GSK2118436) enrolling 14 patients with BRAF V600E-mutated papillary thyroid cancer, 3 out of 9 evaluable patients had a partial response [60]. Vemurafenib and dabrafenib are currently FDA approved for the treatment of BRAF V600E metastatic melanoma. Clinical trials of single-agent vemurafenib and dabrafenib as well as combination treatments are ongoing in patients with BRAF V600E-mutated thyroid cancer (NCT01286753, NCT01723202), and several other BRAF inhibitors are in development.

RAS

Between 20 % and 50 % of patients with follicular thyroid adenomas or carcinomas and 0–15 % of patients with PTC have point mutations in codon 61 of RAS [61,62]. Additionally, in patients with RET mutation-negative sporadic medullary thyroid cancer, RAS mutations can be found in up to 68 % of patients [63]. The farnesyltransferase inhibitor tipifarnib prevents farnesylation of RAS which is required to anchor RAS to the inner surface of the cell membrane, where it functions in signal transduction. A phase 1/2 study of tipifarnib given in combination with the multi-kinase inhibitor sorafenib reported objective responses in 6 of 35 patients, with an additional 12 patients having stable disease for at least 6 months [64].

MEK

MEK is an important downstream effector of RAF, RAS, and RET signaling via the MAPK pathway. Liu and colleagues reported that MEK inhibition was effective only in thyroid cancer cell lines with mutations in BRAF, with minimal or no activity in cell lines with wild-type BRAF [65]. Synergy has been observed in vitro when MEK inhibitors are used in combination other kinase inhibitors [1,15]. The MEK inhibitor, selumetinib, resensitized eight patients (40 %) with radioiodine-refractory (RAI) tumors and reduction in tumor size was seen in all of them following administration of iodine-131 [66]. The MEK inhibitor, trametinib, is being tested in combination with dabrafenib in a randomized phase 2 trial (NCT01723202).

PIK3

Phosphoinositide-3-kinase (PI3K) is an important signal transducer via the AKT pathway. Activating mutations and amplifications of the PI3K subunits are common in human malignancies, and approximately 31 % of follicular adenomas, 55 % of FTC, 24 % of PTC, and 58 % of ATC harbor at least one abnormality in PIK3 or the associated tumor-suppressor PTEN [67]. Furuya and colleagues [22] treated a cohort of mice that developed spontaneous follicular-like thyroid cancer with the PI3K inhibitor LY294002 and reported

Table 105.2 Ongoing clinical trials enrolling patients with advanced thyroid cancer

Treatment	Mechanism	Phase	Title	Clinical trial ID
Cytotoxic chemotherapy				
Bevacizumab + doxorubicin	Anti-VEGF, topoisomerase II inhibitor	Phase 2	Avastin and doxorubicin postoperatively for patients with anaplastic thyroid cancer	NCT00804830
Crolibulin + cisplatin	Microtubule inhibitor, DNA cross-linking	Phase 1/2	A phase I/II trial of crolibulin (EPC2407) plus cisplatin in adults with solid tumors with a focus on anaplastic thyroid cancer (ATC)	NCT01240590
Pemetrexed + paclitaxel	Antimetabolite, microtubule inhibitor	Phase 2	Pemetrexed + paclitaxel in patients with recurrent/advanced thyroid cancer	NCT00786552
Small-molecule targeted inhibitors				
Cediranib +/– lenalidomide	Multi-kinase inhibitor, multiple mechanisms	Phase 2	Cediranib maleate with or without lenalidomide in treating patients with thyroid cancer	NCT01208051
Dabrafenib + lapatinib	BRAF inhibitor, EGFR and HER-2 tyrosine kinase inhibitor	Phase 1	Dabrafenib and lapatinib ditosylate in treating patients with refractory thyroid cancer that cannot be removed by surgery	NCT01947023
Dabrafenib +/– trametinib	BRAF inhibitor with or without a MEK inhibitor	Phase 2	Dabrafenib with or without trametinib in treating patients with recurrent thyroid cancer	NCT01723202
Everolimus	mTOR inhibitor	Phase 2	RAD001 for patients with radioiodine-refractory thyroid cancer	NCT00936858
		Phase 2	Everolimus in treating patients with locally advanced or metastatic thyroid cancer	NCT01164176
		Phase 2	Everolimus in treating patients with progressive or recurrent, unresectable, or metastatic thyroid cancer	NCT01118065
Everolimus + sorafenib	mTOR inhibitor, multi-kinase inhibitor	Phase 2	Study of everolimus and sorafenib in patients with advanced thyroid cancer who progressed on sorafenib alone	NCT01263951
		Phase 2	Evaluating the combination of everolimus and sorafenib in the treatment of radioactive iodine-refractory thyroid cancer	NCT01141309
Pasireotide + everolimus	Somatostatin analogue, mTOR inhibitor	Phase 2	A trial of pasireotide and everolimus in adult patients with radioiodine-refractory differentiated and medullary thyroid cancer	NCT01270321
Pazopanib	Multi-kinase inhibitor	Phase 2	Pazopanib in treating patients with advanced thyroid cancer	NCT00625846
Ponatinib	Multi-kinase inhibitor	Phase 2	Ponatinib for advanced medullary thyroid cancer	NCT01838642
Sunitinib	Multi-kinase inhibitor	Phase 2	Sutent adjunctive treatment of differentiated thyroid cancer	NCT00668811
Temsirolimus + sorafenib	mTOR inhibitor, multi-kinase inhibitor	Phase 2	Combination of temsirolimus and sorafenib in the treatment of radioactive iodine-refractory thyroid cancer	NCT01025453
Vandetanib + bortezomib	Multi-kinase inhibitor, proteasome inhibitor	Phase 1/2	A targeted Ph I/II trial of ZD6474 (vandetanib; ZACTIMA) plus the proteasome inhibitor, bortezomib (velcade (registered trademark)), in adults with solid tumors with a focus on hereditary or sporadic, locally advanced, or metastatic medullary thyroid Ca (MTC)	NCT00923247
Vemurafenib	BRAF inhibitor	Phase 2	A study of RO5185426 in patients with metastatic or unresectable papillary thyroid cancer positive for the BRAF V600 mutation	NCT01286753
Gene therapy				
rAd-p53	Gene therapy	Phase 4	rAd-p53 gene therapy for advanced malignant thyroid tumors	NCT00902122
Epigenetic modulation/radioiodine resensitization				
Alpha-lipoic acids	Redifferentiation agent	Phase 2	Redifferentiation therapy using alpha-lipoic acid in thyroid cancer	NCT01396733
Panobinostat	Deacetylase inhibitor	Phase 2	Trial of LBH589 in metastatic thyroid cancer	NCT01013597
Pazopanib + iodine I-131	Multi-kinase inhibitor	Phase 1	Iodine I 131 and pazopanib hydrochloride in treating patients with recurrent and/or metastatic thyroid cancer previously treated with iodine I 131 that cannot be removed by surgery	NCT01413113
Valproic acid	Histone deacetylase inhibitor	Phase 2	A phase II trial of valproic acid in patients with advanced thyroid cancers of follicular cell origin	NCT01182285
Other				
Lithium	Multiple	Phase 2	An initial study of lithium in patients with medullary thyroid cancer	NCT00582712

decreased tumor cell growth and impaired metastatic spread of the tumor. A separate report suggested that treatment of papillary thyroid cancer cells with LY294002 increases expression of the sodium iodide symporter (NIS) with associated increases in radioiodide uptake [23]. Several PIK3 inhibitors are in development for human malignancies.

AKT

Mutations in AKT are uncommon in thyroid cancer, but AKT activation via aberrant activation of upstream signaling pathways, such as PIK3 overexpression, PTEN inactivation, and RAS GTPase activity, occurs frequently in advanced thyroid malignancies [68]. Thyroid cancer cell lines characterized by mutations which upregulate AKT activity were sensitive to treatment with the direct AKT inhibitor MK2206; cell lines lacking AKT pathway-specific mutations did not respond to treatment [2]. Salaun and colleagues [28] pursued an alternative approach by transfecting follicular thyroid cancer cells with a nonfunctional form of the AKT co-signaling molecule FOXO3a, resulting in tumor growth arrest in a murine model. Thus, FOXO3a may be an additional target in suppressing AKT signaling.

mTOR

AKT signaling is mediated in part via the mTOR pathway, which is known to be important in thyroid cancer. Patients with medullary thyroid cancer and aggressive variants of papillary thyroid cancer have been shown to demonstrate increased levels of activation of mTOR-associated signaling proteins [18]. Treatment of medullary thyroid cancer cells with mTOR inhibitors such as rapamycin and everolimus has been shown to result in cell death and tumor inhibition, and case responses have also suggested potential activity of everolimus in patients with medullary thyroid cancer [18,19]. A phase 2 trial with everolimus in locally advanced or metastatic thyroid cancer of all histologies showed disease control rate in 31 (81 %) patients >12 weeks with two patients (5 %) having a partial response (one papillary and one follicular thyroid cancer) [69].

ALK

Mutations in the ALK gene are characteristic of anaplastic T-cell lymphoma and ALK rearrangements are seen in a small subset of patients with non-small cell lung cancer. Murugan and Xing [3] identified activating mutations in ALK in 11 % of patients with anaplastic thyroid cancer; similar mutations were not seen in well-differentiated thyroid cancers. ALK inhibition has proved to be of clinical benefit in non-small cell lung cancer [70], and further investigation is merited in thyroid cancer.

p53

p53 is a critical regulator of the cell cycle and functions as a tumor-suppressor gene. The COSMIC database of somatic mutations in cancer reports p53 mutations in approximately 16 % of patients with thyroid cancer and up to 65 % of patients with anaplastic thyroid cancer [71]. Thyrocyte-specific inactivation of both p53 and PTEN results in spontaneous development of undifferentiated anaplastic-like thyroid cancers in a mouse model [72]. Messina and colleagues [20] were able to restore the activity of mutant p53 in undifferentiated thyroid cancer cell lines with the small molecule Prima-1, upregulating p53 target genes and increasing the sensitivity of the treated cell lines to cytotoxic chemotherapy with doxorubicin or cisplatin. A clinical trial of p53 gene therapy in thyroid cancer is ongoing (NCT00902122).

Epigenetic Modulation

Promoter hypermethylation and histone deacetylation are at least partially responsible for the loss of radioiodine sensitivity in certain differentiated thyroid cancers [73–78]. Hypermethylation of tumor suppressors is also very common, affecting PTEN in 46 % of papillary thyroid carcinomas and 85 % of follicular adenomas and carcinomas, p16 in nearly 30 % of DTC, RAS association family 1A tumor-suppressor gene in roughly 38 % of all thyroid carcinomas, and Rap1 GTPase-activating protein (Rap1GAP) in up to 71 % of PTC [79–82]. Preclinical assessments of the activity of deacetylase inhibitors have been promising [8–10], but clinical activity in an early-phase clinical trial of the histone deacetylase inhibitor vorinostat was limited, with no patient showing an objective response; one of three patients with papillary thyroid cancer did demonstrate reacquisition of radioiodine uptake [83]. Further investigation is ongoing.

Other Targets

Preclinical work has identified multiple other potential therapeutic targets, including estrogen receptor blockade [6], HIF-1 alpha and HSP90 inhibition [11], HMG CoA reductase inhibition [12,13], proteasome blockade [24,25], microRNA targeting and inhibition [16,17], PPARγ inhibition [21], and lithium response pathways [14]. Several of these are currently being investigated in clinical trials.

Summary

The last 10 years has seen an explosion in understanding the molecular pathophysiology of thyroid cancer. Targeted therapies are currently being investigated intensively, with multiple novel agents entering human clinical trials. Such work has led to the recent approval of vandetanib and cabozantinib in advanced medullary thyroid cancer, the first targeted therapies to be approved by the FDA for thyroid cancer. For a continuing updated list of thyroid cancer clinical trials, the reader is directed to www.cancer.gov and www.clinicaltrials.gov. For recent abstracts or preclinical and clinical studies in progress, the research meeting proceedings of the American Association for Cancer Research can be searched at www.aacr.org and of the American Society of Clinical Oncology www.asco.org.

References

1. Liu R, Liu D, Xing M. The Akt inhibitor MK2206 synergizes, but perifosine antagonizes, the BRAFV600E inhibitor PLX4032 and the MEK1/2 inhibitor AZD6244 in the inhibition of thyroid cancer cells. J Clin Endocrinol Metab. 2011.
2. Liu R, et al. The Akt-specific inhibitor MK2206 selectively inhibits thyroid cancer cells harboring mutations that can activate the PI3K/Akt pathway. J Clin Endocrinol Metab. 2011;96(4):E577–85.
3. Murugan AK, Xing M. Anaplastic thyroid cancers harbor novel oncogenic mutations of the ALK gene. Cancer Res. 2011;71(13):4403–11.
4. Nehs MA, et al. Late Intervention with anti-BRAFV600E therapy induces tumor regression in an orthotopic mouse model of human anaplastic thyroid cancer. Endocrinology. 2011.
5. Nucera C, et al. Targeting BRAFV600E with PLX4720 displays potent antimigratory and anti-invasive activity in preclinical models of human thyroid cancer. Oncologist. 2011;16(3):296–309.
6. Somjen D, et al. Anti-thyroid cancer properties of a novel isoflavone derivative, 7-(O)-carboxymethyl daidzein conjugated to N-t-Boc-hexylenediamine in vitro and in vivo. J Steroid Biochem Mol Biol. 2011;126(3–5):95–103.
7. Hong ZY, et al. Inhibition of Akt/FOXO3a signaling by constitutively active FOXO3a suppresses growth of follicular thyroid cancer cell lines. Cancer Lett. 2012;314(1):34–40.
8. Catalano MG, et al. Cytotoxic activity of the histone deacetylase inhibitor panobinostat (LBH589) in anaplastic thyroid cancer in vitro and in vivo. Int J Cancer. 2012;130(3):694–704.
9. Chen ST, et al. Down-regulation of matrix metalloproteinase-7 inhibits metastasis of human anaplastic thyroid cancer cell line. Clin Exp Metastasis. 2012;29(1):71–82.
10. Borbone E, et al. Histone deacetylase inhibitors induce thyroid cancer-specific apoptosis through proteasome-dependent inhibition of TRAIL degradation. Oncogene. 2010;29(1):105–16.
11. Mo JH, et al. HIF-1alpha and HSP90: target molecules selected from tumorigenic papillary thyroid carcinoma cell line. Cancer Sci. 2011.
12. Shui HA, et al. Proteomics and bioinformatics analysis of lovastatin-induced differentiation in ARO cells. J Proteomics. 2011.
13. Zeybek ND, et al. Rosuvastatin induces apoptosis in cultured human papillary thyroid cancer cells. J Endocrinol. 2011;210(1):105–15.
14. Adler JT, et al. Inhibition of growth in medullary thyroid cancer cells with histone deacetylase inhibitors and lithium chloride. J Surg Res. 2010;159(2):640–4.
15. Koh YW, et al. Sorafenib and Mek inhibition are synergistic in medullary thyroid carcinoma in vitro. Endocr Relat Cancer. 2011.
16. Xiong Y, et al. MiR-886-3p regulates cell proliferation and migration, and is dysregulated in familial non-medullary thyroid cancer. PLoS One. 2011;6(10):e24717.
17. Geraldo MV, Yamashita AS, Kimura ET. MicroRNA miR-146b-5p regulates signal transduction of TGF-beta by repressing SMAD4 in thyroid cancer. Oncogene. 2011.
18. Kouvaraki MA, et al. Activation of mTOR signaling in medullary and aggressive papillary thyroid carcinomas. Surgery. 2011;150(6):1258–65.
19. Faggiano A, et al. Everolimus is an active agent in medullary thyroid cancer: a clinical and in vitro study. J Cell Mol Med. 2011.
20. Messina RL, et al. Reactivation of p53 mutants by p53 reactivation and induction of massive apoptosis in thyroid cancer cells. Int J Cancer. 2011.
21. Dobson ME, et al. Pioglitazone induces a proadipogenic antitumor response in mice with PAX8-PPARgamma fusion protein thyroid carcinoma. Endocrinology. 2011;152(11):4455–65.
22. Furuya F, et al. Inhibition of phosphatidylinositol 3-kinase delays tumor progression and blocks metastatic spread in a mouse model of thyroid cancer. Carcinogenesis. 2007;28(12):2451–8.
23. Kogai T, et al. Phosphoinositide-3-kinase inhibition induces sodium/iodide symporter expression in rat thyroid cells and human papillary thyroid cancer cells. J Endocrinol. 2008;199(2):243–52.
24. Du ZX, et al. Proteasome inhibition induces a p38 MAPK pathway-dependent antiapoptotic program via Nrf2 in thyroid cancer cells. J Clin Endocrinol Metab. 2011;96(5):E763–71.
25. Gao YY, et al. Implication of oxygen-regulated protein 150 (ORP150) in apoptosis induced by proteasome inhibitors in human thyroid cancer cells. J Clin Endocrinol Metab. 2010;95(11):E319–26.
26. Goncalves AP, et al. Orthovanadate-induced cell death in RET/PTC1-harboring cancer cells involves the activation of caspases and altered signaling through PI3K/Akt/mTOR. Life Sci. 2011;89(11–12):371–7.
27. Raouane M, et al. Synthesis, characterization, and in vivo delivery of siRNA-squalene nanoparticles targeting fusion oncogene in papillary thyroid carcinoma. J Med Chem. 2011;54(12):4067–76.
28. Salaun PY, et al. Toxicity and efficacy of combined radioimmunotherapy and bevacizumab in a mouse model of medullary thyroid carcinoma. Cancer. 2010;116(4 Suppl):1053–8.
29. Viglietto G, et al. RET/PTC oncogene activation is an early event in thyroid carcinogenesis. Oncogene. 1995;11(6):1207–10.
30. Soh EY, et al. Thyroid-stimulating hormone promotes the secretion of vascular endothelial growth factor in thyroid cancer cell lines. Surgery. 1996;120(6):944–7.
31. Soh EY, et al. Vascular endothelial growth factor expression is higher in differentiated thyroid cancer than in normal or benign thyroid. J Clin Endocrinol Metab. 1997;82(11):3741–7.
32. Capp C, et al. Increased expression of vascular endothelial growth factor and its receptors, VEGFR-1 and VEGFR-2, in medullary thyroid carcinoma. Thyroid. 2010;20(8):863–71.
33. Tuttle RM, et al. Serum vascular endothelial growth factor levels are elevated in metastatic differentiated thyroid cancer but not increased by short-term TSH stimulation. J Clin Endocrinol Metab. 2002;87(4):1737–42.
34. Pasieka Z, et al. Evaluation of the levels of bFGF, VEGF, sICAM-1, and sVCAM-1 in serum of patients with thyroid cancer. Recent Results Cancer Res. 2003;162:189–94.
35. Lennard CM, et al. Intensity of vascular endothelial growth factor expression is associated with increased risk of recurrence and decreased disease-free survival in papillary thyroid cancer. Surgery. 2001;129(5):552–8.
36. Dhar DK, et al. Tumor vascularity predicts recurrence in differentiated thyroid carcinoma. Am J Surg. 1998;176(5):442–7.
37. Cohen EE, et al. Axitinib is an active treatment for all histologic subtypes of advanced thyroid cancer: results from a phase II study. J Clin Oncol. 2008;26(29):4708–13.

38. Exelixis. Exelixis' cabozantinib meets primary endpoint in phase 3 clinical trial for medullary thyroid cancer. 24 Oct 2011; Available from: http://www.exelixis.com/investors-media/press-releases.
39. Sherman SI, et al. Motesanib diphosphate in progressive differentiated thyroid cancer. N Engl J Med. 2008;359(1):31–42.
40. Schlumberger MJ, et al. Phase II study of safety and efficacy of motesanib in patients with progressive or symptomatic, advanced or metastatic medullary thyroid cancer. J Clin Oncol. 2009;27(23):3794–801.
41. Lam ET, et al. Phase II clinical trial of sorafenib in metastatic medullary thyroid cancer. J Clin Oncol. 2010;28(14):2323–30.
42. Carr LL, et al. Phase II study of daily sunitinib in FDG-PET-positive, iodine-refractory differentiated thyroid cancer and metastatic medullary carcinoma of the thyroid with functional imaging correlation. Clin Cancer Res. 2010;16(21):5260–8.
43. Wells S, et al. Vandetanib (VAN) in locally advanced or metastatic medullary thyroid cancer (MTC): a randomized, double-blind phase III trial (ZETA). J Clin Oncol. 2010;28:15s: p. abstr 5503.
44. Mukherji SK. Bevacizumab (Avastin). AJNR Am J Neuroradiol. 2010;31(2):235–6.
45. Eng C, et al. The relationship between specific RET proto-oncogene mutations and disease phenotype in multiple endocrine neoplasia type 2. International RET mutation consortium analysis. JAMA. 1996;276(19):1575–9.
46. Moura MM, et al. Correlation of RET somatic mutations with clinicopathological features in sporadic medullary thyroid carcinomas. Br J Cancer. 2009;100(11):1777–83.
47. Vitagliano D, et al. The tyrosine kinase inhibitor ZD6474 blocks proliferation of RET mutant medullary thyroid carcinoma cells. Endocr Relat Cancer. 2010;18(1):1–11.
48. Kondo T, Ezzat S, Asa SL. Pathogenetic mechanisms in thyroid follicular-cell neoplasia. Nat Rev Cancer. 2006;6(4):292–306.
49. Nikiforov YE. RET/PTC rearrangement in thyroid tumors. Endocr Pathol. 2002;13(1):3–16.
50. Tallini G, Asa SL. RET oncogene activation in papillary thyroid carcinoma. Adv Anat Pathol. 2001;8(6):345–54.
51. Santoro M, Melillo RM, Fusco A. RET/PTC activation in papillary thyroid carcinoma: European Journal of Endocrinology Prize Lecture. Eur J Endocrinol. 2006;155(5):645–53.
52. Cohen Y, et al. BRAF mutation in papillary thyroid carcinoma. J Natl Cancer Inst. 2003;95(8):625–7.
53. Kimura ET, et al. High prevalence of BRAF mutations in thyroid cancer: genetic evidence for constitutive activation of the RET/PTC-RAS-BRAF signaling pathway in papillary thyroid carcinoma. Cancer Res. 2003;63(7):1454–7.
54. Nikiforova MN, et al. BRAF mutations in thyroid tumors are restricted to papillary carcinomas and anaplastic or poorly differentiated carcinomas arising from papillary carcinomas. J Clin Endocrinol Metab. 2003;88(11):5399–404.
55. Trovisco V, et al. BRAF mutations are associated with some histological types of papillary thyroid carcinoma. J Pathol. 2004;202(2):247–51.
56. Xing M. BRAF mutation in thyroid cancer. Endocr Relat Cancer. 2005;12(2):245–62.
57. Begum S, et al. BRAF mutations in anaplastic thyroid carcinoma: implications for tumor origin, diagnosis and treatment. Mod Pathol. 2004;17(11):1359–63.
58. Soares P, et al. BRAF mutations typical of papillary thyroid carcinoma are more frequently detected in undifferentiated than in insular and insular-like poorly differentiated carcinomas. Virchows Arch. 2004;444(6):572–6.
59. Flaherty KT, et al. Inhibition of mutated, activated BRAF in metastatic melanoma. N Engl J Med. 2010;363(9):809–19.
60. Falchook GS, et al. Dabrafenib in patients with melanoma, untreated brain metastases, and other solid tumours: a phase 1 dose-escalation trial. Lancet. 2012;379(9829):1893–901.
61. Vasko V, et al. Specific pattern of RAS oncogene mutations in follicular thyroid tumors. J Clin Endocrinol Metab. 2003;88(6):2745–52.
62. Motoi N, et al. Role of ras mutation in the progression of thyroid carcinoma of follicular epithelial origin. Pathol Res Pract. 2000; 196(1):1–7.
63. Moura MM, et al. High prevalence of RAS mutations in RET-negative sporadic medullary thyroid carcinomas. J Clin Endocrinol Metab. 2011;96(5):E863–8.
64. Hong DS, et al. Inhibition of the Ras/Raf/MEK/ERK and RET kinase pathways with the combination of the multikinase inhibitor sorafenib and the farnesyltransferase inhibitor tipifarnib in medullary and differentiated thyroid malignancies. J Clin Endocrinol Metab. 2011;96(4):997–1005.
65. Liu D, et al. BRAF mutation-selective inhibition of thyroid cancer cells by the novel MEK inhibitor RDEA119 and genetic-potentiated synergism with the mTOR inhibitor temsirolimus. Int J Cancer. 2010;127(12):2965–73.
66. Ho AL, et al. Selumetinib-enhanced radioiodine uptake in advanced thyroid cancer. N Engl J Med. 2013;368(7):623–32.
67. Hou P, et al. Genetic alterations and their relationship in the phosphatidylinositol 3-kinase/Akt pathway in thyroid cancer. Clin Cancer Res. 2007;13(4):1161–70.
68. Viglietto G, et al. Contribution of PKB/AKT signaling to thyroid cancer. Front Biosci. 2011;16:1461–87.
69. Lim SM, et al. A multicenter, phase II trial of everolimus in locally advanced or metastatic thyroid cancer of all histologic subtypes. Ann Oncol. 2013;24(12):3089–94.
70. Kwak EL, et al. Anaplastic lymphoma kinase inhibition in non-small-cell lung cancer. N Engl J Med. 2010;363(18):1693–703.
71. Forbes SA, et al. COSMIC: mining complete cancer genomes in the Catalogue of Somatic Mutations in Cancer. Nucleic Acids Res. 2011;39(Database issue):D945–50.
72. Antico Arciuch VG, et al. Thyrocyte-specific inactivation of p53 and Pten results in anaplastic thyroid carcinomas faithfully recapitulating human tumors. Oncotarget. 2011;2:1109–26.
73. Venkataraman GM, et al. Restoration of iodide uptake in dedifferentiated thyroid carcinoma: relationship to human Na+/I-symporter gene methylation status. J Clin Endocrinol Metab. 1999;84(7):2449–57.
74. Xing M, et al. Methylation of the thyroid-stimulating hormone receptor gene in epithelial thyroid tumors: a marker of malignancy and a cause of gene silencing. Cancer Res. 2003;63(9):2316–21.
75. Hoque MO, et al. Quantitative assessment of promoter methylation profiles in thyroid neoplasms. J Clin Endocrinol Metab. 2005; 90(7):4011–8.
76. Xing M. Gene methylation in thyroid tumorigenesis. Endocrinology. 2007;148(3):948–53.
77. Furuya F, et al. Histone deacetylase inhibitors restore radioiodide uptake and retention in poorly differentiated and anaplastic thyroid cancer cells by expression of the sodium/iodide symporter thyroperoxidase and thyroglobulin. Endocrinology. 2004;145(6):2865–75.
78. Puppin C, et al. Effects of histone acetylation on sodium iodide symporter promoter and expression of thyroid-specific transcription factors. Endocrinology. 2005;146(9):3967–74.
79. Alvarez-Nunez F, et al. PTEN promoter methylation in sporadic thyroid carcinomas. Thyroid. 2006;16(1):17–23.
80. Elisei R, et al. Genetic and epigenetic alterations of the cyclin-dependent kinase inhibitors p15INK4b and p16INK4a in human thyroid carcinoma cell lines and primary thyroid carcinomas. Cancer. 1998;83(10):2185–93.
81. Nakamura N, et al. RASSF1A and NORE1A methylation and BRAFV600E mutations in thyroid tumors. Lab Invest. 2005;85(9):1065–75.
82. Zuo H, et al. Downregulation of Rap1GAP through epigenetic silencing and loss of heterozygosity promotes invasion and progression of thyroid tumors. Cancer Res. 2010;70(4):1389–97.
83. Woyach JA, et al. Lack of therapeutic effect of the histone deacetylase inhibitor vorinostat in patients with metastatic radioiodine-refractory thyroid carcinoma. J Clin Endocrinol Metab. 2009;94(1):164–70.

Part XIV

Additional Resources

106 Prophylaxis Against Radiation Exposure from Radioiodine

Arthur B. Schneider and James M. Smith

Introduction

The major cause of accidental exposure to radioactive iodine that would endanger a sizable population of individuals is its release from the core of a functioning nuclear power-generating facility. Because the half-lives of the iodine radionuclides of interest are 8 days or shorter, an accident at a reactor that has been inactive for a relatively brief period or a nuclear storage facility would not create a risk to the thyroid. For similar reasons, it is not likely that a terrorist act involving a "dirty bomb" would require prophylactic measures to protect the thyroid gland. The discussion that follows applies primarily to large populations exposed to volatile radioiodines rather than individuals who might be exposed in the setting of a scientific laboratory.

Protection against a nuclear accident includes sheltering from fallout, avoiding ingestion of contaminated food, and evacuation from the contaminated area. Milk is especially important because grazing animals harvest fallout from large areas and iodine is concentrated by the mammary glands into milk. In Belarus following the Chernobyl accident, a median of about 90 % of the thyroid radioactive iodine exposure in children came through the ingestion of milk [1]. Countermeasures, however, may be insufficient or too slow to provide complete thyroid protection, whereas blockade of thyroid iodine uptake by a sufficiently high blood level of stable iodide can be achieved quickly and even in advance of exposure. KI, of course, will only protect the thyroid gland and only against internal radiation from radioactive iodine.

The accident in 1986 at Chernobyl in the USSR (now Chornobyl in Ukraine) has provided answers to several questions: whether a nuclear power accident can indeed result in thyroid cancer, the magnitude of the risk from internal thyroid radiation, and whether high doses of potassium iodide (KI) can be safely administered to a large population [2, 3]. Fallout in the Bryansk oblast of Russia, more than 50 miles at its closest point to the Chornobyl reactor, has been associated with thyroid cancer in children [4]. This is well beyond the 10-mile radius recommended by the US Nuclear Regulatory Commission for the pre-distribution of potassium iodide (KI) tablets. Dose-response analyses from several studies indicate that the risk from internal radiation is similar in magnitude to that of external radiation [5, 6]. One case-control study showed an approximately threefold reduction in risk for children who were given potassium iodide whether they lived in areas with low or high soil iodine levels [7]. Side effects after administration of KI to millions of children and adults in Poland were uncommon, mild, and reversible [3]. Furthermore, as much as 30 % of thyroid radiation received by children who were evacuated from Pripyat, the closest village, and in other children as far away as Poland has been attributed to inhalation [3, 8]. A portion of the inhaled radionuclides can be radioiodines with half-lives measured in hours. Since this exposure would occur over a shorter time, it is possible that it would have a higher oncogenic potential for a given amount of radiation than the major component, ^{131}I [9].

Pharmacology of KI

The major blocking effect of excess iodine on thyroid iodine accumulation occurs at the basal membrane of the thyroid follicular cell [10]. The active transport of the

A.B. Schneider, MD, PhD (✉)
Section of Endocrinology, Diabetes and Metabolism, University of Illinois at Chicago, 1819 W Polk (MC 640), Chicago, IL 60612, USA
e-mail: abschnei@uic.edu

J.M. Smith, PhD
Division of Environmental Health, Emory University, Rollins School of Public Health, 518 Clifton Road, NE, Atlanta, GA 30322, USA
e-mail: jsmith9@emory.edu

L. Wartofsky, D. Van Nostrand (eds.), *Thyroid Cancer*, DOI 10.1007/978-1-4939-3314-3_106

very small physiological concentration of iodide by the Na/I symporter is overwhelmed by the much higher concentration derived from the recommended doses of KI (see below). The 100 mg of iodine in a 130 mg tablet of KI exceeds the normal dietary iodine intake (about 200 μg) by nearly three orders of magnitude. In addition, excess iodine near the apical cell membrane interferes with organification of thyroglobulin and thyroid hormone formation, and any iodide that enters the cell is rapidly excreted [11]. A third effect of excess iodine interferes with thyroid hormone release from the gland but this does not effectively compromise the major beneficial effect on iodine accumulation.

Potassium iodide, as a tablet or liquid, is rapidly absorbed from the intestinal tract and rapidly excreted in the urine [12]. As shown in Table 106.1, largely as predicted by modeling iodine kinetics, the greatest protection is provided when KI is given 1 h before exposure but is still substantial if it is given within 8 h after exposure [13, 14]. A more recent experimental study, using ^{123}I to estimate the effects of KI on ^{131}I, found somewhat smaller reductions of thyroid absorbed dose than shown in the table [15]. Specifically, given 2 h after ^{131}I, the new study finds that the averted dose is about 60 %, rather than 80 %, and at 8 h it is about 25 %, rather than 40 %. Of importance, the new data show that younger subjects have a more rapid clearance of iodine from the circulation, reducing the effect of KI in them. Therefore, the authors conclude, prompt administration of KI is especially important in younger people, presumably including children. For ongoing exposure to ^{131}I, daily administration of KI is needed for continued protection.

KI is currently available without a doctor's prescription as 130 mg and 65 mg tablets in individually sealed, lightproof wrapping and an oral solution containing 65 mg per ounce [16]. The tablets have an FDA-approved shelf life of 7 years and the US Nuclear Regulatory Commission believes that it is safe to take it beyond that [17, 18]. For infants (see below) smaller doses must be prepared, either by dissolving the tablet or diluting an available iodide solution. Detailed information for home preparation of solutions from 130 to 65 mg tablets have been provided on the Food and Drug Administration web site [19].

Table 106.1 KI protection against a single ^{131}I exposure

Hours between KI and ^{131}I ingestion	−96	−48	−1	0	2	3	8
Percent protection	Very little	≈80	Highest	98	80	60	40

Data at 0 and 3 h are experimental (see ref. [13]). Other data are derived from models (see Ref. [14])

Side Effects

Potential side effects of KI are thyroid-related (hypothyroidism, hyperthyroidism, neonatal goiter), gastrointestinal (nausea, vomiting, diarrhea, pain), allergy related (angioedema, arthralgia, eosinophilia, urticaria), and skin rashes.

Among 12,040 children living in Poland at the time of the Chornobyl accident, most of whom received a single dose of KI (15 mg for newborn infants, 50 mg for children under 5 years, 70 mg for others) but some of whom had multiple doses and a few of whom had been given tincture of iodine, non-thyroid side effects were mild and infrequent [3]. The most common were vomiting in 2.38 % and skin rashes in 1.07 %. Among 5,061 adults, most of whom had received one dose of 70 mg KI, vomiting was reported in 0.85 % and skin rashes in 1.24 %. It was estimated that only about 0.2 % of the population receiving KI had medically significant adverse reactions. Two adults with chronic obstructive lung disease and known sensitivity to iodides were hospitalized for acute respiratory distress.

In attempting to evaluate the occurrence of thyroid-related side effects in follow-up studies in Poland [3], no significant change in the prevalence of thyroid disease or abnormal thyroid function was detected except in the case of newborn infants. In 3,214 infants given KI during the first days of life and tested during the 3rd to 5th days, 12 (0.37 %) had elevated TSH. Although TSH returned to normal by the 16th to 20th day of life and follow-up in the second to third year of life detected no abnormality, the possibility of a subtle effect on cognitive development was not excluded.

Radiation Guidelines

As a result of the Chornobyl experience, the World Health Organization in 1999 [20] and the US Food and Drug Administration in 2001 [21] revised their published guidelines for iodine prophylaxis in radiation emergencies. Their recommendations are summarized in Table 106.2. Both organizations provide considerable background information and justification for their recommendations as part of their guidelines.

The differences are in the estimated thyroid radiation dose triggering KI administration to children and the KI dose to use for adolescent children. Both conclude that adults over 40 year should receive KI only to prevent thyroid gland damage by a high radiation dose. This is because their risk of radiation-induced thyroid cancer is very low and their risk of KI-induced thyroid-related side effects, especially transient hypo- and hyperthyroidism, is relatively high. The FDA Guidelines emphasize the safety of KI in children and young

Table 106.2 WHO and FDA guidelines for KI use in a radiation emergency

	Radiation dose threshold (cGy)[a]		KI dose (mg)	
	WHO 1999	FDA 2001	WHO 1999	FDA 2001
Adults >40 years	500	500	130	130
18–40 years	10	10	130	130
Pregnant or lactating	1	5	130	130
Adolescents	1	5	130	65–130[b]
Children 3–12 years	1	5	65	65
>1 month to 3 years	1	5	32	32
<1 month	1	5	16	16

[a]1 cGy, or 10 mGy is equivalent to 1 rad
[b]Dose can vary with age or body size

adults [21]. The infant's thyroid and probably the fetal thyroid after the first few months of gestation are both particularly susceptible to the carcinogenic effects of radiation, as well as to radiation-induced hypothyroidism. Because of their small size, the relative uptake of radioactive iodine (quantity per unit mass) is high. Therefore, it is especially important to provide protection with KI in these cases, but the lowest effective KI dose should be used [22].

In lactating mothers, the amount of iodide secreted in the milk is too low to protect the infant, so both mother and child should be given KI [23]. The US Centers for Disease Control and Prevention recommends "Women who are breastfeeding should take only one dose of KI if they have been internally contaminated with (or are likely to be internally contaminated with) radioactive iodine. Because radioactive iodine quickly gets into breast milk, CDC recommends that women internally contaminated with (or are likely to be internally contaminated with) radioactive iodine stop breastfeeding and feed their child baby formula or other food if it is available. If breast milk is the only food available for an infant, nursing should continue" [24, 24a].

An important element of any radiological emergency preparation plan is to have the capability to perform at least two major functions. First, the emergency response team should possess the capability of radiological monitoring to track the extent and progress of the environmental contamination. Secondly, those responsible for the response should have the capability (or ready access to those who do) of predicting radiation exposures to people who work or live in the vicinity of the accident, even those who might be exposed hundreds of miles or more from the accident site.

Predicting "downwind" radiation exposures to people involves specialists such as health physicists providing relevant input parameters into computer models. These programs, for example, as provided by the National Atmospheric Release Advisory Center, can furnish estimates of the dispersal of the radioactivity in air, at least within a broad range of likely values [25]. With this knowledge, other models can be used to project what quantity of the radioactivity will be inhaled from the passing plume or ingested from the contaminated water or foodstuff [26]. All such models, of course, require not only demographic information but also a myriad of assumptions about diets and lifestyles for the local populations and are therefore often highly uncertain. However, the underlying purpose of using models is to bring together with some rigor all that is known or can be reasonably assumed about the situation in order to arrive at best quantitative estimates of attained or predicted radiation doses to people.

Much has been learned over the years about significant pathways of intake for the radioiodines. Models, and tables derived from them, have been developed to describe how the isotopes are distributed to the thyroid and to estimate the radiation dose that the thyroid will likely receive. The International Commission on Radiological Protection (ICRP) provides "dose coefficients" by gender and age for radionuclides including those of iodine. The dose coefficient expresses the radiation dose over time ("committed dose") that the thyroid will receive for a unit intake of a radioiodine isotope, and the coefficients are listed for inhalation and ingestion pathways separately [27, 28].

As an example, suppose a radioactive plume of ^{131}I is released from a nuclear power plant accident. The health physicists incorporate the measured or estimated ^{131}I released at the site into a computer model that takes into account the local terrain and weather patterns at the time of the accident. The program then projects approximate radioactive concentrations of ^{131}I in the plume as it passes over a town downwind of and a known distance from the plant. Those results can link into other software programs to estimate the inhaled quantity of ^{131}I for those working or living in the town.

The last step is that of using the tabulated dose coefficients referred to above (thyroid dose from a unit of ^{131}I intake) to compute likely ranges of radiation dose to the thyroid of hypothetical individuals. If the predicted thyroid radiation dose is greater than the thresholds listed in Table 106.2, specific actions such as evacuation or KI administration can be recommended with some degree of confidence to officials in charge of the emergency operations. In the USA the responsibility of deciding what actions to take rests with the individual states and local governments [29].

KI Availability and Distribution

It is evident that, for KI prophylaxis to be effective, it must be available within hours of the time of need, that the public must be adequately informed in advance, and that the appropriate health and radiation agencies must give timely and accurate information to the populace. There are strong differences of opinion between those who believe that KI should be provided, and those who believe it should not. The latter cite the following to support their view: (a) Nuclear reactors in the USA and most other countries are designed better than the one at Chornobyl. They are less likely to have an accident, are able to mitigate an accident, and are strong enough to withstand most foreseeable terrorist acts. The events in Fukushima now make this argument questionable. (b) The provision of KI has serious legal and logistical problems. In fact some organizations including schools have rejected storing KI for these reasons [23]. (c) Some people may misunderstand the role of KI and not evacuate contaminated areas.

On the other hand, based on the evidence reviewed above, many organizations have endorsed the use of KI distribution programs in planning for nuclear power accidents. Those include in the USA the American Thyroid Association, the American Academy of Pediatrics, the Endocrine Society, and the American Association of Clinical Endocrinology. As a result of these differing views, it is not surprising that there is a great disparity between countries and between localities within countries regarding whether or how they have planned for KI use [23].

The US Nuclear Regulatory Commission has long required that KI be made available in and immediately surrounding a nuclear power station for staff and for people who cannot be evacuated. It now requires that states with population within a 10-mile radius of the station should consider KI in its emergency planning. The federal government provides KI tablets if they are requested but planning for its distribution and/or its stockpiling is a prerogative of the state.

As required by a congressional mandate to assess strategies for distribution and administration of KI, a committee of the US National Academy of Sciences published a detailed report in 2004 [23]. Although the committee confirmed the safety and the usefulness of KI, it concluded that the geographic and logistic diversity among the states was too great to accommodate a uniform national program. It recommended instead that KI distribution plans should be developed by the states with federal support, and it provided detailed suggestions for program development. It also recommended that the federal government should maintain KI stockpiles sufficient to ensure that an adequate supply of KI tablets is available for the target population and should develop a distribution system to supplement the states' programs. It further recommended development of a national program to evaluate the different KI distribution plans that are developed and to assess health effects of KI use in the case that KI administration is implemented after an emergency.

Legislation in the USA in 2002 required distribution of KI within the 20 miles surrounding a nuclear power plant. However, in 2007 the President, acting through the Office of Science and Technology Policy, exercised his authority contained in the legislation, resulting in reducing the area to a 10-mile radius [30]. Of the 34 states in the USA that are within 10 miles of a nuclear power plant, 25 have requested and/or received KI tablets through the US Nuclear Regulatory Commission [30]. The Commission no longer supplies KI solution, suitable for pediatric use [30]. As a result it is necessary for households to obtain the liquid form privately or prepare it from tablets [19]. What subsequently happens with respect to distribution and the efforts to achieve it varies from state to state. There is relatively little data on the success of KI distribution programs. In New Jersey, a state that instituted pre-distribution around two nuclear power plants in 2002, a survey was conducted about 2.5 years later [31]. In eligible communities the range of households supplied with KI was 1–60 %. An encouraging result, one demonstrating an additional benefit the KI distribution program, was the higher number of survey questions answered correctly by members of households with KI. The survey appears to show that in the event of a radiological emergency, there could be a rush to hospitals and other facilities to obtain KI, adding to the problems created by a general unawareness about how to obtain information and respond.

Reports about the events at Fukushima show that each radiological emergency will have its own characteristics [32]. The accidents at Chernobyl and Fukushima both released massive amounts of radioiodines, with the former about ten times more than the latter. In contrast to Chernobyl, where acknowledgement of the accident was long delayed, in Japan evacuation in the closest areas began immediately, even before the releases escalated due to hydrogen explosions in the reactors, some of the airborne radioactivity went out over the sea, and food containing iodine isotopes was controlled. Thus, according to a World Health Organization report "The exposure pathways that contribute most to thyroid dose vary with location and distance from the site. In the more affected regions, inhalation from the cloud and the external dose from groundshine are important, but with increasing distance from the site (i.e. when overall exposure is very low) the ingestion of food becomes the main contributor" [33]. KI had not been distributed before the accident, and for the most part, it was not administered. Concern over low levels of ^{131}I in water led to a study which showed that boiling would not remove it [34]. However, two types of water filters, both containing activated charcoal, could [35].

A more general review of the potential health effects from the Fukushima nuclear power plant accident has been published by the World Health Organization [33].

Summary

KI provides a safe and effective means to protect the thyroid gland from internal radiation following an accident that releases radioiodines. Knowledge derived from the Chornobyl accident has shown that provision of KI is necessary for the public's safety. However, pre-distribution of KI to those living in the vicinity of active nuclear power plants is not universally accepted. The WHO, the FDA and the Nuclear Regulatory

Commission in the USA, and the governments of most of the developed nations have promulgated guidance and regulations for KI use in radiation emergencies.

References

1. Drozdovitch V, Khrouch V, Maceika E, Zvonova I, Vlasov O, Bratilova A, et al. Reconstruction of radiation doses in a case-control study of thyroid cancer following the Chernobyl accident. Health Phys. 2010;99:1–16.
2. Cardis E, Hatch M. The Chernobyl accident – an epidemiological perspective. Clin Oncol (R Coll Radiol). 2011;23:251–60.
3. Nauman J, Wolff J. Iodide prophylaxis in Poland after the Chernobyl reactor accident: benefits and risks. Am J Med. 1993;94:524–32.
4. Davis S, Stepanenko V, Rivkind N, Kopecky KJ, Voillequc P, Shakhtarin V, et al. Risk of thyroid cancer in the Bryansk oblast of the Russian federation after the Chernobyl power station accident. Radiat Res. 2004;162:241–8.
5. Ron E, Lubin JH, Shore RE, Mabuchi K, Modan B, Pottern LM, et al. Thyroid cancer after exposure to external radiation: a pooled analysis of seven studies. Radiat Res. 1995;141:259–77.
6. Ron E. Thyroid cancer incidence among people living in areas contaminated by radiation from the Chernobyl accident. Health Phys. 2007;93:502–11.
7. Cardis E, Kesminiene A, Ivanov V, Malakhova I, Shibata Y, Khrouch V, et al. Risk of thyroid cancer after exposure to ^{131}I in childhood. J Natl Cancer Inst. 2005;97:724–32.
8. Balonov M, Kaidanovsky G, Zvonova I, Kovtun A, Bouville A, Luckyanov N, et al. Contributions of short-lived radioiodines to thyroid doses received by evacuees from the Chernobyl area estimated using early in vivo activity measurements. Radiat Prot Dosim. 2003;105:593–9.
9. Schneider AB, Robbins J. Ionizing radiation and thyroid cancer. In: Fagin J, editor. Thyroid cancer. Boston: Kluwer Academic Publishers; 1998. p. 27–57.
10. Verger P, Aurengo A, Geoffroy B, Le Guen B. Iodine kinetics and effectiveness of stable iodine prophylaxis after intake of radioactive iodine: a review. Thyroid. 2001;11:353–60.
11. Wolff J. Iodide prophylaxis for reactor accidents. In: Nagataki S, Yamashita S, editors. Nagasaki symposium radiation and human health: proposal from Nagasaki. Amsterdam: Elsevier Science B.V; 1996. p. 227–37.
12. Takamura N, Hamada A, Yamaguchi N, Matsushita N, Tarasiuk I, Hashi T, et al. Urinary iodine kinetics after oral loading of potassium iodine. Endocr J. 2003;50:589–93.
13. Blum M, Eisenbud M. Reduction of thyroid irradiation from 131-I by potassium iodide. JAMA. 1967;200:1036–40.
14. Zanzonico PB, Becker DV. Effects of time of administration and dietary iodine levels on potassium iodide (KI) blockade of thyroid irradiation by I-131 from radioactive fallout. Health Phys. 2000;78:660–7.
15. Hanscheid H, Reiners C, Goulko G, Luster M, Schneider-Ludorff M, Buck AK, et al. Facing the nuclear threat: thyroid blocking revisited. J Clin Endocrinol Metab. 2011;96:3511–6.
16. U.S. Food and Drug Administration. Frequently asked questions on Potassium Iodide (KI). http://www.fda.gov/Drugs/EmergencyPreparedness/BioterrorismDrugPreparedness/ucm072265.htm. Accessed 15 Aug 2013.
17. U.S. Nuclear Regulatory Commission. Frequently asked questions about potassium iodide (Reviewed/Updated, 11 Dec 2012). http://www.nrc.gov/about-nrc/emerg-preparedness/about-emerg-preparedness/potassium-iodide/ki-faq.html. Accessed 15 Aug 2013.
18. U.S. Food and Drug Administration Center for Drug Evaluation Branch. Guidance for federal agencies and state and local governments: potassium iodide tablets shelf life extension. www.fda.gov/downloads/Drugs/GuidanceComplianceRegulatoryInformation/Guidances/ucm080549.pdf. Accessed 15 Aug 2013.
19. U.S. Food and Drug Administration. Home preparation procedure for emergency administration of potassium iodide Tablets to infants and small children (Updated: 12 Nov 2012). http://www.fda.gov/Drugs/EmergencyPreparedness/BioterrorismDrugPreparedness/ucm072248.htm. Accessed 15 Aug 2013.

19a. Spallek L, Krille L, Reiners C, Schneider R, Yamashita S, Zeeb H. Adverse effects of iodine thyroid blocking: a systematic review. Radiat Prot Dosimetry. 2012 Jul;150(3):267-77. doi: 10.1093/rpd/ncr400. Epub 2011 Oct 20. Review. PubMed PMID: 22021061.

20. World Health Organization. Guidelines for iodine prophylaxis following radiation accidents: update 1999. Geneva: World Health Organization; 1999.
21. U.S. Food and Drug Administration Center for Drug Evaluation Branch. Guidance: potassium iodide as a thyroid blocking agent in radiation emergencies. Rockville; 2001.
22. Delange F. Iodine prophylaxis following nuclear accidents. Concern for the neonate? Cell Mol Biol (Noisy-le-Grand). 2001;47:417–8.
23. Committee to Assess the Distribution and Administration of Potassium Iodide in the Event of a Nuclear Incident. Distribution and administration of potassium iodine in the event of a nuclear incident. Washington, DC: National Research Council of the National Academies, National Academies Press; 2004.
24. Centers for Disease Control and Prevention. Fact sheet: potassium iodide (KI). http://www.bt.cdc.gov/radiation/ki.asp. Accessed 15 Aug 2013.

24a. Schneider AB, Smith JM. Potassium iodide prophylaxis: what have we learned and questions raised by the accident at the Fukushima Daiichi Nuclear Power Plant. Thyroid. 2012;22:344–6.

25. Overview of national atmospheric release advisory center. https://narac.llnl.gov/narac_overview.html. Accessed 15 Aug 2013.
26. Eisenbud M, Gesell T. Environmental radioactivity from natural, industrial, and military sources. 4th ed. New York: Academic; 1997. p. 63–134.
27. ICRP. Age-dependent doses to members of the public from intake of radionuclides – part 1. ICRP Publication 56. Ann ICRP; 1990. p. 20.
28. ICRP. Age-dependent doses to members of the public from intake of radionuclides – part 4 Inhalation dose coefficients. ICRP Publication 71. Ann ICRP; 1995. p. 25.
29. U.S. Dept. Homeland Security. National response framework, second edition: May 2013. http://www.fema.gov/media-library/assets/documents/32230?id=7371. Accessed 15 Aug 2013.
30. U.S. Nuclear Regulatory Commission. Consideration of potassium iodide in emergency planning. http://www.nrc.gov/about-nrc/emerg-preparedness/about-emerg-preparedness/potassium-iodide.html. Accessed 12 Aug 2013.
31. Blando J, Robertson C, Pearl K, Dixon C, Valcin M, Bresnitz E. Assessment of potassium iodide (KI) distribution program among communities within the emergency planning zones (EPZ) of two nuclear power plants. Health Phys. 2007;92:S18–26.
32. Facts on Fukushima: session 1. Radioactive contamination of the environment and radiation doses to the public. http://www.ustream.tv/recorded/17196685. Accessed 21 Sept 2011.
33. World Health Organization. Health risk assessment from the nuclear accident after the 2011 Great East Japan earthquake and tsunami, based on a preliminary dose estimation. Geneva: World Health Organization; 2013. p. 39.
34. Tagami K, Uchida S. Can we remove iodine-131 from tap water in Japan by boiling? – Experimental testing in response to the Fukushima Daiichi Nuclear Power Plant accident. Chemosphere. 2011;84:1282–4.
35. Higaki S, Hirota M. Decontamination efficiencies of pot-type water purifiers for ^{131}I, ^{134}Cs and ^{137}Cs in rainwater contaminated during Fukushima Daiichi nuclear disaster. PLoS One. 2012;7:e37184.

Low-Iodine Diets

107

Kenneth D. Burman

Introduction

In patients with thyroid cancer, radioactive iodine scans and treatment must be performed in conjunction with thyrotropin (TSH) stimulation [1–9]. Classically, serum TSH elevations and stimulation of thyroid cells by TSH have been achieved by withdrawing the patient from thyroid hormone supplementation, thereby allowing the patient to become hypothyroid. Alternatively, TSH elevations can be accomplished by the administration of recombinant human TSH [10]. Regardless of the method, to maximize efficacy, it is important that the accompanying radioactive iodine scan (or treatment) be performed when the patient's total-body iodine stores are relatively depleted [4, 11–13].

Administered radioactive iodine competes with the unlabeled serum iodine concentrations for available sites in thyroid follicular cells by affecting iodide uptake and transport by the sodium-iodide symporter (NIS). Consequently, as the competition provided by unlabeled iodine in the serum decreases, the transport of radioiodine and avidity of the thyroid tissue for the radioactive iodine increase [14–21]. Also, a general principle is that unlabeled ^{127}I (naturally occurring) and labeled radioactive iodine (^{123}I or ^{131}I) are handled identically by the body and thyroid tissue. In the starkest example, administration of a radiocontrast agent that contains a large amount of unlabeled iodine can provide such an excess of iodine that the ability of thyroid tissue to trap radioactive iodine is compromised to less than 1 %. The mechanism of this decreased radioactive iodine uptake is thought mainly to be related to downregulation of NIS but is also related to the competition of both labeled and unlabeled iodine for the thyroid NIS [14–21].

In contrast, decreased iodine stores in the body and lowered serum iodine are thought to enhance the action of NIS. This principle lies at the center of the rationale for low-iodine diets. This belief, yet unproven, is that a low-iodine diet can benefit ultimate outcome and prognosis in relation to increasing thyroidal radioiodine uptake and improving the long-term effect of radiation on residual thyroid tissue. This rule guides most centers managing patients with thyroid cancer to recommend that patients undergoing diagnostic radioiodine scans or treatment adhere to a low-iodine diet for at least 2 weeks prior to study.

Iodine Metabolism

Iodine* is a chemical element found in a wide variety of foods and chemical agents (e.g., radiocontrast dye). The nonradioactive form of iodine has a molecular weight of 127 (i.e., ^{127}I), and the most common radioisotopes in clinical use are ^{123}I and ^{131}I, with the former used only for diagnostic purposes and the latter for both diagnosis and treatment.

In normal subjects, dietary iodine is absorbed through the small intestine and transported in the plasma to the thyroid, where it is concentrated, oxidized, and then incorporated into thyroglobulin as thyroxine (T4), triiodothyronine (T3), and inactive lesser iodinated analogs. When the stored thyroid hormones are needed, partly under the influence of TSH stimulation, thyroglobulin is subjected to proteolysis, and the stored thyroid hormones are then released. Following secretion into the blood, the predominant thyroid hormones, T4 and T3, are deiodinated by specific enzymes located mainly in the liver and kidney; thus, free iodine is released. Serum iodine is then passively filtered through the kidney, where it is excreted. Under normal conditions, the thyroid gland traps about 10–30 % of the iodine that is available, and the normal thyroid gland contains approx 5–10 mg of iodine,

K.D. Burman, MD (✉)
Director, Divisions of Endocrinology, Washington Hospital Center and Georgetown University Hospital, 110 Irving Street NW 2A-72, Washington, DC 20010, USA
e-mail: kenneth.d.burman@medstar.net

L. Wartofsky, D. Van Nostrand (eds.), *Thyroid Cancer*, DOI 10.1007/978-1-4939-3314-3_107

most of which is stored, as noted in colloid (i.e., in thyroglobulin) as T4 and T3.

As described, the thyroid gland avidly traps iodine because of the presence of NIS, and a small amount of iodine is similarly trapped by the salivary glands. The kidneys passively filter and excrete the iodine in the blood; the breasts trap and secrete a small amount of iodine, especially during lactation [14–21]. Renal excretion varies with filtered load and reflects 97 % of dietary intake, with less than about 3 % excreted in the stool. Renal iodide is passively reabsorbed and depends on the glomerular filtration rate. Patients with significant renal disease excrete less iodine in their urine.

The protein responsible for iodide transport, NIS, is located at the basolateral plasma membrane of thyrocytes. TSH and iodine deficiency upregulate NIS, and iodine excess suppresses it [14–16, 19–24].

In subjects with an intact thyroid gland, excess iodine can cause hyperthyroidism (primarily in the setting of underlying autonomous function, as in Graves' disease or toxic nodular disease), and deficient iodine exposure can cause goiters and hypothyroidism. The range of iodine intake that may be related to thyroid dysfunction is highly variable and partially depends on genetic factors.

The National Health and Nutrition Examination Survey (NHANES III) demonstrated that the median national urinary iodine excretion in the United States in samples collected between 1988 and 1994 was 145 μg/L. Iodine intake had been higher in the previous decades. The median urine excretion in men was 160 μg/L and in women, 130 μg/L. Less than 50 μg/L of iodine was excreted by 8.1 % of men and 15.1 % of women. For women of childbearing age (14–44 years), urinary iodine concentration in the 2.5–97.5 percentiles was 18–650 μg/L. For pregnant women, the range was 42–550 μg/L [25–29]. The iodine content in the US diet varies based on various nonmedical reasons and according to a 2007 publication, is thought to be adequate in most nonpregnant adults [30, 31].

Thyroid Cancer

When patients with thyroid cancer are prepared for ^{131}I therapy, they have already had most or all of their thyroid gland removed surgically, and their 24 h radioactive iodine uptake typically ranges from approx 0.1 % to 10 % [2, 4, 9, 32]. As noted above, there is a virtual equilibrium between the amounts of nonradioactive iodine ingested daily in food, drink, and other exogenous sources and that ultimately excreted in the urine per day. Therefore, measuring urine iodine content can accurately reflect what the dietary consumption has been for the previous time period, probably about 7–14 days. Either the 24 h urine iodine can be measured or a random urine sample can be assessed with the urine concentration estimated by conversion to microgram per liter. This latter measurement is adequate (and much easier) for thyroid cancer patients because only an estimate is needed, and most patients excrete about 1 L of urine daily. Typically, the urine iodine excretion is expressed per gram of urine creatinine. In customary circumstances, every thyroid cancer patient prepared for a radioactive scan and/or treatment should have a urine iodine measurement to ensure the subsequent radioactive iodine therapy will be administered under optimal conditions. Adherence to a low-iodine diet for about 2 weeks can decrease the urine iodine concentration to less than 200 μg/L and possibly even less than 50 μg/L.

Iodine exists ubiquitously in the environment in food, water, chemicals, and medications. Significant iodine deficiency that lasts for several months may cause goiter and/or hypothyroidism, especially in individuals with underlying autoimmune thyroid disease [33–36]. If newborns are born to mothers with significant iodine deficiency, the neonates may display goiters and profound hypothyroidism, including mental retardation [37–41]. The minimum daily requirement for iodine has been set at 150 μg/day for those living in the United States; however, pregnant and lactating women should probably increase their intake further to at least 220 and 290 μg/day, respectively. However, in select circumstances, such as preparation for ^{131}I scan and/or therapy in a thyroid cancer patient, judicious use of a low-iodine diet for a short period of time is not considered detrimental. Of course, the issue of iodine deficiency is not relevant to the thyroid cancer patient who no longer has a thyroid gland and is taking exogenous thyroid hormone.

Iodine Sources

Amiodarone is an antiarrhythmic agent widely used in both Europe and the United States [42]. The drug contains 37.2 % iodine and is typically prescribed in doses of 300–1,200 mg/day, providing 100–400 mg of iodine and an estimated 900 μg of free iodide. In the setting of iodine-induced thyroid disease or to reduce iodine intake to facilitate scanning and therapy, the drug usually cannot be discontinued because of medical reasons. Amiodarone therapy will completely abrogate the ability to treat a patient with radioactive iodine. In fact, even if it can be stopped, it takes months or years for the urine iodine to decrease sufficiently to allow radioactive iodine therapy. Radioactivity should not be administered to pregnant or lactating women or women who have recently lactated.

Additionally, the various intravenous contrast dyes contain significant amounts of iodine and should be avoided for at least 6–8 weeks prior to starting a low-iodine diet [43–46]. Radiocontrast dyes contain approximately 180,000–320,000 μg of iodine. The majority of this iodine is organic iodine, but significant quantities of free iodide are present or are released via hepatic deiodination and generation of free iodide.

It is unknown how long it takes to dissipate this iodine following radiocontrast dye administration or ingestion. In individuals with normal renal function, it probably requires about 4–8 weeks, but this issue has not been adequately studied.

The most practical manner to ensure the body's iodine stores are decreased is to assess urine iodine content. The usual contrast agent employed for magnetic resonance imaging (e.g., gadolinium) does not contain iodine.

A wide variety of other substances contain significant iodine, such as medication pills or tablets coated with red dye. It is important to examine the contents of food and medications to determine if that particular agent contains considerable amounts of iodine. Common iodide-containing drugs are listed in Tables 107.1, 107.2, and 107.3. Antitussives contain 15–325 mg of iodine per teaspoon and may provide about 90–3,900 mg per day. Patients should also be asked whether they are taking any so-called "alternative" medications that may contain iodine and multivitamins, which are often supplemented with iodine [47, 48].

Iodochlorhydroxyquin may be contained in topical antifungal and bacteriostatic creams or solutions. Povidone-iodine solution (Betadine) is commonly used as a topical antiseptic. High blood iodide levels have been reported following topical and intravaginal application of povidone. Antiamebic drugs with the active compound iodoquinol contain organic iodine. In typical dosages, they provide 19.5 mg of iodine daily, usually for a 20-day course.

Table 107.1 Common sources of iodine in North America

Dietary iodine	Daily intake (μg)
Dairy products, grains, meat, mixed dishes, vegetables, desserts, eggs, iodized salt	52, 78, 31, 26, 20, 20, 10, 380

Table 107.2 General food types to avoid or use when adhering to a low-iodine diet

Food items	Avoid	Permitted
Drinks	Soda, hot chocolate, and vegetable juices	Coffee, tea, and other juices
Breads	Commercial pastries, breads, and dough	Homemade pastries prepared properly
Meat	Canned and processed meats and dinners	Fresh unsalted meat
Fruits	Canned or preserved fruits	Fresh fruits
Vegetables	Canned or frozen vegetables	Fresh vegetables
Cereals	Dry or hot cereals	Puffed wheat and rice
Dairy products	Eggs and cream	Milk, yogurt, and nondairy creamer
Spices	Pickles, soy sauce, mustard, and ketchup	Nonpreserved herbs and spices

Low-Iodine Diet

The types of food to avoid include iodized salt and processed, packaged, or preserved canned foods [6–8] (Table 107.2). Salt, per se, does not have to be avoided. Only iodized salt and non-iodized salt are readily available in most food stores. It is critically important that the patient reads all food labels to avoid those that contain iodized salt. Even water may contain iodine, as it is known to be bactericidal and added to water in the US public park system; distilled water is therefore most desirable. Potassium iodate is commonly used in flour as a dough conditioner or preservative, and pastry food or mixes should also be avoided. Unsalted butter or margarine is also preferable. Even fresh fish may contain large amounts of iodine, and kelp (seaweed) should definitely be avoided. Dairy products, particularly milk, may contain significant quantities of iodine, possibly because of the use of iodophors used in the procurement process or iodine antisepsis of dairy farm equipment.

There are multiple appropriate methods to employ a low-iodine diet prior to radioiodine scan and/or treatment. We generally initiate the low-iodine diet approximately 2 weeks prior to the diagnostic scan and continue until 1–2 days after the radioiodine treatment.

With the advent of the ability to perform diagnostic scans or therapies with recombinant human TSH stimulation, rather than after T4 withdrawal, the issue of iodine contained within the L-T4 molecule arose. Thus, the patients will be continuing to take exogenous L-T4 with its significant iodine content during a Thyrogen-stimulated radioiodine scan or treatment. The iodine generated from the T4 therapy constitutes an added burden (Table 107.3). Consequently, it is strongly urged that these patients maintain a low-iodine diet prior to their isotopic studies. L-T4 contains approx 66 % iodine, and if a patient takes 150 μg L-T4 daily, then this medication will contribute about 100 μg of iodine intake, in addition to that from dietary intake. Therefore, patients taking L-T4 therapy while maintaining a low-iodine diet will necessarily have a higher iodine intake than if they showed similar dietary adherence in preparation for a withdrawal scan. Another option is to switch the patients from T4 to T3 (which contains one less iodine molecule) during the interval for the scan and/or therapy. In either case, the amount of iodine provided by the thyroid hormone, together with that in a strict low-iodine diet [48], will still be relatively low, and the radioactive iodine scan and treatment should be effective. We typically continue the patient on levothyroxine therapy during recombinant human TSH stimulation without switching to triiodothyronine. In summary, adherence to a low-iodine diet seems prudent for a thyroid cancer patient being prepared for radioiodine scan and treatment. Further studies are needed that assess the efficacy of these recommendations, with a focus on the optimal goal of 24 h iodine intake, as expressed by urine measurements.

Table 107.3 Iodine content of radiocontrast dyes and medications

Substance	Iodine content	Usual dose	Total dose of iodine (mg)
Radiologic contrast dyes			
Cholecystographic dyes			
Iopanoate, ipodate, tyropanoate, iodoxamate	55–70 %	3–9 g	1,650–6,300
Diatrizoate, iodamide, iothalamate	45–60 %	1–70 g	450–4,200
Lymphangiographic dye			
Lipiodol (iodized poppy-seed oil)	45–60 %	1–70 g	450–4,200
Myelographic dye			
Metrizamide	48 %	5–15 mL	1,100–3,000
Iodide-containing drugs			
Oral agents			
Amiodarone	75 mg/200 mg tablet	300–1,200 mg/day (initial)	75–300/day
Benziodarone	49 mg/100 mg tablet	100–200 mg/day	49–98/day
Iodine-containing cough medications	15–325 mg/teaspoon	1–2 teaspoon/q4h	90–3,900/day
Potassium iodide			
Calcium iodide			
Iodinate glycerol			
Iodochlorhydroxyquin (antiamebic)	104 mg/tablet	600–650 mg tid × 20 day	312/day
Iodine-containing vitamins (prenatal vitamins)	0.15 mg/tablet	1/day	0.15/day
Quadrinal (KI)	320 mg/tablet	1 tablet qid or 10 mL q4h	1,280–1,920/day
	160 mg/5 mL		
Kelp tablets	0.15 mg/tablet	1 or more/day	≥0.15/day
Antithyroidal preparations			
Lugol solution	8.4 mg/drop*	15 drops qid	378/day*
SSKI	38 mg/drop*	5 drops qid	760/day*
Topical iodine preparations			
Iodohydroxyquinolone	12 mg/g	4 g/day	4,800/day
Povidone-iodine (Betadine)	10 mg/mL	Variable	
Ophthalmic solution			
Echothiophate iodide	5–40 μg/drop*	2 drops qid	0.40–0.320/day*
Idoxuridine solution	18 μg/drop*	2 drops qid	0.144/day*

*Depending on drop size [49]

References

1. Haugen BR, et al. A comparison of recombinant human thyrotropin and thyroid hormone withdrawal for the detection of thyroid remnant or cancer. J Clin Endocrinol Metab. 1999;84(11):3877–85. In Process Citation, MEDLINE record in process.
2. Mazzaferri EL, Jhiang SM. Long-term impact of initial surgical and medical therapy on papillary and follicular thyroid cancer. Am J Med. 1994;97(5):418–28.
3. Bal C, et al. Prospective randomized clinical trial to evaluate the optimal dose of 131 I for remnant ablation in patients with differentiated thyroid carcinoma. Cancer. 1996;77(12):2574–80.
4. Burman KD. Low iodine diet. In: Van Nostrand D, Bloom G, Wartofsky L, editors. Thyroid cancer: a guide for patients. Baltimore: Keystone Press; 2004. p. 83–8.
5. Kim HK, et al. Daily urine iodine excretion while consuming a low-iodine diet in preparation for radioactive iodine therapy in a high iodine intake area. Clin Endocrinol (Oxf). 2011;75(6):851–6.
6. Morsch EP, et al. Two weeks of a low-iodine diet are equivalent to 3 weeks for lowering urinary iodine and increasing thyroid radioactive iodine uptake. Thyroid. 2011;21(1):61–7.
7. Sawka AM, et al. Dietary iodine restriction in preparation for radioactive iodine treatment or scanning in well-differentiated thyroid cancer: a systematic review. Thyroid. 2010;20(10):1129–38.
8. Bahn RS, et al. Hyperthyroidism and other causes of thyrotoxicosis: management guidelines of the American Thyroid Association and American Association of Clinical Endocrinologists. Thyroid. 2011;21:593–646.
9. American Thyroid Association Guidelines Task Force on Thyroid Nodules and Differentiated Thyroid Cancer. Haugen BR, Alexander EK, Bible KC, Doherty GM, Mandel SJ, Nikiforov YE, Pacini F, Randolph GW, Sawka AM, Schlumberger M, Schuff KG, Sherman SI, Sosa JA, Steward DL, Tuttle RM, Wartofsky L. 2015 American Thyroid Association Management Guidelines for Adult Patients with Thyroid Nodules and Differentiated Thyroid Cancer. Thyroid 2016; 26:1–133.
10. Ladenson PW, et al. Comparison of administration of recombinant human thyrotropin with withdrawal of thyroid hormone for radioactive iodine scanning in patients with thyroid carcinoma. N Engl J Med. 1997;337(13):888–96.
11. Ain KB, et al. Low-iodine tube-feeding diet for iodine-131 scanning and therapy. Clin Nucl Med. 1994;19(6):504–7.
12. Maxon HR, et al. Low iodine diet in I-131 ablation of thyroid remnants. Clin Nucl Med. 1983;8(3):123–6.

13. Goslings BM. Proceedings: effect of a low iodine diet on 131-I therapy in follicular thyroid carcinomata. J Endocrinol. 1975; 64(3):30P.
14. Baker CH, Morris JC. The sodium-iodide symporter. Curr Drug Targets Immune Endocr Metabol Disord. 2004;4(3):167–74.
15. Haberkorn U, et al. Iodide kinetics and dosimetry in vivo after transfer of the human sodium iodide symporter gene in rat thyroid carcinoma cells. J Nucl Med. 2004;45(5):827–33.
16. Ward LS, et al. Low expression of sodium iodide symporter identifies aggressive thyroid tumors. Cancer Lett. 2003;200(1):85–91.
17. Rudnicka L, et al. Expression of the Na(+)/I(-) symporter in invasive ductal breast cancer. Folia Histochem Cytobiol. 2003;41(1): p. excretion data from National Health and Nutrition Examination Surveys I and III (1971–1974 and 1988–1994) [see comments]. J Clin Endocrinol Metab. 1998;83(10):3401–8.
18. Upadhyay G, et al. Functional expression of sodium iodide symporter (NIS) in human breast cancer tissue. Breast Cancer Res Treat. 2003;77(2):157–65.
19. Dohan O, et al. The sodium/iodide symporter (NIS): characterization, regulation, and medical significance. Endocr Rev. 2003;24(1):48–77.
20. Wagner S, et al. Regulation of sodium-iodide-symporter gene expression in human thyrocytes measured by real-time polymerase chain reaction. Exp Clin Endocrinol Diabetes. 2002;110(8):398–402.
21. Smyth PP. The thyroid, iodine and breast cancer. Breast Cancer Res. 2003;5(5):235–8.
22. Lacroix L, et al. Expression of the apical iodide transporter in human thyroid tissues: a comparison study with other iodide transporters. J Clin Endocrinol Metab. 2004;89(3):1423–8.
23. Smit JW, et al. Iodide kinetics and experimental (131)I therapy in a xenotransplanted human sodium-iodide symporter-transfected human follicular thyroid carcinoma cell line. J Clin Endocrinol Metab. 2002;87(3):1247–53.
24. Vanderpump MP, et al. Iodine status of UK schoolgirls: a cross-sectional survey. Lancet. 2011;377(9782):2007–12.
25. Hollowell JG, et al. Serum TSH, T(4), and thyroid antibodies in the United States population (1988 to 1994): National Health and Nutrition Examination Survey (NHANES III). J Clin Endocrinol Metab. 2002;87(2):489–99.
26. Hollowell JG, et al. Iodine nutrition in the United States. Trends and public health implications: iodine excretion data from National Health and Nutrition Examination Surveys I and III (1971–1974 and 1988–1994). J Clin Endocrinol Metab. 1998;83(10):3401–8. see comments.
27. Oddie TH, et al. Iodine intake in the United States: a reassessment. J Clin Endocrinol Metab. 1970;30(5):659–65.
28. Soldin OP, Soldin SJ, Pezzullo JC. Urinary iodine percentile ranges in the United States. Clin Chim Acta. 2003;328(1–2):185–90.
29. Hollowell JG, Haddow JE. The prevalence of iodine deficiency in women of reproductive age in the United States of America. Public Health Nutr. 2007;10(12A):1532–9. discussion 1540–1.
30. Spencer CA, et al. National Health and Nutrition Examination Survey III thyroid-stimulating hormone (TSH)-thyroperoxidase antibody relationships demonstrate that TSH upper reference limits may be skewed by occult thyroid dysfunction. J Clin Endocrinol Metab. 2007;92(11):4236–40.
31. Haddow JE, et al. Urine iodine measurements, creatinine adjustment, and thyroid deficiency in an adult United States population. J Clin Endocrinol Metab. 2007;92(3):1019–22.
32. Mazzaferri EL, Jhiang SM. Differentiated thyroid cancer long-term impact of initial therapy. Trans Am Clin Climatol Assoc. 1994;106:151–68. discussion 168–70.
33. Heinisch M, et al. Goiter prevalence and urinary iodide excretion in a formerly iodine-deficient region after introduction of statutory Iodization of common salt. Thyroid. 2002; 12(9):809–14.
34. Azizi F, Navai L, Fattahi F. Goiter prevalence, urinary iodine excretion, thyroid function and anti-thyroid function and anti-thyroid antibodies after 12 years of salt iodization in Shahriar, Iran. Int J Vitam Nutr Res. 2002;72(5):291–5.
35. Wu T, et al. Iodised salt for preventing iodine deficiency disorders. Cochrane Database Syst Rev. 2002;3:CD003204.
36. Zimmermann MB, et al. Urinary iodine concentrations in swiss schoolchildren from the Zurich area and the Engadine valley. Schweiz Med Wochenschr. 1998;128(20):770–4.
37. Delange F, et al. Iodine deficiency during infancy and early childhood in Belgium: does it pose a risk to brain development? Eur J Pediatr. 2001;160(4):251–4.
38. Delange F. The disorders induced by iodine deficiency. Thyroid. 1994;4(1):107–28.
39. Klett M, et al. Effect of iodine supply on neonatal thyroid volume and TSH. Acta Paediatr Suppl. 1999;88(432):18–20.
40. Liesenkotter KP, et al. Earliest prevention of endemic goiter by iodine supplementation during pregnancy. Eur J Endocrinol. 1996;134(4):443–8.
41. Glinoer D, et al. A randomized trial for the treatment of mild iodine deficiency during pregnancy: maternal and neonatal effects. J Clin Endocrinol Metab. 1995;80(1):258–69.
42. Bartalena L, et al. Treatment of amiodarone-induced thyrotoxicosis, a difficult challenge: results of a prospective study. J Clin Endocrinol Metab. 1996;81(8):2930–3.
43. Henzen C, Buess M, Brander L. Iodine-induced hyperthyroidism (iodine-induced Basedow's disease): a current disease picture. Schweiz Med Wochenschr. 1999;129(17):658–64.
44. Kamel N, et al. Sodium ipodate in the treatment of toxic diffuse goiter. Short-term and long-term effects on thyrotoxicosis. Endocrinologie. 1988;26(2):99–105.
45. Laurberg P. Multisite inhibition by ipodate of iodothyronine secretion from perfused dog thyroid lobes. Endocrinology. 1985; 117(4):1639–44.
46. Laurberg P. The effect of some iodine-containing radiocontrast agents on iodothyronine secretion from the perfused canine thyroid. Endocrinology. 1982;111(6):1904–8.
47. Leung AM, Pearce EN, Braverman LE. Iodine content of prenatal multivitamins in the United States. N Engl J Med. 2009;360(9):939–40.
48. Pearce EN, et al. Sources of dietary iodine: bread, cows' milk, and infant formula in the Boston area. J Clin Endocrinol Metab. 2004;89(7):3421–4.
49. Nuovo J, Wartofsky L. In: Becker KL, editor. Principles and practice of endocrinology and metabolism. Philadelphia: Lippincott Williams and Wilkins; 2002.

Appendix A: Books and Manuals

Gary Bloom

Textbooks for Physicians and Professionals

Management of Thyroid Cancer and Related Nodular Disease. McDougall IR, New York. Springer, 2006.

Practical Management of Thyroid Cancer. Mazzeferri EL, Harmer C, Mallick UK, Kendall-Taylor P, New York. Springer, 2006.

Essentials of Thyroid Cancer Management. Amdur RJ, Mazzeferri EL, New York. Springer, 2005.

Thyroid Cancer. Biersack HJ, Grunwald F. New York: Springer Verlag, 2005, 2nd Edition.

Thyroid Cancer: **Diagnosis and Treatment**. Clark OH, Noguchi S. Quality Medical Publishing, 2000.

Thyroid Cancer. Fagin JA. Springer, New York, 1998.

Werner and Ingbar's The Thyroid: A Fundamental and Clinical Text. Braverman LE, Cooper DS. Wolters Kluwer, 2012, 10th Edition.

Thyroid Disease: The Facts. Vanderpump, MPJ, Tunbridge WMG. Oxford University Press, New York, NY, 2008, 4th edition.

Radiation Oncology: Rationale, Technique, Results. Cox JD, Ang KK. St. Louis, MO: C.B. Mosby, 2010, 9th edition.

Cancer: Principles and Practice of Oncology. DeVita Jr VT, Lawrence TS, Rosenberg SA. Philadelphia, Wolters Kluwer, 2014, 10th Edition.

Publications for Patients, Family, and Friends

Thyroid Cancer: A Guide for Patients. Van Nostrand D, Wartofsky L, Bloom G, Kulkarni K, editors. Baltimore, MD: Keystone Press, 2010, 2nd Edition. Available through ThyCa: Thyroid Cancer Survivors' Association, Inc. (www.thyca.org) and all major book stores.

Thyroid Cancer Basics. ThyCa: Thyroid Cancer Survivors' Association, Inc., 2012, 1st edition. www.thyca.org

Anaplastic Thyroid Cancer. ThyCa: Thyroid Cancer Survivors' Association, Inc., 2013, 1st edition.

Medullary Thyroid Cancer. ThyCa: Thyroid Cancer Survivors' Association, Inc., 2014, 1st edition.

Low-Iodine Cookbook. Guljord L, editor. ThyCa: Thyroid Cancer Survivors' Association, Inc., 8th edition, 2016.

Light of Life Foundation Cookbook. 2014, 2nd edition.

What You Need to Know About Thyroid Cancer. Online pamphlet available at: http://www.cancer.gov/publications/patient-education/wyntk-thyroid-cancer.

The Official Patient's Sourcebook on Thyroid Cancer. A reference manual for self-directed patient research. Parker JN, Parker PM. San Diego, CA: ICON Health Publications. 2002.

The Thyroid, Cancer and You. Wolfe A. Xlibris Corp, 2003 (www.xlibris.com).

Thyroid for Dummies. Rubin AL. New York, NY: For Dummies, Inc., 2006, 2nd edition.

Your Thyroid: A Home Reference. Wood LC, Cooper DS, Ridgway EC. Ballantine Books, Boston, MA, 2006, 4th edition.

The Thyroid Cancer Book. Rosenthal MS. St. Victoria, B.C.: CreateSpace Independent Publishing Platform, 2006, 2nd Edition.

The Thyroid Sourcebook for Women. Rosenthal MS. McGraw-Hill Education, Columbus, OH, 2005, 2nd Edition.

The Thyroid Sourcebook: Everything You Need to Know. Rosenthal MS. McGraw-Hill Education, Lincolnwood, IL, 2005, 2nd Edition.

L. Wartofsky, D. Van Nostrand (eds.), *Thyroid Cancer*, DOI 10.1007/978-1-4939-3314-3

Could It Be My Thyroid? Rubenfeld SM. Evans & Company, Houston, TX, 2003.

The Thyroid Guide. Ditkoff BA, Lo Gerfo PL. William Morrow Paperbacks, New York, NY, 2000.

The Thyroid Gland: A Book for Thyroid Patients. Hamburger JI. Privately published, 1991, 7th Edition.

Twenty-first Century Complete Medical Guide to Thyroid Cancer. Authoritative Government Documents and Clinical References, and Practical Information for Patients and Physicians, CD-rom, Progressive Management. This is a CD-rom of official public domain US federal government files, much of which is already available free through the federal government at www.cancer.gov and other websites noted in Appendix B. 2002.

The Harvard Medical School Guide to Overcoming Thyroid Problems. Garber JR, White S. McGraw-Hill, New York, NY, 2005.

A large portion of this appendix was reproduced from *Thyroid Cancer: A Guide for Patients*, with permission from Keystone Press, Inc.

Appendix B: Additional Sources of Information

Gary Bloom

Thyroid and/or Cancer Professional Organizations

American Thyroid Association, Inc.: A professional medical society of physicians and scientists dedicated to the advancement, prevention, diagnosis and treatment of thyroid disorders and thyroid cancer.
Address:
6066 Leesburg Pike, Suite 550
Falls Church, VA 22041
Communication data:
Office: 703-998-8890
Fax: 703-998-8893
E-mail: thyroid@thyroid.org
Website: www.thyroid.org
Services:
For general endocrinologist referrals and general thyroid information

American Association of Clinical Endocrinologists (AACE): This is a professional medical organization of more than 2500 clinical endocrinologists. The American Association of Clinical Endocrinologists is a professional community of physicians specializing in endocrinology, diabetes, and metabolism committed to enhancing the ability of its members to provide the highest quality of patient care.
Address:
245 Riverside Ave., Suite 200
Jacksonville, FL 32202
Communication data:
Telephone: 904-353-7878
Fax: 904-353-8185
Website: www.aace.com
To find an endocrinologist, go to www.aace.com/resources/find-an-endocrinologist
Clinical guidelines: www.aace.com/publications/guidelines
Services:
Find an endocrinologist
Clinical guidelines

The Endocrine Society
Address:
2055 L Street NW, Suite 600
Washington, DC 20036
Communication data:
Office: 888-363-6274 or 202-971-3636
Fax: 202-736-9705
E-mail: societyservices@endo-society.org
Website: www.endo-society.org
Service:
The world's oldest, largest, and most active organization of 18,000 members devoted to research on hormones and the clinical practice of endocrinology. The Society works to foster a greater understanding of endocrinology among the general public and practitioners of complementary medical disciplines and to promote the interests of all endocrinologists at the national scientific research and health policy levels of government.

Thyroid Disease Manager: An up-to-date analysis of thyrotoxicosis, hypothyroidism, thyroid nodules and cancer, thyroiditis, and all aspects of human thyroid disease and thyroid physiology. It provides physicians, researchers, and trainees (as well as patients) around the world with an authoritative, current, complete, objective, free, and downloadable source on the thyroid. This website is directed to helping physicians care for their patients with thyroid problems.
Address:
Endocrine Education, Inc.
Box P-94
South Dartmouth, MA 02748
Communication data:
E-mail: ldegroot@earthlink.net
Website: www.thyroidmanager.org

L. Wartofsky, D. Van Nostrand (eds.), *Thyroid Cancer*, DOI 10.1007/978-1-4939-3314-3

A large portion of this appendix was reproduced from *Thyroid Cancer: A Guide for Patients*, with permission from Keystone Press, Inc.

Information Regarding Clinical Trials

National Institutes of Health (developed by the National Library of Medicine): ClinicalTrials.gov offers up-to-date information for locating federally and privately supported clinical trials for a wide range of diseases and conditions. A clinical trial (also clinical research) is a research study in human volunteers to answer specific health questions. Interventional trials determine whether experimental treatments or new ways of using known therapies are safe and effective under controlled environments. Observational trials address health issues in large groups of people or populations in natural settings.
Website: www.clinicaltrials.gov

National Cancer Institute:
Website: www.cancer.gov/clinicaltrials/

Patient Support Groups and Information Sources

Hormone Health Network: The Hormone Health Network is a leading source of hormone-related health information for the public, physicians, allied health professionals, and the media. Our mission is to serve as a resource for the public by promoting the prevention, treatment, and cure of hormone-related conditions through outreach and education.
Address:
8401 Connecticut Avenue, Suite 900
Chevy Chase, MD 20815–5817
Communication data:
Telephone: 1-800-HORMONE
Fax: 301-941-0259
E-mail: hormone@endocrine.org
Website: www.hormone.org
Services:
Information on Clinical Trials
Patient information factsheets and brochures
Find an endocrinologist in your area; physician referral database

ThyCa: Thyroid Cancer Survivors' Association, Inc. (ThyCa): An international, nonprofit organization of thyroid cancer survivors, family members, and health professionals advised by nationally recognized leaders in the field of thyroid cancer, dedicated to education, communication, and support for thyroid cancer survivors, families, and friends.
Address:
P.O. Box 1545
New York, NY 10159–1545
Communication data:
Telephone: 1-877-588-7904 (toll free) Fax: 1-630-604-6078
E-mail: thyca@thyca.org
Website: www.thyca.org
Services (more information available through the website or the above communication data):
Local support groups by region below
E-mail discussion groups, Facebook, Inspire, Instagram, Twitter, Yahoo!Groups
Person-to-person support with toll-free survivors' telephone line
Website with over 650 pages plus extensive links list free low-iodine-diet cookbook
Thyroid Cancer Basics, Anaplastic Thyroid Cancer, and Medullary Thyroid Cancer handbooks and other free publications
Newsletter, which is free online
National conference and regional workshops
Thyroid cancer awareness materials
Help develop thyroid cancer support groups
Thyroid Cancer Awareness Month
Thyroid Cancer Research Funds

States with local ThyCa support groups are: Alabama, Arizona, Arkansas, California, Colorado, Connecticut, Delaware, District of Columbia, Florida, Georgia, Hawaii, Idaho, Illinois, Indiana, Iowa, Kansas, Kentucky, Maine, Maryland, Massachusetts, Michigan, Minnesota, Mississippi, Missouri, Nebraska, Nevada, New Hampshire, New Jersy, New Mexico, New York, North Carolina, Ohio, Oklahoma, Oregon, Pennsylvania, South Carolina, Tennessee, Texas, Utah, Vermont, Virginia, Washington, and Wisconsin.

Countries with local ThyCa support groups are: Australia, The Bahamas, Canada, Costa Rica, Greece, United Kindom, and the Philippines

Thyroid Cancer Canada (Cancer de la thyroide Canada): Formed by a group of Canadian thyroid cancer patients who came together in a common search for information and support in dealing with treatment, recovery, and long-term monitoring of thyroid cancer. Offers information and support to those affected by thyroid cancer through our website and through an online discussion forum. The forum allows thyroid cancer patients, regardless of whether they are newly diagnosed, on the road to recovery, or long-term survivors, as well as their caregivers, friends, or family, to give and receive emotional support. Here they can post messages, listen, ask questions, and/or exchange experiences and information with those who have "been there."

Address:
P.O. Box 23007
550 Eglinton Ave. West
Toronto, ON M5N 3A8 CANADA
Communication data:
Telephone: 416-487-8267 (during office hours only)
Fax: 416-487-0601
E-mail: info@thyroidcancercanada.org
Website: www.thyroidcancercanada.org

Light of Life Foundation: This foundation improves the quality of life of thyroid cancer patients through continual education of the lay public and the medical community and by promoting research and development to improve thyroid cancer care.
Address:
P.O. Box 163
Manalapan, NJ 07726
Communication data:
Telephone: 609-409-0900
Fax: 609-409-0902
Website: www.checkyourneck.com
E-mail: info@checkyourneck.com

Thyroid Foundation of America: Provides health education and support to thyroid patients.
Communication data:
Website: www.allthyroid.org

Thyroid Foundation of Canada (La Fondation canadiennne de la Thyroide): The Thyroid Foundation of Canada (TFC) is the oldest North American patient education association. The TFC promotes awareness and education about thyroid disease including thyroid cancer.
Address:
P.O. Box 298
Bath, ON K0H 1G0 CANADA
Communication data:
Office: 1-800-267-8822
Website: www.thyroid.ca

Thyroid Federation International: A worldwide network of affiliated thyroid patient organizations.
Address:
P.O. Box 471
Bath, ON K0H 1G0 CANADA
Communication data:
E-mail: tfi@thyroid-fed.org
Website: www.thyroid-fed.org

American Cancer Society
Communication data:
Telephone: 1-800-227-2345
Website: www.cancer.org: Select the Learn About Cancer button, and then select Thyroid Cancer under "select a cancer type".
Information on cancer, employment, insurance, law, Americans with Disabilities Act, diet, vitamins/supplements, and complementary treatment approaches.

National Cancer Institute at the National Institutes of Health
Address:
BG 9609 MSC 9760
9609 Medical Center Drive
Bethesda, MD 20892–9760
Communication data:
Telephone: 800-4-Cancer (800-422-6237)
Website: www.cancer.gov
Click on Thyroid Cancer listed under "Cancer Types." Or under find a cancer type, click on "T." Then click on thyroid cancer.
Radiation Therapy Website: www.cancer.gov/Publications/patient-education/radiation-therapy-and-you
Services:
Information on types of cancers, treatment, clinical trials, and research.

National Coalition for Cancer Survivorship: Advocates for quality cancer care for all people touched by cancer and provides tools that empower people to advocate for themselves.
Address:
1010 Wayne Avenue, Suite 315
Silver Spring, MD 20910
Communication data:
Office: 877-NCCS-YES (877-6227-937)
E-mail: info@canceradvocacy.org
Website: www.canceradvocacy.org

Pharmaceutical Companies

AbbVie Inc. (manufacturer of Synthroid®)
Address:
AbbVie Inc.
1 North Waukegan Road
North Chicago, IL 60064
Communication data:
Websites: www.synthroid.com

Akrimax Pharamaceutical, LLC (Manufacturer of Tirosint ®)

Address:
11 Commerce Drive, Suite 100
Cranford, NJ 07016
Communication data:
Telephone: 908-372-0506
Website: www.tirosint.com

Pfizer (manufacturer of Levoxyl® and Cytomel®)

Address:
Pfizer
235 East 42nd Street
New York, NY 10017
Communication data:
Telephone: 800-Try-First (800-879-3477) or 212-733-2323
Website: www.levoxyl.com

Genzyme Corporation (manufacturer of Thyrogen®)

Address:
500 Kendall Square
Cambridge, MA 02142
Communication data:
Telephone: 800-745-4447, option 2 or 617-768-9000
Website: www.thyrogen.com
Information about Thyrogen:
Genzyme's Patient Information Kit provides understanding about Thyrogen.

AstraZeneca (manufacturer of Caprelsa®)

Address:
1800 Concord Pike
Wilmington, DE 19803
Communication data:
Telephone: 800-236-9933
Website: www.caprelsa.com
Information about Caprelsa:
Caprelsa is for some patients with advanced medullary thyroid cancer.
Caprelsa® Patient Access Support (CPAS) Program
Call: 800-367-4999
AstraZeneca, the maker of Caprelsa, is committed to helping patients with advanced medullary thyroid cancer (MTC). Once your health care team has prescribed Caprelsa for you, CPAS can provide the following: (1) Insurance Verification, including benefit verification, and help with facilitating prior authorization process, and (2) Patient access programs, including Caprelsa Patient Savings Program for eligible insured patients, and identification of possible alternate coverage options for qualified underinsured and uninsured patients. For Safety Information: caprelsa.com/caprelsa-resources.aspx#isi

Bayer HealthCare Pharamaceuticals, Inc. and Amgen (manufacturer of Nexavar®)

Address:
Bayer HealthCare
100 Bayer Boulevard
P.O. Box 915
Whippany, NJ 07981–0915
Communication data:
Telephone: 866-Nexavar (866-639-2827)
Website: www.nexavar-us.com
Information about Nexavar:
Nexavar is for some patients with advanced differentiated thyroid cancer.
Nexavar® – REACH (Resource for Expert Assistance and Care Helpline)
Call: 866-639-2827
REACH (Resource for Expert Assistance and Care Helpline) is a valuable resource for Bayer Oncology patients. Once patients have been prescribed one of the oncology drugs from Bayer (Nexavar®), REACH reimbursement counselors are able to provide access to financial support for eligible patients, including co-pay assistance, patient education, and guidance from a team of nurses, along with specialty pharmacy provider (SPP) assistance.
Enrollment forms are available online at www.Nexavar-us.com

or

Amgen
One Amgen Center Drive
Thousands Oaks, CA 91320-1799

Eisai Co, Ltd. (manufacturer of Lenvima®)

Address:
100 Tice Boulevard
Woodcliff Lake, NJ 07677
Communication data:
Telephone: 201-692-1100
Fax: 201-692-1804
Website: www.lenvima.com
Information about Lenvima:
Lenvima® is for some patients with advanced differentiated thyroid cancer.
Lenvima® Eisai Assistance and Support for you (E.A.S.Y.™) program
Call: 1-855- Eisai-4-U (1-855-347-2448)
Eisai is committed to providing assistance to you for access and reimbursement issues through the E.A.S.Y. program.

Exelixis, Inc. (manufacturer of Cometriq®)

Address:

210 East Grand Avenue

So. San Francisco, CA 94080

Communication data:

Telephone: 855-253-3273 or 650-837-7000

Website: www.cometriq.com

Information about Cometriq:

Cometriq is for some patients with advanced medullary thyroid cancer.

Exelixis® Access Services (EAS)

Call: 1-855-253-EASE (3273), available 8:00 am to 11:00 pm ET, Monday through Friday

Exelixis® Access Services (EAS) offers a full range of services to meet the needs of MTC patients. Their trained professionals can help you with insurance coverage questions, financial assistance, and coordinating delivery of Cometriq®.

Miscellaneous Websites

American Cancer Society (ACS)	www.cancer.org
American Medical Association	www.ama-assn.org
American Medical Women's Association	www.amwa-doc.org
Cancer.Gov (National Cancer Institute)	www.cancer.gov
Cancer Information Service (NIH)	www.cancer.gov/aboutnci/contact.center
Cancer Medicine Textbook (Holland and Frei)	www.ncbi.nlm.nih.gov/books/nbk
Cancernetwork.com	www.cancernetwork.com
Centers for Disease Control and Prevention (CDC)	www.cdc.gov
Centers for Medicare and Medicaid Services (CMS)	www.cms.gov
Clinical Trials.gov	www.clinicaltrials.gov
CNN Health	www.cnn.com/health/
Doctor's Guide	www.docguide.com/general-practice/popular/US.30days
Food and Drug Administration (FDA)	www.fda.gov
Health Finder	www.healthfinder.gov
The Office of Disease Prevention and Health Promotion	www.health.gov
Health Resources and Services Administration (HRSA)	www.hrsa.gov
Health Sciences Library (University of Washington)	www.hsl.uw.edu
Martindale's Health Science Guide	www.martindalecenter.com
MedicineNet.com	www.medicinenet.com
Medline Plus	www.nlm.nih.gov/medlineplus/
MedNews	www.mednews.com
Medscape	www.medscape.com
MedWeb	www.medweb.com
Merck Manual Home Health Handbook	www.merckmanuals.com/home/
Merck Manual of Diagnosis and Therapy	www.merckmanuals.com/professional/
Merck Manual of Geriatrics	www.merckmanuals.com/professional/geriatrics/approach_to_the_geriatric_patient/introduction_to_geriatrics.html
National Center for Complementary and Integrative Medicine	www.nccih.nih.gov
National Health Information Center	www.health.gov/nhic/
National Institutes of Health (NIH)	www.nih.gov
National Institutes of Mental Health	www.nimh.nih.gov
US National Library of Medicine	www.nlm.nih.gov
Health National Institutes of Health – Health Topics	www.health.nih.gov/see_all_topics.aspx
Office of the Surgeon General	www.surgeongeneral.gov
OncoLink	www.oncolink.org
PubMed	www.ncbi.nlm.nih.gov/pubmed
Reuters Health	www.reuters.com/news/health
University of Iowa Hospitals and Clinics	www.uihealthcare.org
USA.Gov: Government Made Easy	www.usa.gov
WebMD	www.webmd.com
Yahoo Health News	news.yahoo.com/health

Appendix C: Examples of Various Forms and Instructions for Patients Treated with ^{131}I

John Glenn and Richard J. Vetter

The following four examples may be copied or adapted for your use when treating patients with ^{131}I.

Example 1: Release Following ^{131}I Therapy

Written instructions to the patient who will recover at home

The main protection for family and friends is for you to avoid close contact for about 3 days after coming home. This time period may vary by factors such as the amount of ^{131}I administered, the amount of uptake of ^{131}I in your thyroid tissue and the adopted guidelines of your treating facility.

The most critical person who is at potential risk of harm is an infant or small child. Nursing an infant or small child after receiving radioactive iodine will transfer the radioactive iodine from the mother to the child in the milk. Radioactive iodine ingested by the child will expose the thyroid of the child to potentially harmful levels of radiation. Lifelong medication may be required to prevent serious effects, both mentally and physically, if the child's thyroid receives a high dose of radiation.

Although there is no evidence that the amount of radiation received by other people coming close to you will do detectable harm, it is reasonable to take certain precautions for at least 3 days following release.

Once you get home:

1. Keep a safe distance from other people.
   (a) Sleep alone for three nights.
   (b) Avoid kissing and sexual intercourse for 7 days.
   (c) Minimize time in public places, including public transportation, theaters, and sporting events for 3 days. You can eat meals with your family during this time.
   (d) Stay at least 3 ft away from people if you will be involved with them for more than 1 h in the first 3 days.
2. You may care for children during this time, but time spent holding a child on a lap or lying next to you should be minimized.
3. Breastfeeding must be avoided, because it could seriously harm the infant.
4. Wash hands frequently for several days. Sweat contains a small amount of radioactive iodine.
5. Wash bed linens and clothes separately for 3 days. After 3 days, resume normal care.
6. Use a separate bathroom for 3 days, if possible. Urine contains excreted radioactive iodine. Flush twice when using the toilet. If separate facilities are not available, good hygiene habits are adequate to minimize radioactive contamination.

These guidelines will limit exposure to others far below acceptable levels. Radioactive iodine will disappear completely through your own body excretions and as part of the physical nature of radioactive decay. If you wish to be very cautious, maintain these restrictions for 7 days.

Example 2: Hospitalization Following Radioiodine Therapy

Information concerning your hospitalization

1. There will be restrictions on visitors during your hospitalization. Minors (under age 18) and pregnant women will not be permitted to visit unless the doctor gives permission. All visits will be restricted to a few minutes, and persons must remain a marked distance away. You are encouraged to tell friends and family not to visit.
2. Any personal belongings that you bring will be checked for radioactive iodine before you leave. Belongings that cannot be cleaned to acceptable release levels, such as radios, magazines, books, and so on, may have to be held for you until the radioactive iodine has decayed. Therefore, you should not bring any belongings with you that you cannot afford to be without for possibly a few weeks.
3. Nurses will be able to provide normal medical care but will use gloves and shoe covers when entering your room.
4. Housekeeping will be limited in your room. Housekeeping personnel are not permitted to enter the room, and all items must be measured using radiation detection instruments before leaving the room.

L. Wartofsky, D. Van Nostrand (eds.), *Thyroid Cancer*, DOI 10.1007/978-1-4939-3314-3

5. You may use the toilet without concern about the radioactive iodine. Men should sit while urinating to minimize splashing. All other normal sanitary practices should be followed. The toilet should be flushed three times with the lid down.

Example 3: Information to Consider When Releasing a Patient After ^{131}I Treatment

Questionnaire concerning hospitalization for patients administered ^{131}I

By answering the following questions and agreeing to follow the guidelines, you may be able to be released earlier because of your limited contact with other people:

1. Are you a woman nursing a small child or infant?
   Yes ____ **No** ____
   Note: Nursing an infant or small child after receiving radioactive iodine will transfer the radioactive iodine from the mother to the child through the milk. Radioactive iodine ingested by the child will expose the thyroid of the child to potentially harmful levels of radiation. Lifelong medication may be required to prevent serious effects both mentally and physically if the child's thyroid receives a high dose of radiation. **If you are nursing a child and choose not to stop, inform Nuclear Medicine personnel, and your administration will be at a later date after you have permanently ceased nursing this child.**

2. Can you take care of yourself except for brief visits and not be in the same room with another person for more than 3 h total during each of the first 3 days?
   Yes ____ **No** ____ If no, briefly explain circumstances:
   ____

3. Will you be able to maintain distance from other people, including: Sleeping alone for at least one night (recommend 3 nights)? Avoiding kissing and sexual intercourse for at least 3 days? Staying at least 3 ft away from people if you will be involved with them for more than 1 h a day in the first 3 days?
   Yes ____ **No** ____
   If no, briefly explain circumstances: ____________
   ____

4. Will you avoid travel by airplane or mass transit for the first day?
   Yes ____ **No** ____ If no, briefly explain circumstances:
   ____

5. Will you avoid prolonged travel in an automobile with others for the at least first 2 days?
   Yes ____ **No** ____ If no, briefly explain circumstances:
   ____

6. Will you have sole use of a bathroom for at least 2 days?
   Yes ____ **No** ____ If no, briefly explain circumstances:
   ____

I have read these guidelines, understand the instructions, and agree to avoid contacts in accordance with my answers to items 2 through 6. (*Note:* If you cannot manage at home and avoid close contact, it may be necessary for you to remain in the hospital up to an additional 24 h.)

Signature: ____________________ Date: ________
(Patient or other person in accordance with hospital informed consent policy.)

Example 4: Estimating Radiation Dose to Members of the Public

Determination of acceptable dose for release of patients administered ^{131}I regulatory limit

10 CFR 35.75 permits release of patients if the total effective dose equivalent to any other individual from exposure to the released individual is not likely to exceed 5 millisieverts (0.5 rem).

Acceptable Methods

The dose to any other individual may be estimated by calculation. Acceptable methods are described in Appendix B of Regulatory Guide 8.39 "Release of Patients Administered Radioactive Materials." Appendix B contains procedures for performing patient-specific dose calculations and describes how various factors may be considered in the calculations. The latest information on patient release should be reviewed before releasing patients based on this method (www.nrc.gov).

Calculations

Calculations are based on Equation B-1 from Regulatory Guide 8.39, which includes consideration of the time the person spends near the patient and the distance from the patient. Taken together, the time and distance interaction are called the occupancy factor, E. Our purpose here is to point out that the estimate will vary depending on the value of E.

$E = 0.25$ or 0.125 depending on the patient's circumstances. Interview the patient carefully to determine the most appropriate occupancy factor. Previous measurements of doses to family members and considerations of normal human behavior suggest that an occupancy factor of 0.25 at 1 m will produce a conservative estimate of the dose to family members when instructions on minimizing doses to others are given. An occupancy factor of 0.125 may be appropriate when the patient lives alone for at least the first 2 days or has few visits by family or friends for at least the first 2 days.

1. If the patient has not submitted information about possible contacts with other people, we can assume without further justification the occupancy factor is 0.25. [Reference: Regulatory Guide 8.39 "Release of Patients Administered Radioactive Materials" and 10 CFR 35.75]
2. If the patient has submitted information about possible contacts with other people and has answered yes to all questions 2–6 of the questionnaire, we can assume the occupancy factor is 0.125. [Reference: Section B.1.2, "Occupancy Factors to Consider for Patient-Specific Calculations," Regulatory Guide 8.39 "Release of Patients Administered Radioactive Materials."]
3. If the patient has submitted information about possible contacts with other people but has answered no to any of the questions 2–6 of the questionnaire, the Radiation Safety Officer will make the determination of acceptable occupancy factor. [Reference: Section B.1.2, Regulatory Guide 8.39 "Release of Patients Administered Radioactive Materials."]

Index

L. Wartofsky, D. Van Nostrand (eds.), *Thyroid Cancer*, DOI 10.1007/978-1-4939-3314-3

C

M

S

T

U

V

W

Printed by Printforce, the Netherlands